DOA	Dead on arrival	**GFR**	Glomerular filtration rate
DOB	Date of birth	**GI**	Gastrointestinal
DOE	Dyspnea on exertion	**Grav I, II, etc.**	Pregnancy one, two, three, etc.
DPT	Diphtheria-pertussis-tetanus		(*Gravida*)
DRG	Diagnosis-related group	**GSW**	Gunshot wound
DT	Delirium tremens	**gtt**	Drops (*guttae*)
DTR	Deep tendon reflex	**GU**	Genitourinary
D5W	Dextrose 5% in water	**Gyn**	Gynecology
Dx	Diagnosis	**H & P**	History and physical
EBV	Epstein-Barr virus	**HAV**	Hepatitis A virus
ECF	Extended care facility; extra-cellular fluid	**Hb; Hgb**	Hemoglobin
		HBV	Hepatitis B virus
ECG	Electrocardiogram, electrocardiograph	**HCG**	Human chorionic gonadotropin
		HCT	Hematocrit
ECHO	Echocardiography	**HDL**	High-density lipoprotein
ECT	Electroconvulsive therapy	**HEENT**	Head, eye, ear, nose, and throat
ED	Emergency department; erythema dose; effective dose	**Hg**	Mercury
		Hgb	Hemoglobin
EDD	Estimated date of delivery (formerly EDC, estimated date of confinement)	**HIV**	Human immunodeficiency (AIDS) virus
		h/o	History of
EEG	Electroencephalogram, electroencephalograph	**H_2O_2**	Hydrogen peroxide
		HPI	History of present illness
EENT	Eye, ear, nose, and throat	**HR**	Heart rate
EKG	Electrocardiogram; electrocardiograph	**HSV**	Herpes simplex virus
		HT; HTN	Hypertension
ELISA	Enzyme-linked immunosorbent assay	**hx; Hx**	History
		I & O	Intake and output
EMG	Electromyogram	**IBW**	Ideal body weight
EMS	Emergency medical service	**ICP**	Intracranial pressure
ENT	Ear, nose, and throat	**ICU**	Intensive care unit
ER	Emergency room (hospital); external resistance	**IDDM**	Insulin-dependent diabetes mellitus
		Ig	Immunoglobulin
ERV	Expiratory reserve volume	**IM**	Intramuscular; infectious mononucleosis
ESR	Erythrocyte sedimentation rate		
ESRD	End stage renal disease	**IPPB**	Intermittent positive-pressure breathing
FBS	Fasting blood sugar		
Fe	Iron	**IRV**	Inspiratory reserve volume
FEV	Forced expiratory volume	**I.U.**	International Unit
FH, Fhx	Family history	**IUD**	Intrauterine device
FHR	Fetal heart rate	**IV**	Intravenous
FTT	Failure to thrive	**IVP**	Intravenous pyelogram, intravenous push
FUO	Fever of unknown origin		
fx	Fracture	**K**	Potassium
GB	Gallbladder	**KCl**	Potassium chloride
GC	Gonococcus or gonorrheal		

MOSBY'S POCKET DICTIONARY

of Medicine, Nursing, & Allied Health

THIRD EDITION

Kenneth N. Anderson

Lois E. Anderson

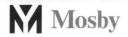

St. Louis Baltimore Boston Carlsbad Chicago Minneapolis New York Philadelphia Portland
London Milan Sydney Tokyo Toronto

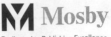
Dedicated to Publishing Excellence

A Times Mirror
Company

Vice President and Publisher: Nancy L. Coon
Editor-in-Chief: N. Darlene Como
Senior Developmental Editor: Laurie Sparks
Project Manager: Deborah Vogel
Poduction Editor: Mary Drone
Designer: Bill Drone
Manufacturing Manager: Linda Ierardi

Printed in the United States of America
Composition by Clarinda Company
Printing/binding by R.R. Donnelley & Sons Company

Mosby, Inc.
11830 Westline Industrial Drive
St. Louis, Missouri 63146

Library of Congress Cataloging in Publication Data

Mosby's pocket dictionary of medicine, nursing & allied health /
  [edited by] Kenneth N. Anderson, Lois E. Anderson. — 3rd ed.
    p. cm.
  Abridgement of: Mosby's medical, nursing & allied health
dictionary / revision editor, Kenneth N. Anderson. 5th ed. c1998.
  ISBN 0-8151-3166-6
  1. Medicine—Dictionaries. 2. Nursing—Dictionaries. 3. Health-
-Dictionaries.   I. Anderson, Kenneth, 1921-   . II. Anderson, Lois
E. III. Mosby's medical, nursing & allied health dictionary.
  [DNLM: 1. Dictionaries, Medical. 2. Nursing dictionaries.
3. Allied Health Occupations dictionaries.   W 13 M8942 1998]
R121.M892   1998
610'.3—dc21
DNLM/DLC
for Library of Congress   98-3311
                                             CIP

98 99 00 01 02 / 9 8 7 6 5 4 3 2 1

Contents

Consultants

The following individuals assisted in the development of this dictionary by acting as consultants to *Mosby's Medical, Nursing, and Allied Health Dictionary*, ed. 5, from which this dictionary is derived:

Mary A. Allen, RN, MSN
Aris J. Andrews, RN, MS
Bert Atsma
Emilie J. Aubert, MA, PT
Edward S. Bennett, OD, MS, MEd
Barbara Billek-Sawhney, MS, PT
Christine Bolwell, RN, MSN
Barbara Broome, RN, MSN, CNS
Jerri Bryant, RN, MPH
Bernadette Butler, RN(C), EdD
William Callaway, BA, RT(R)
Gayle K. Campbell, RN, BSN, BHSA
Toni Cascio, RN, MN
Peggy S. Cass, RN, PhD
Carol J. Chancey, RN, MS
Michael S. Clement, MD
Charlene D. Coco, RN, MN
Jeffrey A. Cokely, PhD
Mary Boudreau Conover, RN, BSN
John C. Conroy, MSc, PhD
Ted T. Crites, BS
Sharon Bartz Croft, RN, MSN
Bernadette D. Curry, RN, PhD
Pat Czar
Rick Daniels, RN, PhD
Patricia O'Brien Dardis, RN, MS, CS, FNP
Mardell Davis, RN, MSN, CETN
Kamela O. Deel, RN, BSN, MEd
George DeMaagd, PharmD, BCPS
Hetty Lucienne DeVroom, RN, BSN, CNRN
Clarice L. Dietrich, RDH, MA
Kathleen A. Dietz, RN, MA, MS, AOCN
James P. Embrey, PhD
Deborah Oldenburg Erickson, BSN, MSN
Linda Fasciani, RN, BSN, MSN
Michael A. Fiedler, MS, CRNA
Katherine M. Fortinash, RN, MSN, CS
Donna G. Friedman, PhD
Yvonne S. Garner, RN, MA, EdS
Florencetta H. Gibson, RN, MEd, MSN
Theresa N. Grabo, PhD, CRNP
Lucille I. Grimm, RN, EdD
Linda B. Haas, RN, PhC, CDE
Diane Hamilton, RN, PhD
Wendy B. Hamilton, RN, BA, MEd

E. Charles Healey, PhD
Toni Lee Hebda, RNC, BSN, MNEd, PhD, MSIS
Mary Lou Aguilar Hernandez, RN, MS
Peggy O'Neill Hewlett, RN, PhD
Sandra K. Highsmith, DMD
Beth Hogan-Quigley, RN, MSN, CRNP
Mildred O. Hogstel, RN(C), PhD
Stuart S. Howards, MD
Michael S. Hudecki, PhD, DSc
Patrick Jackson, RPN, BGS, BSc, PhD
Trudi James-Parks, RT(R)
Frank E. Johnson, MD
Eleftheria T. Karapas, RN, MS
Karen Kelly, RN, EdD, CNAA
Patricia T. Ketcham, RN, MSN
Carl A. Kirton, RN, MA, ACRN, ANP-CS
Diane Langevin, CDA, RDH, MA
Yolanda Lonsford, RN, MS, MSN
Ruth Ludwick, RNC, PhD
Janis Luft, NP, MS
Ann Marriner-Tomey, BS, MS, PhD
Lori A. Martell, PhD
Sheryl Martz, RN, MSN, CS, NP-C
Cindy Mascara
Mary N. McAlindon, RN, EdD, CNAA
Donna McCarthy-Beckett
Edwina A. McConnell, RN, PhD, FRCNA
Mary S. Merchant, RN, MSN
Patricia Mezinskis, RN, MSN, CS
Vicky Minninger, RN, MSN
Diane Moro, MSRN
Patricia Morrison-Sasso, RNC, BSN, MA, CS, NP
Joyce L. Muholland, MA, MS, RNC, ANP
Helen K. Mussallem, CC, BN, MA, EdD, LLD, DSc, FRCN, MRSH
Dean Nelson, PhD
Connie Neuburger, RN, BSN, MS, MN
Kim Neudorf, BSN
Ainslie T. Nibert, RN, MSN, CCRN
Noreen Heer Nicol, RN, MS, INP
Patricia A. Nutz, RN, MSN, MEd
Kathleen Deska Pagana, RN, PhD
Charlane Pehoski, ScD, OTR/L
Joyce Powers, RN, MSN, CS

Foreword

The complexity and continuing evolution of health science vocabularies require that students and professionals alike have an affordable, compact, yet thorough quick reference to the language of their fields. *Mosby's Pocket Dictionary of Medicine, Nursing, & Allied Health* provides students and practitioners of the health sciences with a succinct and portable abridgement of *Mosby's Medical, Nursing, & Allied Health Dictionary,* which has been used by hundreds of thousands of nurses, allied health professionals, and physicians in their education and practice. The first edition of *Mosby's Pocket Dictionary of Medicine, Nursing, & Allied Health,* published in 1990, was the first pocket dictionary to address the broad spectrum of health science terminology in the medical, nursing, and allied health professions.

To reflect new developments in many facets of health care, approximately 5000 new entries have been added to this edition. In addition, all new and former entries were reviewed by experts and updated, as needed, to reflect current knowledge and practice. To assist out readers in recognizing alternate spellings, selected British spellings have been added where appropriate.

New to this edition is a list of abbreviations commonly used in health care. This list may be found on the front and back endsheets.

The extensive vocabulary of the larger dictionary has been retained by restructuring and condensing its many encyclopedic entries while retaining the essential content of the definitions. An example can be seen in a comparison of the entries for drugs. The pocket edition defines the drug and relates the indications for its use, whereas the parent volume includes further information on contraindications and adverse effects.

In the pocket dictionary, the user will continue to find many of the valuable features of our larger dictionary, including clear pronunciations and etymologies for thousands of terms.

Development of this third edition of our pocket dictionary has taken the effort of many people. We gratefully acknowledge and appreciate the work of all who participated. The valuable contributions by all who were involved in the parent work and in particular the authors whose works were consulted and the writers and editors are also gratefully acknowledged.

The extremely positive response to the first two editions leads us to believe that *Mosby's Pocket Dictionary of Medicine, Nursing, & Allied Health* will remain an eminently useful and usable resource. We welcome your comments and suggestions for improving future editions.

Guide to the Dictionary

A. Alphabetic order

The entries are alphabetized in dictionary style, that is, letter by letter, disregarding spaces or hyphens between words:

analgesic	**artificial lung**
anal	**artificially acquired**
membrane	**immunity**
analog	**artificial pacemaker**

The alphabetization is alphanumeric: words and numbers form a single list with numbers positioned as though they were spelled-out numerals: Nilstat / 90-90 traction / ninth nerve. (An example of the few exceptions to this rule is the sequence 17-hydroxycorticosteroid / 11-hydroxyetiocholanolone / 5-hydroxyindoleacetic acid, which can be found between the entries hydroxochloroquine sulfate and hydroxyl, not, as may be expected, 17-. . . in letter "S," 11-. . . in letter "E," and 5-. . . in letter "F.")

Small subscript and superscript numbers are disregarded in alphabetizing: No / N$_2$O / nobelium.

Compound headwords are given in their natural word order: abdominal surgery, not surgery, abdominal; achondroplastic dwarf, not dwarf, achondroplastic. There are few exceptions to this natural word order; nearly all of these concern formal classifications, for example: "comfort, alteration in: pain, a NANDA-accepted nursing diagnosis . . ."

(NOTE: In this guide, the term "headword" is used to refer to any alphabetized and nonindented definiendum, be it a single-word term or a compound term.)

In some cases, there may be one or more terms that are synonymous with a headword or derived from a headword. If the synonym or derivation would immediately precede or follow the definition, it is not included as a separate entry. Therefore, if a term is not listed at the expected place, the reader might find it among the boldface terms of the immediately preceding or immediately following entry.

B. Etymology

ETYMOLOGY is shown for principal entries and in other instances where it contributes immediately to a better understanding of the meaning: "lysergide, . . . Also called LSD (an abbreviation of the original German name, *Lyserg-Säure-Diäthylamid*), lysergic acid diethylamide, *(slang)* acid." "hangnail, . . . painful . . . (Hang is not related to the verb but is an old English word for pain.) . . ."

C. Pronunciation

All sounds, both English and non-English, are represented by letters or combinations of letters of the alphabet with few adaptations, and with the schwa (/ə/), the neutral vowel. Pronunciations are shown between slants. The following pronunciation key shows the symbols used:

Vowels

SYMBOLS	KEY WORDS
/a/	hat
/ä/	father
/ā/	fate
/e/	flesh
/ē/	she
/er/	air, ferry
/i/	sit
/ī/	eye
/ir/	ear
/o/	proper
/ō/	nose
/ô/	saw
/oi/	boy
/o͞o/	move
/o͝o/	book
/ou/	out
/u/	cup, love
/ur/	fur, first
/ə/	(the neutral vowel, always unstressed, as in) ago, focus
/ər/	teacher, doctor
/œ/	as in (French) feu /fœ/; (German) schön /shœn/
/Y/	as in (French) tu /tY/; (German) grün /grYn/

/N/   This symbol does not represent a sound but indicates that the preceding vowel is a nasal, as in French bon /bôN/, or international /aNternäsyōnäl′/.

Consonants

SYMBOLS	KEY WORDS
/b/	book
/ch/	chew
/d/	day
/f/	fast
/g/	good
/h/	happy
/j/	gem
/k/	keep
/l/	late
/m/	make
/n/	no
/ng/	sing, drink
/ng·g/	finger
/p/	pair
/r/	ring
/s/	set
/sh/	shoe, lotion
/t/	tone
/th/	thin
/th/	than
/v/	very
/w/	work
/y/	yes
/z/	zeal
/zh/	azure, vision
/kh/	as in (Scottish) loch /lokh/; (German) Rorschach /rôr′shokh/
/kh/	as in (German) ich /ikh/ (or, approximated, as in English fish: /ish/, /rĭsh/)
/nyə/	Occurring at the end of French words, this symbol is not truly a separate syllable but an /n/ with a slight /y/ (similar to the sound in "onion") plus a near-silent /ə/, as in Bois de Boulogne /bo͞olō′nyə/

ACCENTS: Pronunciation is shown with primary and secondary accents. A raised dot shows that two vowels (or occasionally, two consonants) are pronounced separately.

Many of the numerous *Latin* terms in this dictionary are not given with pronunciation, mainly because there are different ways (all of them understood) in which Latin is pronounced by the English speaker and may be pronounced by speakers elsewhere. However, guidance is given in many cases, often to reflect common usage.

LATIN AND GREEK PLURALS: The spelling of Latin and Greek plurals is shown in most instances. However, when the plural formation is regular according to Latin and Greek rules, the pronunciation is usually not included.

NOTE: Notwithstanding the listing of Latin and Greek plurals in this dictionary, and the rules of Latin and Greek pluralization, in most instances it is acceptable or even preferable to pluralize Latin and Greek words according to the rules of English words. (For certain kinds of entries, both the English and the foreign plurals are given in this dictionary, usually showing the English form first, as, for example, in nearly all -oma nouns: hematoma, pl. hematomas, hematoma.)

a, symbol for **arterial blood.**

A, 1. abbreviation for **accommodation. 2.** symbol for alveolar gas. **3.** abbreviation for **ampere. 4.** abbreviation for **anterior. 5.** abbreviation for **atomic weight (mass). 6.** abbreviation for **axial. 7.** symbol for **mass number.**

A68, symbol for a protein found in the brain tissue of Alzheimer's disease patients. It is also found in the developing normal brains of fetuses and infants but begins to disappear by the age of 2 years.

AA, 1. abbreviation for **achievement age. 2.** abbreviation for **Alcoholics Anonymous. 3.** abbreviation for **amplitude of accommodation. 4.** abbreviation for **anesthesiologist's assistant.**

/amaa,/ama/ama, /amA/amA, (in prescriptions) abbreviation for *ana,* indicating an equal amount of each ingredient to be compounded.

AAAI, abbreviation for **American Academy of Allergy and Immunology.**

AACN, 1. abbreviation for **American Association of Colleges of Nursing. 2.** abbreviation for **American Association of Critical Care Nurses.**

AAFP, abbreviation for American Academy of Family Practice.

AAI, abbreviation for **ankle-arm index.**

AAIN, abbreviation for **American Association of Industrial Nurses.**

AAL, abbreviation for **anterior axillary line.**

AAMC, abbreviation for **American Association of Medical Colleges.**

AAMI, abbreviation for **Association for the Advancement of Medical Instrumentation.**

AAN, abbreviation for **American Academy of Nursing.**

AANA, abbreviation for **American Association of Nurse Anesthetists.**

AANN, 1. abbreviation for **American Association of Neuroscience Nurses. 2.** abbreviation for **American Association of Neurological Nurses.**

AANNT, abbreviation for **American Association of Nephrology Nurses and Technicians.**

AAOHN, abbreviation for *American Association of Occupational Health Nurses.*

AAOMS, abbreviation for *American Association of Oral and Maxillofacial Surgeons.*

AAPA, abbreviation for **American Academy of Physicians' Assistants.**

AAPB, abbreviation for **American Association of Pathologists and Bacteriologists.**

AAPMR, abbreviation for **American Academy of Physical Medicine and Rehabilitation.**

Aaron's sign [Charles D. Aaron, American physician, 1866–1951], a diagnostic sign in appendicitis indicated by pain or distress when pressure is applied over McBurney's point in the epigastric region.

AARP, abbreviation for **American Association of Retired Persons.**

AART, abbreviation for **American Association for Respiratory Therapy.**

AAUP, abbreviation for **American Association of University Professors.**

AAV, abbreviation for **adenoassociated virus.**

Ab, abbreviation for **antibody.**

abacterial /ab′aktir′ē·əl/, any atmosphere or condition free of bacteria; literally, without bacteria.

abaissement /ä′bāsmäN′/ [Fr, a lowering], **1.** a falling or depressing. **2.** (in ophthalmology) the displacement of a lens.

abalienation /abāl′yənā′shən/, **1.** a state of physical deterioration or mental decay. **2.** a state of insanity.—**abalienate,** *v.,* **abalienated,** *adj.*

A band, the area between two I bands of a sarcomere, marked by partial overlapping of actin and myosin filaments.

abandonment of care /əban′dənment/, (in law) wrongful cessation of the provision of care to a patient, usually by a physician or a nurse.

abapical /abap′əkəl/, opposite the apex.

abarognosis /aber′agnō′sis/, [Gk, *a,* not, *baros,* weight, *gnosis,* knowledge], an inability to judge or compare the weight of objects, particularly those held in the hand.

abarticular /ab′ärtik′yŏŏlər/, **1.** pertaining to a condition that does not affect a joint. **2.** pertaining to a site or structure remote from a joint.

abarticular gout [L, *ab,* away from, *articulus,* joint], gout symptoms that affect tissues other than joints, such as ligaments.

abarticulation /ab'ärtik'yəlā'shən/, **1.** dislocation of a joint. **2.** a synovial joint.

abasia /əbā'zhə/, [Gk, *a, basis,* not step], the inability to walk, caused by lack of motor coordination.—**abasic, abatic,** *adj.*

abate /əbāt'/ [ME, *abaten,* to beat down], to decrease or reduce in severity or degree.

abatement /əbāt'mənt/, a decrease in severity of symptoms.

abatic, pertaining to an inability to walk.

abaxial /abak'sē-əl/ [L, *ab, axis* from axle], **1.** pertaining to a position outside the axis of a body or structure. **2.** pertaining to a position at the opposite extremity of a structure.

Abbe-Estlander operation /ab'ē-est'/, [Robert Abbe, American surgeon, 1851–1928; Jakob A. Estlander, Finnish surgeon, 1831–1881], a surgical procedure that transfers a full-thickness section of one oral lip to the other lip.

Abbe-Zeiss apparatus /äbā'tsīs'/ [Ernst K. Abbe, German physicist, 1840–1905; Carl Zeiss, German optician, 1816–1885], an apparatus for calculating the number of blood cells in a measured amount of blood.

Abbott-Miller tube [William Abbott, American physician, 1902–1943; T.G. Miller, American physician, 1886–1981], a double-lumen tube with an inflatable balloon at one end used in the diagnosis and treatment of small bowel obstructions.

Abbott pump /ab'ət/, a trademark for a small portable pump that can be adjusted and finely calibrated to deliver precise amounts of medication in solution through an intravenous infusion set.

ABC, abbreviation for **aspiration biopsy cytology.**

Abdellah, Faye Glenn, a nursing theorist who introduced a typology of 21 nursing problems in 1960 in *Patient-Centered Approaches to Nursing.* The concepts of nursing, nursing problems, and the problem-solving process are central to Abdellah's work. The typology provided a scientific body of knowledge unique to nursing, making it possible to move away from the medical model of educating nurses. The nursing diagnosis classification system may be considered an outgrowth of Abdellah's typology.

abdomen /ab'dəmən, abdō'mən/ [L, belly], the part of the body between the thorax and the pelvis. The abdominal cavity contains the inferior part of the esophagus, the stomach, the intestines, the liver, the spleen, the pancreas, and other organs. —**abdominal** /abdom'-/, *adj.*

abdominal adhesion /abdom'inəl/, the binding together of tissue surfaces of abdominal organs, usually involving the intestines and causing obstruction. The condition may result from trauma or inflammation and may form after abdominal surgery. The patient experiences abdominal distension, pain, nausea, vomiting, and increased pulse rate. Surgery may be required.

abdominal aorta, the part of the descending aorta that passes from the aortic hiatus of the diaphragm into the abdomen. It supplies blood to abdominal structures such as the testes, ovaries, kidneys, and stomach. Its branches are the celiac, superior mesenteric, inferior mesenteric, middle suprarenal, renal, testicular, ovarian, inferior phrenic, lumbar, middle sacral, and common iliac arteries.

abdominal aortography, the process of producing a radiograph of the abdominal aorta using a radiopaque contrast medium.

abdominal aponeurosis, the conjoined tendons of the oblique and transverse skeletal muscles of the abdomen.

abdominal bandage, a broad absorbent bandage commonly used after abdominal surgery.

abdominal binder, a bandage or elasticized wrap that is applied around the lower part of the torso to support the abdomen. It is sometimes applied after abdominal surgery to decrease discomfort.

abdominal breathing, a pattern of inhalation and exhalation in which most of the ventilatory work is done with the abdominal muscles.

abdominal cavity, the space within the abdominal walls between the diaphragm and the pelvic area, containing the liver, stomach, intestines, spleen, gallbladder, kidneys, and associated tissues and vessels.

abdominal decompression, an obstetric technique to reduce pressure on the abdomen during the first stage of labor. The abdomen is enclosed in a chamber that permits surrounding pressure to be controlled.

abdominal delivery, the delivery of a child through a surgical incision in the abdomen. The procedure may be any of the several kinds of cesarean section.

abdominal examination, the physical assessment of a patient's abdomen by visual inspection and the use of auscultation, percussion, and palpation. Visual inspection of the normally oval shape of the abdominal surface while the patient is supine may reveal abnormal surface features indicating effects of disease or injury. Subsurface tumors, fluid accumulation, or hypertrophy of the liver or spleen may be observed as an abnormal surface feature. Auscultation may reveal vascular sounds that provide information about arterial disorders such as aortic aneurysms, as well as bowel sounds that are indicative of intestinal function. If the patient is pregnant, auscultation can detect the fetal heart beat and the circulation of blood in the placenta. Percussion involves gently striking the abdominal wall at various points to produce vibrations. The vibrations, in turn, help detect the condition of internal organs. In palpation, indirect exploration of the abdomen is performed by using the examiner's sense of touch to detect areas of tenderness or rigidity, muscle tone, and skin condition, as well of shapes and sizes of subsurface organs.

abdominal fistula, an abnormal passage from an abdominal organ to the surface of the abdomen. In a colostomy, a passage from the bowel to an opening on the surface of the abdomen is created surgically.

abdominal gestation, the implantation of a fertilized ovum outside the uterus but within the peritoneal cavity.

abdominalgia /abdom'ənal'jə/ [L, *abdomen,* belly; Gk, *algos,* pain], a pain in the abdomen.

abdominal girth, the circumference of the abdomen, usually measured at the umbilicus.

abdominal hernia, a hernia in which a loop of bowel protrudes through the abdominal musculature, often through the site of an old surgical scar.

abdominal hysterectomy, the excision of the uterus through the abdominal wall.

abdominal inguinal ring, an opening of the inguinal canal on the abdominal wall through which the male spermatic cord and the female round ligament pass.

abdominal muscles, the set of muscles that make up the ventral abdominal wall, including the external oblique *(obliquus externus abdominis),* internal oblique *(obliquus internus abdominis),* transversalis *(transversus abdominis),* rectus abdominis, and pyramidalis. Broad and thin, the external oblique muscle is the largest and most superficial of the abdominal muscles. The abdominal muscles compress the abdominal contents during urination, defecation, vomiting, parturition, and forced expiration.

abdominal nephrectomy [L, *abdominis,* belly; Gk, *nephr,* kidney, *ektome,* cutting out], the surgical removal of a kidney through an abdominal incision.

abdominal pain, acute or chronic localized or diffuse pain in the abdominal cavity. Abdominal pain is a significant symptom because its cause may require immediate surgical or medical intervention. The most common causes of severe abdominal pain are inflammation, perforation of an intraabdominal structure, circulatory obstruction, intestinal or ureteral obstruction, or rupture of an organ located within the abdomen. Specific conditions include appendicitis, perforated gastric ulcer, strangulated hernia, superior mesenteric arterial thrombosis, and small and large bowel obstruction. Conditions producing acute abdominal pain that may require surgery include appendicitis, acute or severe and chronic diverticulitis, acute and chronic cholecystitis, cholelithiasis, acute pancreatitis, perforation of a peptic ulcer, various intestinal obstructions, abdominal aortic aneurysms, and trauma affecting any of the abdominal organs. Gynecologic causes of acute abdominal pain that may require surgery include acute pelvic inflammatory disease, ruptured ovarian cyst, and ectopic pregnancy. Abdominal pain associated with pregnancy may be caused by the weight of the enlarged uterus; rotation, stretching, or compression of the round ligament; or squeezing or displacement of the bowel. Chronic abdominal pain may be functional or may result from overeating or excessive air swallowing (aerophagia). Organic sources of abdominal pain include peptic ulcer, hiatus hernia, gastritis, chronic cholecystitis and cholelithiasis, chronic pancreatitis, pancreatic carcinoma, chronic diverticulitis, intermittent low-grade intestinal obstruction, and functional indigestion.

abdominal paracentesis [L, *abdominis,* belly; Gk, *para,* near, *kentesis,* puncturing], the surgical puncturing of the abdominal cavity to remove fluid for diagnosis or treatment.

abdominal pregnancy, an extrauterine pregnancy in which the conceptus develops in the abdominal cavity after being extruded from the fimbriated end of the fallopian tube or through a defect in the tube or uterus. The placenta may implant on the abdominal or visceral peritoneum. Abdominal pregnancy may be suspected when the abdomen has enlarged but the uterus has remained small for the length of gestation. Abdominal pregnancies constitute approximately 2% of ectopic pregnancies and approximately 0.01% of all pregnancies. The condition results in perinatal death of the fetus in most cases and maternal death in approximately 6%. Because of its rarity, the condition may be unsuspected, and diagnosis is often delayed. Surgical removal of the placenta, sac, and embryo or fetus is necessary if attached to the posterior part of the tube, ovary, broad ligament, and uterus.

abdominal pulse, the pulse of the abdominal aorta.

abdominal quadrant, any of four topographic areas of the abdomen divided by two imaginary lines, one vertical and one horizontal, intersecting at the umbilicus. The divisions are the left upper quadrant (LUQ), the left lower quadrant (LLQ), the right upper quadrant (RUQ), and the right lower quadrant (RLQ).

abdominal reflex, a superficial neurologic reflex obtained by firmly stroking the skin of the abdomen, normally resulting in a brisk contraction of abdominal muscles in which the umbilicus moves toward the site of the stimulus. This reflex is lost in diseases of the pyramidal tract.

abdominal regions, the nine topographic subdivisions of the abdomen, determined by four imaginary lines, in a tic-tac-toe pattern, imposed over the anterior surface. The upper horizontal line passes along the level of the cartilages of the ninth rib; the lower along the iliac crests. The two vertical lines extend on each side of the body from the cartilage of the eighth rib to the center of the inguinal ligament. The lines divide the abdomen into three upper, three middle, and three lower zones: right hypochondriac, epigastric, and left hypochondriac regions (upper zones); right lateral (lumbar), umbilical, and left lateral (lumbar) regions (middle zones); right inguinal (iliac), pubic (hypogastric), and left inguinal (iliac) regions (lower zones).

abdominal splinting, a rigid contraction of the abdominal wall muscles. It usually occurs as an involuntary reaction to the pain of a visceral disease or disorder or postoperative discomfort.

abdominal sponge [L, *abdominis,* belly; Gk, *spongia,* sponge], a special type of gauze pad used as absorbent and covering for the viscera.

abdominal surgery, any operation that involves an incision into the abdomen. Some kinds of abdominal surgery are **appendectomy, cholecystectomy, colostomy, gastrectomy, herniorrhaphy,** and **laparotomy.**

abdominal wound, a break in the continuity of the abdominal wall. A wound that exposes or penetrates the viscera raises the danger of infection or peritonitis.

abdominocardiac reflex /-kär′dē·ək/, an immediate, involuntary response of the heart to stimulation of the abdominal viscera. The reflex is mediated through the vagus nerve.

abdominocyesis /abdom′inōsī·ē′sis/, an abdominal pregnancy.

abdominogenital /-jen′itəl/, pertaining to the abdomen and reproductive system.

abdominohysterotomy /-his′tərot′əmē/, hysterotomy through an abdominal incision.

abdominopelvic cavity /-pel′vik/, the space between the diaphragm and the groin. There is no structurally distinct separation between the abdomen and pelvic regions.

abdominoperineal /-per′inē′əl/, pertaining to the abdomen and the perineum, including the pelvic area, female vulva and anus, and male anus and scrotum.

abdominoplasty, a surgical procedure to tighten the abdominal muscles.

abdominoscopy /abdom′inos′kəpē/ [L, *abdomen;* Gk, *skopein,* to view], a procedure for examining the contents of the peritoneum in which an electrically illuminated tubular device is passed through a trocar into the abdominal cavity.

abdominoscrotal /-skrō′təl/, pertaining to the abdomen and scrotum.

abdominothoracic arch /-thôras′ik/, the lower boundary of the front of the thorax.

abdominovaginal /-vaj′inəl/, pertaining to the abdomen and vagina.

abdominovesical /-ves′ikəl/, pertaining to the abdomen and bladder.

abducens /abdoo͞′sənz/ [L, drawing away], pertaining to a movement away from the median line of the body.

abducens muscle, the extraocular lateral rectus muscle that moves the eyeball outward.

abducens nerve [L, *abducere,* to take away], either of a pair of the sixth cranial nerves. It controls the lateral rectus muscle, turning the eye outward.

abduct /abdukt′/, to move away from the median plane of the body.

abduction [L, *abducere,* to take away], movement of a limb away from the body.

abduction boots, a pair of orthopedic casts for the lower extremities, available in both short-leg and long-leg configurations, with a bar incorporated at ankle level to provide hip abduction.

abductor /abduk′tər/ [L, *abducere*], a muscle that draws a body part away from the midline, or one part from another.

abembryonic /ab′embrē·on′ik/, opposite the position of the embryo.

Abernethy's sarcoma. /ab′ərnē′thēz/ [John Abernethy, British surgeon, 1764–1831], a malignant neoplasm of fat cells, usually occurring on the trunk.

aberrant /aber′ənt/ [L, *aberrare,* to wander], **1.** pertaining to a wandering from the usual or expected course, such as various ducts, nerves, and vessels in the body. **2.** (in botany and zoology) pertaining to an abnormal individual, such as certain atypical members of a species.

aberrant goiter, an enlargement of a supernumerary or ectopic thyroid gland.

aberrant ventricular conduction (AVC), the temporary abnormal intraventricular conduction of a supraventricular impulse. It is usually associated with a change in cycle length.

aberration /ab′ərā′shən/ [L, *aberrare,* to wander], **1.** any departure from the usual course or normal condition. **2.** abnormal growth or development. **3.** (in psychology) an illogical and unreasonable thought or belief, often leading to an unsound mental state. **4.** (in genetics) any change in the number or structure of the chromosomes. **5.** (in optics) any imperfect image formation caused by unequal refraction or focalization of light rays through a lens.

abetalipoproteinemia /əbā′təlip′ōprō′tinē′mē-ə/ [Gk, *a, beta,* not beta, *lipos,* fat, *proteios,* first rank, *haima,* blood], a rare inherited disorder of fat metabolism, characterized by acanthocytosis, low or absent serum beta-lipoproteins, and hypocholesterolemia.

abeyance /əbā′əns/, a state of inaction or interruption of function.

ABG, abbreviation for **arterial blood gas.**

ABI, abbreviation for **ankle-brachial index.**

abient /ab′ē-ənt/ [L, *abire,* to go away], characterized by a tendency to move away from stimuli. —**abience,** *n.*

ability /əbil′itē/, the capacity to act in a specified way because of the possession of appropriate skills and mental or physical fitness.

abiogenesis /ab′ē-ōjen′əsis/ [Gk, *a + bios,* not life, *genein,* to produce], spontaneous generation; the theory that organic life can originate from inorganic, inanimate matter. —**abiogenetic,** *adj.*

abiosis /ab′ē-ō′sis/ [Gk, *a + bios* not life], a nonviable condition or a situation that is incompatible with life. —**abiotic,** *adj.*

abiotrophy /ab′ē-ot′rəfē/ [Gk, *a + bios + trophe* nutrition], a premature depletion of vitality or the deterioration of certain cells and tissues, especially those involved in genetic degenerative diseases. —**abiotrophic** /ab′ē-ətrō′fik/, *adj.*

ablastemic /ab′lastem′ik/, nongerminal or not germinating.

ablate /ablāt′ [L, *ab + latus,* carried away], to cut away or remove.

ablation /ablā′shən/ [L, *ab + latus,* carried away], an amputation, an excision of any part of the body, or a removal of a growth or harmful substance.

ablepharia /ab′ləfer′ēə/, a defect characterized by partial or total absence of the eyelids.

ablepsia /əblep′sē-ə/ [Gk, *a + blepein,* not to see], the condition of being blind.

abluent, pertaining to the ability of a substance to cleanse or wash away.

ablution /ablōō′shən/, the act of washing or bathing.

ABMS, abbreviation for *American Board of Medical Specialties.*

abnerval current /abnur′vəl/ [L, *ab,* from; Gk, *neuron,* nerve], an electrical current that passes from a nerve to and through muscle.

abneural /abnōōr′əl/, away from the central nervous system or the neural axis.

abnormal behavior /abnôr′məl/ [L, *ab + norma,* away from rule], maladaptive acts or activities detrimental to the individual or to society.

abnormality /ab′nôrmal′itē/ [L, *ab,* away from, *norma,* the rule], a condition that differs from the usual physical or mental state.

abnormal psychology, the study of any behavior that deviates from culturally accepted norms.

abnormal tooth mobility, excessive movement of a tooth within its socket as a result of injury or disease in the supporting tissues.

ABO blood groups, a system for classifying human blood based on the antigenic components of red blood cells and their corresponding antibodies. The ABO blood group is identified by the presence or absence of two different antigens, A and B, on the surface of the red blood cell. The four blood types in this grouping, A, B, AB, and O, are determined by and named for these antigens. Type AB indicates the presence of both antigens; type O the absence of both.

aboiement /ä′bô-ämaN′/, an involuntary making of abnormal, animal-like sounds such as barking. Aboiement may be a clinical sign of Gilles de la Tourette's syndrome.

abort /əbôrt′/ [L, *ab,* away from, *oriri,* to be born], **1.** to deliver a nonviable fetus; to miscarry. **2.** to terminate a pregnancy before the fetus has developed enough to live outside the uterus. **3.** to terminate in the early stages or to discontinue before completion, as to arrest the usual course of a disease, to stop growth and development, or to halt a project.

aborted systole, a contraction of the heart that is usually weak and is not associated with a radial pulse.

abortifacient /əbôr′tifā′shənt/, **1.** producing abortion. **2.** an agent that causes abortion.

abortion /əbôr′shən/ [L, *ab* + *oriri*], the spontaneous or induced termination of pregnancy before the fetus has developed to the stage of viability. Kinds of abortion include **habitual abortion, infected abortion, septic abortion, threatened abortion,** and voluntary abortion.

abortionist, a person who performs abortions.

abortion on demand, a concept promoted by prochoice health advocates that it is the right of a pregnant woman to have an abortion performed at her request.

abortion pill. See **mifepristone.**

abortive infection /əbôr′tiv/, an infection in which some or all viral components have been synthesized, but no infective virus is produced.

abortus /əbôr′təs/, any incompletely developed fetus that results from an abortion, particularly one weighing less than 500 g.

abortus fever, a form of brucellosis, the only one endemic to North America. It is caused by *Brucella abortus,* an organism so named because it causes abortion in cows. Infection in humans results from the ingesting contaminated milk from cows infected with *B. abortus.*

abouchement /ä′bōōshmäN′/ [Fr, a tube connection], the junction of a small blood vessel with a large blood vessel.

ABP, abbreviation for **arterial blood pressure.**

ABPM, abbreviation for **ambulatory blood pressure monitoring.**

ABR, abbreviation for **auditory brainstem response.**

abrachia /əbrā′kē-ə/ [Gk, *a* + *brachion,* without arm], the absence of arms. **—abrachial,** *adj.*

abrachiocephalia /əbrā′kē-ōsəfā′lyə/ [Gk, *a,* not, *brachion,* arm, *kephale,* head], a fetal anomaly in which both the head and the arms are missing.

abrade /əbrād′/, to remove the epidermis or other skin layers, usually by scraping or rubbing.

abrasion /əbrā′zhən/ [L, *abradere,* to scrape off], a scraping, or rubbing away of a surface, such as skin or teeth, by friction. Abrasion may be the result of trauma such as a skinned knee; of therapy, as in dermabrasion of the skin for removal of scar tissue; or of normal function, such as the wearing down of a tooth by mastication. **—abrade,** *v.,* **abrasive,** *adj.*

abrasive, 1. pertaining to a substance that can grind or wear down another substance. **2.** an object or surface that can cause an abrasion.

abreact /ab′rē·akt′/, **1.** to release a repressed emotion. **2.** to work off by catharsis effects of a repressed disagreeable experience. **3.** to mentally relive or bring into consciousness repressed experiences.

abreaction /ab′rē·ak′shən/ [L, *ab,* from, *re,* again, *agere,* to act], an emotional release resulting from mentally reliving or bringing into consciousness, through the process of catharsis, a long-repressed, painful experience.

abrosia /əbrō′zhə/ [Gk, fasting], a condition caused by fasting or abstaining from food.

abruption [L, *ab,* away from, *rumpere,* rupture], a sudden breaking off or tearing apart.

abruptio placentae [L, *ab,* away from, *rumpere,* to rupture], separation of the placenta implanted in normal position in a pregnancy of 20 weeks or more or during labor before delivery of the fetus. It occurs in approximately 1 in 200 births, and, because it often results in severe hemorrhage, it is a significant cause of maternal and fetal mortality. Cesarean section must be performed immediately and rapidly. If the pregnancy is near term, labor may be permitted or induced by amniotomy. A premature pregnancy may be allowed to continue under close observation of the mother at bed rest.

abs feb, abbreviation for *absente febre,* a Latin phrase meaning in the absence of fever.

abscess /ab′səs/ [L, *abscedere,* to go away], **1.** a cavity containing pus and surrounded by inflamed tissue, formed as a result of suppuration in a localized infection (characteristically, a staphylococcal infection). Healing usually occurs when an abscess drains or is incised. **2. dental abscess,** an abscess that develops anywhere along the root length of a tooth.

abscess of liver [L, *abscedere,* to go away; AS, *lifer*], an abscess in the liver cells, usually caused by an amebic infection, bacterial infection, or trauma, characterized by sweats and chills, pain, nausea, and vomiting.

abscissa /absis′ə/ [L, *ab,* away; *scindere,* to cut], a point on a horizontal Cartesian coordinate plane measured from the *y-* (or vertical) axis running perpendicular to the plane, or *x*-axis.

abscission /absish′ən/ [L, *abscinere,* to cut away], the process of cutting away, such as, in corneal abscission, removal of the prominence of the cornea.

absconsio abskon′shō/ [L, *ab,* away from, *condo,* hidden], a cavity or fossa.

abscopal /abskō′pəl/, pertaining to the effect of irradiated tissue on remote tissue not exposed to radiation.

absence seizure, an epileptic seizure characterized by a sudden, momentary loss of consciousness. Occasionally it is accompanied by minor myoclonus of the neck or upper extremities, slight symmetric twitching of the face, or loss of muscle tone. The seizures usually occur many times a day without a warning aura and are most frequent in children and adolescents, especially at puberty. The patient experiencing a typical seizure has a vacant facial expression and ceases all voluntary motor activity; with the rapid return of consciousness, the patient may resume conversation at the point of interruption without realizing what occurred.

absenteeism /ab'səntē'izəm/, (for health or related reasons) absence from work. The most common causes of absenteeism include influenza and occupationally related skin diseases.

absent without leave (AWOL) /ā'wôl/ [L, *absentia*], a term used to describe a patient who departs from a psychiatric facility without authorization.

Absidia /absid'ē-ə/, a genus of fungus belonging to the class Phycomycetes. Several species have been found to cause infections of otosclerosis and pulmonary and general mycosis in humans.

absolute, unconditional, unrestricted, or independent of arbitrary standards.

absolute agraphia [L, *absolutus,* set loose; Gk, *a,* not, *graphein,* to write], a complete inability to write caused by a central nervous system lesion. The person is unable to write even the letters of the alphabet.

absolute discharge /ab'səloot/ [L, *absolutus,* set free], a final and complete termination of the patient's relationship with a caregiving agency.

absolute growth, the total increase in size of an organism or a particular organ or part, such as the limbs, head, or trunk.

absolute humidity, the actual mass or content of water in a measured volume of air. It is usually expressed in grams per cubic meter or pounds per cubic foot or cubic yard.

absolute temperature, temperature that is measured from a base of absolute zero on the Kelvin or Rankine scale.

absolute threshold [L, *absolutus,* set loose; AS, *therscold*], the lowest point at which a stimulus can be perceived.

absolute zero, the temperature at which all molecular activity ceases. It is a theoretic value derived by calculations and projections from experiments with the behavior of gases at extremely low temperatures.

absolutum glaucoma /ab'səloo'təm/ [L, *abolutus* + Gk, *cataract*], complete blindness in which a glaucoma-induced increase in intraocular pressure results in permanent vision loss. The optic disc is white and deeply excavated, and the pupil is usually widely dilated and immobile.

absorb /absôrb', əbzôrb'/ [L, *absorbere,* to swallow], **1.** the act of drinking in, wholly engulfing, assimilating, or taking up various substances; for example, the tissues of the intestines absorb fluids. **2.** the energy transferred to tissues by radiation, such as an absorbed dose of radioactivity.

absorbable gauze /əbsôr'bəbəl/, a material produced from oxidized cellulose that can be absorbed. It is applied directly to tissue to stop bleeding.

absorbable surgical suture, [L, *absorbere,* to suck up; Gk, *cheirourgos,* surgery; L, *sutura*], a suture made from material that can be completely removed by the body's phagocytes.

absorbance /əbsôr'bəns/, the degree of absorption of light or other radiant energy by a medium through which the radiant energy passes.

absorbed dose, (in radiotherapy) the energy imparted by ionizing radiation per unit mass of irradiated material at the place of interest. The SI unit of absorbed dose is the gray, which is 1 J/kg and equals 100 rad.

absorbent /absôr'bənt/ [L, *absorbere,* to suck up], **1.** capable of attracting and absorbing substances into itself. **2.** a product or substance that can absorb liquids or gases.

absorbent dressing, a dressing of any material applied to a wound or incision to absorb secretions.

absorbent gauze, a fabric or pad with various forms, weights, and uses. It may be a rolled, single-layered fine fabric for spiral bandages; or it may be a thick, multilayered pad for a sterile pressure dressing. There may also be an adhesive backing.

absorbifacient /absôr'bifā'shənt/ [L, *absorbere* + *facere,* to make], **1.** any agent that promotes or enhances absorption. **2.** causing or enhancing absorption.

absorption /absôrp'shən/ [L, *absorbere*], **1.** the incorporation of matter by other matter through chemical, molecular, or physical action, such as the dissolving of a gas in a liquid or the taking up of a liquid by a porous solid. **2.** (in physiology) the passage of substances across and into tissues, such as the passage of digested food molecules into intestinal cells or the passage of liquids into kidney tubules. **3.**

absorption coefficient (in radiology) the process of absorbing radiant energy by living or nonliving matter with which the radiation interacts.

absorption coefficient, (in radiology) the fractional loss in intensity of electromagnetic energy as it interacts with an absorbing material. It is usually expressed per unit of thickness or per unit mass.

absorption rate constant, a value describing how much drug is absorbed per unit of time.

absorption spectrum, the range of electromagnetic energy that is used for spectroanalysis, including both visible light and ultraviolet radiation; also, a graph of the spectrum for a specific compound.

absorptivity /ab'sôrptiv'itē/, absorbance at a particular wavelength divided by the product of the concentration of a substance and the sample path length.

abstinence /ab'stinəns/, voluntary avoidance of a substance or the performance of an act, such as a method of birth control.

abstinence syndrome [L, abstinere, to hold back; Gk, syn, together, dromos, course], the withdrawal symptoms experienced by a chemically dependent person who is suddenly deprived of a regular intake of alcohol or other addictive substance.

abstract /ab'strakt, abstrakt'/, **1.** a condensed summary of a scientific article, literary piece, or address. **2.** to collect data such as from a medical record.

abstraction /abstrak'shən/ [L, abstrahere, to drag away], a condition in which the teeth or other maxillary and mandibular structures are below their normal position or away from the occlusal plane.

abstract thinking, the final, more complex stage in the development of the cognitive thought processes. It is characterized by adaptability, flexibility, and the use of concepts and generalizations.

abulia /əboo'lyə/ [Gk, a + boule, without will], a loss of the ability or reduced capacity to exhibit initiative or make decisions.

abuse /abyoōs'/ [L, abuti, to waste], **1.** improper use of equipment, a substance, or a service, such as a drug or program, either intentionally or unintentionally. **2.** to physically or verbally attack or injure. An example is **child abuse.**

abused person [Fr, abuser, to disuse, persone, a character acted], an individual who has been harmed or maltreated by another person or by a situation.

abuse of the elderly. See **elder abuse.**

Abuse Protection: Child, a Nursing Interventions Classification defined as identification of high-risk, dependent child relationships and actions to prevent possible or further infliction of physical, sexual, or emotional harm or neglect of basic necessities of life.

Abuse Protection: Elder, a Nursing Interventions Classification defined as identification of high-risk, dependent elder relationships and actions to prevent possible or further infliction of physical, sexual, or emotional harm; neglect of basic necessities of life; or exploitation.

abutment /əbut'mənt/ [Fr, abouter to place end to end], a tooth, root, or implant that serves to support and provide retention for a fixed or movable prosthesis.

abutment tooth, a tooth selected to support a prosthesis.

ABVD, an anticancer drug combination of doxorubicin, bleomycin, vinblastine, and dacarbazine.

Ac, symbol for the element **actinium.**

AC, 1. abbreviation for **alternating current. 2.** abbreviation for *accommodative convergence.*

a.c., (in prescriptions) abbreviation for *ante cibum,* a Latin phrase meaning "before meals."

A-C, abbreviation for *alveolar-capillary.*

acacia gum, a dried, gummy exudate of the acacia tree *(Acacia senegal)* used as a suspending or emulsifying agent in medicines.

academic ladder /ak'ədem'ik/ [Gk, akademeia, school], the hierarchy of faculty appointments in a university through which a faculty member must advance from the rank of instructor to assistant professor to associate professor to professor.

acalculia /a'kalkoo'lyə/ [Gk, a, not; L, calculare, to reckon], a type of aphasia characterized by the inability to perform simple mathematic calculations.

acampsia /əkamp'sē·ə/ [Gk, a + kampsein, not to bend], a condition in which a joint is rigid.

acantha /əkan'thə/ [Gk, akantha, thorn], a spine or a spinous projection. **—acanthoid,** adj.

acanthamebiasis /əkan'thəmēbī'əsis/, a potentially fatal meningoencephalitis infection caused by strains of **Acanthamoeba.** It is commonly acquired by bathing in water contaminated by the microorganism.

Acanthamoeba /əkan'thəmē'bə/, a genus of free-living amebas typically found in soil and water. The organisms may invade and colonize the skin, lung, genitourinary system, brain, and central nervous system.

acanthesia /al'anthē'zhə/, pin prick paresthesia; an abnormality of cutaneous sensory perception that causes a simple touch to be felt as a painful pin prick.

acanthiomeatal line /əkan'thē·ō'mē·ā'təl/, a hypothetic line extending from the external auditory meatus to the acanthion. In dentistry a full maxillary denture is constructed so that its occlusal plane is parallel with this line.

acanthion, a point at the center of the base of the anterior nasal spine.

Acanthocheilonema perstans /akan′thōkī′ lənē′mə/, a threadworm usually found in Africa. It commonly infects wild and domestic animals and occasionally invades the bloodstream of humans, causing a skin rash, muscle and joint pains, and various neurologic disorders.

acanthocyte /əkan′thəsīt′/ [Gk, *akantha* + *kytos,* cell], an abnormal red blood cell with spurlike projections.

acanthocytosis /akan′thōsītō′sis/ [Gk, *akantha* + *kytos* + *osis,* condition], the presence of acanthocytes in the circulating blood.

acanthoid, resembling a spinous process.

acanthoma /ak′anthō′mə/ [Gk, *akantha* + *oma,* tumor], localized hypertrophy arising from the prickle-cell layer of the epidermis. It may be benign or malignant.

acanthoma fissuration, development of a fissure bordered by increased thickening at sites of friction of the prickle-cell level of epidermis.

acanthorrhexis, the rupture of intercellular bridges of the prickle-cell layer of epidermis, as in eczema or contact dermatitis.

acanthosis /ak′ənthō′sis/ [Gk, *akantha* + *osis,* condition], an abnormal thickening of the prickle-cell layer of the skin, as in eczema and psoriasis. —acanthotic, *adj.*

acanthosis nigricans /nē′grikanz′/, a skin disease characterized by hyperpigmented, velvety thickening of the skin, common in the neck, axilla, and groin.

acapnia /əkap′nē·ə/, a deficiency of carbon dioxide in the blood. The condition is usually the result of hyperventilation.

AC/A ratio, (in ophthalmology) the proportion between accommodative convergence (AC) and accommodation (A), or the amount of convergence automatically resulting from the dioptric focusing of the eyes at a specified distance. The ratio of accommodative convergence to accommodation is usually expressed as the quotient of accommodative convergence in prism diopters divided by the accommodative response in diopters.

acarbia /akär′bē·ə/ [Gk, *a,* not; L, *carbo,* coal], **1.** a decrease in the bicarbonate level in the blood. **2.** any condition that lowers the bicarbonate level in the blood.

acardia /akär′dē·ə/ [Gk, *a* + *kardia,* without heart], a rare congenital anomaly in which the heart is absent. It is sometimes seen in a conjoined twin whose survival depends on the circulatory system of its twin. —acardiac, *adj.*

acardius acephalus, an acardiac fetus that lacks a head and most of the upper part of the body.

acardius acormus, an acardiac fetus that has a grossly defective trunk.

acardius amorphus, an acardiac fetus with a rudimentary body that does not resemble the normal form.

acariasis /ak′ərī′əsis/ [Gk, *akari,* mite, *osis,* condition], any disease caused by an acarid such as scrub typhus that is transmitted by trombiculid mites.

acarid /ak′ərid/, one of the many mites that are members of the order Acarina, which includes a great number of parasitic and free-living organisms. Important as vectors of scrub typhus and other rickettsial agents are the six-legged larvae of trombiculid mites, which are parasitic of humans, many other mammals, and birds.

acarodermatitis /ak′ərōdur′mətī′tis/ [Gk, *akari,* mite, *derma,* skin, *itis,* inflammation], a skin inflammation caused by mites or ticks.

acarophobia -fō′bē·ə/, a morbid dread of tiny parasites or the delusion that tiny insects such as mites have invaded the skin.

acaudal /ākôr′dəl/ [Gk, *a,* without; L, *cauda,* tail], without a tail.

acc, Acc, abbreviation for **accommodation.**

accelerated idiojunctional rhythm /aksel′ ərā′tid id′ē·ō·ō-/, an automatic junctional rhythm at a rate exceeding the normal firing rate of the junction but slower than 100 beats/min (60 to 99 beats/min).

accelerated idioventricular rhythm (AIVR), an automatic ectopic ventricular rhythm, faster than the normal rate of the His-Purkinje system but slower than 100 beats/min (50 to 99 beats/min) and without retrograde conduction to the atria.

accelerated junctional rhythm, an ectopic junctional heart rhythm with a rate that exceeds the normal firing rate of junctional tissue, with or without retrograde atrial conduction.

accelerated respiration, an abnormally rapid rate of breathing, usually more than 25 breaths per minute.

acceleration /aksel′ərā′shən/ [L, *accelerare,* to quicken], an increase in the speed or velocity of an object or reaction. —accelerator, *n.*

acceleration-deceleration injury, injury resulting from a collision between a body part and another object while both are in motion.

acceleration phase, (in obstetrics) the first period of active labor, stage I, characterized by an increased rate of dilation of the cervical canal as charted on a Fried-man curve.

accelerator /aksel′ərā′tər/ [L, *accelerare,* to quicken], **1.** a nerve or muscle that increases the rate of performance of some function. **2.** an agent or apparatus that is used to increase the rate at which a substance acts or a function proceeds.

accentuation /aksen′chōō·ā′shən/ ′L, *ac-centus,* accent], an increase in distinct-ness or *loudness,* as in heart sounds.

acceptable daily intake (ADI) /aksep′ təbəl/, the maximum amount of any sub-stance that can be safely ingested by a hu-man. Ingestion that exceeds this amount may cause toxic effects.

acceptance of individuality /aksep′təns/, (in psychiatry) an index of family health in which differentiation or individuation is a valued goal.

acceptance of separation, an indicator of mental well-being in which a loss is mourned in a healthy manner.

acceptor /aksep′tər/ [L, *accipere,* to re-ceive], **1.** an organism that receives from another person or organism living tissue such as transfused blood or a trans-planted organ. **2.** a substance or com-pound that combines with a part of another substance or compound.

access, a means of approach, such as the space needed for the manipulation of den-tal or surgical instruments.

access cavity /ak′ses/ [L, *accedere,* to ap-proach], a coronal opening to the center of a tooth, required for effective cleaning, shaping, and filling of the pulp canal and chamber.

accessory /akses′ərē/ [L, *accessonis,* ap-pendage], **1.** a supplement used chiefly for convenience or for safety, such as the electric elevator mechanisms for hospital beds. **2.** a structure that serves one of the main anatomic systems such as the acces-sory organs of the skin, the hair, the nails, and the skin glands.

accessory diaphragm, a congenital de-fect in which a second diaphragm or part of a diaphragm develops in the chest. It may be separated from the true diaphragm by a lobe of a lung.

accessory gland, glandular tissue that contributes in a secondary way to the function of a similar gland, which may be nearby or some distance away.

accessory ligament [L, *accessionis,* a thing added, *ligare,* to bind], a ligament that helps strengthen a union between two bones, even though it is not part of a joint capsule.

accessory movements, joint movements that are necessary for a full range of mo-tion but that are not under direct voluntary

control of the individual. Examples in-clude rotation and gliding motions.

accessory muscle, a relatively rare ana-tomic duplication of a muscle that may ap-pear anywhere in the muscular system.

accessory muscles of respiration [L, *supplementary*], additional or reinforc-ing muscles, such as muscles of the neck, back, and abdomen, that may play a more prominent role in respiration during a breathing disorder or during exercise.

accessory nasal sinuses [L, *accessus,* ex-tra, *nasus,* nose, *sinus,* hollow], the para-nasal sinuses that occur as hollows within the skull but open into the nasal cavity and are lined with a mucous membrane that is continuous with the nasal mucous mem-brane.

accessory nerve, either of a pair of cra-nial nerves essential for speech, swallow-ing, and certain movements of the head and shoulders. Each nerve has a cranial and a spinal part, communicates with cer-tain cervical nerves, and connects to the nucleus ambiguus of the brain.

accessory organ, an organ or other dis-tinct collection of tissues that contributes to the function of another organ, such as the ocular muscles and eyelids, which contribute to the function of the eye.

accessory pancreas [L, *accessionis,* a thing added; Gk, *pan,* all, *kreas,* flesh], small clusters of pancreas cells detached from the pancreas and sometimes found in the wall of the stomach or intestines.

accessory pancreatic duct, a small duct opening into the pancreatic duct or duode-num near the mouth of the common bile duct.

accessory pathway, an abnormal con-duction connection between an atrium and a ventricle that is outside the normal con-duction system.

accessory phrenic nerve, the nerve that joins the phrenic nerve at the root of the neck or in the thorax, forming a loop around the subclavian vein.

accessory placenta [L, *accessionis,* a thing added, *placenta,* flat cake], a small pla-centa that may develop attached to the main placenta by umbilical blood vessels.

accessory root canal, a lateral branching of the pulp canal in a tooth, usually occur-ring in the apical third of the root.

accessory sign, a sign that is not typical or characteristic of a particular disease.

accessory spleen [L, *accessus,* extra; Gk, *splen*], small nodules of spleen tissue that may occur in the gastrosplenic ligament, greater omentum, or other visceral sites.

accessory thymus [L, *accessus,* extra; Gk, *thymos,* thymelike], a nodule of thymus tissue that is isolated from the gland.

accessory tooth, a supernumerary tooth that does not resemble a normal tooth in size, shape, or position.

ACCH, abbreviation for **Association for the Care of Children's Health.**

accident /ak′sidənt/ [L, *accidere,* to happen], any unexpected or unplanned event that may result in death, injury, property damage, or a combination of serious effects.

accident-prone, describing a person who experiences accidents and accompanying injuries at a much greater than average rate.

acclimate /aklī′mit, ak′limāt/ [L, *ad,* toward; Gk, *klima,* region], to adjust physiologically to a different climate or environment or to changes in altitude or temperature. **acclimation, acclimatization,** *n.*

acclimatization to heat [L, *ad,* toward; Gk, *klima,* region], a process whereby the body adapts to an environment with warmer temperatures.

accommodation (A, acc, Acc) /əkom′ədā′shən/ [L, *accommodatio,* adjustment], **1.** the state or process of adapting or adjusting one thing or set of things to another. **2.** the continuous process or effort of the individual to adapt or adjust to surroundings to maintain a state of homeostasis, both physiologically and psychologically. **3.** the adjustment of the eye to variations in distance. **4.** (in sociology) the reciprocal reconciliation of conflicts between individuals or groups concerning habits and customs, usually through a process of compromise, arbitration, or negotiation.

accommodation reflex, an adjustment of the eyes for near vision, consisting of pupillary constriction, convergence of the eyes, and increased convexity of the lens.

accommodative strabismus /əkom′ədā′tiv/ [L, *accommodatio,* adjustment; Gk, *strabismos,* squint], **1.** strabismus resulting from abnormal demand on accommodation, such as convergent strabismus, uncorrected hyperopia, or divergent strabismus uncorrected myopia. **2.** strabismus resulting from the act of accommodation in association with a high AC/A ratio.

accomplishment quotient /əkom′plishmənt/, a numeric evaluation of a person's achievement age compared with mental age, expressed as a ratio multiplied by 100.

accountability /əkoun′təbil′itē/, being accountable or responsible for the moral and legal requirements of proper patient care.

accreditation /əkred′itā′shən/, a process whereby a professional association or nongovernmental agency grants recognition to a school or institution for demonstrated ability to meet predetermined criteria.

accrementition /ak′rəmentish′ən/, growth or increase in size by the addition of similar tissue or material, as in cellular division, simple fission, budding, or gemmation.

accretio cordis /əkrē′shē·ō/ [L, *accrescere,* to increase, *cordis,* heart], an abnormal condition in which the pericardium adheres to a structure around the heart.

accretion /əkrē′shən/ [L, *accrescere,* to increase], **1.** growth or increase by the addition of material of the same nature that is already present. **2.** the adherence or growing together of parts that are normally separated. **3.** the accumulation of foreign material, especially within a cavity. —**accrete,** *v.,* **accretive,** *adj.*

acculturation /əkul′chərā′shən/, the process of adopting the cultural traits or social patterns of another population group.

accumulated dose equivalent /əkyōō′ myəlā′tid/, an estimate of an individual's absorbed dose of radiation over a lifetime. The unit used to express this absorbed dose is the rem. Occupationally exposed persons are allowed no more than 5 rem per year.

accuracy /ak′yərəsē′/, the extent to which a measurement is close to the true value.

accurate empathy /ak′yərit/, a communication technique used by a nurse to convey an understanding of the patient's feelings and experiences.

ACE, abbreviation for **angiotensin-converting enzyme.**

acebutolol /as′əbōō′təlol/, a beta-adrenergic blocking agent prescribed in the treatment of hypertension, angina pectoris, cardiac arrhythmias, and other cardiovascular disorders.

acedia /əsē′dē·ə/ [Gk, *akedia,* apathy], a condition of listlessness and a form of melancholy, marked by indifference and sluggish mental processes.

ACE inhibitor. See **angiotensin-converting enzyme inhibitor.**

acellular /āsel′yələr/, without cells.

acentric /āsen′trik/ [Gk, *a, kentron,* not center], **1.** having no center. **2.** (in genetics) describes a chromosome fragment that has no centromere.

ACEP, abbreviation for **American College of Emergency Physicians.**

acephalobrachia /asef′əlōbrā′kē·ə/ [Gk, *a* + *kephale,* without head, *brachion,* arm], a congenital anomaly in which a fetus lacks both arms and a head.

acephalocardia /-kär′dē·ə/ [Gk, *a,* not, *kephale,* head, *cardia,* heart], congenital absence of both head and heart.

acephalus /əsef′ələs/ [Gk, *a*, not, *kephale*, head], a headless fetus.

acephaly /əsef′əlē/ [Gk, *a, kephale*, without head], a congenital defect in which the head is absent or not properly developed. —**acephalic,** *adj*.

acerola /as′ərō′lə/, a small, cherrylike fruit of the genus *Malpigia* that grows in tropical climates. It is a richer source of vitamin C than any other known fruit.

acesulfame-K /as′əsul′fām/, a synthetic noncaloric sweetener. It is approximately 200 times sweeter than sucrose. Heat does not affect its sweetening ability, an advantage over aspartame.

acet, abbreviation for an acetate carboxylate anion.

acetabular /as′ətab′yələr/ [L, *acetabulum*, little saucer], pertaining to the acetabulum, the cup-shaped hip socket into which the head of the femur is set.

acetabular notch, an indentation in the margin of the acetabulum, the cup-shaped socket of the hip bone.

acetabuloplasty /as′ətab′yəlōplas′tē/, plastic surgery performed on the acetabulum.

acetabulum /as′ətab′yələm/, *pl.* **acetabula** [L, vinegar cup], the large, cup-shaped cavity at the juncture of the ilium, the ischium, and the pubis, in which the ball-shaped head of the femur articulates.

acetal, 1. a colorless liquid, C_2H_4 $(OC_2H_5)_2$, sometimes used as a hypnotic. **2.** any compound with the general formula $R_2C(OR)_2$ or $RCH(OR)_2$, in which R indicates an alkyl or aryl group.

acetaldehyde /as′ətəldē′hīd/, a colorless, volatile liquid with a pungent odor produced by the oxidation of ethyl alcohol. In the human body acetaldehyde is produced in the liver by the action of alcohol dehydrogenase and other enzymes.

acetaminophen /əset′əmin′əfin/, an analgesic and antipyretic drug used in many nonprescription pain relievers. It has no antiinflammatory properties. It is often prescribed for mild to moderate pain and fever.

acetaminophen poisoning, a toxic reaction to the ingestion of excessive doses of acetaminophen. In adults dosages exceeding 10 to 15 g can produce liver failure, and doses above 25 g can be fatal. Large amounts of acetaminophen metabolites can overwhelm the glutathione-detoxifying mechanism of the liver, resulting in progressive necrosis of the liver within 5 days. The onset of symptoms may be marked by nausea and vomiting, profuse sweating, pallor, and oliguria.

acetate /as′itāt/, a salt of acetic acid.

acetate kinase, an enzyme that catalyzes the transfer of a phosphate group from adenosine triphosphate to acetate.

acetazolamide /as′ətəzō′ləmīd/, a carbonic anhydrase inhibitor diuretic agent prescribed for edema, glaucoma, and epilepsy (primarily petit mal).

Acetest, a trademark for a product used to test for the presence of abnormal quantities of acetone in the urine of patients with diabetes mellitus or other metabolic disorders.

acetic /əsē′tik, əset′ik/ [L, *acetum*, vinegar], pertaining to substances having the sour properties of vinegar or acetic acid; also, chemical compounds possessing the radical CH_3CO—.

acetic acid, a clear, colorless, pungent liquid that is miscible with water, alcohol, glycerin, and ether and that constitutes 3% to 5% of vinegar.

acetic fermentation, the production of acetic acid or vinegar from a weak alcoholic solution.

acetoacetic acid /as′ətō·əsē′tik, əsē′tō-/, a colorless, oily keto acid produced by the metabolism of lipids and pyruvates. It is excreted in trace amounts in normal urine and in elevated levels in diabetes mellitus.

acetohexamide /-hek′səmīd/, a sulfonylurea oral antidiabetic prescribed in the treatment of type II noninsulin-dependent diabetes mellitus (NIDDM).

acetol kinase, an enzyme that catalyzes the transfer of a phosphate group from adenosine triphosphate to hydroxyacetone.

acetone /as′ətōn/, a colorless, aromatic, volatile liquid ketone body found in small amounts in normal urine and in larger quantities in the urine of persons with diabetes who are experiencing ketoacidosis or starvation. Commercially prepared acetone is used to clean the skin before injections.

acetone in urine test, a test for the presence of dimethylketone in the urine of patients, used as a laboratory indication of ketosis and the severity of diabetes mellitus. Chemically treated test paper strips or sticks are exposed to urine. If acetone is present in the urine as the result of incomplete breakdown of fatty and amino acids in the body, the test strips change color. A similar test uses a compound added directly to a urine sample.

acetonide grouping, an acetone-based ketal or ketone-alcohol derivative present in some corticosteroid drugs.

acetonuria /as′ətōnŏŏr′ē·ə/, the presence of acetone and diacetic bodies in the urine.

acetpyrogall /as′ətpī′rəgal/, a topical irritant used as a caustic and keratolytic agent.

acetyl (CH_3CO), a monovalent radical

associated with derivatives of acetic acid, sometimes indicated by the symbol Ac.

acetylcholine (ACh) /as′ətilkō′lēn, əsē′-til-/, a direct-acting cholinergic neurotransmitter agent widely distributed in body tissues, with a primary function of mediating synaptic activity of the nervous system and skeletal muscles. Its active phase is transient because it is rapidly destroyed by acetylcholinesterase. Its activity also can be blocked by atropine at junctions of nerve fibers with glands and smooth muscle tissue.

acetylcholinesterase (AChE) /-kō′lines′-tərās/, an enzyme that inactivates the neurotransmitter acetylcholine by hydrolyzing the substance to choline and acetate. The action reduces or prevents excessive firing of neurons at neuromuscular junctions.

acetylcoenzyme A /əsē′til-kō·en′zīm, as′-ətil-/, a molecule that is formed in the course of several important metabolic processes. The formation of acetylcoenzyme A is the critical intermediate step between anaerobic glycolysis and the citric acid cycle.

acetylcysteine /-sis′tēn/, a mucolytic and acetaminophen antidote prescribed in the treatment of chronic pulmonary disease, acute bronchopulmonary disease, atelectasis resulting from mucous obstruction, and acetaminophen poisoning.

acetylsalicylic acid. See **aspirin.**

acetylsalicylic acid poisoning /əsē′təlsal′-isil′ik, as′itəl-/, toxic effects of overdosage of the commonly used antipyretic and analgesic drug aspirin. Early symptoms of overdosage include dizziness, ringing in the ears, changes in body temperature, gastrointestinal discomfort, and hyperventilation. Severe poisoning is marked by respiratory alkalosis, which may lead to metabolic acidosis. Children are particularly vulnerable to the potential toxic effects of salicylates.

acetyltransferase /-trans′fərās/, any of several enzymes that transfer acetyl groups from one compound to another.

ACG, abbreviation for **apexcardiography.**

ACh, abbreviation for **acetylcholine.**

ACH, abbreviation for **adrenocortical hormone.**

achalasia /ak′əlā′zhə/ [Gk, a + chalasis without relaxation], an abnormal condition characterized by inability of a muscle to relax, particularly the cardiac sphincter of the stomach.

Achard-Thiers syndrome /ash′ärtērz′/ [Emile C. Achard, French physician, 1860–1941; Joseph Thiers, French physician, b. 1885], a hormonal disorder seen in postmenopausal women with diabetes, characterized by growth of body hair in a masculine distribution.

ache /āk/ [OE, acan, to hurt], **1.** a pain characterized by persistence, dullness, and usually moderate intensity. An ache may be localized, as a stomach ache, headache, bone ache, or general ache, as in the myalgia that accompanies a viral infection or a persistent fever. **2.** to suffer from a dull, persistent pain of moderate intensity.

AChE, abbreviation for **acetylcholinesterase.**

acheiria /əkī′rē·ə/ [Gk, a, not, cheir, hand], congenital absence of one or both hands.

acheiropody /al′īrop′ədē/ [Gk, a, not, cheir, hand, pous, foot], absence of hands and feet.

achievement age /əchēv′mənt/, the level of a person's educational development as measured by an achievement test and compared with the normal score for chronologic age.

achievement quotient (AQ), a numeric expression of a person's achievement age determined by various achievement tests, divided by the chronologic age and expressed as a multiple of 100.

achievement test, a standardized test for the measurement and comparison of knowledge or proficiency in various fields of vocational or academic study.

Achilles tendon /əkil′ēz/ [Achilles, Greek mythologic hero], the common distal tendon of the soleus and gastrocnemius muscles of the leg. It is the thickest and strongest tendon in the body and begins near the middle of the posterior part of the leg.

Achilles tendon reflex, a deep tendon reflex consisting of plantar flexion of the foot when a sharp tap is given directly to the tendon of the gastrocnemius muscle at the back of the ankle. This reflex is often absent in people with peripheral neuropathies or diabetes.

achiral, pertaining to the absence of chirality in a compound, as in stereochemical isomers.

achlorhydria /ā′klôrhī′drē·ə/ [Gk, a + chloros, not green, hydor, water], an abnormal condition characterized by the absence of hydrochloric acid in the gastric juice. Achlorhydria occurs most commonly in atrophy of the gastric mucosa, gastric carcinoma, and pernicious anemia involving metabolism and absorption of intrinsic and extrinsic factors. It is also found in severe iron deficiency anemia.— achlorhydric, adj.

achloropsia /ā′klôrop′sē·ə/ [Gk, a, not,

chloros, green, *opsis,* vision], an inability to see green; green blindness.

acholia /əkō'lē·ə/ [Gk, *a* + *chole,* bile], **1.** the absence or decrease of bile secretion. **2.** any condition that suppresses the flow of bile into the small intestine. —**acholic,** *adj.*

acholuria /ak'əlŏŏr'ē·ə/ [Gk, *a* + *chole,* without bile, *ouron,* urine], the absence or lack of bile pigments in the urine.

achondrogenesis /ākon'drōjen'əsis/, a form of dwarfism characterized by gross limb shortening and hydropic head and trunk.

achondroplasia /ākon'drōplā'zhə/ [Gk, *a* + *chondros,* without cartilage, *plassein,* to form], a disorder of the growth of cartilage in the epiphyses of the long bones and skull. It results in premature ossification, permanent limitation of skeletal development, and dwarfism typified by protruding forehead and short, thick arms and legs on a normal trunk.

achondroplastic dwarf /-plas'tik/, the most common type of dwarf, characterized by disproportionately short limbs; a normal-sized trunk; a large head with a depressed nasal bridge; and a small face, stubby hands, and lordosis.

achroma akrō'mə/ [Gk, *a,* without, *chroma,* color], lack of color.

achromatic, **1.** free of color. **2.** color blind. **3.** a substance not colored by common staining agents.

achromatic lens /ak'rəmat'ik/, [Gk, *a,* without, *chroma,* color; L, *lentil*], a lens in which the focal lengths for red and blue colors of the spectrum are the same, refracting light without decomposing it into its component colors.

achromatic vision. See **color blindness.**

achromia /akrō'mēə/ [Gk, *a* + *chroma,* without color], the absence or loss of normal skin pigment.

Achromobacter, akrō'mōbak'tər/, a genus of gram-negative, rod-shaped, and flagellated bacteria that do not form pigment on agar. The species are generally saprophytic, nonpathogenic organisms found in water, soil, and the human digestive tract.

achromocyte /ākrō'məsīt/, a sickle-shaped, abnormally pale erythrocyte.

achylia /ākī'lē·ə/ [Gk, *a, chylos,* not juice], an absence or severe deficiency of hydrochloric acid and pepsinogen (pepsin) in the stomach. This condition may also occur in the pancreas when the exocrine part of that gland fails to produce digestive enzymes.

achylous /əkī'ləs/, **1.** pertaining to a lack of gastric juice or other digestive secretions. **2.** pertaining to a lack of chyle.

acicular /əsik'yələr/ [L, *aciculus,* little needle], needle-shaped, such as certain leaves and crystals.

acid /as'id/ [L *acidus* sour], **1.** a compound that yields hydrogen ions when dissociated in solution. Acids turn litmus red, have a sour taste, and react with bases to form salts. Acids have chemical properties essentially opposite to those of bases. **2.** *slang.* lysergic acid diethylamide (LSD). **3.** sour or bitter to the taste.

acidalbumin, a substance formed by the action of mild acid solutions on albumin.

acid-base balance, a condition existing when the net rate at which the body produces acids or bases equals the net rate at which acids or bases are excreted. The result of acid-base balance is a stable concentration of hydrogen ions in body fluids.

Acid-Base Management, a Nursing Interventions Classification defined as promotion of acid-base balance and prevention of complications resulting from acid-base imbalance.

Acid-Base Management: Metabolic Acidosis, a Nursing Interventions Classification defined as promotion of acid-base balance and prevention of complications resulting from serum HCO_3 levels lower than desired.

Acid-Base Management: Metabolic Alkalosis, a Nursing Interventions Classification defined as promotion of acid-base balance and prevention of complications resulting from serum HCO_3 levels higher than desired.

Acid-Base Management: Respiratory Acidosis, a Nursing Interventions Classification defined as promotion of acid-base balance and prevention of complications resulting from serum pCO_2 levels higher than desired.

Acid-Base Management: Respiratory Alkalosis, a Nursing Interventions Classification defined as promotion of acid-base balance and prevention of complications resulting from serum pCO_2 levels lower than desired.

acid-base metabolism, the metabolic processes that maintain the balance of acids and bases essential in regulating the composition of body fluids. Metabolic buffer systems within the body maintain this ratio, and, when the ratio is upset, either acidosis or alkalosis results.

Acid-Base Monitoring, a Nursing Interventions Classification defined as collection and analysis of patient data to regulate acid-base balance.

acid bath, a bath taken in water containing a mineral acid to help reduce excessive sweating.

acid burn, damage to tissue caused by

exposure to an acid. The severity of the burn is determined by the strength of the acid and the duration and extent of exposure. Emergency treatment includes irrigating the affected area with large amounts of water.

acid dust, an accumulation of highly acidic particles of dust. Such substances accumulate in the atmosphere and account for much of the smog hanging over large metropolitan areas. Many respiratory illnesses, such as lung cancer and asthma, may be aggravated or caused by such dust.

acid dyspepsia, a digestive disorder associated with excessive stomach acidity.

acid-fast bacillus (AFB), a type of bacillus that resists decolorizing by acid after accepting a stain. Examples include *Mycobacterium tuberculosis* and *M. leprae.*

acid-fast stain, a method of staining used in bacteriology in which a smear on a slide is treated with carbol-fuchsin stain, decolorized with acid alcohol, and counterstained with methylene blue to identify acid-fast bacteria.

acid flush, a runoff of precipitation with a high acid content, as may occur during thaws.

acidify /asid'əfī/, **1.** to make a substance acidic, as through the addition of an acid. **2.** to become acidic.

acidity /asid'itē/ [L, *acidus,* sour], the degree of sourness, sharpness of taste, or ability of a chemical to yield hydrogen ions in an aqueous solution.

acidity of the stomach, the degree of gastric acid in the stomach. The acidity varies during any 24-hour period but averages in the range of pH 0.9 to 1.5. The main source of stomach acidity is hydrochloric acid secreted by gastric glands of the stomach.

acid mist, mist containing a high concentration of acid or particles of any toxic chemical, such as carbon tetrachloride or silicon tetrachloride.

acid mucopolysaccharide, a major chemical constituent of ground substance in the dermis.

acidophil /as'idōfil, əsid'əfil/ [L, *acidus* + Gk, *philein,* to love], **1.** a cell or cell constituent with an affinity for acid dyes. **2.** an organism that thrives in an acid medium. —**acidophilic,** *adj.*

acidophilic adenoma, a tumor of the pituitary gland characterized by cells that can be stained red with an acid dye. Gigantism and acromegaly can be caused by an acidophilic adenoma.

acidophilus mllk /as'idof'ələs/, milk inoculated with cultures of *Lactobacillus acidophilus,* used in various enteric disorders to change the bacterial flora of the gastrointestinal tract.

acidosis /as'idō'sis/ [L, *acidus* + Gk, *osis,* condition], an abnormal increase in hydrogen ion concentration in the body, resulting from an accumulation of an acid or the loss of a base. The various forms of acidosis are named for their cause; for example, respiratory acidosis results from respiratory retention of CO_2. Treatment depends on diagnosis of the underlying abnormality and correction of the acid-base imbalance. —**acidotic,** *adj.*

acidosis dialysis, a type of metabolic acidosis that may develop when contaminating bacteria alter the pH of the dialysis bath.

acidotic, pertaining to acidosis, either depletion of base or accumulation of acid.

acid-perfusion test, a test to demonstrate sensitivity of the esophagus to acid, a condition suggestive of reflux esophagitis (heartburn). A weak hydrochloric acid solution and normal saline solution are dripped alternately into the esophagus via a nasal-esophageal tube without telling the patient which solution is being infused. A positive response is pain with acid but not with saline solution.

acid phosphatase, an enzyme found in the kidneys, serum, semen, and prostate gland. It is elevated in serum in cancers of the prostate and in trauma.

acid poisoning, a toxic condition caused by the ingestion of a toxic acid agent such as hydrochloric, nitric, phosphoric, or sulfuric acid, some of which are ingredients in cleaning compounds. Emergency treatment includes giving copious amounts of water, milk, or beaten eggs to dilute the acid. Vomiting is not induced, and mild solutions of alkali are not given.

acid rain, the precipitation of moisture, as rain, with high acidity caused by release into the atmosphere of pollutants from industry, motor vehicle exhaust, and other sources.

acid rebound, a condition of hypersecretion of gastric acid that may occur after the initial buffering effect of an antacid.

acid salt, a salt that is formed from only partial replacement of hydrogen ions from the related acid, leaving some degree of acidity. An example is sodium bicarbonate.

acid therapy, a method for removing warts, which uses plaster patches impregnated with acid, such as 40% salicylic acid.

acidulous /əsid'yələs/, slightly acidic or sour.

aciduria [L, *acidus* + Gk, *ouron* urine, the presence of acid in the urine. The condition may be caused by a diet rich in meat proteins or certain fruits, the introduction of a medication for the treatment of a urinary tract disorder, an inborn error of metabolism, or ketoacidosis.

acinar cell /as'inər/ [L, *acinus,* grape], a cell of the tiny lobules of a compound gland or similar saclike structure such as an alveolus.

Acinetobacter /as'inē' təbak'tər/, a genus of nonmotile, aerobic bacteria of the family Neisseriaceae that often occurs in clinical specimens.

acinic cell adenocarcinoma /asin'ik/ [L, *acinus,* grape], an uncommon low-grade malignant neoplasm that develops in the secreting cells of racemose glands, especially the salivary glands.

aciniform [L, *acinus,* form] /asin'ifôrm/, shaped like a cluster of grapes, particularly used to refer to glandular tissue.

acinitis /as'inī'tis/, any inflammation of the tiny, grape-shaped parts of certain glands.

acinotubular gland /as'inōt(y)ōōb'yələr/, grape-shaped, a gland in which the acini are tube-shaped.

acinus /as'inəs/, *pl.* **acini** [L, grape], **1.** any small saclike structure, particularly one found in a gland. **2.** a subdivision of the lung consisting of the tissue distal to a terminal bronchiole.

AC J, abbreviation for *acromioclavicular joint.*

ACLS, abbreviation for **advanced cardiac life support.**

ACMC, abbreviation for **Association of Canadian Medical Colleges.**

acme /ak'mē/, the peak or highest point, such as the peak of intensity of a uterine contraction during labor.

acne /ak'nē/ /ak'nē/ [Gk, *akme,* point], a disease of the skin common where sebaceous glands are numerous (face, upper back, and chest). Characteristic lesions include open (blackhead) and closed (whitehead) comedo, papule, pustule, and nodule. It seems to result from thickening of the follicular opening, increased sebum production, the presence of bacteria, and the host's inflammatory response. Treatment includes the use of topical and oral antibiotics, topical and oral retinoids, benzoyl peroxide, and azelaic acid.

acne atrophica /atrof'ikə/, a skin disorder characterized by small scars or pits left by an earlier occurrence of acne vulgaris.

acne cachecticorum, an eruption or irritation of the skin that may occur in patients who are very weak and debilitated. It is characterized by soft, mildly infiltrated pustular lesions.

acne conglobata /kong'glōbā'tə/, a se-

vere form of acne with abscess, cyst, scar, and keloid formation.

acneform /ak'nifôrm/, resembling acne.

acneform drug eruption, any of various skin reactions to a drug characterized by papules and pustules resembling acne.

acne fulminans, a form of severe cystic acne characterized by inflamed nodules and plaques that can result in skin ulcers and severe scarring.

acnegenic /ak'nijen'ik/ [Gk, *akme* + *genein,* to produce], causing or producing acne.

acne keloid [Gk, *akme,* point, *kelis,* spot, *eidos,* form], excessive scar tissue that has developed at the site of an acne lesion.

acne necrotica miliaris, a rare, chronic type of folliculitis of the scalp, occurring mostly in adults and characterized by tiny pustules.

acne neonatorum, a skin condition of newborns caused by sebaceous gland hyperplasia and characterized by the formation of grouped comedones on the nose, cheeks, and forehead.

acne papulosa, a common skin condition that develops small papular lesions. It is considered a papular form of acne vulgaris.

acne pustulosa, a form of acne in which the predominant lesions are pustular and may result in scarring.

acne rosacea., See **rosacea.**

acne urticaria /ur'tiker'ē·ə/, a form of acne marked by papules that are predominantly edematous and wheallike and that have been aggravated by scratching.

ACNM, abbreviation for *American College of Nurse-Midwives.*

ACOG, abbreviation for **American College of Obstetricians and Gynecologists.**

acognosia /ak'og·nō'zhə/, a knowledge of remedies.

acorea /ā'kôrē'ə/ [Gk, *a,* without, *kore,* pupil], an absence of the pupil of the eye.

acoria /akôr'ē·ə/ [Gk, *a,* without, *koros,* satiety], a condition characterized by constant hunger and eating, even when the appetite is small.

acorn-tipped catheter, a flexible catheter with an acorn-shaped tip used in various diagnostic procedures, especially in urology.

acousma /əkooz'mə/ [Gk, *akousma,* something heard], a hallucinatory impression of strange sounds.

acoustic /əkoos'tik/ [Gk, *akouein,* to hear], pertaining to sound or hearing.

acoustic apparatus, the various components of the sense of hearing.

acoustic cavitation, a potential biologic effect of ultrasonography, marked by large-amplitude oscillations of microscopic gas bubbles.

acoustic center, the part of the brain in the temporal lobe of the cerebrum in which the sense of hearing is located.

acoustic-immittance audiometry, hearing testing used to evaluate the status of the outer and middle ears and the acoustic-reflex arc. It includes tympanometry, static-compliance testing, and acoustic reflex measures.

acoustic impedance, the effect of interference with the passage of sound waves, such as those generated by ultrasound equipment, by objects in the path of the sound wave. Testing of middle ear impedance is part of audiologic evaluation batteries to detect middle ear problems.

acoustic meatus [Gk, *akoustikos,* hearing; L, *meatus,,* a passage], the external or internal canal of the ear.

acoustic microscope, a microscope in which the object being viewed is scanned with sound waves and its image reconstructed with light waves.

acoustic nerve. See **vestibulocochlear nerve.**

acoustic neuroma, a benign unilateral or bilateral tumor that develops from the eighth cranial (vestibulocochlear) nerve and grows within the auditory canal. Tinnitus, progressive hearing loss, headache, facial numbness, papilledema, dizziness, and an unsteady gait may result.

acoustic reflex, contraction of the stapedius muscle in the middle ear in response to a loud sound. The acoustic reflex threshold is the lowest level of sound that will elicit an acoustic reflex and is in the range of 85 to 90 dB HL in individuals with normal hearing.

acoustics /əkōōs′tiks/ [Gk, *akoustikos,* hearing], the science of sound.

acoustic shadow, an ultrasound image produced by the presence of dense material such as calculi in a scan of soft tissue.

acoustic trauma, a sudden loss of hearing, partial or complete, caused by an extremely loud noise, a severe blow to the head, or other trauma. It may be temporary or permanent.

acoustooptics /əkōōs′tō-op′tiks/, a field of physics that studies the generation of light waves by ultra high–frequency sound waves.

ACP, **1.** abbreviation for *American College of Pathologists.* **2.** abbreviation for **American College of Physicians. 3.** abbreviation for **American College of Prosthodontists.**

acquired /əkwī′ərd/ [L, *acquiere,* obtain], pertaining to a characteristic, condition, or disease originating after birth, not caused by hereditary or developmental factors but by a reaction to environmental influences outside of the organism.

acquired hypogammaglobulinemia [L, *acquirere,* to obtain; Gk, *hypo,* a deficiency, *gamma,* third letter of Greek alphabet; L, *globulus,* small globe; Gk, *haima,* blood], an acquired deficiency of the gamma globulin blood fraction.

acquired immunity, any form of immunity that is not innate and is obtained during life. It may be natural or artificial and actively or passively induced. Naturally acquired immunity is obtained by the development of antibodies resulting from an attack of infectious disease or by the transmission of antibodies from the mother through the placenta to the fetus or to the infant through the colostrum. Artificially acquired immunity is obtained by vaccination or by the injection of antiserum.

acquired immunodeficiency syndrome (AIDS) /ādz/, a syndrome involving a defect in cell-mediated immunity that has a long incubation period, follows a protracted and debilitating course, is manifested by various opportunistic infections, and has a poor prognosis. The disorder originally was found in homosexual men and intravenous drug users but now occurs increasingly among heterosexual men and women and children of those with the disease. AIDS is caused by either of two varieties of the human immunodeficiency virus, designated HIV-1 and HIV-2. HIV is a retrovirus that attracts and kills CD4+ lymphocytes (T helper cells), weakening the immune system's ability to prevent infection. The virus may also invade macrophages, in which it replicates freely, undetected by the immune system. HIV is not spread by casual contact but rather by sexual intercourse or exposure to contaminated blood, semen, breast milk, or other body fluids of infected persons. A patient may be diagnosed as having AIDS if he or she is infected with HIV, has a CD4+ count below 200 to 500/ml, and exhibits one or more of the following signs and symptoms: extreme fatigue, intermittent fever, night sweats, chills, lymphadenopathy, enlarged spleen, anorexia and consequent weight loss, severe diarrhea, apathy, and depression. As the disease progresses, characteristics are a general failure to thrive, anergy, and any of a variety of recurring infections, most commonly *Pneumocystis carinii* pneumonia, tuberculosis, meningitis, and encephalitis caused by aspergillosis, candidiasis, cryptococcosis, cytomegalovirus, toxoplasmosis, or herpes simplex. Most patients with AIDS are susceptible to malignant neoplasms, especially Kaposi's sarcoma, Burkitt's lymphoma, and non-Hodgkin's lymphoma, that both cause and result from immunodeficiency. Treatment consists primarily of combined chemotherapy to counteract the opportunistic infections. Although there is no known cure for AIDS, the antiviral drug zidovudine has been shown to slow the progress of the disease and prolong the lives of patients. Alternative antiviral drugs include didanosine (ddi), stavudine (d4T), and zalcitabine (ddc).

acquired pellicle, an amorphous, acellular membranous layer that forms over exposed tooth and gingival surfaces, restorations, and dental calculus.

acquired sterility [L, *acquiere, to obtain, sterilis,* barren], the failure to conceive after once bearing a child.

acquired trait [L, *acquiere,* to obtain + *trahere,* to draw], a physical characteristic that is not inherited but may be an effect of the environment or a mutation.

ACR, abbreviation for **American College of Radiology.**

acral /ak'rəl/ [Gk, *akron,* extremity], pertaining to the arms and legs.

acrid /ak'rid/, sharp or pungent, bitter and unpleasant to the smell or taste.

acridine /ak'ridēn/, a dibenzopyridine compound used in the synthesis of dyes and drugs.

acrimony /ak'rəmō'nē/ [L, *acrimonia,* pungency], a quality of bitterness, harshness, or sharpness.

acrocentric /ak'rōsen'trik/ [Gk, *akron,* extremity, *kentron,* center], pertaining to a chromosome in which the centromere is located near one of the ends so that the arms of the chromatids are extremely uneven. Compare **metacentric, submetacentric, telocentric.**

acrochordon /ak'rōkôr'don/, a benign, pedunculated growth commonly occurring on the eyelids, neck, axilla, or groin.

acrocyanosis /ak'rōsī'ənō'sis/ [Gk, *akron* + *kyanos,* blue], a condition characterized by blue discoloration, coldness, and sweating of the extremities, especially the hands. It may be caused by arterial spasm and may be precipitated by cold or by emotional stress. Another kind of acrocyanosis is **peripheral acrocyanosis of the newborn.**

acrodermatitis /-dur'mətī'tis/ [Gk, *akron* + *derma,* skin, *itis* inflammation], any eruption of the skin of the hands and feet caused by a parasitic mite belonging to the order Acarina.

acrodermatitis enteropathica /en'tərōp-ath'ikə/, a rare, chronic disease of infants characterized by vesicles and bullae of the skin and mucous membranes, alopecia, diarrhea, and failure to thrive.

acrodynia /ak'rōdin'ē·ə/ [Gk, *akron* + *odyne,* pain], a disease that occurs in infants and young children. Symptoms include edema, pruritus, generalized skin rash, pink coloration of the extremities and scarlet coloration of the cheeks and nose, profuse sweating, digestive disturbances, photophobia, polyneuritis, extreme irritability alternating with periods of listlessness and apathy, and failure to thrive.

acroesthesia /ak'rō·esthē'zhə/ [Gk, *akron,* extremity, *aisthesis,* sensation], a condition of unpleasant feelings in the hands or feet.

acrokeratosis verruciformis /ak'rōker'-ətō'sis/, an inherited skin disorder characterized by the appearance of flat wart-like lesions on the dorsum of the hands and feet and occasionally on the wrists, forearms, and knees.

acrokinesis /-kīnē'sis/ [Gk, *akron,* extremity, *kinesis,* motion], a state in which the limbs possess an abnormally wide range of motion.

acromegalic eunuchoidism, /-məgal'ik/, a rare disorder characterized by genital atrophy and the development of female secondary sex characteristics, occurring in men with advanced acromegaly caused by a tumor in the anterior pituitary gland.

acromegaly /ak'rəmeg'əlē/ [Gk, *akron* + *megas,* great], a chronic metabolic condition characterized by a gradual marked enlargement and elongation of the bones of the face, jaw, and extremities. The condition is caused by the overproduction of growth hormone. —**acromegalic,** *adj.*

acromial process /əkrō·mē·əl/ [Gk, *akron,* extremity, *omos,* shoulder], a flat, triangular lateral extension of the scapula.

acromicria /ak'rəmik'rē·ə/, an anomaly characterized by abnormally small hands and feet. The person may also possess unusually small facial features such as nose and ears.

acromioclavicular articulation /-mī'ōklavik'yələr/, the gliding joint between the acromial end of the clavicle and the medial margin of the acromion process of the scapula.

acromiocoracoid /-kôr'əkoid/, pertaining to the acromion and coracoid processes.

acromiohumeral /-hyōō'mərəl/, pertaining to the acromion and the humerus.

acromion /əkrō'mē·ən/ [Gk, *akron* + *omos,* shoulder], the lateral extension of the spine of the scapula, forming the highest point of the shoulder and connecting with the clavicle at a small oval surface in the middle of the spine. It gives attachment to the deltoideus and trapezius muscles. —**acromial,** *adj.*

acromioscapular /-skap′yələr/, pertaining to the acromion process and the scapula.

acroosteolysis /ak′rō·os′tē·ol′isis/, an occupational disease that mainly affects people who work with polyvinylchloride (PVC) plastic materials. It is characterized by Raynaud's phenomenon, loss of bone tissue in the hands, and sensitivity to cold temperatures.

acroparesthesia /ak′rōpar′isthē′zhə/ [Gk, akron + para, near, aisthesis, feeling], **1.** an extreme sensitivity at the tips of the extremities of the body, caused by nerve compression in the affected area or by polyneuritis. **2.** a disease characterized by tingling, numbness, and stiffness in the extremities, especially in the fingers, hands, and forearms.

acrophobia [Gk, akron + phobos, fear], a pathologic fear or dread of high places that results in extreme anxiety.

acrosomal reaction /ak′rəsō′məl/, the pattern of various chemical changes that occur in the anterior of the head of the spermatozoon in response to contact with the ovum and that lead to the sperm's penetration and fertilization of the ovum.

acrosome /ak′rəsōm′/ [Gk, akron + soma, body], the caplike structure surrounding the anterior end of the head of a spermatozoon. —acrosomal, adj.

acrotic /əkrot′ik/ [Gk, a + krotos, not beating], **1.** pertaining to the surface or to the skin glands. **2.** pertaining to the absence or the weakness of a pulse.

acrylate, an anion, salt, ester, or conjugate base of acrylic acid.

acrylic acid (CH$_2$COOH), a corrosive liquid used in the production of plastic materials used in medical and dental procedures.

acrylic resin base /əkril′ik/, (in dentistry) a denture base made of acrylic resin.

acrylic resin dental cement, a dental cement for restoring or repairing damaged teeth.

ACS, 1. abbreviation for American Cancer Society. **2.** abbreviation for American Chemical Society. **3.** abbreviation for American College of Surgeons. **4.** abbreviation for anodal closing sound.

ACSM, abbreviation for American College of Sports Medicine.

ACTH, abbreviation for adrenocorticotropic hormone.

actigraph /ak′tigraf′/, any instrument that records changes in the activity of a substance or an organism and produces a graphic record of the process, such as an electrocardiograph machine, which produces a record of electrical cardiac activity.

actin, a protein forming the thin fibrils in muscle fibers that are pulled on by the myosin cross-bridges to cause a muscle contraction and muscle relaxation.

acting out, the expression of intrapsychic conflict or painful emotion through overt behavior that is usually pathologic, defensive, and subconscious and that may be destructive or dangerous.

actinic /aktin′ik/ [Gk, aktis, ray], pertaining to radiation, such as sunlight or x-rays.

actinic burn, a burn caused by exposure to sunlight or other source of ultraviolet radiation.

actinic conjunctivitis [Gk, actis, ray, + L, conjunctivus, connecting; Gk, itis, inflammation], an eye inflammation caused by exposure to the ultraviolet (UV) radiation of sunlight or other UV sources, such as acetylene torches, therapeutic lamps (sun lamps), and klieg lights.

actinic dermatitis, a skin inflammation or rash resulting from exposure to sunlight, x-ray, or atomic particle radiation. Chronic or recurrent actinic dermatitis can predispose to skin cancer.

actinic keratosis, a slowly developing, localized thickening of the outer layers of the skin as a result of chronic, prolonged exposure to the sun. Treatment of this premalignant lesion includes surgical excision, cryotherapy, and topical chemotherapy.

actinism, the ability of sunlight or similar forms of radiation to produce chemical changes.

actinium (Ac), a rare, radioactive metallic element. Its atomic number is 89; its atomic weight (mass) is 227. It occurs in some ores of uranium.

Actinobacillus /ak′tinōbasil′əs/, a genus of small, gram-negative bacillus, with members that are pathogenic for humans and other animals. The species Actinobacillus actinomycetemcomitans is the cause of actinomycosis in humans.

Actinomyces /ak′tinōmī′sēz/ [Gk, aktis, ray, mykes, fungus], a genus of anaerobic, gram-positive bacteria. Species that may cause disease in humans, such as Actinomyces israelii, are normally present in the mouth and throat.

actinomycin A /-mī′sin/, the first of a group of chromopeptide antibiotic agents derived from soil bacteria. Most are derivatives of phenoxazine and contain actinocin. They are generally active against gram-positive bacteria, fungi, and neoplasms.

actinomycin B, an antibiotic antineoplastic agent derived from Actinomyces antibioticus.

actinomycin D. See **dactinomycin.**

actinomycosis /ak'tinōmīkō'sis/, a chronic, systemic disease characterized by deep, lumpy abscesses that extrude a thin, granular pus through multiple sinuses. The most common causative organism in humans is *Actinomyces israelii*, a normal inhabitant of the bowel and mouth. Disease occurs after tissue damage, usually in the presence of another infectious organism. There are four principal forms of actinomycosis. Cervicofacial actinomycosis occurs with the spread of the bacterium into the subcutaneous tissues of the mouth, throat, and neck as a result of dental or tonsillar infection. Thoracic actinomycosis may represent proliferation of the organism from cervicofacial abscesses into the esophagus, or it may result from inhalation of the bacterium into the bronchi. Abdominal actinomycosis usually follows an acute inflammatory process in the stomach or intestines, such as appendicitis, diverticulum of the large bowel, or a perforation of the stomach. Generalized actinomycosis may involve the skin, brain, liver, and urogenital system.

actinotherapy, the use of ultraviolet, other parts of the spectrum of the sun's rays, or x-rays to treat various disorders, particularly skin diseases.

action, activity used to carry out a function or produce an effect.

action level, the level of concentration at which an undesirable or toxic component of a food is considered dangerous enough to public health to warrant government prohibition of the sale of that food. The U. S. Food and Drug Administration tests foods for action levels.

action potential, an electrical impulse consisting of a self-propagating series of polarizations and depolarizations, transmitted across the plasma membranes of a nerve fiber during the transmission of a nerve impulse and across the plasma membranes of a muscle cell during contraction or other activity.

action tremor, [L, *agere*, to do, *tremor*, shaking], a tremor that occurs or is evident during voluntary movements.

activate /ak'tǝvāt/, [L, *activus*, active], to induce or prolong an activity or render optimal action.

activated charcoal, a general-purpose emergency antidote and a powerful pharmaceutic adsorbent prescribed in the treatment of acute poisoning and the control of flatulence.

activated partial thromboplastin time (APTT), a timed blood test that determines the efficacy of various clotting factors used in the diagnosis of coagulation disorders. The normal value in venous blood is 32 to 51 seconds.

activating enzyme, an enzyme that promotes or sustains an activity, such as catalyzing the combining of amino acids to form peptides or proteins.

activation, the promotion or production of an activity, such as the generation of a catalyst, protein synthesis, or enzymatic function.

activation energy /ak'tivā'shǝn/ [L, *activus,* active], the energy required to convert reactants to transition-state species that will spontaneously proceed to products.

activation factor. See **factor XII.**

activator /ak'tivā'tǝr/, **1.** a substance, force, or device that stimulates activity in another substance or structure, especially a substance that activates an enzyme. **2.** a substance that stimulates the development of an anatomic structure in the embryo. **3.** an internal secretion of the pancreas. **4.** an apparatus for making substances radioactive, such as a cyclotron or neutron generator. **5.** (in dentistry) a removable orthodontic appliance that functions as a passive transmitter and stimulator of the perioral muscles.

active anaphylaxis [Gk, *ana,* up, *phylaxis,* protection], a condition of hypersensitivity caused by the reaction of the immune system of the body to injection of a foreign protein.

active assisted exercise [L, *activus*], the movement of the body or any of its parts primarily through the individual's own efforts but accompanied by the aid of a therapist or some device such as an exercise machine.

active carrier [OFr, *carier*], a person without signs or symptoms of an infectious disease who carries the causal microorganisms.

active electrode [Gk, *elektron,* amber, *hodos,* way], an electrode that is applied at a specific point to produce stimulation in a concentrated area in electrotherapy.

active exercise, repetitive movement of a part of the body as a result of voluntary contraction and relaxation of the controlling muscles.

active expiration [L, *expirare,* to breathe out], forced exhalation, using the abdominal wall, intracostal muscles, and diaphragm.

active hyperemia [L, *activus* + Gk, *hyper,* excessive, *haima,* blood], the increased flow of blood into a particular body part.

active immunity, a form of long-term, acquired immunity; it protects the body against a new infection as the result of antibodies that develop naturally after an initial infection or artificially after a vaccination.

active labor [L, *activus,* active, *labor,* work], the normal progress of the birth process, including uterine contractions, dilation of the cervix, and descent of the fetus into the birth canal.

Active Listening, a Nursing Interventions Classification defined as attending closely to and attaching significance to a patient's verbal and nonverbal messages.

active movement, muscular action at a joint as a result of voluntary effort.

active-passive, (in psychiatry) a concept that characterizes persons as either actively involved in shaping events or passively reacting to them.

active play, any activity from which one derives amusement, entertainment, enjoyment, or satisfaction by taking a participatory rather than a passive role.

active range of motion (AROM), the range of movement through which a joint can be moved without assistance.

active resistance exercise, the movement or exertion of the body or any of its parts performed totally through the individual's own efforts against a resisting force.

active resistance training (ART), a conditioning or rehabilitation program designed to enhance a patient's muscular strength, power, and endurance through progressive active resistance exercises and muscle overloading.

active sensitization [L, *agere,* to do, *sentire,* to feel], the condition that results when a specific antigen is injected into a person known to be susceptible.

active site, the place on the surface of an enzyme where its catalytic action occurs.

active specific immunotherapy, a therapy in which a cancer patient is exposed to irradiated tumor cells. The injected cells stimulate the production of antibodies that destroy the tumor cells.

active transport, the movement of materials across the membrane of a cell by means of chemical activity that allows the cell to admit otherwise impermeable molecules against a concentration gradient. Expediting active transport are carrier molecules within the cell that bind and enclose themselves to incoming molecules. Active transport is the means by which the cell absorbs glucose and other substances needed to sustain life and health.

activities of daily living (ADL) /aktiv′itēz/, the activities usually performed in the course of a normal day in the person's life, such as eating, toileting, dressing, bathing, or brushing the teeth. The ability to perform the activities of daily living may be compromised by a variety of causes, including chronic illnesses and accidents. An ADL checklist is often used before discharge from a hospital. If any activities cannot be adequately performed, arrangements are made with an outside agency, such as a visiting nurse service, or with family members to provide the necessary assistance.

activity, the action of an enzyme on an amount of substrate that is converted to product per unit of time under defined conditions.

activity coefficient, a proportionality constant, γ, relating activity, α, to concentration, expressed in the equation, $\alpha = \gamma c$.

activity intolerance, a NANDA-accepted nursing diagnosis of insufficient physiologic or psychologic energy to endure or complete required or desired daily activities. Defining characteristics include verbal report of fatigue or weakness, abnormal heart rate or blood pressure response to activity, exertional discomfort or dyspnea, and electrocardiographic changes reflecting arrhythmias or ischemia.

activity intolerance, risk for, a NANDA-accepted nursing diagnosis of the risk of experiencing insufficient physiologic or psychologic energy to endure or complete required or desired daily activities. Risk factors are a history of previous intolerance, deconditioned status, presence of circulatory or respiratory problems, and inexperience with activity.

activity theory, a concept proposed by Robert J. Havighurst, an American gerontologist, that continuing activities from middle age promotes well-being and satisfaction in aging.

Activity Therapy, a Nursing Interventions Classification defined as prescription of and assistance with specific physical, cognitive, social, and spiritual activities to increase the range, frequency, or duration of an individual's (or group's) activity.

activity tolerance, the type and amount of exercise a patient may be able to perform without undue exertion or possible injury.

actomyosin /ak′təmī′əsin/, a complex consisting of parallel threads of actin and myosin proteins in muscle fibers. When a muscle fiber contracts, the two proteins slide past each other, shortening the fiber while increasing its apparent thickness.

actual cautery /ak′choo·əl/ [L, *actus,* act], the application of heat, rather than a chemical substance, in the destruction of tissue.

actual charge, the amount actually charged or billed by a practitioner for a service. The actual charge may not be the

actualize /ak'chōō-əlīz'/, the act of fulfilling a potential, as by a person who may develop capabilities through experience and education.

acuity /əkyōō'itē/, the clearness or sharpness of perception, such as visual acuity.

acuminate wart. See **genital wart.**

Acupressure, a Nursing Interventions Classification defined as application of firm, sustained pressure to special points on the body to decrease pain, produce relaxation, and prevent or reduce nausea.

acupressure needles, needles inserted near a source of bleeding to help control blood loss. The needles exert pressure on tissues adjacent to the damaged vessel.

acupuncture /ak'yəpunk'chər/ [L, *acus* + *punctura*, puncture], a traditional Chinese method of producing analgesia or altering the function of a body system by inserting fine, wire-thin needles into the skin at specific sites on the body along a series of lines, or channels, called meridians. —**acupuncturist,** *n.*

acupuncture point, one of many discrete points on the skin along the several meridians, or chains of points of the body. Stimulation of any of the various points may induce an increase or decrease in function or sensation in an area or system of the body.

acus /ā'kəs/ [L], any needlelike structure.

acute /əkyōōt'/ [L, *acutus,* sharp], **1.** (of a disease or disease symptoms) beginning abruptly with marked intensity or sharpness, then subsiding after a relatively short period. **2.** sharp or severe.

acute abdomen, an abnormal condition characterized by the acute onset of severe pain within the abdominal cavity. An acute abdomen requires immediate evaluation and diagnosis because it may indicate a condition that calls for surgical intervention. Information about the onset, duration, character, location, and symptoms associated with the pain is critical in making an accurate diagnosis.

acute abscess, [L, *acutus,* sharp, *abscedere,* to go away], a collection of pus in a body cavity accompanied by localized inflammation, pain, pyrexia, and swelling.

acute air trapping, a condition of bronchiolar construction that results in early airway closure and trapping of air distal to the affected bronchiole. Persons prone to episodes of acute air trapping learn to control exhalations through pursed-lip breathing.

acute alcoholism, drunkenness or intoxication resulting from excessive consumption of alcoholic beverages. The syndrome is temporary and is characterized by depression of the higher nerve centers, causing impaired motor control, stupor, lack of coordination, and often nausea, dehydration, headache, and other physical symptoms.

acute angle, [L, *acutus* + *angulus*], any angle of less than 90 degrees.

acute anicteric hepatitis [Gk, *a,* without, *ikteros,* jaundice, *hepar,* liver, *itis,* inflammation], an acute hepatitis that is not accompanied by jaundice.

acute articular rheumatism [L, *articulare,* to divide into joints; Gk, *rheumatismos,* that which flows], a common form of adult rheumatism, possibly associated with a pyogenic infection in the joints. Symptoms include fever and arthritis.

acute ascending myelitis [L, *ascendere,* to go up; Gk, *myelos,* marrow, *itis,* inflammation], an inflammation of the spinal cord that extends progressively upward with corresponding interference in nerve functions.

acute ascending spinal paralysis, a progressive spinal paralysis that spreads upward toward the brain.

acute atrophic paralysis [Gk, *a, trophe,* without nourishment, *paralyein,* to be palsied], an acute poliomyelitis involving the anterior horns of the spinal cord and resulting in flaccid paralysis of involved muscle groups and later by atrophy.

acute care, a pattern of health care in which a patient is treated for a brief but severe episode of illness, for the sequelae of an accident or other trauma, or during recovery from surgery. Acute care is usually given in a hospital by specialized personnel using complex and sophisticated technical equipment and materials, and it may involve intensive care or emergency care.

acute catarrhal sinusitis [Gk, *kata* + *rhoia,* flow; L, *sinus,* hollow], an inflammation that involves the nose and sinuses.

acute childhood leukemia, a progressive, malignant disease of the blood-forming tissues. It is characterized by the uncontrolled proliferation of immature leukocytes and their precursors, particularly in the bone marrow, spleen, and lymph nodes. It is the most frequent cancer in children, with a peak onset occurring between 2 and 5 years of age. Acute leukemia is classified according to cell type: acute lymphoid leukemia (ALL) includes lymphatic, lymphocytic, lymphoblastic, and lymphoblastoid types; acute nonlymphoid leukemia (ANLL) includes granulocytic, myelocytic, monocytic, myelogenous, monoblastic, and monomyeloblastic types (the myelocytic and monocytic series are abbreviated **AML**). ALL is predominantly a disease of childhood, whereas AML and ANLL occur in all age groups. The exact cause of the disease is unknown, although various factors are implicated, including genetic defects, immune deficiency, viruses, and carcinogenic environmental factors, primarily ionizing radiation.

acute circulatory failure /sur'kyəlɔtôr'ē/, a drop in heart output resulting from cardiac or noncardiac causes and leading to tissue hypoxia. If not controlled immediately, the condition usually progresses to one of shock syndrome.

acute circumscribed edema [L, *circum,* around, *scribere,* to draw; Gk, *oidema,* swelling], a localized edema, often associated with an inflammatory lesion or process.

acute confusional state, a form of central nervous system dysfunction caused by interference with the metabolic or other biochemical processes essential for normal brain functioning. Symptoms may include disturbances in cognition, levels of awareness, memory, and orientation.

acute delirium, an episode of acute organic reaction that is sudden, severe, and transient.

acute diarrhea [Gk, *dia* + *rhein,* to flow], a sudden severe attack of diarrhea.

acute diffuse peritonitis [L, *diffundere,* to pour out; Gk, *peri,* near, *tenein,* to stretch, *itis,* inflammation], an acute widespread attack of peritonitis affecting most of the peritoneum and usually caused by a perforation of an abdominal organ (e.g., stomach or appendix).

acute disease, a disease characterized by a relatively sudden onset of symptoms that are usually severe. An episode of acute disease results in recovery to a state comparable to the patient's condition of health and activity before the disease, in passage into a chronic phase, or in death.

acute disseminated encephalomyelitis, a form of encephalitis that commonly develops after an acute viral infection, such as measles, apparently as an immune attack on the myelin tissue of the nervous system. Early symptoms may include fever, headache, vomiting, and drowsiness and progress to seizures, coma, and paralysis.

acute diverticulitis, a sudden severe, painful disorder of the intestinal tract, resulting from inflammation of one or more diverticula, or pouches, in the wall of the bowel. The condition is typically diagnosed through x-rays and treated surgically.

acute endarteritis [Gk, *endon,* within, *arteria,* windpipe, *itis,* inflammation], an

inflamed condition of the cells lining an artery. It may be caused by an infection or the proliferation of fibrous tissue inside the wall of a large artery.

acute epiglottitis, a severe, rapidly progressing bacterial infection of the upper respiratory tract that occurs in young children, primarily between 2 and 7 years of age. It is characterized by sore throat, croupy stridor, and inflamed epiglottis, which may cause sudden respiratory obstruction and possibly death. The infection is generally caused by *Haemophilus influenzae,* type B, although streptococci may occasionally be the causative agent. Transmission occurs by infection with airborne particles or contact with infected secretions.

acute fatigue, a sudden onset of physical and mental exhaustion or weariness, particularly after a period of severe exertion. Physical factors usually include an accumulation of waste products of muscle contractions.

acute fibrinous pericarditis [L, *fibra,* fibrous; Gk, *peri,* near, *kardia,* heart, *itis,* inflammation], an acute inflammation of the endothelial cells of the pericardium with fibers extending into the pericardial sac.

acute goiter, [L, *guttur,* throat], a condition of sudden enlargement of the thyroid gland.

acute granulocytic leukemia (AGL). See **acute myelocytic leukemia (AML).**

acute hallucinatory paranoia, a form of psychosis in which hallucinations are combined with delusions of paranoia.

acute hemorrhagic conjunctivitis, a highly contagious eye disease usually caused by enterovirus type 70. The disease is found primarily in densely populated humid areas, particularly the developing countries or places with a large immigrant population. Clinical features include sudden onset of ocular pain, itching, redness, photophobia, edema of the eyelid, and profuse watery discharge.

acute hemorrhagic pancreatitis [Gk, *haima,* blood, *rhegnynei,* to gush, *pan,* all, *kreas,* flesh], a potentially fatal inflammation of the pancreas characterized by bleeding, tissue necrosis, and digestive tract paralysis.

acute hypoxia, a sudden or rapid depletion in available oxygen at the tissue level. The condition may result from asphyxia, airway obstruction, acute hemorrhage, blockage of the alveoli by edema or infectious exudate, or abrupt cardiorespiratory failure. Clinical signs may include hypoventilation or hyperventilation to the point of air hunger and neurologic deficits ranging from headache and confusion to loss of consciousness.

acute illness, any illness characterized by signs and symptoms that are of rapid onset and short duration; it may be severe and impair normal functioning of the patient.

acute infectious paralysis [L, *inficere,* to stain; Gk, *paralyein,* to be palsied], **1.** an alternative term for acute anterior poliomyelitis. **2.** infectious polyneuritis.

acute intermittent porphyria (AIP), a genetically transmitted metabolic disorder characterized by acute attacks of neurologic dysfunction that can be started by environmental or endogenous factors. Women are affected more frequently than men, and attacks often are precipitated by starvation or severe dieting, alcohol ingestion, bacterial or viral infections, and a wide range of pharmaceutic products. Any part of the nervous system can be affected, and a common effect is mild to severe abdominal pain associated with autonomic neuropathy.

acute lobar pneumonia, a form of pneumonia characterized by lobar distribution of the consolidation of the serofibrous fluid exuded by the alveoli. The condition results from an infection by a virulent type of pneumococcus. Symptoms include a stabbing pain in the side, dry cough, and rusty sputum.

acute lymphocytic leukemia (ALL), a progressive, malignant disease characterized by large numbers of immature cells resembling lymphoblasts in the bone marrow, circulating blood, lymph nodes, spleen, liver, and other organs. The number of normal blood cells is usually reduced. More than three fourths of the cases in the United States occur in children, with the greatest number diagnosed between 2 and 5 years of age. The risk of the disease is increased for people with Down syndrome and for siblings of leukemia patients.

acute myelitis, a sudden, severe inflammation of the spinal cord.

acute myelocytic leukemia (AML), a malignant neoplasm of blood-forming tissues characterized by the uncontrolled proliferation of immature granular leukocytes that usually have azurophilic Auer rods in their cytoplasm. Typical symptoms are spongy bleeding gums, anemia, fatigue, fever, dyspnea, moderate splenomegaly, joint and bone pains, and repeated infections. AML occurs most frequently in adolescents and young adults. The risk of the disease is increased among people who have been exposed to massive doses of radiation and who have certain blood dyscrasias.

acute myocardial infarction (AMI) [L, *acutus,* + Gk, *mys,* muscle, *kardia,* heart; L, *infarcire,* to stuff], the early critical stage of myocardial necrosis caused by blockage of a coronary artery. It is characterized by elevated ST segments in the reflecting leads.

acute necrotizing hemorrhagic encephalopathy, a degenerative brain disease, characterized by marked edema, numerous minute hemorrhages, necrosis of blood vessel walls, demyelination of nerve fibers, and infiltration of the meninges with neutrophils, lymphocytes, and histiocytes. Typical signs are severe headache, fever, and vomiting; convulsions may occur, and the patient may rapidly lose consciousness.

acute necrotizing ulcerative gingivitis (ANUG), a distinct, recurrent periodontal disease that primarily affects the interdental papillae, causing necrosis and ulceration of the gums. There may be fever, bone destruction, a fetid odor, and enlarged lymph nodes in the throat and neck.

acute nephritis, a sudden inflammation of the kidney, characterized by albuminuria and hematuria, but without edema or urine retention. It affects children most commonly and usually involves only a few glomeruli.

acute nicotine poisoning [L, *Nicotiana, potio,* drink], a toxic effect produced by nicotine, usually in the insecticide form. Characteristics include burning sensation in the mouth, nausea and vomiting, diarrhea, palpitations, pulmonary edema, and convulsions that may lead to death.

acute nongonorrheal vulvitis [L, *non,* not; Gk, *gone,* seed, *rhoia,* flow; L, *vulva,* wrapper; Gk, *itis,* inflammation], an inflammation of the vulva resulting from chafing, accumulation of sebaceous material, or other causes that are nonvenereal.

acute nonspecific pericarditis [Gk, *peri,* around, *kardia,* heart, *itis,* inflammation], an inflammation of the pericardium, with or without effusion. It often is associated with myocarditis but usually resolves without complications.

acute pain, severe pain, as may follow surgery or trauma or accompany myocardial infarction or other conditions and diseases. Acute pain occurring in the first 24 to 48 hours after surgery is often difficult to relieve, even with drugs. Acute pain in individuals with orthopedic problems originates from the periosteum, the joint surfaces, and the arterial walls. Muscle pain associated with bone surgery results from muscle ischemia rather than muscle tension.

acute pancreatitis [Gk, *pan,* all, *kreas,*

flesh, *itis,* inflammation], a sudden inflammation of the pancreas caused by autodigestion and marked by symptoms of acute abdomen and escape of pancreatic enzymes into the pancreatic tissues. The condition is associated with biliary disease or alcoholism.

acute paranoid disorder, a psychopathologic condition characterized by a persecutory delusional system of rapid onset, quick development, and short duration, usually lasting less than 6 months. The disorder, which rarely becomes chronic, is most commonly seen in persons who have experienced drastic changes in their environment such as immigrants, refugees, prisoners, and military inductees.

acute pharyngitis, a sudden, severe inflammation of the pharynx.

acute pleurisy, an inflammation of the pleura, often secondary to a lung disease. It is characterized by irritation without recognizable effusion and is localized.

acute primary myocarditis, 1. an inflammation of the heart muscle most commonly caused by a bacterial infection initiated locally or carried through the bloodstream. **2.** a severe inflammation of the heart muscle associated with degeneration in the muscle fibers with the release of leukocytes into the interstitial tissues.

acute promyelocytic leukemia (AProL), a malignancy of the blood-forming tissues, characterized by the proliferation of promyelocytes and blast cells with distinctive Auer rods. Symptoms include severe bleeding and bruises. The patient may also have a low fibrinogen level and platelet count.

acute prostatitis [L, *acutus,* sharp; Gk, *prostates,* one standing before, *itis,* inflammation], a sudden, severe inflammation of the prostate.

acute psychosis, one of a group of disorders in which ego functioning is either impaired or inhibited. The ability to process reality-based information is diminished and disordered. The cause of the particular disorder may be a known physiologic abnormality. In situations in which the physiologic abnormality is not recognized, the functional impairment is still clearly present.

acute pyogenic arthritis, an acute bacterial infection of one or more joints, caused by trauma or a penetrating wound and occurring most frequently in children. Typical signs are pain, redness, and swelling in the affected joint; muscular spasms in the area; chills; fever; diaphoresis; and leukocytosis.

acute rejection [L, *rejicere,* to throw back], the rapid reaction against allograft or xe-

nograph tissue that is incompatible. It occurs after about a week's delay, during which the immune response increases in intensity.

acute respiratory distress syndrome. See **adult respiratory distress syndrome.**

acute respiratory failure (ARF) [L, *acutus* + *respirare,* respiratory, *fallere,* to deceive], a sudden inability of the lungs to maintain normal respiratory function. It may be caused by an obstruction in the airways or failure of the lungs to exchange gases in the alveoli.

acute rheumatic arthritis, arthritis that occurs during the acute phase of rheumatic fever.

acute schizophrenia, a disorder consisting of various degrees of psychosis that is characterized by the sudden onset of personality disorganization. Symptoms include disturbances in thought, mood, and behavior. Episodes appear suddenly in persons whose previous behavior has been relatively normal and are usually of short duration.

acute secondary myocarditis, a sudden severe inflammation of the heart muscle, secondary to a disease of the endocardium or the pericardium or a generalized infection.

acute septic myocarditis [Gk, *septikos,* putrid, *mys,* muscle, *kardia,* heart, *itis,* inflammation], a severe inflammation of the myocardium associated with pus formation, necrosis, and abscess formation.

acute suppurative arthritis [L, *suppurare,* to form pus], a form of arthritis characterized by an invasion of the joint space by pyogenic organisms and the formation of pus in the joint cavity.

acute suppurative sinusitis [L, *acutus,* sharp, *suppurare,* to form pus, *sinus,* hollow; Gk, *itis,* inflammation], a purulent infection of the sinuses. Symptoms are pain over the inflamed area, headache, chills, and fever.

acute tonsillitis [L, *acutus,* sharp, *tonsilla;* Gk, *itis,* inflammation], an inflammation of tonsil(s) associated with a catarrhal exudate over the tonsil or the discharge of caseous or suppurative material from the tonsil crypts.

acute toxicity, the harmful effect of a toxic agent that manifests itself in seconds, minutes, hours, or days after entering the patient.

acute transverse myelitis, an inflammation of the entire thickness of the spinal cord, affecting both the sensory and motor nerves. It can develop rapidly, accompanied by necrosis and neurologic deficit that commonly persist after recovery. Patients in whom spastic reflexes develop soon after the onset of this disease are more likely to recover. This disorder may result from a variety of causes such as multiple sclerosis, measles, pneumonia, and the ingestion of certain toxic agents such as carbon monoxide, lead, and arsenic.

acute tubular necrosis (ATN) [L, *tubulus,* tubule; Gk, *nekros,* dead, *osis,* condition], sudden failure of the kidney tubules. The condition is commonly caused by an interruption of the blood supply to the tubules, resulting in ischemia.

acute urethral syndrome [Gk, *ourethra,* urethra, *syn,* together, *dromos,* course], a group of pelvic area symptoms experienced by women, including dysuria, urinary frequency, urinary tenesmus, lower back pain, and suprapubic aching and cramping. Clinical evidence of a pathogen or other factor to account for the symptoms may be absent.

acyanotic /ā'sī·ənot'ik/ [Gk, *a,* not, *kyanos,* blue], pertaining to absence of a blue appearance of the skin and mucous membranes.

acyanotic congenital defect /āsī'ənot'ik/ [Gk, *a, kyanos,* not blue], a heart defect present at birth that does not produce blue discoloration of the skin and mucous membranes under normal circumstances.

acyclovir /əsī'klōvir/, a herpes simplex virus (HSV-1 or HSV-2) or antiviral agent (acycloguanosine). It is prescribed topically in an ointment for the treatment of herpes simplex keratitis and both topically and systemically in other types of herpes infections, including genital herpes. Acyclovir appears to act selectively by inhibiting the functions of herpesvirus deoxyribonucleic acid molecules.

acyesis /ā'sī·ē'sis/, **1.** the absence of pregnancy. **2.** a condition of sterility in women.

acylation /as'ilā'shən/, the incorporation into a molecule of an organic compound of an acyl group.

a.d., abbreviation for **auris dextra,** or right ear.

AD, Abbreviation for **Alzheimer's disease.**

ADA, **1.** abbreviation for *American Dental Association.* **2.** abbreviation for *American Diabetes Association.* **3.** abbreviation for *American Dietetic Association.* **4.** abbreviation for **adenosine deaminase.**

adactyly /ādak'tilē/ [Gk, *a + daktylos,* not finger or toe], a congenital defect in which one or more digits of the hand or foot are missing.

Adair-Dighton's syndrome [Charles Adair-Dighton, twentieth-century British physician], osteogenesis imperfecta,

type I, the most common and mildest type of failure of normal bone development. The bones are brittle and break easily. The condition is transmitted by an autosomal-dominant gene.

Adam, Evelyn, a Canadian nursing theorist who applied the structure of a conceptual model for nursing in her book, *Être Infirmière* in 1979 (*To Be a Nurse,* 1980). A conceptual model consists of assumptions, beliefs and values, and major units. Adam believes that a theory is useful to more than one discipline, but that a conceptual model for a discipline is useful only to that discipline.

ADAMHA, abbreviation for U.S. *l, Drug Abuse, and Mental Health Administration.*

Adam's apple, *informal,*the bulge at the front of the neck produced by the thyroid cartilage of the larynx.

Adams-Stokes syndrome [Robert Adams, Dublin surgeon, 1791–1875; William Stokes, Dublin physician, 1804–1878], a condition characterized by sudden recurrent episodes of loss of consciousness because of incomplete heart block. Seizures may accompany the episodes.

adaptation /ad'aptā'shən/ [L, *adaptatio,* act of adapting], a change or response to stress of any kind, such as inflammation of the nasal mucosa in infectious rhinitis or increased crying in a frightened child. Adaptation may be normal, self-protective, and developmental.

adaptation model, (in nursing) a conceptual framework that focuses on the patient as an adaptive system, one in which nursing intervention is required when a deficit develops in the patient's ability to cope with the internal and external demands of the environment. These demands are classified into four groups: physiologic needs, the need for a positive self-concept, the need to perform social roles, and the need to balance dependence and independence. Nursing care is planned to promote adaptive responses to cope successfully with the current stress on the patient's well-being.

adapted clothing, clothing that has been modified to permit disabled persons to dress themselves with minimal difficulty.

adapter [L, *adaptatio,* the process of adjusting], a device for joining or connecting two or more parts of a system to enable it to function properly.

adaptive capacity, decreased: intracranial, a NANDA-accepted nursing diagnosis; a clinical state in which intracranial fluid dynamic mechanisms that normally compensate for increases in intracranial volumes are compromised, resulting in repeated disproportionate increases in intra-cranial pressure (ICP) in response to a variety of noxious and nonnoxious stimuli. Defining characteristics include repeated increases in ICP of greater than 10 mm Hg for more than 5 minutes after any of a variety of external stimuli.

adaptive device /adap'tiv/ [L, *adaptatio,* process of adapting; OFr, *devise*], any structure, design, instrument, contrivance, or equipment that enables a person with a disability to function independently.

adaptive hypertrophy [L, *adaptatio,* process of adapting; Gk, *hyper,* excessive, *trophe,* nourishment], a reactive increase in amount of tissue that compensates for a loss of the same or similar tissue so that function is not impaired.

adaptive response, an appropriate reaction to an environmental demand.

ADC, abbreviation for **AIDS-dementia complex.**

ADC Van Disal, /ā'dē'sē'vandī'səl/, a term used as a mnemonic device for recalling the protocol of hospital admission orders. The letters stand for Admission authorization, Diagnosis, Condition, Vital signs, Activity, Drugs, Instructions, Special studies, Allergies, Laboratory tests.

Addams, Jane, (1860–1935) an American social reformer. In Chicago in 1889 she founded Hull House, one of the first social settlements in the United States, where volunteers from many disciplines, including nursing, lived and worked in their professions. She was co-recipient of the Nobel peace prize in 1931.

addict /ad'ikt/ [L, *addicere,* to devote], a person who has become physiologically or psychologically dependent on a chemical such as alcohol or other drugs to the extent that normal social, occupational, and other responsible life functions are disrupted.

addiction /ədik'shən/ [L, *addicere,* to devote], compulsive, uncontrollable dependence on a substance, habit, or practice to such a degree that cessation causes severe emotional, mental, or physiologic reactions.

addictive personality /ədik'tiv/, a personality marked by traits of compulsive and habitual use of a substance or practice in an attempt to cope with psychic pain engendered by conflict and anxiety.

Addis count [Thomas Addis, American physician, 1881–1949], a method for counting red blood cells, white blood cells, epithelial cells, casts, and protein content in a sedimented 12-hour urine sample collected overnight. The count is useful for diagnosing and managing kidney disease.

addisonism, [Thomas Addison, London physician, 1793–1860], a condition characterized by the physical signs of Addison's disease, although loss of adrenocortical functions is not involved. The signs include increase in bronze pigmentation of the skin and mucous membranes caused by increased melanocyte-stimulating hormone, as well as general debility.

Addison's disease [Thomas Addison], a life-threatening condition caused by partial or complete failure of adrenocortical function, often resulting from autoimmune processes, infection (especially tubercular or fungal), neoplasm, or hemorrhage in the gland. All three general functions of the adrenal cortex (glucocorticoid, mineralocorticoid, and androgenic) are lost.

addition [L, *additio,* something added], a chemical reaction in which two complete molecules combine to form a new product, usually by attachment to carbon atoms at a double or triple bond of one of the molecules.

additive /ad'itiv/, any substance added intentionally or indirectly that becomes a part of the food, pharmaceutical, or other product. Additives may be introduced in growing, processing, packaging, storage, or cooking or other final preparation for consumption.

additive effect [L, *additio,* something added, *effectus*], the combined effect of drugs that, when used in combination, produce an enhanced effect that is no greater than the sum of their separately measured individual effects.

adducent /ədoo'sənt/, an agent or other stimulus that causes a limb to be drawn toward the median axis of the body or the fingers or toes to move together.

adduct /ədukt'/ [L, *adducere,* to bring to], to move toward the median axis of the body.

adduction /əduk'shən/ [L, *adducere,* to bring to], movement of a limb toward the axis of the body.

adductor /əduk'tər/, a muscle that draws a part toward the axis or midline of the body.

adductor brevis, a somewhat triangular muscle in the thigh and one of the five medial femoral muscles. It acts to adduct and rotate the thigh medially and to flex the leg.

adductor canal, a triangular channel beneath the sartorius muscle and between the adductor longus and vastus medialis through which the femoral vessels and the saphenous nerve pass.

adductor longus, the most superficial of the three adductor muscles of the thigh and one of five medial femoral muscles. It functions to adduct and flex the thigh.

adductor magnus, the long, heavy triangular muscle of the medial aspect of the thigh. The adductor magnus acts to adduct the thigh. The proximal part acts to rotate the thigh medially and flex it on the hip; the distal part acts to extend the thigh and rotate it laterally.

adenalgia /ad′ənal′jə/ [Gk, aden, gland, algos, pain], a pain in any of the glands.

adenectomy /ad′ənek′təmē/ [Gk, aden + ektome, excision], the surgical removal of any gland.

adenine /ad′ənin/, a purine-base component of the nucleic acids, deoxyribonucleic acid (DNA) and ribonucleic acid (RNA), and a constituent of cyclic adenosine monophosphate (AMP) and the adenosine part of AMP, adenosine diphosphate (ADP), and adenosine triphosphate (ATP).

adenitis /ad′ənī′tis/, an inflammatory condition of a lymph node. Acute adenitis of the cervical lymph nodes may accompany a sore throat and stiff neck. Scarlet fever may cause an acute suppurative cervical adenitis. Swelling of the lymph nodes in the back of the neck is often the result of a scalp infection, insect bite, or infestation by head lice. Inflammation of the lymph nodes of the mesenteric part of the peritoneum often produces pain and other symptoms similar to those of appendicitis.

adenoacanthoma /ad′ənō·ak′anthō′mə/ [Gk, aden + akantha, thorn, oma, tumor], a neoplasm that may be malignant or benign, derived from glandular tissue with squamous differentiation shown by some of the cells.

adenoameloblastoma /ad′ənō·amel′ōblastō′mə/, a benign tumor of the maxilla or mandible composed of ducts lined with columnar or cuboidal epithelial cells. It develops in tissue that normally gives rise to the teeth, and it most often occurs in young people.

adenoassociated virus (AAV) /ad′ənō-/, a defective virus that can reproduce only in the presence of adenoviruses.

adenocarcinoma /ad′ənōkärsinō′mə/ [Gk, aden + karkinos, crab, oma], any one of a large group of malignant epithelial cell tumors of the glands. Specific tumors are diagnosed and named by cytologic identification of the tissue affected; for example, an adenocarcinoma of the uterine cervix is characterized by tumor cells resembling the glandular epithelium of the cervix.—**adenocarcinomatous,** adj.

adenocarcinoma in situ, a localized growth of abnormal glandular tissue that may become malignant. It is most common in the endometrium and large intestine.

adenocele /ad′ənōsēl′/, a cystic, glandular tumor.

adenochondroma /ad′ənōkondrō′mə/ [Gk, aden + chondros, cartilage, oma], a neoplasm of cells derived from glandular and cartilaginous tissues, as a mixed tumor of the salivary glands.

adenocyst /ad′ənōsist′/ [Gk, aden + kytis, bag], a benign tumor in which the cells form cysts. A kind of adenocyst is **papillary adenocystoma lymphomatosum.**

adenocystic carcinoma, a malignant neoplasm composed of cords of uniform small epithelial cells arranged in a sievelike pattern around cystic spaces that often contain mucus. The tumor occurs most frequently in the salivary glands, breast, mucous glands of the upper and lower respiratory tract, and occasionally in vestibular glands of the vulva.

adenoepithelioma /ad′ənō·ep′ithē′lē·ō′mə/ [Gk, aden + epi, on, thele nipple, oma], a neoplasm consisting of glandular and epithelial components.

adenofibroma /ad′ənōfībrō′mə/ [Gk, aden + L, fibra, fiber, oma], a tumor of the connective tissues that contains glandular elements.

adenofibroma edematodes, a neoplasm consisting of glandular elements and connective tissue in which marked edema is present.

adenohypophysis /ad′ənō′hīpof′isis/ [Gk, aden + hypo, beneath, phyein, to grow], the anterior lobe of the pituitary gland. It secretes growth hormone, thyroid-stimulating hormone, adrenocorticotropic hormone, melanocyte-stimulating hormone, follicle-stimulating hormone, luteinizing hormone, prolactin, beta lipotropin molecules, and endorphins. Releasing hormones from the hypothalamus regulate secretions.

adenoid /ad′ənoid/ [Gk, aden + eidos, form], 1. having a glandular appearance, particularly lymphoid. 2. adenoids, the pharyngeal tonsils. —**adenoidal,** adj.

adenoidal speech, an abnormal manner of speaking caused by hypertrophy of the adenoidal tissue that normally exists in the nasopharynx of children. It is often characterized by a muted, nasal quality.

adenoidectomy /ad′ənoidek′təmē/ [Gk, aden + eidos, form, ektome, excision], removal of the lymphoid tissue in the nasopharynx. The surgical procedure may be performed because the adenoids are enlarged, causing obstruction, or chronically infected.

adenoid hyperplasia, a condition in which enlarged adenoid glands cause partial respiratory obstruction, especially in children. Enlarged adenoids are a frequent cause of recurrent otitis media, sinusitis, and conduction deafness.

adenoid hypertrophy [Gk, *aden,* gland, *eidos,* form, *hyper,* excessive, *trophe,* nourishment], an enlargement of the pharyngeal tonsil.

adenoiditis /ad′ənoidī′tis/, inflammation of the adenoids or pharyngeal tonsils.

adenoids, small masses of lymphoid tissue forming the pharyngeal tonsils on the posterior wall of the nasopharynx.

adenoid tissue, the lymphoid tissue that forms the pharyngeal tonsils.

adenoleiomyofibroma /ad′ənōlī′ōmī′ ōfībrō′mə/ [Gk, *aden* + *leios,* smooth, *mys,* muscle; L, *fibra,* fiber; Gk, *oma*], a glandular tumor with smooth muscle, connective tissue, and epithelial elements.

adenolipoma /ad′ənōlipō′mə/ [Gk, *aden* + *lipos,* fat, *oma*], a neoplasm consisting of elements of glandular and fatty tissue.

adenolipomatosis /ad′ənōlipōmətō′sis/, a condition characterized by the growth of adenolipomas in the groin, axilla, and neck.

adenoma /ad′ənō′mə/ [Gk, *aden* + *oma*], a tumor of glandular epithelium in which the cells of the tumor are arranged in a recognizable glandular structure. An adenoma may cause excess secretion by the affected gland, such as acidophilic pituitary adenoma resulting in an excess of growth hormone. **—adenomatous,** *adj.*

adenoma sebaceum /sebā′sē-əm/, an abnormal skin condition consisting of multiple wartlike, yellowish red, waxy papules on the face that are not sebaceous, composed chiefly of fibrovascular tissue. The lesions are usually benign.

adenomatoid /ad′əno′mətoid/ [Gk, *aden* + *oma* + *eidos,* form]. resembling a glandular tumor.

adenomatosis /ad′ənōmətō′sis/, an abnormal condition in which hyperplasia or tumor development affects two or more glands, usually the thyroid, adrenals, or pituitary.

adenomatous goiter /ad′ənō′mətəs/, an enlargement of the thyroid gland caused by an adenoma or numerous colloid nodules.

adenomatous polyp [Gk, *aden,* gland, *oma,* tumor, *polys,* many, *pous,* foot], a tumor that develops in glandular tissue.

adenomatous polyposis coli (APC), a gene associated with familial adenomatous polyposis, an inherited disorder characterized by the development of myriad polyps in the colon, beginning in late adolescence or early adulthood. Untreated, the condition may lead to colon cancer.

adenomyofibroma /ad′ənōmī′ōfībrō′mə/ [Gk, *aden* + *mys,* muscle; L, *fibra,* fiber; Gk, *oma*], a fibrous tumor that contains glandular and muscular components.

adenomyoma /ad′ənōmī-ō′mə/, a tumor of the endometrium of the uterus characterized by a mass of smooth muscle containing endometrial tissue and glands.

adenomyomatosis /ad′ənōmī′ōmətō′sis/, an abnormal condition characterized by the formation of benign nodules resembling adenomyomas, found in the uterus or in parauterine tissue.

adenomyosarcoma /ad′ənōmī′ōsärkō′mə/, a malignant tumor of soft tissue containing glandular elements and striated muscle.

adenomyosis /ad′ənōmī-ō′sis/, **1.** a benign neoplastic condition characterized by tumors composed of glandular tissue and smooth muscle cells. **2.** a malignant neoplastic condition characterized by the invasive growth of uterine mucosa in the uterus, pelvis, colon, or oviducts.

adenopathy /ad′ənop′əthē/ [Gk, *aden* + *pathos,* suffering], an enlargement of any gland. **—adenopathic,** *adj.*

adenopharyngitis /ad′ənōfer′inji′tis/, an inflammation of the adenoid tonsils and the pharynx.

adenosarcoma /ad′ənōsärkō′mə/ [Gk, *aden* + *sarx,* flesh, *oma*], a malignant glandular tumor of the soft tissues of the body.

adenosarcorhabdomyoma /ad′ənōsär′ kōrab′dōmīō′mə/, a tumor composed of glandular and connective tissue, as well as striated muscle elements.

adenosine /əden′əsin, -sēn/, a compound derived from nucleic acid, composed of adenine and a sugar, D-ribose. Adenosine is the major molecular component of the nucleotides adenosine monophosphate, adenosine diphosphate, and adenosine triphosphate and of the nucleic acids deoxyribonucleic acid and ribonucleic acid.

adenosine deaminase (ADA) /dē-am′inās/, an enzyme that catalyzes the conversion of adenosine to the nucleoside inosine through the removal of an amino group. A deficiency of ADA can lead to **severe combined immunodeficiency syndrome (SCIDS).**

adenosine diphosphate (ADP), a product of the hydrolysis of adenosine triphosphate.

adenosine hydrolase, an enzyme that catalyzes the conversion of adenosine into adenine and ribose.

adenosine kinase, an enzyme in the liver and kidney that catalyzes the transfer of a phosphate group from adenosine triphosphate to produce adenosine phosphate.

adenosine monophosphate (AMP), an

ester, composed of adenine-d-ribose and phosphoric acid, that affects energy release in work done by a muscle.

adenosine phosphate, a compound consisting of the nucleotide adenosine attached through its ribose group to one, two, or three phosphate units or phosphoric acid molecules.

adenosine triphosphatase (ATPase), an enzyme in skeletal muscle that catalyzes the hydrolysis of adenosine triphosphate to adenosine diphosphate and inorganic phosphate. Mitochondrial ATPase is involved in obtaining energy for cellular metabolism, and myosin ATPase is involved in muscle contraction.

adenosine triphosphate (ATP), a compound consisting of the nucleotide adenosine attached through its ribose group to three phosphoric acid molecules. It stores energy in muscles; energy is released when it is hydrolyzed to adenosine diphosphate.

adenosis /ad'ənō'sis/, **1.** any disease of the glands, especially a lymphatic gland. **2.** an abnormal development or enlargement of glandular tissue.

adenotomy /ad'ənot'əmē/[Gk, *aden,* gland, *tome,* a cutting], dissection or incision of a gland.

adenotonsillectomy /ad'ənōton'silek'təmē/, surgical removal of the adenoids and tonsils.

adenovirus /ad'ənōvī'rəs/ [Gk, *aden* + L, *virus,* poison], any one of the 33 medium-sized viruses of the Adenoviridae family, pathogenic to humans, that cause conjunctivitis, upper respiratory infection, or gastrointestinal infection. —adenoviral, *adj.*

adenylate /əden'ilāt/, a salt or ester of adenylic acid.

adenylate cyclase, an enzyme that initiates the conversion of adenosine triphosphate to cyclic adenosine monophosphate, a mediator of many physiologic activities.

adenylate kinase, an enzyme in skeletal muscle that makes possible the reaction: ATP + AMP = 2ADP.

adequate and well-controlled studies, clinical and laboratory studies that the sponsors of a new drug are required by law to conduct to demonstrate the truth of the claims made for its effectiveness.

adermia /ədur'mē·ə/ [Gk, *a* + *derma,* without skin], a congenital or acquired skin defect or the absence of skin.

ADH, abbreviation for **antidiuretic hormone.**

ADHA, abbreviation for the **American Dental Hygienists' Association.**

adhere /adhir'/, to stick together or become fastened together, as two surfaces.

adherence /adhir'əns/, **1.** the quality of clinging or being closely attached. **2.** the process in which a person follows rules, guidelines, or standards, especially as a patient follows a prescription and recommendations for a regimen of care.

adherent /adhir'ənt/, [L, *adhaerens,* sticking to], having the tendency to cling, as one substance to the surface of another substance.

adherent pericardium, a condition in which the parietal layer of the pericardium adheres to the epicardium.

adherent placenta [L, *adhaerens,* sticking to, *placenta,* flat cake], a placenta that remains attached to the uterine wall beyond the normal time after birth of the fetus.

adhesin /adhē'sin/, a bacterial product that can split proteins. It combines with epithelial cell glycoproteins or glycolipid receptors.

adhesion /adhē'zhən/ [L, *adhaerens,* sticking to], a band of scar tissue that binds together two anatomic surfaces that normally are separate from each other. Adhesions most commonly occur in the abdomen, where they form after abdominal surgery, inflammation, or injury.

adhesiotomy /adhē'sē·ot'əmē/ [L, *adhaerens* + Gk, *temnein* to cut], the surgical dividing or separating of adhesions, usually performed to relieve an intestinal obstruction.

adhesive /adhē'siv/ [L, *adhaerens,* sticking to], a quality of a substance that enables it to become attached to another substance.

adhesive capsulitis, a condition in a shoulder involving stiffness, pain, and limited range of motion. It most often occurs in midlife.

adhesive pericarditis, a condition characterized by adhesions between the visceral and parietal layers of the pericardium or by adhesions between the pericardium and the mediastinum, diaphragm, or chest wall.

adhesive peritonitis, an inflammation of the peritoneum, characterized by adhesions between adjacent serous surfaces.

adhesive pleurisy, inflammation of the pleura with exudation, causing obliteration of the pleural space through the fusion of the visceral pleural layer covering the lungs and the parietal layer lining the walls of the thoracic cavity.

adhesive skin traction, one of two kinds of skin traction in which the therapeutic pull of traction weights is applied with adhesive straps that stick to the skin over the body structure involved, especially a fractured bone. Adhesive skin traction is used only when continuous traction is desired and skin care for the affected area is easily maintained.

adhesive tape, a strong fabric material covered on one side with an adhesive. Often water-repellent, it may be used to hold bandages and dressings in place, immobilize a part, or exert pressure.

ADI, abbreviation for **acceptable daily intake.**

adiadochokinesia /ā'dē·ad'əkōkinē'zha, ədī'ədō'kō-/, an inability to perform rapidly alternating movements such as pronation and supination or elbow flexion and extension.

adiaphoresis /ā'dē·əfôrē'sis/, an absence or deficiency of sweat.

adiastole /ā'dī·as'təlē/ [Gk, a, not, dia, across, stellein, to set], absence or imperceptibility of the diastolic stage of the cardiac cycle.

adiathermance /a'dī·əthur'məns/ [Gk, a + dia, not across, therme, heat], the quality of being unaffected by radiated heat.

adient /ad'ē-ənt/ [L, adire, moving toward], characterized by a tendency to move toward rather than away from stimuli. —adience, n.

Adie's pupil /ā'dēz/ [William J. Adie, English physician, 1886–1935], an abnormal condition of the eyes marked by one pupil that reacts much more slowly to light changes or to accommodation or convergence than the pupil of the other eye.

Adie's syndrome [William J. Adie], the condition of Adie's pupil accompanied by depressed or absent tendon reflexes, particularly the ankle and knee-jerk reflexes.

adiphenine hydrochloride /ədif'ənin/, an anticholinergic agent with smooth muscle relaxant properties that has been used for spastic disorders of the gastrointestinal and genitourinary tracts.

adipic /ədip'ik/ [L, adeps, fat], pertaining to fatty tissue.

adipocele /ad'ipōsēl'/ [L, adeps + Gk, kele, hernia], a hernia containing fat or fatty tissue.

adipocyte /ad'ipōsīt'/, a fat (adipose) cell.

adipofibroma /ad'ipōfībrō'mə/ [L, adeps + fibra, fiber; Gk, oma], a fibrous neoplasm of the connective tissue with fatty components.

adipokinesis /ad'ipō'kinē'sis/, the mobilization of fat or fatty acids in lipid metabolism.

adipokinin /ad'ipokī'nin/, a hormone of the anterior pituitary that causes mobilization of fat from adipose tissues.

adipometer ad'ipom'ətər/, an instrument for measuring the thickness of a skin area

as a guide to calculating the amount of subcutaneous fat.

adiponecrosis /ad'ipōnikrō'sis/ [L, adeps + Gk, nekros, dead, osis condition], a necrosis of fatty tissue in the body. —**adiponecrotic,** adj.

adiponecrosis subcutanea neonatorum, an abnormal dermatologic condition of the newborn characterized by patchy areas of hardened subcutaneous fatty tissue and a bluish-red discoloration of the overlying skin.

adipose /ad'ipōs/, fatty.

adipose capsule [L, adeps, fat, capsula, little box], a capsule of fatty tissue surrounding the kidney.

adipose tissue [L, adeps, fat; OFr, tissu], a collection of fat cells.

adiposogenital dystrophy /ad'ipō'sōjen' itəl/ [L, adeps + genitalis, generation], a disorder occurring in adolescent boys, characterized by genital hypoplasia and feminine secondary sex characteristics, including female distribution of fat. It is caused by hypothalamic malfunction or by a tumor in the anterior pituitary gland.

adipsia /ādip'sē·ə/ [Gk, a + dipsa, not thirst], absence of thirst.

aditus /ad'itəs/ [L, going to], an approach or an entry.

adjunct /ad'jungkt/ [L, adjungere, to join], (in health care) an additional substance, treatment, or procedure used for increasing the efficacy or safety of the primary substance, treatment, or procedure or for facilitating its performance. —**adjunctive,** adj.

adjunctive group /adjungk'tiv/, a group with specific activities and focuses, such as socialization, perceptual stimulation, sensory stimulation, or reality orientation.

adjunctive psychotherapy, a form of psychotherapy that concentrates on improving a person's general mental and physical well-being without trying to resolve basic emotional problems. Some kinds of adjunctive psychotherapy are **music therapy, occupational therapy, physical therapy,** and **recreational therapy.**

adjunct to anesthesia, one of a number of drugs used to enhance anesthesia that are not in themselves anesthetics. Each drug has a use in anesthetic procedures, as well as a therapeutic indication in other aspects of health care. Adjuncts to anesthesia are used as premedications, as intravenous supplements to hypnotic or analgesic medications, and as neuromuscular blocking agents and therapeutic gases.

adjustable orthodontic band /adjus'təbəl/, a thin metal ring, usually made of stainless steel, equipped with an adjusting screw to allow alteration in size, that is fitted to a tooth and allows the attachment of orthodontic appliances.

adjustment disorder, [L, *adjuxtare,* to bring together], a temporary disorder of varying severity that occurs as an acute reaction to overwhelming stress in persons of any age who have no apparent underlying mental disorders. Symptoms include anxiety, withdrawal, depression, brooding, impulsive outbursts, crying spells, attention-seeking behavior, enuresis, loss of appetite, aches, pains, and muscle spasms.

adjustment, impaired, a NANDA-accepted nursing diagnosis of a state in which the individual is unable to modify his or her life-style/behavior in a manner consistent with a change in health status. Defining characteristics include verbalized nonacceptance of health status change, nonexistent or limited ability to be involved in problem solving or goal setting, lack of movement toward independence, lack of future-oriented thinking, and extended period of shock, disbelief, or anger regarding health status change.

adjuvant /ad'jəvənt/ [L, *ad* + *juvare,* to help], **1.** a substance, especially a drug, added to a prescription to assist in the action of the main ingredient. **2.** (in immunology) a substance added to an antigen that enhances or modifies the antibody response to the antigen. **3.** an additional treatment or therapy.

adjuvant chemotherapy, the use of anticancer drugs after or in combination with another form of cancer treatment, as after apparently complete surgical removal of a cancer. The method is used when there is a significant risk that undetected cancer cells may still be present.

adjuvant therapy, the treatment of a disease with substances that enhance the action of drugs, especially drugs that promote the production of antibodies.

ADL, abbreviation for **activities of daily living.**

adlerian psychology [Alfred Adler, Viennese psychiatrist, 1870–1937], a branch of psychoanalysis that focuses on physical security, sexual satisfaction, and social integration.

ad lib, abbreviation of the Latin phrase *ad libitum,* meaning to be taken as desired.

administration of parenteral fluids /admin'istrā'shən/, the intravenous infusion of various solutions to maintain adequate hydration, restore fluid volume, reestablish lost electrolytes, or provide partial nutrition.

Administration on Aging (AOA), the principal U.S. agency designated to carry out the provisions of the Older Americans Act of 1965. The AOA advises the U.S. Secretary of the Department of Health and Human Services and other federal departments and agencies on the characteristics and needs of older people and develops programs designed to promote their welfare.

admission, 1. the act of being received into a place or class of things. **2.** patient accepted for inpatient service in a hospital. **3.** a concession or acknowledgment.

Admission Care, a Nursing Interventions Classification defined as facilitating entry of a patient into a health care facility.

ADN, abbreviation for **Associate Degree in Nursing.**

ad nauseam [L, *ad,* to; Gk, *nausia,* seasickness], to the extent of inducing nausea and vomiting.

adneural /adnŏŏr'əl/, **1.** located near or toward a nerve or nerve ending. **2.** pertaining to the stage of a nervous disorder in which the symptoms are apparent.

adnexa /adnek'sa/, *sing.* **adnexus** [L, *adnectere,* to tie together], tissue or structures in the body that are adjacent to or near another, related structure. The ovaries and the uterine tubes are adnexa of the uterus. **—adnexal,** *adj.*

adnexal [L, *adnectere,* to tie to], pertaining to accessory organs or tissues, as in the relationship of the fallopian tubes and uterus.

adnexa oculi, the accessory organs of the eye: the eyelids, lashes, eyebrows, conjunctival sac, lacrimal apparatus, and extrinsic muscles of the eye.

adnexa uteri, the uterine appendages: the ovaries, fallopian tubes, and associated ligaments.

adnexectomy /ad'neksek'təmē/ [Gk, *ektome,* cutting out], surgical removal of accessory structures.

adnexitis /ad'neksī'tis/, an inflammation of the adnexal organs of the uterus such as the ovaries or the fallopian tubes.

adnexopexy /adnek'sōpek'sē/, a surgical procedure in which the fallopian tubes and ovaries are elevated and sutured to the abdominal wall.

adolescence /ad'əles'əns/ [L, *adolescere,* to grow up], **1.** the period in development between the onset of puberty and adulthood. It usually begins between 11 and 13 years of age with the appearance of secondary sex characteristics and spans the teen years, terminating at 18 to 20 years of age with the completion of the development of the adult form. During this period the individual undergoes extensive physical, psychologic, emotional, and personality changes. **2.** the state or quality of being adolescent or youthful.

adolescent, 1. pertaining to characteristic of adolescence. **2.** one in the state or process of adolescence; a teenager.

adoption /ədop′shən/ [L, *adoptere,* to choose], a selection and inclusion into an established relationship.

ADP, abbreviation for **adenosine diphosphate.**

adrenal /ədrē′nəl/ [L, *ad,* to, *ren,* kidney], pertaining to the adrenal, or suprarenal glands, which are located on top of the kidneys.

adrenal cortex [L, *ad,* to, *ren,* kidney], the outer and greater part of the adrenal, or suprarenal, gland, fused with the medulla of the gland. It produces mineralocorticoids, androgens, and glucocorticoids, hormones essential to homeostasis.

adrenal cortical carcinoma, a malignant neoplasm of the adrenal cortex that may cause adrenogenital or Cushing syndrome. Such tumors vary in size and may occur at any age. Metastases frequently occur in the lungs, liver, and other organs.

adrenal crisis, an acute, life-threatening state of profound adrenocortical insufficiency in which immediate therapy is required. It is characterized by glucocorticoid deficiency, a drop in extracellular fluid volume, and hyperkalemia. Typically the patient appears to be in shock or coma, with a low blood pressure, weakness, and loss of vasomotor tone.

adrenalectomy /ədrē′nəlek′təmē/ [L, *ad + ren* + Gk, *ektome,* excision], the surgical removal of one or both adrenal glands or the resection of a part of one or both glands. It is performed to reduce the excessive secretion of adrenal hormones when an adrenal tumor or a malignancy of the breast or prostate is present. If both glands are removed, the maintenance dosage of steroids continues for life. Stress and fatigue must be avoided.

adrenal gland, either of two secretory organs perched on top of the kidneys. Each consists of two parts having independent functions: the cortex and the medulla. The adrenal cortex, in response to adrenocorticotropic hormone secreted by the anterior pituitary, secretes cortisol and androgens. Adrenal androgens serve as precursors that are converted by the liver to testosterone and estrogens. Renin from the kidney controls adrenal cortical production of aldosterone. The adrenal medulla manufactures the catecholamines epinephrine and norepinephrine.

adrenal insufficiency [L, *ad,* to, *ren,* kidney, *in,* not, *sufficere,* to suffice], a condition in which the adrenal gland is unable to produce adequate amounts of cortical hormones.

adrenalize /ədrē′nəlīz/, to stimulate or excite.

adrenal medulla, the inner part of the adrenal gland. Adrenal medulla cells secrete epinephrine and norepinephrine when stimulated by the sympathetic division of the autonomic nervous system.

adrenal virilism, a condition characterized by hypersecretion of adrenocortical androgens, resulting in somatic masculinization. Excessive production of the hormone may be caused by a virilizing adrenal tumor, congenital adrenal hyperplasia, or an inborn deficiency of enzymes required to transform endogenous androgenic steroids to glucocorticoids. Girls born with adrenogenitalism may be pseudohermaphroditic with clitoral enlargement and labial fusion in infancy and later have low vocal pitch, acne, amenorrhea, and masculine distribution of hair and muscle development. Boys with congenital adrenogenitalism show precocious development of the penis, the prostate, and pubic and axillary hair; but their testes remain small and immature because negative feedback from the high level of adrenal androgens prevents the normal pubertal increase in pituitary gonadotropin.

adrenarche /ad′rinär′kē/ [L, *ad + ren* + Gk, *arche,* beginning], the intensified activity in the adrenal cortex that occurs at about 8 years of age and increases the elaboration of various hormones, especially androgens.

adrenergic /ad′rinur′jik/ [L, *ad + ren;* Gk, *ergon,* work], pertaining to sympathetic nerve fibers of the autonomic nervous system that liberate norepinephrine at a synapse where a nerve impulse passes.

adrenergic blocking agent. See **antiadrenergic.**

adrenergic bronchodilator, a drug that acts on the beta-2 sympathetic nervous system receptors to relax bronchial smooth muscle cells. Examples include drugs that contain epinephrine, ephedrine, isoproterenol, or albuterol.

adrenergic drug. See **sympathomimetic.**

adrenergic fibers, nerve fibers of the autonomic nervous system that release the neurotransmitter norepinephrine and, in some areas, dopamine. Most postganglionic sympathetic nerve fibers are of this type.

adrenergic receptor [L, *ad + ren,* kidney; Gk, *ergon,* work; L, *recipere,* to receive], a site in a sympathetic effector cell that reacts to adrenergic stimulation. Two types of adrenergic receptors are recognized:

alpha-adrenergic and beta-adrenergic. In general, stimulation of alpha receptors is excitatory of the function of the host organ or tissue, and stimulation of the beta receptors is inhibitory.

adrenocortical /-kôr′tikəl/ [L, *ad* + *ren* + *cortex,* bark], pertaining to the outer or superficial part of the adrenal gland.

adrenocortical hormone (ACH) [L, *ad,* to, *ren,* kidney, *cortex,* bark; Gk, *hormaein,* to set in motion], any of the hormones secreted by the cortex of the adrenal gland, including the glucocorticoids, mineralocorticoids, and sex hormones.

adrenocorticotropic /ədrē′nōkôr′tikōtrop′ ik/ [L, *ad* + *ren* + *cortex,* bark; Gk, *trope,* a turning], pertaining to stimulation of the adrenal cortex.

adrenocorticotropic hormone (ACTH), a hormone of the anterior pituitary gland that stimulates the growth of the adrenal gland cortex and the secretion of corticosteroids. ACTH secretion, regulated by corticotropin-releasing factor from the hypothalamus, increases in response to a low level of circulating cortisol and to stress, fever, acute hypoglycemia, and major surgery.

adrenocorticotropin /-trop′in/, the adrenocorticotropic hormone secreted by the anterior pituitary gland that stimulates secretion of other hormones by the adrenal cortex.

adrenodoxin /ədrē′nōdok′sin/, a nonheme iron protein produced by the adrenal glands that participates in the transfer of electrons within animal cells.

adrenoleukodystrophy (ALD), a rare hereditary childhood metabolic disease that is transmitted as a recessive sexlinked trait and affects only males. It is characterized by adrenal atrophy and widespread cerebral demyelination, producing progressive mental deterioration, aphasia, apraxia, and eventual blindness.

adrenomegaly /-meg′əlē [L, *ad* + *ren,* + Gk, *megaly,* large], an abnormal enlargement of one or both adrenal glands.

adrenomimetic /-mimet′ik/, mimicking the functions of the adrenal hormones.

adrenotropic /-trop′ik/, having a stimulating effect on the adrenal glands.

adromia /ədrō′mē·ə/ [Gk, *a* + *dromos,* not course], the absence of the conductive capacity of any nerve that normally innervates a muscle.

ADRV, abbreviation for **adult rotavirus.**

ADS, abbreviation for **antidiuretic substance.**

Adson's maneuver [Alfred W. Adson, American surgeon, 1887–1951], a test for the thoracic outlet syndrome. The examiner palpates both radial pulses as the

patient takes a deep breath and holds it while extending the neck and turning the head toward the affected side.

adsorb, to attract and hold other material on the surface.

adsorbent /adsôr′bənt/, a substance that takes up another by the process of adsorption, as by the attachment of one substance to the surface of the other.

adsorption /adsôrp′shən/ [L, *ad* + *sorbere,* to suck in], a natural process whereby molecules of a gas or liquid adhere to the surface of a solid. The phenomenon depends on an assortment of factors such as surface tension and electrical charges. Many biologic reactions involve adsorption. In chemistry adsorption is the principle on which chromatography is based and which allows for the separation of a mixture into component fractions for qualitative analysis.

ADT, abbreviation for *Accepted Dental Therapeutics,* a journal published by the Council on Dental Therapeutics of the American Dental Association.

adult /ədult′, ad′ult/ [L, *adultus,* grown up], **1.** one who is fully developed and matured and who has attained the intellectual capacity and the emotional and psychologic stability characteristic of a mature person. **2.** a person who has reached full legal age.

adult day-care center, a facility for the supervised care of older adults, providing such activities as meals and socialization 1 or more days a week during specified daytime hours. The participants return to their homes each evening.

adult ego state, (in psychiatry), a part of the self that analyzes and solves problems using information received from the parent and child ego states.

adulteration /ədul′tərā′shən/ [L, *adulterare,* to defile], the debasement or dilution of the purity of any substance, process, or activity by the addition of extraneous material.

adulthood, the phase of development characterized by physical and mental maturity.

adult nurse practitioner, a registered nurse who has received additional education in the primary health care of adults. The additional education may be obtained through a master's degree program or a nondegree-granting continuing education certificate program.

adult-onset diabetes. See **noninsulin-dependent diabetes mellitus.**

adult respiratory distress syndrome (ARDS), a respiratory disorder characterized by respiratory insufficiency and hypoxemia. Triggers include aspiration of a foreign body, cardiopulmonary bypass surgery, gram-negative sepsis, multiple blood transfusions, oxygen toxicity, trauma, pneumonia, or other respiratory infection. Signs and symptoms of ARDS include breathlessness, tachypnea, hypoxemia, and decreased lung compliance.

adult rotavirus (ADRV), a form of rotavirus that causes severe diarrhea in adults.

advanced cardiac life support (ACLS), emergency medical procedures in which basic life support efforts of cardiopulmonary resuscitation are augmented by establishment of an intravenous fluid line, possible defibrillation, drug administration, control of cardiac arrhythmias, and use of ventilation equipment. The procedures usually require direct or indirect supervision by a physician.

advance directive [Fr, *avancer,* to move forward; L, *dirigere,* to direct], an advance declaration by an individual that states how he or she wishes to be treated if unable to communicate his or her wishes. Kinds of advance directives are **durable power of attorney for health care** and **living will.**

advanced life support. See **Emergency Medical Technician-Advanced Life Support.**

advancement /advans'/ [Fr, *avancer,* to move forward], a surgical technique in which a muscle or tendon is drawn forward.

adventitia /ad'ventish'ə/ [L, *adventitius,* coming from abroad], the outermost layer, composed of connective tissue with elastic and collagenous fibers, of an artery or other structure.

adventitious [L, *adventitius,* from outside sources], **1.** pertaining to an accidental condition or an arbitrary action. **2.** not hereditary. **3.** occurring at an inappropriate place, such as a coating on an artery.

adventitious bursa, an abnormal bursa that develops as a response to friction or pressure.

adventitious crisis, an accidental, uncommon, and unexpected tragedy that may affect an entire community or population, such as an earthquake, flood, or airplane crash.

adventitious sounds, breath sounds that are not normally heard, such as crackles, gurgles, and wheezes.

adverse drug effect /advurs', ad'vers/, a harmful, unintended reaction to a drug administered at normal dosage.

adverse reaction, any harmful or unintended effect of a medication, diagnostic test, or therapeutic intervention.

advocacy /ad'vəkas'ē/, **1.** a process whereby a nurse provides a patient with the information to make certain decisions. **2.** a method by which groups can work together to develop programs that ensure the availability of high-quality health care for a community. **3.** pleading the cause of another, such as when nurses and other health care professionals argue for better care.

adynamia /ad'inā'mē·ə/ [Gk, *a + dynamis,* not strength], lack of physical strength due to a pathologic condition. —**adynamic,** *adj.*

adynamia episodica hereditaria, a condition seen in infancy, characterized by muscle weakness and episodes of flaccid paralysis. It is inherited as an autosomal-dominant trait.

adynamic fever, an elevated temperature with a feeble pulse; nervous depression; and cool, moist skin.

AEA, abbreviation for *above the elbow amputation.* A short AE amputation (near the shoulder) results in the loss of shoulder rotation. After a long AE amputation (just above the elbow), the patient should retain good shoulder function.

Aedes /ā·ē'dēz/ [Gk, *aedes,* unpleasant], a genus of mosquito, prevalent in tropical and subtropical regions. Several species are capable of transmitting pathogenic organisms to humans, including dengue, equine encephalitis, St. Louis encephalitis, tularemia, and yellow fever.

aerate /er'āt/ [Gk, *aer,* air], to charge a substance or a structure with air, carbon dioxide, or oxygen.

aeration [Gk, *aer,* air], **1.** exchange of carbon dioxide for oxygen by blood in the lungs. **2.** a process of exposing a tissue or fluid to air or artificially charging it with oxygen or another gas such as carbon dioxide.

Aerobacter aerogenes. See *Enterobacter cloacae.*

aerobe /er'ōb/ [Gk, *aer + bios,* life], a microorganism that lives and grows in the presence of free oxygen. An aerobe may be **facultative** or **obligate.**

aerobic /erō'bik/, **1.** pertaining to the presence of air or oxygen. **2.** able to live and function in the presence of free oxygen. **3.** requiring oxygen for the maintenance of life. **4.** pertaining to aerobic exercise.

aerobic exercise, any physical exercise that requires additional effort by the heart and lungs to meet the increased demand by the skeletal muscles for oxygen. The exercise generally requires heavier breathing than passive muscular activity and results in increased heart and lung efficiency with a minimum of wasted energy.

aerobic training, prolonged physical exercises designed to require an increased intake and distribution of oxygen within the body. Such exercises involve depletion of the body's normal tissue stores of oxygen by comparatively prolonged exertion and replacement of the oxygen through increased breathing rate. This training can be accomplished by biking, walking, jogging, or other similar activities for at least 20 minutes three times per week.

aerodontalgia /er'ōdontal'jə/ [Gk, *aer* + *odous*, tooth, *algos*, pain], a painful sensation in the teeth caused by a change in atmospheric pressure, as may occur at high altitudes.

aerodynamics, the study of air or other gases in motion or of bodies moving in air.

aerodynamic size, pertaining to the behavior of various aerosol particle sizes and densities.

Aeromonas /er'ōmō'nəs/, a genus of pathogenic rod-shaped gram-negative bacteria found in fresh and salt water and also soil and sewage. Various species affect fish and animals as well as humans, causing wound infections and gastroenteritis.

aerophagy /erof'əjē/ [Gk, *aer* + *phagein*, to eat], the swallowing of air, usually followed by belching, gastric distress, and flatulence.

aerosinusitis /er'ōsī'nəsī'tis/ [Gk, *aer* + L, *sinus*, curve; Gk, *itis*], inflammation, edema, or hemorrhage of the frontal sinuses, caused by expansion of air within the sinuses when barometric pressure is decreased, as in aircraft at high altitudes.

aerosol /er'əsol'/ [Gk, *aer* + *hydor*, water; L, *solutus*, dissolved], **1.** nebulized particles suspended in a gas or air. **2.** a pressurized gas containing a finely nebulized medication for inhalation therapy. **3.** a pressurized gas containing a nebulized chemical agent for sterilizing the air of a room.

aerosol bronchodilator therapy, the use of drugs that relax the respiratory tract smooth muscle tissue when administered as tiny droplets or a mist to be inhaled.

aerospace medicine /er'ōspās/, a branch of medicine concerned with the physiologic and psychologic effects of living and working in an artificial environment beyond the atmospheric and gravitational forces of the earth. The stress of extraterrestrial travel requiring long periods of weightlessness is a major concern.

aerotherapy /er'ōther'əpē/, the use of air in treating disease, as in hyperbaric oxygen treatments.

aerotitis /er'ətī'tis/ [Gk, *aer* + *otikos*, ear, *itis*], an inflammation of the ear caused by changes in atmospheric pressure.

aerotitis media, inflammation or bleeding in the middle ear caused by a difference between the air pressure in the middle ear and that of the atmosphere, as occurs in sudden changes in altitude, in scuba diving, or in hyperbaric chambers. Symptoms are pain, tinnitus, diminished hearing, and vertigo.

Æsculapius /es'kyōōlā'pē·əs/, the ancient Greek god of medicine. Serpents were regarded as sacred by Æsculapius, and he is symbolized in modern medicine by a staff with a serpent entwined about it.

AF, 1. abbreviation for **atrial fibrillation. 2.** abbreviation for **atrial flutter.**

AFB, abbreviation for **acid-fast bacillus.**

afebrile /āfē'bril, āfeb'ril/ [Gk, *a* + *febris*, not fever], without fever.

affect /əfekt'/ [L, *affectus* influence], an outward, observable manifestation of a person's feelings or emotions. —**affective,** *adj.*

affection /əfek'shən/ [L, *affectus,* influence], **1.** an emotional state expressed as by a warm or caring feeling toward another individual. **2.** a morbid process affecting all or a part of the human body.

affective /əfek'tiv/ [L, *affectus*], pertaining to emotion, mood, or feeling.

affective intimacy, a measure of well-being in a family group that focuses on whether members feel close to one another, yet do not lose their individuality.

affective learning, the acquisition of behaviors involved in expressing feelings in attitudes, appreciation, and values.

affective melancholia [L, *affectus,* influence; Gk, *melas,* black, *chole,* bile], a form of severe depression characterized by a lack of interest in normally pleasant activities.

affective psychosis, a psychologic reaction in which the ego's functioning is impaired and the primary clinical feature is a severe disorder of mood or emotions.

affect memory, a particular emotionally expressed feeling that recurs whenever a significant experience is recalled.

afferent /af'ərənt/ [L, *ad* + *ferre,* to carry], proceeding toward a center, as applied to arteries, veins, lymphatics, and nerves.

afferent nerves [L, *ad* + *ferre,* to bear, *nervus*], nerve fibers that transmit impulses from the periphery toward the central nervous system.

afferent pathway [L, *ad* + *ferre,* to bear; AS, *paeth* + *weg*], the course or route taken, usually by a linkage of neurons, from the periphery of the body toward the center.

afferent tract [L, *ad* + *ferre,* to bear, *tractus*], a pathway for nerve impulses traveling inward or toward the brain, the center of an organ, or another body structure.

affidavit /af′idā′vit/ [L, he has pledged], a written statement that is sworn to before a notary public or an officer of the court.

affiliated hospital /əfil′ē-ā′tid/ [L, *ad* + *filius,* to son], a hospital that is associated with a medical school, other health professions, a health program, or other health care institutions.

affinity /əfin′itē/ [L, *affinis,* related], the measure of the binding strength of the antibody-antigen reaction.

affirmation [L, *affirmare,* to make firm], (in psychology) autosuggestion, the point at which a tendency toward positive reaction is observed by the therapist.

affirmative defense /əfur′mətiv/ [L, *affirmare,* to make firm], (in law) a denial of guilt or wrongdoing based on new evidence rather than on simple denial of a charge, as a plea of immunity according to a Good Samaritan law. The defendant bears the burden of proof in an affirmative defense.

afflux /af′luks/ [L, *affluere,* to flow], the sudden flow of blood or other liquid to a part of the body.

affusion /afyoō′zhən/ [L, *affundere,* to pour out], a form of therapy in which water is sprinkled or poured over the body or a particular body part. It is used for pyrexia or other disease conditions.

afibrinogenemia /afī′brinōjenē′mē·ə/ [Gk, *a,* not; L, *fibra,* fiber; Gk, *genein,* to produce, *haima,* blood], a relative lack or absence of fibrinogen in the blood. It may be the result of a primary congenital blood dyscrasia or acquired, as in disseminated intravascular coagulation.

aflatoxins /af′lātok′sins/ [Gk, *a,* not; L, *flavus,* yellow; Gk, *toxikon,* poison], a group of carcinogenic and toxic factors produced by *Aspergillus flavus* food molds.

AFO, abbreviation for **ankle-foot orthosis.**

AFP, abbreviation for **alpha fetoprotein.**

African tick typhus, a rickettsial infection transmitted by ixodid ticks and characterized by fever, maculopapular rash, and swollen lymph nodes.

African trypanosomiasis, a disease caused by the parasite *Trypanosoma brucei gambiense* or *T. brucei rhodesiense,* transmitted to humans by the bite of the tsetse fly.

afterbirth [AS, *aefter* + ME, *burth*], the placenta, the amnion, the chorion, and some amniotic fluid, blood, and blood clots expelled from the uterus after childbirth.

aftercare [AS, *aefter* + *caru*], health care offered a patient after discharge from a hospital or other health care facility.

afterdepolarization /dēpō′lərizā′shən/, a variation of membrane potential second depolarization that follows an action potential. It is thought to be responsible for atrial and ventricular tachycardia, especially in the setting of a long QT interval or digitalis toxicity.

aftereffect, a physical or psychologic effect that continues after the stimulus is removed.

afterimage, a visual sensation that continues after the stimulus ends. The image may appear in colors complementary to those of the stimulus.

afterload [AS, *aefter* + ME, *lod*], the load, or resistance, against which the left ventricle must eject its volume of blood during contraction.

afterloading, (in radiotherapy) a technique in which an unloaded applicator or needle is placed within the patient at the time of an operative procedure and subsequently loaded with the radioactive source under controlled conditions in which health care personnel are protected against radiation exposure.

aftermovement, an involuntary muscle contraction that causes a continued movement of a limb after a strong exertion against resistance has stopped. It is often demonstrated in abduction of the arm.

afterpains [AS, *aefter* + Gk, *poine,* penalty], contractions of the uterus common during the first days after delivery. They tend to be strongest in nursing mothers, in multiparas, and when the uterus has been overdistended. They usually resolve spontaneously but may require analgesia.

afterperception, the apparent perception of a stimulus that continues after the stimulus is removed.

afterpotential wave /-pəten′shəl/, either of two smaller waves, positive or negative, that follows the main spike potential wave of a nerve impulse, as recorded on an oscillograph tracing.

Ag, symbol for the element **silver.**

AGA, abbreviation for **appropriate for gestational age.**

against medical advice (ama), a phrase pertaining to a client's decision to discontinue a therapy despite the advice of medical professionals.

agalactia /ā′gəlak′shə/ [Gk *a* + *gala,* not milk], the inability of the mother to secrete enough milk to breastfeed an infant after childbirth.

agamete /āgam′ēt/ [Gk *a* + *gamos* not marriage], **1.** any of the unicellular organisms, such as bacteria and protozoa, lacking gametes (or sex cells) that reproduce asexually by multiple fission. **2.** any asexual reproductive cell such as a spore or merozoitc that forms a new organism without fusion with another gamete. See also **fungi.**

agametic /āgəmē′tik/, asexual; without recognizable sex organs or gametes.

agamic /āgam′ik/, reproducing asexually, without the union of gametes; asexual.

agammaglobulinemia /agam′əglob′-yoolinē′mē-ə/ [Gk *a* + *gamma,* not gamma (third letter of Greek alphabet); L, *globulus,* small sphere; Gk, *haima,* blood], the absence of the serum immunoglobulin gamma globulin, associated with an increased susceptibility to infection. The condition may be transient, congenital, or acquired.

agamogenesis /əgam′ōjen′əsis/ [Gk, *a* + *gamos,* not marriage, *genein,* to produce], asexual reproduction, as by budding or simple fission of cells; parthenogenesis. —**agamocytogenic, agamogenetic, agamogenic, agamogonic,** *adj.*

aganglionosis /əgang′lē′ənō′sis/ [Gk, *a,* not, *gagglion,* knot, *osis,* condition], absence of parasympathetic ganglion cells in the myenteric plexus, a diagnostic sign of congenital megacolon.

agar-agar /a′gärə′gär/ [Malay], a dried hydrophilic, colloidal product obtained from certain species of red algae. It is widely used as the basic ingredient in solid culture media in bacteriology.

agarose /ag′ärōs/, an essentially neutral fraction of agar used as a medium in electrophoresis, particularly for separation of serum proteins, hemoglobin variants, and lipoprotein fractions.

agastria /əgas′trē-ə/ [Gk, *a* + *gaster,* without stomach], the absence of a stomach.

agastric /āgas′trik/ [Gk, *a* + *gaster,* without stomach], pertaining to lack of a stomach or digestive tract.

AGC, abbreviation for *absolute granulocyte count.*

age [L, *aetus*], a stage of development at which the body has arrived, as measured by physical and laboratory standards to what is normal for a male or female of the same chronologic span of life.

aged /ājd/, a state of having grown older or more mature than others of the population group.

ageism /ā′jizəm/ [L, *aetas,* lifetime], an attitude that discriminates, separates, stigmatizes, or otherwise disadvantages older adults on the basis of chronologic age.

agency [L, *agere,* to do], (in law) a relationship between two parties in which one authorizes the other to act in his or her behalf as agent.

Agency for Health Care Policy and Research (AHCPR), an agency of the U.S. Public Health Service that supports and conducts scientific research, facilitates the development of clinical guidelines, and assesses health care technology.

agenesia corticalis /ā′jenē′zhə/ [Gk, *a* + *genein,* not to produce; L, cortex], the failure of the cortical cells of the brain, especially the pyramidal cells, to develop in the embryo, resulting in infantile cerebral paralysis and severe mental retardation.

agenesis /ājen′əsis/ [Gk, *a* + *genein,* not to produce], **1.** congenital absence of an organ or part, usually caused by a lack of primordial tissue and failure of development in the embryo. **2.** impotence or sterility. —**agenic,** *adj.*

agenetic fracture /ā′jenet′ik/, a spontaneous fracture caused by an imperfect osteogenesis.

ageniocephaly /ājen′ē-ōsef′əlē/ [Gk, *a* + *genein,* not to produce, *kephale,* head], a form of otocephaly in which the brain, cranial vault, and sense organs are intact but the lower jaw is malformed.—**ageniocephalic, ageniocephalous,** *adj.*

agenitalism /ājen′itəliz′əm/, a condition caused by the lack of sex hormones and the absence or malfunction of the ovaries or testes.

agenosomia /əjen′əsō′mē-ə/, a congenital malformation characterized by the absence or defective formation of the genitals and protrusion of the intestines through an incompletely developed abdominal wall.

agenosomus /əjen′əsō′məs/ [Gk, *a* + *genein,* not to produce, *soma,* body], a fetus with agenosomia.

agent [L, *agere,* to do], (in law) a party authorized to act on behalf of another and to give the other an account of such actions.

Agent Orange, a U.S. military code name for a mixture of two herbicides, 2,4-D and 2,4,5-T, used as a defoliant in Southeast Asia during the 1960s war in Vietnam.

age of consent, (in medical jurisprudence) the age at which an individual is legally free to act as an adult, without parental permission for such activities as marriage or sexual intercourse. The specific age of consent varies from 13 to 21, according to local laws.

age of majority, the age at which a person is considered to be an adult in the eyes of the law.

age-specific, data in which the age of the individual is significant for epidemiologic or statistical purposes.

age 30 transition, (in psychiatry), a period between 28 and 33 years of age when an individual may reevaluate the choices made in his or her twenties.

ageusia /əgyōō'sē·ə/ [Gk, *a* + *geusis*, without taste], a loss or impairment of the sense of taste. The degree and cause may vary.

agger /ag'er, aj'ər/, a small mound or eminence of tissue, such as the curved elevation above the atrium of the nose.

agglomerate /əglom'ərāt/ [L, *glomus,* a ball], to collect or gather into a mass, ball, or cluster.

agglomeration [L, *agglomerare,* to gather into a ball], a mass or cluster of individual units.

agglutinant /əglōō'tənənt/ [L, *agglutinare,* to glue], something that causes adhesion, such as an antibody produced in the blood that is stimulated by the presence of an antigen to adhere to it.

agglutination /əglōō'tinā'shən/ [L, *agglutinare,* to glue], the clumping together of cells as a result of interaction with specific antibodies called agglutinins. Agglutinins are used in blood typing and in identifying or estimating the strength of immunoglobulins or immune sera.

agglutination-inhibition test, a serologic technique useful in testing for certain unknown soluble antigens.

agglutination titer, the highest dilution of a serum that will produce clumping of cells or particulate antigens. It is a measure of the concentration of specific antibodies in the serum.

agglutinin /əglōō'tinin/, an antibody that interacts with antigens, resulting in agglutination.

agglutinin absorption, the removal from immune serum of antibody by treatment with homologous antigen, followed by centrifugation and separation of the antigen-antibody complex.

agglutinogen /ag'lōōtin'əjin/ [L, *agglutinare* + Gk, *genein,* to produce], any antigenic substance that causes agglutination (clumping together of cells) by the production of agglutinin.

aggregate /ag'rəgāt/ [L, *ad* + *gregare,* to gather together], the total of a group of substances or components making up a mass or complex.

aggregate anaphylaxis, an exaggerated reaction of immediate hypersensitivity rapidly induced by the injection of an antigen that forms a soluble antigen-antibody complex.

aggregation /ag'rəgā'shən/ [L, *ad* + *gregare,* to gather together], an accumulation of substances, objects, or individuals, as in the clumping of blood cells or the clustering of clients with the same disorder.

aggression /əgresh'ən/ [L, *aggressio,* to attack], a forceful behavior, action, or atti-

tude that is expressed physically, verbally, or symbolically. It may arise from innate drives or occur as a defensive mechanism, often resulting from a threatened ego.

aggressive personality /əgres'iv/, a personality with behavior patterns characterized by irritability, impulsivity, destructiveness, or violence in response to frustration.

aggressive-radical therapy, (in psychiatry) a form of therapy that introduces the political and social viewpoints of the therapist into the therapeutic process.

aging [L, *aetas,* lifetime], the process of growing old, resulting in part from a failure of body cells to function normally or to produce new body cells to replace those that are dead or malfunctioning.

agitated /aj'ətā'təd/ [L, *agitare,* to shake], describing a condition of psychomotor excitement characterized by purposeless, restless activity. Pacing, crying, and laughing sometimes are characteristic and may serve to release nervous tension associated with anxiety, fear, or other mental stress. —**agitate,** *v.,* **agitation,** *n.*

agitated depression, a form of depression characterized by severe anxiety accompanied by continuous physical restlessness and frequently, somatic symptoms.

agitation, a state of chronic restlessness and increased psychomotor activity that is generally observed as an expression of emotional tension.

agitographia /aj'itōgraf'ē·ə/ [L, *agitare* + Gk, *graphein,* to write], a condition characterized by abnormally rapid writing in which words or parts of words are unconsciously omitted.

agitophasia /aj'itōfā'zhə/ [L, *agitare* + Gk, *phasis,* speech], a condition characterized by abnormally rapid speech in which words, sounds, or syllables are unconsciously omitted, slurred, or distorted. The condition is commonly associated with agitographia.

aglossia /əglos'ē·ə/ [Gk, *a* + *glossa,* without tongue], congenital absence of the tongue.

aglycemia /ā'glīsē'mē·ə/ [Gk, *a, glykis,* not sweet, *haima,* blood], an absence of blood sugar.

agnathia /ag·nath'ē·ə/ [Gk, *a, gnathos,* not jaw], a developmental defect characterized by total or partial absence of the lower jaw. —**agnathous,** *adj.*

agnathocephalus /ag·nath'əsef'ələs/, a fetus with agnathocephaly.

agnathocephaly /ag·nath'əsef'əlē/ [Gk, *a* + *gnathos* + *kephale,* head], a congenital malformation characterized by the absence of the lower jaw, defective formation of the mouth, and placement of the eyes low on the face with fusion or approximation of the zygomas and the ears. —**agnathocephalic, agnathocephalous,** *adj.*

agnathus /ag·nath′əs/ [Gk, *a* + *gnathos,* without jaw], a fetus with agnathia.

agnosia /ag·nō′zhə/ [Gk, *a* + *gnosis,* not knowledge], total or partial loss of the ability to recognize familiar objects or persons through sensory stimuli as a result of organic brain damage.

AgNO₃, the chemical formula for silver nitrate.

agonal /ag′ənəl/ [Gk, *agon,* struggle], pertaining to death and dying.

agonal respiration [Gk, *agon,* struggle], a breathing pattern of gasping succeeded by apnea. It generally indicates the onset of respiratory arrest.

agonal thrombus, a mass of blood platelets, fibrin, clotting factors, and cellular elements that forms in the heart in the process of dying.

agonist /ag′ənist/ [Gk, *agon,* struggle], **1.** a contracting muscle whose contraction is opposed by another muscle (an antagonist). **2.** a drug or other substance having a specific cellular affinity that produces a predictable response.

agony /ag′ənē/ [Gk, *agon*], severe physical or emotional anguish or distress, as in pain.

agoraphobia /ag′ərə-/ [Gk, *agora,* marketplace, *phobos,* fear], an anxiety disorder characterized by a fear of being in an open, crowded, or public place, such as a field, tunnel, bridge, congested street, or busy department store, where escape is perceived as difficult or help not available in case of sudden incapacitation.

agranulocyte /āgran′yoolōsīt′/ [Gk, *a,* not; L, *granulum,* small grain; Gk, *kytos,* cell], any leukocyte that does not contain predominant cytoplasmic granules, such as a monocyte or lymphocyte.

agranulocytic /-si′tik/ [Gk, *a,* not, *granule, kytos,* cell], pertaining to a leukocyte or white blood cell that, when stained microscopically, shows no granules in the cytoplasm.

agranulocytosis /āgran′yoolō′sītō′sis/, a severe reduction in the number of white blood cells (basophils, eosinophils, and neutrophils). As a result, neutropenia develops, whereby the body is severely depleted in its ability to defend itself. Fever, prostration, and bleeding ulcers of the rectum, mouth, and vagina may be present.

agraphia /āgraf′ē-ə/ [Gk, *a, graphein,* not to write], a loss of the ability to write, resulting from injury to the language center in the cerebral cortex. —**agraphic,** *adj.*

A : G ratio, the ratio of protein albumin to globulin in the blood serum. On the basis of differential solubility with neutral salt solution, the normal values are 3.5 to 5 g/dl for albumin and 2.5 to 4 g/dl for globulin.

agrypnocoma /agrip′nōkō′mə/ [Gk, *agrypnos,* sleepless], a coma in which there is some degree of wakefulness.

agrypnotic /ag′ripnot′ik/, **1.** insomniac. **2.** a drug or other substance that prevents sleep.

agyria /əjī′rē-ə/, **1.** an abnormal condition caused by excessive absorption and tissue deposition of silver salts. It is marked by a slate-gray coloration of the skin and mucous membranes. **2.** a cerebral cortex abnormality in which the gyri are poorly developed.

AHA, abbreviation for **American Hospital Association.**

"aha" reaction /ähä′/, (in psychology) a sudden realization or inspiration, experienced especially during creative thinking.

AHCPR, abbreviation for **Agency for Health Care Policy and Research.**

AHF, abbreviation for **antihemophilic factor.**

AHH, abbreviation for **aryl hydrocarbon hydroxylase.**

Ahumada-del Castillo syndrome /ä′hōōmä′dädel′ kästē′yō/, [Juan Carlos Ahumada; E. B. del Castillo; twentieth-century Argentine physicians], a form of secondary amenorrhea that may be associated with a pituitary gland tumor.

AI, abbreviation for **artificial intelligence;** abbreviation for **artificial insemination.**

AICD, abbreviation for **automatic implanted cardioverter defibrillator.**

aid, assistance given a person who is ill, injured, or otherwise unable to cope with normal demands of life.

AID, abbreviation for **artificial insemination—donor.**

AIDS /ādz/, abbreviation for **acquired immunodeficiency syndrome.**

AIDS-dementia complex (ADC), a neurologic effect of encephalitis or brain inflammation experienced by nearly one third of all acquired immunodeficiency syndrome (AIDS) patients. The condition is characterized by memory loss and varying levels and forms of dementia. A suggested cause is that the AIDS virus may destroy neurons without actually entering the brain cells. Autopsies indicate that neuron density in AIDS patients may be 40% lower than in the brains of persons who have not experienced AIDS.

AIDS-wasting syndrome, a category of acquired immunodeficiency syndrome

(AIDS). Signs and symptoms may include weight loss, fever, malaise, lethargy, oral thrush, and immunologic abnormalities characteristic of AIDS.

AIH, abbreviation for **artificial insemination—husband.**

ailment [OE, *eglan*], any disease or physical disorder or complaint, generally of a chronic, acute, or mild nature.

air [Gk, *aer*], the colorless, odorless gaseous mixture constituting the earth's atmosphere. It consists of 78% nitrogen; 20% oxygen; almost 1% argon; small amounts of carbon dioxide, hydrogen, and ozone; traces of helium, krypton, neon, and xenon; and varying amounts of water vapor.

air bath, the exposure of the naked body to warm air for therapeutic purposes.

airborne contaminants, materials in the atmosphere that can affect the health of persons in the same or nearby environments. Particularly vulnerable are tissues of the upper respiratory tract and lungs.

airborne precautions, safeguards designed to reduce the risk of airborne transmission of infectious agents. Airborne droplet nuclei consist of small-particle residue (5 μm or smaller in size) of evaporated droplets that may remain suspended in the air for long periods of time. Airborne transmission occurs by dissemination of either airborne droplet nuclei or dust particles containing the infectious agent.

air compressor, a mechanical device that compresses air for storage and is used in handpieces and other air-driven medical and dental tools.

air embolism, the abnormal presence of air in the cardiovascular system, resulting in obstruction of blood flow through the vessel. Air may be inadvertently introduced by injection, during intravenous therapy or surgery, or traumatically, as by a puncture wound.

air entrainment, the movement of room air into the chamber of a jet nebulizer used to treat respiratory diseases. Air entrainment increases the rate of nebulization and the amount of liquid administered per unit of time.

airflow pattern, the pattern of movement of respiratory gases through the respiratory tract, such as laminar, turbulent, or tracheobronchial flow. The pattern is affected by such factors as gas density and viscosity.

air fluidization, the process of blowing warm air through a collection of microspheres to create a fluidlike environment.

air-fluidized bed, a bed with body support provided by thousands of tiny soda-lime glass beads suspended by pressurized temperature-controlled air.

air hunger, a form of respiratory distress characterized by gasping, labored breathing, or dyspnea.

airplane splint, a splint used for immobilizing a fractured humerus during healing. The splint holds the arm in an abducted position at shoulder level, with the elbow bent.

air pollution [L, *polluere*, to defile], contamination of the air by noxious fumes, aromas, or toxic chemicals.

air pump, a pump that forces air into or out of a cavity or chamber.

air sac, a small, terminal cavity in the lung, consisting of the alveoli connected to one terminal bronchiole.

air sickness., a form of motion sickness caused by flying and, in some cases, by traveling on land at high elevations. Symptoms usually include nausea and vomiting and are sometimes accompanied by headache or drowsiness.

air spaces, the alveolar ducts, alveolar sacs, and alveoli of the respiratory system.

air splint, a device for temporarily immobilizing fractured or otherwise injured extremities. It consists of an inflatable cylinder that can be closed at both ends and becomes rigid when filled with air under pressure.

air swallowing, the intake of air into the digestive system, usually involuntary and during eating, drinking, or chewing gum. Air swallowing may also be an effect of anxious behavior. The problem occurs commonly in infants as a result of faulty feeding methods.

air thermometer, a thermometer using air as its expansible medium.

airway [Gk, *aer* + AS, *weg*, way], a tubular passage for movement of air into and out of the lung, trachea, bronchi, and bronchioles; a respiratory anesthesia device; or an oropharyngeal tube used for mouth-to-mouth resuscitation. An airway with a diameter greater than 2 mm is defined as a large, or central, airway; one smaller than 2 mm is called a small, or peripheral, airway.

airway clearance, ineffective, a NANDA-accepted nursing diagnosis of an individual's inability to clear secretions or obstructions from the respiratory tract. Defining characteristics include abnormal breath sounds (crackles, gurgles, wheezes); cough, ineffective or absent; report of difficulty with sputum; report of chest congestion.

airway conductance, the instantaneous volumetric gas flow rate in the airway per unit of pressure difference between the mouth, nose, or other airway opening and the alveoli. It is also the reciprocal of airway resistance.

airway division, one of the 18 segments of the bronchopulmonary system. The segments are usually numbered from 1 to 10 for both the right and left lungs.

Airway Insertion and Stabilization, a Nursing Interventions Classification defined as insertion or assisting with insertion and stabilization of an artificial airway.

Airway Management, a Nursing Interventions Classification defined as facilitation of patency of air passages.

airway obstruction, an abnormal condition of the respiratory system characterized by a mechanical impediment to the delivery or absorption of oxygen in the lungs.

airway resistance, the ratio of pressure difference between the mouth, nose, or other airway opening and the alveoli to the simultaneously measured resulting volumetric gas flow rate. It is the reciprocal of airway conductance.

Airway Suctioning, a Nursing Interventions Classification defined as removal of airway secretions by inserting a suction catheter into the patient's oral airway and/or trachea.

AKA, abbreviation for *above the knee amputation.*

akaryocyte /āker′ē·əsīt′/ [Gk, *a,* not, *karyon,* kernel], a cell without a nucleus, such as an erythrocyte.

akathisia /ak′əthē′zhə/ [Gk, *a* + *kathizein,* not to sit], a pathologic condition characterized by restlessness and agitation, such as an inability to sit still. —**akathisiac,** *adj.*

akeratosis /āker′ətō′sis/, a skin condition in which there is a lack of horny tissue in the epidermis.

akinesia /ā′kinē′zhə, ā′kīnē′zhə/ [Gk, *a, kinesis,* without movement], an abnormal state of motor and psychic hypoactivity or muscular paralysis.—**akinetic** /ā′kinet′ik/, *adj.*

akinesthesia /ākin′esthē′zhə/, a loss of the sense of movement.

akinetic /ā′kinet′ik/ [Gk, *a, kinesis*], without movement], pertaining to a loss of ability to move a part or all of the body.

akinetic apraxia, the inability to perform a spontaneous movement.

akinetic mutism, a state in which a person is unable or refuses to move or to make sounds, resulting from neurologic or psychologic disturbance.

akinetic seizure, a type of seizure disorder observed in children. It is a brief, generalized seizure in which the child suddenly falls to the ground.

Al, symbol for the element **aluminum.**

ala /ā′lə/, *pl.* **alae** [L, wing], **1.** any winglike structure. **2.** the axilla.

Ala, abbreviation for the amino acid **alanine.**

ALA, abbreviation for **aminolevulinic acid.**

ala auris, the auricle of the ear.

ala cerebelli /ser′əbel′ī/, the ala of the central lobule of the cerebellum.

ala cinerea /sinir′ē·ə/, the triangular area on the floor of the fourth ventricle of the brain from which the autonomic fibers of the vagus nerve arise.

ala nasi /nā′sī/, the outer flaring cartilaginous wall of each nostril.

alanine (Ala) /al′ənin/, a nonessential amino acid found in many food protein sources, as well as in the body. It is degraded in the liver to produce pyruvate and glutamate.

alanine aminotransferase (ALT), an enzyme normally present in the serum and tissues of the body, especially the tissues of the liver. This enzyme catalyzes the transfer of an amino group from *l*-alanine to alpha-ketoglutarate.

Al-Anon, an international organization that offers guidance, counseling, and support for the relatives, friends, and associates of alcoholics.

ala of the ethmoid, a small projection on each side of the crista galli of the ethmoid bone. Each ala fits into a corresponding depression of the frontal bone.

ala of the ilium, the upper flaring part of the iliac bone.

ala of the sacrum, the flat extension of bone on each side of the sacrum.

alar /ā′lär/ [L, *ala,* wing], pertaining to a winglike structure, such as the shoulder.

ALARA, an abbreviation for *as low as reasonably achievable.*

alar lamina [L, *ala,* wing, *lamina,* thin plate], the posterolateral area of the embryonic neural tube through which sensory nerves enter.

alar ligament, one of a pair of ligaments that connect the axis to the occipital bone and limit rotation of the cranium.

alar process [L, *ala,* wing, *processus*], a projection of the cribriform plate of the ethmoid bone articulating with the frontal bone.

alarm reaction, the first stage of the general adaptation syndrome. It is characterized by the mobilization of the various defense mechanisms of the body or the mind to cope with a stressful situation of a physical or emotional nature.

alastrim /al′əstrim/ [Port, *alastrar,* to

spread], a mild form of smallpox, with little rash. It is thought to be caused by a weak strain of *Poxvirus variolae.*

Alateen, an international organization that offers guidance, counseling, and support for the children of alcoholics.

ala vomeris /vō'məris/, an extension of bone on each side of the upper border of the vomer.

alba /al'bə/, literally, 'white,' as in *linea alba.*

albedo /albē'dō/ [L, *albus,* white], a whiteness, particularly as a surface reflection.

Albers-Schönberg disease /-shœn'burg, -shōn'-/ [Heinrich E. Albers-Schönberg, Hamburg radiologist, 1865–1921], a form of osteopetrosis characterized by marblelike calcification of bones.

Albert's disease [Eduard Albert, Austrian surgeon, 1841–1900], an inflammation of the bursa that lies between the Achilles tendon and the calcaneus. It is most frequently caused by injury. If treatment is delayed, the inflammation may cause erosion of the calcaneus.

albicans /al'bikənz/ [L, *albus,* white], white or whitish.

albinism /al'biniz'əm/, a congenital hereditary condition characterized by partial or total lack of melanin pigment in the body. Total albinos have pale skin that does not tan, white hair, pink eyes, nystagmus, astigmatism, and photophobia. Lack of skin pigment predisposes the individual to skin cancer.

albinuria /al'binŏōr'ē·ə/, white urine.

Albl's ring, a calcified, ring-shaped shadow visible on a radiograph of an aneurysm of a cerebral artery.

Albright's syndrome /ôl'brīts/ [Fuller Albright, Boston physician, 1900–1969], a disorder characterized by fibrous dysplasia of bone, isolated brown macules on the skin, and endocrine dysfunction. It causes precocious puberty in girls but not in boys.

albumin /albyoo'min/ [L, *albus,* white], a water soluble, heat-coagulable protein. Various albumins are found in practically all animal tissues and in many plant tissues.

albumin A, a blood serum constituent that gathers in cancer cells and is deficient in circulation in cancer patients.

albuminaturia /albyoo'minə tŏōr'ē·ə/, urine that contains an excessive level of a saltlike derivative of albumin and has a low specific gravity.

albumin (human), a plasma-volume expander prescribed in the treatment of hypoproteinemia, hyperbilirubinemia, and hypovolemic shock.

albumin test [L, *albus,* white], any of several tests for the presence of albumin, a class of simple proteins, in the urine, a common sign of renal or functional disorders. One type of albumin test depends on the change in color of a chemically treated strip of paper in the presence of albumin.

albuterol, an adrenergic used as a bronchodilator. It is prescribed in the treatment of bronchospasm in patients with reversible obstructive airway disease.

alcalase, a protein enzyme contained in concentrations of about 60 ppm in certain laundry detergents. It is a cause of enzymatic detergent asthma.

alclometasone dipropionate, a topical corticosteroid prescribed for the relief of symptoms of inflammation and pruritus of corticosteroid-responsive dermatoses.

Alcock's canal [Benjamin Alcock, Irish anatomist, b. 1801], a canal formed by the obturator internus muscle and the obturator fascia through which the pudendal nerve and vessels pass.

alcohol /al'kəhôl/ [Ar *alkohl* subtle essence], **1.** (USP) a preparation containing at least 92.3% and not more than 93.8% by weight of ethyl alcohol, used as a topical antiseptic and solvent. **2.** a clear, colorless, volatile liquid that is miscible with water, chloroform, or ether, obtained by the fermentation of carbohydrates by yeast. **3.** a compound derived from a hydrocarbon by replacing one or more hydrogen atoms with an equal number of hydroxyl (OH) groups. Depending on the number of hydroxyl groups, alcohols are classified as monohydric, dihydric, trihydric.

alcohol bath, a procedure for decreasing an elevated body temperature. A tepid solution of 25% to 50% alcohol in water is sponged lightly on each limb, then on the trunk.

Alcohol, Drug Abuse, and Mental Health Administration (ADAMHA), an agency of the U.S. Department of Health and Human Services with three components—the National Institute on Alcohol Abuse and Alcoholism, the National Institute on Drug Abuse, and the National Institute of Mental Health. It conducts and supports research on the biologic, psychologic, epidemiologic, and behavioral aspects of alcoholism, drug abuse, and mental health and illness.

alcoholic, 1. pertaining to alcohol or its effects on other substances. **2.** a person who has developed a dependency on alcohol through abuse of the substance.

alcoholic ataxia [Ar, *alkohl,* essence; Gk, *ataxia,* disorder], a loss of coordination in performing voluntary movements associated with peripheral neuritis secondary to alcoholism. A similar form of ataxia may occur with neuritis resulting from other toxic agents.

alcoholic blackout, a form of amnesia in which a person has no memory of what occurred during a period of alcohol abuse.

alcoholic cardiomyopathy [Ar, *alkohl,* essence; Gk, *kardia,* heart, *mys,* muscle, *pathos,* disease], a cardiac disease associated with alcohol abuse. It is characterized by an enlarged heart and low cardiac output.

alcoholic coma [Ar, *alkohl* + Gk, *koma,* deep sleep], a state of unconsciousness that results from severe alcoholic intoxication.

alcoholic dementia [Ar, *alkohl* + L, *de,* away, *mens,* mind], a deterioration of normal cognitive and intellectual functions associated with long-term alcohol abuse.

alcoholic dyspepsia, a digestive disorder characterized by abdominal discomfort and provoked by the consumption of alcohol.

alcoholic fermentation, the conversion of carbohydrates to ethyl alcohol.

alcoholic hallucinosis, a form of alcoholic psychosis characterized primarily by auditory hallucinations, abject fear, and persecutory delusions. The condition develops in acute alcoholism as withdrawal symptoms shortly after stopping or reducing alcohol intake.

alcoholic hepatitis, acute toxic liver injury associated with excess ethanol consumption. This is characterized by necrosis, polymorphonuclear inflammation, and in many instances Mallory bodies.

alcoholic ketoacidosis, the fall in blood pH (acidosis), sometimes seen in alcoholics, associated with a rise in serum ketone bodies (acetone, beta-hydroxybutyric acid, and acetoacetic acid).

alcoholic-nutritional cerebellar degeneration, a sudden, severe incoordination in the lower extremity characteristic of poorly nourished alcoholics. The patient walks, if at all, with an ataxic or wide-based gait.

alcoholic paralysis [Ar, *alkohl,* essence; Gk, *paralyein,* to be palsied], a paralysis affecting the peripheral nerves as a result of alcohol consumption.

alcoholic psychosis, any of a group of severe mental disorders, such as pathologic intoxication, delirium tremens, Korsakoff's psychosis, and acute hallucinosis. It is characterized by brain damage or dysfunction that results from excessive use alcohol use.

Alcoholics Anonymous (AA), an international nonprofit organization, founded in 1935, consisting of abstinent alcoholics whose purpose is to stay sober and help others recover from the disease of alcoholism through a 12-step program, including group support, shared experiences, and faith in a higher power.

alcoholic trance, a state of automatism resulting from ethanol intoxication.

alcoholism /al'kəhôliz'əm/, the extreme dependence on excessive amounts of alcohol associated with a cumulative pattern of deviant behaviors. Alcoholism is a chronic illness. The most frequent medical consequences of alcoholism are central nervous system depression and cirrhosis of the liver. The severity of each may be greater in the absence of food intake.

alcohol poisoning, poisoning caused by the ingestion of any of several alcohols, of which ethyl, isopropyl, and methyl are the most common. Ethyl alcohol (ethanol) is found in whiskies, brandy, gin, and other beverages. Ordinarily it is lethal only if large quantities are ingested in a brief period. Isopropyl (rubbing) alcohol is more toxic: Ingestion of 8 ounces may result in respiratory or circulatory failure. Methyl alcohol (methanol) is extremely poisonous: in addition to nausea, vomiting, and abdominal pain, it may cause blindness; and death may follow the consumption of only 2 ounces.

alcohol withdrawal syndrome, the clinical symptoms associated with cessation of alcohol consumption. These may include tremor, hallucinations, autonomic nervous system dysfunction, and seizures.

ALD, abbreviation for **adrenoleukodystrophy.**

aldehyde /al'dəhīd'/ [Ar, *alkohl* + L, *dehydrogenatum,* dehydrogenated], any of a large category of organic compounds derived from oxidation of a corresponding primary alcohol, as in the conversion of ethyl alcohol to acetaldehyde.

aldolase /al'dəlās/, an enzyme found in muscle tissue that catalyzes the step in anaerobic glycolysis involving the breakdown of fructose 1,6-diphosphate to glyceraldehyde 3-phosphate.

aldose /al'dōs/, the chemical form of monosaccharides in which the carbonyl group is an aldehyde.

aldosterone /al'dōstərōn', aldos'tərōn/, a mineralocorticoid steroid hormone produced by the adrenal cortex with action in the renal tubule to retain sodium, conserve water by resorption, and increase potassium excretion in the blood.

aldosteronism /al'dōstərō'nizəm, aldos'-/, a condition characterized by hypersecretion of aldosterone, occurring as a primary disease of the adrenal cortex or, more often, as a secondary disorder in response to various extraadrenal pathologic processes. Primary aldosteronism may be caused by adrenal hyperplasia or by an aldosterone-secreting tumor. Secondary aldosteronism is associated with increased plasma renin activity and may be induced by the nephrotic syndrome, hepatic cirrhosis, idiopathic edema, congestive heart failure, trauma, burns, or other kinds of stress.

aldosteronoma /al'dōstir'əno'mə/, an aldosterone-secreting adenoma of the adrenal cortex that is usually small and occurs more frequently in the left than the right adrenal gland. Hyperaldosteronism with salt retention, expansion of the extracellular fluid volume, and increased blood pressure may occur.

alertness [Fr, *alerte*], a condition of being mentally quick, active, and keenly aware of the environment.

aleukemia, an acute form of leukemia characterized by a diminished total white cell content in the peripheral blood supply, accompanied by a loss of normal bone marrow function.

aleukemic leukemia /ā'lookē'mik/, a type of leukemia in which the total leukocyte count remains within normal limits and few abnormal forms appear in the peripheral blood.

aleukia /āloo'kē·ə/ [Gk, *a* + *leukos*, not white], a marked reduction in or complete absence of white blood cells or blood platelets.

aleukocytosis /āloo'kōsītō'sis/, an extreme decrease or absence of leukocytes in the blood.

Alexander technique, a body-focused alternative health therapy introduced by Frederick Alexander. It focuses on individual variations in body musculature, posture, and the breathing process and on the correction of defects.

alexia /əlek'sē·ə/ [Gk, *a, lexis,* not speech], an inability to comprehend written words.—**alexic,** *adj.*

alexithymia /əlek'sithī'mē·ə, -thim'ē·ə/, an inability to experience and communicate feelings consciously.

alga /al'gə/, *pl.* **algae** /al'jī, al'jē/ [L, seaweed], any of a large group of nonmotile or motile marine plants and protists containing chlorophyll. Many genera and species of algae are found worldwide in fresh water, in salt water, and on land. All belong to the phylum Thallophyta. —**algal,** *adj.*

algid /al'jid/ [L, *algere,* to be cold], chilly or cold.

algid malaria /al'jid/ [L, *algere,* to be cold], a stage of malaria caused by the protozoan *Plasmodium falciparum.* It is

characterized by coldness of the skin, profound weakness, and severe diarrhea.

algodystrophy /al'gōdis'trəfē/, a painful wasting of the muscles of the hands, often accompanied by tenderness and a loss of bone calcium.

algolagnia /al'gōlag'nē·ə/ [Gk, *algos,* pain, *lagneia,* lust], a form of sexual perversion characterized by sadism or masochism.

algology, **1.** the branch of medicine that is concerned with the study of pain. **2.** the branch of science that is concerned with algae.

algophobia [Gk, *algos,* pain, *phobos,* fear], an anxiety disorder characterized by an abnormal, pervasive fear of experiencing pain or of witnessing pain in others.

algor [L, cold], the sensation of cold or a chill, particularly in the first stage of a fever.

algorithm /al'gərith'əm/, **1.** a step-by-step procedure for the solution of a problem by a computer, using specific mathematic or logical operations. **2.** an explicit protocol with well-defined rules to be followed in solving a health care problem.

algor mortis, the reduction in body temperature and accompanying loss of skin elasticity that occur after death.

algospasm /al'gōspaz'əm/, an acute, painful spasm of the muscles.

Alice in Wonderland syndrome, perceptual distortions of space and size, as experienced by the character Alice in the Lewis Carroll story. Similar hallucinogenic experiences have been reported by individuals using drugs of abuse and by patients with certain neurologic diseases.

alien /āl'yən/ [L, *alienare,* to estrange], strange, unusual, or foreign.

alienate /āl'yənāt/ [L, *alienare*], to cause a withdrawal or transference of affection, or detachment.

alienation /āl'yənā'shən/ [L, *alienare,* to estrange], the act or state of being estranged or isolated.

alignment /əlīn'mənt/, **1.** the arrangement of a group of points or objects along a line. **2.** the placing or maintaining of body structures in their proper anatomic positions, such as repairing a fractured bone.

aliment [L, *alimentum,* to nourish], nutrition.

alimentary /al'əmen'tərē/ [L, *alimentum,* nourishment], pertaining to food or nourishment and to the digestive organs.

alimentary duct, the thoracic duct of the lymphatic system.

alimentary system [L, *alimentum,* nourishment; Gk, *systema*], the digestive system.

alimentary tract. See **digestive tract.**

alimentation. nourishment.

aliphatic /al'ifat'ik/ [Gk, *aleiphar,* oil], pertaining to fat or oil, specifically to those hydrocarbon compounds that are open chains of carbon atoms, such as the fatty acids, rather than ring structures.

aliphatic acid, an acid of a nonaromatic hydrocarbon.

aliphatic alcohol, an alcohol that contains an open chain or fatty series of hydrocarbons. Examples include ethyl alcohol and isopropyl alcohol.

alkalemia [Ar, *al + galiy,* wood ash; Gk, *haima,* blood], a condition of increased pH of the blood.

alkali /al'kəlī/ [Ar, *al + galiy,* wood ash], a compound with the chemical characteristics of a base. Alkalis combine with fatty acids to form soaps, turn red litmus blue, and enter into reactions that form water-soluble carbonates.

alkali burn, damage to tissue caused by exposure to an alkaline compound like lye. The victim should be immediately taken to a medical facility if the tissue damage is more than slight and superficial.

alkaline ash /al'kəlīn/, residue in the urine having a pH higher than 7.0.

alkaline ash–producing foods, foods that may be ingested to produce an alkaline pH in the urine, thereby reducing the incidence of acidic urinary calculi, or that may be avoided to reduce the incidence of alkaline calculi. Some foods that result in alkaline ash are milk, cream, and buttermilk.

alkaline bath, a bath taken in water containing sodium bicarbonate, used especially for skin disorders.

alkaline phosphatase, an enzyme present in bone, the kidneys, the intestine, plasma, and teeth. It may be elevated in the serum in some diseases of the bone and liver and in some other illnesses.

alkaline reserve, an additional amount of sodium bicarbonate the body produces to maintain a normal arterial blood pH (7.35 to 7.45) when the carbon dioxide level increases as a result of hypoventilation.

alkalinity /al'kəlin'itē/, pertaining to the acid-base relationship of any solution that has fewer hydrogen ions or more hydroxide ions than pure water, which is an arbitrarily neutral standard with a pH of 7.0.

alkalinize /al'kəlinīz/, **1.** to make a substance alkaline, as through the addition of a base. **2.** to become alkaline.

alkali poisoning, a toxic condition caused by the ingestion of an alkaline agent such as liquid ammonia, lye, and some detergent powders. Emergency treatment includes giving copious amounts of water or milk to dilute the alkali. Vomiting is not induced, and mild acids are not administered. The victim is transported immediately to the hospital.

alkali reserves [Ar, *al + galiy,* the wood ashes,+ L, *reservare,* to save], the volume of carbon dioxide or carbonates at standard temperature and pressure held by 100 ml of blood plasma to be neutralized by lactic or other acids. The principal buffer in blood is bicarbonate, which essentially represents the alkali reserve. Hemoglobin phosphates and additional bases also act as buffers. If the alkali reserve is low, a state of acidosis exists. If the alkali reserve is high, alkalosis exists.

alkaloid /al'kəloid/ [Ar, *al + galiy* + Gk, *eidos,* form], any of a large group of nitrogen-containing organic compounds produced by plants, including many pharmacologically active substances such as atropine, caffeine, cocaine, morphine, nicotine, and quinine.

alkalosis /al'kəlō'sis/ [Ar, *al + galiy* + Gk, *osis,* condition], an abnormal condition of body fluids, characterized by a tendency toward a pH level greater than 7.45, as from an excess of alkaline bicarbonate or a deficiency of acid. Respiratory alkalosis may be caused by hyperventilation, resulting from an excess loss of carbon dioxide and a carbonic acid deficit. Metabolic alkalosis may result from an excess intake or retention of bicarbonate, loss of gastric acid in vomiting, potassium depletion, or any stimulus that increases the rate of sodium-hydrogen exchange.

alkaptonuria /alkap'tōnoor'ē-ə/ [Ar, *al + galiy* + Gk, *haptein* to possess, *ouron* urine], a rare inherited disorder resulting from the incomplete metabolism of tyrosine, an amino acid, in which abnormal amounts of homogentisic acid are excreted as a result of incomplete metabolism of tyrosine, staining the urine dark.—**alkaptonuric,** *adj.*

alkene /al'kēn/, an unsaturated aliphatic hydrocarbon containing one double bond in the carbon chain, such as ethylene.

alkyl /al'kil/, a hydrocarbon fragment derived from alkane by the removal of one of the hydrogen atoms.

alkylamine /al'kiləmīn'/, an amine in which an alkyl group replaces one to three of the hydrogen atoms that are attached to the nitrogen atom, such as methylamine.

alkylating agent /al'kilā'ting/, any substance that contains an alkyl radical and is capable of replacing a free hydrogen atom in an organic compound, or one that acts by a similar mechanism. This type of chemical reaction results in interference with mitosis and cell division, especially in rapidly proliferating tissue. The agents are useful in the treatment of cancer.

alkylation, a chemical reaction in which an alkyl group is transferred from an alkylating agent.

ALL, abbreviation for **acute lymphocytic leukemia.**

allachesthesia /aləkesthē′zhəl/ [Gk, *allache,* elsewhere], a defect of touch sensation in which a stimulus is perceived to be at a point distant from where it is actually applied.

allantoidoangiopagus /al′əntoi′dō·an′ jē·op′əgəs/ [Gk, *allantoeides,* sausagelike, *angeion,* vessel, *pagos,* fixed], conjoined monozygotic twin fetuses of unequal size that are united by the vessels of the umbilical cord. —**allantoidoangiopagous,** *adj.*

allantoin /əlan′tō·in/, a chemical compound (5-ureidohydantoin), $C_4H_6N_4O_3$, that occurs as a white crystallizable substance found in many plants and in the allantoic and amniotic fluids and fetal urine of primates.

allantois /əlan′tois/ [Gk, *allas,* sausage, *eidos,* form], a tubular extension of the endoderm of the yolk sac that extends with the allantoic vessels into the body stalk of the embryo. In human embryos allantoic vessels become the umbilical vessels and the chorionic villi. —**allantoic** /al′əntō′-ik/, *adj.*

allele /əlēl′/, one of two or more alternative forms of a gene that occupy corresponding loci on homologous chromosomes.

allelomorph /əlēl′əmôrf′/, one of two or more contrasting characteristics transmitted by alternative genes.

Allen-Doisy test [Edgar Allen, U.S. endocrinologist, 1892–1943; Edward Doisy, U.S. biochemist and Nobel laureate, 1893–1986], a bioassay test for estrogen and gonadotropins in which ovariectomized mice are injected with an estrogenic substance. The appearance of cornified cells on vaginal smears is regarded as a positive finding.

Allen test, a test for the patency of the radial artery after insertion of an indwelling monitoring catheter.

allergen /al′ərjin/ [Gk, *allos,* other, *ergein,* to work, *genein,* to produce], a substance that can produce a hypersensitive allergic reaction in the body but is not necessarily intrinsically harmful. The body normally protects itself against allergens or antigens by the complex chemical reactions of the humoral immune and the cell-mediated immune systems. Methods to identify specific allergens affecting individuals include a "patch" test, a scratch test, a radioallergosorbent (RAST) test, and a Prausnitz-Küstner (PK) test. —**allergenic,** *adj.*

allergic arthritis, appearance of symptoms of arthritis such as swollen joints after the ingestion of allergenic foods or medications.

allergenic extract, an extract of the protein of a substance to which a person may be sensitive. The extract, which may be prepared from a wide variety of substances from food to fungi, can be used for diagnosis or for desensitization therapy.

allergic /əlur′jik/, **1.** pertaining to allergy. **2.** having an allergy.

allergic asthma, a form of asthma caused by the exposure of the bronchial mucosa to an inhaled airborne antigen. This allergen causes the production of antibodies that bind to mast cells in the bronchial tree. The mast cells then release histamine, which stimulates contraction of bronchial smooth muscle and causes mucosal edema. Psychologic factors may provoke asthma attacks in bronchi already sensitized by allergens.

allergic bronchopulmonary aspergillosis, a form of aspergillosis that occurs in asthmatics when the fungus *Aspergillus fumigatus,* growing within the bronchial lumen, causes a hypersensitivity reaction. The characteristics of the condition are similar to those of asthma, including dyspnea and wheezing.

allergic conjunctivitis, hyperemia of the conjunctiva caused by an allergy. Common allergens that cause this condition are pollen, grass, topical medications, air pollutants, occupational irritants, and smoke. It is bilateral, usually starts before puberty, and lasts about 10 years, commonly recurring in a seasonal pattern.

allergic coryza, acute rhinitis caused by exposure to any allergen to which the person is hypersensitive.

allergic dermatitis [Ger, *allergie,* reaction; Gk, *derma,* skin, *itis,* inflammation], an acute cell-mediated inflammatory response (or reaction) of the skin after exposure of a body area to a contact allergen to which the patient is hypersensitive.

allergic purpura [Gk, *allos,* other, *ergein,* to work; L, *purpura,* purple], a chronic disorder of the skin associated with urticaria, erythema, asthma, and rheumatic joint swellings. Unlike in other forms of purpura, platelet count, bleeding time, and blood coagulation are normal.

allergic reaction, an unfavorable physiologic response to an allergen to which an organism has previously been exposed and to which it has developed antibodies. Subsequent exposure causes the release of chemical mediators and a variety of symptoms, including urticaria, eczema, and bronchospasm. Allergic reactions can be categorized into two basic types: immediate and delayed-type hypersensitivity, depending on the time between exposure to the allergen or antigen and the appearance of symptoms.

allergic rhinitis, inflammation of the nasal passages, usually associated with watery nasal discharge and itching of the nose and eyes, caused by a localized sensitivity reaction to house dust, animal dander, or an antigen, commonly pollen. The condition may be seasonal, as in hay fever, or perennial, as in allergy to dust or animals.

allergic vasculitis, an inflammatory condition of the blood vessels that is induced by an allergen. Allergic cutaneous vasculitis is characterized by itching, malaise, and a slight fever and by the presence of papules, vesicles, urticarial wheals, or small ulcers on the skin.

allergist /al'ərjist/, a physician who specializes in the diagnosis and treatment of allergic disorders.

allergy /al'ərjē/ [Gk, *allos,* other, *ergein,* to work], a hypersensitive reaction to intrinsically common, harmless antigens, most of which are environmental.

Allergy Management, a Nursing Interventions Classification defined as identification, treatment, and prevention of allergic responses to food, medications, insect bites, contrast material, blood, or other substances.

allergy testing, any one of the various procedures used in identifying the specific allergens that afflict a patient. Such tests are helpful in prescribing treatment to prevent allergic reactions or to reduce their severity. The most common is skin testing, which exposes the patient to small quantities of the suspected allergens.

all fours position, the sixth stage in the Rood system of ontogenetic motor patterns. In this stage the lower trunk and lower extremities are brought into a cocontraction pattern while stretching the trunk and limb girdles develops cocontractions of the trunk flexors and extensors.

allied health personnel. See **paramedical personnel.**

alligator forceps, **1.** a forceps with heavy teeth and a double clamp, used in orthopedic surgery. **2.** a forceps with long, thin, angular handles and interlocking teeth.

Allis forceps, curved forceps with serrated edges, used for grasping tissues.

alloantigen /al'ō·an'tijen/ [Gk, *allos,* other], an isoantigen; a substance present in some members of a species that stimulates production of antibodies in other members of the species. An example is blood group antigens.

allodiploid /al'ōdip'loid/ [Gk, *allos,* other, *diploos,* double, *eidos,* form], **1.** pertaining to an individual, organism, strain, or cell that has two genetically distinct sets of chromosomes derived from different ancestral species, as occurs in hybridization. **2.** such an individual, organism, strain, or cell.

allodiploidy /al'ōdip'loidē/, the state or condition of having two genetically distinct sets of chromosomes derived from different ancestral species.

alloesthesia /al'ō·esthē'zhə/, a referred pain or other sensation that is perceived at a remote site on the same or opposite side of the stimulated part of the body.

allogenic /al'ōjen'ik/ [Gk, *allos* + *genein,* to produce], **1.** (in genetics) denoting an individual or cell type that is from the same species but genetically distinct. **2.** (in transplantation biology) denoting tissues, particularly stem cells from either bone marrow or peripheral blood, that are from the same species but antigenically distinct; homologous.

allograft /al'əgraft/ [Gk, *allos,* other + *graphion,* stylus], a nonpermanent graft of tissue between two genetically dissimilar individuals of the same species, such as a tissue transplant between two humans who are not identical twins.

allokeratoplasty /al'ōker'ətoplas'tē/, the repair of a cornea with synthetic transparent material.

allometric growth, the increase in size of different organs or parts of an organism at various rates.

allometron /əlom'itron/, a quantitative change in the proportional relationship of the parts of an organism as a result of the evolutionary process.

allometry /əlom'itrē/ [Gk, *allos* + *metron,* measure], the measurement and study of the changes in proportions of the various parts of an organism in relation to the growth of the whole or within a series of related organisms. —**allometric,** *adj.*

allomorphism /al'ōmôr'fizəm/ [Gk, *allos,* other, *morphe,* form], **1.** a change in crystalline form without a change in chemical composition. **2.** a change in the shape of a group of cells caused by pressure or other physical factors.

allopathic physician /al'ōpath'ik/, a physician who treats disease and injury with active interventions, such as medical and surgical treatment, intended to bring about effects opposite to those produced by the disease or injury.

allopathy /əlop′əthē/ [Gk, *allos* + *pathos,* suffering], a system of medical therapy in which a disease or an abnormal condition is treated by creating an environment that is antagonistic to the disease or condition; for example, an antibiotic toxic to a pathogenic organism is given in an infection, or an iron supplement may be given to increase the synthesis of hemoglobin in iron deficiency anemia.

alloplast /al′ōplast/ [Gk, *allos,* other, *plassein,* to form], a graft made of plastic, metal, or other material foreign to the human body.

alloplastic maneuver [Gk, *allos* + *plassein,* to form], (in psychology) a process that is part of adaptation, involving an adjustment or change in the external environment.

alloplasty /al′ōplas′tē/ [Gk, *allos,* other, *plassein,* to form], plastic surgery in which materials foreign to the human body are implanted.

allopolyploid /al′əpol′iploid/ [Gk, *allos* + *polyplous,* many times, *eidos* form], **1.** pertaining to an individual, organism, strain, or cell that has more than two genetically distinct sets of chromosomes derived from two or more different ancestral species, as occurs in hybridization. **2.** such an individual, organism, strain, or cell.

allopolyploidy /al′əpol′iploi′dē/, the state or condition of having more than two genetically distinct sets of chromosomes from two or more ancestral species.

allopurinol /al′əpyoor′ənôl/, a xanthine oxidase inhibitor uricosuric agent prescribed in the treatment of gout and other hyperuricemic conditions.

allorhythmia /al′ōrith′mē′ə/, an irregular heart rhythm that occurs repeatedly.

all-or-none law, 1. the principle in neurophysiology that if a stimulus is strong enough to trigger a nerve impulse, the entire impulse is discharged. A weak stimulus will not produce a weak reaction. **2.** the principle that the heart muscle, under any stimulus above a threshold level, will respond either with a maximal strength contraction or not at all.

allosteric sites /al′ōster′ik/ [Gk, *allos* + *stereos,* solid], the sites, other than the active site or sites, of an enzyme that bind regulatory molecules.

allotransplantation /al′ō-/, transplantation of an allograft.

allotriodontia /əlot′rē-ōdon′ahə/, **1.** the development of a tooth in an abnormal location, such as a dermoid tumor. **2.** the transplantation of teeth from one individual to another.

allotropic, 1. pertaining to a substance that is changed by digestion to retain some of its nutritive value. **2.** pertaining to an element that may exist in two or more molecular forms, such as carbon in the diamond and graphite forms.

allowable charge /əlou′əbəl/, the maximum amount that a third party, usually an insurance company, will pay to reimburse a provider for a specific service.

allowable costs, components of an institution's costs that are reimbursable as determined by a payment formula. In general, costs of services not considered to be reasonable or necessary to the proper provision of health services are excluded from allowable costs.

allowable dose. See **accumulated dose equivalent.**

allowable error, the amount of error that can be tolerated without invalidating the medical usefulness of the analytic result. Allowable error is defined as having a 95% limit of analytic error; only 1 sample in 20 can have an error greater than this limit.

alloxan /əlok′san/, an oxidation product of uric acid that is found in the human intestine in diarrhea. Alloxan may cause diabetes, destroying the insulin-secreting islet cells of the pancreas.

alloy /al′oi/ [Fr, *aloyer,* to combine metals], a mixture of two or more metals or of substances with metallic properties. A number of alloys have medical applications, such as those used for prostheses and in dental amalgams.

almond oil, an oil expressed from the kernels of the fruit of the sweet almond tree, *Prunus amygdalus.* The fixed oil is a demulcent and mildly laxative. Bitter almond oil is a volatile oil that contains lethal prussic acid.

aloe /al′ō/ [Gk], the inspissated juice of various species of *Aloe* plants, formerly used as a cathartic but generally discontinued because it often causes severe intestinal cramps. It is a component of many topical preparations.

alopecia /al′əpē′shə/ [Gk, *alopex,* fox mange], partial or complete lack of hair resulting from normal aging, endocrine disorder, drug reaction, anticancer medication, or skin disease.

alopecia areata /er′ē-ā′tə/, a disease of unknown cause in which well-defined bald patches occur. The bald areas are usually round or oval and located on the head and other hairy parts of the body. The condition is usually self-limited and often clears completely within 6 to 12 months without treatment.

alopecia congenitalis, congenital baldness in which there may be partial or complete absence of hair at birth.

alopecia neurotica, loss of hair, usually occurring at one site, after a disease or injury involving the nervous system.

alopecia prematura, baldness that occurs early in life, beginning as early as late adolescence.

alopecia senilis, a form of natural hair loss that affects older persons.

alopecia totalis, an uncommon condition characterized by the loss of all the hair on the scalp. The cause is unknown, and the baldness is usually permanent. No treatment is known.

alopecia toxica, a form of hair loss attributed to a febrile illness.

alopecia universalis, a total loss of hair on all parts of the body. The condition is occasionally an extension of alopecia areata.

alpha /al'fə/, A, α, the first letter of the Greek alphabet. It is commonly used as a scientific notation, as in designating a particular physiologic rhythm. It is used in chemical nomenclature to distinguish one variation in a chemical compound from others.

alpha alcoholism, a mild form of alcoholism in which the dependence is psychologic rather than physical.

alpha₁-antitrypsin [Gk, *anti*, against, trypsin], a plasma protein produced in the liver that inhibits the action of proteolytic enzymes such as trypsin. Deficiencies are associated with hepatitis in children and panacinar emphysema in adults. The latter is an inherited condition.

alpha cells [Gk, *alpha,* first letter of the Greek alphabet; L, *cella,* storeroom], cells located in the anterior lobe of the pituitary gland or in the pancreatic islets. In the pancreas they produce glucagon.

alpha error. See **type I error.**

alpha fetoprotein (AFP), a protein normally synthesized by the liver, yolk sac, and gastrointestinal tract of a human fetus but may be found at elevated levels in the sera of adults having certain malignancies.

alpha-fucosidase, a lysosomal enzyme that catalyzes the hydrolysis of fucosides. A deficiency of this enzyme is a cause of fucosidosis.

alpha-galactosidase, an enzyme that catalyzes the conversion of alpha-D-galactoside to D-galactose.

alpha-globulins, one of a group of serum proteins classified as alpha, beta, or gamma on the basis of their electrophoretic mobility. Alpha-globulins have the greatest negative charge, although their anodic mobility is less than that of albumin.

alpha hemolysis, the development of a greenish zone around a bacterial colony growing on blood-agar medium, characteristic of pneumococci and certain streptococci and caused by the partial decomposition of hemoglobin.

alpha₂-interferon /in'tərfir'on/, a protein molecule effective in controlling the spread of common colds caused by rhinoviruses. It is administered as a nasal spray.

alphanumeric, pertaining to a system of characters in which information is coded in combinations of letters and numerals. The characters, which also may include punctuation marks, are used commonly in computer programming to code signals or data.

alpha particle, a particle emitted from an atom during one kind of radioactive decay. It consists of two protons and two neutrons, the equivalent of a helium nucleus.

alpha receptor, any of the postulated adrenergic components of receptor tissues that respond to norepinephrine and to various blocking agents. The activation of the alpha receptors causes such physiologic responses as increased peripheral vascular resistance, dilation of the pupils, and contraction of pilomotor muscles.

alpha redistribution phase, a period after intravenous administration of a drug when the blood level begins to fall from its peak.

alpha state, a condition of relaxed, peaceful wakefulness devoid of concentration and sensory stimulation. It is characterized by the alpha rhythm of brain wave activity, as recorded by an electroencephalograph, and is accompanied by feelings of tranquillity and a lack of tension and anxiety.

Alpha Tau Delta /al'fə tou' del'tə/, a national fraternity of professional nurses.

alpha-tocopherol. See **vitamin E.**

alphavirus /al'favī'rəs/, any of a group of very small togaviruses consisting of a single molecule of single-stranded deoxyribonucleic acid within a lipoprotein capsule.

alpha wave, one of the four types of brain waves, characterized by a relatively high voltage or amplitude and a frequency of 8 to 13 Hz. Alpha waves are the "relaxed waves" of the brain.

Alport's syndrome, [A. C. Alport, South African physician, 1880–1959], a form of hereditary nephritis with symptoms of glomerulonephritis, hematuria, progressive sensorineural hearing loss, and occasional ocular disorders.

alprazolam /al'praz'ələm/, a benzodiazepine antianxiety agent that is prescribed in the treatment of anxiety disorders or the short-term relief of the symptoms of anxiety.

alprostadil, a proprietary form of prostaglandin E_1 used to maintain the patency of the ductus arteriosus in certain neonates. It is recommended as palliative therapy for neonates awaiting surgery to correct congenital heart defects such as tetralogy of Fallot and tricuspid atresia.

ALS, 1. abbreviation for **advanced life support.** See **Emergency Medical Technician—Advanced Life Support. 2.** abbreviation for **amyotrophic lateral sclerosis. 3.** abbreviation for **antilymphocyte serum.**

Alström's syndrome [Carl A. Alström, twentieth century geneticist], an inherited disease characterized by multiple system resistance to hormones. Clinical features include retinal degeneration leading to childhood blindness, vasopressin-resistant diabetes insipidus, and hypogonadism.

ALT, abbreviation for **alanine aminotransferase.**

altered state of consciousness (ASC) [Gk, *alterare,* to change], any state of awareness that differs from the normal awareness of a conscious person. Altered states of consciousness have been achieved, especially in Eastern cultures, by many individuals using various techniques, such as prolonged fasting, deep breathing, whirling, and chanting.

alteregoism /ôl′tərē′gō·iz′əm/, an altruistic feeling for an individual who is similar to or in a similar situation as oneself.

alternans /ôl′tərnənz/ [L, *alternare,* to alternate], a regular rhythm of the heart in which the pulse alternates between strong beats and weak beats (pulsus alternans).

alternate generation /ôl′tərnit/ [L, *alter,* other of two], a type of reproduction in which a sexual generation alternates with one or more asexual generations, as in many plants and lower animals.

alternating current (AC) /ôl′tərnā′ting/, an electric current that reverses direction according to a consistent sinusoidal pattern.

alternating mydriasis, a visual disorder in which there is abnormal dilation of the pupils that affects the left and right eyes alternately.

alternation, the recurrent, successive occurrence of two functions or phases, as when a nerve fiber responds to every other stimulus, or when a heart produces an irregular beat with every other cardiac cycle.

alternation rules, (in psychology) the sociolinguistic rules that establish options available to a person when he or she is speaking to someone else.

alternative inheritance /ôltur′nətiv/, the acquisition of all genetic traits and conditions from one parent, as in self-pollinating plants and self-fertilizing animals.

alternative medicine, any of the systems of medical diagnosis and treatment differing in technique from that of the allopathic practitioner's use of drugs and surgery to treat disease and injury. Examples include faith healing, homeopathy, Indian Ayurvedic medicine, acupuncture, aroma therapy, and therapeutic touch.

alternative pathway of complement activation, a process of antigen-antibody interaction in which activation of the C3 step occurs without prior activation of C1, C4, and C2.

alternator, a device for generating an electric current that changes polarity a specified number of times per second.

alternobaric vertigo, a condition of dysequilibrium caused by unequalized pressure differences in the middle ear, as may be experienced by divers during ascent.

alt hor, (in prescriptions) abbreviation for the Latin phrase *alternis horis,* meaning 'every other hour.'

altitude /ôl′tity ōod/ [L, *altitudo,* height], any location on earth with reference to a fixed surface point, which is usually sea level. Several types of health effects are associated with altitude extremes, including a greater intensity of ultraviolet radiation that results from a thinner atmosphere.

altitude anoxia [L, *altus,* high; Gk, *a,* without, *oxys,* sharp, *genein,* to produce], oxygen deprivation in a high altitude atmosphere.

altitude sickness, a syndrome associated with the relatively low partial pressure (reduced barometric pressure) of oxygen in the atmosphere at altitudes encountered during mountain climbing or travel in unpressurized aircraft. The acute symptoms may include dizziness, headache, irritability, breathlessness, and euphoria.

altruism /al′trōo·iz′əm/, a sense of unconditional concern for the welfare of others. It may be expressed at the level of the individual or the larger social system.

alum /al′əm/ [L, *alumen*], a topical astringent, used primarily in lotions and douches.

alum bath, a bath taken in water containing the mineral salt alum, used primarily for skin disorders.

aluminum (Al) /əlōō′minəm/ [L, *alumen* alum], a widely used metallic element and the third most abundant of all the elements. Its atomic number is 13; its atomic weight (mass) is 26.97. Its compounds are components of many antacids, antiseptics, and astringents. Aluminum hydroxychloride is the most commonly used agent in antiperspirants.

aluminum attenuator, an aluminum filter used to control the hardness of an x-ray beam. The attenuator removes low-energy x-ray photons before they can reach the patient and be absorbed.

aluminum hydroxide gel [L, *alumen,* alum; Gk, *hydor,* water, *oxys,* sharp; L, *gelare,* to congeal], an antacid that works by chemical neutralization and also by adsorption of hydrochloric acid, gases, and toxins.

Alu sequences, a family of repeated sequences in the human genome.

alveobronchitis [L, *alveolus,* little hollow; Gk, *brongchos,* windpipe, *itis,* inflammation], inflammation of the alveoli and bronchioles.

alveolar /alvē′ələr/ [L, *alveolus,* little hollow], pertaining to an alveolus.

alveolar adenocarcinoma [L, *alveolus,* little hollow], a neoplasm in which the tumor cells form alveoli.

alveolar air, the respiratory gases in an alveolus, or air sac, of the lung.

alveolar air equation, a method of calculating the approximate alveolar oxygen tension from the arterial partial pressure of carbon dioxide, the fractional inspired oxygen, and the ratio of carbon dioxide production to oxygen consumption.

alveolar-arterial end-capillary gas pressure difference, the gas pressure difference that exists between alveolar gas and pulmonary capillary blood as the latter leaves the alveolus. It is measured in torr units or mm Hg.

alveolar-arterial gas pressure difference, the difference between the measured or calculated mean partial pressure of a gas, such as CO_2, in the alveoli and the simultaneously measured partial pressure of that gas in systemic arterial blood. It is measured in torr units.

alveolar canal, any of the canals of the maxilla through which the posterior superior alveolar blood vessels and the nerves to the upper teeth pass.

alveolar-capillary membrane, a lung tissue structure, varying in thickness from 0.4 to 2 μm, through which diffusion of oxygen and carbon dioxide molecules occurs during the respiration process.

alveolar cell carcinoma, a malignant pulmonary neoplasm that arises in a bronchiole and spreads along alveolar surfaces. This form of lung cancer is often characterized by a severe cough and copious sputum.

alveolar cleft, a rare form of cleft palate in which the fusion failure extends forward to include the alveolar ridge.

alveolar cyst, an air-filled cavity in the lung or visceral tissues caused by rupture of an alveolar sac.

alveolar distending pressure, the pressure difference between the alveolus and the intrapleural space.

alveolar duct, any of the air passages in the lung that branch out from the respiratory bronchioles. From the ducts arise the alveolar sacs.

alveolar edema, an accumulation of fluid within the alveoli.

alveolar fiber, any one of the many white collagenous fibers of the periodontal ligament that extend from the alveolar bone to the intermediate plexus, where their terminations mix with those of the cemental fibers.

alveolar gas, the gas mixture within the gas-exchange regions of the lungs. It reflects the combined effects of alveolar ventilation and respiratory gas exchange or the expired gas that has come from the alveoli and gas-exchange regions.

alveolar gas volume, the aggregate volume of gas in the lung regions within which respiratory gas exchange occurs. It is indicated by the symbol V_A.

alveolar gingiva, gingiva that covers the alveolar bone and process in the maxilla and mandible. It is firmly attached to the bone.

alveolar macrophages, defense cells within the lungs that act by engulfing and digesting foreign substances inhaled into the alveoli.

alveolar microlithiasis, a disease characterized by the presence of calcium phosphate deposits in the alveolar sacs and ducts. It is familial in about half of cases.

alveolar periosteum [L, *alveolus,* little hollow; Gk, *peri,* near, *osteon,* bone], a dense layer of connective tissue that lines the alveolar cavities of the upper and lower jaws, joining the bones to the horizontal fibers on the cementum of the teeth.

alveolar pressure (P_A), the pressure in the alveoli of the lungs.

alveolar process, the part of the maxilla or mandible that forms the dental arch and serves as a bony investment for the teeth.

alveolar proteinosis, a disorder marked by the accumulation of plasma proteins, lipoproteins, and other blood components in the alveoli of the lungs.

alveolar ridge, the bony ridge of the maxilla or the mandible that contains the alveoli of the teeth.

alveolar sac [L, *alveolus,* little hollow; Gk, *sakkos*], an air sac at one of the terminal cavities of lung tissue.

alveolar socket [L, *alveolus,* little hollow; OFr, *soket*], a cavity in the alveolar bone of the maxilla and mandible that accommodates a tooth.

alveolar soft part sarcoma, a tumor in subcutaneous or fibromuscular tissue, consisting of numerous large round or polygonal cells in a netlike matrix of connective tissue.

alveolar ventilation, the volume of air that ventilates all the perfused alveoli, measured as minute volume in liters. The figure is also the difference between total ventilation and dead space ventilation. The normal average is between 4 and 5 liters per minute.

alveolectomy /al′vē-əlek′təmē/ [L, *alveolus* + Gk, *ektome,* excision], the excision of a part of the alveolar process for aiding the extraction of a tooth or teeth, the modification of the alveolar contour after tooth extraction, or the preparation of the mouth for dentures.

alveoli /alvē′əlī/, small outpouchings of walls of alveolar space through which gas exchange between alveolar air and pulmonary capillary blood takes place.

alveolitis /al′vē-əlī′tis/, an allergic pulmonary reaction to the inhalation of antigenic substances. It is characterized by acute episodes of dyspnea, cough, sweating, fever, weakness, and pain in the joints and muscles.

alveoloplasty /alvē′əlōplas′tē/, reconstruction by plastic surgery of an alveolus.

alveolotomy /al′vē-əlot′əmē/, incision of a dental alveolus performed to drain pus from a dental infection.

alveolus /alvē′ələs/, *pl.* **alveoli** [L, little hollow], a small saclike structure. The term is often used interchangeably with acinus. —**alveolar,** *adj.*

alymphocytosis /alim′fōsītō′sis/ [Gk, *a,* not; L, *lympha,* water; Gk, *kytos,* cell, *osis,* condition], a severe reduction in the total number of circulating lymphocytes in the blood.

Alzheimer's disease (AD) /ôl′zīmərz/ [Alois Alzheimer, German neurologist, 1864–1915], progressive mental deterioration characterized by confusion, memory failure, disorientation, restlessness, agnosia, speech disturbances, inability to carry out purposeful movement, and hallucinosis. The disease sometimes begins in middle life with slight defects in memory and behavior, but the symptoms worsen dramatically after the age of 70. Although it occurs with equal frequency in men and women, the familial risk is four times that of the general population.

Alzheimer's sclerosis [Alois Alzheimer; Gk, *sklerosis,* hardening], the degeneration of small cerebral blood vessels resulting in mental changes.

Am, symbol for the element **americium.**

ama, abbreviation for **against medical advice.**

AMA, abbreviation for **American Medical Association.**

amalgam /əmal′gəm/ [Gk, *malagma,* soft mass], **1.** a mixture or combination. **2.** an alloy of mercury and other metals.

amalgamate, an alloy, usually made with mercury and another metal, in which the proportions of the metal components may be varied according to the desired hardness of the amalgam.

amalgam carrier, (in dentistry) an instrument for carrying plastic amalgam for inserting into a prepared tooth cavity (cavity prep) or mold.

amalgam carver, a dental instrument for shaping plastic amalgam used in some tooth cavity fillings or restorations.

amalgam condenser, (in dentistry) an instrument used for compacting plastic amalgam in filling teeth.

amalgam core, a rigid base for the retention of a cast crown restoration, used in the replacement of a damaged tooth crown.

amalgam tattoo, a discoloration of the gingiva or buccal membrane caused by particles of silver amalgam filling material that becomes embedded under the tissue surface.

Amanita [Gk, *amanitai,* fungus], a genus of mushrooms. Some species, such as *Amanita phalloides,* are poisonous, causing hallucinations, gastrointestinal upset, and pain that may be followed by liver, kidney, and central nervous system damage.

amantadine hydrochloride /əman′tədēn/, an antiviral and antiparkinsonian agent prescribed in the prophylaxis and early treatment of influenza virus A_2 and in treatment of parkinsonism symptoms.

amastia /əmas′tē-ə/ [Gk, *a, mastos,* not breast], absence of the breasts in women caused by a congenital defect, an endocrine disorder resulting in faulty development, lack of development of secondary sex characteristics, or a bilateral mastectomy.

amaurosis /am′ôro′sis/ [Gk, *amaurosin,* to darken], blindness, especially lack of vision resulting from a systemic cause such as disease of the optic nerve or brain, diabetes, or renal disease or after acute gastritis or systemic poisoning produced by excessive use of alcohol or tobacco, rather than from damage to the eye itself. —**amaurotic,** *adj.*

amaurosis fugax /fōō′gaks/, transient episodic blindness.

amaurosis partialis fugax, transitory

partial blindness, usually caused by vascular insufficiency of the retina or optic nerve as a result of carotid artery disease.

amber [Ar, *anbar*], a hard fossilized resin derived from pine trees. An oil of amber, *Oleum succini*, has been used in some pharmaceutical preparations.

amber mutation [Ar, *anbar*, ambergris], (in molecular genetics) a genetic alteration in which a polypeptide chain terminates prematurely because an erroneous code signals the end of the chain.

ambidextrous /am'bēdek'strəs/ [L, *ambo*, both, *dexter*, right], able to use either the left or right hand to perform a task.

ambient /am'bē-ənt/ [L, *ambire*, on both sides], pertaining to the surrounding area or atmosphere.

ambient air standard, the maximum tolerable concentration of any air pollutant such as lead, nitrogen dioxide, sodium hydroxide, or sulfur dioxide.

ambient noise [L, *ambiens*, around; ME, *clamor*], the total noise in a given environment.

ambient pressure, the atmospheric pressure, or pressure in the environment or surrounding area. It is given a reference value of zero (0) cm H_2O.

ambient temperature [L, *ambi*, around, *temperatura*], the temperature of the environment.

ambiguous /ambig'yo͞o·əs/ [L, *ambiguus*, to wander], having more than one direction, development, or interpretation.

ambiguous genitalia [L, *ambigere*, to go around], external genitalia that are not normal and morphologically typical of either sex, as occurs in pseudohermaphroditism.

ambivalence /ambiv'ələns [L, *ambo*, both, *valentia*, strength], **1.** a state in which a person experiences conflicting feelings, attitudes, drives, desires, or emotions, such as tenderness and cruelty or pleasure and pain toward the same person, place, object, or situation. **2.** uncertainty and fluctuation caused by an inability to make a choice between opposites. **3.** a continuous oscillation or fluctuation. —**ambivalent,** *adj.*

ambivalent [L, *ambo*, both, *valentia*, strength], **1.** having equal power on both sides. **2.** (in psychology) having equally strong but opposing emotions, as love and hate for the same person.

ambivert /am'bivurt'/ [L, *ambo*, both, *vertere*, to turn], a person who possesses characteristics of both introversion and extroversion.

amblyopia /am'blē-ō'pē-ə/ [Gk, *amblys*, dull, *ops*, eye], reduced vision in an eye that is not corrected by a manifest refrac-

tion and does not appear to have an obvious pathologic or structural cause.

ambon [Gk, raised stage], a fibrocartilaginous ring that surrounds the cavity of a long bone socket.

ambulance /am'byələns/, an emergency vehicle usually used for the transport of patients to a medical facility in cases of trauma or sudden severe illness.

ambulatory /am'byələtôr'ē/ [L, *ambulare*, to walk about], able to walk, hence describing a patient who is not confined to bed or designating a health service for people who are not hospitalized.

ambulatory automatism, aimless wandering or moving about or performance of mechanical acts without conscious awareness of the behavior.

ambulatory blood pressure monitoring (ABPM), the act of recording a patient's blood pressure at regular intervals under normal living and working conditions.

ambulatory care, health services provided on an outpatient basis to those who visit a hospital or other health care facility and depart after treatment on the same day.

ambulatory schizophrenia, a mild form of psychosis, characterized mainly by a tendency to respond to questions with vague and irrelevant answers. The person also may seem somewhat eccentric and wander aimlessly.

ambulatory surgery center, a medical facility designed and equipped to handle surgery cases such as cataracts, herniorrhaphy, and meniscectomy that do not require overnight hospitalization.

AM care, routine hygienic care that is given patients before breakfast or early in the morning.

amcinonide /amsin'ōnīd/, a topical corticosteroid used to treat inflammatory skin conditions.

amdinocillin /am'dinōsil'in/, a penicillin derivative that is used as a parenteral antibiotic. It is prescribed for the treatment of urinary infections caused by susceptible strains of *Escherichia coli* and various species of *Klebsiella* and *Enterobacter*.

ameba /əmē'bə/ [Gk, *amoibe*, change], a microscopic, single-celled, parasitic organism. Several species may be parasitic in humans, including *Entamoeba coli* and *E. histolytica.*—**amebic,** *adj.*

amebiasis /am'ēbī'əsis/, an infection of the intestine or liver by species of pathogenic amebas, particularly *Entamoeba histolytica*, acquired by ingesting food or water contaminated with infected feces. Mild amebiasis may be asymptomatic; severe infection may cause profuse diarrhea, acute abdominal pain, jaundice, anorexia, and weight loss.

amebic abscess /əmē′bik/, a collection of pus formed by disintegrated tissue in a cavity, usually in the liver, caused by the protozoan parasite *Entamoeba histolytica.*

amebic carrier state, a condition in which a patient may be a carrier of amebic organisms without showing signs or symptoms of an amebic infection. A **precocious carrier** may appear healthy but may subsequently develop the amebic infection.

amebic dysentery, an inflammation of the intestine caused by infestation with *Entamoeba histolytica.* It is characterized by frequent, loose stools flecked with blood and mucus.

amebic hepatitis, an inflammation of the liver caused by an amebic infection, usually after an attack of amebic dysentery.

amebicide /əmē′bəsīd/, a drug or other agent that is destructive to amebae.

ameboid movement /əmē′boid/ [Gk, *amoibe,* ameba, *eidos,* form; L, *movere,* to move], the ameba-like movement of certain types of body cells that can migrate through tissues. The movement generally consists of extension of a part of the cell membrane.

amelanotic /am′ilənot′ik/ [Gk, *a, melas,* not black], pertaining to tissue that is unpigmented because it lacks melanin.

amelanotic melanoma /am′ilənot′/, a melanoma that lacks melanin.

amelia /əmē′lyə/ [Gk, *a, melos,* not limb], **1.** a birth defect marked by the absence of one or more limbs. The term may be modified to indicate the number of legs or arms missing at birth, such as **tetramelia** for the absence of all four limbs. **2.** a psychologic trait of apathy or indifference associated with certain forms of psychosis.

amelification /əmel′ifikā′shən/ [OFr, *amel,* enamel; L, *facere,* to make], the differentiation of ameloblasts, or enamel cells, into the enamel of the teeth.

amelioration [L, *ad,* to, *melior,* better], an improvement in conditions.

ameloblast /am′ilōblast′/ [OFr, *amel* + Gk, *blastos,* germ], an epithelial cell from which tooth enamel is formed, **ameloblastic** /-blas′tik/, *adj.*

ameloblastic fibroma, an odontogenic neoplasm in which simultaneous proliferation of mesenchymal and epithelial tissues occurs without the formation of dentin or enamel.

ameloblastic hemangioma, a highly vascular tumor of cells covering the dental papilla.

ameloblastic odontoma, an odontogenic tumor characterized by an ameloblastoma within an odontoma.

ameloblastic sarcoma, a malignant odontogenic tumor, characterized by the proliferation of epithelial and mesenchymal tissue without the formation of dentin or enamel.

ameloblastoma /am′əlōblastō′mə/ [OFr, *amel* + Gk, *blastos,* germ, *oma*], a highly destructive, malignant, rapidly growing tumor of the jaw.

amelodentinal /am′əlōden′tinəl/ [OFr, *amel* + L, *dens,* tooth], pertaining to both the enamel and the dentin of the teeth.

amelogenesis /am′əlōjen′əsis/ [OFr, *amel* + Gk, *genein,* to produce], the formation of the enamel of the teeth. —**amelogenic,** *adj.*

amelogenesis imperfecta, a hereditary dental defect characterized by a brown coloration of the teeth and resulting from either severe hypocalcification or hypoplasia of the enamel.

amenorrhea /ā′menərē′ə/ [Gk, *a, men,* not month, *rhoia,* to flow], the absence of menstruation. Amenorrhea is normal before sexual maturity, during pregnancy, after menopause, and during the intermenstrual phase of the monthly hormonal cycle; it is otherwise caused by dysfunction of the hypothalamus, pituitary gland, ovary, or uterus; by the congenital absence or surgical removal of both ovaries or the uterus; or by medication. Primary amenorrhea is the failure of menstrual cycles to begin. Secondary amenorrhea is the cessation of menstrual cycles once established. —**amenorrheic,** *adj.*

American Academy of Allergy and Immunology (AAAI), a national organization of physicians specializing in the diagnosis and treatment of allergies and immune system disorders.

American Academy of Nursing (AAN), the honorary organization of the American Nurses Association, created to recognize superior achievement in nursing in order to promote advances and excellence in nursing practice and education. A person elected to membership is given the title of Fellow of the American Academy of Nursing and may use the abbreviation FAAN as an honorific.

American Academy of Physical Medicine and Rehabilitation (AAPMR), a national association of professional health care workers concerned with the diagnosis of physical impairment and the development of therapies and devices to improve physical function.

American Academy of Physicians' Assistants (AAPA), a national organization of physicians' assistants or associates.

American Association for Respiratory Therapy (AART), a national organization of nurses and other health workers in the field of respiratory therapy.

American Association of Colleges of Nursing (AACN), a national organization of baccalaureate and higher degree programs in nursing that was established to address issues in nursing education.

American Association of Critical Care Nurses (AACN), a national organization of nurses working in critical care units.

American Association of Industrial Nurses (AAIN), a national professional association of nurses working in industry and concerned with issues in occupational health.

American Association of Medical Colleges (AAMC), a national organization of faculty members and deans of medical schools and colleges that was established to address issues in medical education.

American Association of Nephrology Nurses and Technicians (AANNT), an organization of nurses and technicians working in the fields of dialysis and renal diseases.

American Association of Neurological Nurses (AANN), a national organization of nurses working in the field of neurology.

American Association of Neuroscience Nurses (AANN), a national organization of nurses working with neurologically impaired patients. The organization is affiliated with the American Association of Neurological Surgeons.

American Association of Nurse Anesthetists (AANA), a professional association of certified registered nurse anesthetists.

American Association of Pathologists and Bacteriologists (AAPB), a national professional organization of specialists in pathology and bacteriology.

American Association of Retired Persons (AARP), a voluntary U.S. organization of older persons, who may or may not be retired, with the goal of improving the welfare of persons over 50 years of age. The AARP advises members of Congress and state legislatures about legislation affecting older individuals.

American Association of University Professors (AAUP), a national organization of faculty members of institutions of higher learning.

American College of Emergency Physicians (ACEP), a national professional organization of physicians specializing in emergency medicine.

American College of Obstetricians and Gynecologists (ACOG), the national organization of obstetricians and gynecologists.

American College of Physicians (ACP), a national professional organization of physicians.

American College of Prosthodontists, an organization of dentists who specialize in restoration of dental or oral structures such as dentures, crowns, and bridges and in diagnosis and treatment of temporomandibular joint and maxillofacial disorders.

American College of Radiology (ACR), a national professional organization of physicians who specialize in radiology.

American College of Surgeons (ACS), a national professional organization of physicians who specialize in surgery.

American Dental Hygienists' Association (ADHA), a national organization of dental hygienists whose purpose is to promote and sustain the art and science of dental hygiene.

American Hospital Association (AHA), a national organization of individuals, institutions, and organizations that works to improve health services for all people.

American Journal of Nursing, the professional journal of the American Nurses Association (ANA). It contains articles of general and specialized clinical interest to nurses and is an important resource regarding the profession in the United States.

American leishmaniasis, a group of mucocutaneous infections caused by various species of *Leishmania,* characterized by disfiguring ulcerative lesions of the nose, mouth, and throat. These infections are most prevalent in forested areas of southern Mexico and in Central and South America.

American Medical Association (AMA), a professional association whose membership is made up of approximately half of the total licensed physicians in the United States, including practitioners in all recognized medical specialties, as well as general primary care physicians. The AMA maintains directories of all qualified physicians (including nonmembers) in the United States, including graduates of foreign medical colleges; evaluates prescription and nonprescription drugs; advises congressional and state legislators regarding proposed health care laws; and publishes a variety of journals.

American National Standards Institute (ANSI), a private nonprofit organization that coordinates voluntary development of standards for medical and other devices in the United States and represents the United States in matters related to international standardization.

American Nurses Association (ANA), the national professional association of registered nurses in the United States. It was founded in 1896 to improve standards of health and the availability of health care given in order to foster high standards for nursing, to promote the professional development of nurses, and to advance the economic and general welfare of nurses. The ANA is made up of 53 constituent associations from the 50 states, the District of Columbia, Guam, and the Virgin Islands, representing more than 900 district associations. ANA publications include *American Nurse, Publications List,* and *The American Journal of Nursing.*

American Nurses Association–Political Action Committee (ANA-PAC), an organization that raises funds for political contributions to candidates for public office at the state and national levels.

American Psychiatric Association (APA), a national professional association for physicians who specialize in psychiatry. It is concerned with the development of standards for psychiatric facilities, the formulation of mental health programs, the dissemination of data, and the promotion of psychiatric education and research. It publishes the *Diagnostic and Statistical Manual of Mental Disorders (DSM).*

American Red Cross, one of more than 120 national organizations that seek to reduce human suffering through various health, safety, and disaster relief programs in affiliation with the International Committee of the Red Cross. The committee and all Red Cross organizations evolved from the Geneva Convention of 1864, following the example and urging of Swiss humanitarian Jean Henri Dunant, who aided wounded French and Austrian soldiers at the Battle of Solferino in 1859. The American Red Cross blood program collects and distributes more blood than any other single U.S. agency and coordinates distribution of blood and blood products to the U.S. Defense Department on request or during national emergencies. The organization annually collects about 4 million blood donations and gives blood to more than 4000 hospitals. American Red Cross nursing and health programs include courses in the home on parenthood, prenatal and postnatal care, hygiene, and venereal disease. Nursing students are enrolled for service in American Red Cross community programs and during disasters. The symbol of the American Red Cross, like that of most other Red Cross societies throughout the world, is a red cross on a field of white; in Switzerland it is a white cross on a red field, in Muslim countries a red crescent, and in Israel a red star of David.

American Registry of Radiologic Technologists (ARRT), a national certifying body for radiologic technologists in the disciplines of radiography, nuclear medicine, radiation therapy, mammography, computed tomography, magnetic resonance imaging, and cardiovascular-interventional technology.

American Sign Language (Ameslan, ASL), a method of manual communication used by some deaf persons. Messages are conveyed by manipulation of the hands and fingers. ASL is a distinct language, with its own grammar and syntax.

American Society of Parenteral and Enteral Nutrition, an organization that provides education, support, and accreditation to persons who specialize in nutrition that is provided through intravenous, enteral, or related types of feeding.

American Speech, Language, and Hearing Association (ASHA), the professional association that certifies audiologists and speech-language pathologists.

Americans With Disabilities Act, legislation approved by the U.S. Congress in July 1990 that would bar discrimination against persons with physical or mental disabilities. The Act defines disability as a condition that "substantially limits" such activities as walking or seeing, and it applies to persons with acquired immunodeficiency syndrome, as well as to alcoholics and drug users undergoing treatment.

American Type Culture Collection (ATCC), a U.S. nonprofit, nongovernmental organization that is concerned with the preservation of specimens of cellular and microbiologic cultures and with the distribution of the cultures to research centers and laboratories in the academic, scientific, and medical communities.

americium (Am) /am′ərish′ē-əm/, a synthetic radioactive element of the actinide group. Its atomic number is 95; its atomic weight (mass) is 243.

Ameslan /am′islan/, abbreviation for American Sign Language.

Ames test /āmz/, a method of testing substances for possible carcinogenicity by exposing a strain of *Salmonella* bacteria to a sample of the substance.

ametropia /am′itrō′pē-ə/ [Gk, *ametros,* irregular, *opsis,* sight], a condition characterized by an optic defect involving an error of refraction such as astigmatism, hyperopia, or myopia. **—ametropic,** *adj.*

AMI, abbreviation for **acute myocardial infarction.**

amicrobic /am′īkrob′ik/, not caused by or related to microbes.

amide, 1. a chemical compound formed from an organic acid by the substitution of an amino (NR$_2$) group for the hydroxyl of a carboxyl (COOH) group. **2.** a chemical compound formed by the deprotonation of an amine, HNR$_2$.

amide local anesthetic, any of more than two dozen compounds that are safe, versatile, and effective local anesthetics. If hypersensitivity to a drug in this group precludes its use, one of the ester-compound local anesthetics may provide analgesia without adverse effect.

amikacin sulfate /am'ikā'sin/, an aminoglycoside antibiotic prescribed in the treatment of various severe infections that are resistant to other antibiotics.

amiloride hydrochloride /am'ilôr'id/, a potassium-sparing diuretic and antihypertensive agent prescribed as adjunctive therapy in the treatment of congestive heart failure or hypertension. It is often given with a thiazide medication.

amine /am'in, əmēn'/ [L, *ammonia*], (in chemistry) a type of organic compound that contains nitrogen.

amine pump, *informal.* an active transport system in the presynaptic nerve endings that takes up released amine neurotransmitters.

amino acid /əmē'nō/, an organic chemical compound composed of one or more basic amino groups and one or more acidic carboxyl groups. Twenty of the more than 100 amino acids that occur in nature are the building blocks of peptide linkages that form polypeptides or proteins. The eight essential amino acids are isoleucine (Ile), leucine (Leu), lysine (Lys), methionine (Met), phenylalanine (Phe), threonine (Thr), tryptophan (Trp), and valine (Val). Arginine (Arg) and histidine (His) are essential in infants. Cysteine (Cys) and tyrosine (Tyr) are quasiessential because they may be synthesized from methionine (Met) and phenylalanine (Phe), respectively. The main nonessential amino acids are alanine (Ala), asparagine (Asn), aspartic acid (Asp), glutamine (Glm), glutamic acid (Glu), glycine (Gly), proline (Pro), and serine (Ser).

amino acid group, a category of organic chemicals containing the monovalent amine radical NH$_2$, an acid or COOH, and a group idiosyncratic to that particular amino acid group.

aminoaciduria /ame'nō·as'idōōr'ē·ə/, the abnormal presence of amino acids in the urine that usually indicates an inborn metabolic defect, as in cystinuria.

aminobenzoic acid /-benzō'ik/, a metabolic product of the catabolism of the amino acid tryptophan.

aminocaproic acid /əmē'nōkəprō'ik, am'inō-/, a hemostatic prescribed to stop excessive bleeding that results from hyperfibrinolysis.

aminolevulinic acid (ALA) /am'inōlev'ōōlin'ik/, the aliphatic precursor of heme. It may be detected in the urine of some patients with porphyria, liver disease, and lead poisoning.

aminophylline /am'ənōfil'in, əmē'nō-/, a bronchodilator prescribed in the treatment of bronchial asthma, emphysema, and bronchitis.

aminophylline poisoning, an adverse reaction to an excessive intake of a methylxanthine drug such as caffeine or theophylline. Symptoms may include nausea, diarrhea, vomiting, abdominal pain, and gastrointestinal bleeding; headache, tinnitus, thirst, delirium, and seizures; and tachycardia and blood pressure changes.

aminopyrine /-pī'rin/, a white chemical compound with analgesic and antipyretic effects. Its continued or excessive use may lead to agranulocytosis.

aminotransferase /-trans'fərās/, an enzyme that catalyzes the transfer of an amino group from an alpha-amino acid to an alpha-keto acid, with pyridoxal phosphate and pyridoxamine phosphate acting as coenzymes. Aspartate amino transferase (AST), normally present in serum and various tissues, is released by damaged cells. A high serum level of AST may be diagnostic in myocardial infarction or hepatic disease. Alanine aminotransferase (ALT), a normal constituent of serum and various tissues, is released by injured tissue and may be present in high concentrations in the sera of patients with acute liver disease.

amiodarone hydrochloride, an oral antiarrhythmic drug prescribed for the treatment of life-threatening recurrent ventricular fibrillation and recurrent, hemodynamically unstable ventricular tachycardia refractory to other drugs.

amitosis /am'ətō'sis/ [Gr, *a, mitos,* not thread], direct cell division in which there is simple fission of the nucleus and cytoplasm (e.g., bacterial fission). It does not involve the complex stages of chromatin separation of the chromosomes that occur in mitosis. —**amitotic,** *adj.*

amitriptyline /am'itrip'tilin/, a tricyclic antidepressant prescribed in the treatment of depression.

AML, abbreviation for **acute myelocytic leukemia.**

ammonia /amō'nē·ə/ [Gk, *ammoniakos,* salt of Ammon, Egyptian god], a colorless pungent gas consisting of nitrogen and hydrogen, produced by the decomposition of nitrogenous organic matter. Some of its many uses are as an aromatic stimulant, a detergent, and an emulsifier.

ammoniacal fermentation /am'ənī'əkəl/, the production of ammonia and carbon dioxide from urea by the enzyme urease.

ammonia intoxication, an adverse reaction to ammonia, which is formed as a product of amino acid and nucleic acid catabolism. Ammonia is converted to urea in the liver and excreted by the kidneys. In liver diseases such as cirrhosis, ammonia may accumulate in the blood, resulting in neurologic damage.

ammonium ion, an NH_4^+ ion formed by the reaction of ammonia (NH_3) with a hydrogen ion (H^+).

ammonuria /am'ōnoŏr'ē-ə/, urine that contains an excessive amount of ammonia.

amnesia /amnē'zhə/ [Gk, a, mnasthai, to forget], a loss of memory caused by brain damage or by severe emotional trauma. Kinds of amnesia include **anterograde amnesia, posttraumatic amnesia,** and **retrograde amnesia.**

amnesiac /amnē'sē-ək/, a person with a loss of memory caused by brain damage or severe emotional trauma.

amnesic /amnē'sik/ [Gk, a, mnasthai, to forget], in a state of forgetfulness or showing signs of memory loss or impairment.

amnesic aphasia [Gk, a, mnasthai + a, phasis, without speech], an inability to remember spoken words or to use words for names of objects, circumstances, or characteristics.

amnestic apraxia /amnes'tik/, the inability to carry out a movement in response to a request because of a lack of ability to remember the request.

amniocentesis /am'nē-ōsentē'sis/ [Gk, amnos, lamb's caul, kentesis, pricking], an obstetric procedure in which a small amount of amniotic fluid is removed for laboratory analysis. It is usually performed between the sixteenth and twentieth weeks of gestation to aid in the diagnosis of fetal abnormalities.

amniography /am'nē og'rəfē/, a procedure used to detect placement of the placenta by x-ray examination.

Amnioinfusion, a Nursing Interventions Classification defined as infusion of fluid into the uterus during labor to relieve umbilical cord compression or to dilute meconium-stained fluid.

amnion /am'nē-on/ [Gk, amnos, lamb's caul], a membrane, continuous with and covering the fetal side of the placenta, that forms the outer surface of the umbilical cord.

amnionitis /am'nē-ōnī'tis/, an inflamma-

tion of the amnion. The condition may develop after early rupture of the fetal membranes.

amnioscopy /am'nē-os'kəpē/, direct visual examination of the fetus and amniotic fluid with an endoscope that is inserted into the amniotic cavity through the uterine cervix or an incision in the abdominal wall.

amniotic /am'nē-ot'ik/, pertaining to the amnion.

amniotic band disruption sequence syndrome, an abnormal condition of fetal development characterized by the development of fibrous bands within the uterus that entangle the fetus, leading to deformities in structure and function.

amniotic cavity [Gk, amnion, fetal membrane; L, cavum], the fluid-filled cavity of the amniotic sac surrounding the fetus.

amniotic fluid, a liquid produced by the fetal membranes and the fetus. It surrounds the fetus throughout pregnancy, protecting it from trauma and temperature variations, providing freedom of fetal movements, and helping to maintain the fetal oxygen supply. The volume totals about 1000 ml at term. In addition to providing the fetus with physical protection, the amniotic fluid is a medium of active chemical exchange. Amniotic fluid itself is clear, although desquamated fetal cells and lipids give it a cloudy appearance.

amniotic fluid embolism [Gk, amnion; L, fluere, to flow; Gk, embolos, plug], a quantity of amniotic fluid that enters the maternal blood system during labor and/or delivery and becomes lodged in a vessel. It is usually fatal to the mother if it is a pulmonary embolism.

amniotic fold, an embryonic growth feature observed in many vertebrates, particularly birds and reptiles. It consists of flaps of ectoderm and mesoderm that grow over the back of an embryo to form the amnion.

amniotic sac, a thin-walled bag that contains the fetus and amniotic fluid during pregnancy. It has a capacity of 4 to 5 L at term. The wall of the sac extends from the margin of the placenta. The amnion, chorion, and decidua that make up the wall are each a few cell layers thick. The intact sac and its fluid provide for the equilibration of hydrostatic pressure within the uterus. During labor the sac effects the uniform transmission of the force of uterine contractions to the cervix for dilation.

amniotomy /am'nē-ot'əmē/, the artificial rupture of the fetal membranes (ARM). It is usually performed to stimulate or accelerate the onset of labor. The procedure is painless.

amobarbital /am'ōbär'bətal/, a barbiturate sedative-hypnotic prescribed for the relief of anxiety and insomnia and as an anticonvulsant.

A-mode, the amplitude modulation display in diagnostic ultrasonography. It represents the time required for the ultrasound beam to strike a tissue interface and return its signal to the transducer.

A-mode ultrasound [L, *ultra,* beyond, *sonus,* sound], a display of ultrasonic echoes in which the horizontal axis of the cathode ray tube display represents the time required for the return of the echo and the vertical oscilloscope trace represents the strength of the echo. The mode is used in echoencephalography.

amok [Malay, *amoq,* furious], a psychotic frenzy with a desire to kill anybody encountered. The murderous episodes may follow periods of severe depression.

amorph /ā'môrf, əmôrf'/ [Gk, *a, morphef,* not shape], **1.** inactive gene; a mutant allele that has little or no effect on the expression of a trait. **2.** abbreviation for *amorphous,* such as amorph IZS (amorphous insulin zinc suspension).

amorphic, (in genetics) pertaining to a gene that is inactive or nearly inactive so that it has no determinable effect.

amorphous [Gk, *a,* not, *morphe,* form], **1.** describing an object that lacks definite visible shape or form. **2.** (in chemistry) a substance that is not crystalline.

amorphous crystals /əmôr'fəs/, shapeless, ill-defined crystals, usually phosphates.

amoxapine /əmok'sepin/, an antidepressant similar to the tricyclics. It is prescribed in the treatment of mental depression.

amoxicillin /əmok'səsil'in/, a beta-lactam semisynthetic oral penicillin antibiotic similar to ampicillin. It is prescribed in the treatment of infections caused by a susceptible gram-negative or gram-positive organism.

AMP, abbreviation for **adenosine monophosphate.**

ampere (A) /am'pēr/ [André M. Ampere, French physicist, 1775–1836], a unit of measurement of the amount of electric current. An ampere, according to the meter-kilogram-second (MKS) system, is the amount of current passed through a resistance of 1 ohm by an electric potential of 1 volt.

amperometry /am'parom'ətrē/, the measurement of current at a single applied potential.

amphetamine poisoning, toxic effects of overdosage of amphetamines. Symptoms usually include excitement, tremors,

tachycardia, hallucinations, delirium, convulsions, and circulatory collapse. Emergency first aid requires gastric lavage with tap water or induced emesis.

amphetamines /amfet'əmēnz/, a group of nervous system stimulants, including amphetamine and its chemical congeners dextroamphetamine and methamphetamine, that are subject to abuse because of their ability to produce wakefulness and euphoria. Abuse leads to compulsive behavior, paranoia, hallucinations, and suicidal tendencies.

amphetamine sulfate, a colorless watersoluble salt of amphetamine that stimulates the central nervous system. It has been used to treat certain respiratory complaints, to reduce fatigue, and to treat narcolepsy. It formerly was used to treat obesity.

amphidiarthrodial joint /am'fēdī'ärthrō'dē·əl/ [Gk, *amphi,* both kinds], a type of joint that combines amphiarthrosis with diarthrosis, permitting movement in more than one direction, such as that of the lower jaw.

amphigenetic /am'fijənet'ik/ [Gk, *amphi,* both sides, *genein,* to produce], **1.** produced by the union of gametes from both sexes. **2.** bisexual; having both testicular and ovarian tissue.

amphigenous inheritance /amfij'ənəs/, the acquisition of genetic traits and conditions from both parents.

amphigonadism /am'figō'nədiz'əm/, true hermaphroditism; presence of both testicular and ovarian tissue. —**amphigonadic,** *adj.*

amphigony /amfig'ənē/ [Gk, *amphi + gonos,* generation], sexual reproduction. —**amphigonic** /am'figon'ik/, *adj.*

amphikaryon /am'fiker'ē·on/ [Gk, *amphi + karyon,* nucleus], a nucleus containing the diploid number of chromosomes. —**amphikaryotic,** *adj.*

amphimixis /am'fimik'sis/ [Gk, *amphi + mixis,* mingling], **1.** the union of germ cells in reproduction so that both maternal and paternal hereditary characteristics are derived; interbreeding. **2.** (in psychoanalysis) the union and integration of oral, anal, and genital libidinal impulses in the development of heterosexuality.

amphipathic /-path'ik/ [Gk, *amphi + pathos* suffering], pertaining to a molecule having two sides with characteristically different properties, such as a detergent, which has both a polar (hydrophilic) end and a nonpolar (hydrophobic) end but is long enough so that each end demonstrates its own solubility characteristics.

amphoric breath sound /amfôr'ik/ [Gk, *amphoreus,* jug], an abnormal, resonant, hollow blowing sound heard with a stethoscope. It indicates a cavity opening into the bronchus or a pneumothorax.

amphoteric /am'fōter'ik/ [Gk, *amphoteros,* pertaining to both], a substance that can have a positive, zero, or negative charge, depending on conditions.

amphotericin B /am'fəter'əsin/, an antifungal medication prescribed for topical or systemic use in the treatment of fungal infections.

amphotericin methyl ester (AME), an antiviral drug used in experimental treatment of human deficiency virus infections.

amphoterism /-ter'izəm/ [Gk, *amphoteros,* both], a quality of a chemical compound that permits it to act as an acid or a base.

ampicillin /am'pəsil'in/, a semisynthetic aminopenicillin prescribed in the treatment of infections caused by a broad spectrum of sensitive gram-negative and gram-positive organisms.

ampicillin sodium, the sodium salt of ampicillin, prescribed as an antibiotic to treat gram-positive organisms and some gram-negative organisms.

amplification /am'plifikā'shən/ [L, *amplificare,* to make wider], **1.** (in molecular genetics) a process in which the amount of plasmid deoxyribonucleic acid (DNA) is increased in proportion to the amount of bacterial DNA by treatment with certain substances, including chloramphenicol. **2.** the replication in bulk of an entire gene library. **—amplify,** *v.*

amplifier, a device that controls power from a mechanical, electrical, hydraulic, or other source so that the output is greater than the input.

amplitude /am'plityōōd/ [L, *amplus,* wide], width or breadth of range or extent, such as amplitude of accommodation or amplitude of convergence.

amplitude of accommodation (AA), the total accommodative power of the eye, determined by the difference between the refractive power for farthest vision and that for nearest vision.

amplitude of convergence, the difference in the power needed to turn the eyes from their far point to their near point of convergence.

ampule /am'pyōōl/ [Fr, *ampoule,* phial], a small, sterile glass or plastic container that usually contains a single dose of a solution.

ampulla /ampōōl'ə/ [L, flasklike bottle], a rounded, saclike dilation of a duct, canal, or any tubular structure, such as the lacrimal duct, semicircular canal, uterine tube, rectum, or vas deferens.

ampulla of rectum, a flask-shaped dilation near the end of the rectum.

ampullary tubal pregnancy /ampōō'lərē/, am'pəler'ē/, a kind of tubal pregnancy in which implantation occurs in the ampulla of one of the fallopian tubes.

ampullula /ampōōl'yələ/, a spheric dilation of a minute lymph or blood vessel or duct.

amputation /am'pyōōtā'shən/ [L, *amputare,* to excise], the surgical removal of a part of the body or a limb or part of a limb. It is performed to treat recurrent infections or gangrene in peripheral vascular disease, to remove malignant tumors, and to treat severe trauma. With the patient under anesthesia, the part is removed, and a shaped flap is cut from muscular and cutaneous tissue to cover the end of the bone. A section may be left open for drainage if infection is present.

Amputation Care, a Nursing Interventions Classification defined as promotion of physical and psychologic healing after amputation of a body part.

amputation flap, a flap of skin used to cover the end of an amputation stump.

amputation neuroma, a form of traumatic neuroma that may develop near the stump after the amputation of an extremity.

amputation-stump bandage, an elastic figure-of-eight bandage applied to cover the stump after an amputation.

amputee /am'pyətē'/, a person who has had one or more extremities traumatically or surgically removed.

AMRA, abbreviation for *American Medical Records Association.*

amrinone lactate /am'rinōn/, an intravenous cardiac inotropic drug prescribed in the short-term management of congestive heart failure in patients who do not respond to therapy with digitalis, diuretics, and vasodilators.

Amsler grid [Marc Amsler, Swiss ophthalmologist, 1891–1968], a checkerboard grid of intersecting dark horizontal and vertical lines with one dark spot in the middle. To discover a visual field defect, the person simply covers or closes one eye and looks at the spot with the other.

AMT, abbreviation for *American Medical Technologists.*

amu, abbreviation for **atomic mass unit.**

amusia /əmyōō'sē·ə/, a loss of the ability to recognize melodies.

amyelia /am'ī·ēl'yə/ [Gk, *myelos,* marrow], the absence of a spinal cord.

amyelinic neuroma /amī'əlin'ik/ [Gk, *a, myelos,* without marrow, *neuron,* nerve, *oma*], a tumor that contains only nonmyelinated nerve fibers.

amygdala /amig'dələ/ [Gk, *amygdale,* almond], an almond-shaped mass of gray matter in the front part of the temporal lobe of the brain.

amygdalin /əmig′dəlin/ [Gk, *amygdale,* almond], a naturally occurring cyanogenic glycoside obtained from bitter almonds and apricot pits. It has been promoted as a potential cancer remedy under the trademark of Laetrile.

amygdaloid /-dəloid/, resembling a tonsil.

amygdaloid fossa [Gk, *amylon, eidos,* starchlike; L, *fossa,* ditch], a space in the wall of the oropharynx, between the pillars of the fauces, that is occupied by the palatine tonsil.

amygdaloid nucleus [Gk, *amygdale,* almond, *eidos,* form; L, *nucleus,* nut], one of the basal nuclei, found in the inferior horn of the lateral ventricle.

amyl alcohol /am′il/ [Gk, *amylon,* starch], a colorless, oily liquid that is only slightly soluble in water but can be mixed with ethyl alcohol, chloroform, or ether.

amylase /am′ilās/ [Gk, *amylon,* starch], an enzyme that catalyzes the hydrolysis of starch into smaller carbohydrate molecules. Alpha-amylase, found in saliva, pancreatic juice, malt, certain bacteria, and molds, catalyzes the hydrolysis of starches to dextrins, maltose, and maltotriose. Beta-amylase, found in grains, vegetables, and malt, is involved in the hydrolysis of starch to maltose.

amylene hydrate /am′əlēn/, a clear, colorless liquid with a camphorlike odor, miscible with alcohol, chloroform, ether, or glycerin and used as a solvent and a hypnotic.

amylic fermentation /əmil′ik/, the formation of amyl alcohol from sugar.

amyl nitrite, a vasodilator prescribed to relieve the vasospasm of angina pectoris and cyanide poisoning.

amyloid /am′iloid/ [Gk, *amylon,* starch, *eidos,* form], **1.** pertaining to or resembling starch. **2.** a starchlike protein-carbohydrate complex that is deposited abnormally in some tissues during certain chronic disease states such as amyloidosis, rheumatoid arthritis, tuberculosis, and Alzheimer's disease.

amyloid liver [Gk, *amylon,* starch, *eidos,* form; AS, *lifer*], liver in which the cells have been infiltrated with amyloid deposits.

amyloidosis /am′iloidō′sis/ [Gk, *amylon* + *eidos,* form, *osis,* condition], a disease in which a waxy, starchlike glycoprotein (amyloid) accumulates in tissues and organs, impairing their function. There are two major forms of the condition. Primary amyloidosis usually occurs with multiple myeloma. Patients with second-

ary amyloidosis usually suffer from another chronic infectious or inflammatory disease such as tuberculosis, osteomyelitis, rheumatoid arthritis, or Crohn's disease. The cause of both types of amyloidosis is unknown. Almost all organs are affected, most often the heart, lungs, tongue, and intestines in primary amyloidosis and the kidneys, liver, and spleen in the secondary type.

amylolysis /am′ēlol′isis/, [Gk, *amylon,* starch, *lysis,* loosening], the digestive process whereby starch is converted into sugars and dextrins by hydrolysis or enzymatic activity.

amyotonia /ā′mī·ōtō′nē·ə/ [Gk, *a, mys,* not muscle, *tonos,* tone], an abnormal condition of skeletal muscle, characterized by a lack of tone, weakness, and wasting, usually the result of motor neuron disease. **—amyotonic,** *adj.*

amyotrophic lateral sclerosis (ALS) /ā′mī·ōtrof′ik/ [Gk, *a, mys* + *trophe,* nourishment], a degenerative disease of the motor neurons, characterized by weakness and atrophy of the muscles of the hands, forearms, and legs, spreading to involve most of the body and face. It results from degeneration of the motor neurons, beginning in middle age and progressing rapidly, causing death within 2 to 5 years.

ana (āa,āā,A̅A̅), (in prescriptions) 'so much of each,' indication of the amount of each ingredient to be compounded; usually written as an abbreviation.

ANA, 1. abbreviation for **American Nurses Association. 2.** abbreviation for **antinuclear antibody.**

anabolic steroid /an′əbol′ik/ [Gk, *anaballein,* to build up], any one of several compounds derived from testosterone or prepared synthetically to promote general body growth, to oppose the effects of endogenous estrogen, or to promote masculinizing effects. All such compounds cause a mixed androgenic-anabolic effect. Anabolic steroids are prescribed in the treatment of aplastic anemia, red-cell aplasia, and hemolytic anemia and in anemias associated with renal failure, myeloid metaplasia, and leukemia.

anabolism /ənab′əliz′əm/ [Gk, *anaballein,* to build up], constructive metabolism characterized by the conversion of simple substances into the more complex compounds of living matter. **—anabolic** /an′-əbol′ik/, *adj.*

anabolite /ənab′ōlīt/ [Gk, *anaballein,* to build up], a product of the process of anabolism.

anacatadidymus /an′əkat′ədid′iməs/ [Gk, *ana,* up, *kata,* down, *didymos,* twin], conjoined twins that are fused in the middle but separated above and below.

anaclisis /an′əklī′sis/ [Gk, *ana* + *klisis,* leaning], **1.** a condition, normal in childhood but pathologic in adulthood, in which a person is emotionally dependent on other people. **2.** a condition in which a person consciously or unconsciously chooses a love object because of a resemblance to the mother, father, or other person who was an important source of comfort and protection in infancy. —**anaclitic** /an′əklit′ik/, *adj.*

anaclitic depression /an′əklit′ik/, a syndrome occurring in infants, usually after sudden separation from the mothering person. Symptoms include apprehension, withdrawal, detachment, incessant crying, refusal to eat, sleep disturbances, and eventually stupor leading to severe impairment of the infant's physical, social, and intellectual development.

anacrotic /an′əkrot′ik/, pertaining to anacrotism, or a pulse with more than one expansion of the artery and observed as a double heartbeat.

anacrotic pulse [Gk, *ana* + *krotos,* stroke], (on a sphygmographic tracing) a pulse characterized by a transient drop in amplitude on the curve of the primary elevation, a notch. It is seen in valvular aortic stenosis.

anacrotism /ənak′rətiz′əm/ [Gk, *ana, krotos,* stroke], a condition characterized by two arterial expansions per heartbeat and observed as a notch on the ascending limb of an arterial pulse pressure tracing.

anacusis /an′əkoo̅′sis/ [Gk, *a, akouein,* not to hear], a total loss of hearing.

anadicrotic pulse /an′ədīkrot′ik/ [Gk, *ana* + *dis,* twice, *krotos,* stroke], (on a sphygmographic tracing) a pulse characterized by two transient drops in amplitude on the curve of primary elevation.

anadidymus /an′ədid′iməs/ [Gk, *ana* + *didymos,* twin], conjoined twins that are united at the pelvis and lower extremities but separated in the upper half.

anadipsia /an′ədip′sē·ə/ [Gk, *ana* + *dipsa,* thirst], extreme thirst, often occurring in the manic phase of bipolar mood disorder. The condition is the result of dehydration caused by the excessive perspiration, continuous urination, and relentless physical activity produced by the intense excitement characteristic of the manic phase.

anaerobe /aner′ōb/ [Gk, *a* + *aer,* not air, *bios,* life], a microorganism that grows and lives in the complete or almost complete absence of oxygen. An example is *Clostridium botulinum.* Anaerobes are widely distributed in nature and in the body.

anaerobic /an′ərō′bik/, **1.** pertaining to the absence of air or oxygen. **2.** able to grow and function without air or oxygen.

anaerobic catabolism, the breakdown of complex chemical substances into simpler compounds, with the release of energy, in the absence of oxygen.

anaerobic exercise, muscular exertion sufficient to result in metabolic acidosis because of accumulation of lactic acid as a product of muscle metabolism.

anaerobic infection, an infection caused by an anaerobic organism, usually occurring in deep puncture wounds that exclude air or in tissue that has diminished oxygen-reduction potential as a result of trauma, necrosis, or overgrowth of bacteria. Kinds of anaerobic infection are **gangrene** and **tetanus.**

anal /ā′nəl/ [L, *anus*], pertaining to the anus.

anal canal, the final part of the alimentary tract, about 4 cm long, between the rectum and the anus.

anal character, (in psychoanalysis) a kind of personality exhibiting patterns of behavior originating in the anal phase of childhood. It is characterized by extreme orderliness, obstinacy, perfectionism, cleanliness, punctuality, and miserliness or their extreme opposites.

anal column, the highly vascular longitudinal folds of the anal canal, in which are found the hemorrhoidal blood vessels.

anal crypt, the depression between rectal columns that encloses networks of veins that, when inflamed and swollen, are called hemorrhoids.

anal eroticism, (in psychoanalysis) libidinal fixation at or regression to the anal stage of psychosexual development, often reflected in such personality traits as miserliness, stubbornness, and overscrupulousness.

anal fissure, a painful linear ulceration or laceration of the skin at the margin of the anus.

anal fistula, an abnormal opening on the cutaneous surface near the anus, usually resulting from a local crypt abscess and also common in Crohn's disease. A perianal fistula may or may not communicate with the rectum.

analgesia /an′əljē′zē·ə/ [Gk, *a, algos,* without pain], a decreased or absent sensation of pain.

analgesic /an′əljē′zik/, **1.** relieving pain. **2.** a drug that relieves pain. The narcotic analgesics act on the central nervous system and alter the patient's perception; they are more often used for severe pain. The nonnarcotic analgesics act primarily at the periphery, do not produce tolerance or dependence, and do not alter the patient's perception; they are used for mild to moderate pain.

Analgesic Administration, a Nursing Interventions Classification defined as use of pharmacologic agents to reduce or eliminate pain.

Analgesic Administration: Interspinal, a Nursing Interventions Classification defined as administration of pharmacologic agents into the epidural or intrathecal space to reduce or eliminate pain.

analgesic nephropathy [Gk, *a, algos,* without pain, *nephros,* kidney, *pathos,* disease], kidney damage resulting from the consumption of excessive amounts of aspirin or similar analgesic medications.

analgia [Gk, *ana,* without, *algos,* pain], an absence of pain.

anal incontinence [L, *anus, incontinentia,* an inability to retain], the lack of voluntary control over fecal discharge.

analog /an'əlog/ [Gk, *analogos,* proportionate], **1.** a substance, tissue, or organ that is similar in appearance or function to another but differs in origin or development, such as the eye of a fly and the eye of a human. **2.** a drug or other chemical compound that resembles another in structure or constituents but has different effects.

analogous /ənal'əgəs/ [Gk, *analogos,* proportionate], similar in function but different in origin or structure, such as wings of birds and flies.

analog signal, a continuous electrical signal representing a specific condition, such as temperature or electrocardiogram waveforms.

analog-to-digital converter, a device for converting analog information, such as temperature or electrocardiogram waveforms, into digital form for processing by a digital computer.

analogy /ənal'əjē/ [Gk, *analogos*], similar to a degree in function or form but different in structure or origin.

anal orifice [L, *orificium,* an opening], **1.** the external opening at the end of the anal canal. **2.** the anus, surrounded by the anal sphincter muscle.

anal reflex, a superficial neurologic reflex obtained by stroking the skin or mucosa of the region around the anus, which normally results in a contraction of the external anal sphincter.

anal sadism, (in psychoanalysis) a sadistic form of anal eroticism, manifested by such behavior as aggressiveness and selfishness.

anal stage, (in psychoanalysis) the pregenital period in psychosexual development, occurring between 1 and 3 years of age, when preoccupation with the function of the bowel and the sensations associated with the anus are the predominant source of pleasurable stimulation.

anal verge [L, *anus* + *vergere,* to bend], the area between the anal canal and the perianal skin.

analysand /ənal'isand'/, a person undergoing psychoanalysis.

analysis /ənal'əsis/ [Gk, *ana* + *lyein,* to loosen], **1.** the separation of substances into their constituent parts and the determination of the nature, properties, and composition of compounds. In chemistry, **qualitative analysis** is the determination of the elements present in a substance; **quantitative analysis** is the determination of how much of each element is present in a substance. **2.** an informal term for **psychoanalysis.** —**analytic,** *adj.* **analyze,** *v.*

analysis of variance (ANOVA), a series of statistical procedures for determining whether the differences among two or more groups of scores are attributable to chance alone.

analyst /an'əlist/, **1.** a psychoanalyst. **2.** a person who analyzes the chemical, physical, or other properties of a substance or product.

analyte /an'əlīt/, any substance that is measured. The term is usually applied to a component of blood or other body fluid.

analytical chemistry, a branch of chemistry that deals with identification (qualitative) and measurement (quantitative) of the components of chemical compounds or mixtures of compounds.

analytic psychology /an'əlit'ik/, **1.** the system in which phenomena such as sensations and feelings are analyzed and classified by introspective rather than experimental methods. **2.** a system of analyzing the psyche according to the concepts developed by Carl Gustav Jung. It differs from the psychoanalysis of Sigmund Freud in stressing a "collective unconscious" and a mystic, religious factor in the development of the personal unconscious while minimizing the role of sexual influence on early emotional and psychologic development.

analyzing /an'əlī'zing/, (in five-step nursing process) a category of nursing behavior in which the health care needs of the client are identified and the goals of care are defined. The nurse interprets data; identifies problems involving the client, the client's family, and significant others; defines goals and establishes priorities; integrates the information; and projects the expected outcomes of nursing activities.

anamnesis /an'amnē'sis/ [Gk, *anamimneskein,* to recall], **1.** remembrance of the past. **2.** the accumulated data concerning a medical or psychiatric patient and the patient's background, including family, previous environment, experiences, and particularly recollections, for use in analyzing his or her condition.

anamnestic /an'amnes'tik/, **1.** pertaining to amnesia or memory. **2.** pertaining to the immunologic memory and the immune response to an antigen to which immunocompetent cells have been exposed.

ANA-PAC, abbreviation for **American Nurses Association-Political Action Committee.**

anaphase /an'əfāz/ [Gk, *ana* + *phainein*, to appear], the third of four stages of nuclear division in mitosis and in each of the two divisions of meiosis. In mitosis and the second meiotic division, the centromeres divide, and the two chromatids, which are arranged along the equatorial plane of the spindle, separate and move to the opposite poles of the cell, forming daughter chromosomes. In the first meiotic division the pairs of homologous chromosomes separate from each other and move intact to the opposite poles of the spindle.

anaphia /ənā'fē·ə/, an inability to perceive tactile stimuli.

anaphoresis, (in electrophoresis) the movement of anions in a solution or suspension toward the anode.

anaphylactic /an'əfilak'tik/ [Gk, *ana*, up, *phylaxis*, protection], pertaining to anaphylaxis.

anaphylactic hypersensitivity, an immunoglobulin (Ig)E- or IgG-dependent, immediate-acting humoral systemic hypersensitivity response to an exogenous antigen. Many substances can trigger anaphylaxis in a susceptible person.

anaphylactic reactions [Gk, *ana, phylaxis,* protection; L, *re, agere,* to act], acute allergic responses involving IgE-mediated antigen-stimulated mast cell activation. Exposure to the antigen may result in dyspnea, airway obstruction, shock, urticaria, and, in some cases, death.

anaphylactic shock, a severe and sometimes fatal systemic hypersensitivity reaction to a sensitizing substance such as a drug, vaccine, specific food, serum, allergen extract, insect venom, or chemical. This condition may occur within seconds to minutes from the time of exposure to the sensitizing factor (allergen) and is commonly marked by respiratory distress and vascular collapse. The quicker the systemic atopic reaction occurs in the individual after exposure, the more severe the associated shock is likely to be. The involved allergen enters the systemic circulation and triggers an incomplete humoral

response that allows the allergen to combine with immunoglobulin (Ig) E and cause the release of histamine. Also entering into the reaction are IgG and IgM, which cause the release of complement fractions, further stimulating histamine action.

anaphylatoxin /an'əfī'lətok'sin/, a polypeptide derived from complement. It mediates changes in mast cells leading to the release of histamine and other immunoreactive or inflammatory reactive substances.

anaphylaxis /an'əfilak'sis/ [Gk, *ana* + *phylaxis,* protection], an exaggerated, life-threatening hypersensitivity reaction to a previously encountered antigen. The response, which is mediated by antibodies of the immunoglobulin (Ig)E or IgG class of immunoglobulins, causes the release of chemical mediators from the mast cells. The reaction may be a localized wheal and flare of generalized itching, hyperemia, angioedema, and, in severe cases, vascular collapse, bronchospasm, and shock. The severity of symptoms depends on the original sensitizing dose of the antigen, the amount and distribution of antibodies, and the route of entry and size of the dose of antigen producing anaphylaxis.—**anaphylactic,** *adj.*

anaplasia /an'əplā'zhə/ [Gk, *ana* + *plassein,* to shape], a change in the structure and orientation of cells, characterized by a loss of differentiation and reversion to a more primitive form. Anaplasia is characteristic of malignancy.—**anaplastic** /an'-əplas'tik/, *adj.*

anaplastic [Gk, *ana,* backward, *plassein,* to mold], pertaining to anaplasia.

anapnea /anap'nē·ə/ [Gk, *ana, pnoia,* breath], respiration or restoration of breathing.

anarthria /anär'thrē·ə/ [Gk, *a, arthron,* not joint], a loss of control of the muscles of speech, resulting in the inability to articulate words. The condition is usually caused by damage to a central or peripheral motor nerve.

anasarca /an'əsär'kə/ [Gk, *ana* + *sarx,* flesh], severe generalized, massive edema. Anasarca often occurs in edema associated with renal disease when fluid is retained for an extended period. —**anasarcous,** *adj.*

anastomose /ənas'təmōs/ [Gk, *anastomoein,* to provide a mouth], to open a channel or passage between two vessels or cavities that are normally separate.

anastomosis /ənas'tōmō'sis/ *pl.* **anastomoses** [Gk, *anastomoein,* to provide a mouth], **1.** a connection between two vessels. **2.** a surgical joining of two ducts, blood vessels, or bowel segments to allow flow from one to the other. A vascular anastomosis may be performed to bypass an aneurysm or a vascular or arterial occlusion.

anastomosis at elbow joint, a convergence of blood vessels at the elbow joint, consisting of various veins and parts of the brachial and deep brachial arteries and their branches.

anastomotic /ənas'təmot'ik/, pertaining to or resembling an anastomosis.

anastrozole, an aromatase inhibitor prescribed in the treatment of advanced breast cancer for postmenopausal women whose disease has not responded to treatment with tamoxifen.

anatomic [Gk, *ana* + *temnein,* to cut], pertaining to the structure of the body.

anatomic age, the estimated age of an individual based on the stage of development or deterioration of the body as compared to that of other persons of the same chronologic age.

anatomic crown, the part of the dentin of a tooth, covered by enamel.

anatomic curve, the curvature of the different segments of the vertebral column. In the lateral contour of the back, the cervical and lumbar curves appear concave, and the thoracic and sacral curves appear convex.

anatomic height of contour, an imaginary line that encircles and designates the greatest convexity of a tooth.

anatomic neck of the humerus [Gk, *ana,* up, *temnein,* to cut; AS, *hnecca;* L, *humerus,* shoulder], the part of the humerus where there is a slight constriction adjoining the head.

anatomic pathology [Gk, *ana,* up, *temnein,* to cut, *pathos,* disease, *logos,* science], the study of the effects of disease on the structure of the body.

anatomic position, a position of the body, as if standing erect, facing directly forward, feet pointed forward slightly apart, arms hanging down at the sides with palms facing forward. This is the standard neutral position of reference used to describe sites or motions of various parts of the body.

anatomic snuffbox, a small, cuplike depression on the back of the hand near the wrist formed by the tendons reaching toward the thumb and index finger as the thumb is abducted, the wrist flexed, and the digits extended.

anatomic topography [Gk, *ana* + *temnein,* to cut, *topos,* place, *graphein,* to write], a system of identification of a body part in terms of the region in which it is located and its nearby structures.

anatomic zero joint position, the beginning point of a joint range of motion.

anatomy /ənat'əmē/ [Gk, *ana* + *temnein,* to cut], **1.** the study, classification, and description of structures and organs of the body. **2.** the structure of an organism.

anatripsis /an'ətrip'sis/, a therapy that involves rubbing or friction with or without a simultaneous application of a medicine.

ANC, abbreviation for *absolute neutrophil count.*

A.N.C., abbreviation for **Army Nurse Corps.**

ancestor [L, *antecessorem*], one from whom a person is descended, through the mother or the father. The term assumes a direct lineal line of descent, excluding collateral family members of previous generations.

anchorage [Gk, *agkyra,* anchor], surgical fixation of a movable body organ.

ancillary /an'səler'ē/, pertaining to something that is subordinate, auxiliary, or supplementary.

anconeus /angkō'nē·əs/ [Gk, *agkon,* elbow], one of seven superficial muscles of the posterior forearm. A small triangular muscle, it originates on the dorsal surface of the lateral condyle of the humerus and inserts in the olecranon process of the ulna. It functions to extend the forearm.

ancrod /ang'krod/, the venom of the Malayan pit viper, used to remove fibrinogen from the circulation to prevent clotting of the blood.

Ancylostoma /ang'kilos'təmə/ [Gk, *agkylos,* crooked, *stoma,* mouth], a genus of nematode that is an intestinal parasite and causes hookworm disease.

ancylostomiasis /an'səlos'təmī'əsis/, hookworm disease, more specifically that caused by *Ancylostoma duodenale, A. braziliense,* or *A. caninum.* Infection by *A. duodenale* is generally more harmful and less responsive to treatment than that by *Necator americanus,* which is the hookworm most often found in the southern United States.

Andersen's disease [Dorothy H. Andersen, American pediatrician, 1901–1963], a rare glycogen storage disease characterized by a genetic deficiency of branching enzyme (amylo-1:4, 1:6 transglucosidase), causing the deposition in tissues of abnormal glycogen with long inner and outer chains.

androgamone /an'drōgam'ōn/ [Gk, *andros,* man, *gamos,* marriage], a gamone secreted by the male gamete.

androgen /an'drəjin/ [Gk, *andros* + *genein,* to produce], any steroid hormone that increases male characteristics. Natural hormones such as testosterone and its esters and analogs are primarily used as substitutional therapy during the male climacteric.—**androgenic** /an'drōjen'ik/, adj.

androgynous /androj'inəs/, **1.** (of a man or woman) having some characteristics of both sexes. Social role, behavior, personality, and appearance are reflections of individuality and are not determined by gender. **2.** hermaphroditic.—**androgyny** /-droj'ənē/, n.

android [Gk, andros + eidos, form], pertaining to something that is typically masculine, or manlike, such as an android pelvis.

android pelvis, a type of pelvis with a structure characteristic of the male. It is not uncommon in women. The bones are thick and heavy, and the inlet is heart-shaped.

andrology /androl'əjē/ [Gk, aner, man, logos, science], the study of the health of males.

andropause /an'drəpôs/, a change of life for males that may be expressed in terms of a career change, divorce, or reordering of life. It is associated with a decline in androgen levels that occurs in men during their late forties or early fifties.

androsterone /andros'tərōn/ [Gk, andros + stereos, solid], originally believed to be the principal male sex hormone. The greater potency of several other male sex hormones has relegated androsterone largely to historic biochemical interest.

anecdotal /an'əkdot'əl/ [Gk, anekdotos, unpublished], pertaining to knowledge based on isolated observations and not yet verified by controlled scientific studies.

anecdotal records, medical findings usually based on one or a few observed episodes of patient care, as distinguished from results compiled in a large-scale scientific or systematic study.

anechoic /an'ekō'ik/, (in ultrasonography) free of echoes or without echoes.

anemia /anē'mē-ə/ [Gk, a + haima, without blood], a decrease in hemoglobin in the blood to levels below the normal range of 4.2 million/mm^3 to 6.1 million/mm^3. Anemia may be caused by a decrease in red cell production, an increase in red cell destruction, or a loss of blood. Depending on the severity, anemia may be accompanied by clinical findings that stem from the diminished oxygen-carrying capacity of the blood. Signs and symptoms include fatigue, exertional dyspnea, dizziness, headache, insomnia, and pallor.

anemia of chronic disease, a decrease in the number of circulating erythrocytes as a result of a chronic inflammatory state.

anemia of pregnancy, a condition of pregnancy characterized by a reduction in the concentration of hemoglobin in the blood. It may be physiologic or pathologic. In physiologic anemia of pregnancy, the reduction in concentration results from dilution because the plasma volume expands more than the red blood cell volume. In pathologic anemia of pregnancy, the oxygen-carrying capacity of the blood is deficient because of disordered erythrocyte production or excessive loss of erythrocytes through destruction or bleeding.

anemic /anē'mik/ [Gk, a, without, haima, blood], pertaining to anemia.

anemic anoxia, a condition characterized by an oxygen deficiency in body tissues, resulting from a decrease in the number of erythrocytes in the blood or in the amount of hemoglobin.

anencephaly /an'ensef'əlē/ [Gk, a + egkephalos, without brain], congenital absence of major partions of the brain and malformation of the brainstem. The cranium does not close, and the vertebral canal remains a groove. Transmitted genetically, anencephaly is not compatible with life.—**anencephalous**, adj.

anephrogenesis /anef'rōjen'əsis/ [Gk, a, without, nephros, kidney, genein, to produce], condition of being born without kidneys.

anergia /ənur'jə/, **1.** a condition of lethargy or lack of physical activity. **2.** a diminished or absent sensitivity to commonly used test antigens.

anergic /ənur'jik/, pertaining to a lack of energy or activity.

anergic stupor /ənur'jik/, a kind of dementia characterized by quietness, listlessness, and nonresistance.

anergy /an'ərjē/ [Gk, a, ergon, not work], **1.** lack of activity. **2.** an immunodeficient condition characterized by a lack of or diminished reaction to an antigen or group of antigens. This state may be seen in advanced tuberculosis and other serious infections, acquired immunodeficiency syndrome, and some malignancies. —**anergic**, adj.

aneroid /an'əroid/, not containing a liquid; used especially to describe a device in contrast to one that performs a similar function that does contain liquid, such as an aneroid sphygmomanometer, which does not contain a column of liquid mercury.

aneroid barometer, a device consisting of a flexible spring in a sealed, evacuated metal box that is used to measure atmospheric pressure. It is less accurate than a mercury barometer and is generally used for nonscientific work.

anesthesia /an'esthē'zhə/ [Gk, anaisthesia, lack of feeling], the absence of normal sensation, especially sensitivity to pain, as induced by an anesthetic substance or by hypnosis or as occurs with traumatic or pathophysiologic damage to nerve tissue. Anesthesia induced for medical or surgical purposes may be topical, local, regional, or general and is named for the anesthetic agent used, the method or procedure followed, or the area or organ anesthetized.

Anesthesia Administration, a Nursing Interventions Classification defined as preparation for and administration of anesthetic agents and monitoring of patient responsiveness during administration.

anesthesia machine, an apparatus for administering inhalation anesthetic agents and needed medical gases.

anesthesia patients, classification of, the system by which the American Society of Anesthesiologists classifies patients in five categories by physical status class. Class I includes patients who are healthy; who are without organic, physiologic, biochemical, or psychiatric problems; and for whom anesthesia is required only for a local condition, such as an inguinal hernia or fibroid uterus. Class II includes patients who have mild to moderate systemic disease, whether involving or extraneous to the condition requiring anesthesia, such as anemia, mild diabetes, moderate hypertension obesity, or chronic bronchitis. Class III includes patients who have severe systemic disturbances or disease, whether or not related to the procedure requiring surgical anesthesia. Class IV includes patients who have severe systemic disease that is a constant threat to life that may or may not be related to the intended surgical procedure. Class V includes the moribund patient who is not expected to survive more than 24 hours with or without surgical intervention, such as a person in shock with a ruptured abdominal aneurysm or a massive pulmonary embolus. The letter *E* is added to the roman numeral to indicate an emergency procedure, as when the condition of a patient scheduled for an elective herniorrhaphy requires emergency treatment when the hernia ruptures.

anesthesia screen, a metal, inverted U-shaped frame that attaches to the sides of an operating table, 12 to 18 inches above a patient's upper chest. It is covered with a sheet to prevent contamination of an operative site on the chest or abdomen by airborne infection from the patient or the anesthetist and to provide a wide sterile field for the surgeon.

anesthesia shock, [Gk, *anaisthesia;* Fr, *choc*], a condition of shock produced by an overdose of anesthetic.

anesthesiologist /an′əsthē′zē·ol′əjist/, a physician who completes an accredited 4-year residency in anesthesia. Although anesthesiologists do administer anesthesia directly, they more often supervise nurse anesthetists in the delivery of anesthesia, act as consultants, head anesthesia departments or divisions, or direct intensive care units or pain management clinics.

anesthesiologist's assistant (AA), an allied health professional who assists the anesthesiologist in collecting preoperative data, such as taking an accurate health history and performing an appropriate physical examination; in performing various preoperative tasks, such as the insertion of intravenous and arterial lines, central venous pressure monitors, special catheters; in managing the airway and administering drugs for induction and maintenance of anesthesia; in administering supportive therapy, such as intravenous fluids and vasodilators; in providing recovery room care and in performing other functions and tasks relating to care in an intensive care unit or pain clinic; in providing anesthesia monitoring services; and in performing administrative functions and tasks, such as staff education.

anesthesiology /-ol′əjē/, the branch of medicine that is concerned with the relief of pain and with the administration of medication to relieve pain during surgery.

anesthetic /an′esthet′ik/, a drug or agent that is capable of producing a complete or partial loss of feeling (anesthesia).

anesthetist /ənes′thətist/, **1.** a person who administers anesthesia. **2.** an anesthesiologist.

anesthetize /ənes′thətīz/ [Gk, *anaisthesia,* lack of feeling], to induce a state of anesthesia.

anetoderma /an′ətōdur′mə/ [Gk, *anetos,* relaxed, *derma,* skin], an idiopathic clinical change produced by focal damage to elastin fibers that results in looseness of skin.

aneuploid /an′yo͞oploid/ [Gk, *a, eu,* not good, *ploos,* fold, *eidos,* form], **1.** pertaining to an individual, organism, strain, or cell that has a chromosome number that is not an exact multiple of the normal, basic haploid number characteristic of the species. **2.** such an individual, organism, strain, or cell.

aneuploidy /an′yo͞oploi′dē/, any variation in chromosome number that involves individual chromosomes rather than entire sets. There may be fewer chromosomes, as in Turner syndrome (only one chromosome), or more chromosomes, as in Down's syndrome (trisomy 21).

aneurysm /an′yo͞oriz′əm/ [Gk, *aneurysma,*

widening], a localized dilation of the wall of a blood vessel. It is usually caused by atherosclerosis and hypertension, or less frequently by trauma, infection, or a congenital weakness in the vessel wall. Aneurysms are common in the aorta but also occur in peripheral vessels. They are fairly common in the lower extremities of older people, especially in the popliteal arteries. A sign of an arterial aneurysm is a pulsating swelling that produces a blowing murmur on auscultation. An aneurysm may rupture, causing hemorrhage, or thrombi may form in the dilated pouch and give rise to emboli that may obstruct smaller vessels. —aneurysmal /an'yooriz'məl/, adj.

aneurysmal bone cyst, a cystic lesion that tends to develop in the metaphyseal region of long bones but may occur in any bone, including the vertebrae. It may produce pain and swelling.

aneurysmal thrill, a vibration that can be felt over an aneurysm. In arterial aneurysms the vibration is felt only in systole, but in arteriovenous aneurysms it is felt during both systole and diastole.

aneurysmal varix [Gk, aneurysma, a widening; L, varix, a dilated vein], a varicose vein in which the enlargement is due to an acquired communication with an adjacent artery.

aneurysm needle, a needle equipped with a handle, used to ligate aneurysms.

ANF, 1. abbreviation for American Nurses Foundation. **2.** abbreviation for Australian Nursing Federation.

anger [L, angere, to hurt], an emotional reaction characterized by extreme displeasure, rage, indignation, or hostility. It is considered to be of pathologic origin when such a response does not realistically reflect a person's actual circumstances.

Anger Control Assistance, a Nursing Interventions Classification defined as facilitation of the expression of anger in an adaptive nonviolent manner.

angiitis /anjē-ī'tis/ [Gk, angeion, vessel, itis], an inflammatory condition of a vessel, chiefly a blood or lymph vessel.

angina /anji'nə, an'jinə/ [L, angor, quinsy (strangling)], **1.** a spasmodic, cramplike choking feeling. **2.** a term now used primarily to denote cardiac pain caused by anoxia of the myocardium. **3.** a descriptive feature of various diseases characterized by a feeling of choking, suffocation, or crushing pressure and pain. —**anginal,** adj.

angina decubitus, a condition characterized by periodic attacks of cardiac pain that occur when the person is lying down.

anginal, pertaining to angina.

angina pectoris, a paroxysmal thoracic pain caused most often by myocardial anoxia as a result of atherosclerosis or spasm of the coronary arteries. The pain usually radiates down the inner aspect of the left arm and is frequently accompanied by a feeling of suffocation and impending death. Attacks of angina pectoris are often related to exertion, emotional stress, and exposure to intense cold.

angina sine dolore /sē'nə dolôr'ə, sī'nē/, a painless episode of coronary insufficiency.

angioblastic meningioma /an'jē-ōblas'tik/, a tumor of the blood vessels of the meninges covering the spinal cord or the brain.

angioblastoma /an'jē-ōblastō'mə/ [Gk, angeion, vessel, blastos, germ, oma], a tumor of blood vessels in the brain. Kinds of angioblastomas are **angioblastic meningioma** and **cerebellar angioblastoma.**

angiocardiogram /an'jē-ōkär'dē-ōgram'/, a series of radiographic images of the heart taken in rapid succession during and immediately after injection of a radiopaque contrast medium into coronary blood vessels.

angiocardiography /-kär'dē-og'rəfē/ [Gk, angeion + kardia, heart, graphein, to record], the process of producing a radiograph of the heart and great vessels of the heart. A radiopaque contrast medium is injected directly into the heart by a catheter introduced through the antecubital veins.

angiocardiopathy /-kär'dē-op'əthē/ [Gk, angeion, vessel, kardia, heart, pathos, disease], a disease of the blood vessels of the heart.

angiocarditis /-kärdī'tis/, an inflammation of the heart and large blood vessels.

angiocatheter /an'jē-ōkath'ətər/, a hollow, flexible tube inserted into a blood vessel to withdraw or instill fluids.

angiochondroma /an'jē-ōkondrō'mə/ [Gk, angeion + chondros, cartilage, oma], a cartilaginous tumor characterized by an excessive formation of blood vessels.

angioedema /an'jē-ō'idē'mə/, an acute, painless, dermal, subcutaneous, or submucosal swelling of short duration. It involves the face, neck, lips, larynx, hands, feet, genitalia, or viscera. It may result from food or drug allergy, infection, or emotional stress; or it may be hereditary.

angiofibroma /an'jē-ōfībrō'mə/ [Gk, angeion + L, fibra, fiber; Gk, oma], an angioma containing fibrous tissue.

angiogenesis /an'jē-ōjen'əsis/ [Gk, angeion + genesis, origin], the ability to evoke blood vessel formation, a property of malignant tissue. The presence of angiogenesis in breast tissue is regarded as a precursor of histologic evidence of breast cancer.

angiogenin /an'jē-ōjen'in/, a protein that mediates the formation of blood vessels. Angiogenin is used experimentally to stimulate the development of new blood vessels in wound healing, stroke, or coronary heart disease.

angioglioma /an'jē-ōglē-ō'mə/ [Gk, *angeion* + *glia*, glue, *oma*], a highly vascular tumor composed of neuroglia.

angiogram /an'jē-əgram/ [Gk, *angeion*, vessel, *gramma*, writing], a radiographic image of a blood vessel into which contrast medium has been injected.

angiograph /an'jē-əgraf/ [Gk, *angeion*, vessel, *graphein*, to record], an instrument that records the patterns of pulse waves.

angiography /an'jē·og'rəfē/ [Gk, *angeion* + *graphein*, to record], the x-ray visualization of the internal anatomy of the heart and blood vessels after the intravascular introduction of radiopaque contrast medium. —**angiographic,** *adj.*

angiokeratoma /an'jē-ōker'ətō'mə/ [Gk, *angeion* + *keras*, horn, *oma*], a vascular, horny neoplasm on the skin, characterized by clumps of dilated blood vessels, clusters of warts, and thickening of the epidermis, especially the scrotum and the dorsal aspect of the fingers and toes.

angiokeratoma circumscriptum, a rare skin disorder characterized by discrete papules and nodules in small patches on the legs or on the trunk.

angiokeratoma corporis diffusum, an uncommon familial disease in which phospholipids are stored in many parts of the body, especially the blood vessels, causing vasomotor, urinary, and cutaneous disorders and, in some cases, muscular abnormalities.

angiolipoma /an'jē-ōlipō'mə/ [Gk, *angeion* + *lipos*, fat, *oma*], a benign neoplasm containing blood vessels and tissue.

angioma /an'jē-ō'mə/ [Gk, *angeion*, vessel, *oma* tumor], any benign tumor with blood vessels (hemangioma) or lymph vessels (lymphangioma). Most angiomas are congenital; some, such as cavernous hemangiomas, may disappear spontaneously.

angioma arteriale racemosum /ärtir'ē-ā'lē ras'əmō'səm/ [Gk, *angeion* + *oma* + L, *arteria,* airpipe, *racemus,* grape], a vascular neoplasm characterized by the intertwining of many small, newly formed, dilated blood vessels.

angioma cutis, a nevus composed of a network of dilated blood vessels.

angioma serpiginosum /sərpij'inō'səm/ [Gk, *angeion* + *oma* + L, *serpere,* to

creep], a cutaneous disease characterized by rings of tiny vascular points appearing as red dots.

angiomatosis /an'jē-ōmətō'sis/, a condition characterized by numerous vascular tumors.

angiomyoma, [Gk, *angeion* + *mys,* muscle, *oma*], a tumor composed of vascular and muscular tissue elements.

angiomyosarcoma /an'jē-ōmī'ōsärkō'mə/ [Gk, *angeion* + *mys* muscle, *sarx,* flesh, *oma*], a tumor containing vascular, muscular, and connective tissue elements.

angioneurotic anuria /-nōōrot'ik ənyōōr'ē·ə/ [Gk, *angeion* + *neuron,* nerve, *a* + *ouron,* not urine], an abnormal condition characterized by an almost complete absence of urination caused by destruction of tissue in the renal cortex.

angioneurotic gangrene, [Gk, *angeion* + *neuron,* nerve, *gaggraina*], the death and putrefaction of tissue caused by an interruption of the blood supply resulting from thrombotic arteries or veins.

angiopathy /an'jē-op'əthē/ [Gk, *angeion,* vessel, *pathos,* disease], a disease of the blood vessels.

angioplasty /an'jēōplas'tē/ [Gk, *angeion,* vessel, *plassein,* to mold], the reconstruction of blood vessels damaged by disease or injury.

angiopoiesis /-poi·ē'sis/ [Gk, *angeion,* vessel, *poien,* to make], the process of blood vessel formation.

angiorrhaphy /an'jē-ôr'əfē/ [Gk, *angeion,* vessel, *rhaphe,* suture], the repair by suture of any blood vessel.

angiosarcoma /an'jē-ōsärkō'mə/, a rare, malignant tumor consisting of endothelial and fibroblastic tissue that proliferates and eventually surrounds vascular channels.

angiosclerosis /-sklerō'sis/ [Gk, *angeion,* vessel, *skleros,* hard, *osis,* condition], a thickening and hardening of the walls of the blood vessels.

angioscope /an'jē-əskōp'/, a type of microscope that permits inspection of the capillary vessels.

angiospasm /an'jē-ōspaz'əm/, a sudden, transient constriction of a blood vessel.

angiotensin /an'jē-ōten'sin/ [Gk, *angeion* + L, *tendere,* to stretch], a polypeptide in the blood that causes vasoconstriction, increased blood pressure, and the release of aldosterone from the adrenal cortex. Angiotensin is formed by the action of renin on angiotensinogen, an alpha-2-globulin that is produced in the liver and constantly circulates in the blood.

angiotensin-converting enzyme (ACE), a protein (dipeptidyl carboxypeptidase) that catalyzes the conversion of angiotensin I to angiotensin II by splitting two terminal amino acids.

angiotensin-converting enzyme (ACE) inhibitor, serum protease inhibitor that blocks the formation of angiotensin II and decreases the degradation of bradykinin and other kinins. ACE inhibitors cause a decrease in sodium and water retention, a decrease in blood pressure, an improvement in cardiac output, and a decrease in heart size.

angiotensinogen /-tensin'əjən/, a serum globulin produced in the liver that is the precursor of angiotensin.

angiotensin sensitivity test (AST), a test for sensitivity to angiotensin II by infusion of angiotensin II amide into the right cubital vein.

angle /ang'gəl/ [L, *angulus*], **1.** the space or the shape formed at the intersection of two lines, planes, or borders. The divergence of the lines, planes, or borders may be measured in degrees of a circle. **2.** (in anatomy and physiology) the geometric relationships between the surfaces of body structures and the positions affected by movement.

angle board, (in dentistry) a device used for facilitating the establishment of reproducible angular relationships between a patient's head, the x-ray beam, and the x-ray film.

angle former, (in dentistry) one of a series of paired cutting instruments having cutting edges at an angle other than a right angle in relation to the axis of the blade.

angle of convergence, an angle formed between the visual axis of an eye focused on an object and a median line.

angle of incidence, the angle at which an ultrasound beam hits the interface between two different types of tissues, such as the facing surfaces of bone and muscle.

angle of iris, the angle formed between the cornea and the iris at the periphery of the anterior chamber of the eye. The aqueous fluid normally drains through this angle, which may be blocked in glaucoma.

angle of Louis [Pierre C A Louis, French physician, 1787–1872], the sternal angle between the manubrium and the body of the sternum.

angle of mandible, the measure in degrees of the relationship between the body and the ramus of the mandible.

angle of refraction [L, *angulus* + *refringere*, to break apart], the angle that a refracted ray of light makes with a line perpendicular to the refracting surface at the point of refraction.

angle of Treitz /trīts/ [Wenzel Treitz, Czech physician, 1819–1872], a sharp curve or flexure at the junction of the duodenum and jejunum.

Angle's Classification of Malocclusion [Edward Hartley Angle, American orthodontist, 1855–1930], a classification of the various types of malocclusion. Classification is based on the relation of different teeth in the upper and lower jaws, such as the maxillary and the mandibular first molars and the incisors.

angor /ang'gôr/, a condition of extreme distress, usually occurring in abdominal or pectoral angina or during a sudden attack of blindness.

angstrom (Å) /ang'strəm/ [Anders J. Angström, Swedish physicist, 1814–187], a unit of measure of length equal to 0.1 millimicron (1/10,000,000 meter), or 10^{-10} meter.

angular gyrus /ang'gyələr/ [L, *angulus* + Gk, *gyros*], a folded convolution in the inferior parietal lobe where it unites with the temporal lobe of the cerebral cortex.

angular movement [L, *angularis*, sharply bent], one of the four basic movements allowed by the various joints of the skeleton. It is a movement in which the angle between two adjoining bones is decreased, as in flexion, or increased, as in extension.

angular spinal curvature [L, *angulus* + *spina*, backbone, *curvatura*, bend], a sharp bending or sloping of the vertebral column.

angular stomatitis, inflammation at the corner of the mouth.

angular vein, one of a pair of veins of the face, formed by the junction of the frontal and the supraorbital veins.

angulated fracture /ang'gyəlā'tid/, a fracture in which the fragments of bone are at angles.

angulation [L, *angulatus*, bent], **1.** an angular shape or formation. **2.** the discipline of precisely measuring angles, as in mechanical drafting and surveying. **3.** (in radiography) the direction of the primary beam of radiation in relation to the object being radiographed and the film used to record its image.

anhedonia /an'hēdō'nē-ə/ [Gk, *a* + *hedone*, not pleasure], the inability to feel pleasure or happiness in response to experiences that are ordinarily pleasurable. —**anhedonic,** *adj.*

anhidrosis /an'hidrō'sis, an'hī-/ [Gk, *a* + *hidros*, without sweat], an abnormal condition characterized by inadequate perspiration.

anhidrotic /an'hidrot'ik, an'hī-/, **1.** pertaining to anhidrosis. **2.** an agent that reduces or suppresses sweating.

anhydrase /anhī'drās/ [Gk, *a*, not, *hydor*, water], an enzyme that catalyzes the elimination of water molecules from certain compounds, as carbonic anhydrase dehydrates carbonic acid, thereby controlling the amount of carbon dioxide in the blood and lungs.

anhydride /anhī′drīd/ [Gk, *a* + *hydor*, without water], a chemical compound, especially an acid, derived by the removal of water from a substance.

anhydrous /anhī′drəs/ [Gk, *a*, without, *hydor*, water], an absence of water.

anicteric /an′ikter′ik/ [Gk, *a* + *icterus*, not jaundice], pertaining to the absence of jaundice.

anicteric hepatitis, a mild form of hepatitis in which there is no jaundice (icterus). Symptoms include anorexia, gastrointestinal disturbances, and slight fever. Aspartate aminotransferase and alanine aminotransferase are elevated. The infection may be mistaken for flu or be unnoticed.

anidean /anid′ē·ən/ [Gk, *a* + *eidos*, not form], formless; shapeless; denoting an undifferentiated mass, such as an anideus.

anideus /anid′ē·əs/, an anomalous, rudimentary embryo consisting of a simple rounded mass with little indication of the body parts.

aniline /an′ilēn/ [Ar, *alnil*, indigo], an oily, colorless poisonous liquid with a strong odor and burning taste, formerly extracted from the indigo plant and now made synthetically by using nitrobenzene in the manufacture of aniline dyes.

anilingus /ā′niling′gəs/, sexual stimulation of the anus by the tongue or lips.

anilism [Ar, *alnil*, indigo; Gk, *ismos*, state], a condition of poisoning resulting from exposure to aniline compounds. Symptoms generally include cyanosis, weakness, cold sweats, irregular pulse, breathing difficulty, coma, convulsions, and possible sudden heart failure. Treatment includes gastric lavage and induction of emesis.

anima /an′imə/ [L, soul], 1. the soul or life. 2. the active ingredient in a drug. 3. (in Jungian psychology) a person's true, inner, unconscious being or personality, as distinguished from overt personality, or persona. 4. (in analytic psychology) the female component of the male personality.

animal, a living organism capable of movement that subsists on the breakdown of organic substances to a usable form, followed by synthesis of essential-nutrient organic compounds. The distinction between plants and some lower animals is ambiguous.

Animal-Assisted Therapy, a Nursing Interventions Classification defined as purposeful use of animals to provide affection, attention, diversion, and relaxation.

animal pole [L, *anima*], the active, formative part of the ovum protoplasm that contains the nucleus and bulk of the cytoplasm and where the polar bodies form. In mammals it is also the site where the inner cell mass develops and gives rise to germ layers such as the ectoderm.

animation, 1. a state of being alive. 2. an ability to put into action a vivid appearance of life.

animus /an′iməs/ [L, spirit], 1. the active or rational soul; the animating principle of life. 2. (in analytic psychology) the male component of the female personality. 3. (in psychiatry) a deep-seated antagonism that is usually controlled but may erupt with virulence under stress.

anion /an′ī·ən/ [Gk, *ana* + *ion*, backward going], 1. a negatively charged ion that is attracted to the positive electrode (anode) in electrolysis. 2. a negatively charged atom, molecule, or radical.

anion exchange resin, any one of the simple organic polymers with high molecular weights that exchange anions with other ions in solution. Anion exchange resins are used as antacids in treating ulcers.

anion gap, the difference between the concentrations of serum cations and anions, determined by measuring the concentrations of sodium cations and chloride and bicarbonate anions. It is helpful in the diagnosis and treatment of acidosis.

anionic /an′ī·on′ik/ [Gk, *ana*, not, *ion*, going], pertaining to an anion.

anise /an′is/, the fruit of the *Pimpinella anisum* plant. Extract of anise is used in the preparation of carminatives and expectorants.

aniseikonia /an′īsīkō′nē·ə/ [Gk, *anisos*, unequal, *eikon*, image], an abnormal ocular condition in which each eye perceives the same image as being of a different form and size.

anismus /ānis′məs/, extreme contraction of the external sphincter of the anus.

anisocoria /-kôr′ē·ə/, [Gk, *anisos*, unequal, *kore*, pupil], an inequality of the diameter of the pupils of the two eyes.

anisocytosis /anī′sōsītō′sis/ [Gk, *anisos* + *kytos*, cell], an abnormal condition of the blood characterized by excessive red blood cells of variable and abnormal size.

anisogamete /-gam′ēt/ [Gk, *anisos* + *gamos*, marriage], a gamete that differs considerably in size and structure from the one with which it unites, as the macrogamete and microgamete of certain sporozoa. —**anisogametic**, *adj.*

anisogamy /an′īsog′əmē/, sexual conjugation of gametes that are of unequal size and structure, as in certain thallophytes and sporozoa. —**anisogamous**, *adj.*

anisognathic /an'īsōnath'ik/ [Gk, *anisos* + *gnathos*, jaw], pertaining to an abnormal condition in which the maxillary and the mandibular arches or jaws are of significantly different sizes in the same individual.

anisokaryosis /anī'sōker'ē-ō'sis/, significant variation in the size of the nucleus of cells of the same general type. —**anisokaryotic**, *adj.*

anisomastia /anī'sōmas'tē-ə/, a condition in which one female breast is much larger than the other.

anisometropia /anī'sōmetrō'pē-ə/ [Gk, *anisos* + *metron*, measure, *ops*, eye], an abnormal ocular condition characterized by a difference in the refractive powers of the eyes.

anisopia /an'īsō'pē-ə/, a condition in which the visual power of one eye is greater than that of the other.

anisopiesis /-pī-ē'sis/ [Gk, *anisos*, unequal, *piesis*, pressure], a condition of unequal arterial blood pressure on the two sides of the body.

anisotropine methylbromide, an anticholinergic prescribed as adjunctive therapy in the treatment of peptic ulcer.

ankh /ängk/, an ancient Egyptian symbol of life. It resembles a cross with a loop instead of the top beam.

ankle [AS, *ancleow*], **1.** the joint of the tibia and fibula of the leg with the talus of the foot. **2.** the part of the leg where this joint is located.

ankle bandage, a figure-of-eight bandage looped under the sole of the foot and around the ankle. The heel may be covered or left exposed, although covering is preferable because it prevents "window edema."

ankle bone. See *talus*.

ankle-brachial index (ABI), the ratio of ankle systolic blood pressure to arm systolic blood pressure. It is calculated by dividing the highest ankle pressure for each foot by the highest of two brachial artery pressures.

ankle clonus, an involuntary tendon reflex that causes repeated flexion and extension of the foot.

ankle-foot orthosis (AFO), any of a variety of protective external devices that can be applied to the ankle area to prevent injury in a high-risk athletic activity, to protect a previous injury such as a sprain, or to compensate for chronic joint instability.

ankle joint [AS, *ancleow* + L, *jungere*, to join], a synovial hinge joint between the leg and the foot. The rounded malleolar

prominences on each side of the joint form a mortise for the upper surface of the talus.

ankyloglossia /ang'kilōglos'ē-ə/ [Gk, *agkylos*, crooked, *glossa* tongue], an oral defect, characterized by an abnormally short lingual frenum that limits tongue movement and impairs the speech. It may be surgically corrected by a frenotomy or frenectomy.

ankylosed /ang'kilōst/, pertaining to the immobility of a joint resulting from pathologic changes in it or in adjacent tissues.

ankylosing spondylitis /ang'kilō'sing/, a chronic inflammatory disease of unknown origin, first affecting the spine and adjacent structures and commonly progressing to eventual fusion (ankylosis) of the involved joints. In extreme cases a forward flexion of the spine, called a "poker spine" or "bamboo spine," develops.

ankylosis /ang'kilō'sis/ [Gk, *ankylosis*, bent condition], **1.** fixation of a joint, often in an abnormal position, usually resulting from destruction of articular cartilage and subchondral bone, as occurs in rheumatoid arthritis. **2.** also called **arthrodesis, fusion**. Surgically induced fixation of a joint to relieve pain or provide support.

anlage /on'lägə/ [Ger, *Anlage*, disposition, aptitude], (in embryology) the undifferentiated layer of cells from which a particular organ, tissue, or structure develops; primordium rudiment.

ANLL, abbreviation for acute nonlymphocytic leukemia.

anneal [AS, *aelan*, to burn], **1.** a method of tempering metals, glass, or other materials by controlled heating and cooling to make them more malleable and ductile. **2.** a process whereby two separate strands of nucleic acid interact to form a duplex molecule.

annihilation /ənī'əlā'shən/, the total transformation of matter into energy.

annulus /an'yələs/ [L, a ring], any ring-shaped structure, such as the outer edge of an intervertebral disk.

anodal [Gk, *ana* + *hodas*, way], relating to an anode.

anode, the electrode at which oxidation occurs.

anodic stripping voltammetry /ənō'dik/, /anod'ik/, a process of electroanalytic chemistry used to detect trace metals.

anodontia /an'ōdon'tē-ə/ [Gk, *a*, not, *odous*, tooth], a congenital defect in which some or all of the teeth are missing.

anodyne /an'ədīn/ [Gk *a* + *odyne*, not pain], a drug that relieves or lessens pain.

anomaly /ənom'əlē/ [Gk, *anomalos*, irregular], **1.** deviation from what is regarded as normal. **2.** congenital malformation, such as the absence of a limb or the presence of an extra finger. **—anomalous,** *adj.*

anomia /ənō′mē·ə/ [Gk, *a + onoma,* without name], a form of aphasia characterized by the inability to name objects, caused by a lesion in the temporal lobe of the brain.

anomie /an′əmē/, a state of apathy, alienation, anxiety, personal disorientation, and distress resulting from the loss of social norms and goals previously valued.

anoopsia /an′ō·op′sē·ə/ [Gk, *ana,* up, *ops,* eye], a strabismus in which one or both eyes are deviated upward.

Anopheles /ənof′əlēz/ [Gk, *anopheles,* harmful], a genus of mosquito, many species of which transmit malaria-causing parasites to humans.

anopia /anō′pē·ə/ [Gk, *a + ops,* not eye], blindness resulting from a defect in or the absence of one or both eyes.

anoplasty /an′ōplas′tē/ [L, *anus* + Gk, *plassein,* to shape], a restorative operation on the anus.

anorchia /anôr′kē·ə/ [Gk, *a + orchis,* not testis], congenital absence of one or both testes.

anorectal /an′ōrek′təl/, ā′nō- [L, *anus* + *rectus,* straight], pertaining to the anal and rectal parts of the large intestine.

anorectal abscess [L, *anus* + *rectus,* straight, *abscedere,* to go away], an abscess in the area of the anus and rectum.

anorectal stricture [L, *anus* + *rectus,* straight, *strictura,* compression], a narrowing of the anorectal canal. It is sometimes congenital but also may result from surgery to correct a fissure or to remove hemorrhoids.

anorectic /an′ōrek′tik/, **1.** pertaining to anorexia. **2.** lacking appetite. **3.** causing a loss of appetite, as an anorexiant drug.

anorexia /an′ōrek′sē·ə/ [Gk, *a + orexis,* not appetite], lack or loss of appetite, resulting in the inability to eat.

anorexia nervosa, a disorder characterized by a prolonged refusal to eat, resulting in emaciation, amenorrhea, emotional disturbance concerning body image, and fear of becoming obese.

anorexiant, a drug or other agent that suppresses the appetite, such as amphetamine.

anorgasmy /an′ôrgaz′mē/, failure to achieve orgasm.

anorthopia /an′ôrthō′pē·ə/, a visual disorder in which straight lines appear to be curved or angular.

anosigmoidoscopy /an′ōsig′moidos′kəpē/, a procedure in which an endoscope is used for direct examination of the lining of the anus, rectum, and sigmoid colon.

anosmia /anoz′mē·ə/ [Gk, *a + osme,* without smell], loss or impairment of the sense of smell. It usually occurs as a temporary condition resulting from a head cold or respiratory infection or when intranasal swelling or other obstruction prevents odors from reaching the olfactory region. It becomes a permanent condition when the olfactory neuroepithelium or any part of the olfactory nerve is destroyed. **—anosmatic, anosmic,** *adj.*

anosmia gustatoria, the inability to smell foods.

anosmic [Gk, *a + osme,* without smell], pertaining to a loss of the sense of smell.

anosognosia /an′əsog·nō′zhə/ [Gk, *a + nosos,* not disease, *gnosis* knowing], lack of awareness or denial of a neurologic defect, especially paralysis, on one side of the body.

anotia /anō′tē·ə/ [Gk, *a,* without, *ous,* ear], a congenital absence of one or both ears.

ANOVA, abbreviation for **analysis of variance.**

anovaginal /ā′nōvaj′inəl/ [L, *anus + vagina,* sheath], pertaining to the perineal region of the anus and vagina.

anovesical /-ves′ikəl/ [L, *anus + vesicula,* small bladder], pertaining to the anus and bladder.

anovular /anov′yələr/ [Gk, *a,* not, *ovulum*], pertaining to menstrual discharge not associated with the production or release of an ovum.

anovular menstruation [Gk, *a + ovulum,* not egg], menstrual bleeding that occurs although ovulation has not taken place.

anovulation /an′ovyəlā′shən/, failure of the ovaries to produce, mature, or release eggs. The condition may be a result of ovarian immaturity or postmaturity; of altered ovarian function, as in pregnancy and lactation; of primary ovarian dysfunction, as in ovarian dysgenesis; or of disturbance of the interaction of the hypothalamus, pituitary gland, and ovary, caused by stress or disease. **—anovulatory** /anov′yələtôr′ē/, *adj.*

anoxemia /an′okse′mē·ə/, a deficiency of oxygen in the blood.

anoxia /anok′sē·ə/ [Gk, *a + oxys,* not sharp], an abnormal condition characterized by a lack of oxygen. Anoxia may be local or systemic. It may result from an inadequate supply of oxygen to the respiratory system or from an inability of the blood to carry oxygen to the tissues, as in anemic anoxia, or of the tissues to absorb the oxygen from the circulation **—anoxic,** *adj.*

ansa /an′sə/, *pl.* **ansae** [L, handle], (in

anatomy) a looplike structure resembling a curved handle of a vase.

ansa cervicalis, one of three loops of nerves in the cervical plexus, branches of which innervate the infrahyoid muscles.

ANSER system, a pattern of questionnaires for studying developmental defects in children.

ANSI, abbreviation for **American National Standards Institute.**

antacid /antas′id/ [Gk, *anti*, against, *acidus*, sour], **1.** opposing acidity. **2.** a drug or dietary substance that buffers, neutralizes, or absorbs hydrochloric acid in the stomach.

antagonism /antag′əniz′əm/ [Gk, *antagonisma*, struggle], **1.** an inhibiting action between physiologic processes, such as muscle actions. **2.** opposing actions of drugs.

antagonist /antagə′nist/, [Gk, *antagonisma*, struggle], **1.** one who contends with or is opposed to another. **2.** (in physiology) any agent, such as a drug or muscle, that exerts an opposite action to that of another or competes for the same receptor sites. **3.** (in dentistry) a tooth in the upper jaw that articulates during mastication or occlusion with a tooth in the lower jaw. —**antagonistic,** *adj.,* **antagonize,** *v.*

antagonistic reflexes [Gk, *antagonisma* + L, *reflectere*, to bend back], two or more reflexes initiated at the same time that produce opposite effects. The most adaptive or persistent response occurs.

antecedent /an′ti·sē′dənt/ [L, *antecedentem*], a thing or period that precedes others in time or order.

antecubital /-kyoo′bitəl/ [L, *ante*, before, *cubitum*, elbow], in front of the elbow; at the bend of the elbow.

antecubital fossa [L, *ante*, before, *cubitum*, elbow, *fossa*, ditch], a depression at the bend of the elbow.

antecurvature /an′tikur′vəchər/, a slight degree of anteflexion or forward curvature.

anteflexion /-flek′shən/ [L, *ante* + *flectare*, bend], an abnormal position in which an organ is tilted acutely forward, folded over on itself.

antegonial notch /-gō′nē·əl/ [L, *ante* + *gonia*, angle], a depression or concavity commonly present at the junction of the ramus and the mandible, near the attachment of the anterior margin of the masseter.

antegrade /an′təgrād/ [L, *ante*, before, *gredi*, to go], moving forward, or proceeding toward the front.

ante mortem [L, *ante*, before, *mors*, death], before death.

antepartal /an′təpär′təl/ [L, *ante* + *parturire*, to have labor pains], pertaining to the period spanning conception and labor.

antepartal care, care of a pregnant woman during the time in the maternity cycle that begins with conception and ends with the onset of labor.

antepartum hemorrhage [Gk, *ante*, before; L, *parturire*, to have labor pains; Gk, *haima*, blood, *rhegnynai*, to burst forth], bleeding from the uterus during a pregnancy in which the placenta appears to be normally situated, particularly after the 28th week.

antepyretic /-pīret′ik/ [L, *ante*, before; Gk, *pyretos*, fever], before the onset of fever.

anterior (A) /antir′ē·ər/ [L, *ante* + *prior*, foremost], **1.** the front of a structure. **2.** pertaining to a surface or part situated toward the front or facing forward.

anterior atlantoaxial ligament /atlan′tō·ak′sē·əl/, one of five ligaments connecting the atlas to the axis. It is fixed to the inferior border of the anterior arch of the atlas and to the ventral surface of the body of the axis.

anterior atlantooccipital membrane, one of two broad, densely woven fibrous sheets that form part of the atlantooccipital joint between the atlas and the occipital bone.

anterior axillary line (AAL), an imaginary vertical line on the body wall continuing the line of the anterior axillary fold with the upper arm.

anterior cardiac vein, one of several small vessels that return deoxygenated blood from the ventral part of the myocardium of the right ventricle to the right atrium.

anterior cerebral commissure [L, *ante* + *prior*, foremost, *cerebrum*, brain, *commissura*, ajoining], a bundle of fibers in the anterior wall of the forebrain connecting the olfactory bulb and cortex on one side with the similar structures on the other side.

anterior chamber [L, *ante* + *prior*, foremost; Gk, *kamara*, an arched cover], the part of the anterior cavity of the eye in front of the iris. It contains the aqueous humor.

anterior cutaneous nerve, one of a pair of cutaneous branches of the cervical plexus. It arises from the second and third cervical nerves and divides into the ascending and descending branches.

anterior determinants of cusp, (in dentistry) the characteristics of the anterior teeth that determine the cusp elevations and the fossa depressions in restoration of the postcanine teeth.

anterior drawer sign or test, a test for

rupture of the anterior cruciate ligament. The result is positive if there is increased anterior glide of the tibia when the knee is flexed at a 90-degree angle.

anterior fontanel, a diamond-shaped area between the frontal and two parietal bones just above an infant's forehead at the junction of the coronal and sagittal sutures.

anterior guide, (in dentistry) the part of an articulator that is contacted by the incisal guide pin to maintain the selected separation of the upper and lower members of the articulator.

anterior horn cell, a large nerve cell, the body of a motor neuron, in the anterior column of the spinal cord.

anterior horn of the spinal cord [L, *ante* + *prior,* foremost, *cornu,* horn, *spina,* spine; Gk, *chorde,* string], one of the hornlike projections of gray matter into the white matter of the spinal cord. The anterior, or ventral, horn contains efferent fibers innervating skeletal muscle tissue.

anterior longitudinal ligament, the broad, strong ligament attached to the ventral surfaces of the vertebral bodies. It extends from the occipital bone and the anterior tubercle of the atlas to the sacrum.

anterior mediastinal node, a node in one of the three groups of thoracic visceral nodes of the lymphatic system that drains lymph from the nodes of the thymus, the pericardium, and the sternum.

anterior mediastinum, a caudal part of the mediastinum in the middle of the thorax, bounded ventrally by the body of the sternum and parts of the fourth through the seventh ribs and dorsally by the parietal pericardium, extending downward as far as the diaphragm.

anterior nares, the ends of the nostrils that open anteriorly into the nasal cavity and allow the inhalation and exhalation of air. The anterior nares connect with the nasal fossae.

anterior neuropore, the opening of the embryonic neural tube in the anterior part of the forebrain.

anterior-posterior diameter of pelvic outlet, the distance between the middle of the symphysis pubis and the upper border of the third sacral vertebra.

anterior rhizotomy [L, *anterior,* foremost; Gk, *rhiza,* root, *temnein,* to cut], the surgical cutting of the ventral root of a spinal nerve, usually to relieve persistent spasm, involuntary movement, or intractable pain.

anterior tibial artery, one of the two divisions of the popliteal artery, arising in back of the knee, dividing into six branches, and supplying various muscles of the leg and foot.

anterior tibial node, one of the small lymph glands of the lower limb, lying on the interosseous membrane near the proximal part of the anterior tibial vessels.

anterior tooth, any of the incisors or canine central and lateral cuspid teeth.

anterior triangle of neck, a triangular area bounded by the median line of the neck in front, the lower border of the mandible, and a line extending back to the sternocleidomastoid muscle.

anterocclusion /an'tərōklōo'shən/ [L, *ante* + *occludere,* to shut], (in dentistry) a malocclusion in which the mandibular teeth are anterior to their normal position relative to the teeth in the maxillary arch. Compare **anteversion.**

anterograde amnesia [L, *ante* + *prior,* foremost, *gredi,* to go], **1.** the inability to recall events that occur after the onset of amnesia. **2.** the inability to form new memories.

anterograde memory, the ability to recall past events but not recent occurrences.

anteroinferior /an'tərō·infir'ē·ər/, situated in front of but at a lower level, such as the anteroinferior spine of the ilium.

anterolateral /-lat'ərəl/, in front and on each side of another structure or object.

anterolateral thoracotomy, a surgery technique in which entry to the chest is made with an incision below the breast but above the costal margins.

anteroposterior (AP) /an'tərōpostir'ē·ər/ [L, *ante* + *prior,* foremost, *posterus,* coming after], from the front to the back of the body, commonly associated with the direction of the x-ray beam.

anteroposterior vaginal repair, a surgical procedure in which the upper and lower walls of the vagina are reconstructed to correct relaxed tissue.

anterosuperior, situated in front of but at a higher level, such as the anterosuperior spine of the ilium.

anteversion /-vur'shən/ [L, *ante* + *versio,* turning], **1.** an abnormal position of an organ in which it is tilted forward on its axis, away from the midline. **2.** (in dentistry) the tipping or the tilting of teeth or other mandibular structures more anteriorly than normal. **3.** the angulation created in the transverse plane between the neck and shaft of the femur.—**anteverted,** *adj.*

anteverted /an'tivur'tid/, inclined or turned forward.

anthelmintic /ant'helmin'tik/ [Gk, *anti* + *helmins,* against worms], **1.** pertaining to a substance that destroys or prevents the development of parasitic worms, such as filariae, flukes, hookworms, pinworms, roundworms, schistosomes, tapeworms, trichinae, and whipworms. **2.** an anthelmintic drug. An anthelmintic may interfere with the parasites' carbohydrate metabolism, inhibit their respiratory enzymes, block their neuromuscular action, or render them more susceptible to destruction by the host's macrophages.

anthracosis /an'thrəkō'sis/ [Gk, *anthrax,* coal, *osis,* condition], a chronic lung disease characterized by the deposit of coal dust in the lungs and the formation of black nodules on the bronchioles, resulting in focal emphysema.

anthralin /an'thrəlin/, a topical antipsoriatic prescribed in the treatment of psoriasis and chronic dermatitis.

anthrax /an'thraks/ [Gk, *anthrax,* coal, carbuncle], a disease affecting primarily farm animals (cattle, goats, pigs, sheep, and horses), caused by the bacterium *Bacillus anthracis.* Anthrax in animals is usually fatal. Humans most often acquire it when a break in the skin has direct contact with infected animals and their hides, but they may also contract a pulmonary form by inhaling the spores of the bacterium.

anthropoid /an'thrəpoid/ [Gk, *anthropos,* human, *eidos,* form], a noun or adjective generally applied to humanlike apes or other primates; also used to describe a certain kind of pelvis in gynecology and obstetrics.

anthropoid pelvis [Gk, *anthropos,* human, *eidos,* form], a type of pelvis in which the inlet is oval; the anteroposterior diameter is much greater than the transverse. The posterior part of the space in the true pelvis is much greater than the anterior part.

anthropology [Gk, *anthropos,* human, *logos,* science], the science of human beings, from animal-like characteristics to social and environmental aspects.

anthropometry /an'thrəpom'ətrē/ [Gk, *anthropos* + *metron,* measure], the science of measuring the human body as to height, weight, and size of component parts, including skinfolds, to study and compare the relative proportions under normal and abnormal conditions. —**anthropometric,** *adj.*

anthropomorphism /an'thrəpōmôr'fizəm/ [Gk, *anthropos,* human, *morphe,* form], the assignment of human shapes and qualities to other animals.

antiadrenergic /an'ti·ad'rənur'jik, an'tī-/ [Gk, *anti* + L, *ad* + *ren,* to kidney], **1.** pertaining to the blocking of the effects of impulses transmitted by the adrenergic postganglionic fibers of the sympathetic nervous system. **2.** an antiadrenergic agent. Drugs that block the response to norepinephrine bound to alpha-adrenergic

receptors reduce the tone of smooth muscle in peripheral blood vessels, causing increased peripheral circulation and decreased blood pressure.

antiagglutinin /-əglōō'tinin/ [Gk, *anti,* against; L, *agglutinare,* to glue], a specific antibody that counteracts the effects of an agglutinin.

antiamebic /an'ti·əmē'bik/, pertaining to a medication that treats amebic infections.

antianabolic /-an'əbol'ik/, pertaining to drugs or other agents that inhibit or retard anabolic processes, such as cell division and the creation of new tissue by protein synthesis.

antianaphylaxis /-an'əfilak'sis/ [Gk, *anti,* against, *ana,* back, *phylaxis,* protection], a procedure to prevent anaphylactic reactions by injecting a patient with small desensitizing doses of the antigen.

antianemic /-ənē'mik/ [Gk, *anti* + *a* + *haima,* without blood], **1.** pertaining to a substance or procedure that counteracts or prevents a deficiency of erythrocytes. **2.** an agent used to treat or to prevent anemia.

antianginal drug /-anjī'nəl/, any medication that reduces myocardial oxygen consumption or increases oxygen supply to the myocardium to prevent symptoms of angina pectoris.

antiantibody /an'ti·an'tibodē/ [Gk, *anti* + *anti* + AS, *bodig*], an immunoglobulin formed as the result of the administration of an antibody that acts as an immunogen. The antiantibody then interacts with the antibody.

antiantitoxin /-tok'sin/ [Gk, *anti* + *anti* + *toxikon,* poison], an antiantibody that may form in the body during immunization, inhibiting or counteracting the effect of the antitoxin administered.

antiarrhythmic /-ərith'mik/ [Gk, *anti* + *rhythmos,* rhythm], **1.** pertaining to a procedure or substance that prevents, alleviates, or corrects an abnormal cardiac rhythm. **2.** an agent used to treat a cardiac arrhythmia. A defibrillator that delivers a precordial electric shock is often used to restore a normal rhythm to rapid, irregular atrial or ventricular contractions. A pacemaker may be implanted in a patient with an extremely slow heart rate or other arrhythmia. Two of the major antiarrhythmic drugs are lidocaine, which increases the threshold of electrical stimulation in the ventricles during diastole; and a combination of disopyramide, procainamide, and quinidine, which decreases the excitability of the myocardium and prolongs the refractory period. The beta-adrenergic blocking agent propranolol may be used in treating arrhythmias. Verapamil and other calcium blockers control arrhythmias by inhibiting calcium ion influx across the cell membrane of cardiac muscle.

antiarthritic /-ärthrit′ik/ [Gk, *anti,* against, *arthron,* joint, *itis,* inflammation], pertaining to a therapy that relieves symptoms of arthritis.

antibacterial /-baktir′ē-əl/ [Gk, *anti* + *bakterion,* small staff], **1.** pertaining to a substance that kills bacteria or inhibits their growth or replication. **2.** an antibacterial agent. Antibiotics synthesized chemically or derived from various microorganisms exert their bactericidal or bacteriostatic effect by interfering with the production of the bacterial cell wall; by interfering with protein synthesis, nucleic acid synthesis, or cell membrane integrity; or by inhibiting critical biosynthetic pathways in the bacteria.

antibiotic /-bī·ot′ik/ [Gk, *anti* + *bios,* life], **1.** pertaining to the ability to destroy or interfere with the development of a living organism. **2.** an antimicrobial agent, derived from cultures of a microorganism or produced semisynthetically, used to treat infections. The penicillins, derived from species of the fungus *Penicillium* or manufactured semisynthetically, consist of a thiazolidine ring fused to a beta-lactam ring connected to side chains; these agents exert their action by inhibiting mucopeptide synthesis in bacterial cell walls during multiplication of the organisms. Penicillins G and V are widely used in treating many gram-positive coccal infections but are inactivated by the enzyme penicillinase produced by strains of staphylococci; cloxacillin, dicloxacillin, methicillin, nafcillin, and oxacillin are penicillinase-resistant penicillins. Broad-spectrum penicillins effective against gram-negative organisms are ampicillin, carbenicillin, and hetacillin. Aminoglycoside antibiotics, composed of amino sugars in glycoside linkage, interfere with the synthesis of bacterial proteins and are used primarily for treating infections caused by gram-negative organisms. The aminoglycosides include gentamicin derived from *Micromonospora,* semisynthetic amikacin, kanamycin, neomycin, streptomycin, and tobramycin. Macrolide antibiotics, consisting of a large lactone ring and deoxamino sugar, interfere in protein synthesis of susceptible bacteria during multiplication without affecting nucleic acid synthesis. Polypeptide antibiotics derived from species of *Streptomyces* or certain soil bacilli vary in their spectra. Bacitracin and vancomycin are polypeptides used to treat severe staphylococcal infections; capreomycin and vancomycin are antituberculo-

sis agents; and gramicidin is included in ointments for topical infections. Among polypeptide antibiotics effective against gram-negative organisms, colistin and neomycin are administered for diarrhea caused by enteropathogenic *Escherichia coli.* The tetracyclines, including the prototype derived from *Streptomyces,* chlortetracycline, demeclocycline, doxycycline, minocycline, and oxytetracycline, are active against a wide range of gram-positive and gram-negative organisms and some rickettsiae. Antibiotics in this group are primarily bacteriostatic and are thought to exert their effect by inhibiting protein synthesis in the organisms. The cephalosporins, derived from the soil fungus *Cephalosporium* or produced semisynthetically, inhibit bacterial cell wall synthesis and resist the action of penicillinase. They are used in treating infections of the respiratory tract, urinary tract, middle ear, and bones, as well as septicemia caused by a wide range of gram-positive and gram-negative organisms. The group includes cefadroxil, cefamandole, cefazolin, cephalexin, cephaloglycin, cephaloridine, cephalothin, cephapirin, and cephradine. Chloramphenicol, a broad-spectrum antibiotic initially derived from *Streptomyces venezuelae,* inhibits protein synthesis in bacteria.

antibiotic anticancer agents, drugs that may have both antibiotic and anticancer activity. Examples include bleomycin, dactinomycin, daunorubicin, and mitomycin.

antibiotic resistant /-bī·ot′ik/, pertaining to strains of microorganisms that either developed a resistance to antibiotic medications or were never sensitive to the drug.

antibiotic sensitivity test, a laboratory method for determining the susceptibility of bacterial infections to therapy with antibiotics.

antibody (Ab) /an′tibod′ē/ [Gk, *anti* + AS, *bodig*], an immunoglobulin produced by lymphocytes in response to bacteria, viruses, or other antigenic substances. An antibody is specific to an antigen. Each class of antibody is named for its action. Antibodies include agglutinins, bacteriolysins, opsonins, and precipitin.

antibody absorption, the process of removing or tying up undesired antibodies in an antiserum reagent by allowing them to react with undesired antigens.

antibody instructive theory, a theory that each antigenic contact in the life of an individual develops a new antibody, as when a B cell comes in contact with an antigen and subsequently produces plasma cells and memory cells.

antibody-specific theory, (in immunology) a theory of antibody formation proposed in 1955 by F. M. Burnet, stating that preprogrammed, or precommitted, clones of lymphoid cells that are produced in the fetus are capable of interacting with a limited number of antigenic determinants with which the host may have contact. The theory holds that the body contains an enormous number of diverse clones of cells, each genetically programmed to synthesize a different antibody.

antibody therapy, the administration of parenteral immune globulin as a treatment for patients with immunodeficiency diseases.

antibody titer, the concentration of antibodies circulating in the bloodstream of an individual. A rising titer usually indicates the body's response to antigens associated with a developing infection.

anticancer diet /-kan′sər/, a diet, based on recommendations of the American Cancer Society (ACS), National Cancer Institute (NCI), and National Academy of Sciences, to reduce cancer risk factors associated with eating habits.

anticarcinogenic /-kär′sinəjen′ik/ [Gk, *anti,* against, *karkinos,* crab, *oma,* tumor, *genein,* to produce], pertaining to a substance or device that neutralizes the effects of a cancer-causing substance.

anticholinergic /-kō′lənur′jik/ [Gk, *anti* + *chole,* bile, *ergein,* to work], **1.** pertaining to a blockade of acetylcholine receptors that results in the inhibition of the transmission of parasympathetic nerve impulses. **2.** an anticholinergic agent that functions by competing with the neurotransmitter acetylcholine for its receptor sites at synaptic junctions. Anticholinergic drugs are used to treat spastic disorders of the gastrointestinal tract, to reduce salivary and bronchial secretions before surgery, or to dilate the pupil. Many anticholinergic agents reduce parkinsonian symptoms.

anticholinesterase /an′tikol′ənes′tərās/, a drug that inhibits or inactivates the action of acetylcholinesterase. Drugs of this class cause acetylcholine to accumulate at the junctions of various cholinergic nerve fibers and their effector sites or organs, allowing potentially continuous stimulation of cholinergic fibers throughout the central and peripheral nervous systems.

anticipation /antis′ipā′shən/, an appearance before the expected time of a periodic sign or symptom, as a malarial paroxysm or a hereditary disorder.

anticipatory adaptation /antis′əpətôr′ē/ [L, *anticipare,* to receive before], the act of adapting to a potentially distressing situation before actually confronting the problem, as when a person tries to relax before learning the results of a medical examination.

anticipatory grief, feelings of grief that develop before, rather than after, a loss.

anticipatory guidance, the psychologic preparation of a person to help relieve fear and anxiety of an event expected to be stressful. An example is the preparation of a child for surgery by explaining what will happen.

Anticipatory Guidance, a Nursing Interventions Classification defined as preparation of a patient for an anticipated developmental and/or situational crisis.

anticoagulant /-kō·ag′yələnt/ [Gk, *anti* + *coagulare,* curdle], **1.** pertaining to a substance that prevents or delays coagulation of the blood. **2.** an anticoagulant drug. Heparin, obtained from the liver and lungs of domestic animals, is a potent anticoagulant that interferes with the formation of thromboplastin, with the conversion of prothrombin to thrombin, and with the formation of fibrin from fibrinogen.

anticoagulant therapy [Gk, *anti* + L, *coagulare,* to curdle; Gk, *therapeia*], the administration of drugs that reduce the tendency of blood to coagulate, thereby reducing the risk of thrombosis.

anticodon /an′tikō′don/ [Gk, *anti* + *caudex,* book], (in genetics) a sequence of three nucleotides found in transfer ribonucleic acid (RNA). The anticodon pairs complementarily with a specific codon of messenger RNA during protein synthesis that specifies a particular amino acid in the polypeptide chain.

anticomplement, a substance other than an antigen-antibody complex that activates a serum complement, resulting in complement fixation.

anticonvulsant /-kənvul′sənt/ [Gk, *anti* + L, *convellere,* to shake], **1.** pertaining to a substance or procedure that prevents or reduces the severity of epileptic or other convulsive seizures. **2.** an anticonvulsant drug. Hydantoin derivatives, especially phenytoin, apparently exert their anticonvulsant effect by stabilizing the cell membrane and decreasing intracellular sodium, with the result that the excitability of the epileptogenic focus is reduced. Phenacemide and primidone are also used in treating grand mal epilepsy; succinic acid derivatives, valproic acid, paramethadione, and various barbiturates are among the drugs prescribed to limit or prevent petit mal seizures.

antideformity positioning and splinting /-dəfôr′mitē/, the use of splints, braces, or similar devices to prevent or control contractures or other musculoskeletal deformities that may result from disuse, burns, or other injuries.

antidepressant /-dəpres'ənt/, **1.** of or pertaining to a substance or a measure that prevents or relieves depression. **2.** an antidepressant agent. Tricyclic antidepressant agents block reuptake of amine neurotransmitters, but the exact mechanism of the antidepressant action of these drugs is unknown. Monoamine oxidase inhibitors increase the concentration of epinephrine, norepinephrine, and serotonin in storage sites in the nervous system.

antidiabetic /-dī'əbet'ik/, pertaining to an agent that prevents or relieves symptoms of diabetes.

antidiarrheal /-dī'ərē'əl/, a drug or other agent that relieves the symptoms of diarrhea. Antidiarrheals absorb water from the digestive tract, alter intestinal motility, alter electrolyte transport, or adsorb toxins or microorganisms.

antidiuretic /-dī'əret'ik/ [Gk, *anti* + *dia,* through, *ourein,* to urinate], **1.** pertaining to the suppression of urine formation. **2.** an antidiuretic agent. Antidiuretic hormone (vasopressin), produced in hypothalamic nuclei and stored in the posterior lobe of the pituitary gland, suppresses urine formation by stimulating the resorption of water in distal tubules and collecting ducts in the kidneys. —**antidiuresis,** *n.*

antidiuretic hormone (ADH), a hormone that decreases the production of urine by increasing the resorption of water by the renal tubules. ADH is secreted by cells of the hypothalamus and stored in the posterior lobe of the pituitary gland. It is released in response to a decrease in blood volume or an increased concentration of sodium or other substances in plasma, or by pain, stress, or the action of certain drugs.

antidiuretic substance (ADS), any agent that decreases the excretion of urine.

antidotal /-dō'təl/ [Gk, *anti,* against, *dotos,* that which is given], a substance that renders a poison or drug ineffective.

antidote /an'tidōt/ [Gk, *anti* + *dotos,* that which is given], a drug or other substance that opposes the action of a poison.

antidromic conduction /an'tidrom'ik/ [Gk, *anti* + *dromos,* course], the conduction of a neural impulse backward from a receptor in the midpart of an axon. It is an unnatural phenomenon and may be produced experimentally.

antiembolism hose /-em'bəliz'əm/ [Gk, *anti* + *embolos,* plug], elasticized stockings worn to prevent the formation of emboli and thrombi, especially in patients who have had surgery or who have been

restricted to bed. Return flow of the venous circulation is promoted, preventing venous stasis and dilation of the veins, conditions that predispose individuals to varicosities and thromboembolic disorders.

antiemetic /-imet'ik/ [Gk, *anti* + *emesis,* vomiting], **1.** pertaining to a substance or procedure that prevents or alleviates nausea and vomiting. **2.** an antiemetic drug or agent. Belladonna derivatives, bromides, barbiturates and other sedatives, and substances that protect the stomach lining such as lime water or mild gastric astringents have weak antiemetic properties. Chlorpromazine and other phenothiazines are sometimes effective antiemetic agents. In motion sickness scopolamine and antihistamines provide relief.

antiestrogen drug /-es'trəjən/, any of a group of hormone-based products used predominantly in cancer chemotherapy.

antifibrillatory /-fibril'ətôr'ē/, a medication or other agent that suppresses either arterial or ventricular fibrillation.

antifungal /-fung'gəl/, **1.** pertaining to a substance that kills fungi or inhibits their growth or reproduction. **2.** an antifungal, antibiotic drug. Amphotericin B and ketoconazole, both effective against a broad spectrum of fungi, probably act by binding to sterols in the fungal cell membrane and changing the membrane's permeability. Griseofulvin, another broad-spectrum antifungal agent, binds to the host's new keratin and renders it resistant to further fungal invasion. Miconazole inhibits the growth of common dermatophytes, including yeastlike *Candida albicans;* nystatin is effective against yeast and yeastlike fungi.

antigalactic /-gəlak'tik/, pertaining to a drug or other agent that prevents or reduces milk secretion in some mothers of newborns.

anti-GBM disease, an immunologically mediated kidney disorder involving the glomerular basement membrane, which is damaged in the antigen-antibody reaction. The kidney itself may serve as the antigenic target in the reaction.

antigen /an'tijən/ [Gk, *anti* + *genein,* to produce], a substance, usually a protein, that causes the formation of an antibody and reacts specifically with that antigen.

antigen-antibody reaction, a process of the immune system in which immunoglobulin-coated B cells recognize an intruder or antigen and stimulate antibody production. The T cells assist in the antigen-antibody reaction, but the B cells play the key role. Antigen-antibody reactions activate the complement system of the body, amplifying the humoral immunity response of the B cells and causing lysis of the antigenic cells. Antigen-antibody reactions involve the binding of antigens to antibodies to form antigen-antibody complexes that may render the toxic antigen harmless, agglutinize antigens on the surface of microorganisms, or activate the complement system by exposing the complement-binding sites on the antibody molecule. Antigen-antibody reactions normally produce immunity, but they can also produce allergy, autoimmunity, and fetomaternal hematologic incompatibility.

antigen determinant, a small area on the surface of an antigen molecule that fits a combining site of an antibody molecule and binds the antigen in the formation of an antigen-antibody complex. Antigen determinants commonly consist of a sequence of amino acids that determines the shape of these reactive areas.

antigenic /-jen'ik/, provoking an immune response or reacting with antibodies.

antigenic drift [Gk, anti, against, genein, to produce; AS, drifan, drift], the tendency of a virus or other microorganism to alter its genetic makeup, periodically producing a mutant antigen requiring new antibodies and vaccines to combat its effects.

antigenicity /an'tijənis'ətē/, the ability to cause the production of antibodies. The degree of antigenicity depends on the kind and amount of the particular substance and the degree to which the host is sensitive to the antigen and able to produce antibodies.

antigen-presenting cell, a cell that can break down protein antigens into peptides and present them, in conjunction with major histocompatibility complex class II molecules, on the cell surface, where they can interact with T cell receptors.

antigen processing, the steps that occur in an antigenic reaction after a protein is recognized as a foreign, or nonself, substance.

antigen unit, the smallest amount of antigen required to fix one unit of complement.

antiglobulin /an'tiglob'yo͞olin/ [Gk, anti + L, globulus, small globe], an antibody that occurs naturally or is prepared in laboratory animals to be used against human globulin. Specific antiglobulins are used in the detection of specific antibodies, as in blood typing.

antiglobulin test, a test for the presence of antibodies that coat and damage red blood cells as a result of any of several diseases or conditions. The test can detect Rh antibodies in maternal blood and is used to anticipate hemolytic disease of the newborn.

antigravity muscles /-grav'itē/, the muscle groups involved in stabilization of joints or other body parts by opposing the effects of gravity.

antihemophilic factor (AHF) /-hē'mōfil'ik/, blood factor VIII, a systemic hemostatic prescribed in the treatment of hemophilia A, a deficiency of factor VIII.

antihemophilic factor plasma [Gk, anti, against, haima, blood, philein, to love; L, facere, to make; Gk, plassein, to mold], blood plasma that contains the antihemophilic factor VIII.

antihemorrhagic /-hē'mōraj'ik/, any drug or agent used to prevent or control bleeding, such as thromboplastin or thrombin, either of which mediates the blood clotting process.

antihidrotic /-hidrot'ik/ [Gk, anti, + hidros, sweat], an agent that inhibits or prevents the production of sweat.

antihistamine /-his'təmin/ [Gk, anti + histos, tissue, amine (ammonia compound)], any substance capable of reducing the physiologic and pharmacologic effects of histamine, including a wide variety of drugs that block histamine receptors. Many such drugs are readily available as nonprescription medicines for the management of allergies. These substances do not stop the release of histamine, and the ways in which they act on the central nervous system are not completely understood. The antihistamines are divided into histamine H_1 and H_2 blockers, depending on the responses to histamine they prevent.

antihistamine poisoning, an adverse reaction to an excessive intake of antihistamine medication. Symptoms include fatigue, lethargy, delirium, hallucinations, loss of voluntary muscle control, hyperreflexia, tachycardia, dilated pupils, and in severe cases coma. Emergency treatment may include ingestion of activated charcoal, lavage or emesis, administration of oxygen, and artificial respiration.

antihistaminic [Gk, anti + histos, tissue, amine], pertaining to a substance that counteracts the effects of histamine.

antihypercholesterolemic /-hī'pərkō'-leə'tərōlē'mik/, a drug that prevents or controls an increase of cholesterol in the blood. Examples include clofibrate, lovastatin, and colestipol.

antihypertensive /-hī-pərten'siv/, **1.** pertaining to a substance or procedure that reduces high blood pressure. **2.** an antihypertensive agent. Various drugs achieve their antihypertensive effect by depleting tissue stores of catecholamines in peripheral sites, by stimulating pressor receptors in the carotid sinus and heart, by blocking autonomic nerve impulses that constrict blood vessels, by stimulating central inhibitory alpha-adrenergic receptors, or by direct vasodilation. Thiazides and other diuretic agents reduce blood pressure by decreasing blood volume.

antihypotensive /-hī'pōten'siv/, pertaining to any medication or other agent that tends to increase blood pressure.

antiimmune /an'ti·imyo̅o̅n'/ [Gk, anti + L, immunis, free from], pertaining to the prevention or inhibition of immunity.

antiinfectious /-infek'shəs/ [Gk, anti + L, inficere, to stain], pertaining to an agent that prevents or treats infection.

antiinflammatory /-inflam'ətor'ē/ [Gk, anti + L, inflammare, to set afire], 1. pertaining to a substance or procedure that counteracts or reduces inflammation. 2. an antiinflammatory drug or agent. The basis of the antiinflammatory effect of salicylates and nonsteroidal antiinflammatory agents such as ibuprofen, phenylbutazone, and indomethacin appears to involve inhibition of prostaglandin biosynthesis.

antiinitiator /-inish'ē·ātər/, a substance that is a potential cocarcinogen but that may protect cells against cancer development if given before exposure to an initiator.

antileprotic /-leprot'ik/, a drug or other agent that is effective in treating leprosy.

antilipidemic /an'tilip'idē'mik/ [Gk, anti + lipos, fat, haima, blood], 1. pertaining to a regimen, diet, or agent that reduces the amount of lipids in the serum. 2. a drug used to reduce the amount of lipids in the serum.

antilymphocyte serum (ALS) /-lim'fəsīt/, a serum prescribed as an immunosuppressive agent for the reduction of rejection reactions in organ transplantation and as an adjunct in chemotherapy for malignant neoplasms.

antimalarial /-məler'ē·əl/, 1. pertaining to a substance that destroys or suppresses the development of malaria plasmodia or to a procedure that exterminates the mosquito vectors of the disease, such as spraying insecticides or draining swamps. 2. an antimalarial drug that destroys or prevents the development of plasmodia in human hosts.

antimessage, a strand of ribonucleic acid (RNA) that cannot act as messenger RNA because of its negative coding sequence. It must be converted to a positive-strand sequence by a viral transcriptase before it can function as a messenger.

antimetabolite /-mətab'əlīt/ [Gk, anti + metabole, change], a drug or other substance that is an antagonist to or resembles a normal human metabolite and interferes with its function in the body, usually by

competing for the its receptors or enzymes.

antimicrobial /-mīkrō'bē·əl/ [Gk, anti + mikros, small, bios, life], 1. pertaining to a substance that kills microorganisms or inhibits their growth or replication. 2. an agent that kills or inhibits the growth or replication of microorganisms.

antimicrobial drugs [Gk, anti + mikros, small, bios, life, Fr, drogue], drugs that destroy or inhibit the growth of microorganisms.

antimicrobic /-mīkrob'ik/, any agent that prevents or destroys microorganisms or inhibits their growth.

antimitochondrial antibody /-mī'tōkon'drē·əl/, an antibody that acts specifically against mitochondria. These antibodies are not normally present in the blood of healthy people. A laboratory test for the presence of antibodies in the blood is a valuable diagnostic aid in liver disease.

antimitotic /-mītot'ik/, pertaining to the inhibition of cell division.

antimony (Sb) /an'təmō'nē/ [L antimonium], a bluish, crystalline metallic element occurring in nature, both free and as salts. Various antimony compounds are used in the treatment of filariasis, leishmaniasis, lymphogranuloma, schistosomiasis, and trypanosomiasis and as emetics.

antimony poisoning, toxic effect caused by the ingestion or inhalation of antimony or antimony compounds, characterized by vomiting, sweating, diarrhea, and a metallic taste in the mouth. Irritation of the skin or mucous membrane may result from external exposure. Severe poisoning resembles arsenic poisoning.

antimorph /an'təmôrf/ [Gk, anti + morphe, form], a mutant gene that inhibits or antagonizes the normal influence of its allele in the expression of a trait.

antimuscarinic /-mus'kərin'ik/ [Gk, anti + L, musca, fly], inhibiting the stimulation of the postganglionic parasympathetic receptor.

antimutagen /-myoo͞'təjən/ [Gk, anti + L, mutare, to change; Gk, genein, to produce], 1. any substance that reduces the rate of spontaneous mutations or counteracts or reverses the action of a mutagen. 2. any technique that protects cells against the effects of mutagenic agents.—**antimutagenic,** adj.

antineoplastic /-nē'ōplas'tik/ [Gk, anti + neos, new, plasma, something formed], 1. pertaining to a substance, procedure, or measure that prevents the proliferation of malignant cells. 2. a chemotherapeutic agent that controls or kills cancer cells. Drugs used in the treatment of cancer are cytotoxic but are generally more damaging to dividing cells than to resting cells. Cycle-specific antineoplastic agents are more effective in killing proliferating cells than in killing resting cells, and phase-specific agents are most active during a specific phase of the cell cycle. Most anticancer drugs prevent the proliferation of cells by inhibiting the synthesis of deoxyribonucleic acid (DNA) by various mechanisms.

antineoplastic antibiotic, a chemical substance derived from a microorganism or a synthetic analog of the substance, used in cancer chemotherapy.

antineoplastic hormone, a chemical substance produced by an endocrine gland or a synthetic analog of the naturally occurring compound, used to control certain disseminated cancers. Hormonal therapy is designed to counteract the effect of an endogenous hormone required for tumor growth.

antinuclear antibody (ANA) /-nōō'klē-ər/, an autoantibody that reacts with nuclear material. Antinuclear antibodies are found in the blood serum of patients with rheumatoid arthritis, systemic lupus erythematosus, Sjögren's syndrome, polymyositis, and a number of nonrheumatic disorders.

antiodontalgia /an'ti-ō'dontal'jə/, a toothache remedy.

antioncogene /au'ti-on'kəjēn/, a tumor-suppressing gene. It may act by controlling cellular growth. When an antioncogene is inactivated, tumor cellular proliferation begins, and tumor activity accelerates.

antioxidant /-ok'sidənt/, a chemical or other agent that inhibits or retards oxidation of a substance to which it is added. Examples include butylated hydroxyanisole and butylated hydroxytoluene. These substances are added to foods containing fats or oils to prevent oxygen from combining with the fatty molecules, thereby causing them to become rancid.

antioxidation /-ok'sidā'shən/, the prevention of oxidation.

antiparallel /-per'əlal/ [Gk, anti + parallelos, side-by-side], (in molecular genetics) the condition in which molecules such as double-helical strands of deoxyribonucleic acid are parallel but are oriented in opposite directions.

antiparasitic /-per'əsit'ik/ [Gk, anti + parasitos, guest], **1.** pertaining to a substance or procedure that kills parasites or inhibits their growth or reproduction. **2.** an antiparasitic drug such as an amebicide, an anthelmintic, an antimalarial, a schistosomicide, a trichomonacide, or a trypanosomicide.

antiparkinsonian /-pär'kənsəniz'əm/, pertaining to a substance or procedure used to treat parkinsonism. Drugs for this neurologic disorder are of two kinds: those that compensate for the lack of dopamine in the corpus striatum of parkinsonism patients, and anticholinergic agents that counteract the activity of the abundant acetylcholine in the striatum.

antipathic /-path'ik/, pertaining to a strong or excessive aversion or dislike.

antipathy /antip'əthē/ [Gk, anti + pathos, suffering], a strong feeling of aversion or antagonism to particular objects, situations, or individuals.

antiperistalsis /-per'əstal'sis/, a wave of contractions in the digestive tract that moves toward the oral end of the tract. In the duodenum, stomach, or esophagus it results in regurgitation.

antiperistaltic /-per'əstal'tik/ [Gk, anti + peristellein, to wrap around], **1.** pertaining to a substance that inhibits or diminishes peristalsis. **2.** an antiperistaltic agent. Narcotics such as paregoric, diphenoxylate, and loperamide hydrochloride are antiperistaltic agents used to provide symptomatic relief in diarrhea. Anticholinergic (parasympatholytic) drugs reduce spasms of intestinal smooth muscle and are frequently prescribed to decrease excessive gastrointestinal motility.

antiplatelet /-plat'lit/, any agent that destroys platelets or inhibits their function.

antipode /an'tipōd/, something that is diametrically opposite.

antipraxia /prak'sē-ə/, a condition in which functions or symptoms appear to oppose each other.

antiprogestin /-prōjes'tin/, a substance that interferes with the production, uptake, or effects of progesterone.

antiprotease, a substance that is capable of preventing proteolysis.

antiprothrombin /prōthrom'bin/, a substance that inhibits the conversion of prothrombin to thrombin.

antiprotoplasmatic /-prō'təplasmat'ik/, pertaining to agents that damage the protoplasm of cells.

antipruritic /-prōōrit'ik/ [Gk, anti + L, prurire, to itch], **1.** pertaining to a substance or procedure that tends to relieve or prevent itching. **2.** an antipruritic drug. Topical anesthetics, corticosteroids, and antihistamines are used as antipruritic agents.

antipsoriatic /an'tisôr'ē-at'ik/ [Gk, anti + psora, itch], pertaining to an agent that relieves the symptoms of psoriasis.

antipsychotic /-sīkot'ik/ [Gk, anti + psyche, mind, osis, condition], **1.** pertaining to a substance or procedure that counteracts or diminishes symptoms of a psychosis. **2.** an antipsychotic drug. Phenothiazine derivatives are the most frequently prescribed antipsychotics for use in the treatment of schizophrenia and other major affective disorders.

antipyresis /-pīrē'sis/ [Gk, *anti + pyretos,* fever], treatment to reduce and ameliorate fever.

antipyretic /-pīret'ik/ [Gk, *anti + pyretos,* fever], **1.** pertaining to a substance or procedure that reduces fever. **2.** an antipyretic agent. Such drugs usually lower the thermodetection set point of the hypothalamic heat regulatory center, with resulting vasodilation and sweating. A tepid alcohol sponge bath or lukewarm tub bath may decrease an elevated temperature, and hypothermia produced by a cooling blanket is sometimes used for patients with a prolonged high fever.

antipyretic bath, a bath in which tepid water is used to reduce body temperature.

antipyrotic /-pīrot'ik/ [Gk, *anti + pyr,* fire], pertaining to the treatment of burns or scalds.

antirachitic /-rəkit'ik/, pertaining to an agent used to treat rickets.

anti-Rh agglutinin, an antibody to the Rh antigen present on Rh+ red blood cells that causes these cells to clump (agglutinate). This antibody is produced by Rh− persons after exposure to Rh+ red blood cells, as when an Rh− mother is pregnant with an Rh+ fetus.

antirheumatic /-rŏŏmat'ik/ [Gk, *anti + rheumatismos,* that which flows], pertaining to the relief of symptoms of any painful or immobilizing disorder of the musculoskeletal system.

antiseborrheic /-seb'ərē'ik/, pertaining to a drug or agent that is applied to the skin to control seborrhea or seborrheic dermatitis.

antisense /an'tēsens/, (molecular genetics) a ribonucleic acid (RNA) molecule that is complementary to the messenger RNA (mRNA) (sense) molecule produced by transcription of a given gene. The antisense strands of many genes have been synthesized in the laboratory and are useful because they hybridize with the mRNA sense strand and block their translation into amino acids and proteins.

antisepsis /-sep'sis/ [Gk, *anti + sepein,* putrefaction], destruction of microorganisms to prevent infection.

antiseptic /-sep'tik/, **1.** tending to inhibit the growth and reproduction of microorganisms. **2.** a substance that tends to inhibit the growth and reproduction of microorganisms.

antiseptic dressing, a fabric or pad treated with a solution and applied to a wound or an incision to prevent or treat infection.

antiseptic gauze, a dressing permeated with a solution to prevent infection, sometimes packaged in individual sealed packets.

antiserum /an'tisir'əm/, *pl.* **antisera, antiserums** [Gk, *anti* + L, whey], serum of an animal or human containing antibodies against a specific disease, used to confer passive immunity to that disease. Antisera do not provoke the production of antibodies. There are two types of antiserum: antitoxin is an antiserum that neutralizes the toxin produced by specific bacteria, but it does not kill the bacteria; antimicrobial serum acts to destroy bacteria by making them more susceptible to the leukocytic action.

antiserum anaphylaxis, an exaggerated reaction of hypersensitivity in a normal person after the injection of serum from a sensitized individual.

antishock garment, trousers designed to apply pressure on circulation in the lower part of the body, thereby increasing the amount of blood in the upper part.

antisialogogue /-sī·al'əgŏg'/ [Gk, *anti* + *sialon,* saliva, *agogos,* leading], a drug that reduces saliva secretion.

antisocial personality /-sō'shəl/ [Gk, *anti* + L, *socius,* companion], a person who exhibits attitudes and overt behavior contrary to the customs, standards, and moral principles accepted by society.

antisocial personality disorder, a condition characterized by repetitive behavioral patterns that are contrary to usual moral and ethical standards and cause a person to experience continuous conflict with society. Symptoms include aggressiveness, callousness, impulsiveness, irresponsibility, hostility, a low frustration level, a marked emotional immaturity, and poor judgment.

antispasmodic /-spazmod'ik/, a drug or other agent that prevents smooth muscle spasms, as in the uterus, digestive system, or urinary tract.

antistreptolysin-O test (ASOT, ASO, ASLT) /an'tistrep'təlī'sinō'/, a streptococcal antibody test for finding and measuring serum antibodies to streptolysin-O, an exotoxin produced by most group A and some group C and G streptococci. The test is often used as an aid in the diagnosis of rheumatic fever.

antithrombin /-throm'bin/, a substance that inhibits the action of thrombin.

antithrombotic /-thrombot'ik/, preventing or interfering with the formation of a thrombus or blood coagulation.

antithymocyte globulin (ATG) /an'tithī'məsīt/, a gamma globulin fraction rendered immune to T lymphocytes.

antithyroid drug /-thī'roid/, a preparation that inhibits the synthesis of thyroid hormones and is commonly used in the treatment of hyperthyroidism. The major antithyroid drugs are thioamides, such as propylthiouracil, and methimazole. In the body such substances interfere with the incorporation of iodine into the tyrosyl residues of thyroglobulin required for the production of the hormones thyroxine and triiodothyronine.

antitoxin /-tok'sin/ [Gk, anti + toxikon, poison], a subgroup of antisera usually prepared from the serum of horses immunized against a particular toxin-producing organism, such as botulism antitoxin given therapeutically in botulism and tetanus and diphtheria antitoxin given prophylactically to prevent those infections.

antitrismus /-tris'məs/, a tonic muscular spasm that forces the mouth to open.

antitrust /-trust'/, (in law) against the operation, establishment, or maintenance of a monopoly in the manufacture, production, or sale of a commodity, provision of a service, or practice of a profession.

antitrypsin /-trip'sin/, a protein produced in the liver that blocks the action of trypsin and other proteolytic enzymes.

antitubercular /-toōbur'kyələr/, any agent or group of drugs used to treat tuberculosis. At least two drugs, and usually three, are required in various combinations in pulmonary tuberculosis therapy.

antitumor antibodies, natural products that interfere with deoxyribonucleic acid in such a way as to prevent its further replication and the transcription of ribonucleic acid.

antitussive /an'titus'iv/ [Gk, anti + L, tussive, cough], 1. against a cough. 2. any of a large group of narcotic and nonnarcotic drugs that act on the central and peripheral nervous systems to suppress the cough reflex. Because the cough reflex is necessary for clearing the upper respiratory tract of obstructive secretions, antitussives should not be used with a productive cough.

antivenin /an'tiven'in/ [Gk, anti + L, venenum, poison], a suspension of venom-neutralizing antibodies prepared from the serum of immunized horses. Antivenin confers passive immunity and is given as a part of emergency first aid for various snake and insect bites.

antiviral, destructive to viruses.

antivitamin [Gk, anti + L, vita, life, amine], a substance that inactivates a vitamin.

Anton's syndrome [Gabriel Anton, German neuropsychiatrist, 1858–1933], a form of anosognosia in which a person with partial or total blindness denies being visually impaired, despite medical evidence to the contrary.

antral gastritis [Gk, antron, cave], an abnormal narrowing of the antrum, or distal part, of the stomach. The narrowing is not a true gastritis, but a radiographic finding that may represent gastric ulcer or tumor.

antrectomy /antrek'təmē/, the surgical excision of the pyloric part of the stomach.

antrum, pl. **antra** [Gk, antron, cave], a hollow body area usually surrounded by bone. The cardiac antrum is a dilation of the esophagus. The fluid-filled cavity in a mature graafian follicle is also termed an antrum.

antrum cardiacum /an'trəm/, a constricted passage from the esophagus to the stomach, lying just inside the opening formed by the cardiac sphincter.

ANUG, abbreviation for **acute necrotizing ulcerative gingivitis.**

anular /an'yələr/ [L, annulus, ring], describing a ring-shaped lesion surrounding a clear, normal, unaffected disk of skin.

anular ligament, a ligament that encircles the head of the radius and holds it in the radial notch of the ulna. Distal to the notch, the anular ligament forms a complete fibrous ring.

anulus /an'yələs/, a ring of circular tissue, such as the whitish tympanic anulus around the perimeter of the tympanic membrane.

anuria /ənŏŏr'ē·ə/ [Gk, a, ouron, not urine], the cessation of urine production or a urinary output of less than 100 ml per day. Anuria may be caused by kidney failure or dysfunction, a decline in blood pressure below that required to maintain filtration pressure in the kidney, or an obstruction in the urinary passages. A rapid decline in urinary output, leading ultimately to anuria and uremia, occurs in acute renal failure.—**anuric, anuretic,** adj.

anus /ā'nəs/, the opening at the terminal end of the anal canal.

anxietas /angzī'ətas/ [L, anxiety], a state of anxiety, nervous restlessness, or apprehension, often accompanied by a feeling of oppression in the epigastrium. Kinds of anxietas are **anxietas presenilis** and **restless legs syndrome.**

anxietas presenilis [L, anxietas + prae, before, senex, aged], a state of extreme anxiety associated with the climacteric period of life.

anxiety /angzī'ətē/ [L anxietas], anticipation of impending danger and dread accompanied by restlessness, tension, tachycardia, and breathing difficulty not associated with an apparent stimulus.

anxiety, a NANDA-accepted nursing diagnosis defined as a vague, uneasy feeling, the source of which is often nonspecific or unknown to the individual. Defining characteristics of anxiety may be subjective or objective. Subjective characteristics include increased tension, apprehension, persistent increased helplessness, and feelings of uncertainty, fear, distress, and impending doom. Objective characteristics include increased heart rate, dilated pupils, restlessness, poor eye contact, trembling, increased perspiration, and expressed concern regarding life events.

anxiety attack, an acute psychobiologic reaction manifested by intense anxiety and panic. Symptoms vary according to the individual and the intensity of the attack but typically include palpitations, shortness of breath, dizziness, faintness, profuse sweating, pallor of the face and extremities, gastrointestinal discomfort, and a vague feeling of imminent doom or death.

anxiety disorder, a disorder in which anxiety is the most prominent feature. The symptoms range from mild, chronic tenseness, with feelings of timidity, fatigue, apprehension, and indecisiveness, to more intense states of restlessness and irritability that may lead to aggressive acts, persistent helplessness, or withdrawal.

anxiety dream, a dream that is accompanied by restlessness and a gradual increase in pulse rate.

anxiety hysteria [L, *anxietas;* Gk, *hystera,* womb], a disorder characterized by symptoms of both anxiety and hysteria.

anxiety reaction [L, *anxietas + re, agere,* to act], a clinical characteristic in which anxiety is the predominant feature or is experienced by a person facing a dreaded situation to the extent that his or her functioning is impaired. The reaction may be expressed as a panic disorder, a phobia, or a compulsion.

Anxiety Reduction, a Nursing Interventions Classification defined as minimizing apprehension, dread, foreboding, or uneasiness related to an unidentified source of anticipated danger.

anxiety state [L, *anxietas + state*], a mental or emotional reaction characterized by apprehension, uncertainty, and irrational fear. Anxiety states may be accompanied by physiologic changes such as rapid heartbeat, dilated pupils, and dry mouth.

anxiolytic /angk′sē-ōlit′ik/, a sedative or minor tranquilizer used primarily to treat episodes of anxiety. Kinds of anxiolytics include barbiturates, benzodiazepines,

chlormezanone, hydroxyzine, meprobamate, and tybamate.

AOA, abbreviation for **Administration on Aging.**

AORN, abbreviation for **Association of Operating Room Nurses.**

aorta /ā·ôr′tə/ [Gk, *aerein,* to raise], the main trunk of the systemic arterial circulation, comprising four parts: the ascending aorta, the arch of the aorta, the thoracic part of the descending aorta, and the abdominal part of the descending aorta. It starts at the aortic opening of the left ventricle, rises a short distance, bends over the root of the left lung, descends within the thorax on the left side of the vertebral column, and passes through the aortic hiatus of the diaphragm into the abdominal cavity.

aortic /ā·ôr′tik/ [Gk, *aerein,* to raise], pertaining to the aorta.

aortic aneurysm, a localized dilation of the wall of the aorta caused by atherosclerosis, hypertension, or, less frequently, syphilis. The lesion may be a saccular distension, a fusiform or cylindroid swelling of a length of the vessel, or a longitudinal dissection between the outer and middle layers of the vessel wall.

aortic angiogram, a set of radiographic images of the aorta, taken after the injection of an iodinated contrast medium.

aortic arch syndrome, any of a group of occlusive conditions of the aortic arch producing a variety of symptoms related to obstruction of the large branch arteries. Such conditions as atherosclerosis, Takayasu's arteritis, and syphilis may cause aortic arch syndrome. The symptoms include syncope, temporary blindness, hemiplegia, aphasia, and memory loss.

aortic atresia [Gk, *aeirein + a, tresis,* a boring], a congenital anomaly in which the left side of the heart is defective and there is an imperforation of the aortic valve.

aortic notch [Gk, *aeirein,* to raise; OFr, *enochier*], the dicrotic notch on the descending limb of an arterial pulse sphygmogram. It marks the closure of the aortic valve and immediately precedes the dicrotic wave.

aortic obstruction [L, *obstruere,* to build against], a blockage or impediment that interrupts the flow of blood in the aorta.

aortic regurgitant murmur [Gk, *aeirein,* to raise; L, *re,* again, *gurgitare,* to flow, *murmur,* humming], a high-pitched, early diastolic heart murmur that is a sign of aortic incompetence. A failure of the aortic valves to close completely during ventricular diastole allows some blood to flow back into the left ventricle.

aortic regurgitation, the blood flow during systole from the aorta back into the left ventricle.

aortic sinus [Gk, *aeirein,* to raise; L, *sinus,* little hollow], any of three dilations, one anterior and two posterior, between the aortic wall and the semilunar cusps of the aortic valve.

aortic stenosis (AS) [Gk, *aeirein* + *stenos,* narrow, *osis,* condition], a cardiac anomaly characterized by a narrowing or stricture of the aortic valve. It is secondary to congenital malformation or of fusion of the cusps, as may result from rheumatic fever. Aortic stenosis obstructs the blood flow from the left ventricle into the aorta, causing decreased cardiac output and pulmonary vascular congestion.

aortic thrill [Gk, *aeirein,* to raise; AS, *thyrlian*], a palpable chest vibration caused by stenosis of the aortic valve or by an aortic aneurysm. It is usually felt or palpated in the second intercostal space to the right of the sternum in systole, by using the flat of the hand or the fingertips.

aortic valve, a valve in the heart between the left ventricle and the aorta. It is composed of three semilunar cusps that close in diastole to prevent blood from flowing back into the left ventricle from the aorta.

aortitis /ā′ôrtī′tis/, an inflammatory condition of the aorta. It occurs most frequently in tertiary syphilis and occasionally in rheumatic fever.

aortocoronary /ā·ôr′tōkôr′əner′ē/ [Gk, *aeirein* + L, *corona,* crown], pertaining to the aorta and coronary arteries.

aortocoronary bypass [AS, *bi,* alongside; Fr, *passer*], a surgical procedure for treatment of angina pectoris or coronary vessel disease, in which a saphenous vein, mammary artery, or other blood vessel or a synthetic graft is used to build a shunt from the aorta to one of the coronary arteries to bypass a circulatory obstruction.

aortogram /ā-ôr′təgram/ [Gk, *aeirein* + *gramma,* record], a radiographic image of the aorta made after the injection of a radiopaque medium in the blood.

aortography /ā-ôrtog′rəfē/ [Gk, *aeirein* + *graphein,* to record], a radiographic process in which the aorta and its branches are injected with any of various contrast media for visualization. —**aortographic,** *adj.*

aortopulmonary fenestration /ā-ôr′tōpul′mənər′ē/ [Gk, *aerein* + L, *pulmoneus,* lung, *fenestra,* window], a congenital anomaly characterized by an abnormal fenestration in the ascending aorta and the pulmonary artery cephalad to the semilunar valve, allowing oxygenated and unoxygenated blood to mix.

AOTA, abbreviation for American Occupational Therapy Association.

AOTCB, abbreviation for *American Occupational Therapy Certification Board.*

AOTF, abbreviation for *American Occupational Therapy Foundation.*

AP, abbreviation for **anteroposterior.**

APA, 1. abbreviation for **American Psychiatric Association. 2.** abbreviation for *American Psychological Association.*

APACHE /əpach′ē/, an acronym for *Acute Physiology and Chronic Health Evaluation,* a system of classifying severity of illnesses in intensive care patients.

apareunia /ā′pərо̄о̄′nē-ə/, an inability to perform sexual intercourse caused by a physical or psychologic sexual dysfunction.

apathetic hyperthyroidism /ap′əthet′ik/, a form of thyrotoxicosis that tends to affect mainly older adults who have stereotyped "senile" physical features and whose behavior is apathetic and inactive rather than hyperkinetic.

apathy /ap′əthē/ [Gk, *a, pathos,* not suffering], an absence or suppression of emotion, feeling, concern, or passion; an indifference to stimuli found generally to be exciting or moving. —**apathetic,** *adj.*

apatite /ap′ətīt/ [Gk, *apate,* deceit], an inorganic mineral composed of calcium and phosphate that is found in the bones and teeth.

APC, 1. abbreviation for **aspirin, phenacetin, caffeine. 2.** abbreviation for *atrial premature contraction.* **3.** abbreviation for **adenomatous polyposis coli.**

APD, abbreviation for adult polycystic disease.

apepsia /āpep′sē-ə/ [Gk, *a,* without, *pepsis,* digestion], a condition involving a failure of the digestive functions.

aperient /əpir′ē-ənt/ [L., *aperire,* to open], a mild laxative.

aperistalsis /āper′istal′sis/ [Gk, *a,* without, *peristellein,* to clasp], a failure of the normal waves of contraction and relaxation that move contents through the digestive tract.

aperitive /əper′itiv/ [L, *aperere,* to open], a stimulant of the appetite.

Apert's syndrome /äperz′/ [Eugene Apert, French pediatrician, 1868–1940], a rare condition characterized by an abnormal craniofacial appearance in combination with partial or complete fusion of the fingers and toes.

aperture /ap′ərchər/ [L, *apertura,* an opening], an opening or hole in an object or anatomic structure.

aperture of frontal sinus, an external opening of the frontal sinus into the nasal cavity.

aperture of glottis, an opening between the true vocal cords and the arytenoid cartilages.

aperture of larynx, an opening between the pharynx and larynx.

aperture of sphenoid sinus, a round opening between the sphenoid sinus and nasal cavity, situated just above the superior nasal concha.

apex /ā′peks/, *pl.* **apices** /ā′pisēz/ [L, tip], the top, end, or tip of a structure, such as the apex of the heart or the apices of the teeth.

apex beat, a pulsation of the left ventricle of the heart, palpable and sometimes visible at the fifth intercostal space.

apexcardiogram (ACG) /-kär′dē-əgram′/, a graphic representation of the pulsations of the chest over the heart in the region of the cardiac apex.

apexcardiography (ACG) /-kär′dē-og′-rəfē/, the recording of heart pulsations obtained from the cardiac apex.

apex cordis [L, *apex + cordis,* of the heart], the pointed lower border of the heart. It is directed downward, forward, and to the left and is usually located at the level of the fifth intercostal space.

apexification /-if′ikā′shən/ [L, *apex + facere,* to make], (in dentistry) the process of induced tooth root development or apical closure of the root by the placement of hard material after an apicoectomy.

apexigraph /āpek′sigraf′/, (in dentistry) a device used for determining the position of the apex of a tooth root.

apex murmur [L, *apex,* summit, *murmur,* humming], a sound heard best at the apex of the heart.

apex of the lung, the highest point of the lung as it extends to the level of the first rib at the base of the neck.

apex pneumonia [L, *apex,* summit; Gk, *pnemon,* lung], pneumonia in which consolidation is limited to the upper lobe of one lung.

apex pulmonis /pəlmō′nis/ [L, *apex + pulmoneus,* lung], the rounded upper border of each lung, projecting above the clavicle.

Apgar score /ap′gär/ [Virginia Apgar, American anesthesiologist, 1909–1974], the evaluation of an infant's physical condition, usually performed 1 minute and again 5 minutes after birth, based on a rating of five factors that reflect the infant's ability to adjust to extrauterine life. The infant's heart rate, respiratory effort, muscle tone, reflex irritability, and color are scored from a low value of 0 to a normal value of 2. The five scores are combined, and the totals at 1 minute and 5 minutes are noted; for example, Apgar 9/10 is a score of 9 at 1 minute and 10 at 5 minutes.

APHA, abbreviation for *American Public Health Association.*

aphagia /əfā′jē-ə/ [Gk, *a + phagein,* not to eat], a condition characterized by the loss of the ability to swallow as a result of organic or psychologic causes.

aphagia algera, a condition characterized by the refusal to eat or swallow because doing so causes pain.

aphakia /əfā′kē-ə/ [Gk, *a, phakos,* not lens], (in ophthalmology) a condition in which part or all of the crystalline lens of the eye is absent, usually because it has been surgically removed, as in the treatment of cataracts. **—aphakic, aphacic,** *adj.*

aphasia /əfā′zhə/ [Gk, *a + phasis,* not speech], an abnormal neurologic condition in which language function is defective or absent because of an injury to certain areas of the cerebral cortex. The deficiency may be sensory or receptive, in which language is not understood, or expressive or motor, in which words cannot be formed or expressed.

aphasic, pertaining to **aphasia.**

aphemia /əfē′mē-ə/, a loss of the ability to speak. The term is applied to emotional disorders, as well as neurologic causes.

apheresis /əfer′əsis, af′ərē′sis/ [Gk, *aphairesis,* removal], a procedure in which blood is temporarily withdrawn, one or more components are selectively removed, and the rest of the blood is reinfused into the donor. The process is used in treating various disease conditions in the donor, for obtaining blood elements for treatment of other patients, or for research purposes.

aphonia /āfō′nē-ə/ [Gk, *a, phone,* without voice], a condition characterized by loss of the ability to produce normal speech sounds that results from overuse of the vocal cords, organic disease, or psychologic causes such as anxiety. **—aphonic, aphonous,** *adj.*

aphonia paralytica /par′əlit′ikə/, a condition characterized by a loss of the voice caused by paralysis or disease of the laryngeal nerves.

aphonia paranoica, an inability to speak that lacks an organic basis and that is characteristic of some forms of mental illness.

aphonic pectoriloquy /āfon′ik/, the abnormal transmission of voice sounds through a cavity or a serous pleural effusion detected during auscultation of a lung.

aphonic speech, abnormal speech in which vocalizations are whispered.

aphoria /əfôr′ē-ə/, a condition in which

physical weakness is not lessened as a result of exercise.

aphrasia /əfā′zhə/, a form of aphasia in which a person may be able to speak or understand single words but is not able to communicate with words that are arranged in meaningful phrases or sentences.

aphronia /əfrō′nē·ə/ [Gk, *a, phronein,* not to understand], (in psychiatry) a condition characterized by an impaired ability to make common-sense decisions. **—aphronic,** *n., adj.*

aphthae /af′thē/ [Gk, *aphtha,* eruption], a common condition of shallow, painful ulcerations that usually affect the oral mucosa. Aphthae occasionally may affect other body tissues, including the gastrointestinal tract and the external genitalia.

aphthous [Gk, *aphtha,* eruption], pertaining to aphthae.

aphthous stomatitis /af′thəs/ [Gk, *aptha,* eruption; *stoma,* mouth, *itis* inflammation], a recurring condition characterized by the eruption of painful ulcers (commonly called canker sores) on the mucous membranes of the mouth.

APIC, abbreviation for **Association for Practitioners of Infection Control.**

apical /ap′ikəl, ā′pi-/ [L, *apex,* tip], **1.** pertaining to the summit or apex. **2.** pertaining to the end of a tooth root.

apical curettage [L, *apex;* Fr, scraping], (in dentistry) debridement of the apical surface of a tooth and removal of diseased soft tissues in the surrounding bony crypt.

apical fiber, one of the many fibers of the periodontal ligament. These fibers radiate around the apex of the tooth extending into the bone at the bottom of the alveolus.

apical lordotic view /lôrdot′ik/, a radiograph made by positioning the patient leaning backward at an angle of approximately 45 degrees.

apical odontoid ligament /ōdon′toid/, a ligament connecting the axis to the occipital bone. It extends from the process of the axis to the anterior margin of the foramen magnum.

apical periodontitis [L, *apex,* summit; Gk, *peri,* near, *odous, tooth, itis,* inflammation], an inflammation around the apex of the root of a tooth.

apical pulse, the heart rate as auscultated with a stethoscope placed on the chest wall adjacent to the cardiac apex.

apicectomy /ap′isek′təmē/ [L, *apex* + Gk, *ektome* excision], the surgical removal of the apex or the apical part of a tooth root, usually in conjunction with apical curettage or root canal therapy.

apicitis /ap′isī′tis/, an inflammation of the apex of a body structure, such as the apex of a lung or root of a tooth.

apicoectomy /ā′pikō·ek′təmē/, surgical removal of the apex of a tooth root.

apicotomy /ā′pikot′əmē/, a surgical incision into the apex of a body structure.

apituitarism /ā′pityoo′itəriz′əm/ [Gk, *a,* without; L, *pituita,* phlegm; Gk, *ismos,* a state], an absence or loss of function of the pituitary gland.

APKD, abbreviation for *adult polycystic kidney disease.*

aplasia /əplā′zhə/ [Gk, *a, plassein,* not to form], **1.** a developmental failure resulting in the absence of an organ or tissue. **2.** (in hematology) a failure of the normal process of cell generation and development.

aplasia cutis congenita [Gk, *a, plassein;* L, *cutis,* skin, *congenitus* born with], the congenital absence of a localized area of skin. It is usually covered by a thin, translucent membrane or scar tissue, or it may be raw and ulcerated.

aplastic /āplas′tik/ [Gk, *a, plassein,* not to form], **1.** pertaining to the absence or defective development of a tissue or organ. **2.** failure of a tissue to produce normal daughter cells by mitosis.

aplastic anemia, a deficiency of all of the formed elements of blood, representing a failure of the cell-generating capacity of bone marrow. Neoplastic disease of bone marrow and destruction of bone marrow by exposure to toxic chemicals, ionizing radiation, or some antibiotics or other medications are common etiologies.

Apley's scratch test, a method for assessing the range of motion of the shoulders. The patient is asked to scratch his or her back while reaching over the head with one hand and behind the back with the other hand. The test requires abduction and lateral rotation of one shoulder and adduction and medical rotation of the other shoulder.

APMA, abbreviation for *American Podiatric Medical Society.*

apnea /apnē′ə, ap′nē·ə/ [Gk, *a* + *pnein,* not to breath], an absence of spontaneous respiration. Types of apnea include **cardiac apnea, deglutition apnea, periodic apnea of the newborn, primary apnea, reflex apnea, secondary apnea,** and **sleep apnea. —apneic,** *adj.*

apnea alarm mattress [Gk, *a* + *pnein,* not to breathe], a bed surface for infants, designed to sound an alarm if the child stops breathing for a given period of time.

apnea monitoring, the act of closely observing the respiratory activity of individuals, particularly infants. The procedure may involve the use of electronic devices that detect changes in thoracic or abdominal movements and heart rate. Apneic detection devices may include an alarm that sounds if breathing stops.

apneustic breathing /apnōō'stik/ [Gk, *a, pneusis,* not breathing], a pattern of respirations characterized by a prolonged inspiratory phase followed by expiration apnea.

apneustic center, an area of nerve tissue in the lower part of the pons that controls the inspiratory phase of respiration.

apocrine /ap'əkrīn, -krin/ [Gk, *apo,* from, *krinein,* to separate], **1.** pertaining to a gland that loses part of its substance during secretion. **2.** pertaining to sweat glands, which are most numerous in the axilla and groin.

apocrine secretion [Gk, *apo + krinein;* L, *secernere,* to separate], a mammary gland type of secretion in which the end of the secreting cell is broken off and its contents expelled. Thus the secretion contains cellular granules in addition to fluid.

apocrine sweat gland [Gk, *apo,* from, *krinein,* to separate], one of the large dermal exocrine glands located in the axillary, anal, genital, and mammary areas of the body. The apocrine glands become functional only after puberty. They secrete sweat containing nutrients consumed by skin bacteria.

apoenzyme /ap'ō·en'zīm/ [Gk, *apo + en,* into, *zyme,* ferment], the protein part of a holoenzyme. The nonprotein part is the prosthetic group, which is usually permanently attached to the apoenzyme.

apogee /ap'əjē/ [Gk, *apo + ge,* earth], the climax of a disease or the period of greatest severity of signs and symptoms, usually followed by a crisis.

apolipoprotein /ap'ōlip'ōprō'tēn/ [Gk, *apo + lipos,* fat, *protos,* first], the protein component of lipoprotein complexes.

apolipoprotein A-I, a protein component of lipoprotein complexes found in high-density lipoprotein (HDL) and chylomicrons.

apolipoprotein A-II, a protein component of lipoprotein complexes found in high-density lipoprotein (HDL) and chylomicrons.

apolipoprotein B, a protein component of lipoprotein complexes found in low-density lipoprotein (LDL), very low–density lipoprotein (VLDL), and intermediate-density lipoprotein (IDL). It is elevated in the plasma of patients with familial hyperlipoproteinemia.

apolipoprotein E, a protein component of lipoprotein complexes found in very low–density lipoprotein (VLDL), high-density lipoprotein (HDL), chylomicrons, and chylomicron remnants. It is elevated

in patients with type III hyperlipoproteinemia.

aponeurosis /ap'ōnōōrō'sis/, *pl.* **aponeuroses** [Gk, *apo + neuron,* nerve, sinew], a strong sheet of fibrous connective tissue that serves as a tendon to attach muscles to bone or as fascia to bind muscles together.

aponeurosis of the external abdominal oblique, the strong membrane that covers the entire ventral surface of the abdomen and lies superficial to the rectus abdominis. Fibers from both sides of the aponeurosis interlace in the midline to form the linea alba.

aponeurotic fascia /-nōōrot'ik/ [Gk, *apo,* from, *neuron,* tendon], a thickened layer of connective tissue that provides attachment to a muscle.

apophyseal fracture, a fracture that separates a projection (apophysis) of a bone from the main osseous tissue at a point of strong tendinous attachment.

apophysis /əpof'isis/ [Gk, a growing away], any small projection, process, or outgrowth, usually on a bone.

apophysitis /əpof'əsī'tis/, a condition characterized by the inflammation of an outgrowth, projection, or swelling, especially a bony outgrowth that is not separated from the bone.

apoprotein /ap'ōprō'tēn/, a polypeptide chain not yet complexed to its specific prosthetic group.

apoptosis /ā'pōtō'sis, ā'poptō'sis/ [Gk, *apo,* away, *ptosis,* falling], the sloughing off of a scab or other skin crust.

aposia /āpō'shə/ [Gk, *a,* not, *posis,* thirst], a complete lack of thirst.

apothecaries' measure /əpoth'əker'ēz/ [Gk, *apotheke,* store], a system of graduated liquid volumes originally based on the minim, formerly equal to 1 drop of water but now standardized to 0.06 ml; 60 minims equals 1 fluid dram, 8 fluid drams equals 1 fluid ounce, 16 fluid ounces equals 1 pint, 2 pints equal 1 quart, 4 quarts equals 1 gallon.

apothecaries' weight, a system of graduated amounts arranged in order of heaviness and based on the grain, formerly equal to the weight of a plump grain of wheat but now standardized to 65 mg; 20 grains equals 1 scruple, 3 scruples equals 1 dram, 8 drams equals 1 ounce, 12 ounces equals 1 pound.

apothecary /əpoth'əker'ē/ [Gk, *apotheke,* store], a pharmacist.

apparatus /ap'ərat'əs/ [L, *ad,* toward, *parare,* to make ready], a device or a system composed of different parts that act together to perform some special function.

appendage /əpen'dij/ [L, *appendere,* to add

something], an accessory structure attached to another part or organ.

appendectomy /ap'əndek'təmē/ [L, *appendere* + Gk, *ektome*, excision], the surgical removal of the vermiform appendix, most often through an incision in the right lower quadrant of the abdomen. The operation is performed in acute appendicitis to remove an inflamed appendix before it ruptures.

appendical reflex /əpen'dikəl/, extreme tenderness at McBurney's point on the abdomen, a diagnostic finding in appendicitis.

appendiceal /ap'endish'əl/, pertaining to the vermiform appendix.

appendicectomy /əpen'disek'təmē/, **1.** surgical removal of the vermiform appendix. **2.** surgical removal of an appendage.

appendicitis /əpen'disī'tis/ [L, *appendere* + Gk, *itis*], inflammation of the vermiform appendix, usually acute, which, if undiagnosed, leads rapidly to perforation and peritonitis. The most common symptom is constant pain in the right lower quadrant of the abdomen around McBurney's point, which the patient describes as having begun as intermittent pain in midabdomen. To decrease the pain, the patient keeps knees bent to prevent tension of abdominal muscles. Appendicitis is characterized by vomiting, a low-grade fever of 99° to 102° F, an elevated white blood count, rebound tenderness, a rigid abdomen, and decreased or absent bowel sounds. Appendicitis is most likely to occur in teenagers and young adults and is more frequent in males.

appendicitis pain [L, *appendere*, to hang upon, *poena*, penalty], severe general abdominal pain that develops rapidly and usually becomes localized in the lower right quadrant. It is accompanied by extreme tenderness over the right rectus muscle with rebound pain at McBurney's point. Occasionally the pain is on the left side.

appendicular /ap'əndik'yələr/, **1.** pertaining to the vermiform appendix. **2.** pertaining to the limbs of the skeleton.

appendicular abscess, 1. an abscess on a limb. **2.** an abscess of the vermiform appendix.

appendicular skeleton, the bones of the limbs and their girdles, attached to the axial skeleton.

appendix /əpen'diks/, *pl.* **appendixes, appendices,** an accessory part of a main structure.

appendix dyspepsia [L, *appendere* + Gk, *dys,* difficult, *peptein,* to digest], an abnormal condition characterized by impairment of the digestive function associated with chronic appendicitis.

appendix epididymidis /ep'ididim'idis/, a cystic structure sometimes found on the head of the epididymis. It represents a remnant of the mesonephros.

appendix epiploica /əp'iplô'ikə/, *pl.* **appendices epiploicae** [L, *appendere* + Gk, *epiploon,* caul], one of the fat pads scattered through the peritoneum along the colon and the upper part of the rectum, especially along the transverse and the sigmoid parts of the colon.

apperception /ap'ərsep'shən/ [L, *ad,* toward, *percipere,* to perceive], **1.** mental perception or recognition. **2.** (in psychology) a conscious process of understanding or perceiving in terms of a person's previous knowledge, experiences, emotions, and memories. **—apperceptive,** *adj.*

appestat /ap'əstat/, a center in the brain that controls the appetite.

appetite /ap'ətīt/ [L, *appetere,* to long for], a natural or instinctive desire, such as for food.

apple picker's disease, an allergic reaction with respiratory complaints, associated with the handling of apples that have been treated with a fungicide.

apple sorter's disease, a form of contact dermatitis caused by chemicals used in washing apples.

appliance /əplī'əns/ [L, *applicare,* to apply], a device or instrument designed for a specific purpose, such as a dental orthodontic appliance.

application /ap'likā'shən/, a computer procedure or problem to be processed, such as payroll, inventory, data about patients, scheduling of procedures and activities, pharmacy requisition and control, recording of nursing notes, and care planning.

applicator /ap'lika'tər/, a rodlike instrument with a piece of cotton on the end, used for the local application of medication.

applied anatomy /əplīd'/, the study of the structure of the organs of the body as it relates to the diagnosis and treatment of disease.

applied chemistry, the application of the study of chemical elements and compounds to industry and the arts.

applied psychology, 1. the interpretation of historical, literary, medical, or other data according to psychologic principles. **2.** any branch of psychology that emphasizes practical rather than theoretic approaches and objectives, such as clinical psychology, child psychology, industrial psychology, and educational psychology.

AP portable chest radiograph, a radiographic examination of the chest performed with a portable x-ray machine in the room of an immobilized patient. The film holder is placed behind the patient with the x-ray tube in front.

apposition /ap′əsish′ən/ [L, *apponere*, to put to], the placing of objects in proximity, as in the layering of tissue cells or juxtapositioning of facing surfaces side-by-side.

appositional growth, an increase in size by the addition of new tissue or similar material at the periphery of a particular part or structure, as in the addition of new layers in bone and tooth formation.

apposition suture, a suture that holds the margins of an incision close together.

approach, the steps in a particular surgical procedure, from division of the most superficial parts of the anatomy through exposure of the operation site.

approach-approach conflict [L, *ad* + *propiare*, to draw near], a conflict resulting from the simultaneous presence of two or more incompatible impulses, desires, or goals, each of which is desirable.

approach-avoidance conflict, a conflict resulting from the presence of a single goal or desire that is both desirable and undesirable.

appropriate for gestational age (AGA) infant /əprō′prē·it/ [L, *ad,* toward, *proprius,* ownership], a newborn whose size, growth, and maturation are normal for gestational age, whether delivered prematurely, at term, or later than term.

approximal /əprok′siməl/ [L, *approximare,* to approach], close, or very near.

approximate /əprok′simāt/ [L, *ad* + *proximare,* to come near], to draw two tissue surfaces close together as in the repair of a wound or to draw the bones of a joint together as in physical therapy.

approximator /əprok′səmā′tər/, a medical instrument used to draw together the edges of divided tissues, as in closing a wound or repairing a fractured rib.

apraxia /əprak′sē·ə/ [Gk, *a* + *pressein,* not to act], an impairment in the ability to perform purposeful acts or to manipulate objects in the absence or loss of motor power sensation or coordination. **Ideational apraxia** is characterized by impairment caused by a loss of the perception of the use of an object. **Motor apraxia** is characterized by an inability to use an object or perform a task, although it is understood. **Amnestic apraxia** is characterized by an inability to perform the function because of an inability to remember the command to perform it. Apraxia of speech is an articulatory disorder caused by brain damage and results in an inability to program the position of speech muscles and the sequence of muscle movements necessary to produce understandable speech. —**apraxic,** *adj.*

aprobarbital /ap′rōbär′bital/, an intermediate-acting barbiturate prescribed as a sedative-hypnotic for sedation and induction of sleep on a short-term basis.

aprosody /āpros′odē/ [Gk, *a* + *prosodia,* not modulated voice], a speech defect characterized by the absence of the normal variations in pitch, loudness, intonation, and rhythm of word formation.

aprosopia /ā′prəsō′pē·ə/ [Gk, *aprosopos,* faceless], a congenital absence of part or all of the facial structures. The condition is usually associated with other malformations.

APTA, abbreviation for *American Physical Therapy Association.*

aptitude /ap′tətyo͞od/ [L, *aptitudo,* ability], a natural ability, tendency, talent, or capability to learn, understand, or acquire a particular skill; mental alertness.

aptitude test, any of a variety of standardized tests for measuring an individual's ability to learn certain skills.

apyretic /ā′pīret′ik/ [Gk, *a* + *pyretos,* without fever], an afebrile condition.

apyrexia /ā′pīrek′sē·ə/ [Gk, *a* + *pyrexis,* without fever], an absence or remission of fever.

AQ, abbreviation for **achievement quotient.**

aqua (aq) /ä′kwə/, the Latin word for water.

aquaphobia /ä′kwəfō′bē·ə/ [L, *aqua,* water; Gk, *phobos,* fear], fear of water.

aquapuncture /-pungk′chər/ [L, *aqua,* water, *punctura,* puncture], the injection of water under the skin or spraying of a fine jet of water onto the skin surface to relieve a mild irritation.

aquathermia pad, /-thur′ mē·ə/, a waterproof plastic or rubber pad that can be applied to areas of muscle sprain, edema, or mild inflammation. The pad contains channels through which heated or cooled water flows. The device is connected by hoses to a bedside control unit that contains a temperature regulator, a motor for circulating the water, and a reservoir of distilled water.

aqueduct /-dukt/ [L, *aqua,* water, *ductus,* act of leading], any canal, channel, or passage through or between body parts, as the cerebral aqueduct in the brain.

aqueductus /ak′wəduk′təs/, the Latin word for canal.

aqueous /ā′kwē·əs, ak′wē·əs/ [L, *aqua*], **1.** watery or waterlike. **2.** a medication prepared with water.

aqueous chambers [L, *aqua,* water; Gk, *kamara,* something with an arched cover], the anterior and posterior chambers of the eye, containing the aqueous humor.

aqueous extract, a water-based preparation of plant or animal substance containing the biologically active part without the cellular residue.

aqueous humor, the clear, watery fluid circulating in the anterior and posterior chambers of the eye.

aqueous phase, a fluid stage of a substance that may also exist in other forms during cycles of change, such as the occurrence of water in a liquid state and at other times as ice or water vapor.

aqueous solution [L, *aqua,* water + *solutus,* dissolved], a homogenous liquid preparation of any substance dissolved in water.

Ar, symbol for the element **argon.**

AR, abbreviation for *assisted respiration.*

arachidonic acid /ar′əkidon′ik/ [L, *arachos,* a legume], an essential long-chain fatty acid that is a component of lecithin and a basic material in the biosynthesis of some prostaglandins.

arachnid [Gk, *arachne,* spider], pertaining to the animal class of Arachnida, which includes spiders, scorpions, mites, and ticks.

arachnitis /ar′əknī′tis/, inflammation of the arachnoid membrane covering the brain.

arachnodactyly /ərak′nōdak′tilē/ [Gk, *arachne,* spider, *dactylos,* finger], a congenital condition of having long, thin, spiderlike fingers and toes. It is seen in Marfan's syndrome.

arachnoid /ərak′noid/ [Gk, *arachne,* spider, *eidos,* form], resembling a cobweb or spiderweb, such as the arachnoid membrane. —**arachnoidal,** *adj.*

arachnoidism /ərak′noidiz′əm/ [Gk, *arachne,* spider, *eidos,* form], the condition produced by the bite of a venomous spider.

arachnoid membrane, a thin, delicate membrane enclosing the brain and the spinal cord, interposed between the pia mater and the dura mater.

arachnoid villi /vil′ī/ [Gk, *arachne,* spider, *villus,* shaggy hair], projections of fibrous tissue from the arachnoid membrane.

arachnophobia /ərak′nōfō′bē·ə/, a morbid fear of spiders.

Aran-Duchenne muscular atrophy /aran′-dōōshen′/ [François A. Aran, French physician, 1817–1861; Guillaume B. A. Duchenne, French neurologist, 1806–1875], a form of amyotrophic lateral sclerosis affecting the hands, arms, shoulders, and legs at the onset before becoming more generalized.

arbitrary inference /är′bitrer′ē in′fərəns/, a form of cognitive distortion in which a judgment based on insufficient evidence leads to an erroneous conclusion.

arbitrator /är′bətrā′tər/ [L, *arbiter,* umpire], an impartial person appointed to resolve a dispute between parties. —**arbitration,** *n.*

arbovirus /är′bōvī′rəs/, any one of more than 300 arthropod-borne viruses that cause infections characterized by a combination of two or more of the following: fever, rash, encephalitis, and bleeding into the viscera or skin. Dengue, yellow fever, and equine encephalitis are three common arboviral infections.

arc [L, *arcus,* bow], a part of the circumference of a circle.

ARC, See **AIDS-wasting syndrome.**

arcade [L, *arcus,* bow], an arch or series of arches.

arch, any anatomic structure that is curved or has a bowlike appearance.

arch bar, any one of various types of wires, bars, or splints that conform to the arch of the teeth, used in the treatment of fractures of the jaws and in the stabilization of injured teeth.

archenteron /arken′təron/, *pl.* **archentera** [Gk, *arche,* beginning, *enteron,* intestine], the primitive digestive cavity formed by the invagination into the gastrula during the embryonic development of many animals.—**archenteric,** *adj.*

arches of the foot [L, *arcus,* bow; AS, *fot*], the bony arches of the instep, including the longitudinal (anteroposterior) and the transverse arches.

archetype /är′kətīp′/ [Gk, *arche* + *typos,* type], **1.** an original model or pattern from which a thing or group of things is made or evolves. **2.** (in analytic psychology) an inherited primordial idea or mode of thought derived from the experiences of the human race and present in the unconscious of the individual in the form of drives, moods, and concepts. —**archetypal, archetypic, archetypical,** *adj*

archiblastoma /är′kiblastō′mə/ [Gk, *arche* + *blastos,* germ, *oma*], a tumor composed of cells derived from the layer of tissue surrounding the germinal vesicle.

architectural barriers /är′kətek′chərəl/, architectural features of homes and public buildings that limit access and mobility of disabled persons.

architis /ärkī′tis/ [Gk, *archos,* anus, *itis,* inflammation], an inflammation of the anus.

arch length /ärch/, the distance from the distal point of the most posterior tooth on one side to the same point on the other side, usually measured through the points of contact between adjoining teeth.

arch length deficiency, the difference in any dental arch between the required length to accommodate all the natural teeth and the actual space available.

arch of the aorta, one of the four parts of the aorta, giving rise to three arterial branches called the innominate (brachiocephalic), left common carotid, and left subclavian arteries.

arch width, the width of a dental arch, which varies in all diameters between the left and right opposite teeth and is determined by direct measurement between the canines, the first molars, and the second premolars.

arch wire, an orthodontic wire fastened to two or more teeth through fixed attachments, used to cause or guide tooth movement.

arcing spring contraceptive diaphragm /är'king/, a kind of contraceptive diaphragm in which the flexible metal spring that forms the rim is a combination of a flexible coil spring and a flat band spring made of stainless steel.

arcuate /är'kyōō·at/ [L, *arcuatus,* bowed], an arch or bow shape.

arcuate scotoma [L, *arcuatus* bowed; Gk, *skotoma,* darkness], an arc-shaped blind area that may develop in the field of vision of a person with glaucoma. It is caused by damage to nerve fibers in the retina.

arcus senilis /senē'lis/ [L, bow, aged], an opaque ring, gray to white in color, that surrounds the periphery of the cornea. It is caused by deposits of fat granules in the cornea or hyaline degeneration and occurs primarily in older persons.

ARDS, abbreviation for **adult respiratory distress syndrome.**

area /er'ē·ə/ [L, space], (in anatomy) a limited anatomic space that contains a specific structure of the body or within which certain physiologic functions predominate, such as the aortic area and the association areas of the cerebral cortex.

Area Restriction, a Nursing Interventions Classification defined as limitation of patient mobility to a specified area for purposes of safety or behavior management.

areata /erē·ā'tə/, occurring in patches, such as hair loss in alopecia areata.

area under the concentration curve (AUC), a method of measurement of the bioavailability of a drug based on a plot of blood concentrations sampled at frequent intervals. It is directly proportional to the total amount of unaltered drug in the patient's blood.

areflexia /ā'rēflek'sē·ə/, the absence of the reflexes.

Arenavirus /er'inəvī'rəs/, a genus of viruses usually transmitted to humans by contact with the excreta of wild rodents. Individual arenaviruses are identified with specific geographic areas, such as **Bolivian hemorrhagic fever, Lassa fever,** and **Argentine hemorrhagic fever.** Arenavirus infections are characterized by slow onset, fever, muscle pain, rash, petechiae, hemorrhage, delirium, hypotension, and ulcers of the mouth.

areola /erē'ōlə/, *pl.* **areolae, 1.** a small space or a cavity within a tissue. **2.** a circular area of a different color surrounding a central feature, such as the discoloration about a pustule or vesicle. **3.** the part of the iris around the pupil.

areola mammae /mam'ē/, the pigmented, circular area surrounding the nipple of each breast.

areolar /erē'ələr/ [L, *areola,* little space], pertaining to an areola.

areolar gland, one of the large sebaceous glands in the areolae encircling the nipples of the breasts of women. The areolar glands secrete a lipoid fluid that lubricates and protects the nipple.

areolar tissue, a kind of connective tissue having little tensile strength and consisting of loosely woven fibers and areolae.

areolitis /er'ē·əlī'tis/, an inflammation of the areolas of the breasts.

ARF, abbreviation for **acute respiratory failure.**

Arg, abbreviation for the amino acid **arginine.**

argentaffin cell /är'jentaf'in/ [L, *argentum,* silver, *affinitas,* affinity], a cell containing granules that stain readily with silver and chromium. Such cells occur in most regions of the gastrointestinal tract.

argentaffinoma /är'jentaf'inō'mə/, a carcinoid tumor arising most often from argentaffin cells in epithelium of the crypts of Lieberkühn in the digestive tract.

Argentine hemorrhagic fever, an infectious disease caused by an arenavirus transmitted to humans by the ingestion of food contaminated by the excreta of infected rodents and by personal contact.

arginase /är'jinās/, an enzyme that catalyzes the hydrolysis of arginine during the urea cycle, producing urea and ornithine.

arginine (Arg) /är'jinin/, an amino acid produced by the digestion or hydrolysis of proteins, formed during the urea cycle by the transfer of a nitrogen atom from aspartate to citrulline.

argininemia /är'jininē'mē·ə/, an autosomal-recessive disorder characterized by an increased amount of arginine in the blood caused by a deficiency of arginase. Without arginase, ammonia cannot be metabolized into urea.

argininosuccinic acidemia /är′jin′inō′-suksin′ik/, an inherited amino acid metabolism disorder in which the lack of an enzyme, argininosuccinase, results in an excess of argininosuccinic acid in the blood. The condition is characterized by seizures and mental retardation.

argon (Ar) /är′gon/ [Gk, argos, inactive], a colorless, odorless, chemically inactive gas and one of the six rare gases in the atmosphere. Its atomic weight (mass) is 39.95; its atomic number is 18. It forms no compounds.

Argyll Robertson pupil [Douglas M.C.L. Argyll Robertson, Scottish ophthalmologist, 1837–1909], a pupil that constricts on accommodation but not in response to light. It is most often seen with miosis and in advanced neurosyphilis.

argyria /ärjī′rē·ə/, [Gk, argyros, silver], a dull blue or gray coloration of the skin, conjunctiva, and internal organs caused by prolonged exposure to silver salts.

argyrophil /ärji′rəfil/ [Gk, argyros, silver, philein, to love], a cell or other object that is easily stained or impregnated with silver.

ariboflavinosis /ārī′bōflā′vinō′sis/ [Gk, a, not, ribose; L, flavus, yellow; Gk, osis], a condition caused by deficiency of riboflavin (vitamin B_2) in the diet. It is characterized by lesions at the corners of the mouth, on the lips, and around the nose and eyes; by seborrheic dermatitis, and by various visual disorders.

Arica therapy, an alternative mental health treatment introduced by Oscar Ichazo that focuses on altered states of consciousness with a goal of increasing the powers of the mind.

Arkansas stone /är′kənsô/, a fine-grained stone of novaculite used to sharpen surgical instruments.

arm [L, armus], 1. the part of the upper limb of the body between the shoulder and the elbow. 2. nontechnical. the arm and the forearm.

ARM, abbreviation for artificial rupture of the (fetal) membranes.

armamentarium /är′məmenter′ē·əm/ [L, armamentum, implement], the total therapeutic assets of a physician or medical facility, including medicines and equipment.

arm board, 1. a board used to position the affected arm of a hemiplegic person. It fastens to the arm rest of a wheelchair, supporting the arm in the correct position to subluxate the shoulder and flaccid arm and to prevent edema. 2. a board used to keep the arm still to permit the drawing of

blood or starting of an intravenous needle.

arm cylinder cast, an orthopedic device of plaster of paris or fiberglass, used for immobilizing the upper limb from the wrist to the upper arm.

Army Nurse Corps (ANC), a branch of the U.S. Army, founded February 2, 1901, with headquarters in Falls Church, Virginia.

Arneth's classification of neutrophils [Joseph Arneth, German physician, 1873–1953], a system expressed in chart form in which neutrophils are divided into five classes according to the number of segments of their nuclei and are further subdivided according to the shape of the nuclei. Immature neutrophils with a single-lobed nucleus are placed on the far left side of the chart; those with multilobed nuclei are placed on the far right side.

Arnold-Chiari malformation /är′nəldkē·är′ē/ [Julius Arnold, German pathologist, 1835–1915; Hans Chiari, French pathologist, 1851–1916], a congenital herniation of the brainstem and lower cerebellum through the foramen magnum into the cervical vertebral canal.

Arnold, Friedrich, [German anatomist, 1803–1890], investigator of structures and functions of the brain and nervous system, including the nerve center of the cough reflex.

AROM, abbreviation for active range of motion.

aroma [Gk, spice], any agreeable odor or pleasing fragrance, especially of food, drink, spices, or medication.

aromatic /er′ōmat′ik/ [Gk, aroma, spice], 1. pertaining to a strong but agreeable odor such as a spicy odor. 2. a stimulant or spicy medicine.

aromatic alcohol, a fatty alcohol in which part of the hydrogen of the alcohol radical is replaced by a phenyl hydrocarbon.

aromatic ammonia spirit, a strongly fragrant solution of ammonium carbonate in dilute liquid ammonia, oils, alcohol, and water. It is used as a reflex stimulus, an antacid, and a carminative to relieve flatulence.

aromatic bath, a medicated bath in which aromatic substances or essential oils are added to the water.

aromatic compounds, organic compounds that contain a benzene, naphthalene, or analogous ring. Many of these compounds have agreeable odors, which accounts for the use of this term for such compounds.

aromatic elixir [Ar, al-iksir, philosopher's stone], a pleasant smelling flavor agent added to some medications.

aromatic hydrocarbon [Gk, *aroma,* spice; *hydor,* water; L, *carbo,* coal], an organic compound that has a benzene or quinoid ring, as distinguished from an open-chain aliphatic compound.

arousal [OE, to rise], a state of responsiveness to sensory stimulation.

arousal level, the state of sensory stimulation needed to induce active wakefulness in a sleeping infant. Arousal levels range from deep sleep to a drowsy state.

array, [ME, *aray,* preparation], an arrangement or order of components or other objects, usually according to a predetermined system or plan.

arrest [L, *ad, resistare,* to withstand], to inhibit, restrain, or stop, as to arrest the course of a disease.

arrested dental caries, dental decay in which the area of decay has stopped progressing and infection is not present but in which the demineralized area in the tooth remains as a cavity.

arrested development, the cessation of one or more phases of the developmental process in utero before normal completion, resulting in congenital anomalies.

arrested labor [L, *ad* + *restare,* to withstand, *labor,* work], an interruption in the labor process that may be caused by lack of uterine contractions.

arrhenoblastoma /erē′nōblastō′mə/ [Gk, *arrhen,* male, *blastos,* germ, *oma,* tumor], an ovarian neoplasm, the cells of which mimic those in testicular tubules and secrete male sex hormone, causing virilization in females.

arrhenogenic /erē′nōjen′ik/, producing only male offspring.

arrhenokaryon /erē′nōker′ē·on/ [Gk, *arrhen,* male, *karyon,* nucleus], an organism that is produced from an egg that has only paternal chromosomes.

arrhythmia /ərith′mē·ə, ərith′mē·ə/ [Gk, *a* + *rhythmos,* without rhythm], any deviation from the normal pattern of the heartbeat. —**arrhythmic, arrhythmical,** *adj.*

ARRT, abbreviation for **American Registry of Radiologic Technologists.**

arsenic (As) /är′sənik/ [Gk, *arsen,* strong], an element that occurs throughout the earth's crust in metal arsenides, arsenious sulfides, and arsenious oxides. Its atomic number is 33; its atomic weight (mass) is 74.92. This element has been used for centuries as a therapeutic agent and as a poison and continues to have limited use in some trypanosomicidal drugs such as melarsoprol and tryparsamide.—**arsenic** /ärsen′ik/, *adj.*

arsenic poisoning, toxic effect caused by the ingestion or inhalation of arsenic or a substance containing arsenic, an ingredient in some pesticides, herbicides, dyes, and medicinal solutions. Small amounts absorbed over a period of time may result in chronic poisoning, producing nausea, headache, coloration and scaling of the skin, hyperkeratoses, anorexia, and white lines across the fingernails. Ingestion of large amounts of arsenic results in severe gastrointestinal pain, diarrhea, vomiting, and swelling of the extremities.

arsenic stomatitis [Gk, *arsen,* strong; *stoma,* mouth, *itis,* inflammation], an abnormal oral condition associated with arsenic poisoning, characterized by dry, red, painful oral mucosa; ulceration; purpura; and mobility of teeth.

arsine (AsH₃), a colorless poisonous gas with an unpleasant odor. It occurs in various industries, particularly where scrap metal is used or produced.

ART, abbreviation for **active resistance training.**

arterectomy /är′tərek′təmē/, the surgical removal of a segment of an artery.

arterial /ärtir′ē·əl/ [Gk, *arteria,* airpipe], pertaining to an artery.

arterial bleeding [Gk, *arteria,* airpipe; ME, *blod*], loss of blood from an artery. The event is usually characterized by blood that is bright red and spurting.

arterial blood gas (ABG), the oxygen and carbon dioxide in arterial blood, measured by various methods to assess the adequacy of ventilation and oxygenation and the acid-base status.

arterial blood pressure (ABP), the pressure of the blood in the arterial system, which depends on the heart's pumping pressure, the resistance of the arterial walls, the blood quantity, and its viscosity.

arterial capillaries, microscopic blood vessels (capillaries) extending beyond the terminal ends of arterioles.

arterial catheter [Gk, *arteria,* airpipe, *katheter,* a thing lowered into], a tubular instrument that can be inserted into an artery either to draw blood or to measure blood pressure directly.

arterial circulation [Gk, *arteria* + L, *circulare,* to go around], the movement of blood through the arteries directed away from the heart to the tissues, as opposed to venous circulation away from the tissues to the heart.

arterial hemorrhage, the loss of blood from an artery, often associated with vessel trauma, or the blood loss that accompanies removal of a large-bore arterial catheter.

arterial insufficiency, inadequate blood flow in arteries. It may be caused by occlusive atherosclerotic plaques or emboli;

damaged, diseased, or intrinsically weak vessels; arteriovenous fistulas; aneurysms; hypercoagulability states; or heavy use of tobacco. Signs of arterial insufficiency include pale, cyanotic, or mottled skin over the affected area; absent or decreased sensations; tingling; diminished sense of temperature; muscle pains; reduced or absent peripheral pulses; and, in advanced disease, atrophy of muscles of the involved extremity.

arterial insufficiency of lower extremities, a condition characterized by hardening, thickening, and loss of elasticity of the walls of peripheral arteries. It causes decreased circulation, sensation, and function. Symptoms include sharp, cramping pain during exercise or rest at night; numbness; skin changes ranging from pallor to ulceration; and loss of hair on the legs. Pedal and popliteal pulses may be diminished or absent.

arterial line (A-line), an arterial blood monitoring system consisting of a catheter inserted into an artery and connected to pressure tubing, a transducer, and a monitor. The device permits continuous direct blood pressure readings, as well as access to the arterial blood supply when samples are needed for analysis.

arterial murmur, a sound produced by blood moving through an artery.

arterial nephrosclerosis [Gk, *arteria,* airpipe, *nephros,* kidney, *sklera,* hard, *osis,* condition], arteriosclerosis of the kidney arteries leading to deprivation of oxygenated blood to the kidney tissues and their destruction.

arterial palpitation [Gk, *arteria,* airpipe; L, *palpitare,* to flutter], a beating felt in an artery.

arterial pH, the hydrogen ion concentration of arterial blood. Normal range is 7.35 to 7.45. The figure represents a ratio of 20:1 of bicarbonate ions to carbon dioxide dissolved in the blood.

arterial pressure, the stress exerted by circulating blood on the artery walls. It is the product of the cardiac output and the systemic vascular resistance.

arterial rete /rē′tē/ [Gk, *arteria,* airpipe; L, *rete,* net], a network of arteries and arterioles.

arterial sclerosis [Gk, *arteria,* airpipe, *sklerosis,* hardening], a thickening of the arteries.

arterial tension, the pressure on artery walls caused by the force of blood being squeezed into the systemic circulation by contraction of the heart's left ventricle.

arterial thrill, a vibration that can be felt over an artery.

arterial wall, the fibrous and muscular wall of vessels that carry oxygenated blood from the heart to structures throughout the body, and of the pulmonary arteries that carry deoxygenated blood from the heart to the lungs. The wall of an artery has three layers: the **tunica intima,** the inner coat; the **tunica media,** the middle coat; and the **tunica adventitia,** the outer coat.

arteriectomy /ärtir′ē·ek′təmē/ [Gk, *arteria* + *ektome,* cutting out], the surgical removal of a part of an artery.

arteriofibrosis /ärtir′ē·ōfībrō′sis/, an inflammatory fibrous thickening of the walls of the arteries and arterioles, resulting in a narrowing of the lumen of the vessels.

arteriogram /ärtir′ē·əgram′/, an x-ray film of an artery injected with a radiopaque medium. See also **arteriography.**

arteriography /ärtir′ē·og′rəfē/ [Gk, *arteria,* airpipe, *graphein,* to record], a method of radiologic visualization of arteries performed after a radiopaque contrast medium is introduced into the bloodstream or into a specific vessel by injection or through a catheter. —**arteriographic,** *adj.*

arteriole /ärtir′ē·ōl/ [L, *arteriola,* little artery], the smallest of the arteries. Blood flowing from the heart is pumped through the arteries, to the arterioles, to the capillaries, into the veins, and returned to the heart. The muscular walls of the arterioles constrict and dilate in response to both local factors and neurochemical stimuli; thus arterioles play a significant role in peripheral vascular resistance and in regulation of blood pressure.

arteriolosclerosis /ärtir′ē·ō′ləsklərō′sis/, pathologic thickening, hardening, and loss of elasticity of the arteriole walls.

arteriopathy /ärtir′ē·op′əthē/ [Gk, *arteria* + *pathos,* suffering], a disease of an artery.

arterioplasty /ärtir′ē·əplas′tē/ [Gk, *arteria* + *plassein,* to mold], plastic surgery of an artery. The procedure is often performed to correct an aneurysm.

arteriosclerosis /ärtir′ē·ō′sklərō′sis/ [Gk, *arteria* + *sklerosis,* hardening], a common arterial disorder characterized by thickening, loss of elasticity, and calcification of arterial walls. It results in a decreased blood supply, especially to the cerebrum and lower extremities. The condition often develops with aging and in hypertension, nephrosclerosis, scleroderma, diabetes, and hyperlipidemia. Typical signs and symptoms include intermittent claudication, changes in skin temperature and color, altered peripheral pulses, bruits over an involved artery, headache, dizziness, and memory defects.

arteriosclerosis obliterans [Gk, *arteria* + *skleros* + L, *obliterare*, efface], a gradual narrowing of the arteries with degeneration of the intima and thrombosis. The condition may lead to complete occlusion of the artery and subsequent gangrene.

arteriosclerotic /-sklərot'ik/ [Gk, *arteria* + *skleros*, hard], pertaining to a thickening and hardening of the arterial wall.

arteriosclerotic heart disease (ASHD), a thickening and hardening of the walls of the coronary arteries.

arteriosclerotic retinopathy [Gk, *arteria*, airpipe, *sklerosis*, hardening; L, *rete*, net; Gk, *pathos*, disease], a disorder of the retina associated with hardening and thickening of the arteries supplying that part of the eye. It often accompanies hypertension.

arteriospasm /ärtir'ē-ōspaz'əm/ [Gk, *arteria* + *spasmos*, spasm], a spasm of an artery.

arteriostenosis /-stənō'sis/, a narrowing of an artery.

arteriotomy /ärtir'ē-ot'əmē/, a surgical incision in an artery.

arteriovenous /-vē'nəs/ [Gk, *arteria* + L, *vena*, vein], pertaining to arteries and veins.

arteriovenous anastomosis [Gk, *arteria* + L, *vena*; Gk, *anastomoein*, to form a mouth], a communication between an artery and a vein, either as a congenital anomaly or as a surgically produced link between vessels.

arteriovenous aneurysm, a dilation affecting both an artery and a vein, often as an abnormal linkage between a vein and artery.

arteriovenous angioma of the brain, a congenital tumor consisting of a tangle of coiled, usually dilated arteries and veins, islets of sclerosed brain tissue, and occasionally cartilaginous cells.

arteriovenous fistula, an abnormal communication between an artery and vein. It may occur congenitally or result from trauma, infection, arterial aneurysm, or a malignancy.

arteriovenous oxygen (a-vo₂) difference, the arterial oxygen content minus the central venous oxygen content.

arteriovenous shunt (AV shunt), a passageway, artificial or natural, that allows blood to flow from an artery to a vein without going through a capillary network.

arteritis /är'tərī'tis/ [Gk, *arteria* + *itis*], an inflammatory condition of the inner layers or the outer coat of one or more arteries. It may occur as a clinical entity or accompany another disorder, such as rheumatoid arthritis, rheumatic fever, polymyositis, or systemic lupus erythematosus.

arteritis umbilicalis, a septic inflammation of the umbilical artery in newborns, usually by the bacteria of the species *Clostridium tetani.*

artery /är'tərē/ [Gk, *arteria*, airpipe], one of the large blood vessels carrying blood in a direction away from the heart.

artery forceps, any forceps used for grasping, compressing, and holding the end of an artery during ligation. Generally self-locking, its handles are scissorslike.

arthralgia /ärthral'jə/ [Gk, *arthron*, joint, *algos*, pain], joint pain. —**arthralgic,** *adj.*

arthritis /ärthrī'tis/ [Gk, *arthron*, joint, *itis*], any inflammatory condition of the joints, characterized by pain, swelling, heat, redness, and limitation of movement.

arthrocentesis /är'thrōsintē'sis/ [Gk, *arthron* + *kentesis*, pricking], the puncture of a joint with a needle and the withdrawal of fluid, performed to obtain samples of synovial fluid for diagnostic purposes.

arthrogram /är'thrəgram/, a radiogram of a joint after injection of a contrast medium.

arthrography [Gk, *arthron*, joint, *graphein*, to record], a method of radiographically visualizing the inside of a joint.

arthrogryposis multiplex congenita [Gk, *arthron* + *gryposis*, joint curve; L, *multus*, many, *plica*, fold, *congenitus*, born with], fibrous stiffness of one or more joints, present at birth. It is often associated with incomplete development of the muscles that move the involved joints and degenerative changes of the motor neurons that innervate those muscles.

arthrokinematic /är'thrəkin'əmat'ik/, pertaining to the movement of bone surfaces within a joint.

arthron /är'thron/ [Gk], a joint, including its various components of bones, cartilaginous inserts, all soft tissue structures intervening between the rigid skeletal parts, and the adjacent muscular elements.

arthropathy /ärthrop'əthē/ [Gk, *arthron* + *pathos*, suffering], any disease or abnormal condition affecting a joint. —**arthropathic,** *adj.*

arthroplasty /är'thrəplast'ē/ [Gk, *arthron* + *plassein*, to shape], the surgical reconstruction or replacement of a painful, degenerated joint to restore mobility in osteoarthritis or rheumatoid arthritis or to correct a congenital deformity. Either the bones of the joint are reshaped and soft tissue or a metal disk is placed between the reshaped ends, or all or part of the joint is replaced with a metal or plastic prosthesis.

arthropod /är'thrəpod'/ [Gk, *arthron* + *pous*, foot], a member of the Arthropoda, a large phylum of animal life that includes crabs and lobsters as well as mites, ticks, spiders, and insects.

arthroscope /-skōp'/ [Gk, *arthron* + *skopein*, to watch], a type of endoscope used to examine joints.

arthroscopy /ärthros'kəpē/ [Gk, *arthron* + *skopein*, to watch], the examination of the interior of a joint performed by inserting a specially designed endoscope through a small incision. The procedure, used chiefly in knee problems, permits biopsy of cartilage or synovium, diagnosis of a torn meniscus, and, in some instances, removal of loose bodies in the joint space. —**arthroscopic,** *adj.*

arthrous /är'thrəs/ [Gk, *arthron*], **1.** pertaining to joints or articulation of bones. **2.** pertaining to a disease of a joint.

Arthus reaction /ärtoōs'/ [Nicholas M. Arthus, French physiologist, 1862–1945], a rare, severe, immediate nonatopic hypersensitivity reaction to injection of a foreign substance, which is usually not irritating but in certain individuals is antigenic.

articular /ärtik'yələr/ [L, *articulare,* to divide into joints], relating to a joint or the involvement of joints.

articular capsule [L, *articulare,* to divide into joints], an envelope of tissue that surrounds a freely moving joint, composed of an external layer of white fibrous tissue and an internal synovial membrane.

articular cartilage [L, *articulare* + *cartilago*], a type of hyaline connective tissue that covers the articulating surfaces of bones within synovial joints.

articular disk, the platelike cartilaginous end of certain bones in movable joints, sometimes closely associated with surrounding muscles or with cartilage.

articular fracture, a fracture involving the articular surfaces of a joint.

articular head, a projection on a bone that forms a joint with another bone.

articular muscle, a muscle that is attached to the capsule of a joint.

articular process of vertebra, a bony outgrowth on a vertebra that forms a joint with an adjoining vertebra.

articulate /ärtik'yələt/ [L, *articulare,* to divide into joints], **1.** to form a joint. **2.** to use speech that is distinct and connected.

articulated /ärtik'yəlā'tid/, **1.** united by

a movable joint. **2.** expressed in clear speech.

articulation of the pelvis /ärtik'yəlā'shən/, any one of the connections between the bones of the pelvis, involving four groups of ligaments. The first group connects the sacrum and the ilium; the second, the sacrum and the ischium; the third, the sacrum and the coccyx; and the fourth, the two pubic bones.

articulator /ärtik'yəlā'tər/ [L, *articulare,* to divide into joints], (in dentistry) a mechanical device used in the fabrication and testing of dental prostheses. It represents the temporomandibular joints and jaw members to which maxillary and mandibular casts may be attached.

artifact /är'təfakt/ [L, *ars,* skill, *facere,* to make], anything extraneous, irrelevant, or unwanted, such as a substance, structure, or piece of data or information. In radiologic imaging, spurious electronic signals may appear as an artifact in an image, thereby confusing the radiologist and the results of any examination.

artifactual modification /är'təfak'choō·əl/, a change in protein structure caused by in vitro manipulation.

artificial /är'tifish'əl/ [L, *artificium,* not natural], **1.** made by human work as a substitute for something that is natural. **2.** simulated, resulting from art in imitation of nature.

artificial abortion, an abortion that is produced deliberately.

artificial airway [L, *artificiosum,* skillfully made], a plastic or rubber device that can be inserted into the upper or lower respiratory tract to facilitate ventilation or the removal of secretions.

Artificial Airway Management, a Nursing Interventions Classification defined as maintenance of endotracheal and tracheostomy tubes and prevention of complications associated with their use.

artificial ankylosis, a surgical procedure in which two or more parts of a joint are fixed so that the joint becomes immovable.

artificial anus, a surgical opening into the bowel, as in a colostomy.

artificial assists, any prosthetic devices or contrivances that may enable a physically challenged person to function. Examples include heart pacemakers, crutches, and artificial limbs.

artificial classification of cavities, any cavity that may be classified in one of six groups, the first five of which are those proposed by G. V. Black. Class 1: cavities associated with structural tooth defects in the occlusal surfaces of posterior teeth and lingual surfaces of anterior teeth, such as pits and fissures; class 2: cavities in the proximal surfaces of premolars and molars; class 3: cavities in the proximal surfaces of the canines and incisors that do not involve removal and restoration of the incisal angle; class 4: cavities in the proximal surfaces of canines and incisors that require the removal and restoration of the incisal angle; class 5: cavities, except pit cavities, in the gingival third of the labial, buccal, or lingual surfaces of the teeth; class 6: cavities on the incisal edges and cusp tips of the teeth.

artificial crown, a dental prosthesis that restores part or all of the coronal part of a natural tooth.

artificial eye, a prosthetic device resembling a normal eyeball that is fitted into the socket of an eye that has been removed.

artificial fever, an elevated body temperature produced by artificial means, such as the injection of malarial parasites or a vaccine known to produce fever symptoms or application of heat to the body. An artificial fever may be prescribed for a patient to arrest a disease that is sensitive to elevated body temperatures.

artificial heart, a mechanical device of molded polyurethane, consisting of two ventricles implanted in the body and powered by an air compressor located outside the body. The first artificial heart for humans was implanted in December 1982.

artificial insemination (AI), the introduction of semen into the vagina or uterus by mechanical or instrumental means rather than by sexual intercourse. The procedure is planned to coincide with the expected time of ovulation so that fertilization can occur.

artificial insemination—donor (AID), artificial insemination in which the semen specimen is provided by an anonymous donor. The procedure is used primarily in cases in which the husband is sterile.

artificial insemination—husband (AIH), artificial insemination in which the semen specimen is provided by the husband. The procedure is used primarily in cases of impotency, low sperm count, or a vaginal disorder or when the husband is incapable of sexual intercourse because of some physical disability.

artificial intelligence (AI), a system that makes it possible for a machine to perform functions similar to those performed by human intelligence, such as learning, reasoning, self-correcting, and adapting. Computer technology produces many instruments and systems that mimic and surpass some human capabilities, as speed of counting, correlating, sensing, and deducing.

artificial kidney, a device used to remove the body waste in circulating blood, commonly excreted in urine. It usually consists of a set of tubes or catheters that pass the blood through a dialysate solution where wastes are removed by osmosis and diffusion.

artificial labor [L, *artificiosus,* artificial, *labor,* work], induced labor, as when started with drugs or mechanical devices.

artificial menopause [L, *artificiosus,* artificial, *men,* month; Gk, *pauein,* to cease], the termination of menstrual periods by surgery, radiation, or other methods.

artificial saliva [L, *artificialis,* artifice, *saliva,* spittle], a mixture of carboxymethylcellulose, sorbitol, sodium and potassium chloride in an aqueous solution. It is available in a spray container for the treatment of xerostomia, or dry mouth.

artificial selection, the process by which the genotypes of successive plant and animal generations are determined through controlled breeding.

artificial stone, a calcined gypsum derivative similar to but stronger than plaster of paris, used for making dental casts and dies.

artificial tears, a pharmaceutical preparation of various polymers that can be instilled in the eyes of patients suffering from dry eye or keratoconjunctivitis sicca.

artificial ventilation, the process of supporting respiration by manual or mechanical means when normal breathing is inefficient or has stopped. Effective ventilation of the lungs may fail because of bronchial obstruction by swelling, a foreign body, increased secretions, neuromuscular weakness, status asthmaticus, exhaustion, pharmacologic depression, or trauma to the chest wall. Before an attempt to administer artificial ventilation, the airway is tested, and any obstruction removed.

art therapy, a type of adjunctive mental health treatment in which the patient is encouraged to express his or her feelings through various forms of artwork.

Art Therapy, a Nursing Interventions Classification defined as facilitation of communication through drawings or other art forms.

aryepiglottic folds /er′ē·ep′iglot′ik/, folds of mucous membrane that extend around the margins of the larynx from a junction with the epiglottis. They function as a sphincter during swallowing.

aryl hydrocarbon hydroxylase (AHH), an enzyme that converts carcinogenic chemicals in tobacco smoke and in polluted air into active carcinogens within the lungs.

As, symbol for the element **arsenic.**

AS, abbreviation for **aortic stenosis.**

a.s., abbreviation for **auris sinistra.**

ASA, 1. abbreviation for *American Society of Anesthesiologists.* 2. abbreviation for **aspirin** (acetylsalicylic acid).

ASAHP, abbreviation for *American Society of Allied Health Professionals.*

ASAP, abbreviation for *as soon as possible.*

asaphia /āsä′fē-ə/ [Gk, *asapheia,* obscurity], indistinct speech.

asbestos /asbes′təs/ [Gk, *asbestos,* unquenchable], a group of fibrous impure magnesium silicate minerals. Inhalation of the fibers can lead to pulmonary fibrosis if the fibers accumulate in terminal bronchioles. Continued exposure to asbestos fibers can result in lung cancer.

asbestos body, an asbestos fiber engulfed by a macrophage or a mass of spicules coated with calcium, iron salts, and other substances, as found in the lungs of asbestosis patients.

asbestosis [Gk, *asbestos,* inextinguishable, *osis,* condition], a chronic lung disease caused by the inhalation of asbestos fibers that results in the development of alveolar, interstitial, and pleural fibrosis. Asbestos miners and workers are most frequently affected, but the disease sometimes occurs in other people who have been exposed to asbestos building materials.

ASC, abbreviation for **altered state of consciousness.**

ascariasis /as′kərī′əsis/ [Gk, *askaris,* intestinal worm, *osis,* condition], an infection caused by a parasitic worm, *Ascaris lumbricoides,* that migrates through the lungs in its larval stage. The eggs are passed in human feces, contaminating the soil and allowing transmission to the mouths of others through hands, water, or food. After hatching in the small intestine, the larvae travel through the wall of the intestine and are carried by the lymphatics and blood to the lungs.

Ascaris /as′kəris/, a genus of large parasitic intestinal roundworms, such as *Ascaris lumbricoides,* a cause of ascariasis, found throughout temperate and tropic regions.

ascending aorta /asen′ding/ [L, *ascendere,* to climb], one of the four main sections of the aorta, branching into the right and left coronary arteries.

ascending colon, the segment of the colon that extends from the cecum in the lower right side of the abdomen to the transverse colon at the hepatic flexure on the right side.

ascending neuritis [L, *ascendere,* to rise; Gk, *neuron,* nerve, *itis,* inflammation], a nerve inflammation that begins on the periphery and moves upward along a nerve trunk.

ascending neuropathy, a disease of the nervous system that begins at a lower place in the body and spreads upward.

ascending paralysis, a condition in which there is successive flaccid paralysis of the legs, then the trunk and arms, and finally the muscles of respiration. Causes include poliomyelitis, infectious polyneuritis, and exposure to toxic chemicals.

ascending pharyngeal artery, one of the smallest arteries that branch from the external carotid artery, deep in the neck. It supplies various organs and muscles of the head, such as the tympanic cavity, the longus capitis, and the longus colli.

ascending poliomyelitis [L, *ascendere,* to rise; Gk, *polios,* gray, *myelos,* marrow, *itis,* inflammation], poliomyelitis that begins in the legs and spreads upward to involve the trunk and respiratory muscles.

ascending tract [L, *tractus*], a nervous system pathway found in the spinal cord that carries impulses toward the brain.

asceticism /aset′isiz′əm/ [Gk, *askein,* to exercise], (in psychiatry) a defense mechanism that involves repudiation of all instinctual impulses.

Aschoff bodies [Karl A.L. Aschoff, German pathologist, 1866–1942; AS, *bodig*], tiny rounded or spindle-shaped nodules containing multinucleated giant cells, fibroblasts, and basophilic cells. The are found in joints, tendons, the pleura, and the cardiovascular system of rheumatic fever patients.

ascites /əsī′tēz/ [Gk, *askos,* bag], an abnormal intraperitoneal accumulation of a fluid containing large amounts of protein and electrolytes. The condition may be accompanied by general abdominal swelling, hemodilution, edema, or a decrease in urinary output. Ascites is a complication, for example, of cirrhosis, congestive heart failure, nephrosis, malignant neoplastic disease, peritonitis, or various fungal and parasitic diseases. **—ascitic,** *adj.*

ascites praecox /prē′koks/ [Gk, *askos* + L, premature], an abnormal accumulation of fluid within the peritoneal cavity preceding the generalized edema associated with pericarditis.

ascitic fluid /əsit′ik/ [Gk, *askos,* bag], a watery fluid containing albumin, glucose, and electrolytes that accumulates in the peritoneal cavity in association with certain diseases such as liver disease or congestive heart failure. The fluid occurs as leakage from the veins and lymphatics into extravascular spaces.

ascorbemia /as′kôrbē′mē-ə/ [Gk, *a,* not; AS, *scurf,* scurvy; Gk, *haima,* blood], the presence of ascorbic acid in the blood in amounts greater than normal, usually reflecting only an excess of ascorbic acid intake.

ascorbic acid /əskôr′bik/ [Gk, *a,* not; AS, *scurf,* scurvy], a water-soluble, white crystalline vitamin present in citrus fruits, tomatoes, berries, potatoes, and fresh green and leafy vegetables. It is essential for the formation of collagen and fibrous tissue for normal intercellular matrices in teeth, bone, cartilage, connective tissue, and skin and for the structural integrity of capillary walls. Severe deficiency results in scurvy.

ascorburia /as′kôrby oŏr′ē·ə/ [Gk, *a,* not; AS, *scurf,* scurvy; Gk, *ouron,* urine], the presence of ascorbic acid in the urine in amounts greater than normal. It usually reflects only an excess ascorbic acid intake.

ascribed role /əskrībd′/, an assigned role in society, based on age, sex, or other factors about which the individual has no choice.

ASD, abbreviation for **atrial septal defect.**

asepsis /āsep′sis/ [Gk, *a, sepsis,* not decay], **1.** the absence of germs. **2. medical asepsis,** procedures used to reduce the number of microorganisms and prevent their spread. **3.** surgical asepsis, procedures used to eliminate any microorganisms; sterile technique. —**aseptic,** *adj.*

aseptic /āsep′tik/ [Gk, *a,* without, *sepsis,* decay], pertaining to a condition free of living pathogenic organisms or infected material.

aseptic-antiseptic, both aseptic and antiseptic.

aseptic body image, an awareness by operating room personnel of body, hair, makeup, clothing, jewelry, and placement with regard for maintenance of a sterile environment. The body image also includes an awareness of changing proximities between sterile and contaminated areas as a field becomes progressively contaminated.

aseptic bone necrosis, a type of bone and joint damage that may occur in workers exposed to repeated compressed-air environments, as in diving or tunneling occupations.

aseptic fever, a fever not associated with infection. Mechanical trauma, as in a crushing injury, can cause fever even when no pathogenic microorganism is present.

aseptic gauze, any gauze that is sterile and therefore free of microorganisms.

aseptic meningitis, an inflammation of the meninges that is caused by one of a number of viruses, including coxsackievi-

ruses, nonparalytic polioviruses, echoviruses, and mumps.

aseptic necrosis [Gk, *a, sepsis,* without decay, *nekros,* dead, *osis,* condition], cystic and sclerotic degenerative changes in tissues, as may follow an injury in the absence of infection.

aseptic peritonitis [Gk, *a, sepsis,* without decay, *peri,* near, *teinein,* to stretch, *itis,* inflammation], peritonitis in which inflammation of the peritoneum is caused by chemicals, radiation, or injury, rather than by an infectious agent.

aseptic surgery [Gk, *a, sepsis,* without decay, *cheirourgos,* surgeon], the prevention of contamination during surgical procedures.

aseptic technique, any health care procedure in which added precautions are used to prevent contamination of a person, object, or area by microorganisms.

asexual /āsek′shoo·əl/ [Gk, *a,* not; L, *sexus,* male or female]. **1.** not sexual. **2.** pertaining to an organism that has no sexual organs. **3.** pertaining to a process that is not sexual. —**asexuality,** *n.*

asexual dwarf, an adult dwarf whose genital organs are underdeveloped.

asexual generation, any type of reproduction that occurs without the union of male and female gametes, such as fission, budding, sporulation, or parthenogenesis.

asexualization /āsek′shoo·əlīzā′shən/, the process of making one incapable of reproduction; sterilization of an individual or animal by castration, vasectomy, removal of the ovaries, or use of chemicals.

asexual reproduction, a type of reproduction found in plants and lower animals in which new organisms are formed without the union of gametes, as occurs in budding, fission, and spore formation.

ASHA, abbreviation for **American Speech, Language, and Hearing Association.**

ASHD, abbreviation for **arteriosclerotic heart disease.**

Asherman syndrome, secondary amenorrhea in a hormonally normal woman, caused by obliteration of the endometrial cavity by adhesions that form as a result of curettage or infection.

asiderosis /ā′sidərō′sis/, an iron deficiency and a cause of anemia.

ASL, abbreviation for **American Sign Language.**

ASLT, abbreviation for **antistreptolysin-O test.**

ASMT, abbreviation for *American Society for Medical Technology.*

Asn, abbreviation for the amino acid **asparagine.**

asocial /āsō′shəl/ [Gk, *a,* without; L, *so-*

cius, companion], withdrawn or disengaged from normal contacts with other individuals.

asoma /āsō′mə/ [Gk, *a,* not, *soma,* body], a fetus with an incomplete trunk and head.

ASOT, abbreviation for **antistreptolysin-O test.**

asparaginase /aspar′əjinās/ [Gk, *asparagos,* asparagus], an enzyme that catalyzes the hydrolysis of asparagine to asparaginic acid and ammonia.

asparagine (Asn) /aspar′əjin/, a nonessential amino acid found in many proteins in the body.

aspartame /aspär′tām, as′pərtām/, a white, almost odorless crystalline powder that is used as an artificial sweetener. Excessive use of this nonnutritive sweetener should be avoided by patients with phenylketonuria (PKU) because the substance hydrolyzes to form aspartylphenylalanine.

aspartate aminotransferase (AST) /aspär′tāt/, an enzyme normally present in body serum and in certain body tissues, especially those of the heart and liver. This enzyme affects the intermolecular transfer of an amino group from aspartic acid to alpha-ketoglutaric acid, forming glutamic acid and oxaloacetic acid.

aspartate kinase, an enzyme that catalyzes the transfer of a phosphate group from adenosine triphosphate to aspartate to produce phosphoaspartate.

aspartic acid (Asp) /aspär′tik/, a nonessential amino acid present in sugar cane, beet molasses, and breakdown products of many proteins.

aspastic /āspas′tik/, not characterized by spasms.

aspect [L, *aspectus,* a look], the appearance, look, facing, or fronting of a person or object.

aspergillic acid /as′pərjil′ik/, an antibiotic substance derived from *Aspergillus flavus,* an aflatoxin-producing mold found on corn, grain, and peanuts.

aspergillosis /as′pərjilō′sis/ [L, *aspergere,* to sprinkle; Gk, *osis,* condition], an infection caused by a fungus of the genus *Aspergillus* that can cause inflammatory, granulomatous lesions on or in any organ.

Aspergillus /as′pərjil′əs/ [L, *aspergere,* to sprinkle], a genus of fungi that is a common contaminant in the laboratory and a cause of nosocomial infection.

aspurmatic /ā′spurmat′ik/, pertaining to an inability to secrete or ejaculate semen.

aspermia /āspur′mē-ə/ [Gk, *a, sperma,* without seed], lack of formation or ejaculation of semen.

aspermatogenesis /āspur′mətōjen′əsis/,

a failure of the male genitals to produce spermatozoa.

asphyxia /asfik′sē-ə/ [Gk, *a + sphyxis,* without pulse], severe hypoxia leading to hypoxemia and hypercapnia, loss of consciousness, and, if not corrected, death. Some of the more common causes of asphyxia are drowning, electrical shock, aspiration of vomitus, lodging of a foreign body in the respiratory tract, inhalation of toxic gas or smoke, and poisoning. —**asphyxiate,** *v.,* **asphyxiated,** *adj.*

asphyxia livida /liv′ədə/, an abnormal condition in which a newborn's skin is cyanotic, the pulse is weak and slow, and the reflexes are slow or absent.

asphyxia neonatorum, a condition in which a newborn does not breathe spontaneously. The asphyxia may develop before or during labor or immediately after delivery.

asphyxia pallida /pal′ədə/, an abnormal condition in which a newborn appears pale and limp, shows signs of apnea, and suffers from bradycardia as marked by a heartbeat of 80 beats/min or less.

asphyxiate /asfik′sē-āt/ [Gk, *a + sphyxis,* without pulse], to induce an inability to breathe. Causes may include circulatory congestion, chemical poisoning, electrical shock, or physical suffocation.

asphyxiation [Gk, *a + sphyxis,* without pulse], a state of asphyxia or inability to breathe.

aspirant /as′pirənt/, the fluid, gas, or solid particles that are withdrawn from the body by aspiration methods.

aspirant maneuver, a procedure used in making x-ray films of the laryngopharyngeal area. The patient exhales completely and then slowly inhales while making a harsh, high-pitched sound.

aspirate /-rāt/ [L, *aspirare,* to breathe upon], to withdraw fluid or air from a cavity. The process is usually aided by use of a syringe or a suction device.

aspirating needle, a long hollow needle used to remove fluid from a cavity, vessel, or structure of the body.

aspirating syringe /-rā′ting/, (in dentistry) a hypodermic syringe used in the injection of local anesthetics. Checking for blood in the cartridge before injecting ensures that the anesthetic solution is not being deposited in a blood vessel.

aspiration /as′pirā′shən/, **1.** the act of taking a breath, inhaling. **2.** the act of withdrawing a fluid, such as mucus or serum, from the body by a suction device. —**aspirate,** *n.*

aspiration biopsy, the removal of living tissue for microscopic examination by suction through a fine needle attached to a syringe. The procedure is used primarily to obtain cells from a lesion containing fluid or when fluid is formed in a serous cavity.

aspiration biopsy cytology (ABC), a microscopic examination of cells obtained directly from living body tissue by aspiration through a fine needle.

aspiration drug abuse, the inhalation of a liquid, solid, or gaseous chemical into the respiratory system for nontherapeutic purposes.

aspiration of vomitus, the inhalation of regurgitated gastric contents into the pulmonary system.

aspiration pneumonia, an inflammatory condition of the lungs and bronchi caused by inhaling foreign material or vomitus containing acid gastric contents.

Aspiration Precautions, a Nursing Interventions Classification defined as prevention or minimization of risk factors in the patient at risk for aspiration.

aspiration, risk for, a NANDA-accepted nursing diagnosis of a state in which an individual is at risk for entry of gastric secretions, oropharyngeal secretions, or exogenous food or fluids into tracheobronchial passages caused by dysfunction or absence of normal protective mechanisms. Risk factors include reduced level of consciousness, depressed cough and gag reflexes, presence of a tracheostomy or an endotracheal tube, overinflated tracheostomy or endotracheal tube cuff, inadequate inflation of a tracheostomy or endotracheal tube cuff, gastrointestinal tubes, and bolus tube feedings or medication administration.

aspirator /as'pirā'tər/ [L, *aspirare*, to breathe upon], any instrument that removes a substance from body cavities by suction, such as a bulb syringe, piston pump, or hypodermic syringe.

aspirin (ASA) /as'pirin/, an analgesic, antipyretic, and antirheumatic prescribed to reduce fever and relieve pain and inflammation.

aspirin poisoning. See **salicylate poisoning.**

asplenia /āsplē'nē·ə/ [Gk, *a*, without, *spleen*], absence of a spleen. The condition may be congenital or result from surgical removal.

ASRT, abbreviation for *American Society of Radiologic Technologists.*

assault /əsôlt'/ [L, *assilirere*, to leap upon], 1. an unlawful act that places another person, without that person's consent, in fear of immediate bodily harm or battery. 2. the act of committing an assault. 3. to threaten a person with bodily harm or injury.

assay /asā', as'ā/ [Fr, *essayer*, to try], the

analysis of the purity or effectiveness of drugs and other biologic substances, including laboratory and clinical observations.

assertiveness /əsur'tivnes/, behavior directed toward claiming one's rights without denying those of others.

Assertiveness Training, a Nursing Interventions Classification defined as assistance with the effective expression of feelings, needs, and ideas while respecting the rights of others.

assertive training /əsur'tiv/ [L, *asserere*, to join to oneself], a therapeutic technique to help individuals become more self-assertive and self-confident in interpersonal relationships.

assessing /əses'ing/ [L, *assidere*, to sit beside], (in five-step nursing process) a category of nursing behavior that includes the gathering, verifying, and communicating of information related to the client. The nurse collects information from verbal interactions with the patient, the patient's family, and significant others; examines standard data sources for information; systematically checks for symptoms and signs; determines the patient's ability to perform self-care activities; assesses the patient's environment; and identifies reactions of the staff (including the nurse who is performing the assessment) to the patient and to the patient's family and significant others.

assessment /əses'mənt/ [L, *assidere*, to sit beside], (in medicine and nursing) 1. an evaluation or appraisal of a condition. 2. the process of making such an evaluation. 3. (in a problem-oriented medical record) an examiner's evaluation of the disease or condition based on the patient's subjective report of the symptoms and course of the illness or condition and the examiner's objective findings, including data obtained through laboratory tests, physical examination, and medical history.—**assess,** *v.*

assessment of the aging patient, an evaluation of the changes characteristic of advancing years exhibited by an elderly person.

assimilate /əsim'əlāt/ [L, *assimilare*, to make alike], to absorb nutritive substances from the digestive tract to the circulatory system and convert them into living tissues.

assimilation [L, *assimulare*, to make alike], 1. the process of incorporating nutritive material into living tissue; the end stage of the nutrition process, after digestion and absorption or simultaneous with absorption. 2. (in psychology) the incorporation of new experiences into a person's pattern of consciousness. 3. (in sociology) the process in which a person or a group of people of a different ethnic background become absorbed into a new culture. —assimilate, v.

assist-control mode, a system of mechanical ventilation in which the patient is allowed to initiate breathing, although the ventilator delivers a set volume with each breath.

assisted breech [L, *assistere,* to stand by], an obstetric operation in which a baby being born feet or buttocks first is permitted to deliver spontaneously as far as its umbilicus and is then extracted.

assisted circulation [L, *assistere,* to stand, *circulare,* to go around], a method of treating patients with severe circulatory deficiencies by introducing a mechanical pumping system to aid the blood flow.

assisted death, a form of euthanasia in which an individual expressing a wish to die prematurely is helped to accomplish that goal by another person, either by counseling and/or by providing a poison or other lethal instrument. The assisted death may be regarded as a homicide or suicide by local authorities, and the person giving assistance may be held responsible for the death. In most cases, the deceased was a terminally ill patient.

assisted reproductive technology, the manipulation of egg and sperm in treating infertility. The processes include the administration of drugs to induce ovulation, fertilization, gamete intrafallopian transfer, zygote intrafallopian transfer, and cryopreservation of gametes.

assisted suicide, a form of euthanasia in which a person wishes to commit suicide but feels unable to perform the act alone because of a physical disability or lack of knowledge about the most effective means. An individual who assists a suicide victim in accomplishing that goal may or may not be held responsible for the death, depending on local laws.

assisted ventilation, the use of mechanical or other devices to help maintain respiration, usually by delivering air or oxygen under positive pressure.

associated antagonist, one of a pair of muscles or group of muscles that pull in opposite directions but whose combined action results in moving a part in one direction.

Associate Degree in Nursing (ADN) /əsō′shē·āt/ [L, *associare,* to unite], an academic degree awarded on satisfactory completion of a 2-year course of study, usually at a community or junior college. The recipient is eligible to take the national licensing examination to become a registered nurse. An associate degree in nursing is not available in Canada.

associate nurse, 1. (in primary nursing, United States) a nurse who is responsible for implementing a primary nurse's care plans. **2.** in some states, a registered nurse who holds a diploma from a hospital school of nursing or an associate degree.

association /əsō′shē·ā′shən/ [L, *associare,* to unite], **1.** a connection, union, joining, or combination of things. **2.** (in psychology) the connection of remembered feelings, emotions, sensations, thoughts, or perceptions with particular persons, things, or ideas.

association area, any part of the cerebral cortex involved in the integration of sensory information.

Association for Practitioners of Infection Control (APIC), a national professional organization of nurses working in the field of infection control.

Association for the Advancement of Medical Instrumentation (AAMI), a nonprofit organization involved in education and standards relating to biomedical engineering.

Association for the Care of Children's Health (ACCH), an international interdisciplinary organization concerned with the psychosocial needs of children and their families in health care settings.

associationist model of learning /əsō′shē·ā′shənist/, a theory that defines learning as behavioral change that is a result of reinforced practice. If the response has not been reinforced repeatedly, an alternative behavior may be substituted.

Association of Canadian Medical Colleges (ACMC), a Canadian organization of the deans and faculty members of the nation's 16 medical schools.

association of ideas, a mental connection established between similar or simultaneously occurring ideas, feelings, or perceptions.

Association of Operating Room Nurses (AORN), a national organization of operating room nurses.

Association of Women's Health, Obstetric, and Neonatal Nurses (AWHONN), an organization of nurses working in obstetrics and gynecology in the United States.

association paralysis, a motor neuron disease in which wasting, weakness, and fasciculation of the tongue, facial muscles, pharynx, and larynx occur.

association test, a technique used in psychiatric diagnosis and in educational and psychologic evaluation in which a person is asked to respond to a stimulus word with the first word that comes to mind.

associative looseness /əsō'shətiv/, a form of thought disorder in which the patient is unable to maintain consistent thought for more than a few minutes and jumps from thought to thought in a conversation.

associative play, a form of play in which a group of children participate in similar or identical activities without formal organization, group direction, group interaction, or a definite goal.

assortive mating, the matching of males and females for reproduction in a manner that eliminates natural selection.

assumed role /əs(y)oomd'/, a role in life that an individual usually selects or achieves by choice, such as one's role in marriage or employment.

AST, abbreviation for **aspartate aminotransferase.**

astasia /astā'zhə/, a lack of motor coordination marked by an inability to stand or sit without assistance.

astasia-abasia [Gk, a, stasis, not stand, a, basis, not step], a form of ataxia in which the patient is unable to stand or walk because of lack of motor coordination but able to carry out natural leg movements when sitting or lying down.

astatine (At) [Gk, astasis, unsteady], a very unstable, radioactive element that occurs naturally in tiny amounts. Its atomic number is 85; its atomic weight (mass) is 210.

asteatosis /as'tē-ətō'sis/ [Gk, a, stear, without tallow, osis, condition], a dry skin condition caused by a deficiency of sebaceous gland secretions. Scales and fissures may result from the dryness.

astereognosis /əstir'ē-og·nō'sis/ [Gk, a, stereos, not solid, gnosis, knowledge], an inability to identify objects by touch.

asterixis /as'tərik'sis/ [Gk, a, sterixis, not fixed position], a hand-flapping tremor, often accompanying metabolic disorders.

asteroid body [Gk, aster, star, eidos, form], an irregular star-shaped structure that develops in the giant cells in certain diseases, including sarcoidosis, actinomycosis, and nocardiosis.

asthenia /asthē'nē·ə/ [Gk, a + sthenos, without strength], **1.** the lack or loss of strength or energy; weakness; debility. **2.** (in psychiatry) lack of dynamic force in the personality.—**asthenic,** adj.

asthenic /asthen'ik/ [Gk, a + sthenos, without strength], pertaining to a condition of weakness, feebleness, or loss of vitality.

asthenic habitus [Gk, a + sthenos, without strength; L, habere, to have], a body structure characterized by a slender build with long limbs, an angular profile, and prominent muscles or bones.

asthenic personality, a personality characterized by low energy, lack of enthusiasm, depressed emotions, and oversensitivity to physical and emotional strain.

asthenopia /as'thənō'pē-ə/ [Gk, a, sthenos + ops, eye], a condition in which the eyes tire easily because of weakness of the ocular or ciliary muscles. Symptoms include pain in or around the eyes, headache, dimness of vision, dizziness, and slight nausea.

asthma /az'mə/ [Gk, panting], a respiratory disorder characterized by recurring episodes of paroxysmal dyspnea, wheezing on expiration/inspiration caused by constriction of the bronchi, coughing, and viscous mucoid bronchial secretions. The episodes may be precipitated by inhalation of allergens or pollutants, infection, cold air, vigorous exercise, or emotional stress.

asthma in children, a chronic inflammatory disorder of the airways. The inflammation causes symptoms associated with obstructive airflow and characterized by recurring attacks of paroxysmal dyspnea, wheezing, prolonged expiration, and an irritative cough that is a common, chronic illness in childhood. Onset usually occurs between 3 and 8 years of age. Asthmatic attacks are caused by constriction of the large and small airways resulting from bronchial smooth muscle spasm, edema, inflammation of the bronchial wall, or excessive production of mucus. It is a complex disorder involving biochemical, immunologic, infectious, endocrinologic, and psychologic factors. Asthma attacks in the past were classified as either extrinsic or intrinsic. Most extrinsic attacks in children were associated with an allergenic hypersensitivity to a foreign substance such as airborne pollen, mold, house dust, certain foods, animal hair and skin, feathers, insects, smoke, and various chemicals or drugs. In infants, especially those with a family history of allergic reactions, food allergy is a common precipitating factor.

asthmatic breathing /azmat'ik/ [Gk, asthma, panting; AS, braeth], breathing marked by prolonged wheezing on exhalation caused by spasmodic contractions of the bronchi.

asthmatic bronchitis, an inflammation and swelling of the mucous membrane of the bronchi in a patient with asthma.

asthmatic cough [Gk, asthma + AS, cohhetan], a wheezing cough accompanied by signs of breathing difficulty.

asthmatic eosinophilia, a form of eosinophilic pneumonia, characterized by allergic bronchospasm, expectoration of bronchial casts containing eosinophils and mycelium, and cough and fever. The condition usually occurs in the fourth or fifth decade of life and is twice as common in women as in men. It is a result of hypersensitivity to *Aspergillus fumigatus* or *Candida albicans.*

astigmatic /as'tigmat'ik/ [Gk, *a, stigma,* without point], pertaining to astigmatism, or an error of refraction in which a ray of light is not sharply focused on the retinal tissue but is spread over a more diffuse area. Astigmatism is due to differences in curvature in the various meridians of the cornea and lens of the eye.

astigmatism /əstig'mətiz'əm/ [Gk, *a, stigma,* without point], an abnormal condition of the eye in which the light rays cannot be focused clearly in a point on the retina because the spheric curve of the cornea is not equal in all meridians. Vision is typically blurred; if uncorrected, it often results in visual discomfort or asthenopia. The person cannot accommodate to correct the problem. The condition usually may be corrected with contact lenses or with eyeglasses ground to neutralize the condition.

astringent /əstrin'jənt/ [Gk, *astringere,* to tighten], **1.** a substance that causes contraction of tissues on application, usually used locally. **2.** having the quality of an astringent.—**astringency,** *n.*

astringent bath, a bath in which alum, tannic acid, or another astringent is added to the water.

astringent douche, a cleansing stream containing substances such as alum that can contract the mucous membrane of the vagina.

astroblastoma /as'trōblastō'mə/ [Gk, *aster,* star, *blastos,* germ, *oma,* tumor], a malignant neoplasm of the brain and spinal cord. Cells of an astroblastoma lie around blood vessels or around connective tissue septa.

astrocyte /as'trōsīt'/ [Gk, *aster + kytos,* cell], a large, star-shaped neuroglial cell found in certain tissues of the nervous system.

astrocytoma /as'trōsītō'mə/ [Gk, *aster, kytos + oma*], a primary tumor of the brain composed of astrocytes and characterized by slow growth, cyst formation, invasion of surrounding structures, and often development of a highly malignant glioblastoma within the tumor mass.

astrocytosis /as'trōsītō'sis/ [Gk, *aster + kytos + osis,* condition], an increase in the number of neuroglial cells with fibrous or protoplasmic processes frequently observed in an irregular area adjacent to degenerative lesions, such as abscesses, certain brain neoplasms, and encephalomalacia.

asylum /əsī'ləm/ [Gk, *asylon,* inviolable], an institution for the care of physically or mentally handicapped persons judged incapable of caring for themselves.

asymmetric /ā'simet'rik, as'imet'rik/ [Gk, *a + symmetria,* without proportion], (of the body or parts of the body) unequal in size or shape; different in placement or arrangement about an axis. —**asymmetry** /āsim'itrē, asim'-/, *n.*

asymptomatic /āsimp'təmat'ik/ [Gk, *a,* without, *symptoma,* that which happens], without symptoms.

asymptomatic neurosyphilis [Gk, *a,* without, *symptoma, neuron,* nerve; Fr, *syphilide*], a form of neurosyphilis characterized by pathologic changes in the cerebrospinal fluid, although there are no symptoms of nervous system damage. Asymptomatic neurosyphilis may occur many years before actual nervous system damage is noticeable.

asynclitism /āsing'klitiz'əm/ [Gk, *a + syn,* not together, *kleisis,* to lean], presentation of a parietal aspect of the fetal head to the maternal pelvic inlet in labor. The sagittal suture is parallel to the transverse diameter of the pelvis but anterior or posterior to it. Anterior asynclitism, in which the anterior part presents, is called Nägele obliquity. Posterior asynclitism is called Litzmann obliquity.

asyndesis /əsin'dəsis/, a mental disorder marked by an inability to assemble related ideas or thoughts into one coherent concept.

asynergy /āsin'ərjē/ [Gk, *a + syn + ergein,* to work], **1.** a condition characterized by faulty coordination among groups of organs or muscles that normally function harmoniously. **2.** the state of muscle antagonism found in cerebellar disease.

asyntaxia /ā'sintak'sē-ə/ [Gk, *a + syn + taxis,* arrangement], any interference with the orderly sequence of growth and differentiation of the fetus during embryonic development, resulting in one or more congenital anomalies.

asyntaxia dorsalis, failure of the neural tube to close during embryonic development.

asystole /āsis'təlē/ [Gk, *a + systole,* not contraction], a life-threatening cardiac condition characterized by the absence of electrical and mechanical activity in the heart. Clinical signs include lack of pulse and breathing. —**asystolic** /ā'sistol'ik/, *adj.*

asystolic cardiac rhythm /ā'sistol'ik/, an electrocardiographic recording that appears as a flat line, indicating cardiac arrest.

At, symbol for the element **astatine.**

Atabrine stomatitis, an abnormal oral condition that may be associated with the use of Atabrine (quinacrine hydrochloride), characterized by oral changes that simulate lichen planus.

ataractic /at'ərak'tik/ [Gk, *ataraktos,* quiet], pertaining to a drug or other agent that has a tranquilizing or sedating effect.

ataraxia /at'ərak'sē'ə/ [Gk, *a,* not, *tarakos,* disturbed], a state of mental tranquility.

atavism /at'əviz'əm/ [L, *atavus,* ancestor], the appearance in an individual of traits or characteristics more like those of a grandparent or earlier ancestor than of the parents. Atavistic data may offer clues to an examining physician of genetic or familial health factors.—**atavistic,** *adj.*

ataxia /ətak'sē·ə/ [Gk, without order], an abnormal condition characterized by impaired ability to coordinate movement. A staggering gait and postural imbalance are caused by a lesion in the spinal cord or cerebellum.—**ataxial, ataxic,** *adj.*

ataxiaphasia /-fā'zhə/ [Gk, *ataxia,* without order], a state in which a person is unable to connect words properly as needed to form a sentence.

ataxia-telangiectasia syndrome [Gk, *ataxia* + *telos,* end, *angeion,* vessel, *ektasis,* expansion], a rare genetic disorder involving deficits in immunoglobulin metabolism that is transmitted as an autosomal-recessive trait. The onset usually occurs in infancy and progresses slowly with increasing cerebellar degeneration (ataxia) to severe disability. Telangiectasias are most prominent on skin surfaces exposed to the sun.

ataxic breathing, a type of breathing associated with a lesion in the medullary respiratory centers and characterized by a series of inspirations and expirations.

ataxic dysarthria, abnormal speech characterized by faulty formation of sounds because of neuromuscular dysfunction of the cerebellum.

ATCC, abbreviation for **American Type Culture Collection.**

atelectasis /at'ilek'təsis/ [Gk, *ateles,* incomplete, *ektasis,* expansion], an abnormal condition characterized by the collapse of the alveoli, preventing the respiratory exchange of carbon dioxide and oxygen. Symptoms may include diminished breath sounds, a mediastinal shift toward the side of the collapse, fever, and increasing dyspnea.

ateliosis /ətē'lē·ō'sis/ [Gk, *ateles,* incomplete, *osis,* condition], a form of dwarfism caused by the absence or destruction of eosinophil cells of the adenohypophysis. The person may appear childlike and have poorly developed muscles.

ateliotic dwarf /at'əlē·ot'ik/, a dwarf whose skeleton is incompletely formed as a result of the nonunion of the epiphyses and diaphyses during bone development.

atelorachidia /at'əlôr'əkid'ē·ə/ [Gk, *ateles,* incomplete, *rhachis,* spine], a defective, incomplete formation of the spinal column.

atenolol /aten'əlôl/, a beta₁ blocker prescribed for the treatment of hypertension.

ATG, abbreviation for **antithymocyte globulin.**

athelia /āthē'lē·ə/ [Gk, *a,* not, *thele,* nipple], an absence of nipples.

atherectomy /ath'ərek'təmē/, surgical removal of an atheroma in a major artery.

atherectomy catheter, a specially designed catheter for cutting away atheromatous plaque from the lining of an artery. The catheter is positioned and monitored by fluoroscopy.

atheroembolic renal disease /ath'ərō·embol'ik/, a condition of gradual or rapid kidney failure resulting from obstruction of the renal arteries by atheromas and emboli.

atheroembolism /ath'ərō·em'bəliz'əm/, obstruction of a blood vessel by a cholesterol-containing embolism originating from an atheroma in a major artery.

atherogenesis [Gk, *athere,* porridge, *oma,* tumor, *genein,* to produce], the formation of subintimal plaques in the lining of arteries.

atheroma /ath'ərō'mə/ [Gk, *athere,* meal, *oma,* tumor], an abnormal mass of fat or lipids, as in a sebaceous cyst or in deposits in an arterial wall. —**atheromatous,** *adj.*

atheromatosis /ath'ərōmətō'sis/, the development of many atheromas.

atheromatous plaque, a yellowish raised area on the lining of an artery formed by fatty deposits.

atherosclerosis /ath'ərōsklərō'sis/ [Gk, *athere,* meal, *sklerosis,* hardening], a common arterial disorder characterized by yellowish plaques of cholesterol, lipids, and cellular debris in the inner layers of the walls of large and medium-sized arteries. The condition begins as a fatty streak and gradually builds to a fibrous plaque or atheromatous lesion. The vessel walls become thick, fibrotic, and calcified, and the lumen narrows, resulting in reduced blood flow to organs normally supplied by the artery. Atheromatous lesions are major causes of coronary heart disease, angina pectoris, myocardial infarction, and other cardiac disorders. The disorder usually occurs with aging and is often associated with tobacco use, obesity, hypertension, elevated low-density lipoprotein cholesterol levels, and diabetes mellitus.

atherosclerotic aneurysm /-ot′ik/ [Gk, *athere* + *skleros*, hard, *aneurysma*, a widening], a dilation that results from atherosclerotic weakening of an arterial wall.

atherothrombosis /ath′ərō′thrombō′sis/, a thrombus originating in an atheromatous blood vessel.

athetoid /ath′ətoid/, pertaining to athetosis.

athetosis /ath′ətō′sis/ [Gk, *athetos*, not fixed], a neuromuscular condition characterized by slow, writhing, continuous, and involuntary movement of the extremities, as seen in some forms of cerebral palsy and in motor disorders resulting from lesions in the basal ganglia, tabes dorsalis, or other conditions.

athiaminosis /əthī′əminō′sis/, a condition resulting from lack of thiamine in the diet.

athlete's heart /ath′lēts/, the typical normal but enlarged heart of an athlete trained for endurance. It is characterized by a slow heart rate, an increased pumping capacity, and a greater-than-average ability to deliver oxygen to skeletal muscles.

athletic habitus /athlet′ik/, a physique characterized by a well-proportioned muscular body with broad shoulders, thick neck, deep chest, and flat abdomen.

athletic trainer, an allied health professional who, with the consultation and supervision of attending physicians, is an integral part of the health care system associated with sports. Through both academic preparation and practical experience, the athletic trainer provides a variety of services, including injury prevention and recognition, immediate care, treatment, and rehabilitation of athletic trauma. Standards for recognition of athletic training as an allied health occupation were approved by the American Medical Association in 1990.

atlantal /ətlan′təl/, pertaining to the atlas, the first cervical vertebra.

atlantoaxial /ətlan′tō·ak′sē·əl/ [Gk, *atlas*, to bear, *axis*, pivot], pertaining to the first two cervical vertebrae.

atlantooccipital joint /-oksip′itəl/ [Gk, *atlas*, to bear; L, *ob*, against, *caput*, head], one of a pair of condyloid joints formed by the articulation of the atlas of the vertebral column with the occipital bone of the skull.

atlas [Gk, *Atlas*, a mythical giant, compelled to uphold the world], the first cervical vertebra, articulating with the occipital bone and the axis.

ATLS, abbreviation for *advanced trauma life support.*5

atm, 1. abbreviation for **atmosphere. 2.** abbreviation for **atmospheric.**

atman /ät′män/, (in psychiatry) a concept derived from Eastern Indian philosophy that the highest value is knowledge of one's true self.

atmosphere (atm) /at′məsfir/ [Gk, *atmos*, vapor, *sphaira*, sphere], **1.** the natural body of air, composed of approximately 20% oxygen, 78% nitrogen, and 2% carbon dioxide and other gases, that covers the surface of the earth. **2.** an envelope of gas, which may or may not duplicate the natural atmosphere in chemical components. **3.** a unit of gas pressure that is usually defined as being equivalent to the average pressure of the earth's atmosphere at sea level, or about 14.7 pounds per square inch. —**atmospheric,** *adj.*

atmospheric pressure /-fer′ik/, the pressure exerted by the weight of the atmosphere.

ATN, abbreviation for **acute tubular necrosis.**

atom /at′əm/ [Gk, *atmos*, indivisible], **1.** (in physics) the smallest division of an element that exhibits all the properties and characteristics of the element. It comprises neutrons, electrons, and protons. The number of protons in the nucleus of every atom of any given element is the same and is called its atomic number. **2.** *nontechnical.* the amount of any substance that is so small that further division is not possible. —**atomic,** *adj.*

atomic mass. See **atomic weight.**

atomic mass unit (amu) /ətom′ik/, the mass of a neutral atom of an element, expressed as $^1/_{12}$ of the mass of carbon, which has an arbitrarily assigned value of 12. The energy equivalent of 1 amu is 931.2 MeV. The mass equivalent of 1 amu is $1.66(10^{-24}$ g).

atomic number, the number of protons, or positive charges, in the nucleus of an atom of a particular element. In a neutral atom, the atomic number equals the number of electrons, and their number and arrangement determine the chemical characteristics of the atom, with the exception of its atomic weight (mass) and radioactivity.

atomic theory [Gk, *atmos*, indivisible, *theoria*, speculation], the concept that all matter is composed of submicroscopic atoms that are in turn composed of protons, electrons, and neutrons. A chemical element is identified by the number of protons in its atoms.

atomic weight (A, at. wt.), the relative mass of a specific isotope of an element compared with a standard carbon atom isotope with an assigned atomic mass of 12.

atomizer /at′əmī′zər/, a device used to

reduce a liquid and eject it as a fine spray or vapor.

atonia /ătō′ne̅·ə/ [Gk, *a* + *tonos,* without tone], decreased or absent muscle tone.

atonic /əton′ik/, **1.** weak. **2.** lacking normal tone, as in the case of a muscle that is flaccid. **3.** lacking vigor, such as an atonic ulcer, which heals slowly. —**atony** /at′onē/, *n.*

atonic constipation, constipation caused by the failure of the colon to respond to the normal stimuli for evacuation caused by loss of muscle tone. It may occur in elderly or bedridden patients or after prolonged dependence on laxatives.

atonicity [Gk, *a* + *tonos,* without tone], a condition of atony or lack of muscle tone or tension.

atopic /ātop′ik/ [Gk, *a* + *topos,* not place], pertaining to a hereditary tendency to experience immediate allergic reactions such as asthma, atopic dermatitis, or vasomotor rhinitis because of the presence of an antibody (atopic reagin) in the skin and sometimes the bloodstream. —**atopy** /at′opē/, *n.*

atopic allergy [Gk, *a,* not, *topos,* place], a form of allergy that afflicts persons with a genetic predisposition to hypersensitivity to certain allergens. Examples include asthma and food allergies.

atopic dermatitis, an intensely pruritic, often excoriated inflammation commonly found on the face and antecubital and popliteal areas of allergy-prone (atopic) individuals.

atopognosia /ātop′əgnō′zhə/ [Gk, *a, topos,* not place, *gnosis,* knowledge], a form of agnosia in which a person is unable to locate a tactile sensation correctly.

ATP, abbreviation for **adenosine triphosphate.**

ATPase, abbreviation for **adenosine triphosphatase.**

ATPD, abbreviation for *ambient temperature, ambient pressure, dry.*

ATPS, abbreviation for *ambient temperature, ambient pressure, saturated* (with water vapor).

atransferrinemic anemia /ā′transfer′inē′-mik/, an iron-transport deficiency disease characterized by a failure of iron to move from the liver or other storage sites to tissues in which erythrocytes develop.

atraumatic /ā′trômat′ik/ [Gk, *a,* without, *trauma*], pertaining to therapies or therapeutic instruments and devices that are unlikely to cause tissue damage.

atresia /ətrē′zhə/ [Gk, *a, tresis,* not perforation], the absence of a normal body opening, duct, or canal, such as of the anus, vagina, or external ear canal. —**atresic, atretic,** *adj.*

atresic teratism /ətrē′sik/ [Gk, *a, tresis* + *tera,* monster], a congenital anomaly in which any of the normal openings of the body, such as the mouth, nares, anus, or vagina, fails to form.

atrial fibrillation (AF) /ā′trē-əl/, a cardiac arrhythmia characterized by disorganized electrical activity in the atria accompanied by an irregular ventricular response that is usually rapid. The atria quiver instead of pumping in an organized fashion, resulting in compromised ventricular filling and reduced stroke volume. Atrial fibrillation is associated with rheumatic heart disease (left atrial dilation), mitral stenosis, acute myocardial infarction, and heart surgery; or it may be idiopathic (lone atrial fibrillation).

atrial flutter (AF), a type of atrial tachycardia with rates from 230 to 380/min. Two kinds, typical and atypical, have been identified and are distinguished from each other by their rates and electrocardiographic (ECG) patterns. During typical atrial flutter the atrial rate is 290 to 310/min and produces "fence post" or "sawtooth" ECG waves.

atrial gallop, an abnormal cardiac rhythm in which a low-pitched extra heart sound is heard late in diastole, just before the S_1, on auscultation of the heart.

atrial myxoma, a benign, pedunculated, gelatinous tumor that originates in the interatrial septum of the heart. The tumor is characterized by palpitations, disseminated neuritis, nausea, weight loss, fatigue, dyspnea, fever, and occasional sudden loss of consciousness.

atrial premature complex (APC), a premature heart contraction that arises from a focal point in the atrium.

atrial septal defect (ASD), a congenital cardiac anomaly characterized by an abnormal opening between the atria. The severity of the condition depends on the size and location of the defect, which are related to the stage at which embryonic development of the septum was arrested. The defects are classified as ostium secundum defect, in which the aperture in the septum secundum (second septum) of the fetal heart fails to close; ostium primum defect, in which there is inadequate development of the endocardial cushions of the first septum of the heart; and sinus venosus defect, in which the superior part of the atrium fails to develop.

atrial septum [L, *atrium,* hall, *saeptum,* fence], a partition between the left and right atria of the heart.

atrial standstill, a condition of complete failure of the atria to contract. Generally a junctional escape pacemaker maintains continuation of ventricular activity during atrial standstill. P waves are absent in all electrocardiogram surface leads, and A waves are absent in the jugular venous pulse and right atrial pressure tracings.

atrial systole, the contraction of the atria of the heart, which precedes ventricular contraction by a fraction of a second.

atrial tachycardia [L, *atrium,* hall; Gk, *tachys,* quick, *kardia,* heart], rapid beating of the atria caused by abnormal automaticity, triggered activity, or intraatrial reentry. Atrial tachycardia may be either nonparoxysmal (common form) or paroxysmal (uncommon form). The atrial rate is usually less than 200 beats/min; however, when the cause is digitalis excess, the atrial rate increases gradually (130 to 250 beats/min) as the digitalis is continued.

atrichia /ātrik'ē-ə/ [Gk, *a,* not, *thrix,* hair], **1.** pertaining to a group of bacteria that lack flagella. **2.** the absence of hair.

atrichosis /ā'trikō'sis/ [Gk, *a* + *trichia* without hair, *osis,* condition], a congenital absence of hair.

atrioventricular (AV) /ā'trē-ōventrik'-yələr/ [L, *atrium,* hall, *ventriculus*], pertaining to a connecting conduction event or anatomic structure between the atria and ventricles.

atrioventricular block (AVB) [L, *atrium* + *ventriculus,* little belly], a disorder of cardiac impulse transmission that reflects prolonged, intermittent, or absent conduction of the impulse between the atria and ventricles. It commonly occurs at the AV node or within the bundle branch system.

atrioventricular (AV) bundle, a band of atypical cardiac muscle fibers with few contractile units. It arises from the distal part of the AV node and extends across the AV groove to the top of the intraventricular septum, where it divides into the bundle branches.

atrioventricular (AV) dissociation, a breakdown in the normal conduction of excitation through the heart, allowing the atria and ventricles to beat independently under the control of their own pacemakers.

atrioventricular (AV) junction [L, *jungere,* to join], the region of the heart that separates the atria from the ventricles. It includes the AV bundle (bundle of His) and surrounds the AV node.

atrioventricular (AV) node, an area of specialized cardiac muscle that receives the cardiac impulse from the sinoatrial node and conducts it to the AV bundle and thence to the Purkinje fibers and walls of the ventricles. The AV node is located in the septal wall between the left and right atria.

atrioventricular (AV) septum, a small part of membrane that separates the atria from the ventricles of the heart.

atrioventricular (AV) valve, a valve in the heart through which blood flows from the atria to the ventricles. The valve between the left atrium and left ventricle is the mitral (bicuspid) valve; the right AV valve is the tricuspid valve.

at risk, the state of an individual's or population's being vulnerable to a particular disease or event. The factors determining risk may be environmental, psychosocial, psychologic, or physiologic.

atrium /ā'trē-əm/, *pl.* **atria** [L, hall], a chamber or cavity, such as the right and left atria of the heart or the nasal cavity.

atrium of ear, the external part of the ear, including the auricle and the tubular part of the external auditory meatus.

atrium of the heart, one of the two upper chambers of the heart. The right atrium receives deoxygenated blood from the superior vena cava, the inferior vena cava, and the coronary sinus. The left atrium receives oxygenated blood from the pulmonary veins.

atrophic /ātrof'ik/ [Gk, *a,* without, *trophe,* nourishment], characterized by a wasting of tissues, usually associated with general malnutrition or a specific disease state.

atrophic catarrh [Gk, *a, trophe,* without nourishment, *kata,* down, *rhoia,* flow], an abnormal condition characterized by inflammation and discharge from the mucous membranes of the nose, accompanied by the loss of mucosal and submucosal tissue.

atrophic cirrhosis [Gk, *a* + *trophe,* without nourishment, *kirrhos,* yellowish coloration], a form of advanced portal cirrhosis with massive shrinking of the liver.

atrophic fracture, a spontaneous fracture caused by bone atrophy, as in the bones of an elderly person.

atrophic gastritis, a chronic inflammation of the stomach, associated with degeneration of the gastric mucosa. Seen in elderly patients and in persons with pernicious anemia, it rarely causes epigastric pain.

atrophic glossitis, a pathologic condition in which the various papillae are lost from the dorsum of the tongue, resulting in a very sore and highly sensitive surface that makes eating difficult.

atrophic rhinitis [Gk, *a* + *trophe,* without nourishment, *rhis,* nose, *itis,* inflammation], a nasal condition in which there is atrophy of the mucous membrane of the nose, resulting in failure of the ciliary function and drying and crusting of the lining of the nasal passages. This may alter olfactory sensation.

atrophic vaginitis [Gk, *a* + *trophe,* without nourishment; L, *vagina,* sheath; Gk, *itis,* inflammation], degeneration of the vaginal mucous membrane after menopause.

atrophied /at'rōfīd/ [Gk, *a* + *trophe,* without nourishment], decreased in size because of disuse or disease, as an organ, tissue, or body part.

atrophoderma /at'rōfədur'mə/ [Gk, *a* + *trophe* + *derma,* skin], the wasting away or decrease in thickness of the skin. The atrophy may affect the entire body surface or only localized areas.

atrophy /at'rəfē/ [Gk, *a* + *trophe,* without nourishment], a wasting or diminution of size or physiologic activity of a part of the body because of disease or other influences. A skeletal muscle may undergo atrophy as a result of lack of physical exercise or neurologic or musculoskeletal disease. Cells of the brain and central nervous system may atrophy in old age because of restricted blood flow to those areas. —**atrophic,** *adj.,* **atrophy,** *v.*

atrophy of disuse [Gk, *a, trophe* + L, *dis,* opposite of, *usus*], a shrinkage of tissues resulting from immobility or lack of exercise.

atropine /at'rōpin/ [Gk, *Atropos,* one of the three Fates], an alkaloid from *Atropa belladonna* and *Datura stramonium* plants.

atropine sulfate, an antispasmodic and anticholinergic prescribed in the treatment of gastrointestinal hypermotility, inflammation of the iris or the uvea, cardiac arrhythmias, and certain kinds of poisoning and as an adjunct to anesthesia.

atropine sulfate poisoning [Gk, *Atropos,* fate; L, *sulphur* + *potio,* drink], toxic effects of an overdose of a drug sometimes used as an adjunct to general anesthesia. Symptoms include tachycardia, hot and dry flushed skin, dry mouth with thirst, restlessness and excitement, urinary retention, constipation, and a burning pain in the throat. Treatment includes gastric lavage and administration of barbiturates, as well as physostigmine and pilocarpine if the eyes are involved.

attachment [Fr, *attachement*], **1.** the state or quality of being affixed or attached. **2.** (in psychiatry) a mode of behavior in which one individual relates in an affiliative or dependent manner to another; a feeling of affection or loyalty that binds one person to another. **3.** (in dentistry) any device, such as a retainer or artificial crown, used to secure a partial denture to a natural tooth in the mouth.

attachment apparatus, the combination of tissues that invest and support the teeth, such as the cementum, the periodontal ligament, and the alveolar bone.

Attachment Promotion, a Nursing Interventions Classification defined as facilitation of the development of the parent-infant relationship.

attack, an episode in the course of an illness, usually characterized by acute and distressing symptoms.

attending [L, *attendo,* to notice], (in psychology) pertaining to an aroused readiness to perceive, with an adjustment of the brain and sense organs to focus on a situation.

attending physician [L, *attendere,* to stretch], the physician who is responsible for a particular patient. In a university setting, an attending physician often also has teaching responsibilities and holds a faculty appointment.

attention [L, *attendere,* to stretch], the element of cognitive functioning in which the mental focus is maintained on a specific issue, object, or activity.

attention deficit disorder, a syndrome affecting children, adolescents, and adults characterized by short attention span, hyperactivity, and poor concentration. The symptoms may be mild or severe and are associated with functional deviations of the central nervous system without signs of major neurologic or psychiatric disturbance.

attention deficit hyperactivity disorder, a childhood mental disorder with onset before 7 years of age and involving impaired or diminished attention, impulsivity, and hyperactivity.

attenuated /əten'yōō·ā'tid/ [L, *attenuare,* to make thin], pertaining to the dilution of a solution or the reduction in virulence or toxicity of a microorganism or a drug by weakening it.

attenuated virus [L, *attenuare,* to make thin, *virus,* poison], a strain of virus whose virulence has been lowered by physical or chemical processes or by repeated passage through the cells of another species. Vaccines made by attenuated strains are used to prevent tuberculosis, smallpox, measles, mumps, rubella, polio, and yellow fever.

attenuation /əten'yōō·ā'shən/ [L, *attenuare,* to make thin], the process of reduction, such as attenuation of an x-ray beam by reducing its intensity, weakening of the degree of virulence of a disease organism, or culturing under unfavorable conditions.

attenuation coefficient, (in positron emission tomography) a number that represents the difference between the number

A

attenuator /əten'yoō-ā'tər/ [L, *attenuare,* to make thin], an agent that weakens the toxicity of a poisonous substance or the virulence of a microorganism.

attitude /at'ətyoōd, -toōd/, 1. a body position or posture, particularly the fetal position in the uterus, as determined by the degree of flexion of the head and extremities. 2. (in psychiatry) any of the major integrative forces in the development of personality that gives consistency to an individual's behavior.

attitudinal isolation /at'ətyoō'dənəl/ [L, *attitudo,* posture], a type of social isolation that results from a person's own cultural or personal values.

attitudinal reflex, any reflex initiated by a change in position of the head or by a change in position of the head with respect to the position of the body. Kinds of attitudinal reflexes include **tonic neck reflex** and **tonic labyrinthine reflex.**

attraction [L, *attrahere,* to draw to], a tendency of the teeth or other maxillary or mandibular structures to become elevated above their normal position.

attrition /ətrish'ən/ [L, *atterere,* to wear away], the process of wearing away or wearing down by friction.

at. wt., abbreviation for **atomic weight.**

atypia /ātip'ēə/ [Gk, *a + typos,* without type], a condition of being irregular or nonstandard.

atypical /ātip'əkəl/ [Gk, *a + typos,* without type], a condition or object that is not of a usual or standard type.

atypical measles syndrome (AMS), a form of measles (rubeola) that tends to infect persons previously immunized by killed measles vaccine or live, diluted measles vaccine that may have been stored improperly. Symptoms differ from those of typical measles, beginning with a sudden high fever, headache, abdominal pain, and coughing.

atypical *Mycobacterium* [Gk, *a + typos,* without type, *mykes,* fungus, *bakterion,* small staff], a group of mycobacteria, including pathogenic and nonpathogenic forms, that are classified according to their ability to produce pigments, growth characteristics, and reactions to chemical tests.

atypical pneumonia [Gk, *a + typos,* without type, *pneumon,* lung, *ia,* condition], a group of relatively mild symptoms of chills, headache, muscular pains, moderate fever, and coughing, but without evidence of a bacterial infection. Chest x-ray film may show mottling at the bases. Eaton

agent, or *Mycoplasma pneumoniae,* may be the cause of the symptoms.

atypical somatoform disorder, an abnormal condition marked by physical symptoms and complaints that appear related to a preoccupation with an imagined defect in one's personal appearance or ability.

Au, symbol for the element **gold.**

audible /ô'dəbəl/ [L, *audire,* to hear], capable of being heard. Some animals are able to hear sounds of higher or lower frequencies and different intensities than those audible to most humans.

audioanalgesia /ô·dē·ō·an'əljē'sē·a [L, *audire,* to hear; Gk, *a, algos,* not pain], the use of music to enhance relaxation and distract a patient's mind from pain, as during dentistry.

audiogram /ô'dē·əgram'/ [Gk, *audire + gramma,* record], a chart showing the faintest level at which an individual is able to detect sounds of various frequencies, usually in octaves from 125 Hz to 8000 Hz.

audiologist /-ol'əjist/ [L, *audire,* to hear; Gk, *logos,* science], a health professional with a master's degree in audiology who studies the sense of hearing, detects and evaluates hearing loss, and works to rehabilitate individuals with hearing loss.

audiology /-ol'əjē/ [L, *audire* + Gk, *logos,* science], a field of research and clinical practice devoted to the study of hearing disorders, assessment of hearing, hearing conservation, and aural rehabilitation. —**audiologic,** *adj.*

audiometer /ô'dē·om'ətər/ [L, *audire* + Gk, *metron,* measure], an electric device for testing hearing.

audiometrist /ô'dē·om'ətrist/, a technician who has received special training in the use of pure tone audiometry equipment. An audiometrist conducts the hearing tests selected and interpreted by an audiologist.

audiometry /ô'dē·om'ətrē/, the testing of the sensitivity of the sense of hearing. Various audiometric tests determine the lowest intensity of sound at which an individual can perceive auditory stimuli (hearing threshold) and distinguish different speech sounds.—**audiometric,** *adj.*

audiovisual /ô'dē·ōvizh'əl/, pertaining to communication that uses both sight and sound messages.

audit /ô'dit/, 1. a final statement of account. 2. a review and evaluation of health care procedures.

auditory /ô'dətôr'ē/ [L, *auditorius,* hearing], pertaining to the sense of hearing and the hearing organs involved.

auditory amnesia [L, *auditorius,* hearing;

Gk, *amnesia,* forgetfulness], a loss of memory for the meaning of sounds.

auditory area [L, *auditorium,* hearing], the sound perception area of the cerebral cortex. It is located in the floor of the lateral fissure and on the dorsal surface of the superior temporal gyrus.

auditory brainstem response (ABR), an electrophysiologic test used to measure hearing sensitivity and evaluate the integrity of ear structures from the auditory nerve through the brainstem. It is also used to screen hearing of newborns.

auditory epilepsy, a reflex form of epilepsy provoked by sounds.

auditory hair [L, *audire,* to hear; AS, *haer*], one of the cells with hairlike processes in the spiral organ of Corti. The hairs, or cilia, function as sensory receptors.

auditory hallucination [L, *audire,* to hear, *alucinari,* a wandering mind], a subjective experience of hearing voices or other sounds despite the absence of an actual reality based external stimulus to account for the phenomenon.

auditory meatus [L, *audire,* to hear, *meatus,* passage], **1.** the external auditory meatus, a tubelike channel of the external ear extending from the auricle to the tympanum of the middle ear. **2.** the internal auditory meatus, a short channel extending from the petrous part of the temporal bone to the fundus near the vestibule. It contains the eighth cranial nerve.

auditory nerve, See **vestibulocochlear nerve.**

auditory ossicles [L, *audire* + *ossiculum,* little bone], the malleus, the incus, and the stapes, three small bones in the middle ear that articulate with each other. As the tympanic membrane vibrates, it transmits sound waves through the ossicles to the cochlea.

auditory system assessment, an evaluation of the patient's ears and hearing and an investigation of present and past diseases or conditions that may be responsible for an auditory impairment.

auditory threshold [L, *audire,* to hear; AS, *threscold*], the lowest intensity at which a sound may be heard.

auditory vertigo [L, *audire,* to hear, *vertigo,* dizziness], a form of vertigo associated with ear disease. It is characterized by sensations of gyration and, when severe, with prostration and vomiting.

Auerbach's plexus [Leopold Auerbach, German anatomist, 1828–1897; L, *plexus,* plaited], the myenteric plexus, a group of autonomic nerve fibers and ganglia located in the muscle tissue of the intestinal tract.

Auer rod /ou′ər/ [John Auer, American physiologist, 1875–1948], an abnormal, needle-shaped or round, pink-staining inclusion in the cytoplasm of myeloblasts and promyelocytes in acute myelogenous or myelomonocytic leukemia. These inclusions contain enzymes such as acid phosphatase, peroxidase, and esterase and may represent abnormal derivatives of cytoplasmic granules.

augmentation /ôg′məntā′shən/ [L, *augmentare,* to increase], **1.** a process in which a substance or mechanism can stimulate an increased rate of biologic activity, such as faster cell division or heartbeat. **2.** breast augmentation.

augmentation mammoplasty, a surgical procedure to enlarge the breasts.

aura /ôr′ə/ [L, breath], *pl.* **aurae** /ôr′ē/, **1.** a sensation, as of light or warmth, that may precede an attack of migraine or an epileptic seizure. **2.** *pl.* **auras,** an emanation of light or color surrounding a person as seen in Kirlian photography and studied in current nursing research in healing techniques.

aural /ôr′əl/, pertaining to the ear or hearing. —**aurally,** *adv.*

aural, pertaining to an aura.

aural forceps, a dressing forceps with fine, bent tips used in surgery.

aural rehabilitation, a form of therapy in which hearing-impaired individuals are taught to improve their ability to communicate. Methods taught include, but are not limited to, speech-reading, auditory training, use of hearing aids, and use of assistive listening devices such as telephone amplifiers.

auramine /ôr′əmēn/, a yellow aniline dye used in the manufacture of paints, textiles, and rubber products. The experimental carcinogen in animals has been identified as a cause of bladder cancer in humans. Also called *dimethyl aniline.*

auramine O, a fluorescent, yellow aniline dye used as a stain for the tubercle bacillus and for deoxyribonucleic acid .

auranofin /ôr′ənof′in/, an oral gold antiarthritic drug prescribed for the treatment of rheumatoid arthritis.

aurantiasis cutis /ôr′əntī′əsis/ [L, *aurantium,* orange; Gk, *osis,* condition; L, *cutis,* skin], a yellowish skin pigmentation that results from eating excessive amounts of foods containing carotene, such as carrots.

auricle /ôr′ikəl/ [L, *auricula,* little ear], **1.** also called **pinna.** the external ear. **2.** the left or right cardiac atrium, so named because of its earlike shape.

auricular /ôrik′yələr/, **1.** pertaining to the auricle of the ear. **2.** otic.

auricularis anterior, one of three extrinsic muscles of the ear. It functions to move the auricula forward and upward.

auricularis posterior, one of three extrinsic muscles of the ear. It serves to draw the auricula backward.

auricularis superior, a thin, fan-shaped muscle that is one of three extrinsic muscles of the ear. It acts to draw the auricula upward.

auricular line, a hypothetic line passing through the external auditory meatuses and perpendicular to the Frankfort horizontal plane.

auricular point, the center of the external auditory meatus.

auriculin /ôrik'yəlin/, a hormonelike substance with diuretic activity produced in the atria of the heart.

auriculocranial /-krā'nē-əl/, pertaining to the auricle of the ear and the cranium.

auriculotemporal /-tem'pərəl/, pertaining to the auricle of the ear and the temporal area of the skull.

auriculoventriculostomy /ôrik'yəlōventrik'yəlos'təmē/ [L, auricula + ventriculus, little belly; Gk, stoma, opening], a surgical procedure that directs cerebrospinal fluid into the general circulation in the treatment of hydrocephalus, usually in the newborn. In this procedure a polyethylene tube is passed from the lateral ventricle through a bur hole in the parietal skull area under the scalp and into the jugular vein or abdomen for the discharge of cerebrospinal fluid.

auris dextra (a.d.), the Latin term for right ear.

auris sinistra (a.s.), the Latin term for left ear.

aurothioglucose /ôr'ōthī'ōglōō'kōs/, an organic gold antiarthritic used in chrysotherapy. It is prescribed for adjunctive treatment of adult and juvenile rheumatoid arthritis.

auscult /ôs'kult/ [L, auscultare, to listen], to practice auscultation, or to listen and interpret sounds produced within the body.

auscultation /ôs'kəltā'shən/ [L, auscultare, to listen], the act of listening for sounds within the body to evaluate the condition of the heart, blood vessels, lungs, pleura, intestines, or other organs or to detect the fetal heart sound. Auscultation may be performed directly with the unaided ear; but most commonly a stethoscope is used to determine the frequency, intensity, duration, and quality of the sounds. —**auscultate,** v., **auscultatory** /ôskul'tətôr'ē/, adj.

Austin Flint murmur [Austin Flint, American physiologist, 1812–1886], a low-pitched sound characteristic of severe aortic regurgitation without mitral valve

disease. It is typically heard during ventricular middiastole at the apex.

Australia antigen, hepatitis B surface antigen (HBsAg), found in the serum of a person who has acute or chronic hepatitis B. Medical personnel must take adequate precautions to prevent autoinoculation, especially in dialysis units, blood banks, and laboratories. Blood banks routinely screen for Australia antigen to prevent causing active hepatitis B infection in a transfusion recipient.

Australian lift, a type of shoulder lift used to move a patient who is unable to assume a sitting position on a bed or other surface.

autacoid /ô'təkoid/, any of a group of substances, as hormones, that are produced in one organ and transported via blood or lymph as a means to control a physiologic process in another part of the body.

authenticity /ô'thəntis'itē/, (in psychiatry) emotional and behavioral openness; a quality of being genuine and trustworthy.

authoritarian personality, a group of behavioral traits characteristic of one who advocates obedience and strict adherence to rules.

authority /ôthôr'ətē/, a relationship between two or more persons or groups characterized by the influence one may exercise over the other through ideas, commands, suggestions, or instructions.

authority figure, a person who by virtue of status, strength, knowledge, or other recognized superiority exerts influence over others.

autism [Gk, autos, self], a mental disorder characterized by extreme withdrawal and an abnormal absorption in fantasy, accompanied by delusion, hallucination, and inability to communicate verbally or otherwise relate to people.—**autistic,** adj.

autistic disorder /ôtis'tik/ [Gk, autos, self], a pervasive developmental disorder with onset in infancy or childhood, characterized by impaired social interaction, impaired communication, and a restricted repertoire of activities and interests.—**autistic,** adj.

autistic phase, a period of preoedipal development, according to Mahler's system of personality stages. It lasts from birth to around 1 month and is considered normal.

autistic thought, a form of thinking that is internally stimulated in which the ideas have a private meaning to the individual. Autistic thinking is a symptom in patients with schizophrenia. Fantasy life may be interpreted as reality.

autoactivation /-ak'tivā'shən/ [Gk, autos,

self, *activus,* active], a process of self-activation, as when a gland is stimulated by its own secretions.

autoagglutination /-əglōō'tənā'shən/ [Gk, *autos,* self; L, *agglutinare,* to glue], **1.** the agglutination or clumping of red blood cells by the serum of the same individual. **2.** the agglutination or clumping together of certain antigens such as bacteria.

autoamputation /-amp'yōōtā'shən/, the spontaneous detachment of a body part, usually the fourth or fifth toe, as occurs among the males of some African peoples. The condition is usually painless and has no other symptoms.

autoantibody /ô'tō·an'tibod'ē/ [Gk, *autos* + *anti,* against; AS, *bodig,* body], an immunoglobulin that reacts against native tissue because of the failure to recognize "self." Normal body proteins may be converted to autoantigens by chemicals, infectious organisms, or therapeutic drugs. Some examples of autoantibodies are those found against gastric parietal cells in pernicious anemia, against platelets in autoimmune thrombocytopenia, and against antigens on the surface of erythrocytes in autoimmune hemolytic anemia.

autoantigen /ô'tō·an'tijin/ [Gk, *autos* + *anti,* against, *genein,* to produce], an endogenous body constituent that stimulates the production of autoantibodies and a resulting autoimmune reaction.

autoantitoxin /-an'titok'sin/, an antibody produced as protection against a toxin resulting from infection, such as *Escherichia coli* endotoxin.

autoaugmentation /-ôg'məntā'shən/, a surgical procedure in which the detrusor muscle of the bladder is removed, leaving the bladder epithelium otherwise intact.

autoblast /ô'təblast/, an independent microorganism.

autocatheterization /-kath'əter'izā'shən/ the insertion of a catheter by the patient.

autochthonous /ôtok'thənəs/, [Gk, *autos,* self, *chthon,* earth], **1.** relating to a disease or other condition that appears to have originated in the part of the body in which it was discovered. **2.** (in psychology) describing the sudden appearance of a system of delusions.

autochthonous idea /ôtok'thənəs/ [Gk, *autos* + *chthon,* earth], an idea that originates in the unconscious and arises spontaneously in the mind, independently of the conscious train of thought.

autoclassis /ôtok'ləsis/ [Gk, *autos,* self, *klassis,* breaking], the rupturing or breaking of a part of the body caused by a force or agent arising from within the body itself.

autoclave /ô'təklāv/, an appliance used to sterilize medical instruments or other objects with steam under pressure.

autocrine /ô'təlrin/, denoting the effect of a hormone on cells that produce it.

autodigestion, a condition in which gastric juices in the pancreas or stomach digest the organ's own tissues.

autodiploid /ô'tōdip'loid/ [Gk, *autos* + *diploos,* double, *eidos,* form], **1.** pertaining to an individual, organism, strain, or cell containing two genetically identical or nearly identical chromosome sets that are derived from the same ancestral species and result from the duplication of the haploid set. **2.** such an individual, organism, strain, or cell.

autodiploidy /ô'tōdip'loidē/, the state or condition of having two genetically identical or nearly identical chromosome sets from the same ancestral species. Such a state enables cell division to occur in a normal manner.

autoeroticism /-irot'əsiz'əm/ [Gk, *autos* + *eros,* love], **1.** sensual, sexual gratification of the self, usually obtained through the stimulus of one's own body without the participation of another person. **2.** sexual feeling or desire occurring without any external stimulus. **3.** (in Freudian psychoanalytic theory) an early phase of psychosexual development, occurring in the oral and the anal stages. —autoerotic, *adj.*

autoerythrocyte sensitization /ô'tō-ərith'rəsīt/ [Gk, *autos* + *erythros,* red, *kytos,* cell], hypersensitivity to the patient's own red blood cells resulting in the spontaneous appearance of painful, hemorrhagic spots on the anterior aspects of the arms and legs.

autogenesis /ô'tōjen'əsis/ [Gk, *autos* + *genein,* to produce], **1.** abiogenesis. **2.** self-produced condition; a condition originating from within the organism. —autogenetic, autogenic, *adj.*

autogenic therapy /-jen'ik/, a mental health therapy introduced by Wolfgang Luthe. It is based on the concept that natural forces in the brain are able to remove disturbing influences so that functional harmony can be restored in the mind and body.

Autogenic Training, a Nursing Interventions Classification defined as assisting with self-suggestions about feelings of heaviness and warmth for the purpose of inducing relaxation.

autogenous /ôtoj'ənəs/, **1.** self-generating. **2.** originating from within the organism, as a toxin or vaccine.

autogenous graft [Gk, *autos,* self, *genein,* to produce, *graphion,* stylus], a skin

A

autogenous vaccine [Gk, *autos*, self, *genein*, to produce; L, *vaccinus*, cow], a vaccine prepared from cultures of the microorganism taken from a lesion of the patient to be treated.

autograft /ô'təgraft'/ [Gk, *autos* + *graphion*, stylus], surgical transplantation of any tissue from one part of the body to another location in the same individual. Autografts are used in several kinds of plastic surgery, most commonly to replace skin lost in severe burns.

autohemolysis /-hēmol'isis/ [Gk, *autos*, self, *haima*, blood, *lysein*, to loosen], the destruction of erythrocytes by hemolytic agents found in an individual's own blood.

autohypnosis [Gk, *autos*, *hypnos*, sleep], the self-induction of hypnosis by an individual who concentrates on one subject to attain an altered state of consciousness. It may also occur in a person who has become sensitized to the process by undergoing hypnosis a number of times.

autoimmune /-imyōōn'/ [Gk, *autos* + L, *immunus*, exempt], pertaining to the development of an immune response to one's own tissues.

autoimmune disease, one of a large group of diseases characterized by the subversion or alteration of the function of the immune system of the body, resulting in the production of antibodies against the body's own cells. Autoantigens normally present in the internal cells stimulate the development of autoantibodies, which, unable to distinguish antigens of the internal cells from external antigens, act against the internal cell to cause localized and systemic reactions. These reactions affect the epithelial and connective tissues of the body, causing a variety of diseases. There are known or suspected hematologic, rheumatologic, neurologic, and endocrine disorders associated with autoimmunity.

autoimmune theory, a concept that as one ages defects occur in the body's autoimmune system. As a result of the defects, a person's antibody cells can no longer distinguish between tissues that are "self" and "nonself." One's own body cells are then misidentified as foreign protein matter to be attacked by the antibodies.

autoimmunity /-imyōō'nitē/, an abnormal characteristic or condition in which the body reacts against constituents of its own tissues. Autoimmunity may result in hypersensitivity and autoimmune disease.

autoimmunization /-im'yənizā'shən/, the process whereby an individual's immune system develops antibodies against one or more of the person's own tissues.

autoinfection, an infection by disease organisms already present in the body but developing in a different body part.

autoinfusion /-infyōō'zhən/, a technique for forcing blood from the extremities to the body core by applying bandages. It may be used to control bleeding and, in surgery, to create a relatively bloodless surgical field.

autoinoculation /-inok'yəlā'shən/ [Gk, *autos* + L, *inoculare*, to graft], the inoculation of a microorganism obtained by contact with a lesion on one's own body, producing a secondary infection.

autointoxication /-intok'sikā'shən/ [Gk, *autos* + L, *in;* Gk, *toxikon*, poison], a condition of poisoning by substances generated by one's own body, as by toxins resulting from a metabolic disorder.

autokeratoplasty /-ker'ətoplas'tē/, the surgical transfer of corneal tissue from one eye of a patient to repair the cornea of the other.

autokinesia /-kinē'zhə/, voluntary movement.

autolesion /-lē'zhən/, a self-inflicted injury.

autolet /ô'tōlet/, a small, sharp instrument, as a lancet, that is used to obtain a capillary blood specimen.

autologous /ôtol'əgəs/ [Gk, *autos* + *logos*, ratio], pertaining to a tissue or structure occurring naturally and derived from the same individual.

autologous graft [Gk, *autos*, *logos*, *graphion*, stylus], the transfer of tissue from one site to another on the same body.

autologous transfusion, a procedure in which blood is removed from a donor and stored for a variable period before it is returned to the donor's circulation.

autolysis /ôtol'isis/, the spontaneous destruction of tissues by intracellular enzymes. It generally occurs in the body after death.

automatic implanted cardioverter defibrillator (AICD), a surgically implanted device that automatically detects and corrects potentially fatal arrhythmias.

automatic infiltration detector /ô'təmat'ik/ [Gk, *automatismos*, self-action], a temperature-sensitive device that activates an alarm and automatically stops an intravenous infusion when the intravenous fluid passes into tissue. The device detects any cooling of the skin at the intravenous site, a common sign of infiltration.

automaticity /ô'tōmatis'itē/, a property of specialized excitable tissue that allows self-activation through spontaneous development of an action potential, as in the pacemaker cells of the heart.

automatic speech, speech composed of

or containing words or phrases spoken without much conscious thought, often consisting of expletives, profanities, and greetings.

automation /ô'təmā'shən/, use of a machine designed to follow a predetermined sequence of individual operations repeatedly and automatically.

automatism /ôtom'ətiz'əm/ [Gk, *automatismos,* self-action], **1.** (in physiology) involuntary function of an organ system independent of apparent external stimuli, such as the beating of the heart, or dependent on external stimuli but not consciously controlled, such as the dilation of the pupil of the eye. **2.** (in philosophy) the theory that the body acts as a machine and that the mind, whose processes depend solely on brain activity, is a noncontrolling adjunct of the body. **3.** (in psychology) mechanical, repetitive, and undirected behavior that is not consciously controlled, as seen in psychomotor epilepsy, hysterical states, and such acts as sleepwalking.

automnesia /ô'tômnē'zhə/, the recollection of a previous experience.

autonomic /ô'tənom'ik/ [Gk, *autos* + *nomos,* law], **1.** having the ability to function independently without outside influence. **2.** pertaining to the autonomic nervous system.

autonomic-active bronchodilators, a category of drugs with actions that dilate bronchiolar smooth muscle tissue by acting on the autonomic nervous system. Examples include adrenergic drugs such as epinephrine and anticholinergic products such as atropine sulfate.

autonomic drug, any of a large group of drugs that mimic or modify the function of the autonomic nervous system.

autonomic dysreflexia, a dysreflexia that is the result of impaired function of the autonomic nervous system caused by simultaneous sympathetic and parasympathetic activity. It occurs in quadriplegics and some paraplegics.

autonomic ganglion [Gk, *autos,* self, *nomos,* law, *ganglion,* knot], a physical grouping of autonomic neuron cell bodies.

autonomic hyperreflexia, a neurologic disorder characterized by a discharge of sympathetic nervous system impulses as a result of stimulation of the bladder, large intestine, or other visceral organs.

autonomic imbalance [Gk, *autos,* self, *nomos,* law; L, *in,* not, *bilanx,* having two scales], a disruption of a segment of the autonomic nervous system, as in autonomic ataxia.

autonomic nerve [Gk, *autos,* self, *nomos,* law, *neuron,* nerve], a nerve of the autonomic nervous system, which includes both the sympathetic and parasympathetic nervous systems. It possesses the ability to function independently and spontaneously as needed to maintain optimal status of body activities.

autonomic nervous system, the part of the nervous system that regulates involuntary function, including the activity of the cardiac muscle, smooth muscles, and glands. It has two divisions. The sympathetic nervous system accelerates heart rate, constricts blood vessels, and raises blood pressure; the parasympathetic nervous system slows heart rate, increases intestinal peristalsis and gland activity, and relaxes sphincters.

autonomic reflex, any of a large number of normal reflexes governing and regulating the functions of the viscera. Autonomic reflexes control such activities of the body as blood pressure, heart rate, peristalsis, sweating, and urination.

autonomy /ôton'əmē/ [Gk, *autos* + *nomos,* law], the quality of having the ability or tendency to function independently. —**autonomous,** *adj.*

autonomy drive, a behavioral trait characterized by the attempt of an individual to master the environment and to impose his or her purposes on it.

autophagia /-fā'jə/, **1.** a mental disorder characterized by the biting or eating of one's own flesh, as may occur in Lesch-Nyan syndrome. **2.** the automatic consumption of one's own tissues by fasting or dieting. **3.** the metabolic action of catabolism.

autoplastic maneuver /-plas'tik/, (in psychology) a process that is part of adaptation, involving an adjustment within the self.

autoplasty /ô'təplas'tē/ [Gk, *autos* + *plassein,* to shape], a plastic surgery procedure in which autografts, or parts of the patient's own tissues, are used to replace or repair body areas damaged by disease or injury.

autoploid /ô'təploid/, having homologous chromosome sets, or two or more copies of a single haploid set.

autopodium /-pō'dē·əm/, the distal major subdivision of a hand or foot.

autopolyploid /ô'tōpol'iploid/ [Gk, *autos* + *polyploos,* many times, *eidos* form], **1.** pertaining to an individual, organism, strain, or cell that has more than two genetically identical or nearly identical sets of chromosomes that are derived from the same ancestral species. **2.** such an individual, organism, strain, or cell.

autopolyploidy /ô'tōpol'iploi'dē/, the state or condition of having more than two identical or nearly identical sets of chromosomes.

autopsy /ô′topsē/ [Gk, *autos* + *opsis,* view], a postmortem examination performed to confirm or determine the cause of death.—**autopsic, autopsical,** *adj.,* **autopsist,** *n.*

autopsy pathology, the study of disease by the examination of the body after death by a pathologist.

autoregulation [Gk, *autos,* self; L, *regula,* rule], an intrinsic capacity of tissues to regulate their own blood flow or metabolic activity. The former process is due to the self-excitable contractile process of smooth muscle that acts to constrict and dilate vessels. It allows organ systems to maintain constant blood flow despite variations in systemic arterial pressure and is an essential mechanism to meet the metabolic needs of an organ.

autosensitization /-sen′sətīzā′shən/ [Gk, *autos,* self; L, *sentire,* to feel], the sensitization of an individual by humoral antibodies or a delayed cellular reaction to substances in his or her own body tissues.

autosepticemia /-sep′tisē′mē-ə/, a systemic infection in which pathogens are present in the circulating bloodstream, developing from an infection within the body.

autoserous treatment /ô′təsir′əs/ [Gk, *autos* + L, *serum,* whey], therapy of an infectious disease by inoculating the patient with the patient's own serum.

autosite /ô′təsīt/ [Gk, *autos* + *sitos,* food], the larger, more normally formed member of unequal or asymmetric conjoined twins on whom the other smaller fetus depends for various physiologic functions and for nutrition and growth. —**autositic.** *adj.*

autosmia /ôtoz′mē-ə/ [Gk, *autos,* self, *osme,* smell], awareness of one's own body odor.

autosomal /ô′təsō′məl/ [Gk, *autos* + *soma,* body], **1.** pertaining to or characteristic of an autosome. **2.** pertaining to any condition transmitted by an autosome.

autosomal-dominant inheritance, a pattern of inheritance in which the transmission of a dominant gene on an autosome causes a characteristic to be expressed. Affected individuals have an affected parent unless the condition is the result of a new mutation. Achondroplasia, osteogenesis imperfecta, polydactyly, Marfan's syndrome, and some neuromuscular disorders are autosomal-dominant disorders.

autosomal inheritance, a pattern of inheritance in which the transmission of traits depends on the presence or absence of certain genes on the autosomes. The pattern may be dominant or recessive, and

males and females are usually affected with equal frequency. The majority of hereditary disorders are the result of a defective gene on an autosome.

autosomal-recessive inheritance, a pattern of inheritance in which the transmission of a recessive gene on an autosome results in a carrier state if the person is heterozygous for the trait (Aa) and will show the trait if homozygous (aa) for it. One fourth of the children of two heterozygous parents (Aa) are affected. All of the children of two homozygous affected parents (aa) are affected. Cystic fibrosis, phenylketonuria, and galactosemia are examples of traits that result from autosomal-recessive inheritance.

autosomatognosis /sō′mətognō′sis/, a phantom sensation that an amputated part of the body is still attached.

autosome /ô′təsōm/, any chromosome that is not a sex chromosome and that appears as a homologous pair in the somatic cell. Humans have 22 pairs of autosomes, which are involved in transmitting all genetic traits and conditions other than those that are sex-linked.

autosplenectomy /ô′tōsplinek′təmē/ [Gk, *autos* + *splen,* spleen, *ektome,* excision], a progressive shrinking of the spleen that may occur in sickle cell anemia. The spleen is replaced by fibrous tissue and becomes nonfunctional.

autosuggestion [Gk, *autos* + L, *suggerere,* to suggest], an idea, thought, attitude, or belief suggested to oneself, often as a formula or incantation, as a means of controlling one's behavior.

autotopagnosia /ô′tōtop′əg·nō′zhə/ [Gk, *autos* + *topos,* place, *a* + *gnosis,* without knowledge], the inability to recognize or localize the various body parts because of organic brain damage.

autotoxemia /-toksē′mē-ə/, a form of poisoning caused by substances generated within the body as a result of the pathologic alteration of the person's own tissues.

autotoxic. pertaining to autotoxins.

autotransfusion /-transfyoo′zhən/, the collection, anticoagulation, filtration, and reinfusion of blood from an active bleeding site. It may be used in cases of major trauma or in major surgery when blood can be collected from a sterile site.

Autotransfusion, a Nursing Interventions Classification defined as collecting and reinfusing blood that has been lost during or after surgery from clean wounds.

autovaccination, a second vaccination in which a virus from the first vaccine sore is used.

autozygous /-zī′gəs/, pertaining to genes

in a homozygote that are copies of the same ancestral gene as a result of a consanguineous mating.

auxanology /ôks'ənol'əjē/ [Gk, *auxein,* to grow, *logos,* science], the scientific study of growth and development. —**auxanologic,** *adj.*

auxcardia [Gk, *auxein,* increase, *kardia,* heart], an enlarged heart.

auxesis /ôksē'sis/, *pl.* **auxeses** [Gk, *auxein* + *osis,* condition], an increase in size or volume because of cell expansion rather than an increase in the number of cells or tissue elements; hypertrophy. —**auxetic,** *adj., n.*

auxiliary /ôksil'yərē/ [L, *auxilium,* aid], an individual or group serving in assistive, supporting, or complementary tasks in a clinical setting.

auxiliary enzyme [L, *auxilium,* assist], an enzyme that links the enzyme being measured with an indicator enzyme.

auxotonic /ôk'sōton'ik/, pertaining to muscle contractions that increase in force as resistance is encountered.

auxotox [Gk, *auxein,* increase, *toxikon,* poison], a chemical with a particular atomic grouping that, if added to a relatively benign substance, increases the toxic characteristics of the mixture.

AV, abbreviation for *arteriovenous, atrioventricular.*

available arch length /əvā'ləbəl/ [ME, *availen,* to be of use], the length or space in a dental arch that is available for all the natural teeth of an individual.

avalvular /āvalv'yələr/ [Gk, *a,* without; L, *valva,* valve], an absence of one or more valves.

avascular /āvas'kyələr/ [Gk, *a,* without; L, *vasculum,* vessel], **1.** (of a tissue area) not receiving a sufficient supply of blood. **2.** (of a kind of tissue) not having blood vessels.

avascular graft [Gk, *a,* without; L, *vasculum,* vessel; Gk, *graphion,* stylus], a tissue graft in which there is no infiltration of blood vessels.

avascularization [Gk, *a,* without; L, *vasculum,* vessel], pertaining to a diversion of blood flow away from tissues.

AVB, abbreviation for **atrioventricular block.**

average, (in mathematics) a value established by dividing the sum of a series by the number of its units.

aversion therapy /əvur'zhən/ [L, *aversus,* a turning away], a form of behavior therapy in which punishment or an unpleasant or painful stimulus such as electric shock or drugs that induce nausea is used to suppress undesirable behavior.

aversive stimulus /əvur'siv/, an undesir-

able stimulus, such as electric shock, that causes psychic or physical pain.

avian tuberculosis /ā'vē-ən/, a strain of tuberculosis in birds, caused by *Mycobacterium avium.* The organism is also pathogenic in humans and is especially problematic in the immunocompromised, such as those with human immunodeficiency virus infection.

aviation medicine /āv'ē-ā'shən/, a branch of medicine that is concerned with the health effects of travel by aircraft, including such aspects as jetlag, restricted body movement for long periods, and reaction to violent aircraft movement in turbulent weather.

aviation physiology, a branch of physiology that is concerned with the effects on humans and animals exposed for long periods to pressurized cabins, radiation hazards at high altitudes, weightlessness, disturbances of biologic rhythms, acceleration, and mental functions under stressful flying conditions.

avidin, a glycoprotein in raw egg white that interacts with biotin to make it unavailable to the body. Cooking destroys avidin.

avidity /avid'itē/ [L, *avidus,* eager], an inexact measure of the binding strength of antibodies to multiple antigenic determinants on natural antigens.

A-V interval [L, *intervallum,* space between ramparts], a term used in pacing terminology to identify the specific time interval between the atrial (A) beat and the ventricular (V) beat.

avirulent /āvir'yələnt/ [Gk, *a,* not; L, *virus,* poison], not virulent; not pathogenic.

avitaminosis /āvī'təminō'sis/ [Gk, *a,* not; L, *vita,* life, amine, *osis,* condition], a condition resulting from a deficiency of or lack of absorption or use of one or more vitamins in the diet.

AV nicking, a vascular abnormality on the retina of the eye, visible on ophthalmologic examination, in which a vein is compressed by an arteriovenous crossing. The vein appears "nicked" as a result of constriction or spasm. It is a sign of hypertension, arteriosclerosis, or other vascular conditions.

Avogadro's law /av'ōgad'rōz/ [Amedeo Avogadro, Italian physicist, 1776–1856], a law in physics stating that equal volumes of all gases at a given temperature and pressure contain the identical number of molecules.

Avogadro's number [Amedeo Avogadro], the number of atoms in exactly 12 g of the isotope of carbon C_{12}, or 6.02×10^{23}. One mole of any monoatomic element contains this number of atoms, and one mole of any polyatomic element or molecule contains this number of molecules.

avoidance [ME, *avoiden,* to empty], (in psychiatry) a conscious or unconscious defense mechanism, physical or psychologic, by which an individual tries to avoid or escape from unpleasant stimuli, conflicts, or feelings such as anxiety, fear, pain, or danger.

avoidance-avoidance conflict, a conflict resulting from the confrontation of two or more alternative goals or desires that are equally aversive and undesirable.

avoidance conditioning, the establishment of certain patterns of behavior to avoid unpleasant or painful stimuli.

avoidant personality, a personality disorder characterized by hypersensitivity to rejection and a reluctance to start a relationship because of a fear of not being accepted uncritically.

avoirdupois weight /av'ərdəpoiz'/ [OF, *avoir de pois,* property of weight], the English system of weights in which there are 7000 grains, 256 drams, or 16 ounces to 1 pound. One ounce in this system equals 28.35 g, and 1 pound equals 453.59 g.

avulsed teeth /əvulst/ [L, *avulsio,* a pulling away], teeth that have been forcibly displaced from their normal position.

avulsion /əvul'shən/ [L, *avulsio,* a pulling away], the separation, by tearing, of any part of the body from the whole. —**avulse,** *v.*

avulsion fracture, a fracture caused by the tearing away of a fragment of bone where a strong ligamentous or tendinous attachment forcibly pulls the fragment away from osseous tissue.

awake anesthesia [ME, *awakenen*], an anesthetic procedure in which analgesia and anesthesia are accomplished without loss of consciousness. Dental procedures, surgery on a limb or an extremity, scopic examinations, and certain kinds of head surgery are performed using awake anesthesia.

AWHONN, abbreviation for **Association of Women's Health, Obstetric, and Neonatal Nurses.**

AWOL /ā'wôl/, abbreviation for **absent without leave.**

axial (A) /ak'sē-əl/ [Gk, *axon,* axle], **1.** pertaining to or situated on the axis of a body structure or part. **2.** (in dentistry) relating to the long axis of a tooth.

axial current, the central part of the blood current.

axial gradient, 1. the variation in metabolic rate in different parts of the body. **2.** the development toward the body axis or

its parts in relation to the metabolic rate in the various parts.

axial skeleton [L, *axis,* axle; Gk, *skeletos,* dried up], the bones forming the axis of the skeleton, including the skull, vertebrae, ribs, and sternum.

axial spillway, a groove that crosses a cusp ridge or a marginal ridge and extends onto an axial surface of a tooth.

axifugal /aksif'yəgəl/ [L, *axis,* axle, *fugere,* to flee], extending away from an axis or axion.

axilla /aksil'ə/, *pl.* **axillae** [L, wing], a pyramid-shaped space forming the underside of the shoulder between the upper arm and the side of the chest. —**axillary,** *adj.*

axillary abscess [L, *axilla,* wing, *abscedere,* to go away], an abscess in the armpit.

axillary artery /ak'sələr'ē/ [L, *axilla,* wing], one of a pair of continuations of the subclavian arteries that starts at the outer border of the first rib and ends at the distal border of the teres major, where it becomes the brachial artery.

axillary line, an imaginary vertical line on the body wall, passing through a point midway between the anterior and posterior folds of the axilla.

axillary nerve, one of the last two branches of the posterior cord of the brachial plexus before the posterior cord becomes the radial nerve.

axillary node, one of the lymph glands of the axilla that help fight infections in the chest, armpit, neck, and arm and drain lymph from those areas. The 20 to 30 axillary nodes are divided into the lateral group, the anterior group, the posterior group, the central group, and the medial group.

axillary temperature [L, *axilla,* wing, *temperatura*], the body temperature as recorded by a thermometer placed in the armpit. The reading is generally 0.5° to 1° less than the oral temperature.

axillary vein, one of a pair of veins of the upper limb that becomes the subclavian vein at the outer border of the first rib.

axillofemoral bypass graft /ak'silōfem'ərəl/, a synthetic artery that is surgically anastomosed to the axillary and common femoral arteries. The graft shunts blood between those arteries, increasing blood flow to the lower extremities.

axion /ak'sē-on/, **1.** the brain and spinal cord. **2.** the cerebrospinal axis.

axis, *pl.* **axes** /ak'sēz/ [Gk, *axon,* axle], **1.** (in anatomy) a line that passes through the center of the body, or a part of the body, such as the frontal axis, binauricular axis, and basifacial axis. **2.** the second cervical vertebra, about which the atlas rotates, allowing the head to be turned, extended, and flexed.

axis artery, one of a pair of extensions of the subclavian arteries, running into and supplying the upper limb, continuing into the forearm as the palmar interosseous artery.

axis deviation, an electrocardiogram trace in which the QRS axis of the heart in the frontal plane lies outside the usual range of −30 to 110 degrees. It represents an abnormal direction of ventricular depolarization.

axis traction, 1. the process of pulling a baby's head with obstetric forceps in a direction in line with the path of least resistance, following the curve of Carus through the mother's birth canal. **2.** *informal.* any mechanical device attached to obstetric forceps to facilitate pulling in the proper direction.

axoaxonic synapse /ak'sō-akson'ik/ [Gk, *axon,* axle (to) *axon,* axle], a type of synapse in which the axon of one neuron comes in contact with the axon of another neuron.

axodendrosomatic synapse /-den'drōsō-mat'ik/, a type of synapse in which the axon of one neuron comes in contact with both the dendrites and the cell body of another neuron.

axolysis /aksol'isis/, the degeneration of the axon of a nerve cell.

axon /ak'son/ [Gk, axle], usually a long, slender extension of a neuron capable of conducting action potentials or self-propagating nervous impulses.

axon flare, vasodilation, reddening, and increased sensitivity of skin surrounding an injured area, caused by an axon reflex.

axonography /ak'sənog'rəfē/, the recording of electrical activity in the axon of a nerve cell.

axonotmesis /ak'sənotmē'sis/ [Gk, *axon* + *temnein,* to cut], an interruption of the axon from nerve injury, with subsequent wallerian degeneration of the distal nerve segment.

axon reflex [Gk, *axon,* axle], a neuron reflex in which an afferent impulse travels along a nerve fiber away from the cell body until it reaches a branching, where it is diverted to an end organ without entering the cell body. It does not involve a complete reflex arc, and therefore it is not a true reflex.

axon sheath [Gk, *axon* + AS, *scaeth*], a laminated myelin sheath that is interrupted at intervals by nodes of Ranvier.

axoplasm /ak'sōplaz'əm/, cytoplasm of an axon.

axoplasmic flow /ak'sōplaz'mik/ [Gk, *axon* + *plassein,* to shape], the continuous pulsing, undulating movement of the cytoplasm between the cell body of a neuron, where protein synthesis occurs, and the axon fiber to supply it with the substances vital for the maintenance of activity and for repair.

axosomatic synapse /ak'sōsōmat'ik/ [Gk, *axon* + *soma,* body], a type of synapse in which the axon of one neuron comes in contact with the cell body of another neuron.

axotomy /ak'sōplaz'əm/, surgical transection of an axon.

azatadine maleate /azat'ədēn/, an antihistamine with antiserotonin, anticholinergic, and sedative effects. It is used in the treatment of allergic rhinitis and chronic urticaria.

azathioprine /az'əthī'ōprēn/, an immunosuppressive prescribed to prevent organ rejection after transplantation and to treat lupus erythematosus and other systemic inflammatory diseases.

azithromycin, an antibiotic that suppresses the formation of protein by bacteria, retards bacterial growth, or causes death of the microorganisms. It is prescribed in the treatment of mild to moderate infections by certain bacteria in adults, including respiratory tract infections, skin disorders, and sexually transmitted diseases.

azlocillin sodium /az'lōsil'in/, a semisynthetic penicillin antibiotic prescribed for lower respiratory tract, urinary tract, skin, and bone and joint infections and bacterial septicemia caused by susceptible strains of microorganisms, mainly *Pseudomonas aeruginosa.*

azo compounds /ā'zō/ [Fr, *azote,* nitrogen], one of many organic aromatic compounds containing the divalent chromophore, -N = N-. They are produced by the alkaline reduction of nitro compounds.

azo dye, a type of nitrogen-containing compound used in commercial coloring materials. Some forms of the chemical are potential carcinogens.

azoic /āzō'ik/ [Gk, *a,* not, *zoe,* life], devoid of organic life.

azoospermia /āzō'əspur'mē-ə/ [Gk, *a, zoon,* not animal, *sperma* seed], lack of spermatozoa in the semen. It may be caused by testicular dysfunction, chemotherapy combination, or blockage of the tubules of the epididymis; or it may be induced by vasectomy.

azoprotein /ā'zōprō'tēn/, a protein coupled to another substance through a diazo (N=N—) linkage. Azoproteins are often used in immunochemical procedures.

azotemia /az'ōtē'mē·ə/ [Fr, *azote,* nitrogen; Gk, *haima,* blood], retention of excessive amounts of nitrogenous compounds in the blood. This toxic condition is caused by failure of the kidneys to remove urea from the blood and is characteristic of uremia. —**azotemic,** *adj.*

azoturia /az'ōtŏŏr'ēə/ [Fr, *azote,* nitrogen; Gk, *ouron,* urine], an excess of nitrogenous compounds, including urea in the urine.

azure /āzhər/, one of a group of basic blue methylthionine or phenothiazine dyes used in staining blood and cell nuclei.

azurophil, a substance that stains readily with an azure blue dye.

azurophilia /āzh'ŏŏrəfil'yə/, a condition in which the blood contains some cells that have granules that stain readily with azure (blue) dye.

azygography /az'īgog'rəfē/, the radiographic imaging of the azygos venous system after injection of an iodinated contrast medium.

azygospore /az'igəspô'r/ [Gk, *a* + *zygon,* not yoke, *sporos,* seed], a spore that is produced directly from a gamete that does not undergo conjugation, as in certain algae and fungi.

azygous /az'əgəs/ [Gk, *a* + *zygon,* not yoke], occurring as a single entity or part, such as any unpaired anatomic structure; not part of a pair. —**azygos** /az'əgos'/, *n.*

azygous lobe, a congenital anomaly of the lung caused by a fold of pleural tissue carried by the azygous vein during descent into the thorax during embryonic development. It produces an extra lobe in the right upper lung.

azygous vein, one of the seven veins of the thorax. Beginning opposite the first or second lumbar vertebra, it rises through the aortic hiatus in the diaphragm and ends in the superior vena cava.

B, β, See **beta.**

B, symbol for the element **boron.**

B6 bronchus sign, an artifact in a lung radiograph in which an air bronchogram appears in the lower lobe as a result of consolidation of atelectasis.

B19 virus, a strain of human parvovirus associated with a number of diseases, including hemolytic anemia, erythema infectiosum, fifth disease, and symptoms of arthritis and arthralgia.

Ba, symbol for the element **barium.**

BA, abbreviation for *Bachelor of Arts.*

babbling, a stage in speech development characterized by the production of strings of speech sounds in vocal play.

Babcock's operation [William W. Babcock, American surgeon, 1872–1963], the removal of a varicosed saphenous vein by insertion of an acorn-tipped sound, tying the vein to the sound and drawing it out.

babesiosis /bəbē′sē·ō′sis/ [Victor Babes, Romanian bacteriologist, 1854–1926], an infection caused by protozoa of the genus *Babesia.* The parasite is introduced into the host through the bite of ticks of the species *Ixodes dammini* and infects red blood cells.

Babinski's reflex /bəbin′skēz/ [Joseph F.F. Babinski, French neurologist, 1857–1932], dorsiflexion of the big toe with extension and fanning of the other toes elicited by firmly stroking the lateral aspect of the sole of the foot. The reflex is normal in newborns and abnormal in children and adults.

Babinski's sign [Joseph Babinski], a series of partial responses that are pathognomonic of different degrees of upper motor neuron disease, including (1) absence of an ankle jerk in sciatica; (2) an extensor plantar response, with an extension of the great toe and adduction of the other toes; (3) a more pronounced concentration of platysma on the unaffected side during blowing or whistling; (4) pronation that occurs when an arm affected by paralysis is placed in supination; and (5) when a patient in a supine position with arms crossed over the chest attempts to assume a sitting position, the thigh on the affected side is flexed and the heel is raised, whereas the leg on the unaffected side remains flat.

baby [ME, *babe*], **1.** an infant or young child, especially one who is not yet able to walk or talk. **2.** to treat gently or with special care.

baby bottle tooth decay, a dental condition that occurs in children between 12 months and 3 years of age as a result of being given a bottle at bedtime, resulting in prolonged exposure of the teeth to milk or juice. Caries are formed because pools of milk or juice in the mouth break down to lactic acid and other decay-causing substances. Preventive measures include elimination of the bedtime feeding or substitution of water for milk or juice in the nighttime bottle.

Baby Jane Doe regulations, rules established in 1984 by the U.S. Health and Human Services Department requiring state governments to investigate complaints about parental decisions involving the treatment of handicapped infants. The controversial regulations have been found illegal by a federal court. The popular name for the federal rules was taken from the name "Jane Doe" given to an infant born in New York with an open spinal column and other defects who became the object of a campaign to force lifesaving surgery for the child over parental objections.

baby talk, **1.** the speech patterns and sounds of young children learning to talk, characterized by mispronunciation, imperfect syntax, repetition, and phonetic modifications such as lisping or stuttering. **2.** the intentionally oversimplified manner of speech, imitative of young children learning to talk, used by adults in addressing children or pets. **3.** the speech patterns characteristic of regressive stages of various mental disorders, especially schizophrenia.

BAC, abbreviation for **bronchoalveolar carcinoma.**

bacampicillin hydrochloride, a semisynthetic penicillin prescribed in the treatment of respiratory tract, urinary tract, skin, and gonococcal infections.

Bachelor of Science in Nursing (BSN) /bach′ələr/, an academic degree awarded on satisfactory completion of a 4-year

Bacillaceae /bas′əlā′si-ē/ [L, *bacillum,* small rod], a family of Schizomycetes of the order Eubacteriales, consisting of gram-positive, rod-shaped cells that can produce cylindric, ellipsoid, or spheric endospores. Some are parasitic on insects and animals and pathogenic.

bacillary angiomatosis′ /bas′əler′ē/, a condition of multiple angiomata caused by an infection of *Bartonella.* The infectious agent is also the cause of cat-scratch fever. It is manifested in human immunodeficiency virus/Ninfected patients as small hemangioma-like lesions of the skin but may also involve the lymph nodes and viscera. The skin lesions are often mistaken for Kaposi's sarcoma.

bacille Calmette-Guérin (BCG) /kalmet′-gāraN′/ [Léon C.A. Calmette, French bacteriologist, 1863–1933; Camille Guérin, French bacteriologist, 1872–1961], an attenuated strain of tubercle bacilli used in many countries as a vaccine against tuberculosis, most often administered intradermally with a multiple-puncture disk. It appears to prevent the more serious forms of tuberculosis and to give some protection to persons living in areas where tuberculosis is prevalent.

bacille Calmette-Guérin vaccine. See BCG vaccine.

bacillemia /bas′əlē′mē-ə/, a condition in which bacilli are circulating in the blood.

bacilli /bəsil′ī/, *sing.* **bacillum** [L, *bacillum,* small rod], any rod-shaped bacteria.

bacilliform /bəsil′ifôrm/, rod-shaped, like a bacillus.

bacillosis /bas′əlō′sis/, a condition in which bacilli have invaded tissues, inducing symptoms of an infection.

bacilluria /bas′əlōōr′ē-ə/ [L, *bacillum* + Gk, *ouron,* urine], the presence of bacilli in the urine.

bacillus, a gram-positive aerobic or facultatively anaerobic, spore-bearing, rod-shaped microorganism of the family Bacillaceae.

Bacillus /bəsil′əs/, a genus of aerobic, gram-positive spore-producing bacteria in the family Bacillaceae, order Eubacteriales. The genus includes 33 species, 3 of which are pathogenic, and the rest saprophytic soil forms.

Bacillus anthracis,, a species of gram-positive, facultative anaerobe that causes anthrax.

Bacillus cereus, a species of bacilli found in the soil. It causes food poisoning (an emetic type and a diarrheal type) by the formation of an enterotoxin in contaminated foods. It can also cause infections such as ocular infections.

bacitracin /bas′itrā′sin/ [L, *bacillum* + *Tracy,* surname of patient in whom toxin-producing bacillus species was isolated], an antibacterial prescribed for skin infections sensitive to bacitracin.

back [AS, *baec*], the posterior or dorsal part of the trunk of the body between the neck and pelvis. The back is divided by a middle furrow that lies over the tips of the spinous processes of the vertebrae. The skeletal part of the back includes the thoracic and lumbar vertebrae and both scapulae. The nerves that innervate the various muscles of the back arise from the segmental spinal nerves.

backache /bak′āk/ [AS, *baec* + ME, *aken*], a pain in the lumbar, lumbosacral, or cervical region of the back, varying in sharpness and intensity. Causes may include muscle strain or other muscular disorders or pressure on the root of a nerve, such as the sciatic nerve, caused in turn by a variety of factors, including a herniated vertebral disk. Treatment may include heat, ultrasound, and devices to provide support for the affected area.

back-action condenser, (in dentistry) an instrument for compacting amalgams that has a U-shaped shank to develop the condensing force from a pulling motion rather than the more common pushing motions.

backboard, a long, flat, rigid piece of wood or other material that is placed under an accident victim with possible spinal injury. It is used to transport the patient to a hospital.

backbone, the vertebral column.

backcross [AS, *baec* + *cruc,* cross], **1.** (in genetics) the mating (cross) between a heterozygote and a homozygote. **2.** the organism or strain produced by such a cross.

background radiation [AS, *baec* + OE, *grund,* ground], naturally occurring radiation emitted by materials in the soil, groundwater, and building material; radioactive substances in the body, especially potassium 40 (^{40}K); and cosmic rays from outer space. Each year the average person is exposed to 44 millirad (mrad) of cosmic radiation, 44 mrad of external terrestrial radiation, and 18 mrad of naturally occurring internal radioactive sources.

back pressure [AS, *baec* + L, *premere,* to press], pressure that builds in a vessel or a cavity as fluid accumulates.

baclofen, an antispastic agent prescribed for the alleviation of spasticity.

bacteremia /bak′tirē′mē-ə/ [Gk, *bakterion,* small staff, *haima,* blood], the presence of bacteria in the blood. —**bacteremic,** *adj.*

bacteria /baktir'ē·ə/, *sing.* **bacterium** [Gk, *bakterion,* small staff], any of the small unicellular microorganisms of the class Schizomycetes. The genera vary morphologically, being spheric (cocci), rod-shaped (bacilli), spiral (spirochetes), or comma-shaped (vibrios).

bacterial adherence /baktir'ēəl/, the process whereby bacteria attach themselves to cells or other surfaces before proliferating. Some mononuclear phagocytes are able to adhere to surfaces other than living tissues such as glass or plastic.

bacterial aneurysm, a localized dilation in the wall of a blood vessel caused by the growth of bacteria. It often follows septicemia or bacteremia and usually occurs in peripheral vessels.

bacterial endocarditis, an acute or subacute bacterial infection of the endocardium or the heart valves or both. The condition is characterized by heart murmur, prolonged fever, bacteremia, splenomegaly, and embolic phenomena.

bacterial enzyme, an enzyme produced by a bacterium.

bacterial food poisoning, a toxic condition resulting from the ingestion of food contaminated by certain bacteria. Acute infectious gastroenteritis caused by various species of *Salmonella* is characterized by fever, chills, nausea, vomiting, diarrhea, and general discomfort beginning 8 to 48 hours after ingestion and continuing for several days. Food poisoning caused by the neurotoxin of *Clostridium botulinum* is characterized by gastrointestinal symptoms, disturbances of vision, weakness or paralysis of muscles, and, in severe cases, respiratory failure.

bacterial inflammation [L, *bacterium* + *inflammare,* to set afire], any inflammation that is part of a body's response to a bacterial infection.

bacterial kinase, 1. a kinase of bacterial origin. 2. a bacterial enzyme that activates plasminogen, the precursor of plasmin.

bacterial laryngitis, a form of laryngitis caused by a bacterial agent and usually associated with rhinosinusitis or laryngotracheal bronchitis. Signs of a bacterial infection are a cough and purulent rhinorrhea.

bacterial plaque, a film composed of microorganisms that attaches with acquired pellicle to the teeth and causes dental caries and infections of the gingival tissue. Mucin secreted by the salivary glands is also a component of plaque.

bacterial prostatitis, a bacterial infection of the prostate. Acute bacterial infections usually involve gram-negative bacilli such as *Escherichia coli.* Most cases are treated with broad-spectrum antimicrobial drugs. Abscesses may be associated with anaerobic bacteria. Chronic bacterial prostatitis is usually caused by gram-negative bacilli. It is less common and may be characterized by low back pain, dysuria, and perineal discomfort.

bacterial protein, a protein produced by a bacterium.

bacterial resistance, the ability of certain strains of bacteria to develop a tolerance toward specific antibiotics.

bacterial toxin [Gk, *bakterion,* small staff, *toxikon,* poison], any poisonous substance produced by a bacterium. Kinds of bacterial toxins include **endotoxin** and **exotoxin.**

bacterial vaccine, a saline solution suspension of a strain of attenuated or killed bacteria prepared for injection into a patient to stimulate development of active immunity to that strain.

bacterial vaginosis [Gk, *bakterion,* small staff; L, *vagina,* sheath; Gk, *osis,* condition], a chronic inflammation of the vagina caused by a bacterium, *Gardnerella vaginalis.*

bacterial virus, a virus with the ability to destroy bacteria.

bactericidal /baktir'isī'dəl/, destructive to bacteria.

bactericidal antibiotic [Gk *bakterion* + *caedere,* to kill; Gk, *anti,* against, *bios,* life], an antibiotic drug that kills bacteria.

bactericide /baktir'əsīd/ [GK, *bakterion* + L, *caedere,* to kill], any drug or other agent that kills bacteria.

bactericidin [Gk, *bakterion* + L, *caedere,* to kill], an antibody that kills bacteria in the presence of complement.

bacteriocin /baktir'ē·əsin/, protein produced by certain species of bacteria that are toxic to related strains of those bacteria.

bacteriocinogenic /baktir'ēəsin'əjen'ik/, pertaining to an organism capable of producing bacteriocins.

bacteriogenic /baktir'ē·əjen'ik/, 1. capable of producing bacteria. 2. derived from or originating in bacteria.

bacteriologic /baktir'ē·əloj'ik/ [Gk, *bakterion*], pertaining to **bacteriology.**

bacteriologic sputum examination, a laboratory procedure to determine the presence or absence of bacteria in a specimen of a patient's sputum. Part of the specimen is stained and examined microscopically on a glass slide, and part is mixed with culture medium and allowed to incubate for more specific examination later.

bacteriologist /baktir′ē·ol′əjist/, a specialist in the scientific study of bacteria.

bacteriology /-ol′əjē/ [Gk, *bakterion* + *logos,* science], the scientific study of bacteria.

bacteriolysin /baktir′ē·əlī′sin/ [Gk, *bakterion* + *lyein,* to loosen], an antibody that causes the breakdown of a particular species of bacterial cell.

bacteriolysis /baktir′ē·ol′əsis/, the intracellular or extracellular breakdown of bacteria. **—bacteriolytic,** *adj.*

bacteriophage /baktir′ē·əfāj′/ [Gk, *bakterion* + *phagein,* to eat], any virus that causes lysis of host bacteria, including the blue-green algae. Bacteriophages resemble other viruses in that each is composed of either ribonucleic acid or deoxyribonucleic acid. **—bacteriophagic,** *adj.,* **bacteriophagy** /-of′əjē/, *n..*

bacteriophage typing, the process of identifying a species of bacterium according to the type of virus that attacks it.

bacteriospermia /baktir′ēəspur′mē·ə/, the presence of bacteria in semen.

bacteriostasis /baktir′ē·os′təsis/ [Gk, *bakterion* + Gk, *stasis,* standing still], a state of suspended growth and/or reproduction of bacteria.

bacteriostatic /baktir′ē·əstat′ik/ [Gk, *bakterion* + *statikos,* standing], tending to restrain the development or the reproduction of bacteria.

bacteriuria /baktir′ēyŏŏr′ē·ə/, the presence of bacteria in the urine.

bacteroid /bak′təroid/, **1.** pertaining to or resembling bacteria. **2.** a structure that resembles a bacterium. **—bacteroidal, bacterioidal,** *adj.*

Bacteroides /bak′təroi′dēz/ [Gk, *bakterion,* small staff, *eidos,* form], a genus of obligate anaerobic bacilli normally found in the colon, mouth, genital tract, and upper respiratory system. Severe infection may result from the invasion of the bacillus through a break in the mucous membrane.

BAER, abbreviation for **brainstem auditory evoked response.**

baffling, the process of removing large water particles from suspension in a jet nebulizer so that the particles entering the patient's airways are of a uniform therapeutic size.

bag [AS, *baelg*], a flexible or dilatable sac or pouch designed to contain gas, fluid, or semisolid material such as crushed ice. Several types of bags are used in medical or surgical procedures to dilate the anus, vagina, or other body openings.

bagasse /bəgas′/, [Fr, cane trash], the crushed fibers or the residue of sugarcane.

bagassosis /bag′əsō′sis/, a self-limited lung disease caused by an allergic response to bagasse, the fungi-laden, dusty debris left after the syrup has been extracted from sugarcane.

bagging, *informal.* the artificial ventilation performed with a ventilator or respirator bag. The bag is squeezed to deliver air to the patient's lungs through a mask or an endotracheal tube.

bag lady/man, a homeless indigent person who carries all of his or her personal possessions in a portable container.

bag of waters, the membranous sac of amniotic fluid surrounding the fetus in the uterus of a pregnant woman.

bag-valve-mask resuscitator, a device consisting of a manually compressible container with a plastic bag of oxygen at one end and at the other a one-way valve and mask that fit over the mouth and nose of the person to be resuscitated.

Bainbridge reflex [Francis A. Bainbridge, English physiologist, 1874–1921], a cardiac reflex consisting of an increased pulse rate, resulting from stimulation of stretch receptors in the wall of the left atrium.

Baker's cyst [William M. Baker, British surgeon, 1839–1896], a cyst that forms at the back of the knee. It is often associated with rheumatoid arthritis and may appear only when the leg is straightened.

baker's itch [AS, *giccan,* to bake], a rash that may develop on the hands and forearms of bakery workers, probably as an allergic reaction to flours or other ingredients in bakery products.

BAL, **1.** abbreviation for *British antilewisite.* See **dimercaprol. 2.** abbreviation for **bronchoalveolar lavage.**

balance [L, *bilanx,* having two scales], **1.** an instrument for weighing. **2.** a normal state of physiologic equilibrium. **3.** a state of mental or emotional equilibrium. **4.** to bring into equilibrium.

balanced anesthesia, *informal.* a highly variable technique of general anesthesia in which no single anesthetic agent or preset proportion of the combination of agents is used; rather, an individualized mixture of anesthetics is administered according to the needs of a particular patient for a particular operation.

balanced articulation, the simultaneous contacting of the upper and lower teeth as they glide over each other when the mandible is moved from centric relation to various eccentric relations.

balanced diet, a diet containing all the essential nutrients that cannot be synthesized by the body in amounts adequate for growth, energy needs, nitrogen equilibrium, repair, and maintenance of normal health.

balanced occlusion, **1.** an occlusion of

the teeth that presents a harmonious relation of the occluding surfaces in centric and eccentric positions within the functional range of mandibular positions and tooth size. 2. the simultaneous contacting of the upper and lower teeth on both sides and in the anterior and posterior occlusal areas of the jaws.

balanced polymorphism, in a population, the recurrence of an equalized mixture of homozygotes and heterozygotes for specific genetic traits, which are maintained from generation to generation by the forces of natural selection.

balanced suspension, a system of splints, ropes, slings, pulleys, and weights for suspending the lower extremities of the body, used as an aid to healing and recuperation from fractures or from surgical intervention.

balanced traction, a system of balanced suspension that supplements traction in the treatment of fractures of the lower extremities or after various operations affecting the lower parts of the body.

balanced translocation, the transfer of segments between nonhomologous chromosomes in such a way that there are changes in the configuration and total number of chromosomes, but each cell or gamete contains no more or no less than the normal amount of diploid or haploid genetic material.

balancing side, (in dentistry) the side of the mouth opposite the working side of dentition or a denture.

balanic /bəlan′ik/ [Gk, *balanos,* acorn], pertaining to the glans penis or the glans clitoridis.

balanitis /bal′ənī′tis/ [Gk, *balanos + itis*], inflammation of the glans penis.

balanitis diabetica, an inflammation of the glans penis or glans clitoridis caused by the sugar content of the urine and commonly seen in diabetics.

balanitis xerotica obliterans /zirot′ikə oblit′ərans/ [Gk, *balanos + itis + xeros,* dry, *tokos,* labor; L, *obliterare,* to efface], a chronic skin disease of the penis, characterized by a white indurated area surrounding the meatus.

balanoplasty /bal′ənōplas′tē/ [Gk, *balanos + plassein,* to shape], an operation involving plastic surgery of the glans penis.

balanoposthitis /bal′ənōposthī′tis/ [Gk, *balanos + posthe,* penis, foreskin, *itis*], a generalized inflammation of the glans penis and prepuce. It is characterized by soreness, irritation, and discharge, which occurs as a complication of bacterial or fungal infection.

balanopreputial /bal′ənōpripyoo′shəl/ [Gk, *balanos + L, praeputium,* foreskin], pertaining to the glans penis and the prepuce.

balanorrhagia /bal′ənōrā′jē·ə/ [Gk, *balanos + rhegnynai,* to burst forth], balanitis in which pus is discharged copiously from the penis.

balantidiasis /bal′əntidī′əsis/, an infection caused by ingestion of cysts of the protozoan *Balantidium coli.* In some cases the organism is a harmless inhabitant of the large intestine, but infection with *B. coli* usually causes diarrhea.

Balantidium coli /bal′əntid′ē·əm/ [Gk, *balantidion,* little bag, *kolon,* colon], the largest and the only ciliated protozoan species that is pathogenic to humans, causing balantidiasis.

baldness [ME, *balled*], absence of hair, especially from the scalp.

Balint's syndrome [Rudolph Balint, Hungarian neurologist, 1874–1929], a group of visual symptoms characterized by agnosia and optic ataxia. The patient experiences nystagmus, or loss of control of eye movements, simultaneously with loss of perceptive ability. The patient may begin to follow a moving object but lose it. The cause is bilateral disease of the parietotemporal areas of the brain.

Balkan traction frame, an overhead rectangular frame attached to the bed and used for attaching splints, suspending or changing the position of immobilized limbs, or providing continuous traction with weights and pulleys.

Balkan tubulointerstitial nephritis /too′-byəlō·in′tərstish′əl/, a chronic kidney disorder marked by renal insufficiency, proteinuria, tubulointerstitial nephritis, and anemia. The disease is endemic in the Balkans but is not hereditary.

ball [ME, *bal*], a relatively spheric mass, such as one of the chondrin balls embedded in hyaline cartilage.

Ballance's sign [Charles A. Ballance, English surgeon, 1856–1936], a dull percussion resonance sound heard on the right flank of a patient lying in the left decubitus position. The sound may shift with the patient's change of position. The condition is attributed to rupture of the spleen, which causes an accumulation of liquid blood on the right side and coagulated blood on the left.

ball-and-socket joint, a synovial joint in which the globular (ball-shaped) head of an articulating bone is received into a cuplike cavity, allowing the distal bone to move around an indefinite number of axes with a common center, such as in hip and shoulder joints.

ball-catcher position, a position of the hands for making a radiograph to diagnose rheumatoid arthritis. The hands are held with the palms upward and the fingers cupped, as if to catch a ball.

ballism /bôl′izəm/ [Gk, *ballismo,* dancing], an abnormal neuromuscular condition characterized by uncoordinated swinging of the limbs and jerky movements.

ballistic movement /bəlis′tik/, a high-velocity musculoskeletal movement, such as a tennis serve or boxing punch, requiring reciprocal organization of agonistic and antagonistic synergies.

ballistics /bəlis′tiks/ [Gk, *ballein,* to throw], the study of the motion, trajectory, and impact of projectiles, including bullets and rockets.

ballistocardiograph [Gk, *ballein,* to throw, *kardia,* heart, *graphein,* to record], an apparatus for recording body movements caused by the thrust of the heart during systolic ejection of the blood into the aorta and the pulmonary arteries.

ballistocardiography /balis′tōkär′dē·og′-rə fē/, the recording of body movements in reaction to the beating of the heart and the circulation of the blood.

ball of the foot, the part of the foot composed of the distal heads of the metatarsals and their surrounding fatty fibrous tissue pad.

balloon angioplasty /bəlo͞on′/, a method of dilating or opening an obstructed blood vessel by threading a small balloon-tipped catheter into the vessel. The balloon is inflated to widen the blood vessel.

balloon bezoar [Fr, *ballon,* a large ball; Ar, *bazahr,* counterpoison], a balloon that is inserted into the stomach and inflated to create a sensation of fullness, used as a therapy for obesity.

balloon compression, a percutaneous therapy for trigeminal neuralgia. A balloon is inflated to compress the gasserian ganglion and produce trigeminal injury.

balloon tamponade, [Fr, tamponnade], a procedure whereby a flexible inflatable device with a triple-lumen tube and two inflatable balloons is inserted into a passageway and expanded to block the flow of blood or to force open a stenosis.

balloon-tip catheter, a catheter bearing a nonporous inflatable sac around its far end. After insertion of the catheter, the sac can be inflated with air or sterile water introduced via injection into a special port at the near end of the catheter.

ballottable /bəlot′əbəl/ [Fr, *balloter,* a shaking about], pertaining to a use of palpation to detect movement of objects suspended in fluid, such as a fetus in amniotic fluid.

ballottable head [Fr, *ballotage,* shaking up], a fetal head that has not descended and become fixed in the maternal bony pelvis.

ballottement /bä′lôtmäN′, bəlot′ment/ [Fr, tossing], a technique of palpating an organ or floating structure by bouncing it gently and feeling it rebound.

ball thrombus, a relatively round, coagulated mass of blood, containing platelets, fibrin, and cellular fragments, that may obstruct a blood vessel or an orifice, usually the mitral valve of the heart.

ball-valve action, the intermittent opening and closing of an orifice by a buoyant, ball-shaped mass, which acts as a valve. Some kinds of objects that may act in this manner are kidney stones, gallstones, and blood clots.

balm /bäm/ [Gk, *balsamon,* balsam], **1.** a healing or a soothing substance such as any of various medicinal ointments. **2.** an aromatic plant of the genus *Melissa* that relieves pain.

balneology /bal′nē·ol′əjē/ [L, *balneum,* bath; Gk, *logos,* science], a field of medicine that deals with the chemical compositions of various mineral waters and their healing characteristics, especially in baths. —**balneologic,** *adj.*

balneotherapy /bal′nē·ōther′əpē/ [L, *balneum* + Gk, *therapeia,* treatment], use of baths in the treatment of many diseases and conditions.

balsam /bôl′səm/ [Gk, *balsamon*], any of a variety of resinous saps, generally from evergreens, usually containing benzoic or cinnamic acid. Balsam is sometimes used in rectal suppositories and dermatologic agents as a counterirritant.

Baltimore Longitudinal Study of Aging, a long-range examination of interrelations between cerebral physiologic changes of advancing age and psychologic capacities and psychiatric symptoms of men over 65 years of age. Men selected for the original study (1955) were of varied backgrounds in categories of religion, country of birth, education, occupation, retirement and employment, and householder status (ranging from independent to nursing home) in order to explore uncontrolled factors that might lead to new knowledge regarding aging. Numerous other studies are being done..

Bamberger's sign [Heinrich Bamberger, Austrian physician, 1822–1888], **1.** a neural disorder characterized by the feeling of a tactile stimulation at a corresponding point on the opposite side of the body. **2.** pericardial effusion signs at the level of the scapula that disappear when the patient leans forward.

bamboo spine /bambo͞o′/ [Malay, *bambu*],

the characteristically rigid spine of advanced ankylosing spondylitis.

band [ME, *bande*, strip], **1.** (in anatomy) a bundle of fibers, as seen in striated muscle, that encircles a structure or binds one part of the body to another. **2.** (in dentistry) a strip of metal that fits around a tooth and serves as an attachment for orthodontic components. **3.** the immature form of a segmented granulocyte characterized by a sausage-shaped nucleus.

band adapter, an instrument for aiding in the fitting of a circumferential orthodontic band to a tooth.

bandage /ban'dij/ [ME, *bande,* strip], **1.** a strip or roll of cloth or other material that may be wound around a part of the body in a variety of ways to secure a dressing, maintain pressure over a compress, or immobilize a limb or other part of the body. **2.** to apply a bandage.

bandage shears, a sturdy pair of scissors used to cut through bandages. The blades of most bandage shears are angled to the shaft of the instrument, and the lower blade is rounded and blunt to facilitate insertion under the bandage without harming the patient's skin.

band cell, a developing granular leukocyte in circulating blood, characterized by a curved or indented nucleus.

banding [ME, *bande,* strip], (in genetics) any of several techniques of staining chromosomes with fluorescent stains or chemical dyes that produce a series of lateral light and dark areas whose intensity and position are characteristic of each chromosome.

bandpass, (in radiology) a measure of the number of times per second an electron beam can be modulated. It is a factor that influences horizontal resolution on a cathode-ray tube.

band pusher, an instrument used for adapting metal orthodontic bands to the teeth.

band remover, an instrument used to help take orthodontic bands off of the teeth.

bank blood [It, *banca,* bench; AS, *blod*], anticoagulated preserved blood collected from donors, usually in units of 500 ml, and stored under refrigeration for future use.

Banting, Sir Frederick G. [Canadian physician, 1891–1941], co-winner, with John J. Macleod, of the 1923 Nobel prize for medicine and physiology for their research, with the Canadian physiologist Charles H. Best, showing the link between the pancreas and insulin in the control of diabetes.

Banti's syndrome /ban'tēz/ [Guido Banti,

Italian pathologist, 1852–1925], a progressive disorder involving several organ systems, characterized by portal hypertension, splenomegaly, anemia, leukopenia, gastrointestinal tract bleeding, and cirrhosis of the liver.

BAO, abbreviation for **basal acid output.**

bar, (in physical science) a measure of air pressure. It is equal to 1000 millibars, or 10^6 dyne/cm^2, or approximately 1 standard atmosphere (1 atm).

baralyme /ber'əlīm/ [Gk, *barys,* heavy; AS, *lim,* lime], a mixture of calcium and barium compounds used to absorb exhaled carbon dioxide in an anesthesia rebreathing system.

barbiturate /bärbichŏŏrāt, -ərit/ [Saint Barbara, drug discovered on day of the saint, 1864], a derivative of barbituric acid that acts as a sedative or hypnotic. These derivatives act by depressing the respiratory rate, blood pressure, temperature, and central nervous system.

barbiturate coma [Ger, Saint Barbara's Day, Gk, *koma,* deep sleep], an effect of barbituric acid or its derivatives, which may be rapid-acting sedatives, hypnotics, and respiratory depressants. Death may result from intentional or accidental overdosage.

barbiturism /bärbich'əriz'əm/, **1.** acute or chronic poisoning by any of the derivatives of barbituric acid. **2.** addiction to a barbiturate.

bar clasp arm, (in prosthetic dentistry) a clasp arm that originates from the denture base and serves as an extracoronal retainer.

Bard-Pic's syndrome /bärd'pik'/ [Louis Bard, French anatomist, 1857–1930; Adrian Pic, French physician, b. 1863], a condition characterized by progressive jaundice, enlarged gallbladder, and cachexia, associated with advanced pancreatic cancer.

Bard's sign [Louis Bard], the increased oscillations of the eyeball in organic nystagmus when the patient tries to visually follow a target moved from side to side across the line of sight.

bare lymphocyte syndrome, an immune deficiency condition caused by defective beta-2 microglobulin, one of the major histocompatibility antigens on cell surfaces. It is inherited as an autosomal-recessive trait.

baresthesia /bär'esthē'zhə/, sensitivity to weight or pressure.

bar graph [OF, *barre*], a graph in which frequencies are represented by bars extending from the ordinate or the abscissa, allowing the distribution of the entire sample to be seen at once.

bariatrics /ber′ē·at′riks/ [Gk, *baros,* weight, *iatros,* physician], the field of medicine that focuses on the treatment and control of obesity and diseases associated with obesity.

baritosis /ber′ətō′sis/, a benign form of pneumoconiosis caused by an accumulation of barium dust in the lungs. The condition is most likely to affect persons involved in the mining and processing of barite, a barium product used in the manufacture of paints.

barium (Ba) /ber′ē·əm/ [Gk, *barys,* heavy], a pale yellow, metallic element classified with the alkaline earths. Its atomic number is 56; its atomic weight (mass) is 137.36.

barium enema, a rectal infusion of barium sulfate, a radiopaque contrast medium, which is retained in the lower intestinal tract during roentgenographic studies for diagnosis of obstruction, tumors, or other abnormalities.

barium meal, the ingestion of barium sulfate, a radiopaque contrast medium, for the radiographic examination of the esophagus, stomach, and intestinal tract in the diagnosis of such conditions as dysphagia, peptic ulcer, and fistulas.

barium poisoning, a condition characterized by a severe, rapid decrease in plasma potassium levels and a shift of potassium into cells caused by the ingestion of soluble barium salts. The patient may experience nausea, vomiting, abdominal cramps, bloody diarrhea, dizziness, ringing in the ears, cardiac arrest, and respiratory failure.

barium sulfate, a radiopaque medium used as a diagnostic aid in roentgenology. It is prescribed for x-ray examination of the gastrointestinal tract.

barium swallow [Gk, *barys* heavy; AS, *swelgan,* to swallow], the oral administration of a radiopaque barium sulfate suspension to demonstrate possible defects in the esophagus and abnormal borders of the posterior aspects of the heart radiographically.

Barlow's syndrome [John B. Barlow, South African cardiologist, b. 1924], an abnormal cardiac condition characterized by an apical systolic murmur, a systolic click, and an electrocardiogram indicating inferior ischemia.

Barnard, Kathryn E., a nursing theorist who developed the Child Health Assessment Interaction Model. Her model and theory were the outcome of the Nursing Child Assessment Project (1976–1979). Bernard believes that the parent-infant system is influenced by individual characteristics of each member. Those character-

istics are modified to meet the needs of the system by adaptive behavior.

barognosis /ber′əgnō′sis/, *pl.* **barognoses** [Gk, *baros,* weight, *gnosis,* knowledge], the ability to perceive and evaluate weight, especially that held in the hand.

barograph /ber′əgraf′/ [Gk, *baros* + *graphein,* to record], an instrument that continually monitors barometric pressure and records pressure changes on paper.

barometer /bərom′ətər/ [Gk, *baros* + *metron,* measure], an instrument for measuring atmospheric pressure, commonly consisting of a slender tube filled with mercury, sealed at one end, and inverted into a reservoir of mercury. At sea level the normal height of mercury in the tube is 760 mm. —**barometric,** *adj.*

baroreceptor /ber′ōrisep′tər/ [Gk, *baros* + L, *recipere,* to receive], one of the pressure-sensitive nerve endings in the walls of the atria of the heart, the aortic arch, and the carotid sinuses. Baroreceptors stimulate central reflex mechanisms that allow physiologic adjustment and adaptation to changes in blood pressure via changes in heart rate, vasodilation, or vasoconstriction.

barotrauma /ber′ōtrô′mə, -trou′mə/ [Gk, *baros* + *trauma,* wound], physical injury sustained as a result of exposure to increased environmental air pressure such as barotitis media or rupture of the lungs or paranasal sinuses, as may occur among deep-sea divers or caisson workers.

barrel chest, a large, rounded thorax, considered normal in some stocky individuals and certain others who live in high-altitude areas and consequently have increased vital capacity. Barrel chest may also be a sign of pulmonary emphysema.

Barré's pyramidal sign /bärāz′/ [Jean A. Barré, French neurologist, 1880–1971], a diagnostic sign of a prefrontal brain lesion observed as a phenomenon in which the lateral or vertical movement of one leg of a recumbent patient is followed by a similar movement of the other leg.

Barrett's syndrome [Norman R. Barrett, English surgeon, 1903–1979], a disorder of the lower esophagus marked by a benign ulcerlike lesion in columnar epithelium, resulting most often from chronic irritation of the esophagus by gastric reflux of acidic digestive juices.

barrier /ber′ē·ər/ [ME, *barrere*], **1.** a wall or other obstacle that can restrain or block the passage of substances. **2.** something nonphysical that obstructs or separates, such as barriers to communication or compliance. **3.** (in radiography) any device that intercepts beams of x-rays.

barrier creams, ointments, lotions, and

similar preparations applied to exposed areas of the skin to protect skin cells from exposure to various allergens, irritants, and carcinogens, including sunlight.

barrier-free design [AS, *freo,* barreres; L, *designare,* to mark out], the design of homes, workplaces, and public buildings that allows physically challenged individuals to make regular use of such structures.

Barsony-Koppenstein method, a procedure for making radiographic images of the cervical intervertebral foramina.

Barthel Index (BI) [D. W. Barthel, twentieth century American psychiatrist], a disability profile scale developed to evaluate a patient's self-care abilities in 10 areas, including bowel and bladder control. The patient is scored from 0 to 15 points in various categories, depending on his or her need for help.

bartholinitis /bär′təlinī′tis/ [Caspar T. Bartholin, Danish anatomist, 1655–1738; Gk, *itis*], an inflammatory condition of one or both Bartholin's glands, caused by bacterial infection. The condition is characterized by swelling of one or both glands, pain, and development of an abscess in the infected gland.

Bartholin's abscess /bär′təlinz/ [Caspar T. Bartholin; L, *abscedere,* to go away], an abscess of the greater vestibular gland of the vagina.

Bartholin's cyst [Caspar T. Bartholin], a cyst that arises from one of the vestibular glands or from its ducts and fills with clear fluid that replaces the suppurative exudate characteristic of chronic inflammation.

Bartholin's duct [Caspar T. Bartholin], the major duct of the sublingual salivary gland.

Bartholin's gland [Caspar T. Bartholin], one of two small mucus-secreting glands located on the posterior and lateral aspect of the vestibule of the vagina.

Bartholin's gland carcinoma /bär′təlin/ [Caspar T. Bartholin], a rare malignancy that occurs deep in the labia majora. The tumor has overlying skin and some normal glandular tissue.

Barton, Clara, (1821–1912), an American philanthropist, humanitarian, and founder of the American National Red Cross. During the U.S. Civil War, she was a volunteer nurse, and at its end she organized a bureau of records to help in the search for missing men. When the Franco-Prussian War erupted, she assisted in the organization of military hospitals in Europe in association with the International Red Cross. This led to her advocacy of establishment of an American Red Cross organization, of which she became the first president.

Bartonella /bär′tənel′ə/ [Alberto Barton, Peruvian bacteriologist, 1871–1950], a genus of small, gram-negative flagellated pleomorphic coccobacilli. Members of the genus are intracellular parasites that infect red blood cells and the epithelial cells of the lymph nodes, liver, and spleen. They are transmitted at night by the bite of a sandfly of the genus *Phlebotomus.*

bartonellosis /bär′tənəlō′sis/, an acute infection caused by *Bartonella bacilliformis,* transmitted by the bite of a sandfly. It is characterized by fever, severe anemia, bone pain, and, several weeks after the first symptoms are observed, multiple nodular or verrucose skin lesions.

Barton's fracture [John R. Barton, American surgeon, 1794–1871], a fracture of the distal articular surface of the radius, which may be accompanied by the dorsal dislocation of the carpus on the radius.

Bartter's syndrome /bär′tərz/ [Frederick C. Bartter, American physiologist, 1914–1983], a rare hereditary disorder, characterized by hyperplasia of the juxtaglomerular area and secondary hyperaldosteronism.

basal /bā′səl/ [Gk, *basis,* foundation], pertaining to the fundamental or basic, as basal anesthesia, which produces the first stage of unconsciousness, and the basal metabolic rate, which indicates the lowest metabolic rate.

basal acid output (BAO), the minimum volume of gastric fluid produced by an individual in a given period. It is used in the diagnosis of various diseases of the stomach and intestines.

basal anesthesia [Gk, *basis,* foundation, *anaisthesia,* lack of feeling], **1.** a state of unconsciousness just short of complete surgical anesthesia in depth, in which the patient does not respond to words but reacts to pinprick or other noxious stimuli. **2.** narcosis produced by injection or infusion of potent sedatives alone, without added narcotics or anesthetic agents. **3.** any form of anesthesia in which the patient is completely unconscious, in contrast to awake anesthesia.

basal body temperature, the temperature of the body taken in the morning, orally or rectally, after at least 8 hours of sleep and before the patient does anything else, including getting out of bed, smoking a cigarette, moving around, talking, eating, or drinking.

basal body temperature method of family planning, a natural method of family planning that relies on identification of the fertile period of the menstrual cycle by noting the rise in basal body temperature that occurs with ovulation. The progesterone-mediated rise is 0.5° to 1° F; rate and pattern vary greatly from woman to woman and to some extent from cycle to cycle in any one woman. The fertile period is considered to continue until the temperature is above the baseline for 5 days; the rise occurs slowly during all 5 days or increases rapidly, reaching a plateau at which it remains for 3 or 4 days. The days after that period are considered "safe" infertile days.

basal bone, 1. (in prosthodontics) the osseous tissue of the mandible and the maxillae, except for the rami and the processes, which provides support for artificial dentures. **2.** (in orthodontics) the fixed osseous structure that limits the movement of teeth in the creation of a stable occlusion.

basal cell, any one of the cells in the deepest layer of stratified epithelium.

basal cell carcinoma [Gk, *basis* + L, *cella,* storeroom; Gk, *karkinos,* crab, *oma,* tumor], a malignant epithelial cell tumor that begins as a papule and enlarges peripherally, developing a central crater that erodes, crusts, and bleeds. The primary known cause of the cancer is excessive exposure to the sun or to radiation.

basal ganglia [Gk, *basis* + *ganglion,* knot], the islands of gray matter, largely composed of cell bodies, within each cerebral hemisphere. The most important are the caudate nucleus, the putamen, and the pallidum.

basal lamina [Gk, *basis* + L, *lamina,* plate], a thin, noncellular layer of ground substance lying just under epithelial surfaces.

basal membrane, a sheet of tissue that forms the outer layer of the choroid and lies just under the pigmented layer of the retina.

basal metabolic rate (BMR), the amount of energy used in a unit of time by a fasting, resting subject to maintain vital functions. The rate, determined by the amount of oxygen used, is expressed in calories consumed per hour per square meter of body surface area or per kilogram of body weight.

basal metabolism [Gk, *basis* + *metabole,* change], the amount of energy needed to maintain essential body functions, such as respiration, circulation, temperature, peristalsis, and muscle tone. Basal metabolism is measured when the subject is awake and at complete rest, has not eaten for 14 to 18 hours, and is in a comfortable, warm environment.

basal narcosis [Gk, *basis,* foundation, *nar-*

kosis, a benumbing], a narcosis induced with sedatives in a surgical patient before general anesthetic is administered. It is less profound than that of general anesthesia. The patient is unresponsive to verbal stimuli but may respond to noxious stimuli.

basaloid carcinoma /bā′sǝloid/ [Gk, *basis* + *eidos,* form, *karkinos* crab, *oma* tumor], a rare malignant neoplasm of the anal canal containing areas that resemble basal cell carcinoma of the skin.

basal seat, (in dentistry) the oral tissues and structures that support a denture.

basal seat area, the part of the oral structures that is available to support a denture.

basal seat outline, (in dentistry) a profile on the mucous membrane or on a cast of the entire oral area to be covered by a denture.

basal temperature chart [Gk, *basis,* foundation; L, *temperatura* + *charta,* paper], a daily temperature chart, usually including the temperature on awakening. A basal temperature chart is sometimes used by women to establish a date of ovulation, when the temperature may show a sudden increase.

basal tidal volume, the amount of air inhaled and exhaled by a healthy person at complete rest, with all bodily functions at a minimal level of activity, adjusted for age, weight, and sex.

base [Gk, *basis,* foundation], **1.** a chemical compound that increases the concentration of hydroxide ions in aqueous solution. **2.** a molecule or radical that takes up or accepts hydrogen ions. **3.** an electron pair donor. **4.** the major ingredient of a compounded material, particularly one that is used as a medication. **5.** (in radiology) the rigid but flexible foundation of a sheet of x-ray film.

base analog [Gk, *basis* + *analogos,* proportionate], a chemical analog of one of the purine or pyrimidine bases normally found in ribonucleic acid or deoxyribonucleic acid.

Basedow's goiter /bä′sǝdōz/ [Karl A. von Basedow, German physician, 1799–1854], an enlargement of the thyroid gland, characterized by the hypersecretion of thyroid hormone after iodine therapy.

base excess, a measure of metabolic alkalosis or metabolic acidosis (negative value of base excess).

base-forming food, a food that increases the pH of the urine. Base-forming foods mainly are fruits, vegetables, and dairy products, which are sources of sodium and potassium.

baseline /bās′līn/ [Gk, *basis* + L, *linea*], **1.** a known value or quantity with which an unknown is compared when measured or assessed. **2.** (in radiology) any of several basic anatomic planes or locations used for positioning purposes.

baseline behavior, a specified frequency and form of a particular behavior during preexperimental or pretherapeutic conditions.

baseline condition, an environmental condition during which a particular behavior reflects a stable rate of response before the introduction of experimental or therapeutic conditions.

baseline fetal heart rate, the fetal heart rate pattern between uterine contractions.

basement membrane [Fr, *soubassement,* under base], the fragile noncellular layer that secures the overlying epithelium to the underlying tissue.

base of the heart, the part of the heart opposite the apex. It forms the upper border of the heart, lies just below the second rib, and primarily involves the left atrium, part of the right atrium, and the proximal parts of the great vessels.

base of the skull, the floor of the skull, containing the anterior, middle, and posterior cranial fossae and numerous foramina, such as the optic foramen, foramen ovale, foramen lacerum, and foramen magnum.

base pair, a pair of nucleotides in deoxyribonucleic acid but not in ribonucleic acid. One of the pair must be a purine, the other a pyrimidine.

base pairing, (in molecular genetics) the association in nucleic acids of the purine bases adenine and guanine with the pyrimidine bases cytosine, thymine, and uracil.

baseplate [Gk, *basis* + ME, *plate*], a temporary form that represents the base of a denture, used for making records of maxillomandibular relationships, for arranging artificial teeth, or for ensuring a precise fit of a denture by trial placement in the mouth.

base ratio, the ratio of molar quantities of the bases in ribonucleic and deoxyribonucleic acids.

bas-fond /bäfôN′/ [Fr, bottom], the bottom or fundus of any structure, especially the fundus of the urinary bladder.

basic amino acid, an amino acid that has a positive electric charge in solution at a pH of 7.0. The basic amino acids are arginine, histidine, and lysine.

basic group identity, (in psychiatry) the shared social characteristics such as world view, language, values, and ideologic system that evolve from membership in an ethnic group.

basic health services, the minimum degree of health care considered to be necessary to maintain adequate health and protection from disease.

basic human needs, the elements required for survival and normal mental and physical health, such as food, water, shelter, protection from environmental threats, and love.

basic life support (BLS) [Gk, *basis,* foundation; AS, *lif* + L, *supportare,* to bring up to], the role of cardiopulmonary resuscitation and emergency cardiac care in reinstituting circulatory or respiratory function or both in the emergency treatment of a victim of cardiac or respiratory arrest.

basic salt, a salt that contains an unreplaced hydroxide ion from the base generating it, such as Ca(OH)Cl.

basifacial /bā′sifā′shəl/ [Gk, *basis* + L, *facies,* face], pertaining to the lower part of the face.

basilar /bas′ilər/ [Gk, *basis,* foundation], pertaining to a base or a basal area.

basilar artery, the single posterior arterial trunk formed by the junction of the two vertebral arteries at the base of the skull. It extends from the inferior to the superior border of the pons before dividing into the left and right posterior cerebral arteries.

basilar artery insufficiency syndrome, the composite of clinical indicators associated with insufficient blood flow through the basilar artery, a condition that may be caused by arterial occlusion.

basilar artery occlusion, an obstruction of the basilar artery, resulting in dysfunction involving cranial nerves III through XII, cerebellar dysfunction, hemiplegia or quadriplegia, and loss of proprioception.

basilar membrane, the cellular structure that forms the floor of the cochlear duct and is supported by bony and fibrous projections from the cochlear wall.

basilar plexus [Gk, *basis* + L, braided], the venous network interlaced between the layers of the dura mater over the basilar part of the occipital bone.

basilar sulcus [Gk, *basis* + L, furrow], the sulcus that cradles the basilar artery in the midline of the pons.

basilar vertebra, the lowest or last of the lumbar vertebrae.

basilic vein /bəsil′ik/, one of the four superficial veins of the arm, beginning in the ulnar part of the dorsal venous network and running proximally on the posterior surface of the ulnar side of the forearm.

basiloma terebrans /ter′əbrənz/ [Gk, *basis* + *oma* + L, *terebare,* to bore], an invasive basal cell epithelioma.

basin, 1. a receptacle for collecting or

B

holding fluids. A kidney-shaped basin is commonly used as an emesis receptacle. **2.** term used to describe the shape of the pelvis.

basioccipital /bā′si·oksip′ətəl/ [Gk, *basis* + L, *occiput*, back of the head], pertaining to the basilar process of the occipital bone.

basion /bā′sē·on/ [Gk, *basis,* foundation], the midpoint on the anterior margin of the foramen magnum of the occipital bone, opposite the opisthion in the middle of the posterior margin.

basis, the lower part, designating the base of an organ or other structure, such as the base of the cerebrum.

basket cell [L, *bascauda,* dishpan], a cerebral cortex cell with a horizontal axon that sends out branches. Each branch breaks up into a basketlike mesh that surrounds a Purkinje cell.

Basle Nomina Anatomica (BNA), an international system of anatomic terminology adopted at Basel, Switzerland.

basophil /bā′səfil/ [Gk, *basis* + *philein,* to love], a granulocytic white blood cell characterized by cytoplasmic granules that stain blue when exposed to a basic dye. Basophils represent 1% or less of the total white blood cell count.

basophilic adenoma [Gk, *basis* + *philein,* to love, *aden,* gland, *oma*], a tumor of the pituitary gland composed of cells that can be stained with basic dyes.

basophilic leukemia [Gk, *basis* + *philein,* to love, *leukos,* white, *haima,* blood], an acute or chronic malignant neoplasm of blood-forming tissues, characterized by large numbers of immature basophilic granulocytes in peripheral circulation and in tissues.

basophilic stippling [Gk, *basis* + *philein,* to love; D, *stippen,* to prick], the presence of punctate blue nucleic acid remnants in red blood cells, observed under the microscope on a Wright-Giemsa-Gram–stained blood smear. Stippling is characteristic of lead poisoning.

basosquamous cell carcinoma /bā′soskwā′məs/ [Gk, *basis* + L, *squamosus,* scaly], a malignant epidermal tumor composed of basal and squamous cells.

bath [AS, *baeth*], (in the hospital) a cleansing procedure performed daily by or for patients to help prevent infection, preserve the unbroken condition of the skin, stimulate circulation, promote oxygen intake, maintain muscle tone and joint mobility, and provide comfort.

bath blanket, a thin, lightweight cloth used to cover a patient during a bath.

bathesthesia [Gk, *bathys,* deep, *aisthesia,* feeling], sensitivity to deep pressure.

Bathing, a Nursing Interventions Classification defined as cleaning of the body for the purposes of relaxation, cleanliness, and healing.

bathyanesthesia /bath′ēan′esthēzhə/ [Gk, *bathys,* deep, *anaisthesia,* loss of feeling], a loss of deep feeling, such as that associated with organs or structures beneath the body surface or with muscles and joints; a loss of sensitivity to deep structures in the body.

bathycardia /bath′ēkär′dē·ə/ [Gk, *bathys,* deep, *kardia,* heart], a condition in which the heart is located at an abnormally low site in the thorax.

Batten disease [Frederick E. Batten, English neurologist, 1865–1918], a progressive childhood encephalopathy characterized by disturbed metabolism of polyunsaturated fatty acids.

battered woman syndrome (BWS), repeated episodes of physical assault on a woman by the man with whom she lives, often resulting in serious physical and psychologic damage to the woman.

battery [Fr, *batterie*], **1.** a complex of two or more electrolytic cells connected to form a single source providing direct current or voltage. **2.** a series or a combination of tests to determine the cause of a particular illness or the degree of proficiency in a particular skill or discipline. **3.** the unlawful use of force on a person.

Battey bacillus /bat′ē/ [Battey Hospital, in Rome, Georgia, where bacteria strain first isolated], any of a group of atypical mycobacteria, including *Mycobacterium avium* and *M. intracellulare,* that cause a chronic pulmonary disease resembling tuberculosis.

battledore placenta /bat′əldôr′/ [ME, *batyldoure,* a beating instrument; L, *placenta,* flat cake], a condition in which the umbilical cord is attached at the margin of the placenta.

Battle's sign [William H. Battle, English surgeon, 1855–1936], a small hemorrhagic spot behind the ear. It may indicate a fracture of a bone of the lower skull.

Baudelocque's method /bō′dəlok′s/ [Jean I. Baudelocque, French obstetrician, 1746–1810], (in obstetrics) a maneuver used to convert a face presentation to a vertex presentation. The operator flexes the fetal head vaginally and applies counterpressure to the back of the head abdominally while an assistant rotates the fetus in the direction of flexion until the vertex is fixed in the pelvis.

bay, an anatomic depression or recess, usually containing fluid, as the lacrimal bay of the eye.

Bayes' theorem /bāz′/ [Thomas Bayes,

British mathematician, 1702–1761], a mathematic statement of the relationships of test sensitivity, specificity, and the predictive value of a positive test result. The predictive value of the test is the number that is useful to the clinician. A positive result demonstrates the conditional probability of the presence of a disease.

Bayley Scales of Infant Development, [Nancy Bayley, twentieth century American psychologist], a three-part scale for assessing the development of children between the ages of 2 months and 2½ years. Infants are tested for perception, memory, and vocalization on the mental scale; sitting, stair climbing, and manual manipulation on the motor scale; and attention span, social behavior, and persistence on the behavioral scale.

bayonet angle former /bā′ənit/ [Fr, *baionette,* a steel blade], a hoe-shaped, paired cutting instrument for accenting angles in a class 3 tooth cavity.

bayonet condenser [Fr, *baionette*], (in dentistry) an instrument for compacting restorative material.

BBB, 1. abbreviation for **bundle branch block. 2.** abbreviation for **blood-brain barrier.**

B cell, a type of lymphocyte that originates in the bone marrow. A precursor of the plasma cell, it is one of the two lymphocytes that play a major role in the body's immune response.

B cell growth/differentiation factors, substances such as interleukins IL-4, IL-5, and IL-6, derived from T cell cultures, that are necessary for the differentiation of plasma cells and B memory cells and their growth and maturation.

B cell–mediated immunity, the ability to produce an immune response induced by B lymphocytes. Contact with a foreign antigen stimulates B cells to differentiate into plasma cells that release antibodies. Plasma cells also generate memory cells that provide a rapid response if the same antigen is encountered again.

BCG, abbreviation for **bacille Calmette-Guèrin.**

BCG vaccine, an active immunizing agent prepared from bacille Calmette-Guèrin. It is prescribed most commonly for immunization against tuberculosis.

B complex vitamins, a large group of water-soluble nutrients that includes thiamin (vitamin B_1), cyanocobalamin (vitamin B_{12}), niacin (vitamin B_3), pyridoxine (vitamin B_6), riboflavin (vitamin B_2), biotin, folic acid, and pantothenic acid. The B complex vitamins are essential for conversion of simple carbohydrates like glucose into energy; metabolism of fats and proteins; normal functioning of the nervous system; maintenance of muscle tone in the gastrointestinal tract; and the health of skin, hair, eyes, mouth, and liver.

B-DNA, a long, thin form of deoxyribonucleic acid in which the helix is right-handed.

Be, symbol for the element **beryllium.**

BEE, abbreviation for *basal energy expenditure.*

beaded /bē′did/ [ME, *bede*], **1.** having a resemblance to a row of beads. **2.** pertaining to bacterial colonies that develop along the inoculation line in various stab cultures. **3.** pertaining to stained bacteria that develop more deeply stained beadlike granules.

beak, 1. any pointed anatomic structure, as the beak of the sphenoid bone. **2.** a pair of dental pincers used in shaping prostheses. **3.** a radiographic image of a bony protuberance adjacent to a degenerative intervertebral disk.

beak sign, the appearance of abnormal structures on radiographic images of the gastrointestinal tract: a distal esophagus in achalasia and a proximal pyloric canal in pyloric stenosis.

beam [ME, *beem,* tree], **1.** a bedframe fitting for pulleys and weights used in the treatment of patients requiring weight traction. **2.** (in radiology) the primary beam of radiation emitted from the x-ray tube.

BEAM /bēm, bē′ē′ā′em′/, abbreviation for **brain electrical activity map.**

beam alignment, the process of positioning the radiographic tube head so it is aligned properly with the x-ray film.

beam collimation, the restriction of x-radiation to the area being examined or treated by confining the beam with collimators or metal diaphragms or shutters with high radiation absorption power.

beam hardening, the process of increasing the energy level of the x-ray beam spectrum by filtering out the low-energy photons.

BE amputation, an amputation of the arm below the elbow.

beam quality, (in radiology) the energy of the x-ray beam.

beam restrictors, devices that reduce scatter radiation from x-ray equipment.

beam-splitting mirror, a device that allows a radiologist to view a fluoroscopic examination of a patient while the same view is being recorded on film.

bean [ME, *bene*], the pod-enclosed flattened seed of numerous leguminous plants. Beans used in pharmacologic preparations are alphabetized by specific name.

bearing down /ber′ing/ [OE, *beran,* to bear, *adune,* down], a voluntary effort by a woman in the second stage of labor to aid in the expulsion of a fetus. By applying the Valsalva maneuver, the mother increases intraabdominal pressure.

bearing down pains [OE, *beran,* to bear, *adune,* down; L, *poena,* penalty], the pains experienced by a woman during the second stage of labor while performing the Valsalva maneuver to help expel the fetus.

beat, the mechanical contraction or electrical stimulation of the heart muscle, which may be detected and recorded as the pulse.

Beau's lines /bōz′/ [Joseph H.S. Beau, French physician, 1806–1865], transverse depressions that appear as white lines across the fingernails as a sign of an acute severe illness such as malnutrition, a systemic disease, trauma, or coronary occlusion.

Becker's muscular dystrophy, [Peter E. Becker, German geneticist, b. 1908], a chronic degenerative disease of the muscles, characterized by progressive weakness. It occurs in childhood between 8 and 20 years of age. It occurs less frequently, progresses more slowly, and has a better prognosis than the more common pseudohypertrophic form of muscular dystrophy. The pathophysiologic characteristics of the disease are not understood; it is transmitted genetically as an autosomal-recessive trait. Also called benign pseudohypertrophic muscular dystrophy. Compare **Duchenne's muscular dystrophy.**

Beck's Diagnostic Inventory (BDI), [Aaron T. Beck, American psychiatrist, b. 1921], a system of classifying a total of 18 criteria of depressive illness. It was developed by A. T. Beck in the 1970s as a diagnostic and therapeutic tool for the treatment of childhood affective disorders. The BDI is similar to the 21-criteria DSM-IV diagnostic system of the 1980s.

Beck's triad, a combination of three symptoms that characterize cardiac tamponade: high central venous pressure, low arterial pressure, and a small, quiet heart.

Beckwith's syndrome [John B. Beckwith, American pathologist, b. 1933], a hereditary disorder of unknown cause associated with neonatal hypoglycemia and hyperinsulinism. Clinical manifestations include gigantism, macroglossia, omphalocele or umbilical hernia, visceromegaly, and other abnormalities.

beclomethasone dipropionate, a glucocorticoid prescribed in an inhaler in the treatment of bronchial asthma.

becquerel (Bq) /bekrel′, bek′ərel′/ [Antoine H. Becquerel, French physicist, 1852–1908], the SI unit of radioactivity, equal to one radioactive decay per second.

bed [AS, *bedd*], (in anatomy) a supporting matrix of tissue, such as the nail beds of modified epidermis over which the fingernails and the toenails move as they grow.

bed board, a board that is placed under a mattress to give added support to a patient with back problems.

bedbug [AS, *bedd* + ME, *bugge,* hobgoblin], a blood-sucking arthropod of the species *Cimex lectularius* or the species *C. hemipterus* that feeds on humans and other animals. The bite causes itching, pain, and redness.

bed cradle, a frame placed over a bed to prevent sheets or blankets from touching the patient.

Bedford finger stall, a removable finger splint that holds the injured and adjacent finger in a brace or cast.

Bednar's aphthae /bed′närz/ [Alois Bednar, Austrian pediatrician, 1816–1888], the small, yellowish, slightly elevated ulcerated patches that occur on the posterior part of the hard palate of infants who place infected objects in their mouths.

bed pan, a vessel made of metal or plastic that is used to collect feces and urine of bedridden patients.

bed rest, the restriction of a patient to bed for therapeutic reasons for a prescribed period.

Bed Rest Care, a Nursing Interventions Classification defined as promotion of comfort and safety and prevention of complications for a patient unable to get out of bed.

bedridden, describing a person who is confined to bed because of illness or injury.

Bedside Laboratory Testing, a Nursing Interventions Classification defined as performance of laboratory tests at the bedside or point of care.

bedside manner, the behavior of a nurse or doctor as perceived by a patient or peers.

beef tapeworm infection [OF, *buef,* cow; AS, *taeppe, wyrm*], an infection caused by the tapeworm *Taenia saginata,* transmitted to humans when they eat contaminated beef. The infection is rarely found when beef is carefully inspected and thoroughly cooked before eating.

bee sting [AS, *beo* + *stingan*], an injury caused by the venom of bees, usually accompanied by pain and swelling. The stinger of the honeybee usually remains implanted and should be removed. Pain may be alleviated by application of an ice pack or a paste of sodium bicarbonate and water.

behavior /bihā'vyər/ [ME, *behaven*], **1.** the manner in which a person acts or performs. **2.** any or all of the activities of a person, including physical actions, that are observed directly, and mental activity, which is inferred and interpreted.

behavioral isolation /behā'vyərəl/, social isolation that results from a person's socially unacceptable behavior.

behavioral objective, a goal in therapy or research that concerns an act or a specific behavior or pattern of behaviors.

behavioral science, any of the various interrelated disciplines such as psychiatry, psychology, sociology, and anthropology that observe and study human activity, including psychologic and emotional development, interpersonal relationships, values, and mores.

behavior disorder, any of a group of antisocial behavior patterns occurring primarily in children and adolescents, such as overaggressiveness, overactivity, destructiveness, cruelty, truancy, lying, disobedience, perverse sexual activity, criminality, alcoholism, and drug addiction.

behaviorism, a school of psychology founded by John B. Watson that studies and interprets behavior by observing measurable responses to stimuli without reference to consciousness, mental states, or subjective phenomena, such as ideas and emotions.

behaviorist, an advocate of the school of behaviorism.

Behavior Management, a Nursing Interventions Classification defined as helping a patient to manage negative behavior.

Behavior Management: Overactivity/Inattention, a Nursing Interventions Classification defined as provision of a therapeutic milieu that safely accommodates the patient's attention deficit and/or overactivity while promoting optimal function.

Behavior Management: Self-Harm, a Nursing Interventions Classification defined as assisting the patient to decrease or eliminate self-mutilating or self-abusive behaviors.

Behavior Management: Sexual, a Nursing Interventions Classification defined as delineation and prevention of socially unacceptable sexual behaviors.

Behavior Modification, a Nursing Interventions Classification defined as promotion of a behavior change.

Behavior Modification: Social Skills, a Nursing Interventions Classification defined as assisting the patient to develop or improve interpersonal social skills.

behavior systems model, a conceptual framework describing factors that may affect the stability of a person's behavior. The model examines systems of behavior, not the behavior of an individual at any particular time.

behavior therapy, a kind of psychotherapy that attempts to modify observable maladjusted patterns of behavior by substituting a new response or set of responses to a given stimulus.

Behçet's disease /bā'sets/ [Hulusi Behçet, Turkish dermatologist, 1889–1948], a rare and severe illness of unknown cause, mostly affecting young males and characterized by severe uveitis and retinal vasculitis.

BEI, abbreviation for **butanol-extractable iodine.**

bejel /bej'əl/ [Ar, *bajal*], a nonvenereal form of syphilis prevalent among children in the Middle East and North Africa, caused by the spirochete *Treponema pallidum* II. The primary lesion is usually on or near the mouth, appearing as a mucous patch, followed by the development of pimplelike sores on the trunk, arms, and legs.

Békésy audiometry /bek'əsē/ [George von Békésy, Hungarian-American physicist and Nobel laureate, 1899–1972], a type of hearing test in which the subject controls the intensity of the stimulus by pressing a button while listening to a pure tone whose frequency slowly moves through the entire audible range.

bel [Alexander G. Bell, Canadian inventor, 1847–1922], a unit that expresses intensity of sound. It is the logarithm (to the base 10) of the ratio of the power of any specific sound to the power of a reference sound. The most common reference sound has a power of 10^{-16} watts per square centimeter, or the approximate minimum intensity of sound at 1000 cycles per second that is perceptible to the human ear.

belladonna /bel'ədon'ə, belädôn'ä/ [It, fair lady], the dried leaves, roots, and flowering or fruiting tops of *Atropa belladonna*, a common perennial called deadly nightshade, containing the alkaloids hyoscine and hyoscyamine. Hyoscyamine is a source of atropine.

belladonna and atropine poisons [It, *belladonna*, fair lady; Gk, *Atropos*, one of three Fates; L, *potio*, drink], two powerful poisons obtained from solanaceous plants. Atropine, derived from *Atropa belladonna*, blocks the effects of acetylcholine in effector organs supplied by postganglionic cholinergic nerves. Belladonna is obtained from the dried leaves of *Atropa belladonna*, also known as deadly nightshade, or of *Atropa acuminata*, a source of alkaloids that are converted to atropine. Atropine sulfate is commonly used in ophthalmologic applications and as an antispasmodic.

bellows murmur /bel′ōoz/ [AS, *belg,* bag; L, *humming*], a blowing sound, such as that of air moving in and out of a bellows.

bellows ventilator, a respiratory care device in which oxygen and other gases are mixed in a mechanism that contracts and expands. The system pressure is increased or decreased in the chamber surrounding the bellows.

Bell's law [Charles Bell, Scottish surgeon, 1774–1842], an axiom stating that the ventral spinal roots are motor and the dorsal spinal roots are sensory.

Bell's palsy [Charles Bell], a paralysis of the facial nerve. It results from trauma to the nerve, compression of the nerve by a tumor, or, possibly, an unknown infection. The person may not be able to close an eye or control salivation on the affected side. The condition is usually unilateral and can be transient or permanent.

Bell's phenomenon [Charles Bell], a sign of peripheral facial paralysis, manifested by the upward and outward rolling of the eyeball when the affected individual tries to close the eyelid.

Bell's spasm [Charles Bell] a convulsive facial tic.

belly [AS, *beig,* bag], **1.** the central bulging part of a muscle. **2.** See **abdomen.**

belonephobia /bel′ənəfō′bē·ə/, [Gk, *belone,* needle, *phobos,* fear], a morbid fear of objects with sharp points, especially needles and pins.

belt restraint, a device used to secure a patient on a stretcher or in a chair.

Renassi method /bənas′ē/, a positioning procedure for producing x-ray images of the liver.

Bence Jones protein /bens/ [Henry Bence Jones, English physician, 1814–1873], a protein found almost exclusively in the urine of patients with multiple myeloma.

bench research, *informal.* (in medicine) any research done in a controlled laboratory setting using nonhuman subjects.

Bender's Visual Motor Gestalt test [Lauretta Bender, American psychiatrist, 1897–1987; L, *visus,* vision, *movere,* to move; Ger, *Gestalt,* form; L, *testum,* crucible], a standard psychologic test in which the subject copies a series of patterns.

bending fracture, a fracture indirectly caused by the bending of an extremity, such as the foot or the big toe.

bendroflumethiazide /ben′drōfl ōo′məthī′-əzīd/, a diuretic and antihypertensive

prescribed in the treatment of hypertension and edema.

Benedict's qualitative test [Stanley R. Benedict, American biochemist, 1884–1936], a test for sugar in the urine based on the reduction by glucose of cupric ions. Formation of an orange or red precipitate indicates more than 2% sugar (called 4+), yellow indicates 1% to 2% sugar (called 3+), olive green indicates 0.5% to 1% sugar (called 2+), and green indicates less than 0.5% sugar (called 1+).

Benedict's solution [Stanley R. Benedict], a term referring to two reagents (a qualitative and a quantitative) used in the examination of urine specimens. When the solution is heated, the color of the resulting mixture depends on the concentration of glucose in the urine.

beneficiary /ben′əfish′ərē/, a person or group designated to receive certain profits, benefits, or advantages, as the recipient of a will or insurance policy.

benign /binīn′/ [L, *benignus,* kind], (of a tumor) noncancerous and therefore not an immediate threat, even though treatment eventually may be required for health or cosmetic reasons.

benign familial chronic pemphigus [L, *benedicere,* to bless, *familia,* household; Gk, *pemphix,* bubble], a hereditary condition of the skin characterized in the early stages by blisters that break, leaving red, eroded areas followed by crusts.

benign forgetfulness, a temporary memory block in which some fact from the recent or remote past is forgotten but later recalled.

benign hypertension, a misnomer implying an innocent elevation of blood pressure. Because any sustained elevation of blood pressure may adversely affect health, it is incorrect to refer to the condition as "benign."

benign juvenile melanoma, a noncancerous pink or fuchsia raised papule with a scaly surface, usually on a cheek. Occurring most commonly in children between 9 and 13 years of age, it may be mistaken for a malignant melanoma.

benign mesenchymoma [L, *benignare* + Gk, *meso,* middle, *egchyma,* infusion, *oma,* tumor], a benign neoplasm that has two or more definitely recognizable mesenchymal elements in addition to fibrous tissue.

benign neoplasm [L, *benignare* + Gk, *neos,* new, *plasma,* formation], a localized tumor that has a fibrous capsule, limited potential for growth, a regular shape, and cells that are well differentiated. A benign neoplasm does not invade surrounding tissue or metastasize to distant sites.

Some kinds of benign neoplasms are **adenoma, fibroma, hemangioma,** and **lipoma.**

benign nephrosclerosis, a renal disorder marked by arteriolosclerotic (arteriosclerosis affecting mainly the arterioles) lesions in the kidney. It is associated with hypertension.

benign prostatic hypertrophy (BPH), enlargement of the prostate, most common among men over 50 years of age. The condition is not malignant or inflammatory; however, it is usually progressive and may lead to obstruction of the urethra and interference with the flow of urine, possibly causing frequency of urination, need to urinate during the night, pain, and urinary tract infections.

benign stupor, a state of apathy or lethargy, such as occurs in severe depression.

Benner, Patricia, a nursing theorist who confirmed the levels of skill acquisition in nursing practice in *From novice to expert: excellence and power in clinical nursing practice* (1984). Benner used systematic descriptions of five stages: novice, advanced beginner, competent, proficient, and expert. Benner's work describes nursing practice in the context of what nursing actually is and does rather than from context-free theoretic descriptions.

Bennett angle [Norman G. Bennett, English dentist, 1870–1947], (in dentistry) the angle formed by the sagittal plane and the path of the advancing condyle during lateral mandibular movement.

Bennett hand tool test, a test used in occupational therapy and prevocational testing to measure hand function and coordination and speed in performance.

Bennett's fracture [Edward H. Bennett, Irish surgeon, 1837–1907], a fracture that runs obliquely through the base of the first metacarpal bone and into the carpometacarpal joint, detaching the greater part of the articular facet.

bent fracture [ME, *benden*], an incomplete greenstick fracture.

bentonite [Fort Benton, Montana], colloidal, hydrated aluminum silicate used as a bulk laxative and as a base for skin care preparations.

bentonite test, a flocculation test for the presence of rheumatoid factor in patient blood samples. After sensitized bentonite particles are added to the serum, the test result is considered positive for rheumatoid arthritis if adsorption has occurred with 50% of the particles.

benz, abbreviation for a *benzoate carboxylate anion.*

benzalkonium chloride, a disinfectant and fungicide prepared in an aqueous solution in various strengths.

benzene, a colorless, highly flammable liquid hydrocarbon (C_6H_6) derived by fractional distillation of coal tar. The prototypical aromatic compound, it is used in the production of various organic compounds, including pharmaceuticals.

benzene poisoning /ben'zēn/, a toxic condition caused by ingestion of benzene, inhalation of benzene fumes, or exposure to benzene-related products such as toluene or xylene, characterized by nausea, headache, dizziness, and incoordination. In acute cases respiratory failure or ventricular fibrillation may cause death.

benzethonium chloride /ben'zəthō'nē·əm/, a topical antiinfective used for disinfecting the skin and for treating some infections of the eye, nose, and throat. It is also used as a preservative in some pharmaceutical preparations.

benzo(a)pyrene dihydrodiol epoxide (BPDE-I), a carcinogenic derivative of benzo(a)pyrene associated with tobacco smoke.

benzocaine /ben'zəkān/, an ester-type, local anesthetic agent derived from aminobenzoic acid that is most useful when applied topically. It is used in many over-the-counter compounds for pruritus and pain.

benzodiazepine derivative /ben'zōdī·az'-əpin/, one of a group of psychotropic agents, including the tranquilizers chlordiazepoxide, diazepam, oxazepam, lorazepam, and clorazepate, prescribed to alleviate anxiety, and the hypnotics flurazepam and nitrazepam, prescribed in the treatment of insomnia.

benzoic acid /benzō'ik/, a keratolytic agent, usually used with salicylic acid as an ointment in the treatment of athlete's foot and ringworm of the scalp.

benzonatate /benzō'nətāt/, a nonopiate antitussive prescribed to suppress the cough reflex.

benzoyl peroxide /benzō'il/, an antibacterial, keratolytic drying agent prescribed in the treatment of acne.

benzquinamide /benzkwin'əmīd/, an antiemetic prescribed in the treatment of postoperative nausea and vomiting.

benzthiazide /benzthī'əzid/, a diuretic and antihypertensive prescribed in the treatment of hypertension and edema.

benztropine mesylate /benztrō'pēn/, an anticholinergic and antihistaminic agent prescribed as adjunctive therapy in the treatment of all forms of parkinsonism.

benzyl alcohol /ben'zil/, a clear, colorless, oily liquid, derived from certain balsams, used as a topical anesthetic and as a

bacteriostatic agent in solutions for injection.

benzyl benzoate /benzō′āt/, a clear, oily liquid with a pleasant, pervasive aroma. It is used as an agent to destroy lice and scabies, as a solvent, and as a flavor for gum.

bereavement /bərēv′mənt/ [ME, bereven, to rob], a form of depression with anxiety symptoms that is a common reaction to the loss of a loved one. It may be accompanied by insomnia, hyperactivity, and other effects.

Berger's disease [Jean Berger, twentieth-century French nephrologist], a kidney disorder characterized by recurrent episodes of macroscopic hematuria, proteinuria, and a granular deposition of immunoglobulin (IgA) from the glomerular mesangium. The onset of disease is usually in childhood or early adulthood, and males are affected twice as often as females.

Berger's paresthesia [Oskar Berger, nineteenth-century German neurologist; Gk, para, near, aisthesia, sensation], a condition of tingling, prickliness, or weakness and a loss of feeling in the legs without evidence of organic disease. The condition affects young people.

Bergonié-Tribondeau law /ber′gônē′ trā′bônō′/ [Jean A. Bergonié, French radiologist, 1857–1925; Louis F.A. Tribondeau, French physician, 1872–1918], (in radiotherapy) a rule stating that the radiosensitivity of tissue depends on the number of undifferentiated cells, their mitotic activity, and the length of time they are actively proliferating.

beriberi /ber′ēber′ē/ [Sinhalese, beri, weakness], a disease of the peripheral nerves caused by a deficiency of or an inability to assimilate thiamine. It frequently results from a diet limited to polished white rice. Symptoms are fatigue, diarrhea, appetite and weight loss, disturbed nerve function causing paralysis and wasting of limbs, edema, and heart failure.

berkelium (Bk) /burk′lē-əm/ [Berkeley, California], an artificial radioactive transuranic element. Its atomic number is 97; its atomic weight (mass) is 247.

berlock dermatitis [Fr, breloque, bracelet charm], a temporary skin condition, characterized by hyperpigmentation and skin lesions. It is caused by a unique reaction to psoralen-type photosynthesizers commonly used in perfumes, colognes, and pomades, such as oil of bergamot.

Bernard-Soulier syndrome /bernär′ sōōlyā′/, [Jean A. Bernard, French hematologist, b. 1907; Jean-Pierre Soulier, French hematologist, b. 1915], a coagulation disorder characterized by an ab-

sence of or a deficiency in the ability of the platelets to aggregate because of the relative lack of an essential glycoprotein in their membranes.

Bernoulli's principle /bərnōō′lēz/ [Daniel Bernoulli, Swiss scientist, 1700–1782], (in physics) the principle stating that the sum of the velocity and the kinetic energy of a fluid flowing through a tube is constant. The greater the velocity, the less the lateral pressure on the wall of the tube. Thus, if an artery is narrowed by an atherosclerotic plaque, the flow of blood through the constriction increases in velocity and decreases in lateral pressure.

berry aneurysm [ME, berye + Gk, aneurysma, widening], a small, saccular dilation of the wall of a cerebral artery. It occurs most frequently at the junctures of vessels in the circle of Willis.

Bertel method /bur′təl/, a positioning procedure for producing x-ray images of the inferior orbital fissures.

berylliosis /bəril′ē-ō′sis/, poisoning that results from the inhalation of dusts or vapors containing beryllium or beryllium compounds. It is characterized by granulomas throughout the body and by diffuse pulmonary fibrosis, resulting in a dry cough, shortness of breath, and chest pain.

beryllium (Be), a steel-gray, lightweight metallic element. Its atomic number is 4; its atomic weight (mass) is 9.012. Beryllium occurs naturally as beryl and is used in metallic alloys and fluorescent powders.

bestiality /bes′chē-al′itē/, [L, bestia, beast], **1.** a brutal or animal-like character or nature. **2.** conduct or behavior characterized by beastlike appetites or instincts. **3.** sexual relations between a human being and an animal. **4.** sodomy.

beta /bē′tə, bā′tə/, B, β, the second letter of the Greek alphabet, used in scientific notation to denote position of a carbon atom in a molecule, a type of protein configuration, or identification of a type of activity, as beta blocker, beta particle, or beta rhythm. It is used in statistics to define an error in the interpretation of study results.

beta-adrenergic blocking agent. See antiadrenergic.

beta-alaninemia /-al′aninē′mē-ə/, an inherited metabolic disorder marked by a deficiency of an enzyme, beta-alanine-alpha-ketoglutarate aminotransferase. The clinical signs include seizures, drowsiness, and, if uncorrected, death.

beta-blocker, a popular term for beta-adrenergic blocking agent.

beta-carotene [Gk, beta; L, carota, carrot], a vitamin A precursor, ultraviolet screening agent prescribed to ameliorate photosensitivity in patients with erythropoietic protoporphyria.

beta cells, 1. insulin-producing cells situated in the islets of Langerhans. Their insulin-producing function tends to accelerate the movement of glucose, amino acids, and fatty acids out of the blood and into the cellular cytoplasm. 2. the basophilic cells of the anterior lobe of the pituitary gland.

beta decay, a type of radioactivity that results in the emission of beta particles such as electrons or positrons.

beta fetoprotein, a protein found in fetal liver and in some adults with liver disease. It is identical to normal liver ferritin.

beta hemolysis, the development of a clear zone around a bacterial colony growing on blood agar medium, characteristic of certain pathogenic bacteria.

beta-hemolytic streptococci, the pyogenic streptococci of groups A, B, C, E, F, G, H, K, L, M, and O that cause hemolysis of red blood cells in blood agar in the laboratory. These organisms cause most of the acute streptococcal infections seen in humans.

beta-hydroxyisovaleric aciduria, an inherited metabolic disease caused by a deficiency of an enzyme needed to metabolize the amino acid leucine.

beta-lactamase /-lak'tǝmāz/ [*lactam,* a cyclic amide, *ase,* enzyme], an enzyme that catalyzes the hydrolysis of the beta-lactam ring of some penicillins and cephalosporins, producing penicilloic acid and rendering the antibiotic ineffective.

beta-lactamase-resistant antibiotics, antibiotics that are resistant to the enzymatic effects of **beta-lactamase.**

betamethasone, a glucocorticoid prescribed as a topical antiinflammatory agent.

beta-naphthylamine /-nafthil'ǝmēn/, an aromatic amine used in aniline dyes and a cause of bladder cancer in humans.

beta-oxidation, a catabolic process in which fatty acids are used by the body as a source of energy.

beta particle, an electron or positron emitted from the nucleus of an atom during radioactive decay of the atom. Beta particles have a range of 10 m in air and 1 mm in soft tissue.

beta phase, the period immediately following the alpha, or redistribution, phase of drug administration. During the beta phase the blood level of the drug falls more slowly as it is metabolized and excreted from the body.

beta rays, a stream of beta particles, as emitted from atoms of disintegrating radioactive elements. Normally, when the

element is a nuclide with a high ratio of neutrons to protons, the beta particle is an electron; when the nuclide has a higher proportion of protons to neutrons, the beta particle is a positron.

beta receptor, any one of the postulated adrenergic components of receptor tissues that respond to epinephrine and such blocking agents as propranolol. Activation of beta receptors causes various physiologic reactions such as relaxation of the bronchial muscles and an increase in the rate and force of cardiac contraction.

betatron /bā'tǝtron/, a cyclic accelerator that produces high-energy electrons for radiotherapy treatment.

beta wave, one of the four types of brain waves, characterized by relatively low voltage and a frequency of more than 13 Hz. Beta waves are the "busy waves" of the brain, recorded by electroencephalograph from the frontal and the central areas of the cerebrum when the patient is awake and alert with eyes open.

betaxolol hydrochloride /betak'sǝlol/, a topical drug for open-angle glaucoma prescribed for the relief of ocular hypertension and chronic open-angle glaucoma.

bethanechol chloride /bethan'ǝkol/, a cholinergic prescribed in the treatment of fecal and urinary retention and neurogenic atony of the bladder.

Betz cells [Vladimir A. Betz, Russian anatomist, 1834–1894; L, *cella,* storeroom], large pyramidal neurons of the motor cortex with axons that form part of the pyramidal tract associated with voluntary movements.

bevel /bev'ǝl/ [OFr, *baif,* open mouth angle], 1. any angle, other than a right angle, between two planes or surfaces. 2. (in dentistry) any angle other than 90 degrees between a tooth cut and a cavity wall in the preparation of a tooth cavity.

bezoar /bē'zôr/ [Ar, *bazahr,* protection against poison], a hard ball of hair or vegetable fiber that may develop within the stomach of humans. More often it is found in the stomachs of ruminants.

B/F, abbreviation for *black female,* often used in the initial identifying statement in a patient record.

Bh, symbol for the element **Bohrium.**

bhang /bang/ [Hindi, *bag*], an Asian Indian hallucinogenic, composed of dried leaves and the young stems of uncultivated *Cannabis sativa.*

Bi, symbol for the element **bismuth.**

BIA, abbreviation for **bioelectric impedance analysis.**

bias /bī'ǝs/ [MFr, *biais*], 1. an oblique or a diagonal line. 2. a prejudiced or subjective attitude. 3. (in statistics) the distortion of statistical findings. **4.** (in electronics) a voltage applied to an electronic device, such as a vacuum tube or a transistor, to control operating limits.

biased sample /bī'əst/ [OFr, *biais,* slant; L, *exemplum,* sample], (in research), a sample of a group in which all factors or participants are not equally balanced or objectively represented.

biasing /bī'əsing/, a method of treating neuromuscular dysfunction by contracting a muscle against resistance, causing the muscle spindles to readjust to the shorter length.

bibliotherapy, a type of group therapy in which books, poems, and newspaper articles are read in the group to help stimulate thinking about events in the real world and to foster relations among group members.

Bibliotherapy, a Nursing Interventions Classification defined as use of literature to enhance the expression of feelings and the gaining of insight.

bicalutamide, an anticancer chemotherapy agent prescribed in the treatment of prostate cancer. The drug acts by binding to androgen receptors within target cells, preventing androgens from binding to them.

bicameral abscess /bīkam'ərəl/, an abscess with two pockets.

bicarbonate /bīkär'bənāt/ [L, *bis,* twice, *carbo,* coal], an ion of carbonic acid in which only one of the hydrogen atoms has been replaced by a metal or radical, as in sodium bicarbonate ($NaHCO_3$).

bicarbonate precursor, an injection of sodium lactate used in the treatment of metabolic acidosis. It is metabolized in the body to sodium bicarbonate.

bicarbonate therapy, a procedure to increase a patient's stores of bicarbonate when there are signs of severe acidosis.

bicarbonate transport, the route by which most of the carbon dioxide is carried in the bloodstream. Once dissolved in the blood plasma, carbon dioxide combines with water to form carbonic acid, which immediately ionizes into hydrogen and bicarbonate ions.

biceps brachii /bī'seps brā'kē·ī/ [L, *bis,* twice, *caput,* head, *bracchii,* arm], the long fusiform muscle of the upper arm on the anterior surface of the humerus, arising in two heads from the scapula. It flexes the arm and the forearm and supinates the hand.

biceps femoris [L, *bis,* twice, *caput,* head, *femoris,* thigh], one of the posterior femoral muscles. It has two heads at its origin. The biceps femoris flexes the leg and rotates it laterally and extends the

thigh, rotating it laterally. It is one of the **hamstring muscle** group.

biceps reflex, a contraction of a biceps muscle produced when the tendon is tapped with a percussor in testing deep tendon reflexes.

Bichat's membrane /bishäz/ [Marie F.X. Bichat, French anatomist, 1771–1802], an elastic lining beneath the endothelium of an arterial wall.

bicipital groove /bīsip'ətəl/ [L, *bis,* twice, *caput,* head; D, *groeve*], a groove between the greater and lesser tubercles of the humerus for passage of the tendon of the long head of the biceps muscle.

Bickerdyke /bik'ərdīk/, **Mary Ann** (1817–1901), an American nurse who, after taking a short course in homeopathy, cared for the sick and wounded on battlefields during the U.S. Civil War. She insisted on cleanliness, good food, and the best of medical care for her patients.

biclor /bī'klôr/, abbreviation for a *bichloride noncarboxylate anion.*

biconcave /bīkon'kāv/ [L, *bis,* twice, *concavare,* to make hollow], concave on both sides, especially as applied to a lens. —**biconcavity,** *n.*

biconvex /bīkon'veks/ [L, *bis* + *convexus,* vaulted], convex on both sides, especially as applied to a lens. —**biconvexity,** *n.*

bicornate /bīkôr'nāt/ [L, *bis* + *cornu,* horn], having two horns or processes.

bicornate uterus, an abnormal uterus that may be either a single or a double organ with two horns, or branches.

bicuspid /bīkus'pid/ [L, *bis* + *cuspis,* point], **1.** having two cusps or points. **2.** one of the two teeth between the molars and canines of the upper and lower jaws.

bicycle ergometer [L, *bis,* twice; Gk, *kyklos,* circle, *ergon,* work, *metron,* measure], a stationary bicycle dynamometer that measures the strength of an individual's muscle contraction.

b.i.d., (in prescriptions) abbreviation for *bis in die* /dē'ā/, a Latin phrase meaning 'twice a day.'

bidactyly /bīdak'tilē/ [L, *bis* + Gk, *daktylos,* finger], an abnormal condition in which the second, third, and fourth digits on a hand are missing and only the first and fifth are present.—**bidactylous,** *adj.*

bidermoma /bī'dər'mō'mə/ [L, *bis* + Gk, *derma,* skin, *oma,* tumor], a teratoid neoplasm composed of cells and tissues originating in two germ layers.

bidet /bidā'/ [Fr, *pony*], a fixture resembling a toilet bowl, with a rim to sit on and usually equipped with plumbing implements for cleaning the genital and rectal areas of the body.

biduotertian fever /bī′dōō-ətur′shən/ [L, *bis* + *dies,* day, *tertius,* three], a form of malaria characterized by overlapping paroxysms of chills, fever, and other symptoms. It is caused by infection with two strains of *Plasmodium,* each having its own cycle of symptoms, such as in quartan and tertian malaria.

bifid /bī′fid/ [L, *bis* + *findere* to cleave], split into two parts.

bifid tongue [L, *bis* + *findere,* to cleave; AS, *tunge*], a tongue divided by a longitudinal furrow.

bifocal /bīfō′kəl/ [L, *bis* + *focus,* hearth], 1. pertaining to the characteristic of having two foci. 2. (of a lens) having two areas of different focal lengths.

bifocal contact lens, a contact lens that contains corrections for both near and far vision.

bifocal glasses [L, *bis,* twice, *focus,* hearth; AS, *glaes*], eyeglasses in which each lens has two foci to permit both near and far vision.

biforate /bīfôr′āt/ [L, *bis* + *forare,* to pierce twice], having two perforations or foramina.

bifrontal suture /bīfron′təl/ [L, *bis* + *frons,* front, *sutura*], the interlocking lines of fusion between the frontal and parietal bones of the skull.

bifurcate /bīfur′kāt/ [L, *bis,* twice, *furca,* fork], the division or branching of an object into two forks. —**bifurcated,** *adj.*

bifurcation /bī′fərkā′shən/ [L, *bis* + *furca,* fork], a splitting into two branches, such as the trachea, which branches into the two bronchi.

Bigelow's lithotrite /big′əlōz/ [Henry J. Bigelow, American surgeon, 1818–1890; Gk, *lithos,* stone; L, *terere,* to rub], a long-jawed instrument, passed through the urethra, for crushing a calculus in the bladder.

bigeminal /bījem′inəl/ [L, *bis,* twice, *geminus,* twin], pertaining to pairs, twins, or dual events.

bigeminal pregnancy, a twin pregnancy.

bigeminal pulse, an abnormal pulse in which two beats in close succession are followed by a pause during which no pulse is felt.

bigeminal rhythm [L, *bis* + *geminus,* twin; Gk, *rhythmos*], a coupled heartbeat with ventricular or atrial ectopic beats alternating with and precisely coupled to sinus beats; or ventricular ectopics occurring in pairs, such as ventricular tachycardia with 3 : 2 exit block.

bigeminy /bījem′inē/ [L, *bis* + *geminus,* twin], 1. an association in pairs. 2. a cardiac arrhythmia characterized by pairs of beats in which each normal beat is fol-

lowed by a precisely coupled ectopic beat in a repeating manner. —**bigeminal,** *adj.*

bilabe /bī′lāb/ [L, *bis* + *labium,* lip], a narrow forceps used to remove small calculi from the bladder by way of the urethra.

bilaminar /bīlam′ənər/ [L, *bis* + *lamina,* plate], pertaining to or having two layers.

bilaminar blastoderm, the stage of embryonic development before mesoderm formation in which only the ectoderm and entoderm primary germ layers have formed.

bilateral /bilat′ərəl/ [L, *bis* + *lateralis,* side], 1. having two sides. 2. occurring or appearing on two sides. A patient with bilateral hearing loss may have partial or total hearing loss in both ears. 3. having two layers.

bilateral carotid [L, *bis,* twice, *latus,* side; Gk, *karos,* heavy sleep], a main artery to the head and neck that divides into left and right branches and again into external and internal branches.

bilateral lithotomy [L, *bis,* twice, *latus,* side; Gk, *lithos,* stone, *temnein,* to cut], a surgical procedure for removing urinary tract stones from the bladder by making transverse perineal incisions through the lateral lobes of the prostate.

bilateral long-leg spica cast, an orthopedic device of plaster of paris, fiberglass, or other casting material that encases and immobilizes the trunk cranially as far as the nipple line and both legs caudally as far as the toes. A horizontal crossbar to improve immobilization connects the parts of the cast encasing both legs at ankle level.

bilateral strabismus [L, *bis* + *latus,* side; Gk, *strabismos*], an eye disorder, characterized by bilateral squint, which is caused by a failure of ocular accommodation.

bilateral symmetry [L, *bis* + *latus,* side; Gk, *syn,* together, *metron,* measure], similar structure of the halves of an organism.

Bilbao tube /bilbō′ə/, a long, thin, flexible tube that is used to inject barium into the small intestine. The tube is guided with a stiff wire to the end of the duodenum under fluoroscopic control.

bile /bīl/ [L, *bilis*], a bitter, yellow-green secretion of the liver. Stored in the gallbladder, bile receives its color from the presence of bile pigments such as bilirubin. Bile passes from the gallbladder through the common bile duct in response to the cholecystokinin produced in the duodenum in the presence of a fatty meal. Bile breaks these fats into smaller particles and lowers the surface tension), preparing them for further digestion and absorption in the small intestine. **—biliary,** *adj.*

bile acid, a steroid acid of the bile produced during the metabolism of cholesterol. On hydrolysis, bile acid yields glycine and choleic acid.

bile duct abscess, a cavity containing pus and surrounded by inflamed tissue in the bile duct.

bile pigments, a group of substances that contribute to the colors of bile, which may range from a yellowish green to brown. A common bile pigment is bilirubin.

bile salts [L, *bilis,* bile; AS, *sealt*], a mixture of sodium salts of the bile acids and choleic and chenodeoxycholic acids synthesized in the liver as a derivative of cholesterol. Their low surface tension contributes to the emulsification of fats in the intestine.

bile solubility test, a bacteriologic test used in the differential diagnosis of pneumococcal and streptococcal infections.

biliary /bil'ē·er'ē/, pertaining to bile or to the gallbladder and bile ducts, which transport bile. These are often called the **biliary tract** or the biliary system.

biliary abscess, an abscess of the gallbladder or liver.

biliary atresia, congenital absence or underdevelopment of one or more of the biliary structures, causing jaundice and early liver damage.

biliary calculus [L, *bilis,* bile, *calculus,* pebble], a stone formed in the biliary tract, consisting of cholesterol or bile pigments and calcium salts. Biliary calculi may cause jaundice, right upper quadrant pain, obstruction, and inflammation of the gallbladder.

biliary cirrhosis [L, *bilis* + *kirrhos,* yellow, *osis,* condition], an inflammatory condition in which the flow of bile through the ductules of the liver is obstructed.

biliary colic [L, *bilis* + *kolikos,* colon pain], a type of smooth muscle or visceral pain specifically associated with the passing of stones through the bile ducts.

biliary duct, one of the muscular ducts through which bile passes from the liver and gallbladder to the duodenum.

biliary dyskinesia, an abnormal condition caused by a dysfunction of the sphincter of Oddi, disrupting the flow of bile from the gallbladder.

biliary dyspepsia, a digestive upset caused by an inadequate flow of bile into the duodenum.

biliary fistula, an abnormal passage from the gallbladder, a bile duct, or the liver to an internal organ or the surface of the body.

biliary obstruction, blockage of the

common or cystic bile duct, usually caused by one or more gallstones. It impedes bile drainage and produces an inflammatory reaction. Biliary obstruction is characterized by severe epigastric pain, often radiating to the back and shoulder; nausea; vomiting; and jaundice.

biliary tract [L, *bilis,* bile, *tractus*], the pathway for bile flow from the canaliculi in the liver to the opening of the bile duct into the duodenum.

biliary tract cancer, a rare adenocarcinoma in a bile duct often causing jaundice, pruritus, and weight loss. The lesion may be papillary or flat and ulcerated. The tumor is often unresectable at diagnosis.

biligenesis /bil'ijen'əsis/, the process by which bile is produced.

bilingulate /bīling'gyəlit/ [L, *bis,* twice, *lingula,* little tongue], having two tongues or two tonguelike structures.

bilious /bil'yəs/ [L, *bilis,* bile], **1.** pertaining to bile. **2.** characterized by an excessive secretion of bile. **3.** characterized by a disorder affecting bile.

bilirubin /bil'irōō'bin/ [L, *bilis* + *ruber,* red], the orange-yellow pigment of bile, formed principally by the breakdown of hemoglobin in red blood cells after termination of their normal lifespan. In a healthy person about 250 mg of bilirubin is produced daily. The majority of bilirubin is excreted in the stool. The characteristic yellow pallor of jaundice is caused by the accumulation of bilirubin in the blood and in the tissues of the skin.

bilirubinemia /-ē'mē·ə/ [L, *bilis,* bile, *ruber,* red; Gk, *haima,* blood], the presence of bilirubin in the blood.

bilirubinuria /-ōōr'ē·ə/, the presence of bilirubin in urine.

biliuria /bil'iyōōr'ē·ə/ [L, *bilis* + Gk, *ouron,* urine], the presence of bile pigments in the urine.

biliverdin /bil'ivur'din/ [L, *bilis* + *virdis,* green], a greenish bile pigment formed in the breakdown of hemoglobin and converted to bilirubin.

Billings method, a way of estimating ovulation time by changes in the cervical mucus that occur during the menstrual cycle.

Billroth's operation I [Christian A. Billroth, Austrian surgeon, 1829–1894], the surgical removal of the pylorus in the treatment of gastric cancer or peptic ulcer. The proximal end of the duodenum is anastomosed to the stomach.

Billroth's operation II [Christian A. Billroth], the surgical removal of the pylorus and duodenum. The cut end of the stomach is anastomosed to the jejunum through the transverse mesocolon.

Bill's maneuver [Arthur H. Bill, American obstetrician, 1877–1961], an obstetric procedure in which a forceps is used to rotate the fetal head at midpelvis before extraction of the head during birth.

bilobate /bīlō′bāt/ [L, *bis*, twice, *lobus*, lobe], having two lobes.

bilobate placenta [L, *bis*, twice, *lobus*, lobe, *placenta*, flat cake], a placenta with two connected lobes.

bilobulate /bīlob′yəlāt/, having two lobules.

bilocular /bīlok′yələr/ [L, *bis* + *loculus*, compartment], 1. divided into two cells. 2. containing two cells.

bimanual /bīman′yoō·əl/ [L, *bis* + *manus*, hand], pertaining to the functioning of both hands.

bimanual examination, [L, *bis* + *manos*, hand], an examination that requires the use of two hands.

bimanual palpation, the examination of a woman's pelvic organs in which the examiner places one hand on the abdomen and one or two fingers of the other hand in the vagina.

bimanual percussion [L, *bis*, twice, *manus*, hand, *percutere*, to strike through], a diagnostic technique of producing sound vibrations in body cavities by the use of two hands, one serving as the plexor, or "hammer," and the other as the pleximeter, or striking plate.

bimastoid /bīmas′toid/, pertaining to the two mastoid processes of the temporal bone.

bimaxillary /bīmak′siler′ē/ [L, *bis* + *maxilla*, jawbone], pertaining to the right and left maxilla.

bimodal distribution /bīmo′dəl/ [L, *bis* + *modus*, measure], the distribution of quantitative data into two clusters. It is suggestive of two separate, normally distributed populations from which the data are drawn.

bimolecular reaction (E²) /bī′molek′-yələr/, a reaction in which more than one kind of molecule is involved. It may follow first-order, second-order, or more complicated chemical kinetics.

binangle /bin′ang·gəl/ [L, *bini*, twofold, *angulus*, angle], a double-ended surgical or operative instrument that has a shank with two offsetting angles to keep the cutting edge of the instrument within 3 mm of the shaft axis.

binary fission /bī′nərē/ [L, *bini*, twofold, *fissionis*, splitting], direct division of a cell or nucleus into two equal parts. It is the common form of asexual reproduction of bacteria, protozoa, and other lower forms of life.

binary number, a number in the binary system represented by 0s and 1s. For example, the number 2 in the decimal form is written as 10 in the binary form, the decimal number 3 is written as 11, the decimal number 4 is written as 100 in the binary form, and so on.

bind [AS, *binden*], 1. to bandage or wrap in a band. 2. to join together with a band or with a ligature. 3. (in chemistry) to combine or unite molecules by using reactive groups within the molecules or by using a binding chemical.

binder, a bandage made of a large piece of material to fit and support a specific body part.

binding energy, 1. the amount of energy required to separate a nucleus into its individual nucleons. 2. the energy released as the nucleus forms from nucleons.

binding site [ME, *binden* + L, *situs*], the location on the surface of a cell or a molecule where other cell fragments or molecules attach to initiate a chemical or physiologic action.

Binet age /binā′/ [Alfred Binet, French psychologist, 1857–1911], the mental age of an individual, especially a child, as determined by the Binet-Simon tests, which are evaluated on the basis of tested intelligence of the "normal" individual at any given age. The Binet age corresponding to 'profoundly retarded' is 1 to 2 years; to 'severely retarded,' 3 to 7 years; and to 'mildly retarded,' 8 to 12 years.

binocular /bīnok′yələr, bin-/ [L, *bini* + *oculus*, eye], 1. pertaining to both eyes, especially regarding vision. 2. a microscope, telescope, or field glass that can accommodate viewing by both eyes.

binocular fixation, the process of having both eyes directed at the same object at the same time, which is essential for good depth perception.

binocular ophthalmoscope, an ophthalmoscope having two eyepieces used for stereoscopic examination of the eye.

binocular parallax /per′əlaks/ [L, *bini* + *oculus* + Gk, *parallax*, in turn], the difference in the angles formed by the sight lines to two objects situated at different distances from the eyes. Binocular parallax is a major factor in depth perception.

binocular perception, the visual ability to judge depth or distance by virtue of having two eyes.

binocular vision, the simultaneous use of both eyes so that the images perceived by each eye are combined to appear as a single image.

binomial /bīnō′mē·əl/, containing two names or terms.

binomial nomenclature [L, *bis*, twice; Gk, *nomos*, law; L, *nomenclatio*, calling by

name], a system of classification of animals, plants, and other life forms (developed by Carl Linné) that assigns Latinized genus and species names to each, such as *Homo sapiens* for humans.

binovular /bīnov′yələr/ [L, *bini* + *ovum*, egg], developing from two distinct ova, as in dizygotic twins.

binuclear /bīnōō′klē·ər/ [L, *bis*, twice, *nucleus*, nut kernel], having two nuclei, as in the example of a heterokaryon or binucleate hybrid cell.

bioactive [Gk, *bios*, life; L, *activus*, with energy], having an effect on or causing a reaction in living tissue.

bioactivity /-aktiv′itē/, any response from or reaction in living tissue.

bioassay /bī′ō·as′ā, -əsā′/ [Gk, *bios* + Fr, *assayer*, to try], the laboratory determination of the concentration of a drug or other substance in a specimen by comparing its effect on an organism, an animal, or an isolated tissue with that of a standard preparation.

bioastronautics /-as′trōnôt′iks/, the science dealing with the biologic aspects of space travel.

bioavailability /-əvā′libil′itē/ [Gk, *bios* + ME, *availen*, to serve], the degree of activity or amount of an administered drug or other substance that becomes available for activity in the target tissue.

biocenosis /-sənō′sis/, [Fk, *bios*, life, *koinos*, common], an ecologic community.

biochemical marker / kem′ikəl/ [Gk, *bios* + *chemeia*, alchemy], any hormone, enzyme, antibody, or other substance that is detected in the urine or other body fluids or tissues that may serve as a sign of a disease or other abnormality.

biochemistry /-kem′istrē/, the chemistry of living organisms and life processes.

biochemorphics / kemôr′fik/, pertaining to the study of the relationship between chemical structure and biologic function.

biochromatic analysis /-krōmat′ik/ [Gk, *bios* + *chroma*, color], the spectrophotometric monitoring of a reaction at two wavelengths. It is used to correct for background color.

bioclimatology /-klī′mətol′əjē/, the study of the relationship between climate and living organisms and their interactions.

biocybernetics /-sī′bərnet′iks/, the science of communication and control within and among living organisms and their interaction with mechanical or electronic systems.

biodegradable /-digrā′dəbəl/ [Gk, *bios*, life; L, *de*, away, *gradus*, step], the natural ability of a chemical substance to be broken down into less complex compounds or compounds having fewer carbon atoms by bacteria or other microorganisms.

biodynamics /-dīnam′iks/, the study of the effects of dynamic processes such as radiation on living organisms.

bioelectric impedance analysis (BIA) /-ilek′trik/, a method of measuring the fat composition of the body, compared to other tissues, by its resistance to electricity.

bioelectricity /-ilektris′itē/ [Gk, *bios* + *elektron*, amber], electrical current that is generated by living tissues such as nerves and muscles.

bioenergetics /-en′ərjet′iks/ [Gk, *bios* + *energein*, to be active], a system of exercises based on the concept that natural healing will be enhanced by bringing the patient's body rhythms and the natural environment into harmony.

bioequivalent /bī′ō·ikwiv′ələnt/ [Gk, *bios* + L, *aequus*, equal, *valere*, to be strong], **1.** (in pharmacology) pertaining to a drug that has the same effect on the body as another drug, usually one nearly identical in its chemical formulation. **2.** a bioequivalent drug. —**bioequivalence,** *n.*

biofeedback /-fēd′bak/ [Gk, *bios* + AS, *faedan*, food, *baec*, back], a process providing a person with visual or auditory information about the autonomic physiologic functions of his or her body, such as blood pressure, muscle tension, and brain wave activity, usually through use of instruments.

Biofeedback, a Nursing Interventions Classification defined as assisting the patient to modify a body function using feedback from instrumentation.

bioflavonoid /bī′ōflā′vənoid/ [Gk, *bios* + L, *flavus*, yellow; Gk, *eidos*, form], a generic term for any of a group of colored flavones found in many fruits. Bioflavonoids are now considered nonessential nutrients.

biogenesis /bī′ōjen′əsis/ [Gk, *bios* + *genein*, to produce], **1.** also called biogeny /bī·oj′ənē/; the doctrine that living material can originate only from preexisting life and not from inanimate matter. **2.** the origin of life and living organisms, ontogeny and phylogeny. —**biogenetic,** *adj.*

biogenic /bī′ōjen′ik/, **1.** produced by the action of a living organism, such as fermentation. **2.** essential to life and the maintenance of health, such as food, water, and proper rest.

biogenic amine, one of a large group of naturally occurring biologically active compounds, most of which act as neurotransmitters. The most dominant is norepinephrine. These substances are active in regulating blood pressure, elimination, body temperature, and many other centrally mediated body functions.

biogenous /bī·oj'ənəs/, **1.** biogenetic. **2.** biogenic.

biogravics /grav'iks/, the study of the effects of gravitational forces such as weightlessness and gravitational pull (g) forces on living organisms.

biohazard /-haz'ərd/ [Gk, *bios,* life; OFr, *hasard*], anything that is a risk to living organisms, such as exposure to ionizing radiation.

bioinstrument, a sensor or other device implanted into or attached to a living organism for the purpose of recording physiologic data such as brain activity or heart function.

biokinetics /-kinet'iks/ [Gk, *bios,* life, *kinetikos,* moving], a branch of science that deals with movements within developing organisms.

biologic /-loj'ik/ [Gk, *bios + logos,* science], **1.** pertaining to living organisms and their products. **2.** any preparation made from living organisms or their products and used as diagnostic, preventive, or therapeutic agents. Kinds of biologics are **antigens, antitoxins, serums,** and **vaccines.**

biologic activity, the inherent capacity of a substance such as a drug or toxin to alter one or more of the chemical or physiologic functions of a cell, tissue, organ, or entire organism. The capacity has relationships not only to the physical and chemical nature of the substance but also to its concentration and the duration of cellular exposure to it.

biologic armature, the connective tissue–rich aggregate of larger ducts, vessels, and autonomic nerves that in many mammalian exocrine glands serve as an internal framework whose function of support, and often anchorage, resembles that of the armature within a clay sculpture.

biologic death, death attributed to natural causes.

biologic dressing, a dressing for burn injuries that is made from pigskin or synthetic materials with characteristics like those of human skin. The dressing is most effective in treating burns that are of uniform depth and of superficial partial thickness. It should be applied as soon as possible after the injury and should adhere to the wound during healing. Once adherence is established, the wound can be left open, and the patient can bathe and wear clothing over it.

biologic half-life, the time required for the body to eliminate half of an administered dose of any substance by regular physiologic processes.

biologic monitoring, 1. a process of measuring the levels of various physiologic substances, drugs, or metabolites within a patient during diagnosis or therapy. **2.** the measurement of toxic substances in the environment and the identification of health risks to the population.

biologic plausibility, a method of reasoning used to establish a cause and effect relationship between a biologic factor and a particular disease.

biologic psychiatry, a school of psychiatric thought that stresses the physical, chemical, and neurologic causes of and treatments for mental and emotional disorders.

biologic rhythm [Gk, *bios,* life, *logos,* science, *rhythmos*], the periodic recurrence of certain biologic phenomena such as circadian and diurnal rhythms.

biologist /bī·ol'əjist/ [Gk, *bios,* life, *logos,* science], a person who studies the science of life.

biology /bī·ol'əje/, the scientific study of plants, animals, and other life forms. Some branches of biology are **biometry, ecology, evolution, genetics, molecular and cell biology, physiology,** and paleontology.

biolysis /bī·ol'isis/ [Gk, *bios,* life, *lysis,* loosening], the disintegration or dissolution of organic matter resulting from the activity of living organisms, such as bacterial action on living tissue.

biome /bī'ōm/ [Gk, *bios + oma,* tumor, mass], the total group of biologic communities existing in and characteristic of a given geographic region, such as a desert, woodland, or marsh.

biomechanic adaptation /-məkan'ic/, a process in the use of orthotic treatment to enable a disabled person to resume normal function of a body part with the aid of a device such as an ankle-foot brace. The process of adaptation includes the central nervous system input received during therapeutic exercises with the orthotic appliance.

biomechanics [Gk, *bios + mechane,* machine], the study of mechanical laws and their application to living organisms, especially the human body and its locomotor system. —**biomechanic, biomechanical,** *adj.*

biomedical, pertaining to the biologic aspects of medicine and surgery.

biomedical engineering /-med'ikəl/ [Gk, *bios + L, medicare,* to heal], a system of scientific techniques that is applied to biologic processes to often solve practical medical problems or answer questions in biomedical research.

biometry /bī·om'ətrē/, the application of statistical methods in analyzing data obtained in biologic or anthropologic research. See also **biology.**

biomicroscopy /-mīkros'kəpē/, **1.** microscopic examination of living tissue in the body. **2.** ophthalmic examination of the eye by use of a slit lamp and a magnifying lens. See also **slit lamp, slit lamp microscope.**

bionics /bī·on'iks/, the science of applying electronic principles and devices such as computers and solid-state miniaturized circuitry to medical problems, such as artificial pacemakers used to correct abnormal heart rhythms. —**bionic,** adj.

biopharmaceutics /-fär'məsoo'tiks/, the study of the chemical and physical properties of drugs, their components, and their activities in living organisms.

biophore /bī'əfôr'/ [Gk, bios + phora, bearer], according to the German biologist A.F.L. Weismann (1834–1914), the basic hereditary unit contained in the germ plasm from which all living cells develop and all inherited characteristics are transmitted.

biophysics, the application of physical laws and science to life processes of organisms.

biopotentials /-pəten'shəlz/, electrical charges produced by various tissues of the body, particularly muscle tissue during contractions.

biopsy /bī'opsē/ [Gk, bios + opsis, view], **1.** the removal of a small piece of living tissue from an organ or other part of the body for microscopic examination to confirm or establish a diagnosis, estimate prognosis, or follow the course of a disease. **2.** the tissue excised for examination. **3.** informal, to excise tissue for examination. Kinds of biopsy include **aspiration biopsy, needle biopsy, punch biopsy,** and **surface biopsy.** —**bioptic** /bī·op'tik/, adj.

biopsychic /bī'ōsī'kik/ [Gk, bios + psyche, mind], pertaining to mental factors as they relate to living organisms.

biopsychosocial /bī'ōsī'kōsō'shəl/ [Gk, bios + psyche, mind; L, socius, companion], pertaining to the complex of biologic, psychologic, and social aspects of life.

bioptome tip catheter /bī·op'tōm/, a catheter with a special end designed for obtaining endomyocardial biopsy samples. The bioptome tip device is used to monitor heart transplantation patients for early signs of tissue rejection.

biorhythm /bī'ōrithm/ [Gk, bios + rhythmos, rhythm], any cyclic, biologic event or phenomenon, such as the sleep cycle, the menstrual cycle, or the respiratory cycle. —**biorhythmic,** adj.

biosafety, a system for the safe handling of toxic and dangerous biologic and chemical substances. Guidance in biosafety is offered by the U.S. Centers for Disease Control and Prevention, Occupational Safety and Health Administration, and National Institute for Occupational Safety and Health.

biostatistics /-stətis'tiks/, numeric data on births, deaths, diseases, injuries, and other factors affecting the general health and condition of human populations.

biosynthesis /-sin'thəsis/ [Gk, bios + synthesis, putting together], any one of thousands of chemical reactions continually occurring throughout the body in which molecules form more complex biomolecules. —**biosynthetic,** adj.

biosystem, any living organism or complex system of living things.

biotaxis /bī'ōtak'sis/ [Gk, bios + taxis, arrangement], the ability of living cells to develop into certain forms and arrangements. —**biotactic,** adj.

biotaxy /bī'ōtak'sē/, **1.** biotaxis. **2.** the systematic classification of living organisms according to their phenotypic characteristics; taxonomy.

biotechnology /-teknol'əjē/ [Gk, bios + techne, art, logos, science], **1.** the study of the relationships between humans or other living organisms and machinery, such as the health effects of computer equipment on office workers. **2.** the industrial application of the results of biologic research, particularly in fields such as recombinant deoxyribonucleic acids or gene splicing.

biotelemetry /-təlem'ətrē/, the transmission of physiologic data such as electrocardiographic and electroencephalographic recordings, heart rate, and body temperature by radio or telephone systems.

biotherapy, a system of biologic therapy of cancer that uses the effects of alpha and beta interferons and mitogen-stimulated lymphocytes rather than chemical agents.

biotic factors /bī·ot'ik/, environmental influences on living things, as distinguished from climatic or geologic factors.

biotic potential, the possible growth rate of a population of organisms under ideal conditions, including absence of predators and maximum nutrients and space for expansion.

biotin /bī'ətin/ [Gk, bios, life], a colorless, crystalline, water-soluble B complex vitamin that acts as a co-enzyme in fatty acid production and in the oxidation of fatty acids and carbohydrates.

biotin deficiency syndrome, an abnormal condition caused by a deficiency of biotin. It is characterized by dermatitis, hyperesthesia, muscle pain, anorexia, slight anemia, and changes in electrocardiographic activity of the heart.

biotope /bī′ətōp/ [Gk, *bios* + *topos,* place], a specific biologic habitat or site.

biotoxin /bī′ətok′in/, any toxin produced by living organisms.

biotransformation /-trans′fôrmā′shən/ [Gk, *bios* + L, *trans,* across, *formare,* to form], the chemical changes a substance undergoes in the body, such as by the action of enzymes.

Biot's respiration /bē-ōz′/ [Camille Biot, French physician, b. 1878], an abnormal respiratory pattern, characterized by irregular breathing with periods of apnea.

bipalatinoid /bī′palat′inoid, -pal′-/, describing a two-compartment capsule with different medications in each side. It is designed so that the two substances become mixed and activated as the gelatin capsule dissolves.

bipara /bip′ərə/, a woman who has given birth twice in separate pregnancies.

biparietal /bīpərī′ətəl/ [L, *bis,* twice, *paries,* wall], pertaining to the two parietal bones of the head, such as the biparietal diameter.

biparietal diameter (BPD), the transverse distance between the protuberances of the two parietal bones of the skull.

biparietal suture [L, *bis* + *paries,* wall, *sutura*], the interlocking lines of fusion between two parietal bones of the skull.

biparous [L, *bis,* twice, *parere,* to produce], pertaining to the birth of two infants in separate pregnancies.

bipartite /bīpär′tīt/, having two parts.

biped /bī′ped/, 1. having two feet. 2. any animal with only two feet.

bipedal /bīpē′dəl, -ped′əl/ [L, *bis,* twice, *pes,* foot], capable of locomotion on two feet.

bipenniform /bīpen′ifôrm′/ [L, *bis* + *penna,* feather, *forma,* form], (of body structure) having the bilateral symmetry of a feather, such as the pattern formed by the fasciculi that converge on both sides of a muscle tendon in the rectus femoris.

biperiden /bīper′idən/, a synthetic anticholinergic agent prescribed in the treatment of Parkinson's disease and drug-induced extrapyramidal disorders. Biperiden hydrochloride is administered orally, and biperiden lactate is administered intramuscularly or intravenously.

biphasic /bīfā′zik/ [L, *bis* + Gk, *phasis,* appearance], having two phases, parts, aspects, or stages.

bipolar /bīpō′lər/ [L, *bis* + *polus,* pole],

1. having two poles, such as in certain electrotherapeutic treatments using two poles or in certain types of bacterial staining that affect only the two poles of the microorganism under study. 2. (of a nerve cell) having an afferent and an efferent process.

bipolar cell, a cell, such as a retinal neuron, with two main processes arising from the cell body.

bipolar disorder, a major mental disorder characterized by episodes of mania, depression, or mixed mood. One or the other phase may be predominant at any given time, one phase may appear alternately with the other, or elements of both phases may be present simultaneously. Characteristics of the manic phase are excessive emotional displays such as excitement, elation, euphoria, or in some cases irritability accompanied by hyperactivity, boisterousness, impaired ability to concentrate, decreased need for sleep, and seemingly unbounded energy. In the depressive phase, marked apathy and underactivity are accompanied by feelings of profound sadness, loneliness, guilt, and lowered self-esteem.

bipolar lead /lēd/, 1. an electrocardiographic conductor having two electrodes placed on different body regions, with each electrode contributing significantly to the record. 2. *informal.* a tracing produced by such a lead on an electrocardiograph.

bipolar version, a method for changing the position of a fetus in which one hand is placed on the abdomen of the mother and two fingers of the other hand are inserted into the uterus.

bipotentiality /bī′pəten′shē·al′itē/ [L, *bis* + *potentia,* power], the characteristic of acting or reacting according to either of two possible states.

bird face retrognathism, an abnormal facial profile with an underdeveloped mandible, which may be caused by interference of condylar growth associated with trauma or condylar infection.

bird-headed dwarf, a person affected with Seckel's syndrome, a congenital disorder characterized by a short stature; a small head with jaw hypoplasia, large eyes, and a beaklike protrusion of the nose; mental retardation; and various other defects.

birth [ME, *burth*], 1. the event of being born—the entry of a new person out of its mother into the world. 2. the childbearing event—the bringing forth by a mother of a baby. 3. a medical event—the delivery of a fetus by an obstetric attendant.

birth canal, *informal.* the passage that

extends from the inlet of the true pelvis to the vaginal orifice through which an infant passes during vaginal birth.

birth center, a health facility with services limited to maternity care for women judged to be at minimum risk for obstetric complications that would require hospitalization.

birth certificate, a legal document recording information about a birth, including, among other details, the date, time, and location of the event; identity of the mother and father; and identity of the attending physician or licensed midwife.

birth control. See **contraception.**

birth defect. See **congenital anomaly.**

Birthing, a Nursing Interventions Classification defined as delivery of a baby.

birthing chair, a special seat used in labor and delivery to promote the comfort of the mother and the efficiency of birth. The newer birthing chairs allow woman to sit straight up or to recline. The upright position appears to shorten the time in labor, particularly the second or expulsive stage of labor, probably because of gravity and increased participation of the mother. The chair is not suitable for use with anesthesia.

birth injury, trauma suffered by a baby while being born. Some kinds of birth injury are **Bell's palsy, cerebral palsy,** and **Erb's palsy.**

birthmark. See **nevus.**

birth mother, the biologic mother or woman who bears a child. The child may have been conceived in a surrogate mother with sperm of the biologic father.

birth palsy [ME, *burth* + Gk, *paralyein,* to be palsied], a loss of motor or sensory nerve function in some body part caused by a nerve injury during the birth process.

birth parents, the biologic parents, or the combined source of the entire genetic information of a child.

birth rate, the proportion of the number of live births in a specific area during a given period to the total population of that area, usually expressed as the number of births per 1000 of population.

birth trauma, 1. any physical injury suffered by an infant during the process of delivery. 2. the supposed psychic shock, according to some psychiatric theories, that an infant suffers during delivery.

birth weight, the measured heaviness of a baby when born, usually about 3500 g (7.5 pounds). Babies weighing less than 2500 g at term are considered **small for gestational age.** Babies weighing more than 4500 g are considered **large for gestational age** and are often infants of mothers with diabetes.

bisacodyl /bisak'ōdil/, a cathartic prescribed in the treatment of acute or chronic constipation or for emptying of the bowel before or after surgery or before diagnostic radiographic procedures.

bisacromial /bīsəkrō'mē-əl/, pertaining to the two acromions, the triangular, flat, bony plates at the end of the scapula.

bisalbuminemia /bis'albyōōm'inē'mē-ə/, a condition in which two types of albumin exist in an individual. The two types are expressed by heterozygous alleles of the albumin gene and are detected by differences in the mobility of the types on electrophoretic gels.

bisect /bīsekt'/ [L, *bis* + *secare,* to cut], to divide into two equal lengths or parts.

bisexual /bīsek'shōō-əl/ [L, *bis* + *sexus,* male or female], **1.** hermaphroditic; having gonads of both sexes. **2.** possessing physical or psychologic characteristics of both sexes. **3.** engaging in both heterosexual and homosexual activity. **4.** desiring sexual contact with persons of both sexes.

bisexual libido, (in psychoanalysis) the tendency in a person to seek sexual gratification with people of either sex.

bisferial pulse /bisfer'ē-əs/ [L, *bis* + *ferire,* to beat], an arterial pulse that has two palpable peaks, the second of which is slightly weaker than the first. It may be detected in cases of aortic regurgitation and obstructive cardiomyopathy.

bis in die (b.d., b.i.d.) /dē'ā/, a Latin phrase, used in prescriptions, meaning 'twice a day.' It is more commonly used in its abbreviated form.

bismuth (Bi) /biz'məth, bis'-/ [Ger, *wismut,* white mass], a reddish, crystalline, trivalent metallic element. Its atomic number is 83; its atomic weight (mass) is 208.98. It is combined with various other elements such as oxygen to produce numerous salts used in the manufacture of many pharmaceutic substances.

bismuth gingivitis, a symptom of metallic poisoning caused by bismuth administered in the treatment of systemic disease. It is characterized by a dark bluish line along the gingival margin.

bismuth stomatitis, an abnormal oral condition caused by systemic use of bismuth compounds over prolonged periods, characterized by a blue-black line on the inner aspect of the gingival sulcus or pigmentation of the buccal mucosa, sore tongue, metallic taste, and burning sensation in the mouth.

bitartrate /bītär'trāt/, the monoanion of tartaric acid, $C_4H_5O_6$.

bitartrate carboxylate anion, an ionotropic agent used in the treatment of cardiovascular patients.

bite [AS, *bitan*], **1.** the act of cutting, tearing, holding, or gripping with the teeth. **2.** the lingual part of an artificial tooth between its shoulder and incisal edge. **3.** an occlusal record or relationship of upper and lower teeth or jaws.

bitegauge /bīt′gāj′/ [AS, *bitan* + OFr, *gauge*, measure], a prosthetic dental device that helps attain proper occlusion of the teeth rooted in the maxilla and the mandible.

biteguard [AS, *bitan* + OFr, *garder,* to defend], a resin appliance that covers the occlusal and incisal surfaces of the teeth. Its purpose is to stabilize the teeth and provide a platform for the excursive glides of the mandible.

biteguard splint, a device, usually made of resin, for covering the occlusal and incisal surfaces of the teeth and for protecting them from traumatic occlusal forces during immobilization and stabilization processes.

bitelock /bīt′lok′/, a dental device for retaining the occlusion rims in the same relation outside and inside the mouth.

bitemporal /bītem′pərəl/ [L, *bis,* twice, *tempora,* temples], pertaining to both temples or both temporal bones.

bitemporal hemianopia [L, *bis,* twice, *tempora,* temples; Gk, *hemi,* half, *opsis,* vision], a loss of the temporal half of the vision in each eye, usually resulting from a lesion in the chiasmal area such as a pituitary tumor.

biteplane /bīt′plān/, **1.** a plane formed by the biting surfaces of the teeth. **2.** a metal sheet laid across the biting surfaces of mandibular or maxillary teeth to determine the relationship of the teeth to this predetermined plane. **3.** an orthodontic appliance of acrylic resin worn over the maxillary occlusal surfaces and used to treat pain of the temporomandibular joint and adjacent muscles.

biteplate /bīt′plāt/, a device used in dentistry as a diagnostic or a therapeutic aid for prosthodontics or orthodontics.

bite reflex, a swift, involuntary biting action that may be triggered by stimulation of the oral cavity.

bite wing film [AS, *bitan* + ME, *winge*], an adaptation of regular dental x-ray film on which a paper tab is placed so the teeth can hold the film in position during exposure.

bite wing radiograph, a kind of dental radiograph that reveals approximately the coronal parts of maxillary and mandibular teeth and parts of the interdental septa on the same film.

bithionol (TBP) /bithī′ənôl/, a pale gray powder, soluble in acetone, alcohol, or ether, used as a local antiseptic and administered orally in the treatment of infestations of certain flukes that cause parasitic hemoptysis in Asiatic countries.

Bithynia /bəthin′ē-ə/, a genus of snails, species of which act as intermediate hosts to *Opisthorchis.*

biting in childhood, a natural behavior trait and reflex action in infants, acquired at about 5 to 6 months of age in response to the introduction of solid foods in the diet and the beginning of the teething process. The activity represents a significant modality in the psychosocial development of the child, because it is the first aggressive action the infant learns, and through it the infant learns to control the environment.

bitolterol mesylate /bitol′tərol mes′ilāt/, an orally inhaled bronchodilator used in the treatment of bronchial asthma and reversible bronchospasm.

Bitot's spots /bitōz′/ [Pierre Bitot, French surgeon, 1822–1888], white or gray triangular deposits on the bulbar conjunctiva adjacent to the lateral margin of the cornea, a clinical sign of vitamin A deficiency.

bitrochanteric lipodystrophy /bī′trōkən-ter′ik/ [L, *bis* + Gk, *trochanter,* runner; *lipos,* fat, *dys,* bad, *trophe,* nourishment], an abnormal and excessive deposition of fat on the buttocks and the outer aspect of the upper thighs, occurring most commonly in women.

biuret test /bī′yŏŏret/ [L, *bis* + Gk, *ouron,* urine], a method for detecting urea and other soluble proteins in serum.

bivalent /bīvā′lənt/ [L, *bis* + *valere,* to be powerful], (in genetics) a pair of synapsed homologous chromosomes that are attached to each other by chiasmata during the early first meiotic prophase of gametogenesis. The structure serves as the basis for the tetrads from which gametes are produced during the two meiotic divisions. —**bivalence,** *n.*

bivalent antibody, an antibody that has two or more binding sites that can cross-link one antigen to another.

bivalent chromosome, a pair of synapsed homologous chromosomes during the early stages of gametogenesis.

bivalved cast [L, *bis* + *valva,* valve], a cast that is cut in half to detect or relieve pressure underneath, especially when a patient has decreased or no sensation in the part of the body surrounded by the cast.

BK, abbreviation for *below the knee,* a term referring to amputations, amputees, prostheses, and orthoses.

Bk,   symbol for the element **berkelium.**

Blackett-Healy method,   a procedure for positioning a patient for making radiographs of the subscapularis area. The affected shoulder joint is centered to the midline of the film, the arm abducted, and the elbow flexed.

black eye,   contusion around the eye with bruising, discoloration, and swelling.

black measles [AS, *blac* + OHG, *masala*], hemorrhagic measles characterized by a darkened rash caused by bleeding into the skin and mucous membranes.

blackout, *informal,*   a temporary loss of vision or consciousness.

black spots film fault,   a defect in a radiograph, seen as dark spots throughout the image area.

blackwater fever,   a serious complication of chronic falciparum malaria, characterized by jaundice, hemoglobinuria, acute renal failure, and passage of bloody dark red or black urine caused by massive intravascular hemolysis.

Blackwell, Elizabeth, (1821–1910), a British-born American physician, the first woman to be awarded a medical degree. She established the New York Infirmary, a 40-bed hospital staffed entirely by women. Her influence helped establish nursing schools to improve patient care.

black widow spider antivenin,   a passive immunizing agent prescribed in the treatment of black widow spider bite.

black widow spider bite [AS, *blac* + *widewe;* ME, *spithre* + AS, *bitan*], the bite of the spider species *Latrodectus mactans,* a poisonous arachnid found in many parts of the world. Black widow venom contains some enzymatic proteins, including a peptide that affects neuromuscular transmission. The bite is perceived as a sharp pinprick pain, followed by a dull pain in the area of the bite; muscular rigidity in the shoulders, back, and abdomen; restlessness; anxiety; sweating; weakness; and drooping eyelids.

bladder [AS, *blaedre*],   **1.** a membranous sac serving as a receptacle for secretions, such as the gallbladder. **2.** the urinary bladder.

bladder cancer,   the most common malignancy of the urinary tract, characterized by multiple growths that tend to recur in a more aggressive form. Bladder cancer occurs 2.3 times more often in men than in women and is more prevalent in urban than in rural areas. The risk of bladder cancer increases with cigarette smoking and exposure to aniline dyes, beta-naphthylamine, mixtures of aromatic hydrocarbons, or benzidine and its salts. Symptoms of bladder cancer include he-

maturia, frequent urination, dysuria, and cystitis. Urinalysis, excretory urography, cystoscopy, or transurethral biopsy are performed for diagnosis. The majority of bladder malignancies are transitional cell carcinomas; a small percentage are squamous cell carcinomas or adenocarcinomas.

bladder flap, *informal.*   the vesicouterine fold of peritoneum incised during low cervical cesarean section so the bladder can be separated from the uterus to expose the lower uterine segment for incision.

bladder hernia,   a protrusion of the bladder through an opening in the abdominal wall.

bladder irrigation, [AS, *blaedre* + L, *irrigare,* to conduct water],   the washing out of the bladder by a continuous or intermittent flow of saline or a medicated solution. The bladder also may be irrigated by an oral intake of fluid.

Bladder Irrigation,   a Nursing Interventions Classification defined as instillation of a solution into the bladder to provide cleansing or medication.

bladder retraining [AS, *blaedre* + L, *trahere,* to draw],   a system of therapy for incontinence in which a patient in a hospital setting practices withholding urine for intervals that begin with 1 hour and increase over a period of 10 days while maintaining a normal intake of fluid. The patient also learns to recognize and react to the urge to void.

bladder sphincter [AS, *blaedre* + Gk, *sphingein,* to bind],   a circular muscle surrounding the opening of the urinary bladder into the urethra.

Blalock-Taussig procedure /blä′loktô′sig/ [Alfred Blalock, American surgeon, 1899–1964; Helen B. Taussig, American physician, 1898–1986],   surgical construction of a shunt as a temporary measure to overcome congenital pulmonary stenosis and atrial septal defect, as in an infant born with tetralogy of Fallot. The subclavian artery is joined end to end with the pulmonary artery, directing blood from the systemic circulation to the lungs. Thrombosis of the shunt is the major postoperative complication.

blame placing,   the process of placing responsibility for one's behavior on others.

blanch /blanch, blänch/ [Fr, *blanchir,* to become white],   **1.** to cause to become pale, as a spider angiomata may be blanched by using digital pressure. **2.** to whiten or bleach a surface or substance. **3.** to become white or pale, as from vasoconstriction accompanying fear or anger.

blanch test [Fr, *blanchir,* to become white; L, *testum,* crucible],   a test of blood circulation in the fingers or toes. Pressure is applied to a fingernail or toenail until normal color is lost. The pressure is then removed, and, if the circulation is normal, color should return almost immediately, within about 2 seconds.

bland [L, *blandus*], mild or having a soothing effect.

bland aerosols, aerosols that consist of water, saline solutions, or similar substances that do not have important pharmacologic action. They are primarily used for humidification and liquefaction of secretions.

bland diet, a diet that is mechanically, chemically, physiologically, and sometimes thermally nonirritating to the gastrointestinal tract. It is often prescribed in the treatment of peptic ulcer, ulcerative colitis, gallbladder disease, diverticulitis, gastritis, idiopathic spastic constipation, and mucous colitis and after abdominal surgery. Historically it was first called the "white diet" (or Sippy diet, after Dr. Sippy, who developed it). It has progressed to what has been called the "liberal bland diet," which allows all foods except caffeine, alcohol, black pepper, spices, or any other food that could be considered irritating.

blank, a solution containing all of the reagents needed for analysis of a substance except the substance tested.

blanket bath [OFr, *blanchet,* a white garment], the procedure of wrapping the patient in a wet pack and then in blankets.

blast, 1. a primitive cell such as an embryonic germ cell. 2. a cell capable of building tissue, such as an osteoblast in growing bone.

blast cell [Gk, *blastos,* germ], any immature cell such as an erythroblast, lymphoblast, or neuroblast.

blastema /blastē′mə/ [Gk, bud], 1. any mass of living protoplasm capable of growth and differentiation, specifically the primordial undifferentiated cellular material from which a particular organ or tissue develops. 2. in certain animals, a group of cells capable of regenerating a lost or damaged part or creating a complete organism in asexual reproduction. 3. the budding or sprouting area of a plant.— blastemal, blastematic, blastemic, *adj.*

blastic transformation, a late stage in the progress of chronic granulocytic leukemia. Signs of anemia and blood platelet deficiency are present, and half of the blood cells in the bone marrow are immature forms. Blastic transformation indicates that resistance to therapy has developed in the patient who has entered a terminal stage of leukemia.

blastid /blas′tid/ [Gk, *blastos,* germ], the

site in the fertilized ovum where the pronuclei fuse and the nucleus forms.

blastin /blas′tin/ [Gk, *blastanein,* to grow], any substance that provides nourishment for or stimulates the growth or proliferation of cells, such as allantoin.

blastocoele /blas′təsēl′/ [Gk, *blastos,* germ, *koilos,* hollow], the fluid-filled cavity of the blastocyst in mammals and the blastula or discoblastula of lower animals. The cavity increases the surface area of the developing embryo to allow better absorption of nutrients and oxygen.

blastocyst /blas′təsist/ [Gk, *blastos* + *kystis,* bag], the embryonic form that follows the morula in human development. Implantation in the wall of the uterus usually occurs at this stage, on approximately the eighth day after fertilization.

blastocyte /blas′təsīt/ [Gk, *blastos* + *kytos,* cell], an undifferentiated embryonic cell that precedes germ layer formation. — **blastocytic,** *adj.*

blastoderm /blas′tədurm′/ [Gk, *blastos* + *derma,* skin], the layer of cells forming the wall of the blastocyst in mammals and the blastula in lower animals during the early stages of embryonic development. It is produced by the cleavage of the fertilized ovum and gives rise to the primary germ layers, the ectoderm, mesoderm, and endoderm, from which the embryo and all of its membranes are derived. —**blastodermal, blastodermic,** *adj.*

blastodisk /blas′tədisk/, the disklike nonyolk area of the protoplasm surrounding the animal pole where cleavage occurs in a fertilized ovum containing a large amount of yolk, as in birds and reptiles.

blastogenesis /blas′tōjen′əsis/ [Gk, *blastos* + *genein,* to produce], 1. asexual reproduction by budding. 2. the theory of the transmission of hereditary characteristics by the germ plasm, as opposed to the theory of pangenesis. 3. the early development of the embryo during cleavage and formation of the germ layers. 4. the process of transforming small lymphocytes in tissue culture into large blastlike cells by exposure to phytohemagglutinin or other substances, often for the purpose of inducing mitosis. —**blastogenetic,** *adj.*

blastogenic /-jen′ik/, 1. originating in the germ plasm. 2. initiating tissue proliferation. 3. relating to or characterized by blastogenesis.

blastogeny /blastoj′ənē/, the early stages in ontogeny; the germ plasm history of an organism or species, which traces the history of the inherited characteristics.

blastokinin /blas′təkī′nin/ [Gk, *blastos* + *kinein,* to move], a globulin secreted by the uterus in many mammals that may stimulate and regulate the implantation process of the blastocyst in the uterine wall.

blastolysis /blastol'isis/ [Gk, *blastos* + *lysis*, loosening], destruction of a germ cell or blastoderm. —**blastolytic,** *adj.*

blastoma /blastō'mə/ [Gk, *blastos* + *oma,* tumor], a neoplasm of embryonic tissue that develops from the blastema of an organ or tissue. A blastoma derived from a number of scattered cells is pluricentric; one arising from a single cell or group of cells is unicentric. —**blastomatous** /blastom'ətəs/, *adj.*

blastomatosis /blast'tōmətō'sis/ [Gk, *blastos* + *oma,* tumor, *osis,* condition], the development of many tumors from embryonic tissue.

blastomere /blas'təmēr/ [Gk, *blastos* + *meros,* part], any of the cells formed from the first mitotic division of a fertilized ovum (zygote). The blastomeres further divide and subdivide to form the multicellular morula in the first several days of pregnancy. —**blastomeric,** *adj.*

blastomerotomy /-merot'əmē/ [Gk, *blastos* + *meros,* part, *tome,* cut], the destruction or the separation of blastomeres, either caused naturally or induced artificially. —**blastomerotomic,** *adj.*

Blastomyces /blas'tōmī'sēz/ [Gk, *blastos* + *mykes,* fungus], a genus of yeastlike fungus, usually including the species *Blastomyces dermatitidis,* which causes North American blastomycosis, and *Paracoccidioides brasiliensis,* which causes South American blastomycosis.

blastomycosis /blas'tōmīkō'sis/ [Gk, *blastos* + *mykes,* fungus, *osis,* condition], an infectious disease caused by a yeastlike fungus, *Blastomyces dermatitidis.* It usually affects only the skin but may invade the lungs, kidneys, central nervous system, and bones. Skin infections often begin as small papules on the hand, face, neck, or other exposed areas where there has been a cut, bruise, or other injury. The infection may spread gradually and irregularly into surrounding areas. When the lungs are involved, x-ray films of the chest show tumors resembling cancer.

blastopore /blas'təpôr/ [Gk, *blastos* + *poros,* opening], (in embryology) the invagination into a blastula that occurs in the process of becoming a gastrula.

blastula /blas'tyələ/ [Gk, *blastos,* germ], an early stage of the process through which a zygote develops into an embryo, characterized by a fluid-filled sphere formed by a single layer of cells.

blastulation, the transformation of the morula into a blastocyst or blastula by the development of a central cavity, the blastocoele.

BLB mask, abbreviation for **Boothby-Lovelace-Bulbulian mask.**

bleaching agents, medications and over-the-counter preparations used to depigment the skin. The products may be used by persons whose skin has become hyperpigmented through exposure to sunlight and particularly for melasma associated with pregnancy or the use of oral contraceptives.

bleach poisoning, an adverse reaction to ingestion of hypochlorite salts commonly found in household and commercial bleaches. Symptoms include pain and inflammation of the mouth, throat, and esophagus; vomiting; shock; and circulatory collapse. Recommended emergency treatment is to dilute the bleach in the throat and stomach with water, milk, beaten eggs, and melted ice cream. Shock should be treated with intravenous fluids. Vomiting should not be induced, and lavage should not be performed.

bleb /bleb/ [ME, blob], an accumulation of fluid under the skin.

bleed [AS, *blod,* blood], **1.** to lose blood from the blood vessels of the body. **2.** to cause blood to flow from a vein or an artery.

bleeder, *informal.* **1.** a person who has hemophilia or any other vascular or hematologic condition associated with a tendency to hemorrhage. **2.** a blood vessel that bleeds, especially one cut during a surgical procedure.

bleeding, the release of blood from the vascular system as a result of damage to a blood vessel.

bleeding diathesis, a predisposition to abnormal blood clotting.

Bleeding Precautions, a Nursing Interventions Classification defined as reduction of a stimulus that may induce bleeding or hemorrhage in at-risk patients.

Bleeding Reduction, a Nursing Interventions Classification defined as limitation of the loss of blood volume during an episode of bleeding.

Bleeding Reduction: Antepartum Uterus, a Nursing Interventions Classification defined as limitation of the amount of blood loss from the pregnant uterus during third trimester of pregnancy.

Bleeding Reduction: Gastrointestinal, a Nursing Interventions Classification defined as limitation of the amount of blood loss from the upper and lower gastrointestinal tract and related complications.

Bleeding Reduction: Nasal, a Nursing Interventions Classification defined as limitation of the amount of blood loss from the nasal cavity.

Bleeding Reduction: Postpartum Uterus, a Nursing Interventions Classification defined as limitation of the amount of blood loss from the postpartum uterus.

Bleeding Reduction: Wound, a Nursing Interventions Classification defined as limitation of the blood loss from a wound that may be a result of trauma, incisions, or placement of a tube or catheter.

bleeding time, the time required for blood to stop flowing from a tiny wound.

blemish [OFr, *bleme,* to deface], a skin stain, alteration, defect, or flaw.

blended family [ME, *blenden,* to mix], a family formed when parents bring together children from previous marriages.

blending inheritance, the apparent fusion in the offspring of distinct, dissimilar characteristics of the parents, usually of a quantitative nature, such as height, with segregation of the specific traits failing to appear in successive generations.

blennorrhea /blen′ərē′ə/ [Gk, *blennos,* mucus, *rhoia,* flow], excessive discharge of mucus.

bleomycin sulfate /blē-əmī′sin/, an antineoplastic antibiotic prescribed in the treatment of a variety of neoplasms.

blepharal /blef′ərəl/ [Gk, *blepharon,* eyelid], pertaining to the eyelids.

blepharedema /blef′əridē′mə/, a fluid accumulation in the eyelid, causing a swollen appearance.

blepharitis /blef′ərī′tis/ [Gk, *blepharon* + *itis*], an inflammatory condition of the lash follicles and meibomian glands of the eyelids, characterized by swelling, redness, and crusts of dried mucus on the lids. **Ulcerative blepharitis** is caused by bacterial infection. **Nonulcerative blepharitis** may be caused by psoriasis, seborrhea, or an allergic response.

blepharoadenoma /-ad′inō′mə/, a glandular epithelial tumor of the eyelid.

blepharoatheroma /-ath′ərō′mə/, a tumor of the eyelid.

blepharoclonus /blef′ərok′lōnəs/, a condition characterized by muscle spasms of the eyelid.

blepharoncus /blef′ərōn′kəs/ [Gk, *blepharon* + *onkos,* swelling], a tumor of the eyelid.

blepharoplasty /blef′əroplas′tē/ [Gk, *blepharon,* eyelid, *plassein,* to mold], the use of plastic surgery to restore or repair the eyelid and eyebrow.

blepharoplegia /-plē′jē·ə/ [Gk, *blepharon* + *plege,* stroke], paralysis of muscles of the eyelid.

blepharospasm /blef′ərōspaz′əm/ [Gk, *blepharon,* eyelid, *spasmos,* spasm],

the involuntary contraction of eyelid muscles.

Bleuler, Eugen /bloi′lər/ [Swiss psychiatrist, 1857–1939], a pioneer investigator in the fields of autism and schizophrenia. Bleuler introduced the term *schizophrenia* to replace *dementia praecox* and identified four primary symptoms of schizophrenia, known as Bleuler's "4 A's": ambivalence, associative disturbance, autistic thinking, and affective incongruity.

blighted ovum /blī′tid/, a fertilized ovum that fails to develop.

blind [AS, *blind*], the absence of sight. The term may indicate a total loss of vision or may be applied in a modified manner to describe certain visual limitations, as in yellow color blindness (tritanopia) or word blindness (dyslexia).

blind fistula [AS, *blind* + L, pipe], an abnormal passage with only one open end; the opening may be on the body surface or on or within an internal organ or structure.

blind loop [AS, *blind* + ME, *loupe*], a redundant segment of intestine. Blind loops may be created inadvertently by surgical procedures such as side-to-side ileotransverse colostomy.

blind spot, 1. a normal gap in the visual field occurring when an image is focused on the space in the retina occupied by the optic disc. **2.** an abnormal gap in the visual field caused by a lesion on the retina or in the optic pathways or resulting from hemorrhage or choroiditis, often perceived as light spots or flashes.

blink reflex [ME, *blenken* + L, *reflectere,* to bend back], the automatic closure of the eyelid when an object is perceived to be rapidly approaching the eye.

blister, a vesicle or bulla.

bloat [ME, *blout*], a swelling or filling with gas, such as distension of the abdomen that results from swallowed air or intestinal gas.

block [OFr, *bloc*], **1.** a stoppage or obstruction. The term is commonly used to indicate an obstruction to the passage of a nerve impulse, as an alpha block of an impulse on an alpha-adrenergic receptor or a beta block of an impulse to a beta-adrenergic receptor. **2.** an anesthetic injected in a local area, as a spinal block or mandibular block. **3.** a dental device, as a bite block.

blockade /blokād′/, an agent that interferes with or prevents a specific action in an organ or tissue, such as a cholinergic blockade that inhibits transmission of acetylcholine-stimulated nerve impulses along fibers of the autonomic nervous system.

blocked communication, a situation in

which communication with a patient is made difficult because of incongruent verbal and nonverbal messages and messages that contain discrepancies and inconsistencies.

blocking [ME, *blok*], **1.** preventing the transmission of an impulse, such as by the injection of an anesthetic. **2.** interrupting an intracellular biosynthetic process, such as by the action of an antivitamin. **3.** an interruption in the spontaneous flow of speech or thought. **4.** repressing an idea or emotion to prevent it from obtruding into the consciousness.

blocking agent, a substance administered systemically that blocks or diminishes synaptic efficiency. It is usually specific, as with a beta-adrenergic blocking agent.

blocking antibody, an antibody that fails to cross-link and cause agglutination.

blood [AS, *blod*], the liquid pumped by the heart through all the arteries, veins, and capillaries. The blood is composed of a clear yellow fluid called plasma, the formed elements, and a series of cell types with different functions. The major function of the blood is to transport oxygen and nutrients to the cells and to remove carbon dioxide and other waste products from the cells for detoxification and elimination.

blood agar, a culture medium consisting of blood and nutrient agar, used in bacteriology to cultivate certain microorganisms, including *Staphylococcus epidermidis*, *Diplococcus pneumoniae*, and *Clostridium perfringens*.

blood albumin [AS, *blod* + L, *albus*], the plasma protein circulating in blood serum.

blood bank, an organizational unit responsible for collecting, processing, and storing blood for transfusion and other purposes. The blood bank is usually a subdivision of a laboratory in a hospital and is often charged with the responsibility for serologic testing.

blood bank technology specialist, an allied health professional who performs both routine and specialized immunohematologic tests in technical areas of the modern blood bank and who performs transfusion services using methodology that conforms to the *Standards for Blood Banks and Transfusion Services* of the American Association of Blood Banks.

blood-borne pathogens, pathogenic microorganisms that are present in human blood and cause disease in humans. They include, but are not limited to, hepatitis B virus and human immunodeficiency virus.

blood-brain barrier (BBB) [AS, *blod* + *bragen* + ME, *barrere*], an anatomic-physiologic feature of the brain thought to consist of walls of capillaries in the central nervous system and surrounding astrocytic glial membranes. The blood-brain barrier prevents or slows the passage of some drugs and other chemical compounds, radioactive ions, and disease-causing organisms such as viruses from the blood into the central nervous system.

blood buffers [AS, *blod* + ME, *buffe*, to cushion], a system of buffers, composed primarily of dissolved carbon dioxide and bicarbonate ions, that functions in maintaining the proper pH of the blood.

blood capillaries [AS, *blod* + L, *capillaris*, hairlike], the tiny vessels that convey blood between the arterioles and the venules and allow for internal respiration and nourishment of tissues.

blood cell, any of the formed elements of the blood, including red cells (erythrocytes), white cells (leukocytes), and platelets (thrombocytes). Blood cells constitute about 50% of the total volume of the blood.

blood cell casts [AS, *blod* + L, *cella*, storeroom; ONorse, *kasta*], a mass of blood debris released from a diseased body surface or excreted in the urine.

blood circulation [AS, *blod* + L, *circulare*, to go around], the circuit of blood through the body, from the heart through the arteries, arterioles, capillaries, venules, and veins and back to the heart.

blood clot [AS, *blod* + *clott*, lump], a semisolid, gelatinous mass, the final result of the clotting process in blood. Red cells, white cells, and platelets are enmeshed in an insoluble fibrin network of the blood clot.

blood clotting, the conversion of blood from a free-flowing liquid to a semisolid gel. The process usually starts with tissue damage. Within seconds of injury to the vessel wall, platelets clump at the site. If normal amounts of calcium, platelets, and tissue factors are present, prothrombin is converted to thrombin. Thrombin acts as a catalyst for the conversion of fibrinogen to a mesh of insoluble fibrin, in which all the formed elements are immobilized.

blood crossmatching, the direct matching of donor and recipient blood to prevent the transfusion of incompatible blood types. Crossmatching tests for agglutination of (1) donor red blood cells (RBCs) by recipient serum, and (2) recipient RBCs by donor serum.

blood culture medium, a liquid enrichment medium for the growth of bacteria in the diagnosis of blood infections.

blood donor, anyone who donates blood or blood components.

blood dyscrasia [AS, *blod* + Gk, *dys,* bad, *krasis,* mingling], a pathologic condition in which any of the constituents of the blood are abnormal in structure, function, or quality, as in leukemia or hemophilia.

blood fluke, a parasitic flatworm of the class Trematoda, genus *Schistosoma,* including the species *S. haematobium, S. japonicum,* and *S. mansoni.*

blood gas, gas dissolved in the liquid part of the blood. Blood gases include oxygen, carbon dioxide, and nitrogen.

blood gas determination, an analysis of the pH of the blood and the concentration and pressure of oxygen, carbon dioxide, and hydrogen ions in the blood. It can be performed as an emergency procedure to assess acid-base balance and ventilatory status.

blood gas tension, the partial pressure of a gas in the blood.

blood group, the classification of blood based on the presence or absence of genetically determined antigens on the surface of the red cell. Several different grouping systems have been described. These include ABO, Duffy, high-frequency antigens, I, Kell, Kidd, Lewis, low-frequency antigens, Lutheran, MNS, P, Rh, and Xg.

blood island, one of the clusters of mesodermal cells that proliferate on the outer surface of the embryonic yolk sac and give it a lumpy appearance.

blood lactate, lactic acid that appears in the blood as a result of anaerobic metabolism when oxygen delivery to the tissues is insufficient to support normal metabolic demands.

blood lavage [AS, *blod* + L, *lavere,* to wash], the removal of toxic elements from the blood by the injection of serum into the veins.

bloodless, **1.** any organ or body part that lacks blood or appears to lack blood. **2.** a surgical field in which the normal local blood supply has been shunted to other areas.

bloodless phlebotomy [AS, *blod* + ME, *les* + Gk, *phleps,* vein, *tomos,* cutting], a technique of trapping blood in a body region by the application of tourniquet pressure that is less than the pressure needed to interrupt arterial blood flow.

bloodletting, the therapeutic opening of an artery or vein to withdraw blood from a particular area. It is sometimes performed to treat polycythemia and congestive heart failure.

blood level, the concentration of a drug or other substance in a measured amount of plasma, serum, or whole blood.

blood level of glucose [AS, *blod* + OFr,

livel + Gk, *glykys,* sweet], the amount of glucose found in the bloodstream, usually about 70 to 115 mg/dl. Concentrations higher or lower than these can be a sign of a variety of diseases such as diabetes mellitus or pancreatic cancer.

blood osmolality [AS, *blod* + Gk, *osmos,* impulsion], the osmotic pressure of blood. The normal values in serum are 280 to 295 mOsm/L.

blood pH, the hydrogen ion concentration of the blood, a measure of blood acidity or alkalinity. The normal pH values for arterial whole blood are 7.35 to 7.454; for venous whole blood, 7.36 to 7.41; for venous serum or plasma, 7.35 to 7.45.

blood plasma [AS, *blod* + Gk, *plassein,* to mold], the liquid part of the blood, free of its formed elements and particles. Plasma represents approximately 50% of the total volume of blood and contains glucose, proteins, amino acids, and other nutritive materials; urea and other excretory products; and hormones, enzymes, vitamins, and minerals.

blood poisoning. See septicemia.

blood pressure (BP) [AS, *blod* + L, *premere,* to press], the pressure exerted by the circulating volume of blood on the walls of the arteries and veins and on the chambers of the heart. Overall blood pressure is maintained by the complex interaction of the homeostatic mechanisms of the body, moderated by the volume of the blood, the lumen of the arteries and arterioles, and the force of the cardiac contraction. The pressure in the aorta and large arteries of a healthy young adult is approximately 120 mm Hg during systole and 70 mm Hg in diastole. The pulse pressure is approximately 50 mm Hg.

blood pressure monitor [AS, *blod* + L, *premere,* to press, *monere,* to warn], a device that automatically measures blood pressure and records the information continuously. Automatic monitoring of blood pressure is often used in surgery or in an intensive care unit.

Blood Products Administration, a Nursing Interventions Classification defined as administration of blood or blood products and monitoring of patient's response.

blood proteins, [AS, *blod* + Gk, *proteios,* of first rank], the proteins normally in the blood, such as albumin, globulin, hemoglobin, and proteins bound to hormones or other compounds.

blood pump, **1.** a device for regulating the flow of blood into a blood vessel during transfusion. **2.** a component of a heart-lung machine that pumps the blood through the machine for oxygenation and then through the peripheral circulatory system of the body.

blood relative, a related person who shares some of the same genetic material through a common ancestry. Every man and woman is heterozygous for six to eight alleles that could lead to an offspring with a genetically determined disease. In first-cousin marriages, 1:8 of the genes are shared, and the risk of a genetically determined disease is between 3% and 5%, compared with 2% in marriages between a man and woman who are not blood relatives.

bloodshot, a redness of the conjunctiva or sclera of the eye caused by dilation of blood vessels in the tissues.

blood smear, a small specimen of blood that is spread onto a glass microscope slide for examination.

bloodstream, the blood that flows freely through the circulatory system.

blood substitute, a substance used for a replacement or volume expansion for circulating blood. Plasma, human serum albumin, packed red cells, platelets, leukocytes, and concentrates of clotting factors are often administered in place of whole blood transfusions in the treatment of various disorders. Substances that are sometimes used to expand blood volume include dextran, hetastarch, albumin solutions, or plasma protein fraction.

blood sugar, **1.** one of a group of closely related substances such as glucose, fructose, and galactose that are normal constituents of the blood and essential for cellular metabolism. **2.** *nontechnical.* the concentration of glucose in the blood, represented in milligrams of glucose per deciliter of blood.

blood test, any test that yields information about the characteristics or properties of the blood.

blood transfusion [AS, *blod* + L *transfundere,* to pour through], the administration of whole blood or a component, such as packed red cells, to replace blood lost through trauma, surgery, or disease. Blood for transfusion is obtained from a healthy donor or donors whose ABO blood group and antigenic subgroups match those of the recipient and who have an adequate hemoglobin level (above 13.5 g/100 ml for men and above 12.5 g/100 ml for women). Each 500 ml of blood collected from a donor is stored in a plastic bag containing citrate-dextrose or citrate-phosphate. A unit can be stored under refrigeration for only 3 weeks; at that time the leukocytes, platelets, and 20% to 30% of the red cells are nonviable, and the levels of clotting factors V and VIII are low.

blood typing, identification of genetically determined antigens on the surface of the red blood cell used to determine blood groups. Usually a blood bank procedure, typing is the first step in testing blood to be used in transfusion and is followed by crossmatching.

blood urea nitrogen (BUN) [AS, *blod* + Gk, *ouron,* urine, *nitron,* soda, *genein,* to produce], the most prevalent of nonprotein nitrogenous compounds in blood. Urea forms in the liver as the end product of protein metabolism, circulates in the blood, and is excreted through the kidney in urine. The BUN, determined by a blood test, is directly related to the metabolic function of the liver and the excretory function of the kidney.

blood vessel, any one of the network of muscular tubes that carry blood. Kinds of blood vessels are **arteries, arterioles, capillaries, veins,** and **venules.**

blood warming coil, a device constructed of coiled plastic tubing used for the warming of reserve blood for massive transfusions, such as those often required for patients who experience extensive gastrointestinal bleeding.

bloody sputum [AS, *blod* + L, *sputum,* spittle], blood-tinged material expelled from the respiratory passages. The amount and color of blood in sputum expelled by coughing or clearing the throat may indicate the cause and location of the bleeding.

Bloom's syndrome [David Bloom, American physician, b. 1892], a rare genetic disease occurring mainly in Ashkenazi Jews. It is transmitted as an autosomal-recessive trait and is characterized by growth retardation, dilated capillaries of the face and arms, sensitivity to sunlight, and an increased risk of leukemia.

blot, **1.** a technique for transfer of electrophoretically separated components from a gel onto a nitrocellulose membrane, chemically treated paper, or filter for analysis. **2.** the substrate containing the transferred material.

blotch, a skin discoloration that may vary in severity from an area of pigmentation to large pustules or blisters.

blow bottles, a device used in respiratory care to provide resistance to expiration. The bottles are partially filled with water, and the patient is encouraged to blow the water from one bottle to another.

blow-out fracture, a fracture of the floor of the orbit caused by a blow that suddenly increases the intraocular pressure.

BLS, abbreviation for **basic life support.**

blue baby [OFr, *blou* + ME, *babe*], an infant born with cyanosis caused by a congenital heart lesion such as transposition of the great vessels, tetralogy of Fallot, or incomplete expansion of the lungs (congenital atelectasis).

Blue Cross, an independent nonprofit U.S. corporation that functions as a health insurance agency, providing protection for an enrolled patient by covering all or part of the person's hospital expenses. Blue Cross programs vary in different communities because of state laws regulating them.

blue dome cyst, a spheric dilation of a mammary duct in which bleeding has occurred.

blue dot sign, a tender blue or black spot beneath the skin of the testis or epididymis, a sign of testicular torsion of the appendix testis.

blue fever, *informal.* Rocky Mountain spotted fever, so named for the dark cyanotic discoloration of the skin after the initial rickettsial infection.

blue line, a bluish discoloration sometimes observed on the gingival side of the mouth in cases of gingivitis. It is a sign of chronic lead or bismuth poisoning.

blue nevus [OFr, *blou* + L, *naevus,* mole], a sharply circumscribed, usually benign, steel blue skin nodule. It is found on the face or upper extremities, grows very slowly, and persists throughout life. The dark color is caused by large, densely packed melanocytes deep in the dermis of the nevus. Any sudden change in the size of such a lesion demands surgical attention and biopsy.

Blue Shield, an independent nonprofit U.S. corporation that offers patient protection for costs of surgery and other medical services. Although Blue Cross and Blue Shield are technically separate organizations, they generally coordinate their functions in providing benefits covering both hospital costs and physician fees.

blue spot, 1. one of a number of small, grayish-blue spots that may appear near the armpits or around the groins of individuals infested with lice. **2.** one of a number of dark blue round or oval spots that may appear as a congenital condition in the sacral regions of certain children less than 4 or 5 years of age. They usually disappear spontaneously as the affected individual matures.

blunt dissection [ME, *blunt* + L, *dissecare,* to cut apart], a dissection performed by separating tissues along natural lines of cleavage without cutting.

blunt-ended DNA, a double strand of deoxyribonucleic acid in which one or more of the ends have no unpaired bases.

blunthook /blunt′hŏŏk/ [ME, *blunt* + AS,

hoc], **1.** a sturdy hook-shaped bar used in obstetrics for traction between the abdomen and the thigh in cases of difficult breech deliveries. **2.** a hook-shaped device with a blunt end used in embryotomy.

blunting, a decrease in the intensity of emotional expression from the level one would normally expect as a reaction to a specific situation.

blurred film fault /blurd′/, a defect in a photograph or radiograph that appears as an indistinct or blurred image.

blush [ME, *blusshen,* to redden], a brief, diffuse erythema of the face and neck, commonly the result of dilation of superficial small blood vessels in response to heat or sudden emotion.

B/M, abbreviation for *black male,* often used in the initial identifying statement in a patient record.

BMA, abbreviation for **British Medical Association.**

BMD, abbreviation for **Bureau of Medical Devices.**

BMI, abbreviation for **body mass index.**

B-mode, brightness modulation, an imaging technique used in ultrasound scanning in which bright dots on an oscilloscope screen represent echoes and the intensity of the brightness indicates the strength of the echo.

BMR, abbreviation for **basal metabolic rate.**

BNA, abbreviation for *Basle Nomina Anatomica.*

BOA, abbreviation for **born out of asepsis.**

board certification, a process by which physicians are certified in a given medical specialty or subspecialty. Certification is awarded by the 23-member boards of the American Board of Medical Specialties on completion of accredited training and examinations and fulfillment of individual requirements of the board.

board certified, denoting a physician who has completed the certification requirements established by a medical specialty board and has been certified as a specialist in a particular field of medicine.

board eligible, denoting a physician who has completed all of the requirements for admission to a medical specialty board.

boarder baby, an infant abandoned to a hospital because the mother is unable to care for him or her. Many boarder babies are infants born with human immunodeficiency virus (HIV) or to a mother with HIV infection or delivered to mothers who are drug users.

board of health, an administrative body acting on a municipal, county, state, provincial, or national level. Among the tasks

of most boards of health are disease prevention, health education, and implementation of laws pertaining to health.

Boas' test /bō'az/ [Ismar I. Boas, German physician, 1858–1938], **1.** a test for hydrochloric acid in the contents of the stomach. **2.** a test for free hydrochloric acid in the contents of the stomach in which filtered stomach fluid is boiled with a special reagent. **3.** a test for lactic acid in a sample of gastric juice that depends on the oxidation of the lactic acid to aldehyde and formic acid by sulfuric acid and manganese. **4.** a test for gastric motility in which a fasting patient drinks 400 ml of water that has been tinted green by the addition of 20 drops of chlorophyll solution.

bobbing, the act of moving up and down, usually with a jerking motion.

Bodansky unit [Aaron Bodansky, American biochemist, 1887–1961], the quantity of phosphatase in 100 ml of serum needed to liberate 1 mg of phosphorus as phosphate ion from sodium betaglycerophosphate in 1 hour at 37° C. It is used to express the level of certain enzymes, such as acid phosphatase, in the body.

body [AS, *bodig*], **1.** the whole structure of an individual with all the organs. **2.** a cadaver (corpse). **3.** the largest or main part of any structure, such as the body of the stomach.

body burden, the state of activity of a radioactive chemical in the body at a specified time after administration.

body cast [AS, *bodig,* body; ONorse, *kasta*], a molded cast that may extend from the chest to the groin to immobilize the spine.

body cavity, any of the spaces in the human body that contain organs.

body composition, the relative proportions of protein, fat, water, and mineral components in the body. It varies among individuals as a result of differences in body density and degree of obesity. Methods for calculating body composition include underwater weighing and injection of radioactive tracers.

body fluid [AS, *bodig* + L, *fluere,* to flow], fluid contained in the three fluid compartments of the body: the plasma of the circulating blood, the interstitial fluid between the cells, and the cell fluid within the cells.

body image [AS, *bodig* + L, *imago,* likeness], a person's concept of his or her physical appearance. The mental representation, which may be realistic or unrealistic, is constructed from self-observation, the reactions of others, and a complex interaction of attitudes, emotions, memories, fantasies, and experiences, both conscious and unconscious.

body image disturbance, a NANDA-accepted nursing diagnosis of a disruption in the way one perceives one's body. The cause of a disturbance in body image may be a biophysical, cognitive, perceptual, psychosocial, cultural, or spiritual factor. Defining characteristics include verbal or nonverbal responses to a real or perceived change in structure or function, a missing body part, personalization of the missing part by giving it a name, refusal to look at a part of the body, negative feelings about the body, a change in general social involvement or life-style, and a fear of rejection by others.

Body Image Enhancement, a Nursing Interventions Classification defined as improving a patient's conscious and unconscious perceptions and attitudes toward his or her body.

body jacket, an orthopedic cast that encases the trunk of the body but does not extend over the cervical area. It is used to help position and immobilize the trunk for the healing of spinal injuries and scoliosis and after spinal surgery.

body language [AS, *bodig* + L, *lingua,* tongue], a set of nonverbal signals, including body movements, postures, gestures, spatial positions, facial expressions, and body adornment, that give expression to various physical, mental, and emotional states.

body mass index (BMI), a formula for determining obesity. It is calculated by dividing a person's weight in kilograms by the square of the person's height in meters.

body mechanics, the field of physiology that studies muscular actions and the function of muscles in maintaining the posture of the body.

Body Mechanics Promotion, a Nursing Interventions Classification defined as facilitating the use of posture and movement in daily activities to prevent fatigue and musculoskeletal strain or injury.

body movement, motion of all or part of the body, especially at a joint or joints. Some kinds of body movements are **abduction, adduction, extension, flexion,** and **rotation.**

body odor, a fetid smell associated with stale perspiration. Freshly secreted perspiration is odorless, but after exposure to the atmosphere and bacterial activity at the surface of the skin, chemical changes occur to produce the odor.

body of Retzius /ret'sē·əs/ [Magnus G. Retzius, Swedish anatomist, 1842–1919], any one of the masses of protoplasm containing pigment granules at the lower end of a hair cell of the organ of Corti in the internal ear.

body plethysmograph [AS, *bodig* + Gk, *plethynein,* to increase, *graphein* to record], a device for studying alveolar pressures, lung volumes, and airway resistance. The patient sits or reclines in an airtight compartment and breathes normally. The pressure changes in the alveoli are reciprocated in the compartment and recorded automatically.

body position, attitude or posture of the body. Some body positions are **anatomic, decubitus, Fowler's, prone, supine,** and **Trendelenburg.**

body scheme, a piagetian term for a cognitive structure that develops in infants in the sensorimotor period during the first 2 years of life as they learn to differentiate between themselves and the world around them.

body-section radiography, a radiographic technique used to produce a more distinct image of a selected body plane by moving the film and x-ray tube in opposite directions.

body stalk, the elongated part of the embryo that is connected to the chorion. See also **allantois.**

body systems model, (in nursing education) a conceptual framework in which illness is studied in relation to the functional systems of the body. In this model, nursing care is directed to manipulating the patient's environment in such a way that the signs and symptoms of the health problem are alleviated.

body temperature, the level of heat produced and sustained by the body processes. Variations and changes in body temperature are major indicators of disease and other abnormalities. Heat is generated within the body through metabolism of food and lost from the body surface through radiation, convection, and evaporation of perspiration. Heat production and loss are regulated and controlled in the hypothalamus and brainstem. Diseases of the hypothalamus or interference with the other regulatory centers may produce abnormally low body temperatures. Normal adult body temperature, as measured orally, is 98.6° F (37° C). Oral temperatures ranging from 96.5° F to 99° F are consistent with good health, depending on the person's physical activity, the environmental temperature, and that person's usual body temperature. Axillary temperature is usually 1° F lower than the oral temperature. Rectal temperatures may be 0.5° to 1° F higher than oral readings. Body temperature appears to vary 1° to 2° F throughout the day, with lows recorded early in the morning and peaks between 6 and 10 PM.

body temperature, altered, risk for, a NANDA-accepted nursing diagnosis of a state in which the individual is at risk for failure to maintain body temperature within a normal range. Risk factors include extremes of age or weight; exposure to cool-to-cold or warm-to-hot environments; dehydration; inactivity or vigorous activity; medications causing vasoconstriction or vasodilation; altered metabolic rate; sedation; clothing inappropriate for environmental temperature; and illness or trauma affecting temperature regulations.

body type, the general physical appearance of an individual human body. Three commonly used terms for body types are ectomorph, endomorph, and mesomorph.

body-weight ratio, a relation expressed by dividing the body weight in grams by the height in centimeters.

Boerhaave's syndrome /bôr'hävz/ [Hermann Boerhaave, Dutch physician, 1668–1738], a condition marked by spontaneous rupture of the esophagus, leading to mediastinitis and pleural effusion. Clinical manifestations are violent wretching or vomiting. Emergency care with surgery and drainage is needed to save the life of the patient.

Bohr effect [Christian Bohr, Danish physiologist, 1855–1911], the effect of CO_2 and H^+ on the affinity of hemoglobin for molecular O_2. Increasing PCO_2 and H^+ decrease oxyhemoglobin saturation, whereas decreasing concentrations have the opposite effect.

bohrium (Bh). See **element 107.**

boil [AS, *byle,* sore], a skin abscess.

boiling point [ME, *boilen,* to make bubbles; L, *pungere,* to prick], **1.** the temperature at which a substance passes from the liquid to the gaseous state at a particular atmospheric pressure. **2.** the temperature at which the vapor pressure of a liquid equals the external pressure.

bole /bōl/, any of a variety of soft, friable clays of various colors, although usually red from iron oxide. They consist of hydrous silicate of aluminum, are used as pigments, and were once commonly used as absorbents and astringents.

Bolivian hemorrhagic fever /bəliv'ē·ən/, an infectious disease caused by an arenavirus, generally transmitted from infected rodents to humans through contamination of food by rodent urine. The patient experiences chills, fever, headache, muscle ache, anorexia, nausea, and vomiting.

bolus /bō'ləs/ [Gk, *bolos,* lump], **1.** a round mass, specifically a masticated lump of food ready to be swallowed. **2.** a large round preparation of medicinal material for oral ingestion, usually soft and not prepackaged. **3.** a dose of a medication or a contrast material, radioactive isotope, or other pharmaceutic preparation injected all at once intravenously. **4.** (in radiotherapy) material used to fill in irregular body surfaces to improve dose distribution for hyperthermia or to increase the dose to the skin when high-energy photon beams are used. **5.** a clumping in the stomach of ingested foreign material, often the result of habitual behavior.

bolus dose, a relatively large amount of intravenous medication administered rapidly to decrease the response time.

bombard /bämbärd'/, to shower a drug or tissue sample with radioactive particles from a nuclear isotope source.

Bombay phenotype /bombā'/ [Bombay, India, where first reported], a rare genetic trait involving the phenotypic expression of the ABO blood groups. Cells of such individuals are phenotypically of blood type O, and the serum contains anti-A, anti-B, and anti-H antigens.

bond, a strong coulombic force between atoms in a substance.

bonding [ME, *band,* to bind], the attachment process that occurs between an infant and the parents, especially the mother, and is significant in the formation of affectionate ties that later influence both the physical and psychologic development of the child. Perhaps the most important actions for forming positive parent-child attachment are eye contact in the face position and embracing of the infant close to the body.

bonding, (in dentistry) a technique of joining orthodontic brackets or other attachments directly to the enamel surface of a tooth, using orthodontic adhesives.

bond specificity, the nature of enzyme action that causes the disruption of only certain bonds between atoms.

bone [AS, *ban*], **1.** the dense, hard, and somewhat flexible connective tissue constituting the bones of the human skeleton. It is composed of compact osseous tissue surrounding spongy cancellous tissue permeated by many blood vessels and nerves and enclosed in membranous periosteum. **2.** any single element of the skeleton such as a rib, the sternum, or the femur.

bone age [AS, *ban* + L, *aetas*], the stage of development or decline of the skeleton or its segments, as seen in radiographic examination, when compared with x-ray views of the bone structures of other individuals of the same chronologic age.

bone cancer [AS, *ban* + Gk, *karkinos,* crab], a skeletal malignancy occurring as a sarcoma or a myeloma in an area of rapid growth or as metastasis from cancer

elsewhere in the body. Primary bone tumors are rare; the incidence peaks during adolescence, decreases, and then rises slowly after 35 years of age. In adults, bone cancer is linked to exposure to ionizing radiation. Paget's disease, hyperparathyroidism, chronic osteomyelitis, old bone infarcts, and fracture callosities increase the risk of many bone tumors. Most osseous malignancies are metastatic lesions found most often in the spine or pelvis and less often in sites away from the trunk. Bone cancers progress rapidly but are often difficult to detect.

bone cell [AS, *ban* + L, *cella,* storeroom], an osteocyte, a cell with myriad spidery processes embedded in the matrix of bone.

bone cutting forceps, a kind of forceps that has long handles, single or double joints, and heavy blades.

bone cyst [AS, *ban* + Gk, *kytis,* cyst], **1.** an aneurysmal vascular bone cyst, usually eccentrically placed. **2.** osteitis fibrosa cystica, a parathyroid disorder characterized by cyst formation and replacement of bone by fibrous tissue.

bone densitometry, any of several methods of determining bone mass loss by measuring radiation absorption by the skeleton. Common techniques include single-photon absorptiometry of the forearm and heel, dual-photon absorptiometry and dual-energy x-ray absorptiometry of the spine and hip, quantitative computed tomography of the spine and forearm, and radiographic absorptiometry of the hand.

bone graft, the transplantation of a piece of bone from one part of the body to another to repair a skeletal defect.

bone lamella [AS, *ban,* bone, *lamella,* plate], a thin plate of bone matrix, a basic structural unit of mature bone.

bone marrow [AS, *ban* + ME, *marowe*], specialized, semiliquid tissue filling the spaces in cancellous bone of the epiphyses. **Red marrow** is found in many bones of infants and children and in the spongy (cancellous) bone of the proximal epiphyses of the humerus and femur and the sternum, ribs, and vertebral bodies of adults. It is known as myeloid tissue and is essential in the manufacture and maturation of red blood cells, most white blood cells, and platelets. Fatty **yellow marrow** is found in the medullary cavity of most adult long bones.

bone marrow infusion, a method of injecting a fluid substance through an aspiration needle directly into the marrow cavity of a long bone. The substance is absorbed into the general circulation almost immediately.

bone marrow transplant, the transplantation of bone marrow from healthy donors to stimulate production of formed blood cells. The bone marrow is removed from the donor by aspiration and infused intravenously into the recipient.

bone plate [AS, *ban,* bone; OFr, *plate*], a metal plate used to reconstruct a bone that has been fractured. The plate is designed to hold fragments in apposition.

bone recession [AS, *ban* + L, *recedere,* recede], apical progression of the level of the alveolar crest, associated with inflammatory or dystrophic periodontal disease and resulting in decreased bone support for the teeth.

bone scan, the injection of a radioactive substance to enable visualization of a bone via the image produced by emission of radioactive particles.

bone tissue [AS, *ban* + OFr, *tissu*], a hard form of connective tissue composed of osteocytes and a calcified collagenous intercellular substance arranged in thin plates.

Bonwill's triangle [William G.A. Bonwill, American dentist, 1833–1899], an equilateral triangle with 4-inch (10-cm) sides formed by lines from the contact points of the lower central incisors (or the median line of the residual ridge of the mandible) to the condyle on each side and from one condyle to the other.

bony landmark [AS, *ban* + AS, *land, mearc*], a groove or prominence on a bone that serves as a guide to the location of other body structures.

bony thorax [AS, *ban* + Gk, *thorax,* chest], the skeletal part of the chest, including the thoracic vertebrae, ribs, and sternum.

booster injection, the administration of an antigen, such as a vaccine or toxoid, usually in a smaller amount than the original immunization. It is given to maintain the immune response at an appropriate level.

boot, 1. a shoelike prosthetic device for holding a leg or arm during treatment. 2. a basketweave bandage that covers the foot and lower leg. 3. an airtight device in which the arm or leg can be inserted and the air pumped out, creating a partial vacuum to divert blood flow from the surrounding area.

Boothby-Lovelace-Bulbulian   (BLB) mask, an apparatus for the administration of oxygen consisting of a mask fitted with an inspiratory-expiratory valve and a rebreathing bag.

borate /bôr′āt/, any salt of boric acid. Borate salts and boric acid, although formerly used as mild antiseptic irrigant solutions, especially for ophthalmic conditions, are highly poisonous when taken internally or absorbed through a cut, abrasion, or other wound in the skin. Because of the potential for fatal poisoning, such solutions are rarely used now.

borax bath [Ar, *bauraq* + AS, *baeth*], a medicated bath in which borax and glycerin are added to the water.

borborygmus /bôr′bərig′məs/, *pl.,* **borborygmi** [Gk, *borborygmos,* bowel rumbling], an audible abdominal sound produced by hyperactive intestinal peristalsis. Borborygmi are rumbling, gurgling, and tinkling noises heard in auscultation.

border [OFr, *bordure*], an edge or boundary of a body structure.

borderline [OFr, *bordure* + L, *linea*], pertaining to a state of health in which the patient has some of the signs and symptoms of a disease but not enough to justify a definite diagnosis.

borderline personality [OFr, *bordure* + L, *linea* + *personalis*], a personality in which there is a pervasive pattern of instability of self-image, interpersonal relationships, and mood.

Bordetella /bôr′ditel′ə/ [Jules J.B.V. Bordet, Belgian bacteriologist, 1870–1961], a genus of gram-negative coccobacilli, some species of which are pathogens of the respiratory tract of humans, including *Bordetella bronchiseptica, B. parapertussis,* and *B. pertussis.*

boric acid /bôr′ik/, a white, odorless powder or crystalline substance used as a buffer and formerly used as a topical antiseptic and eyewash.

boric acid poisoning, an adverse reaction to the ingestion or absorption through the skin of boric acid, a mild but potentially lethal antiseptic. Symptoms include nausea, vomiting, diarrhea, convulsions, and shock. Emergency first aid measures include inducing vomiting with ipecac and administering large amounts of water. Dialysis may be required in severe cases. Absorption of boric acid from diapers is a threat to infants.

born out of asepsis (BOA), (in a hospital) denoting a newborn who was not delivered in the usual place in an obstetric unit. Depending on the policy of the institution, a BOA-designated infant may have been born on the way to the hospital or in the hospital, on the way to the delivery suite, or in a labor room.

boron (B) /bôr′on/, a nonmetallic element, similar to aluminum. Its atomic number is 5; its atomic weight (mass) is 10.81. Elemental boron occurs in the form of dark crystals and as a greenish-yellow amorphous mass. Certain concentrations of this element are toxic to plant and animal life, but plants need traces of boron for normal growth.

Borrelia /bərel′ē·ə/ [Amédée Borrel, French bacteriologist, 1867–1936], a genus of coarse, unevenly coiled helical spirochetes, several species of which cause tickborne and louseborne relapsing fever. Many animals serve as reservoirs and hosts for *Borrelia*.

Borrelia burgdorferi /burg′dôrfer′ī/, the etiologic agent in Lyme disease. The organism is transmitted to humans by tick vectors, primarily *Ixodes dammini*.

boss [ME, *boce*], a swelling, eminence, or protuberance on an organ, such as a tumor or overgrowth on a bone surface.

Boston exanthem [Boston; Gk, *ex*, out, *anthema*, blossoming], an epidemic disease characterized by scattered, pale red maculopapules on the face, chest, and back, occasionally accompanied by small ulcerations on the tonsils and soft palate. It is caused by echovirus 16 and requires no treatment.

bottle feeding, [OFr, *bouteille* + AS, *faeden*], feeding an infant or young child from a bottle with a rubber nipple on the end as a substitute for or supplement to breastfeeding.

Bottle Feeding, a Nursing Interventions Classification defined as preparation and administration of fluids to an infant via a bottle.

botulinus toxin /boch′əlī′nəs/ [L, *botulus,* sausage; Gk, *toxikon,* poison], any of a group of potent bacterial toxins produced by different strains of *Clostridium botulinum.* The strains are sometimes identified by letters of the alphabet such as A, B, or C.

botulism /boch′əliz′əm/ [L, *botulus,* sausage], an often fatal form of food poisoning caused by an endotoxin produced by the bacillus *Clostridium botulinum.* The toxin is ingested in food contaminated by *C. botulinum,* although it is not necessary for the live bacillus to be present if the toxin has been produced. In rare instances the toxin may be introduced into the human body through a wound contaminated by the organism. Botulism differs from most other types of food poisoning in that it develops without gastric distress and occurs from 18 hours up to 1 week after the contaminated food has been ingested. Botulism is characterized by lassitude, fatigue, and visual disturbances, such as double vision, difficulty in focusing the eyes, and loss of ability of the pupil to accommodate to light. Muscles may become weak, and dysphagia often develops.

Bouchard's node /bŌ̄oshärz′/ [Charles J.

Bouchard, French physician, 1837–1915], an abnormal cartilaginous or bony enlargement of a proximal interphalangeal joint of a finger, usually occurring in degenerative diseases of the joints.

Bouchut's tubes [Jean E.W. Bouchut, French physician, 1818–1891], a set of short cylindric devices used for intubation of the larynx.

bougie /bŌ̄ozhē, bŌ̄ozhē′/ [Fr, candle], a thin cylindric instrument made of rubber, waxed silk, or other flexible material for insertion into canals of the body in order to dilate, examine, or measure them.

boundary /boun′dərē/, (in psychology) an aspect of family health in which the generations are clearly defined and issues dealt with by the appropriate generation.

boundary lubrication, a coating of a thin layer of molecules on each weight-bearing surface of a joint to facilitate a sliding action by the opposing bone surfaces.

boundary maintenance mechanisms, (in psychology) behavior and practices that exclude members of some groups from the customs and values of another group.

bound carbon dioxide, carbon dioxide that is transported in the bloodstream as part of a sodium bicarbonate molecule, as distinguished from dissolved carbon dioxide or bicarbonate ion.

bounding pulse [OFr, *bondir,* to leap; L, *pulsare,* to beat], a pulse that feels full and springlike on palpation as a result of an increased thrust of cardiac contraction or an increased volume of circulating blood within the elastic structures of the vascular system.

Bourdon regulator, a commonly used adjustable mechanism with an attached pressure gauge for cylinders of oxygen or other gases in medical applications.

bouton /bootôn′/ [Fr, button], **1.** a knoblike swelling, such as the expanded end of an axon at a synapse. **2.** a lesion associated with cutaneous leishmaniasis. **3.** a small abscess of the intestinal mucosa in amebic dysentery.

boutonneuse fever /bŌ̄otənŌ̄oz′/ [Fr, *bouton,* button; L, *febris*], an infectious disease caused by *Rickettsia conorii,* transmitted to humans through the bite of a tick. The onset of the disease is characterized by a lesion called a *tache noire* /täshnô·är′/, or black spot, at the site of the infection; fever lasting from a few days to 2 weeks; and a papular erythematous rash that spreads over the body to include the skin of the palms and soles.

boutonnière deformity /bŌ̄otônyer′/ [Fr, buttonhole], an abnormality of a finger marked by the fixed flexion of the proximal interphalangeal joint and the hyperextension of the distal interphalangeal joint.

bovine tuberculosis /bō'vīn/ [L, *bos,* ox, *tuber,* swelling; Gk, *osis,* condition], a form of tuberculosis caused by *Mycobacterium tuberculosis* that primarily affects cattle. Mastitis and pulmonary symptoms can occur.

bowel bypass syndrome, a series of adverse effects that may follow bowel bypass surgery, including chills; fever; joint pain; and skin inflammation on the arms, legs, and thorax.

Bowel Incontinence Care, a Nursing Interventions Classification defined as promotion of bowel continence and maintenance of perianal skin integrity.

Bowel Incontinence Care: Encopresis, a Nursing Interventions Classification defined as promotion of bowel continence in children.

Bowel Irrigation, a Nursing Interventions Classification defined as instillation of a substance into the lower gastrointestinal tract.

Bowel Management, a Nursing Interventions Classification defined as establishment and maintenance of a regular pattern of bowel elimination.

bowel training, /bou'əl/ [OFr, *boel*], a method of establishing regular evacuation by reflex conditioning used in the treatment of fecal incontinence, impaction, chronic diarrhea, and autonomic hyperreflexia. In patients with autonomic hyperreflexia, distension of the rectum and bladder causes paroxysmal hypertension, restlessness, chills, diaphoresis, headache, elevated temperature, and bradycardia.

Bowel Training, a Nursing Interventions Classification defined as assisting the patient to train the bowel to evacuate at specific intervals.

Bowen's disease [John T. Bowen, American dermatologist, 1857–1941], a form of intraepidermal carcinoma (squamous cell). It is characterized by red-brown scaly or crusted lesions that resemble a patch of psoriasis or dermatitis.

Bowman's capsule /bō'mənz/ [William Bowman, English anatomist, 1816–1892], the cup-shaped end of a renal tubule enclosing a glomerulus. With the glomerulus, it is the site of filtration in the kidney.

Bowman's glands [William Bowman; L, *glans,* acorn], glands in the mucous membrane of the mouth.

Bowman's lamina [William Bowman; L, *lamina,* plate], a tough membrane beneath the corneal epithelium.

bowtie filter /bō'tī/, (in radiology) a special bowtie-shaped filter that may be used in computed tomography procedures to compensate for the shape of the patient's head or body.

boxer's fracture [Dan, *bask,* a blow; L, *fractura,* break], a fracture of one or more metacarpal bones, usually the fourth or the fifth, caused by punching a hard object. Such a fracture is often distal, angulated, and impacted.

boxing, (in dentistry) the forming of vertical walls, most commonly made of wax, to produce the desired shape and size of the base of a cast.

Boyle's law /boilz/ [Robert Boyle, English scientist, 1627–1691], (in physics) the law stating that the product of the volume and pressure of a gas contained at a constant temperature remains constant.

BP, abbreviation for **blood pressure.**

BPD, 1. abbreviation for **biparietal diameter. 2.** abbreviation for **bronchopulmonary dysplasia.**

BPDE-I, abbreviation for **benzo(a)pyrene dihydrodiol epoxide.**

BPH, abbreviation for **benign prostatic hypertrophy.**

bpm, abbreviation for *beats per minute.*

Br, symbol for the element **bromine.**

brace [OFr, *bracier,* to embrace], an orthotic device, sometimes jointed, to support and hold any part of the body in the correct position to allow function, such as a leg brace that permits walking and standing.

brachial /brā'kē-əl/ [Gk, *brachion,* arm], pertaining to the arm.

brachial artery, the principal artery of the upper arm that is the continuation of the axillary artery. It has three branches and terminates at the bifurcation of its main trunk into the radial and ulnar arteries.

brachialgia /-al'jē-ə/ [L, *brachium,* arm; Gk, *algos,* pain], a severe pain in the arm, often related to a disorder involving the brachial plexus.

brachialis /brā'kē-al'is/ [Gk, *brachion,* arm], a muscle of the upper arm, covering the anterior part of the elbow joint and the distal half of the humerus. It functions to flex the forearm.

brachial paralysis [L, *brachium,* arm; Gk, *paralyein,* to be palsied], paralysis of an arm or a hand.

brachial plexus [Gk, *brachion* + L, braided], a network of nerves in the neck, passing under the clavicle and into the axilla, originating in the fifth, sixth, seventh, and eighth cervical and first two thoracic spinal nerves. It innervates the muscles and skin of the chest, shoulders, and arms.

brachial plexus anesthesia, an anesthetic block of the upper extremity, performed by injecting local anesthetic near the plexis formed by the last four cervical and first two thoracic nerves.

brachial pulse [Gk, *brachion* + L, *pulsare,* to beat], the pulse of the brachial artery, palpated in the antecubital space.

brachial vein, a vein in the arm that accompanies the brachial artery and drains into the axillary vein.

brachiocephalic, relating to the arm and head.

brachiocephalic artery, first branch of the aortic arch.

brachiocephalic vein, the vein feeding the superior vena cava, collecting blood from the subclavian and jugular veins.

brachiocubital /-kyōō'bitəl/ [Gk, *brachion* + L, *cubitus,* elbow], pertaining to the arm and forearm.

brachioplasty, a surgical procedure to lift and tighten skin of the upper arm.

brachioradialis /-rā'dē-al'is/, the most superficial muscle on the radial side of the forearm. It functions to flex the forearm.

brachioradialis reflex [Gk, *brachion* + L, radial, *reflectare,* to bend backward], a deep tendon reflex elicited by striking the lateral surface of the forearm proximal to the distal head of the radius, characterized by normal slight elbow flexion and forearm supination.

brachybasia /bā'zhə/, abnormally slow walking, with a short, shuffling gait. The condition is associated with cerebral hemorrhage or pyramidal tract disease.

brachycardia /-kär'dē-ə/ [Gk, *brachys,* short, *kardia,* heart], slowness of the heart (less than 60 beats/min).

brachycephaly /-sef'əlē/ [Gk, *brachys,* short, *kephale,* head], a congenital malformation of the skull in which premature closure of the coronal suture results in excessive lateral growth of the head, giving it a short, broad appearance. **brachycephalic** /-səfal'ik/, **brachycephalous** /-sef'ələs/, *adj.*

brachydactyly /-dak'təlē/, a condition in which fingers or toes are abnormally short.

brachytherapy [Gk, *brachys,* short, *therapeia,* treatment], the placement of radioactive sources in contact with or implanted into the tumor tissues to be treated for a specific period.

Bradford frame [Edward H. Bradford, American surgeon, 1848–1926], a rectangular orthopedic frame made of pipes to which heavy movable straps of canvas are attached. The canvas straps run from side to side to support a patient in a prone or supine position. The straps can be removed to permit the patient to urinate or defecate while remaining immobile.

Bradford solid frame, a rectangular

metal orthopedic device covered with canvas that aids in immobilization, especially of children in traction. The main purpose of the device is to assist in maintaining proper immobilization, positioning, and alignment by controlling movement.

Bradford split frame, a rectangular metal orthopedic device covered with two separate pieces of canvas fastened at both ends of the frame. Used especially in pediatrics to aid in the immobilization of children in traction, it is divided in the middle by a large opening designed to accommodate the excretory functions of an incontinent patient in a hip spica cast. The division also allows the upper and lower extremities of the patient to be elevated separately and the cast to be kept clean and dry.

Bradley method [Robert Bradley, twentieth-century American physician], a method of psychophysical preparation for childbirth, comprising education about the physiologic characteristics of childbirth, exercise and nutrition during pregnancy, and techniques of breathing and relaxation for control and comfort during labor and delivery. The father is extensively involved in the classes and acts as the mother's "coach" during labor. Among the advantages of the method are its simplicity, the father's involvement, and the realistic approach to the efforts and discomfort of labor.

bradyarrhythmia /-ərith'mē-ə/ [Gk, *bradys,* slow, *a* + *rhythmos,* without rhythm], an abnormally slow heart rhythm (less than 60 beats/min).

bradycardia /-kär'dē-ə/ [Gk, *bradys,* slow, *kardia,* heart], a condition in which the ventricles beat but at a rate of less than 60 beats/min. Bradycardia takes the form of sinus bradycardia, sinus arrhythmia, and second- or third degree atrioventricular block. Sinus bradycardia is a relatively benign condition. Pathologic bradycardia may be symptomatic of a brain tumor, digitalis toxicity, heart block, or vagotonus

bradycardia-tachycardia syndrome [Gk, *bradys* + *kardia,* + *tachys,* fast, *kardia* + *syn,* together, *dromos,* course], a heart disorder characterized by a heart rate that alternates between abnormally slow and abnormally rapid rhythms.

bradyesthesia /-esthē'zhə/ [Gk, *bradys,* slow, *aisthesis,* feeling], a slowness in perception.

bradykinesia /-kinē'zhə,-kīnē'zhə/ [Gk, *bradys* + *kinesis,* motion], an abnormal condition characterized by slowness of all voluntary movement and speech, such as caused by parkinsonism, other extrapyramidal disorders, and certain tranquilizers.

bradykinin /-ki′nin/ [Gk, *bradys* + *kinein,* to move], a peptide of nonprotein origin containing nine amino acid residues. It is produced from α_2- globulin by kallikrein and is a potent vasodilator.

bradyphagia /-fā′jə/, a habit of eating very slowly.

bradyphasia /-fā′zhə/, an abnormally slow manner of speech, often associated with mental illness.

bradypnea /-pnē′ə/ [Gk, *bradys* + *pnein,* to breath], an abnormally slow rate of breathing.

bradyspermatism /-spur′mətiz′əm/, ejaculation that lacks normal force so that semen trickles slowly from the penis.

bradytachycardia [Gk, *bradys,* slow, *tachy,* fast, *kardia,* heart], a heart rate that alternates between an abnormally slow and an abnormally fast rate, as in *sick sinus syndrome.*

bradyuria /brad′ēyŏŏr′ē-ə/, a condition in which urine is passed very slowly.

Bragg curve [William H. Bragg, English physicist, 1862–1942], (in radiation therapy), the path followed by ionizing particles used in a treatment. Because certain particles reach a peak of potential near the end of their path, the Bragg curve can be used to direct the radiation so that it reaches deep-seated tumors while significantly sparing the normal overlying tissues.

Braille /brāl, brä′yə/ [Louis Braille, French teacher of the blind, 1809–1852], a system of printing for the blind consisting of raised dots or points that can be read by touch.

brain [AS, *bragen*], the part of the central nervous system contained within the cranium. It consists of the cerebrum, cerebellum, pons, medulla, and midbrain.

brain abscess [AS, *bragen* + L, *abscedere,* to go away], a pocket of infection in a part of the brain. It is usually a result of the spread of an infection from another source, such as the skull, sinuses, or other structures in the head. The infection also may be secondary to a disease in the bones, the nervous system outside the brain, or the heart.

brain attack, term for stroke, signifying that it is an emergency situation.

brain concussion [AS, *bragen* + L, *concussus,* a shaking], a bruising to cerebral tissues caused by a violent jarring or shaking or other blunt, nonpenetrating injury to the brain, resulting in a sudden change in momentum of the head. After a mild concussion, there may be a transient loss of consciousness followed, on awakening, by a headache. Severe concussion may cause prolonged unconsciousness and disruption of certain vital functions of the brainstem, such as respiration and vasomotor stability.

brain death [AS, *bragen* + *death*], an irreversible form of unconsciousness characterized by a complete loss of brain function while the heart continues to beat. The legal definition of this condition varies from state to state. The usual clinical criteria for brain death include the absence of reflex activity, movements, and spontaneous respiration. The pupils are dilated and fixed. A diagnosis of brain death may require evaluating and demonstrating that electrical activity of the brain is absent on two electroencephalograms performed 12 to 24 hours apart.

brain electrical activity map (BEAM), a topographic map of the brain created by a computer that is able to respond to the electric potentials evoked in the brain by a flash of light. Potentials recorded at 4-msec intervals are converted into a many-colored map of the brain, showing them to be positive or negative.

brain fever, *informal.* any inflammation of the brain or meninges.

brain scan [AS, *bragen* + L, *scandere,* to climb], a diagnostic procedure using radioisotope imaging techniques to localize and identify intracranial masses, lesions, tumors, or infarcts. Radioisotopes are injected intravenously to circulate to the brain, where they accumulate in abnormal tissue. The radioisotopes are traced and photographed by a scintillator or scanner, and the size and location of the abnormality are determined.

Brain's reflex [Walter R. Brain, English physician, 1895–1966; L, *reflectere,* to bend back], the reflexive extension of the flexed paralyzed arm of a hemiplegia patient when assuming a quadrupedal posture.

brainstem [AS, *bragen* + *stemm*], the part of the brain comprising the medulla oblongata, the pons, and the mesencephalon. It performs motor, sensory, and reflex functions and contains the corticospinal and reticulospinal tracts. The 12 pairs of cranial nerves from the brain arise mostly from the brainstem.

brainstem auditory evoked response (BAER), the electrical activity that may be recorded from the brainstem in the first 10 msec after presentation of an auditory stimulus. A delayed, normally shaped waveform may indicate a hearing loss caused by a middle or inner ear disorder; one or more missing peaks may indicate a neural disorder.

brain syndrome, a group of symptoms resulting from impaired function of the brain. It may be acute and reversible or chronic and irreversible.

brain tumor, an invasive neoplasm of the intracranial part of the central nervous system. Brain tumors cause significant rates of morbidity and mortality but are occasionally treated successfully. In adults 20% to 40% of malignancies in the brain are metastatic lesions from cancers in the breast, lung, gastrointestinal tract, or kidney or a malignant melanoma. The origin of primary brain tumors is not known. Symptoms of a brain tumor are often those of increased intracranial pressure such as headache, nausea, vomiting, papilledema, lethargy, and disorientation. Localizing signs such as loss of vision on the side of an occipital neoplasm may occur. Gliomas, chiefly astrocytomas, are the most common malignancies.

brainwashing, intensive indoctrination, usually of a political or religious nature, applied to individuals to develop in their minds a specific belief and motivation.

brain wave [AS, *bragen* + *wafian*], any of a number of patterns of rhythmic electrical impulses produced in different parts of the brain. Most patterns, identified by the Greek letters alpha, beta, delta, gamma, kappa, and theta, are similar for all normal persons and are relatively stable for each individual. Alpha waves are produced when the person is awake but resting, beta waves signal an active phase of cerebral function, and delta waves are emitted during deep sleep. Brain waves help in the diagnosis of certain neurologic disorders such as epilepsy or brain tumors.

bran, a coarse outer covering or coat of cereal grain such as wheat or rye. It is broken or separated from the meal or flour part of the grain to provide a source of dietary fiber, B vitamins, iron, magnesium, and zinc.

bran bath [OFr, *bren* + AS, *baeth*], a bath in which bran has been boiled in the water. It is used for the relief of skin irritation.

branch, (in anatomy) an offshoot arising from the main trunk of a nerve or blood vessel.

branched tubular gland [OFr, *branche*], one of the many multicellular glands with one excretory duct from two or more tube-shaped secretory branches, such as some of the gastric glands.

branchial /brang′kē-əl/ [Gk, *branchia*, gills], pertaining to body structures of the neck and throat area, particularly the muscles.

branchial arches [Gk, *branchia*, gills; L,

arcus, bow], arched structures in the embryonic pharynx.

branchial cleft [Gk, *branchia*, gills; ME, *clift*], a linear depression in the pharynx of the early embryo opposite a branchial or pharyngeal pouch.

branchial cyst [Gk, *branchia*, gills, *kystis*, bag], a cyst derived from a branchial remnant in the neck.

branchial fistula, a congenital abnormal passage from the pharynx to the external surface of the neck, resulting from the failure of a branchial cleft to close during fetal development.

branchiogenic /brang′kē-ōjen′ik/ [Gk, *branchia*, gills, *genein*, to produce], pertaining to any tissues originating in the branchial cleft or arch.

Brandt-Andrews maneuver [Thure Brandt, Swedish obstetrician, 1819–1895; Henry R. Andrews, English obstetrician, 1871–1942], a method of expressing the placenta from the uterus in the third stage of labor.

brassy cough [AS, *brase*, brassy, *cohhetan*, to cough], a high-pitched cough caused by irritation of the recurrent pharyngeal nerve or by pressure on the trachea.

brawny arm, a swollen arm caused by lymphedema, usually after a mastectomy.

Braxton Hicks version /brak′stənhiks′/ [John Braxton Hicks, English physician, 1823–1897], one of several types of maneuvers sometimes used to turn the fetus from an undesirable position to one that is more likely to facilitate delivery.

BRCA1, symbol for a breast cancer gene. A healthy BRCA1 gene produces a protein that protects against unwanted cell growth. The protein is packaged by the cell's Golgi apparatus into secretory vesicles, which release their contents on the cell's surface. The protein circulates in the intracellular space, attaching itself to neighboring cell receptors. The receptors signal the cell nuclei to stop growing. When the gene is defective, it produces a faulty protein that is unable to prevent proliferation of abnormal cells as they evolve into potentially deadly breast cancer. BRCA1 may also normally inhibit ovarian cancer.

BRCA2, symbol for a breast cancer gene with activity similar to that of BRCA1.

BRCA3, symbol for a breast cancer gene.

breach of contract, the failure to perform as promised or agreed in a contract.

breach of duty, **1.** the failure to perform an act required by law. **2.** the performance of an act in an unlawful way.

break test, a test of a person's muscle strength by application of resistance after the person has reached the end of a range of motion. Resistance is applied gradually in a direction opposite to the line of pull of the muscle or muscle group being tested.

breakthrough, (in psychiatry) a sudden new insight into a problem and its solution after a period of little or no progress.

breakthrough bleeding [AS, *brecan* + ME, *thruh,* across], the escape of uterine blood between menstrual periods, a side effect of using oral contraceptives experienced by some women.

breast [AS, *breast*], **1.** the anterior aspect of the surface of the chest. **2.** a mammary gland.

breast abscess, an abscess of a mammary gland, usually during lactation or weaning.

breast cancer, a malignant neoplastic disease of breast tissue, a common malignancy in women in the United States. The incidence increases with age from the third to the fifth decade and reaches a second peak at age 65. Risk factors include certain genetic abnormalities, a family history of breast cancer, nulliparity, exposure to ionizing radiation, early menarche, late menopause, obesity, diabetes, hypertension, chronic cystic disease of the breast, and, possibly, postmenopausal estrogen therapy. Women who are above 40 years of age when they bear their first child and individuals who have malignancies in other body sites also have an increased risk of development of breast cancer. Initial symptoms, detected in most cases by self-examination, include a small painless lump, thick or dimpled skin, or nipple retraction. As the lesion progresses, there may be nipple discharge, pain, ulceration, and enlarged axillary glands. The diagnosis may be established by a careful physical examination, mammography, and cytologic examination of tumor cells obtained by biopsy.

breast examination, a process in which the breasts and their accessory structures are observed and palpated in assessing the presence of changes or abnormalities that could indicate malignant disease.

breastfeeding [AS, *braest* + ME, *feden*], **1.** suckling or nursing, giving a baby milk from the breast. Breastfeeding encourages postpartum uterine involution and slows the natural return of the menses. **2.** taking milk from the breast.

Breastfeeding Assistance, a Nursing Interventions Classification defined as preparing a new mother to breastfeed her infant.

breastfeeding, effective, a NANDA-accepted nursing diagnosis of a state in which a mother-infant dyad/family exhibits adequate proficiency and satisfaction with the breastfeeding process. Defining characteristics include the mother's ability to position the infant at the breast to promote a successful latch-on response, regular and sustained suckling/swallowing at the breast, infant content after feeding, appropriate infant weight patterns for age, and effective mother-infant communication patterns.

breastfeeding, ineffective, a NANDA-accepted nursing diagnosis of a state in which a mother, infant, and/or family experiences dissatisfaction or difficulty with the breastfeeding process. The major defining characteristic is the unsatisfactory breastfeeding process. Other characteristics include an actual or perceived inadequate milk supply, no observable signs of oxytocin release, persistence of sore nipples beyond the infant's first week of life, and maternal reluctance to put the infant to breast as necessary.

breastfeeding, interrupted, a NANDA-accepted nursing diagnosis of a break in the continuity of the breastfeeding process as a result of inability or inadvisability of putting the baby to the breast for feeding. Defining characteristics include insufficient nourishment by the infant at the breast for some or all feedings, separation of mother and infant, and lack of knowledge about expression and storage of breast milk.

breast implant, the surgical placement of prosthetic material in a breast, either for increasing the breast's size or for performing reconstruction after a mastectomy.

breast milk [AS, *braest* + *meoluc*], human milk. The nurse should counsel mothers that it is easily digested, clean, and warm and that it confers some immunities (bronchiolitis and gastroenteritis are rare in breastfed babies). Infants fed breast milk are less likely to become obese and to have dental malocclusion.

breast milk jaundice, jaundice and hyperbilirubinemia in breastfed infants that occur in the first weeks of life as a result of a metabolite in the mother's milk that inhibits the infant's ability to conjugate bilirubin to glucuronide for excretion.

breast pump, a mechanical or electronic device for withdrawing milk from the breast.

breast shadows, artifacts caused by breast tissue that appear on chest radiographs of women. The shadows accentuate the underlying tissue and may cause the appearance of an interstitial disease process.

breast transillumination [AS, *braest* + L *trans,* through, *illuminare,* to light up], a method of examining the inner structures of the breast by directing light through the outer wall.

breath, the air inhaled and exhaled during ventilation of the lungs.

Breathalyzer /breth'əlī'zər/, trademark for a device that analyzes exhaled air. It is commonly used to test for blood alcohol levels; the test is based on the relationship between alcohol in the breath and alcohol in the blood circulating through the lungs.

breath-holding /breth-/ [AS, *braeth* + ME, *holden*], a form of voluntary apnea that is usually, but not necessarily, performed with a closed glottis. Although breath-holding may be prolonged for several minutes, it is invariably terminated by an involuntary breaking point.

breathing cycle /brē'thing/, a ventilatory cycle consisting of an inspiration followed by the expiration of a volume of gas called the tidal volume. The duration or total cycle time of a breathing cycle is the breathing or ventilatory period.

breathing frequency (f), the number of breathing cycles per a given unit of time.

breathing nomogram [AS, *braeth* + Gk, *nomos,* law, *gramma,* a record], a chart that presents scales of data for body weight, breathing frequency, and predicted basal tidal volume arranged in a pattern. It allows calculation of an unknown value on one scale by drawing a line that connects known values on two other scales.

breathing pattern, ineffective, a NANDA-accepted nursing diagnosis of a state in which the rate, depth, timimg, rhythm, or chest/abdominal wall excursion during inspiration, expiration, or both does not maintain optimal ventilation for the individual. Defining characteristics include dyspnea, shortness of breath; inspiration longer than expiration; irregular breathing rhythm (e.g., apnea, frequent signs, use of accessory muscles of breathing inappropriate to level of activity, asynchronous thoracoabdominal motion); grunting; nasal flaring (infants); paradoxic breathing patterns; use of accessory muscles; and altered chest excursion.

breathing work, the energy required for breathing movements. It is the cumulative product of instantaneous pressure developed by the respiratory muscles and the volume of air moved during a breathing cycle.

breath odor /breth/, an odor usually produced by substances or diseases in the lungs or mouth. Certain specific odors are associated with some diseases such as diabetes, liver failure, uremia, or a lung abscess.

breath sound [AS, *braeth* + L, *sonus*], the sound of air passing in and out of the lungs as heard with a stethoscope.

breath tests, diagnostic tests for intestinal disorders such as bacterial overgrowth, ileal disease, lactase deficiency, and steatorrhea. If lactose absorption is impaired in the small intestine, colonic bacteria ferment the lactose, releasing hydrogen, which is excreted in the breath. Bacterial overgrowth is tested with ^{14}C-cholylglycine, which is normally absorbed by the ileum and recycled via the enterohepatic circulation.

Breckinridge, Mary, (1881–1965), the American nurse who founded the Frontier Nursing Service in Kentucky to improve obstetric care of women living in remote mountainous areas. The service began training midwives and stimulated the establishment of other midwifery schools.

breech birth [ME, *brech* + *burth*], parturition in which the infant emerges feet, knees, or buttocks first. Breech birth is often hazardous: The body may deliver easily, but the aftercoming head may become trapped by an incompletely dilated cervix because infants' heads are usually larger than their bodies.

breech extraction [ME, *brech* + L, *ex,* out, *trahere,* to pull], an obstetric operation in which an infant being born feet or buttocks first is grasped before any part of the trunk is born and delivered by traction.

breech presentation [ME, *brech* + L, *praesentare,* to show], intrauterine position of the fetus in which the buttocks or feet present. It occurs in approximately 3% of labors.

bregma /breg'mə/ [Gk, the front of the head], the junction of the coronal and sagittal sutures on the top of the skull. **—bregmatic,** *adj.*

bregmacardiac reflex /breg'məkär'dē·ək/ [Gk, *bregma,* front of the head], a phenomenon in which pressure on the anterior fontanel of an infant's skull causes the heart to slow.

bremsstrahlung radiation /brems'shträ'lŏong/ [Ger, braking radiation], a type of x-ray in which there is a loss of kinetic energy from interaction with the nucleus of a target atom, resulting in an x-ray photon.

Brenner tumor [Fritz Brenner, German pathologist, b. 1877], an uncommon benign ovarian neoplasm consisting of nests or cords of epithelial cells containing glycogen that are enclosed in fibrous connective tissue. The tumor may be solid or cystic.

bretylium tosylate /britil'ē·əm/, an antiarrhythmic agent prescribed in the treatment of life-threatening ventricular arrhythmias when other measures have not been effective.

brewer's yeast /broo͞oʹərz/ [ME, *brewen,* to boil, *yest,* foam], a preparation containing the dried pulverized cells of a yeast, such as *Saccharomyces cerevisiae,* that is used as a leavening agent and as a dietary supplement. It is a source of the B complex vitamins, many vitamins, and a high grade of protein.

brick dust urine, a sign of precipitated urates in acidic urine in a urinalysis sample.

bridgework, a fixed prosthetic appliance that is cemented permanently to abutment teeth.

bridging [AS, *brycg*], **1.** a nursing technique of positioning a patient so that bony prominences are free of pressure on the mattress by using pads, bolsters of foam rubber, or pillows to distribute body weight over a larger surface. **2.** a nursing technique for supporting a part of the body, such as the testicles in treating orchitis, using a Bellevue bridge made of a towel or other material.

brief psychotherapy, (in psychiatry) treatment directed to the active resolution of personality or behavioral problems rather than to the speculative analysis of the unconscious.

brief reactive psychosis, a short episode, usually less than 2 weeks, of psychotic behavior that occurs in response to a significant psychosocial stressor.

brightness gain /brītʹnes/, (in radiology) the ability of an image intensifier to increase the illumination level of an image.

Brill-Zinsser disease /brilʹzinʹsər/ [Nathan E. Brill, American physician, 1860–1925; Hans Zinsser, American bacteriologist, 1878–1940], a mild form of typhus that recurs in a person who appears to have completely recovered from a severe case of the disease. Some rickettsiae remain in the body after the symptoms of the disease abate, causing the recurrence of symptoms.

brim, the edge of the upper border of the true pelvis, or the pelvic inlet.

Brinnell hardness test [Johann A. Brinnell, Swedish engineer, 1849–1925], a means of determining the surface hardness of a material by measuring the amount of resistance to the impact of a steel ball. The test result is recorded as the Brinnell hardness number. It is commonly used to measure this quality in various materials used in dental restorations, such as amalgams, cements, and porcelains.

Brissaud's dwarf /brisōzʹ/ [Edouard Brissaud, French physician, 1852–1909], a person affected with infantile myxedema

in which short stature is associated with hypothyroidism.

British Medical Association (BMA), a national professional organization of physicians in the United Kingdom.

British Pharmacopoeia (BP), the official British reference work setting forth standards of strength and purity of medications and containing directions for their preparation to ensure that the same prescription written by different doctors and filled by different pharmacists will contain exactly the same ingredients in the same proportions.

British thermal unit (BTU), a unit of heat energy. The amount of thermal energy that must be absorbed by 1 lb of water to raise its temperature by 1° at 39.2° F. It is also equivalent to 1055 joules or 252 calories.

broach, an elongated, tapering dental instrument used in removing pulpal material.

broad beta disease, a familial type of hyperlipoproteinemia in which a lipoprotein, high in cholesterol and triglycerides, accumulates in the blood. The condition is characterized by yellowish nodules (xanthomas) on the elbows and knees, peripheral vascular disease, and elevated serum cholesterol levels.

broad ligament [ME, *brood* + L, *ligare,* to tie], a folded sheet of peritoneum draped over the uterine tubes, the uterus, and the ovaries.

broad ligament of liver [ME, *brod* + L, *ligare,* to bind; AS, *lifer*], a crescent-shaped fold of peritoneum attached to the lower surface of the diaphragm, connecting with the liver and the anterior abdominal wall.

broad-spectrum antibiotic, an antibiotic that is effective against a wide range of infectious microorganisms.

Broca's aphasia /brōʹkəz/ [Pierre P. Broca, French neurologist, 1824–1880], a type of aphasia consisting of nonfluent speech, with a laconic and hesitant, telegraphic quality caused by a large left frontal lesion extending to the fissure of Roland. The patient's agrammatic speech is characterized by abundant nouns and verbs but few articles and prepositions.

Broca's area [Pierre P. Broca], an area involved in speech production situated on the inferior frontal gyrus of the brain.

Broca's fissure [Pierre P. Broca], a cleft or groove encircling Broca's area in the left frontal area of the brain.

Broca's plane [Pierre P. Broca], a plane that extends from the tip of the interalveolar septum between the upper central incisors to the lowest point of the occipital condyle.

Brodie's abscess [Benjamin Brodie, English surgeon, 1783–1862], a form of osteomyelitis consisting of an indolent staphylococcal infection of bone, usually in the metaphysis of a long bone of a child, characterized by a necrotic cavity surrounded by dense granulation tissue.

Brodmann's areas /brod'manz, brōt'mons/ [Korbinian Brodmann, German anatomist, 1868–1918], the 47 different areas of the cerebral cortex that are associated with specific neurologic functions and distinguished by different cellular components.

brom, abbreviation for a *bromide noncarboxylate anion.*

bromhidrosis /brō'midrō'sis/ [Gk, *bromos,* stench, *hidros,* sweat], an abnormal condition in which the apocrine sweat has an unpleasant odor.

bromide /brō'mīd/ [Gk, *bromos,* stench], an anion of bromine. Bromide salts, once widely prescribed as sedatives, are now seldom used for that purpose.

bromide poisoning, an adverse reaction to ingested bromide. Symptoms include nausea, vomiting, an acnelike rash, slurred speech, ataxia, psychotic behavior, and coma.

bromine (Br) /brō'mēn/, a toxic red-brown liquid element of the halogen group. Its atomic number is 35; its atomic weight (mass) is 79.904. Bromine gives off a red vapor that is extremely irritating to the eyes and respiratory tract. Liquid bromine is irritating to the skin.

bromocriptine mesylate /brō'mōkrip'tēn/, a dopamine receptor agonist prescribed for the treatment of amenorrhea and galactorrhea associated with hyperprolactinemia, female infertility, and Parkinson's disease.

bromoderma /brō'mōdur'mə/ [Gk, *bromos,* stench, *derma* skin], an acneiform, bullous, or nodular skin rash, occurring as a hypersensitivity reaction to ingested bromides.

brompheniramine maleate /brom'fənir'əmin/, an antihistamine prescribed in the treatment of hypersensitivity reactions, including rhinitis, skin reactions, and itching.

Brompton's cocktail [Brompton Hospital, England], an analgesic solution containing alcohol, morphine or heroin, and, in some cases, a phenothiazine. The cocktail is administered in the control of pain in the terminally ill patient.

Bromsulphalein (BSP) test /bromsul'-falin/, trademark for sulfobromophthalein, a dye prepared for use in a highly sensitive nonspecific test that measures the ability of liver cells to remove the sulfobromophthalein from the blood.

bronchial /brong'kē-əl/ [Gk, *bronchos,*

windpipe], pertaining to the bronchi or bronchioles.

bronchial breath sound [Gk, *bronchos,* windpipe], a normal sound heard with a stethoscope over the main airways, including trachea and sternum. Expiration and inspiration produce noise of equal duration, which sounds like blowing through a hollow tube.

bronchial cough, a cough associated with bronchiectasis and heard in early stages as hacking and irritating, becoming looser in later stages.

bronchial fremitus, a vibration that can be palpated or auscultated on the chest wall over a bronchus. It results from congestion by secretions that rattle as air passes during respiration.

bronchial hyperreactivity [Gk, *bronchos* + *hyper,* excess; L, *re,* again, *agere,* to act], an abnormal respiratory condition characterized by reflex bronchospasm in response to histamine or a cholinergic drug. It is a universal feature of asthma and is used in the differential diagnosis of asthma and heart disease.

bronchial murmur, a murmur heard as a blowing sound, caused by air flowing in and out of the bronchial tubes.

bronchial secretion, a substance produced in the bronchial tree that consists of mucus secreted by the goblet cells and mucous glands of the bronchi, protein salts released from disintegrating cells, plasma fluid, and proteins, including fibrinogen.

bronchial spasm, an excessive and prolonged contraction of the involuntary muscle fibers in the walls of the bronchi and bronchioles. The contractions may be localized or general.

bronchial toilet, special care that is given patients with tracheostomies and respiratory disorders, including stimulation of coughing, deep breathing, and suctioning of the respiratory tract.

bronchial tree, an anatomic complex of the trachea and bronchi. The bronchi branch from the trachea.

bronchial washing [Gk, *bronchos,* windpipe, ME, *wasshen,* to wash], the irrigation of the bronchi and bronchioles to cleanse them and to collect specimens for laboratory examination.

bronchiectasis /brong'kē-ek'təsis/ [Gk, *bronchos* + *ektasis,* stretching], an abnormal condition of the bronchial tree characterized by irreversible dilation and destruction of the bronchial walls. The condition is sometimes congenital but is more often a result of bronchial infection or of obstruction by a tumor or an aspirated foreign body. Symptoms include a constant cough producing copious purulent sputum, hemoptysis, chronic sinusitis, clubbing of fingers, and persistent moist, coarse crackles.

bronchiolar collapse /brong'kyələr/ [L, *bronchiolus,* little windpipe, *conlabi,* to fall], a condition in which bronchioles become compressed by the pressure of surrounding structures and the lack of inflowing air needed to keep them inflated. The condition occurs in such disorders as emphysema, cystic disease, and bronchiectasis.

bronchiole /brong'kē-ōl/ [L, *bronchiolus,* little windpipe], a small airway of the respiratory system extending from the bronchi into the lobes of the lung. There are two divisions of bronchioles: terminal bronchioles and respiratory bronchioles. —**bronchiolar** /brongkē'ələr/, *adj.*

bronchiolitis /brong'kē-ōlī'tis/ [L, *bronchiolus,* little windpipe; Gk, *itis,* inflammation], an acute viral infection of the lower respiratory tract that occurs primarily in infants less than 18 months of age. It is characterized by expiratory wheezing, respiratory distress, inflammation, and obstruction at the level of the bronchioles. The most common causative agents are the respiratory syncytial viruses and the parainfluenza viruses. *Mycoplasma pneumoniae,* rhinoviruses, enteroviruses, and measles virus are less common causative agents. Transmission occurs by infection with airborne particles or by contact with infected secretions. The diagnosis consists of evidence of hyperinflation of the lungs through percussion or chest x-ray.

bronchiolitis obliterans, a form of bronchiolitis in which the exudate is not expectorated but becomes organized and obliterates the bronchial tubes, causing collapse of the affected part of the lungs.

bronchitis /brongkī'tis/ [Gk, *bronchos,* windpipe, *itis,* inflammation], an acute or chronic inflammation of the mucous membranes of the tracheobronchial tree. **Acute bronchitis** is characterized by a productive cough, fever, hypertrophy of mucus-secreting structures, and back pain. Caused by the spread of upper respiratory viral infections to the bronchi, it is often observed with or after childhood infections such as measles, whooping cough, diphtheria, and typhoid fever. **Chronic bronchitis** is distinguished by an excessive secretion of mucus in the bronchi with a productive cough for at least 3 consecutive months in at least 2 successive years. Additional symptoms are frequent chest infections, cyanosis, hypoxemia, hypercapnia, and a marked tendency to de-

velopment of cor pulmonale and respiratory failure.

bronchoalveolar /-alvē'ələr/ [Gk, *bronchos,* windpipe; L, *alveolus,* little hollow], pertaining to the terminal air sacs at the ends of the bronchioles.

bronchoalveolar carcinoma (BAC), a peripheral well-differentiated neoplasm that spreads locally through the air spaces of the alveoli. A variant of adenocarcinoma, BAC constitutes about 5% of all lung cancers.

bronchoalveolar lavage (BAL), a diagnostic procedure in which small amounts of physiologic solution are injected through a fiberoptic bronchoscope into a specified area of the lung, while the rest of the lung is sequestered by an inflated balloon. The fluid is then aspirated and inspected for pathogenic organisms, malignant cells, and mineral bodies.

bronchoconstriction [Gk, *bronchos,* windpipe; L, *constringere,* to draw tight], a constriction of the bronchi, resulting in a narrowing of the airway lumen.

bronchodilation /-dil'ətā'shən/ [Gk, *bronchos,* windpipe; L, *dilatare,* to widen], an increase in the diameter of the bronchial lumen, allowing increased airflow to and from the lungs.

bronchodilator /-dilā'tər/, a substance, especially a drug, that relaxes contractions of the smooth muscle of the bronchioles to improve ventilation to the lungs. Pharmacologic bronchodilators are prescribed to improve aeration in asthma, bronchiectasis, bronchitis, and emphysema.

bronchogenic /-jen'ik/ [Gk, *bronchos* + *genein,* to produce], originating in the bronchi.

bronchogenic carcinoma, one of the more than 90% of malignant lung tumors that originate in bronchi. Lesions, usually resulting from cigarette smoking, may cause coughing and wheezing, fatigue, chest tightness, and aching joints. In the late stages, bloody sputum, clubbing of the fingers, weight loss, and pleural effusion may be present.

bronchogenic cyst, a cyst that develops in the lung or mediastinum. It may be asymptomatic or cause cough, stridor, wheezing, or dyspnea. It may also become infected or malignant, requiring surgical removal.

bronchography /brongkog'rəfē/, an x-ray examination of the bronchi after they have been coated with a radiopaque substance.

broncholithiasis /-lithī'əsis/, inflammation of the bronchi caused by an accumulation of hard concretions or stones on their lining.

bronchomotor tone, the state of contraction or relaxation of smooth muscle in the bronchial walls that regulates the caliber of the airways.

bronchophony /brongkof'ənē/ [Gk, *bronchos* + *phone,* voice], an increase in intensity and clarity of vocal resonance that may result from an increase in lung tissue density, such as in the consolidation of pneumonia.

bronchopleural fistula /-plo͝or'əl/, an abnormal passageway between a bronchus and the pleural cavity.

bronchopneumonia [Gk, *bronchos* + *pneumon,* lung], an acute inflammation of the lungs and bronchioles, characterized by chills, fever, high pulse and respiratory rates, bronchial breathing, cough with purulent bloody sputum, severe chest pain, and abdominal distension. The disease is usually a result of the spread of bacterial infection from the upper to the lower respiratory tract. Results of the condition are pleural effusion, empyema, lung abscess, peripheral thrombophlebitis, respiratory failure, congestive heart failure, and jaundice.

bronchoprovocation inhalation test, a pulmonary function test performed on patients with a history of asthma who have normal pulmonary function at rest. In a specific test the patient inhales a particular antigen while the forced expiratory volume (FEV) is monitored. In a nonspecific test the patient inhales a substance such as histamine periodically at increasing concentrations while the FEV is measured.

bronchopulmonary /-pul'mōner'ē/ [Gk, *bronchos* + L, *pulmonis,* lung], pertaining to the bronchi and lungs of the respiratory system.

bronchopulmonary dysplasia (BPD) /-po͝ol'mənər'ē/, a chronic respiratory disorder characterized by scarring of lung tissue, thickened pulmonary arterial walls, and mismatch between lung ventilation and perfusion.

bronchopulmonary hygiene, the care and cleanliness of the respiratory tract, including ventilatory/respiratory therapy equipment and natural air passages. Hygienic care also allows for complete assessment of the patient's respiratory condition and of any equipment or devices used to support his or her breathing.

bronchopulmonary lavage [Gk, *bronchos,* windpipe; L, *pulmonis,* lung; Fr, *lavage,* washing out], the irrigation or washing out of the bronchi and bronchioles to remove pulmonary secretions.

bronchoscope /brong'kəskōp'/, a curved, flexible tube for visual examination of the bronchi. It contains fibers that carry light down the tube and project an enlarged image up the tube to the viewer. —**bronchoscopic,** *adj.*

bronchoscopy /brongkos'kəpē/, the visual examination of the tracheobronchial tree, using a bronchoscope. The procedure also may be used for suctioning, for obtaining a biopsy specimen and fluid or sputum for examination, and for removing foreign bodies.

bronchospasm /-spaz'əm/, an abnormal contraction of the smooth muscle of the bronchi, resulting in an acute narrowing and obstruction of the respiratory airway. A cough with generalized wheezing usually indicates the condition.

bronchospirometry /brong'kōspīrom'ətrē/, a technique for the study of the ventilation and gas exchange of each lung separately by the introduction of a catheter into either the left or right mainstem bronchus.

bronchotomogram /-tom'əgram/, an image of the upper respiratory system, from the trachea to the lower bronchi, produced by tomography.

bronchovesicular /-vesik'yələr/, pertaining to the bronchial tubes and the alveoli.

bronchovesicular sounds [Gk, *bronchos,* windpipe; L, *vesicula,* small bladder, *sonus,* sound], normal breath sounds that are between sounds of the bronchial tubes and those of the alveoli, or a combination of the two sounds.

bronchus /brong'kəs/, *pl.* **bronchi** /-kī/ [L; Gk, *bronchos,* windpipe], any one of several large air passages in the lungs through which pass inhaled and exhaled air. Each bronchus has a wall consisting of three layers. The outermost is made of dense fibrous tissue reinforced with cartilage. The middle layer is a network of smooth muscle. The innermost layer consists of ciliated mucous membrane. —**bronchial,** *adj.*

Brönsted acid [Johannes N. Brönsted, Danish physical chemist, 1879–1947], a molecule or an ion that acts as a proton donor.

Brönsted base [Johannes N. Brönsted], a molecule or an ion that acts as a proton acceptor.

broth, **1.** a fluid culture medium such as a solution of lactose or thioglycollate used to support the growth of bacteria for laboratory analysis. **2.** a beverage or other fluid made with meat extract and water.

brow, the forehead, particularly the eyebrow or ridge above the eye.

brown fat [ME, *broun* + AS, *faett,* filled], a type of fat present in newborns and rarely found in adults. Brown fat is a unique source of heat energy for the infant

brownian movement /brou'nyən/ [Robert Brown, Scottish botanist, 1773–1858], a random movement of microscopic particles suspended in a liquid or gas. The movement is produced by the natural kinetic activity of molecules of the fluid that strike the foreign particles.

brown recluse spider, a small poisonous arachnid, *Loxosceles reclusa,* also known as the brown or violin spider, found in both North and South America.

brown recluse spider bite [L, *recludere,* to shut off; ME, *spithre* + AS, *bitan*], the bite of the brown or violin spider, *Loxosceles reclusa,* producing a characteristic necrotic lesion. The venom from its bite usually creates a blister surrounded by concentric white and red circles. There is little or no initial pain, but localized pain develops in about an hour. The patient may experience systemic symptoms. A blood-filled bleb forms that increases in size and eventually ruptures, leaving a black scar.

Brown-Séquard's syndrome /broun' sākär'z/ [Charles E. Brown-Séquard, French physiologist, 1817–1894], a traumatic neurologic disorder resulting from compression of one side of the spinal cord, above the tenth thoracic vertebrae, characterized by spastic paralysis on the body's injured side, loss of postural sense, and loss of the senses of pain and heat on the other side of the body.

brow presentation, an obstetric situation in which the brow, or forehead, of the fetus is the first part of the body to enter the birth canal. Because the diameter of the fetal head at this angle may be greater than that of the mother's pelvic outlet, a cesarean section may be recommended.

brucellosis /broo'səlō'sis/ [David Bruce, English pathologist, 1855–1931], a disease caused by any of several species of the gram-negative coccobacillus *Brucella.* It is primarily a disease of animals (including cattle, pigs, and goats); humans usually acquire it by ingestion of contaminated milk or milk products or through a break in the skin. It is characterized by fever, chills, sweating, malaise, and weakness. Although brucellosis itself is rarely fatal, treatment is important because serious complications such as pneumonia, meningitis, and encephalitis can develop.

Brudzinski's sign /broodzin'skēz/ [Josef Brudzinski, Polish physician, 1874–1917], an involuntary flexion of the arm, hip, and knee when the neck is passively flexed. It occurs in patients with meningitis.

bruit /broo'ē/ [Fr, noise], an abnormal blowing or swishing sound or murmur heard while auscultating a carotid artery, organ, or gland, such as the liver or thyroid. The specific character of the bruit, its location, and the time of its occurrence in a cycle of other sounds are all of diagnostic importance.

Brunnstrom hemiplegia classification, an evaluation procedure that assesses muscle tone and voluntary control of movement patterns in a stroke patient. Results indicate the patient's progress through stages of recovery.

brush biopsy, the use of a catheter with bristles that is inserted through the urethra to collect cells from urinary system tissues.

brush border, microvilli on the free surfaces of certain epithelial cells, particularly the absorptive surfaces of the intestine and the proximal convoluted tubules of the kidney.

Brushfield's spots [Thomas Brushfield, English physician, 1858–1937; ME *spotte* stain], pinpoint white or light yellow spots on the iris of a child with Down's syndrome.

Bruton's agammaglobulinemia [Ogden C. Bruton, American physician, b. 1908], a sex-linked, inherited condition characterized by the absence of gamma globulin in the blood. Those (usually children) affected by the syndrome are deficient in antibodies and susceptible to repeated infections.

bruxism /bruk'sizəm/ [Gk, *brychein,* to gnash the teeth], the compulsive, unconscious grinding and/or clenching of the teeth, especially during sleep or as a mechanism for the release of tension during periods of extreme stress in the waking hours.

Bryant's traction /brī'ənts/ [Thomas Bryant, English physician, 1828–1914; L, *trahere,* to pull], an orthopedic mechanism used to immobilize both lower extremities in the treatment of a fractured femur or in the correction of the congenital dislocation of the hip. This mechanism consists of a traction frame supporting weights, connected by ropes that run through pulleys to traction foot plates.

BSA, 1. abbreviation for body surface area. See **surface area. 2.** abbreviation for *bovine serum albumin.*

BSN, abbreviation for **Bachelor of Science in Nursing.**

BT, abbreviation for **bleeding time.**

BTPD, abbreviation for *body temperature, ambient pressure, dry.*

BTPS, abbreviation for *body temperature, ambient pressure, saturated* (with water vapor).

BTU, abbreviation for **British thermal unit.**

bubble-diffusion humidifier, a device that provides humidified oxygen or other therapeutic gases by allowing the gas to bubble through a reservoir of water.

bubble oxygenator, a heart-lung device that oxygenates the blood while it is diverted outside the patient's body.

bubo /byoo'bō/, *pl.* **buboes** [Gk, *boubon,* groin], a greatly enlarged, tender, inflamed lymph node, usually in the groin, that is associated with diseases such as chancroid, lymphogranuloma venereum, and syphilis.

bubonic plague /byoobon'ik/ [Gk, *boubon,* groin; L, *plaga,* stroke], the most common form of plague. It is characterized by painful buboes in the axilla, groin, or neck; fever often rising to 106° F (41.11° C); prostration with a rapid, thready pulse; hypotension; delirium; and bleeding into the skin from the superficial blood vessels. The symptoms are caused by an endotoxin released by a bacillus, *Yersinia pestis,* usually introduced into the body by the bite of a rat flea that has bitten an infected rat. Conditions favor a plague epidemic when a large infected rodent population lives with a large nonimmune human population in a damp, warm climate.

bucardia /bookär'dē·ə/, extreme enlargement of the heart.

buccal /buk'əl/ [L, *bucca,* cheek], pertaining to the inside of the cheek, the surface of a tooth, or the gum beside the cheek.

buccal administration of medication, oral administration of a drug, usually in the form of a tablet, by placing it between the cheek and the teeth or gum until it dissolves.

buccal bar, a part of an orthodontic appliance that consists of a rigid metal wire extending anteriorly from the buccal side of a molar band.

buccal cavity, the vestibule of the mouth, specifically the area lying between the teeth and lips but more often the teeth and cheeks.

buccal contour [L, *bucca* + *cum,* together with, *tornare,* to turn], the shape of the buccal side of a posterior tooth. It is usually characterized by a slight occlusocervical convexity with its largest prominence at the gingival third of the clinical buccal surface.

buccal fat pad, a fat pad in the cheek under the subcutaneous layer of the skin, over the buccinator. It is particularly prominent in infants and is often called a sucking pad.

buccal flange [L, *bucca* + OFr, *flanche,*

flank], the part of a denture base that occupies the cheek side of the mouth and extends distally from the buccal notch.

buccal glands [L, *bucca,* cheek, *glans,* acorn], small salivary glands located between the buccinator muscle and the mucous membrane in the vestibule of the mouth.

buccal mucosa, the mucous membrane lining the inside of the mouth.

buccal notch, a depression in a denture flange that accommodates the buccal frenum.

buccal smear, a sample of cells removed from the buccal mucosa for purposes of obtaining a karyotype to determine the genetic sex of an individual.

buccal splint, any material, usually plaster, placed on the buccal surfaces of fixed partial denture units to hold the units in position for assembly.

buccinator /buk'sinā'tər/ [L, *buccina,* trumpet], the main muscle of the cheek, one of the 12 muscles of the mouth. The buccinator, innervated by buccal branches of the facial nerve, compresses the cheek, acting as an important accessory muscle of mastication by holding food under the teeth.

buccogingival /buk'ōjinjī'vəl/, pertaining to the internal mouth structures, particularly the cheeks and gums.

buccolinguomasticatory triad /buk'ōling'-wōmas'təkə-tôr'e/ [L, *bucca,* cheek, *lingua,* tongue, *masticare,* to gnash the teeth], a complex of involuntary lip, tongue, jaw, and head movements seen in tardive dyskinesia.

buccopharyngeal /buk'ōfərin'jē·əl/, pertaining to the cheek and pharynx or to the mouth and pharynx.

buccula /buk'yələ/ [L, *bucca,* cheek], a fold of fatty tissue, literally a "little cheek" beneath the chin.

bucket handle fracture [OFr, *buket,* tub; ME, *handel,* part grasped; L, *fractura,* break], a fracture that produces a tear in a semilunar cartilage along the medial side of the knee joint.

bucking, *informal* **1.** gagging on an endotracheal tube. **2.** involuntarily resisting positive pressure ventilation.

buck knife, a periodontal surgical knife with a spear-shaped cutting point, used for an interdental incision associated with a gingivectomy.

Buck's fascia [Gurdon Buck, American surgeon, 1807–1877], the deep fascia encasing the erectile tissue of the penis.

Buck's skin traction [Gurdon Buck], an orthopedic procedure that applies traction to the lower extremity with the hips and the knees extended. It is used in the treatment of hip and knee contractures, in post-operative positioning and immobilization, and in disease processes of the hip and knee.

Buck's traction [Gurdon Buck; L, *trahere,* to pull], one of the most common orthopedic mechanisms by which pull is exerted on the lower extremity with a system of ropes, weights, and pulleys. Buck's traction is used to immobilize, position, and align the lower extremity in the treatment of contractures and diseases of the hip and knee.

Bucky diaphragm [Gustav P. Bucky, American radiologist, 1880–1963; Gk, *diaphragma,* partition], (in radiology) a device consisting of a moving grid that limits the amount of scattered radiation reaching the film and thus obtains increased x-ray film contrast.

buclizine hydrochloride /boo'klazēn/, an antiemetic drug derived from piperazine that has antihistamine properties. It is also used to treat allergies and vertigo.

bud, [ME, *budde*], any small outgrowth that is the beginning stage of a living structure, as a limb bud from which an arm or leg develops.

Budd-Chiari's syndrome /bud'kē·är'ē/ [George Budd, English physician, 1808–1882; Hans Chiari, Czech-French pathologist, 1851–1916], a disorder of hepatic circulation, marked by venous obstruction, that leads to liver enlargement, ascites, extensive development of collateral vessels, and severe portal hypertension.

budding [ME, *budde*], a type of asexual reproduction in which the cell produces a budlike projection containing chromatin that eventually separates from the parent and develops into an independent organism. It is a common form of reproduction in the lower organisms and plants such as sponges, yeasts, and molds.

buddy splint, a splinting technique commonly used after a finger injury requiring immobilization. The injured finger and the adjacent finger are typically taped together to limit the range of motion of the affected finger.

budesonide, a nasal corticosteroid antiinflammatory agent prescribed in the treatment of seasonal or continual inflammation of the mucous membranes of the nasal passages.

Buerger's postural exercises [Leo Buerger, American physician, 1879–1943; L, *ponere,* to place, *exercere,* to continue working], exercises designed to maintain circulation in a limb.

buffalo hump, an accumulation of fat on the back of the neck associated with the prolonged use of large doses of glucocorticoids or the hypersecretion of cortisol caused by Cushing's syndrome.

buffer [ME, *buffe,* to cushion], a substance or group of substances that tends to control the hydrogen ion concentration in a solution by reacting with hydrogen ions when an acid is added to the system and releasing hydrogen ions on the addition of a base. Buffers minimize significant changes of pH in a chemical system. Among the functions carried out by buffer systems in the body is maintenance of the acid-base balance of the blood and of the proper pH in kidney tubules.

buffer anions, the negatively charged bicarbonate, protein, and phosphate ions that comprise the buffer systems of the body.

buffer cations, the positively charged ions of the body's electrolytes, including sodium, calcium, potassium, and magnesium.

buffer solution [ME, *buffet* + L, *solutus,* dissolved], a solution that will minimize changes in pH value despite dilution or addition of a small amount of base or acid.

buffy coat [ME, *buffet* + Fr, *cote*], a grayish-white layer of white blood cells and platelets, mixed with some red blood cells, that accumulates on the surface of sedimented erythrocytes when blood plasma is allowed to stand.

bulb [L, *bulbus,* swollen root], any rounded structure, such as the eyeball, hair roots, and certain sensory nerve endings.

bulbar /bul'bər/ [L, *bulbus*], **1.** pertaining to a bulb. **2.** pertaining to the medulla oblongata of the brain and the cranial nerves.

bulbar ataxia [L, *bulbus,* swollen root; Gk, *ataxia,* without order], a loss of motor coordination caused by a lesion in the medulla oblongata or pons.

bulbar myelitis [L, *bulbus,* swollen root; Gk, *myelos,* marrow, *itis,* inflammation], an inflammation of the central nervous system involving the medulla oblongata.

bulbar palsy [L, *bulbus,* swollen root; Gk, *paralyein,* to be palsied], a form of paralysis resulting from a defect in the motor centers of the medulla oblongata.

bulbar paralysis, a degenerative neurologic condition characterized by progressive paralysis of cranial nerves and involving the lips, tongue, mouth, pharynx, and larynx.

bulbar poliomyelitis [L, *bulbus,* swollen root; Gk, *polios,* gray, *myelos,* marrow, *itis,* inflammation], a form of poliomyelitis that involves the medulla oblongata and gradually progresses to bulbar paralysis, with respiratory and circulatory failure.

bulbiform /bul'bifôrm/, shaped like a bulb.

bulbocavernosus /bul'bōkav'ərnō'səs/ [L, *bulbus,* swollen root, *cavernosum,* full of hollows], a muscle that covers the bulb of the penis in the male and the bulbus vestibuli in the female.

bulbocavernosus reflex, the contraction of the bulbospongiosus muscle when the dorsum of the penis is tapped or the glans penis is compressed.

bulbourethral gland /-yōōrē'thrəl/, one of two small glands located on each side of the prostate, draining to the urethra. Bulbourethral glands secrete a fluid component of the seminal fluid.

bulbous [L, *bulbus,* swollen root], pertaining to a structure that resembles a bulb or that originates in a bulb.

bulb syringe, a device with a bulb that replaces the plunger for instillation or aspiration. Bulb syringes can be used to irrigate an external orifice, such as the auditory canal.

bulimia /byōōlim'ē·ə/ [Gk, *bous,* ox, *limos,* hunger], a disorder characterized by an insatiable craving for food, often resulting in episodes of continuous eating and often followed by purging, depression, and self-deprivation.

bulimic /byōōlim'ik/, pertaining to bulimia.

bulk cathartic [ME, *bulke,* heap; Gk, *kathartikos,* evacuation of bowels], a cathartic that acts by softening and increasing the mass of fecal material in the bowel.

bulla /bōōl'ə, bul'ə/, *pl.* **bullae** [L, bubble], a thin-walled blister of the skin or mucous membranes greater than 1 cm in diameter containing clear, serous fluid. —**bullous,** *adj.*

bulldog forceps, short spring forceps for clamping an artery or vein for hemostasis. The jaws may be padded to avoid injury to vascular tissue.

bullet forceps, a kind of forceps that has thin, curved, serrated blades that are designed for extracting a foreign object, such as a bullet, from the base of a puncture wound.

bullous disease /bōōl'əs/, any disease marked by eruptions of blisters, or bullae, filled with fluid, on the skin or mucous membranes. An example is pemphigus.

bullous impetigo, a form of impetigo in which the skin lesions are bullae instead of vesicles. The crusts are thin and greenish yellow.

bullous myringitis [L, *bulla* + *myringa,* eardrum], an inflammatory condition of the ear, characterized by fluid-filled vesicles on the tympanic membrane and the sudden onset of severe pain in the ear.

bullous pemphigoid [L, *bulla,* bubble; Gk, *pemphix,* bubble, *eidos,* form], a condition characterized by chronic eruptions of skin blisters over multiple body areas.

bumetanide /bōōmet'ənīd/, a loop diuretic related to furosemide. It is prescribed for edema caused by cardiac, hepatic, or renal disease.

BUN, abbreviation for **blood urea nitrogen.**

bundle, a group of nerve fibers or other threadlike structures running in the same direction. See also **fasciculus.**

bundle branch [Dan, *bondel* + Fr, *branche*], a segment of a network of specialized conducting fibers that transmit electrical impulses within the ventricles. Bundle branches are a continuation of the bundle of His, extending from the upper part of the intraventricular septum of the heart.

bundle branch block (BBB), an inability of the cardiac impulse to conduct down the bundle branches, causing an abnormally shaped and widened QRS complex. BBB is commonly seen in high-risk acute anterior wall myocardial infarction. It may be caused by ischemia or necrosis of the bundle branches, trauma (as in surgical manipulation), or mechanical compression of the branches by a tumor. Pacemaker insertion may be performed if further deterioration in conduction is anticipated.

bundle of His., See **atrioventricular (AV) bundle.**

bunion /bun'yən/ [Gk, *bounion,* turnip], an abnormal enlargement of the joint at the base of the great toe. It is caused by inflammation of the bursa. It is characterized by soreness, swelling, thickening of the skin, and lateral displacement of the great toe.

bunionectomy /bun'yənek'təmē/, excision of a bunion.

bunionette /bun'yənet'/, an abnormal enlargement and inflammation of the joint at the base of the small toe.

Bunsen burner /bōō'sən, bun'sən/ [Robert E.W. Bunsen, German chemist, 1811–1899], a standard laboratory gas burner designed to produce nearly complete combustion in a smokeless flame.

Bunyamwera arbovirus /bun'yəmwir'ə/ [Bunyamwera, town in Uganda where the type species was isolated], one of a group of arthropod-borne viruses that infect humans and are carried by mosquitoes from rodent hosts. The virus causes California encephalitis, Rift Valley fever, and other diseases characterized by headache, weakness, low-grade fever, myalgia, and a rash.

B

buoyant density, the thickness or compactness of a substance that allows it to float in a standard fluid.

bupivacaine hydrochloride /byoõpiv'-əkān/, a local anesthetic prescribed for caudal, epidural, peripheral, or sympathetic anesthetic block.

buprenorphine hydrochloride /boõ'-prənôr'fēn/, a parenteral analgesic prescribed for the relief of moderate to severe pain.

bupropion /boõprō'pē·on/, a heterocyclic mood-elevating drug used to treat some types of depression.

burden, a heavy, oppressive load, as a disabling clinical load.

Bureau of Medical Devices (BMD), an agency of the U.S. Food and Drug Administration organized in 1976 with the responsibility of providing standards for and regulation of the manufacture and uses of medical devices.

buret /byoõret'/ [Fr, small jug], a laboratory utensil used to deliver a wide range of volumes accurately.

buried suture [L, *sutura*], a suture that is inserted to draw together soft tissues between the viscus and the skin.

Burkitt's lymphoma /bur'kits/ [Denis P. Burkitt, English surgeon in Africa, b. 1911], a malignant neoplasm composed of undifferentiated lymphoreticular cells that form a large osteolytic lesion in the jaw or, in children, an abdominal mass. The tumor, which is seen chiefly in Central Africa, is characteristically a gray-white mass sometimes containing areas of hemorrhage and necrosis.

burn [AS, *baernan*], any injury to tissues of the body caused by heat, electricity, chemicals, radiation, or gases in which the extent of the injury is determined by the amount of exposure of the cell to the agent and to the nature of the agent. The treatment of burns includes pain relief, careful asepsis, prevention of infection, maintenance of the balance in the body of fluids and electrolytes, and good nutrition.

burn center, a health care facility that is designed to care for patients who have been severely burned. A network of burn centers has been established throughout the United States and Canada to provide sophisticated advanced techniques of care for burn victims.

burner syndrome, a condition of burning pain, especially in the upper extremities, and sometimes accompanied by shoulder girdle weakness. It may be experienced during contact sports such as football as a result of a blow to the head or shoulder. It is attributed to an upper trunk neuropathy of the brachial plexus.

burning drops sign, a sensation of hot liquid dripping into the abdominal cavity caused by a perforated stomach ulcer.

burning feet syndrome, a neurologic disorder characterized by symptoms of a burning sensation in the sole of the foot. The burning tends to be more intense at night and may also involve the hands.

burning pain [AS, *baernan,* to burn; L, *poena,* penalty], the pain experienced as a result of a thermal burn. The term is sometimes used to describe heartburn or myocardial pain.

burnisher /bur'nishər/ [ME, *burnischen,* to make brown], a noncutting dental instrument with one end shaped as a beveled nib, used to smooth out rough edges of restorations.

burnout, a popular term for a mental or physical energy depletion after a period of chronic, unrelieved job-related stress characterized sometimes by physical illness.

burn therapy, the management of a patient burned by flames, hot liquids, explosives, chemicals, or electric current. Partial-thickness burns may be first degree, involving only the epidermis, or second degree, involving the epidermis and corium, whereas full-thickness or third-degree burns involve all skin layers. Second-degree burns covering more than 30% of the body and third-degree burns on the face and extremities or more than 10% of the body surface are critical. In the first 48 hours of a severe burn, vascular fluid, sodium chloride, and protein rapidly pass into the affected area, causing local edema, blister formation, hypovolemia, hypoproteinemia, hyponatremia, hyperkalemia, hypotension, and oliguria. The initial hypovolemic stage is followed by a shift of fluid in the opposite direction, resulting in diuresis, increased blood volume, and decreased serum electrolyte level. Potential complications in serious burns include circulatory collapse, renal damage, gastric atony, paralytic ileus, infections, septic shock, pneumonia, and stress ulcer (Curling's ulcer), characterized by hematemesis and peritonitis.

Burow's solution /byoõr'ōz/ [Karl A. Burow, German physician, 1809–1874], a liquid preparation containing aluminum sulfate, acetic acid, precipitated calcium carbonate, and water used as a topical astringent, antiseptic, and antipyretic for a wide variety of skin disorders.

burp, *informal.* **1.** to belch, or eructate; to expel gas from the stomach through the mouth. **2.** a belch, or eructation.

burr, a rotary instrument fitted into a handpiece and used to cut teeth or bone.

burr cell [ME, *burre* + L, *cella,* storeroom], a form of mature erythrocyte in which the cells or cell fragments have spicules, or tiny projections, on the surface.

burr holes, holes drilled in the skull to drain and irrigate an abscess.

bursa /bur'sə/, *pl.* **bursae** [Gk, *byrsa,* wineskin], **1.** a fibrous sac between certain tendons and the bones beneath them. Lined with a synovial membrane that secretes synovial fluid, the bursa acts as a small cushion that allows the tendon to move over the bone as it contracts and relaxes. **2.** a sac or closed cavity.

bursal abscess /bur'səl/, a collection of pus in the cavity of a bursa.

bursa of Achilles, bursa separating the tendon of Achilles and the calcaneus.

bursectomy /bərsek'təmē/ [Gk, *byrsa,* wine skin, *ektome,* cutting out], the excision of a bursa.

bursitis /bərsī'tis/, an inflammation of the bursa, the connective tissue structure surrounding a joint. Bursitis may be precipitated by arthritis, infection, injury, or excessive or traumatic exercise or effort. The chief symptom is severe pain of the affected joint, particularly on movement. The goals of treatment for bursitis include the control of pain and the maintenance of joint motion.

burst, to break suddenly while under tension or expansion.

bursting fracture [ME, *bersten* + L, *fractura,* break], any fracture that disperses multiple bone fragments, usually at or near the end of a bone.

Burton's line [Henry Burton, English physician, 1799–1849], a dark blue stippled line along the gingival margin, which is a sign of lead poisoning.

buspirone hydrochloride /bōōspir'ōn/, an oral antianxiety drug prescribed for anxiety disorders and the short term relief of anxiety symptoms.

busulfan /bōōsul'fən/, an alkylating agent prescribed in the treatment of chronic myelocytic leukemia.

butabarbital sodium /byōō'təbär'bitôl/, a sedative; intermediate-acting barbiturate. It is prescribed for the relief of anxiety, nervous tension, and insomnia.

butaconazole nitrate /byōō'təkō'nəzōl/, an intravaginal antifungal cream prescribed for the treatment of vulvovaginal fungal infections caused by *Candida* species.

butamben picrate /byōōtam'bən pik'rāt/, a topical local anesthetic for the temporary relief of pain from minor burns.

butane (C_4H_{10}), a colorless petroleum-based gas. It is the fourth member of the paraffin series of hydrocarbons.

butanol-extractable iodine (BEI) /byōō'-tənôl/, iodine that can be separated from plasma proteins by a solvent, as butanol, and measured for analyzing thyroid function.

butaperazine maleate /byōō'təper'əzēn mal'ēblāt/, an antipsychotic prescribed in the treatment of schizophrenia and chronic brain syndrome.

butorphanol tartrate /byōōtôr'fənôl/, a parenteral agonist/antagonist narcotic of the phenanthrene family. It is prescribed for surgical premedication, as an analgesic component of balanced anesthesia, and for prompt relief of moderate to severe pain associated with surgical procedures.

butt, 1. to place two surfaces together to form a joint. **2.** (in dentistry) to place directly against the tissues covering the residual alveolar ridge.

butter, a soft, solid substance, such as the oily mass produced by churning cream.

butterfly bandage [AS, *buttorfleoge*], a narrow adhesive strip with broader winglike ends used to approximate the edges of a superficial wound and to hold the edges together as they heal. It is used in place of a suture in certain cases.

butterfly fracture, a bone break in which the center fragment contained by two cracks forms a triangle.

butterfly rash, an erythematous eruption of both cheeks joined by a narrow band of rash across the nose. It may be seen in lupus erythematosus, rosacea, and seborrheic dermatitis.

buttermilk [Gk, *boutyron,* butter; AS, *meoluc*], **1.** the slightly sour-tasting liquid residue remaining after the solids in cream have been churned into butter. It is nearly fat free and is nutritionally comparable to whole milk. **2.** cultured milk made by the addition of certain organisms to fat-free milk.

butter stools, a fatty fecal discharge from the bowels, as may occur in steatorrhea.

buttock augmentation, a reconstructive procedure in cosmetic surgery for reshaping the buttocks.

buttonhole [OFr, *boton* + AS, *hol*], a small slitlike hole in the wall of a structure or a cavity of the body.

buttonhole fracture, a fracture caused by a straight perforation of a bone, such as by a bullet.

buttonhole stenosis, an extreme narrowing of a vessel. The term usually refers to the mitral valve, in which the valve cusps are contracted to form an opening shaped like a buttonhole.

buttonhook, any of a variety of devices designed to help patients with limited finger range of motion, dexterity, or weakness fasten buttons on clothing.

button suture, a technique in suturing in which the ends of the suture material are passed through buttons on the surface of the skin and tied. It is used to prevent the suture from cutting through the skin.

buttressing, a phenomenon of osteoarthritis in which osteophytes at the hip joint extend across the femoral neck inferior to the femoral head and combine, with a proliferation along the medial aspect of the femoral neck.

buttress plate, a thin, flat metal plate used to provide support in the surgical repair of a fracture.

butyl /byoo′til/ [Gk, *boutyron,* butter, *hyle,* matter], a hydrocarbon radical (C_4H_9), the compounds of which are obtained from petroleum. Butyl compounds, some of which are toxic and irritating, are used in a variety of industrial and medical applications, including anesthesia.

butyl alcohol, a clear, toxic liquid used as an organic solvent. It exists as four isomers, n-butyl, isobutyl, secondary butyl, and tertiary butyl alcohol.

butyric acid /byoo′tir′ik/, a fatty acid occurring in rancid butter, feces, urine, perspiration, and, in trace amounts, spleen and blood. Butyric acid is used in the preparation of flavorings, emulsifying agents, and pharmaceutics.

butyric fermentation, the conversion of carbohydrates to butyric acid.

butyrophenone /byoo′tərōfē′nōn/, one of a small group of major tranquilizers.

They are used in treating psychosis to decrease the choreic symptoms of Huntington's chorea and the tics and coprolalia of Gilles de la Tourette's syndrome.

Buzzard's maneuver [Thomas Buzzard, English neurologist, 1831–191], a modified patellar reflex in which the patient's toes are firmly pressed on the floor while the quadriceps muscle is tapped.

BWS, abbreviation for **battered woman syndrome.**

bypass [AS, *bi,* alongside; Fr, *passer*], **1.** any one of various surgical procedures to divert the flow of blood or other natural fluids from normal anatomic courses. A bypass may be temporary or permanent. Bypass surgery is commonly performed in the treatment of cardiac and gastrointestinal disorders. **2.** a term used by some hospitals to signal that its emergency department lacks the personnel and equipment to handle additional patients, thereby advising that ambulances transporting new patients be diverted to other hospitals.

by-product material, the radioactive waste of nuclear reactors.

byssinosis /bis′inō′sis/ [Gk, *byssos,* flax, *osis,* condition], an occupational respiratory disease characterized by shortness of breath, cough, and wheezing. The condition is an allergic reaction to dust or fungi in cotton, flax, and hemp fibers.

Byzantine arch palate /biz′əntēn/, a congenital anomaly of the roof of the mouth marked by incomplete fusion of the palatal process and the nasal spine.

C

c, 1. symbol for *capillary blood.* 2. abbreviation for **curie.**

C, 1. (in respiratory physiology) symbol for **compliance. 2.** symbol for *concentration of gas in the blood.* 3. symbol for the element **carbon.**

Ca, symbol for the element **calcium.**

CA125, abbreviation for *cancer cell surface antigen 125,* a glycoprotein found in the blood serum of patients with ovarian or other glandular cell carcinomas. Increasing levels of the antigen represent continuing tumor growth, which may indicate a poor prognosis.

CABG, abbreviation for *coronary artery bypass graft.*

cabinet bath [ME, *cabane,* cabin], a bath in which the patient, except his or her head, is enclosed in a cabinet heated by hot air or radiant heat.

Cabot rings /kab'ot/ [Richard C. Cabot, American physician, 1868–1939], threadlike figures, often appearing as loops or rings in red blood cells of patients with severe anemia.

Cabot's splint [Arthur T. Cabot, American surgeon, b. 1852], a metal splint worn behind the thigh and leg for support.

CaC₂, the chemical formula for calcium carbide.

cacao /kəkā'ō/ *cacal,* 1. cocoa. 2. the substance *Theobroma cacao.* 3. the seeds of *Theobroma cacao.*

cacesthesia /kak'əsthē'zhə/ [Gk, *kakos, bad, aisthesis, feeling*], any morbid feeling or disordered sensibility. —cacesthetic, *adj.*

cachectic /kəkek'tik/ [Gk, *kakos,* bad, *hexis,* state], pertaining to a state of generally poor health and malnutrition.

cachet /kāshā'/ [Fr, tablet], any lenticular edible capsule that encloses a dose of medicine.

cachexia /kəkek'sē·ə/ [Gk, *kakos,* bad, *hexis,* state], general ill health and malnutrition, marked by weakness and emaciation, usually associated with severe disease, such as tuberculosis or cancer. —cachectic, *adj.*

cachinnation /kak'ənā'shən/ [L, *cachinnare,* to laugh aloud], excessive laughter with no apparent cause, often part of

the behavioral pattern in schizophrenia. —**cachinnate,** *v.*

CaCl₂, the chemical formula for calcium chloride.

CaCO₃, the chemical formula for calcium carbonate.

CaC₂O₄, the chemical formula for calcium oxalate.

cacodemonomania /kak'ōdē'mənōmā'nē·ə/ [Gk, *kakos + daimon,* spirit, *mania,* madness], an abnormal mental condition in which the patient claims to be possessed by an evil spirit.

cacophony /kəkof'ənē/, *pl.* **cacophonies** [Gk, *kakos + phone,* voice], a harsh or discordant sound or a mixture of confused, different sounds. —**cacophonic, cacophonous,** *adj.*

cacoplastic /kak'əplas'tik/, 1. pertaining to a low or inferior grade of structure or organization. 2. pertaining to a state of morbid growth.

cacosmia /kakoz'mē·ə/ [Gk, *kakos + osme,* odor], the perception of foul odor or stench when none exists. In most instances the condition results from psychologic factors, as in olfactory hallucinations.

CAD, abbreviation for **coronary artery disease.**

cadaver /kədä'vər/ [L, dead body], a corpse used for dissection and study.

cadaver graft, the transfer of tissue from the body of a dead individual to repair a defect in a living person.

cadaveric /kad'äver'ik/, pertaining to or resembling a cadaver.

cadaveric renal transplant (CRT), a kidney transplant from a dead donor.

cadence /kā'dəns/ [L, *cadere,* to fall], a rhythm as in voice, music, or movement, used in a test of the vestibular system.

cadmium (Cd) /kad'mē·əm/(Cd) [Gk, *kadmeia,* zinc ore], a metallic bluish white element that resembles tin. Its atomic number is 48; its atomic weight (mass) is 112.40. Cadmium was formerly included in medications. Such medications have been replaced by less toxic drugs.

cadmium poisoning, poisoning resulting from the inhalation of cadmium in fumes created by welding, smelting, or other industrial processes involving solder. Cad-

183

mium bromide can cause severe gastrointestinal symptoms if swallowed. Cadmium may also cause poisoning by the ingestion of acidic foods prepared and stored in cadmium-lined containers, as lemonade in certain metal cans. The effects may include vomiting, dyspnea, headache, prostration, pulmonary edema, and, possibly, years later, cancer.

caduceus /kədoo′sē-əs/ [L; Gk, *karykeion*, herald], the wand of the god Hermes or Mercury, used as the symbol for the U.S. Army Medical Corps. It is represented as a staff with two serpents coiled around it and is often confused with the staff of Æsculapius, a rod with one snake entwined about it.

café-au-lait spot /kaf′ä-ōlā′/ [Fr, coffee with milk], a pale tan macule, the color of coffee with milk. Simultaneous development of several café-au-lait spots is associated with neurofibromatosis, but occasional café-au-lait spots occur normally.

café coronary /kəfā′/, a collapse of a person who is eating, caused by asphyxiation that results from obstruction of the glottis by a food bolus. Because the signs are similar to those of a heart attack, such episodes are frequently mistaken for coronary occlusions.

caffeine /kafēn′, kaf′ē·in/ [Ar, *qahwah*, coffee], a central nervous system stimulant prescribed to counteract migraine, drowsiness, and mental fatigue.

caffeine poisoning [Ar, *qahwah*, coffee; L, *potio*, drink], a toxic condition caused by the chronic ingestion of excessive amounts of caffeine, which is found in coffee, tea, cola beverages, and certain stimulant drugs. Symptoms include restlessness, anxiety, general depression, tachycardia, tremors, nausea, diuresis, and insomnia.

Caffey's syndrome, [John Caffey, American pediatrician, 1895–1978], the battered baby syndrome, first described by John Caffey in 1946.

CAGE /kāj/, a mnemonic acronym formed by the first letters of four questions designed to screen alcoholic patients: *C*utdown, *A*nnoyed by criticism, *G*uilt about drinking, and *E*ye-opener drinks.

CAH, 1. abbreviation for **chronic active hepatitis. 2.** abbreviation for **congenital adrenal hyperplasia.**

CAHEA, abbreviation for **Committee on Allied Health Education and Accreditation.**

caked /kākt/ [ONorse, *kaka*], formed into a compact mass or crust, as the scab of coagulated blood on a healing wound.

caked breast, an accumulation of milk in the secreting ducts of the breast after childbirth, causing all or a part of the breast to become hardened and the tissues to become engorged.

cal, 1. abbreviation for **small calorie. 2.** abbreviation for a *calcium cation.*

Cal, abbreviation for **kilocalorie, large calorie.**

calabar swelling /kal′əbär/ [Calabar, a Nigerian seaport], an abnormal condition characterized by fugitive, swollen lumps of subcutaneous tissue caused by a parasitic filarial worm endemic to Central and West Africa. The swollen areas migrate with the worm through the body. At times the worm may move under the conjunctiva of the eye and may live in the anterior chamber of the eye.

calamine /kal′əmīn/ [Gk, *kadmeia*, zinc ore], a pink, odorless powdered concoction used as a protectant or an astringent and sometimes prepared as a lotion. It is composed of zinc oxide with 0.5% ferric oxide.

calcaneal /kalkā′nē-əl/ [L, *calcaneum*, heel], pertaining to the calcaneus at the back of the tarsus.

calcaneal epiphysitis, a painful disorder involving the calcaneus at its epiphysis. The condition tends mainly to affect children who are physically active and whose heel bones are still divided by a layer of cartilage.

calcaneal spurs, abnormal, often painful bony outgrowths on the lower surface of the calcaneus, resulting from chronic traumatic pressure on the heel.

calcaneal tuberosity, a transverse elevation on the plantar surface of the calcaneus to which are attached the abductor digiti minimi, the long plantar ligament, and various other muscles.

calcaneodynia /kalkā′nē-ōdin′ē-ə/ [L, *calcaneum* + Gk, *odyne*, pain], a painful condition of the heel.

calcaneus /kalkā′nē-əs/ [L, *calcaneum*, heel], the heel bone. The largest of the tarsal bones, it articulates proximally with the talus and distally with the cuboid. —**calcaneal, calcanean,** *adj.*

calcar /kal′kär/, *pl.* **calcaria,** a spur or a structure that resembles a spur.

calcar avis /ā′vis/ [L, *calcar*, spur, *avis*, bird], a projection on the medial wall of the posterior horn of the lateral ventricle of the brain. It is associated with the lateral extension of the calcarine fissure.

calcareous /kalker′ē-əs/ [L, *calcar*, spur], pertaining to calcium or lime.

calcarine /kal′kərīn/, **1.** having the shape of a spur. **2.** pertaining to the calcar.

calcarine fissure, a groove between the cuneus and the lingual gyrus on the medial surface of the occipital lobe of the brain.

calcereous metastasis, the deposition of calcium salts in visceral organs as a result of hyperparathyroidism, an absorptive disease of the bone, or any cause of hypercalcemia, particularly when associated with hyperphosphatemia.

calcergy /kal'sərjē/, local calcification of soft tissues at the site of injection of certain types of chemicals.

calcifediol /kal'sifē'dē·ol/, a physiologic form of vitamin D prescribed in the treatment of metabolic bone disease associated with chronic renal failure.

calciferol /kalsif'ərôl/ [L, *calx,* lime, *ferre,* to bear], a fat-soluble, crystalline unsaturated alcohol produced by ultraviolet irradiation of ergosterol. It is used as a dietary supplement in the prophylaxis and treatment of rickets, osteomalacia, and other hypocalcemic disorders. Calciferol occurs naturally in milk and fish-liver oils.

calcific /kalsif'ik/ [L, *calx,* lime, *facere,* to make], pertaining to the formation of chalk, lime, or calcium.

calcific aortic disease [L, *calx,* lime], an abnormal condition characterized by small deposits of calcium in the aorta.

calcification [L, *calx* + *facere,* to make], the accumulation of calcium salts in tissues. Normally, about 99% of all the calcium entering the human body is deposited in the bones and teeth; the remaining 1% is dissolved in body fluids such as blood.

calcific tendinitis [L, *calx,* lime, *facere,* to make, *tendo,* tendon; Gk, *itis,* inflammation], a chronic inflammation of a tendon as a result of an accumulation of calcium deposits in the tissue.

calcination /kal'sinā'shən/ [L, *calcinare,* to burn lime], (in dentistry) a process of removing water by heat, used in the manufacture of plaster and stone from gypsum.

calcinosis /kal'sənō'sis/, a condition characterized by abnormal deposits of calcium salts in various tissues. The deposits appear as nodules or plaques.

calcipenia /kal'sipē'nē·ə/, a deficiency of calcium in the body tissues and fluids.

calcitonin /kal'sitō'nin/ [L, *calx* + Gk, *tonos,* tone], a hormone produced in parafollicular cells of the thyroid that participates in regulating the blood level of calcium and stimulates bone mineralization. A synthetic preparation of the hormone is used in the treatment of certain bone disorders.

calcitriol /kalsit're·ôl/, the active form of vitamin D, a regulator of calcium metabolism. It is prescribed in the management of hypocalcemia in patients undergoing chronic renal dialysis.

calcium (Ca) /kal'sē·əm/ [L, *calx,* lime], an alkaline earth metal element. Its atomic number is 20; its atomic weight (mass) is 40.08. Its metallic form is a white flammable solid, somewhat harder than lead. Calcium is the fifth most abundant element in the human body and is mainly present in the bone. The body requires calcium ions for the transmission of nerve impulses, muscle contraction, blood coagulation, cardiac functions, and other processes. It is a component of extracellular fluid and of soft tissue cells. Abnormally high levels of ionized calcium in the extracellular fluid can produce muscle weakness, lethargy, and coma. A relatively small decrease from the normal level of this element can produce tetanic seizures.

calcium carbide (CaC$_2$), a black crystalline compound produced from lime and coke. When mixed with water, it yields acetylene gas (C$_2$H$_2$), which has been used as an anesthetic.

calcium carbonate (CaCO$_2$), 1. precipitated chalk. 2. a white powder sometimes used in antacids.

calcium channel blocker, a drug that inhibits the flow of calcium ions across the membranes of smooth muscle cells. By reduction of the calcium flow, smooth muscle tone is relaxed, and the risk of muscle spasms is diminished. Calcium channel blockers are used primarily in the treatment of heart diseases marked by coronary artery spasms.

calcium chloride (CaCl$_2$), a white granular chemical with an unpleasant taste. It is used in a concentrated solution of the chloride salt of calcium to replenish calcium in the blood. It is prescribed for hypocalcemic tetany and as an antidote for lead or magnesium poisoning or magnesium sulfate overdose.

calcium gluconate (C$_{12}$H$_{22}$CaO$_{14}$), a white odorless, tasteless powder or granules administered orally or intravenously to replenish the body's calcium stores, as after a transfusion.

calcium hydroxide (Ca[OH]$_2$), a bittertasting white powder that may be used in the preparation of treatments for infant diarrhea. Also called *slaked lime.*

calcium hydroxide solution, a clear, colorless liquid sometimes used as an alkali and antidote. Also called *lime water.*

calcium oxalate (CaC$_2$O$_4$), a small, colorless crystal that may be present in urine or that may be a component of renal calculi.

calcium oxide (CaO), a compound formed by the calcination of chalk or marble and sometimes used in the preparation of caustic pastes. Also called calx, quicklime.

calcium phosphate $(Ca_3[PO_4]_2)$, an odorless, tasteless white powder used as a calcium supplement, laxative, and antacid.

calcium pump, a theorized, energy-requiring mechanism for transmitting calcium ions across a plasma membrane from a region of low calcium ion concentration to one of higher concentration.

calcium sulfate $(CaSO_4)$, a white moisture-absorbing powder used for making plaster casts.

calciuria /kal'siŏŏē·ə/ [L, *calx,* lime; Gk, *ouron,* urine], the presence of calcium in the urine.

calcospherite /kal'kəsfir'īt/, a spherical mass of calcium salts and organic matter found in an area of calcification.

calculogenesis /kal'kyəlōjen'əsis/, the formation of calculi.

calculous /kal'kyələs/, **1.** describing a substance that has the hardness of stone. **2.** pertaining to calculus.

calculus /kal'kyələs/, *pl.* **calculi** /kal'kyəlī/ [L, little stone], an abnormal stone formed in body tissues by an accumulation of mineral salts. Calculi are usually found in biliary and urinary tracts.

Caldwell-Moloy pelvic classification /kôl'dwelməloi'/ [William E. Caldwell, American obstetrician, 1880–1943; Howard C. Moloy, American gynecologist, 1903–1953], a system for classifying the structure of the bony pelvis of the female. The types in this system are android, anthropoid, gynecoid, and platypelloid. The sacrum, coccyx, sidewalls, sacrosciatic notch, ischial spines, pubic arch, and ischial tuberosities are the anatomic points of reference used to determine pelvic type.

calefacient /kal'əfā'shənt/ [L, *calare,* to be warm, *facere,* to make], **1.** making or tending to make anything warm or hot. **2.** an agent that imparts a sense of warmth when applied, such as a hot-water bottle or a hot compress.

calf, *pl.* **calves** [ONorse, *kalfi*], the fleshy mass at the back of the leg below the knee, composed chiefly of the gastrocnemius muscle.

calf muscle pump, an action of the calf (soleus) muscles in which the muscles contract and squeeze the popliteal and tibia veins, forcing the blood in those veins to move upward toward the heart.

caliber /kal'ibər/ [Fr, *calibre,* bore of a gun], the diameter of a tube or a canal, as any of the blood vessels.

calibration /kal'ibrā'shən/ [Fr, *calibre,* the bore of a gun], the process of measuring or calibrating against an established standard, such as a deciliter or kilogram.

calibrator, 1. an instrument used to increase the diameter of an opening, as a dilator of a urethral stricture. **2.** an instrument used to measure the size of an opening.

Caliciviridae /kalis'ivir'idē/, a family of plus-stranded ribonucleic acid viruses that have a nonenveloped virion 35 to 40 nm in diameter. It is associated with episodes of gastroenteritis and hepatitis in humans and animals, including exanthema in swine.

caliculus /kalik'yələs/, a cup-shaped structure.

California encephalitis, a common acute viral infection that affects the central nervous system. The mild form is characterized by headache, malaise, gastrointestinal symptoms, and a fever that may reach 104° F. The more severe form may be marked by a sudden onset of fever, vomiting, headaches, lethargy, and signs of neurologic involvement such as loss of reflexes, disorientation, seizure, loss of consciousness, and flaccid paralysis.

californium (Cf) [state of California], an artificial element in the actinide group. Its atomic number is 98; its atomic weight (mass) is 251. Californium-252 isotope is a potent source of neutrons.

caliorraphy /kal'ə·ôr'əfē/, surgical repair of the calyces of the kidney, usually performed to improve urinary drainage into the ureters.

calipers /kal'ipərz/ [Fr, *calibre,* bore of a gun], an instrument with two hinged, adjustable, curved legs, used to measure the thickness or the diameter of a convex or solid body.

caliper splint, a leg splint consisting of two metal rods running from the back of a band around the thigh or from a cushioned ring around the lower part of the pelvis. The rods are attached to a metal plate under the shoe below the arch of the foot.

calisthenics /kal'isthen'iks/, a system of exercise in which emphasis is on movements of muscle groups rather than power and effort. An objective is the acquisition of grace and beauty in exercise.

Calliphoridae /kal'əfôr'ədē/ [Gk, *kallos,* beauty, *pherein,* to bear], a family of medium-sized to large flies that belong to the order Diptera, serve as pathogenic vectors, and may cause intestinal or nasopharyngeal myiasis in humans.

callomania /kal'ōmā'nē·ə/ [Gk, *kallos,* beauty, *mania,* madness], an abnormal psychologic condition characterized by delusions of personal beauty.

callosal fissure /kəlos'əl/ [L, *callosus,* hard, *fissura,* cleft], a groove following the convex aspect of the corpus callosum.

callosomarginal fissure /kəlō'sōmär'jənəl/, a long, irregular groove on the medial surface of a cerebral hemisphere. It divides the cingulate gyrus from the medial frontal gyrus and from the paracentral lobule.

callous ulcer /kal'əs/ [L, *callosus*, hard, *ulcus*, ulcer], an ulcer with a hard indurated base and thick inelastic margins. It lacks a blood supply and is frequently associated with edema of the legs.

callus /kal'əs/ [L, hard skin], **1.** a common, usually painless thickening of the stratum corneum at locations of external pressure or friction. **2.** bony deposit formed between and around the broken ends of a fractured bone during healing. —**callous,** *adj.*

calmative /kä'mətiv/, having a calming or quieting effect.

Calming Technique, a Nursing Interventions Classification defined as reducing anxiety in a patient who is experiencing acute distress.

calmodulin /kalmod'yəlin/, a calcium-binding protein that mediates a variety of biochemical and physiologic processes, including the contraction of muscles and the release of norepinephrine.

calor /kal'ôr/ [L, warmth], heat, as that generated by inflammation of tissues or from the body's normal metabolic processes.

caloric /kalôr'ik/, pertaining to heat or calories.

caloric test, a procedure in which the ear canal is alternately irrigated with warm water or air and cold water or air. The warm irrigation produces a rotatory nystagmus toward the irrigated side. Cold irrigation produces a rotatory nystagmus away from the irrigated side. If the vestibular part of the ear is normal, all irrigations will produce nystagmus that is approximately equal in intensity. If the vestibular part of the ear is diseased, irrigation may produce less nystagmus than the normal ear.

calorie (cal) /kal'ôrē/ [L, *calor,* warmth], the amount of heat required to raise 1 gram of water 1° C at atmospheric pressure. —**caloric,** *adj.*

Calorie (Cal), **1.** the amount of heat (energy) needed to raise the temperature of 1 kilogram of water 1° C. **2.** a unit, equal to the large calorie, used to denote the heat expenditure of an organism and the fuel or energy value of food.

calorific /kal'ərif'ik/, pertaining to the production of heat.

calorigenic /kəlôr'ijen'ik/ [L, *calor,* warmth; Gk, *genein,* to produce], pertaining to a substance or process that produces heat or energy or increases the consumption of oxygen.

calorimeter /kal'ərim'ətər/, a device

used for measuring quantities of heat generated by friction, chemical reaction, or the human body. —**calorimetric,** *adj.*

calorimetry /kal'ərim'ətrē/ [L, *calor,* warmth; Gk, *metron,* measure], the measurement of the amounts of heat radiated and the amounts of heat absorbed. —**calorimetric,** *adj.*

calvaria /kalver'ē-ə/, the skullcap or superior part of the skull, which varies greatly in shape from individual to individual. The fontanels, or soft spots, in the skull of an infant are situated on the surface of the calvaria.

calvities /kalvish'i-ēz/ [L, *calvus,* without hair], baldness. —**calvous,** *adj.*

calyx /kā'liks/, *pl.* **calyces** /kal'isēz/, **calyxes** [Gk, *kalyx,* shell], **1.** a cup-shaped structure within an organ. **2.** a renal calyx. **3.** the wall of an ovarian follicle after expulsion of the ovum at ovulation.

cambium layer [L, *cambire,* to exchange], **1.** the loose inner cellular layer of the periosteum that develops during ossification. **2.** a cellular layer of formative tissue that lies between the wood and the bark in plants.

camera /kam'ərə/ [L, vaulted chamber], (in anatomy) any cavity or chamber, as those of the eye or the heart.

cAMP, abbreviation for **cyclic adenosine monophosphate.**

camphor /kam'fər/ [L, *camphora*], a colorless or white crystalline substance with a penetrating odor and pungent taste that occurs naturally in certain plants, especially *Cinnamomum camphora.*

camphorated oil /kam'fərā'tid/ [Malay, *kapur,* chalk; L, *oleum,* oil], a colorless-to-yellowish liquid with the penetrating, pungent odor of camphor. It is derived from a combination of a dozen organic chemicals, including terpenes, safrole, and acetaldehyde obtained from the camphor laurel plant. It is used mainly as a liniment, counterirritant, and rubefacient.

camphor bath, an air bath in which the air is filled with camphor vapor.

camphor liniment, a pharmaceutic preparation of 12.5% camphor, with alcohol, lavender oil, and ammonia, used as a rubefacient in the relief of rheumatic symptoms.

camphor poisoning, a severe toxic condition resulting from the accidental ingestion of camphorated oils. Symptoms may include headache, hallucinations, nausea, vomiting, diarrhea, convulsions, and kidney failure.

campimeter /kampim'ətər/, (in ophthalmology) an instrument for determining the integrity of the central field of vision.

camptocormia /kamp'tōkôr'mē-ə, a condition in which the back is habitually tilted forward although the spinal column remains flexible. It is frequently diagnosed as a psychologic conversion defense, and there is often a history of trauma.

camptodactyly /kamp'tədak'təlē/ [Gk, *kamptos,* bent, *daktylos,* finger], the permanent flexion of one or more fingers. **—camptodactylic,** *adj.*

camptomelia /kamp'təmē'lyə/ [Gk, *kamptos,* bent, *melos,* arm], a congenital anomaly characterized by bending of one or more limbs, causing permanent bowing or curving of the affected area. **—camptomelic,** *adj.*

Campylobacter [Gk, *campylos,* curved, *bakterion,* small staff], a genus of bacteria found in the family Spirillaceae. The type species is *C. fetus,* which consists of several subspecies that cause human infections, as well as abortion and infertility in cattle.

Campylobacter pylori. See *Helicobacter pylori.*

Camurati-Engelmann disease, [Mario Camurati, Italian physician, 1896–1948; Guido Englemann, twentieth-century Czechoslovakian surgeon] an inherited disorder of bone development marked by an onset of symptoms of muscular pain, weakness, and wasting, mainly in the legs, during childhood. The symptoms vary individually from mild to disabling. In some cases compression of nerve tissue may occur. The symptoms usually subside during early adulthood.

Canadian Association of University Schools of Nursing (CAUSN), a national Canadian organization of baccalaureate and higher-degree programs in nursing in Canada. It includes an accreditation system established in 1987.

Canadian Association of University Teachers (CAUT), a Canadian national organization representing the interests of all who teach in the universities of the provinces and territories of Canada. The official languages of the CAUT are English and French.

Canadian crutch, a wooden or metal device that helps a disabled patient stand or walk. It consists of two uprights with a crosspiece to accommodate the hand and a concave crosspiece that fits the armpit for support.

Canadian Journal of Public Health (CJPH), the official publication of the Canadian Public Health Association.

Canadian Medical Association Journal (CMAJ), the official publication of the Canadian Medical Association.

Canadian Nurses Association (CNA), the official national organization for the professional registered nurses of Canada who are members of the nine provincial nurses' associations, the Northwest Territories Registered Nurses Association, and the Yukon Registered Nurses Association.

Canadian Nurses Association Testing Service (CNATS), the organizational affiliate of the Canadian Nurses Association concerned with testing graduates of approved schools of nursing to qualify them as registered nurses.

Canadian Nurses Foundation (CNF), a national Canadian foundation organized to support scholarship in nursing.

Canadian Nurses Respiratory Society (CNRS), an organization of nurses working with or interested in alleviating the problems of respiratory disease.

Canadian Orthopedic Nurses Association (CONA), a national Canadian organization concerned with the nursing care of orthopedic patients and the continuing education of nurses working in orthopedics.

Canadian Public Health Association (CPHA), a national Canadian organization concerned with issues in public health and epidemiology.

canal /kənal'/ [L, *canalis,* channel], **1.** (in anatomy) a narrow tube or channel. **2.** (in dentistry) one of the accessory root canals and collateral pulp canals in the teeth.

canalicular /kan'əlik'yələr/, pertaining to a small canal.

canaliculus /kan'əlik'yələs/, *pl.* **canaliculi** [L, little channel], a very small tube or channel, such as the microscopic haversian canaliculi throughout bone tissue.

canalization /kan'əlīzā'shən/, the formation of canals or passages through any tissue.

canal of Corti [Alfonso Corti, Italian anatomist, 1822–1888], a space between the inner and outer rods and the basilar membrane of the cochlea in the organ of Corti.

canal of Schlemm /shlem/ [Friedrich Schlemm, German anatomist, 1795–1858], a tiny vein at the angle of the anterior chamber of the eye that connects with the pectinate villi, draining the aqueous humor and funneling it into the bloodstream.

canavanine /kan'əvan'in/, an amino acid antagonist present in alfalfa sprouts that can displace arginine in cellular proteins, thereby rendering them inactive.

cancellous /kan'siləs/ [L, *cancellus,* lattice], (of tissue) latticelike, porous, spongy. Cancellous tissue is normally present in the interior of many bones, where the spaces are usually filled with marrow.

cancellous bone, a latticelike arrangement of bony plates and trabeculae occurring at the ends of the long bones.

cancer /kan'sər/ [L, crab], **1.** a neoplasm characterized by the uncontrolled growth of anaplastic cells that tend to invade surrounding tissue and to metastasize to distant body sites. **2.** any of a large group of malignant neoplastic diseases characterized by the presence of malignant cells. Each cancer is distinguished by the nature, site, or clinical course of the lesion. The basis of cancer is believed to reside in alterations in deoxyribonucleic acid (genes), usually at several loci, but many potential causes are recognized. More than 80% of cancer cases are attributed to cigarette smoking, exposure to carcinogenic chemicals, ionizing radiation, and ultraviolet rays. Many viruses induce malignant tumors in animals; an infectious cause is likely in some human cancers, and *Helicobacter pylori* bacterium probably causes gastric cancer. An excessive rate of malignant tumors in organ transplantation recipients after immunosuppressive therapy indicates that the immune system plays a major role in controlling the proliferation of anaplastic cells. The incidence of different kinds of cancer varies markedly with gender, age, ethnic group, and geographic location. Cancer is second only to heart disease as a cause of mortality in the United States and is a leading cause of death in children between 3 and 14 years of age. In the United States, common sites for the development of malignant tumors are the skin, lung, prostate, breast, and colon. Surgery remains the major form of treatment, but irradiation is widely used as preoperative, postoperative, or primary therapy; chemotherapy, with single or multiple antineoplastic agents, is often highly effective. Many malignant lesions are curable if detected in the early stage.

cancericidal /kan'sərisī'dəl/ [L, *cancer,* crab, *caedere,* to kill], pertaining to a substance or procedure capable of destroying cancer cells.

cancer of the small intestine, a neoplastic disease of the duodenum, jejunum, or ileum. Its characteristics vary, depending on the kind of tumor and the site, but may include abdominal pain, vomiting, weight loss, diarrhea, intermittent bowel obstruction, gastrointestinal bleeding, or a mass in the right abdomen. Adenocarcinomas, the most common tumors, occur more frequently in the duodenum or upper jejunum and form polypoid or constricting napkin-ring growths. Lymphomas, found most often in the lower small intestine, may impair bowel motility by invading nerves and in some cases are associated with a malabsorption syndrome. Surgery, including a wide resection of mesenteric lymph nodes, is typically indicated for adenocarcinomas.

cancerous /kan'sərəs/ [L, crab, *oma,* tumor], pertaining to or resembling a cancer.

cancer staging, a system for describing the size and extent of spread of a malignant tumor, used to plan treatment and predict prognosis. Staging may involve a physical examination, diagnostic procedures, surgical exploration, and histologic examination. The system developed by the American Joint Committee for Cancer Staging and End Results Reporting uses the letter T to represent the tumor, N for the regional lymph node involvement, M for distant metastases, and numeric subscripts in each category to indicate the degree of dissemination.

cancriform /kang'krifôrm'/[L, crab, *forma,* form], pertaining to a lesion resembling a cancer.

cancroid [L, crab; Gk, *eidos,* form], **1.** pertaining to a lesion resembling a cancer. **2.** a moderately malignant skin cancer.

cancrum /kang'krəm/, a gangrenous ulcerative condition, often associated with rhinitis in children.

candicidin /kan'disi'din/, an antifungal antibiotic agent derived from *Streptomyces griseus* and related species. The drug is used in the treatment of vaginal candidiasis, especially that caused by *Candida albicans.*

Candida /kan'didə/ [L, *candidus,* white], a genus of yeastlike fungi, including the common pathogen *Candida albicans.*

Candida albicans /al'bəkanz/, a common budding, yeastlike microscopic fungal organism normally present in the mucous membranes of the mouth, intestinal tract, and vagina and on the skin of healthy people. Under certain circumstances it may cause superficial infections of the mouth or vagina. Infection of the esophagus and invasive systemic infections may occur in persons with human immunodeficiency virus.

candidiasis /kan'didī'əsis/ [L, *candidus* + Gk, *osis,* condition], any infection caused by a species of *Candida,* usually *Candida albicans.* It is characterized by pruritus, a white exudate, peeling, and easy bleeding. Diaper rash, intertrigo, vaginitis, and thrush are common topical manifestations of candidiasis.

Candiru fever /kan'diroo'/, an arbovirus infection transmitted to humans by the bite of a sandfly. It is characterized by an acute fever, headache, and muscle aches.

candle [L, *candela*, light], (in optics) the basic unit of measurement for luminous intensity, equal to 1/60 of the luminous intensity of a square centimeter of a black body heated to 1773.5° C or the solidification temperature of platinum, adopted in 1948 as the international standard of luminous intensity.

candy-striper, *informal.* a hospital volunteer, named for the striped pink and white uniforms traditionally worn by the young people who perform this service.

cane [Ar, *qanah*, reed], a sturdy wooden or metal shaft or walking stick used to give support and mobility to an ambulatory but partially disabled person.

canine fossa /kā'nīn/ [L, *canis*, dog; L, *ditch*], (in dentistry) either of the small depressions on the external surface of each maxilla, superolateral to the canine tooth socket.

canine tooth, any one of the four teeth, two in each jaw, situated immediately lateral to the central incisor teeth in the two human dental arches. The canine teeth are larger and stronger than the incisors and have both anterior and posterior tooth characteristics. Their roots sink deeply into the bones, causing marked prominences on the alveolar arch. The canines erupt as deciduous teeth about 16 to 20 months after birth. The eruption of the permanent canines occurs during the eleventh or twelfth year of life.

canities /kanish'i·ēz/, loss of pigment, as in the graying of hair or the appearance of white streaks in the nails.

canker /kang'kər/ [L, *cancer*, crab], an ulcer or sore in the mouth or genitals.

canker sore, an ulcerous lesion of mouth, characteristic of aphthous stomatitis.

cannabis /kan'əbis/ [Gk, *kannabis*, hemp], a psychoactive herb derived from the flowering tops of hemp plants. It has no currently acceptable clinical use in the United States but has been used in the treatment of glaucoma and as an antiemetic in some cancer patients to counter the nausea and vomiting associated with chemotherapy. Cannabis is controlled under Schedule I of the Controlled Substances Act of 1970. All parts of the plant contain psychoactive substances.

cannabism /kan'əbiz'əm/, a condition associated with excessive or extended use of cannabis (marijuana) drugs. It is characterized by anxiety, disorientation, hallucinations, memory defects, and paranoia.

cannon wave [L, *cane*, tube; AS, *wafian*], a powerful atrial ("A") wave in the jugular venous pulse. Rapid, regular cannon A waves (the "frog sign") are diagnostic of paroxysmal supraventricular tachycardia. Cannon A waves are caused by the contraction of the right atrium against a closed tricuspid valve.

cannula /kan'yələ/ [L, small tube], a flexible tube that may be inserted into a duct or cavity to deliver medication or drain fluid. It may be guided by a sharp, pointed instrument (trocar). A body fluid may be passed through the cannula to the outside. —**cannular, cannulate,** *adj.*

cannulation /kan'yəlā'shən/, the insertion of a cannula into a body duct or cavity, as into the trachea, bladder, or a blood vessel. —**cannulate, cannulize,** *v.*

cantering rhythm [*Canterbury gallop;* Gk, *rhythmos*, beat], a pattern of three heart sounds in each cardiac cycle, resembling the canter of a horse.

cantharis /kan'thäris/, *pl.* **cantharides** /kanther'idēz/ [Gk, *kantharis*, beetle], the dried insect *Cantharis vesicatoria*, which contains cantharidin, formerly used as a topical vesicant.

canthoplasty /kan'thōplas'tē/, a form of plastic surgery used to lengthen the palpebral fissure through the lateral canthus or to restore a defective canthus.

canthorraphy /kanthôr'əfē/, surgery to suture the eyelids at either canthus.

canthus /kan'thəs/, *pl.* **canthi** [Gk, *kanthus*, corner of the eye], the angle at the medial and lateral margins of the eyelids. —**canthic,** *adj.*

Cantor tube [Meyer O. Cantor, American physician, b. 1907], a double-lumen nasoenteric tube with a sealed rubber bag at one end, used to relieve obstructions in the small intestine. One lumen is used to inflate the distal balloon with air, the other to instill mercury to weight the tube. The tube also allows aspiration of intestinal contents.

CaO, chemical formula for calcium oxide.

Ca(OH)$_2$, chemical formula for calcium hydroxide.

CAOT, abbreviation for Canadian Association of Occupational Therapists.

cap, abbreviation for Latin *capiat*, 'let him or her take,' used in prescriptions.

CAP, 1. abbreviation for **College of American Pathologists. 2.** (in molecular genetics) abbreviation for catabolic activator protein. CAP participates in initiating the transcription of ribonucleic acid in organisms without a true nucleus, as bacteria.

capacitance, a measure of electrostatic capacity or the amount of stored electrical charge per unit of electrical potential.

capacitance vessels /kəpas′ətəns/ [L, *capacitas,* capacity], **1.** the blood vessels that hold the major part of the intravascular blood volume. **2.** the veins.

capacitation /kəpas′itā′shən/, the process in which the spermatozoon, after it reaches the ampulla of the fallopian tube, undergoes a series of changes that lead to its ability to fertilize an ovum.

capacity factor /kəpas′itē/ [L, *capacitas + factum,* to make], the ratio of the elution volume of a substance to the void volume in the column.

CAPD, abbreviation for **continuous ambulatory peritoneal dialysis.**

capeline bandage /kap′əlin/ [Fr, hooded cape], a covering applied like a cap. It is used for protecting the head, the shoulder, or a stump.

capillaritis /kap′ilərī′tis/ [L, *capillaris,* hairlike; Gk, *itis,* inflammation], an abnormal condition characterized by a progressive pigmentary disorder of the skin and capillaries without inflammation.

capillary /kap′iler′ē/ [L, *capillaris,* hairlike], one of the microscopic blood vessels (about 0.008 mm in diameter) joining arterioles and venules. The wall consists of a single layer of endothelial cells, which are specialized squamous epithelial cells. Blood and tissue fluids exchange various substances across these walls.

capillary action, the process involving molecular adhesion by which the surface of a liquid in a tube is either elevated or depressed, depending on the cohesiveness of the liquid molecules.

capillary bed, a capillary network.

capillary fracture, any thin hairlike fracture.

capillary fragility, a condition in which weakened capillaries rupture easily when stressed, observed as bleeding under the skin.

capillary hemangioma, a blood-filled birthmark or benign tumor consisting of closely packed small blood vessels. Commonly found during infancy, it first grows, then may spontaneously disappear in early childhood without treatment.

capillary hemorrhage, an oozing of blood from the capillaries.

capillary permeability [L, *capillaris,* hairlike, *permeare,* to pass through], a condition of the capillary wall structure that allows blood elements and waste products to pass through them.

capillary pressure [L, *capillaris,* hairlike, *premere,* to press], the blood pressure within a capillary.

capillary refilling, the process whereby blood returns to a part of the capillary system after being interrupted briefly. A capillary refill of more than 3 seconds is considered a sign of sluggish digital circulation, and a time of 5 seconds is regarded as abnormal.

capillary tufting, an abnormal condition in which pulmonary capillaries project as tufts, or small masses, into the alveoli.

capillus /kəpil′əs/, *pl.* **capilli** [L, filament], one of the hairs of the body, especially one of the hairs of the scalp.

capitate /kap′itāt/, having the shape of a head.

capitate bone [L, *caput,* head; AS, *ban*], one of the largest carpal bones, located at the center of the wrist and having a rounded head that fits the concavity of the scaphoid and the lunate bones.

capitation, a payment method for health care services. The physician, hospital, or other health care provider is paid a contracted rate for each member assigned, regardless of the number or nature of services provided. The contractual rates are usually adjusted for age, gender, illness, and regional differences.

capitulum /kəpich′ələm/, *pl.* **capitula** [L, small head], a small, rounded prominence on a bone where it articulates with another bone.

capitulum humeri /hyoo̅′mərī, hoo̅′mərē/ [L, small head, *humerus,* shoulder], a rounded eminence at the distal end of the humerus that articulates with the radius.

Caplan's syndrome [Anthony Caplan, English physician, 1907–1976], a condition of pneumoconiosis with symptoms of rheumatoid arthritis and radiographic evidence of intrapulmonary nodules.

capnograph /kap′nəgraf′/ [Gk, *kapnos,* smoke, *graphein,* to record], an instrument used in anesthesia, intensive care, and respiratory therapy to produce a capnogram, a tracing that shows the proportion of carbon dioxide in exhaled air.

capnometry /kapnom′ətrē/, the measurement of carbon dioxide in a volume of gas, usually by methods of infrared absorption or mass spectrometry.

capotement /käpōtmäN′, kəpōt′mənt/, a splashing sound made by fluid movements in a dilated stomach.

capping, a process by which cell surface molecules aggregate on a plasma membrane.

capreomycin /kap′rē·ōmī′sin/, an antibiotic prescribed in the treatment of pulmonary infections caused by capreomycin-susceptible strains of *Mycobacterium tuberculosis* when the primary agents are ineffective or cannot be used.

capric acid /kap′rik/ [L, *caper,* goat], a white crystalline substance with a rancid odor, occurring as a glyceride in natural oils.

caprizant /kap′rizant/, describing an irregular leaping or bounding pulse.

caproic acid /kaprō′ik/, a fatty acid present in milk fat and some plant oils. It is used in the production of artificial flavors.

capsicum /kap′sikəm/, the dried ripe fruit of *Capsicum frutescens* of the nightshade (Solanaceae) family, used internally as a gastrointestinal stimulant and externally as a counterirritant.

capsid /kap′sid/ [L, *capsa,* box], the layer of protein enveloping a virion.

capsomere /kap′səmir/, one of the building blocks of a viral capsid. It consists of groups of identical protein molecules and is visible in an electron microscope.

capsular /kap′sələr/ [L, *capsula,* little box], pertaining to or resembling a small container.

capsular cataract [L, *capsula* + Gk, *katarrhaktes,* waterfall], a visual opacity caused by a thickening of the epithelial cells lining the capsule. The condition is frequently the result of the aging process or a disease that involves surrounding eye tissues.

capsular pattern, a series of limitations of joint movement when the joint capsule is a limiting structure. It occurs only in synovial joints that are controlled by muscles and not in joints that depend primarily on ligamentous stability such as the sacroiliac.

capsule /kap′syəl, kap′səl/ [L, *capsula,* little box], **1.** a small soluble container, usually made of gelatin, used for enclosing a dose of medication for swallowing. **2.** a membranous shell surrounding certain microorganisms, such as the pneumococcus bacterium. **3.** a well-defined anatomic structure that encloses an organ or part, such as the capsule of the adrenal gland.

capsulectomy /kap′sələk′təmē/, the surgical excision of a capsule, usually the capsule of a joint or of the lens of the eye.

capsule of the kidney, the fibrous connective enclosure of the kidney.

capsulitis /-ī′tis/ [L, *capsula,* little box; Gk, *itis,* inflammation], an inflammation involving any anatomic capsule.

capsuloma /kap′sələ′mə/, pl. *capsulomas, capsulomata* [L, *capsula* + Gk, *oma,* tumor], a neoplasm of the capsule or the subcapsular area of the kidney.

capsuloplasty /kap′sələplas′tē/, plastic surgery performed on the capsule of a joint.

capsulorraphy /kap′sələr′əfē/, surgical repair of a tear in the capsule of a joint.

capsulorrhexis /kap′sələrek′sis/, a type of cataract operation involving a continuous circular tear in the anterior capsule to allow phacoemulsification of the lens nucleus.

capsulotomy /kap′sələt′əmē/ [L, *capsula* + Gk, *temnein,* to cut], an incision into a capsule, such as in an operation to remove a cataract.

captain-of-the-ship doctrine, the historical medicolegal principle that the physician is ultimately responsible for all patient-care activities; he or she thus may be held accountable and may be sued for negligence or malpractice when the act at issue is performed by an employee or other person under the physician's control, even if not ordered by the physician.

captive reinsurance company, a reinsurance company organized to serve only one client.

captopril /kap′tōpril/, an angiotensin-converting enzyme inhibitor prescribed for the treatment of hypertension and congestive heart failure.

capture, 1. the catching and holding of a nuclear particle, as an electron, or an electrical impulse originating elsewhere. **2.** (in cardiology) the capture of control of the atria or ventricles after a period of independent beating caused by ectopic beats or an atrioventricular block.

capture beat /kap′chər/, the return of atrial control over ventricular contraction, following a period of atrioventricular dissociation.

capture-recapture method, a plan for epidemiologic studies of health problems such as acquired immunodeficiency syndrome, substance abuse, or prostitution. The method provides for comparative analysis of data from various independent sources and adjustment for missing cases.

caput /kā′pət, kap′ət/, pl. *capita* /cap′itə/ [L, head], **1.** the head. **2.** the enlarged or prominent extremity of an organ or part.

caput costae /kos′tē/ [L, head, *costa,* rib], the head of a rib; it articulates with a vertebral body.

caput epididymidis, the head of the epididymis.

caput femoris /fem′əris/, the head of the femur. It articulates with the acetabulum.

caput fibulae /fib′yəlē/, the head of the fibula. It articulates with the lateral condyle of the tibia.

caput humeri /hyoo′mərī/, the head of the humerus. It articulates with the glenoid cavity of the scapula.

caput mallei /mal′ē-ī/, the head of the malleus. It articulates with the incus.

caput mandibulae /mandib′yəlē/, the articular process of the ramus of the mandible.

caput medusae /mədoo′sē/ [L, head of Medusa, a mythical snake-haired Gorgon], a pattern of dilated cutaneous veins radiating from the umbilical area of a newborn. The feature is also observed in cases of cirrhosis of the liver.

caput ossis metacarpalis, the metacarpal head. It articulates with the proximal phalanx of the same digit.

caput phalangis /falan′jis/, the articular head at the distal end of the proximal and middle phalanges.

caput radii /rā′dē-ī/, the head of the radius. It articulates with the capitulum of the humerus.

caput stapedis /stapē′dis/, the head of the stapes.

caput succedaneum /suk′sədənē′əm/ [L, *caput,* head, *succeder,* to replace], a localized pitting edema in the scalp of a fetus that may overlie sutures of the skull. It is usually formed during labor as a result of the circular pressure of the cervix on the fetal occiput.

Carabelli's cusp [Georg Carabelli, Austrian dentist, 1787–1842], an accessory cusp found on the mesiolingual cusp of a maxillary first molar. It may be unilateral or bilateral and varies in size.

caramiphen edisylate /kəram′ifən′ ēdis′-ilāt/, an antitussive prescribed in the treatment of coughs.

carapace /kar′əpās/ [Sp, *carapacho,* hard shell], a horny shield or shell covering the dorsal surface of an animal, such as a turtle.

carb, abbreviation for a *carbonate noncarboxylate anion.*

carbam, abbreviation for a *carbamate carboxylate anion.*

carbamate /kär′bəmāt/, any of a group of anticholinesterase enzymes that cause reversible inhibition of cholinesterase. They are used in certain medications and insecticides. Some carbamates are toxic and may cause convulsions and death through ingestion or skin contact. Atropine is a commonly recommended antidote.

carbamate kinase, a liver enzyme that catalyzes the transfer of a phosphate group from adenosine triphosphate, associated with ammonia and carbon dioxide, to form adenosine diphosphate and carbamoylphosphate.

carbamazepine /kär′bəmaz′əpin/, an anticonvulsant and specific analgesic for trigeminal neuralgia. It is prescribed in the treatment of trigeminal neuralgia and certain seizure disorders.

carbamide peroxide /kär′bəmīd/, a topical antiinfective and ceruminolytic. It is

prescribed to treat canker sores and other minor inflammatory conditions of the gums and mouth and to soften impacted earwax.

carbamino compound /kärbam′inō/, a chemical complex formed by the binding of carbon dioxide molecules to plasma proteins.

carbaminohemoglobin, a chemical complex formed by carbon dioxide and hemoglobin after the release of oxygen by the hemoglobin to a tissue cell. The action is similar to that of the formation of a carbamino compound. It accounts for nearly 25% of the carbon dioxide released in the lung.

carbenicillin disodium /kär′bənəsil′in/, a semisynthetic penicillin antibiotic prescribed in the treatment of certain infections.

carbide, a binary compound of carbon. The various compounds range in stability from explosive copper or silver carbides to hard abrasive compounds, such as silicon carbide.

carbidopa /kär′bidō′pə/, a dopa decarboxylase inhibitor prescribed in combination with levodopa in the treatment of idiopathic Parkinson's disease because it inhibits the degradation of levodopa.

carbinoxamine maleate /kär′bənok′ səmēn/, an antihistamine prescribed in the treatment of hypersensitivity reactions, including rhinitis, skin reactions, and itching.

carbohydrate /kär′bōhī′drit/ [L, *carbo,* coal; Gk, *hydor,* water], any of a group of organic compounds, the most important of which are the saccharides, starch, cellulose, and glycogen. They are classified according to molecular structure as mono-, di-, tri-, poly-, and heterosaccharides. Carbohydrates constitute the main source of energy for all body functions, particularly brain functions, and are necessary for the metabolism of other nutrients. They are synthesized by all green plants and in the body are either absorbed immediately or stored in the form of glycogen. They can also be manufactured in the body from some amino acids and the glycerol component of fats. Symptoms of deficiency include fatigue, depression, breakdown of essential body protein, and electrolyte imbalance.

carbohydrate loading, a dietary practice of some endurance athletes, such as marathon runners, intended to increase glycogen stores in the muscle tissue. The practice is controversial, can produce side effects such as muscle leanness, and is not universally accepted.

carbohydrate metabolism, the sum of

the anabolic and catabolic processes of the body involved in the synthesis and breakdown of carbohydrates, principally galactose, fructose, and glucose. Energy-rich phosphate bonds are produced in many metabolic reactions requiring carbohydrates.

carbolated camphor /kär′bōlā′tid/ [L, *carbo*, coal, *camphora*], a mixture of 1.5 parts camphor with 1 part each of alcohol and phenol, sometimes used as an antiseptic dressing for wounds.

carbol-fuchsin solution /kär′bolfŏŏk′sin/ [L, *carbo*, coal; Leonard Fuchs, German botanist, 1501–1566], a preparation used in the treatment of superficial fungal infections. It contains boric acid, phenol, resorcinol, fuchsin, acetone, and alcohol in water.

carbol-fuchsin stain [L, *carbo*, coal; Leonard Fuchs], a solution of dilute phenol and basic fuchsin used on microorganisms and cell nuclei for microscopic examination.

carbolic acid /kärbol′ik/ [L, *carbo*, coal, *acidus*, sour], a poisonous, colorless-to–pale pink crystalline compound obtained from coal tar distillation and converted to a clear liquid with a strong odor and burning taste by the addition of 10% water.

carbolism /kär′bōliz′əm/, poisoning by phenol, also known as carbolic acid.

carbon (C) /kär′bən/ [L, *carbo*, coal], a nonmetallic, chiefly tetravalent element. Its atomic number is 6; its atomic weight (mass) is 12.011. Carbon occurs in pure form in diamonds, graphite, and fullerenes and is a component of all living tissue. Most of the study of organic chemistry focuses on the vast number of carbon compounds. Carbon is essential to the chemical mechanisms of the body, participating in many metabolic processes and acting as a component of carbohydrates, amino acids, triglycerides, deoxyribonucleic and ribonucleic acids, and many other compounds. Carbon dioxide produced in glycolysis is important in the acid-base balance of the body and in control of respiration.

carbon-11, a radioisotope of carbon with a half-life of 20 minutes. It is produced by a cyclotron and emits positrons.

carbon-14, a beta-emitter with a half-life of about 5700 years. It occurs naturally, arising from cosmic rays, and is used as a tracer in studying various aspects of metabolism and in dating relics that contain natural carbonaceous materials.

carbon arc lamp, an electric lamp producing a strong white light of adjustable intensity from an arc of current between carbon electrodes.

carbonate /kär′bənāt/, a CO_3^- anion. Carbonates are in equilibrium with bicarbonates in water and frequently occur in compounds as insoluble salts such as calcium carbonate.

carbon cycle, the steps by which carbon in the form of carbon dioxide is extracted from and returned to the atmosphere by living organisms. The process starts with the photosynthetic production of carbohydrates by plants, progresses through the consumption of carbohydrates by animals and human beings, and ends with the exhalation of carbon dioxide by those same animals and human beings and with the release of carbon dioxide during the decomposition of dead plants and animals.

carbon dioxide (CO_2) [L, *carbo* + Gk, *dis*, twice, *oxys,* sharp], a colorless, odorless gas produced by the oxidation of carbon. Carbon dioxide, as a product of cell respiration, is carried by the blood to the lungs and exhaled. The acid-base balance of body fluids and tissues is affected by the level of carbon dioxide and its carbonate compounds. Solid carbon dioxide (dry ice) is used in the treatment of some skin conditions.

carbon dioxide bath, a bath taken in water that is saturated with carbon dioxide.

carbon dioxide inhalation, a procedure in which high concentrations of carbon dioxide gas are administered to stimulate breathing in a patient, sometimes as a part of resuscitation efforts. The procedure relies on the characteristic that carbon dioxide excites chemoreceptors that trigger an increase in breathing rate.

carbon dioxide narcosis, a condition of severe hypercapnia, with symptoms of confusion, tremors, convulsions, and possible coma, that may occur if blood levels of carbon dioxide are increased to 70 mm Hg or higher.

carbon dioxide poisoning, toxic effects of inhaling excessive amounts of carbon dioxide. Carbon dioxide is a respiratory stimulant, but it is also an asphyxiant. Concentrations of 10% or greater can cause unconsciousness and death from ventilatory failure. Particularly vulnerable are persons who work in confined spaces with poor air circulation. Faulty home furnaces also have been implicated in many deaths. Home monitors for detection are now available.

carbon dioxide response, the ventilatory reaction to increased concentrations of carbon dioxide gas. Ventilation normally increases linearly up to a concentration of 8% to 10%. The carbon dioxide response curve flattens slightly near the peak and falls off at concentrations of about 20%.

At concentrations around 25%, the person is conscious but unable to perform simple tasks. At concentrations of 30%, carbon dioxide is an anesthetic.

carbon dioxide retention, any increased partial pressure and body stores of carbon dioxide resulting from impaired carbon dioxide elimination. Respiratory acidosis may result from carbon dioxide retention.

carbon dioxide stores, the volume of carbon dioxide contained in the body as a gas and also in the form of carbonic acid, carbonate, bicarbonate, and carbaminohemoglobin. During a steady state of ventilation and aerobic respiration, the carbon dioxide output rate equals the production rate, and the quantity of carbon dioxide stores remains constant.

carbon dioxide tension, the partial pressure of carbon dioxide gas, expressed as PCO_2, which is proportional to its percentage or relative concentration in the blood or lungs. Alveolar PCO_2 directly reflects adequate pulmonary gas exchange in relation to blood flow. A high rate of ventilation causes a lower alveolar PCO_2; a lower rate of breathing leads to higher amounts of alveolar and blood carbon dioxide.

carbon dioxide therapy, the therapeutic inhalation of a low concentration of carbon dioxide gas. Such therapy may be used to dilate the blood vessels, stimulate the cardiovascular brain centers and central nervous system, and overcome hyperventilation.

carbon dioxide titration curve, a line plotted on a graph showing the blood pH and total carbon dioxide concentration changes that result from the addition or removal of carbon dioxide.

carbon fiber, a material consisting of graphite fibers in a plastic matrix used in radiologic devices to reduce patient exposure to x-rays.

carbonic acid (H_2CO_3) /kärbon'ik/ [L, *carbo,* coal, *acidus,* acid], an unstable acid formed by dissolving carbon dioxide in water. It is the basis of carbonated beverages and is related to the carbonate group of compounds.

carbonic anhydrase /anhī'drās/, a zinc-containing enzyme in red blood cells that assists in the hydration of carbon dioxide to carbonic acid in the red blood cell so it can be transported from the tissue cell to the lungs.

carbonic anhydrase inhibitor, a substance that decreases the rate of carbonic acid and H^+ production in the kidney, thereby increasing the excretion of solutes and the rate of urinary output.

carbon monoxide [L, *carbo* + Gk, *monos,* single, *oxys,* sharp], a colorless, odorless, poisonous gas produced by the combustion of carbon or organic fuels in a limited oxygen supply. Carbon monoxide combines irreversibly with hemoglobin, preventing the formation of oxyhemoglobin and reducing the oxygen supply to the tissues.

carbon monoxide poisoning, a toxic condition in which carbon monoxide gas has been inhaled and binds to hemoglobin molecules, thus displacing oxygen from the red blood cells and decreasing the capacity of the blood to carry oxygen to the cells of the body. Headache, dyspnea, drowsiness, confusion, cherry-pink skin, unconsciousness, and apnea occur in sequence as the level of carbon monoxide in the blood increases. The most common source of carbon monoxide is exhaust fumes from an automobile. Treatment includes removal of the victim from the toxic environment, cardiac resuscitation as necessary, and administration of high-flow oxygen.

carbon tetrachloride [L, *carbo* + Gk, *tetra,* four, *chloros,* greenish], a colorless, volatile toxic liquid used as a solvent and in fire extinguishers.

carbon tetrachloride poisoning [L, *carbo,* coal; Gk, *tetra,* four, *chloros,* greenish; L, *potio,* drink], toxic effects of exposure to carbon tetrachloride. It may attack both liver and kidneys. Ingestion of the liquid or inhalation of the fumes usually results in headaches, nausea, central nervous system depression, abdominal pain, and convulsions. In poisoning by inhalation, ventilatory assistance and oxygen may be necessary. In poisoning by ingestion, removal of the poison and gastric lavage are the usual treatments.

carboplatin /kär'bōplat'in/, one of a series of platinum analog drugs used in cancer therapy. It is commonly administered intravenously for the treatment of ovarian cancer.

carboxyfluoroquinolone /kärbok'sēflōō'-ərōkwī'nəlōn/, any of a group of oral quinolone antibiotics that are generally effective against Enterobacteriaceae and show varying activity against *Pseudomonas* and other species. The drugs differ in their oral absorption.

carboxyhemoglobin /kärbok'sēhē'məglō'-bin, -hem'-/ [L, *carbo* + Gk, *oxys,* sharp, *haima,* blood; L, *globus,* ball], a compound produced by the exposure of hemoglobin to carbon monoxide.

carboxyl /kärbok'sil/, a monovalent radical COOH characteristic of organic acids. The hydrogen of the radical can be replaced by metals to form salts.

carboxylation /-lā′shən/, a chemical process in which a carboxyl group (COOH) replaces a hydrogen atom.

carbuncle /kär′bungkəl/ [L, *carbunculus,* little coal], a large site of staphylococcal infection containing purulent matter in deep, interconnecting subcutaneous pockets. Pus eventually discharges to the skin surface through openings. Common sites for carbuncles are the back of the neck and the buttocks.

carbunculosis /karbung′kyəlō′sis/, an abnormal condition characterized by a cluster of deep, painful abscesses that drain through multiple openings onto the skin surface, usually around hair follicles. Carbunculosis is a form of folliculitis, most commonly caused by the coagulase-positive *Staphylococcus aureus.* The lesions caused by this condition may cause fever and malaise.

carcinoembryonic antigen (CEA) /kär′-sənō·em′brēon′ik/ [Gk, *karkinos,* crab, *en,* into, *bryein,* to grow, *anti,* against, *genein,* to produce], an antigen present in very small quantities in adult tissue. A greater than normal amount is suggestive of cancer.

carcinogen /kärsin′əjin/ [Gk, *karkinos* + *genein,* to produce], a substance or agent that causes the development or increases the incidence of cancer.

carcinogenesis /kär′sinəjen′əsis/, the process of initiating and promoting cancer.

carcinogenic /kär′sinəjen′ik/, pertaining to the ability to cause the development of a cancer.

carcinoid /kär′sinoid/ [Gk, *karkinos* + *eidos,* form], a small yellow tumor derived from argentaffin cells in the gastrointestinal mucosa that secrete serotonin and other catecholamines.

carcinoid syndrome, the systemic effects of serotonin-secreting carcinoid tumors manifested by flushing, diarrhea, cramps, skin lesions resembling pellagra, labored breathing, palpitations, and valvular heart disease, especially of the tricuspid and pulmonary valve.

carcinolysis /kär′sinol′isis/ [Gk, *karkinos* + *lysis,* loosening], the destruction of cancer cells. —**carcinolytic,** *adj.*

carcinoma /kär′sinō′mə/, *pl.* carcinomas, carcinomata [Gk, *karkinos* + *oma,* tumor], a malignant epithelial neoplasm that tends to invade surrounding tissue and to metastasize to distant regions of the body. Carcinomas develop most frequently in the skin, large intestine, lungs, stomach, prostate, cervix, or breast. The tumor is firm, irregular, and nodular, with a well-defined border. —**carcinomatous,** *adj.*

carcinoma en cuirasse /äN′kērās′/ [Gk, *karkinos* + *oma* + Fr, breastplate], a rare manifestation of advanced breast cancer characterized by progressive extensive fibrosis and rigidity of the skin of the chest, neck, back, and abdomen.

carcinoma in situ /insit′ōō, insī′tōō [Gk, *karkinos* + *oma* + L, in position], a premalignant neoplasm that has not invaded the basement membrane but shows cytologic characteristics of cancer. Such neoplastic changes in stratified squamous or glandular epithelium frequently occur on the uterine cervix and in the anus, bronchi, buccal mucosa, esophagus, eye, lip, penis, uterine endometrium, and vagina.

carcinoma lenticulare /len′tikōōlär′ə/ [Gk, *karkinos* + *oma* + L, lens], a form of carcinoma tuberosum or scirrhous skin cancer characterized by the development of many small, flat nodules that coalesce to form larger areas resembling a fungous infection.

carcinoma scroti /skrō′tī/, an epithelial cell carcinoma of the scrotum.

carcinoma spongiosum /spon′jē·ō′səm/, a soft and spongy carcinoma with small and large cavities.

carcinoma telangiectaticum /telan′jē-·ektat′ikəm/ [Gk, *karkinos* + *oma* + *telos,* end, *angeion,* vessel, *ektasis,* dilation], a neoplasm of the capillaries of the skin causing dilation of the vessels and red spots on the skin that blanch with pressure.

carcinomatoid /kär′sinō′mətoid/, resembling a carcinoma.

carcinomatous /-om′ətəs/, pertaining to carcinoma.

carcinophilia /kär′sinō′fil′yə/ [Gk, *karkinos* + *philein,* to love], the property in which there is an affinity for carcinomatous tissue. —**carcinophilic,** *adj.*

carcinosarcoma /kär′sinōsärkō′mə/ [Gk, *karkinos* + *sarx,* flesh, *oma,* tumor], a malignant neoplasm composed of carcinomatous and sarcomatous cells. Tumors of this type may occur in the esophagus, thyroid gland, and uterus.

carcinosis /kär′sinō′sis/, *pl.* carcinoses, a condition characterized by the development of many carcinomas throughout the body.

carcinosis pleurae /plōō′rē/, a secondary malignancy of the pleura in which nodules develop throughout the membranes.

carcinostatic /kär′sinōstat′ik/ [Gk, *karkinos* + *statikos,* causing to stand], pertaining to the tendency to slow or halt the growth of a carcinoma.

Cardarelli's sign [Antonio Cardarelli, Italian physician, 1831–1927], a lateral pulsation of the trachea in aneurysm, particularly in dilation of the aortic arch.

cardia /kär′dē-ə/ [Gk, *kardia*, heart], **1.** the opening between the esophagus and the cardiac part of the stomach. **2.** the part of the stomach surrounding the esophagogastric connection, characterized by the absence of acid cells. —**cardiac**, *adj.*

cardiac [Gk, *kardia*, heart], **1.** pertaining to the heart. **2.** pertaining to a person with heart disease. **3.** pertaining to the proximal part of the stomach.

cardiac angiography [Gk, *kardia*, heart, *angeion*, vessel, *graphein*, to record], the radiographic study of the heart and coronary vessels after injection with medium.

cardiac apnea [Gk, *kardia* + *a* + *pnein*, not to breathe], abnormal temporary absence of ventilation, as in Cheyne-Stokes respiration.

cardiac arrest [Gk, *kardia* + L, *ad* + *restare*, to withstand], a sudden cessation of cardiac output and effective circulation. It is usually precipitated by ventricular fibrillation or ventricular asystole. When cardiac arrest occurs, delivery of oxygen and removal of carbon dioxide stop, tissue cell metabolism becomes anaerobic, and metabolic and respiratory acidosis ensue. Immediate initiation of cardiopulmonary resuscitation is required to prevent heart, lung, kidney, and brain damage.

cardiac arrhythmia [Gk, *kardia* + *a* + *rhythmos*, without rhythm], an abnormal cardiac rate or rhythm. The condition is caused by a defect in the sinus node to maintain its pacemaker function or by a failure of the electrical conduction system. Kinds of arrhythmia include **bradycardia, tachycardia, extrasystole, heart block,** and irregular spacing of beats.

cardiac asthma, an attack of asthma associated with heart disease, such as left ventricular failure, and characterized by predominant pulmonary congestion with some bronchoconstriction.

cardiac atrophy, a wasting of heart muscle usually caused by cachexia, aging, or a mediastinal tumor.

Cardiac Care, a Nursing Interventions Classification defined as limitation of complications resulting from an imbalance between myocardial oxygen supply and demand for a patient with symptoms of impaired cardiac function.

Cardiac Care: Acute, a Nursing Interventions Classification defined as limitation of complications for a patient recently experiencing an episode of an imbalance between myocardial oxygen supply and demand resulting in impaired cardiac function.

Cardiac Care: Rehabilitative, a Nursing Interventions Classification defined as promotion of maximum functional activity level for a patient who has suffered an episode of impaired cardiac function that resulted from an imbalance between myocardial oxygen supply and demand.

cardiac catheter, a long, fine catheter designed to be passed into the heart through a blood vessel.

cardiac catheterization, a diagnostic procedure in which a catheter is introduced through an incision into a large vein, usually of an arm or a leg, and threaded through the circulatory system to the heart.

cardiac cirrhosis [Gk, *kardia*, heart, *kirrhos,* yellowish orange, *osis,* condition], an increase of fibrous tissue in the liver resulting from congestive heart failure, chronic myocarditis, or cardiac fibrosis.

cardiac conduction defect, any impairment of the electrical pathways and the specialized muscular fibers that conduct impulses and result in atrial and ventricular contraction.

cardiac cycle [Gk, *kardia* + *kyklos,* circle], the cycle of events during which an electrical impulse is conducted through special fibers, from the sinoatrial node to the atrioventricular node, to the bundle of His and the bundle branches, and to the Purkinje fibers, causing contraction of the atria followed by contraction of the ventricles. Deoxygenated blood enters the right atrium of the heart from the inferior and superior venae cave and is pumped through the tricuspid valve into the right ventricle. From the right ventricle, blood is pumped through the pulmonary valve into the pulmonary artery and the lungs for oxygenation. The contractions of the left and the right atria are nearly simultaneous. Structural, chemical, or electrical abnormalities may cause a large variety of anomalies in electrical conduction, muscular contraction, and blood flow in the heart.

cardiac decompensation, a condition of congestive heart failure in which the heart is unable to fulfill its normal function of ensuring adequate cellular perfusion to all parts of the body without assistance. Causes may include myocardial infarction, increased workload, infection, toxins, or defective heart valves.

cardiac depressant [L, *deprimere,* to press down], an agent that decreases the heart rate and contractility.

cardiac dyspepsia, a digestive disorder associated with heart disease.

cardiac dyspnea [Gk, *dys,* difficult, *pnoia,* breath], breathing distress caused by heart disease, most commonly the result of pulmonary venous congestion.

cardiac edema [Gk, *oidema,* swelling], an accumulation of serum fluid from blood plasma in the interstitial tissues as a result of congestive heart failure. In severe cases the fluid may also accumulate in serous cavities.

cardiac electrical axis, the main direction of electrical current flow in the heart. It may be calculated in the frontal plane (limb leads) or horizontal plane (precordial leads).

cardiac hypertrophy, an abnormal enlargement of the heart muscle. It frequently accompanies long-standing hypertension.

cardiac impulse [Gk, *kardia* + L, *impellere,* to set in motion], the mechanical movement of the thorax, caused by the beating of the heart. It is readily palpable and easily recorded.

cardiac index, a measure of the cardiac output of a patient per square meter of body surface area. It is obtained by dividing the cardiac output in liters per minute by the body surface area.

cardiac insufficiency, the inability of the heart to pump efficiently.

cardiac massage, repeated, rhythmic compression of the heart applied directly, during surgery, or through the intact chest wall in an effort to maintain circulation after cardiac arrest or ventricular fibrillation.

cardiac monitor, a device for the continuous observation of cardiac function.

cardiac monitoring, a continuous check on the functioning of the heart with an electronic instrument that provides an electrocardiographic reading on an oscilloscope.

cardiac murmur, an abnormal sound heard during auscultatory examination of the heart, caused by altered blood flow into a chamber or through a valve. A murmur is classified by time of its occurrence during the cardiac cycle, duration, and intensity of the sound on a scale of I to VI.

cardiac muscle, a special striated muscle of the myocardium, containing dark intercalated disks at the junctions of abutting fibers. Cardiac muscle is an exception among involuntary muscles, which are characteristically smooth. Its contractile fibers resemble those of skeletal muscle but are only one third as large in diameter, are richer in sarcoplasm, and contain centrally located instead of peripheral nuclei.

cardiac output, the volume of blood expelled by the ventricles of the heart, equal to the amount of blood ejected at each beat (the stroke output) multiplied by the heart rate per minute (number of beats in the period of time used in the computation). A normal heart in a resting adult ejects from 4 to 8 L of blood per minute.

cardiac output, decreased, a NANDA-accepted nursing diagnosis of a state in which the amount of blood pumped by the heart is inadequate to meet the metabolic demands of the body's tissues. Defining characteristics include variations in blood pressure readings, arrhythmias, fatigue, jugular vein distension, skin color changes, rales, oliguria, decreased peripheral pulses, dyspnea, restlessness, and chest pain.

cardiac plexus [Gk, *kardia* + L, pleated], one of several nerve complexes situated close to the arch of the aorta. The cardiac plexuses contain sympathetic and parasympathetic nerve fibers that leave the plexuses, accompany the right and left coronary arteries, and enter the heart.

Cardiac Precautions, a Nursing Interventions Classification defined as prevention of an acute episode of impaired cardiac function by minimizing myocardial oxygen consumption or increasing myocardial oxygen supply.

cardiac radionuclide imaging [Gk, *kardia* + L, *radiare,* to shine, *nucleus,* nut kernel, *imago,* image], the noninvasive examination of the heart, using a radiopharmaceutical, such as thallium-201, and a detection device, such as a gamma camera, positron camera, or rectilinear scanner.

cardiac reflex [L, *reflectere,* to bend back], reaction to a pair of stimuli that automatically increase or reduce the heart rate. Stimulation of vagus fibers in the right side of the heart by increased venous return accelerates the heart rate, whereas increased arterial blood pressure stimulates nerve endings in the carotid sinus to slow the heart rate.

cardiac regurgitation [Gk, *kardia,* heart; L, *re* + *gurgitare,* to flow], a backward flow of blood through one or more defective heart valves.

cardiac rehabilitation [Gk, *kardia,* heart; L, *re* + *habilitas,* ability], a supervised program of progressive exercise, psychologic support, education, and training to enable a myocardial infarction patient to resume the activities of daily living on an independent basis. Special training may be needed to enable the patient to adapt to a new occupation and life-style.

cardiac reserve, the potential capacity of the heart to function well beyond its basal level, responding to alterations in physiologic demands.

cardiac rhythm [Gk, *kardia,* heart, *rhythmos*], the recurring beat of the heart.

cardiac souffle [Gk, *kardia,* heart; Fr, puff], a heart murmur.

cardiac sphincter [Gk, *kardia* + *sphingein,* to bind], a ring of muscle fibers at the juncture of the esophagus and stomach.

cardiac standstill, the complete cessation of ventricular contractions and ejection of blood by the heart. Cardiac standstill requires immediate cardiopulmonary resuscitation and pacing.

cardiac stenosis [Gk, *kardia,* heart; Gk, *stenos,* narrow, *osis,* condition], an obstruction of blood flow through any heart chamber that is not valvular in origin. The cause may be a thrombosis or tumor.

cardiac stimulant, a pharmacologic agent that increases the action of the heart. Cardiac glycosides such as digitalis, digitoxin, digoxin, deslanoside, lanatoside, acetyldigitoxin, and ouabain increase the force of myocardial contractions and decrease the heart rate and conduction velocity, allowing more time for the ventricles to relax and become filled with blood. These glycosides are used in the treatment of congestive heart failure, atrial flutter and fibrillation, paroxysmal atrial tachycardia, and cardiogenic shock. Epinephrine, a potent vasopressor and cardiac stimulant, is sometimes used to restore heart rhythm in cardiac arrest. Isoproterenol hydrochloride, which is related to epinephrine, may be used in treating heart block. Amrinone, dobutamine hydrochloride, and dopamine are used in the short-term treatment of cardiac decompensation resulting from depressed contractility.

cardiac syncope [Gk, *kardia,* heart, *syncope,* fainting], a temporary loss of consciousness caused by inadequate cerebral blood flow, which results from a sudden failure in cardiac output for any reason.

cardiac tamponade, compression of the heart produced by the accumulation of blood in the pericardial sac. Signs of cardiac tamponade may include distended neck veins, hypotension, decreased heart sounds, and tachypnea.

cardiac thrombosis [Gk, *kardia,* heart, *thrombos,* lump, *osis,* condition], a blood clot located at a heart valve or in one of the heart chambers. A left ventricular thrombosis may follow a large infarct.

cardiasthenia /kar′dē·asthē′nē·ə/ [Gk, *kardia,* heart, *a,* without, *sthenos,* strength], a form of neurasthenia in which cardiovascular symptoms are prominent.

cardiectomy /kär′dē·ek′təmē/, **1.** removal of the heart. **2.** removal of the cardiac part of the stomach.

cardiectopia /kär′dē·ektō′pē·ə/, abnormal positioning of the heart in the thoracic cavity.

cardinal /kär′dənal/ [L, *cardo,* hinge], so fundamental that other things hinge on it, such as a cardinal trait that influences one's total behavior.

cardinal frontal plane [L, *cardo,* hinge, *frons,* forehead, *planum,* level ground], the plane that divides the body into front and back parts.

cardinal ligament [L, *cardo,* hinge, *ligare,* to bind], a sheet of subserous fascia extending across the female pelvic floor as a continuation of the broad ligament.

cardinal movements of labor, the typical sequence of positions assumed by the fetus as it descends through the pelvis during labor and delivery. The positions are usually designated as engagement, flexion, descent, internal rotation, extension, and external rotation or restitution.

cardinal position of gaze, (in ophthalmology) one of six positions to which the normal eye may be turned. This test evaluates the functioning of the six extraocular muscles and cranial nerves III, IV, and VI. The positions and the corresponding muscles and nerves are as follows: (1) straight nasal: medial rectus and the third cranial nerve; (2) up nasal: inferior oblique and the third cranial nerve; (3) down nasal: superior oblique and the fourth cranial nerve; (4) straight temporal: lateral rectus and the sixth cranial nerve; (5) up temporal: superior rectus and the third cranial nerve; (6) down temporal: inferior rectus and the third cranial nerve.

cardiocatheterization /kär′dē·ōkath′ərī·zā′shən/ [Gk, *kardia,* heart, *katheter,* a thing lowered into], the introduction of a flexible radiopaque catheter through a saphenous or median basilic vein and the superior vena cava to the heart chambers. It may be used to collect samples of blood in the heart and to measure blood pressure in various heart chambers, as well as to illuminate the coronary arteries.

cardiocele /kär′dē·ōsēl′/, protrusion of the heart through an opening in the diaphragm or the abdominal wall.

cardiocirculatory /kär′dē·ōsur′kyŏŏlətôr′ē/ [Gk, *kardia* heart; L, *circulare,* to go around], pertaining to the heart and the circulation.

cardioesophageal reflux /-əsof′əjē′əl/ [Gk, *kardia,* heart, *oisophagos,* gullet; L, *refluere,* to flow back], a backward flow or regurgitation of stomach contents into the esophagus. Repeated episodes of reflux can lead to esophagitis. Among factors contributing to the condition are stomach pressure greater than esophageal pressure, hiatal hernia, and incompetence of the lower esophageal sphincter.

cardiogenic /-jen′ik/, originating in the heart muscle.

cardiogenic shock /kär′dē·ōjen′ik/ [Gk, *kardia* + *genein,* to produce; Fr, *choc*], an abnormal condition characterized by critically low cardiac output associated with acute myocardial infarction and congestive heart failure. Although low cardiac output is a common sign of this disorder, cardiogenic shock may also be associated with normal output. Cardiogenic shock is fatal in about 80% of cases, and immediate therapy is necessary. Depending on the signs, therapy may include diuretics, vasoactive drugs, and the application of various devices.

cardiogram /kär′dē·əgram′/, an electronically recorded tracing of cardiac activity.

cardiography /kär′dē·og′rəfē/, the technique of graphically recording heart movements by means of a cardiograph.

cardiohepatomegaly /-hep′ətōmeg′əlē/, enlargement of the heart and liver.

cardioinhibitory /kär′dē·ō′inhib′itôr′ē/, slowing or inhibiting the function of the heart.

cardiologist /-ol′əjist/, a physician who specializes in the diagnosis and treatment of disorders of the heart.

cardiology /-ol′əjē/ [Gk, *kardia* + *logos,* science], the study of the anatomy, normal functions, and disorders of the heart.

cardiomegaly /kär′dē·ōmeg′əlē/ [Gk, *kardia* + *megas,* large], enlargement of the heart.

cardiomyopathy /kär′dē·ōmī·op′əthē/ [Gk, *kardia* + *mys,* muscle, *pathos,* disease], any disease that affects the structure and function of the heart.

cardiomyopexy /kär′dē·omī′əpek′sē/ [Gk, *kardia* + *mys,* muscle, *pexis,* fixation], a surgical procedure in which the blood supply from the nearby pectoral muscles of the chest is diverted directly to the coronary arteries of the heart.

cardiopathy /kär′dē·op′əthē/ [Gk, *kardia,* heart, *pathos,* disease], a disease of the heart.

cardiopericarditis /-per′ikärdī′tis/, inflammation of both the heart and the pericardium.

cardioplasty /kär′dē·ōplas′tē/, a surgical procedure to correct a defect in the cardiac sphincter of the esophagus that frequently leads to cardiospasm.

cardioplegia /-plē′jə/ [Gk, *kardia* + *plege,* stroke], **1.** paralysis of the heart. **2.** the arrest of myocardial contractions by injection of chemicals, hypothermia, or electrical stimuli for the purpose of performing surgery on the heart.

cardiopulmonary /-pul′məner′ē/ [Gk, *kardia* + L, *pulmo,* lung], pertaining to the heart and lungs.

cardiopulmonary bypass, a procedure used in heart surgery in which the blood is diverted from the heart and lungs by means of a pump oxygenator and returned directly to the aorta.

cardiopulmonary murmur [Gk, *kardia,* heart; L, *pulmo,* lung, *murmur,* humming], a sound heard over the heart during breathing and during the heartbeat. It is caused by vibrations that result when the heart strikes the lung tissue with every beat.

cardiopulmonary resuscitation (CPR), a basic emergency procedure for life support, consisting of artificial respiration and manual external cardiac massage. It is used in cases of cardiac arrest to establish effective circulation and ventilation to prevent irreversible cerebral damage resulting from anoxia. External cardiac massage compresses the heart between the lower sternum and the thoracic vertebral column. During compressions, blood is forced into systemic and pulmonary circulation, and venous blood refills the heart when the compression is released. Mouth-to-mouth breathing or a mechanical form of ventilation is used concomitantly with CPR to oxygenate the blood being pumped through the circulatory system.

cardiorrhaphy /kär′dē·ôr′əfē/ [Gk, *kardia* + *rhaphe,* suture], an operation in which the heart muscle is sutured.

cardioselectivity /-sel′əktiv′itē/, selectivity of a drug, such as a beta-blocker, for heart tissue over other tissues of the body.

cardiospasm /kär′dē·əspaz′əm/ [Gk, *kardia* + *spasmos,* pull], ′ a form of achalasia characterized by a failure of the cardia at the distal end of the esophagus to relax. It causes dysphagia and regurgitation and sometimes requires surgical division of the muscle.

cardiotachometer /kär′dē·ō′təkom′ətər/ [Gk, *kardia* + *tachos,* speed, *metron,* measure], an instrument that continually monitors and records the heartbeat.

cardiotherapy, the treatment of heart disease.

cardiothoracic ratio /thôras′ik/, the ratio between the diameter of the heart at its widest point and the maximum width of the thoracic cavity, assessed by examining a chest x-ray. The normal ratio is 1:2.

cardiotomy /kär′dē·ot′əmē/ [Gk, *kardia* + *temnein,* to cut], **1.** an operation in which the heart is incised. **2.** an operation in which the cardiac end of the stomach or cardiac orifice is incised.

cardiotonic /kär′dē-ōton′ik/ [Gk, *kardia* + *tonos,* tone], **1.** pertaining to a substance that tends to increase the efficiency of contractions of the heart muscle. **2.** a pharmacologic agent that increases the force of myocardial contractions.

cardiotoxic /-tok′sik/ [Gk, *kardia* + *toxikon,* poison], having a toxic or injurious effect on the heart.

cardiovascular /kär′dē-ōvas′kyələr/ [Gk, *kardia* + L, *vasculum,* small vessel], pertaining to the heart and blood vessels.

cardiovascular assessment, an evaluation of the condition, function, and abnormalities of the heart and circulatory system.

cardiovascular disease, any abnormal condition characterized by dysfunction of the heart and blood vessels. Some common kinds of cardiovascular disease are **atherosclerosis, cardiomyopathy, rheumatic heart disease,** syphilitic heart disease, and systemic hypertension. In the United States cardiovascular disease is the leading cause of death.

cardiovascular reflex, a reflex in which heart and circulatory functions are altered in response to changes in heart rate, vascular tone, blood volume, or other variables.

cardiovascular shunt [Gk, *kardia,* heart; L, *vasculum,* small vessel; ME, *shunten*], any abnormal passage between chambers of the heart or between systemic and pulmonary circulatory systems.

cardiovascular system, the network of anatomic structures, including the heart and the blood vessels, that pump blood throughout the body. The system includes thousands of miles of vessels to deliver nutrients and other essential materials to the fluids surrounding the cells and to remove waste products, which are conveyed to excretory organs.

cardiovascular technologist, an allied health professional who performs diagnostic examinations at the request or direction of a physician in one or more of the following three areas: (1) invasive cardiology; (2) noninvasive cardiology; and (3) peripheral vascular study.

cardioversion /-vur′zhən/ [Gk, *kardia* + L, *vertere,* to turn], the restoration of the heart's normal sinus rhythm by delivery of a synchronized electric shock through two metal paddles placed on the patient's chest. Cardioversion is used to slow the heart rate or to restore the heart's normal sinus rhythm when drug therapy is ineffective.

cardiovert, application of electric current

synchronized to the QRS complex to terminate a tachyarrhythmia.

cardioverter /-vur′tər, a defibrillator or other instrument used to convert abnormal heart rhythms into normal rhythms.

carditis /kärdī′tis/, an inflammatory condition of the muscles of the heart, usually resulting from infection. In most cases more than one layer of muscles is involved. Chest pain, cardiac arrhythmia, circulatory failure, and damage to the structures of the heart may occur. Kinds of carditis are **endocarditis, myocarditis,** and **pericarditis.**

Cardiobacterium, a gram-negative genus of facultative anaerobic rod-shaped bacteria that is part of the normal flora of the human nasopharynx region. It is associated with endocarditis.

career ladder, (in nursing education) a pathway for upward mobility that begins with a course of study in practical nursing or a program that grants an **Associate Degree in Nursing.** On completion of this basic level, the candidate may continue up the ladder to earn a **Bachelor of Science in Nursing,** and then to the graduate level to earn a master's degree and a doctoral degree in nursing.

caregiver, one who contributes the benefits of medical, social, economic, or environmental resources to a dependent or partially dependent individual such as a critically ill person.

caregiver role strain, a NANDA-accepted nursing diagnosis of a state in which a caregiver perceives difficulty in performing the family caregiver role. Defining characteristics include the caregiver's report of difficulty in providing specific caregiving activities, inadequate resources to provide required care, worry about the care receiver, feeling that caregiving interferes with other important roles in the caregiver's life, feeling of loss, family conflict, stress, and depression.

caregiver role strain, risk for, a NANDA-accepted nursing diagnosis of a state of vulnerability to experiencing of difficulty in performing the family caregiver role. Risk factors may be physiologic, such as severity of the care receiver's illness; developmental, such as a developmental inability to fulfill the caregiver role; psychosocial, such as psychological or cognitive problems in the care receiver; or situational, such as the presence of abuse or violence.

Caregiver Support, a Nursing Interventions Classification defined as provision of the necessary information, advocacy, and support to facilitate primary patient care by someone other than a health care professional.

care of the chronically ill, medical and nursing services that focus on long-term care of people with chronic diseases or conditions, either at home or in a medical facility. It includes measures specific to the problem, as well as others to encourage self-care, promote health, and prevent loss of function.

care of the sick, (in public health nursing) the care of sick patients in their homes, as distinguished from health supervision. Public health nursing agencies are reimbursed for the nursing services rendered by the nurses according to the kind of service rendered, such as a sick visit or a health supervision visit.

CARF, abbreviation for *Commission on Accreditation of Rehabilitation Facilities.*

caries /ker′ēz/ [L, decay], an infectious disease beginning with progressive destruction of the external surface of the tooth crown and/or exposed root surface. It is characterized by demineralization, disintegration, and destruction of the structure.

carina /kərē′nə/, *pl.* **carinae** [L, keel], any structure shaped like a ridge or keel, such as the carina of the trachea, which projects from the lowest tracheal cartilage.

caring behaviors, actions characteristic of concern for the well-being of a patient, such as sensitivity, comfort, attentive listening, and honesty.

cariocas /kär′ē-ō′kəs/, a form of lateral movement in a gait cycle in which the side-stepping leg is moved successively behind and then in front of the stance leg.

cariogenic /ker′ē-ōjen′ik/, tending to produce caries.

carisoprodol /ker′isōprō′dol/, a skeletal muscle relaxant prescribed for the relief of muscle spasm.

carminative /kärmin′ətiv/ [L, *carminare,* to cleanse], **1.** pertaining to a substance that relieves flatulence and abdominal distension. **2.** an agent that relieves gaseous distension and painful spasms, especially after meals.

carmine dye /kär′min/ [AR, *qirmize* + AS, *deag*], a red coloring substance produced by the addition of alum to an extract of cochineal that is used for staining histologic specimens.

carmustine /kärmus′tin/, a lipid-soluble nitrosourea, 1,3-bis(2-chloroethyl)-*1*-nitrosourea, used as a single antineoplastic agent or with other approved chemotherapeutic agents in the treatment of brain tumors, multiple myeloma, Hodgkin's disease, and non-Hodgkin's lymphomas.

carnal /kär′nəl/ [L, *caro,* flesh], pertaining to the flesh or body, or worldly things, as distinguished from spiritual.

carneous /kär′nē-əs/, having the quality of flesh.

carnitine /kär′nitin/, a substance found in skeletal and cardiac muscle and certain other tissues that functions as a carrier of fatty acids across the membranes of the mitochondria. It is used therapeutically in treating angina and certain deficiency diseases. It has actions that closely resemble those of amino acids and B vitamins.

carnivore /kär′nivôr/ [L, *caro,* flesh, *vorare,* to devour], an animal belonging to the order Carnivora, classified as a flesh eater, with appropriate teeth and a characteristically simple stomach and a short intestine for such a diet. —**carnivorous** /kärniv′ərəs/, *adj.*

carotene /kar′ətin/ [L, *carota,* carrot], a red or orange organic compound found in carrots, sweet potatoes, milk fat, egg yolk, and leafy vegetables. Beta-carotene is a provitamin and in the body is converted into vitamin A.

carotenemia /kar′ətinē′mē-ə/, the presence of high levels of carotene in the blood, which result in an abnormal yellow appearance of the plasma and skin.

carotenoid /kərot′ənoid/, any of a group of red, yellow, or orange highly unsaturated pigments that are found in some animal tissue and in foods such as carrots, sweet potatoes, and leafy green vegetables. Many of these substances, such as carotene, are used in the formation of vitamin A in the body.

carotid /kərot′id/ [Gk, *karos,* heavy sleep], pertaining to the arteries that supply the head and neck.

carotid arch [Gk, *karos,* heavy sleep; L, *arcus,* bow], the third arch of the aorta, the source of the common carotid arteries.

carotid body [Gk, *karos* + AS, *bodig*], a small structure containing neural tissue at the bifurcation of the carotid arteries. It monitors the pressure and oxygen content of the blood and therefore assists in regulating respiration.

carotid-body reflex [Gk, *karos* + AS, *bodig* + L, *reflectere,* to bend back], a normal chemical reflex initiated by a decrease in oxygen concentration in the blood and, to a lesser degree, by increased carbon dioxide and hydrogen ion concentrations that act on chemoreceptors at the bifurcation of the common carotid arteries. The resulting nerve impulses cause the respiratory center in the medulla to increase respiratory activity.

carotid-body tumor, a benign round,

firm growth that develops at the bifurcation of the common carotid artery. The tumor may cause dizziness, nausea, and vomiting if it impedes the flow of blood and pressure is increased in the vascular system.

carotid bruit, a murmur heard over the carotid artery in the neck, suggesting arterial narrowing.

carotid endarterectomy, surgical excision of atheromatous segments of the endothelia and media of the carotid artery, leaving a smooth tissue lining and facilitating blood flow through the vessel.

carotid plexus [Gk, *karos* + L, pleated], any one of three nerve plexuses associated with the carotid arteries.

carotid pulse, the pulse of the carotid artery, palpated by gently pressing a finger in the area between the larynx and the sternocleidomastoid muscle in the neck.

carotid sinus [Gk, *karos* + L, curve], a dilation of the arterial wall at the bifurcation of the common carotid artery. It contains sensory nerve endings from the vagus nerve that respond to changes in blood pressure.

carotid sinus massage, firm rubbing at the bifurcation of the carotid artery at the angle of the jaw. It creates an elevation of blood pressure in the carotid sinus that results in reflex slowing of atrioventricular conduction and sinus rate.

carotid sinus reflex, the decrease in the heart rate resulting from pressure on the carotid artery at the level of its bifurcation.

carotid sinus syndrome, a temporary loss of consciousness that sometimes accompanies convulsive seizures as a result of the intensity of the carotid sinus reflex when pressure builds in one or both carotid sinuses.

carotidynia /kərot′idin′ē-ə/ [Gk, *karos* + *odyne*, pain], a pain along the length of the common carotid artery caused by pressure.

carpal /kär′pəl/ [Gk, *karpos*, wrist], pertaining to the carpus or wrist.

carpal ligaments, four ligaments of the hand: the dorsal ligament, a thick band of white fibrous tissue on the dorsum of the wrist, attached to the lower end of the radius and to the styloid process of the ulna; the **radiate ligament of the wrist,** which projects from the head of the capitate bone to the volar aspects of other carpal bones; the broad, flat **transverse ligament,** which is attached to the tubercle of the scaphoid and the crest of the trapezium; the volar ligament, a superficial part of the flexor retinaculum.

carpal spasm, a sudden, powerful, involuntary contraction observed as a tetanic flexion of the hands and wrists.

carpal tunnel [Gk, *karpos* + Fr, *tonnel*], a conduit for the median nerve and the flexor tendons, formed by the carpal bones and the flexor retinaculum.

carpal tunnel release, a surgical procedure for treating carpal tunnel syndrome.

carpal tunnel syndrome, a common painful disorder of the wrist and hand, induced by compression on the median nerve between the inelastic carpal ligament and other structures within the carpal tunnel. It is often seen in cumulative trauma to the wrist. The median nerve innervates the palm and the radial side of the hand; compression of the nerve causes weakness, pain with opposition of the thumb, and burning, tingling, or aching, sometimes radiating to the forearm and shoulder joint.

carpometacarpal (CMC) joint /-met′ə-kär′pəl/ [Gk, *karpos*, wrist, *meta*, next, *karpos*], any of the joints formed by the distal row of carpal bones and the bases of the metacarpals. The joints are essential for prehensile patterns.

carpopedal [Gk, *karpos*, wrist; L, *pes*, foot], pertaining to the wrist and foot.

carpopedal spasm /-ped′əl/ [Gk, *karpos* + L, *pes*, foot], a spasm of the hand, thumbs, foot, or toes that sometimes accompanies tetany.

carpus /kär′pəs/ [Gk, *karpos*], the wrist, made up of eight bones arranged in two rows. The proximal row consists of the scaphoid, lunate, triangular, and pisiform. The distal row consists of the trapezium, trapezoid, capitate, and hamate.

carrier /ker′ē-ər/ [OFr, *carier*], **1.** a person or animal who harbors and spreads an organism that causes disease in others but does not become ill. **2.** one whose chromosomes carry a recessive gene. **3.** an immunogenic molecule or part of a molecule that is recognized by T cells in an antibody response.

carrier-free, 1. a radioisotope in pure form, free of dilution by stable isotope carriers. **2.** a substance in which every molecule is marked by a radioactive tracer or other tag.

Carroll quantitative test of upper extremity function, a six-part test of a person's ability to grasp and lift objects of different shapes and sizes. It is designed to measure the ability to perform general arm and hand movements required for the activities of daily living.

carrying angle, the angle at which the humerus and radius articulate.

carry-over [L, *carrus,* wagon; AS *ofer*],

contamination of a specimen by the previous one.

car sickness [L, *carrus,* wagon; AS, *seoc*], nausea and vomiting caused by the motion of a vehicle.

cartilage /kär′tilij/ [L, *cartilago*], a nonvascular supporting connective tissue composed of chondrocytes and various fibers. It is found chiefly in the joints, the thorax, and various rigid tubes such as the larynx, trachea, nose, and ear. Temporary cartilage such as sesamoid bones (knee) and those that compose most of the fetal skeleton at an early stage are later replaced by bone. Permanent cartilage remains unossified, except in certain diseases and sometimes in advanced age. —**cartilaginous** /kär′tilaj′inəs/, *adj.*

cartilage graft, the transplantation of cartilage. It is used to correct congenital ear and nose defects in children and to treat severe injuries in adults.

cartilage-hair hypoplasia [L, *cartilago* + AS, *haer* + Gk, *hypo,* under, *plasis,* forming], a genetic disorder characterized by dwarfism caused by hypoplasia of the cartilage, multiple skeletal abnormalities, and excessively sparse, short, fine, brittle hair that is usually light colored.

cartilaginous [L, *cartilago,* cartilage], pertaining to cartilage.

cartilaginous bone, bone that develops by endochondral ossification in a preexisting cartilage.

cartilaginous joint [L, *cartilago* + *junger,* to join], a slightly movable joint in which cartilage unites bony surfaces. Two types of articulation involving cartilaginous joints are synchondrosis and symphysis.

cartilaginous skeleton [L, *cartilago* + Gk, *skeletos,* dried up], the parts of the skeleton that are formed by cartilage.

caruncle /kär′ungkəl/ [L, *caruncula,* small piece of flesh], a small, fleshy projection, as one of the lacrimal caruncles at the inner canthus of the eye or the hymenal caruncles that are the hymenal remnants.

carunculae hymenales [L, *caruncula* + Gk, *hymen,* membrane], remnants of a ruptured hymen that appear as irregular projections of normal skin around the introitus to the vagina.

carve-out, a service not covered in a health insurance contract. It is usually reimbursed according to a different arrangement or rate formula than those services specified under the contract umbrella.

cascade /kaskād′/ [L, *cadere,* to fall], any process that develops in stages, with each stage dependent on the preceding one, often producing a cumulative effect.

cascade humidifier, a bubbling respiratory care device in which gases travel down a tower and pass through a grid into a chamber of heated water.

cascara sagrada /kasker′ə səgrä′də/ [Sp, sacred bark], a stimulant cathartic prepared from the bark of the *Rhamnus purshianus* tree. It is prescribed for constipation.

case [L, *causus,* a happening], **1.** an episode of illness or injury. **2.** a container.

caseation /kā′sē·ā′shən/ [L, *caseus,* cheese], a form of tissue necrosis in which cellular outline is lost and the appearance is that of crumbly cheese. It is typical of tuberculosis. —**caseate,** *v.*

caseation necrosis [L, *caseus,* cheese; Gk, *nekros,* dead, *osis* condition], necrosis that transforms tissue into a dry, cheeselike mass. It occurs primarily in tuberculosis.

case-control study, an investigation using an epidemiologic approach in which previous cases of the condition are used. A group of patients with a particular disease or disorder such as myocardial infarction is compared with a control group of persons who have not had that medical problem.

case fatality rate [L, *causus,* a happening, *fatum,* fate, *(pro) rata*], the number of registered deaths caused by any specific disease, expressed as a percentage of the total number of reported cases of a specific disease.

casefinding, the act of locating individuals with a disease.

case history [L, *causus* + *historia*], a patient's complete medical record before a current illness or injury. The history includes any infectious diseases experienced by the person; all immunizations, hospitalizations, or therapies; information relating to deaths or illnesses of parents and other close family members; allergies; and congenital or acquired physical defects.

casein, a white powder protein that occurs naturally in milk. It contains phosphorus and sulfur and is regarded as a "complete protein" because it contains all essential amino acids. Casein is precipitated when milk turns sour.

case management, 1. a problem-solving process through which appropriate services to individuals and families are ensured. **2.** a method of structuring acute care for all patients in three dimensions: work design, clinical management roles, and concurrent monitoring and feedback. **3.** a client-centered goal-oriented process of assessing the need of an individual for particular services and obtaining those services.

case nursing [L, *casus,* a happening, *nutrix,* nourish], an organizational mode for allocation of nursing staff in which one nurse is assigned to provide total nursing care to one or more patients.

caseous /kā′sē·əs/, cheeselike; describing the mixture of fat and protein that appears in some body tissues undergoing necrosis.

caseous fermentation [L, *caseus,* cheese, *fermentum,* yeast], the coagulation of soluble casein to form insoluble calcium paracaseinate through the action of rennin.

case rate, a pricing method in which a flat amount, often a per diem rate, covers a defined group of procedures and services. It is often used in services such as obstetrics and cardiovascular surgery for exceptions to a relative value scale or resource-based relative value scale.

CaSO₄, the formula for **calcium sulfate.**

cassette /kaset′/ [Fr, little box], a device used in radiography for holding a sheet of x-ray film and a set of screens. A cassette also may have a grid to absorb scattered radiation.

cast [ONorse, *kasta*], **1.** a stiff, solid dressing formed with plaster of paris or other material around a limb or other body part to immobilize it during healing. **2.** a mold of a part or all of a patient's teeth and internal jaw area for fitting prostheses or dentures. **3.** a tiny structure formed by deposits of mineral or other substances on the walls of renal tubules, bronchioles, or other organs. Casts often appear in samples of urine or blood collected for laboratory examination. **4.** the deviation of an eye from the normal parallel lines of vision, such as in strabismus.

cast brace, a combination of a brace within a cast at a joint.

Cast Care: Maintenance, a Nursing Interventions Classification defined as care of a cast after the drying period.

Cast Care: Wet, a Nursing Interventions Classification defined as care of a new cast during the drying period.

cast core [ONorse, *kasta* + L, *cor,* heart], a metal casting, shaped like a stump of a tooth and incorporating a post in the root canal for retaining an artificial tooth crown.

casting, 1. the act of encasing a body part in a cast. **2.** (in dentistry) the process by which crowns, inlays, and other metallic restorations are produced.

casting tape, an adhesive or resin-impregnated tape used for shaping light-weight casts.

castor oil /kas′tər/ [L, beaver, *oleum,* olive oil], an oil derived from *Ricinus communis,* used as a stimulant cathartic. It is prescribed for constipation and for a cleansing preparation of the bowel or colon before examination.

castration /kastrā′shən/ [L, *castrare,* to castrate], the surgical excision of one or both testicles or ovaries, performed most frequently to reduce the production and secretion of certain hormones that may stimulate the proliferation of malignant cells in women with breast cancer or in men with cancer of the prostate.

castration anxiety, 1. the fantasized fear of injury or loss of the genital organs, often as the reaction to a repressed feeling of punishment for forbidden sexual desires. **2.** a general threat to the masculinity or femininity of a person or an unrealistic fear of bodily injury or loss of power.

cast saw, a tool used to cut through a plaster cast.

cast shoe, a shoe worn over a foot that is encased in a plaster cast.

cast stabilization, the use of rods, pins, broom handles, or other devices to lend stability to a cast.

casualty /kazh′əltē/, [L, *casus,* chance], **1.** a serious or fatal accident. **2.** the victims of a serious or fatal accident. **3.** a person, killed, wounded, or otherwise disabled in war.

casuistics /kazh′əwis′tiks/ [L, *casus,* a happening], the recording and study of the cases of any disease.

catabasis /kətab′əsis/, *pl.* **catabases** [Gk, *kata,* down, *bainein,* to go], the phase in which a disease declines. —**catabatic** /kat′əbat′ik/, *adj.*

catabiosis /kat′əbī·ō′sis/, the normal aging of cells. —**catabiotic,** *adj.*

catabolic illness /kat′əbol′ik/, a disorder characterized by weight loss and diminished muscle mass and body fat. Underlying causes include infection, injury, organ system failure, chemotherapy, and uncontrolled diabetes mellitus, particularly type I.

catabolism /kətab′əliz′əm/ [Gk, *kata* + *ballein,* to throw], a metabolic process in which complex substances are broken down by living cells into simple compounds. —**catabolic,** *adj.*

catachronobiology /kat′əkrō′nōbī·ol′əjē/, the study of the harmful effects of time on living systems.

catacrotism /kətak′rətiz′əm/ [Gk, *kata* + *krotein,* to strike], an anomaly of the pulse, characterized by one or more small additional waves in the descending limb of the pulse tracing. —**catacrotic,** *adj.*

catagenesis /kat′əjen′əsis/ [Gk, *kata,* down, *genein,* to produce], a form of evolution that is retrogressive.

catalase /kat′əlās/ [Gk, *katalein,* to dissolve], a heme enzyme, found in almost all biologic cells, that catalyzes the decomposition of hydrogen peroxide to water and oxygen.

catalepsy /kat'əlep'sē/ [Gk, *kata* + *lambanein*, to seize], an abnormal state characterized by a trancelike level of consciousness and postural rigidity. It occurs in hypnosis and in certain organic and psychologic disorders such as schizophrenia, epilepsy, and hysteria.

cataleptic /kat'əlep'tik/, pertaining to mental illness characterized by maintenance of rigid waxlike postures.

catalysis /kətal'əsis/ [Gk, *katalein*, to dissolve], an increase in the rate of a chemical reaction that is caused by a substance that is neither permanently altered nor consumed by the reaction. —**catalytic,** *adj.*

catalyst /kat'əlist/ [Gk, *katalein*, to dissolve], a substance that influences the rate of a chemical reaction without being permanently altered or consumed by the process. Most catalysts, including enzymes in living organisms, accelerate chemical reactions; negative catalysts retard such reactions.

catalyze, to produce catalysis, as speeding up a chemical reaction or physical process.

catamnesis /kat'amnē'sis/ [Gk, *kata* + *men*, month], the medical history of a patient from the onset of an illness.

cataphoria /kat'əfôr'ē·ə/, a tendency of the visual axes of both eyes to assume a low plane after the visual fusional stimuli have been eliminated.

cataphylaxis /kat'əfəlak'sis/ [Gk, *kata* + *phylax*, guard], **1.** the migration of leukocytes and antibodies to the site of an infection. **2.** the deterioration of the natural defense system of the body. —**cataphylactic,** *adj.*

cataplexy /kat'əplek'sē/ [Gk, *kata* + *plexis*, stroke], a condition characterized by sudden muscular weakness and hypotonia, caused by emotions such as anger, fear, or surprise, often associated with narcolepsy. —**cataplectic,** *adj.*

cataract /kat'ərakt/ [Gk, *katarrhakies*, waterfall], an abnormal progressive condition of the lens of the eye, characterized by loss of transparency. A gray-white opacity can be observed within the lens, behind the pupil. Most cataracts are caused by degenerative changes, often occurring after 50 years of age. Congenital cataracts are usually hereditary but may be caused by viral infection during the first trimester of gestation. If cataracts are untreated, sight is eventually lost. Uncomplicated cataracts of old age (**senile cataracts**) are usually treated with excision of the lens and either surgical insertion of an intraocular lens or prescription of special contact lenses or glasses. The soft cataracts of children and young adults may be either incised and drained or fragmented by ultrasound.

cataractogenic /kat'ərak'tōjen'ik/, pertaining to agents that may cause cataracts.

catarrh /kətär'/ [Gk, *kata* + *rhoia*, flow], inflammation of the mucous membranes with discharge, especially inflammation of the air passages of the nose and the trachea. —**catarrhal, catarrhous,** *adj.*

catarrhal conjunctivitis [Gk, *kata* + *rhoia* + L, *conjunctivus*, connecting; Gk, *itis*, inflammation], a simple form of inflammation of the conjunctiva, usually associated with an infection, allergy, exposure to pollution, or physical irritation, as by an eyelash in the eye. It is accompanied by discharge.

catarrhal croup [Gk, *kata* + *rhoia* + Scot, to croak], a severe laryngitis accompanied by a croupy cough.

catarrhal ophthalmia [Gk, *kata* + *rhoia* + *ophthalmos*, eye], a catarrhal inflammation of the conjunctiva with a discharge.

catastrophic care /kat'əstrof'ik/ [Gk, *katastrophe*, sudden downturn; L, *garrire*, to babble], a pattern of medical and nursing care that involves intensive, highly technical life-support care of an acutely ill or severely traumatized patient.

catastrophic health insurance, health insurance that awards benefits to pay for the cost of severe or lengthy disability or illness. Most policies have a limit in total benefits paid, and payment for certain kinds of services may be precluded or limited to a maximum indemnity.

catastrophic illness, any illness that requires lengthy hospitalization, extremely expensive therapies, or other care that would deplete a family's financial resources, unless covered by special medical insurance policies. In Canada catastrophic illness is covered by Medicare.

catastrophic reaction [Gk, *katastrophe*, sudden downturn; L, *re*, again, *agere*, to act], the uncoordinated response to a drastic shock or a sudden threatening condition, as often occurs in the victims of car crashes and disasters.

catatonia /kat'ətō'nē·ə/ [Gk, *kata* + *tonos*, tension], a state of psychologically induced immobility with muscular rigidity at times interrupted by agitation. It is manifested usually as immobility with extreme muscular rigidity or, less commonly, as excessive, impulsive activity. —**catatonic** /kat'əton'ik/, *adj.*

catatonic excitement, a state of extreme

agitation that may occur when a patient is unable to maintain catatonic immobility.

catatonic schizophrenia [Gk, *kata* + *tonos* + *schizein*, to split, *phren*, mind], a form of schizophrenia characterized by alternating periods of extreme withdrawal and extreme excitement. During the withdrawal stage, stupor, muscular rigidity, mutism, blocking, negativism, and catalepsy (cerea flexibilitas) may be seen; during the period of excitement, purposeless and impulsive activity may range from mild agitation to violence.

catatonic stupor, a form of catatonia characterized by a marked decrease in response to the environment with a reduction in spontaneous movement.

CAT-CAM, abbreviation for **contoured adducted trochanteric controlled alignment method.**

catchment area [L, *capere*, to take, *area*, space], the specific geographic area for which a particular institution, especially a mental health center, is responsible.

catch-up growth [L, *capere* + As, *uf, gruowan*], an acceleration of the growth rate following a period of growth retardation caused by a secondary deficiency such as acute malnutrition or severe illness. The phenomenon, which routinely occurs in premature infants, involves rapid increase in weight, length, and head circumference and continues until the normal individual growth pattern is resumed.

cat-cry syndrome [L, *catta*, cat, *quiritare*, to cry out; Gk, *syndromos*, course], a rare, congenital disorder recognized at birth by a kittenlike cry caused by a laryngeal anomaly. The condition is associated with a defect in chromosome 5. Other characteristics include low birth weight, microcephaly, "moon face," wide-set eyes, strabismus, and low-set misshapen ears. Infants are hypotonic; heart defects and mental and physical retardation are common.

catecholamine /kat′əkəlam′in/, any one of a group of sympathomimetic compounds composed of a catechol molecule and the aliphatic part of an amine. Some catecholamines are produced naturally by the body and function as key neurologic chemicals.

catechol-o-methyl transferase (COMT) /kat′əkol′ōmeth′il/, an enzyme that deactivates the catecholamines epinephrine and norepinephrine.

cat-eye syndrome [L, *catta* + AS, *eage* + Gk, *syndromos*, course], a rare congenital autosomal anomaly, marked by the presence of an extra small chromosome 22 and pupils that resemble the vertical pupils of a cat.

categoric data /kat′əgôr′ik/ [Gk, *kategorikos*, affirmation; L, *datus*, giving], (in research) any data that are classified by name rather than by number, such as race, religion, ethnicity, or marital status.

catgut [L, *catta* + AS, *guttas*], a nonabsorbable suture material prepared from the intestines of sheep, used to close surgical wounds.

catharsis /kəthär′sis/, **1.** a cleansing or purging. **2.** the therapeutic release of pent-up feelings and emotions by open discussion of ideas and thoughts. **3.** the process of drawing repressed ideas and feelings into the consciousness by the technique of free association, often in conjunction with hypnosis and use of hypnotic drugs. —**cathartic,** *n.*

cathartic /kəthär′tik/ [Gk, *katharsis,* cleansing], **1.** pertaining to a substance that causes evacuation of the bowel. **2.** an agent that promotes bowel evacuation by stimulating peristalsis, increasing the fluidity or bulk of intestinal contents, softening the feces, or lubricating the intestinal wall. —**catharsis,** *n.*

catheter /kath′ətər/ [Gk, *katheter,* something lowered], a hollow flexible tube that can be inserted into a vessel or cavity of the body to withdraw or instill fluids, monitor types of various information, and visualize a vessel or cavity.

catheter hub, a threaded plastic connection at the end of an intravenous catheter.

catheterization /kath′əturī′zā′shən/, the introduction of a catheter (a hollow flexible tube) into a body cavity or organ to inject or remove a fluid. —**catheterize** /kath′ətərīz/, *v.*

cathexis /kəthek′sis/ [Gk, *kathexis*, retention], the conscious or unconscious attachment of emotional feeling and importance to a specific idea, person, or object. —**cathectic,** *adj*

cathode /kath′ōd/ [Gk, *kata*, down, *hodos,* way], **1.** the electrode at which reduction occurs. **2.** the negative side of the x-ray tube, which consists of the focusing cup and the filament.

cathode ray, a stream of electrons emitted by the negative electrode of a gaseous discharge device when the cathode is bombarded by positive ions, such as in a cathode ray tube or an oscilloscope. The ray itself is usually focused by a series of electromagnets that control its direction and position on a screen coated with a phosphor to create a visible pattern.

cathode ray oscilloscope [Gk, *kata* + *hodos* + L, *radius* + *ocillare*, to swing; Gk, *skopein*, to view], an instrument that produces a visual representation of electrical variations by means of the fluorescent screen of a cathode ray tube. Oscilloscopes have many applications in medicine and nursing, such as the displaying of heartbeats for monitoring and diagnostic purposes.

cathode ray tube (CRT), a vacuum tube that focuses a beam of electrons onto a spot on a screen coated with a phosphor, creating a visible image of information on the face of the tube.

cation /kat′ī·on/ [Gk, *kata,* down, *ion,* going], a positively charged ion.

cation-exchange resin, any one of various insoluble organic polymers with high molecular weights that exchange their cations for other ions in solution.

catling, a long, sharp, double-edged knife used in amputation.

catoptric /kətop′trik/ [Gk, *katoptron,* mirror], pertaining to a reflected image or reflected light, such as from a mirror.

cat scratch fever, a disease that results from the scratch or bite of a healthy cat. Inflammation and pustules are found on the scratched skin, and lymph nodes in the neck, head, groin, or axilla swell later. Fever, headache, and malaise may occur, and symptoms can persist for months.

cat's eye amaurosis [L, *catta* + AS, *aege* + Gk, *amauroin,* to darken], a monocular blindness, with a bright reflection from the pupil caused by a white mass in the vitreous humor resulting from inflammation or a malignant lesion.

Caucasian, pertaining to a person whose ancestors were believed to have in ancient times inhabited the geographic region of the Caucasus in southeastern Europe or whose ancestors were members of the hypothetic Indo-European cultures identified with the Caucasus.

caudad /kô′dad/ [L, *cauda,* tail], toward the tail or end of the body, away from the head.

cauda equina [L, *cauda* + *equus,* horse], the lower end of the spinal cord at the first lumbar vertebra and the bundle of lumbar, sacral, and coccygeal nerve roots that emerge from the spinal cord and descend through the spinal canal of the sacrum and coccyx.

caudal /kô′dəl/, signifying a position toward the distal end of the body.

caudal anesthesia, the injection of a local anesthetic agent into the caudal part of the epidural space through the sacral hiatus to anesthetize sacral and lower lumbar nerve roots. It is now rarely performed except in pediatric anesthesia.

caudal ligaments, bands of fibrous tissue attaching the skin to the coccyx. Remnants of the embryonic notochord, they form a small cup-shaped depression.

caudate /kô′dāt/, having a tail.

caudate lobe of the liver [L, *cauda,* tail; Gk, *lobos,* lobe; AS, *lifer*], a part of the right lobe of the liver that lies near the vena cava.

caudate nucleus [L, *cauda,* tail, *nucleus,* nut kernel], a crescent-shaped mass of gray matter lateral to the thalamus in the floor of the anterior horn and body of the lateral ventricle.

caudate process [L, *cauda* + *processus,* projection], a small elevation of tissue that extends obliquely from the lower extremity of the caudate lobe of the liver to the visceral surface of the right lobe.

caudocephalad /kô′dōsef′əlad/ [L, *cauda,* tail; Gk, *kephale,* head; L, *ad,* toward], movement from the tail toward the head.

caul /kôl/ [ME, *cawel,* basket], the intact amniotic sac surrounding the fetus at birth. The sac usually ruptures or is ruptured during the course of labor or delivery; when it remains intact, it must be torn or cut to allow the baby to breathe.

cauliflower ear [L, *caulis,* cabbage, *fiore,* flower; AS, *eare*], a thickened, deformed pinna and external ear caused by repeated trauma such as that suffered by boxers.

caumesthesia /kô′məsthē′zhə/ [Gk, *kauma,* heat, *aisthesis,* feeling], an abnormal condition in which a patient has a low temperature but experiences a sense of intense heat. **—caumesthetic,** *adj.*

causalgia /kôzal′jə/ [Gk, *kausis,* burning, *algos,* pain], a severe sensation of burning pain, often in an extremity, sometimes accompanied by local erythema of the skin.

causal hypothesis /kô′səl/ [L, *causa,* cause; Gk, *hypotithenia,* foundation], (in research) a hypothesis that predicts a cause-and-effect relationship among the variables to be studied.

causal hypothesis testing study, (in nursing research) an experimental design used in testing a hypothesis that predicts a cause-and-effect relationship within the data to be studied.

causality /kôsal′itē/, (in research) a relationship between one phenomenon or event (A) and another (B) in which A precedes and causes B and the direction of influence and the nature of the effect are predictable and reproducible and may be empirically observed.

causation /kôsā′shən/ [L, *causa*], (in law) the existence of a reasonable connection between the misfeasance, malfeasance, or nonfeasance of the defendant and the injury or damage suffered by the plaintiff.

cause [L, *causa*], any process, substance, or organism that produces an effect or condition.

CAUSN, abbreviation for **Canadian Association of University Schools of Nursing.**

caustic /kôs'tik/ [Gk, *kaustikos,* burning], **1.** any substance that is destructive to living tissue such as silver nitrate, nitric acid, or sulfuric acid. **2.** exerting a burning or corrosive effect.

caustic poisoning, the accidental ingestion of strong acids or alkalis, resulting in burns and tissue damage to the mouth, esophagus, and stomach. The victim experiences immediate pain, swelling, and edema. The pulse may be weak and rapid. Respirations become shallow, and edema may close the airway. Complications, which include circulatory shock, perforation of the esophagus, and pharyngeal edema leading to asphyxia, can be fatal. The victim should be hospitalized or seen by a physician immediately. Administration of "neutralizing" substances is not recommended because of the risk of a heat-producing chemical reaction.

CAUT, abbreviation for **Canadian Association of University Teachers.**

cauterization /kô'tərĭzā'shən/ [Gk, *kauterion,* branding iron], the process of burning a part of the body by cautery.

cauterize /kô'tərīz/ [Gk, *kauterion,* branding iron], to burn tissues by thermal heat, including steam, hot metal, or solar radiation; electricity; or another agent such as dry ice, usually with the objective of destroying damaged or diseased tissues.

cautery /kô'tərē/ [Gk, *kauterion,* branding iron], **1.** a device or agent used in the coagulation of tissue by heat or caustic substances. **2.** a destructive effect produced by a cauterizing agent.

cautery knife, a surgical knife that cuts tissue and seals it to prevent bleeding. The knife is connected to an electric source that generates the heat necessary for cauterization.

Cavell, Edith /kəvel'/, (1865–1915), an English nurse. Trained at London Hospital, in 1907 she was named head of a nurses' training school in Brussels, with the task of raising nursing standards to match those of Britain. After the Germans occupied Belgium in World War I, she nursed or sheltered more than 200 fleeing soldiers and helped them reach Holland. She was arrested by the Germans, tried, and shot on October 12, 1915. Her execution, which she met with courage and fortitude, brought her widespread fame.

cavernous /kav'ərnəs/ [L, *caverna,* hollow place], containing cavities or hollow spaces.

cavernous hemangioma [L, *caverna,* hollow place; Gk *haima,* blood, *oma,* tumor], a benign congenital tumor consisting of large, blood-filled cystic spaces. The scalp, face, and neck are the most common sites.

cavernous sinus [L, *caverna* + *sinus,* curve], one of a pair of irregularly shaped bilateral venous channels between the sphenoid bone of the skull and the dura mater. It is one of the five anterior inferior venous sinuses that drain the blood from the dura mater into the internal jugular vein.

cavernous sinus syndrome, an abnormal condition characterized by edema of the conjunctiva, the upper eyelid, and the root of the nose and by paralysis of the third, fourth, and the sixth cranial nerves. It is caused by a thrombosis of the cavernous sinus.

cavernous sinus thrombosis, a syndrome, usually secondary to infections near the eye or nose, characterized by orbital edema, venous congestion of the eye, and palsy of the nerves supplying the extraocular muscles. The infection may spread to involve the cerebrospinal fluid and meninges.

CAVH, abbreviation for *continuous arteriovenous hemofiltration.*

cavitary /kav'iter'ē/ [L, *cavus,* hollow], **1.** denoting the presence of one or more cavities. **2.** any entozoon having a body cavity or an alimentary canal.

cavitate /kav'itāt/ [L, *cavus,* hollow], the act of rapidly forming and collapsing vapor pockets or bubbles in a flowing fluid with low pressure areas, often causing damage to surrounding structures.

cavitation, **1.** the formation of cavities within the body, such as those formed in the lung by tuberculosis. **2.** any cavity within the body, such as the pleural cavities.

cavity /kav'itē/ [L, *cavus*], **1.** a hollow space within a larger structure, such as the peritoneal or oral cavity. **2.** *nontechnical.* a space in a tooth formed by dental caries.

cavity classification, the taxonomy of carious lesions according to the tooth surfaces on which they occur, such as cervical, proximal, labial, buccal, lingual, or occlusal; type of surface, such as pit and fissure; frequency of occurrence, such as incipient or recurrent; and numeric designation of cavity type.

cavogram /kav'əgram'/ [L, *cavus* + Gk, *gramma,* record], an angiogram of the inferior or superior vena cava.

cavosurface angle /kāv'ōsur'fəs/, (in dentistry) the measure formed by the junction of the wall of a prepared cavity with the external surface of the tooth.

cavosurface bevel [L, *cavus* + *superficies,*

surface; OFr, *baif,* open mouth], the incline of the cavosurface angle of a prepared tooth cavity wall relative to the enamel wall.

cavum /kā′vəm/, *pl.* **cava,** 1. any hollow or cavity. 2. the inferior or superior vena cava.

cavus /kā′vəs/ [L, *cavus,* cavity], an abnormally high arch of the foot.

cayenne pepper. See **capsicum.**

CBA, abbreviation for **cost-benefit analysis.**

CBC, abbreviation for **complete blood count.**

CBF, abbreviation for *cerebral blood flow.*

cc, abbreviation for **cubic centimeter.**

CC, 1. abbreviation for **chief complaint.** 2. abbreviation for *Commission Certified.*

CCK, abbreviation for **cholecystokinin.**

CCPD, abbreviation for **continuous cycling peritoneal dialysis.**

CCRN, 1. abbreviation for *Certified Critical Care Registered Nurse;* 2. trademark of **American Association of Critical-Care Nurses Certified Corporation.**

CCU, abbreviation for **critical care unit.**

Cd, symbol for the element **cadmium.**

cdc, abbreviation for **cell division cycle.**

CDC, abbreviation for **Centers for Disease Control and Prevention.**

CDE, 1. the major symbols used in one system for the nomenclature of the Rh system, in which D is the same as Rh0, the major determining factor of Rh positivity. 2. abbreviation for *common duct exploration.* 3. abbreviation for *Certified Diabetes Educator.*

CDH, abbreviation for **congenital dislocation of the hip.**

CDK, abbreviation for **cyclin-dependent kinase.**

CD4, symbol for a glycoprotein expressed on the surface of most thymocytes and some lymphocytes, including helper T cells. Human CD4 is the receptor that serves as a docking site for human immunodeficiency virus on certain lymphocyte cells. Binding of the viral glycoprotein gp120 to CD4 is the first step in viral entry, leading to the fusion of viral and cell membranes.

CD4 cell count, a measure of "helper" T cells that are responsible to help B cells produce certain antibodies. As the virus binds to CD4 and kills T cells bearing this antigen, the level of CD4 helper T cells in the blood is an indicator of the progress of the infection. The CD4 cell count helps measure effectiveness of clinical trials of human immunodeficiency virus antiviral drugs.

CD4/CD8 count, the ratio of the number of helper T lymphocytes to suppressor and cytotoxic T lymphocytes. The cell numbers are measured with monoclonal antibodies to the surface antigens CD4 on helper T cells and CD8 on suppressor and cytotoxic T cells. In healthy individuals the ratio ranges from 1.6 to 2.2. The ratio is important in monitoring the function of the immune system in patients with viral infections or tissue transplantation.

CD8, symbol for peripheral lymphocyte T cells that secrete large amounts of gamma-interferon, a lymphokine involved in the body's defense against viruses. CD8 cells prevent unnecessary formation of antibodies.

CDR, abbreviation for **computed dental radiography.**

Ce, symbol for the element **cerium.**

CEA, 1. abbreviation for **carcinoembryonic antigen.** 2. abbreviation for **cost-effectiveness analysis.**

ceasmic /sē·az′mik/ [Gk, *keazein,* to split], pertaining to or characterized by a persistent embryonic fissure or abnormal cleavage of parts.

ceasmic teratism [Gk, *keazein* + *teras,* monster], a congenital anomaly, caused by developmental arrest, in which body parts that should be fused remain in their fissured embryonic state, such as in cleft palate.

cecal /sē′kəl/ [L, *caecus,* blind, blind gut], 1. pertaining to the cecum. 2. pertaining to the optic disc or the blind spot in the retina.

cecocolostomy /sē′kōkəlos′təmē/ [L, *caecus,* blind, blind gut; Gk, *kolon,* colon, *stoma,* mouth], 1. a surgical operation that creates an anastomosis between the cecum and the colon. 2. the anastomosis produced by this operation.

cecoileostomy /-il′ē·os′təmē/ [L, *caecus* + *ilia,* intestine, *stoma,* mouth], a surgical operation that connects the ileum with the cecum.

cecopexy /sē′kōpek′sē/ [L, *caecus* + Gk, *pexis,* fix], a surgical operation that fixes or suspends the cecum to correct its excessive mobility.

cecostomy /sēkos′təmē/ [L, *caecus* + Gk, *stoma,* mouth], the surgical construction of an opening into the cecum, performed as a temporary measure to relieve intestinal obstruction in a patient who cannot tolerate major surgery.

cecum /sē′kəm/ [L, *caecus,* blind, blind gut], a pouchlike structure constituting the first part of the large intestine.

cefaclor /sē′fəklôr/, a cephalosporin antibiotic prescribed in the treatment of certain infections.

cefadroxil monohydrate /sē′fədrok′sil/, a cephalosporin antibiotic prescribed in the treatment of certain bacterial infections.

cefamandole nafate /sēfəman′dōlnaf′āt/, a cephalosporin antibiotic prescribed in the treatment of certain bacterial infections.

cefazolin sodium /sēfaz′ōlin/, a cephalosporin antibacterial prescribed in the treatment of infections.

cefonicid sodium /sēfon′isid/, a parenteral cephalosporin-type antibiotic prescribed for infections of the lower respiratory or urinary tract, skin, bones and joints, septicemia, and surgical prophylaxis.

cefoperazone sodium /sē′fōper′əzon/, a cephalosporin antibiotic prescribed in the treatment of respiratory tract, intraabdominal, skin, and female genital tract infections and bacterial septicemia.

ceforanide /sēfôr′anīd/, a parenteral cephalosporin-type antibiotic prescribed for infections of the lower respiratory or urinary tract, skin, or bones and joints; septicemia; endocarditis; and surgical prophylaxis.

cefotaxime sodium /sēfōtak′zēm/, a cephalosporin antibiotic prescribed for lower respiratory tract, genitourinary, gynecologic, intraabdominal, skin, bone and joint, and central nervous system infections and bacterial septicemia caused by strains of microorganisms.

cefotetan disodium /sē′fōtet′ən/, a parenteral cephalosporin antibiotic prescribed for infections of the lower respiratory tract, urinary tract, skin, abdomen, bones or joints, or reproductive organs and for surgical prophylaxis.

cefoxitin sodium /sēfok′sitin/, a cephalosporin antibiotic prescribed in the treatment of certain bacterial infections.

ceftazidime /sēftaz′idēm/, a parenteral cephalosporin-type antibiotic prescribed for treatment of infections of the lower respiratory tract, urinary tract, skin, abdomen, blood, bones and joints, and central nervous system.

ceftibuten, an oral cephalosporin prescribed in the treatment of chronic bronchitis, acute bacterial otitis media, pharyngitis, and tonsillitis.

ceftizoxime sodium /sef′tizok′zēm/, a cephalosporin antibiotic prescribed in the treatment of bacterial infections.

ceftriaxone sodium /sef′trī·ak′sōn/, a parenteral cephalosporin-type antibiotic prescribed for infections of the lower respiratory tract, urinary tract, skin, abdomen, bones, and joints. It is also used to treat gonorrhea, septicemia, and meningi-

tis and in surgical prophylaxis, particularly in coronary bypass operations.

cefuroxime sodium /sef′oorok′zem/, a cephalosporin antibiotic prescribed in the treatment of lower respiratory tract, urinary tract, skin, and gonococcal infections; bacterial septicemia; and meningitis and for the prevention of postoperative infections.

celiac /sē′lē·ak/ [Gk, koilia, belly], pertaining to the abdominal cavity.

celiac artery [Gk, koilia, belly, arteria, airpipe], a thick visceral branch of the abdominal aorta, arising caudal to the diaphragm, usually dividing into the left gastric, common hepatic, and splenic arteries.

celiac disease [Gk, koilia + L, dis, opposite of; Fr, aise, ease], an inborn error of metabolism characterized by the inability to hydrolyze peptides contained in gluten. The disease affects adults and young children who suffer from abdominal distension, vomiting, diarrhea, muscle wasting, and extreme lethargy. A characteristic sign is a pale, foul-smelling stool that floats on water because of its high fat content. Most patients respond well to a high-protein, high-calorie, gluten-free diet.

celiac ganglion, a group of nerve cells located on each side of the crura of the diaphragm. The cells are connected to the celiac plexus.

celiac rickets [Gk, koilia + rhachis, spine, itis, inflammation], arrested growth and osseous deformities resulting from malabsorption of fat and calcium.

celiocolpotomy /sē′lē·ōkəlpot′əmē/ [Gk, koilia + kolpos, vagina, temnein, to cut], an incision into the abdomen through the vagina.

cell [L, cella, storeroom], the fundamental unit of all living tissue. Eukaryotic cells consist of a nucleus, cytoplasm, and organelles surrounded by a plasma membrane. Within the nucleus are the nucleolus (containing ribonucleic acid) and the chromatin (containing protein and deoxyribonucleic acid), which gives rise to chromosomes, wherein are located the determinants of inherited characteristics. Organelles within the cytoplasm include the endoplasmic reticulum, ribosomes, Golgi apparatus, mitochondria, lysosomes, and centrosome. Prokaryotic cells are much smaller and simpler than eukaryocytic cells, even lacking a nucleus. The specialized nature of body tissue reflects the specialized structure and function of its constituent cells.

cella /sel′ə/, pl. cellae [L, storeroom], an enclosed space.

cell bank, a storage facility for frozen tissue samples held for research purposes and for surgical reconstruction of damaged body structures.

cell biology, the science that deals with the structures, living processes, and functions of living cells, especially human cells.

cell body [L, *cella* + AS, *bodig*], the part of a cell that contains the nucleus and surrounding cytoplasm exclusive of any projections or processes, such as the axon and dendrites of a neuron or the tail of a spermatozoon.

cell culture [L, *cella,* storeroom, *colere,* to cultivate], living cells that are maintained in vitro in artificial media of serum and nutrients for the study and growth of certain strains or for experiments in controlling diseases such as cancer.

cell death, 1. terminal failure of a cell to maintain the essential life functions. **2.** the point in the process of dying at which vital functions have ceased at the cellular level.

cell determination, the process by which an undifferentiated embryonic cell undergoes differentiation, developing first into basic endoderm, mesoderm, or ectoderm germ layers and eventually into the specific tissues, specific structures, functioning organs, and complex fluids of the body. The specific ontogenic agent that facilitates the maturation of tissues is unknown.

cell division, the continuous process by which a cell alternates between a long interphase period and mitosis. Mitosis involves four stages: prophase, metaphase, anaphase, and telophase. Cell division does not occur in discrete steps: each phase is part of a continuous process that may require hours for its completion. During the interphase period new deoxyribonucleic acid, ribonucleic acid, and protein molecules are synthesized before the start of the next prophase.

cell division cycle (cdc), the sequence of events that occurs during the growth and division of tissue cells.

cell inclusion [L, *cella,* storeroom, *in* + *claudere,* to shut], pertaining to any foreign matter that is enclosed within a cell.

cell line [L, *cella* + *linea*], a colony of animal cells derived and developed as a subculture from a primary cell culture.

cell mass [L, *cella,* storeroom, *massa*], the embryonic cluster of cells that develops into an individual or a part of an organism.

cell-mediated immune response, a delayed-type intravenous hypersensitivity reaction, mediated primarily by sensitized T cell lymphocytes as opposed to antibodies. Cell-mediated immune reactions are responsible for defense against certain bacterial, fungal, and viral pathogens; malignant cells; and other foreign protein or tissue.

cell organelle [L, *cella,* storeroom; Gk, *organon,* instrument], any of a number of membrane-bound structures within a cell that have specific functions, such as reproduction or metabolism. Examples include mitochondria and Golgi bodies.

cell receptor, a protein located either on a cell's surface, in its cytoplasm, or in its nucleus that binds to a specific ligand, initiating signal transduction and cellular activity.

cells of Paneth /pä′nət, pan′əth/ [Josef Paneth, Austrian physiologist, 1857–1890], large granular epithelial cells found in intestinal glands. They secrete digestive enzymes and bactericidal lysozyme.

cell theory, the proposition that cells are the basic units of all living tissues or organisms and that cellular function is the essential process of living things.

cellular /sel′yələr/ [L, *cella,* storeroom], pertaining to or consisting of cells.

cellular immunity [L, *cellula,* little cell, *immunis,* exempt], the mechanism of acquired immunity characterized by the dominant role of small T cell lymphocytes. Cellular immunity is involved in resistance to infectious diseases caused by viruses and some bacteria and in delayed hypersensitivity reactions, some aspects of resistance to cancer, certain autoimmune diseases, graft rejection, and certain allergies.

cellular infiltration, the migration and grouping of cells within tissues throughout the body.

cellulite /sel′yəlīt/, a nonmedical term for fat and fibrous tissue deposits that result in dimpling of the skin.

cellulitis /sel′yəlī′tis/ [L, *cellula,* little cell; Gk, *itis,* inflammation], a diffuse, acute infection of the skin and subcutaneous tissue characterized most commonly by local heat, redness, pain, and swelling and occasionally by fever, malaise, chills, and headache. Abscess and tissue destruction usually follow if antibiotics are not taken.

cellulose /sel′yŏŏlōs/ [L, *cellula,* little cell], a colorless, insoluble, indigestible transparent solid polysaccharide that is the primary constituent of the cell walls of plants. In the diet it provides the bulk necessary for proper digestive tract functioning.

cell wall, the structure that covers and

protects the plasma membrane in some kinds of cells, such as certain bacteria and all fungi and plant cells.

celosomia /sē′ləsō′mē·ə/ [Gk, *kele*, hernia, *soma*, body], a congenital malformation characterized by a fissure or absence of the sternum and ribs and protrusion of the viscera.

celosomus /sē′ləsō′məs/, a fetus with celosomia.

Celsius (C) /sel′sē·əs/ [Anders Celsius, Swedish scientist, 1701–1744], denoting a temperature scale in which 0° is the freezing point of water and 100° is the boiling point of water at sea level.

cement /siment′/ [L, *caementum*, rough stone], **1.** a sticky or mucilaginous substance that helps neighboring tissue cells stick together. **2.** any of a variety of dental materials used to fill cavities or to hold bridgework or other dental prostheses in place. **3.** a material used in the fixation of a prosthetic joint in adjacent bone, such as methyl methacrylate.

cemental fiber /simen′təl/ [L, *caementum*, rough stone, *fibra*], any one of the many fibers of the periodontal membrane that extend from the cementum to the intermediate plexus.

cement base, (in dentistry) a layer of dental cement material, sometimes medicated, pressed into the bottom of a prepared cavity to protect the pulp, reduce the bulk of metallic restoration, or eliminate undercuts in a tapered preparation.

cementifying fibroma /-ifī′ing/ [L, *caementum* + *facere*, to make, *fibra*, fiber; Gk, *oma*, tumor], **1.** an intraosseous lesion composed of fibrous connective tissue enclosing foci of calcified material resembling cementum. **2.** a rare odontogenic tumor composed of varying amounts of fibrous connective tissue resembling cementum. **3.** central jaw lesion.

cementoblast /simen′təblast/ (in dentistry), a large squamous or cuboidal cell that is responsible for the formation of cementum on the root dentin of a developing tooth.

cementoblastoma /simen′tōblastō′mə/ [L, *caementum* + Gk, *blastos*, germ, *oma*, tumor], an odontogenic fibrous tumor consisting of cells developing into cementoblasts but containing only a small amount of calcified tissue.

cementocyte /simen′təsīt/, a cell found in a bone matrix cavity of cellular cementum.

cementoma /sē′mentō′mə/ [L, *caementum* + Gk, *oma*, tumor], any benign cementum-producing tumor associated with the apices of teeth.

cementopathia /-ōpath′ē·ə/ [L, *caementum* + Gk, *pathos*, disease], an abnormal condition of the teeth caused by necrotic cementum and insufficient cementogenesis.

cementum /simen′təm/, the bonelike connective tissue that covers the roots of the teeth and helps to support them.

cen, abbreviation for **centromere.**

CEN, abbreviation for *Certified Emergency Nurse.*

cenesthesia /sē′nesthē′zhə/ [Gk, *kenos*, empty, *aisthesis*, feeling], the general sense of existing, derived as the aggregate of all the various stimuli and reactions throughout the body at any specific moment to produce a feeling of health or illness.

cenogenesis /sē′nōjen′əsis/ [Gk, *kenos*, empty, *genein*, to produce], the development of structural characteristics that are absent in earlier forms of a species, as an adaptive response to environmental conditions. —**cenogenetic, coenogenetic, caenogenetic,** *adj.*

censor [L, *censere*, to assess], **1.** a person who monitors or evaluates books, newspapers, plays, works of art, speech, or other means of expression to suppress certain kinds of information. **2.** (in psychoanalysis) a psychic suppression that allows unconscious thoughts to rise to consciousness only if they are heavily disguised.

census [L, *censere*, to assess], an enumeration of the population, usually conducted periodically as a function of an official agency. In addition to counting heads, the census often collects information about members of a household and matters relating to the health of the community.

center [Gk, *kentron*], **1.** the middle point of the body or geometric entity, equidistant from points on the periphery. **2.** a group of neurons with a common function such as the accelerating center in the brain that controls the heartbeat.

center of excellence, a tertiary or quaternary health care provider that is identified as the most expert and cost efficient and produces the best outcomes. The term often refers to organ transplantation centers.

center of gravity, the midpoint or center of the weight of a body or object. In the standing adult human the center of gravity is in the midpelvic cavity, between the symphysis pubis and the umbilicus.

Centers for Disease Control and Prevention (CDC), a federal agency of the U.S. government that provides facilities and services for the investigation, identification, prevention, and control of disease. It is concerned with all of the epidemiologic aspects and the laboratory diagnosis of disease. Immunization programs, quarantine regulations and programs, laboratory standards, and community surveillance for disease are among the activities of the CDC, which is located in Atlanta.

centesis /sentē'sis/ [Gk, kentesis, pricking], a perforation or a puncture of a cavity, such as paracentesis or thoracocentesis.

centigram, a mass equal to one hundredth of a gram, or 10 milligrams.

centiliter, a volume equal to one hundredth of a liter, or 10 milliliters.

centimeter (cm) /sen'timē'tər/ [L, centum, hundred; Gk, metron, measure], the metric unit of measurement equal to one hundredth of a meter, or 0.3937 inch.

centimeter-gram-second system (cgs, CGS), the internationally accepted scientific system of expressing length, mass, and time in basic units of centimeters, grams, and seconds. The CGS system is gradually being replaced by the Systeme International d'Unités (SI) or the (International System of Units), based on the meter, kilogram, and second.

centipede bite /sen'təpēd/ [L, centum, hundred, pes, foot], a wound produced by the poison claws and the first body segment of a centipede, an elongate arthropod with many pairs of legs. The bite of a few species, including Scolopendra morsitans in the southern United States, may cause painful local inflammation, fever, headache, vomiting, and dizziness.

centipoise /sen'təpois/ [Jean L.M. Poiseuille, French physiologist, 1797–1869], a measure of the viscosity of a liquid, equal to one hundredth of a poise.

centrad [L, centum, hundred], **1.** pertaining to a central direction. **2.** a unit of measure equal to one hundredth part of a radian. **3.** a measure of the refractive strength of a prism.

central [Gk, kentron, center], pertaining to or situated at a center.

central amaurosis [Gk, kentron + amauroein, to darken], blindness caused by a disease of the central nervous system.

central anesthesia, a loss of feeling or sensation due to a lesion in the central nervous system.

central auditory processing disorder (CAPD), difficulty in processing and interpreting auditory stimuli in the absence of a peripheral hearing loss, usually resulting from a problem in the brainstem or cerebral cortex. Children with CAPD often have difficulty reading and may exhibit other learning disabilities as well.

central biasing /bī'əsing/, a theory of pain modulation in which higher centers such as the cerebral cortex influence the perception of and response to pain.

central canal of spinal cord [Gk, kentron + L, canalis, channel], the conduit that runs the entire length of the spinal cord and contains most of the 140 ml of cerebrospinal fluid in the body of the average individual. The central canal of the spinal cord lies in the center of the cord between the ventral and the dorsal gray commissures and extends toward the cranium into the medulla oblongata, where it opens into the fourth ventricle of the brain.

central catheter [Gk, kentron, central, katheter, a thing lowered into], a catheter inserted into either a central artery or a central vein for diagnostic or therapeutic procedures.

central chemoreceptor, any of the sensory nerve cells or chemical receptors that are located in the medulla of the brain.

central chondrosarcoma [Gk, kentron + chondros, cartilage, sarx, flesh, oma, tumor], a malignant cartilaginous tumor that forms inside a bone.

central electrode, a key part of a radiation detection instrument. It consists of a positively charged rigid wire in the center of a gas-filled cylinder.

central facilitation, (in chiropractic) a model based on neurophysiologic findings that explains the symptoms of subluxogenic pain and discomfort that arise from nonspinal sites.

central incisor, one of the incisors located in the midsagittal plane in the maxillary and mandibular jaws.

central line, an intravenous tubing inserted for continuous access to a central vein for administering fluids and medicines and for obtaining diagnostic information. Keeping the central line in place ensures accessibility to the venous system in case the peripheral veins collapse.

central lobe, one of the lobes constituting each of the cerebral hemispheres, lying hidden in the depths of the lateral sulcus. The central lobe can be seen only if the lips of the sulcus are parted or cut away.

central necrosis [Gk, kentron, central, nekros, dead, osis, condition], death of the central part of a tissue or organ.

central nervous system (CNS) [Gk, kentron + L, nervus, nerve; Gk, systema], one of the two main divisions of the nervous system, consisting of the brain and spinal cord. The central nervous system processes information to and from the peripheral nervous system and is the main network of coordination and control for the entire body. The spinal cord extends various types of nerve fibers from the brain and acts as a switching and relay terminal for the peripheral nervous system. The 12 pairs of cranial nerves emerge directly from the brain. Sensory nerves and motor nerves of the peripheral system leave the spinal cord separately between the vertebrae but unite to form 31 pairs of spinal nerves containing sensory fibers and motor fibers. More than 10 billion neurons constitute but one tenth of the brain cells; the other cells consist of neuroglia. The neurons and the neuroglia form the soft, jellylike substance of the brain, which is supported and protected by the skull. The brain and spinal cord are composed of gray and white matter. The gray matter primarily contains nerve cells and associated processes; the white matter consists predominantly of bundles of myelinated nerve fibers.

central nervous system depressant, any drug that decreases the function of the central nervous system such as alcohol, tranquilizers, barbiturates, and hypnotics. These substances depress excitable tissue throughout the central nervous system by stabilizing neuronal membranes, decreasing the amount of transmitter released by the nerve impulse, and generally depressing postsynaptic responsiveness and ion movement. Central nervous system depressants elevate the seizure threshold and can produce physical dependence in a relatively short period. Sudden withdrawal of general central nervous system depressants that have been used in high doses for prolonged periods is fatal to some individuals.

central nervous system stimulant, a substance that quickens the activity of the central nervous system by increasing the rate of neuronal discharge or by blocking an inhibitory neurotransmitter. Many natural and synthetic compounds stimulate the central nervous system, but only a few are used therapeutically.

central nervous system syndrome (CNS syndrome), a constellation of neurologic and emotional signs and symptoms that results from a massive whole-body dose of radiation.

central nervous system tumor, a neoplasm of the brain or spinal cord that characteristically does not spread beyond the cerebrospinal axis, although it may be highly invasive locally and have widespread effects on body functions. Intracranial neoplasms are about four times more common than those arising in the spinal cord. Many brain tumors are metastatic lesions from primary cancer elsewhere, such as in the breast, lung, gastrointestinal tract, kidney, or a site of melanoma.

central neurogenic hyperventilation

(CNHV) [Gk, *kentron* + *neuron,* nerve, *genein,* to produce], a pattern of breathing marked by rapid and regular ventilations at a rate of about 25 per minute. Increasing regularity, rather than rate, is an important diagnostic sign because it indicates an increasing depth of coma.

central neuronal plasticity, (in chiropractic) the tendency for the neuronal responses to noxious stimuli to spread to other central pathways, producing the symptoms of referred pain.

central pain [Gk, *kentron* + L, *poena,* penalty], pain caused by a lesion in the central nervous system.

central paralysis [Gk, *kentron* + *paralyein,* to be palsied], paralysis caused by a lesion in the central nervous system.

central pathway, a nerve tract in the brain or spinal cord.

central placenta previa [Gk, *kentron* + L, *placenta,* flat cake, *praevius,* preceding], placenta previa in which the placenta is implanted in the lower segment of the uterus and completely covers the internal os of the uterine cervix. In labor, as the cervix dilates, the placenta is gradually separated from the underlying blood vessels in the uterine lining, causing bleeding that usually begins slowly and progresses to hemorrhage that is life-threatening to the mother and baby.

central ray (CR), the part of the x-ray beam that is directed toward the center of the film or of the object being radiographed.

central scotoma [Gk, *kentron* + *skotos,* darkness, *oma,* tumor], an area of blindness or site of depressed vision involving the macula of the retina.

central sensitization, (in chiropractic) a state in which neurons activated by noxious mechanical and chemical stimuli are sensitized by such stimuli and become hyperresponsive to all subsequent stimuli delivered to the neurons' receptive fields.

central sleep apnea, a form of sleep apnea resulting from decreased respiratory center output. It may involve primary brainstem medullary depression.

central sulcus [Gk, *kentron* + L, furrow], a cleft separating the frontal from the parietal lobes of brain.

central tendon, a broad connective tissue sheet that forms the diaphragm. It is composed of interlacing fibers that arise from the lumbar vertebrae, the costal margin, and the xiphoid process of the sternum.

central venous blood pressure, the pressure of blood in the superior vena cava, measured by inserting a catheter attached to a manometer directly outside the right atrium.

central venous catheter, a catheter that is threaded through the internal jugular, antecubital, or subclavian vein, usually with the tip resting in the superior vena cava or the right atrium of the heart.

central venous oxygen saturation (CVSO$_2$), the oxygen saturation in the vena cava. The CVSO$_2$ is measured through a central venous catheter and is useful in measuring cardiac output.

central venous pressure (CVP), the blood pressure in the large veins of the body, as distinguished from peripheral venous pressure in an extremity. It is measured with a water manometer that may be attached to the head of a patient's bed and to a central venous catheter inserted into the vena cava.

central venous pressure (CVP) monitor, a device for measuring and recording the venous blood pressure by means of an indwelling venous catheter and a pressure manometer.

central venous return, the blood from the venous system that flows into the right atrium through the vena cava.

central vertigo [Gk, kentron + L, vertigo, dizziness], vertigo that is caused by a central nervous system disorder.

central vision, vision that results from images falling on the macula of the retina.

centrencephalic /sen'trensifal'ik/ [Gk, kentron + enkephalos, brain], pertaining to the center of the encephalon.

centriciput /sentris'ipŏŏt/, the central part of the head, between the occiput and the sinciput.

centrifugal, 1. denoting a force that is directed outward, away from a central point or axis, such as the force that keeps the moon in its orbit around the earth. **2.** a direction away from the head.

centrifugal analyzer, equipment that uses centrifugal force to mix a sample aliquot, or part, with a reagent and a spinning rotor to pass the reaction mixture through a detector.

centrifugal current, an electrical current in the body with the positive pole near the nerve center and the negative pole at the periphery.

centrifugal force [Gk, kentron + L, fugere, to flee, fortis, strong], a natural force that affects objects undergoing circular motion. The force is the product of the mass and its radial acceleration. In centrifugation, heavier components of a mixture are separated from other components by being thrown to the periphery of the orbit.

centrifuge /sen'trifyoŏj'/ [Gk, kentron + L, fugere, to flee], a device for separating components of different densities contained in liquid by spinning them at high speeds. Centrifugal force causes the heavier components to move to one part of the container, leaving the lighter substances in another. —**centrifugal,** adj., **centrifuge,** v.

centrilobular /sen'trəlob'yələr/ [Gk, kentron + L, lobulus, small lobe], pertaining to the center of a lobule.

centriole /sen'trē-ōl'/ [Gk, kentron], an intracellular organelle, usually as a component of the centrosome. Often occurring in pairs, centrioles are associated with cell division. They appear to aid in the formation of the spindle that develops during mitosis.

centripetal /sentrip'ətəl/ [Gk, kentron + L, petere, to seek], **1.** denoting an afferent direction, such as that of a sensory nerve impulse traveling toward the brain. **2.** denoting the direction of a force pulling an object toward an axis of rotation or constraining an object to a specific curved path.

centripetal current, an electrical current passing through the body from a peripheral positive electrode to a negative pole near the nerve center.

centripetal force, (in radiology) a "center-seeking" electrical force that holds electrons in their orbits around the nucleus of an atom.

centromere /sen'trəmir/ [Gk, kentron + meros, part], the specialized constricted region of the chromosome that joins the two chromatids to each other and attaches to the spindle fiber in mitosis and meiosis. During cell division the centromeres split longitudinally, half going to each of the new daughter chromosomes. —**centromeric,** adj.

centrosome [Gk, kentron + soma, body], a self-propagating cytoplasmic organelle that consists of the centrosphere and the centrioles. It is located near the nucleus and functions as the dynamic center of the cell, especially during mitosis.

centrosphere [Gk, kentron + sphaira, ball], the differentiated, condensed area of cytoplasm surrounding the centrioles in the centrosome of the cell.

centrostaltic /sen'trōstô'tik/, pertaining to the center of movement.

centrum, pl. **centra** [Gk, kentron], any kind of center, especially one related to a body structure, as the centrum semiovale of a cerebral hemisphere.

CEO, C.E.O., abbreviation for **chief executive officer.**

cephalad /sef'əlad/ [Gk, kephale, head], toward the head, away from the end or tail.

cephalalgia /sef'əlal'jə/ [Gk, kephale,

head, *algos*, pain], headache, often combined with another word to indicate a specific type of headache, such as histamine cephalalgia.

cephalea agitata /sef'əlē'ə/, a violent headache that is frequently an early symptom of an infection.

cephaledema /sef'əlidē'mə/, a swelling of the brain caused by fluid accumulation.

cephalexin /sef'əlek'sin/, a cephalosporin antibacterial prescribed orally in the treatment of certain infections.

cephalhematoma /sef'əlhē'mətō'mə,-hem'ətō'mə/, swelling caused by subcutaneous bleeding and accumulation of blood.

cephalic /sifal'ik/, pertaining to the head.

cephalic index [Gk, *kephale*, head, *index*, pointer], a ratio between the breadth and length of the head. It is calculated as 100 times the maximum breadth of the head, measured at the greatest diameter of the cranial vault above the supramastoid crest, divided by the maximum length measured from the most prominent point on the glabella to the opisthocranion.

cephalic presentation, a classification of fetal position in which the head of the fetus is at the uterine cervix. Cephalic presentation is usually further qualified by an indication of the part of the head presenting, such as the occiput, brow, or chin.

cephalic vein, one of the four superficial veins of the upper limb. It receives deoxygenated blood from the dorsal and palmar surfaces of the forearm.

cephalocaudal /sef'əlōkô'dəl/ [Gk, *kephale* + L, *cauda*, tail], pertaining to the long axis of the body, or the relationship between the head and the base of the spine.

cephalocele /sef'əlōsēl'/, the protrusion of a part of the brain through an opening in the skull. The opening may be congenital or may result from an injury.

cephalocentesis /-sentē'sis/, the puncture of the skull with a hollow needle, performed to allow drainage of fluid or an abscess.

cephalomelus /sef'əlom'ələs/ [Gk, *kephale* + *melos*, limb], a deformed individual who has a structure resembling an arm or a leg protruding from the head.

cephalometry /-ɔtrē/, scientific measurement of the head, such as that performed in dentistry to determine appropriate orthodontic procedures for correcting malocclusions and other abnormal conditions. —**cephalometric,** *adj.*

cephalopelvic /-pel'vik/, pertaining to a relationship between the fetal head and the maternal pelvis.

cephalopelvic disproportion (CPD) [Gk,

kephale + L, *pelvis*, basin, *dis*, opposite of, *proportio*, similarity], an obstetric condition in which a baby's head is too large or a mother's birth canal too small to permit normal labor or birth. In relative CPD, the size of the baby's head is within normal limits but larger than average or the size of the mother's birth canal is within normal limits but smaller than average, or both. In absolute CPD, the baby's head is markedly or abnormally enlarged or the mother's birth canal is markedly or abnormally contracted, making vaginal delivery impossible.

cephalopelvimetry /-pelvim'ətrē/, radiographic measurement of the fetal head in utero.

cephalophlebitis, an inflammation of the vena cava.

cephaloridine /sef'əlôr'idēn/, a cephalosporin antibiotic prescribed in the treatment of infections.

cephalosporin /sef'əlōspôr'in/ [Gk, *kephale* + *sporos*, seed], a semisynthetic derivative of an antibiotic originally derived from the microorganism *Cephalosporium falciforme (Acremonium kiliense)*. Cephalosporins are similar in structure to penicillins.

cephalothin sodium /sef'əlō'thin/, a cephalosporin antibacterial prescribed in the treatment of infections.

cephapirin /sef'əprin/, a cephalosporin-type antibiotic prescribed in the treatment of infections caused by cephapirin-susceptible strains of a wide variety of microorganisms that cause septicemia, endocarditis, osteomyelitis, and infections of the respiratory tract, urinary tract, and skin.

cephradine /sef'rədēn/, a cephalosporin antibacterial prescribed in the treatment of certain bacterial infections.

cera, wax. Ordinary yellow beeswax is sometimes identified as cera flava; white beeswax, bleached by exposure to air and sunlight, is known as cera alba.

ceramics /səram'iks/, (in dentistry) the process of making dental restorations from fused porcelain and other glasses.

cercaria /sərker'ē·ə/, *pl.* **cercariae** [Gk, *kerkos*, tail], a minute, wormlike early developmental form of trematode. It develops in a freshwater snail and is released into the water. Cercariae enter the body of the next host by ingestion, by direct invasion through the skin, or through a cut or other break in the skin. They encyst and complete their development in various organs of the body. Each species tends to migrate to one organ, such as *Fasciola hepatica*, which grows to become a liver fluke.

cerclage /serkläzh'/ [Fr, cask hooping],

1. an orthopedic procedure in which the ends of an oblique bone fracture or the chips of a broken patella are bound together with a wire loop or a metal band to hold them in position until healed. **2.** a procedure in which a taut silicone band is applied around the sclera to restore contact between the retina and the choroid when the retina is detached. **3.** an obstetric procedure in which a nonabsorbable suture is used for holding the cervix closed to prevent spontaneous abortion in a woman who has an incompetent cervix.

cerea flexibilitas /sirē′ə flek′sibil′itas/ [L, waxlike flexibility], a cataleptic state, frequently observed in catatonic schizophrenia, in which the limbs maintain the positions in which they are placed for an indefinite period.

cerebellar /ser′əbel′ər/ [L, cerebellum, small brain], pertaining to the cerebellum.

cerebellar angioblastoma [L, cerebellum + Gk, angeion, vessel, blastos, germ, oma], a cystic tumor in the cerebellum composed of a mass of blood vessels. It is frequently associated with von Hippel-Lindau disease.

cerebellar artery occlusion, an obstruction of one of the arteries supplying the cerebellum. It can result in ipsilateral ataxia, facial analgesia, contralateral hemiparesis, and loss of temperature and pain sensations.

cerebellar ataxia [L, cerebellum, small brain; Gk, ataxia, without order], a loss of muscle coordination caused by a lesion in the cerebellum.

cerebellar atrophy [L, cerebellum + Gk, a + trophe, without nourishment], deterioration and wasting of tissues of the cerebellum.

cerebellar cortex, the superficial gray matter of the cerebellum covering the white substance in the medullary core. It consists of two layers, an external molecular layer and an internal granule cell layer.

cerebellar cyst, a cyst that develops in the white matter of the cerebellum and is often associated with an astrocytoma.

cerebellar gait [L, cerebellum, small brain; ONorse, geta, a way], a staggering gait in which the person walks with a wide base and has difficulty turning. The feet are thrown outward, and the person puts his or her weight first on the heel and then on the toes. The condition is caused by a lesion in the cerebellum or cerebellar pathways.

cerebellar inferior peduncle [L, cerebellum, small brain, inferior, lower, pes, foot], a band of nerve fibers that forms the lateral boundary of the bottom part of the fourth ventricle and carries afferent fibers into the cerebellum.

cerebellar middle peduncle [L, cerebellum, small brain, medius + pes, foot], a lateral extension of the transverse nerve fibers of the pons. It consists mainly of fibers from the pontine nuclei to the neocerebellum.

cerebellar notch, 1. anteriorly, a broad depression that lies dorsal to the midbrain and separates the cerebellar hemispheres rostral to the vermis. **2.** posteriorly, a deep depression adjacent to the falx cerebelli.

cerebellar rigidity, a stiffness of the trunk muscles caused by a midline lesion in the cerebellum. In some cases, the limbs may also be rigid and the neck and back arched, as in opisthotonos.

cerebellar speech [L, cerebellum + AS, spaec], abnormal speech characteristic of diseases of the cerebellum. It is characterized by slow, jerky, and slurred articulation that may be intermittent and explosive or monotonous and unvaried in pitch.

cerebellar superior peduncle [L, cerebellum, small brain, superior + pes, foot], a band of nerve fibers that passes from the cerebellum on either side of the superior medullary velum. It includes nerve tracts linking the dentate nucleus to the red nucleus of the midbrain and to the thalamus.

cerebellar tremor [L, cerebellum, small brain, tremor, shaking], an intention tremor or trembling during voluntary movements, caused by lesions in the cerebellum.

cerebellopontine /ser′əbel′ōpon′tīn/ [L, cerebellum + pons, bridge], leading from the cerebellum to the pons varolii.

cerebellospinal /ser′əbel′ōspī′nəl/ [L, cerebellum + spina, backbone], leading from the cerebellum to the spinal cord.

cerebellum /ser′əbel′əm/, pl. **cerebellums, cerebella** [L, small brain], the part of the brain located in the posterior cranial fossa behind the brainstem. It consists of two lateral cerebellar hemispheres, or lobes, and a middle section called the vermis. Three pairs of peduncles link it with the brainstem. Its functions are concerned primarily with coordinating voluntary muscular activity.

cerebral /ser′əbrəl, sərē′brəl/, pertaining to the cerebrum.

cerebral aneurysm [L, cerebrum, brain; Gk, aneurysma, a widening], an abnormal localized dilation of a cerebral artery. It is most commonly the result of congenital weakness of the media or muscle layer of the vessel wall. Cerebral aneurysms may also be caused by infection such as subacute bacterial endocarditis or syphilis and by neoplasms, arteriosclerosis, and trauma. Cerebral aneurysms may occur in infancy or old age. They may be fusiform dilations of the entire circumference of an artery or saccular outcroppings of the side of a vessel, which may be as small as a pinhead or as large as an orange but are usually the size of a pea.

cerebral angiography [L, *cerebrum*, brain; Gk, *angeion*, vessel, *graphein*, to record], a radiographic procedure used to visualize the vascular system of the brain after injection of a radiopaque contrast medium.

cerebral anoxia, a condition in which oxygen is deficient in brain tissue. This state can exist for no more than 4 to 6 minutes before the onset of irreversible brain damage.

cerebral aqueduct [L, *cerebrum* + *aqueductus*, water canal], the narrow conduit, between the third and the fourth ventricles in the midbrain, that conveys the cerebrospinal fluid.

cerebral compression [L, *cerebrum*, brain, *comprimere*, to press together], any abnormal condition, such as hemorrhage, abscess, or tumor, that increases intracranial pressure. If untreated, the compression destroys the brain tissues and causes herniation of the brain.

cerebral cortex [L, *cerebrum* + *cortex*, bark], a layer of neurons and synapses (gray matter) on the surface of the cerebral hemispheres, folded into gyri with about two thirds of its area buried in fissures. It integrates higher mental functions, general movement, visceral functions, perception, and behavioral reactions. It has been classified many different ways. Research has described more than 200 areas on the basis of differences in myelinated fiber patterns and has defined 47 separate function areas with different cell designs.

cerebral depressant [L, *cerebrum*, brain, *deprimere*, to press down], a drug or other agent that has a sedating effect on the brain, reducing activity and alertness and, in some instances, causing a loss of consciousness.

cerebral dominance, the specialization of each of the two cerebral hemispheres in the integration and control of different functions. In 90% of the population, the left cerebral hemisphere specializes in or dominates the ability to speak and write and the capacity to understand spoken and written words. In the other 10% of the population, either the right hemisphere or both hemispheres dominate the speech and writing abilities. The right cerebral hemisphere perceives tactual stimuli and visual spatial relationships better than the left cerebral hemisphere.

cerebral edema [L, *cerebrum* + Gk, *oidema*, swelling], an accumulation of fluid in the brain tissues. Causes include infection, tumor, trauma, or exposure to certain toxins. Early symptoms are changes in level of consciousness: sluggishness, then dilation of pupils, and a gradual loss of consciousness. Cerebral edema can be fatal.

Cerebral Edema Management, a Nursing Interventions Classification defined as limitation of secondary cerebral injury resulting from swelling of brain tissue.

cerebral embolism [L, *cerebrum* + *embolos*, plug], an embolus that blocks blood flow through the vessels of the cerebrum, resulting in tissue ischemia distal to the occlusion.

cerebral fossa, the stem of the lateral sulcus of the cerebrum, which separates the orbital surface of the frontal lobe from the temporal lobe.

cerebral gigantism [L, *cerebrum* + Gk, *gigas*, giant], an abnormal condition characterized by excessive weight and size at birth, accelerated growth during the first 4 or 5 years after birth without any increase in the level of growth hormone, and then reversion to normal growth.

cerebral hemiplegia [L, *cerebrum* + Gk, *hemi*, half, *plege*, stroke], paralysis of one side of the body caused by a brain lesion.

cerebral hemisphere [L, *cerebrum* + Gk, *hemi*, half, *sphaira*, ball], one of the halves of the cerebrum. The two cerebral hemispheres are divided by a deep longitudinal fissure and are connected medially at the bottom of the fissure by the corpus callosum. Prominent grooves subdivide each hemisphere into four major lobes. The hemispheres consist of an external gray layer and an internal white substance that surrounds islands of gray matter called nuclei.

cerebral hemorrhage [L, *cerebrum* + Gk, *haima*, blood, *rhegnynei*, to burst forth], a hemorrhage from a blood vessel in the brain. Three criteria used to classify cerebral hemorrhages are location (subarachnoid, extradural, subdural), kind of vessel involved (arterial, venous, capillary), and origin (traumatic, degenerative). Each kind of cerebral hemorrhage has distinctive clinical characteristics. Most cerebral hemorrhages occur in the region of the basal ganglia and are caused by the rupture of a sclerotic artery as a result of hypertension. Other causes of rupture include congenital aneurysm, cerebrovascular thrombosis, and head trauma.

cerebral infarction [L, *cerebrum*, brain, *infarcire*, to stuff], an area of brain tissue that undergoes necrosis secondary to an interruption of the blood supply, with or without hemorrhage. An infarct may be the result of thrombosis, an embolism, or vasospasm.

cerebral localization, 1. the determination of various areas in the cerebral cortex associated with specific functions, such as the 47 Brodmann's areas. **2.** the diagnosis of a cerebral condition, such as a brain lesion, by determining the area of the brain affected, through analysis of the signs manifested by the patient.

cerebral palsy [L, *cerebrum* + Gk, *para,* beyond, *lysis,* loosening], a motor function disorder caused by a permanent, nonprogressive brain defect or lesion present at birth or shortly thereafter. The neurologic deficit may result in spastic hemiplegia, monoplegia, diplegia, or quadriplegia; athetosis or ataxia; seizures; paresthesia; varying degrees of mental retardation; and impaired speech, vision, and hearing. The disorder is usually associated with premature or abnormal birth and intrapartum asphyxia, causing damage to the nervous system. Abnormalities in breathing, sucking, swallowing, and responsiveness are usually apparent soon after birth, but the characteristic stiff, awkward movements of the infant's limbs may be overlooked for several months. Beginning to walk is usually delayed, and, when it is attempted, the child manifests a typical scissors gait. Early identification of the disorder facilitates the handling of infants with cerebral palsy and the initiation of an exercise and training program.

cerebral peduncle [L, *cerebrum,* brain, *pes,* foot], a pair of cylindric masses of nerve fibers at the upper border of the pons that disappears into the left and right hemispheres. It includes corticopontine and pyramidal-tract fibers.

cerebral perfusion pressure (CPP), a measure of the amount of blood flow to the brain. It is calculated by subtracting the intracranial pressure from the mean systemic arterial blood pressure.

Cerebral Perfusion Promotion, a Nursing Interventions Classification defined as promotion of adequate perfusion and limitation of complications for a patient experiencing or at risk for inadequate cerebral perfusion.

cerebral thrombosis [L, *cerebrum* + Gk, *thrombos,* lump, *osis,* condition], a clotting of blood in any cerebral vessel.

cerebral vertigo [L, *cerebrum,* brain, *vertigo,* dizziness], vertigo that is caused by organic brain disease.

cerebrocerebellar atrophy /ser′əbrōser′ əbel′ər/ [L, *cerebrum,* brain, *cerebellum,*

small brain; Gk, *a + trophe,* without nourishment], a deterioration of the cerebellum caused by certain abiotrophic diseases.

cerebroid /ser′əbroid/ [L, *cerebrum* + Gk, *eidos,* form], resembling the substance of the brain.

cerebroma /ser′əbrō′mə/, any unusual mass of brain tissue.

cerebromeningitis /-men′inji′tis/, an inflammation of the meninges of the brain, characterized by symptoms of fever, headache, vomiting, slow pulse, and effects of cranial nerve involvement such as facial paralysis, ptosis, and squint.

cerebroside /ser′əbrōsīd′/, any of a group of glycolipids found in the brain and other tissue of the nervous system, especially the myelin sheath.

cerebroside sulfatase [L, *cerebrum,* brain, *sulfur,* brimstone, *ase,* enzyme], an enzyme of the hydrolase class that catalyzes the reaction of cerebroside 3-sulfate + H_2O. A deficiency of the enzyme, which is transmitted through an autosomal-recessive gene, causes metachromatic leukodystrophy.

cerebrospinal /ser′əbrōspī′nəl, sərē′brō-/, pertaining to or involving the brain and spinal cord.

cerebrospinal axis [L, *cerebrum,* brain, *spina,* spine, *axle*], a line formed by the brain and spinal cord about which the body turns.

cerebrospinal fluid (CSF), the fluid that flows through and protects the four ventricles of the brain, the subarachnoid spaces, and the spinal canal. It is composed mainly of secretions of the choroid plexi in the lateral ventricles and in the third and the fourth ventricles of the brain.

cerebrospinal ganglion, a cluster of neurons associated with a cranial or spinal nerve. The neurons lack dendrites and have no synapses on their cell bodies.

cerebrospinal nerves, the 12 pairs of cranial nerves and 31 pairs of spinal nerves that originate in the brain and spinal cord.

cerebrospinal pressure [L, *cerebrum* + *spina* + *premere,* to press], the pressure of cerebrospinal fluid in the central nervous system. It usually measures between 100 and 150 mm of H_2O and is measured by a manometer attached to the end of a needle after it has been inserted into the subarachnoid space via lumbar puncture (most commonly)..

cerebrospinal rhinorrhea/otorrhea [L, *cerebrum,* brain, *spina,* backbone; Gk, *rhis,* nose, *rhoia,* flow], a discharge of cerebrospinal fluid (CSF) from the nose or ear.

cerebrovascular /ser′əbrōvas′kyələr, sərē′-

brō-/ [L, *cerebrum* + *vasculum*, little vessel], pertaining to the vascular system and blood supply of the brain.

cerebrovascular accident (CVA), an abnormal condition of the brain characterized by occlusion by an embolus, thrombus, or cerebrovascular hemorrhage, resulting in ischemia of the brain tissues normally perfused by the damaged vessels.

cerebrum /ser'əbrəm, sərē'brəm/, *pl.* **cerebrums, cerebra** [L, brain], the largest and uppermost section of the brain, divided by a longitudinal fissure into the left and right cerebral hemispheres. At the bottom of the groove, the hemispheres are connected by the corpus callosum. The internal structures of the hemispheres merge with those of the diencephalon and further communicate with the brainstem through the cerebral peduncles. The cerebrum performs sensory functions, motor functions, and less easily defined integration functions associated with various mental activities. —**cerebral**, *adj.*

cerium (Ce) /sir'ē·əm/ [L, *Ceres,* Roman goddess of agriculture], a ductile gray rare earth element. Its atomic number is 58; its atomic weight (mass) is 140.13. A compound of cerium, cerium oxalate, is used as a sedative, an antiemetic, and an antitussive.

cerium nitrate, a topical antiseptic used in the treatment of burns to control bacterial and fungal infections.

ceroid /sir'oid/ [L, *cera,* wax; Gk, *eidos,* form], a golden, waxy pigment appearing in the cirrhotic livers of some individuals, in the gastrointestinal tract, in the nervous system, and in the muscles.

ceroma /sirō'mə/ [L, *cera,* wax; Gk, *oma,* tumor], a neoplasm that has undergone waxy degeneration.

certifiable /sur'tif'əbəl/ [L, *certus,* certain, *facere,* to make], 1. a legal term pertaining to a patient with a mental illness who has been found incompetent and requires care by a guardian or in a hospital. 2. pertaining to infectious diseases or dangerous conditions that must be reported to local health authorities.

certificate-of-need or **certificate-of-necessity,** a statement or certificate issued by a governmental agency to the effect that a proposed construction or modification of a health facility will be needed at the time of its completion.

certification [L, *certus,* certain, *facere,* to make], 1. a process in which an individual, an institution, or an educational program is evaluated and recognized as meeting certain predetermined standards. Certification is usually made by a nongov-

ernmental agency. 2. (in nursing) a process in which the professional organization or association verifies that a person who is licensed has met the standards for specialty practice specified by the profession.

certification for excellence, (in nursing) certification that recognizes professional achievement, advanced education, and superior performance in a specialty or subspecialty field of practice.

certification in nursing, one of two processes in which a professional organization formally recognizes the competence of a nurse to practice a subspecialty of nursing. One process, certification for excellence, bases recognition on professional achievement, advanced education, and superior performance. The second process, entry level certification, bases recognition on advanced education in a program approved by the certifying organization.

certified dental assistant /sur'tifīd/, a person who has successfully completed the education, training, and testing of the Dental Assisting National Examination or of the American Dental Assistants' Association.

certified emergency nurse (CEN), a nurse who has had training in emergency nursing and an examination given by the Board of Certification of Emergency Nursing. To remain certified, a CEN must be reexamined every 4 years (or 8 years if specified educational requirements are met within 4 years).

certified milk, raw milk that is obtained, handled, and marketed in compliance with state health laws. The milk must be produced by disease-free cows that are regularly inspected by a veterinarian and milked by sterilized equipment in hygienic surroundings. It must contain less than a specified low bacterial count and must be delivered within 36 hours.

certified nurse-midwife (CNM), (according to the American College of Nurse-Midwives) "an individual educated in the two disciplines of nursing and midwifery, who possesses evidence of certification according to the requirements of the American College of Nurse-Midwives."

certified occupational therapy assistant (COTA) an allied health paraprofessional who, under the direction of an occupational therapist, directs an individual's participation in selected tasks to restore, reinforce, and enhance performance; facilitates learning of skills and functions essential for adaptation and productivity; diminishes or corrects disorders; and promotes and maintains health.

Certified Respiratory Therapy Techni-

cian (CRTT), health care professional who performs routine care, management, and treatment of patients with respiratory disorders. Certification requires completion of an approved 1-year training course and examination by the National Board for Respiratory Care.

certify /sur′tifī/, **1.** to guarantee formally that certain requirements based on expert knowledge of significant, pertinent facts have been met. **2.** to attest, by a legal process, that someone is insane. **3.** to attest to the fact of someone's death in writing, usually on a form required by a local authority. **4.** to declare that a person has satisfied certain requirements for membership or acceptance into a professional or other group. —**certification,** *n.,* **certifiable,** *adj.*

cerulean /siroo′lē·ən/ [L, *caelum,* sky], sky-blue in color.

ceruloplasmin /siroo′lōplaz′min/ [L, *caelum,* sky; Gk, *plassein,* to shape], a blue glycoprotein in plasma that transports 96% of the plasma copper.

cerumen /siroo′mən/ [L, *cera,* wax], a yellowish or brownish waxy secretion produced by vestigial apocrine sweat glands in the external ear canal.

ceruminolytic /siroo′mənolit′ik/, pertaining to a drug or other agent that dissolves cerumen (earwax).

ceruminolytic agent [L, *cera,* wax; Gk, *lysis,* a loosening; L, *agere,* to do], a medication that dissolves or loosens cerumen (earwax) to allow for its removal.

ceruminoma /serō′minō′mə/, an adenocarcinoma in the external auditory meatus.

ceruminosis /siroo′minō′sis/, excessive buildup of cerumen (earwax) in the external auditory canal. It can cause discomfort, symptoms of hearing loss, and local irritation leading to the development of infection.

ceruminous /seroo′minəs/, pertaining to earwax.

ceruminous gland /siroo′minəs/, one of a number of tiny structures in the external ear canal, believed to be modified sweat glands. They secrete a waxy cerumen instead of watery sweat.

cervical /sur′vikəl/ [L, *cervix,* neck], **1.** pertaining to the neck or the region of the neck. **2.** pertaining to the constricted area of a necklike structure, such as the neck of a tooth or the cervix of the uterus.

cervical abortion [L, *cervix* + *ab,* away from, *oriri,* to be born], spontaneous expulsion of a cervical pregnancy.

cervical adenitis [L, *cervix* + Gk, *aden,* gland, *itis,* inflammation], an abnormal condition characterized by enlarged, tender lymph nodes of the neck.

cervical amputation, the removal of the neck of the uterus.

cervical canal, the canal within the uterine cervix, which protrudes into the vagina. The uterine end of the canal is closed at the internal os and, in the nullipara, at the distal end by the external os. The canal is a passageway through which the menstrual flow escapes and, vastly dilated and effaced by labor, through which the infant must pass to be delivered vaginally. Sperm must travel upward through the canal to reach the uterus and fallopian tubes.

cervical cancer, a neoplasm of the uterine cervix that can be detected in the early, curable stage by the Papanicolaou (Pap) test. Factors that may be associated with the development of cervical cancer are coitus at an early age, relations with many sexual partners, genital herpesvirus infections, multiparity, and poor obstetric and gynecologic care. Early cervical neoplasia is usually asymptomatic, but there may be a watery vaginal discharge or occasional spotting of blood; advanced lesions may cause a dark, foul-smelling vaginal discharge, leakage from bladder or rectal fistulas, anorexia, weight loss, and back and leg pains. About 90% of cervical tumors are squamous cell carcinomas, fewer than 10% are adenocarcinomas, and others are mixtures of these kinds, or, in rare cases, sarcomas. Cervical cancer invades the tissues of adjacent organs and may metastasize through lymphatic channels to distant sites, including the lungs, bone, liver, brain, and paraaortic nodes.

cervical cap, a contraceptive device consisting of a small rubber cup fitted over the uterine cervix to prevent spermatozoa from entering the cervical canal.

cervical cauterization, the destruction, usually by heat or electrical current, of abnormal superficial tissues of the cervix.

cervical conization, the excision of a cone-shaped tissue section from the endocervix.

cervical cyst [L, *cervix,* neck; Gk, *kystis,* bag], a mucous cyst of the uterine cervix.

cervical dilation /dil′ətā′shən/ [L, *dilatare,* to widen], the diameter of the opening of the cervix in labor as measured on vaginal examination. It is expressed in centimeters or finger breadths; one finger breadth is approximately 2 cm. At full dilation the diameter of the cervical opening is 10 cm.

cervical disk syndrome, an abnormal condition characterized by compression or irritation of the cervical nerve roots in or near the intervertebral foramina before the roots divide into the anterior and posterior rami. When it is caused by ruptured intervertebral disks, degenerative cervical disk disease, or cervical injuries, it may produce varying degrees of malalignment, causing nerve root compression. Most cervical disk syndromes are caused by injuries that involve hyperextension. Pain, the most common symptom, usually emanates from the cervical area but may radiate down the arm to the fingers and increase with cervical motion. Other signs and symptoms may be paresthesia, headache, blurred vision, decreased skeletal function, and weakened hand grip. Physical examination may reveal varying degrees of muscular atrophy, sensory abnormalities, muscular weakness, and decreased reflexes.

cervical dysplasia, abnormal tissue development of the uterine cervix, with atypical epithelium that may slowly progress to carcinoma.

cervical endometritis, an inflammation of the inner lining of the cervix uteri.

cervical erosion [L, *cervix* + *erodere, to consume*], a condition in which the squamous epithelium of the cervix is abraded as a result of irritation caused by infection or trauma such as childbirth and replaced by columnar epithelium.

cervical fistula, an abnormal passage from the cervix to the vagina or bladder. It may be caused by a malignant lesion, radiotherapy, surgical trauma, or injury during childbirth. A cervical fistula communicating with the bladder permits leakage of urine, causing irritation, odor, and embarrassment.

cervical intraepithelial neoplasia (CIN) /in′trə·ep′ithē′lē·əl/, abnormal changes in the basal layers of the squamous epithelial tissues of the uterus. The disorder is graded according to its pathologic progress, from CIN1 to CIN3; CIN3 represents carcinoma of the cervix. The disorder is associated with human papillomaviruses.

cervical mucus, a secretion of the columnar epithelium lining the upper part of the cervical canal of the uterus.

cervical nerves [L, *cervix*, neck, *nervus*, nerve], the eight pairs of spinal nerves that arise from the cervical segments of the spinal cord, from above the atlas to below the seventh vertebra. The first four supply the head and neck; the other four mainly innervate the upper limbs, scalp, and back.

cervical plexus, the network of nerves formed by the ventral primary divisions of the first four cervical nerves. The plexus is located opposite the cranial aspect of the first four cervical vertebrae. It communicates with certain cranial nerves and numerous muscular and cutaneous branches.

cervical plexus block, nerve block at any point below the mastoid process from the second cervical vertebra to the sixth cervical vertebra. This method is used for operations on the area between the jaw and clavicle.

cervical polyp [L, *cervix* + Gk, *polys,* mean, *pous,* foot], an outgrowth of columnar epithelial tissue of the endocervical canal. It is usually attached to the canal wall by a slender pedicle. Often there are no symptoms, but multiple or abraded polyps may cause bleeding, especially with contact during coitus. Polyps are most common in women above 40 years of age. The cause is not known.

cervical rib, a supernumerary rib that articulates with a cervical vertebra, usually the seventh, but does not reach the sternum.

cervical smear [L, *cervix* + AS, *smero,* grease], a small amount of the secretions and superficial cells of the cervix, secured with a sterile applicator or special small wooden or plastic spatula. For a Papanicolaou's (Pap) smear, it is obtained from the squamocolumnar junction of the uterine cervix and from the vaginal vault and endocervical canal. The specimen is spread on a labeled glass slide and sent for cytologic examination.

cervical spinal fusion surgery, an operation to relieve severe neck pain caused by abnormal movement or adjustment of adjacent vertebrae, a pinched nerve, or spinal compression. The adjacent vertebrae are joined with a metal device or a bone graft made from human bone or a ceramic material.

cervical spondylosis [L, *cervix* + Gk, *spondylos,* vertebra, *osis,* condition], a form of degenerative joint and disk disease affecting the cervical vertebrae and resulting in compression of the associated nerve roots. Symptoms include pain or loss of feeling in the affected arm and shoulder and stiffness of the cervical spine.

cervical stenosis [L, *cervix* + Gk, *stenos,* narrow, *osis,* condition], a narrowing of the canal between the body of the uterus and the cervical os.

cervical traction, a system of traction applied to the cervical spine by applying a force to lift the head.

cervical triangle, one of two triangular areas formed in the neck by the oblique course of the sternocleidomastoideus. The anterior triangle is bounded by the midline of the throat anteriorly, the sternocleidomastoideus laterally, and the body of the mandible superiorly. The posterior triangle is bounded by the clavicle inferiorly and by the borders of the sternocleidomastoideus and the trapezius superiorly.

cervical vertebra, one of the first seven segments of the vertebral column. They differ from the thoracic and lumbar vertebrae through the presence of a vertical foramen in each transverse process. The first cervical vertebra (atlas) has no body; supports the head; and contains a smooth, oval facet for articulation with the dens of the second cervical vertebra. The seventh cervical vertebra has a very long, prominent spinous process that is nearly horizontal and is often used as a palpable reference for locating the other cervical spines.

cervicitis /sur'visī'tis/, acute or chronic inflammation of the uterine cervix. Acute cervicitis is infection of the cervix marked by redness, edema, and bleeding on contact. Symptoms do not always occur but may include any or all of the following: copious, foul-smelling discharge from the vagina; pelvic pressure or pain; scant bleeding with intercourse; and itching or burning of the external genitalia. Chronic cervicitis is a persistent inflammation of the cervix that usually occurs among women in their reproductive years. Symptoms include a thick, irritating, malodorous discharge that may in severe cases be accompanied by significant pelvic pain. The cervix looks congested and enlarged, nabothian cysts are often present, and there are signs of eversion of the cervix and often old lacerations from childbirth.

cervicodynia /sur'vikōdin'ē·ə/, pain in the neck.

cervicogenic dorsalgia, (in chiropractic) pain expressed in the dorsal region and caused by a cervical spine disorder.

cervicogenic headache, (in chiropractic) a condition in which headaches, particularly those classified as muscle tension headaches involving referred pain, are the result of cervical subluxations.

cervicogenicity dysfunction /-jenis'itē/, (in chiropractic) a syndrome of hypomobility, tender points in soft tissues, reduced regional ranges of cervical motion, and static misalignment.

cervicogenic sympathetic syndrome, (in chiropractic) any of a large group of bodily disorders involving the cervical spine and the associated sympathetic trunk of nerve fibers. The effects usually include causalgia and reflex sympathetic dystrophy.

cervicolabial /sur'vikōlā'bē·əl/ [L, *cervix*

+ *labium,* lip], pertaining to or situated on the cheek side of the neck of an incisor or a canine tooth.

cervicoplasty /sur'vikōplas'tē/, plastic surgery performed on either the uterine cervix or the neck.

cervicothoracic /-thôras'ik/, pertaining to the neck and thorax.

cervicotomy /sur'vikot'əmē, a surgical incision into the uterine cervix.

cervicouterine /sur'vikōyōō'tərin/, pertaining to or situated at the cervix of the uterus.

cervicovaginitis /-vaj'inītis/, an inflammation of the cervix and vagina.

cervicovesical /sur'vikōves'ikəl/ [L, *cervix* + *vesica,* bladder], pertaining to the cervix of the uterus and the bladder.

cervix /sur'viks/ [L, neck], the part of the uterus that protrudes into the cavity of the vagina. The cervix is divided into the supravaginal part and the vaginal part. The supravaginal part is separated ventrally from the bladder by the parametrium. The vaginal part of the cervix projects into the cavity of the vagina and contains the cervical canal.

ceryl alcohol /sē'ril/ [L, *cera,* wax; Ar, *alkohl,* essence], a fatty alcohol present in many waxes.

cesarean hysterectomy /sizer'ē·ən/ [L, *Caesar lex,* Caesar's law; Gk, *hystera,* womb, *ektome,* excision], a surgical operation in which the uterus is removed at the time of cesarean section. It is performed most often for complications of cesarean section, usually intractable hemorrhage.

cesarean postmortem section [Caesar's law; L, *post,* after, *mors,* death, *sectio*], the surgical removal of the fetus immediately after the mother's death.

cesarean section [L, *Caesar lex,* Caesar's law, *sectio*], a surgical procedure in which the abdomen and uterus are incised and a baby is delivered transabdominally. It is performed when abnormal maternal or fetal conditions that are judged likely to make vaginal delivery hazardous are present. Maternal indications for the operation include placenta previa or abruptio placentae, and dysfunctional labor. Prior delivery by cesarean section is no longer considered an absolute indication for repeating it in future deliveries. Fetal indications for the operation include fetal distress, cephalopelvic disproportion, and abnormal presentation such as breech and transverse lie. The incision in the skin of the abdomen may be horizontal or vertical, regardless of the kind of internal incision into the uterus.

Cesarean Section Care, a Nursing Interventions Classification defined as preparation and support of a patient who is delivering a baby by cesarean section.

cesium (Cs) /sē'zē·əm/ [L, *caesius,* sky blue], an alkali metal element. Its atomic number is 55; its atomic weight (mass) is 132.9.

cesium 137, a radioactive material with a half-life of 30.2 years that is used in radiotherapy as a sealed source of gamma rays intended for application to various malignancies that are treated by brachytherapy.

cesspool fever, *informal.* typhoid fever.

cestoid /ses'toid/ [Gk, *kestos,* girdle, *eidos,* form], **1.** cestodelike, or resembling a tapeworm. **2.** a tapeworm of the Cestoda subclass.

CET, abbreviation for *Certified Enterostomal Therapist.*

cetyl alcohol /sē'til/ [L, *cetus,* whale; Ar, *alkohl,* essence], a fatty alcohol, derived from spermaceti, used as an emulsifier and stiffening agent in creams and ointments.

cetylpyridinium chloride /sē'təlpī'ridin' ē·əm/, an antiinfective used as a preservative in pharmaceutical preparations and as a topical cleanser. It is prescribed prophylactically to prevent infection of the skin or mucous membranes.

CEU, abbreviation for **continuing education unit.**

Cf, symbol for the element **californium.**

CF test, abbreviation for **complement-fixation test.**

CGC, abbreviation for *Certified Gastrointestinal Clinician.*

cGMP, abbreviation for **cyclic guanosine monophosphate.**

cgs, CGS, abbreviation for **centimeter-gram-second system.**

C_2H_2, chemical formula for acetylene.

C_2H_4, chemical formula for ethylene.

C_6H_6, chemical formula for benzene.

Ch1, symbol for **Christchurch chromosome.**

Chaddock reflex [Charles G. Chaddock, American neurologist, 1861–1936], an abnormal reflex, induced by firmly stroking the ulnar surface of the forearm, characterized by flexion of the wrist and extension of the fingers in fanlike position.

Chaddock's sign [Charles G. Chaddock], a variation of Babinski's reflex, elicited by firmly stroking the side of the foot just distal to the lateral malleolus, characterized by extension of the great toe and fanning of the other toes.

Chadwick's sign /chad'wiks/ [James R. Chadwick, American gynecologist, 1844–1905], the bluish coloration of the vulva and vagina that develops after the sixth week of pregnancy as a normal result of local venous congestion.

chafe [L, *calefacere,* to make warm], an irritation of the skin by friction, such as when rough material rubs against an unprotected area of the body.

chafing, superficial irritation of the skin by friction.

Chagas' disease /chag'əs/ [Carlos Chagas, Brazilian physician, 1879–1934], a parasitic disease caused by *Trypanosoma cruzi,* transmitted to humans by the bite of bloodsucking insects. The acute form is marked by a lesion at the site of the bite, fever, weakness, enlarged spleen and lymph nodes, edema of the face and legs, and tachycardia. The chronic form may be manifested by cardiomyopathy or by dilation of the esophagus or colon.

Chagres fever /chag'ris/ [Chagres River, Panama; L, *febris*], a phlebotomus arbovirus infection transmitted to humans through the bite of a sandfly. The disease is rarely fatal and is characterized by fever, headache, and muscle pains of the chest or abdomen.

chain [L, *catena*], **1.** a length of several units linked together in a linear pattern, such as a polypeptide chain of amino acids or a chain of atoms forming a chemical molecule. **2.** a group of individual bacteria linked together, such as streptococci formed by a chain of cocci. **3.** the serial relationship of certain structures essential to function, such as the chain of ossicles in the middle ear.

chaining, a system of learning behaviors in which each response is a stimulus for the next response.

chain ligature [L, *catena* + *ligare,* to bind], an interlocking ligature that ties off a pedicle at several places by passing a long thread through the pedicle at different points.

chain reaction, 1. (in chemistry) a reaction that produces a compound needed for the reaction to continue. **2.** (in physics) a reaction that perpetuates itself by the proliferating fission of nuclei and the release of atomic particles that cause more nuclear fissions.

chain reflex, a series of reflexes, each stimulated by the preceding one.

chain-stitch suture, a continuous surgical stitch in which each loop of the suture is secured by the next loop.

chalasia /kəlā'zhə/ [Gk, *chalasis,* relaxation], abnormal relaxation or incompetence of the cardiac sphincter of the stomach, resulting in reflux of the gastric contents into the esophagus with subsequent regurgitation.

chalazion /kələ′zion/ [Gk, hailstone], a small, localized swelling of the eyelid resulting from obstruction and retained secretions of the meibomian glands.

chalicosis /kal′ikō′sis/, a type of fibrosis that results from the inhalation of calcium dusts. Respiratory impairment is generally caused by the presence of free silica in the calcium dust.

chalkitis /kalkī′tis/ [Gk, *chalkos*, brass, *itis*, inflammation], an abnormal condition characterized by inflammation of the eyes, caused by rubbing the eyes with the hands after touching or handling brass.

challenge, a method of testing the sensitivity of an individual to a hormone, allergen, or other substance by administering a sample. A small amount may be injected to determine whether the immune system will react by producing appropriate antibodies.

chalone /kā′lōn/ [Gk, *chalan*, to relax], any one of numerous polypeptide inhibitors that are elaborated by a tissue and function like hormones on specific target organs.

chamaeprosopy /kam′əpros′əpē/ [Gk, *chamai*, low, *prosopon*, face], a facial appearance characterized by a low brow and a broad face. —**chamaeprosopic,** *adj.*

chamber [Gk, *kamara*, vaulted enclosure], **1.** a hollow but not necessarily empty space or cavity in an organ, as in the anterior and posterior chambers of the eye or the atrial and ventricular chambers of the heart. **2.** a room or closed space used for research or therapeutic purposes, such as a decompression chamber or hyperbaric oxygen chamber.

Chamberlain's line [W.E. Chamberlain, American radiologist, 1891–1947], a line that extends from the posterior of the hard palate to the dorsum of the foramen magnum.

Chamberlen forceps [Peter Chamberlen, English obstetrician, 1560–1631], one of the earliest kinds of obstetric forceps, introduced in the seventeenth century.

CHAMPUS, abbreviation for **Civilian Health and Medical Programs for Uniformed Services.**

chancre /shang′kər/ [Fr, canker], **1.** a skin lesion, usually of primary syphilis, that begins at the infection site as a papule and develops into a red, bloodless, painless ulcer with a scooped-out appearance. The chancre teems with *Treponema pallidum* spirochetes and is highly contagious. **2.** a papular lesion or ulcerated area of the skin that marks the point of infection of a nonsyphilitic disease such as tuberculosis.

chancroid /shang′kroid/ [Fr, *chancre,* canker; Gk, *eidos,* form], a highly contagious sexually transmitted disease caused by infection with the bacillus *Haemophilus ducreyi.* It characteristically begins as a papule, usually on the skin of the external genitalia; it then grows and ulcerates, other papules form, and, if untreated, the bacillus spreads, causing buboes in the groin.

chancrous /shang′krəs/, describing a condition of chancres or lesions resembling chancres.

change agent, 1. a role in which communication skills, education, and other resources are applied to help a client adjust to changes caused by illness or disability. **2.** a role to help members of an organization adapt to organizational change or to create organizational change.

change of life, *informal.* the female climacteric; menopause.

channel [L, *canalis,* pipe], **1.** a passageway or groove that conveys fluid, such as the central channels that connect the arterioles with the venules. **2.** membrane-bound globular proteins that allow diffusion of specific ions and molecules across a cell membrane.

channeling, referral of increased numbers of patients in exchange for discounted prices; does not apply in Canada.

channel ulcer [L, *canalis,* pipe, *ulcus,* sore], a rare type of peptic ulcer found in the pyloric canal between the stomach and the duodenum.

chaos /kā′əs/, total disorganization with no causal relationships operating.

chaotic atrial tachycardia /kā-ot′ik/, an atrial rhythm of more than 100 beats/min caused by multifocal atrial activity with at least three different shapes of P' waves on the electrocardiogram. The condition is often associated with chronic obstructive lung disease.

Chapman lymphatic reflexes, (in chiropractic) a method of using body wall reflexes to influence the motion of fluids. After a surface locus has been contacted by the tip of the examiner's finger, a firm gentle contact is maintained, and a rotary motion is imparted to the finger to express the fluid content of the locus into the surrounding tissues.

chapped /chapt/ [ME, *chappen,* cracked], pertaining to skin that is roughened, cracked, or reddened by exposure to cold or excessive moisture evaporation. Stinging or burning sensations often accompany the disorder. —**chap,** *v.*

character [Gk, *charassein,* to engrave], the integrated composite of traits and behavioral tendencies that enable a person to react in a relatively consistent way to the customs and mores of society.

character analysis, a systematic investigation of the personality of an individual, with special attention to psychologic defenses and motivations, usually undertaken to improve behavior.

character disorder, a chronic, habitual maladaptive and socially unacceptable pattern of behavior and emotional response.

characteristic curve /ker'əktəris'tik/, (in radiology) the pattern of a plot on a graph representing the relationship between the density or degree of blackness of an x-ray film and the exposure.

characteristic radiation, radiation produced when a projectile electron interacts with an inner-shell electron of a target atom, causing total removal of the electron. It is one of the principles of x-ray production.

Charcot-Bouchard aneurysm /shärkō'-bōōshär'/ [Jean M. Charcot, French neurologist, 1825–1893; Charles J. Bouchard, French physician, 1837–1915], a small, round dilation of a small artery of the cerebral cortex or basal ganglia.

Charcot-Leyden crystal /shärkō'lī'dən/ [Jean M. Charcot; Ernst V. von Leyden, German physician, 1832–1910], any one of the crystalline structures shaped like narrow, double pyramids found in the sputum of persons suffering from bronchial asthma. They are also found in the feces of dysentery patients.

Charcot-Marie-Tooth disease /shärkō'-mərē'tōōth'/ [Jean M. Charcot; Pierre Marie, French neurologist, 1853–1940; Howard H. Tooth, English neurologist, 1856–1925], a progressive hereditary disorder characterized by degeneration of the peroneal muscles of the fibula, resulting in clubfoot, foot drop, and ataxia.

Charcot's fever /shärkōz'/ [Jean M. Charcot], a syndrome characterized by a recurrent fever, jaundice, and abdominal pain in the right upper quadrant that occurs with inflammation of the bile ducts.

Charcot's triad [Jean M. Charcot; Gk, *trias*, three], a set of three signs of brainstem involvement in multiple sclerosis: intention tremor, nystagmus, and scanning speech.

charge nurse, the nurse assigned to manage the operations of the patient care area for the shift. Responsibilities may include staffing, admissions and discharge, and coordination of activities in the patient care area in the absence of the head nurse or nurse manager.

charlatan /shär'lətən/ [Fr, imposter], a totally unqualified individual posing as an expert, especially an individual pretending to be a physician. —**charlatanical,** *adj.*

charley horse /chär'lē hôrs'/, a sudden painful condition of the quadriceps or hamstring muscles characterized by soreness and stiffness. It is the result of a strain, tear, or bruise of the muscle.

chart /chärt/ [L, *charta*, paper], **1.** *informal.* a patient record of data in tabular or graphic form. **2.** to note data in a patient record, usually at prescribed intervals.

charta /kär'tə/, *pl.* **chartae** [L, paper], a piece of paper, especially one treated with medicine, as for external application, or with a chemical for a special purpose such as litmus paper.

charting, the act of compiling data on clinical records or charts. The charts are updated regularly to keep physicians and other health care workers advised of changes in the patient's condition. The data usually include fluctuations in temperature, pulse, respiration, and other variable factors.

chauffeur's fracture /shō'fərz/ [Fr, stoker; L, *fractura*, break], any fracture of the radial styloid, produced by a twisting or a snapping type of injury.

Chaussier's areola /shōsyäz'/ [François Chaussier, French anatomist, 1746–1828; L, little space], an areola of indurated tissue surrounding a malignant pustule.

CHB, abbreviation for **complete heart block.**

CHC, abbreviation for *community health center.*

CHD, abbreviation for **coronary heart disease.**

checkup [Fr, *eschec,* acquire; AS, *uf*], a thorough study or examination of the health of an individual.

Chediak-Higashi's syndrome /ched'ē--ak·higä'shē/ [Moises Chediak, twentieth-century Cuban physician; Ototaka Higashi, twentieth-century Japanese physician], a congenital, autosomal-recessive disorder, characterized by partial albinism, photophobia, pale optic fundi, massive leukocytic inclusions, psychomotor abnormalities, recurrent infections, and early death.

cheek [AS, *ceace*], a fleshy prominence, especially the fleshy protuberances on both sides of the face between the eye and the jaw and the ear and the nose and mouth.

cheesy abscess [AS, *cese* + L, *abscedere,* to go away], an abscess that contains a yellowish semisolid, cheeselike material. It is found in tuberculous abscesses.

cheesy necrosis, tissue death in which the

structures have degenerated into a white, cheesy mass.

cheilectomy /kīlek'tɔmē/, surgical removal of irregular surfaces in the lining of a joint.

cheilitis /kīlī'tis/ [Gk, *cheilos,* lip, *itis,* inflammation], an abnormal condition of the lips characterized by inflammation and cracking of the skin.

cheilocarcinoma /kī'lōkär'sinō'mə/, a malignant epithelial tumor of the lip.

cheiloplasty /kī'ləplas'tē/ [Gk, *cheilos,* lip, *plassein,* to mold], surgical correction of a defect of the lip.

cheilorrhaphy /kīlôr'əfē/ [Gk, *cheilos,* lip, *raphe,* suture], a surgical procedure that sutures the lip, such as in the repair of a congenitally cleft lip or a lacerated lip.

cheilosis /kīlō'sis/, a disorder of the lips and mouth characterized by scales and fissures, resulting from a deficiency of riboflavin in the diet.

cheiralgia /kəral'jə/ [Gk, *cheir* + *algos,* pain], a pain in the hand, especially that associated with arthritis. **—cheiralgic,** *adj.*

cheirognostic /kī'ragnos'tik/ [Gk, *cheir,* hand, *gnostikos,* knowing], able to distinguish between the left and right hands and sides of the body.

cheiromegaly /kī'rōmeg'əlē/ [Gk, *cheir* + *megas,* large], an abnormal condition characterized by excessively large hands. **—cheiromegalic,** *adj.*

cheiroplasty /kī'rōplas'tē/, a surgical procedure to restore an injured or congenitally deformed hand to normal use. **—cheiroplastic,** *adj.*

chelate /kē'lāt/ [Gk, *chele,* claw], **1.** to form a bond, thus creating a ringlike complex. **2.** (in medicine) any coordination compound composed of a central metal ion and an organic molecule with multiple bonds arranged in ring formations, used especially in chemotherapeutic treatments for metal poisoning. **3.** pertaining to chelation.

chelating agent /kē'lāting/, a substance that promotes chelation. Chelating agents are used in the treatment of metal poisoning.

chelation /kēlā'shən/, a chemical reaction in which there is a combination with a metal to form a ring-shaped molecular complex in which the metal is firmly bound and isolated.

chemabrasion /kem'əbrā'zhən/ [Gk, *chemeia,* alchemy; L, *ab* + *radere,* to scrape off], a method of treating scars, chromatosis, or other skin disorders by applying chemicals that remove the surface layers of skin cells.

chemical /kem'əkəl/ [Gk, *chemeia,* alchemy], **1.** a substance composed of chemical elements or a substance produced by or used in chemical processes. **2.** pertaining to chemistry.

chemical action, any process in which natural elements and compounds react with each other to produce a chemical change or a different compound; for example, hydrogen and oxygen combine to produce water.

chemical affinity [Gk, *chemeia,* alchemy; L, *affinis,* related], **1.** an attraction that results in the formation of molecules from atoms. **2.** an attraction between chemicals caused by polarity, as used in chromatography.

chemical agent, any chemical power, active principle, or substance that can produce an effect in the body by interacting with various body substances, such as aspirin, which produces an analgesic effect.

chemical antidote [Gk, *chemeia* + *anti,* against, *dotos,* that which is given], any substance that reacts chemically with a poison to form a compound that is harmless.

chemical burn, tissue damage caused by exposure to a strong acid or alkali such as phenol, creosol, mustard gas, or phosphorus. Emergency treatment includes washing the surface with copious amounts of water to remove the chemical and, if the damage is more than slight and superficial, immediate transport to a medical facility.

chemical carcinogen [Gk, *chemeia,* alchemy, *karkinos,* crab, *oma,* tumor, *genein,* to produce], any chemical agent that can induce the development of cancer in living tissue.

chemical cauterization [Gk, *chemeia* + *kauterion,* branding iron], the corroding or burning of living tissue by a caustic chemical substance such as potassium hydroxide.

chemical disaster, the accidental release of a quantity of toxic chemicals into the environment, resulting in death or injury to workers or members of nearby communities. Examples include the mercury waste poisoning at Minamata, Japan, and the release of methyl isocyanate from a chemical plant in Bhopal, India.

chemical equivalent, a drug or chemical containing similar amounts of the same ingredients as another drug or chemical.

chemical fog, a curtain effect on x-ray film that causes the loss of image quality. It appears as a dull gray discoloration and is usually caused by chemical contamination of the developer.

chemical gastritis, inflammation of the stomach caused by the ingestion of a chemical compound.

chemical indicator, 1. a commercially prepared device that monitors all or part of the physical conditions of the sterilization cycle. **2.** a compound added to a reaction system to show, typically by a change in color, when the process is complete, as in an acid-base titration.

chemical mediator, a neurotransmitter chemical such as acetylcholine.

chemical name, the exact designation of the chemical structure of a drug as determined by the rules of accepted systems of chemical nomenclature.

chemical peel, a therapy to eliminate wrinkles, blemishes, pigment spots, and sun-damaged areas of the skin. Using a chemical solution of phenol, trichloroacetic acid, or alpha hydroxy fruit acid, the top skin layers are peeled away, allowing new, smoother skin with tighter cells to occupy the surface. Immediately after the peel, there may be considerable swelling, which subsides after 7 to 10 days as new skin begins to form.

chemical peritonitis [Gk, *chemeia,* alchemy, *peri,* near, *teinein,* to stretch, *itis,* inflammation], an inflammation of the peritoneum resulting from chemicals, including digestive substances, in the peritoneum.

chemical shift, (in nuclear magnetic response spectrometry) the position of a resonance in the substance of interest relative to the position of the resonance of a standard.

chemical sympathectomy, the removal of a sympathetic nerve tract or ganglion by injection of a corrosive chemical such as phenol.

chemical warfare, the waging of war with poisonous chemicals and gases.

cheminosis /kem'ənō'sis/ [Gk, *chemeia* + *osis,* condition], any disease caused by a chemical substance.

chemist, 1. a person with special education and training in the structures, characteristics, and actions of chemicals. **2.** in Great Britain, a pharmacist.

chemistry /kem'istrē/ [Gk, *chemeia,* alchemy], the science dealing with the elements, their compounds, and the molecular structure and interactions of matter.

chemistry, normal values, the amounts of various substances in the normal human body, determined by testing a large sample of people presumed to be healthy. Normal values are expressed in ranges of numbers, and ranges vary for different age groups and from laboratory to laboratory.

chemodifferentiation /-dif'əren'shē·ā'-shən/, a stage in embryonic development that precedes and controls specialization

and differentiation of the cells into rudimentary organs.

chemonucleolysis /-noo'klē·ol'isis-/ [Gk, *chemeia* + L, *nucleus,* nut kernel; Gk, *lysein,* to loosen], a method of dissolving the nucleus pulposus of an intervertebral disk by the injection of a chemolytic agent such as the enzyme chymopapain.

chemoprophylaxis /-prō'filak'sis/ [Gk, *chemeia* + *prophylax,* advance guard], the use of antimicrobial drugs to prevent the acquisition of pathogens in an endemic area or to prevent their spread from one body area to another.

chemoreceptor /-risep'tər/ [Gk, *chemeia* + L, *recipere,* to receive], a sensory nerve cell activated by chemical stimuli. An example is a chemoreceptor in the carotid artery that is sensitive to the PCO_2 in the blood, signaling the respiratory center in the brain to increase or decrease respiration.

chemoreflex /-rē'fleks/, any reflex initiated by the stimulation of chemical receptors, such as the carotid and aortic bodies, which respond to changes in carbon dioxide, hydrogen ion, and oxygen concentrations in the blood.

chemoresistance, 1. a specific resistance by components of a cell to chemical substances. **2.** the resistance of bacteria or a cancer cell to a chemical designed to treat the disorder.

chemosis /kimō'sis/ [Gk, *cheme,* cockle, *osis,* condition], an abnormal edematous swelling of the mucous membrane covering the eyeball and lining the eyelids. Usually the result of local trauma or infection, chemosis may also occur in acute conjunctivitis.

chemostat /kē'məstat'/, a device that ensures a steady rate of cell division in bacterial populations by maintaining a constant environment.

chemosurgery /-sur'jərē/ [Gk, *chemeia* + *cheirourgos,* surgeon], the destruction of malignant, infected, or gangrenous tissue by the application of chemicals. The technique is used successfully to remove skin cancers.

chemotaxis /-tak'sis/ [Gk, *chemeia* + *taxis,* arrangement], a response involving movement that is positive (toward) or negative (away from) in relation to a chemical stimulus.

chemotherapeutic agent /-ther'əpyoo'tik/, a chemical agent used to treat diseases. The term usually refers to a medication used to treat cancer because it can alter the growth of cancer cells.

chemotherapeutic index, a system for judging the safety and effectiveness of a drug as a ratio between a maximum tolerated (LD$_{50}$) dose per kilogram of body weight balanced against a median effective (ED$_{50}$) or minimal curative dose.

chemotherapy /-ther'əpē/, the treatment of infections and other diseases with chemical agents. The term has been applied over the centuries to a variety of therapies, including malaria therapy with herbs and use of mercury for syphilis. In modern usage chemotherapy usually entails the use of chemicals to destroy cancer cells on a selective basis. The cytotoxic agents used in cancer treatments generally function in the same manner as ionizing radiation; they do not kill the cancer cells directly but instead impair their ability to replicate. Chemotherapeutic agents are often used in combination with radiation treatments for their synergistic effect.

Chemotherapy Management, a Nursing Interventions Classification defined as assisting the patient and family to understand the action and minimize the side effects of antineoplastic agents.

chemotherapy (unsealed radioactive), the oral or parenteral administration of a radioisotope such as iodine 131 (^{131}I) for the treatment of hyperthyroidism or thyroid cancer or phosphorus 32 (^{32}P) for leukemia, polycythemia vera, or peritoneal ascites resulting from widely disseminated carcinoma.

chenodeoxycholic acid /kē'nōdē·ok'sikō'lik/, a secondary bile acid. It is used in vivo to dissolve cholesterol gallstones, particularly in the elderly and poor-risk patients.

cherophobia /kē'rō'fōbē·ə/, a morbid aversion to cheerfulness.

cherry angioma [L, *cerasus* + *angeion,* vessel, *oma,* tumor], a small, bright red, clearly circumscribed vascular tumor on the skin. It occurs most often on the trunk but may appear anywhere on the body. The lesion is common.

cherry red spot, an abnormal red circular area of the choroid, visible through the fovea centralis of the eye and surrounded by a contrasting white edema. It is associated with cases of infantile cerebral sphingolipidosis and sometimes appears in the late infantile form of amaurotic familial idiocy.

cherubism /cher'əbiz'əm/ [Heb, *kerubh*], an abnormal hereditary condition characterized by progressive bilateral swelling at the angle of the mandible, especially in children.

chest [AS, *box*], **1.** the thorax, the cavity enclosed by the ribs, sternum, and diaphragm. **2.** the outside front part of the thoracic cage.

chest bandage, any of several types of fabric dressings for chest injuries, including a three-cornered open chest wrapping, a figure-of-eight roller bandage spica, or a scultetus pattern of narrow strips that can be overlapped and pinned.

chest binder, a broad bandage or girdle, with or without shoulder straps, that encircles the chest and aids in supplying heat or other therapies.

chest drainage, the withdrawal of air, blood, or fluids from the chest cavity through a tube commonly inserted into the pleural space. The tube may be connected to a suction device that helps reinflate a collapsed lung.

chest lead /lēd/, **1.** an electrocardiographic conductor in which the exploring positive electrode is placed on the chest or precordium. The indifferent electrode is placed on the patient's back for a chest back (CB) lead, on the front of the chest for a chest front (CF) lead, on the left arm for a chest left (CL) lead, and on the right arm for a chest right (CR) lead. **2.** *informal.* the tracing produced by such a lead on an electrocardiograph.

chest pain [AS, *cest,* box; L, *poena,* punishment], a physical complaint that requires immediate diagnosis and evaluation. Chest pain may be symptomatic of cardiac disease such as angina pectoris, myocardial infarction, or pericarditis or of pulmonary disease such as pleurisy, pneumonia, or pulmonary embolism or infarction. The source of chest pain may also be musculoskeletal, gastrointestinal, or psychogenic; use of illegal drugs such as cocaine may also cause chest pain. Over 90% of severe chest pain is caused by coronary disease, spinal root compression, or psychologic disturbance. Specific cardiovascular conditions associated with chest pain are myocardial infarction, angina pectoris, pericarditis, and a dissecting aneurysm of the thoracic aorta. Musculoskeletal conditions include rib fractures, swelling of the rib cartilage, and muscle strain. Gastrointestinal conditions associated with chest pain include esophagitis, peptic ulcers, hiatal hernia, gastritis, cholecystitis, and pancreatitis.

Chest Physiotherapy, a Nursing Interventions Classification defined as assisting the patient to move airway secretions from peripheral airways to more central airways for expectorations and/or suctioning.

chest regions, the topographic parts or subdivisions of the chest: presternal, mammary, inframammary, and axillary.

chest thump [AS, *cest,* box, thump echoic], a sharp blow to the chest in the precordial area to restore a normal heartbeat after cardiac arrest.

chest tube, a catheter inserted through

the rib space of the thorax into the chest cavity to restore the negativity to the pleural sac and to remove air or fluid. It is attached to a water-seal chest drainage device.

chewing reflex, a pathologic sign in brain-damaged adults, characterized by repetitive chewing motions when the mouth is stimulated.

Cheyne's nystagmus /shānz/ [John Cheyne, Scottish physician, 1777–1836], an involuntary eyeball movement with a rhythm that resembles that of Cheyne-Stokes respiration.

Cheyne-Stokes respiration (CSR) /chān′ stōks′/ [John Cheyne; William Stokes, Irish physician, 1804–1878; L, *respirare* to breathe], an abnormal pattern of respiration characterized by alternating periods of apnea and deep, rapid breathing. The respiratory cycle begins with slow, shallow breaths that gradually increase to abnormal depth and rapidity. Respiration gradually subsides as breathing slows and becomes shallower, climaxing in a 10- to 20-second period without respiration before the cycle is repeated.

CHF, abbreviation for **congestive heart failure.**

chi /kī/ X, χ [Gk, *chi*], the 22nd letter of the Greek alphabet, sometimes used in scientific notation to designate the 22nd in a series.

ch'i, a Chinese concept of a fundamental life energy that flows in orderly ways along meridians, or channels, in the body.

Chiari-Frommel's syndrome /kē·är′ē-from′əl/ [Johann B. Chiari, German physician, 1817–1916; Richard Frommel, German gynecologist, 1854–1912], a hormonal disorder that occurs after pregnancy in which weaning does not spontaneously end lactation.

chiasm /kī′azəm/ [Gk, *chiasma*, lines that cross], **1.** the crossing of two lines or tracts, as of the optic nerves at the optic chiasm. **2.** (in genetics) the crossing of two chromatids in the prophase of meiosis. —**chiasmal, chiasmic,** *adj.*

chiasma /kī·az′mə/, *pl.* **chiasmata** [Gk, lines that cross], (in genetics) the visible point of connection between homologous chromosomes during the first meiotic division in gametogenesis. The X-shaped configurations form during the late prophase stage and provide the means by which exchange of genetic material occurs. —**chiasmatic, chiasmic,** *adj.*

chiasmapexy /kī·az′məpek′sē/, surgery involving the optic chiasm.

chickenpox /chik′ənpoks′/ [AS, *cicen* + ME, *pokke*], an acute, highly contagious viral disease caused by a herpesvirus, var-

icella zoster virus. It occurs primarily in young children and is characterized by crops of pruritic vesicular eruptions on the skin. The disease is transmitted by direct contact with skin lesions or, more commonly, by droplets spread from the respiratory tract of infected persons, usually in the prodromal period or the early stages of the rash. The vesicular fluid and the scabs are infectious until entirely dry. Indirect transmission through uninfected persons or objects is rare. The diagnosis is usually made by physical examination and by the characteristic appearance of the disease. The virus may be identified by culture of the vesicle fluid.

chiclero ulcer /chikler′ō/ [Mex, *tzictli,* chicle; L, *ulcus*], a kind of American leishmaniasis caused by *Leishmania mexicana.* It is endemic among the workers in the Yucatan and Central America who harvest chicle from the forest. The disease is characterized by cutaneous ulcers on the head that usually heal spontaneously by 6 months, except for those on the pinna of the ear, which may last for years and cause scarring and deformities.

chief cell [Fr, *chef;* L, *cella,* storeroom], **1.** any one of the columnar or cuboidal epithelial cells that line the gastric glands and secrete pepsinogen and intrinsic factor, which are needed for the absorption of vitamin B_{12} and the normal development of red blood cells. Anemia may be caused by the absence of intrinsic factor. **2.** any one of the epithelioid cells with pale-staining cytoplasm and a large nucleus containing a prominent nucleolus. Cords of such cells form the main substance of the pineal body. **3.** any one of the polyhedral epithelial cells, within the parathyroid glands, that contain pale, clear cytoplasm and a vesicular nucleus.

chief complaint (CC), a subjective statement made by a patient describing his or her most significant or serious symptoms or signs of illness or dysfunction.

Chief Executive Officer (CEO, C.E.O.), the most senior official of an organization or institution.

chief resident, a senior resident physician who acts temporarily as the clinical and administrative director of the house staff in a department of the hospital.

chief surgeon, a surgeon appointed or elected head of the surgeons on the staff of a health care facility.

chigger /chig′ər/ [Fr, *chique*], the larva of *Trombicula* mites found in tall grass and weeds. It sticks to the skin and causes irritation and severe itching.

chigoe /chig′ō/, a flea, *Tunga penetrans,* found in tropical and subtropical America and Africa. The pregnant female flea burrows into the skin of the feet, causing an inflammatory condition that may lead to spontaneous amputation of a toe.

chikungunya encephalitis /chik′ən·gun′yə/ [Bantu, to bend upward; Gk, *enkephalos,* brain, *itis,* inflammation], an arbovirus infection characterized by a high fever that begins abruptly, muscle aches, a rash, and pain in the joints. It is transmitted by the bite of a mosquito and occurs mainly in Africa, in Asia, and on some of the Pacific islands.

chilblain /chil′blān/ [AS, *cele,* cold, *bleyn,* blister], redness and swelling of the skin caused by excessive exposure to cold. Burning, itching, blistering, and ulceration similar to those characteristic of a thermal burn may occur.

child [AS, *cild*], **1.** a person of either sex between the time of birth and adolescence. **2.** an unborn or recently born human being; fetus, neonate, infant. **3.** an offspring or descendant; a son or daughter or a member of a particular tribe or clan. **4.** one who is like a child or immature.

child abuse, the physical, sexual, or emotional maltreatment of a child. Child abuse predominantly affects children less than 3 years of age and is the result of multiple and complex factors involving both the parents and the child, compounded by various stressful environmental circumstances such as inadequate physical and emotional support within the family and any major life change or crisis, especially those crises arising from marital strife. Parents at high risk for abuse are characterized as having unsatisfied needs, difficulty in forming adequate interpersonal relationships, unrealistic expectations of the child, and a lack of nurturing experience, often involving neglect or abuse in their own childhoods. Obvious physical marks on a child's body, as burns, welts, or bruises, and signs of emotional distress, including symptoms of failure to thrive, are common indications of some degree of neglect or abuse. Often radiograph films to detect healed or new fractures of the extremities or diagnostic tests to identify sexual molestation are necessary.

childbearing period [AS, *cild* + *beran,* to bear; Gk, *peri,* around, *hodos,* way], the reproductive period in a woman's life, from puberty to menopause. It is the time during which she is physiologically able to conceive children.

childbirth center, a health facility where prenatal care and delivery services are made available to low-risk pregnant women by a team of nurse-midwives, obstetricians, pediatricians, and ancillary health professionals.

Childbirth Preparation, a Nursing Interventions Classification defined as providing information and support to facilitate childbirth and to enhance the ability of an individual to develop and perform the role of parent.

child development, the various stages of physical, social, and psychologic growth that occur from birth through young adulthood.

childhood, **1.** the period in human development that extends from birth until the onset of puberty. **2.** the state or quality of being a child.

childhood aphasia, an inability to process language caused by a brain dysfunction in childhood.

childhood myxedema [AS, *cildhad* + Gk, *myxa,* mucus, *oidema,* swelling], a juvenile form of hypothyroidism characterized by atrophy of the thyroid gland after a severe infection of the gland.

childhood-onset pervasive developmental disorders, disturbances in thought, affect, social relatedness, and behavior that emerge between the ages of 30 months and 12 years of age. An example is autism.

childhood triad, three types of behavior—fire setting, bedwetting, and cruelty to animals—that may predict emerging sociopathy when they occur consistently and in combination.

child neglect, the failure by parents or guardians to provide for the basic human needs of a child by physical or emotional deprivation that interferes with normal growth and development or that places the child in jeopardy.

child psychology, the study of the mental, emotional, and behavioral development of infants and children.

child welfare, a service agency sponsored by the community or special organizations that provide for the physical, social, or psychologic care of children.

chill [AS, *cele*], **1.** the sensation of cold caused by exposure to a cold environment. **2.** an attack of shivering with pallor and a feeling of coldness, often occurring at the beginning of an infection and accompanied by a rapid rise in temperature.

Chilomastix /kī′lōmas′tiks/, a genus of flagellate protozoa, as *Chilomastix mesnili,* a nonpathogenic intestinal parasite of humans.

chimera /kimir′ə, kīmir′ə/ [Gk, *khimaros,* fire-breathing monster], an organism carrying cell populations derived from two or more different zygotes of the same or different species. It may be a natural phenomenon, such as in a bone marrow graft.

chimerism /kimir'izəm/, a state in bone marrow transplantation in which bone marrow and host cells exist compatibly without signs of graft-versus-host rejection disease.

chin, the raised triangular part of the mandible below the lower lip. It is formed by the mental protuberance.

Chinese restaurant syndrome, a group of transient symptoms consisting of tingling and burning sensations of the skin, facial pressure, headache, and chest pain that occur immediately after eating food containing monosodium glutamate, frequently used in Chinese cooking.

chip [AS, *kippen,* to slice], **1.** a relatively small piece of a bone or tooth. **2.** to break off or cut away a small piece.

chip fracture, any small fragmental fracture, usually one involving a bony process near a joint.

chip graft, a transplant consisting of small pieces of cartilage or bone that are packed into defective bone structures.

chiral, (in physical science) describing a compound that cannot be superimposed with its mirror image.

chiralgia /kəral'jə/, a pain in the hand, particularly one that does not result from a nerve injury or disease.

chiropractic /kī'rōprak'tik/ [Gk, *cheir,* hand, *practikos,* efficient], a system of therapy based on the theory that the state of a person's health is determined in general by the condition of his or her nervous system. In most cases treatment provided by chiropractors involves the mechanical manipulation of the spinal column. Some practitioners use radiology for diagnosis, physiotherapy, and diet in addition to spinal manipulation. Chiropractic does not use drugs or surgery, the primary basis of treatment used by medical physicians. A chiropractor is awarded the degree of Doctor of Chiropractic, or D.C., after completing at least 2 years of premedical studies followed by 4 years of training in an approved chiropractic school.

chiropractor /-prak'tər/, a practitioner of **chiropractic.**

chisel fracture, any fracture in which there is oblique detachment of a bone fragment from the head of the radius.

chi square (χ^2) /kī/, (in statistics) a statistical test for an association between observed and expected data represented by frequencies. The test yields a statement of the probability of the obtained distribution having occurred by chance alone.

Chlamydia /kləmid'ē-ə/ [Gk, *chlamys,* cloak], **1.** a microorganism of the genus *Chlamydia.* **2.** a genus of microorganisms

that live as intracellular parasites, have a number of properties in common with gram-negative bacteria, and are currently classified as specialized bacteria. *Chlamydia trachomatis* is responsible for inclusion conjunctivitis, lymphogranuloma venereum, pelvic inflammatory disease, and trachoma. *Chlamydia psittaci* causes a type of pneumonia in humans. *Chlamydia pneumoniae* is responsible for both upper and lower respiratory tract infections and commonly causes community acquired pneumonias. —**chlamydial,** *adj.*

chloasma /klō·az'mə/ /klō·az'mə/ [Gk, *chloazein,* to be green], tan or brown pigmentation, particularly of the forehead, cheeks, and nose, commonly associated with pregnancy or the use of oral contraceptives.

chloasma traumaticum, a pigmentary discoloration that results from friction on the skin.

chloasma uterinum, a skin discoloration that occurs in pregnant women or in diseases of the ovary or uterus.

chloracne /klôrak'nē/ [Gk, *chloros,* green, *akme,* point], a skin condition characterized by small, black follicular plugs and papules on exposed surfaces, especially on the arms, face, and neck of workers in contact with chlorinated compounds such as cutting oils, paints, varnishes, and lacquers.

chloral camphor /klôr'əl/, a mixture of equal parts of camphor and chloral hydrate used externally as a sedative.

chloral hydrate, a sedative and hypnotic prescribed for the relief of insomnia, anxiety, or tension.

chloral hydrate poisoning, an adverse reaction to ingestion of trichloroethylidine glycol, also known as chloral hydrate, which is sometimes used as a hypnotic because of its depressive effects on the central nervous system. Symptoms include irritation of the digestive tract, vomiting, depressed breathing, shock, confusion, and injury to the liver and kidneys.

chlorambucil /klôr'ambōō'sil/, an alkylating agent prescribed in the treatment of a variety of malignant neoplastic diseases, including chronic lymphocytic leukemia and Hodgkin's disease.

chloramphenicol /-amfē'nikol/, an antibacterial and antirickettsia prescribed in the treatment of a wide variety of serious infections.

chlorcyclizine hydrochloride /-sī'klizin/, an antihistamine that has been used for rhinitis, sinusitis, and hay fever. As a cream, it is also used for skin conditions.

chlordiazepoxide /klôr'dī·az'əpok'sīd/, a minor tranquilizer prescribed in the treatment of anxiety, nervous tension, and alcohol withdrawal symptoms.

chlorhexidine /-hek′sidēn/, an antimicrobial agent used as a surgical scrub, hand rinse, and topical antiseptic.

chloride /klôr′īd/ [Gk, *chloros,* green], an anion of chlorine. Metal chlorides are salts of hydrochloric acid; the most common is sodium chloride (table salt).

chloride shift, an exchange of chloride ions in red blood cells in peripheral tissues in response to PCO_2 of blood. The shift reverses in the lungs.

chloridometer /klôr′idom′ətər/, an instrument for measuring the level of chlorides in body fluids.

chloriduria, an excessive level of chlorides in the urine.

chlorinated /klôr′ənā′tid/ [Gk, *chloros,* greenish], pertaining to material that contains or has been treated with chlorine.

chlorinated organic insecticide poisoning, poisoning resulting from the inhalation, ingestion, or absorption of chlorophenothane (DDT) and other insecticides containing chlorophenothane such as heptachlor, dieldrin, and chlordane. It is characterized by vomiting, weakness, malaise, convulsions, tremors, ventricular fibrillation, respiratory failure, and pulmonary edema.

chlorination [Gk, *chloros,* green], the disinfection or treatment of water or other substances with free chlorine.

chlorine (Cl) /klôr′ēn/, a yellowish-green gaseous element of the halogen group. Its atomic number is 17; its atomic weight (mass) is 35.453. It has a strong, distinctive odor; is irritating to the respiratory tract; and is poisonous if ingested or inhaled. It occurs in nature chiefly as a component of sodium chloride in sea water and in salt deposits. It is used as a bleach and as a disinfectant to purify water for drinking or for use in swimming pools.

chlormezanone /-mez′ənōn/, an antianxiety agent prescribed for mild anxiety and for nervous tension.

chloroform /klôr′əfôrm′/ [Gk, *chloros* + L, *formica,* ant], a nonflammable volatile liquid that was the first inhalation anesthetic to be discovered. Chloroform has a low margin of safety and significant toxicity. The drug is not used in the United States.

chloroformism /-iz′əm/, **1.** the practice of inhaling chloroform for its narcotic effect. **2.** the anesthetic effect of chloroform.

chloroleukemia /klôr′ōlo͞okē′mē·ə/ [GK, *chloros,* green, *leukos,* white, *haima,* blood], a kind of myelogenous leukemia in which specific tumor masses are not seen at autopsy but body fluids and organs are green.

chlorolymphosarcoma /-lim′fōsärkō′mə/ [Gk, *chloros* + L, *lympha,* water; Gk, *sarx,* flesh, *oma,* tumor], a greenish neoplasm of myeloid tissue occurring in patients with myelogenous leukemia. The mononuclear cells in the peripheral blood are believed to be lymphocytes rather than myeloblasts, such as found with chloroma.

chloroma /klôrō′mə/, a malignant greenish neoplasm of myeloid tissue that occurs anywhere in the body of patients who have myelogenous leukemia.

chlorophyll /klôr′əfil/ [Gk, *chloros* + *phyllon,* leaf], a plant pigment capable of absorbing light and converting it to energy for the oxidation and reduction involved in photosynthesis of carbohydrates.

chloroprocaine /-prō′kān/, a local anesthetic with a chemical structure similar to that of procaine.

chloroquine /klôr′əkwīn′/, an antimalarial prescribed in the treatment of malaria, extraintestinal amebiasis, rheumatoid arthritis, some forms of lupus erythematosus, and photoallergic reactions.

chlorothiazide /-thī′əzīd/, a diuretic and antihypertensive prescribed in the treatment of hypertension and edema.

chlorotrianisene /-trī·an′isēn/, an estrogen prescribed in the treatment of postpartum breast engorgement, menopausal symptoms, and prostatic cancer.

chlorpheniramine maleate /-fenir′əmēn/, an antihistamine prescribed in the treatment of a variety of hypersensitivity reactions, including rhinitis, skin rash, and pruritus.

chlorpromazine /-prō′məzēn/, a phenothiazine tranquilizer and antiemetic prescribed in the treatment of psychotic disorders, severe nausea and vomiting, and intractable hiccups.

chlorpropamide /-prō′pəmīd/, an oral antidiabetic prescribed in the treatment of noninsulin-dependent diabetes mellitus.

chlorprothixene /-prōthik′sēn/, a thioxanthene antipsychotic agent prescribed in the treatment of psychotic disorders.

chlortetracycline hydrochloride /-tet′rəsī′klēn/, an antibiotic prescribed in the treatment of infections.

chlorthalidone /-thal′idōn/, a diuretic and antihypertensive prescribed in the treatment of high blood pressure and edema.

chlorzoxazone /-zok′səzōn/, a skeletal muscle relaxant prescribed for the relief of muscle spasm.

CHN, abbreviation for *Certified Hemodialysis Nurse.*

choana /kō′ənə/, *pl.* choanae, a funnel-shaped channel.

choanal atresia /kō′ənəl/ [Gk, *choane,* funnel, *a* + *tresis,* not hole], a congenital anomaly in which a bony or membranous occlusion blocks the passageway between the nose and pharynx.

chocolate cyst [Mex, *chocolatl* + Gk, *kystis,* bag], a darkly pigmented cyst sometimes found in the endometrium.

choke [ME, *choken*], to interrupt breathing by compression or obstruction of larynx or trachea.

chokes, a respiratory condition, occurring in decompression sickness, characterized by shortness of breath, substernal pain, and a nonproductive paroxysmal cough caused by bubbles of gas in the blood vessels of the lungs.

choke-saver, a curved forceps that can be inserted into the throat of a person who is choking on a food bolus or similar swallowed object. The tweezerslike device can grasp and retrieve the object.

choking, the condition in which a respiratory passage is blocked by constriction of the neck, an obstruction in the trachea, or swelling of the larynx. It is characterized by decreased movement of air through the airways or sudden coughing and a red face that rapidly becomes cyanotic. The person cannot breathe and clutches his or her throat.

cholagogue /kō′ləgog/ [Gk, *chole,* bile, *agogein,* to draw forth], a drug that stimulates the flow of bile.

cholangiectasis /kōlan′jē·ek′təsis/, dilation of the bile ducts.

cholangiocarcinoma /kōlan′jē·ōkär′sinō′-mə/, a cancer of the biliary epithelium. Risk factors include ulcerative colitis and infestation of liver flukes.

cholangiogram /kōlan′je·əgram′/, an x-ray film of the bile ducts produced after injection of a radiopaque contrast medium.

cholangiography /kōlan′jē·og′rəfē/, a special roentgenographic test procedure for outlining the major bile ducts by the intravenous injection or direct instillation of a radiopaque contrast material.

cholangiohepatoma /kōlan′jē·ōhep′ətō′-mə/, a primary carcinoma of the liver that develops in the bile ducts in which an abnormal mixture of liver cord cells and bile ducts exists.

cholangiolitis /-lī′tis/, an abnormal condition characterized by inflammation of the fine tubules of the bile duct system, which may cause cholangiolitic cirrhosis. —cholangiolitic, *adj.*

cholangioma /kōlan′jē·ō′mə/, a neoplasm of the bile ducts.

cholangioscopy /kōlan′jē·os′kəpē/, direct examination of the bile ducts with a fiberoptic endoscope.

cholangiostomy /kōlan′jē·os′təmē/ [Gk, *chole,* bile, *angeion,* small vessel, *stoma,* mouth], a surgical operation performed to form an opening in a bile duct.

cholangitis /kō′lanjī′tis/, inflammation of the bile ducts, caused either by bacterial invasion or by obstruction of the ducts by calculi or a tumor. The condition is characterized by severe right upper quadrant pain, jaundice (if an obstruction is present), and intermittent fever.

cholate, any salt or ester of cholic acid.

cholecystagogue /kō′ləsis′təgog′/, a drug that stimulates emptying of the gallbladder.

cholecystectomy /kō′lisistek′təmē/ [Gk, *chole* + *kystis,* bag, *ektome,* excision], the surgical removal of the gallbladder, performed to treat cholelithiasis and cholecystitis. The gallbladder is excised, and the cystic duct ligated; the common duct is searched, and any stones found are removed. Cholecystectomy is also done as a laparoscopic procedure.

cholecystic /kō′lisis′tik/, pertaining to the gallbladder.

cholecystitis /kō′lisistī′tis/ [Gk, *chole* + *kystis,* bag, *itis,* inflammation], acute or chronic inflammation of the gallbladder. Acute cholecystitis is usually caused by a gallstone that cannot pass through the cystic duct. Pain is felt in the right upper quadrant of the abdomen, accompanied by nausea, vomiting, eructation, and flatulence. Chronic cholecystitis, the more common type, has an insidious onset. Pain, often felt at night, may follow a fatty meal. Complications include biliary calculi, pancreatitis, and carcinoma of the gallbladder.

cholecystogram /ko′lisis′təgram′/, an x-ray film of the gallbladder, made after the ingestion or injection of a radiopaque substance, usually a contrast material containing iodine.

cholecystography /kō′lisistog′rəfē/, an x-ray examination of the gallbladder. At least 12 hours before the study, the patient has a fat-free meal and ingests a contrast material containing iodine. The iodine, which is opaque to x-rays, is excreted by the liver into the bile in the gallbladder. After the procedure, the patient consumes a fatty meal or cholecystokinin, which stimulates the gallbladder to contract, expelling bile and contrast material into the bile duct.

cholecystoileostomy /kō′lisis′tō·il′ē·os′-təmē/ [Gk, *chole,* bile, *kystis,* bag, *eilein,* to twist, *stoma, mouth],* a surgical procedure performed to connect the gallbladder to the ileum.

cholecystokinin /-kī'nin/ [Gk, *chole* + *kystis*, bag, *kinein*, to move], a hormone produced by the mucosa of the upper intestine that stimulates contraction of the gallbladder and secretion of pancreatic enzymes.

cholecystolithiasis /kō'lisis'tōlithīəsis/, the presence of gallstones in the gallbladder.

cholecystolithotripsy /kō'lisis'tōlith'ətripsē/, a procedure for crushing gallstones in the gallbladder or common bile duct with a lithotrite.

cholecystosonography /kō'lisis'tōsōnog'rəfē/, a method of examining the gallbladder using ultrasound.

choledochal /-dok'əl/ [Gk, *chole*, bile, *dochus*, containing], pertaining to the common bile duct.

choledochojejunostomy /-dok'ōjē'jōōnos'təmē/ [Gk, *chole*, bile, *dochus*, containing; L, *jejunus*, empty; Gk, *stoma*, mouth], a surgical procedure in which the bile duct is connected to the jejunum.

choledocholith /kōed'əkōlith'/, a gallstone in the common bile duct.

choledocholithotomy /-lithot'əmē/ [Gk, *chole* + *dochus*, containing, *lithos*, stone, *temnein*, to cut], a surgical operation to make an incision in the common bile duct to remove a stone.

choledocholithotripsy, a procedure for crushing gallstones in the common bile duct with a lithotrite.

choledocholitis, an inflammation of the common bile duct.

choleic /kōlē'ik/, pertaining to bile.

cholelithiasis /-lithī'əsis/ [Gk, *chole* + *lithos*, stone, *osis*, condition], the presence of gallstones in the gallbladder. The condition affects about 20% of the population above 40 years of age and is more prevalent in women and in persons with cirrhosis of the liver. Many patients complain of unlocalized abdominal discomfort, eructation, and intolerance to certain foods.

cholelithic dyspepsia /kō'lilith'ik/ [Gk, *chole* + *lithos*, stone, *dys*, bad, *peptein* to digest], an abnormal condition characterized by sudden attacks of indigestion associated with dysfunction of the gallbladder.

cholelithotomy /-lithot'əmē/, a surgical operation to remove gallstones through an incision in the gallbladder.

cholera /kol'ərə/ [Gk, *chole* + *rhein*, to flow], an acute bacterial infection of the small intestine, characterized by severe diarrhea and vomiting, muscular cramps, dehydration, and depletion of electrolytes.

The symptoms are caused by toxic substances produced by the infecting organism, *Vibrio cholerae*. The profuse, watery diarrhea, as much as a liter an hour, depletes the body of fluids and minerals.

choleragen /kol'ərəjin/, an exotoxin, produced by the cholera vibrio, that stimulates the secretion of electrolytes and water into the small intestine in Asiatic cholera.

cholera sicca, a form of cholera in which the patient dies of toxemia before the usual symptoms of vomiting and diarrhea develop.

cholera vaccine, an active immunizing agent prescribed as an immunization against cholera.

choleresis /kō'lərē'sis/, the secretion of bile by the liver.

choleretic /kō'ləret'ik/ [Gk, *chole* + *eresis*, removal], **1.** stimulating the production of bile in the liver either by cholepoiesis or by hydrocholeresis. **2.** a choleretic agent.

choleric /kol'ərik, kələr'ik/, having a hot temper or an irritable nature.

choleriform /koler'ifôrm/, resembling cholera.

cholescintigraphy /kō'ləsintig'rəfē/, examination of the gallbladder and bile ducts by scanning with radionuclides.

cholestasis /-stā'sis/ [Gk, *chole* + *stasis*, standing still], interruption in the flow of bile through any part of the biliary system, from liver to duodenum. It is essential for the physician to discover whether the cause is within the liver (intrahepatic) or outside it (extrahepatic). Symptoms of both types of cholestasis include jaundice, pale and fatty stools, dark urine, and intense itching over the skin. —**cholestatic,** *adj.*

cholestatic jaundice, a yellowing of the skin caused by thickening of bile, obstruction of hepatic ducts, or changes in liver cell function.

cholestatic hepatitis /-stat'ik/, a variant of viral hepatitis. Signs are persistent jaundice, itching, and elevated alkaline phosphatase levels. These signs usually abate when the hepatitis remits.

cholesteatoma /kōles'tē·ətō'mə/ [Gk, *chole* + *stear*, fat, *oma*, tumor], a cystic mass composed of epithelial cells and cholesterol that is found in the middle ear and occurs as a congenital defect or as a serious complication of chronic otitis media. The mass may occlude the middle ear, or enzymes produced by it may destroy the adjacent bones, including the ossicles. Surgery is required to remove a cholesteatoma.

cholesterase /kəles'tərās'/ [Gk, *chole* +

aither, air; Ger, *Saure,* acid; *ase,* enzyme suffix], an enzyme in the blood and other tissues that forms cholesterol and fatty acids by hydrolyzing cholesterol esters.

cholesterol /kəles'tərôl/ [Gk, *chole* + *steros,* solid], a waxy lipid found only in animal tissues. A member of a group of lipids called sterols, it is widely distributed in the body. It facilitates the absorption and transport of fatty acids. Cholesterol acts as the precursor for the synthesis of vitamin D at the surface of the skin, of the various steroid hormones, and of the sex hormones. It sometimes crystallizes in the gallbladder to form gallstones. Increased levels of low-density lipoprotein cholesterol may be associated with the pathogenesis of atherosclerosis.

cholesterolemia /-ē'mē-ə/, **1.** the presence of excessive amounts of cholesterol in the blood. **2.** the abnormal condition of the presence of excessive amounts of cholesterol in the blood.

cholesteroleresis /-er'isis/ /kəles'tərôler'-isis/ [Gk, *chole, steros* + *eresis,* removal], the increased elimination of cholesterol in the bile.

cholesterol metabolism, the sum of the anabolic and catabolic processes in the synthesis and degradation of cholesterol in the body. Cholesterol level is increased when cholesterol is ingested and is quickly absorbed. Cholesterol is also synthesized in the liver and can be synthesized by most other body tissues.

cholesterolopoiesis /kəles'tərō'lōpō·ē'sis/ [Gk, *chole* + *steros* + *poiesis,* producing], the elaboration of cholesterol by the liver.

cholesterolosis /kəles'tərəlō'sis/, an abnormal condition in which there are deposits of cholesterol within large macrophages in the submucosa of the gallbladder.

cholesteryl ester storage disease /kōles-təril/, an inherited disorder in which there is an accumulation of neutral lipids such as cholesterol esters and glycerides in body tissues. A form of the disorder affecting infants, with symptoms in the first weeks after birth, is Wolman's disease.

cholestyramine /-tir'əmēn/, a substance that acts on the liver's bile acids. It interrupts the bile-acid cycle and increases the function of low-density lipoprotein receptors, thereby increasing cellular cholesterol uptake and lowering blood cholesterol levels.

cholestyramine resin, an ion-exchange resin and antihyperlipoproteinemic agent prescribed for hyperlipoproteinemia and for pruritus resulting from partial biliary obstruction.

cholic acid, a bile acid synthesized in the liver from cholesterol. Cholan-24-oic acid is stored in the liver bound to coenzyme A and converted to glycine and taurine bile salts before secretion into bile.

choline /kō'lēn/ [Gk, *chole,* bile], a lipotropic substance sometimes included in the vitamin B complex as essential for the metabolism of fats in the body. Choline is a primary component of acetylcholine, the neurotransmitter, and functions with inositol as a basic constituent of lecithin. It prevents fat deposits in the liver and facilitates the movement of fats into the cells.

choline esters, a group of cholinergic drugs that act in body sites where acetylcholine is the neurotransmitter. Examples include bethanechol, carbachol, and methacholine.

cholinergic /-ur'jik/ [Gk, *chole* + *ergon,* to work], **1.** pertaining to nerve fibers that liberate acetylcholine at the myoneural junctions. **2.** the tendency to transmit or to be stimulated by or to stimulate the elaboration of acetylcholine.

cholinergic blocking agent, any agent that blocks the action of acetylcholine and substances similar to acetylcholine. Such agents, in effect, block the action of cholinergic nerves that transmit impulses by the release of acetylcholine at their synapses.

cholinergic crisis, a pronounced muscular weakness and respiratory paralysis caused by excessive acetylcholine, often apparent in patients suffering from myasthenia gravis as a result of overmedication with anticholinesterase drugs.

cholinergic fibers [Gr, *chole,* bile, *ergon,* work; L, *fibra*], nerve fibers of the autonomic nervous system that release the neurotransmitter acetylcholine. They include all preganglionic fibers, all postganglionic sympathetic fibers to sweat glands, and efferent fibers innervating skeletal muscle.

cholinergic nerve, a nerve that releases the neurotransmitter acetylcholine at its synapse. The cholinergic nerves include all the preganglionic sympathetic and preganglionic parasympathetic nerves, the postganglionic parasympathetic nerves, the somatic motor nerves to skeletal muscles, and some nerves to sweat glands and to certain blood vessels.

cholinergic receptor [Gk, *chole,* bile, *ergein,* to work; L, *recipere,* to receive], a specialized sensory nerve ending that responds to the stimulation of acetylcholine.

cholinergic urticaria [Gk, *chole* + *ergon,* to work; L, *urtica,* nettle], an abnormal and usually temporary vascular reaction of the skin, often associated with sweating in susceptible individuals subjected to stress, strong exertion, or hot weather. The condition is characterized by small, pale, itchy papules.

cholinesterase /kō'lines'tərās/, an enzyme that acts as a catalyst in the hydrolysis of acetylcholine to choline and acetate.

choliopancreatography /kō'lē·ōpan'krē·-ātog'rəfē/ [Gk, *chole* + *pan*, all, *kreas*, flesh, *graphein*, to record], the x-ray visualization of the bile and pancreatic ducts.

chondral /kon'drəl/, pertaining to cartilage.

chondralgia /kondral'jē·ə/, pain that appears to originate in cartilage.

chondrectomy /kondrek'təmē/, the surgical excision of a cartilage.

chondrial bone [Gk, *chondros,* cartilage; AS, *ban,* bone], pertaining to bone that forms under the periosteal membrane.

chondriocont /kon'drē·ōkont'/, a threadlike or rod-shaped mitochondrion.

chondriome /kon'drē·ōm/ [Gk, *chondros,* cartilage], the total mitochondria content of a cell, taken as a unit.

chondriomite /kon'drē·ōmīt'/ [Gk, *chondros* + *mitos,* thread], a single granular mitochondrion or a group of such organelles that appear in a chain formation.

chondritis /kondrī'tis/, any inflammatory condition affecting the cartilage.

chondroangioma /kon'drō·an'jē·ō'mə/ [Gk, *chondros* + *angeion,* vessel, *oma,* tumor], a benign mesenchymal tumor containing vascular and cartilaginous elements.

chondroblast /kon'drōblast/ [Gk, *chondros* + *blastos,* germ], any one of the cells that develop from the mesenchyma and form cartilage.

chondroblastoma /kon'drōblastō'mə/, chondroblastomata, a benign tumor, derived from precursors of cartilage cells, that develops most frequently in epiphyses of the femur and humerus.

chondrocalcinosis /kon'drōkal'sinō'sis/ [Gk, *chondros* + L, *calyx,* lime; Gk, *osis,* condition], an arthritic disease in which calcium deposits are present in the peripheral joints. It resembles gout and often occurs in patients over 50 years of age who have osteoarthritis or diabetes mellitus.

chondrocarcinoma /kon'drōkär'sinō'mə/ [Gk, *chondros* + *karkinos,* crab, *oma,* tumor], a malignant epithelial tumor in which cartilaginous metaplasia is present.

chondroclast /kon'drōklast'/ [Gk, *chondros* + *klasis,* breaking], a giant multinucleated cell associated with the resorption of cartilage. —**chondroclastic,** *adj.*

chondrocostal /kon'drōkos'təl/ [Gk, *chon-*dros + L, *costa,* rib], pertaining to the ribs and costal cartilages.

chondrocyte /kon'drəsīt/ [Gk, *chondros* + *kytos,* cell], any one of the polymorphic cells that form the cartilage of the body. —**chondrocytic,** *adj.*

chondrodysplasia /kon'drōdisplā'zhə/ [Gk, *chondros* + *dys,* bad, *plassein,* to form], an inherited disease characterized by abnormal growth at the ends of bones, particularly the long bones of the arms and legs.

chondrodysplasia punctata, an inherited form of dwarfism characterized by skin lesions, radiographic evidence of epiphyseal stippling, and a pug nose. There are two types of the anomaly: a benign Conradi-Hunermann form and a lethal rhizomelic form.

chondrodystrophia calcificans congenita /-distrō'fē·ə/ [Gk, *chondros* + *dys,* bad, *trophe,* nourishment; L, *calyx,* lime, *congenitus,* born with], an inherited defect characterized by many small opacities in the epiphyses of the long bones. Dwarfism; contractures; cataracts; mental retardation; and short, stubby fingers develop as the infant grows into childhood.

chondrodystrophy /kon'drōdis'trəfē/ [Gk, *chondros* + *dys,* bad, *trophe,* nourishment], a group of disorders in which there is abnormal conversion of cartilage to bone, particularly in the epiphyses of the long bones.

chondroectodermal dysplasia /kon'-drō·ek'tədur'məl/, an inherited form of dwarfism marked by distal limb shortening, postaxial polydactyly, and cardiovascular abnormalities.

chondroendothelioma /kon'drō·en'dōthē'lē·ō'mə/ [Gk, *chondros* + *endon,* within, *thele,* nipple, *oma,* tumor], a benign mesenchymal tumor containing cartilaginous and endothelial components.

chondrofibroma /kon'drōfibrō'mə/, a fibrous tumor that contains cartilaginous components.

chondrogenesis /kon'drōjen'əsis/, the development of cartilage. —**chondrogenetic,** *adj.*

chondroid /kon'droid/, resembling cartilage.

chondrolipoma /kon'drōlipō'mə/, a benign mesenchymal tumor containing fatty and cartilaginous components.

chondroma /kondrō'mə/, a benign, fairly common tumor of cartilage cells that grows slowly within cartilage (enchondroma) or on the surface (ecchondroma). —**chondromatous,** *adj.*

chondromalacia /kon'drōmələ'shə/ [Gk, *chondros* + *malakia,* softness], a softening of cartilage. **Chondromalacia fetalis**

is a lethal congenital form of the condition in which a stillborn infant has soft and pliable limbs. **Chondromalacia patellae** occurs in young adults after knee injury and is characterized by swelling, pain, and degenerative changes, which are revealed on x-ray examination.

chondromatosis /kon′drōmətō′sis/, a condition characterized by the presence of many cartilaginous tumors. A kind of chondromatosis is synovial chondromatosis.

chondromere /kon′drōmir/ [Gk, *chondros* + *meros,* part], a cartilaginous embryonic vertebra and its costal component.

chondromyoma /kon′drōmī·ō′mə/ [Gk, *chondros* + *mys,* muscle, *oma,* tumor], a benign mesenchymal tumor containing myomatous and cartilaginous tissue.

chondromyxofibroma /kon′drōmik′sōfī-brō′mə/ [Gk, *chondros* + *myxa,* mucus; L, *fibra,* fiber, *oma,* tumor], a benign tumor that develops from cartilage-forming connective tissue. The lesion, typically a firm, grayish-white mass, tends to occur in the knee and small bones of the foot.

chondromyxoid /kon′drōmik′soid/ [Gk, *chondros* + *myxa,* mucus, *eidos,* form], composed of cartilaginous and myxoid elements.

chondrophyte /kon′drōfīt′/ [Gk, *chondros* + *phyton,* growth], an abnormal mass of cartilage. —**chondrophytic,** *adj.*

chondroplasia /-plā′zhə/ [Gk, *chondros,* cartilage, *plassein,* to form], the formation of cartilage.

chondroplasty /kon′drōplas′tē/ [Gk, *chondros* + *plassein,* to form], the surgical repair of cartilage.

chondrosarcoma /kon′drōsärkō′mə/ [Gk, *chondros* + *sarx,* flesh, *oma,* tumor], a malignant neoplasm of cartilaginous cells or their precursors that occurs most frequently in long bones, the pelvic girdle, and the scapula. —**chondrosarcomatous,** *adj.*

chondrosarcomatosis /kon′drōsär′kōmə-tō′sis/, a condition characterized by multiple malignant cartilaginous tumors.

chondrosis /kondrō′sis/, 1. the development of the cartilage of the body. 2. a cartilaginous tumor.

chondrotomy /kondrot′əmē/, a surgical procedure for dividing a cartilage.

chopping, a therapeutic exercise to improve the strength and coordination of upper trunk nerves and muscles by lifting the arms overhead and lowering them in a chopping or slashing movement.

chorda /kôr′də/, a cordlike filament such as a nerve or tendon.

chordae tendineae /kô′dētendin′i·ē/, *sing.*

chorda tendinea /kô′dätendin′ē·ä/, the strands of tendon that anchor the cusps of the mitral and tricuspid valves to the papillary muscles of the ventricles of the heart, preventing prolapse of the valves into the atria during ventricular contraction.

chordee /kôr′dē, kôr′dā/ [Gk, *chorde,* cord], a congenital defect of the genitourinary tract resulting in a ventral curvature of the penis, caused by presence of a fibrous band of tissue instead of normal skin along the corpus spongiosum.

chordencephalon /kôrd′ensef′əlon/ [Gk, *chorde* + *enkephalos,* brain], the part of the central nervous system that develops in the early weeks of pregnancy from the neural tube and includes the mesencephalon, the rhombencephalon, and the spinal cord. —**chordencephalic,** *adj.*

chorditis /kôrdī′tis/, 1. inflammation of a spermatic cord. 2. inflammation of the vocal cords or of the vocal folds.

chordoid /kôr′doid/ [Gk, *chorde* + *eidos,* form], resembling the notochord or notochordal tissue.

chordoma /kôrdō′mə/, a rare tumor that develops from the fetal notochord.

chordotomy /kôrdot′əmē/ [Gk, *chorde* + *temnein,* to cut], surgery in which the anterolateral tracts of the spinal cord are surgically divided to relieve pain.

chorea /kôrē′ə/ [Gk, *choreia,* dance], a condition characterized by involuntary purposeless, rapid motions, as flexing and extending of the fingers, raising and lowering the of shoulders, or grimacing. —**choreic** /kôrā′ik/, *adj.*

chorea gravidarum /kôr′ē·əgrav′idär′əm/, Sydenham's chorea that occurs during the early months of pregnancy with or without a previous history of rheumatic disease.

choreic ataxia /kôrē′ik/ [Gk, *choreia,* dance, *ataxia,* without order], a form of ataxia in which patients lack muscular coordination and movements are marked by involuntary twitching and abrupt jerking.

choreiform /kərē′əförm′/, resembling the rapid jerky movements associated with chorea.

choreiform spasm [Gk, *chorea,* dance; L, *forma* + Gk, *spasmos*], a condition of involuntary muscle contractions that result in dancing motions. In one type powerful contractions of the leg muscles cause a leaping, jumping action. It can also involve arm, shoulder, and neck muscles.

choreoathetoid cerebral palsy /kôr′-ē·ō·ath′ətoid/, a form of cerebral palsy characterized by choreiform (jerky, ticlike twitching) and athetoid (slow, writhing) movements.

choreoathetosis /kô′ē·ō·ath′ətō′sis/ [Gk, *choreia,* dance, *athetos,* not fixed], irregular involuntary movements that may involve the face, neck, trunk, extremities, or respiratory muscles, giving an appearance of restlessness. The writhing movements may vary from subtle to wild and ballistic and are commonly associated with administration of levodopa in parkinsonism.

chorioadenoma /kərē′ō·ad′inō′mə/ [Gk, *chorion,* skin, *aden,* gland, *oma,* tumor], an epithelial cell tumor of the outermost fetal membrane that is intermediate in the malignant development of a hydatid mole to invasive choriocarcinoma.

chorioadenoma destruens /des′trōō·əns/ [Gk, *chorion* + *aden* + *oma* + L, *destruere,* to pull down], an invasive hydatidiform mole in which the chorionic villi of the mole penetrate into the myometrium and parametrium of the uterus and metastasize to distant parts of the body.

chorioamnionic /-am′nē·ot′ik/, pertaining to the chorion and the amnion.

chorioamnionitis /-am′nē·ōnī′tis/ [Gk, *chorion* + *amnion,* fetal membrane, *itis,* inflammation], an inflammatory reaction in the amniotic membranes caused by bacteria or viruses in the amniotic fluid.

choriocarcinoma /kôr′ē·ōkär′sinō′mə/, an epithelial malignancy of fetal origin that develops from the chorionic part of the products of conception. The primary tumor usually appears in the uterus as a soft, dark red, crumbling mass; may invade and destroy the uterine wall; and may metastasize through lymph or blood vessels.

choriocele /kôr′ē·əsēl′/ [Gk, *chorion* + *kele,* hernia], a hernia or protrusion of the tissue of the choroid layer of the eye.

choriogenesis /kôr′ē·ōjen′əsis/, the development of the chorion, which is first evident in the first month of pregnancy. —**choriogenetic,** *adj.*

chorion /kôr′ē·on/ [Gk, *chorion,* skin], (in biology) the outermost extraembryonic membrane composed of trophoblast lined with mesoderm. It develops villi about 2 weeks after fertilization and is vascularized by allantoic vessels 1 week later. It gives rise to the placenta and persists until birth as the outer of the two layers of membrane containing the amniotic fluid and the fetus.

chorionic gonadotropin (CG) /kôr′ē·on′ik gon′ədōtrop′in/ [Gk, *chorion* + *gone,* seed, *trophe,* nutrition], a chemical component of the urine of pregnant women and pregnant mares. This glycoprotein hormone is secreted by the placental trophoblastic cells. It is composed of two subunits, alpha and beta human chorionic gonadotropin. The alpha subunit is nearly identical to similar subunits of the follicle-stimulating, luteinizing, and thyroid-stimulating hormones. The specific hormonal effects of chorionic gonadotropin are activated by the beta part. They include stimulation of the corpus luteum to secrete estrogen and progesterone and to decrease lymphocyte activation.

chorionic plate [Gk, *chorion* + *platys,* flat], the part of the fetal placenta that gives rise to chorionic villi, which attach to the uterus during the early stage of formation of the placenta.

chorionic sac [Gk, *chorion,* skin, *sakkos,* sack], the saclike membrane that develops from the blastocyst wall to envelop the embryo.

chorionic villi [Gk, *chorion* + L, *villus,* shaggy hair], tiny vascular fibrils on the surface of the chorion that infiltrate the maternal blood sinuses of the endometrium and help form the placenta.

chorionic villi sampling [Gk, *chorion,* skin; L, *villus,* shaggy hair, *exemplum,* sample], a procedure for obtaining prenatal evaluation data early in a pregnancy by withdrawing a chorionic villi sample from the fetal membranes. The sample is obtained through a catheter inserted into the uterus.

chorioretinitis /kôr′ē·ōret′inī′tis/, an inflammatory condition of the choroid and retina of the eye, usually as a result of parasitic or bacterial infection. It is characterized by blurred vision, photophobia, and distorted images.

chorioretinopathy /kôr′ē·ōret′ənop′əthē/ [Gk, *chorion* + L, *rete,* net; Gk, *pathos,* disease], a noninflammatory process caused by disease that involves the choroid and the retina.

choroid /kôr′oid/ [Gk, *chorion* + *eidos,* form], a thin, highly vascular layer of the eye between the retina and sclera.

choroidal malignant melanoma /kôroi′dəl/ [Gk, *chorion* + *eidos* + L, *malignus,* ill-disposed; Gk, *melas,* black, *oma,* tumor], a tumor of the choroid coat of the eye that grows into the vitreous humor, causing detachment and degeneration of the overlying retina.

choroiditis /kôr′oidī′tis/, an inflammatory condition of the choroid membrane of the eye.

choroid membrane, a vascular layer of tissue between the retina and the sclera of the eye.

choroidocyclitis /kôroi′dōsiklī′tis/ [Gk, *chorion* + *eidos* + *kyklos,* circle, *itis,* inflammation], an abnormal condition characterized by inflammation of the choroid and the ciliary processes.

choroidopathy /kôr'oidop'əthē/, noninflammatory degeneration of the choroid.

choroid plexectomy /pleksek'təmē/ [Gk, *chorion* + *eidos* + L, *plexus,* pleated; Gk, *ektome,* excision], a surgical procedure for the reduction of cerebrospinal fluid production in the ventricles of the brain in hydrocephalus, usually in the newborn.

choroid plexus [Gk, *chorion* + *eidos* + L, pleated], any one of the tangled masses of tiny blood vessels contained within the third, the lateral, and the fourth ventricles of the brain, responsible for producing cerebrospinal fluid.

Christchurch chromosome (Ch1) [Christchurch, city on South Island of New Zealand], an abnormally small acrocentric chromosome of the karyotype G group, involving any members of chromosome pairs 21 or 22, in which the short arms are missing or partially deleted.

Christian Science, a religious system founded in 1879 by Mary Baker Eddy [1821–1910], based on the metaphysical teachings of Phineas P. Quimby. It holds that healing should be achieved through spiritual means, that sickness and death are illusions, and that one can overcome illness by refusing to think about it.

Christian-Weber disease [Henry A. Christian, American physician, 1876–1951; Frederick Parkes Weber, English physician, 1863–1962], a rare form of panniculitis characterized by nodular formations in the subcutaneous tissues and prolonged intermittent relapsing fever.

chromaffin /krō'məfin/ [Gk, *chroma,* color; L, *affin,* affinity], having an affinity for strong staining with chromium salts.

chromaffin cell, any one of the special cells that compose the paraganglia and are connected to the ganglia of the celiac, renal, suprarenal, aortic, and hypogastric plexuses. The chromaffin cells of the adrenal medulla secrete two catecholamines, epinephrine and norepinephrine, that affect smooth muscle, cardiac muscle, and glands in the same way as sympathetic stimulation, by increasing and prolonging sympathetic effects.

chromate (CrO$_4^{2-}$), any salt of chromic acid.

chromatic /krōmat'ik/ [Gk, *chroma,* color], **1.** pertaining to color. **2.** stainable by a dye. **3.** pertaining to chromatin.

chromatic asymmetry of iris [Gk, *chroma,* color, *a* + *symmetria,* commensurability, *iris,* rainbow], a difference in color of the two irides.

chromatic dispersion [Gk, *chroma* + L, *dis,* apart, *spargere,* to scatter], the splitting of light into its various component wavelengths or frequencies, such as with a prism.

chromatid /krō'mətid/ [Gk, *chroma,* color], one of the two identical threadlike filaments of a chromosome.

chromatid deletion, the breakage of a chromatid. The breakage may be caused by a single-hit effect produced by radiation. The fragments are isochromatids.

chromatin /krō'mətin/ [Gk, *chroma,* color], the material within the cell nucleus from which the chromosomes are formed. It consists of fine, threadlike strands of deoxyribonucleic acid attached to a protein base, usually histone. During cell division, parts of the chromatin condense and coil to form the chromosomes. —**chromatinic,** adj.

chromatin-negative, pertaining to or descriptive of the nuclei of cells that lack sex chromatin, specifically characteristic of the normal male but also present in certain chromosomal abnormalities.

chromatin-positive, pertaining to or descriptive of the nuclei of cells that contain sex chromatin, specifically characteristic of the normal female, but also present in certain chromosomal abnormalities.

chromatism /krō'mətiz'əm/, **1.** an abnormal condition characterized by hallucinations in which the affected individual sees colored lights. **2.** abnormal pigmentation.

chromatogram /krōmat'əgram'/, **1.** the record produced by the separation of gaseous substances or dissolved chemical substances moving through a column of absorbent material that filters out the various absorbates in different layers. **2.** any graphic record produced by any chromatographic method.

chromatography /krō'mətog'rəfē/, any one of several processes for separating and analyzing various gaseous or dissolved chemical materials according to differences in their absorbency with respect to a specific substance and according to their different pigments. —**chromatographic,** adj.

chromatopsia /krō'mətop'sē·ə/ [Gk, *chroma* + *opsis,* vision], **1.** an abnormal visual condition that makes colorless objects appear tinged with color. **2.** a form of color blindness characterized by the imperfect perception of various colors. It may be caused by a deficiency in one or more of the retinal cones or by defective nerve circuits that convey color-associated impulses to the cerebral cortex. The most common defect in color sense is the inability to distinguish red from green.

chromatosis /-ō'sis/, condition of abnormal skin pigmentation in any part of the body.

chromaturia /-ŏŏr'ē-ə/ [Gk, *chroma,* color, *ouron,* urine], urine that has an abnormal color.

chromesthesia /krō'misthē'zhə/ [Gk, *chroma* + *aisthesis,* feeling], **1.** the color sense that depends on the mixture of wavelengths in the light that enters the eye and the response of the different types of retinal cones associated with color vision. **2.** an abnormal condition characterized by the confusion of other senses such as taste and smell with imagined sensations of color.

chromhidrosis /krō'midrō'sis/ [Gk, *chroma* + *hidros,* sweat], a rare, functional disorder in which apocrine sweat glands secrete colored sweat.

chromic catgut /krō'mik/ [Gk, *chroma,* color; L, *catta;* AS, *guttas*], surgical catgut that has been treated with chromium trioxide to strengthen it.

chromic myopia, a kind of color blindness characterized by the ability to distinguish colors of only those objects that are close to the eye.

chromium (Cr) /krō'mē-əm/ [Gk, *chroma,* color], a hard, brittle metallic element. Its atomic number is 24; its atomic weight (mass) is 51.99. It does not occur naturally in pure form but exists in combination with iron and oxygen in chromite. Traces of chromium occur in plants and animals, and there is evidence that this element may be important in human nutrition, especially in carbohydrate metabolism. Chromium 51 isotope is used in blood studies.

chromium alum, a chemical commonly used to fix, or harden, the emulsion of an x-ray film during manual processing.

chromobacteriosis /krō'məbaktir'ē-ō'sis/, an extremely rare, usually fatal systemic infection caused by a gram-negative bacillus *Chromobacterium violaceum.* It is found in fresh water in tropic and subtropic regions and enters the body through a break in the skin.

chromoblastomycosis /krō'mōblas'tō-mīkō'sis/ [Gk, *chroma* + *blastos,* germ, *mykes,* fungus, *osis,* condition], a chronic infectious skin disease caused by any of a variety of fungi and characterized by the appearance of pruritic, warty nodules that develop in a cut or other break in the skin.

chromogen /krō'mōjən/, a substance that absorbs light, producing color.

chromomere /krō'məmir/ [Gk, *chroma* + *meros,* part], any of the series of beadlike structures that lie along the chromonema of a chromosome during the early stages of cell division.

chromonema /krō'mənē'mə/ [Gk, *chroma* + *nema,* thread], the coiled filament along which the chrommeres lie that forms the central part of the chromatid of the chromosome during cell division. —**chromonemal, chromonematic, chromonemic,** *adj.*

chromophilic /krō'məfil'ik/ [Gk, *chroma* + *philein,* to love], denoting a cell, tissue, or microorganism that is easily stained, particularly certain leukocytes.

chromophobia /krō'məfō'bē·ə/ [Gk, *chroma* + *phobos,* fear], **1.** the resistance of certain cells and tissues to stains. **2.** a morbid aversion to colors. —**chromophobe,** *n.*

chromophobic /krō'məfō'bik/, denoting a cell, tissue, or microorganism that is not easily stained, particularly certain cells of the anterior lobe of the pituitary gland.

chromophobic adenoma, a tumor of the pituitary gland composed of cells that do not stain with acid or basic dyes.

chromosensitive, descriptive of a substance that is affected by and responds to changes in chemical composition.

chromosomal aberration /-sō'məl/ [Gk, *chroma* + *soma,* body; L, *aberrare,* to wander], any change in the structure or number of any of the chromosomes for a given species, which can result in anomalies of varying severity. In humans a number of physical disabilities and disorders are directly associated with chromosomal defects of both the autosomes and the sex chromosomes, including Down's, Turner's, and Kleinfelter's syndromes.

chromosomal nomenclature, a standard nomenclature that serves to identify the complement of chromosomes in an individual according to the number of chromosomes, sex, and deletion or addition of a specific chromosome or part of a chromosome. Complement in a normal human female is recorded as 46,XX and for a normal male, 46,XY. Chromosomal aberrations are designated by indicating the total chromosomal number, sex complement, and group or specific chromosome in which the addition or deletion occurs. The short arm of a chromosome is designated *p,* the long arm is *q,* and a translocation is *t.*

chromosomal sex [Gk, *chroma,* color, *soma,* body; L, *sexus,* male or female], in mammals the sex of an individual as determined by the presence or absence of the Y chromosome.

chromosome /krō'məsōm/ [Gk, *chroma* + *soma,* body], any one of the threadlike nucleoprotein structures in the nucleus of a cell that function in the transmission of genetic information. Each consists of a double strand of deoxyribonucleic acid (DNA), which is coiled in a helix formation and attached to a protein base, usually a histone. The genes, which contain the genetic material that controls the inheritance of traits, are arranged in a linear pattern along the entire length of each DNA strand. Each species has a characteristic number of chromosomes in the somatic cell, which in humans is 46 and includes 22 homologous pairs of autosomes and 1 pair of sex chromosomes, with one member of each pair derived from each parent. —**chromosomal,** *adj.*

chromosome coil, the spiral formed by the coiling of two or more chromonemata of the chromatid within the chromosome.

chromosome complement, the normal number of chromosomes found in the somatic cell of any given species. In humans it is 46, consisting of 22 pairs of homologous autosomes and 1 pair of sex chromosomes.

chromosome puff, a band of accumulated chromatic material located at a specific site on a giant chromosome. It is indicative of gene activity, specifically deoxyribonucleic acid and ribonucleic acid synthesis, for the particular locus.

chromosome walking, a molecular genetic technique by which overlapping molecular clones that span large chromosomal intervals are isolated.

chromotherapy /krō'məther'əpē/, a system of treating disease with colored lights chosen from specific regions of the spectrum.

chromotrope /krō'mətrōp/ [Gk, *chroma* + *trepein,* to turn], **1.** a component of tissue that stains metachromatically with metachromatic dyes. **2.** any one of several dyes differentiated by numeric suffixes. —**chromotropic,** *adj.*

chronaxy /krō'naksē/ [Gk, *chronos,* time, *axia,* value], (in electroneuromyography) a measure of the shortest duration of an electrical stimulus needed to excite nerve or muscle tissue.

chronic /kron'ik/ [Gk, *chronos,* time], (of a disease or disorder) developing slowly and persisting for a long period, often for the remainder of a person's lifetime.

chronic abscess [Gk, *chronos,* time; L, *abscedere,* to go away], a slowly developing abscess that produces pus but shows little or no inflammation, redness, or pain. It is often a tuberculous abscess.

chronic active hepatitis (CAH), a potentially fatal form of hepatitis complicated by portal inflammation and extending into the parenchyma. There may be progressive destruction of the liver lobule with necrosis and fibrosis leading to scarring and cirrhosis. Possible causes include viral infections, drugs, and autoimmune reactions.

chronic airway obstruction, a type of pulmonary disorder in which the patient, when at rest, breathes at a normal rate and may have prolongation of the expiratory phase with pursed-lip breathing.

chronic alcoholism, a pathologic condition resulting from the habitual use of alcohol in excessive amounts. Symptoms of the disease include anorexia, diarrhea, weight loss, neurologic and psychiatric disturbances (most notably depression), and fatty deterioration of the liver, sometimes leading to cirrhosis.

chronic anterior poliomyelitis, an inflammation of the gray matter in the spinal cord, resulting in atrophy of muscles of the upper extremities and neck, with long periods of remission of symptoms.

chronic appendicitis, a type of appendicitis characterized by thickening or scarring of the vermiform appendix, caused by previous inflammation.

chronic bacterial prostatitis, a prolonged but relatively mild bacterial infection of the prostate. Symptoms may include pain, fever, and dysuria, but they are less intense than in acute prostatitis.

chronic bronchitis, a very common debilitating pulmonary disease, characterized by greatly increased production of mucus by the glands of the trachea and bronchi and resulting in a cough with expectoration for at least 3 months of the year for more than 2 consecutive years.

chronic carrier, an individual who acts as host to pathogenic organisms for an extended period without displaying any signs of disease.

chronic delirium [Gk, *chronos,* time; L, *delirare,* to rave], a form of delirium in which the patient shows signs of psychosis but is afebrile. The condition is sometimes associated with exhaustion, malnutrition, and wasting.

chronic disease, a disease that persists over a long period as compared with the course of an acute disease. The symptoms of chronic disease are sometimes less severe than those of the acute phase of the same disease.

chronic endoarteritis [Gk, *chronos,* time, *endon,* within, *arteria,* airpipe, *itis,* inflammation], an inflammatory condition of the tunica intima lining of an artery wall. It may be accompanied by fatty degeneration of arterial tissue and calcium deposits.

chronic endocarditis [Gk, *chronos,* time, *endon,* within, *kardia,* heart, *itis,* inflammation], an inflammatory condition of the endocardium lining the heart. It usually follows an attack of acute endocarditis, syphilis, or an atheroma. It frequently involves the cardiac valves, making them incompetent.

chronic fatigue syndrome (CFS), a condition characterized by disabling fatigue, accompanied by a constellation of symptoms, including muscle pain, multijoint pain without swelling, painful cervical or axillary adenopathy, sore throat, headache, impaired memory or concentration, and unrefreshing sleep. The disorder often persists for years; spontaneous resolution occurs in fewer than 40% of cases.

chronic glomerulonephritis, a noninfectious disease of the glomerulus of the kidney characterized by proteinuria, hematuria, edema, and decreased production of urine.

chronic gout [Gk, *chronos,* time; L, *gutta,* drop], a persistent condition of purine metabolism, characterized by abnormally high levels of serum uric acid and attacks of arthritis, with deposits of urates in the joints. The disorder may be familial and, if untreated, can lead to renal failure.

chronic hepatitis [Gk, *chronos,* time, *hepar,* liver, *itis,* inflammation], a state in which symptoms of hepatitis continue for several months and may increase in severity. In some cases of hepatitis B, the patient may become a lifelong carrier of the antigen and may show prolonged evidence of the infection.

chronic hyperplastic rhinitis [Gk, *chronos,* time, *hyper,* excess, *plassein,* to form, *rhis,* nose, *itis,* inflammation], chronic inflammation of the mucous membranes of the nose, with polyp formation.

chronic hyperplastic sinusitis [Gk, *chronos,* time, *hyper,* excess, *plassein,* to form; L, *sinus,* hollow; Gk, *itis,* inflammation], chronic sinus inflammation, with polyp formation in the nose and sinuses.

chronic hypertrophic rhinitis [Gk, *chronos,* time, *hyper,* excess, *trophe,* nourishment, *rhis,* nose, *itis,* inflammation], a condition of chronic inflammation of the nasal mucosa associated with enlargement of the mucous membrane.

chronic hypoxia, a usually slow, insidious reduction in tissue oxygenation resulting from gradually destructive or fibrotic lung diseases, congenital or acquired heart disorders, or chronic blood loss. The person experiences persistent mental and physical fatigue, shows sluggish mental

responses, and complains of a loss of ability to perform physical tasks.

chronic illness, any disorder that persists over a long period and affects physical, emotional, intellectual, social, or spiritual functioning.

chronic intractable pain [Gk, *chronos,* time; L, *intractabilis* + *poena,* penalty], persistent pain that fails to respond to nonnarcotic analgesics and other treatment measures.

chronicity /krōnis'itē/, a state of being chronic.

chronic leg ulcer [Gk, *chronos,* time; ONorse, *leggr* + L, *ulcus,* ulcer], a slow-healing ulcer of the leg (usually the lower leg). Typically it is associated with varicose veins, deep venous insufficiency, or a similar circulatory obstacle.

chronic lingual papillitis [Gk, *chronos* + L, *lingua,* tongue, *papilla,* nipple; Gk, *itis*], an inflammatory disorder of the tongue, sometimes extending to the buccal mucosa and palate. It is characterized by irregularly scattered red patches, thinning of the lingual papillae, severe burning pain, and shedding of epidermal tissue.

chronic low blood pressure, systolic and diastolic blood pressures that are consistently below normal.

chronic lymphocytic leukemia (CLL) [Gk, *chronos* + L, *lympha,* water; Gk, *kytos,* cell, *leukos,* white, *haima,* blood], a neoplasm of blood-forming tissues characterized by a proliferation of small, long-lived lymphocytes, chiefly B cells, in bone marrow, blood, liver, and lymphoid organs. The disease has an insidious onset and progresses to cause malaise, ready fatigability, anorexia, weight loss, nocturnal sweating, lymphadenopathy, and hepatosplenomegaly.

chronic mountain sickness [Gk, *chronos,* time; L, *montana;* AS, *soec*], a form of altitude sickness in which the increased production of red cells results in polycythemia. Some symptoms, such as headache, weakness, and limb aches, occasionally develop in indigenous mountain dwellers as well as in persons who had become acclimatized to the higher altitudes.

chronic mucocutaneous candidiasis, a rare form of candidiasis, characterized by candidal infection lesions of the skin, mucous membranes, gastrointestinal tract, and respiratory tract. This disease usually occurs during the first year of life but can develop at any time. It affects both males and females and may be associated with an inherited defect of the cell-mediated immune system that allows autoantibodies to develop against target organs. The humoral immune system functions normally in this disease. The onset of infections associated with the disease may precede endocrinopathy.

chronic myelocytic leukemia (CML), a malignant neoplasm of blood-forming tissues, characterized by a proliferation of granular leukocytes and often of megakaryocytes. The disease occurs most frequently in mature adults and begins insidiously. Its progress is marked by malaise, fatigue, heat intolerance, bleeding gums, purpura, skin lesions, weight loss, hyperuricemia, abdominal discomfort, and massive splenomegaly.

chronic myocarditis [Gk, *chronos,* time, *mys,* muscle, *kardia,* heart, *itis,* inflammation], an inflammatory condition of the myocardium that persists after an acute bacterial attack. Chronic myocarditis is characterized by degeneration of muscle tissue and fibrosis or infiltration of interstitial tissues.

chronic nephritis [Gk, *chronos,* time, *nephros,* kidney, *itis,* inflammation], a form of kidney inflammation usually secondary to another disease such as chronic pyelonephritis. In chronic interstitial nephritis the kidney becomes small and granular with thickening of arteries and arterioles and proliferation of interstitial tissue. There may be functional abnormalities such as urea retention, hematuria, and casts.

chronic nephropathy, a kidney disorder characterized by generalized or local damage to the tubulointerstitial areas of the kidney. The condition frequently results from more than a single cause, such as diabetes and a bacterial infection. Symptoms include polyuria, renal acidosis, edema, proteinuria, and blood in the urine.

chronic obstructive pulmonary disease (COPD), a progressive and irreversible condition characterized by diminished inspiratory and expiratory capacity of the lungs. The person complains of dyspnea with physical exertion, difficulty in inhaling or exhaling deeply, and sometimes a chronic cough.

chronic pain, pain that continues or recurs over a prolonged period, caused by various diseases or abnormal conditions such as rheumatoid arthritis. Chronic pain may be less intense than acute pain. The person with chronic pain does not usually display increased pulse and rapid respiration because these autonomic reactions to pain cannot be sustained for long periods.

chronic pancreatitis [Gk, *chronos,* time, *pan,* all, *kreas,* flesh, *itis,* inflammation], chronic inflammation of the pancreas with fibrosis and calcification of the gland. It

may follow repeated acute attacks and can lead to diabetes.

chronic peritonitis [Gk, *chronos,* time, *peri,* near, *tenein,* to stretch, *itis,* inflammation], a form of peritonitis in which the peritoneum thickens and ascites develop. The condition is usually associated with another disorder, such as pericarditis or polyserositis.

chronic pharyngitis [Gk, *chronos,* time, *pharynx,* throat, *itis,* inflammation], a form of throat inflammation that may be associated with the lymphoid granules in the pharyngeal mucosa.

chronic prostatitis [Gk, *chronos,* time, *prostates,* one standing before, *itis,* inflammation], a persistent inflammatory condition of the prostate characterized by dull, aching pain in the lower back or perineal area, dysuria, fever, and discharge from the penis.

chronic rejection, rejection of transplanted tissue caused by antibody activity that may continue for several months.

chronic rheumatism [Gk, *chronos,* time, *rheumatismos,* that which flows], a chronic nonspecific painful condition of the musculoskeletal tissues, including nonarticular forms of arthritis.

chronic synovitis [Gk, *chronos,* time, *syn,* together; L, *ovum,* egg; Gk, *itis,* inflammation], chronic inflammation of the synovial membrane of a joint.

chronic tetanus [Gk, *chronos,* time, *tetanos,* convulsive tension], **1.** a form of tetanus with a delayed onset, slow progression of the disease, and milder than usual symptoms. **2.** a reactivated tetanus infection in a healed wound.

chronic tuberculous mastitis, a rare infection of the breast resulting from extension of tuberculosis of underlying ribs.

chronic undifferentiated schizophrenia, a condition marked by the symptoms of more than one of the classic types of schizophrenia —simple, **paranoid, or catatonic.**

chronograph /kron′əgraf/ [Gk, *chronos* + *graphein,* to record], a device that records small intervals of time, such as a stopwatch. **—chronographic,** *adj.*

chronologic /kron′əloj′ik/ [Gk, *chronos* + *logos,* reason], **1.** arranged in time sequence. **2.** pertaining to chronology.

chronologic age, the age of an individual expressed as time that has elapsed since birth. The age of an infant is expressed in hours, days, or months; the age of children and adults is expressed in years.

chronopsychophysiology /kron′ōsī′kofis′-ē·ol′əjē/, the science of physiologic cyclic processes in the body.

chronotherapeutics /kron′ōther′əpyo͞o′-

tiks/, a branch of medicine concerned with effects of circadian rhythms in human health, such as the hour of the day when asthma symptoms or heart attacks are most likely to occur and the best time of day for treating certain complaints.

chronotropism /krənot'rəpiz'əm/ [Gk, *chronos* + *trepein*, to turn], the act or process of affecting the regularity of a periodic function, especially interference with the rate of heartbeat. —**chronotropic,** *adj.*

chrysarobin /kris'ərō'bin/, a substance obtained from the wood of araboa trees and used as an irritant in the treatment of parasitic skin diseases and psoriasis.

chrysiasis /krəsī'əsis/ [Gk, *chrysos,* gold, *osis,* condition], an abnormal condition that may develop after gold therapy. The condition is characterized by the deposition of gold in body tissues.

chrysotherapy /kris'ōther'əpē/ [Gk, *chrysos* + *therapeia,* treatment], the treatment of any disease with gold salts. —**chrysotherapeutic,** *adj.*

Chua K'a, a holistic counseling system of muscle tension release that emphasizes clarification and cleansing of the mind and emotions.

Churg-Strauss's syndrome /churg'strous'/, [Jacob Churg, twentieth-century American pathologist; Lotte Straus, twentieth-century American pathologist], an allergic disorder marked by granulomatosis, usually of the lungs and often involving the circulatory system.

Chvostek's sign /khvôsh'teks/ [Franz Chvostek, Austrian surgeon, 1835–1884], an abnormal spasm of the facial muscles elicited by light taps on the facial nerve in patients who are hypocalcemic. It is a sign of tetany.

chyle /kīl/ [Gk, *chylos,* juice], the cloudy liquid products of digestion taken up by the small intestine. Consisting mainly of emulsified fats, chyle passes through fingerlike projections in the small intestine. —**chylous,** *adj.*

chylemia /kīlē'mē·ə/, a condition in which chyle appears in the blood.

chylocele /kī'ləsēl/, a cystic lesion caused by an effusion of chylous fluid into the tunica vaginalis of the testes.

chyloid /kī'loid/, resembling the chyle that fills the lacteals of the small intestine during the digestion of fatty foods.

chylomediastinum /kī'lōmē'dē·astī'nəm/ [Gk, *chylos,* juice; L, *mediastinus,* midway], the presence of chyle in the mediastinum.

chylomicron /kī'lōmī'kron/ [Gk, *chylos* + *mikros,* small], minute droplets of lipoproteins measuring less than 0.5 μm in diameter. Chylomicrons consist of about 90% triglycerides with small amounts of cholesterol, phospholipids, and protein. They are synthesized in the gastrointestinal tract and carry dietary glycerides from the intestinal mucosa via the thoracic lymphatic duct into the plasma.

chylothorax /kī'lōthôr'aks/ [Gk, *chylos* + *thorax,* chest], a condition marked by the effusion of chyle from the thoracic duct into the pleural space.

chylous /kī'ləs/ [Gk, *chylos,* juice], pertaining to or resembling chyle.

chylous ascites, an abnormal condition characterized by an accumulation of chyle in the peritoneal cavity.

chyluria /kīlŏŏr'ē·ə/ [Gk, *chylos* + *ouron,* urine], a condition characterized by milky appearance of the urine caused by the presence of chyle.

chymase /kī'mās/, a serine proteinase present in human mast cells, most prominent in skin and connective tissue, where it can cleave angiotensin and stimulate mucous glands.

chyme /kīm/ [Gk, *chymos,* juice], the viscous, semifluid contents of the stomach present during digestion of a meal. Chyme then passes through the pylorus into the duodenum, where further digestion occurs.

chymopapain /kī'mōpəpā'ēn/ [Gk, *chymos* + Sp, *papaya*], a proteolytic enzyme isolated from the fruit of *Carica papaya* and related to papain.

chymotrypsin /kī'mōtrip'sin/ [Gk, *chymos* + *tryein,* to rub, *pepsin,* digestion], **1.** a proteolytic enzyme, produced by the pancreas, that catalyzes the hydrolysis of casein and gelatin. **2.** a yellow crystalline powder prepared from an extract of ox pancreas, which is used in treating digestive disorders.

chymotrypsinogen /kī'mōtripsin'əjən/, a substance, produced in the pancreas, that is the zymogen precursor to the enzyme chymotrypsin. It is converted to chymotrypsin by trypsin.

Ci, abbreviation for **curie.**

CI, abbreviation for **Colour Index.**

cibophobia /sē'bə-/ [L, *cibus,* food; Gk, *phobos,* fear], an abnormal or morbid aversion to food or eating.

CIC, abbreviation for *Certified Infection Control.*

cicatricial alopecia /sisətrish'əl/, a form of baldness produced by scar formation in dermatoses such as lupus erythematosus, usually progressing to permanent baldness.

cicatricial scar [L, *cicatrix,* scar; Gk, *eschara,* scab], a fibrous scar that remains after a wound has healed.

cicatricial stenosis [L, *cicatrix,* scar; Gk, *stenos,* narrow, *osis,* condition], the narrowing of a duct or tube caused by the formation of scar tissue.

cicatrix /sik′ətriks, sikā′triks/, *pl.* **cicatrices** /sik′ətrī′sēz/ [L, scar], scar tissue that is avascular, pale, contracted, and firm after the earlier phase of skin healing characterized by redness and softness. —**cicatricial** /sik′ətrish′əl/, *adj.* —**cicatrize,** *v.*

cicatrize /sik′ətrīz/ [L, *cicatrix,* scar], to heal so as to form a scar.

ciclopirox /sī′kləpī′roks/, an antifungal agent prescribed in the treatment of tinea and candidiasis.

cicutism /sik′yŏŏtiz′əm/ [L, *Cicuta,* hemlock; Gk, *ismos,* process], poisoning caused by water hemlock, resulting in cyanosis, dilated pupils, convulsions, and coma.

CID, abbreviation for **cytomegalic inclusion disease.**

cigarette drain [Sp, *cigarro* + AS, *dranen*], a surgical drain fashioned from a section of gauze or surgical sponge drawn into a tube of gutta-percha.

cigarette smoking, the inhalation of the gases and hydrocarbon vapors generated by slowly burning tobacco in cigarettes. The practice stems partly from the effect on the nervous system of the nicotine contained in the smoke. In addition to nicotine, nearly 1000 other chemicals have been identified in cigarette smoke.

ciguatera poisoning /sē′gwəter′ə/ [Sp, *cigua,* sea snail; L, *potio,* drink], a nonbacterial food poisoning that results from eating fish contaminated with the ciguatera toxin. Characteristics of ciguatera poisoning are vomiting, diarrhea, tingling or numbness of extremities and the skin around the mouth, itching, muscle weakness, pain, and respiratory paralysis.

cilia /sil′ē·ə/, *sing.* **cilium** [L, eyelids or eyelashes], **1.** the eyelids or eyelashes. **2.** small, hairlike processes on the outer surfaces of some cells, aiding metabolism by producing motion, eddies, or current in a fluid. —**ciliary,** *adj.*

ciliary /sil′ē·er′ē/ [L, *cilia*], pertaining to the eyelashes or eyelids.

ciliary body [L, *cilia*], the thickened part of the vascular tunic of the eye that joins the iris with the anterior part of the choroid.

ciliary canal, the spaces of the iridocorneal angle.

ciliary ganglion, a small parasympathetic ganglion in the orbit of the eye that controls pupillary and accommodative reflexes.

ciliary gland, one of the numerous tiny, modified sweat glands arranged in several rows near the free margins of the eyelids.

ciliary margin, the peripheral border of the iris, continuous with the ciliary body.

ciliary movement, the waving motion of the hairlike processes projecting from the epithelium of the respiratory tract and from certain microorganisms.

ciliary mucus transport, the movement of particles from the upper respiratory tract by means other than exhalation. It occurs particularly through the constant wave motion of microscopic cilia lining the tract and the mucous layer.

ciliary muscle, a semitransparent circular band of smooth muscle fibers attached to the choroid of the eye, the chief agent in adjustment of the eye to view near objects.

ciliary process, any one of about 80 tiny fleshy projections on the posterior surface of the iris, forming a frill around the margin of the crystalline lens of the eye.

ciliary ring, a small grooved band of tissue, about 4 mm wide, that forms the posterior part of the ciliary body of the eye.

ciliary zone, an outer circular area on the anterior surface of the iris, separated from the inner circular area by the angular line. The ciliary zone contains the stroma of the iris.

Ciliata /sil′ē·ā′tə/, a class of protozoa of the subphylum Ciliophora, characterized by cilia throughout the life cycle.

ciliate /sil′ē·it/, of or having cilia, as certain epithelial cells of the body or protozoa of the class Ciliata.

ciliated epithelium /sil′ē·ā′tid/ [L, *cilia* + Gk, *epi,* upon, *thele,* nipple], any epithelial tissue that projects cilia from its surface, such as parts of the epithelium in the respiratory tract.

ciliospinal /sil′ē·ōspī′nəl/, pertaining to a relationship between the ciliary body of the eye and the spinal cord.

ciliospinal reflex /sil′ē·ōspī′nəl/ [L, *cilia* + *spina,* backbone, *reflectere,* to bend backward], a normal brainstem reflex initiated by scratching or pinching the skin of the neck or face, causing dilation of the pupil.

cimbia /sim′bē·ə/, a girdlelike band of white fibers that extends across the surface of the cerebral peduncle.

cimetidine /simet′idēn/, a histamine H_2-receptor antagonist. It is prescribed to inhibit the production and secretion of acid in the stomach in the treatment of duodenal ulcer, pancreatitis, and hypersecretory conditions.

CIN, abbreviation for **cervical intraepithelial neoplasia.**

cinchona /singkō′nə, chinchō′nə/ [countess of Chinchon, Peru], the dried bark of the stem or root of species of *Cinchona*, containing the alkaloids quinine and quinidine.

cinchonism /sin'kōniz'əm/, a condition resulting from excessive ingestion of cinchona bark or its alkaloid derivatives. Cinchonism is characterized by hearing loss, headache, ringing in the ears, and signs of cerebral congestion.

cineangiocardiogram /sin'ē·an'jē·ōkär'-dē·əgram'/, a radiograph of the cardiovascular system obtained by special instruments that use a combination of radiographic, fluoroscopic, and motion-picture techniques.

cineangiocardiography /sin'ē·an'jē·ōkär'-dē·og'rəfē/ [Gk, *kinesis*, movement, *angeion*, vessel, *kardia*, heart, *graphein*, to record], the filming of fluorescent images of the cardiovascular system by a combination of fluoroscopic, radiographic, and motion-picture techniques.

cineangiogram /sin'ē·an'jē·əgram'/, a movie film record of a blood vessel or a part of the cardiovascular system, obtained by injecting a patient with a nontoxic radiopaque medium and filming the action of the vessels through which it courses.

cineangiograph /sin'ē·an'jē·əgraf'/, a special movie camera for recording fluorescent images of the cardiovascular system.

cine film /sin'ē/, a special type of motion picture film used in cineradiography, usually in cardiac catheterization or gastrointestinal studies.

cineradiography /sin'irā'dē·og'rəfē/ [Gk, *kinesis*, movement; L, *radiere*, to shine; Gk, *graphein*, to record], the filming with a movie camera of the images that appear on a fluorescent screen, especially those images of body structures that have been injected with a nontoxic radiopaque medium.

cingulate /sing'gyəlit/ [L, *cingulum*, girdle], **1.** having a zone or girdle, usually with transverse markings. **2.** pertaining to a cingulum.

cingulectomy /sing'gyŏŏlek'təmē/ [L, *cingulum* + Gk, *ektome*, excision], the surgical excision of a part of the cingulate gyrus in the frontal lobe of the brain and the immediately surrounding tissue.

cingulotomy /sing'gyŏŏlot'əmē/ [L, *cingulum* + *temnein*, to cut], a procedure in brain surgery to alleviate intractable pain by producing lesions in the tissue of the cingulate gyrus of the frontal lobe.

cinnamon /sin'əmən/ [Gk, *kinnamomon*], the aromatic inner bark of several species of *Cinnamomum*, a tree native to the

East Indies and China. Saigon cinnamon is commonly used as a carminative, an aromatic stimulant, and a spice. —**cinnamic**, *adj.*

CIPM, abbreviation for **Comité International des Poids et Mesures.**

circa [L, *circa*, about], approximate, as an approximate date or number.

circadian dysrhythmia /sərkā'dē·ən, sur'-kədē'ən/ [L, *circa*, about, *dies*, day; Gk, *dys*, bad, *rhythmos*], the biologic and psychologic stress effects of jet lag, or rapid travel through several time zones. In addition to a shift in normal eating and sleeping patterns, disruption of medication schedules and other therapies may occur.

circadian rhythm [L, *circa*, about, *dies*, day; Gk, *rhythmos*], a pattern based on a 24-hour cycle, especially the repetition of certain physiologic phenomena, as sleeping and eating.

circinate /sur'sināt/ [L, *circinare*, to make round], having a ring-shaped outline or formation; annular.

circle [L, *circulus*], (in anatomy) a circular or nearly circular structure of the body, as the circle of Willis and circle of Zinn. —**circular**, *adj.*

circle of least confusion, (in optics) a disk representing the image of a theoretic point made by a lens.

circle of Willis [Thomas Willis, English physician, 1621–1675], a vascular network at the base of the brain. It is formed by the interconnection of the internal carotid, anterior cerebral, posterior cerebral, basilar, anterior communicating, and posterior communicating arteries.

CircOlectric (COL) bed, trademark for an electronically controlled bed that can be vertically rotated 210 degrees and allows the patient to move vertically from the prone to supine position.

circuit /sur'kit/ [L, *circuitus*, going around], a course or pathway, particularly one through which an electric current passes. Current passes through a closed or continuous circuit and stops if the circuit is open, interrupted, or broken.

circuit training, a method of physical exercise in which activities are arranged in sets so that the participant moves quickly from one to another with a minimum of rest between sets.

circular bandage /sur'kyələr/ [L, *circularis*, round], a bandage wrapped around an injured part, usually a limb.

circular fiber, any one of the many fiber in the free gingiva that encircle the teeth

circular fold, one of the numerous annular projections in the small intestine. The vary in size and frequency and are formed by mucous and submucous tissue.

circulation /sur'kyəlā'shən/ [L, *circulatio*, to go around], movement of an object or substance through a circular course so that it returns to its starting point, such as the circulation of blood through the circuitous network of arteries and veins.

circulation rate [L, *circulatio*, to go around, *ratum*, calculation], the velocity of blood flow, usually measured in the amount of blood pumped through the heart per minute. The rate varies with such factors as blood volume and cardiac contractility.

circulation time, normal, the time required for blood to flow from one part of the body to another. Timing a particle of blood involves injecting a traceable dye or radioisotope into a vein and timing its reappearance in an artery at the point of injection.

Circulatory Care, a Nursing Interventions Classification defined as promotion of arterial and venous circulation.

Circulatory Care: Mechanical Assist Device, a Nursing Interventions Classification defined as temporary support of the circulation through the use of mechanical devices or pumps.

circulatory failure /sur'kyələtôr'ē/ [L, *circulatio* + *fallere*, to deceive], inability of the cardiovascular system to supply the cells with enough oxygenated blood to meet metabolic demands.

circulatory overload [L, *circulatio*, to go around; AS, *ofer* + ME, *lod*], an effect of increased blood volume, as by transfusion, that raises the blood pressure. The condition can lead to heart failure or pulmonary edema.

Circulatory Precautions, a Nursing Interventions Classification defined as protection of a localized area with limited perfusion.

circulatory system, the network of channels through which the nutrient fluids (blood) of the body circulate.

circulus arteriosus minor [L, circle; Gk, *arteria*, airpipe; L, less], the small artery encircling the outer circumference of the iris.

circumanal /sur'kəmā'nəl/ [L, *circum*, around, *anus*], pertaining to the area surrounding the anus.

circumcision /-sizh'ən/ [L, *circum*, around, *cadere*, to cut], a surgical procedure in which the prepuce of the penis or the prepuce of the clitoris is excised. Ritual circumcision is required by the religions of approximately one sixth of the world's population.

circumcorneal /-kôr'nē-əl/, pertaining to the area of the eye surrounding the cornea.

circumduction /sur'kəmduk'shən/ [L, *cir-cum* + *ducere*, to lead], **1.** one of the four basic movements allowed by the various joints of the skeleton. It is a combination of abduction, adduction, extension, and flexion. **2.** the circular movement of a limb or the eye.

circumference /surkum'fərens/ [L, *circum*, around, *ferre*, to bear], **1.** the perimeter or periphery of a circle. **2.** a circular plane surface of a joint.

circumferential, encircling; pertaining to a circumference or perimeter.

circumferential fibrocartilage /sərkum'-fərən'shəl/ [L, *circum* + *ferre*, to bring, *fibra*, fiber, *cartilago*], a structure made of fibrocartilage, in which fibrocartilaginous rims surround the margins of various articular cavities, as the glenoid labra of the hip and the shoulder.

circumflex /sur'kəmfleks/ [L, *circum*, around, *flexere*, to bend], pertaining to blood vessels or nerves that wind around other body structures.

circumlocution /-lōkoo'shən/, the use of pantomime or nonverbal communication or word substitution by a patient to avoid revealing that a word is difficult to say or has been forgotten.

circumoral /sur'kəmôr'əl/ [L, *circum* + *os*, mouth], pertaining to the area of the face around the mouth.

circumoral pallor [L, *circum*, around, *os*, mouth, *pallor*, paleness], paleness of the skin area around the mouth, a possible sign of scarlet fever.

circumscribed /-skrībd'/ [L, *circum*, around, *scribere*, to draw], within a well-defined area, or in one with definite boundaries or limits.

circumscribed abscess [L, *circum*, around, *scribere*, to draw, *abscedere*, to go away], an abscess separated from surrounding tissues by a wall of fibroblasts.

circum-speech [L, *circum* + AS, *spaec*], (in psychiatry) behavioral characteristics associated with conversation. The characteristics include body language, maintenance of personal space between individuals, hand sweeps, head nods, and task-oriented activities such as walking or knitting while carrying on a conversation.

circumstantiality /-stan'shē-al'ite/ [L, *circum* + *stare*, to stand], (in psychiatry) a speech pattern in which a patient has difficulty separating relevant from irrelevant information while describing an event.

circus movement, **1.** an unusual and involuntary rolling or somersaulting caused by injured neurologic mechanisms that control body posture, such as the cerebral pedicles or the vestibular apparatus. **2.** an unusual circular gait caused by injury to the brain or basal nerve centers. **3.** a mechanism associated with the excitatory wave of the atrium of the heart and atrial flutter or fibrillation.

cirrhosis /sirō'sis/ [Gk, *kirrhos*, yellow-orange, *osis*, condition], a chronic degenerative disease of the liver in which the lobes are covered with fibrous tissue, the parenchyma degenerates, and the lobules are infiltrated with fat. Gluconeogenesis, detoxification of drugs and alcohol, bilirubin metabolism, vitamin absorption, gastrointestinal function, hormonal metabolism, and other functions of the liver deteriorate. Cirrhosis is most commonly the result of chronic alcohol abuse and sometimes nutritional deprivation, hepatitis, cardiac problems, or other causes. The symptoms of cirrhosis are the same, regardless of the cause: nausea, fatigue, anorexia, weight loss, ascites, varicosities, and spider angiomas.

cis configuration /sis/, **1.** the presence of the dominant alleles of two or more pairs of genes on one chromosome and the recessive alleles on the homologous chromosome. **2.** the presence of the mutant genes of a pair of pseudoalleles on one chromosome and the wild-type genes on the homologous chromosome. **3.** (in chemistry) a form of isomerism in which two substituent groups are on the same side of a double bond.

cisplatin /sisplat'in/, an antineoplastic prescribed in the treatment of neoplasms, such as metastatic testicular, prostatic, and ovarian tumors.

cistern /sis'tərn/ [L, *cisterna*, vessel], a storage reservoir for fluids.

cisterna /sistur'nə/, *pl.* **cisternae** [L, vessel], a cavity that serves as a reservoir for lymph or other body fluids.

cisterna chyli [L, vessel, *chylos*, juice], a dilation at the beginning of the thoracic duct. It receives the two lumbar lymphatic trunks and the intestinal lymphatic trunk.

cisternal puncture /sistur'nəl/ [L, vessel, *punctura*, a piercing], the insertion of a needle into the cerebellomedullary cistern to withdraw cerebrospinal fluid for examination. The puncture is made between the atlas and the occipital bone.

cisterna subarachnoidea [L, vessel, *sub*, under; Gk, *arachne*, spider, *eidos*, form], any one of many small subarachnoid spaces that serve as reservoirs for cerebrospinal fluid.

cistron /sis'tron/ [L, *cis*, this side, *trans*, across], a fragment or part of deoxyribonucleic acid that codes for a specific polypeptide. It is the smallest unit functioning as a transmitter of genetic information. In modern molecular genetics the cis-tron is essentially synonymous with the gene. —**cistronic,** *adj.*

cisvestitism /sisves'titiz'əm/ [L, *cis*, this side, *vestis*, garment], the practice of wearing attire appropriate to the sex of the individual involved but not suitable to the age, occupation, or status of the wearer.

cit, abbreviation for *citrate carboxylate anion.*

citicoline /sit'ikō'lin/, a natural substance that is a component of cell membranes. A pharmaceutic version is used to help stroke victims by inducing injured membranes to repair themselves, limiting cell death.

citrate /sit'rāt, sī'trāt/ [L, *kitron*, citron], **1.** an anion of citric acid. **2.** the act of treating with a citrate or citric acid. —**citration,** *n.*

citric acid /sit'rik/ [Gk, *kitron*, citron; L, *acidus*, sour], a white, crystalline organic acid soluble in water and alcohol. It is extracted from citrus fruits, especially lemons and limes, or obtained by fermentation of sugars and is used as a flavoring agent in foods, carbonated beverages, and certain pharmaceutic products, especially laxatives.

citric acid cycle [Gk, *kitron*, citron; L, *acidus*, sour; Gk, *kyklos*, circle], a sequence of enzymatic reactions involving the metabolism of carbon chains of sugars, fatty acids, and amino acids to yield carbon dioxide, water, and high-energy phosphate bonds. The cycle is initiated when pyruvate combines with coenzyme A (CoA) to form a two-carbon unit, acetyl-CoA, which enters the cycle by combining with four-carbon oxaloacetic acid to form six-carbon citric acid. In subsequent steps isocitric acid, produced from citric acid, is oxidized to oxalosuccinic acid, which loses carbon dioxide to form alpha-ketoglutaric acid. Succinic acid, resulting from the oxidative decarboxylation of alpha-ketoglutaric acid, is oxidized to fumaric acid, and its oxidation regenerates oxaloacetic acid, which condenses with acetyl-CoA, closing the cycle. The citric acid cycle provides a major source of adenosine triphosphate energy.

citrin /sit'rin/ [Gk, *kitron*, citron], a crystalline flavonoid concentrate that is used as a source of bioflavonoid.

citrulline /sitrul'ēn/ [L, *Citrullus*, watermelon], an amino acid produced from ornithine during the urea cycle. It is subsequently transformed to arginine by the transfer of a nitrogen atom from aspartate

citrullinemia /-ē'mē-ə/, a disorder of amino acid metabolism caused by a deficiency of an enzyme, argininosuccinic acid synthetase. The clinical features include vomiting, convulsions, and coma.

Civilian Health and Medical Programs for Uniformed Services (CHAMPUS), a health care insurance system for military dependents and members of the military services when certain kinds of care are not available through the usual U.S. military medical service.

CJPH, abbreviation for *Canadian Journal of Public Health.*

C/kg, a unit of radiation exposure in the SI system. It represents coulombs per kilogram of air, as in the relationship, 1 roentgen (R) = 2.58×10^{-4} C/kg of air.

Cl, symbol for the element **chlorine.**

claim, (in indemnity insurance) a demand for payment for care that has been provided.

claims-made policy [L, *clamere,* to cry out; ME, *maken* + L, *politicus,* the state], a professional liability insurance policy that covers the holder for the period in which a claim of malpractice is made.

clairvoyance /klervoi'əns/, the alleged power or ability to perceive or to be aware of objects or events without the use of the physical senses.

clamp [AS, *clam,* to hold together], an instrument with serrated tips and locking handles, used for gripping, holding, joining, supporting, or compressing an organ or vessel.

clang association /klang/ [L, *clangere,* to resound, *associare,* to unite], the mental connection between dissociated ideas made because of similarity in the sounds of the words used to describe the ideas.

clap, a colloquial term for gonorrhea.

clapping [AS, *cloeppan,* to beat], (in massage) the procedure of making percussive movements on a patient's body, usually on the chest wall, by lowering the cupped palms alternately in a series of rapid, stimulating blows.

Clapton's line [Edward Clapton, English physician, 1830–1909], a greenish line at the base of the teeth, indicative of copper poisoning.

clarification /kler'ifikā'shən/ [L, *clarus,* clear, *facere,* to make], (in psychology) an intervention technique designed to guide the patient in focusing on and recognizing gaps and inconsistencies in his or her statements.

clarify /kler'əfī/, (in chemistry) to clear a turbid liquid by allowing any suspended matter to settle, by adding a substance that precipitates any suspended matter, or by heating. —**clarification,** *n.*

Clark's rule [Cecil Clark, twentieth-century British physician; L, *regula,*

model], a method of calculating the approximate pediatric dosage of a drug for a child by using this formula: weight in pounds/150 × adult dose.

clasp [ME, *clippen,* to embrace], **1.** (in dentistry) a sleevelike fitting that is fastened over a tooth to hold a partial denture in place. **2.** (in surgery) any device for holding together tissues, especially bones.

clasp-knife reflex, an abnormal sign in which a spastic limb resists passive motion and then suddenly gives way, similar to the motion of the blade of a jackknife.

clasp torsion, the twisting of a dental retentive clasp arm on its long axis of a removable partial denture.

class II biologic safety cabinet, a container that recirculates air through a high-efficiency filter. It is usually located in a hospital pharmacy and is used to prepare chemotherapeutic agents in an environment that protects personnel from exposure.

classical conditioning, a form of learning in which a previously neutral stimulus begins to elicit a given response through associative training.

classic cesarean section [L, *classicus,* first-class, *Caesar lex,* Caesar's law, *sectio,* a cutting], a method for surgically delivering a baby through a vertical midline incision of the upper segment of the uterus.

classic tomography [L, *classicus* + Gk, *tome,* section, *graphein,* to record], a method that moves the x-ray source and the x-ray plate during an exposure to produce an image in which all but a particular plane is blurred out.

classification /klas'ifikā'shən/ [L, *classis,* collection, *facere,* to make], (in research) a process in data analysis in which data are grouped according to previously determined characteristics. —**classify,** *v.*

classification of caries [L, *classis,* collection, *facere,* to make, *caries,* decay], a system of defining dental caries according to the affected part of the tooth. The system, devised by G. V. Black, defines class I caries as pits and fissures on the occlusal surfaces of molars and premolars (bicuspids), in facial and lingual surfaces of molars, and in the lingual surfaces of maxillary incisors; class II as proximal surfaces of premolars and molars, not broken through from proximal to occlusal; class III as proximal surfaces of incisors and canines, not including the incisal angles; class IV as proximal surfaces of incisors and canines that include the incisal angles; and class V as cervical one third of facial or lingual surfaces, not pits and fissures.

classification of malocclusion [L, *classis,*

collection, *mallus*, bad, *occludere*, to close up], a system developed by E. H. Angle for defining malposition and contact of the maxillary and mandibular teeth. The system: class I (neutroclusion), a normal anteroposterior relationship of the jaws. The buccal groove of the mandibular first molar occludes with the mesiobuccal cusp of the maxillary first molar. Class II (distoclusion). The buccal groove of the mandibular first molar is distal to the mesiobuccal cusp of the maxillary first permanent molar by at least the width of a premolar. Class III (mesioclusion). The buccal groove of the mandibular first molar is mesial to the mesiobuccal cusp of the maxillary first molar.

classification schemes, systems of organizing data or information, usually involving categories of items with similar characteristics. An example is the *International Classification of Diseases (ICD)* compiled by the World Health Organization (WHO), in which basic disease categories are assigned a three-digit code with optional digits for specific disease entities. Other classification schemes include that of the North American Nursing Diagnoses Association (NANDA) and the *Diagnostic and Statistical Manual of Mental Disorders (DSM)*, prepared by the American Psychiatric Association.

claudication /klô′dikā′shən/ [L, *claudicatio*, a limping], cramplike pains in the calves caused by poor circulation of the blood to the leg muscles. The condition is commonly associated with atherosclerosis.

claustrophobia /klôs′trə-/ [L, *claustrum*, a closing; Gk, *phobos*, fear], a morbid fear of being in or becoming trapped in enclosed or narrow places.

claustrum /klôs′trəm/, *pl.* **claustra** [L, a closing], **1.** a barrier, as a membrane that partially closes an aperture. **2.** a thin sheet of gray matter, composed chiefly of spindle cells, situated lateral to the external capsule of the brain and separating the internal capsule from white matter of the insula.

clavicle /klav′ikəl/ [L, *clavicula*, little key], a long, curved, horizontal bone directly above the first rib, forming the ventral part of the shoulder girdle. It articulates medially with the sternum and laterally with the acromion of the scapula and accommodates the attachment of numerous muscles.

clavicular /kləvik′yələr/, pertaining to the clavicle (collarbone).

clavicular notch [L, *clavicula* + OFr, *enochier*], one of a pair of oval depressions at the superior end of the sternum.

clawhand [AS, *clawu* + *hand*], an abnormal condition of the hand characterized by extreme flexion of the middle and distal phalanges and hyperextension of the metacarpophalangeal joints.

claw-type traction frame, an orthopedic apparatus that holds various pieces of traction equipment, such as pulleys, ropes, and the weights by which traction is applied to various parts of the body or by which various parts of the body are suspended.

clean-catch specimen, a urine specimen that is as free of bacterial contamination as possible without the use of a catheter.

cleansing enema, an enema, usually composed of soapsuds, administered to remove all formed fecal material from the colon.

clearance /klir′əns/ [L, *clarus*, clear], the removal of a substance from the blood via the kidneys. Kidney function can be tested by measuring the amount of a specific substance excreted in the urine in a given length of time.

clear cell [L, *clarus* + *cella*, storeroom], **1.** a type of cell found in the parathyroid gland that does not take on a color with the ordinary tissue stains used for microscopic examination. **2.** the principal cell of most renal cell carcinomas and occasionally of ovarian and parathyroid tumors. **3.** a specific type of epidermal cell, probably of neural origin, that has a dark-staining nucleus but clear cytoplasm with hematoxylin and eosin stain.

clear cell carcinoma, **1.** a malignant tumor of the tubular epithelium of the kidney. Characteristically the malignant cells contain abundant clear cytoplasm. **2.** an uncommon ovarian neoplasm characterized by cells with clear cytoplasm.

clearing agent, a chemical, such as ammonium thiosulfate, used in the processing of exposed x-ray film to remove unexposed and undeveloped silver halide from the emulsion.

clearing test, a range of motion test that moves the joint to its limits, stretching the capsule and other soft tissues in an attempt to reproduce symptoms. If the range of motion is normal and no symptoms are produced, the joint is cleared as a cause of a musculoskeletal disorder.

clear-liquid diet [L, *clarus* + *liquere*, to flow], a diet that supplies fluids and provides minimal fiber. The diet is nutritionally inadequate and should not be used for more than 24 hours.

cleavage /klē′vij/ [AS, *cleofan*, to split], **1.** the series of repeated mitotic cell divisions that occur in the ovum immediately after fertilization to form a mass of cells that transforms the single-celled zygote into a multicellular embryo capable of growth and differentiation. At this initial stage, as the zygote remains uniform in size, the cleavage cells, or blastomeres, become smaller with each division. **2.** the act or process of cleaving or splitting, primarily the splitting of a complex molecule into two or more simpler molecules.

cleavage fracture, any fracture that splits cartilage with the avulsion of a small piece of bone from the distal part of the lateral condyle of the humerus.

cleavage line, any one of a number of linear striations in the skin that delineate the general structural pattern and tension of the subcutaneous fibrous tissue. They correspond closely to the crease lines on the surface of the skin and are present in all areas of the body but are visible only in certain sites, as the palms of the hands and soles of the feet.

cleavage plane, 1. the area in a fertilized ovum where cleavage takes place; the axis along which any cell division occurs. **2.** any plane within the body where organs or structures can be separated with minimal damage to surrounding tissue.

cleave /klēv/ [AS, *cleofan*], segment or divide, as in cell division or the splitting of a complex molecule into simpler molecules.

cleft [ME, *clift*], **1.** divided. **2.** a fissure, especially one that originates in the embryo, such as the branchial cleft or the facial cleft.

cleft cheek, a transverse facial cleft, appearing as an abnormally large mouth. It is caused by the failure of the maxillary and mandibular processes to fuse during embryonic facial development.

cleft foot, an abnormal condition in which the division between third and fourth toes extends into the metatarsus of the foot.

cleft hand, a hand that develops in two parts because of the failure of a digit and metacarpal to form normally during embryonic development.

cleft jaw, an abnormal jaw resulting from failure of the left and right mandibles to fuse properly during embryonic development.

cleft lip, a congenital anomaly consisting of one or more clefts in the upper lip that result from the failure in the embryo of the maxillary and median nasal processes to close.

cleft-lip repair, the surgical correction of a unilateral or bilateral congenital interruption of the upper lip, usually resulting from the embryologic failure of the me-

dian nasal and maxillary processes to unite.

cleft palate, a congenital defect characterized by a fissure in the midline of the palate, resulting from the failure of the two sides to fuse during embryonic development. The fissure may be complete, extending through both the hard and soft palates into the nasal cavities, or it may show any degree of incomplete or partial cleft.

cleft-palate repair, the surgical correction of a congenital fissure in the midline of the partition separating the oral and nasal cavities. Palatine clefts range from a simple separation in the uvula to an extensive fissure involving the soft and hard palates and extending forward unilaterally or bilaterally through the alveolar ridge. A cleft lip often accompanies a cleft palate. Repair of a cleft palate is usually undertaken in the child's second year.

cleft sternum, a fissure in the sternum caused by a failure in embryonic development.

cleft tongue [ME, *clift* + AS, *tunge*], a tongue divided by a longitudinal fissure.

cleft uvula, an abnormal congenital condition in which the uvula is split into halves as a result of the failure of the posterior palatine folds to unite.

cleidocranial dysostosis /klē′dōkrā′nē·əl/ [Gk, *kleis*, key, *kranion*, skull, *dys*, bad, *osteon*, bone], a rare abnormal hereditary condition characterized by defective ossification of the cranial bones and by the complete or partial absence of the clavicles. The defective ossification of the cranial bones delays the closing of the cranial sutures and produces large fontanels.

clemastine /klemas′tēn/, an antihistaminic agent prescribed in the treatment of symptoms of allergic rhinitis, pruritus, or lacrimation.

click [Fr, *cliquer*, to clash], (in cardiology) an extra heart sound that occurs during systole.

client /klī′ənt/ [L, *clinare*, to lean], **1.** a person who is recipient of a professional service. **2.** a recipient of health care, regardless of the state of health. **3.** a recipient of health care who is not ill or hospitalized. **4.** a patient.

client-centered therapy, a nondirective method of group or individual psychotherapy, originated by Carl Rogers, in which the therapist's role is to listen to and then reflect or restate without judgment or interpretation the words of the client.

client/server system, a computer configuration in which the workload is divided between a client computer and a server, as might be used in a health care management plan.

climate /klī′mit/ [Gk, *klima,* inclination], a composite of the prevailing weather conditions that characterize any particular geographic region. **—climatic,** *adj.*

climax /klī′maks/ [Gk, *klimax,* ladder], a peak of intensity, such as a sexual orgasm or the high point of a fever.

climbing fiber [ME, *climben* + L, *fibra*], a type of nerve fiber that carries impulses to the Purkinje cells of the cerebellar cortex.

clindamycin hydrochloride /klin′dəmī′sin/, an antibacterial prescribed in the treatment of certain serious infections (including anaerobic and some gram-positive organisms).

clinic [Gk, *kline,* bed], **1.** a department in a hospital where persons who do not require hospitalization may receive medical care. **2.** a group practice of doctors. **3.** a meeting place for doctors and medical students where instruction can be given at the bedside of a patient or in a similar setting. **4.** a seminar or other scientific medical meeting. **5.** a detailed published report of the diagnosis and treatment of a health care problem.

clinical /klin′ikəl/ [Gk, *kline,* bed], **1.** pertaining to a clinic. **2.** pertaining to direct bedside medical care. **3.** pertaining to materials or equipment used in the care of a sick person.

clinical analysis, the use of laboratory data, including blood tests, urinalysis, and microscopic tissue studies, in determining a diagnosis and treatment regimen.

clinical assessment, an evaluation of a patient's physical condition and prognosis based on information gathered from physical and laboratory examinations and the patient's medical history.

clinical crown, 1. the part of a tooth that is covered by enamel and visible in the mouth. **2.** the part of a tooth that is occlusal to the deepest part of the gingival crevice.

clinical-crown/clinical-root ratio, the proportion between the length of the part of the teeth lying coronal to the epithelial attachment and the length of the part of the root lying apical to the epithelial attachment. The ratio is useful in the diagnosis and prognosis of periodontal disease.

clinical cytogenetics, the branch of genetics that studies the relationship between chromosomal abnormalities in cells and pathologic conditions.

clinical diagnosis, a diagnosis made on the basis of knowledge obtained by medical history and physical examination

alone, without benefit of laboratory tests or x-ray films.

clinical disease, a stage in the history of a pathologic condition that begins with anatomic or physiologic changes that are sufficient to produce recognizable signs and symptoms of a disease.

clinical epidemiology, the application of the science of epidemiology in a clinical setting. Emphasis is on a medically defined population, as opposed to statistically formulated disease trends derived from examination of larger population categories.

clinical genetics, a branch of genetics that studies inherited disorders and investigates the possible genetic factors that may influence the occurrence of any pathologic condition.

clinical horizon, the imaginary line above which detectable signs and symptoms of a disease first begin to appear.

clinical humidity therapy, respiratory therapy in which water is added to the therapeutic gases to make breathing them more comfortable.

clinical judgment, the application of information based on actual observation of a patient, combined with laboratory findings and the health care workers' training and experience in determining a diagnosis.

clinical laboratory, a laboratory in which tests directly related to the care of patients are performed.

clinical medicine, a system of health maintenance based on direct observation of and communication with a patient.

clinical nurse specialist (CNS), a registered nurse who holds a master's degree in nursing and who has acquired advanced knowledge and clinical skills in a specific area of nursing practice.

clinical-pathologic conference, a teaching conference in which a case is presented to a clinician, who then demonstrates the process of reasoning that leads to his or her diagnosis. A pathologist then presents an anatomic diagnosis, based on the study of tissue removed at surgery or obtained in autopsy.

clinical pathology, the laboratory study of disease by a pathologist using techniques appropriate to the specimen being studied.

clinical pathway, a description of practices likely to result in favorable outcomes for a particular diagnosis that uses prospectively defined resources to minimize cost. It may be based on research, literature, or common practice.

clinical pelvimetry, a process used to assess the size of the birth canal by means of the systematic vaginal palpation of specific bony landmarks in the pelvis and an estimation of the distances between them. Findings are commonly recorded in terms such as adequate, borderline, or inadequate, rather than in centimeters or inches.

clinical psychology, the branch of psychology concerned with the diagnosis, treatment, and prevention of a wide range of personality and behavioral disorders.

clinical research center, an organization, often associated with a medical school or a teaching hospital, that studies, analyzes, correlates, and describes medical cases. Such centers usually have extensive laboratory facilities and specialized staffs of physicians and medical technicians.

clinical specialist, a physician or nurse who has advanced training in a particular field of practice, as a nurse-midwife, pediatrician, or radiologist.

clinical thermometer [Gk, *kline*, bed, *therme*, heat, *metron*, measure], a thermometer designed for measuring body temperature.

clinical thermometry, a method for determining temperature in heated tissue.

clinical trial exemption (CTX), authorization to administer an investigational agent to patients or volunteer subjects under specified conditions of a particular research study in a clinical setting.

clinical trials, organized studies to provide large bodies of clinical data for statistically valid evaluation of treatment.

clinician /klinish'ən/, a health professional whose practice is based on direct observation and treatment of a patient, as distinguished from other types of health workers, such as laboratory technicians and those employed in research.

clinic without walls, a health care system formed by the merger of selected functions, such as administrative, billing and collections, purchasing, personnel, and payroll of various physician groups, without the merger of any physical facilities. The physician practices remain geographically separate, thus offering shared services at lower cost over a wider geographic area.

clinocephaly /klī'nōsef'əlē/ [Gk, *klinein*, to bend, *kephale*, head], a congenital anomaly of the head in which the upper surface of the skull is saddle shaped or concave. —**clinocephalic, clinocephalous,** *adj.*

clinodactyly /klī'nōdak'təlē/ [Gk, *klinein* + *daktylos*, finger], a congenital anomaly characterized by abnormal lateral or medial bending of one or more fingers or toes. —**clinodactylic, clinodactylous,** *adj.*

clinoid processes /klī'noid/ [Gk, *kline*, bed, *eidos*, form; L, *processus*], the anterior, middle, and posterior processes of the sphenoid bone at the base of the skull.

clinometer /klīnom'ətər/, an instrument used to measure angular convergence of the eyes or the degree of paralysis of extraocular muscles.

clip [AS, *clyppan*, to embrace], a surgical device used for grasping the skin to align the edges of a wound and to stop bleeding, especially of the smaller blood vessels. It is also used in radiography for localization.

clitoridectomy /klit'əridek'təmē/, the excising of all or part of the clitoris, and sometimes part of the labia, a form of ritual mutilation performed on over 100 million girls and women in more than 40 countries. It is usually performed at 4 to 12 years of age, without anesthesia, with crude cutting tools, and with few or no precautions against infection. The reasons for this ancient practice are very complex, including the male desire to control female sexuality. As of June 1996, the U.S. Board of Immigration Appeals recognized genital mutilation as a form of persecution and a basis for asylum for girls and women.

clitoridotomy, an incision into the clitoris.

clitoris /klit'əris/ [Gk, *kleitoris*], the vaginal erectile structure homologous to the corpora cavernosa of the penis. It consists of two corpora cavernosa within a dense layer of fibrous membrane, joined along their inner surfaces by an incomplete fibrous septum.

clitoritis /klit'ôrī'tis/, inflammation of the clitoris.

clivus /klī'vəs/ [L, slope], an inclined surface, as on the sphenoid bone.

CLL, abbreviation for **chronic lymphocytic leukemia.**

cloaca /klō·ā'kə/, *pl.* **cloacae** [L, sewer], **1.** (in embryology) the end of the hindgut before the developmental division into the rectum, the bladder, and the primitive genital structures. **2.** (in pathology) an opening into the sheath of tissue around a necrotic bone.

cloacal membrane /klō·ā'kəl/, a thin sheath that separates the internal and external parts of the cloaca in the developing embryo.

clobetasol propionate /klōbet'əsol prō'-pyōnāt/, a topical corticosteroid prescribed for the short-term treatment of inflammation and pruritus associated with certain moderate to severe types of dermatitis.

clocortolone pivalate /klōkôr'təlōn piv'-

əlāt/, a topical corticosteroid used as an antiinflammatory agent.

clofibrate /klō'fəbrāt/, an antihyperlipoproteinemic prescribed in the treatment of high blood levels of cholesterol, triglycerides, or both.

clomiphene citrate /klō'məfēn/, a nonsteroidal antiestrogen that acts to stimulate ovulation. It is prescribed principally in the treatment of anovulation and oligoovulation in women.

clomiphene stimulation test, a test used to evaluate gonadal function in males who show signs of abnormal pubertal development. Clomiphene, a nonsteroidal analog of estrogen, stimulates the hypothalamic-pituitary system to raise follicle-stimulating hormone and luteinizing hormone levels of the blood.

clonal /klō'nəl/, pertaining to a clone.

clonal marker, a defective or functionally unidentified sequence of deoxyribonucleic acid in a clone of cancer cells. Such sequences are used to monitor the growth of cancer cells after chemical or other treatments.

clonazepam /klōnaz'əpam/, a benzodiazepine anticonvulsant prescribed in the prevention of seizures in petit mal epilepsy and other convulsive disorders.

clone [Gk, klon, a plant cutting], a group of genetically identical cells or organisms derived from a single common cell or organism through mitosis.

clonic /klon'ik/ [Gk, klonos, tumult], pertaining to increased reflex activity, as in upper motor neuron lesions when repetitive muscular contractions and relaxations in rapid succession are induced by stretching.

clonic convulsion [Gk, klonos, tumult; L, convulsio, cramp], a form of convulsion characterized by rhythmic alternate involuntary contraction and relaxation of muscle groups.

clonicity /klōnis'itē, a state of clonus.

clonic spasm [Gk, klonos, tumult, spasmos], involuntary alternating contractions and relaxations of muscles.

clonidine hydrochloride /klō'nədēn/, an antihypertensive prescribed for the reduction of high blood pressure.

cloning /klō'ning/, a procedure for producing multiple copies of genetically identical organisms or of individual genes. Organisms may be cloned by transplanting blastocysts from one embryo into an empty zona pellucida or nuclei from the cells of one individual into enucleated oocytes. Genes may be cloned by isolating them from the genome of one organism and incorporating them into the genome of an asexually reproducing organism such as a bacterium or a yeast.

clonogenic cell /klō'nōjen'ik/, a cell that can proliferate into a colony of genetically identical cells.

clonorchiasis /klō'nôrkī'əsis/, an infestation of liver flukes.

Clonorchis sinensis /klōnôr'kis sinen'sis/, the Chinese or Oriental liver fluke, a form of trematode that is acquired by humans who eat raw or imperfectly cooked fish that is the intermediate host of the parasite.

clonus /klō'nəs/ [Gk, klonos, tumult], an abnormal pattern of neuromuscular activity, characterized by rapidly alternating involuntary contraction and relaxation of skeletal muscle. **—clonic,** adj.

C-loop, a surgically formed loop of bowel with a C-shape.

clor, abbreviation for a chloride noncarboxylate anion.

clorazepate dipotassium /klôraz'əpāt dī-/, a benzodiazepine tranquilizer prescribed in the treatment of anxiety, nervous tension, and alcohol withdrawal.

closed amputation [L, claudere, to shut, amputare, to cut away], a kind of amputation in which one or two broad flaps of muscular and cutaneous tissue are retained to form a cover over the end of the bone. It is performed only when no infection is present.

closed bite [L, claudere + AS, bitan], a decrease in the occlusal vertical dimension produced by various factors such as tooth abrasion and insufficient eruption of supportive posterior teeth.

closed-chain, (in organic chemistry) pertaining to a compound in which the carbon atoms are bonded to form a closed ring.

closed-chain exercise, exercise in which the distal aspect of the extremity is in contact with a support surface such as the floor or a balance board.

closed-circuit breathing, any breathing system in which a contained gas mixture is rebreathed, either directly or after recirculation through a water or carbon dioxide absorbing unit. An example is a spirometer.

closed-circuit helium dilution, a technique for measuring residual lung volume and functional residual capacity in which a patient breathes through a spirometer containing a known concentration of helium.

closed dislocation [L, claudere, to shut, dis, apart, locare, to place], a dislocation not accompanied by a skin break at the joint.

closed fracture [L, claudere, to shut, fractura], a bone fracture not accompanied by a break in the skin.

closed group, a group in which all members are admitted at the same time and vacancies that occur in the membership are not filled.

closed loop, a biologic feedback system in which a substance produced affects its own output.

closed-panel HMO, (in the United States) a health maintenance organization in which physicians have few if any private patients.

closed physician-hospital organization (PHO), (in the United States) an organization of selected physicians on a hospital medical staff who have proved to be high-quality, cost-effective practitioners.

closed reduction of fractures [L, *claudere*, to shut, *reducere*, to lead back, *fractura*], the manual reduction of a fracture without incision.

closed system, a system that does not interact with its environment.

closed-system helium dilution method, a technique for measuring functional residual capacity and residual volume.

closed-wound suction, any one of several techniques for draining potentially harmful fluids such as blood, pus, serosanguineous fluid, and tissue secretions from surgical wounds. The technique is used as an aid to many operations such as mastectomies, augmentations, plastic and reconstructive procedures, and urologic and urogenital procedures. Closed-wound suction devices usually consist of disposable transparent containers attached to suction tubes and portable suction pumps.

closing capacity (CC), (in respiratory therapy) the sum of the closing volume and the residual volume of gas in the lungs.

closing volume (CV), the volume of gas remaining in the lungs when the small airways begin to close during a controlled maximum exhalation.

clostridial /klostrid'ē·əl/ [Gk, *kloster*, spindle], pertaining to anaerobic spore-forming bacteria of the genus *Clostridium*.

Clostridium /-ē·əm/ [Gk, *kloster*, spindle], a genus of spore-forming anaerobic bacteria of the Bacillaceae family involved in gas gangrene, botulism, food poisoning, cellulitis, wound infections, and tetanus.

Clostridium botulinum [Gk, *kloster*, spindle], a species of anaerobic bacteria that cause botulism in humans and botulism-like diseases in other animals. Botulinus food poisoning results from ingesting food containing preformed toxins produced by the species. It is a proteolytic pathogen commonly present in soil, where its endospores can survive for years. Their resistance to heat makes them an impor-

tant source of poisoning in improperly cooked or canned foods.

Clostridium difficile, /difis'ilē/ a pathogenic species of anaerobic bacteria found in the feces of newborns. The strain is a cause of colitis and diarrhea, particularly after the patient has received antibiotic therapy, and is a frequent cause of nosocomial diarrhea.

Clostridium perfringens [Gk, *kloster*, spindle], a species of anaerobic gram-positive bacteria capable of causing gas gangrene in humans and various digestive and urinary tract diseases in livestock.

closure /klō'zhər/ [L, *claudere*, to shut], **1.** the surgical closing of a wound by suture or staple. **2.** a visual phenomenon in which the mind sees an entire figure when only a part is actually visible.

closylate /klos'ilāt/, a contraction for *p*-chlorobenzenesulfonate.

clot retraction, the shrinking of a semisolid mass formed by coagulation of blood, lymph, or other fluid. The rate of retraction of a normal standing blood clot is about 24 hours, depending on such factors as the number of platelets in the clot.

clotrimazole /klōtrim'əzōl/, a broad-spectrum antifungal agent of the imidazole group used in topical applications to treat fungal and yeast infections.

clotting time [AS, *clott*], the time required for blood to form a clot, tested by collecting 4 ml of blood in a glass tube and examining it for clot formation.

cloud baby [AS, *clud* + *babe*], a newborn who appears well and healthy but is a carrier of infectious bacterial or viral organisms. The infant may contaminate the surrounding environment as airborne droplets from the respiratory tract form clouds of the organisms.

clouding of consciousness, a mental state in which a patient is confused about or is not fully aware of the immediate surroundings.

clove /klōv/ [L, *clavus*, nail], the dried flower bud of *Eugenia caryophyllata*. It contains the lactone caryophyllin and a volatile oil used as a dental analgesic, a germicide, and a salve.

clove-hitch sling, a bandage that begins with a clove-hitch knot at the center. The loop made is fitted to the hand. The two loose ends are extended over and behind the shoulders and tied beside the neck.

cloverleaf nail /klō'vərlēf'/ [AS, *clafre* + *leaf* + *nagel*], a surgical nail shaped in cross section like a cloverleaf, used especially in the repair of fractures of the femur.

cloverleaf skull deformity, a congenital defect characterized by a trilobed skull resulting from the premature closure of multiple cranial sutures during embryonic development.

cloxacillin sodium /klok'səsil'in/, an antibacterial prescribed in the treatment of serious infections, primarily those caused by penicillin-resistant strains of staphylococci.

clubbed penis, [ME, *clubbe* + L, *penis*], a penis that is curved or twisted or both. The abnormality may be accompanied by epispadias or hypospadias.

clubbing [ME, *clubbe*], an abnormal enlargement of the distal phalanges. It usually is associated with cyanotic heart disease or advanced chronic pulmonary disease but sometimes occurs with biliary cirrhosis, colitis, chronic dysentery, and thyrotoxicosis. Clubbing occurs in all the digits but is most easily seen in the fingers.

clubfoot [ME, *clubbe* + AS, *fot*], a congenital deformity of the foot, sometimes resulting from intrauterine constriction and characterized by unilateral or bilateral deviation of the metatarsal bones of the forefoot. Ninety-five percent of clubfoot deformities are equinovarus, characterized by medial deviation and plantar flexion of the forefoot, but a few are calcaneovalgus, or calcaneovarus, characterized by lateral deviation and dorsiflexion either outward from or inward toward the midline of the body.

club hair, a hair in the resting or final stage of the growth cycle.

cluster analysis [AS, *clyster*, growing together; Gk, *analyein*, to loosen], (in statistics) a complex technique of data analysis of numeric scale scores that produces clusters of variables related to one another. The technique is performed with a computer.

cluster breathing, a breathing pattern in which a closely grouped series of respirations is followed by apnea. The activity is associated with a lesion in the lower pontine region of the brainstem.

cluster headache, a migrainelike condition characterized by attacks of intense pain that is unilateral in nature. The pain occurs most often over the eye and forehead. It is accompanied by flushing and watering of the eyes and nose. The attacks occur in groups with a duration of several hours.

cluster-of-differentiation (CD) antigen, one of a group of cell membrane molecules that are used to classify leukocytes into subsets.

cluttering [ME, *clotter*], a speech defect characterized by a rapid, confused, nervous delivery with uneven rhythmic patterns and omission or transposition of various letters or syllables.

clysis /klī'sis/ [Gk, *klyster*, washout], the nonoral insertion or injection of a fluid into the body, such as the administration of an enema..

cm, abbreviation for **centimeter.**

Cm, symbol for the element **curium.**

cm², abbreviation for **square centimeter.**

cm³, abbreviation for **cubic centimeter.**

CMA, abbreviation for *Canadian Medical Association.*

CMAJ, abbreviation for *Canadian Medical Association Journal.*

CMC, abbreviation for **carpometacarpal.**

CMF, an anticancer drug combination of cyclophosphamide, methotrexate, and flurorouracil.

CMHC, abbreviation for **community mental health center.**

CML, abbreviation for **chronic myelocytic leukemia.**

cmm, c mm, cu mm, mm³, abbreviation for **cubic millimeter.**

CMRNG, abbreviation for *chromosomally mediated resistant Neisseria gonorrhoeae.*

CMT, abbreviation for *Certified Medical Transcriptionist.*

CMV, abbreviation for **cytomegalovirus.**

CNA, 1. abbreviation for **Canadian Nurses Association.** 2. abbreviation for certified nurse administrator.

CNAA, abbreviation for certified nurse administrator, advanced.

CNATS, abbreviation for **Canadian Nurses Association Testing Service.**

CNF, abbreviation for **Canadian Nurses Foundation.**

CNHV, abbreviation for **central neurogenic hyperventilation.**

Cnidaria, a phylum of marine animals that includes jellyfish, sea anemones, hydroids, and corals.

CNM, abbreviation for **Certified Nurse-Midwife.**

CNOR, abbreviation for *Certified Nurse, Operating Room.*

CNP, abbreviation for **community nurse practitioner.**

CNRN, abbreviation for *Certified Neuroscience Registered Nurse.*

CNRS, abbreviation for **Canadian Nurses Respiratory Society.**

CNS, 1. abbreviation for **central nervous system.** 2. abbreviation for **Clinical Nurse Specialist.**

CNSN, abbreviation for *Certified Nutrition Support Nurse.*

CNS sympathomimetic, a drug, such as cocaine or an amphetamine, whose effect mimic those of sympathetic nervous system stimulation.

Co, symbol for the element **cobalt.**

CO, 1. formula for **carbon monoxide. 2.** abbreviation for **cardiac output.**

CoA, abbreviation for **coenzyme A.**

CO₂, formula for **carbon dioxide.**

coagglutination /kō′əglōō′tənā′shən/ [L, *cum* + *agglutinare,* to glue], a clumping of red blood cells by mixtures of protein antigens and their antisera.

coagulability /kō·ag′yələbil′itē/ [L, *coagulare,* to curdle], the state of being able to coagulate or form blood clots.

coagulant /kō·ag′yələnt/ [L, *coagulare,* to curdle], an agent that causes a coagulum, or blood clot, to form.

coagulase /kō·ag′yəlās/ [L, *coagulare,* to curdle], an enzyme produced by bacteria, particularly *Staphylococcus aureus,* that promotes the formation of fibrin from fibrinogen to form thrombi.

coagulate /kō·ag′yəlāt/, to undergo or cause to undergo the chemical process whereby a fluid becomes curdled or clotted.

coagulated /kō·ag′yəlā′tid /, curdled; changed to a clotted state.

coagulation /kō·ag′yəlā′shən/ [L, *coagulare,* to curdle], **1.** the process of transforming a liquid into a solid, especially of the blood. **2.** (in colloid chemistry) the transforming of the liquid dispersion medium into a gelatinous mass. **3.** the hardening of tissue by some physical means, as by electrocoagulation or photocoagulation.

coagulation current, an electric current delivered by a needle ball or variously shaped points to bind tissues together.

coagulation factor, one of the factors in the blood, the interactions of which are responsible for the process of blood clotting. The factors, using standardized numeric nomenclature, are factor I, fibrinogen; factor II, prothrombin; factor III, tissue thromboplastin; factor IV, calcium ions; factors V and VI, proaccelerin or labile factor; factor VII, proconvertin or stable factor; factor VIII, antihemophilic globulin; factor IX, plasma thromboplastin component (PTC); factor X, Stuart-Power factor; factor XI, plasma thromboplastin antecedent (PTA); factor XII, Hageman factor or glass factor or contact factor; factor XIII, fibrin-stabilizing factor or fibrinase or Laki-Lorand factor.

coagulative /kō·ag′yəlā′tiv/, **1.** causing blood clot formation. **2.** an agent that assists the transformation of blood clots.

coagulopathy /kō·ag′yəlop′əthē/, a pathologic condition that affects the ability of the blood to coagulate.

coalesce /kō′əles′/ [L, *coalescere,* to grow together], to grow together.

coal tar, a topical antieczematic prescribed in the treatment of chronic skin diseases such as eczema and psoriasis.

Coanda effect, a phenomenon of fluid movement similar to the Bernoulli effect in which passage of a stream of gas next to a wall results in a pocket of turbulence between the wall and the gas flow. The turbulence forms a low-pressure bubble that makes the gas stream adhere to the wall. The principle is used in fluidic ventilators.

coaptation splint /kō′aptā′shən/ [L, *coaptare,* to fit together; ME *splinte*], a small splint fitted to a fractured limb to prevent overriding of the fragments of bone.

coarct /kō·ärkt′/ [L, *coarctare,* to press together], the act of narrowing or constricting, especially the lumen of a blood vessel.

coarctate retina /kō·ärk′tāt/ [L, *coartare,* to press together, *rete,* net], a funnel-shaped retina caused by a leakage of fluid between the retina and the choroid.

coarctation /kō′ärktā′shən/, a stricture or contraction of the walls of a vessel such as the aorta.

coarctation of the aorta, a congenital cardiac anomaly characterized by a localized narrowing of the aorta. It results in increased pressure proximal to the defect and decreased pressure distal to it. Symptoms of the condition are directly related to the pressure changes created by the constriction. Clinical manifestations include dizziness, headaches, fainting, epistaxis, reduced or absent femoral pulses, and muscle cramps in the legs from tissue anoxia during increased exercise.

coarse /kôrs/ [ME, *cors,* common], (in physiology) involving a wide range of movements, such as those associated with tremors and other involuntary motions of the skeletal muscle.

coarse crackle [ME, *cors,* common, *krakelen*], an abnormal breathing sound caused by air moving through an excessive amount of fluid in an airway, as in pulmonary edema.

coarse fremitus, a rough, loud, tremulous vibration of the chest wall noted on palpation of the chest during a physical examination as the person inhales and exhales.

coarse tremor [ME, *cors,* common; L, *tremor,* shaking], a tremor in which the movements are relatively slow and may involve larger muscle groups.

coat [ME, *cote*], **1.** a membrane that covers the outside of an organ or part. **2.** one of the layers of a wall of an organ or part, especially a canal or vessel.

coated tablet [ME, *cote* + Fr, *tablette*], a solid disc of one or more pharmaceutical agents coated with sugar or a flavoring to mask the taste or by a substance that resists dissolution in the stomach but allows release of the medication in the intestine.

coated tongue [ME, *cote* + AS, *tunge*], a tongue with a white, yellow, or brown furred surface, representing a possible accumulation of mycelia, bacteria, food debris, or desquamated epithelial cells. There are many possible causes, ranging from a fungal infection to sleeping with the mouth open.

cobalamin /kōbōl′əmin/ [Ger, *kobold*, mine goblin], a generic term for a chemical part of the vitamin B_{12} group.

cobalt (CO) /kō′bôlt/ [Ger, *kobold*, mine goblin], a metallic element that occurs in the minerals cobaltite, smaltite, and linnaeite. Its atomic number is 27; its atomic weight (mass) is 58.9. Cobalt is a component of vitamin B_{12}, is found in most common foods, and is readily absorbed by the gastrointestinal tract. This element is common in the human diet, but the precise daily intake requirement is not known, and cobalt deficiency in humans has not been seen. Some amounts of cobalt stimulate the production of erythropoietin, but large doses depress erythrocyte production.

cobalt-60 (^{60}Co), (in radiotherapy) a radioactive isotope of the silver-white metallic element cobalt with a mass number of 60 and a half-life of 5.2 years. ^{60}Co emits high-energy gamma rays and is the most frequently used radioisotope in radiotherapy.

COBRA /kō′brə/, abbreviation for **Consolidated Omnibus Reconciliation Act.**

cobra venom solution [L, *colubra*, snake, *venenum*, venom, *solutus*, dissolved], a sterile physiologic salt solution containing minute amounts of cobralysin, the hemolytic substance in cobra venom.

coca, a species of South American shrubs native to Bolivia and Peru and cultivated in Indonesia. It is a natural source of cocaine.

cocaine baby /kōkān′/, an infant with birth defects caused by exposure to cocaine in utero.

cocaine hydrochloride, a white crystalline powder used as a local anesthetic. It was originally derived from coca leaves but can also be prepared synthetically. Cocaine is a Schedule II drug under the Controlled Substances Act of 1970. In solution the drug is sometimes used as a topical anesthetic applied to mucous membranes. Its vasoconstrictive action slows bleeding and limits absorption. Prolonged or frequent use may damage the mucous membranes.

cocaine hydrochloride poisoning [Sp, *coca* + *HCl* + L, *potio*, drink], toxic effects of exposure to the colorless crystalline alkaloid derived from coca leaves. Although used as a local analgesic for a century, cocaine is highly toxic with moderate vasoconstrictor activity and serious psychotropic effects. Symptoms include nervous excitement, restlessness, incoherent speech, fever, hypertension, and cardiac arrhythmias, leading to convulsions, collapse, respiratory arrest, and death. The euphoric effect of cocaine lasts about 30 minutes.

cocarcinogen /kōkär′sənəjən/ [L, *cum*, together with; Gk, *karkinos*, crab, *genein*, to produce], an agent that alone does not transform a normal cell into a cancerous state but in concert with another agent can effect the transformation.

Coccidia, a subclass of parasitic protozoa found in humans and other vertebrates and also some invertebrates. Among species of Coccidia pathogenic to humans is *Cyclospora cayatanensis.*

coccidian, pertaining to *Coccidia.*

coccidioidomycosis /koksid′ē·oi′dōmīkō′sis/ [Gk, *kokkos*, berry, *eidos*, form, *mykes*, fungus, *osis*, condition], an infectious fungal disease caused by the inhalation of spores of the bacterium *Coccidioides immitis*, which is carried on windborne dust particles. The disease is endemic in hot, dry regions of the southwestern United States and Central and South America. It is an opportunistic disease associated with human immunodeficiency virus infection. Primary infection is characterized by symptoms resembling those of the common cold or influenza. Secondary infection, occurring after a period of remission, is marked by low-grade fever, anorexia and weight loss, cyanosis, dyspnea, hemoptysis, focal skin lesions resembling erythema nodosum, and arthritic pain in the bones and joints.

coccidiosis /kok′sidē·ō′sis/ [Gk, *kokkos* + *osis*, condition], a parasitic disease of tropical and subtropical regions caused by the ingestion of oocysts of the protozoon *Isospora belli* or *I. hominis.* Symptoms include fever, malaise, abdominal discomfort, and watery diarrhea.

coccoid /kok′oid/ [Gk, *kokkos*, berry, *eidos*, form], having a spheric shape.

coccus /kok′əs/, *pl.* **cocci** /kok′sī, kok′ī/ [Gk, *kokkos*, berry], a bacterium that is round, spheric, or oval, as gonococcus, pneumococcus, staphylococcus, streptococcus. —**coccal**, *adj.*

coccyalgia /kok′si·al′jə/, a pain in or near the coccyx.

coccygeal body /koksij'ē·əl/ [Gk, *kokkyx,* cuckoo's beak; AS, *bodig*],   the coccyx.

coccygeal vertebra, one of the four segments of the vertebral column that fuse to form the adult coccyx. They are considered rudimentary vertebrae and have no pedicles, laminae, or spinous processes.

coccygeus /koksij'ē·əs/ [Gk, *kokkyx,* cuckoo's beak], one of two muscles in the pelvic diaphragm. Stretching across the pelvic cavity like a hammock, it is a triangular sheet of muscle and tendinous fibers. It acts to draw the coccyx ventrally, helping to support the pelvic floor.

coccygodynia /kok'sigōdin'ē·ə/, a pain in the coccygeal area.

coccyx /kok'siks/, *pl.* **coccyges** /koksī'jēz, kok'sijēz/ [Gk, *kokkyx,* cuckoo's beak], the beaklike bone joined to the sacrum by a disk of fibrocartilage at the base of the vertebral column. It is formed by the union of three to five probably vestigial rudimentary vertebrae. —**coccygeal** /koksij'ē·əl/, *adj.*

cochineal /koch'inēl'/ [L, *coccineus,* bright red], a red dye prepared from the dried female insects of the species *Coccus cacti* containing young larvae. During the preparation of the dye the larvae are extracted with an aqueous solution of alum, and the resulting dye has been used in coloring medicines.

cochlea /kok'lē·ə/ [L, snail shell], a conic bony structure of the inner ear, perforated by numerous apertures for passage of the cochlear division of the vestibulocochlear nerve. Part of the osseous labyrinth, it is a spiral tunnel about 30 mm long with two full and three quarter turns, resembling a tiny snail shell. —**cochlear,** *adj.*

cochlear canal /kok'lē·ər/, [L *cochlea* + *canalis* channel], a bony spiral tunnel within the cochlea of the internal ear. It contains one opening that communicates with the tympanic cavity, a second that connects with the vestibule, and a third that leads to a tiny canal opening on the inferior surface of the temporal bone.

cochlear implant, an electronic device that is surgically implanted into the cochlea of a deaf individual. It may be implanted in the middle ear, the cochlear window, or the inner ear. Although the implant does not transmit speech clearly, it allows the individual to be aware of sounds that would not otherwise be audible to him or her and to use those sounds along with other environmental cues to improve communication.

cochlear nerve [L, *cochlea,* snail shell, *nervus,* nerve], one of the main divisions of the eighth cranial nerve, with fibers that arise in spiral ganglion cells of the spiral

organ and terminate in the dorsal and ventral cochlear nuclei of the brainstem.

cochlear toxicity, poisonous effects of drugs that may result in hearing disorders such as sensorineural hearing loss and tinnitus.

cochleovestibular /kok'lē-ō'westib'yələr/, pertaining to the cochlea and vestibule of the ear.

cockroach, the common name of members of the Blattidae family of insects that infest homes, workplaces, and other areas inhabited by humans. Cockroaches transmit a number of disease agents, including bacteria, protozoa, and eggs of parasitic worms.

cockscomb papilloma /kok'skōm/ [AS, *cocc* + *camb* + L, *papilla,* nipple; Gk, *oma,* tumor], a benign small red lesion that may project from the uterine cervix during pregnancy; it regresses after delivery.

cocktail [AS, *cocc* + *toegel*], *informal.* an unofficial mixture of drugs, usually in solution, combined to achieve a specific purpose.

cockup splint, a splint used to immobilize the wrist and leave the fingers free.

coconsciousness /kōkon'shənəs/, (in psychiatry) conscious states of which the patient is not aware because they are not in the focus of attention but at the fringe of the content of consciousness.

cocontraction /kō'kəntrak'shən/, the simultaneous contraction of agonist and antagonist muscles around a joint to hold a position.

COD, abbreviation for *cause of death.*

code [L, *caudex,* book], **1.** (in law) a published body of statutes, as a civil code. **2.** a collection of standards and rules of behavior, as a dress code. **3.** a symbolic means of representing information for communication or transfer, as a genetic code. **4.** a system of notation that allows information to be transmitted rapidly, such as Morse code, or in secrecy, such as a cryptographic code. **5.** *informal.* a discreet signal used to summon a special team to resuscitate a patient. **6.** to enter data by use of a given programming language into a computer.

Code for Nurses, a set of rules of conduct for the nursing profession adopted by the American Nurses Association in 1976.

codeine /kō'dēn, kō'dē·in/ [Gk, *kodeia,* poppyhead], a narcotic analgesic and antitussive used to treat mild to moderate pain, diarrhea, and cough.

codeine phosphate, a narcotic analgesic and antitussive prescribed to suppress cough and to relieve mild to moderate pain.

codeine sulfate, a water-soluble salt of monomethylmorphine, an alkaloid derived from opium. It is used as a mild hypnotic, an analgesic, and a cough reflex suppressant.

Code Management, a Nursing Interventions Classification defined as coordination of emergency measures to sustain life.

code of ethics, a statement encompassing the set of rules to which practitioners of a profession are expected to conform.

codependent, a state of close association with a person who is dependent on or addicted to a potentially destructive behavior such as substance abuse, gambling, or smoking. The codependent person facilitates the behavior of the dependent one.

code team, a specially trained and equipped team of physicians, nurses, and technicians that is available to provide cardiopulmonary resuscitation when summoned by a code set by the institution.

coding [L, *caudex,* book], the process of organizing information into categories, which are assigned codes for the purposes of sorting, storing, and retrieving the data.

cod-liver oil, a pale-yellow fatty oil extracted from the fresh livers of the codfish and other related species. It is a rich source of fat-soluble vitamins A and D.

Codman's exercise [Ernest A. Codman, American surgeon, 1869–1940; L, *exercere,* to keep at work], mild exercises for restoring range of motion and function in the arms or shoulders after injury and immobilization of the limbs.

codominant /kōdom'ənənt/ [L, *cum,* together with, *dominari,* to rule], pertaining to the equal degree of dominance of two alleles or traits fully expressed in a phenotype, as when a person inherits both the A and B genes of the ABO blood group and has AB type blood. —**codominance,** *n.*

codominant inheritance, the transmission of a trait or condition in which both alleles of a pair are given full expression in a heterozygote, such as in the AB or MNS blood group antigens and the leukocyte antigens.

codon /kō'don/, a unit of three adjacent nucleotides along a deoxyribonucleic acid or messenger ribonucleic acid molecule that designates a specific amino acid in the polypeptide chain during protein synthesis.

coefficient /kō'efish'ənt/ [L, *cum,* together with, *efficere,* to effect], a mathematic relationship between factors that can be used to measure or evaluate a characteristic under specified conditions.

coelenteron /sēlen'təron/, *pl.* **coelentera** [Gk, *koilos,* hollow, *enteron,* intestine],

the digestive cavity of members of the phylum Cnidaria, such as the hydra and jellyfish.

coelom /sē'ləm/ [Gk, *koilos,* hollow], the body cavity of the developing embryo. —**coelomic, celomic,** *adj.*

coelosomy /sē'ləsō'mē/ [Gk, *koilos* + *soma,* body], a congenital anomaly characterized by protrusion of the viscera from the body cavity.

coenzyme /kō·en'zīm/ [L, *cum,* together with, *en,* in, *zyme,* ferment], a nonprotein substance that combines with an apoenzyme to form a complete enzyme or holoenzyme. Coenzymes include some of the vitamins, such as B_1 and B_2, and have smaller molecules than enzymes.

coenzyme A (CoA) [L, *cum* + *en,* into, *zyme,* ferment], an important metabolite in the citric acid cycle. Although not a true enzyme, it plays a significant role in the transfer of acetyl groups and the metabolism of acids and amino acids.

coenzyme Q (CoQ), a designation for quinones with polymer side chains that mediate electron transfer between cytochrome beta and cytochrome c. It is chemically similar to tocopherols, including vitamin E.

coffee [Ar, *qahwah*], the dried and roasted ripe seeds of *Coffea arabica, C. liberica,* and *C. robusta* trees that grow in almost all tropical areas. Coffee contains the alkaloid caffeine.

coffee-ground vomitus, dark brown vomitus the color and consistency of coffee grounds, composed of gastric juices and old blood and indicative of slow upper gastrointestinal bleeding.

cognition /kognish'ən/ [L, *cognoscere,* to know], the mental process characterized by knowing, thinking, learning, understanding, and judging.

cognitive /kog'nitiv/, pertaining to the mental processes of comprehension, judgment, memory, and reasoning, as contrasted with emotional and volitional processes.

cognitive development, the developmental process by which an infant becomes an intelligent person, acquiring knowledge with growth and improving his or her ability to think, learn, reason, and abstract.

cognitive dissonance [L, *cognoscere,* to know, *dis,* opposite of, *sonare,* to sound], a state of tension resulting from a discrepancy in a person's emotional and intellectual frame of reference for interpreting and coping with his or her environment.

cognitive function, an intellectual process by which one becomes aware of, perceives, or comprehends ideas.

cognitive learning, 1. learning that i

concerned with acquisition of problem-solving abilities and with intelligence and conscious thought. **2.** a theory that defines learning as behavioral change based on the acquisition of information about the environment.

cognitive psychology, the study of the development of thought, language, and intelligence in infants and children.

cognitive restoration, an intervention technique designed to restore cognitive functioning.

cognitive restructuring, a change in attitudes, values, or beliefs that impacts a person's self-expression; it occurs as a result of insight or behavioral achievement.

Cognitive Restructuring, a Nursing Interventions Classification defined as challenging a patient to alter distorted thought patterns and view self and the world more realistically.

Cognitive Stimulation, a Nursing Interventions Classification defined as promotion of awareness and comprehension of surroundings by utilization of planned stimuli.

cognitive structuring, the process of reviewing with a patient the changes that have occurred in his or her thinking to instill a sense of change and of his or her role in bringing about that change.

cognitive therapy, any of the various methods of treating mental and emotional disorders that help a person change attitudes, perceptions, and patterns of thinking.

cogwheel respiration, a breathing pattern characterized by a repeated series of brief interruptions of inhalation and exhalation.

cogwheel rigidity [ME, *cugge,* tooth on a gear; AS, *hweol* + L, *rigiditas,* unbending], an abnormal rigor in muscle tissue, characterized by jerky movements when the muscle is passively stretched.

cohabitate /kōhab′ıtāt/, to live together in a relationship when not married.

cohere /kōhir′/ [L, *cohaerere,* to cling together], to stick together, as similar molecules of a common substance.

coherence /kōhir′əns/, **1.** the property of sticking together, as the molecules within a common substance. **2.** (in psychology) the logical pattern of expression and thought evident in the speech of a normal, stable individual. —**coherent,** *adj.*

cohesive bandage /kōhē′siv/, a dressing material that will adhere to itself but not to other surfaces.

cohesiveness /kōhē′sivnəs/ [L, *cohaerere,* to cling together], **1.** (in psychiatry) a force that attracts members to a group and causes them to remain in it. **2.** (in dentistry) a property of annealed pure

gold that allows it to be used as a filling material.

cohesive termini, (in molecular genetics) the complementary single-stranded ends projecting from a double-stranded deoxyribonucleic acid segment that can be joined by molecular genetic techniques to introduced fragments. Also called *sticky ends.*

COHN, abbreviation for *Certified Occupational Health Nurse.*

cohort /kō′hôrt/ [L, *cohortem,* large group], (in statistics) a collection or sampling of individuals who share a common characteristic, such as members of the same age or sex.

cohort study, (in research) a study concerning a specific subpopulation, such as the children born between December and May in 1975 and those born in the same months in 1955.

coiled tubular gland [L, *colligere,* to gather together, *tubulus,* small tube, *glans,* acorn], one of the many multicellular glands that contain a coiled, tube-shaped secretory part, such as the sweat glands.

coil-spring contraceptive diaphragm, a kind of contraceptive diaphragm in which the flexible metal spring that forms the rim is a coiled, circular spring.

coincidence counting /kō·in′sidəns/ [L, *coincidere,* to occur together], (in radiotherapy) the detection of two photons that arrive at separate counters simultaneously as the result of annihilation of a positron (created during a radioactive decay) and an electron. As an imaging technique, the coincidence counting of two photons greatly reduces the significance of any background radiation.

coital headache /kō′itəl/, an uncommon type of headache, mainly affecting men, that begins during or immediately after coitus.

coitus /kō′itəs/ [L, *coire,* to come together], the sexual union of two people of opposite sex in which the penis is introduced into the vagina, typically resulting in mutual excitation and usually orgasm. —**coital,** *adj.*

colation /kōlā′shən/ [L, *colare,* to strain], the act of filtering or straining, as urine is often strained for medical examination.

colchicine /kol′chəsēn/ [Gk, *kolchikon*], a gout suppressant prescribed in the treatment of acute gout and prophylaxis of recurrent gouty arthritis.

cold [AS, *kald*], **1.** the absence of heat. **2.** a contagious viral infection of the upper respiratory tract, usually caused by a strain of rhinovirus. It is characterized by rhinitis, tearing, low-grade fever, and malaise and is treated symptomatically with rest, mild analgesia, decongestants, and increased fluid intake.

COLD /kōld/, abbreviation for *chronic obstructive lung disease.*

cold abscess, a site of infection that does not show common signs of heat, redness, and swelling.

cold agglutinin, a nonspecific antibody, found on the surface of red blood cells in certain diseases, that may cause clumping of the cells at temperatures below 36° C and may cause hemolysis. The phenomenon does not occur at body temperature. Mycoplasma pneumonia, infectious mononucleosis, and many lymphoproliferative disorders are associated with cold agglutinins.

cold agglutinin disease [AS, *kald* + L, *agglutinare,* to glue, *dis,* without; Fr, *aise,* ease], a disorder characterized by circulating antibodies that can agglutinate red cells at less than normal body temperatures. They occur in the sera of patients with atypical pneumonia and blood diseases, particularly hemolytic anemia. The disease also tends to affect elderly patients.

cold bath, a bath in which the water temperature is approximately 50° F (10° C) to 65° F (18° C), used primarily to reduce body temperature.

cold-blooded, unable to regulate body heat, as fishes, reptiles, and amphibians, which have internal temperatures that are close to the temperatures of the environments in which they live.

cold caloric irrigation, a procedure for testing the integrity of brainstem function. It is carried out by irrigating the external auditory canal of the patient with a cold saline solution while the head is flexed at approximately 30 degrees, after checking the patency of the ear canal. The stimulus results in jerky but regular eye movements in a normal patient.

cold compress [AS, *kald* + L, *comprimere,* to press together], a pad of damp, thickly folded, soft absorbent cloth, dipped into cold water, wrung out, and applied to a body part for the relief of pain or reduction of inflammation.

cold environment, a human environment arbitrarily designated as one in which the temperature is below 10° C (50° F). The human body generally begins to experience some functional impairment when unprotected in temperatures below 15° C (59° F). The body's hemostatic mechanism reacts with vasoconstriction, reducing heat loss to the environment. When vasoconstriction no longer eases the thermal strain between the skin and the environment, muscular hypertonus and shivering become mechanisms for maintaining body temperature.

cold injury, any of several abnormal and often serious physical conditions caused by exposure to cold temperatures, such as frostbite and hypothermia.

cold-pressor test, a test for the tendency to develop essential hypertension. One hand of the individual is immersed in ice water for about 60 seconds. An excessive rise in the blood pressure or an unusual delay in the return of normal blood pressure when the hand is removed from the water is believed to indicate that the individual is at risk for hypertension.

cold-sensitive mutation, a genetic alteration resulting in a gene that functions only at high temperature.

cold sore. See **herpes simplex (HSV-I).**

cold ulcer, a small gangrenous ulceration on an extremity caused by poor circulation.

cold urticaria [AS, *kald* + L, *urtica,* nettle], wheals caused by exposure to cold temperatures.

cold-wet-sheet pack, a form of somatic therapy for agitated patients. The patient is swathed in cold, wet sheets, which are then warmed by body heat. The warmth and immobilization are reported to be soothing to very agitated patients.

colectomy /kəlek'təmē/ [Gk, *kolon,* colon, *ektome,* excision], surgical excision of part or all of the colon performed to treat cancer of the colon, diverticulitis, or severe chronic ulcerative colitis.

coleotomy /kō'lē-ot'əmē/, a surgical incision into the pericardium or vagina.

colestipol hydrochloride /kōles'tipol/, an antihyperlipoproteinemic that acts by sequestering bile acids in the intestine, thus reducing plasma levels of cholesterol. It is prescribed in the treatment of hypercholesterolemia and xanthoma.

colic /kol'ik/ [Gk, *kolikos,* colon pain], **1.** sharp visceral pain resulting from torsion, obstruction, or smooth muscle spasm of a hollow or tubular organ, such as a ureter or the intestines. **2.** pertaining to the colon. —**colicky,** *adj.*

colicinogen /kol'isin'əjən/ [(*E.*) *coli* + L, *caedere,* to kill; Gk, *genein,* to produce], an episome in some strains of *Escherichia coli* that induces secretion of a colicin, a protein lethal to other strains of the bacterium.

coliform /kol'ifôrm/ [(*E.*) *coli* + L, *forma,* form], **1.** pertaining to the colon-aerogenes group, or the *Escherichia coli* species of microorganisms, which comprises most of the intestinal flora in humans and other animals. **2.** having the characteristic of a sieve or cribriform structure, such as some of the porous bones of the skull.

colistimethate sodium /kō'listim'əthāt/, an antibacterial prescribed in the treatment of gastrointestinal infections caused by certain gram-negative microorganisms and as a topical medication.

colistin sulfate /kōlis'tin/, an antibacterial prescribed topically in the treatment of infections of the outer ear and systemically for the treatment of serious gram-negative infections and gastroenteritis caused by *Escherichia coli* infections.

colitis /kōlī'tis/, an inflammatory condition of the large intestine. Inflammatory bowel disease is characterized by severe diarrhea, bleeding, and ulceration of the mucosa of the intestine. Weight loss and pain are significant. —**colitic,** *adj.*

collaborative power structure /kəlab'-ərətiv'/, an arrangement whereby adult members of a functional family make major decisions and are in agreement about power distribution.

collagen /kol'əjən/ [Gk, *kolla,* glue, *genein,* to produce], a protein consisting of bundles of tiny reticular fibrils that combine to form the white glistening inelastic fibers of the tendons, ligaments, and fascia. —**collagenous** /kəlaj'ənəs/, *adj.*

collagenase ointment /kəlaj'ənās/, a medication used in the treatment of decubitus ulcers, burns, and other epidermal lesions. It is an enzyme preparation derived from the fermentation of *Clostridium histolyticum.*

collagen disease, an abnormal condition characterized by extensive disruption of the connective tissue, such as inflammation and fibrinoid degeneration. Some collagen diseases are polyarteritis nodosa, systemic lupus erythematosus, and rheumatoid arthritis,

collagen injection, a reconstructive technique in cosmetic surgery to enhance the lips or fatten sunken facial skin.

collagenoblast /kəlaj'ənōblast'/ [Gk, *kolla* + *genein* + *blastos,* germ], a cell that differentiates from a fibroblast and functions in the formation of collagen. It can also transform into cartilage and bone tissue by metaplasia.

collagenous fiber /kəlaj'ənəs/, any one of the tough, white protein fibers that constitute much of the intercellular substance and the connective tissue of the body.

collagen shield, a material derived from porcine scleral tissue, used in cataract surgery and in promotion of corneal healing. The shield enhances the penetration and effective time of subconjunctival antibiotics and corticosteroids administered during the surgical procedure. The collagen shield is designed to dissolve within 12 hours.

collagen vascular disease, any of a group of acquired disorders that have in common diffuse immunologic and inflammatory changes in small blood vessels and connective tissue. Common features of most of these entities include arthritis, skin lesions, iritis and episcleritis, pericarditis, pleuritis, subcutaneous nodules, myocarditis, vasculitis, and nephritis.

collapse /kəlaps'/ [L, *collabi,* to fall], **1.** *nontechnical.* a state of extreme depression or a condition of complete exhaustion caused by physical or psychosomatic problems. **2.** an abnormal condition characterized by shock. **3.** the abnormal sagging of an organ or the obliteration of its cavity.

collapse of the lung [L, *collabi,* to fall together; AS, *lungen*], a reduction in the volume of the lung and the amount of air in it. The condition results from increased intrapleural pressure caused by accumulation of air or fluid in the pleural cavity or from a loss of internal pressure and elastic recoil of the lung.

collar [L, *collum,* neck], any structure that encircles another, usually around its neck, such as the periosteal bone collars that form around the diaphyses of young bones.

collarbone. See **clavicle.**

collateral /kōlat'ərəl/ [L, *cum,* together with, *lateralis,* side], **1.** secondary or accessory. **2.** (in anatomy) a small branch, such as any one of the arterioles or venules in the body.

collateral circulation [L, *cum* + *latus,* side, *circulare,* to go around], a redundant blood pathway developed through enlargement of secondary vessels after obstruction of a main channel.

collateral fissure, a fissure separating the subcalcarine and subcollateral gyri of the cerebral hemisphere.

collateral pulp canal, (in dentistry) a branch of the pulp canal that emerges from the root at a place other than the apex.

collateral ventilation, the ventilation of pulmonary air spaces (alveoli) through indirect pathways, such as anastomosing bronchioles.

collateral vessel [L, *cum* + *latus,* side, *vascellum,* small vase], a branch of an artery or vein used as an accessory to the blood vessel from which it arises.

collecting tubule [L, *colligere,* to gather, *tubulus,* small tube], any one of the many relatively large straight tubules of the kidney that funnel urine into the renal pelvis. The collecting tubules play an important role in maintaining the fluid balance of the body by allowing water to osmose through their membranes into the interstitial fluid in the renal medulla.

collective bargaining /kəlek′tiv/, the use of collective action by employees in negotiating working conditions and economic issues with their employer.

collective unconscious [L, *colligere,* to gather; AS, *un,* not; L, *conscious,* aware], (in analytic psychology) that part of the unconscious common to all humans.

collector, (in medicine) a device with various modifications, used for gathering secretions from the bronchi and esophagus for bacteriologic and cytologic examination.

college [L, *collegium,* society], **1.** an institution of higher learning. **2.** an organization of individuals with common professional training and interests such as the American College of Nurse-Midwives, the American College of Cardiology, or the American College of Surgeons.

College of American Pathologists (CAP), a national professional organization of physicians who specialize in pathology.

Colles' fascia /kol′ēz/ [Abraham Colles, Irish surgeon, 1773–1843; L, band], the deep layer of the subcutaneous fascia of the perineum, constituting a distinctive structure in the urogenital region of the body. It is a strong, smooth sheet of tissue containing elastic fibers that give it a characteristic yellow tint.

Colles' fracture [Abraham Colles], a fracture of the radius at the epiphysis within 1 inch of the joint of the wrist, which causes displacement of the hand to a dorsal and lateral position.

colligative /kol′igā′tiv/ [L, *colligere,* to gather], (in physical chemistry) pertaining to those properties of matter that depend on the concentration of particles, such as molecules and ions, rather than the chemical properties of any substance.

collimate [L, *collineare,* to align], to make parallel.

collimator /kol′imā′tər/ [L, *collinare,* to bring into alignment], (in radiotherapy) a device for limiting the size and shape of a radiation beam. It is used to reduce scatter radiation, thereby decreasing the patient dose needed and increasing radiographic quality.

colliquation /kol′ikwā′shən/ [L, *cum,* together with, *liquifacere,* to make liquid], the degeneration of a body tissue to a liquid state, usually associated with necrotic tissue.

colliquative /kol′ikwā′tiv/, characterized by a profuse fluid discharge as in suppurating wounds and body structures that are infected.

collision tumor /kəlizh′ən/ [L, *cum,* together with, *laedere,* to strike], a tumor formed as two separate growths, developing close to each other, join.

collodion /kəlō′dē·ən/ [Gk, *kolla,* glue, *eidos,* form], a clear or slightly opaque, highly inflammable liquid composed of pyroxylin, ether, and alcohol. It dries to a strong, transparent film that is used as a surgical dressing.

collodion baby, an infant whose skin at birth is covered with a scaly, parchment-like membrane.

colloid /kol′oid/ [Gk, *kolla,* glue, *eidos,* form], a state or division of matter in which large molecules or aggregates of molecules (1 to 100 nm in size) do not precipitate and are dispersed in another medium.

colloidal solution /koloi′dəl/ [Gk, *kolla,* glue, *eidos,* form; L, *solutus,* dissolved], a solution in which small particles such as large polymeric molecules are homogenously dispersed through a liquid medium.

colloidal sulfur, a form of very finely divided sulfur that is used in the treatment of acne and other skin disorders.

colloid bath, a bath taken in water that contains such substances as bran, gelatin, and starch, used to relieve irritation and inflammation.

colloid chemistry, the science dealing with the composition and nature of chemical colloids.

colloid corpuscle, an amyloid body.

colloid cyst [Gk, *kolla,* glue, *eidos,* form, *kystis,* bag], **1.** a thyroid gland follicle distended with thyroid secretion. **2.** a cyst in the third ventricle, leading to hydrocephalus.

colloid goiter, a greatly enlarged, soft thyroid gland in which the follicles are distended with colloid.

colloid substance, a jellylike substance formed in the deterioration of the protoplasm of tissues.

colloid suspension [Gk, *kolla,* glue, *eidos,* form; L, *suspendere,* to hang], a system of solids dispersed in a liquid medium, with particles generally smaller than 100 nm.

collum /kol′əm/, the anatomic neck structure between the head and shoulders.

columella, 1. a small column **2.** the fleshy terminal part of the nasal septum.

column, any elongated anatomic structure. It is usually oriented vertically and may provide structural support.

collateral innervation, reinnervation of denervated neurons caused by sprouting of uninjured axons in the vicinity.

collyrium /kolir′ē·əm/, an ophthalmic

liquid containing medications to be instilled into the eye.

coloboma /kol′əbō′mə/ [Gk, *koloboma*, defect], a congenital or pathologic defect in the ocular tissue of the body, usually affecting the iris, ciliary body, or choroid by forming a cleft that extends inferiorly. Colobomas are usually the result of the failure of part of the fetal fissure to close. —**colobomatous,** *adj.*

colon /kō′lən/ [Gk, *kolon*], the part of the large intestine extending from the cecum to the rectum. It has four segments: ascending colon, transverse colon, descending colon, and sigmoid colon. —**colonic** /kəlon′ik/, *adj.*

colonic fistula [Gk, *kolon* + L, pipe], an abnormal passage from the colon to the surface of the body or an internal organ or structure.

colonic irrigation, a procedure for washing the inner wall of the colon by filling it with water and then draining it. It is not considered an enema, but rather a technique for removing any material that may be present high in the colon.

colonization /kol′ənīzā′shən/, the presence and multiplication of microorganisms without tissue invasion or damage.

colonoscope /kō′lənōskōp′/ [Gk, *kolon* + *skopein*, to watch], a long, flexible endoscope, usually fiberoptic, that permits examination of the interior of the entire colon.

colonoscopy /kō′lənos′kəpē/, the examination of the mucosal lining of the colon using a colonoscope, an elongated endoscope.

colony /kol′ənē/ [L, *colonia*], **1.** (in bacteriology) a mass of microorganisms in a culture that originates from a single cell. Some kinds of colonies, according to different configurations, are smooth colonies, rough colonies, and dwarf colonies. **2.** (in cell biology) a mass of cells in a culture or in certain experimental tissues such as a spleen colony.

colony counter, a device used for counting colonies of bacteria growing in a culture. It usually consists of an illuminated, transparent plate divided into sections of known area.

colony-stimulating factor (CSF), a cellular growth factor required for cells to pass a restriction point in their reproductive cycle. It is no longer needed after cells have entered the deoxyribonucleic acid synthesis phase.

coloproctectomy /kō′ləproktek′təmē/, surgical removal of the colon and rectum..

coloproctitis /kō′ləprakti′tis/, an inflammation of both the colon and rectum.

coloptosis /kō′lopto′sis/ [Gk, *kolon* + *pto-*

sis, fall], the prolapse or downward displacement of the colon.

Colorado tick fever, a relatively mild, self-limited arbovirus infection transmitted to humans by the bite of a tick. Symptoms, occurring in two phases separated by a period of remission, include chills, fever, and headache; pain in the eyes, legs, and back; and sensitivity to light.

color blindness [L, color; AS *blint*], an abnormal condition characterized by an inability to distinguish colors of the spectrum clearly. In most cases it is not a blindness but a weakness in perceiving colors distinctly. There are two forms of color blindness: **Daltonism,** the more common form, is characterized by an inability to distinguish reds from greens. It is an inherited, sex-linked disorder. Total color blindness, or **achromatic vision,** is characterized by an inability to perceive any color at all. Only white, gray, and black are seen. It may be the result of a defect in or absence of the cones in the retina.

color dysnomia /disnō′mē·ə/ [L, color; Gk, *dys*, difficult, *onoma*, name], an inability to name colors despite an ability to match and distinguish them. It may be caused by expressive dysphasia.

colorectal cancer /kō′lərek′təl/ [Gk, *kolon*, colon; L, *rectus*, straight], a malignant neoplastic disease of the large intestine characterized by a change in bowel habits and the passing of blood (melena). Malignant tumors of the large bowel usually occur after 50 years of age, are slightly more frequent in women than in men, and are common in the Western world. The risk of large bowel cancer is increased in patients with chronic ulcerative colitis, villous adenomas, and especially familial adenomatous polyposis of the colon. People who have a high-fat diet, a high consumption of alcohol, and low activity levels; those who smoke tobacco; and those who have inhaled asbestos fibers or who have been irradiated are more likely than others to have colorectal cancer.

colorimetry /kol′ərim′ətrē/, **1.** measurement of the intensity of color in a fluid or substance. **2.** measurement of color in the blood by use of a colorimeter to determine hemoglobin concentration. —**colorimetric,** *adj.*

color vision, a recognition of color as the result of changes in the pigments of the cones in the retina that react to varying intensities of red, green, and blue light.

colosigmoidoscopy /kō′ləsig′moidos′kəpē/ [Gk, *kolon* + *sigma*, S-shaped, *eidos*, form, *skopein*, to look], the direct examination of the sigmoid part of the colon with a sigmoidoscope.

colostomate /kəlos'təmāt/ [Gk, *kolon* + *stoma,* mouth; L, *atum,* one acted upon], a person who has undergone a colostomy.

colostomy /kəlos'təmē/ [Gk, *kolon* + *stoma,* mouth], surgical creation of an artificial anus on the abdominal wall by incising the colon and drawing it out to the surface, performed for cancer of the colon, benign obstructive tumors, and severe abdominal wounds. A colostomy may be single-barreled, with one opening, or double-barreled, with distal and proximal loops open onto the abdomen.

colostomy irrigation, a procedure used by colostomates to clear the bowel of fecal matter and to help establish an evacuation schedule.

colostrum /kəlos'trəm/ [L, first milk after birth], the fluid secreted by the breast during pregnancy and the first days after delivery before lactation begins. It consists of immunologically active substances (maternal antibodies) and white blood cells, water, protein, fat, minerals, vitamins, and carbohydrate in a thin, yellow serous fluid.

colotomy /kōlot'əmē/, a surgical incision into the colon, usually performed through the abdominal wall.

Colour Index (C.I.), a publication of dyers, colorists, and textile chemists that specifies all the standard industrial pigments and stains according to five-digit numbers associated with chemical coloring materials.

colovaginal /kō'lōvaj'inəl/ [Gk, *kolon,* colon; L, *vagina,* sheath], pertaining to the colon and vagina, or to a communication between the two structures.

colpalgia /kolpal'jə/, a pain in the vagina.

colpectomy /kolpek'təmē/, the surgical excision of the vagina.

colpitis /kolpī'tis/, an inflammation of the vagina.

colpocystitis /kol'pōsistī'tis/, an inflammation of the vagina and urinary bladder.

colpocystocele /kol'pəsis'təsēl/ the prolapse of the urinary bladder into the vagina, usually through the anterior vaginal wall.

colpohysterectomy /-his'tərek'təmē/ [Gk, *kolpos,* vagina, *hystera,* womb, *ektome,* excision], vaginal hysterectomy.

colporrhaphy /kolpôr'əfē/ [Gk, *kolpos* + *raphe,* suture], a surgical procedure in which the vagina is sutured, as for the purpose of narrowing it.

colposcope /kol'pəskōp/, a lighted instrument with lenses for direct examination of the surfaces of the vagina and cervix.

colposcopy /kolpos'kəpē/ [Gk, *kolpos* + *skopein,* to watch], an examination of the vagina and cervix with an optical magnifying instrument (colposcope).

colpotomy /kolpot'əmē/ [Gk, *kolpos* + *temnein,* to cut], any surgical incision into the wall of the vagina.

columnar cell /kəlum'nər/ [L, *columna,* column, *cella,* storeroom], an epithelial cell that appears long and narrow when sectioned along its long axis.

columnar epithelium [L, *columna,* column; Gk, *epi,* upon, *thele,* nipple], a type of epithelial cell that resembles a hexagonal prism.

columnar layer [L, *columna,* column; AS, *lecgan*], the layer of rods and cones in the retina.

column chromatography [L, *columna* + Gk, *chroma,* color, *graphein* to record], the process of separating and analyzing a group of substances according to the differences in their absorption affinities for a given absorbent as evidenced by pigments deposited during filtration through the same absorbent contained in a glass cylinder or tube. The substances are dissolved in a liquid that is passed through the absorbent. The absorbates move down the column at different rates and leave behind a band of pigments that is subsequently washed with a pure solvent to develop discrete pigmented bands that constitute a chromatograph.

coma /kō'mə/ [Gk, *koma,* deep sleep], a state of profound unconsciousness characterized by the absence of spontaneous eye openings, response to painful stimuli, and vocalization. The person cannot be aroused. Coma may be the result of trauma, space-occupying brain tumor, hematoma, toxic metabolic condition, acute infectious disease with encephalitis, vascular disease, or brain ischemia.

comatose /kō'mətōs/, pertaining to a state of coma, or abnormally deep sleep, caused by illness or injury.

combat fatigue [L, *com,* together, *battuere,* to beat, *fatigare,* to tire], any of a variety of psychoneurotic disorders resulting from exhaustion, the stress of combat, or the cumulative emotions and psychologic strain of warfare or similar situations. It is characterized by anxiety, depression, irritability, memory and sleep disorders, and various related symptoms.

combination chemotherapy /kom'binā'shən/, the simultaneous use of two or more anticancer drugs.

combined carbon dioxide [L, *com,* together, *bini,* twofold], the part of the total carbon dioxide that is contained in blood carbonate; it can be calculated as the difference between the total and dissolved carbon dioxide.

combined cycling ventilator, a mechanical ventilator that has more than one mechanism to recycle gases, such as equipment that may have time cycling or pressure cycling as a backup to a volume cycling control device.

combined modality treatment, the use of chemotherapy in combination with surgery or irradiation or both in the treatment of cancer.

combined oxygen, the oxygen that is physically bound to hemoglobin as oxyhemoglobin (HbO_2). One gram-molecular weight of oxygen can combine with 16,700 g of hemoglobin, and each gram of hemoglobin can bind with and carry 1.34 ml of oxygen.

combined patterns, a method of evaluating a patient's neuromuscular functions through tests that reveal the degree of coordination between movement patterns of the trunk and the extremities.

combined system disease, a disorder of the nervous system caused by a deficiency of vitamin B_{12} that results in pernicious anemia and degeneration of the spinal cord and peripheral nerves, marked by increased difficulty in walking, a feeling of vibration in the legs, and a loss of sense of position.

combining sites, 1. concave features on antibody molecules that serve as locations for binding antigens. Because of possible variations in antibody amino acid sequences and molecule configurations, each kind of antibody can provide combining sites for a specific antigen. 2. locations on protein molecules where drugs or other substances may become bound by electrochemical attraction.

combustion /kəmbus'chen/, the process of burning or oxidation, which may be accompanied by light and heat. Oxygen itself does not burn, but it supports combustion. The rate of combustion is influenced by both oxygen concentration and its partial pressure.

comedo /kom'idō/, pl. **comedones** /komidō'nēz/ [L, comedere, to consume], blackhead, the basic lesion of acne, caused by an accumulation of keratin and sebum within the opening of a hair follicle.

comedocarcinoma /kom'idōkär'sinō'mə/ [L, comedere, to consume; Gk, karkinos, crab, oma, tumor], a malignant intraductal neoplasm of the breast, in which the central cells degenerate and may be easily expressed from the cut surface of the tumor.

comedogenicity /kom'idōjənis'itē/, the ability of certain drugs or agents such as anabolic steroids to produce acne comedones.

comfort measure [L, com, together, fortis, strong], any action taken to promote the soothing and relief of a patient, as a back rub, a change in position, or the prewarming of a stethoscope or bedpan.

comfort zone [ME, comforten + Gk, zone, belt], the boundaries of temperature, humidity, wind velocity, and solar radiation within which a person dressed in a specified manner can perform certain tasks without discomfort.

Comité International des Poids et Mesures (CIPM) /kômitä' aNternäsyōnäl' dä pô·ä' ä mesYr'/, a group of scientists who meet periodically to define the international (SI) units of physical quantities, as the volume of a liter, the length of a meter, or the precise amount of time in a minute.

command automatism, a condition characterized by an abnormal mechanical responsiveness to commands, usually followed without critical judgment, such as may be seen in hypnosis and certain psychotic states.

command hallucination, a condition in which individuals hear and obey voices that command them to perform certain acts.

commensal /kəmen'səl/ [L, com, together, imensa, table], (two different species) living together in an arrangement that is not harmful to either and may be beneficial to both.

commensalism /kəmen'səliz'əm/, a state of symbiosis in which one or both of the organisms may gain some benefits from the arrangement, but neither is harmed.

comminuted /kom'inyoo'tid/ [L, comminuere, to break into pieces], crushed or broken into a number of pieces.

comminuted fracture, a fracture in which there are several breaks in the bone, creating numerous fragments.

comminution /kom'nyoo'shən/, a fracture in which the bone is broken in several pieces or shattered.

commissure /kom'isōōr, -syōōr/ 1. a band of nerve fiber or other tissue that crosses from one side of the body to the other, usually connecting two structures or masses of tissue. 2. a site of union of two anatomic parts, as the corner of the eye, lips, or labia.

commissurotomy /kom'ishōōrot'əmē/ [L, commissura, a connection; Gk, temnein, to cut], the surgical division of a fibrous band or ring connecting corresponding parts of a body structure.

commitment [L, *committere,* to entrust], **1.** the placement or confinement of an individual in a specialized hospital or other institutional facility. **2.** the legal procedure of admitting a mentally ill person to an institution for psychiatric treatment. **3.** a pledge or contract to fulfill some obligation or agreement, used especially in some forms of psychotherapy or marriage counseling.

common bile duct [L, *communis,* common, *bilis,* bile, *ducere,* to lead], the duct formed by the juncture of the cystic and hepatic ducts.

common carotid artery [L, *communis* + Gk, *karos,* heavy sleep, *arteria,* airpipe], one of the major arteries supplying blood to the head and neck. Each divides into an external common carotid and an internal common carotid. Branches of the external carotid supply the face, scalp, and most of the neck and throat tissues.

common carotid plexus, a network of nerves on the common carotid artery, supplying sympathetic fibers to the head and the neck, with branches that accompany the cranial blood vessels.

common hepatic artery, the visceral branch of the celiac trunk of the abdominal aorta, passing posterior to the pylorus and dividing into five branches.

common iliac artery, a division of the abdominal aorta, starting to the left of the fourth lumbar vertebra and dividing into external and internal iliac arteries.

common iliac node, a node in one of the seven groups of parietal lymph nodes serving the abdomen and the pelvis.

common iliac vein, one of the two veins that are the sources of the inferior vena cava, formed by the union of the internal and external iliac veins.

commune /kom′yo͞on/, a small community of people who share certain social and economic objectives. Members may also share property ownership and control local political leadership.

communicability period /kəmyo͞o′-nəkəbil′itē/, the usual time span during which contact with an infected person is most likely to result in spread of the infection.

communicable /kəmyo͞o′nəkəbəl/ [L, *communis,* common], contagious; transmissible by direct or indirect means, as a communicable disease.

communicable disease, any disease transmitted from one person or animal to another directly, by contact with excreta or other discharges from the body; or indirectly, via substances or inanimate objects such as contaminated drinking glasses, toys, or water; or via vectors such as flies, mosquitoes, ticks, or other insects. Many communicable diseases, by law, must be reported to the local health department.

communicating hydrocephalus /kəmyo͞o′-nikā′ting/ [L, *communicans* + Gk, *hydor,* water, *kephale,* head], a form of hydrocephalus in which there is an increase in cerebrospinal fluid that involves the entire ventricular system and the subarachnoid space. It is caused by an abnormality in the ability to absorb fluid in the subarachnoid space.

communication /kəmyo͞o′nikā′shən/ [L, *communis,* common], any process in which a message containing information is transferred, especially from one person to another, via any of a number of media.

communication channels, (in communication theory) any gesture, action, sound, written word, or visual image used in transmitting messages.

Communication Enhancement: Hearing Deficit, a Nursing Interventions Classification defined as assistance in accepting and learning alternate methods for living with diminished hearing.

Communication Enhancement: Speech Deficit, a Nursing Interventions Classification defined as assistance in accepting and learning alternate methods for living with impaired speech.

Communication Enhancement: Visual Deficit, a Nursing Interventions Classification defined as assistance in accepting and learning alternate methods for living with diminished vision.

communication, impaired verbal, a NANDA-accepted nursing diagnosis of a state in which an individual experiences a decreased or absent ability to use or understand language in human interaction. Defining characteristics include slurring, stuttering, difficulty in forming words or sentences, problem in expressing thoughts verbally, inappropriate verbalization, dyspnea, and disorientation. The critical defining characteristics, one of which must be present for the diagnosis to be made, are an inability to speak the dominant language of the culture, a difficulty in speaking or verbalizing, or the absence of speech.

communication theme, (in psychiatry) a recurrent concept or idea that ties together components of communication. Kinds of communication themes include content theme, in which a single concept links varied topics of discussion; mood theme, in which the underlying idea is the emotion communicated by the individual; and interaction theme, in which a particular idea best describes the dynamics between communicating participants.

communication theory, an hypothesis that describes a model of a system of information transfer consisting of a source of information (the sender), a transmitter, a communication channel, a source of noise (interference), a receiver, and a purpose for the message.

community /kəmyoo′nitē/ [L, *communis,* common], a group of species who reside in a designated geographic area and who share common interests or bonds.

community-acquired infection, an infection contracted from the environment, including those acquired indirectly from the use of medications. Community-acquired infections are distinguished from nosocomial, or hospital-acquired, diseases by the types of organisms that affect patients who are recovering from a disease or injury.

community coping, ineffective, a NANDA-accepted nursing diagnosis of a pattern of community activities for adaptation and problem solving that is unsatisfactory for meeting the demands or needs of the community. Defining characteristics include a community's inability to meet its own expectations, deficits of community participation, deficits in communication methods, excessive community conflicts, and stressors perceived as excessive.

community coping, potential for enhanced, a NANDA-accepted nursing diagnosis of a pattern of community activities for adaptation and problem solving that is satisfactory for meeting the demands or needs of the community but can be improved for management of current and future problems/stressors. The major defining characteristics include deficits in one or more characteristics that indicate effective coping.

community health nursing, a field of nursing that is a blend of primary health care and nursing practice with public health nursing. The community health nurse conducts a continuing and comprehensive practice that is preventive, curative, and rehabilitative.

community medicine, a branch of medicine that is concerned with the health of the members of a community, municipality, or region.

community mental health, a treatment philosophy based on the social model of psychiatric care that advocates that a comprehensive range of mental health services be readily accessible to all members of the community.

community mental health center (CMHC), a community-based center

that provides comprehensive mental health services, including ambulatory and inpatient care. The specific services to be provided are defined in an act of the U.S. Congress, the Community Mental Health Centers Act.

community nurse practitioner (CNP), a nurse who has completed a postbaccalaureate program in community nursing.

community psychiatry, the branch of psychiatry concerned with the development of an adequate and coordinated program of mental health care for residents of specified catchment areas.

community rating system, a program of health maintenance organizations (HMOs) that uses revenues and membership targets to determine health insurance premium rates. The HMO uses its own history in the calculation of rates.

community reintegration, the return and acceptance of a disabled person as a participating member of the community.

Comolli's sign /kōmō′lē/ [Antonio Comolli, Italian pathologist, b. 1879], a triangular swelling corresponding to the shape of the scapula after a fracture of that bone.

comorbidity, two or more coexisting medical conditions or unrelated disease processes.

compact bone /kompakt/ [L, *compingere,* to put together], hard, dense bone that is usually found at the periphery of skeletal structures, as distinguished from spongy cancellous bone.

companion animal, a dog, cat, or other pet that provides health benefits to a person. Companion animals may help to relieve stress or serve a more active role, as do guide dogs for blind persons and dogs trained to detect telephone or doorbell sounds for deaf persons.

companionship /kəmpan′yənship′/ [L., *com,* together, *panis,* food], (in psychiatric nursing) the assignment of a staff member or of another patient to stay with a disturbed patient to provide support and to protect the patient from self-harm or harm to others.

comparative anatomy /kəmper′ətiv/ [L, *com* + *par,* equal], the study of the morphologic characteristics of all living animals.

comparative embryology, the study of the similarities and differences among various organisms during the embryologic period of development.

comparative method, the analytic method to which the test method is compared in the comparison-of-methods experiment.

comparative physiology, the study of the

similarities and differences of the vital processes found in various species of living organisms to determine fundamental physiologic relationships.

comparative psychology, 1. the study of human behavior as it relates to or differs from animal behavior. 2. the study of the psychologic and behavioral differences among various peoples.

compartment model /kəmpärt′mənt/, a mathematic representation of the body or an area of the body created to study physiologic or pharmacologic kinetic characteristics. A compartment model can simulate all of the biologic processes involved in the kinetic behavior of a drug after it has been introduced into the body, leading to a better understanding of its pharmacodynamic effects.

compartment syndrome [L, com + partiri, to share], a pathologic condition caused by the progressive development of arterial compression and reduction of blood supply.

compatibility /kəmpat′əbil′itē/ [L, compatibilis, agreeable], 1. the quality or state of existing together in harmony; congruity. 2. the orderly, efficient integration of the elements of one system with those of another. 3. the formation of a stable chemical or biochemical system, specifically in medication, so that two or more drugs can be administered at the same time without producing undesired side effects or without canceling or affecting the therapeutic effects of the others. 4. (in immunology) the degree to which the body's defense system tolerates the presence of foreign material, such as transfused blood, grafted tissue, or transplanted organs, without an immune reaction. 5. (in blood grouping or crossmatching) the lack of reaction between blood groups so that there is no agglutination when the red blood cells of one sample are mixed with the serum of another sample; no reaction from transfused blood. —**compatible,** adj.

compendium /kəmpen′dē·əm/, pl. **compendia** [L, compendere, to weigh], a collected body of information on the standards of strength, purity, and quality of drugs. The official compendia in the United States are the United States Pharmacopoeia, the Homeopathic Pharmacopoeia of the United States, and their supplements.

compensated acidosis /kom′pənsā′tid/ [L, compensare, to balance, acidus, sour; Gk, osis, condition], a condition in which the pH of the blood is maintained within normal limits (adult/child: 7.35 to 7.45) although the blood bicarbonate level is below normal or the PCO_2 is above normal.

compensated alkalosis, a condition in which the blood bicarbonate is increased or the PCO_2 is decreased but buffering keeps the blood pH within the normal range.

compensated flowmeter [L, compensare, to balance], a gas therapy device with a scale that is calibrated against a constant pressure of 50 psi instead of the atmosphere.

compensated gluteal gait, one of the more common abnormal gaits associated with a weakness of the gluteus medius. It is a variation of the Trendelenburg gait. It involves the dropping of the pelvis on the unaffected side of the body during the walking cycle between the moment of heel strike on the affected side and before the moment of heel strike on the unaffected side.

compensated heart failure, an abnormal cardiac condition in which heart failure is compensated for by such mechanisms as increased sympathetic adrenergic stimulation of the heart, fluid retention with increased venous return, increased end-diastolic ventricular volume and fiber length, and hypertrophy.

compensating current /kom′pənsā′ting/, an electric current that neutralizes the intensity of a muscle current.

compensating curve, the curvature of alignment of the occlusal surfaces of the teeth, developed to compensate for the paths of the condyles as the mandible moves from centric to eccentric positions.

compensating filter, (in radiology) a device, such as a wedge fashioned from aluminum or plastic, that is positioned over a body area to compensate for differences in radiopacity.

compensation /kom′pənsā′shən/ [L, compensare, to balance], 1. the process of counterbalancing any defect in body structure or function. 2. (in cardiology) the process of maintaining an adequate blood flow through such normal cardiac and circulatory mechanisms as tachycardia, fluid retention with increased venous return, and hypertrophy. Failure of the heart to compensate and to provide the required cardiac output indicates a diseased heart muscle. 3. (in psychiatry) a complex defense mechanism that allows one to avoid the unpleasant or painful emotional stimuli that result from a feeling of inferiority or inadequacy. 4. (in chiropractic) changes in structural relationships that accommodate foundation disturbances and maintain balance.

compensator /kom′pənsā′tər/, a device used in radiotherapy to correct for irregularities in body surfaces by providing a

C

differential attenuation of the beam before it reaches the patient.

compensatory hypertrophy /kəmpen'-sətôr'ē/ [L, *compensare,* to balance], an increase in the size or function of an organ or part to counteract a structural or functional defect.

compensatory pause, a pause noted on an electrocardiogram after a premature complex; it precedes the next normal complex.

competence /kom'pətəns/ [L, *competentia,* capable], **1.** (in embryology) the total capacity of an embryonic cell to react to determinative stimuli with various types of differentiation. **2.** the ability of bacteria to take up donor deoxyribonucleic acid molecules.

competent community /kom'pətənt/, a population that is aware of resources and alternatives, can make reasoned decisions about issues facing the group, and can cope adaptively with problems. It parallels the concept of positive mental health.

competitive-binding assay /kompet'itiv/ [L, *competere,* to come together], an analytic procedure based on the reversible binding of a ligand to a binding protein.

competitive displacement, the tendency of one drug to displace another at a protein-binding site when both drugs are taken at the same time. The bound drug becomes less pharmacologically active than the free drug.

competitive identification, the unconscious modeling of one's personality on that of another as a means of outdoing or bettering the other person.

competitive inhibitor, an inhibitor of an enzyme reaction that competes with the substrate by binding at the active site.

complaint [L, *complangere,* to beat the breast], **1.** (in law) a pleading by a plaintiff made under oath to initiate a suit, It is a statement of the formal charge and the cause for action against the defendant. **2.** *informal.* any ailment, problem, or symptom identified by the client, patient, member of the person's family, or other knowledgeable person.

complement /kom'pləmənt/ [L, *complementum,* that which completes], one of 11 complex, enzymatic serum proteins. In an antigen-antibody reaction, complement causes lysis.

complement abnormality, an unusual condition characterized by deficiencies or dysfunctions of any of the nine functional components of the enzymatic proteins of blood serum. The components are labeled C1 through C9. The most common abnormalities are C2 and C3 deficiencies and C5 familial dysfunction. Patients with

complement deficiencies or dysfunctions may be more susceptible to infections and to collagen vascular diseases. Studies indicate that primary complement deficiencies may be inherited. Secondary complementary deficiencies may stem from immunologic reactions such as drug-induced serum disease, which depletes complement.

complemental inheritance /kom'pləmen'təl/, the acquisition or expression of a trait or condition as a result of the presence of two independent pairs of nonallelic genes. Both of the genes must be present for the characteristic to appear in the phenotype.

complementary feeding /kom'pləmen'tərē/ [L, *complementum,* that which completes], a supplemental feeding given an infant who is still hungry after breastfeeding.

complementary gene, either member of two or more nonallelic gene pairs that interact to produce an effect not expressed in the absence of any of the pairs.

complement cascade, a biochemical process involving the C1 to C9 complement components in which one complement interacts with another in a specific sequence called a complement pathway. The reaction sequence is C1, 4, 2, 3, 5, 6, 7, 8, 9 (the first complements are out of numeric sequence for historical reasons). The cascade effect leads to an accumulation of fluid in a cell and finally lysis of the membrane, causing the cell to rupture.

complement fixation, an immunologic reaction in which an antigen combines with an antibody and its complement, causing the complement factor to become inactive or fixed.

complement-fixation test (C-F test), any serologic test in which complement fixation is detected, indicating the presence of a particular antigen. Specific C-F tests are used to aid in the diagnosis of amebiasis, Rocky Mountain spotted fever, trypanosomiasis, and typhus.

complement protein molecule [L, *complementum* + *proteios,* first rank], any of the protein molecules that are chief humoral mediators of antigen-antibody reactions in the immune system. Nine are involved in the "classical pathway" cascade that results in the lysis of antibody-coated bacteria. They are designated C_1 to C_9.

complete abortion [L, *complere,* to fill up], termination of pregnancy in which the conceptus is expelled or removed in its entirety.

complete bed bath, a bath in which the entire body of a patient is washed while the he or she is in bed.

complete blood count (CBC), a determination of the number of red and white blood cells per cubic millimeter of blood. Most laboratories use an electronic counter for reporting numbers of red and white blood cells. Platelets are more difficult to count automatically, and many laboratories currently count them manually. Many electronic blood counters also automatically determine hemoglobin or hematocrit and include this value in the complete blood count.

complete breech, a fetal presentation in which the buttocks present with the legs folded on the thighs and the thighs on the abdomen. The position of the fetus is the same as in a normal vertex presentation but upside down.

complete dislocation [L, *complere,* to fill up, *dis,* apart, *locare,* to place], a dislocation in which the articular surfaces of the joint are completely separated.

complete fistula, an abnormal passage from an internal organ or structure to the surface of the body or to another internal organ or structure.

complete fracture, a bone break that completely disrupts the continuity of osseous tissue across the entire width of the bone involved.

complete health history, a health history that includes a history of the present illness, a health history, social history, occupational history, sexual history, and family health history.

complete heart block (CHB) [L, *complere,* to fill up; Gk, *kardia,* heart; OFr, *bloc*], a condition of total failure of the conduction of all impulses from the atria to the ventricles so they beat independently.

complete hernia [L, *complere,* to fill up, *hernia,* rupture], a hernia characterized by protrusion of the hernial sac and abdominal contents through the abdominal wall.

complete paralysis [L, *complere,* to fill up; Gk, *paralyein,* to be palsied], paralysis characterized by a complete loss of motor function.

complete protein, a protein that contains all the essential amino acids in appropriate amounts. Examples are casein (milk protein) and egg whites.

complete rachischisis, a rare congenital fissure of the entire vertebral column and spinal cord, resulting from failure of the embryonic neural tube to close.

complete response (CR), (in oncology) the total disappearance of a tumor.

complex /kom′pleks, kəmpleks′/ [L, *complexus,* an embrace], **1.** a group of items, as chemical molecules, that are related in structure or function as are the iron and protein parts of hemoglobin or

the cobalt and protein parts of vitamin B_{12}. **2.** a combination of signs and symptoms of disease that forms a syndrome. **3.** (in psychology) a group of associated ideas with strong emotional overtones that affect a person's attitudes.

complex carbohydrate, a polysaccharide, such as a carbohydrate that is composed of a large number of glucose molecules, so called to distinguish it from a simple sugar.

complex cavity, a cavity that involves more than one surface of a tooth.

complex protein, a protein that contains a simple protein and at least one molecule of another substance, as a glycoprotein, lipoprotein, nucleoprotein, or hemoglobin.

Complex Relationship Building, a Nursing Interventions Classification defined as establishing a therapeutic relationship with a patient who has difficulty in interacting with others.

complex spatial relations, the perceptual relationship of one figure or part of a figure to another.

complex sugars, sugar molecules that can be hydrolyzed or digested to yield two molecules of the same or different simple sugars, such as sucrose, lactose, and maltose.

compliance /kəmplī′əns/ [L, *complere,* to complete], **1.** fulfillment by a patient of a caregiver's prescribed course of treatment. **2.** (in respiratory physiology) a measure of distensibility of the lung volume produced by a unit pressure change.

compliance factor, a measure of the amount of trapped tidal volume in a mechanical ventilating system associated with expansion of the flexible tubing when pressure is applied.

complicated dislocation [L, *complicare,* to fold together, *dis,* apart, *locare,* place], a dislocation complicated by damage to other tissues.

complicated fracture, a fracture accompanied by injury to neighboring soft tissues such as nerves and blood vessels.

complicated labor [L, *complicare,* to fold together, *labor,* work], any labor that is made more difficult or complex by a deviation from the normal procedure.

complication [L, *complicare,* to fold together], a disease or injury that develops during the treatment of a preexisting disorder. An example is a bacterial infection that is acquired by a person weakened by a viral infection. The complication frequently alters the prognosis.

component /kəmpō′nənt/ [L, *componere,* to assemble], a significant part of a larger unit.

component drip set, a device used for delivering intravenous fluids, especially whole blood. It includes plastic tubing and a combination drip-chamber and filter.

component syringe set, a device used for delivering intravenous fluids. It includes plastic tubing, two slide clamps, a Y-connector, and a syringe.

component therapy, a transfusion of specific blood components instead of whole blood. Packed red cells or platelet-rich plasma suspensions may be transfused in larger quantities than would be possible if whole blood were used.

composite core /kəmpos'it/ [L, *componere,* to assemble], a buildup of composite resin, designed and installed to retain an artificial tooth crown.

composite graft, a transplantation that involves more than one type of tissue, such as skin and cartilage.

composite odontoma, an odontogenic tumor composed of abnormally arranged calcified enamel and dentin.

compos mentis /kom'pōs men'tis/, having a sound mind.

compound [L, *componere,* to assemble], **1.** /kom'pound/ (in chemistry) a substance composed of two or more different elements, chemically combined in definite proportions, that cannot be separated by physical means. **2.** /kom'pound/ any substance composed of two or more different ingredients. **3.** /kəmpound'/ to make a substance by combining ingredients, such as a pharmaceutic. **4.** denoting an injury characterized by multiple factors, such as a compound fracture.

compound aneurysm, a localized dilation of an arterial wall in which some of the layers are distended and others are ruptured or dissected.

compound dislocation [L, *componere,* to assemble, *dis,* apart, *locare,* to place], a dislocation in which a break in the skin is associated with the affected joint.

compound fracture, a fracture in which the broken end or ends of the bone have torn through the skin.

compound joint [L, *componere,* to assemble, *jungere,* to join], any joint that involves more than two bones.

compound microscope [L, *componere,* to assemble; Gk, *mikros,* small, *skopein,* to view], a microscope with two or more simple or complex lens systems.

compound monster, a fetus in which some of the parts or organs are duplicated but not fully developed.

compound tubuloalveolar gland /too'-byəlō'alvē'ələr/, one of the many multicellular glands with more than one secretory duct that contains both tube-shaped

and sac-shaped parts, such as the salivary glands.

Comprehensive Health Manpower Act of 1971, legislation passed by the U.S. Congress to provide educational funding for nurse-practitioner and physician-assistant programs.

Comprehensive Health Planning (CHP) and Public Health Services Amendments, legislation passed by the U.S. Congress in 1966 that emphasized regional planning and introduced the concept that each person has a "right to health care."

comprehensive medical care, a health care program that provides for preventive medical care and rehabilitative services in addition to traditional chronic and acute illness services.

compress /kom'pres/ [L, *comprimere,* to press together], a soft pad, usually made of cloth, used to apply heat, cold, or medication to the surface of a body area. A compress also may be applied over a wound to help control bleeding.

compressibility factor /kəmpres'ibil'itē/, a measure of the amount of tidal volume that may be trapped in a mechanical ventilator system in relation to the water pressure applied. It is expressed in milliliters of gas per centimeter of water pressure.

compressible volume /kəmpres'əbəl/, a part of the tidal volume of gas produced by a mechanical ventilator that is prevented from reaching a patient by compression of the gas and expansion of the flexible tubing in the equipment.

compression /kəmpresh'ən/ [L, *comprimere,* to press together], the act of pressing, squeezing, or otherwise applying pressure to an organ, tissue, or body area. Kinds of pathologic compression include **compression fracture,** in which bone surfaces are forced against each other, causing a break, and **compression paralysis,** marked by paralysis of a body area caused by pressure on a nerve.

compression fracture, a bone break, especially in a short bone, that disrupts osseous tissue and collapses the affected bone.

compression neuropathy, any of several disorders involving damage to sensory nerve roots or peripheral nerves, caused by mechanical pressure or localized trauma. It is characterized by paresthesia, weakness, or paralysis.

compression paralysis [L, *comprimere,* to press together; Gk, *paralyein,* to be palsied], a paralysis that is caused by sustained pressure on a peripheral nerve. The condition can be temporary or permanent, depending on the duration and intensity of pressure.

compressions, (in physical science) regions of high molecular density, such as a great amount of ultrasound energy, within a longitudinal wave.

compressive atelectasis /kəmpres′iv/, a loss of the lung's ability to move air in and out of the atelectatic region as a result of intrathoracic pressures that compress the alveoli. The condition may result from a pulmonary embolism.

compressor naris /kompres′ôr nät′is/, the transverse part of the nasalis muscle that serves to depress the cartilage of the nose and to draw the ala toward the septum.

compromise /kom′prəmīs/ [L, *com,* together, *promittere,* to promise], an action that may involve a change in a person's behavior, as in substituting goals or delaying satisfaction of needs in one area to reduce stress in another.

compromise body image, a new body image acquired by a patient as part of his or her adjustment to a physical dysfunction. A compromise body image incorporates and modifies unacceptable features of the condition through psychologic defense mechanisms.

compromised host, a person who is less than normally able to resist infection because of immunosuppressive therapy, immunologic defect, severe anemia, or concurrent disease or condition, including human immunodeficiency virus infection, metastatic malignancy, cachexia, or severe malnutrition.

Compton scatter [Arthur H. Compton, American physicist, 1892–1962], the principal interaction process of photons with tissue in the diagnostic and therapeutic radiology energy range.

compulsion [L, *compellere,* to urge], an irresistible, repetitive irrational impulse to perform an act that is usually contrary to one's ordinary judgments or standards yet results in overt anxiety if it is not completed. **—compulsive,** *adj.*

compulsion need [L, *compellere,* to urge; Gk, *neuron,* nerve, *osis,* condition], an irresistible, irrational urge to perform certain acts repeatedly in spite of conscious recognition that doing so is abnormal behavior. The compulsive act may have symbolic significance to the patient.

compulsive /kəmpul′siv/ [L, *compellere,* to urge], pertaining to an act repeatedly performed under the stress of pathologic, intense need.

compulsive idea [L, *compellere,* to urge], a recurring irrational idea that persists in the mind, usually generating an irresistible urge to perform an inappropriate act.

compulsive personality, a type of character structure with a pattern of chronic and obsessive adherence to rigid standards of conduct. The person is usually excessively conscientious and inhibited, is extremely inflexible, has an extraordinary capacity for work, and lacks a normal ability to relax and to relate to other people.

compulsive personality disorder, a condition in which an irrational preoccupation with order, rules, ritual, and detail interferes with everyday functioning and normal behavior.

compulsive polydipsia, a compelling urge to drink excessive amounts of liquid. Extreme cases can result in death from water intoxication and electrolyte imbalance.

compulsive ritual, a series of acts a person feels must be carried out, even though he or she recognizes that the behavior is useless and inappropriate.

computed dental radiography (CDR), a method using a digital computer for projecting radiographic images of the teeth and jaws of a patient onto a video monitor. CDR may expose a patient to less radiation than conventional dental radiography.

computed tomography (CT) /kəmpyoo′-tid/, a radiographic technique that produces a film that represents a detailed cross section of tissue structure. The procedure is painless and noninvasive and requires no special preparation. Because modern CT equipment does not involve motion of the x-ray tube, heat loading is not a problem, and multilevel images can be acquired in a very short time, sometimes during a single held breath; during a period of two held breaths as many as 40 continuous tomographic images can be produced in a single-slice mode.

CONA, abbreviation for **Canadian Orthopedic Nurses Association.**

conation /kōnā′shən/ [L, *conari,* to attempt], the mental process characterized by desire, impulse, volition, and striving. **—conative,** *adj.*

concanavalin A /kon′kənav′əlin/, a hemagglutinin, isolated from the meal of the jack bean, that reacts with polyglucosans in the blood of mammals and causes agglutination.

concatenates /kənkat′ənāts/, long molecules formed by continuous repeating of the same molecular subunit.

concave [L, *concavare,* to make hollow], curved like the interior of an arched circle.

concave-convex joint relationship /kon′-kāv, konkāv′/, the relative shape of each component of a joint's articulating surfaces. One surface is usually concave, and the other convex.

concave spherical lens [L, *concavare,* to make hollow; Gk, *sphaira,* ball; L, *lentil*], a lens that has curved, depressed surfaces that cause the rays of light to diverge. It is used for the management of myopia.

concavity /kən'kav'itē/, a deep depression or inward curving surface of an organ or body structure.

concealed accessory pathway /kənsēld/ [L, *con*, together, *celare*, to hide], (in cardiology) an atrioventricular connection that is present but is capable of retrograde conduction only.

concealed hemorrhage, the escape of blood from a ruptured vessel into internal organs or cavities.

concealed junctional extrasystole, an impulse that arises in and discharges the nodo-His region or His bundle but fails to reach either atria or ventricles. It is identified by its blocking or delaying effect on subsequent atrioventricular conduction.

conceive /kənsēv'/ [L, *concipere*, to take together], to become pregnant.

concentrate /kon'səntrāt/ [L, *con* + *centrum*, center], **1.** to decrease the bulk of a liquid mixture and increase the quantity of dissolved substances per unit of volume by the removal of solvent through evaporation or other means. **2.** a substance, particularly a liquid, that has been strengthened and reduced in volume through such means.

concentration gradient, a gradient across a membrane that separates a high concentration of a particular ion from a low concentration of the same ion.

concentric /kənsen'trik/ [L, *con* + *centrum*, center], describing two or more circles that have a common center.

concentric contraction, a common form of muscle contraction that occurs in rhythmic activities when the muscle fibers shorten as tension develops.

concentric fibroma, a fibrous tumor surrounding the uterine cavity.

concentric hypertrophy [L, *con* + *centrum*, center; Gk, *hyper*, excessive, *trophe*, nourishment], a type of tissue overgrowth in which the walls of an organ continue to increase but the exterior size remains the same and the internal size diminishes.

concept [L, *concipere*, to take together], a construct or abstract idea or thought that originates and remains within the mind. —**conceptual,** *adj.*

conception /kənsep'shən/ [L, *concipere*, to take together], **1.** the beginning of pregnancy, usually taken to be the instant that a spermatozoon enters an ovum and forms a viable zygote. **2.** the act or process of fertilization. **3.** the act or process of creating an idea or notion. **4.** the idea or notion created; a general impression resulting

from the interpretation of a symbol or set of symbols.

conceptional age, in fetal development the number of weeks since conception. It is assumed to be 2 weeks less than gestational age.

conceptive /kənsep'tiv/ [L, *concipere*, to take together], **1.** able to become pregnant. **2.** pertaining to or characteristic of the mental process of forming ideas or impressions.

conceptual disorder /kənsep'choo·əl/ [L, *concipere*, to take together], a disturbance in thought processes, cognitive activities, or ability to formulate concepts.

conceptual framework, a group of concepts that are broadly defined and systematically organized to provide a focus, a rationale, and a tool for the integration and interpretation of information.

conceptus /kənsep'təs/ [L, *concipere*, to take together], the product of conception; the fertilized ovum and its enclosing membranes at all stages of intrauterine development, from implantation to birth.

concha /kong'kə/, a body structure that is shell-shaped, as the cavity in the external ear that surrounds the external auditory canal meatus.

conchitis /kongkī'tis/, an inflammation of a concha of the ear or nose.

concoction /kənkok'shən/ [L, *con* + *coquere*, to cook], a remedy prepared from a mixture of two or more drugs or substances that have been heated.

concomitant /konkom'itənt/ [L, *con* + *comitari*, to accompany], designating one or more of two or more things, occurring simultaneously, that may or may not be interrelated or produced as a result of the others; accompanying.

concomitant strabismus, a condition of crossed eyes in which the angle of squint is the same in all directions of gaze.

concomitant symptom, any symptom that accompanies a primary symptom.

concordance /kənkôr'dəns/ [L, *concordare*, to agree], (in genetics) the expression of one or more specific traits in both members of a pair of twins. —**concordant,** *adj.*

concreteness /kənkrēt'nes/ [L, *concrescere*, to be formed], the content of a communication that includes specific feelings, behaviors, and experiences or situations.

concrete operation /kon'krēt, konkrēt'/, a thought process based on tangible rather than abstract points of reference.

concrete thinking, a stage in the development of the cognitive thought processes in the child. During this phase thought becomes increasingly logical and coherent so that the child is able to classify, sort, order, and organize facts while still being incapable of generalizing or dealing in abstractions.

concurrent infection [L, *concurrere,* to run together, *inficere,* to stain], a condition during which a person has two or more simultaneous infections.

concurrent review, part of a utilization management program in which inpatient or home health care is reviewed as it is provided. Reviewers, usually nurses, monitor appropriateness of the care, the setting, and the progress of discharge plans.

concurrent sterilization, a method of preparing an infant-feeding formula in which all ingredients and equipment are sterilized before mixing.

concurrent validity, validity of a test or a measurement tool that is established by simultaneously applying a previously validated tool or test to the same phenomenon, or data base, and comparing the results.

concussion /konkush′ən/ [L, *concutere,* to shake violently], **1.** damage to the brain caused by a violent jarring or shaking, such as a blow or an explosion. **2.** *informal.* **brain concussion.**

condensation /kon′dənsā′shən/ [L, *condensare,* to make thick], **1.** a reduction to a denser form, such as from water vapor to a liquid. **2.** (in psychology) a process often present in dreams in which two or more concepts are fused so that a single symbol represents the multiple components.

condensation nuclei, neutral particles, such as dust, in the atmosphere that are able to absorb or adsorb water and grow. At relatively high humidities they form fogs or hazes. Condensation nuclei consisting of sulfuric or nitric acid vapors or nitrogen oxides may be a source of respiratory irritants.

condensed milk, a thick liquid prepared by the evaporation of half of the water content of cow's milk.

condenser, (in dentistry) an instrument for compacting restorative material into a prepared tooth cavity. It has a working end, or nib, with a flat or serrated face.

condition /kəndish′ən/ [L, *condicere,* to make arrangements], **1.** a state of being, specifically in reference to physical and mental health or well-being. **2.** anything that is essential to or restricts or modifies the appearance or occurrence of something else. **3.** to train the body or mind, usually through specific exercises and repeated exposure to a particular state or thing. **4.** (in psychology) to subject a person or animal to conditioning or associative learning so that a specific stimulus always elicits a particular response.

conditional discharge /kəndish′ənəl/, a specified leave of absence or liberty from a psychiatric hospital in which certain behaviors are expected from the patient and the original commitment order remains in effect.

conditioned avoidance response, a learned reaction that is performed either consciously or unconsciously to avoid an unpleasant or painful stimulus.

conditioned escape response, a learned reaction that is performed either consciously or unconsciously to stop or escape from an aversive stimulus.

conditioned orientation response (COR), the desired response in an audiometry technique used in hearing tests for children less than 2 years of age. A toy mounted on a loudspeaker moves or lights up after presentation of a test tone. If later test sounds are audible to the child, he or she will look toward the toy after hearing a tone.

conditioned reflex, a reflex developed gradually by training in association with a specific repeated external stimulus.

conditioned response, an automatic reaction to a stimulus that does not normally elicit such response but has been learned through training. Such responses can be physical or psychologic and are produced by repeated association of some physiologic function or behavioral pattern with an unrelated stimulus or event.

conditioned stimulus [L, *conditio* + *stimulus,* goad], any stimulus to which a reflex response has been conditioned by previous training or experience.

conditioning /kəndish′əning/ [L, *condicere,* to make arrangements], a form of learning based on the development of a response or set of responses to a stimulus or series of stimuli.

condom /kon′dəm/, a soft, flexible sheath that covers the penis and prevents semen from entering the vagina in sexual intercourse and is used to prevent transmission of an infection and conception.

condom catheter, a tube attached to a sheath for the penis. It is used to carry urine to a collecting bag.

conduct disorder /kon′dukt/, (in psychiatry) behavior in an adolescent or child that is unacceptable in the social environment.

conduction /kənduk′shən/ [L, *conducere,* to lead], **1.** (in physics) a process in which heat is transferred from one substance to another because of a difference in temperature; a process in which energy is transmitted through a conductor. **2.** (in physiology) the process by which a nerve impulse is transmitted.

conduction anesthesia, a loss of sensation, especially pain, in a region of the body, produced by injecting a local anesthetic along the course of a nerve or nerves to inhibit the conduction of impulses to and from the area supplied by that nerve or nerves.

conduction aphasia, a dissociative speech phenomenon in which a patient has no difficulty in comprehending words seen or heard and no dysarthria, yet has problems in self-expression. The patient may substitute words similar in sound or meaning for the correct ones but is unable to repeat from dictation, to spell, and to read aloud.

conduction pathway, the route followed by nerve impulses propagated along synaptically connected neurons.

conduction system, specialized tissue that carries electrical impulses, such as bundle branches and Purkinje fibers.

conduction system of the heart, the network of highly specialized muscle tissue that transmits the electrical impulses needed for a heartbeat. It includes the sinoatrial and atrioventricular (AV) nodes, the AV bundle (bundle of His), the left and right bundle branches, and the Purkinje fibers.

conduction velocity, the speed with which an electrical impulse can be transmitted through excitable tissue, as in the movement of an action potential through His-Purkinje fibers of the heart.

conductive hearing loss /kənduk′tiv/ [L, conducere, to lead], a form of hearing loss in which sound is inadequately conducted through the external or middle ear to the sensorineural apparatus of the inner ear. Sensitivity to sound is diminished, but clarity (interpretation of the sound) is not changed as long as the sound is sufficiently loud.

conductivity, pertaining to the ability of an electrical or other system to transmit sound, heat, light, or electromagnetic energy.

conductor, 1. any substance through which electrons flow readily. 2. (in psychiatry) a family therapist who uses his or her own personality to give direction to patients in therapy.

conduit /kon′dit, kon′doo·it/, 1. an artificial channel or passage that connects two organs or different parts of the same organ. 2. a tube or other device for conveying water or other fluids from one region to another.

condylar fracture /kon′dilər/ [Gk, kondylos, knuckle], any fracture of the round end of a hinge joint, usually occurring at the distal end of the humerus or femur,

that frequently detaches a small bone fragment that includes the condyle.

condylar guide, a mechanical device on a dental articulator, designed to guide articular movement similar to that produced by the paths of the condyles in the temporomandibular joints.

condyle /kon′dīl/ [Gk, kondylos, knuckle], a rounded projection at the end of a bone that anchors muscle ligaments and articulates with adjacent bones.

condyloid /kon′diloid/ [Gk, kondylos, knuckle], resembling a knuckle.

condyloid joint [L, kondylos + eidos, form], a synovial joint in which a condyle is received into an elliptic cavity, as the wrist joint. A condyloid joint permits no axial rotation but allows flexion, extension, adduction, abduction, and circumduction.

condyloma /kon′dilō′mə/, pl. condylomata, [Gk, kondyloma, a knob], a wartlike growth on the anus, vulva, or glans penis, usually sexually transmitted.

condyloma latum, pl. condylomata lata, a flat, moist papular growth that appears in secondary syphilis in the coronal sulcus of the perineum or on the glans penis.

cone /kōn/ [Gk, konos, cone], 1. a photoreceptor cell in the retina of the eye that enables a person to visualize colors. There are three kinds of retinal cones, one each for the colors blue, green, and red; other colors are seen by stimulation of more than one type of cone. 2. a cone-shaped device attached to radiologic equipment to focus x-rays on a small target of tissue. —conic /kon′ik/, conical, adj.

cone biopsy, surgical removal of a cone-shaped segment of the cervix, including both epithelial and endocervical tissue.

cone cutting, the interference by a radiographic cone with an x-ray beam caused by misalignment of the tube, cone, and film.

cone of light, 1. a triangular reflection observed during an ear examination when the light of an otoscope is focused on the image of the malleus. 2. the group of light rays entering the pupil of the eye and forming an image on the retina.

confabulation /kənfab′yəlā′shən/ [L, con + fabulari, to speak], the fabrication of experiences or situations, often recounted in a detailed and plausible way to fill in and cover up gaps in memory.

confession /kənfesh′ən/, an act of seeking expiation through another from guilt for a real or imagined transgression.

confidentiality, /kon′fiden′shē·al′itē/ the nondisclosure of certain information except to another authorized person.

confinement /kənfīn′mənt/ [L, confinis,

common boundary], **1.** a state of being held or restrained within a specific place to hinder or minimize activity. **2.** the final phase of pregnancy during which labor and childbirth occur.

confinement deprivation, an emotional disorder that may result when an individual is separated from familiar surroundings or denied contact with familiar persons or objects. It may occur when one is confined to a single room.

conflict /kon'flikt/ [L, *conflictere,* to strike together], **1.** a mental struggle, either conscious or unconscious, resulting from the simultaneous action of opposing or incompatible thoughts, ideas, goals, or emotional forces, such as impulses, desires, or drives. **2.** a painful state of consciousness caused by the arousal of such opposing forces and the inability to resolve them. **3.** (in psychoanalysis) the unconscious emotional struggle between the demands of the id and those of the ego and superego or between the demands of the ego and the restrictions imposed by society.

confluence of the sinuses /kon'flōō·əns/ [L, *confluere,* to flow together], the wide junction of the superior sagittal, straight, and occipital sinuses with the two large transverse sinuses of the dura mater.

confluent /kon'flōō·ənt/ [L, *confluere,* to flow together], running together, such as the sinuses of the dura mater or some skin eruptions.

confrontation test /kon'frəntā'shən/ [L, *con* + *frons,* forehead], a method of assessing a patient's visual field by moving an object into the periphery of each of the visual quadrants. The test is conducted while one eye is covered and the vision of the other is fixed on a point straight ahead. The patient reports when the moving object is first detected at the edge of the visual field.

confusion /kənfyōō'shən/ [L, *confundere,* to mingle], a mental state characterized by disorientation regarding time, place, person, or situation. It causes bewilderment, perplexity, lack of orderly thought, and inability to choose or act decisively and perform the activities of daily living. —**confusional,** *adj.*

confusion, acute, a NANDA-accepted nursing diagnosis defined as the abrupt onset of a cluster of global, transient changes and disturbances in attention, cognition, psychomotor activity, level of consciousness, and/or sleep/wake cycle. Defining characteristics include fluctuation in cognition, sleep/wake cycle, level of consciousness, or psychomotor activity; increased agitation or restlessness; misper-

ceptions; and lack of motivation to initiate or follow through with goal-directed or purposeful behavior.

confusional state, a mild form of delirium. It may occur in any age group or may accompany preexisting brain disease. The confusion may be characterized by failure to perform activities of daily living, memory deficits, disruptive behavior, and inappropriate speech.

confusion, chronic, a NANDA-accepted nursing diagnosis defined as an irreversible long-standing and/or progressive deterioration of intellect and personality characterized by decreased ability to interpret environmental stimuli and decreased capacity to perform intellectual thought processes; it is manifested by disturbances of memory, orientation, and behavior. Defining characteristics include clinical evidence of organic impairment, altered interpretation of or response to stimuli, and progressive or long-standing cognitive impairment, unchanged level of consciousness, impaired socialization, impaired memory (short- and long-term), and altered personality.

congener /kon'jənər/ [L, *con* + *genus,* origin], one of two or more things that are similar or closely related in structure, function, or origin. Examples of congeners are muscles that function identically and chemical compounds similar in composition and effect. —**congenerous** /kənjen'ərəs/, *adj.*

congenital /kənjen'itəl/ [L, *congenitus,* born with], present at birth, as a congenital anomaly or defect.

congenital absence of sacrum and lumbar vertebrae, an abnormal condition present at birth and characterized by varying degrees of deformity, ranging from the absence of the lower segment of the coccyx to the absence of the entire sacrum and all lumbar vertebrae.

congenital adrenal hyperplasia, a group of disorders that have in common an enzyme defect resulting in low levels of cortisol and increased secretion of adrenocorticotropic hormone. During intrauterine life the disorder leads to pseudohermaphroditism in female infants and macrogenitosomia in male infants.

congenital amputation, the absence of a fetal limb or part at birth. The condition previously was attributed to amputation by constricting bands in utero but now is regarded as a developmental defect.

congenital anomaly, any abnormality present at birth, particularly a structural one, which may be inherited genetically acquired during gestation, or inflicted during parturition.

congenital aspiration pneumonia [L, *congenitus*, born with, *aspirare*, to breathe upon; Gk, *pneumon*, lung], a neonatal lung inflammation caused by the aspiration of fluid or meconium during labor.

congenital cardiac anomaly, any structural or functional abnormality or defect of the heart or great vessels present at birth. Congenital heart disease is a major cause of neonatal distress and is the most common cause of death in the newborn other than problems related to prematurity. Congenital heart defects may result from genetic causes or environmental factors such as maternal infection or exposure to radiation or noxious substances during pregnancy. Most defects are probably caused by some interaction between genetic and environmental factors that results in arrested embryonic development. Congenital heart anomalies are classified broadly according to the resulting alteration in circulation as acyanotic, in which no unoxygenated blood mixes in the circulatory system, or cyanotic, in which unoxygenated blood enters the system. The general effects of cardiac malformations on cardiovascular functioning are increased cardiac workload, increased pulmonary vascular resistance, inadequate cardiac output, and decreased oxygen saturation that results from the direct shunting of unoxygenated blood into the circulatory system. The general physical symptoms of these pathophysiologic alterations are growth retardation, decreased exercise tolerance, recurrent respiratory infections, dyspnea, tachypnea, tachycardia, cyanosis, tissue hypoxia, and murmurs.

congenital cyanosis [L, *congenitus*, born with; Gk, *kyanos*, blue, *osis*, condition], cyanosis present at birth caused by a congenital heart disease or atelectasis of the lungs.

congenital cyst [L, *congenitus*, born with; Gk, *kystis*, bag], a cyst present at birth, as a dermoid cyst resulting from an embryonic defect in the skin or midline structures.

congenital dermal sinus, a channel present at birth, extending from the surface of the body and passing between the bodies of two adjacent lumbar vertebrae to the spinal canal.

congenital dislocation of the hip, an orthopedic defect, present at birth, in which the head of the femur does not articulate with the acetabulum as a result of an abnormal shallowness of the acetabulum.

congenital erythropoietic porphyria [L, *congenitus*, born with; Gk, *erythros*, red, *poein*, to make, *porphyros*, purple], a rare autosomal-recessive trait caused by a defect in hemoglobin synthesis in erythrocytes and release of porphyrin from normoblasts in the bone marrow. The porphyrin is excreted in the urine. Symptoms may include dermatitis, enlarged spleen, and hemolytic anemia.

congenital glaucoma, a rare form of glaucoma affecting infants and young children, which results from a congenital closure of the iridocorneal angle by a membrane that obstructs the flow of aqueous humor and increases the intraorbital pressure. The condition is progressive, is usually bilateral, and may damage the optic nerve.

congenital goiter, an enlargement of the thyroid gland at birth. It may be caused by a deficiency of enzymes or iodine required for the production of thyroxine.

congenital hernia [L, *congenitus*, born with, *hernia*, rupture], a hernia caused by a defect present at birth, as an umbilical hernia.

congenital hypogammaglobulinemia [L, *congenitus*, born with; Gk, *hypo*, deficiency, *gamma*, third letter of Greek alphabet; L, *globus*, small globe, *haima*, blood], a genetic disease characterized by a deficiency of gamma globulin and antibody in the serum. The cause may be a genetic defect leading to a failure of development of a normal β-lymphocyte system and immune responses.

congenital immunity [L, *congenitus*, born with, *immunis*, free from], the immunity one has at birth that is acquired from the mother's antibodies as they pass through the placenta.

congenital jaundice [L, *congenitus*, born with; Fr, *jaune*, yellow], jaundice present at birth or during the first 24 hours of life. It is usually caused by poorly developed bile ducts.

congenital laryngeal stridor [L, *congenitus*, born with; Gk, *larynx* + L, *stridens*, a grating noise], a harsh respiratory sound that some infants make the first weeks after birth.

congenital nonspherocytic hemolytic anemia, a group of blood disorders made up of a number of similar inherited diseases, each with a deficiency of one of the enzymes of red cell glycolysis. Most are associated with varying degrees of hemolysis.

congenital pulmonary arteriovenous fistula, a direct connection between the arterial and venous systems of the lung present at birth that results in a right-to-left shunt and permits unoxygenated blood to enter the systemic circulation. The fistula may be single or multiple and may occur in any part of the lung.

congenital scoliosis, an abnormal condition present at birth, characterized by a lateral curvature of the spine. It results from specific congenital rib and vertebral anomalies. The etiologic and pathologic characteristics of congenital scoliosis are divided into six categories. Category I is associated with partial unilateral failure of the formation of a vertebra. Category II is associated with complete unilateral failure of the formation of a vertebra. Category III is associated with bilateral failure of segmentation with the absence of disk space. Category IV is associated with the unilateral failure of segmentation with the unsegmented bar. Category V is associated with the fusion of ribs. Category VI is associated with any condition not covered in the other categories. Category IV scoliosis seems to progress more rapidly and cause the greatest degree of deformity.

congenital short neck syndrome, a rare congenital malformation of the cervical spine in which the cervical vertebrae are fused, usually in pairs, into one mass of bone; this fusion causes decreased neck motion and decreased cervical length, sometimes with neurologic involvement. When the deformity involves nerve-root compression, symptoms of peripheral nerve involvement such as pain or a burning sensation may be evident, accompanied by paralysis, hyperesthesia, or paresthesia.

congenital syphilis [L, *congenitus,* born with; Gk, *syn,* together, *philein,* to love], a form of syphilis acquired in utero. It is generally characterized by osteitis, rashes, coryza, and wasting in the first months of life. Later childhood signs of the infection include interstitial keratitis, deafness, and notches in the incisor teeth. Some infected infants may appear disease free at birth; but typical signs of the disease develop in adolescence.

congested, having an excessive accumulation of a substance such as blood. The condition may be the result of increased production and/or outflow of the substance. It also can result from a decreased ability of the heart to pump.

congestion /kənjes′chən/ [L, *congerere,* to accumulate], an abnormal accumulation of fluid in an organ or body area. The fluid is often mucus, but it may be bile or blood.

congestive, /kənjes′tiv/ pertaining to congestion.

congestive atelectasis [L, *congerere* + Gk, *ateles,* incomplete, *ektasis,* stretching], severe pulmonary congestion characterized by diffuse injury to alveolar-capillary membranes, resulting in hemorrhagic edema, stiffness of the lungs, difficult ventilation, and respiratory failure.

congestive cardiomyopathy [L, *congerere,* to accumulate; Gk, *kardia,* heart, *mys,* muscle, *pathos,* disease], a heart muscle disease characterized by heart failure and enlargement.

congestive dysmenorrhea [L, *congerere,* to accumulate; Gk, *dys,* difficult, *men,* month, *rhein,* to flow], a form of secondary dysmenorrhea caused by pelvic congestion, which arises from an increased blood supply in the area caused by a pelvic disease.

congestive heart failure, an abnormal condition that reflects impaired cardiac pumping. It is caused by myocardial infarction, ischemic heart disease, or cardiomyopathy. Failure of the ventricle to eject blood efficiently results in volume overload, chamber dilation, and elevated intracardiac pressure. Retrograde transmission of increased hydrostatic pressure from the left side of the heart causes pulmonary congestion; elevated pressure from the right side of the heart causes systemic venous congestion and peripheral edema.

congestive splenomegalia [L, *congerere,* to accumulate; Gk, *splen* + *megas,* large], an enlarged spleen associated with gastric hemorrhage, anemia, portal hypertension, and cirrhosis of the liver.

conglomerate silicosis /kənglom′ərit/ [L, *con* + *glomerare,* to wind into a ball], a severe form of silicosis marked by conglomerate masses of mineral dust in the lungs, causing acute shortness of breath, coughing, and production of sputum. Cor pulmonale usually develops.

Congress for Nursing Practice, a unit of the American Nurses Association whose activities concern the scope of nursing practice, legal aspects of nursing practice, public recognition of the significance of nursing practice in health care, and implications of health care trends for nursing practice.

congruent communication /kong′-groo·ənt/, a communication pattern in which the person sends the same message on both verbal and nonverbal levels.

conization /kon′īzā′shən/, the removal of a cone-shaped sample of tissue, as in a cone biopsy.

conjoined manipulation /kənjoind′/ [L, *con* + *jungere,* to yoke together], the use of both hands in obstetric and gynecologic procedures, with one positioned in the vagina and the other on the abdomen

conjoined twins, two fetuses developed from the same ovum who are physically united at birth. Conjoined twins result when separation of the blastomeres in early embryonic development does not oc cur until a late cleavage phase and is incomplete, causing the fused condyle.

conjoint family therapy, /kənjoint/ a form of psychotherapy in which a therapist sees a single nuclear family and addresses the issues and problems raised by family members.

conjugata /kon'jəgā'tə [L, *conjugere,* to yoke together], pertaining to the combined diameters of the pelvis.

conjugate /kon'jəgit/ [L, *con* + *jungere,* to yoke together], (in pelvimetry) the measurement of the female pelvis to determine whether the presenting part of a fetus can enter the birth canal.

conjugated estrogen /kon'jəgā'tid/, a mixture of sodium salts of estrogen sulfates, chiefly those of estrone, equilin, and 17-alpha-dihydroequilin, blended to approximate the average composition of estrogenic substances in the urine of pregnant mares. Conjugated estrogens may be prescribed to relieve postmenopausal vasomotor symptoms such as hot flushes; to treat atrophic vaginitis, female hypogonadism, and primary ovarian failure; and to provide palliation in advanced prostatic carcinoma and metastatic breast cancer.

conjugate deviation [L, *conjugere,* to yoke together, *deviare,* to turn aside], pertaining to movements of the two eyes in which their visual axes function in parallel. The cause is a dysfunction of the ocular muscles, which allows the eyes to diverge to the same side when at rest.

conjugated protein, a compound that contains a protein molecule united to a nonprotein substance.

conjugate paralysis [L, *conjugere,* to yoke together; Gk, *paralyein,* to be palsied], a condition of paralysis of the conjugate movements of the two eyes, up or down or to the right or left. There is no diplopia. The cause is a cranial nerve lesion.

conjugation /kon'jəgā'shən/, (in genetics) a form of sexual reproduction in acellular organisms. In *Paramecium,* for example, both partners swap micronuclear material so that each partner exchanges (or sends) "male" pronuclei to the recipient "female." This genetic material is incorporated, recombined, and then passed on to the progeny through replication.

conjugon /kon'jōōgon/, an episome that induces bacterial conjugation.

conjunctiva /kon'jungktī'və/ [L, *conjunctivus,* connecting], the mucous membrane lining the inner surfaces of the eyelids and anterior part of the sclera. The palpebral conjunctiva lines the inner surface of the eyelids and is thick, opaque, and highly vascular. The bulbar conjunctiva is loosely connected, thin, and transparent, covering the sclera of the anterior third of the eye.

conjunctival burns /-ī-vəl/, chemical burns of the conjunctiva. Emergency treatment involves irrigating the eye with copious amounts of water for as long as 30 minutes or until the chemical has been neutralized. Emergency medical care should be sought.

conjunctival reflex, a protective mechanism of the eye in which the eyelids close whenever the conjunctiva is touched.

conjunctival ring, a narrow ring at the junction of the conjunctiva and the periphery of the cornea.

conjunctival sac [L, *conjunctivus,* connecting; Gk, *sakkos*], the space enclosed by the conjunctiva and the eyelids.

conjunctival test, a procedure used to identify offending allergens by instilling the eye with a dilute solution of the allergenic extract.

conjunctivitis /kənjungk'tivī'tis/, inflammation of the conjunctiva caused by bacterial or viral infection, allergy, or environmental factors. Red eyes, thick discharge, sticky eyelids in the morning, and inflammation without pain are characteristic.

conjunctivitis of newborn [L, *conjunctivus,* connecting, *itis,* inflammation; ME, *newe* + *borne*], a condition characterized by a purulent discharge from the eyes of an infant during the first 3 weeks of life. Frequent causes include maternal gonococcal and chlamydial infections, which may lead to blindness if untreated.

connecting fibrocartilage [L, *con* + *nectere,* to bind], a disk of fibrocartilage found between many joints, especially those with limited mobility, such as the spinal vertebrae. Each disk is composed of concentric rings of fibrous tissue separated by cartilaginous laminae.

connective /kənek'tiv/ [L, *cum,* together with, *nectere,* to bind], pertaining to a binding or connection.

connective tissue, tissue that supports and binds other body tissue and parts. It derives from the mesoderm of the embryo and is dense, containing large numbers of cells and large amounts of intercellular material. The intercellular material is composed of fibers in a matrix or ground substance that may be liquid, gelatinous, or solid, such as in bone and cartilage. Kinds of connective tissue are **bone, cartilage, fibrous,** and loose connective tissue.

Conn's syndrome [Jerome W. Conn, American physician, b. 1907; Gk, *syn,* together, *dromos,* course], primary hyperaldosteronism, characterized by excessive secretion of aldosterone with symptoms of headache, fatigue, nocturia, and increased urination. The patient may also experience hypertension, hypokalemic alkalosis potassium depletion, and hypervolemia.

consanguinity /kon'sang·gwin'itē/ [L, *con* + *sanguis,* blood], a hereditary or "blood" relationship between persons that results from a common parent or ancestor.

conscience [L, *conscientia,* to be privy to information], **1.** the moral, self-critical sense of what is right and wrong. **2.** (in psychoanalysis) the part of the superego system that monitors thoughts, feelings, and actions and measures them against internalized values and standards.

conscious /kon'shəs/ [L, *conscire,* to be aware], **1.** (in neurology) capable of responding to sensory stimuli; awake, alert; aware of one's external environment. **2.** (in psychiatry) that part of the psyche or mental functioning in which thoughts, ideas, emotions, and other mental content are in complete awareness.

consciousness /kon'shəsnes/, a clear state of awareness of self and the environment in which attention is focused on immediate matters.

conscious proprioception, the conscious awareness of body position and movement of body segments. It is regulated by the lemniscal system through pathways that begin in joint receptors and end in the parietal lobe of the cerebral cortex; it enables the cortex to refine voluntary movements.

conscious sedation, the administration of central nervous system depressant drugs and/or analgesics to supplement topical, local, or regional anesthesia during surgical or diagnostic procedures. It is most often used to supplement analgesia, relieve anxiety, and/or provide amnesia for the event. Consciousness is depressed, and the patient may fall asleep but is not unconscious. Anesthetic monitoring during conscious sedation includes, at a minimum, monitoring of blood pressure, electrocardiography, and pulse oximetry.

consensual /konsen'choo·əl/ [L, *con* + *sentire,* to feel], pertaining to a reflex action in which stimulation of one body part results in a response in another.

consensual light reflex, a normally present crossed reflex in which light directed at one eye causes the opposite pupil to contract. In monocular blindness the pupil of the blind eye reacts consensually with stimulation of the seeing eye but does not cause constriction of the pupil of either eye.

consensually validated symbols, symbols that are accepted by enough people that they have an agreed-on meaning.

consensual reaction, contraction of the pupil of one eye when the contralateral

retina is stimulated. It is a common reflex.

consensual validation, a mutual agreement by two or more persons about a particular meaning that is to be attributed to verbal or nonverbal behavior.

consensus sequence /kənsen'səs/, (in molecular genetics) a sequence in a strand of ribonucleic acid (RNA) nucleotides that is used as a site for the insertion of a splice of an RNA sequence from another source into the segment.

consent /kənsent'/ [L, *consentire,* to agree], to give approval, assent, or permission.

consenting adult, an adult who willingly agrees to participate in an activity with one or more other adults. The term is usually applied to sexual activity.

consequences /kon'səkwen'səs/, stimulus events that follow a behavior that strengthen or weaken it. They may be either reinforcers or punishers.

conservation of energy /kon'sərvā'shən/ [L, *conservare,* to preserve], (in physics) a law stating that in any closed system the total amount of energy is constant.

conservation of matter, (in physics) a law stating that matter can be neither created nor destroyed and that the amount of matter in the universe is finite.

conservation principles of nursing, a conceptual framework for nursing that is directed to maintaining the wholeness or integrity of the patient when the normal ability to cope is disturbed or exceeded by stress. Nursing intervention is determined by the patient's need to conserve energy and to maintain structural, personal, and social integrity. The nurse acts as a "conservationist."

Consolidated Omnibus Budget Reconciliation Act (COBRA), legislation that provides for limited continuation of health coverage for individuals and families at the individual's own expense when the individual terminates employment from an organization that provides health insurance.

consolidation /kənsol'idā'shən/ [L, *consolidare,* to make solid], **1.** the combining of separate parts into a single whole. **2.** a state of solidification. **3.** (in medicine) the process of becoming solid, as when the lungs become firm and inelastic in pneumonia.

consolidation of individuality and emotional constancy, (in psychiatry) the fourth and final subphase in Mahler's system of the separation-individuation phase of preoedipal development. It begins toward the end of the second year.

constancy /kon'stənsē/, an absence of variation in quality of distinctive features despite location, rotation, size, or color of an object.

constant pressure generator, a machine that provides or generates a constant gas pressure throughout the inspiratory cycle of breathing. The pressure may range from a low value, such as 12 cm H_2O, to a high value of as much as 3500 cm H_2O, as required.

constant region, an area of an immunoglobulin molecule in which the amino acid sequence is relatively constant.

constant touch, a technique to diagnose the sensitivity of an injured body part such as a hand by pressing the eraser end of a pencil or another object in various areas to determine the person's ability to detect the pressure.

constipation /kon'stipā'shən/ [L, *constipare,* to crowd together], difficulty in passing stools or incomplete or infrequent passage of hard stools. Among the organic causes are intestinal obstruction, diverticulitis, and tumors. Functional impairment of the colon may occur in elderly or bedridden patients who fail to respond to the urge to defecate. —**constipated,** *adj.*

constipation, a NANDA-accepted nursing diagnosis of a condition with causes that include less than adequate intake and bulk, less than adequate physical activity, medication side effects, chronic use of medications and enemas, gastrointestinal obstructive lesions, neuromuscular or musculoskeletal impairment, and weak abdominal musculature. Defining characteristics include decreased frequency of elimination; a hard, formed stool; a palpable rectal mass; straining at stool; decreased bowel sounds; and reported feeling of abdominal or rectal fullness or pressure.

constipation, colonic, a NANDA-accepted nursing diagnosis of a state in which an individual's pattern of elimination is characterized by hard, dry stool that results from a delay in passage of food residue. Defining characteristics include decreased frequency, hard dry stool, straining at stool, painful defecation, abdominal distension, and a palpable mass.

constipation, perceived, a NANDA-accepted nursing diagnosis of a state in which an individual makes a self-diagnosis of constipation and ensures a daily bowel movement through use of laxatives, enemas, and suppositories. The defining characteristic is an expectation of a daily bowel movement, which may be expected at the same time every day, with the resulting overuse of laxatives, enemas, and suppositories.

constipation, rectal, a NANDA-accepted nursing diagnosis of a state in which an individual's pattern of elimination is characterized by stool retention, normal stool consistency, and delayed elimination that results from biopsychosocial disruptions. Abdominal discomfort, rectal fullness, and a change in flatus also occur.

constitution, the general bodily health of an individual, expressed by the person's physical and mental abilities to function adequately in adverse circumstances.

constitutional delay /kon'stityoo'shənəl/ [L, *constituere,* to establish], a period in a child's development during which growth may be interrupted. In some cases constitutional delay may be associated with an illness or stressful event.

constitutional disease [L, *constituere,* to set up; Gk, *dis,* without; Fr, *aise,* ease], any disease associated with the inborn physical condition of the client, such as a hereditary susceptibility.

constitutional psychology, the study of the relationship of individual psychologic makeup to body morphologic characteristics and organic functioning.

constitutive resistance /kənstich'ootiv/, the bacterial resistance to antibiotics that is contained in the deoxyribonucleic acid molecules of the organism. The trait can be passed on to daughter cells through cell division.

constriction /kənstrik'shən/ [L, *constringere,* to draw tight], an abnormal closing or reduction in the size of an opening or passage of the body, as in vasoconstriction of a blood vessel.

constriction ring, a band of contracted uterine muscle that forms a stricture around part of the fetus during labor, usually after premature rupture of the membranes and sometimes impeding labor.

constrictive cardiomyopathy /kənstrik'tiv/ [L, *constringere,* to draw tight; Gk, *kardia,* heart, *mys,* muscle, *pathos, dis,* ease], a heart disorder in which there is decreased diastolic compliance of the ventricles, imitating constrictive pericarditis.

constrictive pericarditis, a fibrous thickening of the pericardium caused by gradual scarring or fibrosis of the membrane. The pericardium gradually becomes a rigid membrane that resists the normal dilation of the heart chambers during the blood-filling phases of the cardiac cycle.

constrictor /kənstrik'tər/, a muscle that causes a narrowing of an opening, as the ciliary body fibers that control the size of the pupil.

constructional apraxia /kənstruk'shənəl/ [L, *construere,* to build], a form of apraxia characterized by the inability to copy drawings or to manipulate objects to form patterns or designs. It is caused by a right hemisphere lesion.

constructive aggression /kənstruk′tiv/, an act of self-assertiveness in response to a threatening action for purposes of self-protection and preservation.

constructive interference, (in ultrasonography) an increase in amplitude of sound waves that results when multiple waves of equal frequency are transmitted precisely in phase.

construct validity /kon′strəkt/, validity of a test or measurement tool that is established by demonstrating its ability to identify the variables that it proposes to identify.

consultant /kənsul′tənt/ [L, *consultare,* to deliberate], a person who by training and experience has acquired a special knowledge in a subject area that has been recognized by a peer group.

consultation /kon′səltā′shən/ [L, *consultare,* to deliberate], a process in which the help of a specialist is sought to identify ways to handle problems in patient management or in planning and implementing health care programs.

consultee-centered communication /kon′-sultē′/, expert advice or guidance that is given a consultee (health care worker) to improve the consultee's capacity to function more effectively in working with patients.

contact [L, *contingere,* to touch], **1.** the touching or drawing together of two surfaces, as those of upper and lower teeth. **2.** the moving together, either directly or indirectly, of two individuals so as to allow the transmission of an infectious organism from one to the other. **3.** a person who has been exposed to an infectious disease.

contact allergy, hypersensitivity to a substance that produced a reaction in a previous contact or that is structurally similar to another substance that produced such a reaction.

contact dermatitis, skin rash resulting from exposure to a primary irritant or to a sensitizing antigen. In the nonallergic type a primary irritant such as an alkaline detergent or an acid causes a lesion similar to a thermal burn. In the allergic type sensitizing antigens cause an immunologic change in certain lymphocytes. Subsequent exposure to the antigen causes the lymphocytes to release irritating chemicals, leading to inflammation, edema, and vesiculation.

contact factor. See **factor XII.**

contact hour, a 50-minute "hour" used to measure time for continuing education programs.

contact lens, a small, curved lens, pri-

marily plastic in composition, shaped to fit the person's eye either to correct refractive error or to enhance appearance. The two primary forms of contact lenses are (1) rigid gas-permeable lenses, and (2) soft lenses.

contactor /kəntak′tər/, a switching device that is part of the timer for the control of voltage across an x-ray tube.

Contact Precautions, safeguards designed to reduce the risk of transmission of epidemiologically important microorganisms by direct or indirect contact. Direct-contact transmission involves skin-to-skin contact and physical transfer of microorganisms to a susceptible host from an infected or colonized person (having the presence of microorganisms, but without clinical signs or symptoms of infection). This can occur when health care personnel perform patient-care activities that require physical contact. Indirect-contact transmission involves contact of a susceptible host with a contaminated intermediate object, usually inanimate, in the patient's environment.

contact shield, a protective device constructed of metal or other material that is positioned directly over the eyes or gonads of a patient to be exposed to an x-ray beam.

contagion /kəntā′jən/ [L, *contingere,* to touch], the transmission of a disease by direct contact with a person who has it or by indirect contact through handling of clothing, bedding, dishes, or other objects the person has used.

contagious /kəntā′jəs/ [L, *contingere,* to touch], communicable, such as a disease that may be transmitted by direct or indirect contact. —**contagion,** *n.*

contagious pustular dermatitis [L, *contingere,* to touch, *pustula,* pustules; Gk, *derma,* skin, *itis,* inflammation], a skin disease normally affecting sheep but transmitted to humans who handle infected animals. It is caused by a pox virus and results in lesions on the hands and occasionally on the face.

contaminant /kəntam′inənt/ [L, *contaminare,* to bring in contact], an agent that causes contamination, pollution, or spoilage, such as a mold spore that makes food unsafe to eat.

contaminated culture, a bacterial culture that has acquired unwanted foreign microorganisms.

contamination /-ā′shən/ [L, *contaminare,* to pollute], a condition of being soiled, stained, touched, or otherwise exposed to harmful agents, making an object potentially unsafe for use as intended or without barrier techniques.

content validity, validity of a test or

measurement as a result of the use of previously tested items or concepts within the tool.

context [L, *contexere,* to weave together], (in communications theory) the setting, meaning, and language of a message.

continence /kon'tinəns/ [L, *continere,* to contain], **1.** the ability to control bladder or bowel function. **2.** the use of self-restraint, particularly in regard to sexual intercourse.

continent ileostomy /kon'tinənt/, an ileostomy that drains into a surgically created pouch or reservoir in the abdomen. Involuntary discharge of intestinal contents is prevented by a nipple valve created from the ileum.

contingency contracting /kəntin'jənsē/ [L, *contingere,* to touch], a formal agreement between a psychotherapist and a patient undergoing behavior therapy regarding the consequences of certain actions by both parties.

contingency management, any of a group of techniques used in behavior therapy that attempts to modify a behavioral response by controlling the consequences of that response.

continuing care nurse /kəntin'yoo·ing/, [L, *continuare,* to unite], a nurse who specializes in coordination of the overall needs of the patient with the potential health care resources of the community. Continuing care nursing responsibilities and discharge planning ideally begin at the time a patient is admitted to a hospital.

continuing education, (in nursing) formal educational programs designed to promote the knowledge, skills, and professional attitudes of nurses. Continuing education is required for relicensure in many states. It is not to be confused with academic degree-granting programs, such as advanced education or graduate education.

continuing education unit (CEU), a point awarded to a professional person by a professional organization for having attended an educational program relevant to the goals of the organization.

continuity theory /kon'tinyoo'itē/, a concept that an individual's personality does not change as the person ages, with the result that his or her behavior becomes more predictable.

continuous ambulatory peritoneal dialysis /kəntin'yoo·əs/ [L, *continuare,* to unite, *ambulare,* to walk about; Gk, *peri,* near, *tenein,* to stretch, *dia,* through, *lysis,* loosening], a maintenance system of peritoneal dialysis in which an indwelling catheter permits fluid to drain into and out of the peritoneal cavity by gravity.

continuous anesthesia [L, *continuare,* to

unite], a method for maintaining regional nerve block in anesthesia for surgical operations or labor in which an anesthetic solution is infused either at intervals or at a low rate of flow. The procedure is named according to the area infiltrated: continuous epidural, caudal, spinal, or brachial plexus block.

continuous cycling peritoneal dialysis (CCPD), a type of dialysis in which the patient is attached to an automatic cycler for short exchanges while sleeping at night.

continuous fever, a fever that persists steadily for a prolonged period.

continuous flow analyzer, a device that automatically analyzes a series of samples of biologic materials that are continuously pumped into tubes along with appropriate reagents.

continuous murmur [L, *continuare,* to unite, *murmur,* humming], an uninterrupted heart murmur or cervical venous hum that characteristically begins in systole and persists through diastole.

continuous negative chest wall pressure, a negative pressure (below ambient pressure) that is applied to the chest wall during the entire respiratory cycle, thus increasing transpulmonary pressure.

continuous passive motion (CPM), a technique for maintaining or increasing the amount of movement in a joint, using a mechanical device that applies force to produce joint motion without normal muscle function.

continuous phase [L, *continuare,* to unite; Gk, *phasis,* appearance], the phase of a colloidal solution corresponding to that of the solvent of a true solution.

continuous positive airway pressure (CPAP), (in respiratory therapy) a method of noninvasive ventilation assisted by a flow of air delivered at a constant pressure throughout the respiratory cycle. It is performed for patients who can initiate their own respirations but who are not able to maintain adequate arterial oxygen levels without assistance. CPAP may be given through a ventilator and endotracheal tube, through a nasal cannula, or into a hood over the patient's head.

continuous positive-pressure ventilation, a positive pressure above ambient pressure maintained at the upper airway throughout the breathing cycle. The term is usually applied to positive end expiratory pressure and mechanical ventilation.

continuous reinforcement, a schedule of strengthening or rewarding behavior in which omission of a response is followed by a reinforcing event or behavior.

continuous tremor, fine, rhythmic, purposeless movements that persist during rest but sometimes disappear briefly during voluntary movements.

continuous tub bath, a therapeutic bath, usually prescribed in the treatment of some dermatologic conditions, in which the patient lies supported in a medicated solution of tepid water.

continuous wave (CW), 1. an uninterrupted flow of energy, such as a beam of laser light, as opposed to pulsed emission of energy. **2.** sound intensity that remains constant while ultrasound energy is being produced 100% of the time throughout the procedure.

continuum /kəntin'yōo·əm/, *pl.* **continua, 1.** a continuous series or whole. **2.** (in mathematics) a system of real numbers.

contoured adducted trochanteric controlled alignment method (CAT-CAM) /kon'tōord/, a design for an artificial lower limb for persons who have undergone above the knee amputations.

contra bevel [L, *contra,* against; OFr, *baif,* open mouth], **1.** (in dentistry) the angle between a cutting blade and the base of the periodontal pocket when the blade is held so that it separates the sulcular epithelium from the external epithelium of the gingiva. **2.** (in dentistry) an external bevel of a tooth preparation extending onto a buccal or lingual cusp from an intracoronal restoration.

contraception /kon'trəsep'shən/ [L, *contra + concipere,* to take in], a process or technique for preventing pregnancy by means of a medication, device, or method that blocks or alters one or more of the processes of reproduction in such a way that sexual union can occur without impregnation. Kinds of contraception include **cervical cap, condom, contraceptive diaphragm, intrauterine device, natural family planning method, oral contraceptive,** spermicide, and **sterilization.**

contraceptive /kon'trəsep'tiv/, [L, *contra + concipere,* to take in], any device or technique that prevents conception.

contraceptive diaphragm a contraceptive device consisting of a hemisphere of thin rubber bonded to a flexible ring and inserted into the vagina together with spermicidal jelly or cream so that spermatozoa cannot enter the uterus, thus preventing conception.

contraceptive diaphragm fitting, a procedure, performed in an office or clinic, in which a contraceptive diaphragm is selected according to the clinical assessment of anatomic factors specific to the woman being fitted.

contraceptive effectiveness, the effectiveness of a method of contraception in preventing pregnancy. It is sometimes represented as a percentage but more accurately as the number of pregnancies per 100 woman-years. A contraceptive method that results in a pregnancy rate of fewer than 10 pregnancies per 100 woman-years is considered highly effective.

contraceptive jelly [L, *contra,* opposed, *concipere,* to take in, *gelare,* to congeal], a gelatinous preparation containing a spermicide to be introduced into the vagina to prevent conception.

contraceptive method, any act, device, or medication for avoiding conception or a viable pregnancy.

contract [L, *con + trahere,* to draw], /kon' trakt/ **1.** an agreement or a promise that meets certain legal requirements, including competence of both or all parties to the contract, proper lawful subject matter, mutuality of agreement, mutuality of obligation, and consideration (the exchange of something of value in payment for the obligation undertaken). **2.** /kəntrakt'/, to make such an agreement or promise. —**contractual** /kəntrak'chōo·əl/, *adj.*

contracted kidney, a kidney that is greatly reduced in size and function as a result of an overgrowth of fibrous tissue and a diminished blood supply. The condition occurs in arteriolar nephrosclerosis and glomerulonephritis.

contractile /kəntrak'tíl/ [L, *con,* with, *trahere,* to draw], capable of becoming reduced in size or length or of being drawn together in response to some stimulus.

contractile ring dysphagia [L, *con + trahere,* to draw; AS, *hring*], an abnormal condition characterized by difficulty in swallowing caused by an overreactive interior esophageal sphincteric mechanism that induces painful sticking sensations under the lower sternum.

contractility /kon'traktil'itē/, (in cardiology) a property of muscle tissue, particularly cardiac muscle, that allows it to contract by shortening the sarcomeres.

contraction /kəntrak'shən/ [L, *con + trahere,* to draw], **1.** a reduction in size, especially of muscle fibers. **2.** an abnormal shrinkage. **3.** (in labor) a rhythmic tightening of the musculature of the upper uterine segment that begins as mild tightening and becomes very strong late in labor, occurring as frequently as every 2 minutes and lasting over 1 minute. **4.** abnormal smallness of the birth canal or part of it, a cause of dystocia. Inlet contraction exists if the anteroposterior diameter is 10 cm or less or if the transverse diameter is 11.5 cm or less. Midpelvic contraction exists if the sum of the measurements in centimeters of the interspinous diameter (nor mally 10.5 cm) and the posterior sagittal diameter (normally 5 cm) is 13.5 cm or less. Outlet contraction exists if the intertuberous diameter is 8 cm or less.

contractions stress test (CST), ultrasound monitoring of the fetal heart rate during uterine contractions induced by oxytocin administration or nipple stimulation.

contract-model HMO, a model in which the health maintenance organization (HMO) contracts with individual physicians rather than groups of providers for services not produced directly by the HMO.

contracture /kəntrak′chər/ [L, *contractura,* a pulling together], an abnormal, usually permanent condition of a joint, characterized by flexion and fixation and caused by atrophy and shortening of muscle fibers or by loss of the normal elasticity of the skin, such as from the formation of extensive scar tissue over a joint.

contraindicate /kon′trə·in′dikāt/ [L, *contra,* against; *indicare,* to make known], to report the presence of a disease or physical condition that makes it impossible or undesirable to treat a particular client in the usual manner or to prescribe medicines that might otherwise be suitable.

contraindication /in′dikā′shən/ [L, *contra,* against, *indicare,* to make known], a factor that prohibits the administration of a drug or the performance of an act or procedure in the care of a specific patient.

contralateral /-lat′ərəl/ [L, *contra* + *lateralis,* side], affecting or originating in the opposite side of a point or reference, such as a point on a body.

contralateral reflexes [L, *contra,* against, *latus,* side, *reflectere,* to bend back], an overflow phenomenon of the nervous system in which a reflex is elicited on one side of the body by a stimulus to the opposite side.

contrast /kon′trast/ [L, *contra,* against, *stare,* to stand], a measure of the differences in radiographic density between two adjacent areas in an image. Contrast may be based on differences in optic density, differences in radiation transmission, or other parameters.

contrast bath, a bath in which the patient alternately immerses a part of the body, usually the hands or feet, in hot and cold water for a specified period. The procedure is used to increase the blood flow to a particular area.

contrast examination, the use of radiopaque materials to make internal organs visible on x-ray film.

contrast medium, a radiopaque substance that is injected into the body, introduced via catheter, or swallowed to facilitate radiographic imaging of internal structures that otherwise are difficult to visualize on x-ray films.

contrasuppressor cell, one of a group of T cells that inhibit the function of T suppressor cells.

contrecoup injury /kôntrekoo′/ [L, *contra,* against; Fr, *coup,* blow; L, *injuria*], an injury, usually involving the brain, in which the tissue damage is on the side opposite the trauma site, as when a blow to the left side of the head results in brain damage on the right side.

contributory negligence, a legal term describing a situation in which both the plaintiff and the defendant share in the negligence that caused injury to the plaintiff.

control [Fr, *controler,* to register], to exercise restraint or maintain influence over a situation, as in self-control, the conscious limitation or suppression of impulses.

control cable, a stainless steel wire, usually contained in a flexible stainless steel housing, used to move or lock a prosthesis into place.

control gene, (in molecular genetics) a gene such as the operator gene or regulator gene that controls the transcription of the amino acid sequence in the structural gene by either inducing or repressing protein synthesis.

controlled area, a part of a hospital or other health facility that is occupied primarily by personnel who work with radioactive materials. It is designed with barrier shielding to confine the radiation.

controlled association, 1. a direct connection of relevant ideas that results from a specific stimulus. **2.** a process of drawing repressed ideas into the consciousness in response to words spoken by a psychoanalyst.

controlled oxygen therapy, the administration of oxygen to a patient on a dose-response basis in which oxygen is regarded as a drug and only the smallest amount of gas is used to obtain a desired therapeutic effect.

controlled substance [Fr, *controle,* to register; L, *substantia,* essence], any drug defined in the five categories of the federal **Controlled Substances Act of 1970.** The categories, or schedules, cover opium and its derivatives, hallucinogens, depressants, and stimulants.

Controlled Substances Act, a U.S. law enacted in 1970 that regulates the prescribing and dispensing of psychoactive drugs, including stimulants, depressants, and hallucinogens. The act lists five categories of restricted drugs, organized by their medical acceptance, abuse potential, and ability to produce dependence.

controlled ventilation, the use of an intermittent positive-pressure breathing unit or other respirator that has an automatic cycling device that replaces spontaneous respiration.

control of hemorrhage, the limitation of the flow of blood from a break in the wall of a blood vessel. Some of the methods for controlling hemorrhage are direct pressure, use of a tourniquet, and application of pressure on pressure points proximal to the wound. Direct pressure with a thick compress is applied in such a way that the edges of the wound are drawn together. A tourniquet is applied proximal to the site of bleeding only in the most extreme emergency because the limb may then have to be removed as a result of tissue anoxia stemming from the use of the tourniquet. Firm manual pressure is applied to a pressure point over the main artery supplying the wound. Points used to obtain the pulse may be used as pressure points to stop hemorrhage.

control process, a system of establishing standards, objectives, and methods and measuring actual performance, comparing results, reinforcing strengths, and taking necessary corrective action.

contuse, to injure a body part without breaking the skin.

contusion /kənt(y)ōo′zhən/ [L, *contundere,* to bruise], an injury that does not disrupt the integrity of the skin, caused by a blow to the body and characterized by swelling, discoloration, and pain. The immediate application of cold may limit the development of a contusion.

convalescence /kon′vəles′əns/ [L, *convalescere,* to grow strong], the period of recovery after an illness, injury, or surgery.

convalescent carrier, a person who has recovered from the symptoms of an infectious disease but is still capable of transmitting pathogens to others.

convection /kənvek′shən/ [L, *convehere,* to bring together], (in physics) the transfer of heat through a gas or liquid by the circulation of heated particles.

convergence /kənvur′jəns/ [L, *convergere,* to bend together], the movement of two objects toward a common point, such as the turning of the eyes inward to see an object close to the face.

convergent evolution, the adaptation of nonhomologous organs in different phylogenetic species in response to similar environmental conditions.

convergent nystagmus, an intermittent spasmodic movement of the eyes in which they move rhythmically toward each other and slowly return to the original position. It is usually caused by a tumor of the anterior aqueduct of Silvius, third ventricle, or midbrain.

conversion /kənvur′zhən/ [L, *convertere,* to turn around], **1.** changing from one form to another, transmutation. **2.** (in obstetrics) the correction of a fetal position during labor. **3.** (in psychiatry) an unconscious defense mechanism by which emotional conflicts that ordinarily cause anxiety are repressed and transformed into symbolic physical symptoms that have no organic basis.

conversion disorder, an abnormality in which repressed emotional conflicts are changed into sensory, motor, or visceral symptoms with no underlying organic cause such as blindness, anesthesia, hypesthesia, hyperesthesia, paresthesia, involuntary muscular movements, paralysis, aphonia, mutism, hallucinations, catalepsy, choking sensations, or respiratory difficulties.

conversion factor, a dollar value multiplied by a procedure's unit value, from the **Current Procedural Terminology (CPT)** codes or a relative value scale, used to calculate the payment amount for contracted services or to set a price for a service.

conversion reaction, an ego defense mechanism whereby intrapsychic conflict is expressed symbolically through physical symptoms.

convex [L, *convextus,* vaulted], having a surface that curves outward.

convoluted [L, *convolutus,* rolled together], twisted, rolled together, with one part over another in a scroll. Also **convolute.**

convoluted kidney tubules /kon′vəlōo′tid/ [L, *convolutus,* rolled together; ME, *kidenei;* L, *tubulus*], pertaining to the convoluted part of the nephron that leads from the glomerulus to the connecting ducts. The proximal and distal sections are convoluted, whereas the ascending and descending limbs of Henle's loop are relatively straight.

convoluted seminiferous tubules, the long threadlike tubes in the areolar tissue of the testes. The testes also contain straight segments of seminiferous tubules.

convulsion. See **seizure.**

convulsive seizure /kənvul′siv/ [L, *convulsio,* cramp; OFr, *seisir*], a sudden onset of a disease characterized by convulsions, palpitations, and other symptoms. The term is sometimes applied to an attack of an epileptic disorder.

convulsive tic, a disorder of the facial nerve, causing involuntary spasmodic contractions of the facial muscles supplied by that nerve.

Coolidge tube, William D. Coolidge, American physician, 1873–1977], a basic type of hot-cathode x-ray tube that, with modern refinements, has been used by radiologists since it was invented in 1913.

cooling [AS, *colian*, cool],   reducing body temperature by the application of a hypothermia blanket, cold moist dressings, ice packs, or an alcohol bath.

cooling rate,   the rate at which temperature decreases with time (° C/minute) immediately after the completion of hyperthermia treatment.

Coombs' positive hemolytic anemia /kōōmz/ [Robin R. A. Coombs, British immunologist, b. 1921],   a form of anemia that results from premature destruction of circulating red blood cells.

cooperative play /kō·op′erətiv′/,   any organized recreation among a group of children in which activities are planned for the purpose of achieving some goal.

coordinated reflex /kō·ôr′dinā′tid/ [L, *co-ordinare*, to arrange],   a sequence of muscular actions that occur in a purposeful, orderly progression, such as the act of swallowing.

copayment /kō′pāmənt/,   (in the United States) an amount paid for each office or emergency room visit or purchase of prescription drugs by a health insurance plan enrollee for specific services such as immunizations or physical examinations.

COPD, abbreviation for **chronic obstructive pulmonary disease.**

coping [Gk, *kolaphos*, buffet],   a process by which a person deals with stress, solves problems, and makes decisions. The process has two components, cognitive and noncognitive. The cognitive component includes the thought and learning necessary to identify the source of the stress.

coping, defensive, a NANDA-accepted nursing diagnosis of a state in which an individual has a falsely positive self-evaluation based on a self-protective pattern that defends against underlying perceived threats to positive self-regard. Defining characteristics include denial of obvious problems, projection of blame, rationalization of failures, hypersensitivity in response to a slight or criticism, a superior attitude toward others, difficulty in establishing or maintaining relationships, hostile laughter or ridicule of others, difficulty in reality-testing perceptions, and lack of follow through or participation in treatment or therapy.

coping, family: potential for growth, a NANDA-accepted nursing diagnosis de-

fined as effective managing of adaptive tasks by the family member involved with the client's health challenge, who now is exhibiting desire and readiness for enhanced health and growth in regard to self and in relation to the client.

coping, ineffective family: compromised, a NANDA-accepted nursing diagnosis of a lack or absence of emotional and psychologic support for the client that is usually available from a family member or other supportive person, a deficiency that causes the client further difficulty in coping with the current health problem. Defining characteristics include expression by the client that support is lacking or expression by the supportive person that fear, anticipatory grief, anxiety, or another reaction is interfering with the ability to give support to the client.

coping, ineffective family: disabling, a NANDA-accepted nursing diagnosis of the detrimental attitudes and behavior of a family, a family member, or another person who is important to the client. The cause of the problem is often the disablement of the significant person by grief, anxiety, guilt, hostility, or despair. Defining characteristics include neglect in the care of the client, intolerance, rejection or abandonment, adoption of the client's symptoms, disregard of the client's needs, and marked distortion of reality in regard to the client's health problem.

coping,   ineffective   individual, a NANDA-accepted nursing diagnosis defined as impairment of a person's adaptive behaviors and problem-solving abilities in meeting life's demands and roles. The problem may result from situational crises, maturational or developmental crises, or personal vulnerability. Defining characteristics include an inability to meet the expectations of a role, an inability to meet one's basic needs, or an alteration in ability to participate in society. The critical defining characteristics, one of which must be present for the diagnosis to be made, are an inability to ask for help, an inability to solve problems, and verbalization of the inability to cope.

coping mechanism, any effort directed to stress management, including task-oriented and ego defense mechanisms; the factors that enable an individual to regain emotional equilibrium after a stressful experience.

coping resources,   the characteristics of a person, group, or environment that are helpful in assisting individuals in adapting to stress.

coping style,   the cognitive, affective, or

behavioral responses of a person to problematic or traumatic life events.

COPP, an anticancer drug combination of cyclophosphamide, procarbazine, and prednisone.

copper (Cu) [L, *cuprum*], a malleable, reddish-brown metallic element. Its atomic number is 29; its atomic weight (mass) is 63.55. It is a component of several important enzymes in the body and is essential to good health. Copper deficiency is rare because only 2 to 5 mg daily, easily obtained from a variety of foods, is sufficient for a proper balance. Copper accumulates in individuals with Wilson's disease, primary biliary cirrhosis, and occasionally chronic extrahepatic biliary tract obstruction.

copperhead /kop'ərhed'/ [L, *cuprum* + ME, *hed*], a poisonous pit viper found mainly in the southeastern United States. The reddish brown, darkly banded snake is responsible for nearly 40% of the snakebites in the United States; few bites are fatal. Pain, swelling, fang marks, and a bruise are usually present.

coprolalia /kop'rōlā'lyə/ [Gk, *kopros,* dung, *lalein,* to babble], the excessive use of obscene language.

coprolith, a hard mass of feces in the intestinal tract usually caused by excessive absorption of water from the large intestine.

coproporphyria /kop'rōpôrfir'ē·ə/ [Gk, *kopros* + *porphyros,* purple], a rare hereditary metabolic disorder in which large quantities of nitrogenous substances, called porphyrins, are excreted in the feces. Attacks, with varying gastrointestinal and neurologic symptoms, may be precipitated by certain drugs.

coproporphyrin /kop'rōpôr'firin/ [Gk, *kopros* + *porphyros,* purple], any of the nitrogenous organic substances normally excreted in the feces that are products of the breakdown of bilirubin from hemoglobin decomposition.

CoQ, abbreviation for **coenzyme Q.**

cor /kôr/, **1.** the heart. **2.** relating to the heart.

coracoacromial /kôr'əkō·əkro'mē·əl/, pertaining to the coracoid process and the acromion of the scapula.

coracobrachialis /kôr'əkōbrā'kē·al'is/, a muscle with its origin on the scapula and its insertion on the inner side of the humerus. It functions to adduce the shoulder.

coracoid process /kôr'əkoid/ [Gk, *korax,* crow, *eidos,* form; L, *processus*], the thick, curved extension of the superior border of the scapula, to which the pectoralis minor is attached.

coral snake, a poisonous snake with transverse red, yellow, and black bands that is native to the southern United States. Bites are rare; pain does not always result, but neuromuscular and respiratory effects may be severe.

cord [Gk, *chorde,* string], any long, rounded, flexible structure. The body contains many different cords, such as the spermatic, vocal, spinal, neural, umbilical, and hepatic cords. —**cordal,** *adj.*

cordal, pertaining to a cord, such as the umbilical cord.

cord blood, blood taken from the umbilical cord vein or artery of the fetus. Like bone marrow, cord blood is rich in peripheral blood stem cells. It can be frozen and stored for later transfusion.

cord blood transplantation, the removal of blood from the umbilical cord of a fetus or its placenta for the treatment of blood diseases.

corditis /kôrdī'tis/ [Gk, *chorde* + *itis,* inflammation], an abnormal inflammation of the spermatic cord, accompanied by pain in the testis, often caused by an infection originating in the urethra or by tumor, hydrocele, or varicocele.

core [L, *cor,* heart], (in dentistry) a section of a mold, usually of plaster, made over assembled parts of a dental restoration to record and maintain their relationships so that the parts can be reassembled in their original position.

core temperature [L, *cor,* heart, *temperatura*], the temperature of deep structures of the body such as the liver, as compared to that of peripheral tissues.

Cori cycle [Carl F. Cori, American physician, 1896–1984; Gerty T. Cori, American biochemist, 1896–1957; co–Nobel laureates in 1947], a physiologic mechanism whereby lactate, produced by glycolysis of glucose in contracting muscle, is converted back to glucose in the liver and returned via the circulation to the muscles.

Cori's disease /kôr'ēz/ [Carl F. Cori; Gerty T. Cori], a rare type of glycogen storage disease, in which the lack of an enzyme results in abnormally large deposits of glycogen in the liver, skeletal muscles, and heart. Signs are an enlarged liver, hypoglycemia, acidosis, and, occasionally stunted growth.

corkscrew esophagus /kôrk'skroo/ [ME, *cork* bark; L, *scrofa,* sow]; Gk, *oisophagos,* gullet], a neurogenic disorder in which normal peristaltic contractions of the esophagus are replaced by spastic movements that occur spontaneously or with swallowing or gastric acid reflux.

corn [L, *cornu,* horn], a horny mass of

condensed epithelial cells overlying a bony prominence. Corns result from chronic friction and pressure.

cornea /kôr′nē·ə/ [L, *corneus,* horny], the convex, transparent anterior part of the eye, comprising one sixth of the outermost tunic of the eye bulb. It is a fibrous structure with five layers: the anterior corneal epithelium, continuous with that of the conjunctiva; the anterior limiting layer (Bowman's membrane); the substantia propria; the posterior limiting layer (Descemet's membrane); and the endothelium of the anterior chamber (keratoderma). It is dense, uniform in thickness, and nonvascular.

corneal abrasion /kôr′nē·əl/ [L, *corneus* horny, *abrasio* scraping], the rubbing off of the outer layers of the cornea.

corneal corpuscle, one of the fixed flattened connective tissue cells between the lamellae of the cornea.

corneal grafting, transplantation of corneal tissue from one human eye to another, performed to improve vision in corneal scarring or distortion or to remove a perforating ulcer. The affected area is excised, using an operating microscope; an identical section of clear cornea is cut from the donor eye and sutured in place, using an operating microscope. After surgery the eye is covered with a protective metal shield. The patient is cautioned against coughing, sneezing, vomiting, sudden movement, and lifting.

corneal loupe, (in ophthalmology) a magnifying lens designed especially for examining the cornea.

corneal reflex, a protective mechanism for the eye in which the eyelids close when the cornea is touched.

corneoblepharon, adhesion of the eyelid to the cornea.

cornification /kôr′nlfikā′shən/, the conversion of cells into the horny layer of the skin.

corn pad, a device that helps relieve the pressure and pain of a corn on the toes of the feet by transferring the pressure to surrounding unaffected areas. Corn pads are constructed of pliable fabric and fashioned in various ways to accommodate different conditions.

cornua /kôr′nōō·ə/, an anatomic structure that resembles a horn.

cornual pregnancy /kôr′nyōō·əl/ [L, *cornu,* horn, *praegnans,* child bearing], an ectopic pregnancy in one of the straight or curved extensions of the body of the uterus. The signs include a uterus that is asymmetric and tender, as well as cramping and spotting. The cornu of the uterus

usually ruptures between 12 and 16 weeks of the pregnancy unless the condition is treated surgically.

corona /kərō′nə/ [L, crown], **1.** a crown. **2.** a crownlike projection or encircling structure, such as a process extending from a bone. **—coronal, coronoid,** *adj.*

coronal section [L, *corona,* crown, *sectio*], a section of the body cut in the plane of the coronal suture, or parallel to it.

coronal suture, the serrated transverse suture between the frontal bone and the parietal bone on each side of the skull.

corona radiata, *pl.* **coronae radiatae** [L, crown; *radiare* to emit rays], **1.** a network of fibers that weaves through the internal capsule of the cerebral cortex and intermingles with the fibers of the corpus callosum. **2.** an aggregate of cells that surrounds the zona pellucida of the ovum.

coronary /kôr′əner′ē/ [L, *corona,* crown], **1.** (in anatomy) pertaining to encircling structures such as the coronary arteries; pertaining to the heart. **2.** *nontechnical.* myocardial infarction or occlusion.

coronary arteriovenous fistula, an unusual congenital abnormality characterized by a direct communication between a coronary artery, usually the right, and the right atrium or ventricle, the coronary sinus, or the vena cava. A large shunt may result in growth failure, limited exercise tolerance, dyspnea, and anginal pain.

coronary artery, one of a pair of arteries that branch from the aorta, including the left and right coronary arteries. Because these vessels and their branches supply the heart, any dysfunction or disease that affects them can cause serious, sometimes fatal complications. The branches of the coronary arteries are affected by many different disorders such as embolic, neoplastic, inflammatory, and noninflammatory diseases.

coronary artery disease, any one of the abnormal conditions that may affect the heart's arteries and produce various pathologic effects, especially the reduced flow of oxygen and nutrients to the myocardium. Any of the coronary artery diseases, such as coronary atherosclerosis, coronary arteritis, or fibromuscular hyperplasia of the coronary arteries, may produce the common characteristic symptom of angina pectoris. The most common kind of coronary artery disease is coronary atherosclerosis, now the leading cause of death in the Western world. Coronary atherosclerosis occurs most frequently in populations with regular diets high in calories, total fat, saturated fat, cholesterol, and refined carbohydrates. Other risk factors include cigarette smoking, hypertension, serum cholesterol levels, coffee intake, alcohol intake, deficiencies of vitamins C and E, water hardness, hypoxia, carbon monoxide, social overcrowding, heredity, climate, and viruses. Atherosclerosis develops with the formation of fatty fibrous plaques that narrow the lumen of the coronary arteries and may lead to thrombosis and myocardial infarction. Although no single cause of atherosclerosis has been found, development of the disease is closely associated with plasma lipids and the lipoproteins that transport plasma lipids from one tissue to another.

coronary artery fistula, a congenital anomaly characterized by an abnormal communication between a coronary artery and the right side of the heart or the pulmonary artery.

coronary bypass, open heart surgery in which a prosthesis or a section of a blood vessel is grafted onto one of the coronary arteries, bypassing a narrowing or blockage in a coronary artery. The operation is performed in coronary artery disease to improve the blood supply to the heart muscle and to relieve anginal pain.

coronary care nursing, the nursing care provided in a hospital in a coronary care unit. Nursing in this setting requires technical knowledge, judgment, and skills, as well as ability to give emotional support to patients and their families during the acute stage of cardiac dysfunction.

coronary care unit. See **critical care unit (CCU).**

coronary collateralization, the spontaneous development of new blood vessels in or around areas of restricted blood flow to the heart.

coronary heart disease (CHD), a term formerly used for coronary artery disease, a condition causing reduced flow of oxygen and nutrients to the heart.

coronary occlusion, an obstruction of an artery that supplies the heart. When complete, it causes myocardial infarction; when incomplete, it may cause angina. The underlying pathophysiologic characteristic is the atherosclerotic plaque, which usually slowly develops by buildup of lipid and macrophage complexes. Rapid plaque accumulation is frequently caused by hemorrhage within a plaque. If the plaque ruptures, platelets aggregate, fibrin deposits itself, spasm occurs, and a thrombus develops, resulting in acute myocardial infarction. Treatment includes prompt intravenous thrombolysis and administration of heparin; primary percutaneous transvenous coronary angioplasty can achieve prompt reperfusion.

coronary plexus, [L, *corona,* crown, *plexus,* plaited], a network of autonomic nerve fibers located near the base of the heart.

coronary sinus, the wide venous channel, about 2.25 cm long, situated in the coronary sulcus and covered by muscular fibers from the left atrium. It drains five coronary veins: the great cardiac vein, the small cardiac vein, the middle cardiac vein, the posterior vein of the left ventricle, and the oblique vein of the left atrium.

coronary thrombosis, a development of a thrombus that blocks a coronary artery, often causing myocardial infarction and death. Coronary thromboses commonly develop in segments of arteries with atherosclerotic lesions.

coronary valve [L, *corona,* crown, *valva,* folding door], the valve of the coronary sinus, a semicircular fold of endocardium, leading into the right atrium.

coronary vein, one of the veins of the heart that drain blood from the capillary beds of the myocardium through the coronary sinus into the right atrium.

Coronaviridae, a family of four antigenic groups of single-stranded ribonucleic acid viruses. Some strains of the organism are associated with upper respiratory infections in humans.

coronavirus /kôr′ənəvī′rəs/ [L, *corona + virus,* poison], a member of a family of viruses that includes several types capable of causing acute respiratory illnesses.

coroner /kôr′ənər/ [L, *corona,* crown], a public official who investigates the causes and circumstances of deaths that occur within a specific legal jurisdiction or territory, especially those that may have resulted from unnatural causes.

coronoid fossa /kô′rənoid/ [L, *corona + Gk, eidos,* form; L, *fossa,* ditch], a small depression in the distal dorsal surface of the humerus that receives the coronoid process of the ulna when the forearm is flexed.

coronoid process of mandible, a prominence on the anterior surface of the ramus of the mandible to which each temporal muscle attaches.

coronoid process of ulna, a wide, flaring projection of the proximal end of the ulna. The proximal surface of the process forms the lower part of the trochlear notch.

corporate practice of medicine, (in the United States) the role of nonpracticing physicians or nonprofessional corporations in employment relationships with physicians engaged in providing health care. Laws governing corporate practice of medicine vary among different states but generally they require practitioner control over diagnosis and treatment, practitioner setting of fees, a reasonable relationship between services provided by layperson or corporation and amounts charged to the practitioner, and an unaltered practitioner-patient relationship.

corpse /kôrps/ [L, *corpus,* body], the body of a dead human.

corpulence [L, *corpus,* body], obesity.

corpulent /kôr′pyələnt/, obese.

cor pulmonale /kôr pŏŏl′mənal′ē/ [L, heart + *pulmoneus,* lungs], enlargement of the heart's right ventricle caused by primary lung disease. It eventually results in right ventricular hypertrophy and then right ventricular failure. Pulmonary hypertension associated with this condition is caused by some disorder of the pulmonary parenchyma or of the pulmonary vascular system between the origin of the left pulmonary artery and the entry of the pulmonary veins into the left atrium. Chronic cor pulmonale commonly increases the size of the right ventricle, which cannot accommodate an increase in pressure as easily as the left ventricle. In some patients, however, the disease also increases the size of the left ventricle.

corpus albicans /kôr′pəs/ a pale white spot on the surface of the ovary that arises from the corpus luteum if conception does not occur.

corpus callosum, a transverse band of nerve fibers joining the cerebral hemispheres. It is located at the bottom of the longitudinal fissure between the two hemispheres and is covered by the cingulate gyrus.

corpus cavernosum [L, body + *caverna* hollow place], a type of spongy erectile tissue within the penis or clitoris. The tissue becomes engorged with blood during sexual excitement.

corpuscle /kôr′pəsəl/ [L, *corpusculum,* little body], **1.** any cell of the body. **2.** a red or white blood cell. —**corpuscular,** *adj.*

corpuscular radiation /kôrpəs′kyələr/ [L, *corpusculum* + *radiare,* to emit rays], the radiation associated with subatomic particles, such as electrons, protons, neutrons, or alpha particles, which travel in streams at various velocities.

corpus luteum /kôr′pəs lōō′tē·əm/, *pl.* **corpora lutea** [L, *corpus,* body, *luteus,* yellow], an anatomic structure on the ovary surface, consisting of a spheroid of yellowish tissue 1 to 2 cm in diameter that grows within the ruptured ovarian follicle after ovulation. During a woman's reproductive years a corpus luteum forms after every ovulation. It acts as a short-lived en-

docrine organ that secretes progesterone, which serves to maintain the decidual layer of the uterine endometrium in the richly vascular state necessary for implantation and pregnancy. If conception occurs, the corpus luteum grows and secretes increasing amounts of progesterone.

corpus spongiosum /spon′jē·ō′səm/, one of the cylinders of spongy tissue that, with the corpora cavernosa, form the penis.

corrected pressure [L, *corrigere,* to make straight], a method of applying Boyle's law of gas pressures to adjust simultaneously for changes in both pressure and humidity.

corrective emotional experience /kərek′tiv/, a process by which a patient gives up old behavior patterns and learns or relearns new patterns by reexperiencing early unresolved feelings and needs.

correlation /kôr′əlā′shən/ [L, *com* + *relatio,* a carrying back], (in statistics) a relationship between variables that may be negative (inverse), positive, or curvilinear.

correlative differentiation /kərel′ətiv/, (in embryology) specialization or diversification of cells or tissues caused by an inductor or other external factor.

correspondence, (in ophthalmology) the relationship between corresponding points on each retina. The simultaneous stimulation of the points results in the sensation of viewing a single object.

Corrigan's pulse [Dominic J. Corrigan, Irish physician, 1802–1880], a bounding pulse in which a great surge is felt, followed by a sudden and complete absence of force or fullness in the artery. It occurs in excited emotional states, in various abnormal cardiac conditions, and as a result of systemic arteriosclerosis.

corrosion, /kərō′zhen/ a result of an oxidation-reduction reaction, or deterioration of a substance by a destructive agent.

corrosion of surgical instruments [L, *corrodere,* to gnaw away], the rusting of surgical instruments or the gradual wearing away of their polished surfaces caused by oxidation and the action of contaminants. It usually results from inadequate cleaning and drying of surgical instruments after use, sterilization with solutions that eat into the surface, overexposure to such solutions, or a faulty autoclave.

corrosive /kərō′siv/ [L, *corrodere,* to gnaw away], **1.** eating away a substance or tissue, especially by chemical action. **2.** an agent or substance that eats away a substance or tissue. —**corrode,** *v.,* **corrosion,** *n.*

corrosive gastritis, an acute inflammatory condition of the stomach caused by the ingestion of an acid, alkali, or other corrosive chemical in which the lining of the stomach is eaten away by the corrosive substance.

corrugator supercilii /kôr'əgā'tər soo'pərsil'ē-ī/ [L, *corrugare*, to wrinkle; *super*, above, *cilium*, eyelash], one of the three muscles of the eyelid. It functions to draw the eyebrow downward and inward, as if to frown.

cortex, *pl.* **cortices** /kôr'tisēz/ [L, bark], the outer layer of a body organ or other structure, as distinguished from the internal substance.

cortical blindness /kôr'tikəl/ [L, *cortex* + AS, *blind*], loss of vision that results from a lesion in the visual center of the cerebral cortex of the brain.

cortical bone, bone that is 70% to 90% mineralized.

cortical fracture [L, *cortex* + *fractura*, break], any fracture that involves the cortex of the bone.

corticosteroid /kôr'tikōstir'oid/ [L, *cortex* + *steros*, solid], any one of the natural or synthetic hormones elaborated by the adrenal cortex (excluding the sex hormones of adrenal origin) that influence or control key processes of the body. These processes include carbohydrate and protein metabolism, maintenance of serum glucose levels, electrolyte and water balance, and functions of the cardiovascular system, the skeletal muscle, the kidneys, and other organs. The corticosteroids synthesized by the adrenal glands include the glucocorticoids and the mineralocorticoids. The principal glucocorticoids are cortisol and corticosterone. The only physiologically important mineralocorticoid in humans is aldosterone.

corticotropin-releasing factor (CRF) /kôr'tikōtrop'in/, a polypeptide secreted by the hypothalamus into the bloodstream. It triggers the release of adrenocorticotropic hormone from the pituitary gland.

cortisol /kôr'təsôl/, a steroid hormone that occurs naturally in the body and is produced synthetically for pharmacologic use. It is prescribed for inflammation.

cortisone /kôr'təsōn/, a glucocorticoid produced in the liver and made synthetically. It is prescribed for inflammation.

Corynebacterium /kôr'inē'baktir'ē-əm/ [Gk, *koryne*, club, *bakterion*, small staff], a common genus of rod-shaped curved bacilli that includes many species. The most common pathogenic species are *Corynebacterium acnes,* commonly found in acne lesions, and *C. diphtheriae,* the cause of diphtheria.

cosine law, a rule that optimal irradiation occurs when the source of radiation is at right angles to the center of the area being irradiated.

cosmesis, the use of cosmetics or surgery for preserving or enhancing appearance.

cosmetic dermatitis, a form of irritant or allergic contact dermatitis caused by ingredients in cosmetic products. The meaning is commonly broadened to include soaps, shampoos, deodorants, and depilatories, in addition to perfumes, coloring agents, and toiletries.

cosmetic surgery /kosmet'ik/ [Gk, *kosmesis,* adornment], reconstruction of cutaneous or underlying tissues, performed to improve and correct a structural defect or to remove a scar, birthmark, or normal evidence of aging. Kinds of cosmetic surgery include **blepharoplasty, rhinoplasty, rhytidoplasty.**

cosmic radiation /kos'mik/, high-energy particles with great penetrating power that originate in outer space and reach the earth as normal background radiation. The rays consist partly of high-energy atomic nuclei.

costa /kos'tə/, *pl.* **costae** /kos'tē/, a rib.

costal /kos'təl/ [L, *costa,* rib], **1.** pertaining to a rib. **2.** situated near a rib or on a side close to a rib.

costal arch [L, *costa* + *arcus,* bow], an arch formed by the shafts of the ribs.

costal cartilage, the cartilage at the anterior end of each rib.

costalgia /kostal'jē-ə/ [L, *costa,* rib; Gk, *algos,* pain], a pain in the ribs.

costal notch, an indentation beside a costal cartilage on the side of the sternum.

cost analysis [L, *costare,* to stand firm; Gk, *ana,* again, *lyein,* to loosen], an analysis of the disbursements of an activity, agency, department, or program.

COSTAR /kō'stär/, abbreviation for *COmputer STored Ambulatory Record* system, an on-line interactive computerized information system for the public health field.

cost-based value, a relative value scale used to determine the total units of services provided by a medical practice. The total cost of running the practice and the total units of service are then used to calculate the costs for each service provided.

cost-benefit analysis (CBA), a type of economic evaluation of medical care expense. It compares the monetary benefit derived from different health interventions with the cost of providing each of the interventions.

cost-benefit ratio, a mathematic representation of the relationship of the cost of an activity to the benefit of its outcome or product.

cost cap, *informal.* a limit on the amount

of money that an agency, department, or institution may spend.

cost center, a department, division, or other subunit of an institution established within its accounting system so that the income and expenses of the subunit can be separated from the income or expenses of other centers and monitored for cost and benefit.

cost control, the process of monitoring and regulating the expenditure of funds by an agency or institution.

costectomy /kostek'təmē/, surgical removal of a rib.

cost effectiveness, the extent to which an activity is thought to be as valuable as it is expensive. A public-assistance program that issued vouchers for nutritious foods in pregnancy might be considered cost-effective if it lowered the costly incidence of perinatal morbidity.

cost-effectiveness analysis (CEA), a type of economic evaluation used to determine the best use of money available for medical care. It compares different kinds of interventions with similar but not identical effects on the basis of the cost per unit achieved.

cost model, (in the United States)a managed care system in which all components of patient care are defined as costs as opposed to sources of revenue.

costocervical /kos'tōsur'vikəl/ [L, costa, rib, cervix, neck], pertaining to or involving the ribs and the neck.

costochondral /kos'təkon'drəl/ [L, costa + Gk, chondros, cartilage], pertaining to a rib and its cartilage.

costochondritis, an inflammation of the costal cartilage of the anterior chest wall. It is characterized by pain and tenderness.

costoclavicular /ˌklavik'yələr/ [L, costa + clavicula, little key], pertaining to or involving the ribs and the clavicle.

costoclavicular line, an imaginary vertical line between the sternal and midclavicular lines.

costophrenic (CP) angle /-fren'ik/ [L, costa + phrenicus, diaphragm], the angle at the bottom of the lung where the diaphragm and chest wall meet.

costosternal /-stur'nəl/, pertaining to or involving the ribs and the sternum.

costotransverse articulation /-transvurs'/ [L, costa + transversus, a cross direction], any of the 20 gliding joints between the ribs and associated vertebrae, except the eleventh and twelfth ribs.

costovertebral /-vur'təbrəl/, of or relating to a rib and the vertebral column.

costovertebral angle (CVA), one of two angles that outline a space over the kidneys. The angle is formed by the lateral

and downward curve of the lowest rib and the vertical column of the spine itself.

cost-sharing program, (in the United States) a financial risk-management strategy often used by insurance companies and self-insured employers in which employees share the cost of health services, such as through deductibles and co-insurance.

cost shifting, (in the United States) a mechanism for reducing inpatient costs by providing services in outpatient setting. The inpatient cost per case is reduced, but the overall cost to the organization does not change.

cost-utility analysis (CUA), a type of economic evaluation of different approaches to managed health care costs. It compares the degree to which quality of life is improved per dollar spent. A quality-of-life index is used to compare interventions, including quality adjusted life years.

cosyntropin /kō'sintrop'in/, a synthetic form of adrenocorticotropic hormone that is used in the diagnosis and treatment of adrenal hypofunction disorders such as Addison's disease.

COTA, abbreviation for **Certified Occupational Therapy Assistant.**

cottonmouth, a poisonous pit viper commonly found near water and swamps of the southeastern part of the United States. The symptoms of the bite of a cottonmouth are rapid swelling, severe pain, skin discoloration at bite marks, and weakness.

Cotton's fracture, a trimalleolar fracture involving medial, lateral, and posterior malleoli.

cotton-wool exudate [Ar, qutun + AS, wull + ME, spot], a soft-white exudate observed on the retina of patients with certain systemic conditions, such as acquired immunodeficiency syndrome, hypertension, and lupus. It can also be observed in retinal infections.

cotyledon /kot'ilē'don/ [Gk, kotyledon, cup-shaped], one of the visible segments on the maternal surface of the placenta. A typical placenta may have 15 to 28 cotyledons, each consisting of fetal vessels, chorionic villi, and intervillous space.

cotyloid /kot'iloid/, cup-shaped, as the acetabulum.

cough /kôf/ [AS, cohhetan], a sudden, audible expulsion of air from the lungs. Coughing is preceded by inspiration, the glottis is partially closed, and the accessory muscles of expiration contract to expel the air forcibly from the respiratory passages. Coughing is an essential protective response that serves to clear the lungs, bronchi, and trachea of irritants and secretions or to prevent aspiration of foreign material into the lungs. It is a common symptom of diseases of the chest and larynx.

cough fracture, any fracture of a rib, usually the fourth to eighth rib, caused by violent coughing.

cough syncope [AS, *cohhetan* + Gk, *syncope,* fainting], a temporary loss of consciousness caused by an interruption in cerebral blood flow during coughing.

coulomb /kōō′lōm/ [Charles A. de Coulomb, French physicist, 1736–1806], the SI unit of electricity equal to the quantity of charge transferred in 1 second across a conductor in which there is a constant current of 1 ampere, or 1 ampere-second.

Coulomb's law [Charles A. de Coulomb], (in physics) a law stating that the force of attraction or repulsion between two electrically charged bodies is directly proportional to the strength of the electrical charges and inversely proportional to the square of the distance between them.

coulometry /kōōlom′ətrē/, a type of electroanalytic chemistry in which a reagent generated at the surface of an electrode reacts with a substance to be measured. The substance, usually a metal ion, is measured in terms of the coulombs required for the reaction.

coumarin /kōō′mərin/, an anticoagulant prescribed for prophylaxis and treatment of thrombosis and embolism.

counseling [L, *consulere,* to consult], the act of providing advice and guidance to a patient or his or her family. It helps the patient recognize and manage stress and that facilitates interpersonal relationships.

count [L, *computere,* to calculate], a computation of the number of objects or elements present per unit of measurement.

counterclaim [L, *contra,* against, *clamere,* to cry out], (in law) a claim made by a defendant establishing a cause for action in his or her favor against a plaintiff.

counterconditioning, a process used in behavioral therapy in which a learned response is replaced by an alternative response that is less disruptive.

countercurrent, a change in the direction of flow of a fluid. An example is the countercurrent in the ascending branch of a kidney tubule where osmolality undergoes a reversal after a gradual change in sodium chloride concentrations.

counterinjunction /-injungk′shən/, (in transactional analysis) an overt message from the parent ego state of the mother or father that may be difficult to follow if it conflicts with earlier parental instructions.

counterphobic behavior /-fō′bik/, an expression of reaction to a phobia by a patient who actively seeks exposure to the type of situation that precipitates phobic symptoms.

counterpulsation /-pulsā′shən/ [L, *contra* + *pulsare,* to beat], **1.** the action of a circulatory-assist pumping device that is synchronized with cardiac systole and diastole to decrease the work of the heart. **2.** the process of increasing the intraaortic pressure in diastole by inflation of an intraaortic balloon and deflation of the balloon immediately before the next systole.

countershock [L, *contra* + Fr, *choc*], (in cardiology) a high-intensity, short-duration electric shock applied to the area of the heart, resulting in total cardiac depolarization.

counterstain, a second stain added to a previously stained tissue sample to make cellular details more distinct.

countertraction /-trak′shən/ [L, *contra* + *trahere,* to pull], a force that counteracts the pull of traction, especially in orthopedics, such as the force of body weight resulting from the pull of gravity.

countertransference /-transfur′əns/, the conscious or unconscious emotional response of a psychotherapist or psychoanalyst to a patient.

countertransport /-trans′pôrt/ [L, *contra* + *trans,* across, *portare,* carry], the simultaneous transport of two different substances across the same membrane, each in the opposite direction.

counting cell hemocytometer [OFr, *conter* + L, *cella,* storeroom; Gk, *haima,* blood, *metron,* measure], a device for counting the number of cells in a volume of blood or other fluid. It consists of a microscope slide with a counting chamber. The chamber has a known volume, and the slide has a ruled area to help count the cells.

counts per minute (cpm), a measure of the rate of ionizing emissions by radioactive substances.

coup /kōō/ [Fr, blow], any blow or stroke or the effects of such a blow to the body, usually used with a French word identifying a type of stroke: **1. coup de sabre** /kōōdəsäb′r(ə)/, a wound resembling a sword cut. **2. coup de soleil.** See **sunstroke. 3. coup sur coup** /kōōsYrkōō′/, administration of a drug in small amounts over a short period rather than in a single larger dose. **4. contre coup** /kôNtrəkōō′/, an injury most often associated with a blow to the skull in which the force of the impact is transmitted through the skull bones to the opposite side of the head, where the bruise, fracture, or other sign of injury appears.

couples' therapy, psychotherapy in which couples, who may be married or unmarried but living together, undergo therapy together.

coupling /kup′ling/ [L, *copula*, bonding], **1.** the act of coming together, joining, or pairing. **2.** (in genetics) the situation in linked inheritance in which the nonalleles of two or more mutant genes are located on the same chromosome and are close enough that they are likely to be inherited together. **3.** (in radiation therapy) the efficiency of transfer of power from an applicator to the treatment site.

coupling interval, the interval between the dominant heartbeat and a linked ectopic beat.

Courvoisier's law /kōōrvô·ä·zē·āz′/ [Ludwig Courvoisier, Swiss surgeon, 1843–1918], a statement that the gallbladder is smaller than usual if a gallstone blocks the common bile duct but is dilated if the common bile duct is blocked by something other than a gallstone, such as pancreatic cancer.

couvade /kōōväd′/, a custom in some non-Western cultures whereby the husband goes through mock labor while his wife is giving birth.

Couvelaire uterus /kōōvəler′/ [Alexandre Couvelaire, French obstetrician, 1873–1948], a hemorrhagic process in uterine musculature that may accompany severe abruptio placentae. Extravasated blood effuses between the muscle fibrils and under the uterine peritoneum. The uterus takes on a purplish color and does not contract well.

covalent bond, a chemical bond that forms by the sharing of two, four, or six electrons between two atoms.

coverage /kuv′ərij/, the extent to which services rendered by a health care program cover the potential need for them.

covered benefit, a health service included in the premium of a policy paid by or on behalf of the enrolled patient.

Cowden's disease [Cowden, family name of the first recorded case], an autosomal-dominant disorder characterized by hypertrichosis, gingival fibromatosis, facial papules, hemangiomas, and postpubertal fibroadenomatous breast enlargement.

Cowper's gland /kou′pərz/ [William Cowper, English surgeon, 1666–1709], either of two round, pea-sized glands embedded in the urethral sphincter of the male.

cowpox /kou′poks/ [AS, *cu* + ME, *pokkes*], a mild infectious disease characterized by a pustular rash, caused by the vaccinia virus transmitted to humans from infected cattle. Cowpox infection usually confers immunity to smallpox because of the similarity of the variola and vaccinia viruses.

coxa /kok′sə/, *pl.* **coxae** [L, hip], the hip joint; the head of the femur and the acetabulum of the innominate bone.

coxal articulation /kok′səl/ [L, *coxa* + *articularis,* relating to the joints], the ball-and-socket joint of the hip, formed by the articulation of the head of the femur into the cup-shaped cavity of the acetabulum.

coxa magna, an abnormal widening of the head and neck of the femur.

coxa valga, a hip deformity in which the angle formed by the axis of the head and neck of the femur and the axis of its shaft is significantly increased.

coxa vara, a hip deformity in which the angle formed by the axis of the head and neck of the femur and the axis of its shaft is decreased.

coxa vara luxans, a fissure or crack in the neck of the femur with dislocation of the head, caused by coxa vara.

coxsackievirus /koksak′ē-/ [Coxsackie, New York; L, *virus,* poison], any of 30 serologically different enteroviruses associated with a variety of symptoms and primarily affecting children during warm weather. Among the diseases associated with coxsackievirus infections are herpangina, hand-foot-and-mouth disease, epidemic pleurodynia, myocarditis, pericarditis, aseptic meningitis, and several exanthems.

CP, 1. abbreviation for *candle power.* **2.** abbreviation for **cerebral palsy. 3.** abbreviation for *chemically pure.*

CPAN, abbreviation for *Certified Post-Anesthesia Nurse.*

CPAP, abbreviation for **continuous positive airway pressure.**

CPD, 1. abbreviation for **cephalopelvic disproportion. 2.** abbreviation for childhood polycystic disease. **3.** abbreviation for *congenital polycystic disease.*

C peptide, a biologically inactive residue of insulin formation in the beta cells of the pancreas.

CPHA, abbreviation for the **Canadian Public Health Association.**

CPK, abbreviation for *creatine phosphokinase.*

CPK isoenzyme fraction, one of several blood-borne enzymes that are released after myocardial necrosis. The isoenzyme of creatine phosphokinase (CPK) is identified as MB isoenzyme, or MB-CPK, and is a diagnostic clue to heart damage.

cpm, abbreviation for **counts per minute.**

CPNP/A, abbreviation for *Certified Pediatric Nurse Practitioner/Associate.*

CPPB, abbreviation for *continuous positive-pressure breathing.*

CPPD, abbreviation for *calcium pyrophosphate dihydrate.*

CPPV, abbreviation for **continuous positive-pressure ventilation.**

CPR, abbreviation for **cardiopulmonary resuscitation.**

CPRAM, abbreviation for *controlled partial rebreathing anesthesia method.*

cps, abbreviation for **cycles per second.** See **hertz.**

CPT, abbreviation for *Current Procedural Terminology.*

CPT codes, a coding system, defined in the publication *Current Procedural Terminology (CPT),* for medical procedures that allows for comparability in pricing, billing, and utilization review.

Cr, symbol for the element **chromium.**

CR, abbreviation for *controlled respiration.*

crab louse [AS, *crabba* + *lus*], a species of body louse, *Pthirus pubis,* that infests the hairs of the genital area. It is often transmitted between persons by venereal contact.

crack [ME, *craken*], a street drug made by chemically converting cocaine hydrochloride to a form that can be smoked.

crack baby, an infant who was exposed to effects of cocaine in utero by a mother who used the "crack" form of the drug while pregnant.

cracked-pot sound [ME, *craken* + *pott* + L, *sonus,* sound], a sound sometimes heard on percussion over a cavity with an opening to a bronchus.

crackle, a common abnormal respiratory sound heard on auscultation of the chest during inspiration, characterized by discontinuous bubbling noises.

cradle cap [AS, *cradel* + *caeppe*], a common seborrheic dermatitis of infants, which consists of thick, yellow greasy scales on the scalp. Treatment includes application of oil or ointment to soften the scales and frequent shampoos.

cramp [AS, *crammian,* to fill], **1.** a spasmodic and often painful contraction of one or more muscles. **2.** a pain resembling a muscular cramp.

cranial bones /krā′nē·əl/ [Gk, *kranion,* cranium; AS, *ban*], the bones of the skull, particularly the part of the cranium that encloses the brain.

cranial cavity, the cavity of the skull containing the brain and other tissues.

cranial nerves [Gk, *kranion,* skull; L, *nervus*], the 12 pairs of nerves emerging from the cranial cavity through various openings in the skull. Beginning with the most anterior, they are designated by Roman numerals and named (I) olfactory, (II) optic, (III) oculomotor, (IV) trochlear, (V) trigeminal, (VI) abducens, (VII) facial, (VIII) vestibulocochlear (acoustic), (IX) glossopharyngeal, (X) vagal, (XI) accessory, (XII) hypoglossal. The cranial nerves originate in the base of the brain and carry impulses for such functions as smell, vision, ocular movement, pupil contraction, muscular sensibility, general sensibility, mastication, facial expression, glandular secretion, taste, cutaneous sensibility, hearing, equilibrium, swallowing, phonation, tongue movement, head movement, and shoulder movement.

cranial sutures, the interlocking lines of fusion of the bones forming the skull. The lines gradually become less prominent as a person matures.

craniectomy /krā′nē·ek′təmē/ [Gk, *kranion,* cranium, *ektome,* excision out], the surgical removal of a part of the cranium.

craniocervical /-sur′vikəl/ [Gk, *kranion* + L, *cervix,* neck], pertaining to the junction of the skull and neck, particularly the area of the foramen magnum.

craniodidymus /krā′nē·ōdid′iməs/ [Gk, *kranion* + *didymos,* twin], a two-headed fetus in which the bodies are fused.

craniofacial /-fā′shəl/ [Gk, *kranion,* cranium; L, *facies,* face], pertaining to the cranium and the face.

craniofacial dysostosis [Gk, *kranion* + L, *facies,* face; Gk, *dys,* bad, *osteon,* bone], an abnormal hereditary condition characterized by acrocephaly, exophthalmos, hypertelorism, strabismus, parrot-beaked nose, and hypoplastic maxilla with relative mandibular prognathism.

craniohypophyseal xanthoma /krā′nē·ōhī′pōfiz′ē·əl/ [Gk, *kranion* + *hypo,* deficient, *phyein,* to grow, *xanthos,* yellow, *oma,* tumor], a condition in which cholesterol deposits are formed around the hypophyses of the bones, as in Hand-Schüller-Christian's disease.

craniology /krā′nē·ol′əjē/, the study of the shape, size, proportions, and other features of the human skull. It is usually associated with anthropologic research.

craniometaphyseal dysplasia /-met′əfiz′ē·əl/, an inherited bone disorder characterized by paranasal overgrowth, thickening of the skull and jaw, and entrapment of cranial nerves. The patient may experience nasorespiratory infections associated with bone overgrowth at the sinuses, as well as malocclusion of the jaws.

craniopagus /krā′nē·op′əgəs/ [Gk, *kranion* + *pagos,* fixed], conjoined twins united at the heads. Fusion can occur at the frontal, occipital, or parietal region.

craniopharyngeal /krā′nē·ōfərin′jē·əl/ [Gk, *kranion* + *pharynx,* throat], pertaining to the cranium and pharynx.

craniopharyngioma /krā′nē-ō-fərin′jē-ō′mə/, a congenital pituitary tumor, appearing most often in children and adolescents, that arises in cells derived from Rathke's pouch or the hypophyseal stalk. The tumor may interfere with pituitary function, damage the optic chiasm, disrupt hypothalamic control of the autonomic nervous system, and cause hydrocephalus.

cranioplasty /krā′nē-ōplast′tē/, plastic surgery performed on the skull.

craniostenosis /krā′nē-ō′stənō′sis/ [Gk, kranion + stenos, narrow, osis, condition], a congenital deformity of the skull that results from premature closure of the sutures between the cranial bones. —**craniostenotic**, adj.

craniostosis /krā′nē-ostō′sis/ [Gk, kranion + osteon, bone, osis, condition], premature ossification of the sutures of the skull, often associated with other skeletal defects. The sutures close before or soon after birth. Without surgical correction the growth of the skull is inhibited, the head is deformed, and the eyes and brain are often damaged.

craniotabes /krā′nē-ōtā′bēz/ [Gk, kranion + L, tabes, wasting], benign congenital thinness of the top and back of the skull of a newborn. The condition is common because the rate of brain growth exceeds the rate of calcification of the skull during the last month of gestation.

craniotomy /kran′ē-ot′əmē/ [Gk, kranion, skull, temnein, to cut], any surgical opening into the skull, performed to relieve intracranial pressure, to control bleeding, or to remove a tumor.

craniotubular /-tōōb′yələr/, pertaining to a bossing, or overgrowth, of bone that produces an abnormal contour and increased bone density.

cranium /krā′nē-əm/ [Gk, kranion, skull], the bony skull that holds the brain. It is composed of eight bones: the frontal, occipital, sphenoid, ethmoid, and paired temporal and parietal bones. —**cranial**, adj.

crankcase-spool catheter /krangk′kās/, a special elastic catheter stored within a plastic spool to facilitate its insertion, especially for hyperalimentation. When fully inserted, the crankcase-spool catheter is usually lodged in the subclavian vein. The catheter is highly flexible, and each revolution of the spool feeds about 5 inches of the catheter into the vein involved.

crash cart, a cart carrying emergency equipment such as medications, antiarrhythmics, vasopressors, suction devices, sutures, scalpels, surgical needles, sponges, swabs, retractors, hemostats, forceps, airways, O_2 supplies, IV supplies, tracheal tubes, and often a defibrillator. Hospital emergency rooms and intensive care units usually have several crash carts equipped according to prescribed specifications.

crater, a pitlike depression, as results where an ulcer has been surgically removed.

cravat bandage /krəvat′/ [Fr, cravate, scarf, bande, strip], a triangular bandage folded lengthwise. It may be used as a circular, figure-of-eight, or spiral bandage to control bleeding or to tie splints in place.

cravat bandage for clenched fist, a pressure dressing made by folding the points of a triangular bandage to form a band about the fist.

cravat bandage for fracture of clavicle, a sling dressing that includes a 2-by-4-inch soft pad in the armpit. The triangular bandage is placed with the center point on the affected shoulder. The hand and wrist are laid against it. The opposite ends are lifted to cover and support the arm. The bandage ends are drawn together and tied at the back.

cravat elbow bandage, a triangular dressing that holds the elbow at a 45-degree angle, beginning with the center over the point of the elbow. The bandage is completed with one end around the forearm and the other around the upper arm.

cravat sling bandage, a support for a fractured arm prepared by laying the wrist on the center of the triangular bandage while the forearm is at a right angle. The two ends of the bandage are carried around the neck and tied.

C-reactive protein (CRP) /-rē·ak′tiv/, a protein not normally detected in the serum but present in many acute inflammatory conditions and with necrosis. CRP appears in the serum before the erythrocyte sedimentation rate begins to rise, often within 24 to 48 hours of the onset of inflammation. After a myocardial infarction it is present in 24 hours. CRP disappears when an inflammatory process is suppressed by salicylates, steroids, or both.

cream [Gk, chrima, oil], **1.** the part of milk rich in butterfat. **2.** any fluid mixture of thick consistency, often used as a method of applying medication to the surface of the body.

crease [ME, creste, crest], an indentation or margin formed by a doubling back of tissue, such as the folds on the palm of the hand and sole of the foot.

creatine /krē′ətēn, -tin/ [Gk, kreas, flesh], an important nitrogenous compound produced by metabolic processes in the body. Combined with phosphorus, it forms high-energy phosphate.

creatine kinase (CK), an enzyme of the transferase class in muscle, brain, and other tissues. It catalyzes the transfer of a phosphate group from adenosine triphosphate to creatine, producing adenosine diphosphate and phosphocreatine.

creatine phosphate [Gk, *kreas,* flesh; Du, *potasschen*], an enzyme that increases in blood levels when muscle damage has occurred, as in pseudohypertrophic muscular dystrophy.

creatinine /krē·at′inēn, -nin/, a substance formed from the metabolism of creatine, commonly found in blood, urine, and muscle tissue.

creatinine clearance test, a diagnostic test for kidney function. It measures the rate at which creatinine is cleared from the blood by the kidney. It is calculated on the basis of a urine volume in milliliters per minute times the amount of milligrams per liter of urinary creatinine excreted in 24 hours. The resulting figure is divided by the amount of serum creatinine in milligrams per deciliter.

creatinine height index (CHI), a measurement of a 24-hour urinary excretion of creatinine, which is generally related to the patient's muscle mass and is an indicator of malnutrition, particularly in young males.

credentialing, examination and review of the credentials of health care providers employed or certified by a clinic or other facility to ensure that they have the training and licensure necessary to deliver care.

credentials /kriden′shelz/, a predetermined set of standards, such as licensure or certification, establishing that a person or institution has achieved professional recognition in a specific field of health care.

Credé's maneuver [Karl S. Credé, German physician, 1819–1892], a technique for aiding the expulsion of the placenta. The uterus is pushed toward the birth canal by pressure exerted by the thumb of one hand on the posterior surface of the abdomen and the other hand on the anterior surface.

Credé's method /kredāz′/ [Karl S. Credé], a technique for promoting the expulsion of urine by manual compression of the bladder through pressure on the lower abdominal wall.

Credé's prophylaxis [Karl S. Credé], the instillation of a 1% silver nitrate solution into the conjunctiva of newborns to prevent ophthalmia neonatorum.

creep, a rheologic effect of metals and other solid materials that may become elongated or deformed as a result of a load being applied for a long period. For example, creep can occur in silver amalgam fillings that have been in place for some time.

creeping eruption [AS, *creopan,* bent; L, *erumpere,* to burst forth], a skin lesion characterized by irregular, wandering red lines made by the burrowing larvae of hookworms and certain roundworms.

cremaster /krimas′tər/ [Gk, *kremastos,* hanging], a thin muscular layer that spreads out over the spermatic cord in a series of loops. It is a continuation of the obliquus internus. It functions to draw the testis up toward the superficial inguinal ring in response to cold or to stimulation of the nerve.

cremasteric reflex /krē′məster′ik/, a superficial neural reflex elicited by stroking the skin of the upper inner thigh in a male. This action normally results in a brisk retraction of the testis on the side of the stimulus.

crematorium, a facility for the disposal of dead bodies by burning.

crenation /krinā′shən/ [L, *crena,* notch], the formation of notches or leaflike scalloped edges on an object. Red blood cells exposed to a hypertonic saline solution acquire a notched, shriveled surface as a result of the osmotic effect of the solution. They are then called crenated red blood cells. —**crenate, crenated,** *adj.*

creosol /krē′əsol/, an oily liquid that is one of the active constituents (phenol) of creosote. It should not be confused with cresol.

creosote /krē′əsōt/, a flammable oily liquid with a smoky odor that is used primarily as a wood preservative. It can cause a wide variety of health problems, ranging from cancer and corneal damage to convulsions.

crepitant /krep′itənt/ [L, *crepitans,* crackling], pertaining to the feel or sound of crackling or rattling, or of rough surfaces being rubbed together.

crepitant crackle [L, *crepitans,* crackling], an abnormal breathing sound produced at the end of inspiration and caused by air entering collapsed alveoli that contain fibrous exudate. It occurs in cases of pneumonia, tuberculosis, and pulmonary edema.

crepitus /krep′itəs/ [L, crackling], **1.** flatulence or the noisy discharge of fetid gas from the intestine through the anus. **2.** a sound or feel that resembles the crackling noise associated with gas gangrene, rubbing of bone fragments, air in superficial tissues, or crackles of a consolidated area of the lung in pneumonia.

crescendo angina /krishen′dō/ [L, *cres-*

cere, to increase], a form of anginal discomfort associated with ischemic electrocardiographic changes, marked by increased frequency, provocation, intensity, or character.

crescendo murmur [L, *crescere,* to increase, *murmur,* humming], a murmur of steadily increasing intensity to a sudden termination.

crescent bodies, 1. (in a blood smear) large, pale, crescent-shaped cells produced from fragile erythrocytes as the blood film preparation is made. **2.** large, round bodies with pink crescentlike margins found in blood of some anemia patients.

cresol /krē'sol/, a mixture of three isomers in a liquid with a phenolic odor. It is derived from coal tar and used in synthetic resins and disinfectants. Cresol is a potentially lethal protoplasmic poison that can be absorbed through the skin. Symptoms of chronic poisoning include skin eruptions, digestive disorders, uremia, jaundice, nervous disorders, vertigo, and mental changes.

crest, a narrow elongated elevation, as the iliac crest.

CREST syndrome /krest/, abbreviation for *calcinosis, Raynaud's phenomenon, esophageal dysfunction, sclerodactyly, and telangiectasis,* which may occur for varying periods in patients with scleroderma.

cretin dwarf /krē'tən/, a person in whom short stature is caused by infantile hypothyroidism and severe deficiency of thyroid hormone.

cretinism /krē'təniz'əm/ [Fr, *cretin,* idiot], a congenital condition characterized by severe hypothyroidism and often associated with other endocrine abnormalities. Typical signs of cretinism include dwarfism, mental deficiency, puffy facial features, dry skin, large tongue, umbilical hernia, and muscular incoordination. The disorder occurs usually in areas in which the diet is deficient in iodine and goiter is common. —**cretinoid, cretinous,** *adj.,* **cretin,** *n.*

cretinoid, resembling a cretin or the state of cretinism.

Creutzfeldt-Jakob's disease /krots'felt-yä'kôp/ [Hans G. Creutzfeldt, German neurologist, 1885–1964; Alfons M. Jakob, German neurologist, 1884–1931], a rare fatal encephalopathy caused by an as yet unidentified slow virus. The disease occurs in middle age; symptoms are progressive dementia, dysarthria, muscle wasting, and various involuntary movements such as myoclonus and athetosis.

crevice /krev'is/, a cleft or fissure such as that between the gum and the neck of a tooth.

CRF, abbreviation for **corticotropin-releasing factor.**

cribriform /krib'rifôrm'/ [L, *cribum,* sieve], describing a structure with many perforations or punctures, as in the cribriform plate of the ethmoid bone.

cricoid /krī'koid/ [Gk, *krikos,* ring, *eidos,* form], **1.** having a ring shape. **2.** a ring-shaped cartilage connected to the thyroid cartilage by the cricothyroid ligament at the level of the sixth cervical vertebra.

cricoidectomy /-ek'təmē/ [Gk, *krikos* + *eidos* + *ektome,* excision], a surgical procedure for removing the cricoid cartilage.

cricoid pressure, a technique to reduce the risk of the aspiration of stomach contents during induction of general anesthesia. The cricoid cartilage is pushed against the body of the sixth cervical vertebra, compressing the esophagus to prevent passive regurgitation.

cricopharyngeal /krī'kōfərin'jē-əl/ [Gk, *krikos* + *pharynx,* throat], pertaining to the cricoid cartilage and the pharynx.

cricopharyngeal incoordination, a defect in the normal swallowing reflex. The cricopharyngeus muscle ordinarily serves as a sphincter to keep the top of the esophagus closed except when the person is swallowing, vomiting, or belching. The trachea remains open for breathing, but air normally does not enter the esophagus during respiration. When the series of neuromuscular actions is not properly coordinated as a result of disease or injury, the patient may choke, swallow air, regurgitate fluid into the nose, or experience discomfort in swallowing food.

cricothyroid membrane /-thī'roid/, a fibroelastic membrane, including the cricothyroid ligament that connects the cricoid and thyroid cartilages.

cricothyrotomy /krī'kōthīrot'əmē/ [Gk, *krikos* + *thyreos,* shield, *eidos,* form, *temnein,* to cut], an emergency incision into the larynx performed to open the airway in a person who is choking. A small vertical midline cut is made just below the Adam's apple and above the cricoid cartilage. The incision is opened further with a transverse cut through the cricothyroid membrane, and the wound is spread open. The new opening must be held open with a tube that is open at both ends to allow air to move in and out.

Crigler-Najjar's syndrome /krig'lərnaj'är/ [John F. Crigler, Jr., American pediatrician, b. 1919; Victor A. Najjar, Lebanese-born American microbiologist, b. 1914], a congenital familial autosomal anomaly, in which glucuronyl transferase, an enzyme, is deficient or absent. The condition is characterized by nonhemolytic jaundice, an accumulation of unconjugated bilirubin in the blood, and severe disorders of the central nervous system.

crime [L, *crimen*], any act that violates a law and may have criminal intent.

Crimean-Congo hemorrhagic fever /krīmē'ən/, an arbovirus infection transmitted to humans through the bite of a tick, characterized by fever, dizziness, muscle ache, vomiting, headache, and other neurologic symptoms.

criminal psychology, the study of the mental processes, motivational patterns, and behavior of criminals.

crisis /krī'sis/ [Gk, *krisis,* turning point], **1.** a transition for better or worse in the course of a disease, usually indicated by a marked change in the intensity of signs and symptoms. **2.** a turning point in events affecting the emotional state of a person, such as death or divorce.

crisis intervention, (in psychiatry) a short-term intense therapy that emphasizes identification of the event that triggered the emotional trauma. Focus is on neutralizing the trauma.

crisis-intervention unit, a group trained in emergency medical treatment and in various methods for rendering psychiatric therapeutic assistance to a person or group of persons during a period of crisis, especially instances involving suicide attempts or drug abuse.

crisis resolution, (in psychiatry) the development of effective adaptive and coping devices to resolve a crisis.

crisis theory, a conceptual framework for defining and explaining the phenomena that occur when a person faces a problem that appears to be insoluble.

crisscross inheritance [*Christ cross; L, in + hereditas,* in heredity], the acquisition of genetic characteristics or conditions from the parent of the opposite sex.

crista supraventricularis /kris'tə soo' prəven'trik'yələr'is/ [L, *crista,* ridge; *supra,* above, *ventriculus,* little belly], the muscular ridge on the interior dorsal wall of the right ventricle of the heart.

criterion /krītir'ē·ən/, *pl.* **criteria** [Gk, *kriterion,* a means for judging], a standard or rule by which something may be judged, such as a health condition or a diagnosis established. Criteria are sets of rules or principles against which something may be measured, such as health care practices.

critical care. See **intensive care.**

critical care unit (CCU), a specially equipped hospital area designed for the treatment of patients with sudden, life-threatening conditions. These units contain resuscitation and monitoring equipment and are staffed by personnel specially trained and skilled in recognizing and immediately responding to cardiac emergencies.

critical organs /krit'ikəl/ [Gk, *krisis,* turning point, *organon,* instrument], tissues that are the most sensitive to irradiation, such as the gonads, lymphoid organs, and intestine. The skin, cornea, oral cavity, esophagus, vagina, cervix, and optic lens are the next most sensitive organs to irradiation.

critical pathway. See **clinical pathway.**

critical period [Gk, *kritikos,* critical, *peri,* near, *hodos,* way], a period during a developmental or rehabilitation crisis. Examples are the brief period in which a zygote may be formed, in which a patient may survive a myocardial infarction, or when an embryo is most vulnerable to effects of medications used by the mother.

critical period of development, a specific time during which the environment has its greatest impact on an individual's development.

critical point, the temperature and pressure at which, in a sealed system, the densities of the liquid and gas forms of a substance are equal and the two are not visibly separated.

critical pressure, the pressure exerted by a vapor in a closed system at the critical temperature.

critical temperature, the highest temperature at which a substance can exist as a liquid outside a sealed system.

CRNA, abbreviation for *certified registered nurse anesthetist.*

CRNI, abbreviation for *certified registered nurse, intravenous.*

crocodile shagreen, a rare degenerative disorder involving either of two membranes of the cornea in which the tissues acquire the appearance of crocodile leather. The disorder may affect Descemet's deep membrane or Bowman's superficial membrane.

Crohn's disease /krōnz/ [Burrill B. Crohn, American physician, 1884–1983], a chronic inflammatory bowel disease of unknown origin, usually affecting the ileum, the colon, or another part of the gastrointestinal tract. Diseased segments may be separated by normal bowel segments. Crohn's disease is characterized by frequent attacks of diarrhea, severe abdominal pain, nausea, fever, chills, weakness, anorexia, and weight loss.

cromolyn sodium /krom'əlin/, an antiasthmatic that acts by inhibiting allergic histamine release. It is prophylactically prescribed in the treatment of bronchial asthma.

Cronkhite-Canada's syndrome /krong′ kīt/ [Leonard W. Cronkhite, American physician, b. 1919; Wilma J. Canada, twentieth-century American radiologist], an abnormal familial condition characterized by gastrointestinal polyposis accompanied by ectodermal defects such as nail atrophy, alopecia, and excessive skin pigmentation. In some individuals it is also accompanied by protein-losing enteropathy; malabsorption; and deficiency of blood calcium, potassium, and magnesium.

cross [L, *crux*], (in genetics) any method of crossbreeding or any individual, organism, or strain produced from crossbreeding.

cross-bite tooth [L, *crux* + AS, *bitan, toth*], any of the posterior teeth that allow the modified buccal cusps of the upper teeth to be positioned in the central fossae of the lower teeth.

crossbreeding [L, *crux* + *bredan*], the production of offspring by the mating of plants or animals of different varieties, strains, or species; hybridization.

crossed amblyopia [L, *crux*, cross; Gk, *amblys*, dull, *ops*, eyes], a visual disorder in which the patient is unable to see on one side of the visual field, associated with hemianesthesia of the opposite side of the body.

crossed extension reflex, one of the spinally mediated reflexes normally present in the first 2 months of life. It is demonstrated by the adduction and extension of one leg when the foot of the other leg is stimulated.

crossed grid, (in radiography) an assembly of two parallel x-ray grids that are rotated at right angles to each other.

crossed reflex, any neural reflex in which stimulation of one side of the body results in a response on the other, such as the consensual light reflex.

cross-eye. See **esophoria.**

cross fertilization, 1. (in zoology) the union of gametes from different species or varieties to form hybrids. **2.** (in botany) the fertilization of the flower of one plant by the pollen from a different plant, as opposed to self-fertilization.

cross infection [L, *crux*, cross, *inficere*, to stain], the transmittal of an infection from one patient in a hospital or health care setting to another patient in the same environment.

crossing over, the exchange of sections of chromatids between homologous pairs of chromosomes during the prophase stage of the first meiotic division.

crossmatching of blood [L, *crux* + AS, *ge- maecca*, matching], a procedure used to determine compatibility of a donor's blood with that of a recipient after the specimens have been matched for major blood type. Serum from the donor's blood is mixed with red cells from the recipient's blood, and cells from the donor are mixed with serum from the recipient. If agglutination occurs, an antigenic substance is present, and the bloods are not compatible.

crossover /kros′ovər/ [L, *crux* + AS, *ofer*], the result of the recombination of genes on homologous pairs of chromosomes during meiosis.

cross-reacting antibody [L, *crux,* cross, *re* + *agere,* to act; Gk, *anti* + AS, *bodig,* body], an antibody that reacts with antigens that are similar to but different from the specific antigens with which it originally reacted.

cross resistance, the resistance to a particular antibiotic that also results in resistance against a different antibiotic to which the bacteria may not have been exposed.

cross section, 1. a transverse section cut through a structure. **2.** (in nuclear physics) of a specific atom or particle at a specific radiation, the area perpendicular to the direction of the radiation that one attributes to the atom or particle.

cross-sectional [L, *crux* + *secare,* to cut], (in statistics) pertaining to the comparative data of two groups of persons at one point in time.

cross-sectional anatomy, the study of the relationship of the structures of the body by the examination of cross sections of the tissue or organ.

cross sensitivity, a sensitivity to one substance that predisposes an individual to sensitivity to other substances that are related in chemical structure.

cross-sequential /-sikwen′shəl/ [L, *crux* + *sequi,* to follow], (in statistics) pertaining to data that compare several cohorts at different points in time.

cross-species transplant, a tissue or organ from an animal of one species that has been implanted into an animal of another species. Also called xenotransplant.

cross-tolerance, a tolerance to other drugs that develops after exposure to only one agent. An example is the cross tolerance that develops between alcohol and barbiturates.

crotamiton /krōtam′iton/, a scabicide prescribed in treating scabies and other pruritic skin diseases.

croup /kroop/ [Scot, to croak], an acute viral infection of the upper and lower respiratory tracts that occurs primarily in infants and young children 3 months to 3 years of age after an upper respiratory tract infection. It is characterized by hoarseness; irritability; fever; a distinctive harsh, brassy cough; persistent stridor during inspiration; and dyspnea and tachypnea resulting from obstruction of the larynx. The most common causative agents are the parainfluenza viruses, especially type 1, followed by the respiratory syncytial viruses (RSVs) and influenza A and B viruses. —**croupous, croupy,** *adj.*

Croupette /kro͞opet′/,   trademark for a device that provides cool humidification with the administration of oxygen or of compressed air.

Crouzon's disease /kro͞ozonz′/ [Octave Crouzon, French neurologist, 1874–1938; L, *dis* + Fr, *aise,* ease],   a familial disease characterized by a malformed skull and various ocular disorders, including exophthalmos, divergent squint, and optic atrophy.

crowing inspiration /krō′ing/ [ME, *crouen* + L, *inspirare,* to breathe in],   a harsh, noise audible on inhalation caused by an acute obstruction in the larynx.

crown [L, *corona*],   **1.** the upper part of an organ or structure, such as the top of the head. **2.** the part of a human tooth that is covered by enamel.

crown-heel length [L, *corona* + AS, *hela, lengthu*],   the length of an embryo, fetus, or newborn as measured from the crown of the head to the heel. It is compared to the standing height of an older individual.

crowning [L, *corona*],   (in obstetrics) the phase at the end of labor in which the fetal head is seen at the introitus of the vagina. The labia are stretched in a crown around the head just before birth.

crown/root ratio,   the relation of the clinical crown to the clinical root of a tooth.

crown-rump length,   the length of an embryo, fetus, or newborn as measured from the crown of the head to the prominence of the buttocks.

crown static,   an x-ray film artifact caused by a buildup and discharge of electrons in the film emulsion. It is most likely to appear during periods of low environmental humidity.

CRP,   abbreviation for **C-reactive protein.**

CRRN,   abbreviation for *Certified Rehabilitation Registered Nurse.*

CRT,   1. abbreviation for **cadaveric renal transplant. 2.** abbreviation for **cathode-ray tube.**

CRTT,   abbreviation for **Certified Respiratory Therapy Technician.**

crucial anastomosis /kro͞o′shəl/ [L, *crux,* cross; Gk, *anastomoein,* to provide a mouth],   an anastomosis in the upper part

of the thigh, formed between the first perforating branch of the profunda femoris artery, the inferior gluteal artery, and the lateral and medial circumflex arteries.

cruciate ligament of the atlas [L, *crux,* cross, *ligare,* to bind],   a crosslike ligament attaching the atlas to the base of the occipital bone above and the posterior surface of the body of the axis below.

crucible /kro͞o′səbəl/,   a cone-shaped vessel made of a refractory material, used in chemistry to melt or calcine materials at temperatures too high for other laboratory equipment to tolerate.

cruciform /kro͞o′sifôrm/ [L, *crux,* cross], in the shape of a cross.

cruciform ligament,   any cross-shaped band of white fibrous tissue connecting bones and forming a joint capsule.

crude birth rate [L, *crudus,* raw; ME, *burth* + L, *reri,* to reckon],   the number of births per 1000 people in a population during 1 year.

cruor /kro͞o′ôr/ [L, blood],   a blood clot containing erythrocytes.

crura anthelicis /kro͞or′ə anthel′isis, ant·hē′lisis/ [L, *crus,* leg; Gk, *anti,* against, *helix,* coil],   the two ridges on the external ear marking the superior termination of the anthelix and bounding the triangular fossa.

crural /kro͞o′rəl/,   pertaining to the leg, particularly the upper leg or thigh.

crural hernia [L, *crus,* leg, *hernia,* rupture],   a hernia that protrudes behind the posterior layer of the femoral sheath.

crural ligament,   a band of fibrous tissue that spans the gap between the anterior superior iliac spine and the pubic tubercle.

crus /krus/, *pl.* **crura** /kro͞or′ə/ [L, leg], **1.** the leg, from knee to foot. **2.** a structure resembling a leg, such as the crura anthelicis.

crus cerebri /ser′əbrī, -brē/ [L, *crus* + *cerebrum,* brain],   the ventral part of the cerebral peduncle, composed of the descending fiber tracts passing from the cerebral cortex to form the longitudinal fascicles of the pons.

crushing wound /krush′ing/ [ME, *crushen* + AS, *wund*],   a break in the external surface of the body caused by a severe force applied against the tissues. The body structures may be crushed without signs of external bleeding.

crush syndrome [ME, *crushen*],   a severe, life-threatening condition caused by extensive crushing trauma, characterized by destruction of muscle and bone tissue, hemorrhage, and fluid loss resulting in hypovolemic shock, hematuria, renal failure, and coma.

crust [L, *crusta,* shell],   a solidified, hard

outer layer formed by the drying of a body exudate, common in dermatologic conditions such as eczema, impetigo, seborrhea, and favus and during the healing of burns and lesions; a scab.

crutch [AS, *cryce*], a wooden or metal staff, the most common kind of which reaches from the ground almost to the axilla, to aid a person in walking. A padded, curved surface at the top fits under the arm; a grip in the form of a crossbar is held in the hand at the level of the palms to support the body.

Crutchfield tongs [William G. Crutchfield, American neurosurgeon, b. 1900; ME, *tonges*], an instrument inserted into the skull to hyperextend the head and neck of patients with fractured cervical vertebrae. The tongs are inserted into small burr holes drilled in each parietal region of the skull; the surrounding skin is sutured and covered with a collodion dressing. A weight is suspended from a rope extending from the center of the tongs over a pulley attached to the head of the bed.

crutch gait, a gait achieved by a person on crutches by alternately bearing weight on one or both legs and on the crutches. The gait selected and learned is determined by the physical and functional abilities of the patient and the diagnosis.

crutch palsy, the temporary or permanent loss of sensation or muscle control resulting from pressure on the radial nerve by a crutch.

Cruveilhier-Baumgarten's syndrome /krYvāyā'-boum'gätən/ [Jean Cruveilhier, French pathologist, 1791–1874; Paul Baumgarten, German pathologist, 1848–1928], recanalization of the paraumbilical veins with cirrhosis of the liver, portal hypertension, and splenomegaly.

crux /kruks, krŏŏks/, 1. cross. 2. a difficult problem. 3. a vital, basic, or decisive point.

cry [OFr, *crier*], 1. a sudden, loud voluntary or automatic vocalization in response to pain, fear, or a startle reflex. 2. weeping, as a reaction or an emotional response to depression or grief.

crying vital capacity (CVC), a measurement of the tidal volume while an infant is crying. The CVC may be valuable in monitoring infants with lung diseases that cause changes in functional residual capacity.

cryoanesthesia /krī'ō·an'isthē'zhə/ [Gk, *kryos,* cold, *aisthesis,* feeling], the freezing of a part of the body to achieve adequate deadening of neural sensitivity to pain during brief minor surgical procedures.

cryocautery /krī'ōkô'tərē/ [Gk, *kryos* +

kauterion, branding iron], the application of any substance, such as solid carbon dioxide, that destroys tissue by freezing.

cryogen /krī'əjən/ [Gk, *kryos* + *genein,* to produce], 1. a chemical that induces freezing, used to destroy diseased tissue without injury to adjacent structures. Cell death is caused by dehydration after cell membranes rupture. 2. (in magnetic resonance imaging [MRI]) a chemical used to cool the MRI electromagnet so that higher energies can be achieved. —**cryogenic,** *adj.*

cryoglobulin /krī'ōglob'yŏŏlin/ [Gk, *kryos* + L, *globulus,* small sphere], an abnormal plasma protein that precipitates and coalesces at low temperatures and dissolves and disperses at body temperature.

cryoglobulinemia /krī'ōglob'yŏŏlinē'mē·ə/ [Gk, *kryos* + L, *globulus,* small sphere; Gk, *haima,* blood], the presence of cryoglobulins in the blood.

cryonics /krī·on'iks/ [Gk, *kryos,* cold], the techniques in which cold is applied for a variety of therapeutic goals, including brief local anesthesia, destruction of superficial skin lesions, and preservation of cells, tissue, organs, or the entire body. —**cryonic,** *adj.*

cryoprecipitate /-prisip'itāt/, 1. any precipitate formed on cooling of a solution. 2. a preparation rich in factor VIII needed to restore normal coagulation in hemophilia. It is collected from fresh human plasma that has been frozen and thawed.

cryopreservation /krī'ōpres'ərvā'shən/ a method of preserving tissues and organs in a viable state at extremely low temperatures.

cryostat /krī'ōstat/ [Gk, *kryos* + *statos,* standing], a device used in surgical treatment of pathologic disorders that consists of a special microtome used for freezing and slicing sections of tissue for study by a surgical pathologist.

cryosurgery /-sur'jərē/ [Gk, *kryos* + *cheirourgos*], use of subfreezing temperature to destroy tissue. Cryosurgery is performed to destroy the ganglion of nerve cells in the thalamus in the treatment of Parkinson's disease, to destroy the pituitary gland to halt the progress of some kinds of metastatic cancer, and to treat various cancers and lesions of the skin. The process is also used in ophthalmology to cause the edges of a detached retina to heal and to remove cataracts. The coolant is circulated through a metal probe, chilling it to as low as −160° C (−320° F).

cryotherapy /krī'ōther'əpē/ [Gk, *kryos* + *therapeia*], a treatment using cold as a destructive medium for some of the common skin disorders. Solid carbon dioxide or liquid nitrogen is applied briefly with a sterile cotton-tipped applicator.

crypt /kript/ [Gk, *kryptos,* hidden], a blind pit or tube on a free surface. Some kinds of crypts are **anal crypt, dental crypt,** and **synovial crypt.**

cryptic /krip′tik/ [Gk, *kryptos,* hidden], pertaining to something concealed.

cryptocephalus /krip′tōsef′ələs/ [Gk, *kryptos* + *kephale,* head], a malformed fetus that has a small, underdeveloped head. —**cryptocephalic, cryptocephalous,** *adj.,* **cryptocephaly,** *n.*

cryptococcosis /krip′tōkokō′sis/, an infectious disease caused by a fungus, *Cryptococcus neoformans,* which spreads from the lungs to the brain and central nervous system, skin, skeletal system, and urinary tract. It is characterized by the development of nodules or tumors filled with a gelatinous material in visceral and subcutaneous tissues. Initial symptoms may include coughing or other respiratory effects because the lungs are a primary site of infection. After the fungus spreads to the meninges, neurologic symptoms, including headache, blurred vision, and difficulty in speaking, may develop.

Cryptococcus /-kok′əs/, a genus of yeastlike fungi that reproduce by budding rather than producing spores. Certain pathogenic species exist; *C. neoformans* is the most important.

Cryptococcus neoformans, a species of yeastlike fungus that causes cryptococcosis, a potentially fatal infection that can affect the lungs, skin, and brain.

cryptodidymus /krip′tōdid′əməs/ [Gk, *kryptos* + *didymos,* twin], conjoined twins; one fetus is small, underdeveloped, and concealed within the body of the other, more fully formed autosite.

crypt of iris, any one of the small pits in the iris along its free margin encircled by the circulus arteriosus minor.

cryptogenic /-jen′ik/ [Gk, *kryptos,* hidden, *genein,* to produce], **1.** pertaining to a disease of unknown cause. **2.** a parasitic organism living within another organism.

cryptogenic infection, a disease caused by pathogenic microorganisms of obscure or unknown origin.

cryptogenic septicemia, a systemic infection in which pathogens are present in the bloodstream but no primary focus of infection can be identified.

cryptomenorrhea /krip′tōmenôrē′ə/ [Gk, *kryptos* + L, *mens,* month; Gk, *rhoia,* flow], an abnormal condition in which the products of menstruation are retained within the vagina because of an imperforate hymen, or, less often, within the uterus because of an occlusion of the cervical canal. —**cryptomenorrheal,** *adj.*

cryptophthalmos /krip′tофthal′mos/ [Gk, *kryptos* + *ophthalmos,* eye], a developmental anomaly characterized by complete fusion of the eyelids, usually with defective formation or lack of eyes.

cryptorchidism /kriptôr′kidiz′əm/ [Gk, *kryptos,* hidden, *orchis,* testis], a developmental defect characterized by failure of one or both of the testicles to descend into the scrotum. They are retained in the abdomen or inguinal canal.

cryptosporidiosis, a gastrointestinal disease caused by a waterborne parasitic protozoon, *Cryptosporidium parvum.* The disease was relatively unknown as a human pathogen before a 1993 epidemic in the Milwaukee, Wisconsin, area, where 400,000 persons were stricken with diarrhea after drinking water contaminated with the parasite. In addition to contaminated drinking water, sources of infection include raw or undercooked foods contaminated with *Cryptosporidium* oocysts and direct contact with infected humans or animals. Symptoms of watery diarrhea, abdominal cramps, nausea, vomiting, and low-grade fever may appear 2 to 10 days after infection.

cry reflex, a normal infantile reaction to pain, hunger, or need for attention. The reflex may be absent in an infant born prematurely or in poor health.

crystal /kris′təl/ [Gk, *krystallos*], a solid inorganic substance, the atoms or molecules of which are arranged in a regular, repeating three-dimensional pattern, which determines the shape of a crystal. —**crystalline,** *adj.*

crystalline, describing material with a regular geometric shape. Crystalline substances have a very narrow melting point range.

crystalline lens /kris′təlin, -līn/ [Gk, *krystallos* + L, lentil], a transparent structure of the eye, enclosed in a capsule, situated between the iris and the vitreous humor, and slightly overlapped at its margin by the ciliary processes. It refracts light to focus images on the retina. The lens is a transparent biconvex structure with the posterior surface more convex than the anterior. It is composed of a soft cortical material, a firm nucleus, and concentric laminae.

crystallization /kris′təlīzā′shən/ [Gk, *krystallos,* rock crystal], the production of crystals, either by cooling a liquid or gas to a solid state or by cooling a solution until the solute precipitates as a crystalline deposit.

crystalloid /kris′təloid/ [Gk, *krystallos* +

eidos, form], a substance in a solution that can diffuse through a semipermeable membrane.

crystalluria /kris′tǝlŏŏr′ē·ǝ/, the presence of crystals in the urine. The condition may be a source of urinary tract irritation; adequate intake of alkali can prevent it.

Cs, symbol for the element **cesium.**

CS, abbreviation for **cesarean section.**

CSF, 1. abbreviation for **cerebrospinal fluid. 2.** abbreviation for **colony-stimulating factor.**

CSN, abbreviation for *certified school nurse.*

CSR, abbreviation for **Cheyne-Stokes respiration.**

c-src, a cellular oncogene or protooncogene present in some animals. It hybridizes with oncogenes of the highly virulent Rous sarcoma virus.

CST, abbreviation for **contraction stress test.**

CT, abbreviation for **computed tomography.**

C3 nephritic factor, a C3 complement protein molecule that may be deposited in glomerular capillary walls and mesangial tissues, precipitating or contributing to local immune inflammatory injury and kidney damage.

Cu, symbol for the element **copper.**

CUA, abbreviation for **cost-utility analysis.**

cubic centimeter (cm³) [Gk, *kybos* + L, *centum,* hundred; Gk, *metron,* measure], a theoretic cube or its equivalent, each edge of which is 1 centimeter long. One cubic centimeter is equivalent to 1 milliliter.

cubic millimeter (cmm, c mm, cu mm, mm³), a unit of volume equal to one millionth of a liter.

cubital /kyōō′bitǝl/, pertaining to the elbow or the forearm.

cubital fossa, a depression in the front of the elbow, immediately lateral to the tendon of the biceps brachii muscle.

cubitus /kyōō′bitǝs/, **1.** the elbow. **2.** the forearm.

cuboidal epithelium /kyōōboi′dǝl/ [Gk, *kybos,* cube, *eidos,* form, *epi,* above, *thele,* nipple], simple epithelial cells that are generally cube-shaped and one layer thick.

cuboid bone /kyōō′boid/ [Gk, *kybos,* cube, *eidos,* form], the cuboidal tarsal bone on the lateral side of the foot, proximal to the fourth and fifth metatarsal bones.

cu cm, abbreviation for **cubic centimeter.**

cue /kyōō/, a stimulus that determines or may prompt the nature of a person's response.

cuff [ME], an inflatable elastic tube that

is placed around the upper arm and inflated with air to restrict arterial circulation during blood pressure examination.

cuffed endotracheal tube, an endotracheal tube with a balloon at one end that may be inflated to tighten its fit in the lumen of the airway. The balloon forms a cuff that prevents gastric contents from passing into the lungs and gas from leaking back from the lungs.

cuffing, a pathologic condition in which cufflike borders of leukocytes form around small blood vessels, as in certain infections.

cuirass /kwiras′/ [Fr, *cuirasse,* breastplate], **1.** a negative-pressure full-body respirator. An electrically driven pump is adjusted to match the timing of the patient's spontaneous breathing. **2.** a tightly fitted chest bandage.

cul-de-sac /kul′dǝsak, kYdesok′/, *pl.* **culs-de-sac, cul-de-sacs** [F, bottom of the bag], a blind pouch or cecum, such as the conjunctival cul-de-sac or the dural cul-de-sacs.

cul-de-sac of Douglas [James Douglas, Scottish anatomist, 1675–1742], a pouch formed by the caudal part of the parietal peritoneum.

culdocentesis /kul′dōsentē′sis/, the use of needle puncture or incision through the vagina to remove intraperitoneal fluid, including purulent material.

culdoplasty /kul′dōplas′tē/ [Fr, *cul-de-sac,* bottom of the bag; Gk, *plassein,* to mold], plastic surgery to correct a defect in the posterior fornix of the vagina.

culdoscope /kul′dǝskōp′/, an endoscope with an attached light that can be inserted through the posterior wall of the vagina for examination of the pelvic viscera.

culdotomy /kuldot′ǝmē/, incision or needle puncture of cul-de-sac of Douglas by way of the vagina.

Culex /kōō′leks/, a genus of humpbacked mosquitoes. It includes species that transmit viral encephalitis and filariasis.

Cullen's sign [Thomas S. Cullen, American gynecologist, 1868–1953], the appearance of faint, irregularly formed hemorrhagic patches on the skin around the umbilicus. Cullen's sign may appear 1 to 2 days after the onset of anorexia and the severe, poorly localized abdominal pains that are characteristic of acute pancreatitis.

cult, a specific complex of beliefs, rites, and ceremonies associated with some particular person or object, which is maintained by a social group. A cult is often considered as having magical significance.

cultural event, a communication of meaning that takes place each time one member of a society interacts with another member.

cultural healer, a member of an ethnic or cultural group who uses traditional methods of healing rather than modern scientific methods to provide health care for other members of the group or members of another ethnic minority group.

culturally relativistic perspective, an ability to understand the behavior of transcultural patients (those who move from one culture to another) within the context of their own culture.

cultural relativism, a concept that health and normality emerge within a social context and that the content and form of mental health will greatly vary from one culture to another.

culture /kul′chər/ [L, *colere,* to cultivate], **1.** (in microbiology) a laboratory test involving the cultivation of microorganisms or cells in a special growth medium. **2.** (in psychology) a set of learned values, beliefs, customs, and behavior that is shared by a group of interacting individuals.

culture-bound, pertaining to a health condition that is specific to a particular culture, such as a belief in the effects of certain kinds of prayer or the "evil eye."

Culture Brokerage, a Nursing Interventions Classification defined as bridging, negotiating, or linking the orthodox health care system with a patient and family of a different culture.

culture procedure, (in bacteriology) any of several techniques for growing colonies of microorganisms to identify a pathogen and to determine its sensitivity to various antibiotics. Usually a specimen is secured, and a small amount is placed into or on one or more culture media, because different organisms are nourished by different nutrients and grow best at different specific pH levels.

culture shock, the psychologic effect of a drastic change in the cultural environment of an individual. The person may exhibit feelings of helplessness, discomfort, and disorientation in attempting to adapt to a different cultural group with dissimilar practices, values, and beliefs.

cum /kŏŏm/, together with.

cu mm, abbreviation for **cubic millimeter.**

cumulative /kyōō′myəlā′tiv/ [L, *cumulare,* to pile on], increasing by incremental steps with an eventual total that may exceed the expected result.

cumulative action, 1. the increased activity of a therapeutic measure or agent when administered repeatedly. **2.** the increased activity demonstrated by a drug

when repeated doses accumulate in the body and exert a greater biologic effect than the initial dose.

cumulative dose, the total dosage that accumulates as a result of repeated exposure to radiation or a radiopharmaceutic product.

cuneate /kyōō′nē·āt/ [L, *cuneus,* wedge], (of tissue) wedge-shaped; especially in relation to cells of the nervous system.

cuneiform /kyōōnē′əfôrm′/ [L, *cuneus,* wedge, *forma*], (of bone and cartilage) wedge-shaped.

cuneiform cartilage [L, *cuneus,* wedge, *forma* + *cartilago*], an elongated elastic laryngeal cartilage at the edge of the aryepiglottic fold, above and anterior to the corniculate cartilage.

cuneus /kyōō′nē·əs/, a wedge-shaped region of the cerebral cortex lying between the parieto-occipital and postcalcarine sulci.

cunnilingus /kun′əling′gəs/, the oral stimulation of the female genitalia.

cup arthroplasty of the hip joint [L, *cupa,* cask; Gk, *arthron,* joint, *plassein,* to form], the surgical replacement of the head of the femur by a metal or plastic mold to relieve pain and increase motion in arthritis or to correct a deformity. The damaged or diseased bone is removed, and the acetabulum and the head of the femur are reshaped. A cup is inserted between the two and becomes the articulating surface of the femur. After surgery the patient's leg is placed on an abduction pillow to hold it in a position of abduction extension and internal rotation to keep the disk in place in the acetabulum.

cup/disc ratio, (in ophthalmology) the mathematic relationship between the horizontal or vertical diameter of the physiologic cup and the diameter of the optic disc.

cupping, a counterirritant technique of applying a suction device to the skin to draw blood to the surface of the body.

cupping and vibrating, the procedures to help remove mucus and fluid from the lungs using the techniques of manual percussion and vibration to dislodge and mobilize the secretions. Cupping is performed by the rhythmic percussion of the affected segments of the lungs or bronchi by the practitioner's cupped hands placed over the affected area and tensing and contracting the muscles of the hand, arm, and, mainly, shoulder.

cupric /kyōō′prik/ [L, *cuprum,* copper], pertaining to copper in its divalent form, as cupric sulfate. Also termed copper (II), as in copper (II) sulfate.

cupula, /kyōō′pələ/ any cup- or dome-shaped structure, such as the top of a lymphatic bundle in the small intestine.

cupulolithiasis /kyōō´pyōōlōlithī´əsis/ [L, *cupula,* little cup; Gk, *lithos,* stone], a severe, long-lasting vertigo brought on by movement of the head to certain positions. Among the many possible causes are otitis media, ear surgery, and injury to the inner ear. In addition to extreme dizziness, signs are nausea, vomiting, and ataxia.

curare /kyōōrä´rē/ [S. Am. Indian, *ourari*], a substance derived from tropical plants of the genus *Strychnos.* It is a potent neuromuscular blocker that acts by preventing transmission of neural impulses across the myoneural junctions. A large dosage can cause complete paralysis, but action is usually reversible with anticholinergics.

curariform /kyōōrä´rifôrm´/ [*curare* + L, *forma*], **1.** chemically similar to curare. **2.** having the effect of curare.

cure /kyōōr/ [L, *cura*], **1.** restoration to health of a person afflicted with a disease or other disorder. **2.** the favorable outcome of the treatment of a disease or other disorder. **3.** a course of therapy, a medication, a therapeutic measure, or another remedy used in treatment of a medical problem, as faith healing, fasting, rest cure, or work cure.

curet /kyōōret´/ [Fr, *curette,* scoop], **1.** a surgical instrument shaped like a spoon or scoop for scraping and removing material or tissue from an organ, cavity, or surface. **2.** to remove tissue or debris with such a device.

curettage /kyōōr´ətäzh´/ [Fr, *curette,* scoop], scraping of material from the wall of a cavity or other surface, performed to remove tumors or other abnormal tissue or to obtain tissue for microscopic examination. Curettage also refers to clearing unwanted material from fistulas and areas of chronic infection.

curie (c, Ci) /kyōōr´ē/ [Marie S. Curie, Polish-born chemist and physicist, 1867–1934; Pierre Curie, French chemist and physicist, 1859–1906; both Nobel laureates], a unit of radioactivity used before adoption of the becquerel (Bq) as the SI unit. It is equal to 3.70×10^{10} Bq.

curium (Cm) /kyōō´rē·əm/ [Marie S. Curie; Pierre Curie], a radioactive metallic element. Its atomic number is 96; its atomic weight (mass) is 247.

Curling's ulcer [Thomas B. Curling, English surgeon, 1811–1888], a duodenal ulcer that develops in people who have suffered severe stress.

CURN, abbreviation for *Certified Urological Registered Nurse.*

currant jelly clot /kur´ənt/ [ME, *corauns* + L, *gelare,* to congeal; AS, *clott*], a red,

jellylike blood clot that is rich in hemoglobin from erythrocytes in the clot.

current /kur´ənt/ [L, *currere,* to run], **1.** a flowing or streaming movement. **2.** a flow of electrons along a conductor in a closed circuit; an electric current. **3.** certain physiologic electrical activity and characteristics of blood circulation. Physiologic currents include abnerval, action, axial, centrifugal, centripetal, compensating, demarcation, and electrotonic currents.

current of injury, an abnormal current flow to and from injured myocardium. It results from reduced membrane potential in the injured area compared to that of the normal fibers.

Current Procedural Terminology (CPT), a system developed by the American Medical Association for standardizing the terminology and coding used to describe medical services and procedures.

curriculum vitae (CV) /kərik´ələm wē´tī, vē´tē/, *pl.* **curricula vitae** [L, *curriculum,* course, *vita,* life], a summary of educational and professional experiences, including activities and honors, to be used in applications for employment, for biographic citations on professional meeting programs, or for related purposes.

Curschmann's spiral /kōōrsh´mon/ [Heinrich Curschmann, German physician, 1846–1910; Gk, *speira,* coil], coiled fibril of mucus occasionally found in the sputum of persons with bronchial asthma.

curtain effect /kur´tən/, (in radiology) an x-ray film artifact caused by chemical processing stains, which are produced when chemicals are not properly squeezed from the film during development.

curvature, a bending or curving of a line from the course of a straight line.

curvature myopia /kur´vəchər/, a type of nearsightedness caused by refractive errors associated with an excessive curvature of the cornea.

curve [L, *curvare,* to bend], (in statistics) a straight or curved line used as a graphic method of demonstrating the distribution of data collected in a study or survey.

curve of Carus [Karl G. Carus, German anatomist, 1789–1869], the normal axis of the pelvic outlet.

curve of occlusion, 1. a curved occlusal surface that simultaneously contacts the major part of the incisal and occlusal prominences of the existing teeth. **2.** the curve of dentition on which lie the occlusal surfaces of the teeth.

curve of Spee /shpā, spē/ [Ferdinand Graf von Spee, German embryologist, 1855–1937], **1.** the anatomic curvature of the occlusal alignment of the teeth, beginning at the tip of the lower canine, following the buccal cusps of the natural premolars and molars, and continuing to the anterior border of the ramus. **2.** the curve of the occlusal surfaces of the arches in vertical dimension, produced by a downward dipping of the mandibular premolars, with a corresponding adjustment of the upper premolars.

curvilinear /cur'vilin'ē·ər/ [L, *curvus*, bent, *linea*, line], pertaining to a curved line.

curvilinear trend [L, *curvus*, bent, *linea*, line; AS, *trendan*, to turn], (in statistics) a trend in which a graphic representation of the data yields a curved line.

cushingoid /kōōsh'ingoid/ [Harvey W. Cushing, American surgeon, 1869–1939; Gk, *eidos*, form], having the habitus and facies characteristic of Cushing's disease: fat pads on the upper back and face, ruddy complexion, striae on trunk, thin legs, and excess facial hair.

Cushing's disease /kōōsh'ingz/ [Harvey W. Cushing], a metabolic disorder characterized by abnormally increased secretion of adrenocortical steroids caused by increased amounts of adrenocorticotropic hormone secreted by the pituitary, such as by a pituitary adenoma. Excess adrenocortical hormones result in accumulations of fat on the chest, upper back, and face and occurrence of edema, hyperglycemia, increased gluconeogenesis, muscle weakness, purplish striae on the skin, decreased immunity to infection, osteoporosis with susceptibility to bone fractures, acne, and facial hair growth in women.

Cushing's syndrome [Harvey W. Cushing], a metabolic disorder resulting from the chronic and excessive production of cortisol by the adrenal cortex or by the administration of glucocorticoids in large doses for several weeks or longer. When occurring spontaneously, the syndrome represents a failure in the body's ability to regulate the secretion of cortisol or adrenocorticotropic hormone (ACTH). (Normally cortisol is produced only in response to ACTH, and ACTH is not secreted in the presence of high levels of cortisol.) The most common cause of the syndrome is a pituitary tumor that increases secretion of ACTH. The patient with Cushing's syndrome has a decreased glucose tolerance; central obesity; round "moon" face; supraclavicular fat pads; an overhanging, striae-covered pad of fat on the chest and abdomen; buffalo hump; scant menstrual periods or decreased testosterone levels; muscular atrophy; edema; and hypokalemia.

cushion [OFr, *coissin*], any anatomic structure that resembles a pad or pillow.

cusp [L, *cuspis*, point], **1.** a sharp projection or a rounded eminence that rises from the chewing surface of a tooth, such as the two pyramidal cusps that arise from the premolars. **2.** any one of the small flaps on the valves of the heart, as the ventral, dorsal, and medial cusps attached to the right atrioventricular valve.

cuspid /kus'pid/ [L, *cuspis*, point], **1.** having but one cusp, or point. **2.** canine tooth.

cuspless tooth /kusp'les/, a tooth without cuspal prominences on its occlusal surface, possibly as a result of attrition.

custodial care /kəstō'dē·əl/ [L, *custodia*, guarding, *garrire*, to chatter], services and care of a nonmedical nature provided on a long-term basis, usually for convalescent and chronically ill individuals.

customary and reasonable charge, (in the United States) a fee usually established by health insurance or government agencies that is considered to be the "usual" cost of a specific medical service. The fee is commonly based on the amount the company or agency will pay for that service and may vary with geographic area.

cut, (in molecular genetics) a fissure or split in a double strand of deoxyribonucleic acid in contrast to a nick in a single strand.

cutaneous /kyōōtā'nē·əs/ [L, *cutis*, skin], pertaining to the skin.

cutaneous absorption, the taking up of substances through the skin.

cutaneous anaphylaxis, a localized exaggerated reaction of hypersensitivity in the form of a wheal and flare caused by an antigen injected into the skin of a sensitized individual, as a test of sensitivity to various allergens.

cutaneous horn, a hard, skin-colored projection of the epidermis, usually on the head or face.

cutaneous larva migrans, a skin condition caused by a hookworm, *Ancylostoma braziliense*, a parasite of cats and dogs. Its ova are deposited in the ground with the feces of infected animals, develop into larvae, and invade the skin of people, particularly bare feet, although any skin may be involved. As they migrate through the epidermis, a trail of inflammation follows the burrow, causing severe pruritus. Secondary infections often occur if the skin has been broken by scratching.

cutaneous nerve, any mixed peripheral nerve that supplies a region of the skin.

cutaneous nevus [L, *cutis*, skin, *naevus*, birthmark], a congenital discoloration of a skin area, such as a strawberry birthmark.

cutaneous papilloma, a small brown o

flesh-colored outgrowth of skin, occurring most frequently on the neck of an older person.

cutaneous sensation [L, *cutis,* skin, *sentire,* to feel], a sensation experienced in or arising from receptors of the skin.

Cutaneous Stimulation, a Nursing Interventions Classification defined as stimulation of the skin and underlying tissues for the purpose of decreasing undesirable signs and symptoms such as pain, muscle spasm, or inflammation.

cutdown [ME, *cutten* + *doun*], an incision into a vein and the insertion of a catheter for intravenous infusion. It is performed when an infusion cannot be started by venipuncture for total parenteral nutrition.

cuticle /kyōō′təkəl/ [L, *cuticula,* little skin], **1.** epidermis. **2.** the sheath of a hair follicle. **3.** the thin edge of cornified epithelium at the base of a nail.

cuticula /kyōōtik′yələ/, the cuticle, a narrow region of epidermis that covers the proximal surface of a fingernail or toenail.

cutis laxa /kyōō′təs/ [L, skin, *laxus,* loose], abnormally loose, relaxed skin resulting from an absence of elastic fibers in the skin, usually a hereditary condition.

cutis marmorata, skin that has a "marbled" appearance caused by conspicuous dilation of small vessels.

cutting oil dermatitis, a skin disorder that affects machinists and others who use cutting oils as coolants and lubricants. Exposure to the oil obstructs hair follicles, sweat ducts, and sebaceous glands, leading to development of comedones and folliculitis.

cuvette /kyōōvet′/ [Fr, *cuva,* tub], a small, transparent tube or container with specific optical properties. It is used in laboratory research and analyses such as photometric evaluations, colorimetric determinations, and turbidity studies.

CVA, 1. abbreviation for **cerebrovascular accident. 2.** abbreviation for **costovertebral angle.**

CVB, abbreviation for *chorionic villus biopsy.*

CVP, 1. abbreviation for **central venous pressure. 2.** an anticancer drug combination of cyclophosphamide, vincristine, and prednisone.

CW, abbreviation for **continuous wave.**

cyanide poisoning /sī′ənid, -nīd/ [Gk, *kyanos,* blue], poisoning resulting from the ingestion or inhalation of cyanide from such substances as bitter almond oil, wild cherry syrup, prussic acid, hydrocyanic acid, or potassium or sodium cyanide. Characterized by tachycardia, drowsiness, seizures, headache, apnea, and cardiac ar-

rest, it may caused death within 1 to 15 minutes.

cyanocobalamin /sī′ənōkōbal′əmin/ [Gk, *kyanos* + Ger, *kobald,* mine goblin], a red crystalline, water-soluble substance that is the common pharmaceutic form of vitamin B_{12}. It is involved in the metabolism of protein, fats, and carbohydrates; normal blood formation; and neural function. Deficiency is usually caused by the absence of intrinsic factor (produced in the stomach), which is necessary for the absorption of cyanocobalamin from the gastrointestinal tract and causes pernicious anemia and brain damage. Symptoms of deficiency include nervousness, neuritis, numbness and tingling in the hands and feet, poor muscular coordination, unpleasant body odor, and menstrual disturbances.

cyanogenetic glycosides /sī′ənōjənet′ik/, chemical compounds contained in foods that release hydrogen cyanide when chewed or digested. The act of chewing or digestion disrupts the structure of the substances, causing cyanide to be released. Although human poisoning by cyanogenetic glycosides is rare, cases of cyanide poisoning by certain varieties of lima beans, cassava, and bitter almond have been reported.

cyanomethemoglobin /sī′ənō′met·hē′-məglō′bin/ [Gk, *kyanos* + *meta,* together with, *haima,* blood; L, *globus,* ball], a hemoglobin derivative formed during nitrite therapy for cyanide poisoning.

cyanopsia /sī′ənop′sē·ə/, a visual condition in which everything appears to have a blue tint.

cyanosed /sī′ənōst/, having a bluish discoloration of the skin, fingernails, and mucous membranes caused by a deficiency of oxygen in the blood.

cyanosis /sī′ənō′sis/ [Gk, *kyanos,* blue, *osis,* condition], bluish discoloration of the skin and mucous membranes caused by an excess of deoxygenated hemoglobin in the blood or a structural defect in the hemoglobin molecule, such as in methemoglobin. —**cyanotic,** *adj.*

cyanotic congenital defect /sī′ənot′ik/, an inborn heart defect that allows the mixing of unsaturated (venous) blood with saturated (arterial) blood to produce cyanosis.

cyberknife /sī′bənīf/, an automated gamma radiation beam used to treat brain tumors. The beam is directed to the tumor from many different angles. The separation of the multiple low-level beams reduces potential for harm to brain tissue as the target is irradiated.

cybernetics /sī′bərnet′iks/, the science of control and communication in living and nonliving systems, as in comparative study of electronic computers and the living brain.

cyclacillin /sī′kləsī′lin/, a penicillin antibiotic prescribed in the treatment of certain bacterial infections.

cyclamate /sī′kləmāt/, an artificial nonnutritive sweetener formerly used in the form of calcium or sodium salt.

cyclandelate /sīklan′dəlāt/, a vasodilator prescribed in the treatment of muscular ischemia and peripheral vascular obstruction or spasm.

cyclarthrosis /sīklärthrō′sis, sik′-/, a pivot joint, capable of rotation.

cycle [Gk, *kyklos,* circle], a series of events that recurs at specified intervals.

cyclencephaly /sīk′lənsef′əlē/ [Gk, *kyklos,* circle, *enkephalos,* brain], a developmental anomaly characterized by the fusion of the two cerebral hemispheres. —**cyclencephalic, cyclencephalous,** *adj.,* **cyclencephalus,** *n.*

cycles per second (cps). See **hertz (Hz).**

cyclic adenosine monophosphate (cAMP) /sik′lik, sī′klik/, a cyclic nucleotide formed from adenosine triphosphate by the action of adenyl cyclase. This cyclic compound, known as the "second messenger," participates in the action of catecholamines, vasopressin, adrenocorticotropic hormone, and many other hormones.

cyclic guanosine monophosphate (cGMP), a substance that mediates the action of certain hormones in a manner similar to that of cyclic adenosine monophosphate (cAMP).

cyclic vomiting, periodic episodes of vomiting associated with migraine and usually accompanied by headaches and symptoms of ketosis. The episodes may begin in childhood.

cyclin /sī′klin/, one of a class of intracellular proteins that appear during the eukaryotic cell cycle. The cyclin concentration increases during the cycle until halfway to the mitosis stage, when it drops to zero.

cyclin-dependent kinase (CDK), a protein kinase that is activated by cyclin.

cyclitis /siklī′tis/ [Gk, *kyklos + itis*], inflammation of the ciliary body that causes redness of the sclera adjacent to the cornea of the eye.

cyclizine hydrochloride /sī′klizēn/, an antihistamine prescribed in the treatment or prevention of motion sickness.

cyclobenzaprine hydrochloride, /sī′-kləben′zəprēn/, a muscle relaxant prescribed in the short-term treatment of muscle spasm.

cyclodestructive /sī′klədistruk′tiv/, (in ophthalmology) a procedure to damage the ciliary body in order to diminish the production of aqueous fluid in the treatment of glaucoma.

cyclodialysis /-dī·al′isis/, a surgical procedure performed on patients with glaucoma. A pathway is opened between the anterior chamber of the eye and the suprachoroidal space, allowing excess fluid to drain and reducing intraocular pressure.

cycloduction /-duk′shən/, (in ophthalmology) the range of rotation of an eye around its visual axis, which allows binocular single vision to be maintained.

cyclophosphamide /-fos′fəmīd/, an alkylating agent prescribed in the treatment of neoplasms and as an immunosuppressant in organ transplantation.

cyclopia /sīklō′pē·ə/ [Gk, *Cyclops,* mythic one-eyed giant], a developmental anomaly characterized by fusion of the orbits into a single cavity containing one eye. —**cyclops,** *n.*

cycloplegia /sī′kləplē′jə/ [Gk, *kyklos + plege,* stroke], paralysis of the ciliary muscles, as induced by certain ophthalmic drugs to allow examination of the eye.

cycloplegic /sī′kləplē′jik/, **1.** pertaining to a drug or treatment that causes paralysis of the ciliary muscles of the eye. **2.** one of a group of anticholinergic drugs used to paralyze the ciliary muscles of the eye for ophthalmologic examination or surgery. Any of the cycloplegics may cause adverse effects in persons sensitive to anticholinergics.

cycloserine /sī′klōser′ēn/, an antibiotic prescribed in the treatment of active pulmonary and extrapulmonary tuberculosis.

Cyclospora cayetanensis, a pathogenic protozoan that causes diarrhea, cramps, and fever in humans. The microorganism, a coccidian parasite about 0.01 mm in diameter, was not identified scientifically until 1979, after the first known cases of the infection were diagnosed. Before 1996 only three outbreaks of *Cyclospora* infection had been reported in the United States. In May and June 1996, clusters of cases were reported in 10 states and in Ontario, Canada. Although *Cyclospora* is transmitted by the fecal-oral route, person-to-person transmission is unlikely because excreted oocytes require days to weeks under favorable conditions to become infectious.

cyclosporin /-spôr′in/, any of a group of biologically active metabolites of *Tolypocladium inflatum gams* and certain other fungi. The major forms are cyclosporin A and C, which are cyclic oligopeptides with immunosuppressive, antifungal, and antipyretic effects. As immunosuppressants

cyclosporins primarily affect the T cell lymphocytes.

cyclosporine /-spôr′ēn/, an alternative term for cyclosporin A.

cyclothymic disorder /-thīm′ik/ [Gk, kyklos + thymos, mind], a disorder of mood, wherein the essential feature is a chronic mood disturbance of at least 2 years' duration, involving numerous periods of depression and hypomania, but not of sufficient severity and duration to meet the criteria for a major depressive or manic episode.

cyclothymic personality, a personality characterized by swings in mood from elation to depression.

cyclotomy /sīklot′əmē/, a surgical procedure for the correction of a defect in the ciliary muscle of the eye.

cyclotron /sī′klətron/ [Gk, kyklos + electron, amber], a device used to accelerate charged particles or ions. The particles bombard special targets, where they create radioactive species to be used as radiopharmaceuticals or to make neutrons that can be used for radiotherapy.

cyclotropia /sī′klōtrō′pəe·ə/, (in ophthalmology) a condition in which the ocular position of one eye is rotated around its axis with respect to the other eye.

cyesis /sī-ē′sis/ [Gk, kyesis, pregnancy], pregnancy.

cylinder, a solid body having a circular transverse section.

cylindrical grasp /silin′drikəl/, the normal position of the hand and fingers when holding cylindrical objects. The fingers close and flex around the object, which is stabilized against the palm of the hand. It occurs as a reflex action in infants and later develops into a voluntary gross grasp.

cylindroma /sil′indrō′mə/ [Gk, kylindros, cylinder], a tumor that appears to have cylinders of stroma surrounded by epithelial cells.

cyma line /sī′mə/, an S-shaped line seen on radiographs at the articulation of the talonavicular and calcaneocuboid bones of the foot.

cypionate /sī′pyōnāt/, contraction of cyclopentanepropionate.

cyproheptadine hydrochloride /sī′prōhep′tədēn/, an antihistamine prescribed in the treatment of hypersensitivity reactions, including rhinitis, skin rash, and pruritus.

Cys, abbreviation for **cysteine.**

cyst /sist/ [Gk, kystis, bag], a closed sac in or under the skin lined with epithelium and containing fluid or semisolid material, for example, a **sebaceous cyst.**

cystadenocarcinoma /sis′tədē′nəkär′sinō′mə/, a type of pancreatic tumor that evolves from a mucus cystadenoma. Clinical features include epigastric pain and a palpable abdominal mass.

cystadenoma /sis′tədinō′mə/ [Gk, kystis + aden, gland, oma, tumor], **1.** an adenoma associated with a cystoma. **2.** an adenoma containing multiple cystic structures. The cysts may be serous, containing serum; or pseudomucinous, containing clear serous fluid or thick, viscid fluid.

cystathioninemia /sis′təthī′aninē′mē·ə/, an inherited metabolic disorder caused by a deficiency of the enzyme cystathionase that causes an excess of the amino acid methionine. Some patients may be asymptomatic, whereas others show signs of mental retardation.

cystectomy /sistek′təmē/ [Gk, kystis + ektome, excision], a surgical procedure in which all or a part of the urinary bladder is removed, as may be required in treating bladder cancer.

cysteamine bitartrate, a urinary tract product for treatment of kidney disease. It is prescribed in the treatment of an inherited amino acid metabolic disease affecting the kidneys.

cysteine (Cys) /sis′tēn/, a nonessential amino acid found in many proteins in the body, including keratin. It is a metabolic precursor of cystine and an important source of sulfur for various body functions.

cystic /sis′tik/ [Gk, kystis, bag], **1.** pertaining to a cyst. **2.** pertaining to a fluid-filled sac, such as the gallbladder or urinary bladder.

cystic bile, concentrated bile stored in the gallbladder.

cystic carcinoma, a malignant neoplasm containing closed cavities or saclike spaces. These tumors may occur in the breast and ovary.

cystic duct, the duct through which bile from the gallbladder passes into the common bile duct.

cysticercosis /sis′tisərkō′sis/ [Gk, kystis + kerkos, tail, osis, condition], an infection and infestation by the larval stage of the pork tapeworm Taenia solium or the beef tapeworm T. saginata. The eggs are ingested and hatch in the intestine; the larvae invade the subcutaneous tissue, brain, eye, muscle, heart, liver, lung, and peritoneum. The invasive, early phase of the infection is characterized by fever, malaise, muscle pain, and eosinophilia. Years later epilepsy and personality change may appear if the brain is affected.

cysticercus /sis′tisur′kəs/, a larval form of tapeworm. It consists of a single scolex enclosed in a bladderlike cyst.

cystic fibroma, a fibrous tumor in which cystic degeneration has occurred.

cystic fibrosis, an inherited autosomal-recessive disorder of the exocrine glands, causing those glands to produce abnormally thick secretions of mucus, elevation of sweat electrolytes, increased organic and enzymatic constituents of saliva, and overactivity of the autonomic nervous system. The glands most affected are those in the pancreas, the respiratory system, and the sweat glands. Cystic fibrosis is usually recognized in infancy or early childhood, chiefly among whites. The earliest manifestation is meconium ileus, an obstruction of the small bowel by viscid stool. Other early signs are a chronic cough; frequent, foul-smelling stools; and persistent upper respiratory infections. The most reliable diagnostic tool is the sweat test, which shows elevations of levels of both sodium and chloride.

cystic goiter, an enlargement of the thyroid gland containing cysts resulting from mucoid or colloid degeneration, or liquefaction.

cystic kidney [Gk, *kystis,* bag; ME, *kidenei*], pertaining to any of several kidney disorders in which cysts form, including congenital polycystic disease, solitary renal cysts, or cortical cysts associated with nephrosclerosis.

cystic lymphangioma, a cystic growth formed by lymph vessels, usually congenital and occurring most frequently in the neck, axilla, or groin of children.

cystic mastitis, a form of mammary dysplasia with inflammation and the formation of nodular cysts in the breast tissue. The cysts contain a turbid fluid. Symptoms may vary with individual breast changes that occur during the menstrual cycle.

cystic myxoma, a tumor of connective tissue that has undergone cystic degeneration.

cystic neuroma, a neoplasm of nerve tissue that has degenerated and become cystic.

cystic tumor, a tumor with cavities or sacs containing a semisolid or a liquid material.

cystine /sis′tin/, a nonessential amino acid found in many proteins in the body, including keratin and insulin. Cystine is a product of the oxidation of two cysteine molecules.

cystinosis /sis′tinō′sis/ [*cystine* + Gk, *osis,* condition], a congenital disease characterized by glucosuria; proteinuria; cystine deposits in the liver, spleen, bone marrow, and cornea; rickets; excessive amounts of phosphates in the urine; and retardation of growth.

cystinuria /sis′tinŏŏr′ē-ə/ [*cystine* + Gk, *ouron,* urine], **1.** abnormal presence of the amino acid cystine in the urine collected in a 24-hour specimen. **2.** an inherited defect of the renal tubules, characterized by excessive urinary excretion of cystine and several other amino acids. The disorder is caused by an autosomal-recessive trait that impairs cystine resorption by the kidney tubules. In high concentration cystine tends to precipitate in the urinary tract and form kidney or bladder stones.

cystitis /sistī′tis/ [Gk, *kystis* + *itis,* inflammation], an inflammatory condition of the urinary bladder and ureters characterized by pain, urgency and frequency of urination, and hematuria. It may be caused by a bacterial infection, calculus, or tumor.

cystocele /sis′təsēl′/ [Gk, *kystis* + *kele,* hernia], a herniation or protrusion of the urinary bladder through the wall of the vagina.

cystochromoscopy /sis′təkrōmos′kəpē/, examination of the bladder after administration of a colored dye performed as an investigation of renal function and urinary system condition.

cystofibroma /-fībrō′mə/, a fibrous tumor that contains a cyst.

cystogram /sis′təgram′/ [Gk, *kystis* + *gramma,* record], a graphic record of the urinary bladder, usually a series of x-ray films, obtained as a part of any excretory urographic procedure, such as in retrograde pyelography or retrograde cystoscopy.

cystography /sistog′rəfē/, the radiographic examination of the bladder after introduction of a radiopaque contrast medium.

cystoid /sis′toid/ [Gk, *kystis,* bag + *eidos,* form], pertaining to or resembling a cyst or bladder.

cystojejunostomy /-ji′jōōnos′təmē/, drainage of a cyst, such as a pancreatic pseudocyst, into the jejunum.

cystolithalopaxy /-lith′əlōpek′sē/, removal of a kidney stone from the bladder by crushing, then extracting the particles via irrigation.

cystolithotomy /-lithot′əmē/, surgical opening of the urinary bladder and removal of a kidney stone.

cystoma /sistō′mə/ [Gk, *kystis* + *oma,* tumor], any tumor or growth containing cysts, especially one in or near the ovary.

cystometer /sistom′ətər/ /sistom′ətər/, an instrument that measures bladder capacity in relation to changing urine pressure.

cystometrogram /sis′tōmet′əgram′/, the

graphic results of the measurements made by a cystometer.

cystometography /sis'tōmətog'rəfē/, a urologic procedure that measures the amount of pressure exerted on the bladder at varying degrees of capacity.

cystometry /sistom'ətrē/ [Gk, *kystis* + *metron,* measure], the study of bladder function by use of a cystometer.

cystoprostatectomy /-pros'tətek'təmē/, surgical removal of the bladder, prostate gland, and seminal vesicle.

cystosarcoma phyllodes /sis'tōsärkō' məfilō'dēs/, a malignant stromal breast tumor that grows rapidly and tends to recur if not adequately excised.

cystoscope /sis'təskōp'/ [Gk, *kystis* + *skopein,* to look], an instrument for examining and treating lesions of the urinary bladder, ureter, and kidney. It consists of an outer sheath with a lighting system, a viewing obturator, and a passage for catheters and operative devices.

cystoscopy /sistos'kəpē/, the direct visualization of the urinary tract by means of a cystoscope inserted into the urethra. The procedure is usually performed with the patient under sedation or anesthesia in the lithotomy position. The bladder is distended with air or water when the patient is in a fasting state. —**cystoscopic,** *adj.*

cystostomy /sistos'təmē/, an opening made in the bladder for drainage, usually through a catheter.

cystotomy /sistot'əmē/, incision of the urinary bladder, often performed for removal of a calculus.

cystoureterography /sis'təyŏŏr'ətərog'rəfē/, the process of producing a radiographic image of the bladder and ureters after introduction of an iodinated contrast medium.

cystourethrogram /sis'tə·yŏŏrē'thrəgram'/, a radiograph of the urinary bladder and urethra, usually performed with use of an iodinated contrast medium to make the structures visible.

cystourethrography /sis'təyŏŏr'ēthrog'rəfē/, the process of obtaining a radiographic image of the urethra and urinary bladder after introduction of an iodinated contrast medium.

cysts of liver, small single, simple watery cysts, usually secondary to another disorder such as cystic kidney disease.

cytarabine /siter'əbēn/, an antineoplastic agent prescribed in the treatment of acute and chronic myelocytic leukemia, acute lymphocytic leukemia, and erythroleukemia.

cytoanalyzer /sī'tō·an'əlī'zər/, an electronic device that screens samples of smears of suspected malignancies.

cytoarchitectonic /sī'tō·är'kitekton'ik/ /sī' tō-/ [Gk, *kytos,* cell; L, *architectura,* architecture], pertaining to the cellular arrangement within a tissue or structure.

cytoarchitecture /-är'kitek'chər/, the typical pattern of cellular arrangement within a particular tissue or organ, as in the cerebral cortex.—**cytoarchitectural,** *adj.*

cytochemism /sī'tōkem'izəm/ [Gk, *kytos* + *chemeia,* alchemy], the chemical activity within the living cell, specifically the various reactions to and affinity for chemical substances.

cytochemistry /-kem'istrē/, the study of the various chemicals within a living cell and their actions and functions.

cytochrome /sī'tōkrōm/ [Gk, *kytos,* cell, *chroma,* color], **1.** a class of hemoproteins whose function is electron transport. These proteins have the ability to reverse the valence of heme-iron compounds, alternating between ferrous and ferric states. **2.** proteins involved in mitochondrial exudative electron transport systems associated with adenosine triphosphate production.

cytochrome P-450 [Gk, *kytos,* cell, *chroma,* color], a cytochrome protein involved with extramitochondrial electron transport in the liver and during drug detoxification.

cytocide [Gk, *kytos* + L, *caedere,* to kill], any substance that is destructive to cells. —**cytocidal,** *adj.*

cytoclesis /sī'tōklē'sis/ [Gk, *kytos* + *klesis,* calling for], the influence exerted by one cell on the action of other cells; the vital principle of all living tissue. —**cytocletic, cytobiotactic,** *adj.*

cytoctony /sītok'tənē/ [Gk, *kytos* + *ktonos,* killing], the destruction of cells, specifically the killing of cells in culture by viruses.

cytode /sī'tōd/ [Gk, *kytos* + *eidos,* form] the simplest type of cell, consisting of a protoplasmic mass without a nucleus, such as a bacterium.

cytodiagnosis /-dī'əgnō'sis/, diagnosis of a suspected pathologic tissue by a microscopic examination of the cells in the sample.

cytodieresis /sī'tōdī·er'isis/, *pl.* **cytodiereses** [Gk, *kytos* + *diairesis,* separation], cell division, especially the phenomena involving the division of the cytoplasm.— **cytodieretic,** *adj.*

cytodifferentiation /-dif'əren'shē·ā'shən/ [Gk, *kytos* + L, *differentia,* difference], **1.** a process by which embryonic cells acquire biochemical and morphologic properties essential for specialization and diversification. **2.** the total and gradual transformation from an undifferentiated to a fully differentiated state.

cytofluorograph /-flôr′əgraf/, a diagnostic instrument used to measure the level of CD4 T lymphocytes in human immunodeficiency virus–positive patients. The lymphocytes are stained with specific monoclonal antibodies.

cytogene /sī′təjēn/ [Gk, *kytos* + *genein*, to produce], a particle within the cytoplasm of a cell that is self-replicating, derived from the genes in the nucleus and capable of transmitting hereditary information.

cytogenesis /sī′tōjen′əsis/ [Gk, *kytos* + *genein*, to produce], the origin, development, and differentiation of cells. —**cytogenetic, cytogenic,** *adj.*

cytogeneticist /sī′tōjənet′isist/, one who specializes in cytogenetics.

cytogenetics /sī′tōjənet′iks/, the branch of genetics that studies the cellular constituents concerned with heredity, primarily the structure, function, and origin of the chromosomes.—**cytogenetic,** *adj.*

cytogenic /-jen′ik/, pertaining to the formation of cells.

cytogenic gland, a glandular organ that secretes living cells, specifically the testes and ovary.

cytogenic reproduction, the formation of a new organism from a unicellular germ cell, either sexually through the fusion of gametes to form a zygote or asexually by means of spores.

cytogeny /sītoj′ənē/, **1.** cytogenetics. **2.** the origin and development of the cell. —**cytogenic, cytogenous,** *adj.*

cytogony /sītog′ənē/, cytogenic reproduction.

cytohistogenesis /sī′tōhis′tōjen′əsis/ [Gk, *kytos* + *histos,* tissue, *genein,* to produce], the structural development and formation of cells. —**cytohistogenetic,** *adj.*

cytoid /sī′toid/ [Gk, *kytos* + *eidos,* form], like a cell.

cytoid body, a small white spot on the retina of each eye that is seen by using an ophthalmoscope in examining the eyes of a patient affected with systemic lupus erythematosus.

cytokerastic /sī′tōkəras′tik/ [Gk, *kytos* + *kerastos,* mixed], pertaining to or characteristic of cellular development from a lower to a higher form or from a simple to a more complex arrangement.

cytokine /sī′təkīn/, one of a large group of low-molecular-weight proteins secreted by various cell types and involved in cell-to-cell communication, coordinating antibody and T cell immune interactions, and amplifying immune reactivity. Cytokines include colony-stimulating factor, interfer-

ons, interleukins, and lymphokines, which are secreted by lymphocytes.

cytokine network /sī′təkīn/, a group of cytokines that modulate and regulate signaling between cells during immune responses. According to the immune network theory, T cells and B cells mutually interact, responding to cytokines as well as antigens. This interaction allows the cytokine to direct T cells to antiviral or antitumor functions or to promote allergic reactions.

cytokinesis /sī′tōkinē′sis, -kīnē′sis/ [Gk, *kytos* + *kinesis,* movement], the division of the cytoplasm, exclusive of nuclear division, that occurs during the final stages of mitosis and meiosis to form daughter cells; the total of all the changes that occur in the cytoplasm during mitosis, meiosis, and fertilization. —**cytokinetic,** *adj.*

cytologic map [Gk, *kytos* + *logos,* science; L, *mappa,* table napkin], the graphic representation of the location of genes on a chromosome, based on correlating genetic recombination test-crossing results with the structural analysis of chromosomes that have undergone such changes as deletions or translocations as detected by banding techniques.

cytologic sputum examination, a microscopic examination of a specimen of bronchial secretions, including a search for cells that may be cancerous or otherwise abnormal.

cytologist /sītol′əjist/, one who specializes in the study of cells, specifically one who uses cytologic techniques in the differential diagnosis of neoplasms.

cytology /sītol′əjē/ [Gk, *kytos* + *logos,* science], the study of cells, including their formation, origin, structure, function, biochemical activities, and pathologic characteristics. —**cytologic, cytological,** *adj.*

cytolysin /sītol′isin/ [Gk, *kytos* + *lyein,* to loosen], an antibody that dissolves antigenic cells. Kinds of cytolysin are **bacteriolysin** and **hemolysin.**

cytolysis /sītol′isis/, *pl.* **cytolyses** [Gk, *kytos* + *lyein,* to loosen], the destruction or breakdown of the living cell, primarily by the disintegration of the outer membrane. —**cytolytic,** *adj.*

cytomegalic /sī′tōmegal′ik/, describing a condition characterized by abnormally large cells.

cytomegalic inclusion disease (CID) [Gk, *kytos* + *megas,* large; L, *in, claudere,* in enclosure], a viral infection caused by the cytomegalovirus, a member of the herpesviruses family. It is characterized by malaise, fever, lymphadenopathy, pneumonia, hepatosplenomegaly, and superinfection with various bacteria and fungi as a result of the depression of immune response characteristic of herpesviruses. It is primarily a congenitally acquired disease of newborns, transmitted in utero. Results may range from spontaneous abortion or fatal neonatal illness to birth of a normal infant.

cytomegalovirus (CMV) /sī'tōmeg'əlōvī'rəs/ [Gk, *kytos* + *megas*, large; L, *virus*, poison], a member of a group of large species-specific herpes-type viruses with a wide variety of disease effects.

cytometer /sītom'ətər/ [Gk, *kytos* + *metron*, measure], a device for counting and measuring the number of cells within a specified amount of fluid, such as blood, urine, or cerebrospinal fluid.

cytometry /sītom'ətrē/, the counting and measuring of cells, specifically blood cells. —**cytometric,** *adj.*

cytomitome /sī'təmī'tōm/ [Gk, *kytos* + *mitos*, thread], the fibrillary network within the cytoplasm of a cell, as contrasted with that in the nucleoplasm.

cytomorphology /-môrfol'əjē/ [Gk, *kytos* + *morphe*, shape, *logos*, science], the study of the various forms of cells and the structures contained within them. —**cytomorphologic, cytomorphological,** *adj.,* **cytomorphologist,** *n.*

cytomorphosis /sī'tōmôr'fəsis/, *pl.* **cytomorphoses** [Gk, *kytos* + *morphosis*, shaping], the various changes that occur within a cell during the course of its life cycle, from the earliest undifferentiated stage until destruction.

cytopathic /-path'ik/, pertaining to the effect of disease or another disorder on a cell, such as damage from a virus or nuclear radiation.

cytopathogenic effect /-path'əjen'ik/, the morphologic changes in a cultured cell caused by cytopathic damage.

cytopathology /-pathol'əjē/, the study of changes at the cellular level caused by disease.

cytopenia /-pē'nē·ə/, [Gk, *kytos* + *penes*, poor], a deficiency of cells in the blood.

cytophagy /sītof'əjē/, cell destruction by phagocytes.

cytopheresis /sī'tōfer'əsis/ [Gk, *kytos* + *aphairesis*, withdrawal], **1.** a therapeutic technique to remove red or white blood cells or platelets from patients with certain blood disorders. **2.** a laboratory procedure for separating specific components, such as white blood cells or platelets, from donor blood by centrifugation.

cytophotometer /sī'tōfətom'ətər/ [Gk, *kytos* + *phos*, light, *metron*, measure], an instrument for measuring light density

through stained parts of cytoplasm, used for locating and identifying chemical substances within cells.

cytophotometry /sī'tōfətom'ətrē/, the identification of chemical substances within cells, using a cytophotometer. —**cytophotometric,** *adj.*

cytophysiology /-fis'ē·ol'əjē/ [Gk, *kytos* + *physis*, nature, *logos,* science], the study of the biochemical processes involved in the functioning of an individual cell, as contrasted with the functioning of organs or tissues. —**cytophysiologic, cytophysiological,** *adj.,* **cytophysiologist,** *n.*

cytoplasm /sī'təplaz'əm/ [Gk, *kytos* + *plassein,* to mold], all of the substance of a cell other than the nucleus.

cytoplasmic inheritance /sī'tōplaz'mik/, the acquisition of traits or conditions controlled by self-replicating substances within the cytoplasm, such as mitochondria or chloroplasts, rather than by the genes. The phenomenon occurs in plants and lower animals but has not yet been demonstrated in humans.

cytoscopy /sītos'kəpē/ [Gk, *kytos* + *skopein,* to watch], the diagnostic study of cells obtained from patient specimens with the aid of microscopes and other laboratory equipment.

cytosine /sī'təsin/, a major pyrimidine base found in nucleotides and a fundamental constituent of deoxyribonucleic acid and ribonucleic acid. In free or uncombined form it occurs in trace amounts in most cells.

cytosis /sītō'sis/, a condition in which there is a greater than normal number of cells in a tissue or organ.

cytoskeleton /-skel'ətən/ [Gk, *kytos* + *skeletos,* dried body], the cytoplasmic elements, including the tonofibrils, keratin, and other microfibrils, that function as a supportive system within a cell, especially an epithelial cell.

cytosome /sī'təsōm/, a multilayered membrane-bound lamellar body found in type II pneumocytes. It is a precursor of pulmonary surfactant.

cytotechnologist /teknol'əjist/, an allied health professional who specializes in the study of the structure and function of cells. Cytotechnologists prepare cellular samples for study under the microscope and assist in the diagnosis of disease by the examination of the samples. Using the findings of the cytotechnologist, the physician is able to detect cancer and other diseases at a very early stage.

cytotoxic /tok'sik/ [Gk, *kytos* + *toxikon,* poison], pertaining to a pharmacologic compound or other agent that destroys or damages tissue cells.

cytotoxic drug, any pharmacologic compound that inhibits the proliferation of cells within the body. Such compounds as the alkylating agents and the antimetabolites are designed to destroy abnormal cells selectively; they are commonly used in chemotherapy.

cytotoxic hypersensitivity [Gk, *kytos* + *toxikon,* poison, *hyper,* above; L, *sentire,* to feel], an immunoglobulin (Ig) G or an IgM complement-dependent, immediate-acting hypersensitive humoral response to foreign cells or to alterations of surface antigens on the cells.

cytotoxic killer T cells, a subset of the T lymphocytes that have the ability to cause lysis of specific target cells such as those containing viral antigens.

cytotoxin /sī'tōtok'sin/ [Gk, *kytos* + *toxikon,* poison], a substance that has a toxic effect on certain cells. An antibody may act as a cytotoxin.—**cytotoxic,** *adj.*

cytotrophoblast /sī'tōtrof'əblast'/ [Gk, *kytos* + *trophe,* nutrition, *blastos,* germ], the inner layer of cells of the trophoblast of the early mammalian embryo that gives rise to the outer surface and villi of the chorion. —**cytotrophoblastic,** *adj.*

cytotropism /sī'tōtrop'izm/, a characteristic of some living cells and agents that enables them to approach other cells or selectively bind them.

CY-VA-DIC, an anticancer drug combination of cyclophosphamide, vincristine, doxorubicin, and dacarbazine.

d, symbol for one tenth.

D, 1. symbol for *dead space gas.* **2.** symbol for **diffusing capacity. 3.** abbreviation for *diopter.* **4.** abbreviation for *dexter,* meaning 'right.'

da, symbol for the multiple 10.

DA, abbreviation for **developmental age.**

daboia /dəboi′ə/ [Hind, *dabna,* to lurk], a local name for Russell's viper, a large, very poisonous snake indigenous to India and Southeast Asia. Its venom is used as a coagulant in cases of hemophilia.

dacarbazine /dekär′bəzēn/, an alkylating agent used as an antineoplastic. It is prescribed primarily in the treatment of malignant melanoma, sarcoma, and Hodgkin's disease.

Dacron cuff, a sheath of Dacron surrounding an atrial or a venous catheter to prevent accidental displacement.

dacryoadenitis /dak′rē-ō-ad′ənī′tis/, an inflammation of the lacrimal gland.

dacryocyst /dak′re-ōsist′/ [Gk, *dakryon,* tear, *kytis,* bag], a lacrimal sac at the medial angle of the eye.

dacryocystectomy /dak′rē-ōsistek′təmē/ [Gk, *dakryon* + *kytis,* bag, *ektome,* excision], partial or total excision of the lacrimal sac.

dacryocystitis /dak′rē-ōsistī′tis/, an infection of the lacrimal sac caused by obstruction of the nasolacrimal duct. It is characterized by tearing and discharge from the eye.

dacryocystorhinostomy /dak′rē-osis tōrī-nos′təmē/ [Gk, *dakryon* + *kytis,* bag, *rhis,* nose, *stoma,* mouth], a surgical procedure for restoring drainage into the nose from the lacrimal sac when the nasolacrimal duct is obstructed.

dacryostenosis /dak′rē-ōstinō′sis/ [Gk, *dakryon* + *stenos,* narrow, *osis,* condition], an abnormal stricture of the nasolacrimal duct, occurring either as a congenital condition or as a result of infection or trauma.

dactinomycin /dak′tinōmī′sin/, an antibiotic used as an antineoplastic agent in the treatment of a variety of malignant neoplastic diseases, including Wilms' tumor and rhabdomyosarcoma in children.

dactyl /dak′til/ [Gk, *dactylos,* finger], a digit (finger or toe). —**dactylic** /daktil′ik/, *adj.*

dactyledema /dak′tilidē′mə/, edema of the fingers or toes.

dactylion /daktil′ē-on/, a condition of complete or partial webbing of fingers.

dactylitis /dak′tilī′tis/, a painful inflammation of the fingers or toes, usually associated with sickle cell anemia or certain infectious diseases, particularly syphilis or tuberculosis.

DAI, abbreviation for **diffuse axonal injury.**

daily adjusted progressive resistance exercise (DAPRE), a program of isotonic exercises that allows for individual differences in the rate at which a patient regains strength in an injured or diseased body part.

Daily Reference Values (DRVs), a set of dietary standards for eight nutrients and food compartments: total fat, saturated fat, cholesterol, total carbohydrates, dietary fiber, protein, potassium, and sodium. They are part of the U.S. Food and Drug Administration Daily Value label reference.

dairy food substitute, a group of foods that includes imitation cream, coffee whitener, cheese, and ice cream. Although similar in taste and texture to genuine dairy products, nondairy products can differ markedly in composition from products they resemble. Some substitutes may contain milk components despite nondairy claims.

Dakin's solution [Henry D. Dakin, American biochemist, 1880–1952; L, *solutus* dissolved], an antiseptic solution containing boric acid and 0.4% to 0.5% of sodium hypochlorite.

dalteparin sodium, a low–molecular weight heparin prescribed to prevent deep vein thrombosis in adults undergoing abdominal surgery who are at risk for clotting.

dalton [John Dalton, English chemist and mathematician, 1766–1844], **1.** an unofficial unit of atomic mass, based on ¹⁄₁₆ of the gram mass of hydrogen. **2.** (in biochemistry) unit (kilodaltons) that expresses the molecular weight (mass) of proteins and nucleic acids.

daltonism /dôl'təniz'əm/ [John Dalton], *informal.* a form of red-green color blindness. It is genetically transmitted as a sex-linked autosomal-recessive trait.

Dalton's law of partial pressures /dôl'tənz/ [John Dalton], (in physics) a law stating that the total pressure exerted by a mixture of gases is equal to the sum of the pressures that could be exerted by the gases if they were present alone in the container.

dam, a barrier to the flow of fluid, as a dam placed around a tooth to protect it from saliva during restoration.

damages /dam'ijəs/ [L, *damnum,* loss], (in law) a sum of money awarded to a plaintiff by a court as compensation for any loss, detriment, or injury to the plaintiff's person, property, or rights caused by the malfeasance or negligence of the defendant. Actual damages are awarded to reimburse the plaintiff for the loss or injury sustained. Nominal damages are awarded to show that a legal wrong has been committed, although no recoverable loss can be determined. Punitive damages exceed the actual cost of injury or damage and are awarded when the defendant has acted with malice or reckless disregard of the plaintiff's rights.

damp [AS, vapor], a potentially lethal atmosphere in caves and mines. Black damp or choke damp is caused by absorption of the available oxygen by coal seams. Fire damp is composed of methane and other explosive hydrocarbon gases. White damp is another name for carbon monoxide.

damping [AS, vapor], (in cardiology) a diminishing of the amplitude of a series of waves or oscillations, as in damping of the arterial pressure waveform.

danazol /dan'əzol/, a synthetic androgen that acts to suppress the output of gonadotropins from the pituitary. It is prescribed in the treatment of endometriosis.

dance reflex [ME, *dauncen* + L, *reflectere,* to bend back], a normal response in the neonate to simulate walking by a reciprocal flexion and extension of the legs when held in an erect position and inclined forward, with the soles touching a hard surface.

dance therapy, (in psychology) the use of rhythmic body movements or dance to release expression of feelings.

dander, dry scales shed from the scalp.

dandruff /dan'druf/, an excessive amount of scaly material composed of dead, keratinized epithelium shed from the scalp that may be a mild form of seborrheic dermatitis.

Dandy-Walker cyst [Walter E. Dandy, American neurosurgeon, 1886–1946; Arthur E. Walker, American surgeon, b. 1907], a cystic malformation of the fourth ventricle of the brain, resulting from hydrocephalus.

danthron /dan'thron/, a stimulant laxative prescribed in the treatment of constipation or for bowel evacuation before radiologic or surgical procedures.

dantrolene sodium /dan'trəlēn/, a skeletal muscle relaxant prescribed in the treatment of muscle spasticity resulting from injury to the spinal cord or cerebrum. It is not indicated in treatment of spasm from rheumatic disorders.

DAPRE, abbreviation for **daily adjusted progressive resistance exercise.**

dapsone (DADPS) /dap'sōn/, a bacteriostatic sulfone derivative prescribed in the treatment of lepromatous leprosy and dermatitis herpetiformis.

Darier's sign /dīryāz'/ [Jean F. Darier, French dermatologist, 1856–1938], a burning or itching sensation induced by stroking skin lesions in cases of urticaria pigmentosa.

dark adaptation, a normal increase in sensitivity of the retinal rod cells of the eye to detect any light that may be available for vision in a dimly lighted environment. The process is accompanied by an adjustment of the pupils to allow more light to enter the eyes.

dark-field microscopy [AS, *deorc,* hidden, *feld,* field; Gk, *mikros,* small, *skopein,* to look], examination with a darkfield microscope in which the specimen is illuminated by a peripheral light source. Organisms in specimens that have been prepared for use with a darkfield microscope appear to glow against a dark background.

dark-film fault [AS, *deorc,* hidden, *filmen,* skin; L, *fallere,* to disappoint], a defect in a photograph or radiograph that appears as an excessively darkened image and image area.

darkroom, a room in a hospital or similar facility for the storage and processing of light-sensitive materials such as x-ray film.

darwinian ear /därwin'ē·ən/ [Charles R. Darwin, English naturalist, 1809–1882], an external ear with an upper border that projects upward in a flat, sharp edge.

darwinian theory [Charles R. Darwin], the hypothesis of Charles Darwin that organic evolution results from the process of natural selection of those variants of plants and animals best suited to survive in their environmental surroundings. —**darwinian,** *adj., n.*

DASE, abbreviation for **Denver Articulation Screening Examination.**

data /dā′tə, dat′ə, dä′tə/, *sing.* **datum** [L, *datum,* giving], pieces of information, especially those that are part of a collection to be used in an analysis of a problem.

data acquisition system (DAS), a radiation detection system that measures the amount of radiation passing through a patient.

data analysis, (in research) the phase of a study that includes classifying, coding, and tabulating information needed to perform quantitative or qualitative analyses according to the research design and appropriate to the data.

data clustering, the grouping of related information from a patient's health history, physical examination, and laboratory results as part of the process of making a diagnosis.

data collection, (in research) the phase of a study that includes the gathering of information and identification of sampling units as directed by the research design.

data retrieval, the recovery of information from an organized filing system such as a computer data base, an index card file, or color-coded record folders.

data source, the origin of information relevant to a patient's level of wellness and health patterns.

data validation, the process of determining whether information gathered during the process of data collection is complete and accurate.

date/acquaintance rape, a sexual assault or rape by a person known to the victim, such as a date, employer, friend, or casual acquaintance.

daughter cell [ME, *doughter,* female, child; L, *cella,* storeroom], one of the cells produced by the division of a parent cell.

daughter chromosome [ME, *doughter,* female, child; Gk, *chroma,* color, *soma,* body], either of the paired chromatids that during the anaphase stage of mitosis separate and migrate to opposite ends of the cell before division. Each contains the complete genetic information of the original chromosome.

daughter cyst, a small parasitic cyst, usually a derivative of a hydatid cyst.

daughter element, an element that results from the radioactive decay of a parent element. An example is technetium-99, which is the daughter element created by the decay of an atom of molybdenum-99.

daunorubicin hydrochloride /dô′nŏrōō′- bisin/, an anthracycline antibiotic antineoplastic agent prescribed in the treatment of cancer, particularly the leukemias and neuroblastoma.

Davidson regimen [Edward C. Davidson, American physician, 1894–1933; L, direc-

tion], a method of treating chronic constipation in children, developing regular bowel habits, and identifying individuals with functional bowel disease or obstructive disorders. The child is then given mineral oil in increasing doses, until four or five loose bowel movements occur daily. Some children, especially those less than 2 years of age, require supplementation with fat-soluble vitamins to maintain proper nutrition. The child is placed on a potty-chair at a specific time each day for 5 to 15 minutes, and, as regular habits develop, the mineral oil is gradually withdrawn over a period of several weeks.

DAWN /dôn/, abbreviation for **Drug Abuse Warning Network.**

dawn phenomenon [ME, *daunen* + Gk, *phainomenon,* anything seen], a tendency for persons with insulin-dependent diabetes mellitus to require an increased insulin dose in the early morning hours as a result of an increase in plasma glucose concentration.

day care [OE, *doeg* + L, *garrire,* to chatter], a specialized program or facility that provides care for preschool children, usually within a group framework, either as a substitute for or an extension of home care, particularly for single parents or for two parents, both employed outside the home.

daydream, a usually nonpathologic reverie that occurs while a person is awake. The content is usually the imagined fulfillment of wishes that are not disguised.

day health care services, the provision of hospitals, nursing homes, or other facilities for health-related services to adult patients who are ambulatory or can be transported and who regularly use such services for a certain number of daytime hours but do not require continuous inpatient care.

day hospital [OE, *doeg* + L, *hospes,* guest], a psychiatric facility that offers a therapeutic program during daytime hours for patients.

dB, abbreviation for **decibel.**

Db, symbol for the element **dubnium.**

d/c, abbreviation for *discontinue.*

DC, abbreviation for **direct current.**

D&C, abbreviation for **dilation and curettage.**

D&E, abbreviation for **dilation and evacuation.**

DD, abbreviation for **developmental disability.**

ddC, symbol for 2′3-dideoxycytidine, an antiretroviral drug used in the treatment of acquired immunodeficiency syndrome. It is related chemically to DDI.

D

DDD pacing, one of the three-letter codes for electrical heart pacemakers. The letters indicate *D*ual chamber paced for both chambers, *D*ual chamber activity sensing, and *D*ual response.

DDI, 1. abbreviation for 2′,3′-dideoxyinosine, an antiretroviral medication. **2.** abbreviation for **dideoxyinosine.**

DDS, abbreviation for *Doctor of Dental Surgery.*

DDST, abbreviation for **Denver Developmental Screening Test.**

DDT (dichlorodiphenyltrichloroethane), a nondegradable water-insoluble chlorinated hydrocarbon once used worldwide as a major insecticide, especially in agriculture. In recent years knowledge of its adverse impact on the environment has led to restrictions in its use. It is still used as a pediculicide where epidemic-scale delousing is justified, as in barracks and refugee camps.

DE, abbreviation for **dose equivalent.**

DEA, 1. abbreviation for *Drug Enforcement Administration.* **2.** abbreviation for **Drug Enforcement Agency.**

deactivation /dē·ak′tivā′shən/ [L, *de,* from, *activus,* active], the process of becoming or making something inactive or inoperable.

dead, pertaining to absence of all vital functions in a previously living organism.

dead-end host [AS, *dead* + *ende* + L, *hospes,* guest], any animal from which a parasite cannot escape to continue its life cycle. Humans are dead-end hosts for trichinosis, because the larvae encyst in muscle and human flesh is unlikely to be a source of food for other animals susceptible to this parasite.

dead fetus syndrome, a condition in which the fetus has died but has remained in the uterus for some time. The condition leads to a blood coagulation disorder and the eventual delivery is usually accompanied by massive bleeding.

dead space [AS, dead; L, *spatium*], **1.** a cavity that remains after the incomplete closure of a surgical or traumatic wound, leaving an area in which blood can collect and delay healing. **2.** the amount of lung in contact with ventilating gases but not with pulmonary blood flow. Alveolar dead space is characterized by alveoli that are ventilated by the pulmonary circulation but are not perfused. Anatomic dead space is an area in the trachea, bronchi, and air passages containing air that does not reach the alveoli during respiration. **Physiologic dead space** is an area in the respiratory system that includes the anatomic dead space together with the space in the alveoli occupied by air that does not

contribute to the oxygen-carbon dioxide exchange.

dead space effect, any of several potential adverse effects of dead space resulting from mechanical ventilation, particularly when there is alveolar dead space. In hospitalized patients it causes hypoxemia and hypercarbia. A pulmonary embolism can also produce a dead space effect; blood flow in the pulmonary arteries is reduced without impeding ventilation.

deaf [AS], **1.** unable to hear; hard of hearing. **2.** people who are unable to hear or who have hearing impairment. —**deafness,** *n.*

deafferentation /dē·af′ərəntā′shən/ [L, *de,* from, *ad + ferre,* to bear], the elimination or interruption of afferent nerve impulses.

deafness, a condition characterized by a partial or complete loss of hearing. In assessing deafness the ears are examined for drainage, crusts, accumulation of cerumen, or structural abnormality. It is determined whether the hearing loss is conductive or sensory, temporary or permanent, and congenital or acquired in childhood, adolescence, or adulthood. The effect of aging is evaluated. A psychosocial assessment is conducted to ascertain whether the individual is well adjusted to hearing loss or reacts to the disability with fear, anxiety, frustration, depression, anger, or hostility. In all cases the degree of loss and the kind of impairment causing it are determined.

deaminase /dē·am′inās/ [L, *de,* away, *amine,* ammonia; Fr, *diastase,* enzyme], one of the subclasses of enzymes that catalyze the hydrolysis of the NH_2 bond in amino compounds. The enzymes are usually named according to the substrate, such as **adenosine deaminase, guanine deaminase,** or **guanosine deaminase.**

deamination /dē′aminā′shən/, the removal, usually by hydrolysis, of the NH_2 radical from an amino compound.

dean [L, *decanus,* chief of ten], chief executive and educational officer of a unit of a university, school, or college.

dean's tax, a part of physician practice plan income in an academic medical center that is allocated for the support of the medical school.

dearterialization /dē′ärtir′ē·əlīzā′shən/, **1.** conversion of oxygenated arterial blood into venous blood. **2.** interruption of the supply of arterial blood to an organ or body part.

death [AS], **1.** apparent death, the cessation of life as indicated by the absence of heartbeat or respiration. **2. legal death,** the total absence of activity in the brain and central nervous system, the cardiovascular system, and the respiratory system as observed and declared by a physician.

death instinct, instinctive behavior that tends to be self-destructive.

death mask [AS, *death* + Fr, *masque*], a mask made from a plaster of paris cast of the face of a dead person.

death rate, the number of deaths occurring within a specified population during a particular period, usually expressed in terms of deaths per 1000 persons per year.

death rattle, a sound produced by air moving through mucus that has accumulated in the throat of a dying person after loss of the cough reflex.

death trance, a state in which a person appears to be dead.

"death with dignity" [AS, *death* + L, *dignus,* worthy], the philosophic concept that a terminally ill client should be allowed to die naturally rather than experience a comatose, vegetative life prolonged by mechanical support systems.

debilitating /dibil'itā'ting/, pertaining to a disease or injury that enfeebles, weakens, or otherwise disables a person.

debility /dibil'itē/, feebleness, weakness, or loss of strength.

debride /dibrēd'/ [Fr, *debridle,* remove], to remove dirt, foreign objects, damaged tissue, and cellular debris from a wound or a burn to prevent infection and to promote healing. In treating a wound, debridement is the first step in cleansing. —**debridement** /debrēdmäN'/, *n.*

debris /dəbrē'/, the dead, diseased, or damaged tissue and any foreign material that is to be removed from a wound or other area being treated.

decalcification /dēkal'sifikā'shən/ [L, *de* + *calyx,* lime, *facere,* to make], loss of calcium salts from the teeth and bones caused by malnutrition, malabsorption or other dietary or physiologic factors. It may result from a diet that lacks adequate calcium. Malabsorption may be caused by a lack of vitamin D necessary for the absorption of calcium from the intestine; an excess of dietary fats that can combine with calcium; the presence of oxalic acid, which can combine with calcium; or a relative lack of acid in the digestive tract. Other factors include the parathyroid hormone control of the calcium level in the bloodstream, the ratio of calcium to phosphorus in the blood, and the relative activity of osteoblast cells that form calcium deposits in the bones and teeth and osteoclast cells that absorb calcium from bones and teeth.

decannulation /dēkan'yəlā'shən/ [L, *de,* from, *cannula,* small reed], the removal of a cannula or tube that may have been inserted during a surgical procedure.

decant, the process of separating fluid or solid sediment by pouring off the top liquid layer.

decapitation /dēkap'itā'shən/, literally, cutting off the head, as the head of a bone or the head of a fetus when delivery is not possible otherwise.

decay, 1. a gradual deterioration that accompanies the end of life. **2.** the process of disintegration of a radioactive substance.

decay product /dikā'/ [L, *de* + *cadere,* to fall, *producere,* to produce], (in radiology) a stable or radioactive nuclide formed directly from the radioactive disintegration of a radionuclide or as a result of successive transformation in a radioactive series.

decay time, the period required for a wavelength to go from peak amplitude to 0 volt.

deceleration /dēsel'ərā'shən/ [L, *de* + *accelerare,* to hasten], a decrease in the speed or velocity of an object or reaction.

deceleration injury, an injury resulting from a collision between a rapidly moving body part and a stationary object.

deceleration phase, (in obstetrics) the latter part of active labor, characterized by a decreased rate of dilation of the cervical os on a Friedman curve.

decerebrate /dēser'əbrāt/, **1.** lacking a cerebrum. **2.** lacking neural communication between the cerebrum and lower parts of the central nervous system.

decerebrate posture [L, *de* + *cerebrum,* brain, *ponere* to place], the position of a patient who is usually comatose, in which the arms are extended and internally rotated and the legs are extended with the feet in forced plantar flexion. It is usually observed in patients afflicted by compression of the brainstem at a low level.

decerebration /-brā'shən/ [L, *de,* from, *cerebrum*], the process of removing the brain or cutting the brainstem above the level of the red nucleus, thus eliminating cerebral function.

decibel (dB) /des'əbəl/ [L, *decimus,* one tenth, *bel,* Alexander G. Bell, Canadian inventor, 1847–1922], a unit of measure of the intensity of sound. A decibel is one tenth of 1 bel (B); an increase of 1 B is perceived as a 10-fold increase in loudness, based on a sound-pressure reference level of 0.0002 dyne/cm^2, or 20 micropascals.

decidua /disij'ōō·ə/ [L, *decidere,* to fall off], the epithelial tissue of the endometrium lining the uterus. It envelops the conceptus during gestation and is shed in the puerperium. It is also shed periodically with menstruation.

decidua basalis, the decidua of the endometrium in the uterus that lies beneath the implanted ovum.

decidua capsularis, the decidua of the endometrium of the uterus covering the implanted ovum.

decidual endometritis /disij´o͞o·əl/, an inflammation or infection of any part of the decidua during pregnancy.

decidua menstrualis, the endometrial mucosa shed during menstruation.

decidua vera, the decidua of the endometrium lining the uterus, except for those areas beneath and above the implanted and developing ovum called, respectively, the decidua basalis and the decidua capsularis.

deciduoma /disij´o͞o·ō´mə/, a benign or malignant tumor of endometrial tissue. A deciduoma may develop after a pregnancy, regardless of the outcome. It may be detected on a Papanicolaou's (Pap) smear.

deciduous tooth [L, *decidere,* to fall off; AS, *toth*], any of the set of 20 teeth that appear normally during infancy, consisting of four incisors, two canines, and four molars in each jaw. Deciduous teeth start developing at about the sixth week of fetal life. In most individuals the first deciduous tooth erupts through the gum about 6 months after birth. Thereafter one or more deciduous teeth erupt about every month until all 20 have appeared. The deciduous teeth are usually shed between the ages of 6 and 13.

decigram, a unit of mass in the metric system equal to 100 milligrams or one tenth of a gram.

deciliter, a unit of volume in the metric system equal to 100 milliliters or one tenth of a liter.

decimeter, a unit of length in the metric system equal to 10 centimeters or one tenth of a meter.

decisional conflict, a NANDA-accepted nursing diagnosis of a state of uncertainty about the course of action to be taken when choice among competing actions involves risk, loss, or challenge to personal life values. The diagnosis should specify focus of conflict, such as choices regarding health, family relationships, career, or finances. Defining characteristics include a verbalized feeling of distress related to uncertainty about choices, specification of undesired consequences of alternative actions being considered, delayed decision making, and physical signs of distress or tension such as increased heart rate, increased muscle tension, and restlessness.

decision making, the process of evaluating available information and reaching a judgment or conclusion based on that information.

Decision-Making Support, a Nursing Interventions Classification defined as providing information and support for a patient who is making a decision regarding health care.

decision tree, a systematic method of managing a clinical problem by graphically organizing the probabilities of outcomes of alternative treatments.

declarative memory /dēkler´ətiv/, the mental registration, retention, and recall of past experiences, sensations, ideas, knowledge, and thoughts.

decoction /dikok´shən/ [L, *de* + *coquere,* to cook], a liquid medicine made from an extract of water-soluble substances, usually with the aid of boiling water. Herbal remedies are usually decoctions.

decode /dikōd´/, to interpret coded information into a form usable by a receiver.

decoded message, (in communication theory) a message as translated by a receiver.

decoloration, the natural loss or removal of color, as by bleaching.

decompensation /dē´kəmpənsā´shən/ [L, *de* + *compensare,* to balance], the failure of a system, as cardiac decompensation in heart failure.

decomposition /dē̄´kəmpəsish´ən/ [L, *de* + *componere,* to put together], the dissolution of a substance into simpler chemical forms.

decompression /dē´kəmpresh´ən/ [L, *de* + *comprimere,* to press together], **1.** a technique used to readapt an individual to normal atmospheric pressure after exposure to higher pressures, as in diving. **2.** the removal of pressure caused by gas or fluid in a body cavity, as the stomach or intestinal tract.

decompression sickness, a painful, sometimes fatal syndrome caused by the formation of nitrogen bubbles in the tissues of divers and others who move too rapidly from environments of higher to those of lower atmospheric pressures. Gaseous nitrogen accumulates in the joint spaces and peripheral circulation, impairing tissue oxygenation. Disorientation, severe pain, and syncope follow. Treatment entails rapid return of the patient to an environment of higher pressure (hyperbaric therapy) followed by gradual decompression.

decongestant [L, *de* + *congerere,* to pile up], **1.** pertaining to a substance or procedure that eliminates or reduces congestion or swelling. **2.** a decongestant drug. Adrenergic drugs (α-1 stimulants) such as ephedrine, pseudoephedrine, and phenylpropanolamine hydrochloride, which cause vasoconstriction of nasal mucosa, are used as decongestants.

decontamination /dē'kəntam'inā'shən/, the process of removing foreign material such as blood, body fluids, or radioactivity. It does not eliminate microorganisms but is a necessary step preceding disinfection or sterilization.

decorticate posture /dēkôr'tikāt/ [L, de + cortex, bark, ponere, to place], the position of a comatose patient in which the upper extremities are rigidly flexed at the elbows and wrists. The legs also may be flexed. The decorticate posture indicates a lesion in a mesencephalic region of the brain.

decortication /dēkôr'tikā'shən/ [L, de + cortex, bark], (in medicine) the removal of the cortical tissue of an organ or structure, such as the kidney, the brain, and the lung. —**decorticate,** v., adj.

decrement /dek'rəmənt/ [L, de + crescere, to grow], a decrease or stage of decline, as of a uterine contraction.

decremental conduction /dek'rəmen'təl/, (in cardiology) a transmission, or conveying, that slows progressively as the effectiveness of the propagating impulse gradually decreases.

decrepitate percussion /dēkrep'itit/, a crackling noise produced by tapping the thoracic or abdominal wall of a patient with a respiratory disorder.

decrudescence /dē'krōōdes'əns/ [L, de, from, crudescere, to become bad], a decrease in the severity of symptoms.

decubital /dikyōō'bitəl/ [L, decumbere, to lie down], pertaining to bedsores.

decubitus /dikyōō'bitəs/ [L, decumbere, to lie down], a recumbent or horizontal position, as lateral decubitus, lying on one side.

decubitus posture, the position assumed by a bedridden patient to rest on his or her side to relieve the pressure of body weight on the sacrum, heels, or other areas vulnerable to pressure (decubitus) ulcers.

decubitus projection, (in radiology) a position used in producing a radiograph of the chest or abdomen of a patient who is lying down, with the central ray parallel to the horizon. Variations of the position include left and right anteroposterior oblique, dorsal decubitus, ventral decubitus, and left and right lateral decubitus.

decussate /dəcus'āt/ [L, decussis, intersection], to cross in the form of an "X," as certain nerve fibers from the retina cross at the optic chiasm. —**decussation,** n.

decussation /di'kusā'shən/ [L, decussare, to make a cross], a crossing of central nervous system fibers in the brain, as some

fibers on the left side cross to the right side and vice versa.

decussation of pyramids [L, decussare, to make a cross; Gk, pyramis], the crossing of nerve fibers of the corticospinal motor tract at the ventral side on the lower part of the medulla oblongata.

deductible /dēduk'tibəl/, an amount paid each year by a health insurance plan before benefits begin. It is not synonymous with copayment.

deduction [L, deducere, to lead], a system of reasoning that leads from a known principle to an unknown, or from the general to the specific. Deductive reasoning is used to test diagnostic hypotheses.

deemed status /dēmd/ [AS, deman, to judge; L, status, a standing], a status conferred on a hospital or other organization by a professional standards review organization in formal recognition that the organization's review, continued-stay review, and medical care evaluation programs meet certain effectiveness criteria.

deep brachial artery [As, dyppan, to dip; Gk, brachion, arm, arteria, airpipe], a branch of each of the brachial arteries arising at the distal border of the teres major and supplying the humerus and muscles of the upper arm.

deep breathing and coughing exercises, the movements used to improve aeration or to maintain respiratory function, especially after prolonged inactivity or general anesthesia. Incisional pain after surgery in the chest or abdomen often inhibits normal respiratory excursion.

deep fascia, the most extensive of three kinds of fascia comprising an intricate series of connective sheets and bands that hold the muscles and other structures in place throughout the body, wrapping the muscles in gray, feltlike membranes.

deep heat, the application of heat in the treatment of deep body tissues, particularly muscles and tendons. The thermal effects may be produced with shortwave therapy, phonophoresis, or ultrasound.

deep palmar arch, the termination of the radial artery, joining the deep palmar branch of the ulnar artery in the palm of the hand.

deep reflexes [ME, dep, hollow; L, reflectere, to bend back], any reflexes caused by stimulation of a deep body structure such as a tendon reflex.

deep sensation, the awareness or perception of pain, pressure, or tension in the deep layers of the skin, muscles, tendons, or joints.

deep structure, (in linguistics and neurolinguistics) the deeper experience and meaning to which surface structures in a communication may refer.

deep temporal artery, one of the branches of the maxillary artery on each side of the head. It branches into the anterior and posterior parts.

deep tendon reflex (DTR), a brisk contraction of a muscle in response to a sudden stretch induced by a sharp tap by a finger or rubber hammer on the tendon of insertion of the muscle. Absence of the reflex may be caused by damage to the muscle, peripheral nerve, nerve roots, or spinal cord at that level.

deep vein, one of the many systemic veins that accompany the arteries, usually enclosed in a sheath that wraps both the vein and the associated artery.

deep vein thrombosis, a disorder involving a thrombus in one of the deep veins of the body. Symptoms include tenderness, pain, swelling, warmth, and discoloration of the skin. A deep vein thrombus is potentially life threatening. Treatment is directed to preventing movement of the thrombus toward the lungs.

deep x-ray therapy, the treatment of internal neoplasms such as Wilms' tumor of the kidney, Hodgkin's disease, and other cancers with ionizing radiation from an external source. Deep x-ray therapy frequently causes nausea, malaise, diarrhea, and skin reactions such as blanching, erythema, itching, burning, oozing, or desquamation; but with modern techniques the ray is beamed directly to the site, and the skin can be spared.

defamation /def'əmā'shən/ [L, *diffamare,* to discredit], any communication, written or spoken, that is untrue and that injures the good name or reputation of another or in any way brings that person into disrepute.

default judgment /difôlt'/ [L, *defallere,* to lack, *judicare,* to decide], (in law) a judgment rendered against a defendant as a result of the defendant's failure to appear in court or to answer the plaintiff's claim within the proper time.

defecation /def'ikā'shən/ [L, *defaecare,* to clean], the elimination of feces from the digestive tract through the rectum. —**defecate** /def'ikāt/, *v.*

defecography /def'əkog'rəfē/, a radiographic procedure for evaluating the rectum and anal canal of children with fecal incontinence. The child is examined while sitting on a radiolucent toilet seat or potty.

defective /difek'tiv/ [L, *defectus,* a failing], pertaining to something that is imperfect, or, as in an outdated term, to an individual who may be suffering from any disorder.

defendant /difen'dənt/, (in law) the party

named in a plaintiff's complaint and against whom the plaintiff's allegations are made. The defendant must respond to the allegations.

defense mechanism [L, *defendere,* to repulse, *mechanicus,* machine], an unconscious intrapsychic reaction that offers protection to the self from stress or a threat. Defense mechanisms are of two types: those that diminish anxiety and are used by an individual to integrate more fully into society, and those that do not reduce anxiety but simply postpone the effects of feeling it.

defense reflex, an autonomic defensive response by an animal when threatened.

defensin /difen'sin/, a peptide with natural antibiotic activity found within human neutrophils. Three types of defensins have been identified, each consisting of a chain of about 30 amino acids.

defensive radical therapy /difen'siv/, (in psychology) a view of the therapeutic process in which as a survival tactic the therapist begins at the patient's present state and encourages the patient to avoid self-defeating behavior.

deferens /def'ərenz/ [L], carrying away.

deferoxamine mesylate /dē'fərok'səmēn/, a chelating agent prescribed in the treatment of acute iron intoxication and chronic iron overload.

defervescence /di'fərves'əns/ [L, *defervescere,* to reduce heat], the diminishing or disappearance of a fever. —**defervescent,** *adj.*

defibrillate /difi'brilāt, difib'-/ [L, *de* + *fibrilla,* little thread], to stop fibrillation of the ventricles by delivering an electrical shock through the chest wall.

defibrillation /difi'brilā'shən/, the termination of ventricular fibrillation (involuntary recurrent contraction) by delivery of an electrical shock to the patient's precordium.

defibrillator /difi'brilā'tər, difib'-/, a device that delivers an electrical shock at a preset voltage to the myocardium through the chest wall. It is used for restoring the normal cardiac rhythm and rate when the heart has stopped beating or is fibrillating.

defibrination, the removal of fiber from a body fluid, as removal of fibrin from blood to prevent clotting.

deficiency /difish'ənsē/, a lack or shortage of something.

deficiency disease [L, *de* + *facere,* to make, *dis,* opposite of; Fr, *aise,* ease], a condition resulting from the lack of one or more essential nutrients in the diet or from metabolic dysfunction, impaired digestion or absorption, excessive excretion, or increased biologic requirements.

deficiency of sweating [AS, *swaetan*], a failure of the sweat glands to secrete perspiration in normal amounts. The condition may be the result of a congenital defect, a blockage of the sweat ducts as a sequel to prickly heat, excessive heat, or conditions such as hemorrhage or diarrhea that cause body fluid loss.

deficit /def'isit/, any deficiency or difference from that which is normal, such as an oxygen deficit, a cause of hypoxia.

defined formula diet, nutritional support provided by simple elemental nutritive components that require no further digestive breakdown and thus are readily absorbed.

definitive /difin'ətiv/ [L, *definitivus*, a limiting], **1.** final; clearly established without doubt or question. **2.** (in embryology) fully formed in the final differentiation of a tissue, structure, or organ. **3.** (in parasitology) pertaining to the host in which the parasite undergoes the sexual phase of its reproductive cycle.

definitive host, any animal in which the reproductive stages of a parasite develop. The female *Anopheles* mosquito is the definitive host for malaria. Humans are definitive hosts for pinworms, schistosomes, and tapeworms.

definitive prosthesis, a permanent prosthetic device that replaces an immediate-fit appliance such as a pylon.

definitive treatment, any therapy generally accepted as a specific cure of a disease.

defloration /def'lôrā'shən/ [L, *de* + *flos*, flower, *atio*, process], the rupture of the vaginal hymen. Defloration may occur during sexual intercourse, during a gynecologic examination, through the use of tampons, in athletic sports activity, or by surgery if necessary to remove an obstruction to menstrual flow.

deformity /dıfôr'mıtē/ [L, *deformis*, misshapen], a condition of being distorted, disfigured, flawed, malformed, or misshapen, which may affect the body in general or any part of it. It may be the result of disease, injury, or birth defect.

deg, 1. abbreviation for **degeneration. 2.** abbreviation for **degree.**

degeneration (deg) /dijen'ərā'shən/ [L, *degenerare*, to become unlike others], the gradual deterioration of normal cells and body functions.

degenerative /dijen'ərətiv/, [L, *degenerare*, to become unlike others], pertaining to or involving degeneration or change to a lower or dysfunctional form.

degenerative disease, any disease in which deterioration of structure or function of tissue occurs. Some kinds of degenerative diseases are **arteriosclerosis, cancer,** and **osteoarthritis.**

degenerative lesion [L, *degenerare*, to become unlike others, *laesio*, hurting], an injury or disease state that results in loss of function.

degenerative neuralgia [L, *degenerare*, to become unlike others; Gk, *neuron*, nerve, *algos*, pain], a form of neuralgia caused by degenerative changes in nervous tissue, which usually affects older people.

degenerative neuritis [L, *degenerare*, to become unlike others; Gk, *neuron*, nerve, *itis*, inflammation], an inflammation caused by degenerative changes in nervous tissue.

degloving /dēglov'ing/ [L, *de* + AS, *glof*], **1.** an injury to a finger in which the soft tissue down to the bone, including neurovascular bundles and sometimes tendons, is peeled off. **2.** (in dentistry) the exposure of the bony mandibular anterior or posterior regions by oral surgery. **3.** removal of latex or vinyl hand coverings.

deglutition /di'glootish'ən/ [L, *deglutire*, to swallow], swallowing.

deglutition apnea, the normal absence of respiration during swallowing.

degradation /di'grədā'shən/ [L, *de* + *gradu*, step], the reduction of a chemical compound to a less complex compound, usually by splitting off one or more groups or subgroups of atoms, as in deamination.

degranulation /dēgran'yəlā'shən/, the release of droplets or granules from cells such as mast cells and basophils.

degree (deg) [Fr, *degre*], one of the divisions or intervals marked on a scale of units of measurement.

degrees of freedom (df), a statistical measure of the number of independent observations or choices among members in a sample.

degustation /dē'gəstā'shən/ [L, *degustare*, to taste], the act of tasting.

dehiscence /dihis'əns/ [L, *dehiscere*, to gape], the separation of a surgical incision or rupture of a wound closure.

dehumanization /dihyoo'mənizā'shən/ [L, *de*, from, *humanitas*, human nature], the process of losing altruistic or individual qualities, as may occur in some psychotic states.

dehumidifier /dē'yoomid'ifī'ər/, an apparatus to remove moisture in the atmosphere.

dehydrate /dihī'drāt/ [L, *de* + Gk, *hydor*, water], **1.** to remove or lose water from a substance. **2.** to lose excessive water from the body. —**dehydration,** *n.*

dehydrated alcohol, a clear, colorless, highly hygroscopic liquid with a burning taste, containing at least 99.5% ethyl alcohol by volume.

dehydration /di'hīdrā'shən/, **1.** excessive loss of water from body tissues. Dehydration is accompanied by a disturbance in the balance of essential electrolytes, particularly sodium, potassium, and chloride. Signs of dehydration include poor skin turgor (not a reliable sign in the elderly), flushed dry skin, coated tongue, dry mucous membranes, oliguria, irritability, and confusion. **2.** rendering a substance free from water.

dehydration fever, a fever that frequently occurs in newborns, thought to be caused by dehydration.

dehydration of gingivae, the drying of gum tissue, often the result of mouth breathing, which lowers the resistance of the tissue to infection.

dehydrogenate, to remove hydrogen atoms, as in the oxidation processes.

deinstitutionalization /dē·in'stityoo′ shənəl'īzā'shən/ [L, *de* + *instituere,* to put in place], a change in the location and focus of mental health care from an institutional to a community setting.

Deiters' nucleus /dī'tərz, dē'terz/ [Otto F.C. Deiters, German anatomist, 1834–1863], one of the vestibular nuclei located in the brainstem.

DEJ, abbreviation for **dentinoenamel junction.**

déjà vu /dāzhävY',-vē',-voo'/ [Fr, previously seen], the sensation or illusion that one is encountering a set of circumstances or a place that was previously experienced. The phenomenon results from some unconscious emotional connection with the present experience.

Dejerine-Sottas disease /dezh'ərinsot'əz, -sotäz'/ [Joseph J. Dejerine, French neurologist, 1849–1917; Jules Sottas, French neurologist, 1866–1943], a rare congenital spinocerebellar disorder. It is characterized by the development of palpable thickenings along peripheral nerves, degeneration of the peripheral nervous system, pain, paresthesia, ataxia, and diminished sensation.

del, (in cytogenetics) abbreviation for **deletion.**

Delano, Jane A. (1862–1919), an American nurse who organized the American Red Cross Nursing Service, an association formed to supply nurses to the military forces.

delaviridine, an antiretroviral nonnucleoside analog prescribed in the treatment of human immunodeficiency virus infection.

delayed echolalia [Fr, *delai,* time extension; Gk, *echo,* sound, *lalein,* to babble],

a phenomenon, commonly seen in schizophrenia, involving the meaningless automatic repetition of overheard words and phrases. It occurs hours, days, or even weeks after the original stimulus.

delayed graft [ME, *delaein,* to leave; Gk, *graphein,* stylus], a type of skin graft that is partially elevated and replaced for use in a later transfer.

delayed hypersensitivity, a delayed allergic response of the skin associated with type IV hypersensitivity.

delayed language, failure of language to develop at the expected age. The cause is often unknown.

delayed postpartum hemorrhage, hemorrhage occurring later than 24 hours after giving birth. It is most often caused by retained fragments of the placenta, a laceration of the cervix or vagina that was not discovered or was not completely sutured, or subinvolution of the placental site within the uterus.

delayed sensation, a feeling or impression that is not experienced immediately after a stimulus.

delayed symptom [Fr, *delai* + Gk, *symptoma,* that which happens], a symptom such as shock that may not appear until after the precipitating cause.

delayed treatment seeker, (in psychology) a person who delays seeking treatment for a problematic life event such as a sexual assault until months or years after the event, usually after a precipitating event such as an anniversary reaction.

Delecato-Doman theory, a therapeutic concept that full neurologic organization of a disabled or mentally retarded child requires that the child pass through developmental patterns covering progressively higher anatomic levels of the nervous system.

Delegation, a Nursing Interventions Classification defined as transfer of responsibility for the provision of patient care while retaining accountability for the outcome.

deleterious /del'itir'ē·əs/ [Gk, *deleterios,* destroyer], harmful or dangerous.

deletion (del) /dilē'shən/ [L, *deletionum,* destruction], (in cytogenetics) the loss of a piece of a chromosome that has broken away from the genetic material.

deletion syndrome, any of a group of congenital autosomal anomalies that result from the loss of chromosomal genetic material, because of breakage of a chromatid during cell division, as the cat-cry syndrome, which results from the absence of the short arm of chromosome 5.

deliberate biologic programming /dilib'-ərit/ [L, *deliberare,* to weigh carefully], the Hayflick theory of aging, based on studies showing that human cells contain biologic clocks that predetermine death after undergoing mitosis a finite number of times.

deliberate hypotension, a process used in general anesthesia in which a short-acting hypotensive agent such as sodium nitroprusside or trimethaphan camsylate is given to reduce blood pressure and thus bleeding during surgery.

delinquency /diling'kwənsē/ [L, *delin-quere,* to fail], **1.** negligence or failure to fulfill a duty or obligation. **2.** an offense, fault, misdemeanor, or misdeed; a tendency to commit such acts.

delinquent /diling'kwənt/, **1.** characterized by neglect of duty or violation of law. **2.** one whose behavior is characterized by persistent antisocial, illegal, violent, or criminal acts; a juvenile delinquent.

délire de toucher /dālir'dəto͞oshā'/ [Fr], an abnormal desire or irresistible urge to touch objects.

delirious mania /dilir'ē·əs/, an extreme form of the manic state in which activity is so frenzied, confused, and incoherent that it is difficult to discern any link between affect and behavior.

delirium /dilir'ē·əm/ [L, *delirare,* to rave], **1.** a state of frenzied excitement or wild enthusiasm. **2.** an acute organic mental disorder characterized by confusion; disorientation; restlessness; clouding of the consciousness; incoherence; fear; anxiety; excitement; and often by illusions, hallucinations, usually of visual origin, and at times delusions. The condition is caused by disturbances in cerebral functions that may result from a wide range of metabolic disorders, including nutritional deficiencies and endocrine imbalances; postpartum or postoperative stress; ingestion of toxic substances such as various gases, metals, or drugs, including alcohol; and other causes of physical and mental shock or exhaustion. **—delirious,** *adj.*

delirium constantium, (in psychiatry) a patient's reiteration of a fixed idea.

Delirium Management, a Nursing Interventions Classification defined as provision of a safe and therapeutic environment for a patient who is experiencing an acute confusional state.

delirium of persecution [L, *delirare,* to rave, *persecutor,* to pursue], a state of clouded consciousness or decreased sensorium in which the person believes others are threatening or conspiring against him or her.

delirium tremens (DTs), an acute and sometimes fatal psychotic reaction caused by cessation of excessive intake of alcoholic beverages over a long period. Initial symptoms include loss of appetite, insomnia, and general restlessness, which are followed by agitation; excitement; disorientation; mental confusion; vivid and often frightening hallucinations; acute fear and anxiety; illusions and delusions; coarse tremors of the hands, feet, legs, and tongue; fever; increased heart rate; extreme perspiration; gastrointestinal distress; and precordial pain.

delivery /diliv'ərē/ [L, *de* + *liberare,* to free], (in obstetrics) the birth of a child; parturition.

delivery room, a unit of a hospital used for childbirth and infant resuscitation.

DeLorme technique, a method of exercise with weights for the purpose of strengthening muscles in which sets of repetitions are repeated with rests between sets. The technique involves isotonic exercise and determination of the maximum level of resistance.

delousing /dēlou'sing/ [L, *de,* from; AS, *lus*], to rid a person or object of an infestation of lice.

delta /del'tə/, Δ, δ, fourth letter of the Greek alphabet.

delta agent hepatitis /del'tə/ [L, *agere,* to do; Gk, *hepar,* liver, *itis,* inflammation], an infection caused by a ribonucleic acid virus (δ Ag) associated with the hepatitis B surface antigen in cases of chronic hepatitis and progressive liver damage. The delta agent apparently is able to induce the infection when it is present along with the B surface antigen.

delta-9-tetrahydrocannabinol (THC), a pharmacologically active ingredient of cannabis that has been used in treating some cases of nausea and vomiting associated with cancer chemotherapy.

delta optical density analysis [Gk, *delta,* fourth letter of Greek alphabet, *optikos,* of sight; L, *densus,* thick; Gk, a loosening], a technique used to diagnose anemia in a fetus by measuring the proportion of bilirubin decomposition products in the amniotic fluid. The method involves spectrographic examination of a fluid sample. It measures the bilirubin and bilirubin-products concentration according to the wavelengths of light absorbed by the hemolytic products, as the bilirubin products alter the normal color of the amniotic fluid.

delta wave, 1. also called delta rhythm. the slowest of the four types of brain waves, characterized by a frequency of 4

Hz and a relatively high voltage. Delta waves are "deep-sleep waves" associated with a dreamless state. **2.** (in cardiology) a slurring of the QRS part of an electrocardiogram tracing caused by preexcitation.

deltoid /del′toid/ [Gk, *delta*, triangular, *eidos*, form], **1.** triangular. **2.** pertaining to the deltoid muscle that covers the shoulder.

deltoid ligament [Gk, *delta* + L, *ligamentum*], the medial ligament of the ankle joint.

deltoid muscle, a large, thick triangular muscle that covers the shoulder joint. It is the prime mover of arm abduction. It is also a synergist of arm flexion, extension, and circumduction.

delusion /diloo′zhən/ [L, *deludere*, to deceive], a persistent aberrant belief or perception held inviolable by a person despite evidence that refutes it.

Delusion Management, a Nursing Interventions Classification defined as promoting the comfort, safety, and reality orientation of a patient who is experiencing false, fixed beliefs that have little or no basis in reality.

delusion of being controlled, the false belief that one's feelings, beliefs, thoughts, and acts are governed by some external force, as experienced in various forms of schizophrenia.

delusion of grandeur /grän′dyoor/, the gross exaggeration of one's importance, wealth, power, or talents, as manifested in such disorders as megalomania, general paresis, and paranoid schizophrenia.

delusion of persecution, a morbid belief that one is being mistreated, harassed, or conspired against, as seen in paranoia and paranoid schizophrenia.

delusion of poverty, (in psychology) a false belief of a person that he or she is impoverished.

demand pacemaker [L, *demandere*, to give in charge, *passus*, step; ME, *maken*], a device used to stimulate the heart electrically when the heart's own impulses are not sufficient. Such a device senses the interval between the heart's native beats and fires at a programmed interval.

demarcation /dē′märkā′shən/ [L, *de*, from, *marcare*, to mark], the process of setting limits or boundaries.

demarcation current [L, *de* + *marcare*, to mark], an electrical current that flows from an uninjured to an injured end of a muscle.

deme /dēm/ [Gk, *demos*, common population], a small, local, closely related interbreeding population of organisms or individuals, usually occupying a circumscribed area.

demecarium bromide /dē′məker′ē·əm/, an ophthalmic anticholinesterase agent prescribed in the treatment of open-angle glaucoma.

demeclocycline hydrochloride /dēmek′-lōsī′klēn/, a tetracycline antibiotic prescribed in the treatment of infections, including those in which use of penicillin is contraindicated.

demented /dimen′tid/ [L, *de*, away from, *mens*, mind], a form of mental disorder in which cognitive functions are affected.

dementia /dimen′shə/ [L, *de* + *mens*, mind], a progressive organic mental disorder characterized by chronic personality disintegration; confusion; disorientation; stupor; deterioration of intellectual capacity and function; and impairment of control of memory, judgment, and impulses.

Dementia Management, a Nursing Interventions Classification defined as provision of a modified environment for the patient who is experiencing a chronic confusional state.

demigauntlet bandage /dem′igônt′lit/ [L, *demidus*, half; Fr, *gant*, glove], a glove-like bandage over the hand that leaves the fingers free.

demineralization /dēmin′əral′īzā′shən/ [L, *de* + *minera*, mine], a decrease in the amount of minerals or inorganic salts in tissues, as occurs in certain diseases.

demise /dimīz′/ [OFr, *demettre*], to put away], death, destruction, or end of existence.

democratic style /dem′okrat′ik/, people-centered leadership in which the group participates openly in decision making for group goals.

demography /dəmog′rəfē/ [Gk, *demos*, people, *graphein*, to record], the study of human populations, particularly the size, distribution, and characteristics of members of population groups. Demography is applied in studies of health problems involving ethnic groups, populations of a specific geographic region, or religious groups with special dietary restrictions.

demonstrative /dimon′strətiv/, pertaining to a concept or an action that accompanies and illustrates speech.

demulcent /dimul′sənt/ [L, *demulcere*, to stroke down], **1.** any of several oily substances used for soothing and reducing irritation of surfaces that have been abraded or irritated. **2.** soothing, as a counterirritant or balm.

demyelinate /dēmī′əlināt′/, to remove or destroy the myelin surrounding the axons of nerve cells.

demyelination /dimī′əlinā′shən/ [L, *de* +

Gk, *myelos*, marrow], the process of destruction or removal of the myelin sheath from a nerve or nerve fiber.

denaturation /dēnā′chərā′shən/ [L, *de* + *natura*, natural], **1.** the alteration of the basic nature or structure of a substance. **2.** the process of making a potential food or beverage substance unfit for human consumption, although it may still be used for other purposes, such as a solvent.

denatured alcohol /dēnā′chərd/, ethyl alcohol made unfit for ingestion by the addition of acetone or methanol, used as a solvent and in chemical processes.

denatured protein [L, *de*, from, *natura*, *proteios*, first rank], a protein that has undergone change that causes its original properties to be lost. A protein can be denatured by radiation, heat, strong acids, or alcohol.

dendrite /den′drīt/ [Gk, *dendron*, tree], a slender branching process that extends from the cell body of a neuron and that is capable of being stimulated by a neurotransmitter.

dendritic /dendrit′ik/, **1.** treelike, with branches that spread toward or into neighboring tissues, as dendritic keratitis. **2.** pertaining to a dendrite.

dendritic calculus [Gk, *dendron*, tree, *calculus*, pebble], a large calculus lodged in the pelvis of the kidney and shaped to fit the branches of the calyx.

dendritic cell, a cell that captures antigens and migrates to the lymph nodes and spleen, where it presents the processed antigens to T cells.

dendritic keratitis, a severe herpesvirus infection of the eye. It is characterized by an ulceration of the surface of the cornea resembling a tree with knobs at the ends of the branches. Untreated dendritic keratitis may cause permanent scarring of the cornea with impaired vision or blindness.

dendrodendritic synapse /den′droden-drit′ik/ [Gk, *dendron* + *dendron* + *synaptein*, to join], a type of synapse in which a dendrite of one neuron comes in contact with that of another neuron.

denervated /dēnur′vātid/ [L, *de* + *nervus*, nerve], a condition of having a nerve impulse route interrupted, as by excision or administration of a drug that blocks the pathway. The result is decreased or no transmission of impulses through this pathway.

dengue fever /deng′gē, den′gā/ [Sp, influenza; L, *febris*, fever], an acute arbovirus infection transmitted to humans by the *Aedes* mosquito and occurring in tropic and subtropic regions. The disease usually produces a triad of symptoms: fever; rash; and severe head, back, and muscle pain.

Dengue is a self-limited illness, although recovery may require several weeks.

dengue hemorrhagic fever shock syndrome (DHFS), a grave form of dengue fever characterized by shock with collapse or prostration; cold, clammy extremities; a weak, thready pulse; respiratory distress; and all of the symptoms of dengue fever. Hemorrhage; bruises; small reddish spots indicating bleeding from skin capillaries; and bloody vomit, urine, and feces may be experienced and may precede circulatory collapse.

denial /dinī′əl/ [L, *denegare*, to negate], **1.** refusal or restriction of something requested, claimed, or needed, often causing physical or emotional deficiency. **2.** an unconscious defense mechanism in which emotional conflict and anxiety are avoided by refusal to acknowledge the thoughts, feelings, desires, impulses, or facts that are consciously intolerable.

denial, ineffective, a NANDA-accepted nursing diagnosis of a conscious or unconscious attempt to disavow the knowledge or meaning of an event to reduce anxiety or fear to the detriment of health. The individual delays seeking or refuses medical attention and does not perceive the personal relevance of symptoms or danger. Defining characteristics include the use of home remedies (self-treatment) to relieve symptoms, minimization of symptoms, displacement of the source of symptoms to other organs, and displacement of fear of impact of the condition.

Denis Browne splint [Denis J.W. Browne, twentieth-century Australian surgeon], a splint for the correction of talipes equinovarus (clubfoot), composed of a curved bar attached to the soles of a pair of high-topped shoes.

denitrogenation /dēnī′trōjənā′shən/, the elimination of nitrogen from the lungs and body tissues during a period of breathing pure oxygen.

Denman's spontaneous evolution [Thomas Denman, English physician, 1733–1815; L, *sponte*, voluntarily, *evolvere*, to roll forth], a natural, unassisted turning of the fetus from the transverse presentation. The head rotates back, and, as the breech descends, the shoulder ascends in the pelvis.

dens, *pl.* **dentes** /den′tēz/ [L, tooth], **1.** a tooth or toothlike structure or process. The term is sometimes modified to identify a particular tooth, as dens caninus . **2.** the cone-shaped odontoid process of the axis, or second cervical vertebra.

dense fibrous tissue [L, *densus,* thick], a fibrous connective tissue consisting of compact, strong, inelastic bundles of mostly parallel collagenous fibers that are glistening white.

dens in dente /den′tə/, an anomaly of the teeth, found chiefly in the maxillary lateral incisors and characterized by invagination of the enamel.

densitometer /den′sitom′ətər/ [L, *densus* + Gk, *metron,* measure], **1.** a device that uses a photoelectric cell to detect differences in the density of light transmitted through a medium such as x-ray film or through a liquid. **2.** a device that measures optical density in a radiograph by detecting the intensity of light transmitted through the film.

density /den′sitē/ [L, *densus,* thick], **1.** the amount of mass of a substance in a given volume. The greater the mass in a given volume, the greater the density. **2.** (in radiology) the degree of x-ray film blackening.

density gradient, a variation in the density of a solution caused by a change in concentration of a solute in a confined solution.

dental [L, *dens,* tooth], pertaining to a tooth or teeth.

dental abscess, an abscess that forms in bone or soft tissues of the jaw as a result of an infection that may follow dental caries or injury to a tooth. Symptoms include pain that may be continuous and exacerbated by hot or cold foods or the pressure of closing the jaws firmly.

dental alveolus /alvē′ələs/, a tooth socket in the mandible or maxilla.

dental amalgam, an alloy of silver, tin, and mercury with small amounts of zinc and sometimes copper, used for restoring the function of tooth surfaces affected by dental caries or trauma.

dental anesthesia, any of several numbing procedures used in dental surgery, most commonly injectable local anesthetics to reduce anxiety and pain during treatment. A newer type is electronic anesthesia.

dental ankylosis, solid fixation of a tooth resulting from fusion of the cementum and alveolar bone, with obliteration of the periodontal ligament.

dental anomaly, an aberration in which one or more teeth deviate from the normal in form, function, or position.

dental appliance, any device used by a dentist for a specific purpose, such as an orthodontic device used to correct malocclusion.

dental arch, the curving shape formed by the arrangement of a normal set of teeth.

dental assistant, a person who assists a dentist in the performance of generalized tasks, including chairside aid, clerical work, reception, and some radiography and dental laboratory work.

dental biomechanics, the field of biomechanics, the action of forces, that deals with the biologic effects of dental restoration on oral structures.

dental calculus, a salivary deposit of calcium phosphate and calcium carbonate with organic matter on the teeth or a dental prosthesis.

dental caries, a plaque disease caused by the complex interaction of food, especially starches and sugars, with bacteria that form dental plaque. Plaque adheres to the surfaces of the teeth and provides the medium for the growth of bacteria and the production of organic acids that cause demineralization of enamel. Enzymes produced by the bacteria then attack the protein component of the tooth. This process, if untreated, ultimately leads to the formation of deep cavities and bacterial infection of the pulp chamber, which contains blood vessels and nerves.

dental chart, a simplified graphic representation of the teeth on which clinical, radiologic, and forensic information may be recorded.

dental crypt, the space in the alveolar process occupied by a developing tooth.

dental emergency, an acute disorder of oral health that requires medical attention, including broken, loose, or evulsed teeth caused by traumas; infections and inflammations of the soft tissues of the mouth; and complications of oral sugary such as dry tooth socket.

dental engine, an apparatus consisting of a hand instrument to which various rotating tools or drills can be fitted. It is driven by an electric motor via a continuous cordlike belt over pulleys.

dental erosion, the chemical or mechanochemical destruction of a tooth substance that causes variously shaped concavities at the cementoenamel junctions of teeth. The surfaces of these depressions, unlike those of carious cavities, are hard and smooth.

dental ethics [L, *dens,* tooth; Gk, *ethos,* ethics], a sense of moral obligation and a system of moral principles governing the professional conduct of dental and dental hygienic practices.

dental examination, an inspection of the teeth and surrounding soft tissues of the oral cavity. The examiner generally uses an explorer, a slender steel instrument with a flexible sharp point, to probe the minute indentations on tooth surfaces for signs of demineralization and caries development. Fillings are also inspected, and a radiographic record of the teeth is usually made. The examiner may also insert a periodontal probe into the soft tissue sulcus around each tooth to measure the depth of each sulcus and explore for calculus and root defects.

dental extracting forceps, a type of hand instrument used for grasping teeth during removal from the socket.

dental film, a type of x-ray film made for either intraoral or extraoral exposure. Intraoral films are small, double-emulsion films without screens but with a lead foil backing to reduce patient dose, enclosed in a moisture-resistant envelope. Extraoral films are large, single-emulsion screen films.

dental fistula, an abnormal passage from the apical periodontal area of a tooth to the surface of oral mucous membrane, permitting the discharge of inflammatory or suppurative material.

dental floss, a waxed or unwaxed flavored or unflavored thread used to clean interproximal tooth surfaces or spaces between the teeth.

dentalgia /dental'jē-ə/ [L, *dens,* tooth; Gk, *algos,* pain], toothache.

dental granuloma, a pathologic condition characterized by a mass of granulation tissue that is surrounded by a fibrous capsule attached to the apex of a pulp-involved tooth.

dental handpiece, a device used to drill into teeth.

dental history, a record of a patient's oral health, general health, and medical care, including surgeries and medication use, allergies, childhood diseases, radiographic history, and personal dental care.

dental hygienist, a primary health care professional with special training to provide dental services under the supervision of a dentist. To practice as a Registered Dental Hygienist (RDH), a person must complete at least 2 years of secondary education in an accredited community or dental college or university and be approved by a state or regional board of dental and dental hygiene examiners. Services supplied by a dental hygienist include dental prophylaxis, radiography, administration of medications, and provision of dental education at chairside and in the community.

dental identification [L, *dens,* tooth, *idem,* the same, *facere,* to make], the process of establishing the unique characteristics of the teeth and dental work of an individual, thereby leading to the identification of an individual by comparison with his or her dental charts and records.

dental implant, a plastic or metal device that is implanted into a jawbone to provide permanent support for a fixed bridge or

denture when the bony ridge would provide insufficient support.

dental jurisprudence [L, *dens,* tooth, *juris prudentia,* knowledge of the law], the application of the principles of law as they relate to the practice of dentistry and the relations of dentists to patients, to society, and to each other.

dental laboratory technician, a person who makes dental prostheses and orthodontic appliances as prescribed by a dentist. The dental laboratory technician may have a private laboratory or work in the premises of a dentist.

dental operculum [L, *dens,* tooth, *operculum,* a covering structure], a hood or flap of gingival tissue overlying the crown of an erupting tooth. This tissue usually disappears as the tooth erupts by being chewed away.

dental papilla [L, *dens,* tooth, *papilla,* nipple], a small mass of mesenchymal tissue in the enamel organ, which, during tooth development, differentiates into dentin and dental pulp. The innermost layer consists of a cell-free zone of reticular fibers that form the basement membrane.

dental plate [L, *dens,* tooth; OFr, *plate,* flat structure], a dental prosthesis made to the shape of the maxillary or mandibular jaw to support artificial teeth.

dental prosthesis [L, *dens,* tooth; Gk, *prosthesis,* an addition], a fixed or removable appliance to replace one or more lost or missing natural teeth.

dental public health, the science and art of preventing and controlling dental diseases and promoting dental health through organized community efforts.

dental pulp, a small mass of connective tissue, blood vessels, and nerves located in a chamber within the dentin layer of a tooth.

dental radiograph [L, *dens,* tooth; L, *radire,* to shine; Gk, *graphein,* to record], an intraoral and extraoral x-ray film of teeth and the bone surrounding them.

dental sealants /sē'lənts/, plastic film coatings that are applied and adhere to the caries-free chewing surfaces of teeth to seal pits and fissures where plaque, food, and bacteria usually become trapped.

dental surgeon [L, *dens,* tooth; Gk, *cheirourgos,* surgeon], a dentist who specializes in surgical procedures involving the teeth and surrounding oral tissues. An operative dental surgeon is concerned with the restoration of teeth that have been damaged. An oral and maxillofacial surgeon specializes in surgical reconstruction of facial malformations caused by diseases of the head and neck or traumatic accidents. An oral surgeon specializes in the surgical removal of the teeth and surrounding oral tissues.

dentate fracture /den′tāt/ [L, *dens*], any fracture that causes serrated bone ends that fit together like the teeth of gears.

dentate nucleus, a deep cerebellar nucleus. It receives fibers from the lateral zone of the cerebellar cortex and appears to act as a trigger for the motor cortex, governing intentional movements as well as properties of ongoing movements.

denticle /den′tikəl/, a calcified body in the pulp chamber of a tooth.

denticulate /dentik′yəlit/ [L, *denticulus*, little tooth], having very small teeth or toothlike projections.

dentifrice /den′tifris/ [L, *dens* + *fricare*, to rub], a pharmaceutic compound used with a toothbrush for cleaning and polishing the teeth. It typically contains a mild abrasive, detergent, flavoring agent, and binder.

dentigerous cyst /dentij′ərəs/ [L, *dens* + *gerere*, to bear], one of three kinds of follicular cyst, consisting of an epithelium-lined sac filled with fluid or viscous material that surrounds the crown of an unerupted tooth or odontoma.

dentin /den′tin/ [L, *dens*], the chief material of teeth, surrounding the pulp and situated inside the enamel and cementum. Harder and denser than bone, it consists of solid organic substratum infiltrated with lime salts.

dentin eburnation /ē′burnā′shən/, a change in carious teeth in which softened and decalcified dentin develops a hard, brown, polished appearance.

dentin globule, a small spheric body in peripheral dentin, created by early calcification.

dentinoenamel /den′tinō·inam′əl/ [L, *dens* + OFr, *enesmail*, enamel], pertaining to both the dentin and the enamel of the teeth.

dentinoenamel junction (DEJ), the interface of the enamel and the dentin of a tooth crown, generally conforming to the shape of the crown.

dentinogenesis /den′tinōjen′əsis/ [L, *dens* + Gk, *genein*, to produce], the formation of the dentin of the teeth. —**dentinogenic,** *adj.*

dentinogenesis imperfecta /-jen′əsis/, **1.** a genetic disturbance of the dentin, characterized by early calcification of the pulp chambers, marked attrition, and opalescent hue of the teeth. **2.** a localized form of mesodermal dysplasia affecting the dentin of the teeth. **3.** a genetic condition that produces defective dentin but normal tooth enamel.

dentist [L, *dens*], a person who is quali-

fied by training and licensed by the state or region to diagnose and treat abnormalities of the teeth, gums, and underlying bone, including but not limited to conditions caused by disease, trauma, and heredity. Training requires a minimum of 2 years, preferably 4, in an undergraduate college and a satisfactory score on a Dental Aptitude Test (DAT), followed by 4 years at an American Dental Association–(ADA-) accredited dental college. After completing dental college, a dentist is awarded a degree of either Doctor of Dental Surgery (D.D.S.) or Doctor of Dental Medicine (D.M.D.), which are equivalent.

dentistry /den′tistrē/ [L, *dens*], the art and science of practicing the diagnosis, prevention, and treatment of diseases and disorders of the teeth and surrounding structures of the oral cavity. Responsibilities include the repair and restoration of teeth and replacement of missing teeth, as well as the detection of signs of diseases such as blood dyscrasias and tumors that would require treatment by a dental specialist or physician. There are eight recognized specialties, each requiring additional training after graduation from a dental college: **dental public health, endodontics,** oral and maxillofacial pathology, **oral and maxillofacial surgery, orthodontics and dentofacial orthopedics, pediatric dentistry, periodontics, and prosthodontics.**

dentition /dentish′ən/ [L, *dentire*, to cut teeth], **1.** the development and eruption of the teeth. **2.** the arrangement, number, and kind of teeth as they appear in the dental arch of the mouth. **3.** the teeth of an individual or species as determined by their form and arrangement.

dentoalveolar abscess /den′tō·alvē′ələr/ [L, *dens* + *alveolus*, little hollow, *abscedere*, to go away], the formation and accumulation of pus in a tooth socket or the jawbone around the base of a tooth.

dentofacial /-fā′shəl/, pertaining to an oral or gnathic structure.

dentofacial anomaly, a condition in which an oral or gnathic structure deviates from the normal in form, function, or position.

dentogingival fiber /-jinjī′vəl/ [L, *dens* + *gingiva*, gum], any one of the many peridental fibers that spread like a fan, emerge from the supraalveolar part of the cementum, and terminate in the free gingiva.

dentogingival junction, the junction of the gingival attachment, a nonkeratinized epithelium, and the surface of the teeth.

dentoperiosteal fiber /den′tōper′ē·os′tē·əl/ [L, *dens* + Gk, *peri,* around, *osteon* bone], any one of the many peridental fibers that emerge from the supraalveolar part of the cementum of a tooth and extend apically beyond the alveolar crest into the mucoperiosteum of the attached gingiva.

dentulous /den'tyələs/ [L, *dens,* tooth, *-ulosus,* characterized by], possessing one or more natural teeth.

dentulous dental arch, a dental arch that contains natural teeth.

denture /den'chər/ [L, *dens,* tooth], an artificial tooth or a set of artificial teeth not permanently fixed or implanted.

denture base, 1. the part of a denture that fits the oral mucosa of the basal seat and supports artificial teeth. **2.** the part of a denture that covers the soft tissue of the mouth, commonly made of resin or a combination of resins and metal.

denture flask, a sectional metal case in which plaster of paris or artificial stone is molded, in which dentures or other resin restorations are processed.

denture packing, the laboratory procedure of filling and compressing a denture-base material into a mold in a flask.

denturist /den'chərist/, a person who performs the same type of work as a dental laboratory technician but without a dentist's prescription, providing dental prostheses directly to clients.

denucleated /dēnyoo'klē·ā'tid/ [L, *de,* from, *nucleus,* nut kernel], pertaining to a condition in which the nucleus has been removed.

denudation /den'oodā'shən/ [L, *denudare,* to make bare], **1.** the process of stripping bare. **2.** a condition of losing an outside layer such as an epithelium.

Denver Articulation Screening Examination (DASE), a test for evaluating the clarity of pronunciation in children 2½ to 6 years of age. Each child's performance may be compared with a standardized norm for the age.

Denver classification, the system of identifying and classifying human chromosomes according to the criteria established at the Denver (1960), London (1963), and Chicago (1966) conferences of cytogeneticists. It is based on chromosome size and position of the centromere as determined during mitotic metaphase and is divided into seven major groups, designated A through G, which are arranged according to decreasing length.

Denver Developmental Screening Test (DDST), a test for evaluating development in children from 1 month to 6 years of age. The developmental level of motor, social, and language skills is expressed as a ratio in which the child's age is the denominator and the age at which the norm possesses skills equal to those of the child

being tested is the numerator. The **Denver II,** released in 1990, is a major revision and restandardization of the DDST.

deodorant /dē·ō'dərənt/ [L, *de* + *odor,* smell], **1.** destroying or masking odors. **2.** a substance that destroys or masks odors. Underarm deodorants contain an antiperspirant such as aluminum chloride that forms an obstructive hydroxide gel in sweat ducts. Vaginal deodorant sprays contain a fatty ester emollient, a masking fragrance, and an antimicrobial agent, and are often associated with allergic reactions. Room and breath deodorants contain masking agents such as mint or thyme.

deodorized alcohol /dē·ō'dərīzd'/, a liquid, free of organic impurities, containing 92.5% absolute alcohol.

deodorizing douche, a stream of air or liquid that masks or absorbs foul odors, applied at moderate pressure into a body cavity or onto a body surface.

deontologism /dē'ontol'əgiz'əm/ [Gk, *deon,* obligation, *logos,* science], a doctrine of ethics that states that moral duty or obligation is binding.

deossification /dē·os'ifikā'shən/, the loss of mineral matter from bones.

deoxidizer, an agent that removes oxygen.

deoxygenation /dē·ok'sijənā'shən/ [L, *de,* from; Gk, *oxys,* sharp, *genein,* to produce], the removal of oxygen from a chemical compound.

deoxyribonucleic acid (DNA) /dē·ok'sirī'-bōnookle'ik/, a large double-stranded helical, nucleic acid molecule found principally in the chromosomes of the nucleus of a cell, which is the carrier of genetic information. The genetic information is coded in the sequence of the nucleotides forming the DNA molecule.

Department of Health and Human Services (DHHS), a cabinet-level department of the U.S. government with responsibility for the functions of various federal social welfare and health delivery agencies such as the Food and Drug Administration (FDA). It also directs the U.S. Office of Consumer Affairs, Office of Civil Rights, Administration on Aging, Public Health Service, Indian Health Service, Social Security Administration, and National Institutes of Health.

Department of Transportation (DOT), a cabinet-level department of the U.S. government responsible for national transportation policies, including maritime, aviation, railroad, and highway safety and regulation of the transport of hazardous materials such as medical gases.

dependence /dipen'dəns/ [L, *de* + *pendere,*

to hang upon], **1.** the state of being dependent. **2.** the total psychophysical state of one addicted to drugs or alcohol who must receive an increasing amount of the substance to prevent the onset of withdrawal symptoms.

dependency needs /dipen'dənsē/, the sum of the physical and emotional requirements of an infant for survival, including parenting, love, affection, shelter, protection, food, and warmth. Reliance on others to satisfy these needs decreases with age and maturity.

dependent, pertaining to a condition of being reliant on someone or something else for help, support, favor, and other needs, as a child is dependent on a parent, a narcotics addict is dependent on a drug, or one variable is dependent on another. —**depend,** *v.*

dependent care, health care provided for persons, particularly children and handicapped or elderly individuals, who are dependent on others for part or all of the activities of daily living.

dependent edema [L, *de,* from, *pendere,* to hand; Gk, *oidema,* swelling], a fluid accumulation in the tissues influenced by gravity. It is usually greater in the lower part of the body than in tissues above the level of the heart.

dependent intervention, a therapeutic action based on the written or verbal orders of another health professional.

dependent personality, behavior characterized by excessive or compulsive needs for attention, acceptance, and approval from other people to maintain security and self-esteem.

dependent personality disorder, a mental state characterized by a lack of self-confidence and an inability to function independently.

dependent variable, (in research) a factor that is measured to learn the effect of one or more independent variables.

depersonalization /dēpur'sənəlīzā'shən/ [L, *de* + *persona,* mask], a feeling of strangeness or unreality concerning oneself or the environment, often resulting from anxiety or fatigue.

depersonalization disorder, an emotional disturbance characterized by depersonalization feelings in which a dreamlike atmosphere pervades the consciousness. The body may not feel like one's own, and dramatic and important events may be watched with equanimity.

de Pezzer's catheter /depezäz'/ [Oscar M. de Pezzer, French surgeon, 1853–1917], a self-retaining catheter with a bulbous tip.

depilation /dep'ilā'shən/ [L, *de* + *pilum,* hair], the removal or extraction of hair

from the body, either temporarily by mechanical or chemical means or permanently by electrolysis, which destroys the hair follicle. —**depilate,** *v.*

depilatory /dipil'ətôrē/, **1.** pertaining to a substance or procedure that removes hair. **2.** a depilatory agent.

depilatory techniques [L, *depilare,* to deprive of hair; Gk, *technikos,* skillful], methods of removing unwanted body hair, such as plucking, external application of chemicals, electrolysis, or application of melted wax.

depolarization /dēpō'lərīzā'shən/, the reduction of a membrane potential to a less negative value.

deposition /dep'əzish'ən/ [L, *deponere,* to lay down], (in law) sworn pretrial testimony given by a witness in response to oral or written questions and cross-examination.

depot /dē'pō, dep'ō/ [Fr, depository], **1.** any area of the body in which drugs or other substances such as fat are stored and from which they can be distributed. **2.** (of a drug) injected or implanted to be slowly absorbed into the circulation.

depot injection, an intramuscular injection of a drug in an oil suspension that results in a gradual release of the medication over several days.

depressant /dipres'ənt/ [L, *deprimere,* to press down], **1.** (of a drug) tending to decrease the function or activity of a system of the body. **2.** such a drug; for example, a cardiac depressant, central nervous system depressant, or respiratory depressant.

depressed [L, *deprimere,* to press down], **1.** pertaining to a body structure that has been forced below the surface of surrounding parts, as in a fracture. **2.** pertaining to a condition in which general body activity is diminished, as in depressed urine output during dehydration. **3.** pertaining to an emotional condition, resulting in emotional dejection, loss of initiative, listlessness, loss of appetite, and concentration difficulty.

depressed fracture, any fracture of the skull in which fragments are depressed below the normal surface of the skull.

depression /dipresh'ən/ [L, *deprimere,* to press down], **1.** a depressed area, hollow, or fossa; downward or inward displacement. **2.** a decrease of vital functional activity. **3.** a mood disturbance characterized by feelings of sadness, despair, and discouragement resulting from and normally proportionate to some personal loss or tragedy. **4.** an abnormal emotional state characterized by exaggerated feelings of sadness, melancholy, dejection, worthlessness, emptiness, and hopelessness that are inappropriate and out of proportion to reality. —**depressive,** *adj.*

depression with psychotic features [L, *deprimere,* to press down; Gk, *psyche,* mind, *osis,* condition], a type of depressive disorder or mood disorder in which there are psychotic features, usually of a paranoid or somatic nature.

depressive reaction, a condition of depressive emotional response to an external situation.

depressor /dipres'ər/ [L, *deprimere,* to press down], any agent that reduces activity when applied to nerves and muscles.

depressor reflex [L, *deprimere,* to press down, *reflectere,* to bend back], a reflexive vasodilation, or fall in arterial blood pressure, as may result from stimulation of the carotid sinus.

depressor septi /sep'tī/, one of the three muscles of the nose. It lies between the mucous membrane and the muscular structure of the lip and serves to draw down the ala, constricting the nostril.

deprivation /dep'rivā'shən/ [L, *deprivare,* to deprive], the loss of something considered valuable or necessary by taking it away or denying access to it. In experimental psychology animal or human subjects may be deprived of something desired or expected for study of their reactions.

deprivation of sleep effects [L, *deprivare,* to deprive; ME, *slep* + L, *efficere,* to accomplish], the interference with a basic physiologic urge to sleep, which appears to be governed by sleep centers in the hypothalamus and reticular activating system. Sleep deprivation results in progressive mental aberrations after 30 to 60 continuous hours. After this point boring tasks become intolerable, speech begins to be slurred, and performance becomes increasingly poor. After a week of sleep deprivation, symptoms of psychosis may appear.

depth dose [AS, *diop* + Gk, *dosis,* giving], (in radiotherapy) the relationship between the dose at any depth from a beam of radiation and the dose at the entrance from that beam.

depth perception, the ability to judge depth or the relative distance of objects in space and to orient one's position in relation to them. Binocular vision is essential to this ability.

depth psychology, any approach to psychology that emphasizes the study of personality and behavior in relation to unconscious motivation.

de Quervain's fracture /də kərvānz'/

[Fritz de Quervain, Swiss surgeon, 1868–1940], fracture of the navicular bone of the hand, with dislocation of the lunate bone.

de Quervain's thyroiditis [Fritz de Quervain; Gk, *thyreos,* shield, *otis,* inflammation], an inflammatory condition of the thyroid. It is characterized by swelling and tenderness of the gland, fever, dysphagia, fatigue, and severe pain in the neck, ears, and jaw. The disorder often occurs after a viral infection of the upper respiratory tract. It tends to remit spontaneously and to recur several times.

der, (in cytogenetics) abbreviation for *derivative chromosome.*

derailment /dirāl'mənt/, a pattern of speech in which incomprehensible, disconnected, and unrelated ideas replace logical and orderly thought.

Dercum's disease /dur'kəmz/ [Francis X. Dercum, U.S. neurologist, 1856–1931], a potentially fatal disorder characterized by painful localized fatty swellings and nerve lesions. The disease mainly affects menopausal women.

dereflection /dē'rəflek'shən/ [L, *de* + *reflectere,* to bend back], a technique of logotherapeutic psychology that is directed to taking a person's mind off a certain goal through a positive redirection to another goal, with emphasis on assets and abilities rather than the problems at hand.

dereistic thought /dē'rē·is'tik/ [L, *de* + *res,* thing], a type of mental activity in which fantasy is not modified by logic, experience, or reality.

derivative /dəriv'ətiv/ [L, *derivare,* to turn away], anything that originates in another substance or object; for example, organs and tissues are derivatives of the primordial germ cells.

derived protein /dirivd'/, a small protein obtained by enzymatic or chemical hydrolysis of a larger protein source, such as a proteose, peptone, or peptide.

derived quantity, any secondary quantity such as volume that is derived from a combination of base quantities such as mass, length, and time.

dermabrasion /dur'məbrā'zhən/ [Gk, *derma,* skin; L, *abradere,* to scrape], a treatment for the removal of superficial scars on the skin by the use of revolving wire brushes or sandpaper. An aerosol spray is used to freeze the skin for this procedure.

Dermacentor /dur'məsen'tər/, a genus of ticks. It includes species that transmit Rocky Mountain spotted fever, tularemia, brucellosis, and other infectious diseases.

dermal /dur'məl/ [Gk, *derma,* skin], pertaining to the skin.

dermal graft [Gk, *derma*, skin, *graphion*, stylus], the transplantation of any living skin tissue that contains dermis and thus is capable of regenerating and secreting sweat and sebum and generating new hair growth.

dermal papilla [Gk, *derma*, skin; L, *papilla*, nipple], any small elevation in the dermis, such as the elongated alpine papilla seen in psoriasis.

dermatitis /dur'mətī'tis/ [Gk, *derma* + *itis*, inflammation], an inflammatory condition of the skin. Various cutaneous eruptions occur and may be unique to a particular allergen, disease, or infection.

dermatitis herpetiformis, a chronic, severely pruritic skin disease with symmetrically located groups of red papulovesicular, vesicular, bullous, or urticarial lesions.

dermatocellulitis /dur'mətōsel'yəlī'tis/, an inflammation of the skin and subcutaneous connective tissue.

dermatocyst /dur'mətōsist'/, a cystic tumor of cutaneous tissues.

dermatofibroma /dur'mətōfībrō'mə/ [Gk, *derma* + L, *fibra*, fiber, *oma*, tumor], a cutaneous nodule that is painless, round, firm, gray or red, elevated, and commonly found on the extremities.

dermatofibrosarcoma /-fī'brōsärkō'mə/ [Gk, *derma*, skin; L, *fibra*, fiber; Gk, *sarx*, flesh, *oma*, tumor], a specific type of fibrous tumor of the skin.

dermatoglyphics /dur'mətōglif'iks/ [Gk, *derma* + *glyphe*, a carving], the study of the skin ridge patterns on fingers, toes, palms of hands, and soles of feet. The patterns are used as a basis of identification and also have diagnostic value because of associations between certain patterns and chromosomal anomalies.

dermatographia /dur'mətōgraf'ē·ə/ [Gk, *derma* + *graphein*, to record], a skin condition characterized by wheals that develop from tracing on the skin with the fingernail or a blunted instrument.

dermatologic agent /dur'mətōloj'ik/, a drug used to treat reactions or disorders of the skin.

dermatologist /dur'mətol'əjist/, a physician specializing in disorders of the skin.

dermatology /-ol'əjē/ [Gk, *derma* + *logos*, science], the study of the skin, including its anatomic, physiologic, and pathologic characteristics and the diagnosis and treatment of skin disorders.

dermatoma /dur'mətō'mə, **1.** a skin tumor. **2.** a local path of abnormally thick skin.

dermatome /dur'mətōm/ [Gk, *derma* + *temnein*, to cut], **1.** (in embryology) the mesodermal layer in the early developing embryo that gives rise to the dermal layers of the skin. **2.** (in surgery) an instrument used to cut thin slices of skin for grafting. **3.** an area on the surface of a body innervated by afferent fibers from one spinal root.

dermatomycosis /dur'mətō'mīkō'sis/ [Gk, *derma* + *mykes*, fungus, *osis*, condition], a superficial fungal infection of the skin, characteristically found on parts that are moist and protected by clothing such as the groin or feet. It is caused by a dermatophyte. —**dermatomycotic,** *adj.*

dermatomyositis /dur'mətōmī'ōsī'tis/ [Gk, *derma* + *mys*, muscle, *itis*, inflammation], a disease of the connective tissues characterized by pruritic or eczematous inflammation of the skin and tenderness and weakness of the muscles. Muscle tissue is destroyed, and loss is often so severe that the person may become unable to walk or to perform simple tasks.

dermatopathy /dur'mətop'əthē/, any disorder of the skin.

Dermatophagoides farinae /-fagoi'dēz/ [Gk, *derma* + *phagein*, to eat, *eidos*, form], a ubiquitous species of household dust mite responsible for allergic reactions in sensitive individuals.

dermatophyte /dur'mətōfīt', dərmat'əfīt/, any of several fungi that cause parasitic skin disease in humans.

dermatophytid /dur'mətof'itid, dur'mə-tōfī'tid/ [Gk, *derma* + *phyton*, plant], an allergic skin reaction characterized by small vesicles and associated with dermatomycosis.

dermatophytosis /dur'mətō'fītō'sis/ [Gk, *derma* + *phyton*, plant, *osis*, condition], a superficial fungus infection of the skin caused by *Microsporum, Epidermophyton,* or *Trichophyton* species of dermatophyte. On the trunk and upper extremities it is commonly called "ringworm" infection and is characterized by round or oval scaly patches with slightly raised borders and clearing centers. On the feet small vesicles, cracking, itching, scaling, and often secondary bacterial infections occur and are commonly called "athlete's foot."

dermatoplasty /dur'mətōplas'tē/, a surgical procedure in which skin tissue is transplanted to a body surface damaged by disease or injury.

dermatosclerosis /-sklərō'sis/ [Gk, *derma* + *sklerosis*, hardening], a skin disease characterized by fibrous thickening of the skin.

dermatosis /dur'mətō'sis/ [Gk, *derma* + *osis*, condition], any disorder of the skin, especially those not associated with inflammation.

dermatosis papulosa nigra, a common condition in individuals with darkly pigmented skin. It consists of multiple tiny, benign skin-colored or hyperpigmented papules on the face, neck, and cheeks.

dermis, the layer of the skin just below the epidermis, consisting of papillary and reticular layers and containing blood and lymphatic vessels, nerves and nerve endings, glands, and hair follicles.

dermoid /dur′moid/ [Gk, *derma* + *eidos*, form], **1.** pertaining to the skin. **2.** *informal.* a dermoid cyst.

dermoid cyst, a tumor, derived from embryonal tissues, consisting of a fibrous wall lined with epithelium and a cavity containing fatty material, hair, teeth, bits of bone, and cartilage.

derotation brace /dē′rōtā′shən/, a customized orthosis that provides stability at the knee joint. It consists of a single-joint hinged bar on one side and a rotating dial pad on the opposite side.

DES, abbreviation for **diethylstilbestrol.**

desalination /dēsal′inā′shən/ [L, *de,* from, *sal,* salt], the process of removing salt from water or other substances.

desaturation /dēsach′ərā′shən/ [L, *de,* from, *saturare,* to fill], the formation of an unsaturated chemical compound from a saturated one.

Descemet's membrane /desemāz′/ [Jean Descemet, French physician, 1732–1810], a deep layer of the cornea, between the substantia propria externally and the endothelium internally.

descendens /disen′dənz/, **1.** the descending branch of the hypoglossal nerve. **2.** the cervicalis nerve formed by branches of the second and third cervical nerves.

descending aorta /disen′ding/ [L, *descendere,* to descend; Gk, *aerein,* to raise], the main part of the aorta, consisting of the thoracic aorta and the abdominal aorta, which continues from the aortic arch into the trunk of the body. It supplies many structures, including the esophagus, lymph glands, ribs, stomach, liver, intestines, kidneys, spleen, and reproductive organs.

descending colon, the segment of the colon that extends from the end of the transverse colon at the splenic flexure on the left side of the abdomen down to the beginning of the sigmoid colon in the pelvis.

descending myelitis [L, *descendere,* to descend; Gk, *myelos,* marrow, *itis,* inflammation], a form of myelitis in which the pathologic changes spread downward along the spinal cord.

descending neuritis [L, *descendere,* to descend; Gk, *neuron,* nerve, *itis,* inflammation], a form of neuritis that spreads downward from the upper part of the nervous system.

descending neuropathy [L, *descendere,* to

descend; Gk, *neuron,* nerve, *pathos,* disease], a disease of the peripheral nervous system that spreads downward from the upper part of the body.

descending tract [L, *descendere,* to descend, *tractus*], a nerve tract in the spinal cord that carries impulses away from the brain axis of the body or body part.

descensus /disen′səs/, the process of falling or descending; prolapse.

descriptive anatomy /diskrip′tiv/ [L, *describere,* to write], the study of the morphologic characteristics of the body by systems, such as the vascular system and the nervous system.

descriptive embryology, the study of the changes that occur in cells, tissues, and organs during the progressive stages of prenatal development.

descriptive epidemiology, the first stage of epidemiologic investigation. It focuses on describing disease distribution by characteristics relating to time, place, and person.

descriptive psychiatry, the study of external, readily observable behavior.

DES daughters, a group of women with increased susceptibility to cancer of the vagina and other reproductive organs because their mothers were given an estrogen medication, diethylstilbestrol (DES), from the 1940s through the 1960s to prevent miscarriage. Several other abnormalities have been reported. Sons of women who took DES have an increased risk of undescended testes or other genital disorders.

desensitize /dēsen′sitīz/ [L, *de* + *sentire,* feel], **1.** (in immunology) to render an individual insensitive to any of the various antigens. **2.** (in psychiatry) to relieve an emotionally disturbed person of the stress of phobias and neuroses by encouraging discussion of the anxieties and the stressful experiences that cause the emotional problems involved. **3.** (in dentistry) to remove or reduce the painful response of vital exposed dentin to irritating substances and temperature changes.

deserpidine /disur′pədēn/, a rauwolfia alkaloid prescribed for mild hypertension and mild anxiety.

desiccant /des′ikənt/ [L, *desiccare,* to dry thoroughly], any agent or procedure that promotes drying or causes a substance to dry up.

desiccate /des′ikāt/, **1.** to dry thoroughly. **2.** to preserve by drying, especially food.

designated donor, a person, usually a friend or relative with the same blood type, who has agreed to donate one or more units of blood in advance of a planned surgery. The designated donor blood must undergo the same tests as anonymous donor blood.

designer drugs [L, *de* + *signare,* to mark], synthetic organic compounds that are designed as analogs of illicit drugs, with the same narcotic or other dangerous effects. Because designer drugs are generally not listed as controlled substances by the U.S. Drug Enforcement Agency, prosecution of manufacturers, distributors, or users is frequently difficult.

desipramine hydrochloride /desip′rəmēn/, a tricyclic antidepressant prescribed in the treatment of mental depression.

deslanoside /dislan′əsīd/, a cardiac glycoside prescribed for congestive heart failure and certain arrhythmias.

desmoid tumor /dez′moid/ [Gk, *desmos,* band, *eidos,* form], a fibrous neoplasm that may occur in the head, neck, upper arm, abdomen, or lower extremities. The tumor is usually a firm, rubbery mass.

desmopressin acetate /dez′mōpres′in/, an antidiuretic analog of vasopressin prescribed in the treatment of diabetes insipidus and nocturnal enuresis.

desmosis /dezmō′sis/, any disease of the connective tissue.

desmosome /dez′məsōm/ [Gk, *desmos,* band, *soma,* body], a small, circular, dense area within the intercellular bridge that forms the site of adhesion between certain epithelial cells, especially the stratified epithelium of the epidermis.

desonide /des′ənīd/, a topical corticosteroid prescribed for skin inflammation.

desoximetasone /desok′simet′əson/, a topical corticosteroid prescribed for skin inflammation.

desoxycorticosterone acetate /desok′sikôr′təkōstē′rōn/, a mineralocorticoid hormone prescribed in replacement therapy, in congenital adrenal hyperplasia, and in chronic primary adrenocortical insufficiency to prevent excessive loss of salt from the body.

despair, a feeling of hopelessness and a loss of hope.

desquamation /des′kwəmā′shən/ [L, *desquamare,* to take off scales], a normal process in which the cornified layer of the epidermis is sloughed in fine scales. **—desquamate,** *v.,* **desquamative** /deskwam′ətiv/, *adj.*

desquamative gingivitis, a gingival inflammation, characterized by peeling of the surface epithelium. In its chronic state it is most frequently associated with menopause caused by hormonal changes. It may also be associated with any biologic stress, such as trauma to the epithelium.

desquamative interstitial pneumonia, a respiratory disease characterized by an accumulation of cellular matter in the alveoli and bronchial tubes. It leads to a fibrotic condition with symptoms of coughing, chest pain, weight loss, and dyspnea.

destructive aggression /distruk′tiv/ [L, *destruere,* to destroy, *aggressio,* an attack], an act of hostility unnecessary for self-protection or preservation that is directed at an external object or person.

destructive interference, (in ultrasonography) a phenomenon that results when propagated waves are out of phase so that maximum molecular compression for one wave occurs at the same point as maximum rarefaction for the second wave.

destructive lesion [L, *destruere,* to destroy, *laesio,* a hurting], a disorder that leads to the damage or necrosis of an organ or tissue.

desudation /des′ōōdā′shən/, profuse sweating. It is sometimes followed by a skin rash.

detection bias /ditek′shən/, a potential artifact in epidemiologic data caused by the use of a particular diagnostic technique or type of equipment.

detergent /ditur′jənt/ [L, *detergere,* to cleanse], **1.** a cleansing agent. **2.** (in respiratory therapy) a wetting agent that is administered to mediate the removal of respiratory tract secretions from airway walls.

deterioration /ditir′ē·ərā′shən/ [L, *deterior,* worse], a condition that is gradually worsening.

determinant evolution /ditur′minənt/ [L, *determinare,* to limit], the theory that evolution progresses according to a predetermined course.

determinants of occlusion, (in dentistry) the classifiable factors that influence proper closure of the teeth. The common fixed factors are the intercondylar distance, anatomic characteristics, mandibular centricity, and relationship of the jaws. The common changeable factors are tooth shapes, tooth positions, and vertical dimensions of occlusion, cusp height, and fossa depth.

determinate cleavage /ditur′minit/, mitotic division of the fertilized ovum into blastomeres that are each destined to form a specific part of the embryo. Damage to or destruction of any of these cells results in malformation of an organism.

detoxification /dētok′sifikā′shən/ [L, *de* + Gk, *toxikon,* poison; L, *facere,* to make], the removal of a poison or its effects from a patient.

detoxification service, a hospital service providing treatment to diminish or remove from a patient's body the toxic effects of chemical substances such as alcohol or drugs, usually as an initial step in the treatment of a chemical-dependent person. The service may also be used to remove poisonous substances to which a person may have been exposed.

detoxify /dētok′sifī/ [L, *de,* from; Gk, *toxikon,* poison], to make a poisonous substance harmless or to overcome the effects of a poison.

detrusor urinae muscle /ditrōō′zər/ [L, *detruder,* to thrust; Gk, *ouron,* urine; L, *musculus*], a complex of longitudinal fibers that form the external layer of the muscular coat of the bladder.

deuterium (²H) /dyōōtir′ē-əm/ [Gk, *deuteros,* second], a stable isotope of the hydrogen atom, used as a kinetic tracer.

deutoplasm /dōō′təplaz′əm/ [Gk, *deuteros + plasma,* something formed], the inactive elements of the protoplasm, primarily the stored nutritive material contained in the yolk.

DEV, abbreviation for duck embryo vaccine.

devascularization /dēvas′kyələr′īzā′shən/ [L, *de,* from; *vasculum,* small vessel], the drawing away of blood from a body part or stoppage of blood flow to it.

developer fog, (in radiology) a radiographic image that is dull, washed out, and lacking in contrast. Causes include incorrect developer temperature, immersion time, and developer concentration.

development [Fr, *developper,* to unfold], **1.** the gradual process of change and differentiation from a simple to a more advanced level of complexity. **2.** (in biology) the series of events that occur within an organism from the time of fertilization of the ovum to the adult stage. —**developmental,** *adj.*

developmental age (DA) /divel′əpmen′təl/, an expression of a child's maturational progress stated in age and determined by standardized measurements, as of body size and dimensions; social and psychologic functioning; motor skills; and mental and aptitude tests.

developmental agraphia, a deficiency in a child's ability to learn to form letters and write.

developmental anatomy, the study of the differentiation and growth of an organism from one cell to birth. Also called **embryology.**

developmental anomaly, any congenital defect that results from interference with the normal growth and differentiation of the fetus. Such defects can arise at any stage of embryonic development, vary greatly in type and severity, and are caused by a wide variety of determining

factors, including genetic mutations, chromosomal aberrations, teratogenic agents, and environmental factors.

developmental apraxia [L, *developper,* development; Gk, *a,* not, *prassein,* to do], a condition of ineffective motor planning and execution in children caused by immaturity of their central nervous system.

developmental crisis, severe, usually transient, stress that occurs when a person is unable to complete the tasks of a psychosocial stage of development and is therefore unable to move on to the next stage.

developmental disability (DD), a pathologic condition that starts developing before 18 years of age.

developmental disorder, a form of mental retardation that develops in some children who have progressed normally for the first 3 or 4 years of life.

developmental dyspraxia, a disorder of sensory integration characterized by an impaired ability to plan skilled, nonhabitual coordinated movements.

Developmental Enhancement, a Nursing Interventions Classification defined as facilitating or teaching parents or caregivers to facilitate the optimal gross motor, fine motor, language, cognitive, social, and emotional growth of preschool and school-aged children.

developmental groove, a fine, recessed line in the enamel of a tooth that marks the union of the lobes of the crown in its development.

developmental guidance, (in dentistry) the comprehensive dentofacial orthopedic control over the growth of the jaws and the eruption of the teeth. The control may be needed throughout the entire growth and maturation of the face, beginning at the earliest detection of a developing malformation.

developmental horizon, any of 25 stages in the development of the human embryo from the one-cell stage at conception to the morphologically and physiologically complex organism at the end of the seventh week of gestation.

developmental model, **1.** a conceptual framework devised to be used as a guide in making a diagnosis, in understanding a developmental process, and in forming a prognosis for continued development. **2.** (in nursing) a conceptual framework describing four stages, or processes, of development in the patient during therapy. In the first stage, called *orientation,* the patient begins a relationship with the nurse or other therapist and begins to clarify the problem with his or her help. In the second stage, called *identification,* the patient develops a sense of closeness and attachment to the therapist. In the third stage, called *exploitation,* the patient makes full use of the nursing services offered, begins to assume some control of the interactions, and becomes more independent. During the last stage, called *resolution,* the therapeutic relationship is terminated; the patient is independent and no longer needs the nurse or therapist.

developmental physiology, the study of the physiologic processes as they relate to embryonic development.

developmental quotient (DQ), the numeric expression of a child's developmental level as measured by dividing the developmental age by the chronologic age and multiplying by 100.

developmental sequence [Fr, *developper*; L, *sequi,* to follow], the order in which structure and function change during the process of growth and development of an organism.

developmental task, a physical or cognitive skill that a person must accomplish during a particular age period to continue development. An example is walking, which precedes the development of a sense of autonomy in the toddler period.

developmental theory of aging, a concept based on the premise that traits and characteristics developed early in life tend to continue into the later years.

deviance /dē′vē- əns/ [L, *deviare,* to turn aside], behavior that is contrary to the accepted standards of a community or culture.

deviant /dē′vē-ənt/ [L, *deviare,* to turn aside], pertaining to a person who or object that departs from what is considered normal or standard.

deviant behavior, actions that exceed the usual limits of accepted behavior and involve failure to comply with the social norm of the group.

deviate /dē′vē-it/ [L, *deviare,* to turn aside], **1.** a person or an act that varies from that which is considered standard, such as a social or sexual deviate, or that which is within a statistic norm. **2.** to vary from that which is considered standard or within a statistic norm. —**deviant,** *adj.,* **deviation,** *n.*

deviated septum, a shifted medial partition of the nasal cavity, a condition affecting many adults. The nasal septum more commonly shifts to the left during normal growth, but severe deflection of the septum may significantly obstruct the nasal passages and result in infection, sinusitis, shortness of breath, headache, or recurring nose bleeds.

deviation, axis /dē′vē-ā′shən/ [L, *deviare,* to turn aside, *axle*], (in electrocardiography) an abnormal direction of the mean electrical current of the heart.

deviation from normal, a quality, characteristic, symptom, or clinical finding that is different from what is commonly regarded as normal, such as an elevated temperature, multiple gestation, or an extra digit.

deviation of tongue [L, *deviare,* to turn aside; AS, *tunge*], a tendency of the tongue to turn away from the midline when extended or protruded. The condition is associated with a hypoglossal nerve defect.

device /divīs/ [OFr, *deviser,* to divide], an item other than a drug that has application in the healing arts. The term is sometimes restricted to items used directly by, on, or in the patient, as opposed to surgical instruments or other equipment used for diagnosis and treatment. Devices include orthopedic appliances, crutches, artificial heart valves, pacemakers, prostheses, wheelchairs, cervical collars, hearing aids, and eye glasses.

devitalized /dēvī′təlīzd/, pertaining to tissues with a reduced oxygen supply and blood flow.

dewar /dyoo′ər/, (in nuclear magnetic resonance imaging) a double chamber used to maintain the temperature of superconducting magnet coils at near absolute zero.

dew point /dyoo/, the temperature at which air becomes saturated with water vapor and the water vapor condenses to liquid. In aerosol therapy water may condense on containers, tubing, and other surfaces when the dew point is reached.

DEXA, abbreviation for **dual-energy x-ray absorptiometry.**

dexamethasone /dek′səmeth′əsōn/, a glucocorticoid prescribed in the treatment of inflammatory conditions.

dexchlorpheniramine maleate /deks′-klôrfənir′əmēn mal′ē-it/, an antihistamine prescribed in the treatment of hypersensitivity reactions, including rhinitis, skin rash, and pruritus.

dexrazone, a cardioprotective agent prescribed to protect women from heart problems caused by doxorubicin treatment of breast cancer.

dexter /deks′tər/ [L, *dexter,* right], right side, right.

dexterity /dekster′itē/ [L, *dexteritas*], skillfulness in the use of one's hands or body.

dextrad writing /deks′trad/ [L, *dexter,* right; ME, *writen*], writing that moves from left to right.

dextran fermentation /dek′strən/ [L, *dex-*

ter, right; *fermentare,* to cause to rise], the conversion of dextrose to dextran by the action of *Leuconostoc mesenteroides* dextran (LMD) bacteria.

dextran preparation, any of a group of solutions containing polysaccharides, water, and, in some preparations, electrolytes. These solutions are used as plasma volume extenders in cases of hypovolemia from hemorrhage, dehydration, or another cause.

dextrin, a glucose polymer formed by the hydrolysis of starch. It is a tasteless, colorless, gummy substance, soluble in water. Dextrin is an intermediate during the conversion of starch into monosaccharides, such as glucose.

dextroamphetamine sulfate /deks′trō-amfet′əmēn/, a central nervous system stimulant prescribed in the treatment of narcolepsy and hyperkinetic disorders in children and as an anorexiant in treating exogenous obesity.

dextrocardia /-kär′dē-ə/, the location of the heart in the right hemithorax, either as a result of displacement by disease or as a congenital defect.

dextrocardiogram /-kär′də-ōgram′/ [L, *dexter,* right; Gk, *kardia,* heart, *gramma,* record], an electrocardiogram made from a unipolar electrode facing the right ventricle, producing a complex of a small R wave and a large S wave.

dextromethorphan hydrobromide /-methôr′fən/, an antitussive derived from morphine, but lacking narcotic effects. It is prescribed for the suppression of nonproductive cough.

dextrose /dek′strōs/ [L, *dexter,* right], a glucose available in various solutions for intravenous administration. It is prescribed for calorie deficit, for hypoglycemia, and in solution for fluid deficit.

dextrose and sodium chloride injection, a fluid, nutrient, and electrolyte replenisher. It is available for parenteral use in a variety of concentrations.

dextrothyroxine sodium, an antihyperlipidemic prescribed in the treatment of hyperlipidemia.

df, abbreviation for **degrees of freedom.**

d4T, symbol for **dideoxythymidine.**

dg, abbreviation for **decigram.**

D gene, one of a set of genes lying between the V and J genes, which code for the immunoglobulin heavy chains, or lying in the T cell beta and gamma chain genes.

DHFS, abbreviation for **dengue hemorrhagic fever shock syndrome.**

DHHS, abbreviation for **Department of Health and Human Services.**

dhobie itch /dō′bē/ [Hindi, *dhobie,* laun-

dryman; AS, *giccan*], a form of contact dermatitis associated with the use of laundry marking fluids.

diabetes /dī′əbē′tēz/ [Gk, *diabainein,* to pass through], a clinical condition characterized by the excessive excretion of urine. The excess may be caused by a deficiency of antidiuretic hormone as in diabetes insipidus, or it may be the polyuria resulting from the hyperglycemia that occurs in diabetes mellitus.

diabetes insipidus /insip′idəs/, a metabolic disorder caused by injury of the neurohypophyseal system. It is characterized by copious excretion of urine and excessive thirst caused by deficient production or secretion of the antidiuretic hormone (ADH) or inability of the kidney tubules to respond to ADH. Rarely the symptoms are self-induced by an excessive water intake. The condition may be acquired, familial, idiopathic, neurogenic, or nephrogenic.

diabetes mellitus (DM) /məlī′təs/, a complex disorder of carbohydrate, fat, and protein metabolism that is primarily a result of a deficiency or complete lack of insulin secretion by the beta cells of the pancreas or defects of the insulin receptors. The disease is often familial but may be acquired, as in Cushing's syndrome, as a result of the administration of excessive glucocorticoid. The various forms of diabetes have been organized into categories developed by the National Diabetes Data Group of the National Institutes of Health. Type I diabetes in this classification scheme includes patients dependent on insulin to prevent ketosis. The category is also known as the insulin-dependent diabetes mellitus (IDDM) subclass. Patients with type II, or noninsulin-dependent diabetes mellitus (NIDDM), are those previously designated as having maturity-onset diabetes, adult-onset diabetes, ketosis resistant diabetes, or stable diabetes. Those with gestational diabetes mellitus are women in whom glucose intolerance develops during pregnancy. Secondary diabetes is associated with a pancreatic disease, hormonal changes, adverse effects of drugs, or genetic or other anomalies. A fifth subclass, the impaired glucose tolerance group, includes persons whose blood glucose levels are abnormal although not sufficiently above the normal range to be diagnosed as diabetic. Contributing factors to the development of diabetes are heredity; obesity; sedentary life-style; high-fat, low-fiber diets; hypertension; and aging.

diabetic /dī′əbet′ik/, **1.** pertaining to diabetes. **2.** affected with diabetes. **3.** a person who has diabetes mellitus.

diabetic acidosis [Gk, *diabainein,* to pass through; L, *acidus,* acid; Gk, *osis,* condition], a type of acidosis that may occur in diabetes mellitus as a result of excessive production of ketone bodies during oxidation of fatty acids.

diabetic amaurosis [Gk, *diabainein,* to pass through, *amaurosein,* to darken], blindness associated with diabetes, caused by a proliferative hemorrhagic form of retinopathy that is characterized by capillary microaneurysms and hard or waxy exudates. Cataracts are also common in diabetes.

diabetic center, a cluster of nerve cells on the floor of the fourth ventricle of the brain.

diabetic coma, a life-threatening condition occurring in persons with diabetes mellitus. It is caused by inadequate treatment, failure to take prescribed insulin, excessive food intake, or, most frequently, infection, surgery, trauma, or other stressors that increase the body's need for insulin. Without insulin to metabolize glucose, fats are used for energy, resulting in ketone waste accumulation and metabolic acidosis. Warning signs of diabetic coma include a dull headache, fatigue, inordinate thirst, epigastric pain, nausea, vomiting, parched lips, flushed face, and sunken eyes. The temperature usually rises and then falls; the systolic blood pressure drops, and circulatory collapse may occur.

diabetic diet, a diet prescribed in the treatment of diabetes mellitus. It usually contains limited amounts of simple sugars or readily digestible carbohydrates and increased amounts of proteins, complex carbohydrates, and unsaturated fats. Dietary regulation depends on the severity of the disease and the type and extent of insulin therapy.

diabetic foot and leg care, the special attention given to prevent the circulatory disorders and infections that frequently occur in the lower extremities of diabetic patients. The patient's legs and feet are examined daily for signs of dry, scaly, red, itching, or cracked skin; blisters; corns; calluses; abrasions; infection; blueness and swelling around varicosities; and thickened, discolored nails. The feet are bathed daily in tepid water with mild or superfatted soap and are dried gently but thoroughly with a soft towel. A lanolin-based lotion is then applied.

diabetic gangrene [Gk, *diabainein,* to pass through, *gaggraina*], gangrene, usually involving the lower extremities, that develops secondary to peripheral vascular disease complications related to the diabetic disease process.

diabetic glycosuria [Gk, *diabainein,* to pass through, *glykys,* sweet, *ouron,* urine], excessive excretion of sugar into the urine as an effect of diabetes mellitus.

diabetic ketoacidosis (DKA), diabetic coma, an acute, life-threatening complication of uncontrolled diabetes mellitus. In this condition urinary loss of water, potassium, ammonium, and sodium results in hypovolemia, electrolyte imbalance, extremely high blood glucose levels, and breakdown of free fatty acids, causing acidosis, often with coma. The person appears flushed; has hot, dry skin; is restless, uncomfortable, agitated, and diaphoretic; and has a fruity odor to the breath. Coma, confusion, and nausea are often noted.

diabetic neuropathy, a noninflammatory disease process associated with diabetes mellitus and characterized by sensory and/or motor disturbances in the peripheral nervous system. Patients commonly experience degeneration of sensory nerves and pathways. Early symptoms, which include pain and loss of reflexes in the legs, may occur in patients with only mild hyperglycemia. Diabetes is associated with a wide range of neuropathies, including mononeuritis multiplex, compression and entrapment mononeuropathies, cranial neuropathies, and autonomic and small fiber neuropathies. Differential diagnosis is difficult because not all sensorimotor neuropathies are caused by diabetes.

diabetic polyneuritis, a condition involving many nerves. It usually occurs as a complication in long-term cases of diabetes mellitus.

diabetic polyneuropathy, a long-term complication of diabetes mellitus in which a number of nerves are involved at the same time. Central nervous system, autonomic, and peripheral nerves may be affected. Neuropathic ulcers commonly develop on the feet.

diabetic retinopathy, a disorder of retinal blood vessels. It is characterized by capillary microaneurysms, hemorrhage, exudates, and the formation of new vessels and connective tissue. The disorder occurs most frequently in patients with long-standing, poorly controlled diabetes mellitus. Repeated hemorrhage may cause permanent opacity of the vitreous humor, and blindness may eventually result.

diabetic tabes, a wasting condition associated with diabetic peripheral neuropathy. It may be accompanied by sharp pain, muscle weakness, atrophy of intrinsic foot muscles, and weakness of the toes' extensors and flexors. It may lead to foot drop because of ankle weakness.

diabetic treatment, management of diabetes mellitus by means of a controlled carbohydrate diet, insulin injections, blood sugar level monitoring, or oral hypoglycemic agents such as chlorpropamide, acetohexamide, tolbutamide, and tolazamide.

diabetic vulvovaginitis [Gk, *diabainein,* to pass through; L, *vulva,* wrapper, *vagina,* sheath; Gk, *itis,* inflammation], a form of mycotic inflammation of the vulva and vagina that is associated with diabetes.

diabetic xanthoma, an eruption of yellow papules or plaques on the skin in uncontrolled diabetes mellitus. The lesion disappears as the metabolic functions are stabilized and the disease is controlled.

diabetogenic state /dī′əbet′ōjen′ik/, a health condition manifested by signs and symptoms of diabetes.

diacet, abbreviation for a *carboxylate diacetate anion.*

diacondylar fracture /dī′əkon′dilər/ [Gk, *dia,* through, *kondylos,* knuckle; L, *fractura,* break], any fracture that runs across the line of a condyle.

diadochokinesia /dī·ad′əkōkīnē′zhə/ [Gk, *diadochos,* successor, *kinesis,* motion], the normal ability of the muscles to move a limb alternately in opposite directions by flexion and extension.

diagnose /dī′agnōs/, to determine the type and cause of a health condition on the basis of signs and symptoms of the patient; data obtained from laboratory analysis of fluid, tissue specimens, and other tests; and family and occupational background information.

diagnosis /dī′agnō′sis/, *pl.* **diagnoses** [Gk, *dia + gnosis,* knowledge], **1.** identification of a disease or condition by a scientific evaluation of physical signs, symptoms, history, laboratory test results, and procedures. Kinds of diagnoses are **clinical diagnosis, differential diagnosis, laboratory diagnosis, nursing diagnosis,** and **physical diagnosis. 2.** the art of naming a disease or condition. —**diagnostic,** *adj.,* **diagnose,** *v.*

diagnosis by exclusion [Gk, *dia,* through, *gnosis,* knowledge; L, *excludere,* to shut out], diagnosis made by eliminating other possible causes of disease symptoms.

diagnosis-related group (DRG), a group of patients classified for measuring a medical facility's delivery of care. The classifications, used to determine Medicare payments for inpatient care, are based on primary and secondary diagnosis, primary and secondary procedures, age, and length of hospitalization.

diagnostic /dī′agnos′tik/, pertaining to a diagnosis.

Diagnostic and Statistical Manual of Men-

tal Disorders (DSM), a manual, published by the American Psychiatric Association, listing the official diagnostic classifications of mental disorders. The *DSM* recommends the use of a multiaxial evaluation system as a holistic diagnostic approach. It consists of five axes, each of which refers to a different class of information, including mental and physical data. Axes I and II include all of the mental disorders, classified broadly as clinical syndromes and personality disorders; axis III contains physical disorders and conditions; and axes IV and V provide a coded outline of supplemental information that may be useful for planning individual treatment and predicting its outcome. Each of the classifications of the mental disorders contains a code that provides a reference to the WHO *International Classification of Diseases (ICD).*

diagnostic anesthesia, a procedure in which analgesia is induced to a depth adequate to permit comfortable performance of moderately painful diagnostic procedures of short duration. Awake anesthesia is often used for this purpose.

diagnostician /dī′agnostish′ən/, a person skilled and trained in making diagnoses.

diagnostic medical sonographer, an allied health professional who provides patient services using diagnostic ultrasound under the supervision of a doctor of medicine or osteopathy responsible for the use and interpretation of ultrasound procedures. The sonographer assists the physician in gathering sonographic data necessary to reach diagnostic decisions.

diagnostic peritoneal lavage (DPL), a procedure used to detect intraabdominal bleeding or viscus perforation after abdominal trauma. The open or operative approach allows direct visual examination of the peritoneum when the catheter is inserted. Gastric and bladder decompression must precede performance of DPL.

diagnostic process, the act of determining a patient's health status and evaluating the factors influencing that status.

diagnostic radiology, medical imaging using external sources of radiation.

diagnostic radiopharmaceutical, a radioactive drug administered to a patient as a diagnostic tracer to differentiate normal from abnormal anatomic structures or biochemical or physiologic functions. Most diagnostic radioactive tracers indicate their position within the body by emitting gamma rays. By monitoring the emissions with a collimated external gamma-ray detector, the concentration of the tracer in different organs can be inferred, and low-resolution images of the organs can be obtained. Tracers prepared with tritium, carbon-14, or phosphorus-32, which do not emit gamma rays, are used diagnostically by analyzing the concentration of the isotope in a metabolic end product in the patient's blood, urine, breath, or biopsy samples.

diagnostic services, activities related to the diagnosis made by a physician, which may also be performed by nurses or other health professionals.

diagonal conjugate /dī·ag'ənəl/, a radiographic measurement of the distance from the inferior border of the symphysis pubis to the sacral promontory. The measurement averages around 12.5 to 13 cm in adult women.

diakinesis /dī'əkinē'sis, dī'əkī-/ [Gk, *dia* + *kinesis*, motion], the final stage in the first meiotic prophase in gametogenesis in which the chromosomes achieve maximum contraction and are ready to separate.

dial, a circular diagram with black lines radiating outward across a white background from the center, as is used in tests of astigmatism.

dialect /dī'əlekt/, a variation of a language different from other forms of the same language in pronunciation, syntax, and word meanings.

dialysate /dī·al'isāt/, the solution subjected to dialysis.

dialysis /dī·al'isis/ [Gk *dia* + *lysis* a loosening], **1.** the process of separating colloids and crystalline substances in solution by the difference in their rate of diffusion through a semipermeable membrane. **2.** a medical procedure for the removal of certain elements from the blood or lymph by virtue of the difference in their rates of diffusion through an external semipermeable membrane or, in the case of peritoneal dialysis, through the peritoneum.

dialysis dementia, a neurologic disorder that occurs in some patients undergoing dialysis. The precise cause is unknown, but the effect is believed to be related to chemicals in the dialyzing fluid, drugs administered to the dialysis patient, or both.

dialysis disequilibrium syndrome, a disorder caused by a rapid change in extracellular fluid composition during dialysis. It may be marked by cerebral or neurologic disturbances, cardiac arrhythmias, and pulmonary edema.

dialysis fluid, the solution that flows on the opposite side of a semipermeable membrane to blood.

dialysis shunt [Gk, *dia*, through, *lysis*, loosening; ME, *shunten*], an external artificial link between a peripheral artery

and a vein in an arm or leg for use in hemodialysis.

dialysis technician [Gk, *dia*, through, *lysis*, loosening, *technikos*, skillful], an allied health professional who operates and maintains dialysis equipment for patients with kidney diseases.

dialyzer /dī'əlī'zər/ [Gk, *dia* + *lysis*, loosening], **1.** a machine used in dialysis. **2.** a semipermeable membrane or porous diaphragm in a dialysis machine.

diameter of fetal skull [Gk, *diametros* + L, *fetus* + AS, *skulle*, bowl], the average distances between certain landmarks of the fetal skull as measured at term. These measurements include the following: biparietal, the fetal head between the two parietal eminences, 9.25 cm; occipitofrontal, from the external occipital protuberance to the most prominent point of the frontal midline, 11 cm; occipitomental, from the external occipital protuberance to the midpoint of the chin, 13 cm; and suboccipitobregmatic, from the lowest posterior point of the occipital bone to the center of the anterior fontanel, 9.5 cm.

Diameter-Index Safety System (DISS), a system of standardized connections between cylinders of medical gases and flowmeters or pressure regulators. Each type of gas and connector is assigned a DISS number such as 1040 for nitrous oxide.

Diamond-Blackfan syndrome, a rare congenital disorder evident in the first 3 months of life, characterized by severe anemia and very low reticulocyte count, but normal numbers of platelets and white cells.

diamond burr /dī'(ə)mənd/, (in dentistry) a rotary device that contains diamond chips as an abrasive.

diapedesis /dī'əpidē'sis/ [Gk, *dia* + *pedesis*, an oozing], the passage of red or white blood corpuscles through the walls of the vessels that contain them without damage to the vessels.

diaper rash [ME, *diapre*, patterned fabric], an erythematous, papular, or scaly eruption in the diaper area of infants caused by irritation from feces, moisture, heat, or ammonia produced by the bacterial decomposition of urine. Secondary infection by *Candida albicans* is common.

diaper restraint, a therapeutic device used especially in orthopedics for countertraction with lower-extremity traction when other methods of countertraction are not effective. Diaper restraints are commonly used in treating children with orthopedic diseases and abnormalities and are designed to fit over the pelvic area like diapers, with rings at each of four corners

A webbing strap is threaded through the rings and attached to the top side of the bedspring frame.

diaphanography /dī·af′ənog′rəfē/ [Gk, *diaphanes*, shining through, *graphein*, to record], a type of transillumination used to examine the breast, which uses selected wavelengths of light and special imaging equipment.

diaphanoscopy /dī·af′ənos′kəpē/, examination of an internal structure with a diaphanoscope, an instrument that transilluminates body tissues. It is sometimes used in the diagnosis of breast tumors.

diaphoresis /dī′əfərē′sis/ [Gk, *dia* + *pherein*, to carry], the secretion of sweat, especially the profuse secretion associated with an elevated body temperature, physical exertion, exposure to heat, and mental or emotional stress.

diaphragm /dī′əfram/ [Gk, *diaphragma*, partition], **1.** (in anatomy) a dome-shaped musculofibrous partition that separates the thoracic and abdominal cavities. The convex cranial surface of the diaphragm forms the floor of the thoracic cavity; the concave surface forms the roof of the abdominal cavity. This partition is pierced by various openings through which pass the aorta, esophagus, and vena cava. **2.** *informal.* a contraceptive diaphragm. **3.** (in optics) an opening that controls the amount of light passing through an optical network. **4.** a thin, membranous partition, as that used in dialysis. **5.** (in radiography) a metal plate with a small opening that limits the diameter of the radiographic beam. —**diaphragmatic,** *adj.*

diaphragmatic breathing /dī·əfragmat′ik/ [Gk, *diaphragma*, partition], a pattern of exhalation and inhalation in which most of the ventilatory work is done with the diaphragm. The technique is taught to patients with chronic obstructive pulmonary disease to facilitate respiration.

diaphragmatic flutter, rapid, rhythmic contractions of the diaphragm. The condition may simulate atrial flutter.

diaphragmatic hernia [Gk, *diaphragma*, partition; L, *rupture*], the protrusion of part of the stomach through an opening in the diaphragm, most commonly an abnormally enlarged esophageal hiatus. In some cases the intestines may also herniate into the chest. The enlargement of the normal opening for the esophagus may be caused by trauma, congenital weakness, increased abdominal pressure, or relaxation of ligaments of skeletal muscles; and it permits part of the stomach to slide into the thorax. A sliding hiatal hernia, one of the most common pathologic conditions of the up-

per gastrointestinal tract, may occur at any age but is most frequent in elderly and middle-aged people. A kind of diaphragmatic hernia is **hiatal hernia.**

diaphragmatic node, a node in one of three groups of thoracic parietal lymph nodes, situated on the thoracic side of the diaphragm and consisting of the anterior set, the middle set, and the posterior set.

diaphragmatic peritonitis, an inflammation of the lower surface of the diaphragm.

diaphragmatic pleurisy, inflammation of the pleural covering of the diaphragm, which produces severe pain in the epigastric and hypochondrial regions and occasionally referred pain via the phrenic nerve to the shoulder.

diaphragm stethoscope, an instrument for auscultation of bodily sounds. Originally designed by René Laënnec (1781–1826), it consists of a vibrating disk, or diaphragm, which transmits sound waves through tubing to two earpieces.

diaphyseal aclasis /dī′əfiz′ē·əl ak′ləsis/ [Gk, *dia* + *phyein*, to grow, *a, klasis*, not breaking], a relatively rare abnormal condition that affects the skeletal system. Characterized by multiple exostoses or bony protrusions, it is inherited as a dominant trait.

diaphyseal-epiphyseal fusion, a surgical procedure to eliminate the epiphyseal line and unite the epiphyseal and diaphyseal bones.

diaphysis /dī·af′isis/ [Gk, *dia* + *phyein*, to grow], the shaft of a long bone, consisting of a tube of compact bone enclosing the medullary cavity.

diarrhea /dī′ərē′ə/ [Gk, *dia* + *rhein*, to flow], the frequent passage of loose, watery stools. The stool may also contain mucus, pus, blood, or excessive amounts of fat. Diarrhea is usually a symptom of some underlying disorder. Conditions in which diarrhea is an important symptom are dysenteric disorders, malabsorption syndrome, lactose intolerance, irritable bowel syndrome, gastrointestinal tumors, and inflammatory bowel disease. In addition to stool frequency, patients may complain of abdominal cramps and generalized weakness. Untreated, severe diarrhea may lead to rapid dehydration and electrolyte imbalance. —**diarrheal, diarrheic,** *adj.*

diarrhea, a NANDA-accepted nursing diagnosis in which the causes of the condition include stress and anxiety; dietary intake; side effects of medications; inflammation, irritation, or malabsorption of the bowel; and effects of toxins, contaminants, or radiation. Defining characteristics include abdominal pain, cramping, increased frequency of elimination, increased frequency of bowel sounds, loose or liquid stools, urgency of defecation, and a change in the color of the feces.

Diarrhea Management, a Nursing Interventions Classification defined as prevention and alleviation of diarrhea.

diarticular /dī′artik′yələr/ [Gk, *di,* twice; L, *articulare,* to divide into joints], biarticular, or having two joints.

diastalsis /dī′əstal′sis/, a wave of alternating relaxation and contraction of the smooth muscles lining the walls of the small intestine in response to distension of the intestine.

diastasis /dī·as′təsis/ [Gk, *separation*], the forcible separation of two parts that normally are joined, such as separation of parts of a bone at an epiphysis or of two bones that lack a synovial joint.

diastasis recti abdominis, the separation of the two rectus muscles along the median line of the abdominal wall. In a newborn the condition is the result of incomplete development.

diastatic fermentation /dī′əstat′ik/ [Gk, *diastasis,* separation; L, *fermentare,* to cause to rise], the conversion of starch to glucose by the enzyme ptyalin.

diastema /dī′əstē′mə/ [Gk, *interval*], an abnormally large space between two teeth not caused by the loss of a tooth between them. It is most commonly located between the maxillary central incisors in adults.

diastole /dī·as′tələ/ [Gk, *dia + stellein,* to set], the period between contractions of the atria or the ventricles during which blood enters the relaxed chambers from the systemic circulation and the lungs. Ventricular diastole begins with the onset of the second heart sound and ends with the first heart sound. —**diastolic** /dī′əstol′ik/, *adj.*

diastolic /dī′əstol′ik/, pertaining to diastole, or the blood pressure at the instant of maximum cardiac relaxation.

diastolic augmentation, an increase in arterial diastolic blood pressure produced by a counterpulsation device such as an intraaortic balloon pump.

diastolic blood pressure, the minimum level of blood pressure measured between contractions of the heart. Diastolic pressures for an individual may vary with age, gender, body weight, emotional state, and other factors.

diastolic filling pressure, the blood pressure in the ventricle during diastole.

diastolic murmur [Gk, *dia,* between, *stellein,* to set; L, *murmur,* humming], a noise heard because of a turbulence of blood flow during ventricular relaxation.

With few exceptions, it is caused by organic heart disease.

diastolic thrill, a vibration felt over the heart during ventricular diastole. It may be caused by mitral stenosis, a patent ductus arteriosus, or severe aortic insufficiency.

diastrophic /dī′əstrof′ik/ [Gk, *diastrephein,* to distort], pertaining to a bent or curved condition of bones or distortion of other structures.

diastrophic dwarf, a person in whom short stature is caused by osteochondrodysplasia and is associated with various deformities of the bones and joints, including scoliosis, clubfoot, micromelia, hand defects, multiple joint contractures and subluxations, ear deformities, and cleft palate.

diataxia /dī′ətak′sē·ə/, ataxia affecting both sides of the body.

diathermal /dī′əthur′məl/, pertaining to the use of elevated local temperature in the treatment of a disorder. The raised temperature may be produced by high-frequency electric current, ultrasound, or microwave radiation.

diathermy /dī′əthur′mē/ [Gk, *dia + therme,* heat], the production of heat in body tissues for therapeutic purposes by high-frequency currents that are insufficiently intense to destroy tissues or to impair their vitality. Diathermy is used in treating chronic arthritis, bursitis, fractures, gynecologic diseases, sinusitis, and other conditions.

diathesis /dī·əthē′sis/, *pl.* **diatheses** [Gk, *arrangement*], an inherited physical constitution predisposing to certain diseases or conditions, many of which are believed associated with the Y chromosome because males appear to be more susceptible than females.

diazepam /dī·az′əpam/, a benzodiazepine sedative and tranquilizer prescribed in the treatment of anxiety, nervous tension, and muscle spasm and as an anticonvulsant.

diazoxide /dī′əzok′sīd/, a vasodilator used as an antihypertensive. It is prescribed for the emergency reduction of blood pressure in malignant hypertension and in some cases of hypoglycemia.

dibucaine /dī′bəkān/, a topical anesthetic ointment.

dic, (in cytogenetics) abbreviation for *dicentric.*

DIC, abbreviation for **disseminated intravascular coagulation.**

dicalcium phosphate and calcium gluconate with vitamin D, /dīkal′sē·əm/ a source of calcium and phosphorus. It is prescribed for hypocalcemia, especially in pregnancy and lactation.

dicephaly /dīsef′əlē/ [Gk, *di,* twice, *keph-*

ale, head], a developmental anomaly in which a fetus has two heads. —**dicephalous, dicephalic,** *adj.,* **dicephalus,** *n.*

dichlorphenamide /dī'klôrfen'əmīd/, a carbonic anhydrase inhibitor prescribed in the treatment of chronic glaucoma.

dichotomy /dīkot'əmē/ [Gk, *dicha,* in two, *temnein,* to cut], a division or separation into two equal parts.

dichroic stain /dīkrō'ik/, a radiographic film artifact caused by a colored chemical stain. The color may range from yellow to purple and is usually the result of improper processing.

dichromatic vision /dī'kromat'ik/ [Gk, *di,* twice, *chroma,* color; L, *visio*], a form of color vision in which only two of the three primary colors are perceived.

Dick test [George F. Dick, 1881–1967; Gladys R. H. Dick, 1881–1963; American physicians], a skin test for determining sensitivity to an erythrotoxin produced by the group A streptococci that cause scarlet fever.

dicloxacillin sodium /dī'kloksəsil'in/, a penicillinase-resistant penicillin prescribed in the treatment of staphylococcal infections, especially those caused by penicillinase-producing strains of staphylococci.

dicrotic notch /dīkrot'ik/, a phenomenon observed on the downstroke of the arterial pressure waveform. It represents closure of the aortic valve at the onset of ventricular diastole. Also observed on the pulmonary artery pressure waveform, the interval represents closure of the pulmonic valve.

dicrotic pulse, a pulse with two separate peaks, the second usually weaker than the first.

dicumarol /dīkyōō'mərol/, a synthetic anticoagulant prescribed for the prophylaxis and treatment of thrombosis and embolism.

dicyclomine hydrochloride /dīsī'kləmīn/, an anticholinergic prescribed as an adjunct to ulcer therapy.

didactic /dīdak'tik/ [Gr, *didaskein,* to teach], pertaining to teaching or instruction.

dideoxycytidine (ddC) /dī'dē·ok'sēsī'-tidēn/, an antiretroviral drug that prevents human immunodeficiency virus from multiplying. It is chemically related to **dideoxyinosine (DDI).**

dideoxyinosine (DDI) /dī'dē·oksē·in'ōsēn/, an antiretroviral drug used in the treatment of human immunodeficiency virus infections. DDI inhibits the enzyme reverse transcriptase, thereby restricting viral replication activity. Inside the body DDI is converted to dideoxyadenosine, which be-

comes incorporated into the deoxyribonucleic acid chain, interrupting its normal sequence and making viral replication impossible.

dideoxythymidine (d4T) /dī'dē'oksēthī'midin/, a drug used in the treatment of acquired immunodeficiency virus. Reported toxic effects include anemia and painful peripheral nerves.

didymitis /did'əmī'tis/, an inflammation in a testicle.

didymus /did'iməs/, a testis.

die[1], to cease living.

die[2], (in dentistry) a model of a prepared tooth made from a hard substance, usually dental stone.

diecious /dī·ē'shəs/ [Gk, *di* + *oikos,* house], an animal or plant that is sexually distinct, having either male or female reproductive organs.

dieldrin /dī·el'drin/, a highly toxic pesticide that is also poisonous to humans and animals if ingested, inhaled, or absorbed through the skin. It causes dysfunction of the central nervous system and may be a carcinogen.

diencephalon /dī'ənsef'əlon/ [Gk, *di* + *enkephalon,* brain], the part of the brain between the cerebrum and the mesencephalon. It consists of the hypothalamus, thalamus, metathalamus, and the epithalamus and includes most of the third ventricle.

diener /dē'nər/ [Ger, man-servant], an individual who maintains the hospital laboratory or equipment and facilities.

dienestrol /dī'ines'trôl/, an estrogen prescribed in the treatment of atrophic vaginitis and kraurosis vulvae.

dieresis /dī·er'əsis/, separation of a structure's parts by surgery or other means.

diet /dī'it/ [Gk, *diaita,* way of living], **1.** food and drink considered with regard to their nutritional qualities, composition, and effects on health. **2.** nutrients prescribed, regulated, or restricted as to kind and amount for therapeutic or other purposes. **3.** the customary allowance of food and drink regularly provided or consumed. — **dietetic,** *adj.*

dietary /dī'əter'ē/, pertaining to diet.

dietary amenorrhea [Gk, *diaita,* way of living, *a,* absence, *men,* month, *rhoia,* to flow], an interruption of menstruation caused by malnutrition, starvation, or excessive voluntary dieting.

dietary fiber, a generic term for nondigestible carbohydrate substances found in plant cell walls and surrounding cellular material, each with a different effect on the various gastrointestinal functions such as colon transit time, water absorption, and lipid metabolism. The main dietary fiber components are cellulose, lignin, hemicellulose, pectin, and gums.

dietetic assistant /dī'ətet'ik/, a person who assists in providing food-service supervision and nutritional-care services under the guidance of a registered dietitian. A dietetic assistant is usually required to complete a training program approved by the American Dietetic Association.

dietetic food, 1. a specially prepared low-calorie food, often containing artificial sweeteners. 2. a food prepared for any specific dietary need or restriction, such as salt-free or vegetarian food.

dietetics /dī'itet'iks/, the science of applying nutritional principles to the planning and preparation of foods and regulation of the diet in relation to both health and disease.

dietetic technician, a person qualified by an associate degree program approved by the American Dietetic Association who may assist in providing food service management or nutritional-care services under the supervision of a registered dietitian.

diethylcarbamazine citrate /dī-eth'əl-kärbam'əzēn/, an anthelmintic prescribed in the treatment of ascariasis, filariasis, onchocerciasis, loiasis, and tropical eosinophilia.

diethylpropion hydrochloride /dī-eth'il-prō'pē-on/, an appetite suppressant prescribed in the treatment of exogenous obesity.

diethylstilbestrol (DES) /-stilbes'trol/, synthetic hormone with estrogenic properties.

diethylstilbestrol diphosphate, an antineoplastic agent prescribed for inoperable, progressing prostatic cancer.

dieting syndrome, the extreme practice of following fad diets, often leading to harmful physical and psychologic effects.

Diet Staging, a Nursing Interventions Classification defined as instituting required diet restrictions with subsequent progression of diet as tolerated.

diet therapy, a nutritional therapy based on a person's normal nutritional requirements, but modified for a disease or disorder to provide appropriate changes in amount and form of nutrients, energy value, and texture of solids and liquids.

Dietl's crisis /dē'təlz/ [Joseph Dietl, Polish physician, 1804–1878; Gk, *krisis,* turning point], a sudden excruciating pain in the kidney, caused by distension of the renal pelvis, rapid ingestion of very large amounts of liquid, or kinking of a ureter that produces temporary occlusion of the flow of urine from the kidney.

differential /dif'əren'shəl/, pertaining to or creating a difference.

differential absorption [L, *differentia,* difference], (in radiology) the difference between x-rays absorbed photoelectrically and those not absorbed at all, resulting in the radiographic image.

differential diagnosis, the distinguishing between two or more diseases with similar symptoms by systematically comparing their signs and symptoms.

differential growth, a comparison of the various increases in size or the different rates of growth of dissimilar organisms, tissues, or structures.

differential threshold, the lowest limit at which two stimuli can be differentiated or distinguished.

diffential white blood cell count, an examination and enumeration of the distribution of leukocytes in a stained blood smear. The different kinds of white cells are counted and reported as percentages of the total examined.

diffrentiating agent, a substance such as a retinoid that induces a cell to stop dividing and to differentiate. Such agents may be capable of halting the proliferation of cancer cells.

differentiation /dif'əren'shē-ā'shən/ [L, *differentia,* difference], 1. (in embryology) a process in development in which unspecialized cells or tissues are systemically modified and altered to achieve specific and characteristic physical forms, physiologic functions, and chemical properties. 2. progressive diversification leading to complexity. 3. acquisition of functions and forms different from those of the original. 4. distinguishing of one thing or disease from another, as in differential diagnosis. 5. (in psychology) mental autonomy or separation of intellect and emotions so that one is not dominated by reactive anxiety of a family or group emotional system. 6. the first subphase of the separation-individuation phase in Mahler's system of preoedipal development. —**differentiate,** *v.*

differentiation therapy, a cancer therapy technique in which the malignant cell is regarded as having escaped the normal controls of cell growth and differentiation. The cancer cell is regarded as pathologically arrested at an early stage of differentiation, retaining the ability to proliferate.

diffraction /difrak'shən/ [L, *dis,* opposite of, *frangere,* to break], the bending and scattering of wavelengths of light or other radiation, such as the radiation that passes around obstacles in its path. X-ray diffraction is used in the study of the internal structure of cells. The x-rays are diffracted by cell parts into patterns that are indicative of chemical and physical structure.

diffuse /difyo͞oz/ [L, *diffundere*, to spread out], becoming widely spread, such as through a membrane or fluid.

diffuse abscess, an abscess that spreads into neighboring tissues beyond fibrous walls.

diffuse axonal injury (DAI), a type of brain injury caused by shearing forces that occur between different parts of the brain as a result of rotational acceleration. The corpus callosum and the brainstem are often affected.

diffused light, light in which the precise source cannot be seen while the apparent area of the source is increased.

diffuse erythema, skin redness or inflammation that is spread over a large body surface.

diffse esophageal spasm, abnormal contractions of the esophagus leading to difficult or painful swallowing and chest pain.

diffuse goiter, an enlargement of all parts of the thyroid gland. Symptoms are those of hyperthyroidism.

diffuse hypersensitivity pneumonia, an immunologically mediated inflammatory reaction in the lungs induced by exposure to an allergen or an adverse reaction to a drug. The disorder is characterized by cough, fever, dyspnea, malaise, pulmonary edema, and infiltration of the alveoli with eosinophils and large mononuclear cells.

diffuse idiopathic skeletal hyperostosis, a form of degenerative joint disease in which the ligaments, along the spinal column, become calcified and lose their flexibility.

diffuse myocardial fibrosis, a type of heart disease characterized by a generalized distribution of fibrous tissue that replaces normal heart muscle cells.

diffuse peritonitis [L, *diffundere*, to spread out; Gk, *peri*, near *teinein*, to stretch, *itis*, inflammation], widespread peritonitis affecting most of the peritoneum, usually caused by a ruptured stomach or appendix.

diffuse sclerosis [L, *diffundere*, to spread out; Gk, *sklerosis*, hardening], a form of sclerosis that extends through much of the central nervous system.

diffusing capacity /difyo͞o'sing/, the rate of gas transfer through a unit area of a permeable membrane per unit of gas pressure difference across it. It is affected by specific chemical reactions that may occur in the blood.

diffusing capacity of lungs (D$_L$), the number of milliliters of a gas that diffuse from the lung across the alveolar-capillary (A-C) membrane into the bloodstream each minute for each 1 mm Hg difference in the pressure gradient across the membrane.

diffusion /difyo͞o'zhən/ [L, *diffundere*, to spread out], the process in which particles in a fluid move from an area of higher concentration to an area of lower concentration, resulting in an even distribution of the particles in the fluid.

diffusion constant, a mathematical constant relating to the ability of a substance to spread widely.

diffusion defect, any impairment of alveolar-capillary diffusion caused by pathologic changes in any of the structures of the alveolar-capillary membrane and causing fewer molecules of oxygen to cross the membrane.

diffusion deposition, the impaction of an aerosol particle on the surface of an alveolar membrane or other airway structure, causing it to settle out of a vapor or gas.

diffusion of gases, a natural process, essential in respiration, in which molecules of a gas pass from an area of high concentration to one of lower concentration.

diflorasone diacetate /diflôr'əson dī·os'-ətāt/, a topical corticosteroid prescribed for skin inflammation.

diflunisal /diflo͞o'nisal/, a nonsteroidal antiinflammatory agent prescribed for mild to moderate pain and inflammation in osteoarthritis and other musculoskeletal disorders.

digastricus /dīgas'trikəs/ [Gk, *di*, twice, *gaster*, stomach], one of four suprahyoid muscles having two parts, an anterior belly and a posterior belly. The anterior belly acts to open the jaw and draw the hyoid bone forward. The posterior belly acts to draw back and raise the hyoid bone.

DiGeorge's syndrome /dijôrj'əz/ [Angelo M. DiGeorge, American physician, b. 1921], a congenital disorder characterized by severe immunodeficiency and structural abnormalities, including hypertelorism; notched, low-set ears; small mouth; downward slanting eyes; cardiovascular defects; and absence of the thymus and parathyroid glands.

digest [L, *digerere*, to break down], **1.** /dijest'/ to soften by heat and moisture. **2.** /dijest'/, to break into smaller parts and simpler compounds by mastication, hydrolysis, and action of intestinal secretions and enzymes. **3.** /dī'jəst/, any material that results from digestion or hydrolysis.

digestant /dijes'tənt/, a substance such as pepsin that is added to the diet as an aid to the digestion of food.

digestible /dijes'tibəl/, capable of being digested.

digestion /dijes'chən/ [L, *digerere*, to break down], the conversion of food into absorbable substances in the gastrointestinal tract. Digestion is accomplished through the mechanical and chemical breakdown of food into smaller and smaller molecules, with the help of glands located both inside and outside the gut. —**digestive,** *adj.*

digestive enzyme /dijes′tiv/ [L, *digerere,* to break down; Gk, *en* + *zyme,* ferment], any digestive system enzyme that hydrolyzes fats, proteins, and carbohydrates for absorption.

digestive fever, a slight rise in body temperature that normally accompanies the digestive process.

digestive gland, any one of the many structures that secrete agents involved in the breaking down of food into the constituent absorbable substances needed for metabolism. Some kinds of digestive glands are the salivary glands, gastric glands, intestinal glands, liver, and pancreas.

digestive juice, a thin, colorless secretion of the glands of the human stomach, composed mainly of hydrochloric acid, chymosin, pepsinogen, intrinsic factor, and mucus.

digestive system, the organs, structures, and accessory glands of the digestive tube of the body through which food passes from the mouth to the esophagus, stomach, and intestines. The accessory glands secrete the digestive enzymes, which break down food substances in preparation for absorption into the bloodstream.

digestive tract, a musculomembranous tube, about 9 m long, extending from the mouth to the anus and lined with mucous membrane. Its various parts are the mouth, pharynx, esophagus, stomach, small intestine, and large intestine. The tube, which is part of the digestive system, includes numerous accessory organs.

digital /dij′itəl/ [L, *digitus,* finger], **1.** pertaining to a digit, that is, a finger or toe. **2.** resembling a finger or toe. See also **digitate. 3.** the characterization or measurement of a signal in terms of a series of numbers rather than some continuously varying value.

digital angiography, a technique of producing enhanced radiographic images of the heart and great vessels with computed fluoroscopy equipment.

digital compression [L, *digitus,* finger, *comprimere,* to press together], the act of pressing with the fingers, as when arresting the blood flow from a wound.

digital fluoroscopy, a method of conducting fluoroscopic examinations with an image-intensifier television system combined with a high-speed digital video image processor.

digitalis /dij′ital′is/ [L, *digitus,* finger], a general term for cardiac glycoside. It is prescribed in the treatment of congestive heart failure and certain cardiac arrhythmias.

digitalis poisoning [L, *digitalis,* of the fingers, *potio,* drink], the toxic effects of digitalis medications prescribed for heart disorders such as heart failure and atrial fibrillation. Toxicity may result from the cumulative effect of the drug or from hypokalemia. Symptoms include vomiting, headache, heartbeat abnormalities, and visual color distortions.

digitalis therapy, the administration of a digitalis preparation to a person with a heart disorder to increase the force of myocardial contractions; produce a slower, more regular apical rate; and slow the transmission of impulses through the conduction system. It may be used in treating many cardiac disorders, including atrial fibrillation, atrial septal defect, coarctation of the aorta, congenital heart block, congestive heart failure, endocardial fibroelastosis, great vessel transposition, malformation of the tricuspid valve, myocarditis, paroxysmal atrial tachycardia, and patent ductus arteriosus.

digitalization /dij′ətal′īzā′shən/, the administration of digitalis in doses sufficient to achieve maximum pharmacologic effects without producing toxic symptoms.

digitalized /dij′ətəlīzd′/, having a therapeutic total body level of digitalis, a cardiac glycoside.

digitalizing dose, the amount of digitalis needed to achieve the desired therapeutic effect.

digital radiography (DR) /dij′itəl/, any method of radiographic image formation that uses a computer to store and manipulate data.

digital reflex, 1. a finger-jerk reaction produced by tapping the palmar aspect of the terminal phalanges of the fingers when they are slightly flexed. **2.** sudden flexion of the terminal phalanx of the thumb produced by tapping the terminal phalanx of the middle finger.

digital subtraction angiography (DSA), a method by which radiographic images of blood vessels filled with contrast material are digitized and then subtracted from images stored before the administration of contrast. Thus the background is eliminated, and only the vessels appear.

digital-to-analog converter, a device for translating digital information into a continuous form, as from an ohmmeter or thermometer.

digital tomosynthesis, a system of tomography using a computer and digital fluoroscopy unit, making it possible to synthesize any tomographic plane from a single tomographic pass.

digitate /dij′itāt/ [L, *digitatus,* having fingers], having fingers or fingerlike projections.

digitate wart, a fingerlike horny projection that arises from a pea-shaped base. It is a benign viral infection of the skin and the adjacent mucous membrane.

digitoxin /dig′itok′sin/, a cardiac glycoside obtained from leaves of *Digitalis purpurea.* It is prescribed in the treatment of congestive heart failure and certain cardiac arrhythmias.

digit span test, an examination of the ability of a child to recall a sequence of numbers just spoken.

diglyceride /dīglis′ərīd/, a chemical compound, an ester of glycerol in which the hydrogen in two of the hydroxyl groups is replaced by an acyl radical.

dignathus /dīnath′əs, dignā′thəs/, **1.** a fetus with a double lower jaw. **2.** a person with a cleft of the mandible.

digoxin /digok′sin/, a cardiac glycoside obtained from leaves of *Digitalis lanata.* It is prescribed in the treatment of congestive heart failure and certain cardiac arrhythmias.

digoxin immune Fab, ovine, a parenteral antidote for digoxin toxicity. It is prescribed for life-threatening digoxin or digitoxin toxicity.

dihybrid /dī′hī′brid/ [Gk, *di,* twice; L, *hybrida,* mongrel offspring], (in genetics) pertaining to or describing a person, organism, or strain that is heterozygous for two specific traits.

dihybrid cross, (in genetics) the mating of two individuals, organisms, or strains that have different gene pairs that determine two specific traits or in which two particular characteristics or gene loci are being followed.

dihydric alcohol /dīhī′drik/, an alcohol containing two hydroxyl groups.

dihydroergotamine mesylate /dīhī′drō ərgot′əmēn me′silāt/, an alpha-adrenergic blocking agent prescribed for migraine and vascular headache.

dihydrotachysterol /dīhī′drōtəkis′tərol/, a rapid-acting form of vitamin D prescribed in the treatment of hypocalcemia resulting from hypoparathyroidism and pseudohypoparathyroidism.

dilate /dī′lāt/, to cause a physiologic increase in the diameter of a body opening, blood vessel, or tube.

dilation [L, *dilatare,* to widen], **1.** the condition of being dilated or stretched. **2.** the process of causing a physiologic increase in the diameter of a body opening, blood vessel, or tube.

dilation and curettage (D&C), widening of the uterine cervix and scraping of the endometrium of the uterus. It is done to diagnose disease of the uterus, to correct heavy or prolonged vaginal bleeding, or to empty uterine contents of the products of conception. It is also performed to remove tumors, to rule out carcinoma of the uterus, to remove retained placental fragments after delivery or after an incomplete abortion, and to find the cause of infertility.

dilation and evacuation (D&E) /dīlā′shən/ [L, *dilatare,* to widen, *evacuare,* to empty], the removal of the products of conception, using suction curettage and forceps, during the second trimester of pregnancy; a type of abortion.

dilation of the heart [L, *dilatare,* to widen; AS, *heorte*], an enlargement of the heart caused by stretching of the muscle tissue in the walls as a result of a weakening of the myocardium. The condition is associated with acute pulmonary embolism and heart failure.

dilator /dī′lātər/ [L, *dilatare,* to widen], a device for expanding a body opening or cavity.

dilator naris /dil′ətā′tər/, the alar part of the nasalis muscle that dilates the nostril.

dilator pupillae, a muscle that contracts the iris of the eye and dilates the pupil.

diltiazem /diltī′əzam/, a slow calcium channel blocker or calcium antagonist. It is prescribed for the treatment of vasospastic and effort-associated angina, in addition to hypertension.

diluent /dil′o̅o̅·ənt, dil′yo̅o̅·ənt/ [L, *diluere,* to wash], a substance, generally a fluid, that makes a solution or mixture less concentrated, less viscous, or more liquid.

dilute /dilo̅o̅t′, di′lo̅o̅t/ [L, *diluere,* to wash], **1.** pertaining to a solution that contains a relatively small amount of solute in proportion to solvent. **2.** to make a more concentrated solution less concentrated.

diluting agent /dilo̅o̅′ting/, (in respiratory therapy) a substance that can modify the viscosity of secretions so they can be removed easily. Examples include water and hypotonic saline solution, which can be aerosolized or nebulized.

dimenhydrinate /dim′ənhī′drināt/, an antihistamine prescribed in the treatment of nausea and motion sickness.

dimension, a measure of the width, length, or height of a space, usually described in units of a linear scale.

dimensional stability /dimen′shənəl/, (in

radiology) the rigidity of the polyester base used for radiographic film and its resistance to image distortion from warping or changing size or shape during processing.

dimer /dī'mər/ [Gk, *di,* twice, *meros,* parts], a compound formed by the union of two radicals or two molecules of a simpler compound, as a polymer formed from two or more molecules of a monomer.

dimercaprol /dī'mərkap'rol/, a heavy-metal antagonist. It is prescribed in the treatment of Wilson's disease and acute arsenic, mercury, or gold poisoning, as from an overdosage with mercurial diuretics, arsenics, or gold salts.

dimethindene maleate /dīmeth'indēn/, an antihistamine prescribed in the treatment of hypersensitivity reactions, including rhinitis, skin reactions, and itching.

dimethisterone /dī'məthis'tərōn/, an orally active progestational agent with no androgenic, estrogenic, or anabolic activity.

dimethoxymethylamphetamine (DOM), /dī'məthok'sēmeth'iləmfet'əmēn/ a psychoactive or hallucinogenic agent.

dimethylamine [(CH₃)₂NH], a secondary amine found in guano and decomposing fish.

dimethyl sulfoxide (DMSO) /dīmeth'il/, an antiinflammatory agent and organic solvent. It is prescribed in the treatment of interstitial cystitis and is being investigated as a topical antiinflammatory agent in orthopedic sports injuries.

dimorphous /dīmôr'fəs/ [Gk, *di,* twice, *morphe,* form], (in biology, chemistry, genetics) pertaining to an organism or substance that exists in two distinct forms.

dimple, 1. a slight natural indentation or depression on a body surface, such as on the cheek. **2.** a depression on a body surface resulting from contracting scar tissue or trauma.

dimpled sign, a physical diagnostic test to differentiate between a benign dermatofibroma lesion and a nodular melanoma. On pressure of the examiner's thumb and index finger benign tumors dimple, but malignant growths do not.

dimpling [ME, *dympull*], small, abnormal indentations or depressions on the surface of a body or organ.

dinitrochlorobenzene (DNCB) /dīnī'-trōklôr'ōben'zēn/, a substance applied topically as a test for delayed hypersensitivity reactions. The compound has also been used as an immunotherapeutic agent to treat skin tumors.

dinitrophenol, 1. a dye used in biochemical research into oxidative processes. **2.** a hapten commonly used to induce immune response.

dinucleotide, a compound containing two nucleotides.

diode /dī'od/, (in radiology) an x-ray tube or any electrical or electronic device with two electrodes.

diode laser, a solid-state semiconductor used as a lasing medium.

diolamine /dī·ol'əmēn/, abbreviated form for *diethanolamine.*

Dionysian /dē·onis'ē·ən/ [Gk, *Dionysos,* Greek god of wine], the personal attitude of one who is uninhibited, mystic, sensual, emotional, and irrational and who may seek to escape from the boundaries imposed by the limits of the senses.

diopter /dī·op'tər/ [Gk, *dioptra,* optical measuring instrument], a metric measure of the refractive power of a lens. It is equal to the reciprocal of the focal length of the lens in meters. For example, a lens with a focal length of 0.5 m has a diopter measure of 2.0 (1/0.5) and when prescribed as a corrective lens for the eye should make printed matter most clearly focused when it is held 0.5 m from the eyes.

dioptric power /dī·op'trik/, the refractive power of an optic lens as measured in diopters.

diovulatory /dī·ov'yəlǝtôr'ē/ [Gk, *di,* twice; L, *ovum,* egg], routinely releasing two ova during each ovarian cycle.

dioxide /dī·ok'sīd/ [Gk, *di,* twice, *oxys,* sharp, *genein,* to produce], an oxide that contains two oxygen atoms.

dioxin /dī·ok'sin/, a contaminant of the herbicide 2,4,5-trichlorophenoxyacetic acid (2,4,5-T), widely used throughout the world. Exposure to dioxin is associated with chloracne and porphyria cutanea tarda. Dioxin was a contaminant of the jungle defoliant Agent Orange.

dioxyline phosphate /dī·ok'silēn/, a synthetic antispasmodic and vasodilator prescribed for the relief of angina pectoris and for spasm of blood vessels in arms, legs, or lungs.

DIP, abbreviation for **desquamative interstitial pneumonia.**

dipeptidases /dīpep'tidāz/, the final enzymes in the protein-splitting system of digestion. They complete the task of breaking two-amino-acid dipeptides into single amino acids.

dipeptide, an organic compound formed by the union of two amino acids, with the link provided by the carboxyl group of one molecule and the amine group of the other.

diphasic /dīfā'zik/ [Gk, *di,* twice, *phasis,* appearance], pertaining to something that occurs in two stages or phases.

diphemanil methylsulfate /dīfē'mənil/, an anticholinergic prescribed as an adjunct to ulcer therapy.

diphenadione /dī'fənad'ē-ōn/, an anticoagulant prescribed in the treatment of thrombosis and embolism.

diphenhydramine /dī'fenhī'drəmēn/, an antihistamine that works both centrally and peripherally. A drug with potent anticholinergic effects, it is one of the most commonly used antihistamines.

diphenhydramine hydrochloride, an antihistamine prescribed in the treatment of hypersensitivity reactions, including rhinitis, skin rash, and pruritus, and in the treatment of motion sickness.

diphenidol /dīfē'nidol/, an antiemetic, antivertigo agent prescribed in the treatment of vertigo and vomiting.

diphenoxylate hydrochloride /dī'fənok'-silāt/, an antidiarrheal prescribed in the treatment of noninfectious diarrhea and intestinal cramping.

diphenylpyraline hydrochloride /dī'fenəl-pī'rəlēn/, an antihistamine prescribed in the treatment of hypersensitivity reactions, including rhinitis, skin rash, and pruritus.

2,3-diphosphoglyceric acid (DPG) /dī-fos'fōgliser'ik/, a substance in the erythrocyte that affects the affinity of hemoglobin for oxygen. It is a chief end product of glucose metabolism.

diphtheria /difthir'ē-ə, dipthir'ē-ə/ [Gk, *diphthera,* leather membrane], an acute contagious disease caused by the bacterium *Corynebacterium diphtheriae.* It is characterized by the production of a systemic toxin and a false membrane lining of the mucous membrane of the throat. The toxin is particularly damaging to the tissues of the heart and central nervous system; and the dense pseudomembrane in the throat may interfere with eating, drinking, and breathing. Untreated, the disease is often fatal, causing heart and kidney failure.

diphtheria and tetanus toxoids (DT), an active immunizing agent prescribed for immunization against diphtheria and tetanus.

diphtheria and tetanus toxoids and pertussis vaccine (DTP), an active immunizing agent prescribed for the routine immunization of children less than 6 years of age against diphtheria, tetanus, and pertussis.

diphtheria antitoxin [Gk, *diphtheria,* leather membrane, *anti,* against, *toxikon,* poison], an antitoxin prepared by immunizing horses with diphtheria toxoid and extracting the serum.

diphtherial cough /difthir'ē-əl/, a brassy, noisy, crouplike cough accompanied by stridulous breathing, observed mainly in children with laryngeal diphtheria.

diphtheria toxin [Gk, *diphtheria* + *toxikon,* poison] the filtrate of a broth culture used to prepare an intradermal injectable form of toxin for Schick tests.

diphtheritic croup /dif'thirit'ik/ [Gk, *diphtheria* + Scot, *croak,* to speak hoarsely], a diphtheritic inflammation of the larynx.

diphtheritic laryngitis [Gk, *diphtheria, larynx, itis,* inflammation], an inflammation of the larynx caused by the Klebs-Löffler bacillus *(Corynebacterium diphtheriae).* A serious complication is formation of a false membrane.

diphtheritic membrane, a membrane of coagulated fiber with bacteria and leukocytes. It is usually white or grayish yellow with well-defined margins.

diphtheritic pharyngitis [Gk, *diphtheria* + *pharynx,* throat, *itis,* inflammation], an inflammation of the pharynx caused by an infection of the Klebs-Löffler bacillus *(Corynebacterium diphtheriae)* and associated with the formation of a false membrane.

diphtheritic sore throat, an inflammation of the pharynx or larynx caused by an infection of *Corynebacterium diphtheriae.*

diphtheritic stomatitis, an inflammation of the mucous membrane of the mouth, caused by *Corynebacterium diphtheriae.*

diphtheroid /dif'thəroid'/ [Gk, *diphthera,* leather membrane, *eidos* form], **1.** pertaining to diphtheria. **2.** resembling the bacillus *Corynebacterium diphtheriae.*

Diphyllobothrium /dəfil'ōboth'rē-əm/ [Gk, *di,* twice, *phyllon,* leaf, *bothrion,* pit], a genus of large parasitic intestinal flatworms. The species that most often infects humans is *Diphyllobothrium latum.*

dipivefrin /dī'pivef'rin/, an ophthalmic adrenergic prescribed in the treatment of open-angle glaucoma

diplegia /dīplē'jē-ə/ [Gk, *di,* twice, *plege,* stroke], paralysis of both sides of any body part or of like parts on the opposite sides of the body. A kind of diplegia is **facial diplegia.** —**diplegic,** *adj.*

diplococcus /dip'lokok'əs/, *pl,* **diplococci** /-kok'sī/ [Gk, *diploos,* double, *kokkos* berry], **1.** a member of the Coccaceae family that occurs in pairs. Diplococci are often found as parasites or saprophytes. **2.** describing bacteria of the Coccaceae family, which occur as pairs of cocci.

diploë /dip'lō-ē/, the loose tissue filled with red bone marrow between the two tables of the cranial bones.

diploid /dip'loid/ [Gk, *diploos* + *eidos,* form], pertaining to an individual, organism, strain, or cell that has two complete sets of homologous chromosomes. —**diploidic,** *adj.*

diploidy /dip′loidē/, the state or condition of having two complete sets of homologous chromosomes.

diplokaryon /dip′lōker′ē·on/ [Gk, *diploos* + *karyon,* nut], a nucleus that contains twice the diploid number of chromosomes.

diploma program in nursing, an educational program that is designed to prepare nursing students for entry into practice, usually in 2 or 3 years. The recipient of a diploma is eligible to take the national certifying registration examination to become a registered nurse.

diplomate /dip′ləmāt/, an individual who has earned a diploma or certificate, especially a physician who has been certified by a specialty board.

diplonema /dip′lənē′mə/ [Gk, *diploos,* + *nema,* thread], the looplike formation of the chromosomes in the diplotene stage of the first meiotic prophase of gametogenesis.

diplopagus /diplop′əgəs/ [Gk, *diploos* + *pagos,* something fixed], conjoined twins that are more or less equally developed, although one or several internal organs may be shared.

diplopia /diplō′pē·ə/ [Gk, *diploos* + *opsis,* vision], double vision caused by defective function of the extraocular muscles or a disorder of the nerves that innervate the muscles.

diplornavirus /dī′plôrnəvī′rəs/, a double-stranded ribonucleic acid virus that is the cause of Colorado tick fever. It is related to the reoviruses that are associated with various respiratory infections.

diplosomatia /dip′lōsōmā′shə/ [Gk, *diploos* + *soma,* body], a congenital anomaly in which fully formed twins are joined at one or more areas of their bodies.

diplotene /dip′lətēn/ [Gk, *diploos* + *tainia,* ribbon], the fourth stage in the first meiotic prophase in gametogenesis in which the tetrads exhibit chiasmata between the chromatids of the paired homologous chromosomes and genetic crossing over occurs.

dipodia /dīpō′dē·ə/ [Gk, *di,* twice, *pous,* foot], a developmental anomaly characterized by the duplication of one or both feet.

dipole /dī′pol/, **1.** a molecule whose ends carry opposite partial charges. **2.** a molecule with areas of opposing electrical charges, as hydrogen chloride, which has a predominance of electrons about the chloride part and a positive charge on the hydrogen side.

diprop, abbreviation for a *carboxylate dipropionate anion.*

diprosopus /dīpros′əpəs, dī′prəsō′pəs/ [Gk, *di,* twice, *prosopon,* face], a malformed fetus that has a double face showing varying degrees of development.

dipsesis /dipsē′sis/, extreme thirst.

dipsomania /dip′sōmā′nē·ə/ [Gk, *dipsa,* thirst, *mania,* madness], an uncontrollable, often periodic craving for and indulgence in alcoholic beverages; alcoholism.

dipstick, a chemically treated strip of paper used in the analysis of urine or other fluids.

dipus /dī′pəs/, conjoined twins that have only two feet.

dipygus /dīpī′gəs, dip′əgəs/ [Gk, *di,* twice, *pyge,* rump], a malformed fetus that has a double pelvis, one of which is usually not fully developed.

dipyridamole /dī′pirid′əmōl/, a coronary vasodilator prescribed for the long-term treatment of angina.

direct agglutination test, a test for the presence of antibodies to a specific antigen in which a dilute antiserum is mixed with the antigen in question.

direct antagonist [L, *diregere,* to direct; Gk, *antagonisma,* struggle], one of a pair or a group of muscles that pull in opposite directions, whose combined action prevents the part from moving.

direct blood donation, the donation of a unit of blood for transfusion into a specific individual.

direct calorimetry, the measurement of the amount of heat directly generated by any oxidation reaction, especially one involving a living organism.

direct causal association, a cause-and-effect relationship between a causative factor and a disease with no other factors intervening in the process.

direct contact, mutual touching of two individuals or organisms. Many communicable diseases may be spread by direct contact between an infected and a healthy person.

direct costs, (in managed care) the costs of labor, supplies, and equipment to provide direct patient care services.

direct current (DC), an electric current that flows in one direction only and is substantially constant in value.

direct endometriosis [L, *diregere,* to direct; Gk, *endon,* within, *metra,* womb, *osis,* condition], an invasion of the muscular wall of the uterus by the mucous membrane lining.

direct-exposure film, a type of x-ray film sometimes used to produce images of thin body parts such as the hands and feet that have a high subject contrast.

direct fracture, any fracture occurring at a specific point of injury that is a direct result of that injury.

direct gold, any form of pure gold that may be compacted or condensed directly into a prepared tooth cavity to form a restoration.

direct intervention, hands-on therapy to increase the potential for new motor learning when there are deficits in movement and postural control.

directive therapy [L, *diregere*, to direct, *therapeia*, treatment], a psychotherapeutic approach in which the psychotherapist directs the course of therapy by intervening to ask questions and offer interpretations.

direct laryngoscopy [L, *diregere*, to direct; Gk, *larynx + skopein*, to watch], an examination of the larynx by means of a lighted instrument inserted through the mouth.

direct lead /lēd/, **1.** an electrocardiographic conductor in which the exploring electrode is placed directly onto the surface of the exposed heart. **2.** *informal.* a tracing produced by such a lead on an electrocardiograph.

direct light reflex, the constriction of a pupil receiving increased illumination, as by a flashlight during an ophthalmologic examination.

direct measurement of blood pressure [L, *diregere*, to direct, *mensura*, to measure; ME, *blod + L, premere*, to press], measurement of blood pressure in an artery by inserting a catheter into the blood vessel and recording the pressure directly, as opposed to the indirect method of using a pressure cuff, stethoscope, and sphygmomanometer.

direct nursing care functions, liaison nursing activities that are focused on a particular patient, a patient's family, or a group for whom the nurse is directly responsible and accountable.

direct patient care, (in nursing) care of a patient provided personally by a staff member.

direct provider reimbursement, a method of direct payment for health care services, as fee-for-service.

direct-question interview, an inquiry that usually requires simple one-or two-word responses.

direct reflex, a response that occurs on the same side of the body as the stimulus.

direct retainer, a clasp, attachment, or assembly fastened to an abutment tooth for the purpose of maintaining a removable restoration in its planned position in relation to oral structures.

direct self-destructive behavior (DSDB), any form of suicidal activity such as suicide threats, attempts, or gestures and the act of suicide itself. The person is aware that death is the desired outcome.

direct transfusion [L, *dirigere*, to direct, *transfundere*, to pour through], the transfer of whole blood directly from a vein of the donor to a vein of the recipient.

dirofilariasis /dī′rōfil′ərī′əsis/, a human infestation of the dog heartworm, *Dirofilaria immitis*, which may be transmitted through the bite of any of several species of mosquitoes.

disability /dis′əbil′itē/ [L, *dis*, opposite of, *habilis*, fit], the loss, absence, or impairment of physical or mental fitness.

disablement model /disā′bəlmənt/, an evaluation and treatment model based on specific impairment, functional loss, and attainable quality of life rather than on a medical diagnosis.

disaccharide /dīsak′ərīd/ [Gk, *di*, twice, *sakcharon*, sugar], a general term for simple carbohydrates formed by the union of two monosaccharide molecules.

disadvantaged /dis′ədvan′tijd/ [L, *dis + abante*, superior position], **1.** any group of people who lack money, education, literacy, or another status advantage. **2.** a euphemism for "poor."

disarticulation /dis′ärtik′yəlā′shən/ [L, *dis, articulare*, to divide into joints], separation of a joint without cutting through a bone.

disaster [L, *dis*, apart, *astrum*. a star], any mishap or misfortune that is ruinous, distressing, or calamitous.

disaster-preparedness plan [L, *dis + astrum*, favorable stars, *praeparare*, to prepare], a formal plan of action, usually prepared in written form, for coordinating the response of a hospital staff in the event of a disaster within the hospital or the surrounding community.

discharge [OFr, *deschargier*, to expel], **1.** also **evacuate, excrete, secrete.** to release a substance or object. **2.** to release a patient from a hospital. **3.** to release an electric charge, which may be manifested by a spark or surge of electricity, from a storage battery, condenser, or other source. **4.** to release a burst of energy from or through a neuron. **5.** a release of emotions, often accompanied by a wide range of voluntary and involuntary reflexes, weeping, rage, or other emotional displays. **6.** a substance or object discharged.

discharge abstract /dis′chärj/, items of information compiled from medical records of patients discharged from a hospital, organized and recorded in a uniform format to provide data for statistical studies, reports, or research.

discharge coordinator, an individual who arranges with community agencies and institutions for the continuing care of patients after their discharge from a hospital.

discharge planning, the activities that facilitate a client's movement from one health care setting to another. It is a multidisciplinary process involving physicians, nurses, social workers, and possibly other health professionals; its goal is to enhance continuity of care.

Discharge Planning, a Nursing Interventions Classification defined as preparation for moving a patient from one level of care to another within or outside the current health care agency.

discharge summary, a clinical report prepared by a physician or other health professional at the conclusion of a hospital stay or series of treatments, outlining the patient's chief complaint, diagnostic findings, therapy administered and the patient's response to it, and recommendations on discharge.

discharging lesion [OFr, *deschargier* + L, *laesio,* hurting], an injury or infection of the central nervous system that causes sudden abnormal episodes of discharging nerve impulses.

dischronation /dis'krōnā'shən/, a disorder of time awareness.

disciform keratitis /dis'ifôrm/ [Gk, *diskos,* flat plate; L, *forma,* form; Gk, *keras,* horn, *itis,* inflammation], an inflammatory condition of the eye that often follows an attack of dendritic keratitis; it is believed to be an immunologic response to an ocular herpes simplex infection. The condition is characterized by dislike opacities in the cornea, usually with inflammation of the iris.

disclosing solution [L, *dis* + *claudere,* to close, *solutus,* dissolved], a topically applied dye used in aqueous solution to stain and reveal plaque and other deposits on teeth.

discoblastula /dis'kōblas'tyələ/ [Gk, *diskos,* flat plate, *blastos,* germ], a blastula formed from the partial cleavage that occurs in a fertilized ovum containing a large amount of yolk.

discocyte /dis'kəsīt/ [Gk, *diskos* + *kytos,* cell], a mature normal erythrocyte exhibiting one of many steady-state configurations, such as a biconcave disk without a nucleus.

discoid /dis'koid/ [Gk, *diskos,* flat plate, *eidos,* form], having a flat, round shape.

discoid lupus erythematosus (DLE) [Gk, *diskos* + *eidos,* form; L, *lupus,* wolf; Gk, *erythema,* redness, *osis,* condition], a chronic, recurrent disease, primarily of the skin, characterized by lesions that are covered with scales and extend into follicles. The lesions are typically distributed on the face but may also be present on other parts of the body. The cause of the disease is not established, but there is evidence that it may be an autoimmune disorder, and some cases seem to be induced by certain drugs.

discoid meniscus, an abnormal condition characterized by a discoid rather than semilunar shape of the cartilaginous meniscus of the knee. The condition is a developmental anomaly. Common complaints are that a clicking occurs in the knee joint or that the knee joint gives way. These characteristics are often associated with an injury to the knee but also occur without any history of trauma.

discoid placenta [Gk, *diskos,* quoit, *eidos,* form; L, *placenta,* flat cake], a round placenta.

disconfirmation /diskon'fərmā'shən/, a dysfunctional communication that negates, discounts, or ignores information received from another person.

discordance /diskôr'dəns/ [L, *discordare,* to disagree], (in genetics) the expression of one or more specific traits in only one member of a pair of twins. —**discordant,** *adj.*

discordant twins, twins showing a marked difference in size (greater than 10% in weight) at birth.

discovery /diskov'ərē/ [L, *dis* + *coopiere,* to cover], (in law) a pretrial procedure that allows one party to examine vital witnesses and documents held exclusively by the adverse party.

discrete /diskrēt'/ [L, *discretus,* separated], **1.** individually distinct. **2.** composed of distinct parts.

discrimination /diskrim'inā'shən/ [L, *discrimen,* division], the act of distinguishing or differentiating. The ability to distinguish between touch or pressure at two nearby points on the body is known as two-point discrimination.

discriminator /diskrim'inā'tər/, (in nuclear medicine) an electronic device capable of accepting or rejecting a pulse of energy according to the pulse height of voltage. It is used to separate low- from high-energy radionuclides.

discus articularis /dis'kəs/, a small oval plate between the condyle of the mandible and the mandibular fossa.

disease [L, *dis* + Fr, *aise,* ease], **1.** a condition of abnormal vital function involving any structure, part, or system of an organism. **2.** a specific illness or disorder characterized by a recognizable set of signs and symptoms, attributable to heredity, infection, diet, or environment.

D

disease prevention, activities designed to protect patients or other members of the public from actual or potential health threats and their harmful consequences.

disengagement /dis'engāj'mənt/ [Fr, *disengager*, to release from engagement], **1.** an obstetric manipulation in which the presenting part of the baby is dislodged from the maternal pelvis as part of an operative delivery. **2.** the release or detachment of oneself from other persons or responsibilities. **3.** (in transactional family therapy) a role assumed by a nurse or other therapist in observing and restructuring intervention without becoming actively and directly involved in the problem.

disengagement theory, the psychosocial concept that normally aging individuals and society mutually withdraw from normal interaction.

disequilibrium /disē'kwilib'rē-əm/ [L, *dis*, apart, *aequilibrium*], the loss of balance or adjustment, particularly mental or psychologic balance.

dishpan fracture [AS, *disc*, plate; L, *patina*, dish; *fractura*, break], a fracture that depresses the skull.

disinfect /dis'infekt'/ [L, *dis*, apart, *inficere*, to infect], to eliminate many or all pathogenic microorganisms with the exception of bacterial spores.

disinfectant /dis'infek'tənt/, a liquid chemical that can be applied to objects to eliminate many or all pathogenic microorganisms.

disinfection /dis'infek'shən/, the process of killing pathogenic organisms or rendering them inert.

disinfection of thermometer [L, *dis* + *inficere*, to infect; Gk, *therme*, heat, *metron*, measure], the destruction of infectious organisms that may be present on a clinical glass thermometer. The process usually involves the use of chemical germicides after thorough washing, following the Centers for Disease Control and Prevention guidelines for cleaning, disinfection, and sterilization of hospital equipment.

disinfestation /dis'infestā'shən/ [L, *dis*, apart, *infestare*, to infest], elimination of a threat of infestation by vermin, rodents, lice, or other noxious organisms.

disinhibition /dis'inhibish'ən/ [L, *dis*, apart, *inhibere*, to restrain], the removal of inhibition.

disintegrative psychosis /disin'təgrā'tiv/, a mental disorder of childhood that usually has an onset after 3 years of age and after normal development of speech, social behavior, and other traits. The child becomes irritable and undergoes mental deteriora-

tion, eventually reaching a stage of severe mental retardation. The cause may be a viral infection.

disjunction /disjungk'shən/ [L, *disjungere*, to disjoint], (in genetics) the separation of the paired homologous chromosomes during the anaphase stage of the first meiotic division or of the chromatids of a chromosome during anaphase of mitosis and the second meiotic division.

disk [Gk, *diskos*, flat plate], **1.** also spelled (chiefly in ophthalmology) **disc.** a flat, circular platelike structure, as an articular disk or an optic disc. **2.** *informal.* an intervertebral disk.

diskography /diskog'rəfē/, the radiologic examination of individual intervertebral disks. It involves the injection of a small amount of water-soluble iodinated medium into the center of the disk by a double-needle entry.

dislocation /dis'lōkā'shən/ [L, *dis* + *locare*, to place], the displacement of any part of the body from its normal position, particularly a bone from its normal articulation with a joint. **—dislocate,** *v.*

dislocation fracture, an abnormal displacement associated with a break (fracture) of the bony components of a joint.

dislocation of clavicle [L, *dis*, apart, *locare*, to place, *clavicula*, little key], displacement of the collarbone. It may occur at the sternal end or the acromial or scapular extremity.

dislocation of finger [L, *dis*, apart, *locare*, to place; AS, *finger*], displacement of a finger at a joint as a result of trauma. In the absence of an accompanying fracture, the dislocated finger can usually be reduced by steadying the hand at the wrist and maneuvering the dislocated bone into place.

dislocation of hip [L, *dis*, apart, *locare*, to place; AS, *hype*], a movement of the femoral head out of the hip joint, usually accompanied by pain, rigidity, shortening of the leg, and loss of function. The dislocation may be congenital or acquired and can occur as an obturator dislocation, in which the head of the femur lies in the obturator foramen; a perineal dislocation, in which the head of the femur is displaced into the perineum; a sciatic dislocation, in which the head of the femur is lying in the sciatic notch; or a subpubic dislocation, in which there is anterior displacement of the femoral head.

dislocation of jaw [L, *dis*, apart, *locare*, to place; ME, *jowe*], a displacement of the jaw, which may be unilateral or bilateral, as a result of a blow, a fall, or yawning. The mandible appears fixed in an open position with only the back teeth in contact.

If the mandible appears deviated to one side, the dislocation involves only one side.

dislocation of knee [L, *dis,* apart, *locare,* to place; AS, *cneow*], a displacement of one of the bones of the knee joint. First aid treatment for the dislocation is the same as for a fracture: the joint is immobilized with splints.

dislocation of shoulder [L, *dis* + *locare* + AS, *sculder*], any of several kinds of displacement of the shoulder joint, including acromial joint disruption and separation and dislocation of the glenohumeral joint with the humeral head displaced anteriorly and inferiorly.

dislocation of toe, the abnormal displacement of a metatarsal bone, usually at a joint.

dismiss [L, *dis* + *mittere,* to send], (in law) to discharge or dispose of an action, suit, or motion trial. —**dismissal,** *n.*

disopyramide phosphate /dī′sōpir′əmīd/, a cardiac antiarrhythmic depressant prescribed in the treatment of premature ventricular contractions and ventricular tachycardia.

disorder [L, *dis,* apart, *ordo,* rank], a disruption of or interference with normal functions or established systems, as a mental or nutritional disorder.

disordered metabolism, changes in metabolism that result from disease and medications administered to control diseases. Acquired immunodeficiency syndrome patients may experience severe malnutrition, wasting, weight loss, hypermetabolism, and altered energy metabolism.

disorder of movement [L, *dis,* apart, *ordo,* rank, *movere,* to move], any perverse or abnormal function of muscular action that may result from infection, injury, or congenital disability, such as ataxia, involuntary grimacing, or chorea.

disorder of sleep [L, *dis* + *ordo* + AS, *slaep*], any condition that interferes with normal sleep patterns, such as sleep apnea, phase shift, use of alcohol and certain drugs, excessive sleepiness, sleep walking, nightmares, sleep paralysis, and narcolepsy.

disorganized schizophrenia /disôr′gənīzd/ [L, *dis* + Gk, *organon,* organ], a subtype of schizophrenia characterized by an earlier age of onset, usually at puberty, and a more severe disintegration of the personality than occur in other forms of the disease. The essential features include incoherence, loose associations, gross disorganization of behavior, and flat or inappropriate affect.

disorient /disôr′ē·ənt/, to cause to lose awareness or perception of space, time, or personal identity and relationships.

disorientation /-ā′shən/ [L, *dis* + *orienter,* to proceed from], a state of mental confusion characterized by inadequate or incorrect perceptions of place, time, or identity.

disparate twins /dis′pərāt, disper′it/, twins who are distinctly different from each other in weight and other features.

dispense /dispens′/ [L, *dis,* apart, *pensare,* to weigh], to prepare and issue drugs or drug mixtures from a pharmaceutical outlet or department.

dispersing agent /dispur′sing/ [L, *dis* + *spargere,* to scatter, *agere,* to do], a chemical additive used in pharmaceutics to cause the even distribution of the ingredients throughout the product, such as in dermatologic emulsions containing both oil and water.

dispersion /dispur′shən/, the scattering or dissipation of finely divided material, as when particles of a substance are scattered throughout the volume of a fluid.

displaced fracture /displäst/ [Fr, *deplacement,* to remove], a traumatic bone break in which two ends of a fractured bone are separated. The ends of broken bones in displaced fractures often pierce surrounding skin, as in an open fracture, or may be contained within the skin, as in a closed fracture.

displaced testis [Fr, *deplacement* + L, *testis,* testicle], a testis that is located in the pelvis, inguinal canal, or elsewhere after it normally would have descended into the scrotum.

displacement /displās′mənt/ [Fr, *deplacement,* to remove], **1.** the state of being displaced or the act of displacing. **2.** (in chemistry) a reaction in which an atom, molecule, or radical is removed from combination and replaced by another. **3.** (in physics) the displacing in space of one mass by another, as when the weight or volume of a fluid is displaced by a floating or submerged body. **4.** (in psychiatry) an unconscious defense mechanism for avoiding emotional conflict and anxiety by transferring emotions, ideas, or wishes from one object to a substitute that is less anxiety-producing.

DISS, abbreviation for **Diameter-Index Safety System.**

dissect /disekt′/ [L, *dissecare,* to cut apart], to cut apart tissues for visual or microscopic study using a scalpel, a probe, or scissors. —**dissection,** *n.*

dissecting aneurysm [L, *dissecare,* to cut apart; Gk, *aneurysma,* a widening], a localized dilation of an artery, most commonly the aorta, characterized by a longitudinal dissection between the outer and middle layers of the vascular wall. Blood entering a tear in the intimal lining of the vessel causes a separation of weakened elastic and fibromuscular elements in the medial layer and leads to the formation of cystic spaces filled with ground substance. Rupture of a dissecting aneurysm may be fatal in less than 1 hour.

disseminated /disem'ina'tid/, dispersed or spread throughout, as in an organ or the whole body.

disseminated intravascular coagulation (DIC) [L, *dis* + *seminare,* to sow, *intra,* within, *vasculum,* little vessel, *coagulare,* to curdle], a grave coagulopathy resulting from the overstimulation of clotting and anticlotting processes in response to disease or injury, such as septicemia, acute hypotension, poisonous snakebites, neoplasms, obstetric emergencies, severe trauma, extensive surgery, and hemorrhage. The primary disorder initiates generalized intravascular clotting, which in turn overstimulates fibrinolytic mechanisms; as a result the initial hypercoagulability is succeeded by a deficiency in clotting factors, with hypocoagulability and hemorrhaging.

disseminated myelitis, an inflammation of the spinal cord.

disseminated neuritis, inflammation of peripheral nerves, with pain, tenderness, and loss of function. Lesions may affect the parenchyma of peripheral sensory and motor tracts.

dissent /disent'/ [L, *dis* + *sentire,* to feel], (in law) a statement written by a judge who disagrees with the decision of the majority of the court. The dissent states explicit reasons for the contrary opinion. —**dissenting,** *adj.*

dissociation /disō'shē·ā'shən/ [L, *dis* + *sociare,* to unite], **1.** the act of separating into parts or sections. **2.** an unconscious defense mechanism by which an idea, thought, emotion, or other mental process is separated from the consciousness and thereby loses emotional significance. —**dissociative** /disō'shē·ətiv/, *adj.*

dissociation syndrome, a loss of the ability to sense painful and thermal stimuli, while retaining the sense of touch, tactile discrimination, and position sense.

dissociative anesthesia /disō'shē·ətiv/, an anesthetic procedure characterized by analgesia and amnesia without loss of respiratory function. The patient does not appear to be anesthetized but is "dissociated" from the environment. This form of anesthesia may be used to provide analgesia during brief, superficial operative procedures or diagnostic processes.

dissociative disorder, a category of *DSM-IV* disorder in which emotional conflicts are so repressed that a separation or split in the personality occurs, resulting in an altered state of consciousness or a confusion in identity. Symptoms may include amnesia, somnambulism, fugue, dream state, and dissociative identity disorder.

dissociative identity disorder, a psychiatric disorder characterized by the existence of two or more distinct, clearly differentiated personality structures within the same individual, any of which may dominate at a particular time. Each personality is a complex unit with separate, well-developed emotional and thought processes, behavior patterns, and social relationships.

dissolution /dis'əlo͞o'shən/ [L, *dis* + *solvere,* to loosen], **1.** the separation of a complex chemical compound into simpler molecules. **2.** the dissolving of chemical substances into a homogenous solution. **3.** the loss of mental powers.

dissolve, to disperse the molecules of one substance throughout the bulk of another substance.

dissolved gas /disolvd'/ [L, *dis* + *solvere,* to loosen], gas in a simple physical solution, as distinguished from gas that has reacted chemically with a solvent or other solutes and is chemically combined.

dissonance, the interference between sound waves of different pitches.

distal /dis'təl/ [L, *distare,* to be distant], **1.** away from or the farthest from a point of origin or attachment. **2.** away from or the farthest from the midline or a central point, as a distal phalanx.

distal latency, (in electroneuromyography) the interval between the stimulation of a compound muscle and the observed response.

distal muscular dystrophy, a rare form of muscular dystrophy that usually affects adults. It is characterized by moderate weakness and by wasting that begins in the arms and legs and then extends gradually to the proximal and facial muscles.

distal phalanx, any one of the small distal bones in the third row of phalanges of the hand or foot (second phalanx in the thumb and great toe). The distal phalanx of each of the toes is smaller and more flattened than that of a finger.

distal radioulnar articulation, the pivot-like articulation of the head of the ulna and the ulnar notch on the lower end of the radius, involving two ligaments.

distal renal tubular acidosis (distal RTA), an abnormal condition characterized by excessive acid accumulation and bicarbonate excretion. It is caused by the inability of the kidney's distal tubules to secrete hydrogen ions, thus decreasing the excretion of titratable acids and ammonium and increasing the urinary loss of potassium and bicarbonate. Primary distal RTA occurs mostly in females, adolescents, older children, and young adults. It may occur sporadically or result from hereditary defects. Secondary distal RTA is associated with numerous disorders such as cirrhosis of the liver, malnutrition, starvation, and various genetic abnormalities.

distal sparing, a condition in which the spinal cord remains intact below a lesion. The reflex arc remains but is not modified by supraspinal influences. As a result, spastic movements may occur distal to the level of the lesion.

distal tubule, the part of the nephron lying between the descending Henle's loop and the collecting duct in the kidney.

distance regulation [L, *distantia* + *regula*, rule], behavior that is related to the control of personal space. Most humans establish a quantum of space between themselves and others that offers security from either psychologic or physical threat while not creating a feeling of isolation.

distance vision, the ability to see objects clearly from a distance, usually from more than 20 feet or 6 m away.

distemper /distem'pər/ [L, *dis*, apart, *temperare*, to regulate], **1.** any mental or physical disorder or indisposition. **2.** a potentially fatal viral disease of animals characterized by rhinitis, fever, and a loss of appetite.

distend /distend'/ [L, *distendere*, to stretch], to enlarge or dilate something.

distensibility /disten'sibil'itē/ [L, *distendere*, to stretch], the ability of something to become stretched, dilated, or enlarged.

distension /disten'shən/, the state of being distended or swollen.

distillate /distil'it/ [L, *distillare*, to drop down], the product of distillation.

distillation /dis'tilā'shən/ [L, *distillare*, to drop down], the process of vaporization followed by condensation in another part of the system.

distilled water /distild'/ [L, *distillare,* to drop down; .,S, *waeter*], water that has been purified by being heated to a vapor form and then condensed into another container as liquid water free of nonvolatile solutes.

distogingival /dis'tōjinjī'vəl/, pertaining to the surfaces of a tooth nearest the gum and back of the mouth.

distolabial /dis'tōlā'bē-əl/, pertaining to the surfaces of a tooth nearest the cheek and back of the mouth.

distortion /distôr'shən/ [L, *dis* + *torquere,* to twist], **1.** (in psychology) the process of shifting experience in one's perceptions. Distortions represent personal constructs of truth, validity, and right and wrong. **2.** (in radiology) radiographic image artifacts that may be caused by variations in the size and shape or position of the object.

distractibility /distrak'tibil'itē/ [L, *dis* + *trahere,* to draw apart], a mental state in which attention does not remain fixed on any one subject but wavers or wanders.

distraction /distrak'shən/ [L, *dis* + *trahere,* to draw apart], **1.** a procedure that prevents or lessens the perception of pain by focusing attention on sensations unrelated to pain. **2.** a method of straightening a spinal column by the forces of axial tension pulling on the joint surfaces.

Distraction, a Nursing Interventions Classification defined as purposeful focusing of attention away from undesirable sensations.

distraught /distrôt'/ [OFr, *destrait,* inattentive], a mental state of confusion, distraction, or absentmindedness.

distress /distres'/ [ME, *distressen,* to cause sorrow], an emotional or physical state of pain, sorrow, misery, suffering, or discomfort.

distributing artery, an artery with a tunica media composed of circularly arranged smooth muscle. It receives blood from conducting arteries and distributes the blood to organs and tissues.

distribution, the location of medications in various organs and tissues after administration. The concentration of highly water-soluble drugs may be greater in persons who have less total body water for dilution of the substance. As body fat increases, drugs that are distributed primarily in body fat have a more prolonged effect.

distributive analysis and synthesis /distrib'yətiv/, the system of psychotherapy used by the psychobiologic school of psychiatry. It involves an extensive and systematic investigation and analysis of a person's total past experiences.

distributive care, a pattern of health care that is concerned with environment, heredity, living conditions, life-style, and early detection of pathologic effects.

district [L, *distringere,* to compel], **1.** (in hospital nursing) a group of patients in an area of the unit, usually a subdivision of a ward, for whom a nurse manager or primary nurse is responsible. **2.** the area of a city or town assigned to a public health nurse.

disulfiram /dīsul'firam/, an alcohol-use deterrent prescribed as a deterrent to drinking alcohol in the treatment of chronic alcoholism. It causes severe intestinal cramping, diaphoresis, and nausea if alcohol is ingested.

disuse phenomena /disyo͞os'/ [L, *dis* + *usus,* to make use of; Gk, *phainein,* to show], the physical and psychologic changes, usually degenerative, that result from the lack of use of a part or system of the body. Disuse phenomena are associated with confinement and immobility, especially in orthopedics. The physical changes often induced by continued bed rest constitute problems that affect many key areas and systems of the body, such as the skin, the musculoskeletal system, the gastrointestinal tract, the cardiovascular system, and the respiratory system. Unused muscles lose size and strength, often wasting until they are unable to perform their functions of support and contraction. Contractures are usually caused by flexion, because patients flex knees and hips whenever possible to relax muscles, especially when cold or in pain. The immobilized patient may experience bone demineralization caused by a restricted diet and decreased motility.

disuse syndrome, risk for, a NANDA-accepted nursing diagnosis of a state characterized by potential for deterioration of body systems as the result of prescribed or unavoidable inactivity. Risk factors include paralysis, mechanical immobilization, prescribed immobilization, severe pain, and altered level of consciousness.

diurese /dī'yo͞orēs/, the act of effecting diuresis.

diuresis /dī'yo͞orē'sis/ [Gk, *dia,* through, *ouron,* urine], increased formation and secretion of urine. Diuresis occurs in conditions such as diabetes mellitus, diabetes insipidus, and acute renal failure.

diuretic /dī'yo͞oret'ik/, **1.** (of a drug or other substance) tending to promote the formation and excretion of urine. **2.** a drug that promotes the formation and excretion of urine. The more than 50 diuretic drugs available in the United States and Canada are classified by chemical structure and pharmacologic activity into groups: aldosterone antagonists, carbonic anhydrase inhibitors, loop diuretics, mercurials, osmotics, potassium-sparing diuretics, and thiazides. A diuretic medication may contain drugs from one or more of these groups.

diuretic ceiling effect, the effect of possible increased drug toxicity without additional clinical findings with the administration of more than a certain amount of diuretic drugs in a 24-hour period.

diurnal /dīyo͞or'nəl/ [L, *diurnalis,* of a

day], happening daily, as sleeping and eating.

diurnal enuresis [L, *diurnalis,* of a day; Gk, *enourein,* to urinate], involuntary voiding of urine during daylight hours.

diurnal mood variation, a change in mood that is related to the time of day. Examples are commonly found in differences between "night people" and "morning people."

diurnal rhythm [L, *diurnalis,* of a day; Gk, *rhythmos*], patterns of activity or behavior that follow day-night cycles, such as breakfast-lunch-dinner schedules.

diurnal variation, the range of the output or excretion rate of a substance in a specimen being collected for laboratory analysis over a 24-hour period.

divalproex sodium, an anticonvulsant drug used to treat epilepsy and seizures, controlling simple and complex absence seizures alone or in combination with other anticonvulsant drugs. It is also approved for the treatment of migraines. It is prescribed to prevent or reduce the number of seizures by decreasing the activity of nerve impulses in the brain and central nervous system. Divalproex sodium is converted to valproic acid in the body.

divergence /divur'jəns/ [L, *di* + *vergere,* to incline], a separation or movement of objects away from each other, as in the simultaneous turning of the eyes outward as a result of an extraocular muscle defect.

divergent dislocation /divur'jənt/, the temporary displacement of two bones such as the radius and ulna.

divergent strabismus, /divur'jənt/ [L, *di, vergere,* to incline; ME, *squint*], a visual disorder in which a deviating eye looks outward. The eye often is blind or has defective vision.

diversional activity deficit, a NANDA-accepted nursing diagnosis of a state in which an individual experiences decreased stimulation from or interest or engagement in recreational or leisure activities. The defining characteristics are boredom, a desire for something to do, and an inability to participate in usual hobbies.

diverticular hernia /dī'vurtik'yo͞olər/, the protrusion of a congenital intestinal diverticulum through an opening in the abdominal cavity.

diverticulectomy /dī'vurtik'yo͞olek'təmē/, surgical removal of a diverticulum.

diverticulitis /dī'vurtik'yo͞oli'tis/ [L, *diverticulare,* to turn aside; Gk, *itis,* inflammation], inflammation of one or more diverticula. The penetration of fecal matter through the thin-walled diverticula causes inflammation and abscess formation in the tissues surrounding the colon. With repeated inflammation the lumen of the colon narrows and may become obstructed. During periods of inflammation the patient experiences crampy pain, particularly over the sigmoid colon; fever; and leukocytosis. Barium enemas and proctoscopy are used to rule out carcinoma of the colon, which exhibits some of the same symptoms.

diverticulosis /dī'vurtik'yoōlō'sis/ [L, *diverticulare,* to turn aside; Gk, *osis,* condition], the presence of pouchlike herniations through the muscular layer of the colon, particularly the sigmoid colon. Most patients with this condition have few symptoms except occasional bleeding from the rectum.

diverticulum /dī'vurtik'yoōlǝm/, *pl.* **diverticula** [L, *diverticulare,* to turn aside], a pouchlike herniation through the muscular wall of a tubular organ. A diverticulum may be present in the stomach, the small intestine, or, most commonly, the colon. —**diverticular,** *adj.*

divided dose, a measured fraction of a full dose of a medication given at short intervals so that the full dose is eventually taken within a specified period.

diving, the act of work or recreation in an underwater environment. The main health effects are related to the increased pressure to which the person is subjected as the ambient pressure generally increases by 1 atm (14.7 pounds per square inch) for each 33 feet of descent below the water surface.

diving goiter [AS, *dyypan,* to dip; L, *guttur,* throat], a large movable thyroid gland located at times above the sternal notch and at other times below the notch.

diving reflex, an automatic change in the cardiovascular system that occurs when the face and nose are immersed in cold water. The heart rate decreases, and the blood pressure remains stable or increases slightly, while blood flow to all parts of the body except the brain is reduced.

division [L, *dividere,* to divide], **1.** an administrative subunit in a hospital, such as a division of medical or surgical nursing. **2.** (in public health nursing) an area that encompasses several geographic districts. **3.** the separation of something into two or more parts or sections.

divorce therapy, a type of counseling that attempts to help divorced couples disengage from their former relationship and malicious behavior toward each other or their children.

Dix, Dorothea Lynde (1802–1887), an American humanitarian who achieved fame as a social reformer, primarily for her work in improving prison conditions and care of the mentally ill. During her lifetime she helped to establish mental institutions in 30 states and Canada. During the U.S. Civil War she was appointed superintendent of army nurses for government hospitals.

dizygotic /dī'zīgot'ik/ [Gk, *di,* twice, *zygotos,* yolked together], pertaining to twins from two fertilized ova.

dizygotic twins, two offspring born of the same pregnancy and developed from two ova that were released from the ovary simultaneously and fertilized at the same time. They may be of the same or opposite sex, differ both physically and genetically, and have two separate and distinct placentas and membranes, both amnion and chorion.

dizziness [AS, *dysig,* stupid], a sensation of faintness and whirling or an inability to maintain normal balance in a standing or seated position, sometimes associated with giddiness, mental confusion, nausea, and weakness. A person who experiences dizziness should be carefully lowered to a safe position on a bed, chair, or floor because of the danger of injury from falling.

DKA, abbreviation for **diabetic ketoacidosis.**

dl, dL, abbreviation for **deciliter.**

DLE, abbreviation for **discoid lupus erythematosus.**

DM, abbreviation for **diabetes mellitus.**

D.M.D., abbreviation for *Doctor of Dental Medicine.* It is equivalent to a **D.D.S.** degree.

DMSO, abbreviation for **dimethyl sulfoxide.**

DNA, abbreviation for **deoxyribonucleic acid.**

DNA blotting, the transfer of separated deoxyribonucleic acid fragments from an electrophoretic gel to a nitrocellular sheet.

DNA chimera /kīmē'rǝ/, (in molecular genetics) a recombinant molecule of deoxyribonucleic acid composed of segments from more than one source.

DNA-DNA hybridization, the formation of double-helix deoxyribonucleic acid from two complementary single strands. It is used to compare genome relationships between different species.

DNA fingerprinting, a technique for determining the nucleotide patterns of fragments of deoxyribonucleic acid (DNA). The process follows the restriction endonuclease treatment of DNA from different genomes. The variability between two human chromosomes in the number of times a sequence is repeated is enormous. There is a chance of 1 in 30 billion that two persons would have identical DNA fingerprints. The specificity of the probe makes it applicable to questions of forensic science.

DNA gyrase, an enzyme that catalyzes the breakage, passage, and rejoining of the deoxyribonucleic acid.

DNA helicase, a deoxyribonucleic acid unwinding enzyme that catalyzes the energy-dependent unwinding of the double helix during DNA replication.

DNA library, a collection of multiple nucleotide sequences that are representative of all the deoxyribonucleic acid (DNA) sections in a specific genome. It is also a random assortment of DNA fragments of one organism, linked to vectors and cloned in an appropriate host. After cloning transcribed fragment (axons) and nontranscribed fragments (introns), or spacers, are part of the library system. A DNA probe is used to screen a DNA library to locate a specific sequence. A collection representing the entire genome is called a genomic library.

DNA ligase, an enzyme that can repair breaks in a strand of deoxyribonucleic acid (DNA) by synthesizing a bond between adjoining nucleotides. Under some circumstances the enzyme can join together loose ends of DNA strands, and in some cases it can repair breaks in ribonucleic acid.

DNA polymerase, (in molecular genetics) an enzyme that catalyzes the assembly of deoxyribonucleoside triphosphates into deoxyribonucleic acid, with single-stranded DNA serving as the template.

DNA probe, the process of isolating and labeling a part of a deoxyribonucleic acid (DNA) molecule. Each DNA molecule possesses unique nucleotide sequences, which become "fingerprint" markers. A molecule can be used to detect the presence of a fingerprint in a DNA fragment or bacterial colony.

DNAR, abbreviation for *do not attempt resuscitation*.

DNCB, abbreviation for *dinitrochlorobenzene*.

DNP, abbreviation for **dinitrophenol.**

DNR, abbreviation for *do not resuscitate*.

D.O., abbreviation for *Doctor of Osteopathy*.

DOA, abbreviation for *dead on arrival*.

Dobie's globule /dō'bēz/ [William M. Dobie, English physician, 1828–1915], a very small stainable body in the transparent disk of a striated muscle fiber.

dobutamine hydrochloride /dōbyoo'-təmēn/, a beta-adrenergic stimulating agent prescribed to increase cardiac output in severe chronic congestive heart failure and to provide adjunct in cardiac surgery.

Dock, Lavinia Lloyd (1858–1956), an American public health nurse. She advocated an international public health movement and the improvement of education for nurses. With M. Adelaide Nutting, she wrote *History of Nursing*, a classic in nursing literature.

doctoral program in nursing, an educational program that offers preparation for a doctoral degree in the field of nursing designed to prepare nurses for advanced practice and research. On satisfactory completion of the course of study, the Ph.D. with a major in nursing or D.S.N. (Doctor of Science in Nursing) degree is awarded.

Documentation, a Nursing Interventions Classification defined as recording of pertinent patient data in a clinical record.

docusate /dok'yoosāt/, a stool softener prescribed in the treatment of constipation.

Döderlein's bacillus /dā'dərlīnz, dō'dərlēnz/ [Albert S. Doederlein, German physician, 1860–1941], a gram-positive bacterium present in normal vaginal secretions.

Döhle's inclusion bodies /dā'lə, dōl/ [Karl G.P. Döhle, German pathologist, 1855–1928], blue inclusions in the cytoplasm of some leukocytes in May-Hegglin anomaly and in blood smears from patients with acute viral infections.

doll's-eye reflex, a normal response in newborns to keep the eyes stationary as the head is moved to the right or left. The reflex disappears as ocular fixation develops.

doll's head maneuver, a test for central nervous system brainstem damage in a comatose patient. The head is quickly rotated from side to side. Normally the eyes deviate to the opposite direction. Failure of the eyes to make the movement is an indication of severe brainstem damage.

dolor /dō'lôr/ [L, pain], any condition of physical pain, mental anguish, or suffering from heat. It is one of the four signs of inflammation. The others are calor (heat), rubor (redness), and tumor (swelling).

DOM, abbreviation for **dimethoxymethylamphetamine.**

domain, a region of a protein or polypeptide whose three-dimensional configuration enables it to interact specifically with particular receptors, enzymes, or other proteins.

dome fracture [L, *domus* house, *fractura*, break], any fracture of the acetabulum, specifically involving a weight-bearing surface.

dominance /dom'inəns/ [L, *dominari,* to

rule], (in genetics) a basic principle stating that not all genes determining a given trait operate with equal vigor. If two genes at a given locus produce a different effect, such as eye color, they compete for expression. The gene that is manifest is dominant. —**dominant,** *adj.*

dominant eye /dom′inənt/, the eye that is customarily used for monocular tasks. It may or may not be related to hand preference.

dominant gene [L, *dominari,* to rule; Gk, *genein* to produce], one that produces a phenotypic effect, regardless of whether its allele is the same or different.

dominant group, a social group that controls the value system and rewards in a particular society.

dominant idiotype, a segment of an immunoglobulin molecule that is present on a large proportion of the immunoglobulins generated by a particular antigen.

dominant trait, an inherited characteristic such as eye color that is expressed in an offspring, although it may occur in only one parent.

Donath-Landsteiner syndrome /dō′notland′stīnər/ [Julius Donath, Austrian physician, 1870–1960; Karl Landsteiner, Austrian-American pathologist, 1868–1943], a rare blood disorder marked by hemolysis minutes or hours after exposure to cold. Systemic symptoms include the passage of dark urine, severe pain in the back and legs, headache, vomiting, diarrhea, and moderate reticulocytosis.

Done nomogram, a graph on which a number of variables are plotted so that the value of a dependent variable can be read on the appropriate line when the values of the other variables are given.

Don Juan, a legendary Spanish libertine cited in many works of literature as a seductive and sexually promiscuous man. See also **satyriasis.**

donor /dō′nər/ [L, *donare,* to give], **1.** a human or other organism that gives living tissue to be used in another body, for example, blood for transfusion or a kidney for transplantation. **2.** a substance or compound that gives part of itself to another substance.

donor card [L, *donare,* to give, *charta*], a document in which a person offers to make an anatomic gift of body parts at the time of death for transplantation to recipients needing replacement of vital organs or tissues. The card is often incorporated into a state driver's license so the authorization will be immediately available if the donor dies in a traffic accident.

do not attempt resuscitation (DNAR), an advisory that resuscitation of a patient

should not even be attempted. The order is more strictly defined than the **DNR** *(do not resuscitate),* which may be interpreted as authorizing an attempt at resuscitation.

Donovan bodies /don′əvan/ [Charles Donovan, Irish physician, 1863–1951], encapsulated gram-negative rods of the species *Calymmatobacterium granulomatis,* present in the cytoplasm of mononuclear phagocytes obtained from the lesions of granuloma inguinale.

donut pad /dō′nut/, a pad designed to protect an injured joint. Cut to fit over the site of the injury, it causes the force on the body part to be transferred to surrounding areas.

dopa /dō′pə/, an amino acid produced by oxidation of tyrosine that occurs naturally in plants and animals. It is a precursor of dopamine, epinephrine, and norepinephrine.

dopamine /dō′pəmin/, a naturally occurring sympathetic nervous system neurotransmitter that is the precursor of norepinephrine. It is produced in the substantia nigra and transmitted to the putamen and caudate nucleus. It has an inhibitory effect on movement. A depletion of dopamine produces the symptoms of rigidity, tremors, and bradykinesia that are characteristic of Parkinson's disease.

dopamine hydrochloride, a sympathomimetic catecholamine prescribed in the treatment of shock, hypotension, and low cardiac output.

dopaminergic /dō′pəminur′jik/, having the effect of dopamine.

dopaminergic receptor, a protein on the surfaces of certain cells that binds specifically to the neurotransmitter dopamine. Such receptors on vascular epithelial cells, when stimulated by dopamine, cause the renal mesenteric, coronary, and cerebral arteries to dilate and the flow of blood to increase.

dope [AS, *dyppan,* to dip], *slang,* morphine, heroin, or another narcotic; marijuana; or another substance illicitly bought or sold and often self-administered for sedative, hypnotic, euphoric, or other mood-altering purposes.

Doppler color flow /dop′lər/ [Christian J. Doppler, Austrian physicist and mathematician, 1803–1853], an ultrasonic technique for detecting anatomic details by using color coding of velocity shifts. In cardiographic use of the device, blood directed to the transducer appears as red, and blood moving away from the transducer appears as blue. Doppler color flow is also used in laparoscopic systems for rapid identification and differentiation of ducts and valves in the viscera, particularly in detection and diagnosis of pancreatic and liver tumors and colorectal liver metastases.

Doppler echocardiography [Christian J. Doppler], a technique in which Doppler ultrasound technology is used to evaluate the direction and pattern of blood flow within the heart.

Doppler effect [Christian J. Doppler; L, *effectus*], the apparent change in frequency of sound or light waves emitted by a source as it moves away from or toward an observer. The frequency increases as the source moves toward the observer and decreases as it moves away.

Doppler-guided injection [Christian J. Doppler], the use of a hand-held ultrasound detector in sclerotherapy to guide a needle or syringe for injecting sclerosing fluid.

Doppler probe [Christian J. Doppler], a hand-held diagnostic device that emits an ultrasonic beam into the body. Reflection of the ultrasonic waves from a moving structure causes a change in the frequency.

Doppler scanning [Christian J. Doppler; L, *scandere*, to climb], a technique used in ultrasound imaging to monitor the behavior of a moving substance, such as flowing blood or a beating heart. The frequency of ultrasonic waves reflected from a moving surface is slightly different from that of the incident waves. The detected frequency shift yields information about the moving structure. Fetal heart detectors work on this principle.

Doppler ultrasonography [Christian J. Doppler], a technique for detecting the movement of blood flow. It allows an examiner to hear characteristic alterations in blood flow caused by vessel obstruction in various parts of an extremity. The Doppler shift, the difference between the frequencies transmitted and reflected waves, is audible. The velocities of movements inside the body are converted to sounds, and structures can be identified by their characteristic movements. The technique can also be used to observe fetal heart sounds, localize the placenta, and image heart functions.

dornase /dôr′nās/, a natural proteolytic substance that depolymerizes deoxyribonucleic acid (DNA) molecules. Because as much as 70% of the solid matter of purulent material consists of DNA, dornase is used in respiratory therapy to help break off sputum accumulation in the airways.

dorsal /dôr′səl/ [L, *dorsum*, the back], pertaining to the back or posterior. — **dorsum**, *n*.

dorsal digital vein, one of the communicating veins along the sides of the fingers.

dorsal flexure [L, *dorsalis*, back, *flectere*, to bend], the dorsal convexity of the thoracic region of the spine.

dorsal horns [L, *dorsalis*, back; AS, horn], a pair of slender, crescent-shaped projections of gray matter within the spinal cord, pointing posteriorly. They appear as a horn in transverse sections.

dorsal impaction syndrome, (in sports medicine) dorsal wrist pain after hyperextension weight-bearing activities, as may occur in weight lifting and gymnastics. Treatment requires rest, ice, antiinflammatory drugs, and technique modification.

dorsal inertia posture, a tendency of a debilitated or weak person to slip downward in bed when the head of the bed is raised.

dorsal interventricular artery, the arterial branch of the right coronary artery, branching to supply both ventricles.

dorsalis pedis artery, the continuation of the anterior tibial artery, starting at the ankle joint, dividing into five branches, and supplying various muscles of the foot and toes.

dorsalis pedis pulse, the pulse of the dorsalis pedis artery, palpable between the first and second metatarsal bones on the top of the foot.

dorsal lip, the marginal fold of the blastopore during gastrulation in the early stages of embryonic development of many animals.

dorsal recumbent [L, *dorsalis*, back; *recumbere*, to lie down], lying on the back, as in a supine position.

dorsal recumbent position [L, *dorsalis*, back, *positio*], the supine position with the person lying on the back, head, and shoulders.

dorsal rigid posture, a position in which a patient lying in bed holds one or both legs drawn up to the chest. It often involves only the right leg and is intended to relieve the pain of appendicitis, peritonitis, kidney stones, or pelvic inflammation.

dorsal root [L, *dorsalis*, back; AS, *rot*], the sensory component or posterior root of a spinal nerve, attached centrally to the spinal cord.

dorsal root ganglion [L, *dorsalis* + AS, *rot* + Gk, *ganglion*, knot], a swelling consisting of sensory neuron cell bodies whose axons constitute the dorsal root of a spinal nerve.

dorsal scapular nerve, one of a pair of supraclavicular branches from the roots of the brachial plexus. It supplies the rhomboideus major and the rhomboideus minor and sends a branch to the levator.

dorsiflect /dôr′siflekt/ [L, *dorsum* + *flectere*, to bend], to bend or flex backward as in the upward bending of the fingers, wrist, foot, or toes.

dorsiflexion /dôr'siflek'shən/, flexion toward the back, as accomplished by a muscle.

dorsiflexor /dôr'siflek'sər/, a muscle causing backward flexion of a part of the body, as the hand or foot.

dorsiflexor gait, an abnormal gait caused by the weakness of the dorsiflexors or the ankle. It is characterized by footdrop during the entire gait cycle and excessive knee and hip flexion to allow clearance of the involved extremity during the swing phase.

dorsodynia /dôr'sōdin'ē-ə/, a pain in the back, particularly in the muscles of the upper back area.

dorsolateral /dôr'sōlat'ərəl/, pertaining to the back of the body and the two sides.

dorsolumbar /dôr'sōlum'bər/, pertaining to the back of the body and the lumbar region.

dorsosacral /dôr'sōsā'krəl/, pertaining to the back of the body and the sacrum.

dorsoventral /dôr'sōven'trəl/ [L, *dorsum,* back, *venter,* belly], pertaining to the axis that passes through the back of the body and the abdomen.

dorsum /dôr'səm/ [L, *dorsum,* back], the back of the body; the posterior or upper surface of a body part.

dorsum sellae /sel'ē/, the posterior boundary of the sella turcica of the sphenoid bone. It bears the posterior clinoid process and is an anatomic marker for the location of the pituitary gland at the base of the skull.

dorzolamide hydrochloride, a carbonic anhydrase inhibitor prescribed in the treatment of glaucoma. It reduces intraocular pressure by decreasing the rate of fluid production.

DOS /dos/, abbreviation for *disk operating system.*

dosage [Gk, *didonai,* to give], the regimen governing the size, frequency, and number of doses of a therapeutic agent to be administered to a patient.

dosage compensation /dō'sij/, (in genetics) the mechanism that counterbalances the number of X-linked gene doses in the sex chromosomes so that they are equal in both the male, which has one X chromosome, and the female, which has two. In mammals this is accomplished by genetic activation of only one of the X chromosomes in the somatic cells of females.

dose /dōs/ [GK, *didonai,* to give], the amount of a drug or other substance to be administered at one time.

dose calculations, formulas for adjusting drug dosages for children, elderly adults, or other patients who may lack mechanisms for metabolizing and excreting average adult levels of medications. Infants, for example, have skin that is thin and permeable, a stomach that lacks gastric acid, body temperature that is poorly regulated, and immature liver and kidney . Elderly patients may consume two to eight or more prescription and over-the-counter drugs that may interact with a new medication.

dose equivalent (DE), a quantity used in radiation-safety work that uses a unified scale to equate the amount of radiation dose and the physical damages that it may produce. The unit of dose equivalent is the sievert (Sv) or the rem.

dose-limited side effects, drug reactions that prevent an antineoplastic agent or other drug from being administered in higher doses, thus limiting the effectiveness of the drug.

dose-limiting recommendations, the absorbed dose equivalent limit of radiation exposure, which may vary for different body or organ exposures. For example, the absorbed dose equivalent limit for the skin or forearms of a radiation worker is much higher than the whole-body exposure.

dose rate, (in radiotherapy and fluoroscopy) the amount of delivered radiation absorbed per unit of time.

dose ratemeter /rāt'mētər/, (in radiotherapy and fluoroscopy) an instrument for measuring the dose rate of radiation.

dose response, a range of drug effects between the minimum dose needed to reach the threshold level at which an effect is first observed and a toxic dose level at which adverse effects result.

dose-response relationship, (in radiology) a mathematic relationship between the dose of radiation and the body's reaction to it. In a linear dose-response relationship the response is proportional to the dose.

dose threshold, (in radiotherapy and radiography) the minimum amount of absorbed radiation that produces a detectable degree of a given effect.

dose to skin, (in radiotherapy and radiography) the amount of absorbed radiation at the center of the irradiation field on the skin. It is the sum of the dose in the air and the scatter from body parts.

dosimeter /dōsim'ətər/ [L, *dosis* + Gk, *metron,* measure], an instrument to detect and measure accumulated radiation exposure.

dosimetry /dōsim'ətrē/ [Gk, *dosis,* giving, *metron,* measure], **1.** the determination of the amount, rate, and distribution of radiation or radioactivity from a source of ionizing radiation. **2.** the accurate determination of medicinal doses, based on body size, sex, age, and other factors.

double [L, *duplus*], twice as much in strength, size, or amount.

double bind /bīnd/ [L, *duplus*, double; AS, *bindan*, to bind], a "no win" situation resulting from two conflicting messages from a person who is crucial to one's survival, such as a verbal message that differs from a nonverbal message.

double-blind study, an experiment designed to test the effect of a treatment or substance by using groups of experimental and control subjects in which neither the subjects nor the investigators know which treatment or substance is being administered to which group.

double-blind test [L, *duplus*, double; AS, *blind, testum*, crucible], an experimental design for drug testing in which neither the clients receiving the drugs nor the persons conducting the test know which subjects are receiving a new drug and which are getting a placebo, or sugar pill.

double-channel catheter [L, *duplus*, double; ME, *chanel* + Gk, *katheter*, a thing lowered into], a catheter with two lumens (channels) used to irrigate an internal cavity, with fluid entering one lumen and draining through the other.

double-contrast arthrography, a method of making a radiographic image of a joint by injecting two contrast agents into the capsular space. The technique is most commonly used in radiography of the knee joint.

double-contrast barium enema [L, *duplus*, double, *contra*, against, *stare*, to stand; Gk, *barys*, heavy, *enienai*, to inject], an enema of radiopaque barium followed by evacuation and injection of air. The purpose is to detail radiographically the mucosal lining of the large intestine.

double-emulsion film, x-ray film that is coated with gelatin emulsion on both sides.

double-flap amputation [L, *duplus*, double; ME, *flappe*, flap; L, *amputare*], an amputation in which two flaps are made from the soft tissues to cover an area that has lost its integument in surgery or accident.

double fracture, a fracture consisting of breaks or cracks in two places in a bone, causing more than two bone segments.

double innervation, innervation of effector organs by fibers of the sympathetic and parasympathetic divisions of the autonomic nervous system. The pelvic viscera, bronchioles, heart, eyes, and digestive system are all doubly innervated.

double monster, a fetus that has developed from a single ovum but has two heads, trunks, and multiple limbs.

double-needle entry, a technique for injecting a contrast medium or other agent with two needles, one with a larger bore. In diskography a 20-gauge needle is used to perform a spinal puncture and reach the annulus fibrosus of the disk, after which a longer, 26-gauge needle is passed through the guide needle to the injection target area.

double personality [L, *duplus*, double, *personalis*, of a person], a state of dissociation in which the individual presents personas to associates at different times as two different persons, each with a different name and different personality traits. The two personalities are generally independent, contrasting, and unaware of the existence of the other.

double pneumonia, acute lobar pneumonia affecting both lungs.

double quartan fever, a form of malaria in which paroxysms of fever occur in a repeating pattern of 2 consecutive days followed by 1 day of remission. The pattern is usually the result of concurrent infections by two species of the genus *Plasmodium*, one causing paroxysms every 72 hours and the other every 48 hours.

double setup, a nursing procedure in which an obstetric operating room is prepared for both vaginal delivery and cesarean section. The circulating and scrub nurses lay out the equipment required for both procedures.

double-void, a urinalysis procedure in which the first specimen is discarded and a second, obtained 30 to 45 minutes later, is tested. This method gives a more accurate measure of the amount of glucose in the urine at that particular time.

douche /do͞osh/ [Fr, shower-bath], **1.** a procedure in which a liter or more of a solution of a medication or cleansing agent in warm water is introduced into the vagina under low pressure. The woman often performs the procedure herself, sitting on a toilet seat or semisitting in a bathtub. **2.** to perform a douche.

Douglas's cul-de-sac [James Douglas, Scottish anatomist, 1675–1742; Fr, bottom of the bag], a rectouterine pouch or recess formed by a fold of peritoneum that extends between the rectum and the uterus.

dowager's hump /dow'ijərz/, an abnormal backward curvature of the cervical spine that afflicts some older women.

Downey cells [Hal Downey, American hematologist, 1877–1959], lymphocytes identified in one system of classification of the blood cells of patients with infectious mononucleosis and hepatitis. The cells are designated as Downey I, II, or III lymphocytes.

Down syndrome [John L. Down, English physician, 1828–1896], a congenital condition characterized by varying degrees of mental retardation and multiple defects. It is the most common chromosomal abnormality of a generalized syndrome and is caused by the presence of an extra chromosome 21 in the G group or, in a small percentage of cases, by the translocation of chromosome 14 or 15 in the D group and chromosome 21 or 22. Infants with the syndrome are small and hypotonic, with characteristic microcephaly, brachycephaly, a flattened occiput, and typical facies with a mongoloid slant to the eyes, depressed nasal bridge, low-set ears, and a large, protruding tongue that is furrowed and lacks a central fissure. The hands are short and broad with a transverse palmar or simian crease; the fingers are stubby and show clinodactyly, primarily of the fifth finger. The feet are broad and stubby with a wide space between the first and second toes and a prominent plantar crease. The most significant feature of the syndrome is mental retardation, which varies considerably. The average IQ is in the range of 50 to 60, so that the child is generally trainable and in most instances can be reared at home. The mortality rate is high within the first few years, especially in children with cardiac anomalies.

doxapram hydrochloride /dok′səpram/, a respiratory stimulant prescribed to improve respiratory function after anesthesia, in drug-induced central nervous system depression, and for chronic pulmonary disease associated with acute hypercapnia.

doxepin hydrochloride /dok′səpin/, a tricyclic antidepressant prescribed in the treatment of depression.

doxorubicin hydrochloride /dok′sər ōō′-bisin/, an anthracycline antibiotic prescribed in the treatment of malignant neoplastic diseases.

doxycycline /dok′sisī′klēn/, a tetracycline antibacterial prescribed in the treatment of infections.

doxylamine succinate /dok′silam′ēn/, an antihistamine prescribed for the treatment of acute allergic symptoms produced by the release of histamine.

dp/dt, (in cardiology) the rate of pressure change per unit of time.

DPG, abbreviation for **2,3-diphosphoglyceric acid.**

D.P.H., abbreviation for *Diploma in Public Health.*

D.P.M., abbreviation for *Doctor of Podiatric Medicine.*

DPL, abbreviation for **diagnostic peritoneal lavage.**

DPT vaccine, abbreviation for **diphtheria, tetanus toxoid, and pertussis vaccine.**

DQ, abbreviation for **developmental quotient.**

dr., 1. abbreviation for *drachm.* 2. abbreviation for **dram.**

Dr., abbreviation for *doctor.*

dracunculiasis /drakun′kyŏōlī′əsis/ [Gk, *drakontion,* little dragon, *osis,* condition], a parasitic infection caused by infestation by the nematode *Dracunculus medinensis.* It is characterized by ulcerative skin lesions on the legs and feet that are produced by gravid female worms. People are infected by drinking contaminated water or eating contaminated shellfish.

Dracunculus medinensis /drakun′kyŏō-ləs/, a parasitic nematode of the Mediterranean area that causes dracunculiasis. An American species is *Dracunculus insignis.*

drag-to gait [ME, *dragen* + *gate,* path], a method of walking with crutches in which the feet are dragged rather than lifted with each step.

drain, a tube or other device used to remove air or a fluid from a body cavity or wound. The drain may be a closed system, designed to provide complete protection against contamination, or an open system in which there is a continual exchange of material.

drainage /drā′nij/ [AS, *drachen,* teardrop], the removal of fluids from a body cavity, wound, or other source of discharge by one or more methods. Closed drainage is a system of tubing and other apparatus attached to the body to remove fluid in an airtight circuit that prevents environmental contaminants from entering the wound or cavity. Open drainage is drainage in which discharge passes through an open-ended tube into a receptacle. Suction drainage uses a pump or other mechanical device to assist in extracting a fluid. Tidal drainage is drainage in which a body area is washed out by alternately flooding and then emptying it with the aid of gravity, a technique that may be used in treating a urinary bladder disorder.

drainage tube, a heavy-gauge catheter used for the evacuation of air or a fluid from a cavity or wound in the body.

draining sinus [AS, *drachen,* teardrop; L, *sinus,* hollow], an abnormal channel or fistula permitting the escape of exudate to the outside of the body.

Draize test /drāz/, a controversial method

of testing the toxicity of pharmaceutic and other products to be used by humans by placing a small amount of the substance in the eyes of rabbits. The eye-irritancy potential of a substance is considered a measure of the possible effect of the product on similar human tissues.

dram (dr.) [Gk, *drachme,* weight of the same value], a unit of mass equivalent to an apothecary's measure of 60 grains or ⅛ ounce and to ¹/₁₆ ounce or 27.34 grains avoirdupois.

dramatic play /dramat′ik/ [Gk, *drama,* deed; AS, *plegan,* game], an imitative activity in which a child fantasizes and acts out various domestic and social roles and situations, as rocking a doll, pretending to be a doctor or nurse, or teaching school.

drape [ME, *drap,* cloth], a sheet of fabric or paper, usually the size of a small bed sheet, for covering all or a part of a person's body during a physical examination or treatment. **—drape,** *v.*

Draw-a-Person Test (DAP) [AS, *dragan* + L, *personalis* + *testum,* crucible], a test developed by Karen Machover [American psychologist, b. 1902] based on the interpretation of drawings of human figures of both sexes. Interpretation depends on the subject's verbalizations, self-image, anxiety, and sexual conflicts and other factors.

drawer sign [AS, *dragan* + to drag], a diagnostic sign of a ruptured or torn knee ligament. It is tested by having the patient flex the knee at a right angle while the lower leg is grasped just below the knee and moved first toward, then away from the examiner. The test result is positive for the knee injury if the head of the tibia can be moved more than a half inch from the joint.

drawing, *informal.* a vague sensation of muscle tension.

drawsheet, a sheet that is smaller than a bottom or top sheet of a bed and is usually placed over the middle of the bottom sheet to keep the mattress and bottom linens dry. The drawsheet can also be used to turn or move a patient in bed.

dream [ME, *dreem,* joyful noise], **1.** a sequence of ideas, thoughts, emotions, or images that pass through the mind during the rapid-eye-movement stage of sleep. **2.** the sleeping state in which this process occurs. **3.** a visionary creation of the imagination experienced during wakefulness. **4.** (in psychoanalysis) the expression of thoughts, emotions, memories, or impulses repressed from the consciousness. **5.** (in analytic psychology) the wishes, emotions, and impulses that reflect the personal unconscious and the archetypes that originate in the collective unconscious.

dream analysis, a process of gaining access to the unconscious mind by means of examining the content of dreams, usually through the method of free association.

dream association, a relationship of thoughts or emotions discovered or experienced when a dream is remembered or analyzed.

dream state, a condition of altered consciousness in which a person does not recognize the environment and reacts in a manner opposed to his or her usual behavior, as by flight or an act of violence.

drepanocytic anemia /drep′ənōsit′ik/ [Gk, *drepane,* sickle, *kytos,* cell], sickle cell anemia.

dress code [OFr, *dresser,* to arrange; L, *codex,* book], the standards set by an institution for the appropriate attire of its members.

dressing [OFr, *dresser,* to arrange], a clean or sterile covering applied directly to wounded or diseased tissue for absorption of secretions, protection from trauma, administration of medications, maintaining wound cleanliness, or stopping bleeding.

Dressing, a Nursing Interventions Classification defined as choosing, putting on, and removing clothes for a person who cannot do this for himself or herself.

dressing forceps, a kind of forceps that has narrow blades and blunt or notched teeth designed for dressing wounds, removing drainage tubes, or extracting fragments of necrotic tissue.

Dressler's syndrome /dres′lərz/, [William Dressler, American physician, 1890–1969], an autoimmune disorder that may occur several days to several months after acute coronary infarction, characterized by fever, pericarditis, pleurisy, pleural effusions, and joint pain. It results from the body's immunologic response to a damaged myocardium and pericardium.

DRG, abbreviation for **diagnosis-related group.**

drift [AS, *drifan,* to move forward], a gradual movement away from the original position.

drifting tooth, any one of the teeth that migrate from normal position in the associated dental arch.

Drinker respirator [Philip Drinker, American engineer, 1894–1972], an airtight respirator consisting of a metal tank that encloses the entire body, except the head. Used for long-term therapy, it alternates positive and negative air pressure within the tank, providing artificial respiration.

drip [AS, *dryppan,* to fall in drops], **1.**

the process in which a liquid or moisture forms and falls in drops. **2.** the slow but continuous infusion of a liquid into the body, as into the stomach or a vein. **3.** to infuse a liquid continuously into the body.

drip gavage, a method of feeding a liquid formula diet through a tube inserted through the nostrils to the stomach.

drip system, (in intravenous therapy) an apparatus for delivering specific volumes of intravenous solutions within predetermined periods and at a specific flow rate.

drive [AS, *drifan*, to move forward], a basic, compelling urge. Primary drive refers to one that is innate and in close contact with physiologic processes. A secondary drive is one that evolves during the process of growth and that incites and directs behavior.

dromostanolone propionate /drō'mostan'- əlōn/, a synthetic androgen prescribed for female breast cancer.

dromotropic, an agent that influences the conduction of electrical impulses. A positive dromotropic agent enhances the conduction of electrical impulses to the heart.

dronabinol /drōnab'inol/, an oral antiemetic prescribed for refractory nausea and vomiting caused by cancer chemotherapy.

drop [AS, *dropa*], a small, spheric mass of liquid. A drop may vary in size with differences in temperature, viscosity, and other factors. For therapeutic purposes, a drop is regarded as having a volume of 0.06 to 0.1 ml, or 1 to 1.5 minims.

drop arm test, a diagnostic test for a tear in the supraspinatus tendon. The result is positive if the patient is unable to lower the affected arm from a position of 90 degrees of abduction slowly and smoothly.

drop attack, a form of transient ischemic attack in which a brief interruption of cerebral blood flow causes a person to fall to the floor without losing consciousness. The episode may affect the sense of balance or leg muscle tone.

droperidol /drəper'ədol/, an antipsychotic, sedative drug of the butyrophenone group, used most commonly with a narcotic analgesic (fentanyl) in neuroleptanesthesia.

droplet infection [AS, *dropa* + L, *inficere*, to infect], an infection acquired by the inhalation of pathogenic microorganisms suspended in particles of liquid exhaled, sneezed, or coughed by another infected person or animal.

Droplet Precautions, safeguards designed to reduce the risk of droplet transmission of infectious agents. Droplet transmission involves contact of the conjunctivae or the mucous membranes of the nose or mouth of a susceptible person with large-particle droplets (larger than 5µm in size) containing microorganisms generated from a person who has a clinical disease or is a carrier of the disease. Droplets are generated from the source person primarily during coughing, sneezing, talking, and performance of certain procedures such as suctioning and bronchoscopy. Large-particle droplet transmission requires close contact between source and recipient persons because droplets do not remain suspended in the air and generally travel only short distances (usually 3 feet or less).

dropper, a glass or plastic tube narrowed at one end with a rubber bulb at the other end to dispense a liquid medication one drop at a time.

Drosophila /drōsof'ilə/ [Gk, *drosos,* dew, *philein,* to love], a genus of fly, which includes *Drosophila melanogaster,* the Mediterranean fruit fly. It is useful in genetic experiments because of the large chromosomes found in its salivary glands and its sensitivity to environmental effects, as exposure to radiation.

drowning [ME, *drounen*], asphyxiation caused by submersion in a liquid.

drowsiness, a decreased level of consciousness characterized by sleepiness and difficulty in remaining alert. It may be caused by a lack of sleep, medications, substance abuse, or a cerebral disorder.

drox, abbreviation for a *noncarboxylate hydroxide anion.*

Dr. P.H., abbreviation for *Doctor of Public Health.*

DRSP, abbreviation for **drug-resistant** *Streptococcus pneumoniae.*

drug [Fr, *drogue*], **1.** any substance taken by mouth; injected into a muscle, the skin, a blood vessel, or a cavity of the body; or applied topically to treat or prevent a disease or condition. **2.** *informal.* a narcotic substance.

drug absorption, the process whereby a drug moves from the muscle, digestive tract, or other site of entry into the body toward the circulatory system and the target organ or tissue.

drug abuse, the overuse of a drug for a nontherapeutic effect. Some of the most commonly abused drugs are alcohol, amphetamines, barbiturates, cocaine, methaqualone, narcotics, opium alkaloids, and tranquilizers. Drug abuse may lead to organ damage, addiction, and disturbed patterns of behavior.

Drug Abuse Warning Network (DAWN), a system of collecting information about admissions to emergency treatment facilities for drug abuse.

drug action, the means by which a drug exerts a desired effect.

drug addiction, a condition characterized by an overwhelming desire to continue taking a drug to which one has become habituated through repeated consumption because it produces a particular effect, usually an alteration of mental status. Addiction is usually accompanied by a compulsion to obtain the drug, a tendency to increase the dose, a psychologic or physical dependence, and detrimental consequences for the individual and society.

drug agonist, one of two similar drugs that may affect the same target organ or tissue, producing the same or a similar response.

drug allergy, hypersensitivity to a pharmacologic agent, manifested by reactions ranging from a mild rash to anaphylactic shock, depending on the sensitivity of the individual, the allergen, and the dose.

drug clearance, the elimination of a drug from the body. It is commonly excreted by the kidneys, liver, and lungs. The rate of clearance helps determine the size and frequency of a dosage of a particular medication.

drug compliance, the reliability of the patient in using a prescribed medication exactly as ordered by the physician. Noncompliance occurs when a patient forgets or neglects to take the prescribed dosages at the recommended times or decides to discontinue the drug without consulting the physician.

drug concentration, a relationship between therapeutic and toxic drug levels in a patient. Toxic drug levels may be observed when the body's normal mechanisms for metabolizing and excreting drugs are impaired, as commonly occurs in patients with liver or kidney disorders and in infants with immature organs.

drug dependence, a psychologic craving for, habituation to, abuse of, or physiologic reliance on a chemical substance.

drug dispensing, the preparation, packaging, labeling, record keeping, and transfer of a prescription drug to a patient or an intermediary, such as a nurse, who is responsible for administration of the drug.

drug disposition, the absorption, distribution, metabolism, and excretion of drugs.

drug distribution, the pattern of absorption of drug molecules by various tissues after the chemical enters the circulatory system. Because of differences in pH, cell membrane functions, and other individual tissue factors, most drugs are not distributed equally in all parts of the body.

drug-drug interaction, a modification of the effect of a drug when administered with another drug. The effect may be an increase or a decrease in the action of either substance, or it may be an adverse effect that is not normally associated with either drug.

Drug Enforcement Agency (DEA), an agency of the Drug Enforcement Administration of the federal government, empowered to enforce regulations that control the import or export of narcotic drugs and certain other substances or the traffic of these substances across state lines.

drug fever, a fever caused by the pharmacologic action of a medication, its thermoregulatory action, a local complication of parenteral administration, or, most commonly, an immunologic reaction mediated by drug-induced antibodies. The onset of fever occurs usually between 7 and 10 days after the medication is begun; a return to normal is ordinarily seen within 2 or 3 days of discontinuance of the drug.

drug-food interaction, the effect produced when some drugs and certain foods or beverages are taken at the same time, as in the example of monoamine oxidase inhibitors that can react dangerously with foods containing the amino acid tyramine.

drug holiday, a period of drug withdrawal to reverse long-term adverse effects that may result from chronic treatment. For example, after a 7-to 10-day drug holiday, levodopa responsiveness appears to be enhanced, and lower doses are required.

drug-induced parkinsonism, a reversible syndrome with the clinical features of Parkinson's disease but caused by the acetylcholine-dopamine imbalance of antipsychotic drugs.

drug-induced teratogenesis, congenital anomalies that reflect toxic effects of drugs on the developing fetus.

drug metabolism, the transformation of a drug by the body tissues into a metabolite. Examples include aspirin, which is metabolized to salicylic acid, an analgesic, and codeine, which is converted to morphine.

drug monograph, a statement that specifies the kinds and amounts of ingredients a drug or class of drugs may contain, the directions for the drug's use, the conditions in which it may be used, and the contraindications to its use.

drug overdose (O.D.) [Fr, *drogue,* drug; AS, *ofer;* Gk, *dosis,* giving], an accidental or purposeful dose of a drug large enough to cause severe adverse reactions.

drug potency, a measure of the effect of one drug as compared with a similar medication of the same dosage. The drug that produces the maximum effect with the smallest dose has the greater potency.

drug profile, an outline or summary of the characteristics of a drug or drug family, listing dosage types, pregnancy category, prescription or over-the-counter forms, generics if available, contraindications, and classification if covered by controlled-substance laws.

drug psychosis [Fr, *drogue,* drug; Gk, *psyche,* mind, *osis,* condition], a psychotic state induced by excessive dosage of certain therapeutic drugs, as well as drugs of abuse. Therapeutic drugs often associated with drug-induced psychosis include belladonna, chloral hydrate, paraldehyde, steroids, and isoniazid.

drug rash, a skin eruption, usually an allergic reaction, that is caused by a particular drug. A drug rash that is a sensitivity reaction does not occur the first time the drug is taken; the effect is observed with subsequent uses.

drug reaction [Fr, *drogue,* drug; L, *re, agere,* to act], any adverse effect on the body of therapeutic drugs, drugs of abuse, or the interaction of two or more pharmacologically active agents within a short time span. Drugs most likely to cause adverse reactions include hypnotics, central nervous system stimulants, antidepressants, tranquilizers, and muscle relaxants.

drug receptor, any part of a cell, usually a large protein molecule, with which a drug molecule interacts to trigger a response or effect.

drug rehabilitation center, an agency that provides treatment for a person with a chemical or drug dependency.

drug resistance, the ability of disease organisms to resist effects of drugs that previously were toxic to them. Bacterial resistance to an antibiotic can result from mutation of a strain that has been exposed to an antibiotic or similar agent. Such acquired resistance may result from a chromosomal disruption or acquisition of a stray bit of deoxyribonucleic acid on a resistant plasmid. Alteration or inactivation of the antibiotic is perhaps the most common mechanism of drug resistance. Acquired resistance to beta-lactam antibiotics is determined by the production of enzymes that inactivate the antibiotic. Drug resistance may also result from a change in the target site on which it acts.

drug-resistant *Streptococcus pneumoniae* (DRSP), a widespread strain of respiratory pathogen that is drug resistant. Until the 1960s *S. pneumoniae* was almost uniformly susceptible to penicillin alone. In 1967 resistance to penicillin and other microbial drugs was first reported in Australia; it has since spread worldwide.

drug-seeking behavior (DSB), a pattern of seeking narcotic pain medication or tranquilizers with forged prescriptions, false identification, repeated requests for replacement of "lost" drugs or prescriptions, complaints of severe pain without an organic basis, and abusive or threatening behavior manifested when denied drugs.

drug sequestration, the process by which certain drugs are stored in the body tissues. Examples include tetracycline, which may be stored in bone tissue, and chloroquine, which is stored in the liver.

drug tolerance, a condition of cellular adaptation to a pharmacologically active substance so that increasingly larger doses are required to produce the same physiologic or psychologic effect obtained earlier with smaller doses.

drug trial, the process of determining an adequate and effective therapeutic dose of a specific drug for a particular patient. The trial culminates with (1) an acceptable clinical result, (2) intolerable adverse effects, (3) a poor response after an appropriate blood level is reached, or (4) administration of the drug for a specific time.

drum cartridge catheter technique, a method used in central vein cannulation. The vein is cannulated with an introducer cannula. The needle is removed and replaced by the drum cartridge catheter, which is left in place.

drum electrode, an induction electrode that produces a strong magnetic field, used primarily with pulsed short-wave diathermy.

drusen /drōo'zən/ [Ger, *Druse,* stony granule], small, white hyaline deposits that develop beneath the retinal pigment epithelium, sometimes appearing as nodules within the optic nerve head. They tend to occur most frequently in persons older than 60 years of age.

DRV, abbreviation for **Daily Reference Values.**

dry abscess, a collection of pus that disperses without reaching a point of bursting.

dry catarrh [AS, *dryge* + Gk, *kata,* down, *rhoia,* flow], a dry cough accompanied by almost no expectoration that occurs in severe coughing spells. It is associated with asthma and emphysema in older people.

dry cough, a cough that does not produce sputum.

dry crackle, an abnormal chest sound

produced by air passage through a constricted bronchial tube.

dry dressing, a plain dressing containing no medication, applied directly to an incision or a wound to prevent contamination or trauma or to absorb secretions.

dry eye syndrome, a dryness of the cornea and conjunctiva caused by a deficiency in tear production. It results in a sensation of a foreign body in the eye, burning eyes, keratitis, and erosion of the epithelial layers of the cornea and conjunctiva.

dry gas (D), (in respiratory therapy) a gas that contains no water vapor.

dry heat, a thermal effect produced by adding dry air or reducing the humidity of the environment.

dry heat sterilization [AS, *dryge* + *haetu* + L, *sterilis*], a method of sterilization that uses heated dry air at a temperature of 320° to 356° F (160° to 180° C) for 90 minutes to 3 hours.

dry ice, solid carbon dioxide, with a temperature of about −140° F. It is used in cryotherapy of various skin disorders.

dry labor, *informal.* labor in which amniotic fluid has already escaped. Since amniotic fluid is continually produced, no labor is really dry.

dry pleurisy [AS, *dryge*, dry; Gk, *pleuritis*], an inflammation of the pleura without effusion of serum. The cause may be a localized injury or an early sign of tuberculosis.

Drysdale's corpuscle /drīz′dālz/ [Thomas M. Drysdale, American gynecologist, 1831–1904], one of a number of transparent cells in the fluid of some ovarian cysts.

dry skin, epidermis that lacks moisture or sebum, often characterized by a pattern of fine lines, scaling, and itching. Causes include too-frequent bathing, low humidity, and decreased production of sebum in aging skin.

dry tooth socket, an inflamed condition of a tooth socket (alveolus) after extraction. Normally a blood clot forms over the alveolar bone at the base of the tooth socket after an extraction. If the clot fails to form properly or becomes dislodged, the bone tissue is exposed to the environment and can become infected.

dry vomiting [AS, *dryge* + L, *vomere,* to vomit], nausea with retching that does not produce vomitus.

DSA, abbreviation for **digital subtraction angiography.**

DSB, abbreviation for **drug-seeking behavior.**

DSDB, abbreviation for **direct self-destructive behavior.**

DSM, abbreviation for *Diagnostic and Statistical Manual of Mental Disorders.*

DSN, abbreviation for *Doctor of Science in Nursing.*

DSR, abbreviation for **dynamic spatial reconstructor.**

DT, abbreviation for **diphtheria and tetanus toxoids.**

dTc, abbreviation for *d*-tubocurarine.

DTP vaccine, a combination of diphtheria and tetanus toxoids and killed pertussis vaccine that is administered intramuscularly for active immunization against those diseases.

DTR, abbreviation for **deep tendon reflex.**

DTs, abbreviation for **delirium tremens.**

dual-energy imaging /dyo͞o′əl/, a radiographic imaging technique in which two radiographs are taken of the same target area using two different kilovoltages. One image isolates bone contrast, and the other isolates soft tissue contrast. The combined x-ray films can help to make a more precise identification of an abnormality.

dual-energy x-ray absorptiometry (DEXA), an imaging technique for quantifying bone density for purposes of diagnosis and management of osteoporosis.

dual-focus tube, an x-ray tube used for diagnostic imaging. It has one large and one small focal spot. The large focal spot is used when techniques that produce high heat are required; the small focal spot is used to produce fine, detailed images.

duality of central nervous system control /dyo͞o·al′itē/, a theory that the normal central nervous system is regulated by a check-and-balance feedback program. The theory is based on studies of posture-movement, mobility-stability, flexion-extension synergies, and similar action-reaction examples related to laws of basic physics.

DUB, 1. abbreviation for **dysfunctional uterine bleeding. 2.** a genetically determined human blood factor that is associated with immunity to certain diseases.

Dubin-Johnson syndrome /do͞o′binjon′-sən/ [Isadore N. Dubin, American pathologist, 1913–1980; Frank B. Johnson, American pathologist, b. 1919], a rare chronic hereditary hyperbilirubinemia, characterized by nonhemolytic jaundice, abnormal liver pigmentation, and abnormal function of the gallbladder.

dubnium (Db) [Joint Institute for Nuclear Research at Dubna, Russia], a transuranic element. Its atomic number is 104; its atomic weight (mass) is 260. It is produced by an induced nuclear reaction.

DuBois formula /do͞oboiz′/, a logarithmic method of calculating the number of square meters of body surface area of an individual from the height in centimeters, the weight in kilograms, and a constant, 0.007184.

Dubowitz assessment [Victor Dubowitz, South African-English pediatrician, b. 1931], a system of estimating the gestational age of a newborn according to such factors as posture, ankle dorsiflexion, and arm and leg recoil.

Duchenne-Aran disease /dooˈshenˈäräNˈ/ [Guillaume B.A. Duchenne; François A. Aran, French physician, 1817–1861], muscular atrophy caused by degeneration of the anterior horn cells of the spinal cord and primarily affecting the upper extremities. Chronic muscle wasting and weakness first appear in the hands and advance progressively to the arms and shoulders, eventually affecting the legs and other body areas.

Duchenne's disease /dooˈshenzˈ/ [Guillaume B.A. Duchenne, French neurologist, 1806–1875], a series of three different neurologic conditions: spinal muscular atrophy, **bulbar paralysis,** and **tabes dorsalis.**

Duchenne's muscular dystrophy [Guillaume B.A. Duchenne], an abnormal congenital condition characterized by progressive symmetric wasting of the leg and pelvic muscles. It is an X-linked recessive disease that appears insidiously between 3 and 5 years of age and spreads from the leg and pelvic muscles to the involuntary muscles. Associated muscle weakness produces a waddling gait and pronounced lordosis. Muscles rapidly deteriorate, and calf muscles become firm and enlarged as a result of fatty deposits. Affected children experience contractures, have difficulty climbing stairs, often stumble and fall, and display wing scapulae when they raise their arms.

Duchenne's paralysis [Guillaume B.A. Duchenne; Gk, *paralyein,* to be palsied], a form of motor neuron disease characterized by wasting and weakness in the laryngeal, pharyngeal, tongue, and facial muscles, leading to dysarthria and dysphagia. There may also be pyramidal tract involvement.

duct [L, *ducere,* to lead], a narrow tubular structure, especially one through which material is secreted or excreted.

duct carcinoma, a neoplasm of the epithelium of ducts, especially in the breast or pancreas.

duct ectasia, an abnormal dilation of a duct by lipids and cellular debris.

ductile, having the property of allowing metals to be drawn into the thinness of a wire.

ductility /duktilˈitē/, the property of a material of having a large elastic range and tending to deform before failing from stress.

duction /dukˈshən/, the movement of an individual eyeball from the primary to the secondary or tertiary position of gaze.

ductless gland /duktˈles/, a gland lacking an excretory duct such as an endocrine gland, which secretes hormones directly into blood or lymph.

duct of Rivinus /rivēˈnəs/ [L, *ducere,* to lead; Augustus Q. Rivinus, German anatomist, 1652–1723], one of the minor sublingual ducts.

ductus /dukˈtəs/, *pl.* **ductus** /dukˈtoos/, the Latin term for *duct.*

ductus arteriosus, a vascular channel in the fetus that joins the pulmonary artery directly to the descending aorta.

ductus epididymidis, a tube into which the efferent ductules of the testes empty.

ductus venosus, the vascular channel in the fetus passing through the liver and joining the umbilical vein with the inferior vena cava.

due diligence, efforts made by responsible persons to prevent causing harm to others or their property or organization.

Duke longitudinal study, long-range indepth research into the normal aging process of middle-aged and older men and women conducted at Duke University Medical Center. The Duke studies led to development of the "longevity quotient" used to evaluate an individual's rate of aging. It is calculated by the number of years a person survives beyond a given time divided by the expected number of years derived from actuarial tables.

Dukes' classification, a staging system for colorectal tumors, from A to D, according to the degree of tissue invasion and metastasis. A Dukes' A tumor is one that is confined to the mucosa and submucosa. A B tumor is one that has invaded the musculature but has not involved the lymphatic system. C tumors have invaded the musculature with metastatic involvement of the regional lymph nodes. D tumors are those that have metastasized to distant organ tissues.

dull, 1. blunt. **2.** sluggish. **3.** not sharp, vivid, or intense.

dull pain [ME, *dul,* not sharp; L, *poena,* penalty], a mildly throbbing acute or chronic pain.

dumping syndrome [ME, *dumpen,* to throw down], the combination of profuse sweating, nausea, dizziness, and weakness experienced by patients who have had a subtotal gastrectomy. Symptoms are felt soon after eating, when the contents of the stomach empty too rapidly into the duodenum.

Duncan's mechanism [James M. Duncan, English obstetrician, 1826–1890; Gk, *mechane*, machine], a technique for delivery of the placenta with the maternal surface rather than the fetal surface presenting.

Dunlop skeletal traction, an orthopedic mechanism that helps immobilize the upper limb in the treatment of the contracture or the supracondylar fracture of the elbow. The mechanism uses a system of traction weights, pulleys, and ropes. The system is attached to the bone involved with a pin or wire.

Dunlop skin traction, an orthopedic mechanism that helps immobilize the upper limb in the treatment of contracture and supracondylar fracture of the elbow. The mechanism uses a system of traction weights, pulleys, and ropes, usually applied unilaterally but sometimes bilaterally. Dunlop skin traction may be applied as adhesive or nonadhesive skin traction.

duodenal /doō'ədē'nəl/ [L, *duodeni,* 12 fingers], pertaining to the duodenum.

duodenal bulb, the first part of the superior part of the duodenum, which has a bulblike appearance on radiographic views of the small intestine.

duodenal digestion [L, *duodeni,* 12 fingers, *digere,* to separate], digestion that occurs in the first intestinal segment beyond the pylorus, where secretions of the liver and pancreas are received and mixed with the partially digested food from the stomach. Chyle is formed, fats are emulsified, starch is hydrolyzed, and proteolytic enzymes begin to break down proteins.

duodenal ulcer, an ulcer in the duodenum, the most common type of peptic ulcer.

duodenectomy /doō'ədenek'təmē/ [L, *duodeni,* 12 fingers, Gk, *ektome,* excision], the total or partial excision of the duodenum.

duodenitis /doō'ədenī'tis/ [L, *duodeni,* 12 fingers; Gk, *itis,* inflammation], a condition of inflammation of the duodenum.

duodenography /doō'ədənog'rəfē/ [L, *duodeni,* 12 fingers; Gk, *graphein,* to record], the process of making a radiographic image of the duodenum and pancreas.

duodenoscope /doō'ədē'nəskōp'/, an endoscopic instrument, usually fiberoptic, inserted via the mouth for the visual examination of the duodenum.

duodenoscopy /doō'ədənos'kəpē/, the visual examination of the duodenum by means of an endoscope.

duodenostomy /doō'ədēnos'təmē/ [L, *duodeni,* 12 fingers; Gk, *stoma,* mouth], the surgical creation of a direct opening to the duodenum through the abdominal wall.

duodenum /doō'ədē'nəm, doō·od'inəm/, *pl.* **duodena, duodenums** [L, *duodeni,* 12 fingers], the shortest, widest, and most fixed part of the small intestine, taking an almost circular course from the pyloric valve of the stomach so that its termination is close to its starting point. It is about 25 cm long and is divided into superior, descending, horizontal, and ascending parts.

dup, (in cytogenetics) abbreviation for *duplication.*

duplex scanner /d(y)oō'pleks/, an ultrasound machine that generally combines a 7.5-or 10-MHz imaging probe with a 3-MHz pulsed Doppler to allow visualization of a part of the venous system. The scanner can determine the direction of blood flow within the veins.

duplex transmission [L, *duplex,* twofold], the passage of a neural impulse in both directions along a nerve fiber.

duplex ultrasonography, a combination of real time and Doppler ultrasonography.

duplicating film /doō'plikā'ting/, a single-emulsion film used to copy an existing radiographic image by exposing it to ultraviolet light.

Dupuytren's contracture /dYpY·itraNs', dēpē·itranz'/ [Guillaume Dupuytren, French surgeon, 1777–1835; L, *contractura* drawing together], a progressive painless thickening and tightening of subcutaneous tissue of the palm, causing the fourth and fifth fingers to bend into the palm and resist extension. Tendons and nerves are not involved. Although the condition begins in one hand, both become symmetrically affected.

durable power of attorney for health care /dyoōr'əbəl/, a document that designates an agent or proxy to make health care decisions if the patient is no longer able to make them.

dural sac /dyoōr'əl/ the blind pouch formed by the lower end of the dura mater, at the level of the second sacral segment.

dural sheath, an extension of the dura mater covering the optic nerve and spinal nerve roots.

dura mater /doō'rə mā'tər, dyoō'rə/ [L, *durus,* hard, *mater,* mother], the outermost and most fibrous of the three membranes surrounding the brain and spinal cord. The dura mater encephali covers the brain, and the dura mater spinalis covers the cord.

duration, (in radiology) the length of time a current is flowing.

duress /dyŏŏres'/ [L, *durus,* hard], (in law) an action compelling another person to do what he or she would not do voluntarily. A consent form signed under duress is not valid.

Durham-Humphrey Amendment, a 1952 modification of the 1938 U.S. Food, Drug, and Cosmetic Act. It differentiates between prescription and over-the-counter medications and specifies medications that can or cannot be refilled without a new prescription. It also identifies which original prescriptions and refills can be authorized over the telephone.

Duroziez' murmur /dY'rōzyās, dir'-, dŏŏ'r-/, [Paul L. Duroziez, French physician, 1826–1897; L, *murmur*], a systolic murmur heard over the femoral or other large artery when the artery is compressed. The phenomenon is associated with high arterial pulse pressure or aortic insufficiency. A diastolic murmur may also be heard by increasing pressure on the artery distal to the stethoscope.

dust [AS], any fine, particulate dry matter. Kinds of dust are **inorganic dust** and **organic dust.**

dustborne infection, a disease in which the pathogenic organism is airborne in dust particles, as in coccidioidomycosis.

Dutton's relapsing fever [Joseph E. Dutton, English pathologist, 1877–1905], an infection caused by a spirochete, *Borrelia duttonii,* which is transmitted by a soft tick, *Ornithodoros moubata,* found in human dwellings in tropical Africa. The spirochete enters the lesion through a tick bite, characteristically producing a high fever, chills, rapid heartbeat, headache, joint and muscle pain, vomiting, and neurologic disorders.

duty [ME, *duete,* conduct], (in law) an obligation owed by one party to another. Duty may be established by statute or other legal process, as by contract or oath supported by statute, or it may be voluntarily undertaken.

duty cycle, the percentage of time that ultrasound is being generated (pulse duration) over one pulse period.

Duverney's fracture /dŏŏ'vərnāz'/ [Joseph G. Duverney, French anatomist, 1648–1730], fracture of the ilium just below the anterior superior spine.

dv/dt, (in cardiology) the rate of change of voltage with respect to time.

D.V.M., abbreviation for *Doctor of Veterinary Medicine.*

dwarf /dwôrf/ [AS, *dweorge*], **1.** an ab-

normally short, undersized person, especially one whose body parts are not proportional. **2.** to prevent or retard, for example, normal growth.

dwarfism /dwôrf'izəm/, the abnormal underdevelopment of the body, characterized predominantly by extreme shortness of stature. Dwarfism has multiple causes, including genetic defects; endocrine dysfunction involving either the pituitary or thyroid gland; and chronic diseases such as rickets, renal failure, intestinal malabsorption defects, and psychosocial stress, as in the maternal deprivation syndrome.

dwarf tapeworm infection, a type of intestinal parasitic disease caused by an infestation of *Hymenolepis nana.* It occurs mainly in the southern United States and usually affects children who ingest eggs by placing contaminated materials into the mouth.

Dwayne-Hunt law /dwān'hunt'/, (in radiology) the principle that x-ray energy is inversely proportional to the photon wavelength. As the photon wavelength increases, photon energy decreases, and vice versa. The minimum x-ray wavelength is associated with the maximum x-ray energy.

dwindles, *informal.* a condition of physical deterioration involving several body systems, usually in an elderly person.

Dwyer instrumentation /dwī'ər/, one method for correcting the spinal curvature associated with scoliosis. The Dwyer cable method uses a mechanical device that assists in correcting the curvature. The device is inserted to assist in maintaining the corrected curvature while the fusion heals.

Dy, symbol for the element **dysprosium.**

dyad /dī'ad/ [Gk, *dyas,* two], (in genetics) one of the paired homologous chromosomes, consisting of two chromatids, which result from the division of a tetrad in the first meiotic division of gametogenesis. —**dyadic,** *adj.*

dyadic interpersonal communication /dī·ad'ik/, a process in which two people interact face to face as senders and receivers, as in a conversation.

dyclonine hydrochloride /dī'klənīn/, a local anesthetic, with bactericidal and fungicidal properties, for oral pain, pruritus, insect bites, and minor skin burns and injuries.

dydrogesterone /dī'drəjes'tərōn/, a synthetic oral progestin prescribed for abnormal uterine bleeding, menopausal vasomotor symptoms, pickwickian syndrome, endometrial cancer, and contraception.

dye /dī/ [AS, *deag*], **1.** to apply coloring matter to a substance. **2.** a chemical compound capable of imparting color to a substance to which it is applied. Various dyes are used in medicine as stains for tissues, test reagents, therapeutic agents, and coloring agents in pharmaceutical preparations.

dye laser, a system of highly selective laser destruction of skin blemishes using various dyes at wavelengths at the longer oxygenated hemoglobin absorption peaks to overcome interference from overlying melanin.

Dying Care, a Nursing Interventions Classification defined as promotion of physical comfort and psychologic peace in the final phase of life.

dynamic /dīnam′ik/ [Gk, *dynamis,* force], **1.** tending to change or to encourage change, such as a dynamic nurse-patient relationship. **2.** (in respiratory therapy) a condition of changing volume.

dynamic cardiac work, the energy transfer that occurs during the process of ventricular ejection of blood.

dynamic compliance, the distensibility of the lung, as measured by plethysmography during the breathing cycle.

dynamic equilibrium, the ability of a person to adjust to displacements of the body's center of gravity by changing its base of support.

dynamic ileus, an intestinal obstruction with associated recurrent and continuous muscle spasms.

dynamic imaging, (in ultrasonography) the imaging of an object in motion at a frame rate that does not cause significant blurring of any one image and at a repetition rate sufficient to represent the movement pattern adequately.

dynamic nurse-patient relationship, a conceptual framework in which the interpersonal aspects of the nurse-patient relationship are analyzed. Many factors affect the relationship. Elements in the process include the behavior of the patient, the reaction of the nurse, and the actions of the nurse that are intended to aid the patient.

dynamic psychiatry, the study of motivational, emotional, and biologic factors as determinants of human behavior.

dynamic range, 1. (in radiology) the range of voltage or input signals that result in a digital output. **2.** (in audiology) the range of decibels from the faintest sound a person can hear to the level that causes pain.

dynamic response, the accuracy with which a physiologic monitoring system such as an electrocardiograph simulates the actual event being recorded.

dynamic spatial reconstructor (DSR), a kind of radiographic machine permitting the moving of three-dimensional images

of human organs to be examined visually and from any direction.

dynamic splint [Gk, *dynamis,* force; D, *splinte*], any splint that incorporates springs, elastic bands, or other materials that produce a constant active force to counteract deforming forces of a splint.

dynamometer /dī′nəmom′ətər/ [Gk, *dynamis,* force, *metron,* measure], a device for measuring the degree of force used in the contraction of a group of muscles, such as a squeeze dynamometer, which measures the gross grip strength of the hand muscles.

dyne /dīn/, a unit of force, specifically the force required to accelerate a free mass of 1 g at 1 cm/sec. One dyne equals 10^{-5} newton.

dynode /dī′nōd/, one of a series of platelike elements that amplify electron pulses in a photomultiplier tube. For each electron that strikes each dynode, several secondary electrons are emitted. The dynode gain is the ratio of secondary electrons to incident electrons.

dyphylline /difil′in/, a bronchodilator prescribed in the treatment of bronchospasm in acute bronchial asthma, bronchitis, and emphysema.

dysacusis /dis′əkōō′sis/ [Gk, *dys,* difficult, *akouein,* to hear], a condition in which loud sounds can cause pain or discomfort. It is usually the result of damage to the cochlea.

dysadrenia /dis′adrē′nē-ə/ [Gk, *dys,* bad; L, *ad,* to, *ren,* kidney], abnormal adrenal function characterized by decreased hormone production, as in hypoadrenalism or hypoadrenocorticism, or by increased secretion of the products of the gland, as in hyperadrenalism or hyperadrenocorticism.

dysarthria /disär′thrē-ə/ [Gk, *dys* + *arthroun,* to articulate], difficult, poorly articulated speech resulting from interference in the control over the muscles of speech, usually caused by damage to a central or peripheral motor nerve.

dysarthrosis /dis′ärthrō′sis/ [Gk, *dys,* difficult, *arthron,* joint], any disorder of a joint, including disease, dislocation, or deformity, that makes movement of it difficult.

dysautonomia /disô′tənō′mē-ə/ [Gk, *dys* + *autonomia,* self-government], a dysfunction of the autonomic nervous system that can be a clinical feature of diabetes, parkinsonism, Adie's syndrome, Shy-Drager syndrome, or Riley-Day syndrome. A fairly common effect is orthostatic hypotension with syncope and drop attacks.

dysbarism /dis′bäriz′əm/, a reaction to a sudden change in environmental pressure, such as rapid exposure to the lower atmospheric pressures of high altitudes. It is marked by symptoms similar to those of decompression sickness.

dysbasia /disbā′zhə/, difficulty in walking caused by a nerve lesion or lameness associated with atherosclerosis.

dysbetalipoproteinemia /disbet′əlip′-əprō′tinē′mē-ə/ an accumulation of abnormal beta-lipoprotein in the blood.

dyscholia /diskō′lē-ə/ [Gk, dys + chole, bile], any abnormal condition of the bile, related to either the quantity secreted or the condition of the constituents.

dyschroic film fault /diskrō′ik/, a defect in a radiograph that appears as a pinkish coloration when the film is viewed by transmitted light and as a green coloration when the film is viewed by reflected light.

dyscrasia /diskrā′zhə/ [Gk, dys + krasis, mingling], pertaining to an abnormal condition of the blood or bone marrow such as leukemia, aplastic anemia, or prenatal Rh incompatibility.

dyscrastic fracture /diskrā′sik, diskraz′ik/, any fracture caused by the weakening of a specific bone as a result of a debilitating disease.

dysdiadochokinesia /dis′dī-ədō′kōkinē′-zhə/ [Gk, dys + diadochos, working in turn, kinesis, movement], an inability to perform rapidly alternating movements such as rhythmically tapping the fingers on the knee. The cause is a cerebellar lesion and is related to dysmetria.

dysentery /dis′inter′ē/ [Gk, dys + enteron, intestine], an inflammation of the intestine, especially of the colon, that may be caused by chemical irritants, bacteria, protozoa, or parasites. It is characterized by frequent and bloody stools, abdominal pain, and tenesmus.

dysentery toxin, an exotoxin produced by Shigella dysenteriae.

dysergia /disur′jē-ə/ [Gk, dys + ergon, work], a condition characterized by lack of muscle coordination caused by a defect of efferent nerve impulses.

dysesthesia /dis′esthē′zhə/, a common effect of spinal cord injury characterized by sensations of numbness, tingling, burning, or pain felt below the level of the lesion.

dysfunctional /disfungk′shənəl/ [Gk, dys + L, functio, performance], (of a body organ or system) unable to function normally. —**dysfunction,** n.

dysfunctional communication, a communication that results from inaccurate perceptions, faulty internal filters (personal interpretations of information), and social isolation.

dysfunctional stereotype, a stereotype in

which abnormal or impaired aspects of a culture are emphasized.

dysfunctional uterine bleeding (DUB), abnormal uterine bleeding that is not caused by a tumor, inflammation, or pregnancy. It may be characterized by painless, irregular heavy bleeding or intermenstrual spotting or periods of amenorrhea. The condition is associated with anovulation and unopposed estrogen stimulation.

dysgammaglobulinemia /disgam′əglob′-yəlinē′mē-ə/, an antibody-mediated genetic (primary) immune deficiency disease. As a result of a deficiency of immunoglobulins needed to produce antibodies, the immune response does not adequately protect the client from infection, cancer, or other diseases.

dysgenesis /disjen′əsis/ [Gk, dys + genein, to produce], **1.** defective or abnormal formation of an organ or part, primarily during embryonic development. **2.** impairment or loss of ability to procreate. A kind of dysgenesis is **gonadal dysgenesis.** —**dysgenic,** adj.

dysgenics /disjen′iks/, the study of those factors or situations that are genetically detrimental to the future of a race or species.

dysgenitalism /disjen′itəliz′əm/ [Gk, dys + L, genitalis, belonging to birth], any condition involving the abnormal development of the genital organs.

dysgerminoma /dis′jərminō′mə/ [Gk, dys + L, germen, germ; Gk, oma, tumor], a rare malignant tumor of the ovary that occurs in young women and is believed to arise from the undifferentiated germ cells of the embryonic gonad.

dysgeusia /disgoo′zhə/ [Gk, dys + geusis, taste], an abnormal or impaired sense of taste.

dysglandular /disglan′dyələr/, caused by or related to excessive or inadequate secretion by a gland.

dysgnathic anomaly /disnath′ik/ [Gk, dys + gnathos, jaw], (in dentistry) an abnormality that extends beyond the teeth, affecting the maxilla, the mandible, or both.

dysgraphia /disgraf′ē-ə/ [Gk, dys + graphein, to write], an impairment of the ability to write, caused by a pathologic disorder.

dyskeratosis /dis′kerətō′sis/ [Gk, dys + keras, horn, osis, condition], an abnormal or premature keratinization of epithelial cells.

dyskinesia /dis′kinē′zhə/ [Gk, dys + kinesis, movement], an impairment of the ability to execute voluntary movements. —**dyskinetic** /-et′ik/, adj..

dyskinesia intermittens, a condition of

intermittent limping caused by circulatory impairment.

dyskinetic syndrome /dis'kinet'ik/, a form of cerebral palsy involving a basal ganglion disorder. Clinical features include athetoid movements of the extremities and sometimes the trunk. There may also be choreiform movements that tend to increase with emotional tension and diminish during sleep.

dyslexia /dislek'sē·ə/ [Gk, *dys* + *lexis*, word], an impairment of the ability to read, as a result of a variety of pathologic conditions, some of which are associated with the central nervous system. Dyslexic persons often reverse letters and words, cannot adequately distinguish the letter sequences in written words, and have difficulty determining left from right. —**dyslexic,** *adj.*

dysmaturity /dis'machŏŏr'itē/ [Gk, *dys* + L, *maturare*, to make ripe], **1.** the failure of an organism to develop, ripen, or otherwise achieve maturity in structure or function. **2.** the condition of a fetus or newborn that is abnormally small or large for its age of gestation. Kinds of dysmaturity are **small for gestational age** and **large for gestational age.** —**dysmature,** *adj.*

dysmegalopsia /dis'megəlop'sē·ə/ [Gk, *dys* + *megas*, large, *opsis*, appearance], an inability to judge the size or measure of an object accurately.

dysmelia /dismē'lyə/ [Gk, *dys* + *melos*, limb], an abnormal congenital condition characterized by missing or shortened extremities of the body and associated with abnormalities of the spine in some individuals. It is caused by abnormal metabolism during the development of the embryonic limbs.

dysmenorrhea /dis'menərē'ə/ [Gk, *dys* + *men*, month, *rhein*, to flow], pain associated with menstruation. Primary dysmenorrhea is menstrual pain that results from factors intrinsic to the uterus and the process of menstruation. It is extremely common, occurring at least occasionally in almost all women. If the painful episode is mild and brief, it is considered functional and normal and requires no treatment. In approximately 10% of women dysmenorrhea is sufficiently severe to cause episodes of partial or total disability. Pain occurs typically in the lower abdomen or back and is crampy, occurring in successive waves, apparently in conjunction with intense uterine contractions and slight cervical dilation. Pain usually begins just before, or at the onset of, menstrual flow and lasts from a few hours to 1 day or more. Pain is frequently

associated with nausea, vomiting, and frequent bowel movements with intestinal cramping. Dizziness, fainting, pallor, and obvious distress may also be observed. Secondary dysmenorrhea is menstrual pain that occurs secondary to specific pelvic abnormalities such as endometriosis, adenomyosis, chronic pelvic infection, chronic pelvic congestion, or degenerating fibroid tumors.

dysmetria /dismē'trē·ə/ [Gk, *dys* + *metron*, measure], an abnormal condition that prevents the affected individual from properly measuring distances associated with muscular acts and from controlling muscular action. It is associated with cerebellar lesions and typically characterized by overestimating or underestimating the range of motion needed to place the limbs correctly during voluntary movement.

dysmnesic syndrome /disnē'sik/, a memory disorder characterized by an inability to learn simple new skills, although the person can still perform highly complex skills learned before the onset of the condition. The cause is a disease or injury that affects only certain brain tissues associated with memory.

dysmorphogenesis /dis'môrfōjen'əsis/, the development of ill-shaped or otherwise malformed body structures.

dysmorphophobia /-fō'bē·ə / [Gk, *dys* + *morphe*, form, *phobos*, fear], **1.** a fundamental delusion of body image. **2.** the morbid fear of deformity.

dysorexia /dis'ôrek'sē·ə/, an eating disorder associated with emotional or psychologic impairment.

dysostosis /dis'ostō'sis/ [Gk, *dys* + *osteon*, bone, *osis*], an abnormal condition characterized by defective ossification, especially defects in the normal ossification of fetal cartilages. Kinds of dysostoses include **cleidocranial dysostosis, craniofacial dysostosis, mandibulofacial dysostosis,** metaphyseal dysostosis, and **Nager's acrofacial dysostosis.**

dyspareunia /dis'pərōō'nē·ə/ [Gk, *dys* + *pareunos*, mating], an abnormal pain during sexual intercourse. It may result from abnormal conditions of the genitalia, dysfunctional psychophysiologic reaction to sexual union, forcible coition, or incomplete sexual arousal.

dyspepsia /dispep'sē·ə/ [Gk, *dys* + *peptein*, to digest], a vague feeling of epigastric discomfort felt after eating. There is an uncomfortable feeling of fullness, heartburn, bloating, and nausea. —**dyspeptic,** *adj.*

dysphagia /disfā'jē·ə/ [Gk, *dys* + *phagein*, to swallow], difficulty in swallowing commonly associated with obstructive or motor disorders of the esophagus. Patients with obstructive disorders such as esophageal tumor or lower esophageal ring are unable to swallow solids but can tolerate liquids. Persons with motor disorders such as achalasia are unable to swallow solids or liquids.

dysphagia lusoria, an abnormal condition, characterized by difficulty in swallowing, caused by the compression of the esophagus from an anomalous right subclavian artery that arises from the descending aorta and courses behind or in front of the esophagus.

dysphasia /disfā′zhə/ [Gk, *dys* + *phasis,* speaking], an impairment of speech, not as severe as aphasia, usually the result of an injury to the speech area in the cerebral cortex of the brain.

dysphonia /disfō′nē·ə/ [Gk, *dys* + *phone,* voice], any abnormality in the speaking voice such as hoarseness. Dysphonia puberum identifies the voice changes that occur in adolescent boys.

dysphoria /disfôr′ə·ə/, a disorder of affect characterized by depression and anguish.

dysphylaxia /dis′filek′sē·ə/, a sudden awakening from deep sleep.

dyspigmentation /dispig′məntā′shən/, any abnormality in the production or distribution of skin pigment.

dysplasia /displā′zhə/ [Gk, *dys* + *plassein,* to form], any abnormal development of tissues or organs.

dyspnea /dispnē′ə/ [Gk, *dys* + *pnoia,* breathing], a distressful sensation of uncomfortable breathing that may be caused by certain heart conditions, strenuous exercise, or anxiety. —**dyspneal, dyspneic,** *adj.*

dyspraxia /disprak′sē·ə/ [Gk, *dys* + *prassein,* to do], a partial loss of the ability to perform skilled, coordinated movements in the absence of any associated defect in motor or sensory functions.

dysprosium (Dy) /disprō′sē·əm/ [Gk, *dys* + *prositos,* to approach], a rare-earth metallic element. Its atomic number is 66; its atomic weight (mass) is 162.50. Radioactive isotopes of dysprosium are used in radioisotope scanning.

dysproteinemia /disprō′tēnē′mē·ə/ [Gk, *dys* + *protos,* first, *haima,* blood], an abnormality of the protein content of the blood, usually involving the immunoglobulins.

dysraphia /disrā′fē·ə/ [Gk, *dys* + *raphe,* seam], failure of a raphe to fuse completely, as in incomplete closure of the neural tube.

dysraphic syndrome /disraf′ik/, a developmental disorder, usually involving the spinal cord, such as encephalocele or myelomeningocele.

dysreflexia /dis′riflek′sē·ə/ [Gk, *dys* + L, *reflectere,* to bend back], a NANDA-accepted nursing diagnosis of a state in which an individual with a spinal cord injury at T7 or above experiences or is at risk to experience a life-threatening uninhibited sympathetic response of the nervous system to a noxious stimulus. Defining characteristics include paroxysmal hypertension, bradycardia or tachycardia, diaphoresis above the injury, red splotches on the skin above the injury, pallor below the injury, a headache that is a diffuse pain, chilling, conjunctival congestion, blurred vision, chest pain, metallic taste in the mouth, nasal congestion, and pilomotor reflex. —**dysreflexic,** *adj.*

Dysreflexia Management, a Nursing Interventions Classification defined as prevention and elimination of stimuli that cause hyperactive reflexes and inappropriate responses in a patient with a cervical or high thoracic cord lesion.

dysregulation hypothesis /disreg′yəlā′-shən/, the view that depression and affective disorders do not simply reflect decreased or increased catecholamine activity but that they are failures of the regulation of these systems.

dysrhythmia /disrith′mē·ə/, any disturbance or abnormality in a normal rhythmic pattern, specifically, irregularity in the brain waves or cadence of speech.

Dysrhythmia Management, a Nursing Interventions Classification defined as preventing, recognizing, and facilitating treatment of abnormal cardiac rhythms.

dyssebacea /disibā′shē·ə/ [Gk, *dys* + L, *sebum,* suet], a skin condition characterized by red, scaly, greasy patches on the nose, eyelids, scrotum, and labia.

dyssynergia /dis′inur′jē·ə/ [Gk, *dys* + *syn,* together, *ergein,* work], any disturbance in muscular coordination, as in cases of ataxia.

dystaxia /distak′sē·ə/ [Gk, *dys* + *taxis,* order], partial ataxia such as dystaxia agitans in which a spinal cord irritation causes a tremor but no paralysis.

dysthymia /disthim′ē·ə/ [Gk, *dys* + *thymos,* mind], a form of chronic unipolar depression that tends to occur in elderly persons with debilitating physical disorders, multiple interpersonal losses, and chronic marital difficulties. Several depressive episodes may merge into a low-grade chronic depressive state.

dysthymic disorder /disthim′ik/ [Gk, *dy.* + *thymos,* mind], a disorder of mood in which the essential feature is a chroni disturbance of mood of at least 2 years duration. It involves either depressed mood or loss of interest or pleasure in all or almost all usual activities and pastimes, together with associated symptoms, but not of sufficient severity and duration to meet the criteria for a major depressive episode.

dystocia /distō'shə/ [Gk, *dys* + *tokos,* birth], pathologic or difficult labor that may be caused by an obstruction or constriction of the birth passage or abnormal size, shape, position, or condition of the fetus.

dystonia /distō'nē·ə/ [Gk, *dys* + *tonos,* tone], any impairment of muscle tone. The condition commonly involves the head, neck, and tongue and often occurs as an adverse effect of a medication.

dystonia musculorum deformans, a rare abnormal condition characterized by intense, irregular torsion muscle spasms that contort the body. The muscles of the trunk, shoulder, and pelvis are commonly involved. Muscle power and tone appear normal, but convulsive spasms make the involved muscles relatively useless.

dystonic /diston'ik/, referring to impairments of muscle tone, often excessive increase in tone, when the muscle is in ac-

tion, and to hypotonia when it is at rest, often resulting in postural abnormalities.

dystrophic calcification [Gk, *dys* + *trophe,* nourishment; L, *calx,* lime, *facere,* to make], the pathologic accumulation of calcium salts in necrotic or degenerated tissues.

dystrophin /distrof'in/, a protein that is missing or defective in Duchenne muscular dystrophy, which is localized to the sarcolemma of the muscle cell membrane. Its absence results in abnormal cell permeability, which may lead to cell destruction.

dystrophy /dis'trəfē/ [Gk, *dys* + *trophe,* nourishment], any abnormal condition caused by defective nutrition. It often entails a developmental change in muscles that does not involve the nervous system, such as fatty degeneration associated with increased size but decreased strength. —**dystrophic** /distrof'ik/, *adj.*

dysuria /disyōōr'ē·ə/ [Gk, *dys* + *ouron,* urine], painful urination, usually caused by a bacterial infection or obstructive condition in the urinary tract. The patient complains of a burning sensation when passing urine; and laboratory examination may reveal the presence of blood, bacteria, or white blood cells.

D

E

E, symbol for **expired gas.**

E₁, symbol for **monomolecular elimination reaction.**

E₂, symbol for **bimolecular reaction.**

ea, abbreviation for *each.*

E and GW, abbreviation for **Economic and General Welfare.**

ear [AS, *eare*], one of two organs of hearing and balance, consisting of the external, middle, and internal ear. The external ear includes the skin-covered cartilaginous auricle visible on either side of the head and the part of the external auditory canal outside the skull. The middle ear contains three very small bones, the malleus, incus, and stapes, which transmit vibrations caused by sound waves reaching the tympanic membrane to the oval window of the inner ear. The inner ear contains two separate organs: the vestibular apparatus, which provides the sense of balance, and the organ of Corti, which receives vibrations from the middle ear and translates them into nerve impulses, which are again interpreted by brain cells as specific sounds.

earache /ir′āk/ [AS, *eare* + *acan,* to hurt], a pain in the ear, sensed as sharp, dull, burning, intermittent, or constant. The cause is not necessarily a disease of the ear, because infections and other disorders of the nose, oral cavity, larynx, and temporomandibular joint can produce referred pain in the ear.

Ear Care, a Nursing Interventions Classification defined as prevention or minimization of threats to the ear or to hearing.

eardrop instillation, the instillation of a medicated solution into the external auditory canal of the ear. The patient is asked to turn the head to the side so that the ear being treated faces upward. The orifice is exposed, and the drops of medicine are directed toward the internal wall of the canal.

eardrops [AS, *eare* + *dropa*], a topical, liquid form of medication for the local treatment of various conditions of the ear, such as inflammation or infection of the lining of the external auditory canal or impacted cerumen (earwax).

Early and Periodic Screening Diagnosisand Treatment (EPSDT), a section of the Medicaid program that requires all states to maintain a program to determine the physical and mental defects of persons who are covered by the program and to provide short- and long-range treatment.

ear oximeter [AS, *eare* + Gk, *oxys,* sharp, *genein,* to produce, *metron,* measure], a device placed over the ear lobe that transmits a beam of light through the ear lobe tissue to a receiver. It is a noninvasive method of measuring the level of saturated hemoglobin in the blood; the amount of saturated hemoglobin alters the wavelengths of light transmitted through the ear lobe.

ear speculum [AS, *eare* + L, *speculum,* mirror], a short, funnel-shaped tube attached to an otoscope for examining the ear canal.

ear thermometry, the measurement of the temperature of the tympanic membrane by detection of infrared radiation from the eardrum.

eating disorders, a group of behaviors fueled by unresolved emotional conflicts symptomized by altered food consumption. Disorders include anorexia nervosa, bulimia nervosa, and binge eating.

Eating Disorders Management, a Nursing Interventions Classification defined as prevention and treatment of severe diet restriction and overexercising or bingeing and purging of food and fluids.

Eaton agent, an alternative name for *Mycoplasma pneumoniae,* a common cause of atypical pneumonia in humans.

Eaton-Lambert's syndrome, [Lee M. Eaton, American neurologist; Edward H. Lambert, twentieth-century American physiologist], a form of myasthenia that tends to be associated with lung cancer.

Ebner's glands, [Victor von Ebner, Austrian histologist, 1842–1925], serous glands of the tongue, opening at the bottom of the trough surrounding the circumvallate papillae.

Ebola virus disease /ēbō′lə/ [Ebola River District, Zaire], an infection caused by a species of ribonucleic acid viruses of the *Filovirus* genus. The usually lethal disease is characterized by hemorrhage and fever. There is no known treatment; and i nearly 90% of cases death occurs within 1 week. The Ebola virus is related to the Marburg virus.

EBP, abbreviation for **epidural blood patch.**

Ebstein's anomaly [Wilhelm Ebstein, German physician, 1836–1912; Gk, *anomalia,* irregularity], a congenital heart defect in which the tricuspid valve is displaced downward into the right ventricle. The abnormality is often associated with right-to-left atrial shunting and Wolff-Parkinson-White's syndrome.

EBV, abbreviation for **Epstein-Barr virus.**

ECC, 1. abbreviation for **emergency cardiac care. 2.** abbreviation for *external cardiac compression.*

eccentric /eksen′trik/ [Gk, *ek,* out, *centre,* center], **1.** pertaining to an object or activity that departs from the usual course or practice. **2.** pertaining to behavior that may appear to be odd or unconventional but does not necessarily reflect a disorder.

eccentric contraction, a type of muscle contraction that involves lengthening of the muscle fibers, such as when a weight is lowered through a range of motion. The muscle yields to the resistance, allowing itself to be stretched.

eccentric exercise, a voluntary muscle activity in which there is an overall lengthening of the muscle in response to external resistance.

eccentric implantation [Gk, *ek,* out, *centre,* center], (in embryology) the embedding of the blastocyst within a fold or recess of the uterine wall, which then closes off from the main cavity.

eccentricity /ek′sentris′itē/, behavior that is regarded as odd or peculiar for a particular culture or community, although not unusual enough to be considered pathologic.

eccentric jaw relation, (in dentistry) any jaw relation other than centric relation.

eccentric occlusion [Gk, *ek + centre + L, occludere,* to close up], a closed position of the teeth in which the habitual voluntary closure pattern of the mandible does not coincide with centric relation, resulting in premature tooth contacts.

ecchondroma /ek′əndrō′mə/ [Gk, *ek + chondros,* cartilage, *oma,* tumor], a benign tumor that develops on the surface of a cartilage or under the periosteum of bone.

ecchymoma /ek′imō′mə/, a swelling caused by accumulation of blood on the site of a bruise.

ecchymosis /ek′imō′sis/, *pl.* **ecchymoses** [Gk, *ek + chymos,* juice], bluish discoloration of an area of skin or mucous membrane caused by the extravasation of blood into the subcutaneous tissues as a result of trauma to the underlying blood vessels or fragility of the vessel walls.

ecchymotic mask [Gk, *ek + chymous +* Fr, *masque*], a cyanotic or bluish discoloration of the face of a victim of traumatic asphyxia, as in strangulation or choking. The color is the result of petechial hemorrhages.

ecchymotic rash [Gk, *ek + chymos,* juice; OFr, *rasche,* scurf], a skin eruption characterized by black-blue spots caused by extravasation of blood into the tissues, usually as a result of a contusion.

eccrine /ek′rin/ [Gk, *ekkrinein,* to secrete], pertaining to a sweat gland that secretes outwardly through a duct to the surface of the skin.

eccrine gland, one of two kinds of sweat glands in the dermis. Such glands are unbranched, coiled, and tubular, and they are distributed throughout the dermal covering of the body. They promote cooling by evaporation of their secretion.

ECF, 1. abbreviation for **extended care facility. 2.** abbreviation for **extracellular fluid.**

ECG, 1. abbreviation for **electrocardiogram. 2.** abbreviation for **electrocardiograph.**

ecgonine /ek′gōnēn/, the principal part of the cocaine molecule. It is used as a topical anesthetic.

echinococcosis /ekī′nōkokō′sis/ [Gk, *echinos,* prickly husk, *kokkos,* berry, *osis,* condition], an infestation, usually of the liver, caused by the larval stage of a tapeworm of the genus *Echinococcus.* Humans, especially children, can become infested with larvae by ingesting eggs shed in the stool of infected dogs. Clinical manifestations and prognosis vary, depending on the tissue invaded and the extent of infestation.

Echinococcus /ekī′nōkok′əs/ [Gk, *echinos,* prickly husk, *kokkos,* berry], a genus of small tapeworms that primarily infect canines.

echo /ek′ō/, *informal.* echoradiography

echo beat [Gk, *sound,* AS, *beatan,* to throb], a reciprocal heartbeat, or one that results from the return of an impulse to a chamber of origin.

echocardiogram /ek′ōkär′dē·əgram′/ [Gk, *echo,* sound, *kardia,* heart, *gramma,* record], a graphic outline of movements of the heart structures compiled from ultrasound vibrations that are reflected from these structures.

echocardiography /ek′ōkär′dē·og′rəfē/ [Gk, *echo + kardia,* heart, *graphein,* to record], a diagnostic procedure for

E

studying the structure and motion of the heart. Ultrasonic waves directed through the heart are reflected backward, or echoed, when they pass from one type of tissue to another.

echoencephalogram /ek′ō·ensef′ələgram′/ [Gk, *echo* + *enkephalos*, brain, *gramma*, record], a recording produced by an echoencephalograph.

echoencephalography /ek′ō·ensef′əlog′-rəfē/, the use of ultrasound to study the intracranial structures of the brain. —**echoencephalographic**, *adj.*

echogram /ek′ōgram/ [Gk, *echo*, sound, *gramma*, record], a recording of ultrasound echo patterns of a body structure such as a gravid uterus.

echo home, an independent housing facility for an older person in or near the family home.

echolalia /ek′ōlā′lyə/ [Gk, *echo* + *lalein*, to babble], **1.** (in psychiatry) the automatic and meaningless repetition of another's words or phrases, especially as seen in schizophrenia. **2.** (in pediatrics) a baby's imitation or repetition of sounds or words produced by others. It occurs normally in early childhood development. —**echolalic**, *adj.*

echopraxia /ek′ōprak′sē·ə/ [Gk, *echo* + *prassein*, to practice], imitation or repetition of the body movements of another person, sometimes practiced by schizophrenic patients.

echoradiography /ek′ōrā′dē·og′rəfē/ [Gk, *echo* + L, *radius* ray; Gk, *graphein*, to record], a diagnostic procedure using ultrasonography and various devices for the visualization of internal structures of the body.

echo sign, 1. a repeated sound heard on percussion of a hydatid cyst. **2.** an involuntary repetition of words heard.

echothiophate iodide /-thī′ōfāt/, an anticholinesterase used for ophthalmic purposes. It is prescribed for chronic openangle glaucoma and accommodative esotropia.

ECHO virus /ek′ōvī′rəs/ [*e*nteric cytopathogenic *h*uman *o*rphan + L, *virus*, poison], a picornavirus associated with many clinical syndromes but not identified as the causative organism of any specific disease. There are many ECHO viruses. Bacterial or viral disease may be complicated by ECHO virus infection, as aseptic meningitis accompanying some severe bacterial and viral infections.

Eck's fistula [Nikoli V. Eck, Russian physiologist, 1849–1917], an artificial passage between the end of the hepatic portal vein and the side of the inferior vena cava. It is used to treat esophageal varices in portal hypertension.

eclampsia /iklamp′sē·ə/ [Gk, *ek*, out, *lampein*, to flash], the gravest form of pregnancy-induced hypertension. It is characterized by grand mal seizure, coma, hypertension, proteinuria, and edema. The symptoms of impending seizure often include body temperature of up to 104° F, anxiety, epigastric pain, severe headache, and blurred vision. Convulsions may be prevented by bed rest in a quiet, dimly lit room and parenteral administration of magnesium sulfate and antihypertensive medications.

eclamptogenic toxemia /iklamp′tōjen′ik/ [Gk, *ek* + *lampein*, to flash, *genein*, to produce, *toxikon*, poison, *haima*, blood], a form of septicemia accompanied by convulsions that may occur during pregnancy.

eclectic /iklek′tik/ [Gk, *eklektikos*, selecting], pertaining to a therapy that selects, combines, and incorporates diverse techniques from several systems or theories into an integrated approach.

eclipse scotoma /iklips′/ [Gk, *ekleipsis*, abandoning, *skotos*, darkness, *oma*, tumor], a small central area of depressed or lost vision caused by looking directly at the sun without adequate protection.

ECM, abbreviation for erythema chronicum migrans.

ECMO, abbreviation for **extracorporeal membrane oxygenator.**

E. coli, abbreviation for *Escherichia coli.*

ecologic chemistry /ikəloj′ik/, the study of chemical compounds synthesized by plants that influence ecologic characteristics through chemical communication or toxic effects.

ecologic fallacy, a false assumption that the presence of a pathogenic factor and a disease in a population can be accepted as proof that a particular individual is the cause of the disease.

ecology /ikol′əjē/ [Gk, *oekos*, house, *logos*, science], the study of the interaction between living organisms and their environment.

econazole /ikon′əzōl/, an antifungal agent prescribed in the treatment of tinea and candidiasis.

Economic and General Welfare (E and GW), a structural unit of the American Nurses Association and state nurses' associations whose major goal is to upgrade the salaries, benefits, and working conditions of nurses.

ecosystem /ek′ōsis′təm/, the total of all living and nonliving things that support chain of life events within a particular area.

EC space, abbreviation for *extracellular space.*

ecstasy /ek'stəsē/ [Gk, *ekstasis,* derangement], an emotional state characterized by exultation, rapturous delight, or frenzy. **—ecstatic,** *adj.*

ECT, abbreviation for **electroconvulsive therapy.**

ecthyma /ek'thimə/ [Gk, *ek,* out, *thyein,* to rush], an ulcerative pyoderma characterized by large pustules, crusts, and ulcerations surrounded by erythema. It is caused by a streptococcal infection after a minor trauma.

ectocytic /ek'təsit'ik/ [Gk, *ektos,* outside, *kytos,* cell], outside a cell and not part of its organization.

ectoderm /ek'tədurm/ [Gk, *ektos,* outside, *derma,* skin], the outermost of the three primary cell layers of an embryo. The ectoderm gives rise to the nervous system; the organs of special sense such as the eyes and ears; the epidermis and epidermal tissue such as fingernails, hair, and skin glands; and the mucous membranes of the mouth and anus. **—ectodermal, ectodermic,** *adj.*

ectodermal cloaca /ek'tədur'məl/, a part of the cloaca in the developing embryo that lies external to the cloacal membrane and eventually gives rise to the anus and anal canal.

ectodermoidal /ek'tədərmoi'dəl/ [Gk, *ektos,* outside, *derma,* skin, *eidos,* form], resembling or having the characteristics of ectoderm.

ectomorph /ek'təmôrf'/ [Gk, *ektos* + *morphe,* form], a person whose physique is characterized by slenderness, fragility, and a predominance of structures derived from the ectoderm.

ectoparasite /ek'toper'əsīt/ [Gk, *ektos* + *parasitos,* guest], (in medical parasitology) an organism that lives on the outside of the body of the host, such as a louse.

ectopic /ektop'ik/ [Gk, *ektos* + *topos,* place], **1.** (of an object or organ) situated in an unusual place, away from its normal location, for example, an ectopic pregnancy, which occurs outside the uterus. **2.** (of an event) occurring at the wrong time, as a premature heartbeat or premature ventricular contraction.

ectopic beat, [Gk, *ek,* out, *topos,* place; AS, *beatan*], an impulse that originates in the heart at a site other than the sinoatrial node.

ectopic focus, an area in the heart that produces abnormal beats. Ectopic foci may occur in both healthy and diseased hearts and are usually associated with irritation of a small area of myocardial tissue.

ectopic pregnancy, an abnormal pregnancy in which the conceptus implants outside the uterine cavity. Kinds of ectopic pregnancy are **abdominal pregnancy, ovarian pregnancy,** and **tubal pregnancy.**

ectopic rhythm [Gk, *ek* + *topos,* place, *rhythmos,* beat], an abnormal heart rhythm caused by formation of the impulse in a focus outside the usual pacemaker. Such a rhythm may be protective because of failure or excessive slowing of the sinus node, or it may constitute an active abnormal focus.

ectopic tachycardia [Gk, *ek* + *topos,* place, *tachys,* swift, *kardia,* heart], an abnormally rapid heartbeat resulting from a stimulus from a focus outside the sinoatrial node.

ectopic teratism, a congenital anomaly in which one or more parts are misplaced, such as dextrocardia, palatine teeth, and transposition of the great vessels.

ectopic testis, a testis that has descended from the abdominal cavity and settled in the suprapubic area, the thigh, or the perineum instead of the scrotum. Therapy requires surgery.

ectoplasm, the compact, peripheral part of the cytoplasm of a cell.

ectopy /ek'təpē/ [Gk, *ek,* out, *topos,* place], a condition in which an organ or substance is not in its natural or proper place, such as an ectopic pregnancy that develops outside the uterus or an ectopic heartbeat.

ectrodactyly /ek'trōdak'təlē/ [Gk, *ektrosis,* miscarriage, *daktylos,* finger], a congenital anomaly characterized by the absence of part or all of one or more of the fingers or toes.

ectrogenic teratism /-jen'ik/ [Gk, *ektrosis* + *genein,* to produce, *teras,* monster], a congenital anomaly caused by developmental failure in which one or more parts or organs are missing.

ectrogeny /ektroj'ənē/ [Gk, *ektrosis* + *genein,* to produce], the congenital absence or defect of any organ or part of the body. **—ectrogenic,** *adj.*

ectromelia /ek'trōmē'lyə/ [Gk, *ektrosis* + *melus,* limb], the congenital absence or incomplete development of the long bones of one or more of the limbs. **—ectromelic,** *adj.,* **ectromelus,** *n.*

ectropic /ektrop'ik/, inside-out.

ectropion /ektrō'pē·on/ [Gk, *ek* + *trepein,* to turn], eversion, most commonly of the eyelid, exposing the conjunctival membrane lining the eyelid and part of the eyeball.

ectrosyndactyly /ek'trōsindak'təlē/ [Gk, *ektrosis* + *syn,* together, *daktylos,* finger], a congenital anomaly characterized by the absence of some but not all of the digits, with those that are formed webbed so as to appear fused.

eczema /ek'simə/ [Gk, *ekzein,* to boil over], superficial dermatitis of unknown cause. In the early stage it may be pruritic, erythematous, papulovesicular, edematous, and weeping. Later it becomes crusted, scaly, thickened, and lichenified. —**eczematous,** *adj.*

eczema herpeticum, a generalized vesiculopustular rash caused by herpes simplex virus or vaccinia virus infection of a preexisting rash such as atopic dermatitis.

eczematous conjunctivitis /eksem'ətəs/, conjunctival and corneal inflammation associated with multiple tiny ulcerated vesicles.

ED, abbreviation for **effective dose.**

E.D., abbreviation for **emergency department.**

ED$_{50}$, symbol for **median effective dose.**

edaphon /ed'əfon/, the composite of organisms that live in the soil. —**edaphic,** *adj.*

EDB, 1. abbreviation for **ethylene dibromide.** 2. abbreviation for *expected date of birth.*

EDC, abbreviation for *expected date of confinement.*

EDD, abbreviation for **expected date of delivery.**

eddy currents, small circular electric fields induced when a magnetic field is created. They result in intramolecular oscillation or vibration of tissue contents, causing generation of heat.

edema /idē'mə/ [Gk, *oidema,* swelling], the abnormal accumulation of fluid in interstitial spaces of tissues, such as in the pericardial sac, intrapleural space, peritoneal cavity, or joint capsules. —**edematous, edematose,** *adj.*

edema of glottis [Gk, *oidema,* swelling, *glossa,* tongue], a swelling caused by fluid accumulation in the soft tissues of the larynx. The condition, usually inflammatory, may result from an infection, injury, or inhalation of toxic gases.

edematogenic /ēdem'ətōjen'ik/, causing edema.

edematous /ēdem'ətəs/ [Gk, *oidema,* swelling], pertaining to or resembling edema, or excessive fluid accumulation in the tissues, causing swelling.

edentulous /ēden'chələs/, toothless.

edetate (EDTA) /ed'ətāt/, one of several salts of edetic acid, including calcium disodium edetate and edetate disodium, used as a chelating agent in treating poisoning with heavy metals.

edetate disodium, a parenteral chelating agent prescribed for hypercalcemic crisis, ventricular arrhythmia and heart block resulting from digitalis toxicity, and lead poisoning.

edetic acid (EDTA) /idet'ik/, a chelating agent.

EDG, abbreviation for **electrodynograph.**

edge response function (ERF), the ability of a computed tomography system to reproduce accurately a high-contrast edge, such as the edge of the heart.

edgewise fixed orthodontic appliance, an orthodontic appliance characterized by tooth attachment brackets with a rectangular slot that engages a round or rectangular arch wire. It is used to correct or improve malocclusion.

edible, pertaining to a substance that can be eaten.

EDRF, abbreviation for **endothelial-derived relaxing factor.**

edrophonium chloride /ed'rōfō'nē-əm/, a cholinesterase inhibitor that acts as an antidote to curare and is an aid in the diagnosis of myasthenia gravis. It is prescribed in the treatment of curare toxicity, the diagnosis of suspected myasthenia gravis, and the termination of paroxysmal supraventricular tachycardia.

edrophonium test, a test for myasthenia gravis in which an intravenous solution of edrophonium chloride is injected into a patient.

Edsall's disease [David L. Edsall, American physician, 1869–1945], a cramping condition that is the result of excessive exposure to heat.

EDTA, 1. abbreviation for **edetate.** 2. abbreviation for **edetic acid.**

educational psychology /ej'əkā'shənəl/ [L, *educatus,* to rear; Gk, *psyche,* mind, *logos,* science], the application of psychologic principles, techniques, and tests to educational problems.

EEE, abbreviation for *eastern equine encephalitis.*

EEG, 1. abbreviation for **electroencephalogram.** 2. abbreviation for **electroencephalography.**

EENT, abbreviation for *eyes, ears, nose, and throat.*

EEOC, abbreviation for **Equal Employment Opportunity Commission.**

EFA, abbreviation for **essential fatty acid.**

effacement /ifās'mənt/ [Fr, *effacer,* to erase], the shortening of the vaginal part of the cervix and thinning of its walls as it is stretched and dilated by the fetus during labor.

effect, the result of an agent or cause.

effective compliance /ifek′tiv/ [L, *effectus,* performance], the ratio of tidal volume to peak airway pressure.

effective dose (ED), the dosage of a drug that may be expected to cause a specific desired intensity of effect in the people to whom it is given.

effective half-life (ehl), (in radiotherapy and nuclear medicine) the time required for a radioactive element in an animal body to be diminished 50% as a result of the combined action of radioactive decay and biologic elimination.

effective osmotic pressure, the part of total osmotic pressure of a solution that determines the tendency of the solvent to pass through a boundary, such as a semipermeable membrane.

effective radiating area, the total area of the surface of the transducer that actually produces the sound wave.

effective refractory period, the period after the firing of an impulse during which a cell may respond to a stimulus but the response is not propagated.

effector /ifek′tər/ [L, *efficere,* to accomplish], **1.** an organ that produces an effect, such as glandular secretion, as a result of nerve stimulation. **2.** a molecule such as an enzyme that can start or stop a chemical reaction.

effector cell, **1.** a terminally differentiated leukocyte that performs more than one specific function. **2.** a muscle cell or gland cell.

effeminate /ifem′init/ [L, *effeminare,* to make womanish], womanly or female in physical and mental characteristics, regardless of biologic sex.

efferent /ef′ərənt/ [L, *effere,* to carry out], directed away from a center, such as certain arteries, veins, nerves, and lymphatics.

efferent duct, any duct through which a gland releases its secretions.

efferent nerve, a nerve that transmits impulses away or outward from a nerve center such as the brain or spinal cord, usually causing a muscle contraction or release of a glandular secretion.

efferent pathway [L, *effere,* to carry out; ME, *paeth* + *weg*], **1.** the route of nerve fibers carrying impulses away from a nerve center. **2.** the system of blood vessels that convey blood away from a body part.

effervesce [Gk, *effervescere,* to foam up], to produce small bubbles or foam on the release of gas from a fluid.

effervescence /ef′ərves′əns/ [L, *effervescere,* to foam up], the production of

small bubbles or foam associated with the escape of gas from a fluid.

effervescent /ef′ərves′ənt/, producing and releasing gas bubbles.

efficacy /ef′əkəsē/ [L, *effectus,* performance], (of a drug or treatment) the maximum ability of a drug or treatment to produce a result, regardless of dosage.

efficiency /ifish′ənsē/, **1.** the production of desired results with the minimum waste of time and effort. **2.** the amount of achievement compared with the effort expended. **3.** (in radioassay) the counts perceived by a beta or gamma counter relative to the known disintegration rate of a comparable standard radioactive source.

effleurage /ef′ləräzh′/ [Fr, skimming the surface], a technique in massage in which long, light, or firm strokes are used, usually over the spine and back.

effluent /ef′lo͞o-ənt/, a liquid, solid, or gaseous emission, such as the discharge or outflow from a machine or an industrial process.

effluvium /iflo͞o′vē-əm/ [L, *effluvium,* a flowing out], an outflow of gas or vapor, usually malodorous or toxic.

effort syndrome [Fr, exertion; Gk, *syn,* together, *dromos,* course], an abnormal condition characterized by chest pain, dizziness, fatigue, and palpitations. This condition is often associated with soldiers in combat but occurs also in other individuals. The symptoms of effort syndrome often mimic angina pectoris but are more closely connected to anxiety states.

effort thrombosis, a stress thrombosis involving the subclavian or axillary vein. It follows strenuous exercise and is accompanied by pain, edema, and skin discoloration in the shoulder and upper arm.

effraction /ifrak′shən/, a breaking open or weakening.

effusion /ityo͞o′zhən/ [L, *effundere* to pour out], **1.** the escape of fluid, for example, from blood vessels as a result of rupture or seepage, usually into a body cavity. The condition is usually associated with a circulatory or renal disorder and is often an early sign of congestive heart disease. **2.** the outward spread of a bacterial growth.

eflornithine hydrochloride /eflôr′nithēn/, a drug used to treat *Pneumocystis carinii* pneumonia (PCP).

EFM, abbreviation for **electronic fetal monitor.**

egest /ijest′/ [L, *egerere,* to expel], to discharge or evacuate a substance from the body, especially to evacuate unabsorbed residue of foods from the intestines. —**egesta,** *n. pl.,* **egestive,** *adj.*

eglandulous /ēglan'dyələs, describing an absence of glands.

ego /ē'gō, eg'ō/ [Gk, I or self], **1.** the conscious sense of the self; those elements of a person such as thinking, feeling, and willing that distinguish him or her as an individual. **2.** (in psychoanalysis) the part of the psyche that experiences and maintains conscious contact with reality and tempers the primitive drives of the id and the demands of the superego with the social and physical needs of society.

ego analysis, (in psychoanalysis) the intensive study of the ego, especially the defense mechanisms.

ego boundary, (in psychiatry) a sense or awareness that there is a distinction between the real and unreal.

egocentric /ē'gōsen'trik/ [Gk, ego + kentron, center], **1.** regarding the self as the center, object, and norm of all experience and having little regard for the needs, interests, ideas, and attitudes of others. **2.** a person possessing these characteristics.

ego-dystonic /ē'gōdiston'ik/, describing elements of a person's behavior, thoughts, impulses, drives, and attitudes that are unacceptable to him or her and cause anxiety.

ego-dystonic homosexuality, a psychosexual disorder characterized by discomfort with one's sexuality and a persistent desire to change sexual orientation to heterosexuality.

ego ideal, the image of the self to which a person aspires both consciously and unconsciously and against which he measures himself or herself and judges personal performance.

ego-integrity, an acceptance of self, both successes and failure. It implies a healthy psychologic state.

egoism /ē'gō·iz'əm, eg'-/, **1.** selfishness, an overvaluation of the importance of the self, expressed as a willingness to gain an advantage at the expense of others. **2.** the belief that individual self-interest is, or ought to be, the basic motive for all conscious behavior.

egoist /ē'gō·ist, eg'-/, **1.** a selfish person, one who seeks to satisfy his or her own interests at the expense of others. See also **egotist. 2.** a person who believes in or acts in accordance with the concept that all conscious action is justifiably motivated by self-interest. —**egoistic, egoistical,** adj.

ego libido, (in psychoanalysis) concentration of the libido on the self; self-love, narcissism.

egomania /ē'gōmā'nē·ə/ [Gk, ego, I, mania, madness], a pathologic preoccupa-

tion with the self and an exaggerated sense of one's own importance.

egophony /ēgof'ənē/, (in respiratory therapy) a change in the voice sound as heard on auscultation of a patient with pleural effusion.

ego strength, (in psychotherapy) the ability to maintain the ego by a cluster of traits that together contribute to good mental health.

ego-syntonic /ē'gōsinton'ik/, describing those elements of a person's behavior, thoughts, impulses, drives, and attitudes that are acceptable to him or her and are consistent with the total personality.

egotism /ē'gətiz'əm, eg'-/, vanity, conceit, or overvaluation of the importance of the self and undervaluation or contempt of others. —**egotistic, egotistical,** adj.

egotist /ē'gətist, eg'-/, one who is vain or conceited or who places too much importance on the self and is boastful, egocentric, and arrogant.

EHD, abbreviation for **electrohemodynamics.**

ehl, abbreviation for **effective half-life.**

Ehlers-Danlos's syndrome /ā'lərzdan'ləs/ [Edward Ehlers, Danish physician, 1863–1937; Henri A. Danlos, French physician, 1844–1912], a hereditary disorder of connective tissue, marked by hyperplasticity of skin, tissue fragility, and hypermotility of joints.

Ehrlichia, a genus of small spheric to ellipsoidal, nonmotile gram-negative bacteria. They occur singly or in compact inclusions in circulating mammalian leukocytes. Some species are the etiologic agents of ehrlichiosis and are transmitted by ticks. Two human tickborne diseases have been associated with *Ehrlichia* species: human monocytic ehrlichiosis caused by *E. chaffeensis,* and human granulocytic ehrlichiosis caused by *E. equi.*

ehrlichiosis, a sometimes fatal tickborne infection with symptoms similar to but more severe than those of Lyme disease. The disease usually begins about 10 days after the bite of an infected tick, although some cases have begun abruptly, within hours, with influenza-like symptoms, including painful muscle aches, headaches, fever, chills, loss of appetite, and depressed blood cell counts. Diagnosis is difficult because of the similarities with Lyme disease, and cases of simultaneous infections of both types of bacteria have been reported. Also, one of the organisms associated with ehrlichiosis, *Ehrlichia equi,* is nearly identical to a bacterium that causes fevers in horses.

eicosanoic acid /ī'kōsənō'ik/ [Gk, eikosa, twenty], a fatty acid containing 20 carbon atoms in a straight chain, such as arachidic acid found in peanut oil, butter, and other fats.

EID, abbreviation for **electronic infusion device.**

eidetic /īdet′ik/ [Gk, *eidos,* a form or shape seen], **1.** pertaining to or characterized by the ability to visualize and reproduce accurately the image of objects or events previously seen or imagined. **2.** a person possessing such ability.

eidetic image, an unusually vivid, elaborate, and apparently exact mental image resulting from a visual experience and occurring as a fantasy, dream, or memory.

eighth cranial nerve. See **vestibulocochlear nerve.**

einsteinium (Es) /īnstī′nē·əm/ [Albert Einstein, German-born physicist and Nobel laureate, 1879–1955], a synthetic transuranic metallic element. Its atomic number is 99; its atomic weight (mass) is 254.

Einthoven's formula /īnt′hōvənz/ [Willem Einthoven, Dutch physiologist, scientist and Nobel laureate, 1860–1927; L, *forma,* pattern], the sum of the voltages from ECG lead I, plus those from lead III, minus those from lead II, equals zero (I + III − II = 0). This formula is derived from the mathematical property that the sum of the voltages in any closed path, such as **Einthoven's triangle,** equals zero.

Einthoven's triangle [Willem Einthoven], an equilateral triangle formed by the axes of the three bipolar electrocardiograph (ECG) limb leads I, II, and III. The value of this triangle lies in the principle that the sum of the voltages equals zero. This zero potential is in the center of the triangle and offers a reference point for the unipolar ECG leads.

Eisenmenger's complex /ī′sənmeng′ərz/ [Victor Eisenmenger, German physician, 1864–1932; L, *complexus,* encirclement], a congenital heart disease characterized by a defect of the ventricular septum, a malpositioned aortic root that overrides the interventricular septum, and a dilated pulmonary artery.

ejaculate /ljak′yəlit/, the semen discharged in a single emission. —**ejaculate** /ijak′yəlāt/, v.

ejaculation /-ā′shən/ [L, *ejaculari,* to hurl out], the sudden emission of semen from the male urethra, usually during copulation, masturbation, or nocturnal emission. It is a reflex action. The sensation of ejaculation is commonly called orgasm. —**ejaculatory** /ijak′yəlātôr′ē/, adj.

ejaculatory duct /ijak′yələtôr′ē/, the passage through which semen enters the urethra.

ejection /ijek′shən/ [L, *ejicere,* to cast out], forceful expulsion, as of blood from a ventricle of the heart.

ejection click, a sharp clicking sound from the heart. It may be caused by sudden swelling of a pulmonary artery, abrupt dilation of the aorta, or forceful opening of the aortic cusps.

ejection fraction (EF), the proportion of blood ejected during each ventricular contraction compared with the total ventricular filling volume.

ejection period, the second phase of the ventricular systole. It is the interval when the semilunar valves are open and the blood is being discharged into the aortic and pulmonary arteries.

ejection sound, a sharp clicking noise heard early in systole, coinciding with the onset of either right or left ventricular systolic ejection. It reflects either dilation of the pulmonary artery or aorta or the presence of valvular abnormalities.

EKC, abbreviation for **epidemic keratoconjunctivitis.**

EKG, abbreviation for **electrocardiogram.**

elaborate /ilab′ərāt/ [L, *elaborare,* to work out], (in endocrinology) a process by which a gland synthesizes a complex substance from simpler substances and secretes it, usually under the stimulation of a tropic hormone from the pituitary gland. —**elaboration,** n.

elastance /ilas′təns/ [Gk, *elaunein,* to drive], **1.** the quality of recoiling or returning to an original form after the removal of pressure. **2.** the degree to which an air-or fluid-filled organ such as a lung, bladder, or blood vessel can return to its original dimensions when a distending or compressing force is removed. **3.** the measurement of the unit volume of change in such an organ per unit of decreased pressure change. **4.** the reciprocal of compliance.

elastase, an enzyme that cleaves bonds adjacent to neutral amino acids in elastin.

elastic bandage /ilas′tik/ [Gk, *elaunein,* to drive; Fr, *bande,* strip], a bandage of stretchable fabric that provides support and allows movement.

elastic-band fixation, a method of treatment of fractures of the jaw using rubber bands to connect metal splints or wires that are attached to the maxilla and mandible. Rubber bands are safer than rigid wires in the event of vomiting.

elastic bougie, a flexible bougie that can be passed through angular or winding channels.

elastic cartilage, the most pliant of the three kinds of cartilage, consisting of elastic fibers in a flexible fibrous matrix. It is yellow and is located in various parts of the body, such as the external ear, the auditory tube, and the epiglottis.

elasticity /i'lastis'itē/, the ability of tissue to regain its original shape and size after being stretched, squeezed, or otherwise deformed.

elastic recoil /rē'koil/, the difference between intrapleural and alveolar pressure at a given lung volume under static conditions.

elastic stocking, a type of hosiery that applies pressure to the legs to prevent excessive blood accumulation in the lower extremities caused by faulty vein valves. The stockings are commonly prescribed for patients with varicose veins.

elastic tissue [Gk, *elaunein,* to drive; OFr, *tissu*], a type of connective tissue containing elastic fibers. It is found in ligaments of the spinal column, the cartilage of the external ear, and the walls of some large blood vessels.

elastic traction [Gk, *elaunein* + L, *trahere,* to draw], any therapeutic apparatus that uses an elastic device to pull on a limb.

elastin /ilas'tin/ [Gk, *elaunein,* to drive], a protein that forms the principal substance of yellow elastic tissue fibers.

elastofibroma /ilas'tōfībrō'mə/, a benign nonencapsulated mass of collagenous, fibrous, and elastic tissue that develops in subscapular fatty tissue in older persons.

elation /ilā'shən/ [L, *elatus,* a lifting up], an emotional reaction characterized by euphoria, excitement, extreme joyfulness, optimism, and self-satisfaction.

elbow [AS, *elboga*], the bend of the arm at the joint that connects the upper arm and the forearm.

elbow joint, the hinged articulation of the humerus, ulna, and radius. The elbow joint allows flexion and extension of the forearm and accommodates the radioulnar articulation.

elder abuse, a reportable offense of physical, psychologic, or material abuse, as well as violation of the rights of safety, security, and adequate health care of older adults. Contributing factors may include economic considerations, interpersonal conflicts, health, and dependency. Health care workers are expected to report suspected abuse.

elderly primigravida, a woman who becomes pregnant for the first time after the age of 34.

elective /ilek'tiv/ [L, *eligere,* to choose], pertaining to a procedure that is performed by choice and is not essential, such as elective surgery.

elective abortion, induced termination of a pregnancy, usually before the fetus has developed enough to live if born, deemed necessary by the woman carrying it and performed at her request.

Electra complex /ilek'trə/ (in psychiatry) the libidinous desire of a daughter for her father.

electret /ilek'trət/, an insulator carrying a permanent charge similar to a permanent magnet.

electrical impedance, an opposition to electron flow in a conducting material.

electrically stimulated osteogenesis /ilek'-triklē/ [Gk, *elktron,* amber; L, *stimulare,* to incite; Gk, *osteon,* bone, *genein,* to produce], a bone regeneration process induced by surgically implanted electrodes conveying electrical current, especially at nonunion fracture sites. The process is effective because of the different electrical potentials within bone tissue.

electrical muscle stimulator (EMS), a therapeutic electric current used to stimulate muscle directly, such as when the muscle is denervated and peripheral nerves are not functioning.

electrical potential, the potential difference between charged particles.

electrical potential gradient, the net difference in electrical charge across the membrane of a cell.

electric blood warmer, a device for heating blood before infusions, especially massive transfusions in which cold blood may cause a state of shock.

electric burn, the tissue damage resulting from heat of up to 5000° C generated by an electric current. The points of entrance and exit on the skin are burned, along with the muscle and subcutaneous tissues through which the current passes. Fatal cardiac arrhythmia may result.

electric circuit, the path of the electron flow from a generating source through various components and back to the generating source.

electric current, the net movement of electrons along a conducting medium.

electric field, the lines of force exerted on charged ions in the tissues by the electrodes that cause charged particles to move from one pole to another.

electricity /i'lektris'itē/ [Gk, *elektron,* amber], a form of energy expressed by the activity of electrons and other subatomic particles in motion as in dynamic electricity or at rest as in static electricity. Electricity can be produced by heat; generated by a voltaic cell; or produced by induction, rubbing of nonconductors with dry materials, or chemical activity. Electricity may be negative, when there is a surplus of electrons, or positive, when there is a surplus of protons or a deficiency of electrons.

electric shock, a traumatic physical state caused by the passage of electric current through the body. It usually involves accidental contact with exposed parts of electric circuits in home appliances and domestic power supplies but may also result from lightning or contact with high-voltage wires. The resultant damage depends on the intensity of the electric current, the type of current, and the duration and frequency of current flow. Severe electric shock commonly causes unconsciousness, respiratory paralysis, muscle contractions, bone fractures, and cardiac disorders.

electric spinal orthosis, an electric device that helps control curvature of the spine by stimulating back muscles.

electroanalgesia /ilek′trō-an′əljē′sē-ə/, the use of an electric current to relieve pain.

electroanalytic chemistry /-an′əlit′ik/ [Gk, *elektron* + *analysis*, a loosening, *chemeia*, alchemy], the branch of chemistry concerned with the analysis of compounds by use of electrical properties to produce characteristic observable change in the substance being studied. See also **chemistry.**

electroanesthesia /-an′esthē′zhə/, the use of an electric current to produce local or general anesthesia.

electrocardiogram (ECG, EKG) /-kär′-dē-əgram′/ [Gk, *elektron* + *kardia*, heart, *gramma*, record], a graphic record produced by an electrocardiograph.

electrocardiograph (ECG) /-kär′dē-əgraf′/, a device used for recording the electrical activity of the myocardium to detect transmission of the cardiac impulse through the conductive tissues of the muscle. Electrocardiography allows diagnosis of specific cardiac abnormalities. —**electrocardiographic,** *adj.*

electrocardiographic technician /-kär′dē-ōgraf′ik/, an allied health worker with special training and experience in operating and maintaining electrocardiographic equipment and providing recorded data for diagnostic review by a physician.

electrocardiograph lead /lēd/, **1.** an electrode placed on part of the body and connected to an electrocardiograph. **2.** a record made by the electrocardiograph that varies with the site of the electrode. Electrocardiography is generally performed with the use of six limb leads and six leads placed on the precordium. The peripheral or extremity leads are designated I, II, III, AVR, AVL, and AVF. The chest leads are designated V_1, V_2, V_3, V_4, V_5, and V_6 to indicate the points on the precordium on which the electrodes are placed.

electrocardiography /-kär′dē-og′rəfē/ [Gk, *elektron* + *kardia*, heart, *graphein*, to record], the study of graphs that record electrical activity generated by the heart muscle.

electrocatalysis, the chemical decomposition of tissues caused by the application of electric current to the body.

electrocautery /ilek′trōkô′tərē/ [Gk, *elektron* + *kauterion*, branding iron], the application of a needle or snare heated by electric current for the destruction of tissue, such as for removing warts or polyps and cauterizing small blood vessels to limit blood loss during surgery.

electrochemistry, the study of the electrical effects that accompany chemical action and the chemical activity produced by electrical influence.

electrocoagulation /-kō-ag′yəlā′shən/ [Gk, *elektron* + L, *coagulare*, to curdle], a therapeutic destructive form of electrosurgery in which tissue is hardened by the passage of high-frequency current from an electric cautery device.

electroconvulsive therapy (ECT) /-kənvul′siv/, the induction of a brief convulsion by passing an electric current through the brain for the treatment of affective disorders, especially in patients resistant to psychoactive-drug therapy. ECT is primarily used when rapid definitive response is required for either medical or psychiatric reasons, such as for a patient who is extremely suicidal and when the risks of other treatments outweigh the risk of ECT. A secondary use of ECT is treatment failure of other choices.

electrocution /-kyōō′shən/, death caused by the passage of electric current through the body.

electrode /ilek′trōd/ [Gk, *elektron* + *hodos*, way], **1.** a contact for the induction or detection of electrical activity. **2.** a medium for conducting an electrical current from the body to physiologic monitoring equipment.

electrodermal /-dur′məl/, pertaining to electrical properties of the skin, particularly altered resistance.

electrodermal audiometry [Gk, *elektron* + *derma*, skin; L, *audire*, to hear; Gk, *metron*, measure], a method to determine hearing thresholds in which a harmless electric shock is used to condition the subject to a pure tone; thereafter the tone, coupled with the anticipation of a shock, elicits a brief electrodermal response. The lowest intensity of the sound that produces

E

the skin response is considered the subject's hearing threshold.

electrodesiccation /-des′ikā′shən/ [Gk, *elektron* + *desiccare,* to dry up], a technique in electrosurgery in which tissue is destroyed by burning with an electric spark. It is used primarily for eliminating small superficial growths.

electrodiagnosis /-dī′agnō′sis/ [Gk, *elektron* + *dia,* twice, *gnosis,* knowledge], the diagnosis of disease or injury by electric stimulation of various nerves and muscles.

electrodynamics /-dīnam′iks/, the study of electrostatic charges in motion, such as the flow of electrons in an electric current.

electrodynograph (EDG) /-din′əgraf′/ [Gk, *elektron* + *dynamis,* force, *graphein,* to record], an electronic device used to measure pressures exerted in biologic activity, such as those exerted by the human foot in walking, running, jogging, or climbing stairs.

electroencephalogram (EEG) /ilek′trō-ensef′ələgram′/ [Gk, *elektron* + *enkephalos,* brain, *gramma,* record], a graphic chart on which is traced the electrical potential produced by the brain cells, as detected by electrodes placed on the scalp. The resulting brain waves are called alpha, beta, delta, and theta rhythms, according to the frequencies they produce.

electroencephalograph /ilek′trō-ensef′-ələgram′/, an instrument for receiving and recording the electrical potential produced by the brain cells.

electroencephalographic technologist /ilek′trō-ensef′ələgraf′ik/, a person who is trained in the management of an electroencephalographic laboratory.

electroencephalography (EEG) /ilek′-trō-ensef′əlog′rəfē/, the process of recording brain wave activity. Electrodes are attached to various areas of the patient's head with collodion. During neurosurgery the electrodes can be applied directly to the surface of the brain (intracranial electroencephalography) or placed within the brain tissue (depth electroencephalography) to detect lesions or tumors. —**electroencephalographic,** *adj.*

electrogram /ilek′trōgram′/ [Gk, *elektron* + *gramma,* record], a unipolar or bipolar record of electrical activity of the heart as recorded from electrodes within the cardiac chambers or on the epicardium. Examples are the atrial electrogram, the ventricular electrogram, and the His bundle electrogram.

electrohemodynamics (EHD) /ilek′trō-hē′mōdīnam′iks/ [Gk, *elektron* + *haima,* blood, *dynamis,* force], a technique for noninvasively measuring the mechanical properties of the vascular system and hemodynamic characteristics of the vascular system, including arterial blood pressure, electrical impedance, blood flow, and resistance to blood flow.

electrolysis /il′ektrol′isis/ [Gk, *elektron* + *lysis,* loosening], a process in which electric energy causes a chemical change in a conducting medium, usually a solution or a molten substance, or the decomposition of a substance such as hair follicles. —**electrolytic,** *adj.*

electrolyte /ilek′trōlīt/ [Gk, *elektron* + *lytos,* soluble], an element or compound that, when melted or dissolved in water or another solvent, dissociates into ions and is able to conduct an electric current. Electrolytes differ in their concentrations in blood plasma, interstitial fluid, and cell fluid and affect the movement of substances between those compartments. Proper quantities of principal electrolytes and balance among them are critical to normal metabolism and function. —**electrolytic,** *adj.*

electrolyte balance, the equilibrium between electrolytes in the body.

Electrolyte Management, a Nursing Interventions Classification defined as promotion of electrolyte balance and prevention of complications resulting from abnormal or undesired serum electrolyte levels.

Electrolyte Management: Hypercalcemia, a Nursing Interventions Classification defined as promotion of calcium balance and prevention of complications resulting from serum calcium levels higher than desired.

Electrolyte Management: Hyperkalemia, a Nursing Interventions Classification defined as promotion of potassium balance and prevention of complications resulting from serum potassium levels higher than desired.

Electrolyte Management: Hypermagnesemia, a Nursing Interventions Classification defined as promotion of magnesium balance and prevention of complications resulting from serum magnesium levels higher than desired.

Electrolyte Management: Hypernatremia, a Nursing Interventions Classification defined as promotion of sodium balance and prevention of complications resulting from serum sodium levels higher than desired.

Electrolyte Management: Hyperphosphatemia, a Nursing Interventions Classification defined as promotion of phosphate balance and prevention of complications resulting from serum phosphate levels higher than desired.

E

Electrolyte Management: Hypocalcemia, a Nursing Interventions Classification defined as promotion of calcium balance and prevention of complications resulting from serum calcium levels lower than desired.

Electrolyte Management: Hypokalemia, a Nursing Interventions Classification defined as promotion of potassium balance and prevention of complications resulting from serum potassium levels lower than desired.

Electrolyte Management: Hypomagnesemia, a Nursing Interventions Classification defined as promotion of magnesium balance and prevention of complications resulting from serum magnesium levels lower than desired.

Electrolyte Management: Hyponatremia, a Nursing Interventions Classification defined as promotion of sodium balance and prevention of complications resulting from serum sodium levels lower than desired.

Electrolyte Management: Hypophosphatemia, a Nursing Interventions Classification defined as promotion of phosphate balance and prevention of complications resulting from serum phosphate levels lower than desired.

Electrolyte Monitoring, a Nursing Interventions Classification defined as collection and analysis of patient data to regulate electrolyte balance.

electrolyte solution, any solution containing electrolytes prepared for oral, parenteral, or rectal administration for the replacement or supplementation of ions necessary for homeostasis. Electrolyte solutions containing combinations of calcium, sodium, phosphate, chloride, or magnesium may be given to treat acid-base disturbance. The solutions are available in a wide range of balanced formulas for replacement or maintenance, and most include various trace minerals.

electromagnetic /-magnet'ik/ [Gk, *elektron, Magnesia,* ancient source of lodestone], pertaining to magnetism that is induced by an electric current.

electromagnetic induction [Gk, *elektron* + *magnes,* lodestone; L, *inducere,* to bring in], the production of electric current in a circuit when it is passed through a changing magnetic field.

electromagnetic radiation, radiation that is produced with a combination of magnetic and electrical forces, regarded as a continuous spectrum of energy. It includes a range of energy from that with the shortest wavelength (cosmic rays) to that with the longest (long radio waves).

electromagnetic spectrum, the range of frequencies and wavelengths associated with radiant energy.

electromotive force (EMF) /-mō'tiv/, the electrical potential, or ability of electrical energy to perform work. EMF is usually measured in joules per coulomb, or volts (V). The higher the voltage, the greater the potential of electrical energy.

electromyogram (EMG) /ilek'trōmī'əgram'/, a record of the intrinsic electrical activity in a skeletal muscle. Such data aid the diagnosis of neuromuscular problems and are obtained by applying surface electrodes or by inserting a needle electrode into the muscle.

electromyographic biofeedback /-mī'əgraf'ik/, a therapeutic procedure that uses electronic or electromechanical instruments to measure, process, and feed back reinforcing information with auditory and visual signals accurately. It is used to provide information about muscle activity during ambulation.

electromyographic technician, a health care provider with special training and experience to assist the physician in recording and analyzing muscle action potentials with the use of various electronic devices.

electromyography (EMG) /-mī·og'rəfē/, the process of electrically recording muscle action potentials.

electron /ilek'tron/ [Gk, *elektron,* amber], **1.** a negatively charged elementary particle that has a specific charge, mass, and spin. The number of electrons associated with the nucleus of an atom is equal to the atomic number of the substance. **2.** a negative beta particle emitted from a radioactive substance.

electron capture, a radioactive decay process in which a nucleus with an excess of protons draws an electron into the nucleus, creating a neutron out of a proton, thus decreasing the atomic number of the atom by 1.

electroneurodiagnostic technologist, an allied health professional who specializes in recording and studying the electrical activity of the brain. Working in collaboration with an electroencephalographer, the electroneurodiagnostic technologist takes and abstracts medical histories, applies adequate recording electrodes using electroencephalographic (EEG) and electrophysiologic (EP) techniques, and understands the interface between EEG and EP equipment and other electrophysiologic devices. The responsibilities may also include laboratory management and supervision of EEG technicians.

electroneuromyography /ilek'trōnŏŏr'ōmī·og'rəfē/ [Gk, *elektron* + *neuron,* nerve, *mys,* muscle, *graphein,* to record], a procedure for testing and recording neuromuscular activity by electrical stimulation of nerves. The procedure is helpful in the study of neuromuscular conduction, the extent of nerve lesions, and reflex responses.

Electronic Data Interchange (EDI), a method by which two or more organizations exchange computer-readable transaction data. It is the key factor in achieving automated medical records that can be shared electronically among providers.

electronic fetal monitor (EFM) [Gk, *elektron* + L, *fetus* + *monere,* to warn], a device that allows observation of the fetal heart rate and maternal uterine contractions. It may be applied externally or internally. With an external monitor the fetal heart is detected by an ultrasound transducer positioned on the abdomen. Internal monitoring of the fetal heart rate is accomplished via an electrode clipped to the fetal scalp.

Electronic Fetal Monitoring: Antepartum, a Nursing Interventions Classification defined as electronic evaluation of fetal heart rate response to movement, external stimuli, or uterine contractions during antepartal testing.

Electronic Fetal Monitoring: Intrapartum, a Nursing Interventions Classification defined as electronic evaluation of fetal heart rate response to uterine contractions during intrapartal care.

electronic infusion device (EID), an automated system of introducing a fluid other than blood into a vein. The device may have programmable settings that control the amount of fluid to be infused, rate, low-volume notification level, and a keep-vein-open rate. Some EIDs have titration modes that allow a change in the delivery rate without interrupting fluid flow.

electronic stethoscope, a stethoscope designed and equipped to detect and amplify body sounds.

electronic thermometer, a thermometer that registers temperature by electronic means.

electron microscope, an electronic instrument that scans cell and tissue sections with a beam of electrons, instead of visible light.

electron microscopy, a technique using an electron microscope in which a beam of electrons is focused by an electromagnetic lens and directed onto an extremely thin specimen.

electron volt (eV), a unit of energy equal to the energy acquired by an electron falling through a potential difference of 1 volt. One electron volt equals 1.6×10^{-12} erg or 1.6×10^{-19} J.

electronystagmography /ilek'trōnis'tag-mog'rəfē/ [Gk, *elektron* + *nystagmos,* nodding, *graphein,* to record], a method of assessing and recording eye movements by measuring the electrical activity of the extraocular muscles.

electrophoresis /ilek'trōfərē'sis/ [Gk, *elektron* + *pherein,* to bear], the movement of charged suspended particles through a liquid medium in response to changes in an electrical field. The pattern of migration can be recorded in bands on an **electrophoretogram** /ilek'trōfəret'ōgram/. The technique is widely used to separate and identify serum proteins and other substances. **—electrophoretic,** *adj.*

electrophysiology /-fis'ē·ol'əjē/ [Gk, *elektron* + *physis,* nature, *logos,* science], a branch of biology concerned with the relationship between electrical phenomena and biologic function.

electropiezo activity, changing electrical surface charges of a structure that force the structure to change shape.

electroporation /-pôrā'shən/, a type of osmotic transfection in which an electrical current is used to produce temporary holes in cell membranes, allowing the entry of nucleic acids or macromolecules (a way of introducing new deoxyribonucleic acid into the cell).

electroresection /-risek'shən/ [Gk, *elektron* + L, *re,* again, *secare* to cut], a technique for the removal of bladder tumors by the insertion of an electric wire through the urethra.

electroshock [Gk, *elektron* + Fr, *choc*], a condition of shock caused by accidental contact with an electrical current. The symptoms are similar to those of shock produced by thermal burns, trauma, or coronary thrombosis.

electrosleep therapy [Gk, *elektron* + AS, *slaep* + Gk, *therapeia,* treatment], a technique designed to induce sleep, especially in psychiatric patients, by administering a low-amplitude pulsating current to the brain. The cathode is placed supraorbitally, and the anode is placed over the mastoid process. The current, which is discharged for 15 to 20 minutes, produces a tingling sensation but does not always induce sleep.

electrostatic imaging /-stat'ik/ [Gk, *elektron* + *stasis,* standing still; L, *imago,* image], technique for producing radiographic images in which the ionic charge liberated during the irradiation process is converted to a visible image.

electrostimulation /-stim'yəlā'shən/, the application of electric current to stimulate bone or muscle tissue for therapeutic purposes, such as facilitation of muscle activation and muscle strengthening.

electrosurgery /-sur'jərē/ [Gk, *elektron* + *cheiourgos,* surgeon], surgery performed with various electrical instruments that operate on high-frequency electrical current. Kinds of electrosurgery include **electrocoagulation, electrodesiccation.**

electrotherapeutic current, any of three types of electric current, which, when introduced into biologic tissue, is capable of producing specific physiologic changes. The three types are direct monophasic, alternating biphasic, and pulsed polyphasic electric current.

electrotherapist /-ther'əpist/, a health care provider who has specific training and experience in the therapeutic uses of electricity.

electrotonic current [Gk, *elektron* + *tonos,* tension], a current induced in a nerve sheath without the generation of new current by an action potential.

electrovalence, the valence of an ion, equal to the absolute value of its charge.

eleidin /əlē'ədin/ [Gk, *elaia,* olive tree], a transparent protein substance, resembling keratin, found in the outer stratum lucidum of the epidermis.

element [L, *elementum,* first principle], one of more than 100 primary, simple substances that cannot be broken down by chemical means into any other substance. Each atom of any element contains a specific number of protons in the nucleus and an equal number of electrons outside the nucleus. The nucleus contains a variable number of neutrons.

element 104. See **rutherfordium (Rf).**

element 105. See **dubnium (db).**

element 106. See **seaborgium.**

element 107, an element reportedly synthesized in 1976 by Russian scientists who bombarded isotopes of bismuth with heavy nuclei of chromium-54. The finding was not confirmed by scientists of other nations. Its proposed name is **bohrium (Bh).**

elementary particle, (in physics) a subatomic particle such as an electron, neutron, or proton.

eleoma /ē'lē·ō'mə/, a lipogranuloma, or swelling, usually caused by subcutaneous injection of oil.

elephantiasis /el'əfəntī'əsis/ [Gk, *elephas,* elephant, *osis,* condition], the end-stage lesion of filariasis, characterized by extensive swelling, usually of the external genitalia and the legs. The overlying skin becomes dark, thick, and coarse. Elephantiasis results from filariasis of many years' duration.

elephantine psoriasis /el'əfan'tīn/, a rare form of psoriasis that is characterized by thick, scaly plaques on the hips, thighs, and back.

eleventh cranial nerve. See **accessory nerve.**

eligibility /el'əjəbil'itē/, entitlement of an individual to receive services based on that individual's enrollment in a health care plan.

Eligibility Guarantee Payment, a contract provision for guaranteeing payment from the health maintenance organization to the provider for services already delivered to enrollees whose coverage is terminated retroactively. Not applicable in Canada.

elimination diet /ilim'inā'shən/ [L, *eliminare,* to expel; Gk, *diata,* way of living], a procedure for identifying a food or foods to which a person is allergic by successively omitting from the diet certain foods in order to detect those responsible for the symptoms.

ELISA /əlī'zə/, abbreviation for **enzyme-linked immunosorbent assay.**

elixir /ilik'sər/ [Ar, *il-iksir,* seen as the philosopher's stone], a clear liquid containing water, alcohol, sweeteners, or flavors, used primarily as a vehicle for the oral administration of a drug.

Elliot's position [John W. Elliott, American surgeon, 1852–1925], a supine posture assumed by the patient on the operating table, with a support placed under the lower costal margin to elevate the chest. The position is used in gallbladder surgery.

ellipsis /ilip'sis/, (in psychiatry) the omission by a patient of meaningful thoughts and ideas while undergoing therapy.

ellipsoidal, describing an object that has the shape of a spindle or an ellipse.

elliptocyte /ilip'təsīt/ [Gk, *elleipsis,* ellipse, *kytos,* cell], an oval red blood cell.

elliptocytosis /ilip'tōsītō'sis/ [Gk, *elleipsis* + *kytos* + *osis,* condition], an abnormal condition of the blood characterized by increased numbers of elliptocytes or oval erythrocytes.

elongation /i'longā'shən/ [L, *elongatio,* a prolonging], a state of being lengthened or extended.

elope /ilōp'/ [ME, *gantlopp,* to run away], *informal.* to leave a locked or secured psychiatric institution without notice or permission.

Elopement Precautions, a Nursing Interventions Classification defined as minimizing the risk of a patient's leaving a treatment setting without authorization when departure presents a threat to the safety of the patient or others.

eluate /el'yōō·āt/ [L, *eluere,* to wash out], a solution or substance that results from an elution process.

eluent /el'yōō·ənt/, a solvent or solution used in an elution process, such as column chromatography.

elution /elōō'shən/, the removal of an absorbed substance from a porous bed or chromatographic column by means of a stream of liquid or gas or the application of heat. The term is also applied to the removal of antibodies or radioactive tracers from erythrocytes.

em, abbreviation for **extrinsic muscles.**

EM, abbreviation for **erythema multiforme.**

emaciated /imā'shē·ā'tid/, characterized by an extreme loss of subcutaneous fat that results in a very lean body.

emaciation /imā'shi·ā'shən/ [L, *emaciare,* to make lean], excessive leanness caused by disease or lack of nutrition.

emancipated minor /iman'sipā'tid/ [L, *emancipare,* to set free], a person who is not legally an adult but who, because he or she is married, in the military, or otherwise no longer dependent on the parents, may not require parental permission for medical or surgical care. State and national laws vary in specific interpretations of the rule.

emasculation /imas'kyəlā'shən/, a loss of the testes or penis or both.

embalming /embä'ming/, the practice of applying antiseptics and preservatives to a corpse to retard the natural decomposition of tissues.

Embden-Meyerhof defects /emb'denmī'-ərhof/ [Gustav G. Embden, German biochemist, 1874–1933; Otto F. Meyerhof, German biochemist, 1884–1951], a group of hereditary hemolytic anemias caused by enzyme deficiencies.

embedded tooth, an unerupted tooth, usually completely covered with bone.

embolectomy /em'bəlek'təmē/ [Gk, *embolos,* plug, *ektome,* excision], a surgical incision into an artery for the removal of an embolus or clot, performed as emergency treatment for arterial embolism.

embolic gangrene [Gk, *embolus* + *gaggraina*], the death and putrefaction of body tissues caused by an embolus blocking the blood supply to that part.

embolic necrosis, death of a part of tissue that results from an infarction caused by an embolus.

embolic thrombosis [Gk, *embolos,* plug, *thrombos,* lump, *osis,* condition], a thrombosis that develops at the site of an impacted embolus (foreign body) in a blood vessel.

embolism /em'bəliz'əm/, an abnormal circulatory condition in which a foreign body travels through the bloodstream and becomes lodged in a blood vessel. The symptoms vary with the degree of occlusion that results; the character of the embolus; and the size, nature, and location of the occluded vessel.

embolization agent, a substance used to occlude or drastically reduce blood flow within a vessel. Examples include vasoconstrictors and silicone beads.

embolized atheroma, a fat particle lodged in a blood vessel.

embolotherapy /em'bəlōther'əpē/, a technique of blocking a blood vessel with a balloon catheter. It is used for treating bleeding ulcers and blood vessel defects and for stopping blood flow to a tumor during surgery.

embolus /em'bələs/, *pl.* **emboli** [Gk, *embolos,* plug], a foreign object, a quantity of air or gas, a bit of tissue or tumor, or a piece of a thrombus that circulates in the bloodstream until it becomes lodged in a vessel. —**embolic, emboloid,** *adj.*

Embolus Care: Peripheral, a Nursing Interventions Classification defined as limitation of complications for a patient experiencing, or at risk for, occlusion of peripheral circulation.

Embolus Care: Pulmonary, a Nursing Interventions Classification defined as limitation of complications for a patient experiencing, or at risk for, occlusion of pulmonary circulation.

Embolus Precautions, a Nursing Interventions Classification defined as reduction of the risk of an embolus in a patient with thrombi or at risk for development of thrombus formation.

embolysis /embol'isis/, the dissolution of an embolus, especially one caused by a blood clot.

embrasure /embrā'zhər/, a normally occurring space formed between adjacent teeth as a result of variations in positions and contours. Embrasures provide a spillway for the escape of food during mastication.

embryectomy /em'brē·ek'təmē/ [Gk, *en,* in, *bryein,* to grow, *ektome,* excision], the surgical removal of an embryo, most commonly in an ectopic pregnancy.

embryo /em'brē·ō/ [Gk, *en,* in, *bryein,* to grow], **1.** any organism in the earliest stages of development. **2.** in humans the stage of prenatal development from the time of implantation of the fertilized ovum about 2 weeks after conception until the end of the seventh or eighth week. —**embryonal, embryonoid, embryonic,** *adj.*

embryocidal /em'brē·əsī'dəl/, pertaining to the killing of an embryo.

embryoctony /em′brē-ok′tənē/ [Gk, *en* + *bryein* + *kteinein*, to kill], the intentional destruction of a living embryo or fetus in utero.

embryogenesis /em′brē-ojen′əsis/ [Gk, *en* + *bryein* + *genein*, to produce], the process in sexual reproduction by which an embryo forms from the fertilization of an ovum. —**embryogenetic, embryogenic.** *adj.*

embryologic development /-loj′ik/, the various intrauterine stages and processes involved in the growth and differentiation of the conceptus from the time of fertilization of the ovum until the eighth week of gestation. The stages are related to the biologic status of the unborn child and involve the differentiation of the various cells, tissues, and organ systems and the development of the main external features of the embryo. It occurs from approximately the end of the second week to the eighth week of intrauterine life. The fetal stage follows these stages, beginning at about the ninth week of gestation.

embryologist /em′brē-ol′əjist/, one who specializes in the study of embryology.

embryology /em′brē-ol′əjē/ [Gk, *en, bryein* + *logos*, science], the study of the origin, growth, development, and function of an organism from fertilization to birth. Kinds of embryology include **comparative embryology, descriptive embryology,** and **experimental embryology.** —**embryologic, embryological,** *adj.*

embryoma /em′brē-ō′mə/ [Gk, *en* + *bryein* + *oma,* tumor], a tumor that arises from embryonic cells or tissues.

embryomorph /embrē′əmôrf′/ [Gk, *en* + *bryein* + *morphe,* form], any structure that resembles an embryo, especially a mass of tissue that may represent an aborted conceptus. —**embryomorphous,** *adj.*

embryonal carcinoma /em′brē-ənəl/, a malignant neoplasm derived from germinal cells that usually develops in gonads, especially the testes.

embryonate /em′brē-ənāt′/ [Gk, *en* + *bryein* + L, *atus,* shaped like], **1.** impregnated; containing an embryo. **2.** pertaining to or resembling an embryo.

embryonic abortion, 1. termination of pregnancy before the twentieth week of gestation. **2.** products of conception expelled before the twentieth week.

embryonic anideus [Gk, *en* + *bryein* + *an,* not, *eidos,* form], a blastoderm in which the axial elongation of the primitive streak and primitive groove fail to develop.

embryonic blastoderm, the area of the blastoderm that gives rise to the primitive streak from which the embryonic body develops.

embryonic competence, the ability of an embryonic cell to react normally to the stimulation of an inductor, allowing continued normal growth or differentiation of the embryo.

embryonic disk, the thickened plate from which the embryo develops in the second week of pregnancy.

embryonic layer, one of the three layers of cells in the embryo: endoderm, mesoderm, and ectoderm. From these layers of cells arise all of the structures and organs and parts of the body.

embryonic rest, a part of embryonic tissue that remains in the adult organism.

embryonic stage, (in embryology) the interval of time from the end of the germinal stage, at 10 days of gestation, to the eighth week.

embryonic tissue [Gk, *en* + *bryein,* to grow; OFr, *tissu*], **1.** a loose, gelatinous mass of connective tissue cells. The gelatinous matrix is caused by the presence of mucopolysaccharides. **2.** pertaining to tissue of an embryo.

embryoniform /em′brē-on′ifôrm′/ [Gk, *en* + *bryein* + L, *forma,* form], resembling an embryo.

embryopathy /em′brē-op′əthē/ [Gk, *en* + *bryein* + *pathos,* disease], any anomaly occurring in the embryo or fetus as a result of interference with normal intrauterine development.

embryoplastic /em′brē-ōplas′tik/ [Gk, *en* + *bryein* + *plassein,* to mold], pertaining to the formation of an embryo, usually with reference to cells.

embryoscopy /em′brē-os′kəpē/, the direct examination of an embryo by insertion of a lighted instrument through the mother's abdominal wall and uterus.

embryotome /em′brē-ətōm′/ [Gk, *en* + *bryein* + *temnein,* to cut], a cutting instrument for the removal of a fetus when normal birth is not possible.

embryotomy /em′brē-ot′əmē/ [Gk, *en* + *bryein* + *temnein,* to cut], **1.** the dismemberment or mutilation of a fetus for removal from the uterus when normal delivery is not possible. **2.** the dissection of an embryo for examination and analysis.

embryo transfer, a process of implanting a fertilized ovum in a uterus.

embryotroph /em′brē-ətrof′/ [Gk, *en* + *bryein* + *trophe,* nourishment], the liquefied uterine nutritive material, composed of glandular secretions and degenerative tissue, that nourishes the mammalian embryo until placental circulation is established.

embryotrophy /em′brē-ot′trəfē/, the

E

nourishment of the embryo. —**embryotrophic,** *adj.*

embbryulcia /em'brē·ul'sē·ə/ [Gk, *en* + *bryein* + *elkein*, to draw], the surgical extraction of the embryo or fetus from the uterus.

emergence /imur'jəns/ [L, *emergere,* to come forth], the point in the process of recovery from general anesthesia at which a return of spontaneous respiration, airway reflexes, and consciousness occurs.

emergency /imur'jənsē/ [L, *emergere,* to come forth], a perilous situation that arises suddenly and threatens the life or welfare of a person or group of people, as a natural disaster or a medical crisis.

emergency cardiac care (ECC) [L, *emergens,* generally unexpected; Gk, *kardia* + ME, *caru,* sorrow], the concentration of personnel and facilities organized to sustain the cardiovascular and pulmonary systems when a heart attack occurs. The interventions ensure prompt availability of basic life support (BLS), monitoring and treatment facilities, prevention of complications, and psychologic reassurance. If a heart attack occurs outside a hospital, efforts are devoted to stabilizing the patient's cardiovascular and pulmonary systems before removing the individual to a hospital.

Emergency Care, a Nursing Interventions Classification defined as providing lifesaving measures in life-threatening situations.

Emergency Cart Checking, a Nursing Interventions Classification defined as systematic review of the contents of an emergency cart at established intervals.

emergency childbirth, a birth that occurs accidentally or precipitously in or out of the hospital, without standard obstetric preparations and procedures. Signs and symptoms of impending delivery include increased bloody show, frequent strong contractions, the mother's desire to bear down forcibly or her report that she feels as though she is going to defecate, visible bulging of the bag of waters, and crowning of the baby's head at the vaginal introitus.

emergency department (ED), (in a health care facility) a section of an institution that is staffed and equipped to provide rapid and varied emergency care, especially for those who are stricken with sudden and acute illness or who are the victims of severe trauma.

emergency doctrine, (in law) a doctrine that assumes a person's consent to medical treatment when the he or she is in imminent danger and unable to give informed consent to treatment. Emergency doctrine

assumes that the person would consent if able to do so.

Emergency Medical Service (EMS), a national network of services coordinated to provide aid and medical assistance from primary response to definitive care, involving personnel trained in the rescue, stabilization, transportation, and advanced treatment of traumatic or medical emergencies.

emergency medical technician (EMT), a person trained in and responsible for the administration of specialized emergency care and the transportation of victims of acute illness or injury to a medical facility. EMTs receive ongoing training in new procedures and must qualify for national recertification every 2 years.

emergency medical technician-advanced life support (EMT-ALS), a third-level EMT. The EMT-ALS is locally certified in all the skills of the basic-level EMT and EMT-IV. The EMT-ALS may also administer certain medications following the orders of the hospital physician, with whom radio contact is maintained. An EMT-ALS is also trained in the use of advanced life support systems, including electrical defibrillation equipment.

emergency medical technician-intermediate (EMT-I), a second-level emergency medical technician nationally certified as both an EMT-ALS and an EMT-IV.

emergency medical technician-intravenous (EMT-IV), a second-level emergency medical technician. The EMT-IV is trained and locally certified in intravenous therapy, endotracheal intubation, and use of other antishock techniques.

emergency medical technician-paramedic (EMT-P), an advanced-level emergency medical technician. The EMT-P is nationally certified in all the skills of EMTs of other levels and has additional training in pharmacology and administration of emergency drugs.

emergency medicine, a branch of medicine concerned with the diagnosis and treatment of conditions resulting from trauma or sudden illness.

Emergency Nurses' Association (ENA), a national professional organization of emergency department nurses that defines and promotes emergency nursing practice.

emergency nursing, nursing care provided to prevent imminent severe damage or death or to avert serious injury. Activities that exemplify emergency nursing are basic life support, cardiopulmonary resuscitation, and control of hemorrhage.

emergency readiness, a state of having made advance plans for coping with an unexpected natural disaster, civil disturbance, or military attack that may threaten death and injury to a local population.

emergency room (ER, E.R.), a hospital area specially designed to receive and initially treat patients suffering from sudden trauma or medical problems such as accidental hemorrhage, poisoning, fracture, heart attack, and respiratory failure.

emergent /imur′jənt/ [L, *emergens,* emerging], arising, often unexpectedly, or improving or modifying an existing thing.

emergent evolution, the theory that evolution occurs in a series of major changes at certain critical stages and results from the total rearrangement of existing elements so that completely new and unpredictable characteristics appear within the species.

Emery-Dreifuss's syndrome /em′ərēdrī′-fəs/, [Alan E. H. Emery, British geneticist, b. 1928; F. E. Driefuss, twentieth-century British physician], an X-linked recessive form of scapuloperoneal dystrophy that begins in early childhood and is characterized by joint contractures and cardiac conduction disorders.

emesis basin /em′əsis, əmē′sis/ [Gk, *emesis,* vomiting; Fr, *bassin,* hollow vessel], a kidney-shaped bowl or pan that fits against the neck to collect vomitus.

emesis gravidarum /em′əsis, əmēsis/, vomiting associated with pregnancy.

emetic /imet′ik/, **1.** pertaining to a substance that causes vomiting. **2.** an emetic agent such as apomorphine hydrochloride and syrup of ipecac.

EMG, 1. abbreviation for **electromyogram. 2.** abbreviation for **electromyography. 3.** abbreviation for **exophthalmos, macroglossia, and gigantism.**

EMG syndrome, a hereditary disorder transmitted as an autosomal-recessive trait. Clinical manifestations include exophthalmos, macroglossia, and gigantism, often accompanied by visceromegaly, dysplasia of the renal medulla, and enlargement of the cells of the adrenal cortex.

emissary veins /em′əser′ē/ [L, *emittere,* to send forth], the small vessels in the skull that connect the sinuses of the dura mater with the veins on the exterior of the skull through a series of anastomoses.

emission /imish′ən/ [L, *emittere,* to send out], a discharge or release of something, as a fluid from the body, electronic signals from a radio transmitter, or an alpha or beta particle from an atomic nucleus during radioactive decay.

emission computed tomography (ECT) [L, *emittere,* to send forth; *computare,* to count; Gk, *tome,* section, *graphein,* to record], a form of tomography in which the emitted decay products, as positrons or

gamma rays, of an ingested radioactive pharmaceutical are recorded in detectors outside the body.

emit [L, *emittere,* to send out], to give or send out something, such as energy, sound, heat, or radiation.

emmetropia /em′ətrō′pē·ə/ [Gk, *emmetros,* proportioned, *opsis,* vision], a state of normal vision characterized by the proper relationship between the refractive system of the eyeball and its axial length. This correlation ensures that light rays entering the eye parallel to the optic axis are focused exactly on the retina. —**emmetropic,** *adj.*

Emmet's operation, a surgical procedure for repair of a lacerated perineum or ruptured uterine cervix.

emollient /imol′yənt/ [L, *emolliere,* to soften], a substance that softens tissue, particularly the skin and mucous membranes.

emollient bath, a bath taken in water containing an emollient such as bran to relieve irritation and inflammation.

emotion /imō′shən/ [L, *emovere,* to disturb], the outward expression or display of mood or feeling states. Also, the affective aspect of consciousness as compared with volition and cognition.

emotional abuse /imō′shənəl/, the debasement of a person's feelings that causes the individual to perceive himself or herself as inept, not cared for, and worthless.

emotional age [L, *emovere,* to disturb; L, *aetas,* age], the age of an individual as determined by the stage of emotional development reached.

emotional amalgam, an unconscious effort to deny or counteract anxiety.

emotional amenorrhea, a suppression of menstrual discharge from the uterus caused by psychologic factors

emotional care of the dying patient, the compassionate, consistent support offered to help the terminally ill patient and the family cope with impending death.

emotional deprivation [L, *emovere,* to disturb, *deprivare,* to deprive], a lack of adequate warmth, affection, and interest, especially of a parent or significant nurturer. It is a relatively common problem among institutionalized persons or children from broken homes.

emotional diarrhea, the frequent passage of liquid stools caused by extreme emotional stress.

emotional glycosuria, a temporary increase in the level of sugar excretion in the urine resulting from extreme emotional disturbances.

emotional lability, a condition of excessive emotional reactions and frequent mood changes.

emotional need, a psychologic or mental requirement of intrapsychic origin. It usually centers on such basic feelings as love, fear, anger, sorrow, anxiety, frustration, and depression and involves the understanding, empathy, and support of one person for another. Such needs normally occur in everyone but usually increase during periods of excessive stress or physical and mental illness and during various stages of life, as infancy, early childhood, and old age. If these needs are not routinely met by appropriate, socially accepted means, they can precipitate psychopathologic conditions.

emotional response, a reaction to a particular intrapsychic feeling or feelings, accompanied by physiologic changes that may or may not be outwardly manifested but that motivate or precipitate some action or behavioral response. See also **emotion.**

emotional support, the sensitive, understanding approach that helps patients accept and deal with their illnesses; communicate their anxieties and fears; derive comfort from a gentle, sympathetic, caring person; and increase their ability to care for themselves.

Emotional Support, a Nursing Interventions Classification defined as provision of reassurance, acceptance, and encouragement during times of stress.

empathic /empath'ik/ [Gk, *en,* into, *pathos,* feeling], pertaining to or involving the entering of one person into the emotional state of another while remaining objective and distinctly separate.

empathy /em'pəthē/ [Gk, *en,* in, *pathos,* feeling], the ability to recognize and to some extent share the emotions and states of mind of another and to understand the meaning and significance of that person's behavior. It is an essential quality for effective psychotherapy.—**empathic,** *adj.,* **empathize,** *v.*

emphysema /em'fəsē'mə/ [Gk, *en* + *physema,* a blowing], an abnormal condition of the pulmonary system, characterized by overinflation and destructive changes of alveolar walls. It results in a loss of lung elasticity and decreased gases. When emphysema occurs early in life, it is usually related to a rare genetic deficiency of serum alpha-1-antitrypsin, which inactivates the enzymes leukocyte collagenase and elastase. Acute emphysema may be caused by the rupture of alveoli by severe respiratory efforts, as in acute bronchopneumonia, suffocation, and whooping cough and occasionally during labor. Patients with chronic emphysema may also have a component of chronic bronchitis. Emphysema also occurs after asthma or tuberculosis, conditions in which the lungs are overstretched until the elastic fibers of the alveolar walls are destroyed. In old age the alveolar membranes atrophy and may collapse, producing large air-filled spaces and decreased total surface area of the pulmonary membranes.

emphysematous /em'fisem'ətəs/ [Gk, *en,* in, *physema,* a blowing], pertaining to or affected with emphysema.

emphysematous abscess, an abscess in which air or gas is present.

empiric /empir'ik/ [Gk, *empeirikos,* experimental], pertaining to a method of treating disease based on observations and experience without an understanding of the cause or mechanism of the disorder or the way the therapeutic agent or procedure used effects improvement or cure. The empiric treatment of a new disease may be based on observations and experience gained in the management of analogous disorders.—**empirical,** *adj.*

empirical formula, a chemical formula that shows the smallest ratio of atoms of different elements in a molecule. It does not indicate structural linkage.

empiricism /empir'isiz'əm/, a form of therapy based on the therapist's personal experience and that of other practitioners.—**empiricist,** *n.*

Employment Retirement Income Security Act (ERISA), a federal law, enacted in 1974, regulating employee welfare benefit plans, including group health plans.

emprosthotonos /em'prosthot'ənəs/ [Gk, *emprosthen,* forward, *tenein,* to cut], a position of the body characterized by forward, rigid flexure at the waist. The position is the result of a prolonged involuntary muscle spasm that is most commonly associated with tetanus infection or strychnine poisoning.

empty follicle syndrome, a condition in which oocytes are absent from stimulated follicles.

empty sella syndrome [AS, *oemettig,* unoccupied; L, *sella,* saddle], an abnormal enlargement of the sella turcica in which no pituitary tumor is present; the gland may be smaller than normal, or it may be absent. Signs and symptoms of hormonal imbalance (for example, hypopituitarism) may be present, but some patients may be asymptomatic. The condition is especially frequent in overweight, middle-aged multiparous women.

empyema /em'pī·ē'mə, em'pē·ē'mə/ [Gk, *en* + *ipyon,* pus], an accumulation of pus in a body cavity, especially the pleural space, as a result of bacterial infection such as pleurisy or tuberculosis.

EMS, 1. abbreviation for **electrical muscle stimulator.** 2. abbreviation for **Emergency Medical Service.** 3. abbreviation for **eosinophilia-myalgia syndrome.**

EMS standing orders, routine medical procedures approved in advance for emergency medical services crews to perform before consulting a physician.

EMT, abbreviation for **emergency medical technician.**

EMT-A, abbreviation for *emergency medical technician-ambulance,* a member of an emergency medical services crew.

EMT-ALS, abbreviation for **emergency medical technician-advanced life support.**

EMT-D, abbreviation for *emergency medical technician-defibrillator,* a member of an emergency medical services crew with special training in the use of cardiac defibrillating equipment.

EMT-I, abbreviation for **emergency medical technician-intermediate.**

EMT-IV, abbreviation for **emergency medical technician-intravenous.**

EMT-P, abbreviation for **emergency medical technician-paramedic.**

emulsification /imul′sifikā′shən/, the breakdown of large fat globules into smaller, uniformly distributed particles. Emulsification is the first preparation of fat for chemical digestion by specific enzymes.

emulsifier /imul′sifī′ər/ [L, *emulgere,* to milk out, *facere,* to make], a substance such as egg yolk or gum arabic that can cause oil to be suspended in water.

emulsify [L, *emulgere,* to milk out, *facere,* to make], to disperse a liquid into another liquid, making a colloidal suspension. Soaps and detergents emulsify by surrounding small globules of fat, preventing them from settling out. Bile acts as an emulsifying agent in the digestive tract by dispersing ingested fats into small globules. —**emulsification,** *n.*

emulsion /imul′shən/ [L, *emulgere,* to drain], 1. a system consisting of two immiscible liquids, one of which is dispersed in the other in the form of small droplets. 2. (in photography) a composition sensitive to actinic rays of light, consisting of one or more silver halides suspended in gelatin applied in a thin layer to film.

ENA, abbreviation for **Emergency Nurses' Association.**

enabler /enā′blər/, a significant other of a substance abuser who provides covert support of substance-abusing behavior.

enalapril maleate /enal′əpril/, an an-

giotensin-converting enzyme inhibitor used as an oral antihypertensive drug. It is prescribed in the treatment of hypertension.

enamel /inam′əl/ [OFr, *esmail*], a hard white substance that covers the dentin of the crown of a tooth.

enamel hypocalcification, a hereditary dental defect in which the enamel of the teeth is soft and undercalcified in context yet normal in quantity. It is caused by defective maturation of the ameloblasts.

enamel hypoplasia, a developmental dental defect in which the enamel of the teeth is hard in context but thin and deficient in amount, caused by defective enamel matrix formation with a deficiency in the cementing substance.

enamel niche, either of two depressions on a tooth, located between the lateral dental lamina and the developing dental germ.

enamel organ, a complex epithelial structure on the dental papilla. It produces enamel for the developing tooth.

enanthema /en′anthē′mə/ [Gk, *en* + *anthema,* blossoming], an eruptive lesion of the surface of a mucous membrane.

en bloc /enblok′, äNblôk′/ [Fr, in a block], all together, or as a whole.

encainide /en′kānīd/, a sodium channel antagonist used as an antiarrhythmic agent. It is prescribed in the treatment of life-threatening ventricular arrhythmias and other symptomatic ventricular arrhythmias.

encapsulated /enkaps′yəlā′tid/ [Gk, *en* + L, *capsula,* little box], (of arteries, muscles, nerves, and other body parts) enclosed in fibrous or membranous sheaths.

encephalalgia /ənsef′əlal′jə/, headache.

encephalitis /ensef′əlī′tis/, *pl.* **encephalitides** /-tidez/ [Gk, *enkephalos,* brain, *itis,* inflammation], an inflammatory condition of the brain. The cause is usually an arbovirus infection transmitted by the bite of an infected mosquito, but it may be the result of lead or other poisoning or of hemorrhage. Postinfectious encephalitis occurs as a complication of another infection such as chickenpox, influenza, or measles or after smallpox vaccination. The condition is characterized by headache, neck pain, fever, nausea, and vomiting. Severe inflammation with destruction of nerve tissue may result in a seizure disorder, loss of a special sense or other permanent neurologic problem, or death. Usually the inflammation involves the spinal cord and brain; hence in most cases a more accurate term is *encephalomyelitis.*

encephalocele /ensef′ələsēl′/ [Gk, *en kephalos* + *koilia,* cavity], protrusion of the brain through a congenital defect in the skull; hernia of the brain.

encephalodysplasia, any congenital anomaly of the brain.

encephalogram /ensef'ələgram'/ [Gk, *enkephalos* + *gramma,* record], a radiograph of the brain made during encephalography.

encephalography /ensef'əlog'rəfē/, radiographic delineation of the structures of the brain containing fluid after the cerebrospinal fluid is withdrawn and replaced by a gas such as air, helium, or oxygen. Kinds of encephalography are **pneumoencephalography** and **ventriculography.** —**encephalographic,** *adj.*

encephalomeningitis /-men'inji'tis/ [Gk, *enkephalos,* brain, *meninx,* membrane, *itis,* inflammation], an inflammation of the brain and meninges.

encephalomyelitis /ensef'əlōmī'əlī'tis/ [Gk, *enkephalos* + *myelos,* marrow, *itis*], an inflammatory condition of the brain and spinal cord characterized by fever, headache, stiff neck, back pain, and vomiting. Depending on the cause, the age and condition of the person, and the extent of the inflammation and irritation to the central nervous system, seizures, paralysis, personality changes, a decreased level of consciousness, coma, or death may occur.

encephalomyocarditis /ensef'əlōmī'ōkärdī'tis/ [Gk, *enkephalos* + *mys,* muscle, *kardia,* heart, *itis,* inflammation], an infectious disease of the central nervous system and heart tissue caused by a group of small ribonucleic acid picornaviruses. Symptoms are generally similar to those of poliomyelitis. Most victims recover promptly without sequelae.

encephalon [Gk, *enkephalos,* brain], **1.** the cerebrum and its related structures of cerebellum, pons, and medulla oblongata. **2.** the contents of the cranium.

encephalopathy /ensef'əlop'əthē/ [Gk, *enkephalos* + *pathos,* disease], any abnormal condition of the structure or function of brain tissues, especially chronic, destructive, or degenerative conditions such as Wernicke's encephalopathy or Schilder's disease.

enchondroma /en'kəndrō'mə/ [Gk, *en* + *chondros,* cartilage, *oma,* tumor], a benign, slowly growing tumor of cartilage cells that arises in the extremity of the shaft of tubular bones in the hands or feet.

enchondromatosis /en'kəndrō'mətō'sis/ [Gk, *en* + *chondros,* cartilage, *oma,* tumor, *osis,* condition], a congenital disorder characterized by the proliferation of cartilage within the extremity of the shafts of bones, causing thinning of the cortex and distortion in length.

enchondromatous myxoma /en'kondrō'-mətəs/, a tumor of the connective tissue, characterized by the presence of cartilage between the cells of connective tissue.

enclave /en'klāv, enklāv'/, a detached mass of tissue enclosed in an organ or in a different kind of tissue.

encoded message, (in communication theory) a message as transmitted by a sender to a receiver.

encopresis /en'kōprē'sis/, fecal incontinence. —**encopretic,** *adj.*

encounter [Gk, *en* + L, *contra,* against], (in psychotherapy) the interaction between a patient and a psychotherapist, such as occurs in existential therapy or among several members of a small group such as encounter or sensitivity training groups. In an encounter emotional change and personal growth are effected by participants' expression of strong feelings.

encounter data, information showing use of provider services by health plan enrollees that is used to develop cost profiles of a particular group of enrollees and then to guide decisions about or provide justification for the maintenance or adjustment of premiums.

encounter group, (in psychology) a small group of people who meet to increase self-awareness, promote personal growth, and improve interpersonal communication.

enculturation /enkul'chərā'shən/ [Gk, *en* + L, *cultura,* cultivation], the process of learning the concepts, values, and behavioral standards of a particular culture.

encyst /ensist'/, to form a cyst or capsule. —**encysted,** *adj.*

end /ē'en'dē'/, end/, (in cytogenetics) abbreviation for *endoreduplication.*

endarterectomy /en'därtərek'təmē/ [Gk, *endon,* within, *arteria,* airpipe, *ektome,* excision], the surgical removal of the intimal lining of an artery. The procedure is done to clear a major artery that may be blocked by plaque accumulation. One technique, disobliterative endarterectomy, involves coring the affected segment of the artery, removing the lining along with the obstructive material, but leaving the remaining artery walls as a new passageway for blood flow. Another method is gas endarterectomy, in which carbon dioxide gas is injected between the intimal and medial layers of the artery wall, causing them to separate so the inner lining can be detached.

endarteritis /en'därtərī'tis/ [Gk, *endon* + *arteria* + *itis,* inflammation], an inflammatory disorder of the inner layer of one or more arteries, which may become partially or completely occluded.

endarteritis obliterans, an inflammatory condition of the lining of the arterial walls in which the intima proliferates, narrowing the lumen of the vessels and occluding the smaller vessels.

end artery, a blood vessel that does not join with any other vessel.

end bud [AS, *ende* + Gk, *bolbos,* onion], a mass of undifferentiated cells produced from the remnants of the primitive node and the primitive streak at the caudal end of the developing embryo after formation of the somites is completed.

end-diastolic pressure /-dī·ǝstol'ik/ [AS, *ende* + Gk, *dia* + *stellein,* to set; L, *premere,* to press], the pressure of the blood in the ventricles at the end of diastole and just before the next ventricular systole.

endemic /endem'ik/ [Gk, *endemos,* native], (of a disease or microorganism) the expected or "normal" incidence indigenous to a geographic area or population.

endemic disease, a physical or mental disorder caused by health conditions constantly present within a community. It usually describes an infection that is transmitted directly or indirectly between humans and is occurring at the usual expected rate.

endemic goiter, an enlargement of the thyroid gland caused by the intake of inadequate amounts of dietary iodine. Iodine deprivation leads to diminished production and secretion of thyroid hormone by the gland. Initially the goiter is diffuse; later it becomes multinodular. Endemic goiter occurs occasionally in adolescents at puberty and widely in population groups in geographic areas in which limited amounts of iodine are present in soil, water, and food. A large goiter may cause dysphagia, dyspnea, tracheal deviation, and cosmetic problems.

endemic syphilis, a chronic infectious disease that is closely related to *Treponema pallidum* and is frequently contracted in childhood without venereal contact. It is known as yaws, pinta, and bejel in heavily populated communities of undeveloped nations.

end-feel, the sensation imparted to the examiner's hands at the end point of the available range of motion. It varies according to the limiting structure or tissue. Types of end-feel include capsular, bone-on-bone, spasm, and springy block.

endobronchitis /en'dōbrongkī'tis/, inflammation of the smaller bronchi, often caused by a bronchial mucosal infection.

endocardial, pertaining to the **endocardium.**

endocardial cushion defect /en'dōkär'dē·ǝl/, any cardiac defect resulting from the failure of the endocardial cushions in the embryonic heart to fuse and form the atrial septum.

endocardial cushions, a pair of thickened tissue sections in the embryonic atrial canal.

endocardial fibroelastosis /fī'brō·ē'lastō'sis/ [Gk, *endon* + *kardia,* heart; L, *fibra,* fiber; Gk, *elaunein,* to drive, *osis,* condition], an abnormal condition characterized by the development of a thick fibroelastic endocardium that can cause pump failure.

endocardial murmur, a continuous soft sound made by an abnormality within the heart.

endocarditis /en'dōkärdī'tis/ [Gk, *endon* + *kardia,* heart, *itis,* inflammation], an abnormal condition that affects the endocardium and heart valves and is characterized by lesions caused by a variety of diseases. Kinds of endocarditis are bacterial endocarditis, nonbacterial thrombotic endocarditis, and Libman-Sacks endocarditis. Untreated, all types of endocarditis are rapidly lethal.

endocardium /en'dōkär'dē·ǝm/, *pl.* **endocardia,** the lining of the heart chambers, containing small blood vessels and a few bundles of smooth muscle. It is continuous with the endothelium of the great blood vessels.

endocervical /-sur'fikǝl/ [Gk, *endon* + L, *cervix,* neck], pertaining to the interior of the cervix and uterus.

endocervicitis /en'dōsur'visī'tis/, an abnormal condition characterized by inflammation of the epithelium and glands of the canal of the uterine cervix.

endocervix /en'dōsur'viks/, **1.** the membrane lining the canal of the uterine cervix. **2.** the opening of the cervix into the uterine cavity.

endochondral /·kon'drǝl/ [Gk, *endon,* within, *chondros,* cartilage], pertaining to something within the cartilage.

endocrinasthenia /-krin'asthē'nē·ǝ/, a neural deficit caused by an alteration of the endocrine system.

endocrine /en'dǝkrēn, -krīn/ [Gk, *endon* + *krinein,* to secrete], pertaining to a process in which a group of cells secrete into the blood or lymph circulation a substance (for example, hormone) that has a specific effect on tissues in another part of the body.

endocrine diabetes mellitus [Gk, *endon,* within, *krinein,* to secrete, *diabainein,* to pass through, *mellitus,* honeyed], a form of diabetes associated with diseases of other glands such as the adrenals, pituitary, or thyroid.

endocrine fracture /en'dōkrīn, -krēn/, any fracture that results from weakness of a specific bone caused by an endocrine disorder such as hyperparathyroidism.

endocrine gland, a ductless gland that produces and secretes hormones into the blood or lymph nodes. The hormones exert powerful effects on specific target tissues throughout the body. The endocrine glands include the pituitary, pineal, hypothalamus, thymus, thyroid, parathyroid, adrenal cortex, medulla islets of Langerhans, and gonads. Cells in other structures such as the gastrointestinal mucosa and the placenta also have endocrine functions.

endocrine system [Gk, *endon* + *krinein,* to secrete; *systema*], the network of ductless glands and other structures that elaborate and secrete hormones directly into the bloodstream, affecting the function of specific target organs. Glands of the endocrine system include the thyroid and the parathyroid, the anterior pituitary, the posterior pituitary, the pancreas, the suprarenal glands, and the gonads. The pineal gland is also considered an endocrine gland because it is ductless.

endocrinologist /en'dōkrinol'əjist/, a physician who specializes in the endocrine system and its disorders.

endocrinology /-krinol'əjē/ [Gk, *endon* + *krinein,* to secrete, *logos,* science], the study of the anatomic, physiologic, and pathologic characteristics of the endocrine system and of the treatment of endocrine problems.

endocrinopathy /-krinop'əthē/ [Gk, *endon,* within, *krinein,* to secrete, *pathos,* disease], a disease involving an endocrine gland or a dysfunction that decreases the quality or quantity of its secretion.

endoderm /en'dədurm/ [Gk, *endon* + *derma,* skin], (in embryology) the innermost of the cell layers that develop from the embryonic disk of the inner cell mass of the blastocyst. The endoderm comprises the lining of the cavities and passages of the body and the covering of most of the internal organs.

endodermal /-dur'məl/ [Gk, *endon,* within, *derma,* skin], pertaining to the inner of the three layers of the embryo, the epithelial lining of the respiratory system, the digestive tract, and other tissues.

endodermal cloaca, a part of the cloaca in the developing embryo that lies internal to the cloacal membrane and gives rise to the bladder and urogenital ducts.

endodontics [Gk, *endon,* within, *odous,* tooth], a branch of dentistry that specializes in the diagnosis and treatment of diseases in the dental pulp, tooth root, and its surrounding tissues, and the associated practice of root canal therapy.

endodontist /-don'tist/ [Gk, *endon,* within, *odous,* tooth], a dentist who specializes in the causes, diagnosis, and treatment of diseases of the dental pulp, tooth root, and periapical tissues and performs root canal therapy.

endogenous /endoj'ənəs/ [Gk, *endon* + *genein,* to produce], **1.** growing within the body. **2.** originating from within the body or produced from internal causes, such as a disease caused by the structural or functional failure of an organ or system.—**endogenic,** *adj.*

endogenous carbon dioxide, carbon dioxide produced within the body by metabolic processes.

endogenous infection, an infection caused by the reactivation of previously dormant organisms, as in coccidioidomycosis, histoplasmosis, and tuberculosis.

endogenous obesity, obesity resulting from dysfunction of the endocrine or metabolic system.

endogenous opioid, an opiate-like substance such as an endorphin, produced by the body.

endogenous uric acid [Gk, *endon,* within + *genein,* to produce + *ouron,* urine; L, *acidus*], uric acid produced by the metabolism of purines in the body's own nucleoproteins, as distinguished from metabolism of purine products in foods.

endointoxication /en'dō·intok'sikā'shən/, poisioning caused by a toxin produced within the body, such as from dead and infected tissue in gangrene.

endolymph /en'dəlimf/ [Gk, *endon* + *lympha,* water], the fluid in the membranous labyrinth (cochlear duct) of the internal ear.

endolymphatic duct /-limfat'ik/, a labyrinthine passage joining an endolymphatic sac with the utricle and saccule.

endolymphatic sac, the blind end of an endolymphatic duct.

endomastoiditis /-mas'toidī'tis/, an inflammation within the mastoid cavity and cells.

endometrial /en'dōmē'trē·əl/ [Gk, *endon* + *metra,* womb], **1.** pertaining to endometrium. **2.** pertaining to the uterine cavity.

endometrial biopsy, a microscopic examination of a sample of endometrial tissue to assess corpus luteum function.

endometrial cancer, an adenocarcinoma of the endometrium of the uterus. It is the most prevalent gynecologic malignancy, most often occurring in the fifth or sixth decade of life. Although the cause of endometrial cancer is not clear, some of the risk factors associated with an increased incidence of the disease are a medical his tory of infertility; anovulation, late menopause (>52 years); administration of exogenous estrogen; uterine polyps; and a combination of diabetes, hypertension, and obesity. Abnormal vaginal bleeding, especially in a postmenopausal woman, is the cardinal symptom. Lower abdominal and low back pain may also be present; a large, boggy uterus is often a sign of advanced disease.

endometrial cyst [Gk, *endon,* within, *metra,* womb, *kystis,* bag], **1.** an endometrial tumor. **2.** an ovarian cyst that develops as a distension of an endometrial gland.

endometrial hyperplasia, an abnormal condition characterized by overgrowth of the endometrium resulting from sustained stimulation by estrogen (of endogenous or exogenous origin) that is not opposed by progesterone. Estrogen acts as a growth hormone for the endometrium. Endometrial hyperplasia often results in abnormal uterine bleeding; such bleeding, particularly in older women, constitutes an indication for biopsy or curettage of the endometrium to establish histopathologic diagnosis and to rule out malignancy.

endometrial polyp, a pedunculated overgrowth of endometrium, usually benign. Polyps are a common cause of vaginal bleeding in perimenopausal women and are often associated with other uterine abnormalities such as endometrial hyperplasia or fibroids.

endometrioma /-mē′trē-ō′mə/ [Gk, *endon,* within, *metra,* womb, *oma,* tumor], a tumor or mass of ectopic endometrial tissue that has no function in the uterus.

endometriosis /en′dōmē′trē-ō′sis/ [Gk, *endon + metra,* womb, *osis,* condition], an abnormal gynecologic condition characterized by ectopic growth and function of endometrial tissue. Precise incidence of the disease is unknown, but evidence of it is found in approximately 15% of women who undergo pelvic laparotomy for other indications. The average age of women found to have endometriosis is 37 years. Pregnancy may have an influence in preventing or ameliorating the disease. The causes of endometriosis are unknown.

endometritis /en′dōmitri′tis/ [Gk, *endon + metra,* womb, *itis,* inflammation], an inflammatory condition of the endometrium. It is usually caused by bacterial infection, commonly by gonococci or hemolytic streptococci. The condition is characterized by fever, abdominal pain, malodorous discharge, and enlargement of the uterus. It occurs most frequently after childbirth or abortion and is associated with the use of an intrauterine contraceptive device.

endometrium /en′dōmē′trē-əm/ [Gk, *endon + metra,* womb], the mucous membrane lining of the uterus, consisting of the stratum compactum, the stratum spongiosum, and the stratum basale. The endometrium changes in thickness and structure with the menstrual cycle.

endomorph /en′dəmôrf′/ [Gk, *endon + morphe,* form], a person whose body build is characterized by a soft, round physique with a large trunk and thighs, tapering extremities, an accumulation of fat throughout the body, and a predominance of structures derived from the endoderm.

endomyocarditis /-mī′ōkärdī′tis/ [Gk, *endon,* within, *mys,* muscle, *kardia,* heart, *itis,* inflammation], an inflammation of the lining of the heart.

endoparasite /en′dōper′əsīt/ [Gk, *endon + parasitos,* guest], (in medical parasitology) an organism that lives within the body of the host, such as a tapeworm.

endopathy /endop′əthē/, any disease originating within the person.

endophthalmitis /endof′thalmī′tis/ [Gk, *endon + ophthalmos,* eye, *itis*], an inflammatory condition of the internal eye in which the eye becomes red, swollen, painful, and sometimes filled with pus. This condition may blur the vision and cause vomiting, fever, and headache.

endophthalmitis phacoanaphylactica /fak′ō-an′əfilak′təkə/, an abnormal condition characterized by an acute autoimmune reaction of the eye. It is caused by hypersensitivity of the eye to the protein of the crystalline lens and commonly follows trauma to the crystalline lens or cataract surgery. Associated symptoms include swelling and inflammation of the eye, severe pain, and blurred vision.

endophytic /en′dōfit′ik/ [Gk, *endon + phyton,* plant], pertaining to the tendency to grow inward, such as a tumor that grows into the wall of a hollow organ.

endoplasm /en′doplaz′əm/ [Gk, *endon,* within, *plasma,* plasm], the inner part of cytoplasm.

endoplasmic reticulum /-plaz′mik/ [Gk, *endon + plassein,* to mold], an extensive network of membrane enclosed tubules in the cytoplasm of cells. The structure functions in the synthesis of proteins and lipids and in the transport of these metabolites within the cell.

endoprosthesis /-prosthē′sis, -pros′thəsis/ [Gk, *endon + prosthesis,* addition], a prosthetic device installed within the body, such as dentures or an internal cardiac pacemaker.

end-organ [AS, *ende + Gk, organon,* instrument], a nerve ending in which the terminal nerve filaments are encapsulated.

E

endorphin /endôr'fin/ [Gk, *endon* + *morphe,* shape], any of the neuropeptides composed of many amino acids, elaborated by the pituitary gland, and acting on the central and the peripheral nervous systems to reduce pain. Endorphins are alpha-endorphin, beta-endorphin, and gamma-endorphin, which are chemicals that produce pharmacologic effects similar to those of morphine.

endorsement /endôrs'mənt/ [Gk, *en* + L, *dorsum,* the back], a statement of recognition of the license of a health practitioner in one state by another state.

endoscope /en'dəskōp/ [Gk, *endon* + *skopein,* to look], an illuminated optic instrument for the visualization of the interior of a body cavity or organ. Although the endoscope is generally introduced through a natural opening in the body, it may also be inserted through an incision.—**endoscopic,** *adj.*

endoscopic retrograde cholangiography /en'dəskop'ik/, (in radiology) a diagnostic procedure for outlining the common bile duct. A flexible fiberoptic duodenoscope is placed into the common bile duct.

endoscopy /endos'kəpē/, the visualization of the interior of organs and cavities of the body with an endoscope.

endoskeletal prosthesis /-skel'ətəl/ [Gk, *endon* + *skeletos,* dried up, *prosthesis,* addition], a prosthetic device in which an internal pylon provides the actual support of the body.

endoskeleton, the internal network of bones, to which muscles are attached.

endosteal hyperostosis /endos'tē·əl/, an inherited bone disorder characterized by an overgrowth of the mandible and brow areas. The excessive bone growth can lead to entrapment of cranial nerves, causing facial palsy and loss of hearing.

endothelial /en'dōthē'lē·əl/ [Gk, *endon,* within, *thele,* nipple], pertaining to endothelium.

endothelial cell [Gk, *endon,* within, *thele,* nipple; L, *cella,* storeroom], a lining cell of a body cavity or of the cardiovascular system. It is usually seen as a flat nucleated cell.

endothelial-derived relaxing factor (EDRF), an agent that relaxes smooth muscles and stimulates blood flow in veins.

endothelin (ET) /-thē'lin/, any of a group of vasoconstrictive peptides produced by endothelial cells. Three known endothelins designated as ET-1, ET-2, and ET-3 are chemically related to asp venom. ET-1 is the most potent vasopressor compound yet discovered, being 10 times greater than angiotensin II, previously be-lieved to be the most powerful vasopressor.

endothelium /en'dōthē'lē·əm/ [Gk, *endon* + *thele,* nipple], the layer of simple squamous epithelial cells that lines the heart, the blood and lymph vessels, and the serous cavities of the body.

endothoracic fascia /thôras'ik/, a sheet of connective tissue within the thorax. It separates the parietal pleura from the chest wall and the diaphragm. A thickened part also attaches to the medial border of the first rib.

endotoxin /en'dōtok'sin/ [Gk, *endon* + *toxikon,* poison], a toxin contained in the cell walls of some microorganisms, especially gram-negative bacteria, that is released when the bacterium dies and is broken down in the body.

endotoxin shock [Gk, *endon,* within, *toxikon,* poison; Fr, *choc*], a septic shock in response to the release of endotoxins produced by gram-negative bacteria. The toxin is released on the death of the bacterial cell.

endotracheal /en'dōtrā'kē·əl/ [Gk, *endon* + *tracheia* + *arteria,* airpipe], within or through the trachea.

endotracheal anesthesia, anesthesia that is achieved by the inhalation of an anesthetic gas or mixture of gases through an endotracheal tube into the lungs, where it is absorbed into the bloodstream.

Endotracheal Extubation, a Nursing Interventions Classification defined as purposeful removal of the endotracheal tube from the nasopharyngeal or oropharyngeal airway.

endotracheal intubation, the management of the patient with an airway catheter inserted through the mouth or nose into the trachea. An endotracheal tube may be used to maintain a patent airway, to prevent aspiration of material from the digestive tract in the unconscious or paralyzed patient, to permit suctioning of tracheobronchial secretions, or to administer positive-pressure ventilation that cannot be given effectively by a mask.

endotracheal tube, a large-bore catheter inserted through the mouth or nose and into the trachea to a point above the bifurcation of the trachea. It is used for delivering oxygen under pressure when ventilation must be totally controlled.

endovasculitis /-vas'kyəli'tis/, inflammation of the tunica intima of a blood vessel.

endoxin /endok'sin/, an endogenous analog of digoxin that occurs naturally in humans. It is a hormone that may regulate the excretion of salt.

endplate [AS, *ende* + ME, *plat*], the motor endplate in the nervous system, located at the terminal membrane of an axon and the postjunctional membrane of the adjoining muscle tissue.

end point, 1. (in chemistry) the point at which a physical change associated with the condition of equivalence is observed during a titration. **2.** the point or time at which an activity is finished. **3.** the point at which a chemical indicator changes color.

end-positional nystagmus, a horizontal rhythmic oscillation of the eyes on extreme lateral gaze. It occurs in normal eyes when the fixation point is outside the binocular field.

end-stage disease [AS, *ende* + OFr, *estage* + L, *dis* + Fr, *aise*, ease], a disease condition that is essentially terminal because of irreversible damage to vital tissues or organs. Kidney or renal end-stage disease is defined as a point at which the kidney is so badly damaged or scarred that hemodialysis or transplantation is required for patient survival.

end-tidal capnography /end'tīdəl/, (in respiratory therapy) the process of continuously recording the concentration or percentage of carbon dioxide in expired air. It is used to continuously monitor critically ill patients and in pulmonary function testing.

end-tidal CO₂ determination, the concentration of carbon dioxide in a patient's end-tidal breath.

endurance /endyŏŏr'əns/, the ability to continue an activity despite increasing physical or psychologic stress. Although endurance and strength are different qualities, weaker muscles tend to have less endurance than strong muscles.

enema /en'əmə/ [Gk, *enienai*, to send in], the introduction of a solution into the rectum for cleansing or therapeutic purposes. Enemas may be commercially packed disposable units or reusable equipment prepared just before use.

energy /en'ərjē/ [Gk, *energia*], the capacity to do work or to perform vigorous activity. Energy may occur in the form of heat, light, movement, sound, or radiation. Human energy is usually expressed as muscle contractions and heat production. Chemical energy is that released as a result of a chemical reaction, as in the metabolism of food. **—energetic,** *adj.*

energy conservation, a principle that energy cannot be created or destroyed although, it can be changed from one form into another, as when heat energy is converted to light energy.

energy cost of activities, the metabolic cost in calories or kilojoules of various forms of physical activity. For example,

the average metabolic (MET) equivalent of walking at a rate of 3 km/hr is 2 METs per minute, and the energy cost of walking at a speed of 6 km/hour is 5 METs per minute.

energy field disturbance, a NANDA-accepted nursing diagnosis of a disruption of the flow of energy surrounding a person's being, which causes a disharmony of the body, mind, or spirit. Defining characteristics include temperature change (warmth or coolness), visual changes (image or color), disruption of the field (vacant/hold/spike/bulge), movement (wave/spike/tingling/dense/flowing), and sounds (tone or words).

Energy Management, a Nursing Interventions Classification defined as regulating energy use to treat or prevent fatigue and optimize function.

energy output, the amount of energy expended by work or activity by the body per specified period.

energy-protein malnutrition, a wasting condition resulting from a diet deficient in both calories and proteins.

energy subtraction, (in digital radiographic imaging) a technique in which two different x-ray beams are used alternately to provide a subtraction image resulting from differences in photoelectrical interaction.

enervation /en'ərvā'shən/ [L, *enervare*, to weaken], **1.** reduction or lack of nervous energy; weakness; lassitude; languor. **2.** removal of a complete nerve or a section of nerve.

en face /äNfäs', enfäs'/, "face-to-face"; a position in which the mother's face and the infant's face are approximately 8 inches apart and on the same plane, as when the mother holds the infant up in front of her face or when she nurses the child.

enflurane /en'flŏŏrān/, a nonflammable anesthetic gas of the ether family. It is used for maintenance of general anesthesia. A halogenated volatile liquid, enflurane is administered through calibrated vaporizers, permitting close control of dosage.

engagement /engāj'mənt/ [Fr, a bonding], **1.** fixation of the presenting part of the fetus in the maternal true pelvis. The largest diameter of the presenting part is at or below the level of the ischial spines. **2.** fixation of the fetal head in the maternal midpelvis with the biparietal diameter of the head level with the ischial spines.

engorgement /engôrj'mənt/ [Fr, *engorger,* to fill up], distension or vascular congestion of body tissues, such as the swelling of breast tissue caused by an increased flow of blood and lymph preceding true lactation.

engram /en′gram/, **1.** a hypothetic neurophysiologic storage unit in the cerebrum that is the source of a particular memory. **2.** an interneuronal circuit involving specific neurons and muscle fibers that can be coordinated to perform specific motor activity patterns. **3.** the permanent trace left by a stimulus in nerve tissue.

enhancement /enhans′mənt/ [ME, *enhauncen,* to raise], to improve, heighten, or augment.

enkephalin /enkef′əlin/ [Gk, *enkepalos,* brain, *in,* within], one of two pain-relieving pentapeptides produced in the body. Enkephalins are located in the pituitary gland, brain, and gastrointestinal tract: methionine-enkephalin and isoleucine-enkephalin, each composed of five amino acids, four of which are identical in both compounds. These two neuropeptides can depress neurons throughout the central nervous system.

enkephalinergic neuron /enkef′əlinur′jik/, a nerve cell that releases the peptide neurotransmitter enkephalin.

enol /ē′nol/, an organic compound with an alcohol or hydroxyl group adjacent to a double bond.

enophthalmos /en′əfthal′məs/ [Gk, *en,* in, *ophthalmos,* eye], backward displacement of the eye in the bony socket, caused by traumatic injury or developmental defect.—**enophthalmic,** *adj.*

enriched, 1. (in chemistry) pertaining to a substance containing a proportion of isotope greater than that found in the naturally occurring form of the same element. **2.** (in nutrition) pertaining to foods to which vitamins or minerals have been added within limits specified by the U.S. Food and Drug Administration

enrollee, an individual who has signed up to receive health care under a particular type of plan. Not applicable in Canada.

ENT, abbreviation for *ear, nose, and throat.*

ental /en′tal/ [Gk, *entos,* within], central or inner.

Entamoeba /en′təmē′bə/ [Gk, *entos,* within, *amoibe,* change], a genus of intestinal amebic parasites of which several species are pathogenic to humans.

Entamoeba coli, a common nonpathogenic amebic parasite found in the intestines of humans and other mammals. It is similar to and sometimes confused with *E. histolytica,* the causal agent of amebic dysentery.

Entamoeba gingivalis, a temperature-resistant species of ameba found in the mouth of humans and other mammals. As a causal agent of gingivitis, it is associated with poor dental hygiene.

Entamoeba histolytica /his′təlit′ikə/, a pathogenic species of ameba that causes amebic dysentery and hepatic amebiasis in humans.

enteral /en′tərəl, enter′əl/ /enter′əl/ [Gk, *enteron,* bowel], within the small intestine, or via the small intestine.

enteral feeding, a mode of feeding that uses the gastrointestinal tract, such as oral or tube feeding.

enteral nutrition, the provision of nutrients through the gastrointestinal tract when the client cannot ingest, chew, or swallow food but can digest and absorb nutrients.

enteral tube feeding [Gk, *enteron,* bowel; L, *tubus* + AS, *faedan*], the introduction of nutrients directly into the gastrointestinal tract by feeding tube.

Enteral Tube Feeding, a Nursing Interventions Classification defined as delivering nutrients and water through a gastrointestinal tube.

enterectomy /en′tərek′təmē/ [Gk, *enteron,* intestine, *ektome,* excision], the surgical removal of a part of intestine.

enteric /enter′ik/ [Gk, *enteron,* bowel], pertaining to the intestine.

enteric coating, a layer added to oral medications that are to be absorbed from the intestinal tract. The coating combats the effects of stomach juices, which can interact with or destroy certain drugs.

enteric infection, a disease of the intestine caused by any infection. Symptoms similar to those caused by pathogens may be produced by chemical toxins in ingested foods and by allergic reactions to certain food substances. Among bacteria commonly involved in enteric infections are *Escherichia coli, Vibrio cholerae,* and several species of *Salmonella, Shigella,* and anaerobic streptococci. Enteric infections are characterized by diarrhea, abdominal discomfort, nausea and vomiting, and anorexia.

entericoid fever /enter′ikoid/ [Gk, *enteron* + *eidos,* form], a typhoidlike febrile disease characterized by intestinal inflammation and dysfunction.

enteric orphan virus [Gk, *enteron,* bowel, *orphanos,* bereft; L, *virus,* poison], a gastrointestinal disease virus that has been identified and isolated but was not originally associated with the disease.

enteritis /en′tərī′tis/, inflammation of the mucosal lining of the small intestine, resulting from a variety of causes—bacterial, viral, functional, and inflammatory.

Enterobacter cloacae /en′tirōbak′tər klō-ā′kē, klō-ā′sē/ [Gk, *enteron* + *bakterion* small staff; L, *cloaca,* sewer], a common species of bacteria found in human and animal feces, dairy products, sewage, soil, and water.

Enterobacteriaceae /en'tirōbaktir'ē-ā'si-ē/ [Gk, *enteron* + *bakterion,* small staff], a family of aerobic and anaerobic bacteria that includes both normal and pathogenic enteric microorganisms. Among the significant genera of the family are *Escherichia, Klebsiella, Proteus,* and *Salmonella.*

enterobacterial /-baktir'ē-əl/ [Gk, *enteron* + *bakterion,* small staff], pertaining to a species of bacteria found in the digestive tract.

enterobiasis /en'tirōbī'əsis/ [Gk, *enteron* + *bios,* life, *osis,* condition], a parasitic infestation with *Enterobius vermicularis,* the common pinworm. The worms infect the large intestine, and the females deposit eggs in the perianal area, causing pruritus and insomnia.

Enterobius vermicularis /en'tərō'bē-əs/ [Gk, *enteron* + *bios,* life; L, *vermiculus,* small worm], a common parasitic nematode that resembles a white thread between 0.5 and 1 cm long.

enterocele /en'tirōsēl'/, **1.** a hernia containing intestine. **2.** posterior vaginal hernia.

enteroclysis /en'tərok'lisis/, a radiographic procedure in which a contrast medium is injected into the duodenum to examine the small intestine.

enterococcus /-kokəs/, *pl.* **enterococci** /-kok'sī, -kôk'ē/ [Gk, *enteron* + *kokkos,* berry], any *Streptococcus* that inhabits the intestinal tract.

enterocoele, the abdominal cavity.

enterocolitis /-kōlī'tis/ [Gk, *enteron* + *kolon,* bowel, *itis*], an inflammation involving both the large and small intestines.

enterodynia /-din'ē-ə/, intestinal pain.

enteroenterostomy /en'tərō-en'təros'-təmē/, the surgical creation of an artificial connection between two segments of the intestine.

enteroglucagon / gloo'kəgon/, any of a group of glucagon-like hyperglycemic peptides. It is released by cells in the mucosa in the upper intestine in response to the ingestion of food and stimulates intestinal epithelial cell preparation and renewal.

enterohemorrhagic *Escherichia coli* /-hem'ôraj'ik/, a strain of *E. coli* that causes hemorrhage in the intestines. The organism produces a toxin that damages bowel tissue, causing intestinal ischemia and colonic necrosis. Spread by contaminated beef, the infection can be serious, although there may be no fever. Treatment consists of antibiotics and maintenance of fluid and electrolyte balance.

enterohepatic circulation /en'tərōhə-pat'ik/, a route by which part of the bile produced by the liver enters the intestine, is resorbed by the liver, and then is recycled into the intestine. The remainder of the bile is excreted in feces.

enterokinase /en'tirōkī'nās/ [Gk, *enteron* + *kinesis,* movement, *ase,* enzyme], an intestinal juice enzyme that activates the proteolytic enzyme in pancreatic juice as they enter the duodenum.

enterolith /en'tərōlith'/ [Gk, *enteron* + *lithos,* stone], a stone consisting of ingested material found within the intestine.

enterolithiasis /en'tərōlithī'əsis/, the presence of enteroliths in the intestine.

enteropathic *Escherichia coli* /-path'-əjen'ik/, a strain of *E. coli* that is the cause of epidemic infantile diarrhea.

enteropathy /en'tərop'əthē/, a disease or other disorder of the intestines.

enterostomal therapist /-stō'məl/, a registered nurse who is qualified by education in an accredited program in enterostomal therapy to provide care for patients.

enterostomy /en'təros'təmē/ [Gk, *enteron* + *stoma,* mouth], a surgical procedure that produces an artificial anus or fistula in the intestine by incision through the abdominal wall.

enterotoxigenic /-tok'sijen'ik/ /en'tirōtok'-sijen'ik/, pertaining to an organism or other agent that produces a toxin that causes an adverse reaction by cells of the intestinal mucosa. Examples include bacteria that produce enterotoxins, resulting in intestinal reactions such as vomiting, diarrhea, and other symptoms of food poisoning.

enterotoxigenic *Escherichia coli*, a strain of *E. Coli* that is a frequent cause of diarrhea in travelers.

enterotoxin /-tok'sin/, a toxic substance specific for the cells of the intestinal mucosa, produced usually by certain species of bacteria such as *Staphylococcus.*

enterovirus /-vī'rəs/ [Gk, *enteron* + L, *virus,* poison], a virus that multiplies primarily in the intestinal tract. Kinds of enteroviruses are **coxsackievirus, ECHO virus,** and **poliovirus. —enteroviral,** *adj.*

enthesitis /en'thəsī'tis/, an inflammation of the insertion of a muscle with a strong tendency toward fibrosis and calcification. It is usually only painful when the involved muscle is activated.

entopic /entop'ik/, occurring in the proper place.

entopic phenomena, sensations perceived for mechanical reasons within the eye, such as floaters or flashes caused by retinal changes.

entrainment /entrān′mənt/ [Fr, *entrainer,* to drag along], a phenomenon observed in the microanalysis of sound films in which the speaker moves several parts of the body and the listener responds by moving in ways that are coordinated with the rhythm of the sounds. Entrainment is thought to be an essential factor in the process of maternal-infant bonding.

entrance block /entrans′/ [Fr, *entrer,* to enter; AS, *blok*], (in cardiology) a theoretic zone surrounding a pacemaker focus, protecting it from discharge by an extraneous impulse that might trigger ectopic ventricular contractions.

entrance exposure, (in radiology) the skin dose of radiation. It may be expressed in milliroentgens.

entrapment neuropathy /entrap′mənt/ [OFr, *entraper,* to catch in a trap; Gk, *neuron,* nerve, *pathos,* disease], injury or inflammation of single nerves caused by pressure from surrounding tissues such as ligaments and fascia.

entropion /entrō′pē·on/ [Gk, *en + tropos,* a turning], turning inward or turning toward, usually a condition in which the eyelid turns inward toward the eye. In either the upper or lower eyelid cicatricial entropion can result from scar tissue formation. Spastic entropion results from an inflammation or other factor that affects tissue tone. An inflammation of the eyelid may be the result of an infectious disease or irritation from an inverted eyelash.

entropy /en′trəpē/ [Gk, *en + tropos,* a turning], the tendency of a system to change from a state of order to a state of disorder, expressed in physics as a measure of the part of the energy in a thermodynamic system that is not available to perform work.

ENT specialist, a physician who specializes in the treatment of the ear, nose, and throat.

enucleation /inoo͞′klē·ā′shən/ [L, *e,* without, *nucleus,* nut], **1.** 1. removal of an organ or tumor in one piece. **2.** removal of the eyeball, performed for malignancy, severe infection, extensive trauma, or control of pain in glaucoma.

enucleator /inoo͞′klē·ā′tər/ [L, *e,* without, *nucleus,* nut], a procedure or device for removing a nucleus from a cell.

enuresis /en′yoo͞rē′sis/ [Gk, *enourein,* to urinate], incontinence of urine, especially nocturnal bed-wetting.

envenomation /enven′əmā′shən/, the injection of snake or insect venom into the body.

environment [Gk, *en,* in; L, *viron,* circle], all of the many factors, as physical and psychologic, that influence or affect the life and survival of a person.

environmental carcinogen /envī′rənmen′təl/, any of the natural or synthetic substances that can cause cancer. Such agents may be divided into chemical agents, physical agents, hormones, and viruses.

environmental control units, various apparatus for handicapped persons that control lamps, television, radio, telephone, and alarm systems. Similar to television remote control devices, typically they are switches manipulated by the lips, chin, or other body movements.

environmental health, the total of various aspects of substances, forces, and conditions in and about a community that affect the health and well-being of the population.

environmental health technician, a health care professional who performs technical assistance under professional supervision in monitoring environmental health hazards such as radioactive contamination, air and water pollution, and disposal of chemical wastes of industry.

environmental interpretation syndrome, impaired, a NANDA-accepted nursing diagnosis of a consistent lack of orientation to person, place, time, or circumstances over more than 3 to 6 months, necessitating a protective environment. Defining characteristics include consistent disorientation in known or unknown environments, chronic confusional states, loss of occupation or social functioning resulting from memory decline; inability to follow simple directions or instructions; inability to reason; inability to concentrate; and slowness in responding to questions.

Environmental Management, a Nursing Interventions Classification defined as manipulation of the patient's surroundings for therapeutic benefit.

Environmental Management: Attachment Process, a Nursing Interventions Classification defined as manipulation of the patient's surroundings to facilitate the development of the parent-infant relationship.

Environmental Management: Comfort, a Nursing Interventions Classification defined as manipulation of the patient's surroundings for promotion of optimal comfort.

Environmental Management: Community, a Nursing Interventions Classification defined as monitoring and influencing of the physical, social, cultural, economic, and political conditions that affect the health of groups and communities.

Environmental Management: Safety,

a Nursing Interventions Classification defined as monitoring and manipulation of the physical environment to promote safety.

Environmental Management: Violence Prevention, a Nursing Interventions Classification defined as monitoring and manipulation of the physical environment to decrease the potential for violent behavior directed toward self, others, or environment.

Environmental Management: Worker Safety, a Nursing Interventions Classification defined as monitoring and manipulation of the worksite environment to promote safety and health of workers.

environmental services, a functional unit of a hospital or other health care facility. It has the responsibility for laundry, liquid and solid waste control, safe disposal of materials contaminated by radiation or pathogenic organisms, and general maintenance of safety and sanitation.

enzymatic debridement /en'zīmat'ik/, the use of nonirritating, nontoxic vegetable enzymes to remove dead tissue from a wound without destroying normal tissue.

enzymatic detergent asthma, a type of allergic reaction experienced by persons who have become sensitized to alcalase, an enzyme contained in some laundry detergents.

enzyme /en'zīm/ [Gk, *en,* in, *zyme,* ferment], a complex produced by living cells that catalyzes chemical reactions in organic matter. Most enzymes are produced in tiny quantities and catalyze reactions that take place within the cells.

enzyme commission (EC), a body formed in 1956 by the International Union of Biochemistry, which has standardized the nomenclature for enzymes.

enzyme deficiency anemia, a deficiency of enzymes in the pathways that metabolize glucose and adenosine triphosphate.

enzyme induction [Gk, *en* + *zyme,* ferment; L, *inducere,* to lead in], the increase in the rate of a specific enzyme synthesis from basal to maximum level caused by the presence of a substrate or substrate analog that acts as an inducer. The inducer may be a substance that inactivates a repressor chemical in the cell.

enzyme-linked immunosorbent assay (ELISA), a laboratory technique for detecting specific antigens or antibodies, using enzyme-labeled immunoreactants and a solid-phase binding support such as a test tube. ELISA is nearly as sensitive as radioimmunoassay and more sensitive than complement fixation, agglutination, and other techniques. It is commonly used

in the diagnosis of human immunodeficiency virus infections.

enzymology /en'zīmol'əjē/, the study of enzymes and their actions.

enzymolysis /en'zīmol'isis/ [Gk, *en,* in, *zyme,* leaven, *lysis,* loosening], destruction or change of a substance caused by means of enzymatic action.

enzymopenia /en'zīmōpē'nē-ə/, the deficiency of an enzyme.

enzymuria /en'zīmŏŏr'ē-ə/, the presence of enzymes in urine.

EOA, abbreviation for **esophageal obturator airway.**

EOM, abbreviation for **extraocular muscles.**

eosin /ē'əsin/, a group of red acidic xanthine dyes often used in combination with a blue-purple basic dye such as hematoxylin to stain tissue slides in the laboratory.

eosinopenia /ē'əsinəpē'nē-ə/, an abnormally low number of eosinophil leukocytes in the blood.

eosinophil /ē'əsin'əfil/ [Gk, *eos,* dawn, *philein,* to love], a granulocytic bilobed leukocyte somewhat larger than a neutrophil. It is characterized by large numbers of coarse refractile cytoplasmic granules that stain with the acid dye eosin.—**eosinophilic,** *adj.*

eosinophilia /ē'əsin'ōfil'yə/, an increase in the number of eosinophils in the blood, accompanying inflammatory conditions. Substantial increases are considered a reflection of an allergic response.

eosinophilia-myalgia syndrome, tryptophan-induced, a potentially fatal disorder resulting from ingestion of tryptophan. It is characterized by a symptom complex of severe muscle pain, tenosynovitis, muscle edema, and skin rash lasting several weeks.

eosinophilic /ē'əsin'əfil'ik/, **1.** the tendency of a cell, tissue, or organism to be readily stained by the dye eosin. **2.** pertaining to an eosinophilic leukocyte.

eosinophilic enteropathy, a rare form of food allergy that is characterized by nausea, crampy abdominal pain, diarrhea, urticaria, an elevated eosinophil count in the blood, and eosinophilic infiltrates in the intestine.

eosinophilic granuloma, a simple or multiple growth in the bone or lung characterized by numerous eosinophils and histiocytes. Eosinophilic granulomas occur most frequently in children and adolescents.

eosinophilic leukemia, a malignant neoplasm of the blood-forming tissues in which eosinophils are the predominant cells.

eosinophilic pneumonia, inflammation

of the lungs, characterized by infiltration of the alveoli with eosinophils and large mononuclear cells, pulmonary edema, fever, night sweats, cough, dyspnea, and weight loss.

EP, abbreviation for **evoked potential.**

ependyma /ipen'dimə/ [Gk, an upper garment], a layer of ciliated epithelium that lines the central canal of the spinal cord and the ventricles of the brain. —**ependymal** /ipen'diməl/, *adj.*

ependymal glioma, a large, vascular, fairly solid tumor in the fourth ventricle, composed of malignant glial cells.

ependymitis /ipen'dimī'tis/, an inflammation of the ependymal tissue.

ependymoblastoma /ipen'dimōblastō'mə/, a malignant neoplasm composed of primitive cells of the ependyma.

ependymoma /ipen'dimō'mə/ [Gk, *ependyma,* an upper garment, *oma,* tumor], a neoplasm composed of differentiated cells of the ependyma.

ephapse /ef'aps/ [Gk, *ephasis,* a touching], a point of lateral contact between nerve fibers across which impulses may be transmitted directly through the cell membranes rather than across a synapse.— **ephaptic,** *adj.*

ephaptic transmission /ifap'tik/, the passage of a neural impulse from one nerve fiber, axon, or dendrite to another through the membranes.

ephebiatrics /ēfeb'ē·at'riks/ [Gk, *ephebos,* puberty, *iatros,* physician], a branch of medicine that specializes in the health of adolescents.

ephedrine /ef'ədrēn/, an adrenergic bronchodilator prescribed in the treatment of asthma and bronchitis and used topically as a nasal decongestant.

ephemeral /ifem'ərəl/ [Gk, *epi,* above, *hemera,* day], pertaining to a short-lived condition such as a fever.

ephemeral fever, any febrile condition lasting only 24 to 48 hours that is uncomplicated and of unknown origin.

epiblast /ep'iblast'/ [Gk, *epi,* upon, *blastos,* germ], the primordial outer layer of the blastocyst or blastula, before differentiation of the germ layers, that gives rise to the ectoderm and contains cells capable of forming the endoderm and mesoderm. —**epiblastic,** *adj.*

epicanthus /ep'ikan'thəs/ [Gk, *epi* + *kanthos,* lip of a vessel], a vertical fold of skin over the angle of the inner canthus of the eye. It is a hereditary trait in Asian people and is of no clinical significance. Some infants with Down's syndrome have marked epicanthal folds. —**epicanthal, epicanthic,** *adj.*

epicardia /-kär'dē·ə/ [Gk, *epi,* above, *kardia,* heart], the part of the esophagus that lies between the cardiac orifice of the stomach and the esophageal opening of the diaphragm.

epicardium /ep'ikär'dē·əm/ [Gk, *epi* + *kardia,* heart], one of the three layers of tissue that form the heart wall. The epicardium is the visceral part of the serous pericardium and folds back on itself to form the parietal part of the serous pericardium.—**epicardial,** *adj.*

epicondylar fracture /-kon'dilər/, any fracture that involves the medial or lateral epicondyle of a specific bone, such as the humerus.

epicondyle /ep'ikon'dəl/ [Gk, *epi* + *kondylos,* knuckle], a projection on the surface of a bone above its condyle. —**epicondylar,** *adj.*

epicondylitis /ep'ikon'dilī'tis/, a painful and sometimes disabling inflammation of the muscle and surrounding tissues of the elbow, caused by repeated strain on the forearm near the lateral epicondyle of the humerus, such as from violent extension or supination of the wrist against a resisting force.

epicranial aponeurosis /-krā'nē·əl/ [Gk, *epi* + *kranion,* skull, *apo,* away, *neuron,* tendon], a fibrous membrane that covers the cranium between the occipital and frontal muscles of the scalp.

epicranium /-krā'nē·əm/ [Gk, *epi* + *kranion,* skull], the complete scalp, including the integument, the muscular sheets, and the aponeuroses. —**epicranial,** *adj.*

epicranius [Gk, *epi* + *kranion,* skull], the broad muscular and tendinous layer of tissue covering the top and sides of the skull from the occipital bone to the eyebrows.

epicritic /-krit'ik/, pertaining to the somatic sensations of fine discriminative touch, vibration, two-point discrimination, stereognosis, and conscious and unconscious proprioception.

epidemic /-dem'ik/ [Gk, *epi* + *demos,* people], **1.** affecting a significantly large number of people at the same time. **2.** a disease that spreads rapidly through a demographic segment of the human population, such as everyone in a given geographic area. **3.** a disease or event whose incidence is beyond what is expected.

epidemic diarrhea in newborns [Gk, *epi* above, *demos,* the people, *dia,* through *rhein,* flow; ME, *newe* + *beren*], any severe gastroenteritis epidemic among a community of newborns, as may occur in a hospital nursery.

epidemic encephalitis, any diffuse in

flammation of the brain occurring in epidemic form. Two kinds of epidemic encephalitis are **Japanese encephalitis** and **St. Louis encephalitis.**

epidemic hemorrhagic conjunctivitis [Gk, *epi*, above, *demos*, the people, *haima*, blood, *rhegnynei*, to gush; L, *conjunctivus*, connecting; Gk, *itis*, inflammation], a highly contagious infection, commonly involving an enterovirus, that begins with eye pain accompanied by swollen eyelids and hyperemia of the conjunctiva. It is a self-limiting disorder that has no specific remedy.

epidemic hemorrhagic fever, a severe viral infection marked by fever and bleeding. The disorder develops rapidly and is characterized initially by fever and muscle ache, possibly followed by hemorrhage, peripheral vascular collapse, hypovolemic shock, and acute kidney failure. The arbovirus or other pathogen is believed transmitted by mosquitoes, ticks, or mites.

epidemic keratoconjunctivitis (EKC) [Gk, *epi*, above, *demos*, the people, *keras*, horn; L, *conjunctivus*; Gk, *itis*, inflammation], an acute complex of keratitis and conjunctivitis transmitted by an adenovirus. A highly contagious form of keratoconjunctivitis, it often includes lymph node involvement. It is commonly spread by handling contaminated materials in eye clinics, particularly offices that handle emergency care of eye injuries.

epidemic pleurodynia, an infection caused by a coxsackievirus, mainly affecting children. It is characterized by severe intermittent pain in the abdomen or lower chest, fever, headache, sore throat, malaise, and extreme myalgia.

epidemic typhus, an acute severe rickettsial infection characterized by a prolonged high fever, headache, and dark maculopapular rash that covers most of the body. The causative organism, *Rickettsia prowazekii*, is transmitted indirectly as a result of the bite of the human body louse; the pathogen is contained in feces of the louse and enters the body tissues as the bite is scratched. An intense headache and a fever reaching 40° C (104° F) begin after an incubation period of 10 days to 2 weeks. The rash follows.

epidemic vomiting, an episode of sudden ejection of stomach contents by members of a group of people in close contact. The vomiting, caused by a ribonucleic acid Norwalk virus infection, usually begins without previous signs or symptoms of illness and may continue for several hours, ending abruptly.

epidemiologist /-dē'mē·ol'əjist/, a physician or medical scientist who studies the incidence, prevalence, spread, prevention, and control of disease in a community or a specific group of individuals.

epidemiologist nurse, a registered nurse with special training and experience in the control of infections in the hospital and community.

epidemiology /-dē'mē·ol'əjē/ [Gk, *epi* + *demos*, people, *logos* science], the study of the determinants of disease events in populations. —**epidemiologic,** *adj.*

epidermal nevus /-dur'məl/ [Gk, *epi* + *derma*, skin; L, *naevus*, birthmark], a discrete discolored congenital lesion caused by an overgrowth of epidermis. It may be seen in newborns.

epidermis /ep'idur'mis/ [Gk, *epi* + *derma*, skin], the superficial avascular layers of the skin, made up of an outer dead, cornified part and a deeper living, cellular part. —**epidermal, epidermoid,** *adj.*

epidermitis /ep'idurmī'tis/, an inflammation of the epidermis, the outer layer of the skin.

epidermoid carcinoma /-dur'moid/ [Gk, *epi* + *derma* + *eidos*, form], a malignant neoplasm in which the tumor cells tend to differentiate in the manner of epidermal cells, then form horny cells called prickle cells.

epidermoid cyst, a common benign cavity lined by keratinizing epithelium and filled with a cheesy material composed of sebum and epithelial debris.

epidermolysis bullosa /ep'idərmol'isis/ [Gk, *epi* + *derma* + *lysis*, loosening], a group of rare hereditary skin diseases in which vesicles and bullae develop, usually at sites of trauma.

epidermophytosis /ep'idur'mōfītō'sis/, a superficial fungus infection of the skin.

epididymis /ep'idid'imis/, *pl.* **epididymides** [Gk, *epi* + *didymos*, pair], one of a pair of long tightly coiled ducts that carry sperm from the seminiferous tubules of the testes to the vas deferens.

epididymitis /ep'idid'imī'tis/ [Gk, *epi* + *didymos* + *itis*, inflammation], acute or chronic inflammation of the epididymis. It may result from venereal disease, urinary tract infection, prostatitis, prostatectomy, or prolonged use of indwelling catheters. Symptoms include fever and chills, pain in the groin, and tender, swollen epididymis.

epididymoorchitis /ep'idid'imō'ôrkī'tis/ [Gk, *epi* +, *didymos* + *orchis*, testis, *itis*], inflammation of the epididymis and testis.

epididymovesiculography /ep'idid'-imōves'ikyəlog'rəfē/, a radiologic examination of the seminal ducts. It is usually performed in cases of sterility, cysts, tumors, abscesses, or inflammation.

epidural /ep'ido͞or'əl/ [Gk, epi + dura, hard], outside or above the dura mater.

epidural abscess, a collection of pus between the dura mater of the brain and skull, or between the dura mater of the spinal cord and the vertebral canal.

epidural anesthesia/analgesia, a type of regional block in which a local anesthetic is injected into the epidural space surrounding the dural membrane, which contains cerebrospinal fluid and spinal nerves. Epidurals are most commonly performed in the lumbar area; injections are usually made through a catheter placed in the space with a specialized needle called a Touhy. Epidurals have a wide application in anesthesia and pain management because of their safety and versatility. Epidural anesthesia or analgesia can be tailored to affect an area of the body from the lower extremities up to the upper abdomen.

epidural blood patch (EBP), a treatment for postdural puncture headache in which 15 to 20 ml of a patient's blood is injected into the epidural space at or near the location of a dural puncture. The volume injected displaces cerebrospinal fluid (CSF) from the lumbar CSF space into the area surrounding the brain, often yielding immediate relief.

epidural hemorrhage, a hemorrhage that produces a collection of blood outside the dura mater of the brain or spinal cord.

epidural space, the space immediately above and surrounding the dura mater of the brain or spinal cord, beneath the endosteum of the cranium and the spinal column.

epifolliculitis /ep'ifolik'yəlī'tis/, an inflammation of the hair follicles of the head.

epigastric /-gas'trik/ [Gk, epi, above, gaster, stomach], pertaining to the epigastrium, the area above the stomach.

epigastric hernia, the protrusion of an internal organ through the linea alba.

epigastric node [Gk, epi + gaster, stomach; L, nodus, knot], a node in one of the seven groups of parietal lymph nodes serving the abdomen and pelvis, comprising about four nodes along the caudal part of the inferior epigastric vessels.

epigastric pain [Gk, epi, above, gaster, stomach; L, poena, penalty], pain in the upper middle part of the abdomen.

epigastric reflex [Gk, epi, above, gaster, stomach; L, reflectere, to bend back], a contraction of the rectus abdominis muscle that occurs when the skin surface in the upper and middle abdominal region is stimulated. The reflex also may be induced by stimulation of the axillary region of the fifth and sixth dorsal nerves.

epigastric region, the part of the abdomen in the upper zone between the right and left hypochondriac regions.

epigastric sensation, a weak, sinking feeling of undefined nature that is usually localized in the pit of the stomach but may occur throughout the abdominal region.

epigenesis /ep'ijen'əsis/ [Gk, epi + genein, to produce], (in embryology) a theory of development in which the organism grows from a simple to a more complex form through the progressive differentiation of an undifferentiated cellular unit. —**epigenesist,** n., **epigenetic,** adj.

epiglottis /ep'iglot'is/ [Gk, epi + glossa, tongue], the cartilaginous structure that overhangs the larynx like a lid and prevents food from entering the larynx and the trachea while swallowing.

epiglottitis /ep'iglotī'tis/ [Gk, epi + glossa, tongue, itis, inflammation], an inflammation of the epiglottis. Acute epiglottitis is a severe form of the condition, which primarily affects children. It is characterized by fever, sore throat, stridor, croupy cough and an erythematous, swollen epiglottis. The patient may become cyanotic and require an emergency tracheostomy to maintain respiration.

epilating forceps /ep'ilā'ting/ [L, e + pilus, without hair], a kind of small spring forceps, used for removing unwanted hair.

epilepsy /ep'ilep'sē/ [Gk, epilepsia, seizure], a group of neurologic disorders characterized by recurrent episodes of convulsive seizures, sensory disturbances, abnormal behavior, loss of consciousness, or all of these. Common to all types of epilepsy is an uncontrolled electrical discharge from the nerve cells of the cerebral cortex. Although most epilepsy is of unknown cause, it is sometimes associated with cerebral trauma, intracranial infection, brain tumor, vascular disturbances, intoxication, or chemical imbalance. —**epileptic,** adj., n.

epileptic cry /ep'ilep'tik/, a loud vocalization produced by a person who has epilepsy, often immediately before the onset of a seizure.

epileptic dementia [Gk, epilepsia, seizure; L, de + mens, mind], a loss of cognitive and intellectual functions that develops in some cases of incompletely controlled epilepsy. Symptoms include slowness and circumstantiality of speech and narrowed attention span.

epileptic stupor, the state of unawareness and unresponsiveness that follows an epileptic seizure.

epileptic vertigo [Gk, *epilepsia*, seizure; L, *vertigo*, dizziness], an aura of dizziness that may precede, accompany, or follow an epileptic seizure.

epileptogenic /ep′ilep′tōjen′ik/, causing epileptic seizures.

epimysium /ep′imiz′ē·əm/ [Gk, *epi* + *mys*, muscle], a fibrous sheath that enfolds a muscle and extends between bundles of muscle fibers, as the perimysium.

epinephrine /ep′ənef′rin/ [Gk, *epi* + *nephros*, kidney], an endogenous adrenal hormone and synthetic adrenergic vasoconstrictor. It is prescribed to treat anaphylaxis, acute bronchial spasm, and nasal congestion and to increase the effectiveness of a local anesthetic.

epinephryl borate /-nef′ril/, an adrenergic prescribed in the treatment of primary open-angle glaucoma.

epiotic /ep′ē·ot′ik/, pertaining to the part of the temporal bone that is the ossification center for the mastoid.

epipastic /ep′ipas′tik/ [Gk, *epipassein*, to sprinkle about], dusting powder.

epiphyseal /ep′fiz′ē·əl, ipif′əsē′əl/ [Gk, *epi*, above, *phyein*, to grow], pertaining to or resembling the epiphysis.

epiphyseal fracture [Gk, *epi* + *phyein*, to grow, *fractura*, break], a fracture involving the epiphyseal growth plate of a long bone, which causes separation or fragmentation of the plate.

epiphyseal plate [Gk, *epi*, above, *phyein*, to grow, *platys*, flat], a thin layer of cartilage between the epiphysis, a secondary bone-forming center, and the bone shaft. The new bone forms along the plate.

epiphysis /epif′isis/, pl. **epiphyses** [Gk, *epi* + *phyein*, to grow], the enlarged proximal and distal ends of a long bone.— **epiphyseal** /ipif′əsē′əl/, *adj*.

epiphysitis /ipif′isī′tis/, an inflammation of the epiphysis, usually of a long bone, such as the femur or humerus. The disorder mainly affects children.

epiploic /ep′iplō′ik/, pertaining to the omentum.

epiploic foramen /-plō′ik/ [Gk, *epiploon*, caul; L, *foramen*, a hole], a passage between the peritoneal cavity and the omental bursa. It is lined with peritoneum and is approximately 3 cm in diameter.

episcleritis /ep′isklərī′tis/, inflammation of the outermost layers of the sclera and the tissues overlying its posterior parts.

episcope, a skin surface microscope that uses the technology of epiluminescence microscopy (the application of oil to produce translucence of the epidermis on a skin lesion). The episcope is placed gently over the lesion to observe its general appearance, surface, pigment pattern, border, and depigmentation.

episiotomy /epē′zē·ot′əmē/ [Gk, *episeion*, pubic region, *temnein*, to cut], a surgical procedure in which an incision is made in a woman's perineum to enlarge her vaginal opening for delivery. It is performed most often electively to prevent tearing of the perineum, to hasten or facilitate birth of the baby, or to prevent stretching of perineal muscles and connective tissue.

episode /ep′isōd/ [Gk, *episodion*, coming in besides], an incident or event that stands out from the continuity of everyday life, such as an episode of illness or a traumatic event in the course of a child's development. —**episodic**, *adj*.

episode of hospital care, the services provided by a hospital in the continuous course of care of a patient with a health condition.

episodic care /-sod′ik/, a pattern of medical and nursing care in which services are provided to a person for a particular problem, without an ongoing relationship being established between the person and health care professionals. Emergency rooms provide episodic care.

episome /ep′isōm/ [Gk, *epi* + *soma*, body], (in bacterial genetics) an extrachromosomal replicating unit that exists autonomously or functions with a chromosome.

epispadias /ep′ispā′dē·əs/ [Gk, *epi* + *spadon*, a rent], a congenital defect in which the urethra opens on the dorsum of the penis at some point proximal to the glans. The corresponding defect in women, in which the urethra opens by the separation of the labia minora and a fissure of the clitoris, is quite rare.

epistasis /epis′təsis/ [Gk, a standing], (in genetics) a type of interaction between genes at different loci on a chromosome in which one is able to mask or suppress the expression of the other. —**epistatic**, *adj*.

epistaxis /ep′istak′sis/ [Gk, a dropping], bleeding from the nose caused by local irritation of mucous membranes, violent sneezing, fragility of the mucous membrane or the arterial walls, chronic infection, trauma, hypertension, leukemia, vitamin K deficiency, or, most often, picking the nose.

episternal /ep′istur′nəl/, situated on or over the sternum.

epithalamus /ep′ithal′əməs/ [Gk, *epi* + *thalamos*, chamber], one of the parts of the diencephalon. It includes the trigonum habenulae, the pineal body, and the posterior commissure. —**epithalamic**, *adj*.

epithelial /-thē′lē·əl/ [Gk, *epi*, above, *thele*, nipple], pertaining to or involving the outer layer of the skin.

epithelial cancer [Gk, *epi,* above, *thele,* nipple; L, *cancer,* crab], a carcinoma that develops from epithelium or related tissues in the skin, hollow viscera, and other organs.

epithelial cells, cells arranged in one or more layers that form part of a covering or lining of a body surface. The cells usually adhere to each other along their edges and surfaces.

epithelial debridement [Gk, *epi,* above, *thele,* nipple; Fr, *debridement,* incision], the removal of the entire inner lining and the attachment from the gingival or periodontal pocket in gingival curettage.

epithelialization /-thē′lē·al′izā′shən/ [Gk, *epi,* above, *thele,* nipple; L, *ization,* process], the regrowth of skin over a wound.

epithelial peg [Gk, *epi* + *thele,* nipple], any of the papillary projections of the epithelium that penetrate the underlying stroma of connecting tissue and normally develop in mucous membranes and dermal tissues.

epithelial tissue [Gk, *epi,* above, *thele,* nipple; OFr, *tissu*], a closely packed single or stratified layer of cells covering the body and lining its cavities, with the exception of the blood and lymph vessels.

epithelioblastoma /ep′ithē′lē·ō′blastō′mə/, a tumor composed of epithelial cells.

epithelioid leiomyoma /ep′ithē′lē·oid/ [Gk, *epi* + *thele* + *eidos,* form], an uncommon neoplasm of smooth muscle in which the cells are polygonal in shape. It usually develops in the stomach.

epithelioma /-thē′lē·ō′mə/ [Gk, *epi* + *thele* + *oma,* tumor], a neoplasm derived from the epithelium.

epithelium /-thē′lē·əm/ [Gk, *epi* + *thele,* nipple], the covering of the internal and external organs of the body and the lining of vessels, body cavities, glands, and organs. It consists of cells bound together by connective material and varies in the number of layers and the kinds of cells. The stratified squamous epithelium of the epidermis comprises five different cellular layers. —**epithelial,** *adj.*

epitope /ep′itōp/ [Gk *epi* + *topos,* place], an antigenic determinant that causes a specific reaction by an immunoglobulin. It consists of a group of amino acids on the surface of the antigen.

epitympanic recess /-timpan′ik/ [Gk, *epi* + *tympanon,* drum], the area of the tympanic cavity cranial to the tympanic membrane, which contains the upper half of the malleus and greater part of the incus.

epizootic /ep′izō·ot′ik/, a disease or condition that occurs at about the same time in many of the animals of a species in a geographic area.

EPO, 1. abbreviation for **erythropoietin.** 2. abbreviation for **Exclusive Provider Organization.**

eponym /ep′ənim/ [Gk, *epi,* above, *onyma,* name], a name for a disease, organ, procedure, or body function that is derived from the name of a person, usually a physician or scientist who first identified the condition or devised the object bearing the name. Examples include fallopian tube, Parkinson's disease, and Billing's method.

epoophorectomy /ep′ō·of′ərek′təmē/ [Gk, *epi* + *oophoron,* ovary, *temnein,* to cut], surgical removal of the epoophoron.

epoophoron /ep′ō·of′əron/ [Gk, *epi* + *oophoron,* ovary], a structure that is situated in the mesosalpinx between the ovary and the uterine tube.

epoxy, an organic chemical formula derived from the union of an oxygen atom and two other atoms, usually carbon. Epoxy resins are used as bonding agents.

EPSDT, abbreviation for **Early and Periodic Screening Diagnosis and Treatment.**

epsilon /ep′silon/, E, ε, the fifth letter of the Greek alphabet.

EPSP, abbreviation for *excitatory postsynaptic potential.*

Epstein-Barr virus (EBV) /ep′stīnbär′/ [Michael A. Epstein, b. 1921, English pathologist; Yvonne M. Barr, twentieth-century English virologist; L, *virus,* poison], the herpesvirus that causes infectious mononucleosis, Burkitt's lymphoma, and other lymphoproliferative disorders, especially in transplantation patients.

Epstein's pearls [Alois Epstein, Czechoslovakian physician, 1849–1918; L, *perla,* a mussel], small white pearllike epithelial cysts that occur on both sides of the midline of the hard palate of the newborn.

epulis /epyoo′lis/, *pl.* **epulides** [Gk, *epi* + *oulon,* gum], any tumor or growth on the gingiva.

epulosis /ep′yəlō′sis/, a healing process by scar formation, resulting in the production of a cicatrix.

equal cleavage /ē′kwəl/ [L, *aequare,* to make alike; AS, *cleofan*], mitotic division of the fertilized ovum into blastomeres of identical size, as occurs in humans and most mammals.

equal distribution, a capitation method in which income is distributed equally among providers. It is used when the patient population is geographically and clinically homogeneous. Not applicable in Canada.

Equal Employment Opportunity Com-

equation   421   Erb's point

mission (EEOC), a body appointed by the president of the United States to administer the Civil Rights Act of 1964, particularly to investigate complaints of discrimination in employment in businesses engaged in interstate commerce. Discrimination based on race, color, creed, or national origin is forbidden, but certain kinds of employers and certain conditions of employment allow exceptions to the act.

equation [L, *aequare,* to make equal], an expression in symbols of equality or equivalence.

equatorial plate /ēk′wətôr′ē·əl/ [L, *aequare,* to make alike; Fr, *flat* + *vessel*] the platelike configuration formed by the chromosomes at the center of the spindle during the metaphase stage of mitosis and meiosis.

equianalgesic dose /ē′kwē·an′əljē′sik/, a dose of one analgesic that is equivalent in pain-relieving effects to another analgesic. This equivalence permits substitution of medications to prevent possible adverse effects of one of the drugs. The term is also applied to equivalent alternative dose sizes and routes of administration.

equilibration /ē′kwilibrā′shən/ [L, *aequus,* equal, *libra,* balance], the balancing and integrating of new experiences with those of the past in the psychologic development of an individual.

equilibrium /ē′kwilib′rē·əm/ [L, *aequilibrium*], 1. a state of balance or rest resulting from the equal action of opposing substances such as calcium and phosphorus in the body. 2. (in psychiatry) a state of mental or emotional balance. 3. (in radiotherapy) a point at which the rate of production of a daughter element is equal to the rate of decay of the parent element and the activities of parent and daughter are identical.

equilibrium reaction, any of several reflexes that enable the body to recover balance.

equine encephalitis /ē′kwīn, ek′win/ [L, *equinus,* horse; Gk, *enkephalon,* brain, *itis,* inflammation], an arbovirus infection characterized by inflammation of the nerve tissues of the brain and spinal cord. Other characteristics include high fever; headache; nausea; vomiting; myalgia; and neurologic symptoms such as visual disturbances, tremor, lethargy, and disorientation. The virus is transmitted by the bite of an infected mosquito. Eastern equine encephalitis (EEE) is a severe form of the infection. Western equine encephalitis (WEE) occurs throughout the United States and produces a mild, brief illness, as does Venezuelan equine encephalitis (VEE), which is common in Central and South America, Florida, and Texas.

equine gait [L, *equus,* horse; ONorse, *gata,* a way], a manner of walking characterized by footdrop. The condition is the result of damage to the peroneal nerve, which causes the foot to hang in a toes-downward position.

equinus /ēkwī′nəs/ [L, horse], a condition characterized by tiptoe walking on one or both feet. It is usually associated with clubfoot.

equipotential, 1. (in physics) indicating bodies that have the same electrical potential. **2.** lines of force that have the same electrical potential.

equity model /ek′witē/, an organizational model for medical providers that offers the provider equity in the company instead of cash payments. Not applicable in Canada.

equivalence /ikwiv′ələns/, a state of being equal in value.

equivalent weight [L, *a* + *equs* + *valere,* equal value; AS, *gewiht*], **1.** the weight of an element in any given unit (such as grams) that will displace a unit weight of hydrogen from a compound or combine with or replace a unit weight of hydrogen. **2.** the weight of an acid or base that will produce or react with 1.008 grams of hydrogen ion. **3.** the weight of an oxidizing or reducing agent that will produce or accept one electron in a chemical reaction.

equivocal symptom [L, *aequs,* equal, *vocare,* to call; Gk, *symptoma,* that which happens], a symptom that may be attributed to more than one cause or that may occur in several diseases.

Er, symbol for the element **erbium.**

ER, E.R., abbreviation for **emergency room.**

eradication /irad′ikā′shən/, the process of completely removing or destroying something.

erbium (Er) /ur′bē·əm/ [Ytterby, Sweden], a metallic rare earth element. Its atomic number is 68; its atomic weight (mass) is 167.26.

Erb's muscular dystrophy [Wilhelm H. Erb, German neurologist, 1840–1921], a form of muscular dystrophy that first affects the shoulder girdle and later often involves the pelvic girdle. It is a progressively crippling disease.

Erb's palsy [Wilhelm H. Erb], a kind of paralysis caused by traumatic injury to the upper brachial plexus. It occurs most commonly as a result of forcible traction during childbirth, with injury to one or more cervical nerve roots.

Erb's point Wilhelm H. Erb], a landmark of the brachial plexus on the upper trunk, located about 1 inch (2.5 cm) above the

E

clavicle at about the level of the sixth cervical vertebra.

erectile /irek'til, -tīl/ [L, *erigere,* to erect], capable of being erected or raised to an erect position. The term is usually used to describe spongy tissue of the penis or clitoris that becomes turgid and erectile when filled with blood.

erectile myxoma, an angioma that contains areas of myxomatous tissue.

erection /irek'shən/ [L, *erigere,* to erect], the condition of hardness, swelling, and elevation observed in the penis and to a lesser degree in the clitoris, usually caused by sexual arousal but also occurring during sleep or after physical stimulation. It is needed to enable the penis to enter the vagina and to emit semen.

erector spinae reflex [L, *erigere,* to erect, *spina,* spine, *reflectere,* to bend back], a reflex characterized by contraction of the sacrospinalis and other back muscles when the overlying skin is stimulated.

erg /urg, erg/, a unit of energy in the centimeter-gram-second system equal to the work done by a force of 1 dyne through a distance of 1 cm.

ergastoplasm /ərgas'təplaz'əm/ [Gk, *ergaster,* worker, *plassein,* to mold], a network of cytoplasmic structures that show basophilic staining properties; granular endoplasmic reticulum.

ergogenic, a tendency to increase work output.

ergogenic aid /ur'gōjen'ik/, a substance such as a steroid used by athletes with the expectation that it will provide a competitive edge.

ergoloid mesylate /ur'gōloid/, an adrenergic with psychotropic actions. It is prescribed in the treatment of symptomatic decline in mental capacity with an unknown cause, as in senile dementia.

ergometry /ərgom'ətrē/, the study of physical work activity, including that performed by specific muscles or muscle groups. The studies may involve testing with equipment such as stationary bicycles, treadmills, or rowing machines.

ergonomics /ur'gōnom'iks/ [Gk, *ergon,* work, *nomos,* law], a scientific discipline devoted to the study and analysis of human work, especially as it is affected by individual anatomic, psychologic, and other human characteristics. **—ergonomic,** *adj.*

ergonovine maleate /ur'gōnō'vēn/, an oxytocic ergot alkaloid. It is prescribed to contract the uterus in the treatment or prevention of postpartum or postabortion hemorrhage caused by uterine atony.

ergosterol /ərgos'tərôl/, an unsaturated hydrocarbon of the vitamin D group isolated from yeast, mushrooms, ergot, and other fungi. When treated with ultraviolet irradiation, it is converted into vitamin D_2.

ergot /ur'gət/ [L, *ergota,* a grain fungus], (in pharmacology) the food storage body of a fungus, *Claviceps purpurea,* that commonly infects rye and other cereal grasses. It contains ergot alkaloids.

ergot alkaloid, one of a large group of alkaloids derived from a common fungus, *Claviceps purpurea.* The alkaloids comprise three groups: the amino acid alkaloids typified by ergotamine, the dihydrogenated amino acid alkaloids such as dihydroergotamine, and the amine alkaloids such as ergonovine.

ergotamine tartrate /ərgot'əmēn/, a vasoconstrictor and oxytocic prescribed in the treatment of migraine and postpartum uterine atony.

ergotherapy /ur'gōther'əpē/ [Gk, *ergon,* work, *therapeia,* treatment], the use of physical activity and exercise in the treatment of disease. By extension the therapy includes any procedure that increases the blood supply to a diseased or injured part, such as massage or various types of hot baths. **—ergotherapeutic,** *adj.*

ergotism /ur'gətiz'əm/ [L, *argota,* a grain fungus], **1.** an acute or chronic disease caused by excessive dosages of medications containing ergot. Symptoms may include cerebrospinal manifestations such as spasms, cramps, and dry gangrene. **2.** a chronic disease caused by ingestion of cereal products made with rye flour contaminated by ergot fungus.

ergot poisoning [L, *argota,* a grain fungus; L, *potio,* drink], the toxic effects of ingesting food or medications containing ergot alkaloids, particularly ergotamine.

ergotropic /ur'gōtrop'ik/, **1.** pertaining to an activity or work state involving somatic muscle, sympathetic nervous system, and cortical alpha rhythm activity. **2.** pertaining to the administration of medications or other therapies to energize the power of the body's blood and other tissues to resist infections.

Erickson, Helen C. See **Modeling and Role Modeling.**

ERISA, abbreviation for **Employment Retirement Income Security Act.**

erogenous /iroj'ənəs/ [Gk, *eros,* love, *genein,* to produce], pertaining to the production of erotic sensations or sexual excitement.

erogenous zones, areas of the body in which sexual tension tends to become concentrated and can be relieved by manipulation of the region. The areas include the mouth, anus, and genitals.

Eros /ir'os, er'os/ [Gk, mythic love-inciting

son of Aphrodite], a Freudian term for the drive or instinct for survival, including self-preservation and continuation of the species through reproduction.

erosion /irō′zhən/ [L, *erodere,* to consume], the wearing away or gradual destruction of a surface. For example, a mucosal or epidermal surface may erode as a result of inflammation, injury, or other causes.

erosive gastritis /irō′siv/, an inflammatory condition characterized by multiple erosions of the mucous membrane lining the stomach. Nausea, anorexia, pain, and gastric hemorrhage may occur.

eroticism /irot′isiz′əm/ [Gk, *erotikos,* sexual love], **1.** sexual impulse or desire. **2.** the arousal or attempt to arouse the sexual instinct through suggestive or symbolic means. **3.** the expression of sexual instinct or desire. **4.** an abnormally persistent sexual drive.

erratic /irat′ik/ [L, *erraticus,* wandering], deviating from the normal but with no apparent fixed course or purpose.

error [L, *errare,* to wander], (in research) a defect in the design of a study, in the development of measurements or instruments, or in the interpretation of findings.

ERT, abbreviation for **external radiation therapy.**

erucic acid /eroō′sik/, a fatty acid that has been associated with heart disease. It is present in rapeseed oil.

eructation /ē′ruktā′shən/ [L, *eructare,* to belch], the act of drawing up air from the stomach with a characteristic sound through the mouth.

eruption /irup′shən/ [L, *eruptio,* bursting forth], the appearance of the rapidly forming skin lesion, especially of a viral exanthem, or of a rash that commonly accompanies a drug reaction.

eruptive fever /irup′tiv/ [L, *eruptio,* bursting forth, *febria*], any disease characterized by fever and a rash.

eruptive gingivitis, an inflammation of the gums that may occur concurrently with the breaking through of the permanent teeth.

eruptive xanthoma, a skin disorder associated with elevated triglyceride levels in the blood. Numerous erythematous or pale raised papules suddenly appear on the trunk, legs, arms, and buttocks.

ERV, abbreviation for **expiratory reserve volume.**

erysipelas /er′isip′ələs/ [Gk, *erythros,* red, *pella,* skin], an infectious skin disease characterized by redness, swelling, vesicles, bullae, fever, pain, and lymphadenopathy. It is caused by a species of group A beta-hemolytic streptococci.

erysipeloid /er′isip′əloid/ [Gk, *erhthros* +

pella + *eidos,* form], an infection of the hands characterized by blue-red patches and occasionally by erythema. It is acquired by handling meat or fish infected with *Erysipelothrix rhusiopathiae.*

erythema /er′ithē′mə/ [Gk, *erythros,* red], redness or inflammation of the skin or mucous membranes that is the result of dilation and congestion of superficial capillaries. Examples of erythema are nervous blushes and mild sunburn. —**erythematous,** *adj.*

erythema infectiosum, an acute benign infectious disease, mainly of children. It is characterized by fever and an erythematous rash that begins on the cheeks and later appears on the arms, thighs, buttocks, and trunk.

erythema marginatum, a skin disorder seen in acute rheumatic fever characterized by temporary disk-shaped nonpruritic reddened macules that fade in the center, leaving raised margins.

erythema migrans (EM), a skin lesion that begins as a small papule and spreads peripherally; it is characterized by a raised, red margin and clearing in the center. It may mark the site of a tick bite and is a diagnostic sign of **Lyme disease.**

erythema multiforme (EM) /mul′tifôr′mē, moōl′tēfôr′mā/, any of three major clinical syndromes characterized by lymphocytic infiltrates in the skin that cause keratinocyte necrosis. The patient may experience polymorphous eruption of skin and mucous membranes. Macules, papules, nodules, vesicles or bullae, and target (bull's-eye-shaped) lesions are seen.

erythema neonatorum, a common skin condition of neonates characterized by a pink papular rash frequently superimposed with vesicles or pustules. The rash appears within 24 to 48 hours after birth and disappears spontaneously after several days.

erythema nodosum, a hypersensitivity reaction characterized by bilateral reddened, tender subcutaneous nodules on the shins and occasionally other parts of the body. The nodules last for several days or weeks; never ulcerate; and are often associated with mild fever, malaise, and pain in muscles and joints.

erythema perstans, a persistent local redness of the skin, characteristically annular.

erythematous pemphigus [Gk, *erythros,* red, *pemphix,* bubble], skin disorder characterized by bullous eruptions on the trunk and a facial eruption that resembles that of lupus erythematosus. The condition may be accompanied by seborrheic dermatitis.

erythralgia /er′ithral′jə/ [Gk, *erythros,* red,

algos, pain], a skin disorder characterized by a painful burning sensation, raised skin temperature, and redness, generally of the lower limbs.

erythrasma /er'ithraz'mə/ [Gk, *erythros,* red], a bacterial skin infection common in the axillary or inguinal region, characterized by irregular reddish-brown areas.

erythremia /er'ithrē'mē-ə/ [Gk, *erythros* + *haima,* blood], an abnormal increase in the number of red blood cells.

erythrityl tetranitrate /erith'ritil/, a coronary vasodilator prescribed in the treatment of angina pectoris.

erythroblast /erith'rəblast'/, an immature form of a red blood cell. It is normally found only in bone marrow and contains hemoglobin.

erythroblastoma /-blastō'mə/ [Gk, *erythros,* red, *blastos,* germ, *oma,* tumor], a myeloma tumor (osteolytic neoplasm) in which the cells resemble erythroblasts.

erythroblastosis fetalis /-blastō'sis/ [Gk, *erythros* + *blastos,* germ, *osis,* condition; L, *fetus,* bringing forth], a type of hemolytic anemia in newborns that results from maternal-fetal blood group incompatibility, specifically involving the Rh factor and the ABO blood groups. The condition is caused by an antigen-antibody reaction in the bloodstream of the infant resulting from placental transmission of maternally formed antibodies against the incompatible antigens of the fetal blood. In Rh factor incompatibility the hemolytic reaction occurs only when the mother is Rh negative and the infant is Rh positive. The isoimmunization process rarely occurs in the first pregnancy, but there is increased risk with each succeeding pregnancy.

erythrochromia /-krō'mē-ə/, **1.** a red coloration or stain. **2.** red pigmentation in spinal fluid caused by the presence of blood.

erythrocyanosis /sī'ənō'sis/, a condition characterized by bluish-red discoloration of skin, accompanied by swelling, burning, and itching.

erythrocyte /erith'rəsīt'/ [Gk, *erythros* + *kytos,* cell], mature red blood cell; a biconcave disk about 7 μm in diameter that contains hemoglobin confined within a lipoid membrane. It is the major cellular element of the circulating blood and transports oxygen as its principal function. Erythrocytes originate in the marrow of the long bones. Maturation proceeds from a stem cell (promegaloblast) through the pronormoblast stage to the normoblast, the last stage before the mature adult cell develops.

erythrocyte reinfusion, the process of injecting into an individual's bloodstream red blood cells previously taken from that individual and preserved temporarily by freezing.

erythrocyte sedimentation rate (ESR), the rate at which red blood cells settle out in a tube of unclotted blood, expressed in millimeters per hour. Blood is collected in an anticoagulant and allowed to form a sediment in a calibrated glass column.

erythrocythemia /erith'rōsīthē'mē-ə/ [Gk, *erythros* + *kytos* + *haima,* blood]], an increase in the number of erythrocytes circulating in the blood.

erythrocytopenia /-sī'təpē'nē-ə/ [Gk, *erythros,* red, *kytos,* cell, *penes,* poor], a condition characterized by a deficiency or decrease in number of erythrocytes.

erythrocytosis /erith'rōsītō'sis/ [Gk, *erythros* + *kytos* + *osis,* condition], an abnormal increase in the number of circulating red cells.

erythroderma /erith'rōdur'mə/ [Gk, *erythros* + *derma,* skin], an abnormal redness of the skin.

erythrogenesis, the creation of red blood cells.

erythroid /erith'roid/, **1.** reddish in color. **2.** pertaining to erythrocytes.

erythroleukemia /-lōōkē'mē-ə/ [Gk, *erythros* + *leukos,* white, *haima,* blood], a malignant blood disorder characterized by a proliferation of erythropoietic elements in bone marrow, erythroblasts with bizarre lobulated nuclei, and abnormal myeloblasts in peripheral blood. The disease may have an acute or chronic course.

erythroleukosis, an abnormal increase in numbers of granulocytes and red blood cells.

erythromelalgia /erith'rōmilal'jə/ [Gk, *erythros* + *melos,* limb, *algos,* pain], a rare disorder characterized by a paroxysmal dilation of the peripheral blood vessels. —**erythromelalgic,** *adj.*

erythromycin /erith'rōmī'sin/, an antibacterial antibiotic prescribed in the treatment of many bacterial and mycoplasmal infections, particularly those that cannot be treated with penicillins.

erythron /erith'ron/, the total mass of circulating red blood cells and the red blood cell–forming tissues from which they are derived.

erythropathy /er'ithrop'əthē/, any disease involving the red blood cells (erythrocytes).

erythrophage /erith'rəfāj/, a phagocyte that ingests red blood cells or blood pigment.

erythrophobia /-fō'bē-ə/ [Gk, *erythros* + *phobos,* fear], **1.** an anxiety disorder characterized by an irrational fear of blushing or of displaying embarrassment.

2. a symptom manifested by blushing at the slightest provocation. 3. a morbid fear of or aversion to the color red. —**erythrophobic,** *adj.*

erythroplasia of Queyrat /erith'rōplā'zhə/ [Gk, *erythros* + *plasis,* forming; Louis A. Queyrat, French dermatologist, 1856–1933], a premalignant lesion on the glans or corona of the penis. It is a well-circumscribed reddish patch on the skin.

erythropoiesis /erith'rōpō-ē'sis/ [Gk, *erythros* + *poiein,* to make], the process of erythrocyte production involving the maturation of a nucleated precursor into a hemoglobin-filled nucleus-free erythrocyte that is regulated by erythropoietin, a hormone produced by the kidney. —**erythropoietic,** *adj.*

erythropoietin (EPO) /erith'rōpō-ē'tin/ [Gk, *erythros* + *poiein,* to make], a glycoprotein hormone synthesized mainly in the kidneys and released into the bloodstream in response to anoxia.

Es, symbol for the element **einsteinium.**

ESADDI, abbreviation for **Estimated Safe and Adequate Daily Dietary Intake.**

escape beat [ME, *escapen,* to flee, *beten,* to beat], an automatic beat of the heart that occurs after an interval equal to or longer than the duration of its normal cycle. Escape beats function as safety mechanisms, and anything that produces a long pause in the prevailing heart cycle may allow an escape to occur. Some kinds of pauses in which escape beats occur are caused by sinoatrial (SA) block, atrioventricular (AV) block, and sinus bradycardia.

escape rhythm [OFr, *escaper* + Gk, *rhythmos,* beat], a sustained heartbeat that occurs when the atrioventricular junction or His-Purkinje fiber assumes control because the rate of the sinoatrial node is depressed or blocked, or when the AV node is blocked.

eschar /es'kär/ [Gk, *eschara,* scab], a scab or dry crust that results from trauma, such as a thermal or chemical burn, infection, or excoriating skin disease. —**escharotic,** *adj.*

escharotomy /es'kärot'əmē/, a surgical incision into necrotic tissue resulting from a severe burn. The procedure is sometimes necessary to prevent edema from generating sufficient interstitial pressure to impair capillary filling, causing ischemia.

Escherichia coli (E. coli) /eshirī'kē-ə kō'lī/ [Theodor Escherich, German physician, 1857–1911; Gk, *kolon,* colon], a species of coliform bacteria of the family Enterobacteriaceae, normally present in the intestines and common in water, milk, and soil. *E. coli* is the most frequent cause of urinary tract infection and is a serious gram-negative pathogen in wounds.

escutcheon /eskuch'ən/ [L, *scutum,* shield], the shieldlike pattern of distribution of pubic hair.

Esmarch's bandage /es'märks/ [Johann F. A. von Esmarch, German surgeon, 1823–1908], a broad, flat elastic bandage wrapped around an elevated limb to force blood out of the limb. It is used before certain surgical procedures to create a blood-free field.

ESO, abbreviation for *electrical spinal orthosis.*

esophageal atresia /əsof'əjē'əl, es'ofā'-jē-əl/ [Gk, *oisophagos,* gullet], an abnormal esophagus that ends in a blind pouch or narrows to a thin cord and thus does not provide a continuous passage to the stomach.

esophageal cancer, a rare malignant neoplastic disease of the esophagus. Risk factors associated with the disease are heavy consumption of alcohol, tobacco smoking, betel-nut chewing, Plummer-Vinson syndrome, Barrett's esophagus, and achalasia.

esophageal dysfunction, any disturbance, impairment, or abnormality that interferes with the normal functioning of the esophagus, such as dysphagia, esophagitis, or sphincter incompetence. The condition is one of the primary symptoms of scleroderma.

esophageal lead /lēd/, **1.** an electrocardiographic conductor in which the exploring electrode is placed within the lumen of the esophagus. It is used in identifying cardiac arrhythmias. **2.** *informal.* a tracing produced by such a lead on an electrocardiograph.

esophageal obturator airway, an emergency device that consists of a large tube that is inserted into the mouth through an airtight face mask. The esophagus is blocked by inflating a balloon at the end of the tube. Because of the design, air passes only into the trachea.

esophageal speech [Gk, *oisophagos,* gullet; AS, *spaec*], alaryngeal sounds made by forcing air into and out of the esophagus, causing it to vibrate. It may be produced by a number of methods.

esophageal varices, a complex of longitudinal tortuous veins at the lower end of the esophagus, enlarged and swollen as the result of portal hypertension.

esophageal web, a thin membrane that may develop across the lumen of the esophagus, usually near the level of the cricoid cartilage. The abnormal condition is generally associated with iron deficiency anemia.

esophagectomy /esof'əjek'təmē/ [Gk,

E

oisophagos + *ektome*, excision], a surgical procedure in which all or part of the esophagus is removed, as may be required to treat severe recurrent bleeding esophageal varices or esophageal cancer.

esophagitis /esof'əjī′tis/ [Gk, *oisophagos* + *itis*], inflammation of the mucosal lining of the esophagus caused by infection, irritation from a nasogastric tube, or, most commonly, backflow of gastric juice from the stomach.

esophagocele /esof'əgōsēl′/, a hernia of the mucous membrane through a weakened area in the wall of the esophagus.

esophagogastronomy /esof'əgō'gastron'- əmē/ [Gk, *oisophagos*, gullet, *gaster*, stomach, *stoma*, mouth], the surgical creation of a passage between the esophagus and the stomach.

esophagogastroscopy /-gastros'kəpē/ [Gk, *oisophagos*, gullet, *gaster*, stomach, *skopein*, to watch] the examination of the esophagus and stomach using an endoscope.

esophagogastrostomy /-gastros'təmē/, an artifical anastomosis of the esophagus to the stomach.

esophagojejunostomy /-jij'ōōnos'təmē/ [Gk, *oisophagos*, gullet; L, *jejunum*, empty, *stoma*, mouth], the surgical creation of a direct passage from the esophagus to the jejunum, bypassing the stomach. The procedure is used after total gastrectomy.

esophagomyotomy /-mī'ot'əmē/, a longitudinal incision in the lower part of the esophageal muscle made to treat esophageal achalasia, an obstruction to the passage of food.

esophagoscopy /esof'əgos'kəpē/ [Gk, *oisophagos* + *skopein*, to look], examination of the esophagus with an endoscope.

esophagospasm /esof'əgōspaz'əm/ [Gk, *oisophagos*, gullet, *spasmos*], spasmodic contractions of the walls of the esophagus.

esophagostomy /esof'əgos'təmē/, a surgical opening into the esophagus for enteral tube feeding.

esophagus /esof'əgəs/ [Gk, *oisophagos*], the muscular canal, about 24 cm long, extending from the pharynx to the stomach. It begins in the neck at the inferior border of the cricoid cartilage and descends to the cardiac sphincter of the stomach. The esophagus is composed of a fibrous coat, a muscular coat, and a submucous coat and is lined with mucous membrane. —**esophageal,** *adj.*

esophoria /es'əfôr'ē·ə/ [Gk, *eso*, inward, *pherein*, to bear], the latent deviation of the visual axis of one eye inward and toward that of the other eye in the absence of visual stimuli for fusion. —**esophoric,** *adj.*

esotropia /es'ətrō'pē·ə/ [Gk, *eso* + *tropos*, turning], an inward turning of one eye relative to the other fixating eye. —**esotropic,** *adj.*

ESP, abbreviation for **extrasensory perception.**

espundia /espun'dē·ə/ [Sp, cancerous ulcer], a cutaneous form of American leishmaniasis most common in Brazil, caused by *Leishmania brasiliensis*. The primary lesion often disappears spontaneously, followed by mucocutaneous lesions that destroy the mucosal surface of the nose, pharynx, and larynx.

ESR, abbreviation for **erythrocyte sedimentation rate.**

essential, a necessary part of a thing without which it could not exist.

essential amino acid /esen'shəl/ [L, *essentia*, quality], an organic compound not synthesized in the body that is essential for nitrogen equilibrium in adults and optimal growth in infants and children. Adults require isoleucine, leucine, lysine, methionine, phenylalanine, threonine, tryptophan, and valine. Infants need these amino acids plus arginine and histidine. Cysteine and tyrosine, limited substitutes, respectively, for methionine and phenylalanine, are considered quasi-essential.

essential fatty acid (EFA), a polyunsaturated acid such as linoleic, alpha-linolenic, or arachidonic acid, essential in the diet for proper growth, maintenance, and functioning of the body. A deficiency of EFAs causes changes in cell structure and enzyme function, resulting in decreased growth and other disorders. Symptoms include brittle and lusterless hair, nail problems, dandruff, allergic conditions, and dermatoses, especially eczema in infants.

essential fever, any fever of unknown origin.

essential hypertension, an elevated systemic arterial pressure for which no cause can be found, which is often the only significant clinical finding. Elevated blood pressure is always considered a risk, and individuals with elevated pressures are at risk for cardiovascular disease.

essential nutrient, the carbohydrates, proteins, fats, minerals, vitamins, and water necessary for growth, normal function, and body maintenance.

essential oil, a class of generally aromatic volatile oils extracted from plants for use in flavoring foods, perfumes, and medicines. Some have been used therapeutically for thousands of years.

essential pruritus [L, *essentia*, quality

prurire, to itch], localized or general pruritus that begins without preexisting skin disorder.

essential tremor, an involuntary fine shaking of the hand, the head, and the face, especially during routine body movements. It is a familial disorder inherited as an autosomal-dominant trait and appears during adolescence or in middle age.

essential vertigo [L, *essentia,* quality, *vertigo,* dizziness], a form of vertigo for which no organic cause has been found.

established name, the name assigned to a drug by the U.S. Adopted Names Council. The established name, generally shorter than the chemical name, is the name by which the drug is known to health practitioners.

ester /es′tər/ [Ger, Essigäther acetic ether], a class of chemical compounds formed by the bonding of an alcohol and one or more organic acids. Fats are esters, produced by the bonding of fatty acids with the alcohol glycerol.

esterase /es′tərās/, any enzyme that splits esters.

esterification, the process of combining an organic acid (RCOOH) with an alcohol (ROH) to form an ester (RCOOR).

esterified estrogen /ester′ifīd/, an ester of natural estrogen prescribed for menstrual irregularities, contraception, and menopausal symptoms.

esterify, to convert into an ester.

ester local anesthetic, a class of local anesthetics with an ester group that differentiates it from the amide group of local anesthetics.

esthesia /esthē′zhə/, **1.** capacity for perception. **2.** sensitivity or feeling. **3.** any disorder of the nervous system that affects perception or sensitivity.

esthesiophysiology /esthē′zē-ōfiz′ē-ol′əjē/, the study of sense organ function.

esthetics /esthet′iks/ [Gk, *aisthetikos,* sensitivity], the branch of philosophy dealing with the forms and psychologic effects of beauty. In medicine, esthetics may be applied to dental reconstruction and plastic surgery.

Estimated Safe and Adequate Daily Dietary Intake (ESADDI), nutrient intake recommendations, made by the National Academy of Sciences' Food and Nutrition Board, that give a range of intake for some nutrients because not enough information is available to set recommended dietary allowance. In addition, an ESADDI is used when an exact amount cannot be set because needs vary.

estradiol /es′trədī′ôl/, the most potent naturally occurring human estrogen, also found in hog ovaries and in the urine of pregnant mares.

estramustine phosphate sodium /es′-trəmus′tēn/, an antineoplastic agent prescribed for metastatic or progressive carcinoma of the prostate.

estrangement /estrānj′mənt/ [L, *extraneus,* not belonging], **1.** a psychologic effect of the separation of a mother from her newborn required when the infant is ill or premature or has a congenital defect, thereby diverting the mother from establishing a normal relationship with her child. **2.** the feeling that external objects have a strange, unfamiliar, or unreal quality, caused by a failure of cathexis of the external ego boundary, one of whose functions is to identify external objects as real and familiar.

estriol /es′trē-ôl/, a relatively weak, naturally occurring human estrogen found in high concentrations in urine.

estrogen /es′trojən/ [Gk, *oistros,* gadfly, *genein,* to produce], one of a group of hormonal steroid compounds that promote the development of female secondary sex characteristics. Human estrogen level is elaborated in the ovaries, adrenal cortices, testes, and fetoplacental unit. During the menstrual cycle estrogen renders the female genital tract suitable for fertilization, implantation, and nutrition of the early embryo. Kinds of estrogen are **conjugated estrogen, esterified estrogen, estradiol, estriol,** and **estrone.** —**estrogenic,** *adj.*

estrone /es′trōn/, a relatively potent estrogen prescribed in the treatment of menstrual cycle irregularities, prostatic cancer, and menopausal vasomotor symptoms and in prevention of pregnancy.

estropipate /es′trəpip′āt/, an estrogen prescribed in the treatment of vasomotor symptoms of menopause, atrophic vaginitis, kraurosis vulvae, female hypogonadism, female castration, and primary ovarian failure.

estrus /es′trəs/, the cyclic period of sexual activity in mammals other than primates.

estrus cycle [Gk, *oistros,* gadfly, *kyklos,* circle], the periodic changes in the female body that occur under the influence of sex hormones.

ESWL, abbreviation for **extracorporeal shock-wave lithotripsy.**

eta /ē′tə, ā′tə/, H, η, the seventh letter of the Greek alphabet.

état criblé /ātä′krēblā′/ [Fr, sievelike state], a condition or state of multiple sievelike perforations in swollen lymphatic nodules in the intestine. It is a frequently fatal complication of untreated typhoid fever.

ethacrynic acid /eth′əkrin′ik/, a loop diuretic prescribed to relieve the effects of severe edema and hypertension.

ethambutol hydrochloride /eth'əmbyōō'-təl/, a tuberculostatic antibiotic prescribed in the treatment of pulmonary tuberculosis.

ethanol /eth'ənol/, ethyl alcohol.

ethaverine hydrochloride /eth'əver'ēn/, a smooth muscle relaxant prescribed to relieve spasm of the gastrointestinal or genitourinary tract, arterial vasospasm, and cerebral insufficiency.

ethchlorvynol /ethklôr'vənôl/, a sedative and hypnotic prescribed in the treatment of insomnia.

ether /ē'thər/ [Gk, aither, air], **1.** any of a class of organic compounds in which two hydrocarbon groups are linked by an oxygen atom. **2.** a nonhalogenated volatile liquid no longer used in clinical practice as a general anesthetic.

ethics /eth'iks/ [Gk, ethikos, moral duty], the science or study of moral values or principles, including ideals of autonomy, beneficence, and justice.

Ethics in Patient Referrals Act, a federal law, the Stark Law, enacted in 1989, that prohibits referrals by a physician to a clinical laboratory in which the physician has a financial interest. A 1994 amendment includes other services and equipment such as physical and occupational therapy; radiology and other diagnostic services; radiation therapy; parenteral and enteral nutrients, equipment, and supplies; and home health services.

ethinamate /ethin'əmāt/, a sedative prescribed in the treatment of insomnia.

ethinyl estradiol /eth'inil/, an estrogen prescribed in the treatment of postmenopausal breast cancer, menstrual cycle irregularities, prostatic cancer, and hypogonadism and for contraception and relief of menopausal vasomotor symptoms.

ethionamide /eth'ē·ɘnam'īd/, a tuberculostatic antibacterial prescribed for tuberculosis.

ethmocarditis /eth'mōkärdī'tis/, a chronic inflammation of the cardiac connective tissue.

ethmoid /eth'moid/ [Gk, ethmos, sieve, eidos, form], **1.** pertaining to the ethmoid bone. **2.** having a large number of sievelike openings.

ethmoidal air cell /ethmoi'dəl/ [Gk, ethmos, sieve, eidos, form], one of the numerous small, thin-walled cavities in the ethmoid bone of the skull. The cavities are lined with mucous membrane.

ethmoid bone, the very light and spongy bone at the base of the cranium, also forming the roof and most of the walls of the superior part of the nasal cavity.

ethmoidofrontal suture /eth'moi'dōfron'-təl/, a line in the skull between the cribriform plate of the ethmoid and the orbital plate and posterior margin of the nasal process.

ethmoidolacrimal suture /-lak'rimɘl/, a line in the skull between the orbital plate of the ethmoid and the posterior margin of the lacrimal bone.

ethmosphenoid suture /eth'mōsfē'noid/, a line in the skull between the crest of the sphenoid bone and the perpendicular and cribriform plates of the ethmoid.

ethnic group /eth'nik/, a population of individuals organized on the basis of an assumed common cultural origin.

ethnocentrism /eth'nōsen'trizm/ [Gk, ethnos, nation, kentron, center], **1.** a belief in the inherent superiority of the "race" or group to which one belongs. **2.** a proclivity to consider other ethnic groups in terms of one's own racial origins.

ethoheptazine citrate /eth'ōhep'təzēn/, a nonnarcotic analgesic prescribed to relieve mild to moderate pain.

ethology /ethol'əjē/ [Gk, ethos, character, logos, science], **1.** (in zoology) the scientific study of the behavioral patterns of animals, specifically in their native habitat. **2.** (in psychology) the empiric study of human behavior, primarily social customs, manners, and mores. —**ethologic, ethological,** adj., **ethologist,** n.

ethopropazine hydrochloride /eth'ōprō'-pəzēn/, a phenothiazine anticholinergic agent prescribed in the treatment of extrapyramidal parkinsonism and other nervous system disorders.

ethosuximide /eth'ōsuk'simīd/, an anticonvulsant prescribed in the treatment of petit mal epilepsy.

ethotoin /eth'ōtō'in/, an anticonvulsant prescribed in the treatment of generalized tonic-clonic and complex-partial seizures.

ethyl chloride /eth'il/, a topical anesthetic used in short operations. It is prescribed in the treatment of skin irritations and in minor skin surgery.

ethylene /eth'əlēn/ [Gk, aither, air, hyle, stuff], a colorless flammable gas that is lighter than air and has a slightly sweet odor and taste.

ethylenediamine /eth'əlēndi·am'ēn/, a clear thick liquid having the odor of ammonia. It is used as a solvent, an emulsifier, and a stabilizer with aminophylline injections.

ethylene dibromide (EDB), a volatile liquid used as an insecticide and gasoline additive. Because it has been found to be a cause of cancer in animals, the Environmental Protection Agency has restricted the use of EDB to control insect pests in grains and fruits intended for human use.

ethylene dichloride poisoning, the toxic effects of exposure to ethylene dichloride, a hydrocarbon solvent, diluent, and fumigant, which is one of the most abundant of all chlorinated organic chemicals. It is an eye, ear, nose, throat, and skin irritant. Inhalation or ingestion can lead to serious illness or death.

ethylene glycol poisoning, the toxic reaction to ingestion of ethylene glycol or diethylene glycol, chemicals used in automobile antifreeze preparations. Symptoms in mild cases may resemble those of alcohol intoxication but without the breath odor produced by alcoholic beverages. Vomiting, carpopedal spasm, lumbar pain, renal failure, respiratory distress, convulsions, and coma may also occur.

ethylene oxide, a highly flammable gas used to sterilize surgical instruments and other supplies.

ethylestrenol, an anabolic steroid.

ethylnorepinephrine hydrochloride /eth′-ilnôrep′inef′rin/, a bronchodilator prescribed in the treatment of bronchial asthma.

ethyl oxide, an alternative name for diethyl ether.

ethynodiol diacetate /eth′inōdī′ôl/, a synthetic progestin derivative.

ethynodiol diacetate and ethinyl estradiol, an oral contraceptive prescribed for prevention of pregnancy.

ethynodiol diacetate and mestranol, an oral contraceptive prescribed for contraception.

etidronate disodium /etid′rənāt/, a regulator of calcium metabolism prescribed in the treatment of Paget's disease and heterotopic ossification caused by injury to the spinal cord, and after total hip replacement.

etiology /ē′tē·ol′əjē/ [Gk, *aitia,* cause, *logos,* science], **1.** the study of all factors that may be involved in the development of a disease, including the susceptibility of the patient, the nature of the disease agent, and the way in which the patient's body is invaded by the agent. **2.** the cause of a disease. —**etiologic,** *adj.*

etomidate /etom′idāt/, a short-acting and hypnotic nonbarbiturate intravenous induction agent for general anesthesia.

etopside, an antineoplastic or chemotherapeutic agent and mitotic inhibitor. It is prescribed in the treatment of cancer of the testicles and small cell lung cancer to prevent tumor cells from dividing and spreading.

etretinate /etret′ināt/, a synthetic derivative of vitamin A used as an oral drug to treat psoriasis. It is prescribed for severe recalcitrant psoriasis, including generalized pustular and erythrodermic psoriasis.

etymology [Gk, *etymos,* base; L, *logos,* words], the study of the origin and development of words.

Eu, symbol for the element **europium.**

Eubacterium /yōō′baktir′ē·əm, a genus of gram-positive anaerobic rod-shaped bacteria normally found in soil and water. The organisms are also found in the skin and cavities of humans and other mammals, where they may cause soft-tissue infections.

eubiotics /yōō′bī·ot′iks/ [Gk, *eu,* well, *bios,* life], the science of healthy living.

eucalyptol /yōō′kəlip′tol/, a substance with an aromatic odor obtained from the volatile oil of *Eucalyptus* and used in nasal emollients.

eucatropine hydrochloride /yōōkat′-rəpin/, an ophthalmic anticholinergic prescribed for dilating the pupil in an ophthalmoscopic examination of the eye.

eucholia /yōōkō′lyə/ [Gk, *eu,* well, *chole,* bile], the normal state of the bile as to the quantity secreted and the condition of the constituents.

euchromatin /yōōkrō′mətin/ [Gk, *eu* + *chroma,* color], that part of chromosome material that is active in gene expression during cell division. It stains most deeply during mitosis. —**euchromatic,** *adj.*

eugamy /yōō′gəmē/ [Gk, *eu* + *gamos,* marriage], the union of those gametes that contain the same haploid number of chromosomes. —**eugamic,** *adj.*

eugenics /yōōjen′iks/ [Gk, *eu* + *genein,* to produce], the study of methods for controlling the characteristics of future populations through selective breeding.

euglobulin /yōōglob′yəlin/ [Gk, *eu* + L, *globulus,* small sphere], that fraction of serum globulin that is insoluble in distilled water but soluble in saline solutions. This is one of a number of different properties used to classify proteins.

eugnathic anomaly /yōōnath′ik/ [Gk, *eu* + *gnathos,* jaw, *anomalia,* irregularity], (in dentistry) an abnormality of the teeth and their alveolar supports

eukaryocyte /yōōker′ē·ōsīt′/ [Gk, *eu* + *karyon,* nut, *kytos,* cell], a cell with a true nucleus, found in all higher organisms and in some microorganisms such as amebae, plasmodia, and trypanosomes. —**eukaryotic,** *adj.*

eukaryon /yōōker′ē·on/ [Gk, *eu,* good, *karyon,* nut], **1.** a nucleus that is highly complex, organized, and surrounded by a nuclear membrane, usually characteristic of higher organisms. **2.** an organism containing such a nucleus.

eukaryosis /yoōker'ĭ·ō'sis/ [Gk, *eu* + *karyon*, nut, *osis*, condition], the state of having a highly complex organized nucleus containing organelles surrounded by a nuclear membrane.

eukaryote /yoōker'ē·ot/ [Gk, *eu* + *karyon*, nut], an organism having cells that contain a true nucleus. —**eukaryotic, eucaryotic,** *adj.*

eunuch /yoō'nək/ [Gk, *eune*, couch, *echein*, to guard], a male whose testicles have been destroyed or removed. If this occurs before puberty, secondary sex characteristics fail to develop.

eunuchism /yoō'nəkiz'əm/, the condition of being a eunuch.

eunuchoidism /yoō'nəkoidiz'əm/, deficiency of male hormone function of or formation by the testes. The deficiency leads to sterility and to abnormal tallness, small testes, and immature development of secondary sexual characteristics, libido, and sexual potency.

euphoretic /yoō'fəret'ik/ [Gk, *eu* + *pherein*, to bear], 1. (of a substance or event) tending to produce a condition of well-being or elation. 2. a substance tending to produce a feeling of well-being or elation, as marijuana and other hallucinogenic drugs.

euphoria /yoōfôr'ē·ə/ [Gk, *eu* + *pherein*, to bear], 1. a feeling or state of well-being or elation. 2. an exaggerated or abnormal sense of physical and emotional well-being not based on reality or truth, disproportionate to its cause, and inappropriate to the situation.

euploid /yoō'ploid/ [Gk, *eu* + *ploos*, multiple], 1. pertaining to an individual, organism, strain, or cell that has a chromosome number that is an exact multiple of the normal haploid number characteristic of the species, such as diploid, triploid, tetraploid, or polyploid. 2. such an individual, organism, strain, or cell.

euploidy /yoō'ploidē/, the state or condition of having a variation in chromosome number that is an exact multiple of the characteristic haploid number.

eupnea /yoōp·nē'ə/ [Gk, *eu*, well, *pnein*, to breathe], normal breathing.

europium (Eu) /yoōrō'pē·əm/ [Europe], a metallic rare earth element. Its atomic number is 63; its atomic weight (mass) is 151.96.

eustachian salpingitis /yoōstā'shən/, an inflammation of the eustachian tube.

eustachian tube [Bartolomeo Eustachio, Italian anatomist, 1524–1574; L, *tubus*], a tube lined with mucous membrane that joins the nasopharynx and the middle ear cavity. It is normally closed but opens during yawning, chewing, and swallowing to allow equalization of the air pressure in the middle ear with atmospheric pressure.

eustress /yoō'stres/, 1. a positive form of stress. 2. a balance between selfishness and altruism through which an individual develops the drive and energy to care for others.

euthanasia /yoō'thənā'zhə/ [Gk, *eu* + *thanatos*, death], the deliberate causing of the death of a person who is suffering from an incurable disease or condition. It may be active such as by administration of a lethal drug or passive by withholding of treatment.

euthenics /yoōthen'iks/ [Gk, *eu* + *tithenai*, to place], the science that deals with improvement of the human species through the control of environmental factors such as pollution, malnutrition, disease, and drug abuse.

euthymia, a pleasant, relaxed state of tranquility.

euthymic, pertaining to a normal mood in which the range of emotions is neither depressed nor highly elevated.

euthymism /yoōthī'mizəm/ [Gk, *eu* + *thymos*, thyme flowers], the characteristic of normal mood responses.

euthyroid /yoōthī'roid/ [Gk, *eu*, well, *thyreos*, oblong shield], pertaining to a normal thyroid gland.

evacuant /ivak'yoō·ənt/ [L, *evacuare*, to empty], any medicine or other agent that causes an organ to discharge its contents, as an emetic or laxative.

evacuate /ivak'yoō·āt/ [L, *evacuare*, to empty], 1. to discharge or to remove a substance from a cavity, space, organ, or tract of the body. 2. a substance discharged or removed from the body. —**evacuation,** *n.*

evacuator /ivak'yoō·ā'tər/, an instrument for emptying a cavity, such as removing a calculus from the urinary bladder.

evagination /ēvaj'inā'shən/, the turning inside-out or protrusion of a body part or organ.

evaluating /ival'yoō·ā'shən/ [L, *ex*, away, *valare*, to be strong], (in five-step nursing process) a category of nursing behavior in which the extent to which the established goals of care have been met is determined and recorded. To make this judgment, the nurse estimates the degree of success in meeting the goals, evaluates the implementation of nursing measures, investigates the client's compliance with therapy, and records the client's response to therapy. The nurse evaluates effects of the measures used, the need for change in goals of care, the accuracy of the implementation of nursing measures, and the need for change in the client's environment or in the equipment or procedures used.

Evans blue [Herbert Evans, American anatomist, 1882–1971], a nontoxic blue-green dye. It has been used to determine blood and plasma volumes.

evaporated milk /ivap′ərā′tid/, homogenized whole milk from which 50% to 60% of the water content has been evaporated. It is fortified with vitamin D, canned, and sterilized.

evaporation /ivap′ərā′shən/ [L, *ex + vapor,* steam], the change of a substance from a liquid state to a gaseous state. The process of evaporation is hastened by an increase in temperature and a decrease in atmospheric pressure. —**evaporate,** *v.*

eventration /ē′vəntrā′shən/, the protrusion of the intestines from the abdomen.

event-related potential (ERP) [L, *evenire,* to happen, *relatus,* carry back, *potentia,* power], a type of brain wave that is associated with a response to a specific stimulus, such as a particular wave pattern observed when a patient hears a clicking sound.

evergreen contract, a health care contract that is automatically renewed every year unless it is renegotiated. Not applicable in Canada.

eversion /ivur′zhən/, a turning outward or inside-out, such as a turning of the foot outward at the ankle.

evisceration /ivis′ərā′shən/ [L, *ex + viscera,* entrails], **1.** the removal of the viscera from the abdominal cavity; disembowelment. **2.** the removal of the contents from an organ or an organ from its cavity. **3.** the protrusion of an internal organ through a wound or surgical incision, especially in the abdominal wall. —**eviscerate,** *v.*

evocation /ev′ōkā′shən/ [L, *evocare,* to call forth], (in embryology) a specific morphogenetic change within a developing embryo that results from the action of a single evocator.

evocator /ev′ōkā′tər/ [L, *evocare,* to call forth], a specific chemical substance or hormone that is emitted by the organizer part of the embryonic tissue and acts as a morphogenetic stimulus in the developing embryo.

evoked potential (EP) /ivōkt′/ [L, *evocare,* to call forth, *potentia,* power], an electrical response in the brainstem or cerebral cortex that is elicited by a specific stimulus. The stimulus may affect the visual, auditory, or somatosensory pathway, producing a characteristic brain wave pattern.

evoked response audiometry, a method of testing hearing ability at the level of the brainstem and auditory cortex. Evoked response audiometry is useful in diagnosing possible defects in the vestibulocochlear nerve and brainstem auditory pathways.

evolution /ev′əloo′shən/ [L, *evolvere,* to roll forth], **1.** a gradual, orderly, and continuous process of change and development from one condition or state to another. **2.** (in genetics) the theory of the origin and propagation of all plant and animal species, including humans, and their development from lower to more complex forms through the natural selection of variants produced through genetic mutations, hybridization, and inbreeding. —**evolutionist,** *n.*

evolution of infarction the normal healing process after a myocardial infarction, as demonstrated on successive electrocardiograms.

Ewing's sarcoma /yoo′ingz/ [James Ewing, American pathologist, 1866–1943], a malignant tumor that develops from bone marrow, usually in long bones or the pelvis. It is characterized by pain, swelling, fever, and leukocytosis.

exacerbation /igzas′ərbā′shən/ [L, *exacerbare,* to provoke], an increase in the seriousness of a disease or disorder as marked by greater intensity in the signs or symptoms of the patient being treated.

examination, a critical inspection and investigation, usually following a particular method, performed for diagnostic or investigational purposes.

Examination Assistance, a Nursing Interventions Classification defined as providing assistance to the patient and another health care provider during a procedure or examination.

exanthem /ig′zanthē′mə/ [Gk, eruption], a skin eruption or rash that may have specific diagnostic features of an infectious disease. Chickenpox, measles, roseola infantum, and rubella are usually characterized by a particular type of exanthem. —**exanthematous,** *adj.*

exanthematous /ig′zənthem′ətəs/ [Gk, *ex,* out, *anthema,* blossoming], pertaining to the skin rash that accompanies an infectious disease.

excessive sweat /ikses′iv/ [L, *excedere,* to go out; AS, *swaeaten*], perspiration greater than normal for the ambient environment. It is usually a sign of septic fever, pulmonary tuberculosis, hyperthyroidism, chronic renal disease, or malaria. Abnormal sweating of the hands and feet is often a sign of nervous irritability or other emotional stress.

excess mortality /ikses′/ [L, *excedere,* to go out, *mortalis,* mortal], a premature death, or one that occurs before the average life expectancy for a person of a particular demographic category.

Exchange Lists for Meal Planning, a grouping of foods in which the carbohydrates, fats, proteins, and calories are similar for the serving sizes listed. The lists, published by the American Dietetic Association and the American Diabetes Association, are used in meal planning for various diseases, as well as for weight reduction. Foods are divided into three different groups or lists: carbohydrates, meat and meat substitutes, and fats. The carbohydrate group is subdivided into lists of starch, fruit, milk, other carbohydrates, and vegetables.

exchange transfusion in the newborn /iks·chāng′/ [L, *ex* + *cambire,* to change], the introduction of whole blood in exchange for 75% to 85% of an infant's circulating blood that is repeatedly withdrawn in small amounts and replaced with equal amounts of donor blood. The procedure is performed to improve the oxygen-carrying capacity of the blood in the treatment of erythroblastosis neonatorum by removing Rh and ABO antibodies, sensitized erythrocytes that produce hemolysis, and accumulated bilirubin.

excimer laser /ek′simər/, one of a class of lasers with output in the ultraviolet range of the electromagnetic spectrum. The name is derived from the symbol formed by the combination of xenon atoms (Xe) and halogen atoms (X) to yield xenon-halide compounds as XEX.

excise /iksīz′/ [L, *ex* + *caedere,* to cut], to remove completely, as in the surgical excision of the palatine tonsils.

excision /iksish′ən/ [L, *ex* + *caedere,* to cut], **1.** the process of excising or amputating. **2.** (in molecular genetics) the process by which a genetic element is removed from a strand of deoxyribonucleic acid.

excitability /iksī′təbil′itē/ [L, *excitare,* to arouse], the property of a cell that enables it to react to irritation or stimulation, such as the reaction of a nerve or myocardial cell to an adequate stimulus.

excitant /eksī′tənt/, a drug or other agent that arouses the central nervous system or other body system in a particular manner. Excitants may be drugs or other substances, such as caffeine, or visual or auditory stimuli.

excitation /ek′sitā′shən/ [L, *excitare,* to rouse], a state of mental or physical excitement; nerve or muscle action on impulse.

excitatory amino acids /eksī′tətôr′ē/, amino acids that affect the central nervous system by acting as neurotransmitters and may in some cases act as neurotoxins. Examples include glutamate and aspartate.

excitatory impulse, a sudden force that stimulates activity.

excited state /eksī′tid/ [L, *excitare,* to rouse, *status*], (in chemistry and physics) an energy level of a system that is higher than the ground state. The system decays to the ground state and emits the energy difference, usually in the form of photons.

excitement /eksīt′mənt/, (in psychiatry) a pathologic state marked by emotional intensity, impulsive behavior, anticipation, and arousal. Excitement in schizophrenic inpatients tends to result from blocked communications and hostile feelings between the patients and the hospital staff.

exciting eye, (in sympathetic ophthalmia) the eye that is primarily affected by an injury or infection in a bilateral disorder.

exclusion from base price, a health care contract provision in which high-cost variable items beyond the control of the provider, such as organ procurement costs, are excluded from the base price. Not applicable in Canada.

Exclusive Provider Organization (EPO), a type of managed health care organization in which no coverage is typically provided for services received outside the EPO.

excoriation /ekskôr′ē-ā′shən/ [L, *excoriare,* to flay], an injury to a surface of the body caused by trauma, such as scratching, abrasion, or a chemical or thermal burn.

excrement /eks′krəment/, any waste matter, particularly feces, discharged from the body.

excreta /ekskrē′tə/ [L, *excernere,* to separate], any waste matter discharged from the body.

excrete /ekskrēt′/ [L, *excernere,* to separate], to evacuate a waste substance from the body.

excretion /ekskrē′shən/, the process of eliminating, shedding, or getting rid of substances by body organs or tissues, as part of a natural metabolic activity. Excretion usually begins at the cellular level.

excretory /eks′krətôr′ē/ [L, *excernere,* to separate], relating to the process of excretion, often used in combination with a term to identify an object or procedure associated with excretion, such as **excretory urography.**

excretory duct, a duct that is conductive but not secretory.

excretory organ, an organ that is concerned primarily with the production and discharge of body wastes.

excretory urography, [L, *excernere,* to

separate; Gk, *ouron,* urine, *graphein,* to record], a radiographic examination in which an opaque medium is introduced and its pathways recorded as it is passed through the urinary tract.

excursion /ikskur′zhən/ [L, *ex,* out, *currere,* to run], a departure or deviation from a direct or normal course.

execute /ek′səkyōōt/, (of a computer) to follow a set of instructions to complete a program or specified function.

executive physical /iksek′yətiv/, a physical examination that includes extensive laboratory, radiographic, and other tests that may be provided periodically to management level personnel at employer expense.

exercise /ek′sərsiz/ [L, *exercere,* to exercise], **1.** the performance of any physical activity for the purpose of conditioning the body, improving health, or maintaining fitness or as a means of therapy for correcting a deformity or restoring the organs and body functions to a state of health. **2.** any action, skill, or maneuver that causes muscle exertion and is performed repeatedly to develop or strengthen the body or any of its parts. **3.** to use a muscle or part of the body in a repetitive way to maintain or develop its strength.

exercise amenorrhea, a suppression of menstrual discharge that affects some women who participate in high-intensity athletics.

exercise electrocardiogram (exercise ECG), an electrocardiogram that is recorded as a person walks on a treadmill or pedals a stationary bicycle for a given length of time at a specific rate of speed.

exercise-induced anaphylaxis, a severe allergic reaction brought on by strenuous exercise.

exercise induced asthma /-indyōōst′/, a form of asthma that produces symptoms after strenuous exercise. The effect may be acute but is reversible.

exercise prescription [L, *exercere* + *prae* + *scribere,* to write], an individualized schedule for physical fitness exercises.

Exercise Promotion, a Nursing Interventions Classification defined as facilitation of regular physical exercise to maintain or advance to a higher level of fitness and health.

Exercise Promotion: Stretching, a Nursing Interventions Classification defined as facilitation of systematic slow-stretch-hold muscle exercises to induce relaxation, to prepare muscles/joints for more vigorous exercise, or to increase or maintain body flexibility.

Exercise Therapy: Ambulation, a Nursing Interventions Classification defined as promotion and assistance with walking to maintain or restore autonomic and voluntary body functions during treatment and recovery from illness of injury.

Exercise Therapy: Balance, a Nursing Interventions Classification defined as use of specific activities, postures, and movements to maintain, enhance, or restore balance.

Exercise Therapy: Joint Mobility, a Nursing Interventions Classification defined as use of active or passive body movement to maintain or restore joint flexibility.

Exercise Therapy: Muscle Control, a Nursing Interventions Classification defined as use of specific activity or exercise protocols to enhance or restore controlled body movement.

exercise tolerance, the level of physical exertion an individual may be able to achieve before reaching a state of exhaustion. Exercise tolerance tests are commonly performed on a treadmill under the supervision of a health professional who can stop the test if signs of distress are observed.

exeresis /ekser′əsis [Gk, *ex* + *eresis,* removal], the surgical removal of a part, organ, or body structure.

exertional headache /igzur′shənəl/ [L, *exserere,* to stretch out; AS, *heafod* + *acan,* headache], an acute headache that occurs during strenuous exercise. It usually recedes when the level of effort is reduced, when an analgesic medication is taken, or both.

exfoliation /eksfō′lē·ā′shon/ /eksfō′lē·ā′-shən/ [L, *ex* + *folium,* leaf], peeling and sloughing off of tissue cells. This is a normal process that may be exaggerated in certain skin diseases or after a severe sunburn. —**exfoliative,** *adj.*

exfoliative cytology /eksfo′lē·ətiv/, the microscopic examination of desquamated cells for diagnostic purposes. The cells are obtained from lesions, sputum, secretions, urine, and other material by aspiration, scraping, a smear, or washings of the tissue.

exfoliative dermatitis, any inflammatory skin disorder characterized by excessive peeling or shedding of skin.

exhale /eks·hāl′/ [L, *exhalare,* to breathe out], to breathe out or to let out with the breath. —**exhalation,** *n.*

exhaustion /igzôs′chən/ [L, *exhaurire,* to drain away], a state of extreme loss of physical or mental abilities caused by fatigue or illness.

exhaustion delirium, a delirium that may result from prolonged physical or emotional stress, fatigue, or shock associated with severe metabolic or nutritional problems.

exhaustion psychosis [L, *exhaurire,* to drain out; Gk, *psyche,* mind, *osis,* condition], an abnormal mental condition attributed to physical exhaustion. The main symptom, a delirious state, may develop in some explorers, mountain climbers, persons lost in the wilderness, and terminally ill patients.

exhibitionism /ek'sibish'əniz'əm/ [L, *exhibere,* to exhibit], **1.** the flaunting of oneself or one's abilities to attract attention. **2.** (in psychiatry) a psychosexual disorder that occurs primarily in men in which the repetitive act of exposing the genitals in socially unacceptable situations is the preferred means of achieving sexual excitement and gratification. —**exhibitionist,** *n.*

existential psychiatry /eg'zisten'shəl/ [L, *existere,* to spring forth; Gk, *psyche,* mind, *iatreia,* medical care], a school of psychiatry based on the philosophy of existentialism that emphasizes an analytic, holistic approach in which mental disorders are viewed as deviations within the total structure of an individual's existence rather than as results of any biologically or culturally related factors.

existential therapy, a kind of psychotherapy that emphasizes the development of a sense of self-direction through choice, awareness, and acceptance of individual responsibility.

exit block [L, *exire,* to depart; Fr, *bloc*], (in cardiology) the failure of an expected impulse to emerge from its focus of origin and cause depolarization.

exit dose, (in radiotherapy) the amount of radiation at the side of the body opposite the surface to which the beam is directed.

exocrine /ek'səkrin/ [Gk, *exo,* outside, *krinein,* to secrete], pertaining to the process of secreting outwardly through a duct to the surface of an organ or tissue or into a vessel.

exocrine gland, any of the multicellular glands that open onto the skin surface through ducts in the epithelium, as the sweat glands and the sebaceous glands.

exoenzyme /ek'sō·en'zīm/, an enzyme that does not function within the cells from which it is secreted.

exogenous /igzoj'ənəs/ [Gk, *exo + genein,* to produce], **1.** outside the body. **2.** originating outside the body or an organ of the body or produced from external causes, such as a disease caused by a bacterial or viral agent foreign to the body. —**exogenic,** *adj.*

exogenous hemochromatosis [Gk, *exo,* outside, *genein,* to produce, *haima,* blood, *chroma,* color, *osis,* condition], a condi-

tion of bronzed pigmentation of the skin caused by accumulation of an iron pigment from excessive intake of iron-rich foods or blood transfusions.

exogenous infection [Gk, *exo,* outside, *genein,* to produce; L, *inficere,* to infect], an infection that develops from bacteria normally outside the body that have gained access to the body.

exogenous obesity, obesity caused by a caloric intake greater than needed to meet the metabolic needs of the body.

exogenous uric acid [Gk, *exo,* outside, *genein,* to produce, *ouron,* urine; L, *acidus*], the accumulation of uric acid in the body produced by the metabolism of purine-rich foods.

exon /ek'son/ [Gk, *exo + genein,* to produce], (in molecular genetics) the part of a deoxyribonucleic acid molecule that produces the code for the final messenger ribonucleic acid.

exonuclease /ek'sōnoō'klē·ās/ [Gk, *exo +* L, *nucleus,* nut; *ase,* enzyme], (in molecular genetics) a nuclease that digests deoxyribonucleic acid or ribonucleic acid from the ends of the strands.

exophoria /ek'səfôr'ē·ə/ [Gk, *exo + pherein,* to bear], the latent deviation of the visual axis of one eye outward and away from that of the other eye. It occurs in the absence of visual stimuli for fusion. —**exophoric,** *adj.*

exophthalmia /ek'softhal'mē·ə/ [Gk, *exo + ophthalmos,* eye], an abnormal condition characterized by a marked protrusion of the eyeballs (**exophthalmos, exophthalmus**), usually resulting from the increased volume of the orbital contents caused by a tumor; swelling associated with cerebral, intraocular, or intraorbital edema or hemorrhage; paralysis of or trauma to the extraocular muscles; or cavernous sinus thrombosis. It may also be caused by endocrine disorders such as hyperthyroidism and Graves' disease. —**exophthalmic,** *adj.*

exophthalmic goiter /ek'softhal'mik/, exophthalmos that occurs in association with goiter, as in Graves' disease.

exophthalmometer /ek'səfthalmom'ətər/ [Gk, *exo + ophthalmos,* eye, *metron,* measure], an instrument used for measuring the degree of forward displacement of the eye in exophthalmos.

exophytic /ek'səfit'ik/ [Gk, *exo + phyton,* plant], pertaining to the tendency to grow outward, such as a tumor that grows into the lumen of a hollow organ rather than into the wall.

exophytic carcinoma, a malignant epithelial neoplasm that resembles a papilloma or wart.

exoskeletal prosthesis /ek'səskel'ətəl/ [Gk, *exo* + *skeletos,* dried up, *prothesis,* addition], a prosthetic device in which support is provided by an outside structure (not an implant) such as an artificial limb.

exoskeleton /ek'səskel'ətən/ [Gk, *exo,* outside, *skeletos,* dried up], the hard outer covering of many invertebrates such as crustaceans that lack the bony internal structures of vertebrates.

exostosis /ek'sostō'sis/ [Gk, *exo* + *osteon,* bone], an abnormal benign growth on the surface of a bone. —**exostosed, exostotic,** *adj.*

exostosis cartilaginea [Gk, *ex,* out, *osteon,* bone; L, *cartilago,* cartilage], an outgrowth of cartilage at the ends of long bones.

exoteric /ek'səter'ik/ [Gk, *exoterikos,* external], pertaining to something outside the organism.

exothermic, indicating a chemical process accompanied by the release of heat, such as the loss of body surface heat.

exotoxin /ek'sətok'sin/ [Gk, *exo* + *toxikon,* poison], a toxin that is secreted or excreted by a living microorganism.

expanded role [L, *expandere,* to spread out; OFr, *rolle,* an assumed character], the functions of a nurse that are not specified in the traditional limits of nursing practice legislation. Common roles are primary nurse and nurse practitioner.

expectant treatment /ekspek'tənt/ [L, *exspectare,* to wait for; Fr, *traitment*], application of therapeutic measures to relieve symptoms as they arise in the course of a disease, rather than treatment of the cause of illness.

expectation /eks'pektā'shən/ [L, *exspectare,* to wait for], **1.** (in nursing) anticipation by the staff of a patient's behavior that is based on a knowledge and understanding of the person's abilities and problems. **2.** anticipation of the performance of the nursing staff in defined roles, as role expectation.

expected date of delivery (EDD), the predicted date of a pregnant woman's delivery. Pregnancy lasts approximately 266 days, or 38 weeks from the day of fertilization, but is considered clinically to last 280 days, or 40 weeks, or 10 lunar months, or 9⅓ calendar months from the first day of the last menstrual period (LMP).

expectorant /ikspek'tərənt/ [Gk, *ex,* out, *pectus,* breast], **1.** pertaining to a substance that promotes the ejection of mucus or other exudates from the lung, bronchi, and trachea. **2.** an agent that promotes expectoration by reducing the viscosity of pulmonary secretions or by decreasing the tenacity with which exudates adhere to the lower respiratory tract. —**expectorate,** *v.*

expectoration /ekspek'tərā'shən/, the ejection of mucus, sputum, or fluids from the trachea and lungs by coughing or spitting.

experience rating /ikspir'ē·əns/ [L, *experientia,* testing, *rata*], a system used by an insurance company in the United States to set the premium to be paid by the insured, which is based on the risk to the company of providing the insurance.

experiment, an investigation in which one or more factors may be altered under controlled circumstances to study the effects of altering factors.

experimental design /eksper'imen'təl/ [L, *experimentum* + *designare,* to mark out], (in research) a study design used to test cause-and-effect relationships between variables. The classic experimental design specifies an experimental group and a control group. Subsequent experimental designs have used more groups and more measurements over longer periods.

experimental embryology, the study and analysis through experimental techniques of the factors, mechanisms, and relationships that determine and influence prenatal development.

experimental epidemiology, a type of epidemiologic investigation that uses an experimental model for studies to confirm a causal relationship suggested by observational studies.

experimental medicine, a branch of the practice of medicine in which new drugs or treatments are evaluated for safety and efficacy in a clinical laboratory setting by using animals or, in certain cases, human subjects.

experimental pathology, the study of diseases deliberately induced in laboratory animals.

experimental physiology, a branch of the study of physiology in which the functions of various body systems are evaluated in a clinical laboratory setting by using animals or, in some cases, human subjects.

experimental psychology, the study of mental processes and phenomena by observation in a controlled environment using various tests, manipulations, and experiments.

expertise /eks'pərtēz'/ [L, *experiri,* to try], special skills or knowledge acquired by a person through education, training, or experience.

expert witness /ikspurt', ek'spərt/ [L, *experiri,* to try; AS, *witnes,* knowledge], a person who has special knowledge of a subject about which a court requests testimony.

E

expiration /ik'spirā'shən/ [L, *expirare*, to breathe out], **1.** breathing out, normally a passive process, depending on the elastic qualities of lung tissue and the thorax. **2.** termination or death. —**expire**, *v.*

expiratory /ikspī'rətôr'ē/ [L, *expirare*, to breathe out], pertaining to the expiration of air from the lungs.

expiratory center [L, *expirare*, to breath out; Gk, *kentron*, center], one of several regions of the medulla responsible for control of respiration. It is a subregion specifically involved in carrying out the activity of expiration.

expiratory phase, the part of the respiratory cycle that involves exhalation, or moving air out of the lungs. In a ventilated patient the expiratory phase may be passive.

expiratory reserve volume (ERV), the maximum volume of gas that can be exhaled after a resting volume exhalation.

expiratory retard, (in respiratory care) a mode of mechanical ventilation that mimics the prolonged expiratory phase and pursed-lip breathing of emphysema. The method adds some resistance to expiration.

expire /ikspī'ər/ [L, *expirare*, to breathe out], **1.** to breathe out. **2.** to die.

expired gas (E), any gas exhaled from the lungs.

exploratory /iksplôr'ətôr'ē/ [L, *explorare*, to search out], pertaining to investigation, as in exploratory surgery.

exploratory operation [L, *explorare*, to search out, *operari*, to work], surgical intervention to find the cause of a disorder by opening a body cavity or organ and examining the interior.

explosion, 1. a sudden and violent decomposition of a chemical compound. **2.** a sudden radical breakout.

explosive personality /iksplō'siv/ [L, *ex,* out, *plaudere,* to clap], behavior characterized by episodes of uncontrolled rage and physical abusiveness in reaction to relatively minor stressors.

explosive speech, abnormal speech characterized by slow, jerky articulation interspersed with sudden loud enunciation of words, often seen in brain disorders.

exponent /ikspō'nənt/, a superscript on a number that indicates how many times a number is to be multiplied by itself (for example, $3^4 = 3 \times 3 \times 3 \times 3 = 81$). In medical or scientific reports powers of 10 are commonly used to indicate very large or very small numbers, such as in the examples 10^6 representing 1,000,000 or 10^{-6} representing 1/1,000,000. Exponents also are indicated by prefixes, such as mega- for 10^6 and micro- for 10^{-6}.

exposed pulp [L, *exponere,* to lay out, *pulpa,* flesh], dental pulp that becomes exposed to the external environment and potential bacterial infection. Causes include fracture of the crown through trauma or loss of a tooth crown or penetration of the dentin during restorative preparation.

exposure /ikspō'zhər/ [L, *exponere,* to lay out], (in radiotherapy and radiography) a measure of the ionization of air produced by a beam of radiation. Exposure is defined in coulomb per kilogram of air.

exposure angle, the angle of the arc described by the movement of the radiographic tube and film during tomography while the tube is making an exposure.

exposure switch, (in radiology) a control device designed to interrupt the power automatically when pressure by the operator's hand or foot is released. The purpose is to prevent accidental continuing exposure of the patient to radiation.

exposure unit, any of the conventional or SI units used to measure radiation exposure: roentgen (R), rad, rem, curie (Ci), gray (Gy), sievert (Sv), and becquerel (Bq).

expression /ikspresh'ən/ [L, *exprimere,* to express], **1.** the indication of a physical or emotional state through facial appearance or vocal intonation. **2.** the act of pressing or squeezing to expel something, such as milk from the breast when lactating or the fetus from the uterus by exertion of pressure on the abdominal wall. **3.** (in genetics) the detectable effect or appearance in the phenotype of a particular trait or condition. —**express**, *v.*

expressivity /eks'presiv'itē/ [L, *exprimere,* to make clear], (in genetics) the variability with which basic patterns of inheritance are modified, both in degree and in variety, by the effect of a given gene in people of the same genotype.

expulsive stage of labor /ikspul'siv/ [L, *expellere,* to drive out, *stare,* stand, *labor,* work], the second stage of labor, during which the mother's uterine contractions are accompanied by a bearing-down reflex. It begins after full dilation of the cervix and continues to the complete birth of the infant.

exsanguinate /eksang'gwināt/ [L, *ex, sanguis,* blood], to drain away or deprive an organ of blood.

exsanguination /eksang'gwinā'shən/, a loss of blood.

exstrophy /ek'strōfē/ [Gk, *ekstrephein,* to turn inside out], a congenital malformation in which a hollow organ has its wall turned inside-out, establishing a communication with the exterior.

extended care facility [L, *extendere,* to stretch], an institution devoted to providing medical, nursing, or custodial care for an individual over a prolonged period, such as during the course of a chronic disease or the rehabilitation phase after an acute illness.

extended family, a family group consisting of the biologic or adoptive parents, their children, the grandparents, and other family members. The extended family is the basic family group in many societies.

extended insulin-zinc suspension, a long-acting insulin that is slowly absorbed and slow to act.

extended-wear contact lens, a refractive index device that fits over the cornea, designed to permit air permeation. Oxygen may pass between the lens and the cornea, thereby reducing the risk of corneal irritation.

extender, something that causes an increase in time or size, such as a substance added to a medication to stretch the time required for the drug to be absorbed. A kind of extender is **plasma volume extender.**

extension /iksten'shən/ [L, *extendere,* to stretch], a "straightening" movement allowed by certain joints of the skeleton that increases the angle between two adjoining bones, such as extending the leg, which increases the posterior angle between the femur and the tibia.

extensor /iksten'sər/ [L, *extendere,* to stretch out], any muscle that extends a body part, as the extensor indicis, which extends the index finger.

extensor carpi radialis brevis [L, *extendere* + Gk, *karpos,* wrist; L, *radius,* ray, *brevis,* short], one of the muscles of the posterior forearm. It functions to extend the hand.

extensor carpi radialis longus, one of the seven superficial muscles of the posterior forearm. It serves to extend and flex the hand radially.

extensor carpi ulnaris, one of the muscles of the lateral forearm. It functions to extend and adduct the hand.

extensor digiti minimi, an extensor muscle of the posterior forearm. It functions to extend the little finger.

extensor digitorum, the principal muscle of the medial digits of the posterior forearm. It functions to extend the phalanges and, by continued action, the wrist.

extensor digitorum longus, a penniform muscle located at the lateral part of the anterior leg. It extends the proximal phalanges of the four small toes and dorsally flexes and pronates the foot.

extensor retinaculum of ankle, either of two thick layers of fascia holding tendons in the ankle.

extensor retinaculum of hand, the thick band of antebrachial fascia that wraps tendons of the extensor muscles of the forearm at the distal ends of the radius and the ulna.

extensor retinaculum of wrist, a broad thickening of deep fascia over the back of the wrist, over the extensor tendons.

extensor thrust, a spinal-level reflex present in a human in the first 2 months of life. It is an exaggeration of the positive support reflex and consists of an uncontrolled extension of a flexed leg when the sole of the foot is stimulated.

extern /eks'turn/ [L, *externus,* outward], a medical or dental student who lives outside the institution but provides medical or dental care to patients as an extracurricular activity under the professional supervision of hospital staff members.

external /ikstur'nəl/ [L, *externus,* outward], **1.** being on the outside or exterior of the body or an organ. **2.** acting from the outside, such as an external influence or exogenous factor. **3.** pertaining to the outward or visible appearance.

external abdominal oblique muscle, one of a pair of muscles that are the largest and most superficial of the five anterolateral muscles of the abdomen. Both sides acting together serve to flex the vertebral column, drawing the pubis toward the xiphoid process.

external absorption, the taking up of substances through the mucous membranes or the skin.

external acoustic meatus, the canal of the external ear, composed of bone and cartilage, extending from the auricle to the tympanic membrane.

external aperture of aqueduct of vestibule, an external opening for the small canal extending from the vestibule of the inner ear, located on the internal surface of the petrous part of the temporal bone lateral to the opening for the internal acoustic passage.

external aperture of canaliculus of cochlea, an external opening of the cochlear channel on the margin of the jugular opening in the temporal bone.

external aperture of tympanic canaliculus, the lower opening of the tympanic channel on the inferior surface of the petrous part of the temporal bone.

external carotid artery, one of a pair of arteries with eight major temporal or maxillary branches, rising from the common carotid arteries. It supplies various parts and tissues of the head and neck.

external carotid plexus, a network of

nerves around the external carotid artery, formed by the external carotid nerves from the superior cervical ganglion. It supplies sympathetic fibers associated with branches of the external carotid artery.

external cervical os, an external opening of the uterus that leads into the cavity of the cervix.

external conjugate, the distance measured with obstetric calipers from the depression below the lowest lumbar vertebra posteriorly to the upper border of the symphysis anteriorly (usually about 21 cm).

external counterpulsation, (in cardiology) a noninvasive technique for providing counterpulsation. In one technique the limbs are placed in inflatable trousers. Inflation and deflation are synchronized with the cardiac cycle, generating augmented blood flow during diastole and assisted ejection during systole.

external ear, the outer structure of the ear, consisting of the auricle and the external acoustic meatus.

external fertilization, the union of male and female gametes outside the bodies from which they originated, such as occurs in fish and frogs.

external fistula, an abnormal passage between an internal organ or structure and the cutaneous surface of the body.

external fixation, a method of holding together the fragments of a fractured bone by using transfixing metal pins through the fragments and a compression device attached to the pins outside the skin surface.

external iliac artery, the larger, more superficial division of the common iliac artery, which descends into the thigh and becomes the femoral artery.

external iliac node, a node in one of the seven groups of parietal nodes serving the lymphatic system in the abdomen and the pelvis.

external iliac vein, one of a pair of veins in the lower body that join the internal iliac vein to form the two common iliac veins.

external jugular vein, the more superficial and lateral of a pair of large vessels on each side of the neck that receive most of the blood from the exterior of the cranium and the deep tissues of the face.

external malleolus [L, *externus,* outward, *malleolus,* little hammer], a rounded bony prominence on each side of the ankle joint.

external pacemaker [L, *externus,* outward, *passus,* step; ME, *maken,* to make], **1.** a device used to stimulate the heartbeat electrically by the discharge of impulses through the chest wall, as used in emergency care of significant bradyarrhyth-

mias. **2.** a cardiac pacemaker in which the impulse generator is outside the chest but connected with the heart by wires that pass under the skin.

external pterygoid muscle, one of the four short, thick, somewhat conical muscles of mastication. It functions to open the jaws, protrude the mandible, and move the mandible from side to side.

external radiation therapy (ERT), the therapeutic application of ionizing radiation from an external beam of a kilovoltage radiographic machine; a megavoltage cobalt 60 machine; or a supervoltage linear accelerator, cyclotron, or betatron.

external respiration, the part of the respiratory process that involves the exchange of gases in the alveoli of the lungs.

external rotation, turning outwardly or away from the midline of the body, such as when a leg is externally rotated with the toes turned outward or away from the body's midline.

external shunt, a device for the passage of body fluid from one compartment to another. It consists of a tube or catheter (or a series of such containers) that passes from one compartment or cavity to another over the body surface rather than inside the body.

external version, an obstetric procedure in which a fetus is turned, usually from a breech to a vertex presentation, by external manipulation through the abdominal wall.

exteroceptive /ek'stərōsep'tiv/ [L, *externus,* outside, *recipere,* to receive], pertaining to stimuli that originate from outside the body or to the sensory receptors that they activate.

exteroceptor /ek'stərōsep'tər/ [L, *externus,* outside, *recipere,* to receive], any sensory nerve ending, as those located in the skin, mucous membranes, or sense organs, that responds to stimuli originating outside the body, such as touch, pressure, or sound.

extinction /iksting'shən/, a state of being lost or destroyed.

extirpation /ek'stərpā'shən/ [L, *extirpare,* to root out], the total removal of a diseased organ or body part.

extraarticular /ek'strə-ärtik'yələr/ [L, *extra,* outside, *articulare,* to divide into joints], pertaining to the area outside a joint or within the joint but not involving the joint structures.

extra beat [L, *extra,* outside; AS, *beatan*], an extra systole; an extra heart contraction. It refers to a premature atrial, junctional, or ventricular complex.

extracapsular /-kaps'yələr/ [L, *extra,* outside, *capsula,* little box], pertaining to something outside a capsule, such as the articulare capsule of the knee joint.

extracapsular dendrite [L, *extra* + *capsula* + Gk, *dendron,* tree], pertaining to dendrites of some autonomic nerves that penetrate the capsule boundary and extend some distance from the cell body.

extracapsular fracture [L, *extra* + *capsula,* little box], any fracture that occurs near a joint but does not directly involve the joint capsule. This type of fracture is extremely common in the hip.

extracellular /-sel′yəlor/ [L, *extra* + *cella,* storeroom], occurring outside a cell or cell tissue or in cavities or spaces between cell layers or groups of cells.

extracellular fluid (ECF), the part of the body fluid comprising the interstitial fluid and blood plasma. The adult body contains about 11.2 L of interstitial fluid, constituting about 16% of body weight, and about 2.8 L of plasma, constituting about 4% of body weight.

extracellular matrix, a substance containing collagen, elastin, proteoglycans, glycosaminoglycans, and fluid, produced by cells and the substance in which they are embedded.

extrachromosomal /-krō′məsō′məl/, occurring without direct involvement of the chromosomes.

extracoronal retainer /-kôr′ənəl/ [L, *extra* + *corona,* crown, *retinere,* to hold], **1.** a kind of dental anchor that incorporates a cast restoration lying largely external to the coronal part of a tooth and complements the contour of the tooth crown. **2.** a direct clasp-type retainer that engages an abutment tooth on its external surface, used for the retention and stabilization of a removable partial denture. **3.** a manufactured direct retainer, the protruding part of which is attached to the external surface of a cast crown on an abutment tooth.

extracorporeal /-kôrpôr′ē-əl/ [L, *extra* + *corpus,* body], something that is outside the body, such as extracorporeal circulation in which venous blood is diverted outside the body to a heart-lung machine and returned to the body through a femoral or other artery.

extracorporeal membrane oxygenator (ECMO), a device that oxygenates the blood of a patient outside the body and returns the blood to the patient's circulatory system. The technique may be used to support an impaired respiratory system.

extracorporeal oxygenation, the use of an artificial membrane outside the body to provide for oxygenation in a patient with severe lung disease.

extracorporeal photochemotherapy, a

procedure for treating pemphigus vulgaris by treating the patient's blood outside the body. Certain drugs are first administered to the patient. Some of the patient's blood is then removed temporarily for exposure to ultraviolet light outside the body. The blood, after treatment, is returned to the patient.

extracorporeal shock-wave lithotripsy (ESWL) [L, *extra,* outside, *corpus,* body; Fr, *choc* + AS, *wafian* + Gk, *lithos,* stone, *tribein,* to wear away], use of vibrations of powerful sound waves to break up calculi in the urinary tract.

extracranial /-krā′nē-əl/ [L, *extra,* outside; Gk, *kranion,* skull], pertaining to something outside the skull.

extract [L, *ex,* out, *trahere,* to draw], **1.** /ek′strakt/ a substance, usually a biologically active ingredient of a plant or animal tissue, prepared by the use of solvents or evaporation to separate the substance from the original material. **2.** /ikstrakt′/ to remove a tooth from the oral cavity by means of elevators or forceps or both. /ikstrakt′/ —**extraction,** *n.*

extractor /ikstrak′tər/, a medical instrument such as a forceps, used to remove a foreign body, tissue sample, or medical device placed in a body cavity.

extradural /ek′trədŏŏr′əl/ [L, *extra* + *dura,* hard], outside the dura mater.

extradural anesthesia, anesthetic nerve block achieved by the injection of a local anesthetic solution into the space in the spinal canal outside the dura mater of the spinal cord.

extraembryonic blastoderm /-em′brē-on′-ik/ [L, *extra* + Gk, *en,* in, *bryein,* to grow], the area of the blastoderm outside the embryo that gives rise to the membranes that surround the embryo during gestation.

extraembryonic coelom, a cavity external to the developing embryo that forms between the mesoderm of the chorion and that covering the amniotic cavity and yolk sac.

extraembryonic mesoderm [L, *extra,* outside; Gk, *en* + *bryein,* to grow, *mesos,* middle, *derma,* skin], any mesoderm in the uterus that is not involved with the embryo itself. Included are mesoderms in the amnion, chorion, and yolk sac.

extramammary Paget's disease /-mam′-ərē/ [L, *extra,* outside, *mamma,* breast; James Paget, English surgeon, 1814–1899; L, *dis* + Fr, *aise,* ease], a gradually spreading red, scaly and crusted lesion resembling that of Paget's disease, but not occurring on the breast. A common area is the vulva. The lesions give rise to carcinoma.

extramarital /-mer′itəl/, happening outside a marriage.

extramedullary /-med′yələr′ē/ [L, *extra* + *medulla,* marrow], pertaining to something outside the medulla.

extramedullary myeloma [L, *extra* + *medulla,* marrow], a plasma cell tumor that occurs outside the bone marrow, usually affecting the visceral organs or the nasopharyngeal and oral mucosa.

extramedullary myelopoiesis, the formation and development of myeloid tissue outside the bone marrow.

extraneous /exstrā′nē·əs/ [L, strange], exogenous; originating or entering from outside the organism.

extraocular /-ok′yŏŏlər/ [L, *extra* + *oculus,* eye], outside the eye.

extraocular muscle palsy, an abnormal condition characterized by paralysis of the extrinsic muscles of the eye, such as the superior, inferior, medial, and lateral rectus muscles, and the superior and the inferior oblique muscles.

extraocular muscles (EOM) /·ok′yələr/, the six sets of muscles that control movements of the eyeball. They are the superior rectus and inferior rectus, which move the eye up and down; the medial rectus and the lateral rectus, which move the eye to either side; and the superior oblique and inferior oblique, which move the eye upward and outward, and downward and outward.

extraoral anchorage /-ôr′əl/ [L, *extra* + *oralis,* mouth, *ancora,* hook], an orthodontic holding device outside the mouth, typically linking dental attachments to a wire bow or to hooks extending between the lips and attached by elastic to a cap, a neck strap, or another device outside the mouth.

extraoral orthodontic appliance, a device secured to a part of the face, the neck, or the back of the head to deliver traction force to the teeth or jaws for changing the relative positions of dentitions.

extraperitoneal /-per′itənē′əl/ [L, *extra* + Gk, *peri,* near, around, *teinein* to stretch], occurring or located outside the peritoneal cavity.

extraperitoneal cesarean section, a method for surgically delivering a baby through an incision in the lower uterine segment without entering the peritoneal cavity. The uterus is approached through the paravesical space.

extrapleural /-plŏŏ′əl/, outside the pleural cavity.

extrapleural pneumothorax, a condition in which an air or gas pocket forms between the endothoracic fascia-pleura layer and the adjacent chest wall.

extrapsychic conflict /-sī′kik/ [L, *extra* + Gk, *psyche,* mind; L, *confligere,* to strike together], an emotional conflict that usually occurs when one's inner needs and desires do not coincide with the restrictions of the environment or society.

extrapulmonary /-pul′məner′ē/, outside of or unrelated to the lungs.

extrapulmonary small cell carcinoma, a primary small cell cancer with a histologic diagnosis of small cell carcinoma but located in body areas outside the lungs. It occurs most frequently around the head and neck; in the pancreas, colon, and rectum; and in the genitourinary tract.

extrapyramidal /ek′strəpiram′ədəl/ [L, *extra* + Gk, *pyramis,* pyramid], **1.** pertaining to the tissues and structures outside the cerebrospinal pyramidal tracts of the brain that are associated with movement of the body, excluding motor neurons, the motor cortex, and the corticospinal and corticobulbar tracts. **2.** pertaining to the function of these tissues and structures.

extrapyramidal disease, any of a large group of conditions affecting the extrapyramidal tracts and characterized by involuntary movement, changes in muscle tone, and abnormal posture. Examples include tardive dyskinesia, chorea, athetosis, and Parkinson's disease.

extrapyramidal side effects, side effects that mimic extrapyramidal disease and are caused by drugs that block dopamine receptor sites in the extrapyramidal system tract.

extrapyramidal system, the part of the nervous system that includes the basal nuclei, substantia nigra, subthalamic nucleus, part of the midbrain, and the motor neurons of the spine.

extrapyramidal tracts, the uncrossed tracts of motor nerves from the brain to the anterior horns of the spinal cord, except the crossed fibers of the pyramidal tracts. Within the brain extrapyramidal pathways comprise various relays of motoneurons between motor areas of the cerebral cortex, the basal nuclei, the thalamus, the cerebellum, and the brainstem. The extrapyramidal pathways are functional rather than anatomic units.

extrarenal uremia /-rē′nəl/ [L, *extra* + *ren,* kidney; Gk, *ouron,* urine, *haima,* blood], uremia that may be involved with kidney failure, although the cause is outside the kidney, as in alkalosis that results from excessive alkali ingestion or severe vomiting.

extrasensory /-sen′sərē/ [L, *extra* + *sentire,* to feel], pertaining to alleged awareness of events that cannot be observed by any of the five basic senses. It includes telepathy, clairvoyance, and psychokinesis.

extrasensory perception (ESP) [L, *extra* + *sentire*, to feel, *percipere*, to perceive], alleged awareness or knowledge acquired without using the physical senses.

extrasystole /-sis'təlē/ [L, *extra* + Gk, *systole*, contraction], an abnormal cardiac contraction that results from depolarization by an ectopic inputs.

extrauterine /-yōō'tərin/ [L, *extra* + *uterus*, womb], occurring or located outside the uterus, as an ectopic pregnancy.

extravasation /ikstrav'əsā'shən/ [L, *extra* + *vas*, vessel], **1.** a passage or escape into the tissues, usually of blood, serum, or lymph. **2.** passage or escape into tissue of antineoplastic chemotherapeutic drugs. Signs and symptoms may be sudden onset of localized pain at an injection site, sudden redness or extreme pallor at an injection site, or loss of blood return in an intravenous needle. —**extravasate**, *v.*

extravascular fluid /-vas'kyələr/ [L, *extra*, outside, *vasculum*, small vessel, *fluere*, to flow], fluid in the body that is outside the blood vessels. Examples include lymph and cerebrospinal fluid.

extremity /ikstrem'itē/ [L, *extremitas*], an arm or a leg. The arm may be identified as an upper extremity, and the leg as a lower extremity.

extrinsic /ikstrin'sik/ [L, *extrinsecus*, on the outside], pertaining to anything external or originating outside a structure or organism, including parts of an organ that are not wholly contained within it, as an extrinsic muscle.

extrinsic muscle (em) [L, *extrinsecus*, on the outside], **1.** muscle that is outside the organ it controls, as the extraocular muscles that control eye movements. **2.** muscle that links a limb to the trunk of the body.

extroversion /-vur'zhən/ [L, *extra* + *vertere*, to turn], **1.** the tendency to direct one's interests and energies toward external values or things outside the self. **2.** the state of being totally or primarily concerned with what is outside the self.

extrovert /ik'strəvurt'/, **1.** a person whose interests are directed away from the self and concerned primarily with external reality and the physical environment rather than with inner feelings and thoughts. **2.** a person characterized by extroversion.

extroverted personality /-vur'tid/ [L, *extra*, outside, *vertere*, to turn, *personalis*, of a person], a persona that is directed to a greater degree toward the outer world of people and events rather than the subjective inner world experience.

extrude /ekstrōōd'/ [L, *extrudere*, to push out], to thrust out from a surface or from alignment.

extrusion reflex /ekstrōō'zhən/ [L, *extrudere*, to push out, *reflectere*, to bend back], a normal response in infants to force the tongue outward when touched or depressed. The reflex begins to disappear by about 3 or 4 months of age.

extubation /iks't(y)ōōbā'shən/ [L, *ex*, out, *tuba*, tube], the process of withdrawing a tube from an orifice or cavity of the body. —**extubate**, *v.*

exudate /eks'yōōdāt/ [L, *exsudare*, to sweat out], fluid, cells, or other substances that have been slowly exuded, or discharged, from cells or blood vessels through small pores or breaks in cell membranes.

exudation /eks'yədā'shən/ [L, *exudare*, the discharge of fluid], pus or serum. The exudate may or may not contain fibrous or coagulated material.

exudative /igzōō'dətiv/, relating to the oozing of fluid and other materials from cells and tissues, usually as a result of inflammation or injury.

exudative enteropathy, diarrhea that occurs in diseases characterized by inflammation or destruction of intestinal mucosa.

exudative inflammation [L, *exudare*, to sweat out, *inflammare*, to set afire], an inflammation of a serous or raw cavity in which fluid is released from the inflamed surface.

eye [AS, *eage*], one of a pair of organs of sight, contained in a bony orbit at the front of the skull, embedded in orbital fat, and innervated by four cranial nerves: optic, oculomotor, trochlear, and abducens. Associated with the eye are certain accessory structures such as the muscles, the fasciae, the eyebrow, the eyelids, the conjunctiva, and the lacrimal gland. The bulb of the eye is composed of segments of two spheres with nearly parallel axes that constitute the outside tunic and one of three fibrous layers enclosing two internal cavities separated by the crystalline lens. The smaller cavity anterior to the lens is divided by the iris into two chambers, both filled with aqueous humor. The posterior cavity is larger than the anterior cavity and contains the jellylike vitreous body that is divided by the hyaloid canal. The outside tunic of the bulb consists of the transparent cornea anteriorly and the opaque sclera posteriorly. The intermediate vascular, pigmented tunic consists of the choroid, the ciliary body, and the iris. The internal tunic of nervous tissue is the retina. Light waves passing through the lens strike a layer of rods and cones in the retina, creating impulses that are transmitted by the optic nerve to the brain. Eye movement is controlled by six muscles: the superior and inferior oblique muscles and the superior, inferior, medial, and lateral rectus muscles.

eye bank [AS, *eage* + It, *banca*, bench], a facility for collecting and storing corneas of eyes for transplantation to recipients.

eyebrow [AS, *eage* + *bru*]. **1.** the supraorbital arch of the frontal bone that separates the orbit of the eye from the forehead. **2.** the arch of hairs growing along the ridge formed by the supraorbital arch of the frontal bone.

Eye Care, a Nursing Interventions Classification defined as prevention or minimization of threats to eye or visual integrity.

eyecup, a small vessel or cup that is shaped to fit over the eyeball and used to bathe the exposed surface of the organ.

eye deviation [AS, *eage* + L, *deviare*, to turn aside], **1.** a movement of one or both eyes, singly or jointly, from the median line or from the original direction of fixation. **Manifest deviation** is the number of degrees by which the visual axis of one eye deviates from that of the other in cases of squint, when both eyes are open. **2.** (in strabismus) the departure of the foveal line of sight of one eye from the point of fixation.

eye dominance, an unconscious preference to use one eye rather than the other for certain purposes, such as looking through a telescope.

eyedrops, a liquid medicine that is administered by allowing it to fall in drops onto the conjunctival surface.

eye glasses, transparent lenses held in metal or plastic frames in front of the eyes to correct refractive errors or to protect the eyes from harmful electromagnetic waves or flying objects.

eyeground, the fundus of the eye.

eyelash [AS, *eage* + ME, *lasche*], one of many hairs growing in double or triple rows along the border of the eyelids in front of a row of ciliary glands that are in front of a row of meibomian glands.

eyelid [AS, *eage* + *hlid*], a movable fold of thin skin over the eye, with eyelashes and ciliary and meibomian glands along its margin. The orbicularis oculi muscle and the oculomotor nerve control the opening and closing of the eyelid.

eye patching, 1. placement of a soft patch over a closed eye to restrict lid movement during corneal reepithelialization or a similar healing procedure in progress. **2.** occlusion of the better eye by patch placement in young patients with strabismic amblyopia to force greater use of the amblyopic eye. **3.** patching used in cases of diplopia (double vision).

eye shielding, protection of an injured eye by securing a metal or plastic eye shield or a disposable cup to prevent further injury by rubbing and to reduce stimulation by light and movement.

eye shower, an apparatus for irrigating the eyes after exposure to dust or other debris or chemical contamination. The shower directs one or two streams of water so that they flush over the eyes and lids.

f, **1.** symbol for *breaths per unit time.* **2.** symbol for *respiratory frequency.*

F, **1.** abbreviation for **Fahrenheit. 2.** abbreviation for **farad. 3.** symbol for **fluorine. 4.** abbreviation for **frequency.**

F₁, (in genetics) the symbol for the first filial generation; the heterozygous offspring produced by the mating of two unrelated individuals.

F₂, (in genetics) the symbol for the second filial generation the offspring produced by mating two members of the F₁ generation.

FA, **1.** abbreviation for **fatty acid. 2.** abbreviation for **femoral artery. 3.** abbreviation for **folic acid.**

F.A.A.N., abbreviation for **Fellow of the American Academy of Nursing.**

F_{ab}, the part of an antibody molecule that contains the antigen-binding site, consisting of a light chain and part of a heavy chain. Such fragments are produced when antibodies are digested by enzymes such as the protease papain. F_{ab} fragments are used as an antidote for treating toxicity caused by digoxin, digitoxin, and oleander tea.

Fabere's test /fā′bārāz/, a test for pain or dysfunction in the hip and sacroiliac joints in which overpressure is applied at the knee during flexion, abduction, and external rotation of the hip.

fabrication /fab′rikā′shən/, a psychologic reaction in which false statements are contrived to mask memory defects. It is a clinical feature of Korsakoff's syndrome and other disorders.

FAC, an anticancer drug combination of fluorouracil, doxorubicin, and cyclophosphamide.

F.A.C.C.P., abbreviation for *Fellow of the American College of Chest Physicians.*

F.A.C.D., abbreviation for *Fellow of the American College of Dentists.*

face [L, *facies*], **1.** the front of the head from the chin to the brow, including the skin; the muscles; and the structures of the forehead, eyes, nose, mouth, cheeks, and jaw. **2.** the visage. **3.** to direct the face toward something. —**facial,** *adj.*

face-bow [L, *facies* + AS, *boga*], a device resembling a caliper for measuring the relationship of the maxilla to the tem

poromandibular joints; the measurement is used in the fabrication of denture casts and major restorative procedures involving natural teeth.

face lift, a plastic surgery procedure in which wrinkles and other signs of aging skin are eliminated.

face presentation [L, *facies,* face, *praesentare,* to show], an obstetric presentation in which the chin of the fetus is the point of direction.

facet /fas′it/ [Fr, *facette,* little face], **1.** (in dentistry) a flattened, highly polished wear pattern on a tooth. **2.** a small, smooth-surfaced process for articulation.

facetectomy /fas′itek′təmē/, surgical removal of a facet, particularly the articular facet of a vertebra.

facet joint, synovial joint between articular processes (zygapophytes) of the vertebrae.

facial angle /fāshəl/ [L, *facies* + *angulus,* a corner], an anthropomorphic expression of the degree of protrusion of the lower face.

facial artery, one of a pair of tortuous arteries that arise from the external carotid arteries, divide into four cervical and five facial branches, and supply various organs and tissues in the head.

facial bones, the 14 bones that form the face of the skull. They include two each of the nasal, palatine, inferior nasal concha, maxilla, lacrimal, and zygomatic bones, plus the mandible and vomer.

facial diplegia, a rare neuromuscular condition characterized by bilateral paralysis of various muscles of the face.

facial hemiplegia, paralysis of the muscles of one side of the face.

facial muscle, one of five groups of facial muscles They are the muscles of the scalp, the extrinsic muscles of the ear, the muscles of the nose, the muscles of the eyelid, and the muscles of the mouth.

facial nerve, either of a pair of mixed sensory and motor cranial nerves that arise from the brainstem at the base of the pons and divide in front of the ear into six branches, innervating the scalp, forehead, eyelids, muscles of facial expression, cheeks, and jaw.

facial nerve paralysis, a loss of voluntary control of the muscles of the face, usually on one side.

facial neuralgia, the occurrence of pain in the middle ear and auditory canal caused by inflammation of the otic ganglion.

facial palsy [L, *facies,* face; Gk, *paralyein,* to be palsied], a loss of motor nerve function in the facial muscles.

facial paralysis, an abnormal condition characterized by the partial or total loss of the functions of the facial muscles or the loss of sensation in the face. It may be caused by disease or by trauma.

facial perception, the ability to judge the distance and direction of objects through the sensation felt in the skin of the face. The phenomenon is commonly experienced by those who are blind.

facial tic [L, *facies,* face; Fr, *tic,* twitching], any repetitive, spasmodic, and involuntary contraction of groups of facial muscles.

facial vein, one of a pair of superficial veins that drain deoxygenated blood from the superficial structures of the face.

facies /fā′shē-ēs/, *pl.* **facies** /fā′shē-ēs/ [L, face], 1. the face. 2. the surface of any body structure, part, or organ. 3. facial expression or appearance.

facilitation /fəsil′itā′shən/ [L, *facilitas,* easiness], 1. the enhancement or reinforcement of any action or function so that it can be performed more easily. 2. (in neurology) the phenomenon whereby two or more afferent impulses that individually are not strong enough to elicit a response in a neuron can collectively produce a reflex discharge greater than the sum of the separate responses.

facilitory casting /fəsil′itôr′ē/, a method of making prosthetic casts with materials that increase muscle tone in a specific group while increasing or decreasing range of motion.

faciolingual /fā′shōling′gwəl/, pertaining to the face and tongue.

F.A.C.O.G., abbreviation for *Fellow of the American College of Obstetricians and Gynecologists.*

F.A.C.P., abbreviation for *Fellow of the American College of Physicians.*

F.A.C.S., abbreviation for *Fellow of the American College of Surgeons.*

facsimile (fax), a method of transmitting images or printed matter by electronic means. Images are scanned, converted into electronic signals, and sent to a fax receiver, which reconverts the electronic data into a duplicate of the original image.

F.A.C.S.M., abbreviation for *Fellow of the American College of Sports Medicine.*

factitial /fakti′shəl/ [L, *facticius,* artificial], artificial or self-induced.

factitial dermatitis, a skin rash caused by the patient, usually for secondary gain or as a manifestation of a psychiatric illness.

factitious disorder /faktish′əs/, a *DSM-IV* diagnosis marked by disease symptoms caused by deliberate efforts of a person to gain attention. Such actions may be repeated, even when the individual is aware of the hazards involved.

factor, 1. one of a number of elements contributing to a whole. 2. a number by which another number is exactly divisible. 3. one of a number of elements that effect a specific result.

factor I. See **fibrinogen.**

factor II. See **prothrombin.**

factor III. See **thromboplastin.**

factor IV, a designation for calcium that is involved in the process of blood coagulation.

factor V, an unstable procoagulant needed to convert prothrombin rapidly to thrombin.

factor VI, a hypothetic chemical agent that some suggest is derived from proaccelerin, or factor V, in the process of blood coagulation.

factor VII, a blood procoagulant present in the blood plasma and synthesized in the liver in the presence of vitamin K.

factor VIII, a coagulation factor present in normal plasma but deficient in the blood of persons with hemophilia A.

factor IX, a coagulation factor present in normal plasma but deficient in the blood of persons with hemophilia B.

factor IX complex, a hemostatic containing factors II, VII, IX, and X. It is prescribed in the treatment of hemophilia B. It is a vitamin K–dependent protein synthesized in the liver.

factor X, a coagulation factor that occurs in normal plasma but is deficient in some inherited defects in coagulation.

factor XI, a coagulation factor present in normal plasma. Deficiency results in hemophilia C.

factor XII, a coagulation factor present in normal plasma that triggers the formation of bradykinin and associated enzymatic reactions.

factor XIII, a coagulation factor present in normal plasma that acts with calcium to produce an insoluble fibrin clot.

factor-searching study, (in nursing research) a study design that produces a qualitative narrative description that includes categories or classifications of phenomena.

facultative /fak'əltā'tiv/ [L, *facultus*, capability], not obligatory; having the ability to adapt to more than one condition, such as a facultative anaerobe.

facultative aerobe, an organism able to grow under anaerobic conditions but that develops most rapidly in an aerobic environment.

facultative anaerobe, an organism able to grow under aerobic conditions but that develops most rapidly in an anaerobic environment.

faculty /fak'əltē/ [L, *facultus*, capability], **1.** any normal physiologic function or natural ability of a living organism, such as the digestive faculty or the ability to perceive and distinguish sensory stimuli. **2.** an ability to do something specific, such as learn languages or remember names. **3.** any mental ability or power, such as memory or thought. **4.** a department in an institution of learning or the people who teach in a department of such an institution.

fading time, the time required for a constant stimulus applied to a fixed area of the peripheral visual field to stop.

Faget's sign /fazhāz'/ [Jean C. Faget, French physician, 1818–1884], a falling pulse rate associated with a constant temperature, or a constant pulse associated with a rising temperature.

fagicladosporic acid /faj'iklad'ōspôr'ik/, a toxin produced by *Cladosporium epiphyllum*, a member of a genus of fungi that cause "black spot" in stored meat, tinea nigra, and black degeneration of the brain.

Fahrenheit (F) /fer'ənhīt/ [Daniel G. Fahrenheit, German physicist, 1686–1736], a scale for the measurement of temperature in which the boiling point of water is 212° and the freezing point of water is 32° at sea level.

failed forceps, an attempted mid-forceps operation that is abandoned because there is a greater degree of resistance to rotation or traction than anticipated.

failure to thrive (FTT) /fāl'yər/ [L., *fallere*, to deceive; ME, *thriven*, to grasp], the abnormal retardation of growth and development of an infant resulting from conditions that interfere with normal metabolism, appetite, and activity.

faint [OFr, *faindre*, to feign] *nontechnical,* **1.** to lose consciousness, as in a syncopal attack. **2.** a syncopal attack.

faith healing [L, *fidere*, to trust; AS, *hoelen,* to make whole], alleged healing through the power to cause a cure or recovery from an illness or injury without the aid of conventional medical treatment.

The healer is believed to have been given that power by a supernatural force.

falciform ligament /fal'sifôrm/, a triangular or sickle-shaped ligament of the body.

falciparum malaria /falsip'ərəm/ [L, *falx,* sickle, *forma,* form; It, bad air], the most severe form of malaria, caused by the protozoon *Plasmodium falciparum.* The condition affects red blood cells and is characterized by extremely grave systemic symptoms, mental confusion, enlarged spleen, edema, gastrointestinal symptoms, and anemia.

fallectomy /fəlek'təmē/, the surgical removal of one or both of the fallopian tubes.

fallen arch, a broken down foot arch, which often results in a flat deformity or splay foot. The condition may involve the longitudinal arch, the transverse arch, or both. When the longitudinal arch is involved, the condition is called *flatfoot* or **pes planus.**

fallopian canal [Gabriele Fallopio, Italian anatomist, 1523–1562; L, *canalis*], a passageway for the facial nerve through the petrous bone.

fallopian tube /fəlō'pē-ən/ [Gabriele Fallopio], one of a pair of ducts opening at one end into the uterus and at the other end into the peritoneal cavity, over the ovary. Each tube serves as the passage through which an ovum is carried to the uterus and through which spermatozoa move out toward the ovary.

fallout [AS, *feallan,* to fall, *ut*], the deposition of radioactive debris after a nuclear explosion.

Fall Prevention, a Nursing Interventions Classification defined as instituting of special precautions for a patient at risk for injury from falling.

false ankylosis [L, *fallere,* to deceive; Gk, *agkylosis,* joint stiffness], a type of joint immobility that results from abnormal inflexibility of body parts outside the joint.

false diverticulum [L, *fallere,* to deceive, *diverticulare,* to turn aside], a protrusion of mucous membrane through a muscular coat defect of a hollow organ.

false imprisonment [L, *falsus,* deceptive; ME, *imprisonen*], (in law) the intentional unjustified, nonconsensual detention or confinement of a person for any length of time.

false joint [L, *fallere,* to deceive, *jungere,* to join], a joint that develops at the site of a former fracture.

false negative, an incorrect result of a diagnostic test or procedure that falsely indicates the absence of a finding, condition, or disease.

false-negative rate [L, *fallere,* to deceive, *negare,* to deny, *ratum,* calculate], the rate of occurrence of negative test results in subjects known to have the disease or behavior for which an individual is being tested.

false neuroma, 1. a neoplasm that does not contain nerve elements. 2. a cystic neuroma.

false pelvis, the part of the pelvis superior to a plane passing through the linea terminalis.

false personification, (in psychiatry) the labeling and prejudgment of others without validating evidence.

false positive, a test result that wrongly indicates the presence of a disease or other condition the test is designed to reveal.

false-positive rate [L, *fallere,* to deceive, *positivus + ratum,* calculate], the rate of occurrence of positive test results in tests of individuals known to be free of a disease or disorder for which an individual is being tested.

false suture, an immovable fibrous joint in which rough articulating surfaces form the connection between certain bones of the skull. Two kinds of false sutures are **sutura plana** and **sutura squamosa.**

false transactions, (in transactional analysis), transactions in which communication is stopped or distorted when one individual relates from a different ego state than expected.

false vertebra, one of the vertebral segments that form the sacrum and the coccyx.

false vocal cord, either of two thick folds of mucous membrane in the larynx separating the ventricle from the vestibule.

falx /falks, fôlks/, *pl.* **falces** /fal′sēz, fôl′sēz/ [L, sickle], 1. a sickle-shaped structure. 2. sickle-shaped.

falx cerebelli /ser′əbel′ī/, a small sickle-shaped process of the dura mater attached to the occipital bone above and projecting into the posterior cerebellar notch between the two cerebellar hemispheres.

falx cerebri /ser′əbrī/, a sickle-shaped fold of dura mater membrane extending into and following along the longitudinal fissure of the two hemispheres of the cerebrum.

falx inguinalis, transverse and internal oblique muscles.

falx ligamentosa, the broad ligament of the liver.

FAM, an anticancer drug combination of fluorouracil, doxorubicin, and mitomycin.

famciclovir, an antiviral drug prescribed in the treatment of acute herpes zoster.

familial /fəmi′yəl/ [L, *familia,* household], pertaining to a characteristic, condition, or disease that is present in some families and not others or that occurs in more family members than would be expected by chance.

familial cretinism, a rare genetic disorder caused by an inborn error of metabolism resulting from an enzyme deficiency that interferes with thyroid hormone biosynthesis. Clinical manifestations include lethargy, stunted growth, and mental retardation.

familial histiocytic reticulosis [L, *familia,* household; Gk, *histion,* web, *kytos,* cell; L, *reticulum,* little net; Gk, *osis,* condition], a hereditary disease, transmitted as an autosomal-recessive trait, characterized by anemia, granulocytopenia, and thrombocytopenia. Phagocytosis of blood cells and infiltration of bone marrow by histocytes commonly cause death in childhood.

familial hypercholesterolemia, an inherited disorder transmitted as a dominant trait and characterized by a high level of serum cholesterol, tendinous xanthomas, and early evidence of atherosclerosis, especially of the coronary arteries. Affected individuals at 50 years of age have 3 to 10 times greater risk of ischemic heart disease than the general population. In type IIA familial hypercholesterolemia, only low-density lipoprotein (LDL) level is elevated, whereas in type IIB LDL and very low–density lipoprotein levels are increased.

familial periodic paralysis [L, *familia,* household; Gk, *peri,* near, *hodos,* way, *paralysein,* to be palsied], a rare inherited disorder in which clients suffer attacks of general flaccid paralysis after attacks of hypokalemia (potassium depletion). The episodes may follow administration of glucose and are relieved by administration of potassium chloride.

familial polyposis, an abnormal condition characterized by multiple polyps in the colon and rectum. The disease has high malignancy potential and is inherited. A kind of familial polyposis is **Gardner's syndrome.**

family [L, *familia,* household], 1. a group of people related by heredity, such as parents, children, and siblings. The term sometimes is broadened to include persons related by marriage or those living in the same household who are emotionally attached, interact regularly, and share concerns for the growth and development of the group and its individual members. 2. a group of persons having a common surname, such as the Anderson family. 3. a category of animals or plants situated on a taxonomic scale between order and genus. Humans are members of the genus *Homo sapiens,* which is a part of the hominid family, which, in turn, is a division of the primate order of mammals. —**familial,** *adj.*

family Apgar, a family therapy rating system in which the name Apgar contains the first letters of five words—*a*daptability, *p*artnership, *g*rowth, *a*ffection, and *re*solve—that represent the questionnaire categories. Each family member indicates a degree of satisfaction in each of the five categories on a scale of 0 to 2. The system is used most frequently in studies of families with a geriatric member.

family care leave, absence from a job that is permitted for an employee to care for a family member who is ill, disabled, or pregnant. The U.S. Family and Medical Leave Act of 1993 provides 12 weeks of unpaid leave per year from a job for the birth or adoption of a child; for the care of a seriously ill child, spouse, or parent; or for a serious illness affecting the employee. The law applies only to companies with 50 or more employees. Employers must guarantee that a worker can return to the same or a comparable job.

family-centered care, primary health care that includes an assessment and implementation of actions needed to maintain or improve the health of the family unit and its members.

family-centered maternity care, a system for the delivery of safe, high-quality health care adapted to the physical and psychosocial needs of the patient, the patient's entire family, and the newly born offspring.

family-centered nursing care, nursing care directed to improving the potential health of a family or any of its members.

family counseling, a program of providing information and professional guidance to members of a family concerning specific health matters, such as the care of a severely retarded child or the risk of transmitting a known genetic defect.

family disorganization, a breakdown of a family system. It may be associated with parental overburdening or loss of support systems for family members. Family disorganization can contribute to the loss of social controls that families usually impose on their members.

family dynamics, the forces at work within the family that produce particular behaviors or symptoms.

family functions, processes by which the family operates as a whole, including communication and manipulation of the environment for problem solving.

family history, an essential part of a patient's medical history in which he or she is asked about the health of members of the immediate family in a series of specific questions to discover any disorders to which the patient may be particularly vulnerable.

Family Integrity Promotion, a Nursing Interventions Classification defined as promotion of family cohesion and unity.

Family Integrity Promotion: Childbearing Family, a Nursing Interventions Classification defined as facilitation of the growth of individuals or families who are adding an infant to the family unit.

Family Involvement, a Nursing Interventions Classification defined as facilitating family participation in the emotional and physical care of the patient.

family medicine, the branch of medicine that is concerned with the diagnosis and treatment of health problems in people of either sex and any age. Practitioners of family medicine are often called family practice physicians, or family physicians. They often act as the primary health care providers.

Family Mobilization, a Nursing Interventions Classification defined as use of family strengths to influence patient's health in a positive direction.

family myths, myths that are constructed to deny the reality of family situations.

family nurse practitioner (FNP), a nurse practitioner possessing skills necessary for the detection and management of acute self-limiting conditions and management of chronic stable conditions. An FNP provides primary ambulatory care for families in collaboration with primary care physicians.

family of origin, the family into which a person is born.

family of procreation, the family a person forms through marriage and/or childbearing.

family physician, a medical practitioner of the specialty of family medicine.

Family Planning: Contraception, a Nursing Interventions Classification defined as facilitation of pregnancy prevention by provision of information about the physiologic characteristics of reproduction and methods to control contraception.

Family Planning: Infertility, a Nursing Interventions Classification defined as management, education, and support of the patient and significant other undergoing evaluation and treatment for infertility.

Family Planning: Unplanned Pregnancy, a Nursing Interventions Classification defined as facilitation of decision making regarding pregnancy outcome.

F

family practice [L, *familia*, household; Gk, *praktikos*, ready for action], a medical specialty that encompasses several branches of medicine, including internal medicine, preventive medicine, pediatrics, surgery, psychiatry, and obstetrics and gynecology; includes client management, counseling, and problem solving; and coordinates total health care delivery to all members of a family, regardless of sex or age.

family practice physician, a practitioner of family medicine, usually one who has completed a residency program in the specialty.

family processes, altered, a NANDA-accepted nursing diagnosis of the state in which a family that normally functions effectively experiences a dysfunction. Defining characteristics include the inability of the family system to meet the physical, emotional, spiritual, or security needs of its members; the inability of family members to communicate adequately, to express or accept a wide range of feelings, or to relate to each other for mutual growth and maturation; ineffective decision-making processes; inappropriate or poorly communicated family rules, rituals, or symbols; and unexamined family myths.

family processes, altered: alcoholism, a NANDA-accepted nursing diagnosis of the state in which the psychosocial, spiritual, and physiologic functions of the family unit are chronically disorganized, leading to conflict, denial of problems, resistance to change, ineffective problem solving, and a series of self-perpetuating crises. Defining characteristics include a wide range of feelings, roles and relationships, and behaviors. Feelings include decreased self-esteem, anger, frustration, powerlessness, anxiety, distress, insecurity, responsibility for the alcoholic's behavior, resentment, and shame or embarrassment. Roles and relationships include disturbed family dynamics, ineffective spouse communication, altered role function, inconsistent parenting, family denial, intimacy dysfunction, and chronic family problems. Behaviors include inappropriate expression of anger, difficulty with intimate relationships, loss of control of drinking, ineffective problem-solving skills, enabling of alcoholic to maintain drinking, manipulation, dependency, criticizing, and inadequate understanding or knowledge of alcoholism.

Family Process Maintenance, a Nursing Interventions Classification defined as minimization of family process disruption effects.

family structure, the composition and membership of the family and the organization and patterning of relationships among individual family members. In planning health care for a family member or the entire family, an awareness of that family's structure may be important.

Family Support, a Nursing Interventions Classification defined as promotion of family values, interests, and goals.

family therapy, (in psychiatry) a therapy modality that focuses treatment on the process between family members that supports and perpetuates symptoms; a way of conceptualizing human relationship problems that focuses on the context in which an emotional problem is generated.

Family Therapy, a Nursing Interventions Classification defined as assisting family members to move their family toward a more productive way of living.

famotidine /famot'idēn/, an oral and parenteral antiulcer drug prescribed in treatment of duodenal ulcer and pathologic hypersecretory conditions such as Zollinger-Ellison syndrome.

fan beam, a geometric pattern that results from collimating a spatially extended x-ray beam with a long, narrow slit.

FANCAP, *U.S.* a mnemonic device for helping student nurses learn to assess, provide, and evaluate direct patient care. It stands for fluids, aeration, nutrition, communication, activity, and pain.

Fanconi's anemia /fankō'nēs/ [Guido Fanconi, Swiss pediatrician, 1892–1979], a rare, usually congenital disorder transmitted as an autosomal-recessive trait, characterized by aplastic anemia in childhood or early adult life, bone abnormalities, chromatin breaks, and developmental anomalies.

Fanconi's syndrome, [Guido Fanconi], a group of disorders that includes renal tubular function, glycosuria, phosphaturia, and bicarbonate wasting. The condition is often marked by osteomalacia, acidosis, rickets, and hypokalemia. Idiopathic Fanconi's syndrome is inherited and usually accompanies other genetic disorders such as Wilson's disease. Acquired Fanconi's syndrome is usually the result of toxicity from various sources, including ingestion of outdated tetracycline.

fango /fän'gō/ [It, mud], mud taken from thermal springs at Battaglia, Italy, and used to treat gout and other rheumatic diseases.

fan lateral projection, a technique for making a radiographic image of the hand without superimposition of the phalanges. The patient places the fingers around a sponge wedge designed so that each finge appears separately, in a fanlike pattern, on the x-ray film.

fantasy /fan'təsē/ [Gk, *phantasia,* imagination], **1.** the unrestrained free play of the imagination; fancy. **2.** a mental image, usually distorted or grotesque, that is often the result of the action of drugs or a disease of the central nervous system. **3.** the mental process of transforming undesirable experiences into imagined events.

F.A.O.T.A., abbreviation for *Fellow of the American Occupational Therapy Association.*

F.A.P.T.A., abbreviation for *Fellow of the American Physical Therapy Association.*

farad (F) /fer'ad/ [Michael Faraday, English scientist, 1791–1871], a unit of capacitance that increases the potential difference between the plates of a capacitor by 1 volt with a charge of 1 coulomb.

Faraday cage /fer'ədā/, (in nuclear magnetic resonance imaging) a wire-mesh cage that surrounds the magnetic resonance scanner to shield it from stray radiofrequency waves.

Farber test, a microscopic examination of newborn meconium for lanugo and squamous cells. The absence of hair or skin cells is suggestive of intestinal obstruction or atresia and requires further evaluation.

Far Eastern hemorrhagic fever, a form of epidemic hemorrhagic fever, indigenous to Asia, that is transmitted by a virus carried by an Asian rodent. The infection is characterized by chills, fever, headache, abdominal pain, nausea, vomiting, anorexia, and extreme thirst.

farmer's lung [L, *firmare,* to make firm], a respiratory disorder caused by the inhalation of actinomycetes or other organic dusts from moldy hay. It is a form of hypersensitivity pneumonitis.

far point [ME, *farr* + L, *punctus,* pricked], **1.** the farthest distance from the eye at which an object can be seen clearly when the eye is at rest and accommodation is fully relaxed. **2.** the point at which the visual axes of the two eyes meet when at rest.

F²ARV, abbreviation for Fear/Frustration (F²), Anger, Rage, and Violence, a highly volatile emotional reaction that escalates from fear or frustration and proceeds sequentially through anger and rage to violence.

FAS, abbreviation for **fetal alcohol syndrome.**

fascia /fash'ē-ə/, *pl.* **fasciae** [L, band], the fibrous connective tissue of the body that may be separated from other specifically organized structures such as tendons, aponeuroses, and ligaments. It varies in thickness and density and in the amounts of fat, collagenous fiber, elastic fiber, and tissue fluid it contains. —**fascial,** *adj.*

fascia bulbi, a thin membranous socket that envelops the eyeball from the optic nerve to the ciliary region and allows it to move freely.

fascial cleft /fash'ē-əl/ [L, *fascia* + ME, *clift*], a place of cleavage between two contiguous fascial surfaces, such as the deep fasciae and the subcutaneous fasciae.

fascial compartment, a part of the body that is walled off by fascial membranes, usually containing a muscle or group of muscles or an organ.

fascial membrane lamination, a pad of connective tissue that contains fat and an occasional blood vessel or lymph node.

fascia thoracolumbalis, the extensive subdivision of the vertebral fascia that sheaths the sacrospinalis muscle.

fascicular /fəsik'yələr/ [L, *fasciculus,* little bundle], pertaining to something arranged in bundles, such as groups of nerve or muscle fibers.

fascicular neuroma, a neoplasm composed of myelinated nerve fibers.

fasciculation /fasik'yŏŏlā'shən/ [L, *fasciculus,* little bundle, *atio,* process], a localized uncoordinated, uncontrollable twitching of a single muscle group innervated by a single motor nerve fiber or filament that may be palpated and seen under the skin. Fasciculation of the heart muscle is known as fibrillation. —**fascicular,** *adj.,* **fasciculate,** *v.*

fasciculus /fəsik'yələs/, *pl.* **fasciculi** [L, little bundle], a small bundle of muscle, tendon, or nerve fibers. —**fascicular,** *adj.*

fasciitis /fas'ē-ī'tis/, **1.** an inflammation of the connective tissue that may be caused by streptococcal or other types of infection, an injury, or an autoimmune reaction. **2.** an abnormal benign growth (*Pseudosarcomatous fasciitis*) resembling a tumor that develops in the subcutaneous oral tissues, usually in the cheek.

fasciodesis /fā'sē-ōdē'sis/, a surgical procedure in which a fascia is attached to another fascia or to a tendon.

fascioliasis /fas'ē-ōlī'əsis/ [L, *fasciola,* little bundle; Gk, *osis,* condition], infection by the liver fluke *Fasciola hepatica.* It is characterized by epigastric pain, fever, jaundice, eosinophilia, urticaria, and diarrhea; fibrosis of the liver is a consequence of prolonged infection.

fasciolopsiasis /fas'ē-ōlopsī'əsis/ [L, *fasciola,* little band; Gk, *opsis,* appearance, *osis,* condition], an intestinal infection prevalent in Asia. It is characterized by abdominal pain, diarrhea, constipation, eosinophilia, ascites, and sometimes edema.

It is caused by the fluke *Fasciolopsis buski.*

Fasciolopsis buski /fas′ē-əlop′sis bus′kē/, a species of fluke that is an important intestinal parasite endemic in Asia and the tropics. In the United States and other countries it is occasionally found in imported food products.

fascioscapulohumeral muscular dystrophy /fas′ē-ōskap′yəlōhyōō′mərəl/ [L, *fasciculus,* little bundle, *scapula,* shoulder blade, *humerus,* shoulder], an abnormal congenital condition that is one of the main types of muscular dystrophy. It is characterized by progressive symmetric wasting of the skeletal muscles, especially the muscles of the face, the shoulders, and the upper arms, without any associated neural or sensory disorders.

fasciotomy /fas′ē-ot′əmē/, a surgical incision into an area of fascia.

F.A.S.R.T., abbreviation for *Fellow of the American Society of Radiologic Technologists.*

fast [AS, *faest,* firm], **1.** resistant to change, especially to the action of a specific drug or chemical, as a staining agent. **2.** abstinence from all or certain foods.

fast-acting insulin, one of a group of insulin preparations in which the onset of action is approximately 1 hour and the duration of the action is approximately 6 to 14 hours. Fast-acting insulins include **insulin regular, prompt insulin zinc suspension,** and **semilente.**

fast brushing, the use of a battery-powered brush to stimulate C fibers (group IV afferent neurons), which send many collaterals to the reticular activating system.

fastigial nucleus /fastij′ē-əl/, one of a group of deep cerebellar nuclei that receive input from the medial zone of the cerebellum. It is involved in the control of posture and equilibrium.

fastigium /fastij′ē-əm/ [L, ridge], **1.** the highest point in the course of a fever, or the most symptomatic point in the course of an illness. **2.** the angle at the top of the roof of the fourth ventricle in the brain.

fasting [AS, *foestan,* to observe], the act of abstaining from food for a specific period, usually for therapeutic or religious purposes.

fast neutron therapy, a radiotherapeutic technique used in the treatment of certain soft tissue sarcomas.

fast pain, a localized sensation of discomfort felt immediately after a noxious stimulus is delivered.

fast smear, a cytologic sample of tissue scrapings from the vaginal-cervical area, smeared on a microscope slide and fixed immediately for routine screening.

fast-twitch (FT) fiber, a muscle fiber that can develop high tension rapidly.

fat [AS, *faett*], **1.** a substance composed of lipids or fatty acids and occurring in various forms or consistencies ranging from oil to tallow. **2.** a type of body tissue composed of cells containing stored fat (depot fat). Stored fat is usually identified as white fat, which is found in large cellular vesicles, or brown fat, which consists of lipid droplets. Stored fat contains more than twice as many calories per gram as sugars and serves as a source of quickly mobilized body energy.

fatal /fā′təl/ [L, *fatum,* what has been spoken], leading inevitably to death.

fatality /fātal′itē/, [L, *fatalis,* preordained], **1.** an individual case of death. **2.** a condition, disease, or disaster resulting in death.

fatality rate, the death rate observed in a specified group of people involved in a simultaneous event.

fat embolism, a circulatory condition characterized by the blocking of an artery by a plug of fat. The embolus enters the circulatory system after the fracture of a long bone or, less commonly, after traumatic injury to adipose tissue or to a fatty liver. Fat embolism usually occurs suddenly 12 to 36 hours after an injury and is characterized by symptoms related to the site occluded, such as severe chest pain, pallor, dyspnea, tachycardia, delirium, prostration, and in some cases coma.

father complex [L, *pater+ complecti,* to embrace], *nontechnical.* a repressed desire for an incestuous relationship with one's father.

father fixation, an arrest in psychosexual development characterized by an abnormally persistent, close, and often paralyzing emotional attachment to one's father.

fatigability /fat′igəbil′itē/, a tendency to become tired or exhausted quickly or easily. It may occur in certain types of cells that undergo periods of excessive activity.

fatigue /fətēg′/ [L, *fatigare,* to tire], a state of exhaustion or a loss of strength or endurance, such as may follow strenuous physical activity. **2.** loss of ability of tissues to respond to stimuli that normally evoke muscular contraction or other activity. **3.** an emotional state associated with extreme or extended exposure to psychic pressure, as in battle or combat fatigue.

fatigue, a NANDA-accepted nursing diagnosis of an overwhelming sense of exhaustion and decreased capacity for physical and mental work, regardless of adequate sleep. Defining characteristics include verbalization of fatigue or lack of energy, inability to maintain usual routines, a perceived need for additional energy to accomplish routine tasks, an increase in physical complaints, impaired ability to concentrate, decreased performance, and decreased libido.

fatigue fever, a benign episode of fever and muscle pain after overexertion. The symptoms are caused by an accumulation of the metabolic waste products of muscle contractions.

fatigue fracture, any fracture that results from excessive physical activity and not from any specific injury, as commonly occurs in the metatarsal bones of runners.

fatigue state [L, *fatigare,* to tire, *status,* condition], the state of lowest energy of a system.

fat injection, transplantation of a patient's own fat to other areas on the body, as to the face to minimize wrinkles or to the lips or penis to augment size.

fat metabolism, the biochemical process by which fats are broken down, incorporated, and used by the cells of the body. Fats provide more food energy than carbohydrates; the catabolism of 1 g of fat provides 9 kcal of heat as compared with 4.1 kcal yielded in the catabolism of 1 g of carbohydrate. Before the final reactions in fat catabolism can occur, fats must be hydrolyzed into fatty acids and glycerol. The body can synthesize only saturated fatty acids. Essential unsaturated fatty acids can be supplied only by diet. Certain hormones such as insulin, growth hormone, adrenocorticotropic hormone, and the glucocorticoids control fat metabolism.

fat necrosis [AS, *faett* + Gk, *nekros,* dead, *osis,* condition], a condition caused by trauma or infection in which neutral fats are broken down into fatty acids and glycerol. Fat necrosis occurs most commonly in the breasts and subcutaneous areas. It also may develop in the abdominal cavity after an episode of pancreatitis causes a release of enzymes from the pancreas.

fat overload syndrome, a condition of hepatosplenomegaly, anemia, gastrointestinal disturbances, and very high triglyceride levels resulting from intravenous administration of fat emulsion.

fat pad, a mass of closely packed fat cells surrounded by fibrous tissue septa. Fat pads may be generously supplied with capillaries and nerve endings. Intraarticular fat pads are also covered by a layer of synovial cells.

fatty acid [AS, *faett* + L, *acidus,* sour], any of several organic acids produced by the hydrolysis of neutral fats. Essential fatty acids are unsaturated molecules that

cannot be produced by the body and must therefore be included in the diet. Some kinds of are **arachidonic** and **linoleic.**

fatty alcohol, a hydroxy derivative of a hydrocarbon from the paraffin series.

fatty cirrhosis [AS, *faett* + Gk, *kirrhos,* yellow, *osis,* condition], a form of cirrhosis that develops over a long period of poor nutrition, resulting in fatty infiltration of the liver.

fatty degeneration [AS, *faett* + L, *degenerare,* to deviate], the abnormal deposition of fat within cells or the fatty tissue invasion of organs.

fatty diarrhea, the excretion of fatty, foul-smelling stools that float on water. The condition is associated with chronic pancreatic disease and other malabsorption disorders.

fatty infiltration, a normal phase of breast development characterized by accumulation of increased amounts of fat around the parenchymal breast tissue.

fatty infiltration of heart [AS, *faett* + L, *in* + *filtrare* + AS, *heorte*], an accumulation of large amounts of fat within the cells of the heart. The heart muscle may be marked by irregular streaks of pale areas of fatty infiltration. It is sometimes associated with severe and prolonged anemia.

fatty liver, an accumulation of triglycerides in the liver. The causes include obesity, diabetes, excessive consumption of alcohol, intravenous administration of drugs such as tetracycline and corticosteroids, and exposure to toxic substances such as carbon tetrachloride and yellow phosphorus.

fatty stool [AS, *faett* + *stol,* seat], a stool containing an abnormally large amount of fat, as indicated by its floating on water.

fatty tissue [AS, *faett* + OFr, *tissu*], loose connective tissue with many cells that contain fat vacuoles.

fauces /fô′sēz/ [L, *faux,* throat], the opening of the mouth into the pharynx. The anterior pillars of the fauces form the glossopalatine arch; the posterior pillars form the pharyngopalatine arch.

faucial isthmus /fô′shəl/, an aperture between the pharynx and the mouth.

faulty restoration /fôl′tē/ [L, *fallere,* to deceive, *restaurare,* to renew], any dental filling or fabrication that contains flaws, such as overhanging or incomplete fillings and incorrect anatomic characteristics of occlusal and marginal ridge areas.

favism /fä′vizəm/ [It, *fava,* bean], an acute hemolytic anemia caused by ingestion of the beans or inhalation of the pollen from the *Vicia faba* (fava) plant. Symptoms include dizziness, headache,

F

vomiting, fever, jaundice, eosinophilia, and often diarrhea.

favus /fā′vəs/ [L, honeycomb], a fungal infection of the scalp, skin, or nails, more common in children than adults. It is caused by *Trichophyton* fungi. Favus is characterized by thick yellow crusts with suppuration, a honeycomb appearance, a distinct "mousy" odor, permanent scars, and alopecia.

fax, abbreviation for **facsimile.**

F.C.A.P., abbreviation for *Fellow of the College of American Pathologists.*

FCC, abbreviation for **Federal Communications Commission.**

F$_c$ fragment, a part of a molecule of an antibody that has been split by a proteolytic enzyme. The F$_c$ part is sometimes identified as the crystallizable fragment.

FDA, abbreviation for **Food and Drug Administration.**

FDI numbering system [Fr, Fédération Dentaire Internationale], an internationally used two-digit system for identifying and referring to teeth established through the FDI, headquartered in Paris, France.

Fe, symbol for the element **iron.**

fear [ME, *fer,* danger], a NANDA-accepted nursing diagnosis of a feeling of dread related to an identifiable source that the client is able to validate. The defining characteristic is an ability to identify the source of fear.

fear-tension-pain syndrome, a concept formulated by Grantly Dick-Read, M.D., to explain the pain commonly expected and reported in childbirth. The concept proposes that attitudes induce anxiety before labor and cause fear in labor. He advocated education, exercise, and warm emotional and physical support in labor to counteract the syndrome and coined the term *natural childbirth* for a labor or delivery in which the woman participates in a natural experience.

febrifacient /feb′rifāshənt/, an agent that induces a fever.

febrile /fē′bril, feb′ril/ [L, *febris,* fever], pertaining to or characterized by an elevated body temperature, such as a febrile reaction to an infectious agent. **—febrility,** *n.*

febrile delirium [L, *febris,* fever, *delirare,* to rave], a symptom of disordered central nervous system function, with excitement, restlessness, and disorientation accompanying some acute fevers.

febrile seizure, a seizure associated with a febrile illness. Treatment depends on the age of the patient and the number of seizures. Generalized recurrent febrile seizures in children may be treated as grand mal epilepsy.

febrile state [L, *febris,* fever, *status,* condition], a significant increase in body temperature accompanied by increased pulse and respiration rates, anorexia, constipation, insomnia, headache, pains, and irritability.

febrile urine, a deep orange–colored strong-smelling urine of a patient with a fever, usually caused by concentration of the urine as a result of dehydration.

fecal fistula [L, *faex,* waste matter, *fistula,* pipe], an abnormal passage from the colon to the external surface of the body, discharging feces.

fecal impaction, an accumulation of hardened or inspissated feces in the rectum or sigmoid colon that the individual is unable to move. Diarrhea may be a sign of fecal impaction, since only liquid material is able to pass the obstruction. Persons who are dehydrated, nutritionally depleted, on long periods of bed rest; receiving constipating medications; or undergoing barium radiographic studies are at risk of developing fecal impaction.

fecalith /fē′kəlith/ [L, *faex* + Gk, *lithos,* stone], a hard, impacted mass of feces in the colon.

fecal softener, a drug that lowers the surface tension of the fecal mass, allowing the intestinal fluids to penetrate and soften the stool.

feces /fē′sēz/ [L, *faex,* waste matter], waste or excrement from the digestive tract that is formed in the intestine and expelled through the rectum. Feces consist of water, food residue, bacteria, and secretions of the intestines and liver. **—fecal,** *adj.*

fecundation /fē′kəndā′shən, fek′-/ [L, *fecundare,* to make fruitful], impregnation or fertilization; the act of fertilizing. **—fecundate,** *v.*

fecundity /fikun′ditē/, the ability to produce offspring, especially in large numbers and rapidly; fertility. **—fecund** /fek′ənd, fē′kənd/, *adj.*

Federal Communications Commission (FCC), a U.S. federal agency that assigns frequencies for all radio transmitters in the United States, including diathermies.

federally qualified HMO, a health maintenance organization that is qualified to receive federal funding as defined under U.S. regulations.

Federal Register, a document published by the U.S. government each working day to inform the public of executive regulations, presidential orders, hearings and meeting schedules of various federal agencies, and related matters. The *Federal Register* contains announcements of the

Food and Drug Administration, the Environmental Protection Agency, and other government bureaus that regulate matters of health and safety.

Federal Tort Claims Act, a statute passed in 1946 that allows the U.S. federal government to be sued for the wrongful action or negligence of its employees.

Federal Trade Commission (FTC), an agency in the executive branch of the U.S. federal government created to promote trade and to prevent practices that restrain free enterprise and competition, including the area of health care.

Federation Licensing Examination (FLEX), the standardized licensing examination for state licensure of physicians. Developed by the U.S. Federation of State Medical Boards, the examination is based on National Board of Medical Examiners test materials.

feedback [AS, *faedan* + *baec*], (in communication theory) information produced by a receiver and perceived by a sender that informs the sender of the receiver's reaction to the message.

feedforward control, an anticipatory correction in motor behavior. During movement various brain centers depend on feedback from receptors to control motor behavior. If the actual and intended motor behaviors do not match, an error signal is generated, and alterations are made.

feeding [AS, *faedan*], the act or process of taking or giving food or nourishment. Kinds of feeding include **breastfeeding** and **tube feeding.**

Feeding, a Nursing Interventions Classification defined as providing nutritional intake for a patient who in unable to feed self.

fee-for-service [AS, *feoh,* property; L, *servitum,* slavery], **1.** a charge made for a professional activity, such as a physical examination, the fitting of a contraceptive diaphragm, or the monitoring of a person's blood pressure. **2.** a system for the payment of professional services in which the practitioner is paid for the particular service rendered, rather than receiving a salary.

fee-for-service equivalent, (in U.S. managed care) a specialty capitation method in which a fee schedule is developed for service and providers are paid a percentage of the fee schedule.

feeling, 1. a quality of mood. **2.** a subjective experience caused by stimulation of a sensory nerve.

fee schedule, (in U.S. managed care) the specific dollar amount to be charged for each service offered.

fee screen system, a method of establishing payment for physician services that is based on the usual, customary, or reasonable charge according to a regional evaluation.

FEF, abbreviation for **forced expiratory flow.**

Fehling's solution /fā'lingz/ [Hermann C. von Fehling, German chemist, 1812–1885], a solution containing cupric sulfate with sodium hydroxide and potassium sodium tartrate, used for testing for the presence of glucose and other reducing substances in the urine.

Feingold diet /fīn'gōld/, a diet developed by the American pediatrician Benjamin Feingold for treating hyperactive children. The diet excludes foods manufactured with synthetic colorings, flavorings, and preservatives and limits the intake of fruits and vegetables that contain salicylates.

Feldenkrais therapy /fel'dənkrīs/, (in psychiatry) an alternative therapy based on establishment of a good self-image through awareness and correction of body movements.

feldspar /feld'spär/ [Ger, *feld,* field, *spath,* spar], a crystalline mineral of aluminum silicate with potassium, sodium, barium, and calcium. It is an important component of dental porcelain.

fellatio /fəlā'shō/, oral stimulation of the male genitalia.

fellow [AS, *feolaga,* friendly association], **1.** a member of a learned society. **2.** a graduate student who holds a position in a university or college. **3.** a peer, associate, or person of the same class or rank.

Fellow of the American Academy of Nursing (F.A.A.N.), a member of the American Academy of Nursing.

fellowship /fel'ōship/ [As, *feolaga,* friendly association], a grant given to a person to pay for study or training or to allow payment for work on a special project.

felon /tel'ən/ [L, *fel, venom*], a suppurative abscess on the distal phalanx of a finger.

felony /fel'ənē/, (in criminal law) a crime declared by statute to be more serious than a misdemeanor and deserving of a more severe penalty.

Felty's syndrome /fel'tēz/ [Augustus R. Felty, American physician, 1895–1963], hypersplenism that occurs with adult rheumatoid arthritis, characterized by splenomegaly, leukopenia, and frequent infections.

female [L, *femella,* young woman], **1.** pertaining to the sex that has the ability to become pregnant and bear children; feminine. **2.** a female person.

female catheterization, a procedure for removing urine by means of a urinary catheter introduced through the urinary meatus and urethra into the bladder. The procedure is performed for relief of distension if voluntary micturition is not possible (such as after trauma or surgery), as a preparation for and during anesthesia, or if a specimen of urine from the bladder is required or medication is to be instilled into the bladder. A straight catheter or a retention catheter with a balloon may be used.

female circumcision, the surgical excision of the prepuce of the clitoris.

female genital mutilation, the ritual practice in some cultures of excising the entire clitoris without anesthetic, sometimes as part of a maturity initiation rite.

female pseudohermaphroditism, a form of the congenital gonadal disorder in which ovaries are present, irrespective of the condition of the external genitals.

female reproductive system assessment, an evaluation of a patient's genital tract and breasts with an investigation of past and present disorders that may be factors in the individual's current gynecologic condition.

female sexual dysfunction, impaired or inadequate ability of a woman to engage in or enjoy satisfactory sexual intercourse and orgasm. Causes include anxiety, fear, negative emotions associated with sexual arousal and intercourse, and interpersonal problems. Treatment is focused on eliminating physical problems and sexual anxieties and on enhancing erotic sensitivities.

female sterility [L, *femella,* young woman, *sterilis,* barren], a condition of being an infertile woman. The inability to reproduce may result from congenital defects in the reproductive system such as failure of the uterus to develop normally or disease, injury, or corrective surgery that affects functioning of the ovaries, fallopian tubes, uterus, cervix, or vagina.

feminist therapy, an alternative therapy that is both a philosophic approach to the conduct of therapy and a specific type of therapy. The focus of both types is a consciousness raising that focuses on the presence of sexism and sex role stereotyping in society.

feminization /fem'inīzā'shən/ [L, *femina,* woman], **1.** the normal development or induction of female secondary sex characteristics. **2.** the induction of female sex characteristics in a genotypic male. Testicular feminization may be caused by the inability of target tissues to respond to endogenous or administered androgen.

feminizing adrenal tumor /fem'inī'zing/, a rare neoplasm of the adrenal cortex, characterized in males by gynecomastia, hypertension, diffuse pigmentation, a high level of estrogen in urine, and loss of potency.

femoral /fem'ərəl/ [L, *femur,* thigh], pertaining to the femur or the thigh.

femoral artery, an extension of the external iliac artery into the lower limb, starting immediately distal to the inguinal ligament and ending at the junction of the middle and lower thirds of the thigh.

femoral condyle, one of a pair of large flared prominences on the distal end of the femur.

femoral epiphysis, a secondary bone-forming center of the femur, separated from the main part of the bone by cartilage during the period of bone immaturity.

femoral hernia, a hernia in which a loop of intestine descends through the femoral canal into the groin.

femoral nerve, the largest of the seven nerves stemming from the lumbar plexus and the main nerve of the anterior part of the thigh.

femoral pulse, the pulse of the femoral artery, palpated in the groin.

femoral reflex [L, *femur,* thigh, *reflectere,* to bend back], an extension of the knee and a plantar flexion of the toes of the foot that occurs when the skin on the upper anterior third of the thigh is stimulated.

femoral torsion, an extreme lateral or a medial twisting rotation of the femur on its longitudinal axis, which may be caused by the action of the gluteal muscles.

femoral vein, a large vein in the thigh originating in the popliteal vein and accompanying the femoral artery in the proximal two thirds of the thigh. Its distal part lies lateral to the artery; its proximal part, deeper to the artery. Near its termination it is joined by the great saphenous vein.

femur /fē'mər/, *pl.* **femora, femurs** [L, thigh], the thigh bone, which extends from the pelvis to the knee. It is largely cylindric and is the longest and strongest bone in the body. In an erect posture it inclines medially, drawing the knee joint near the line of gravity of the body.

fenestra /fines'trə/, *pl.* **fenestrae** [L, window], **1.** an aperture, as in a bandage or cast, that is cut out to relieve pressure or to administer regular skin care. **2.** a microscopic opening in certain capillaries specialized in filtration, as in the glomerular capillaries of the kidney.

fenestrated /fen'əstrā'tid/ [L, *fenestra,* window], having numerous small holes or openings.

fenestrated drape, a drape with a round or slitlike opening in the center.

fenestration /fen'əstrā'shən/ [L, *fenestra,* window], **1.** a surgical procedure in which an opening is created to gain access to the cavity within an organ or a bone. **2.** an opening created surgically in a bone or organ of the body. **3.** (in dentistry) a procedure to expose a root tip of a tooth to permit drainage of exudate. —**fenestrate,** v.

fenfluramine hydrochloride /fenfloor'-əmēn/, a sympathomimetic anorectic agent prescribed to decrease the appetite in exogenous obesity.

fenoprofen calcium /fē'nəprō'fen/, a nonsteroidal antiinflammatory agent and analgesic prescribed in the treatment of arthritis and other painful inflammatory conditions.

fenoterol /fen'ōter'ol/, a beta-adrenergic drug used in respiratory therapy.

fentanyl, a potent narcotic analgesic, used most commonly with the sedative and antipsychotic drug droperidol as an adjunct in anesthesia.

fentanyl citrate /fen'tənil/, a narcotic analgesic prescribed as an adjunct to general anesthesia, as a preoperative and postoperative analgesic, and as a component in neuroleptanesthesia and analgesia.

Ferguson's reflex, a contraction of the uterus after the cervix is stimulated. The reflex is an important function of labor.

fermentation /fur'məntā'shən/ [L, *fermentare,* to cause to rise], a chemical change that is brought about in a substance by the action of an enzyme or microorganism, especially the anaerobic conversion of foodstuffs to certain products.

fermentative dyspepsia /fərmen'tətiv/, an abnormal condition characterized by impaired digestion associated with the fermentation of digested food.

fermium (Fm) /fur'mē·əm/ [Enrico Fermi, Italian physicist, 1901 1954], a synthetic transuranic metallic element. Its atomic number is 100, its atomic mass (weight) is 257.

ferning test /fur'ning/ [AS, *faern,* fern; L, *testum,* crucible], a technique used to determine the presence of estrogen in the uterine cervical mucus. It is often used to test for ovulation; high levels of estrogen cause the cervical mucus to dry in a fernlike pattern on a slide.

ferredoxin, a nonheme protein containing equal amounts of iron and sulfur. Ferredoxins are involved in electron transport in photosynthesis and nitrogen fixation.

ferric /fer'ik/, pertaining to a cation of iron in which the metal is trivalent, as in ferric chloride and ferric hydroxide.

ferritin /fer'itin/ [L, *ferrum,* iron], an iron compound formed in the intestine and stored in the liver, spleen, and bone marrow for eventual incorporation into hemoglobin molecules. Serum ferritin levels are used as an indicator of the body's iron stores.

ferrokinetics /fer'ōkinet'iks/, the study of iron metabolism.

ferromagnetic /fer'ōmagnat'ik/, pertaining to substances such as iron, nickel, and cobalt that are strongly affected by magnetism.

ferrotherapy /fer'ōther'əpē/, the use of iron and iron compounds in the treatment of illness.

ferrous, pertaining to a compound of iron in which the metal is divalent, such as ferrous ammonium sulfate.

ferrous sulfate /fer'əs/, a hematinic agent prescribed in the treatment of iron deficiency anemia.

fertile /fur'təl/ [L, *fertilis,* fruitful], **1.** capable of reproducing or bearing offspring. **2.** (of a gamete) capable of inducing fertilization or being fertilized. **3.** prolific; fruitful; not sterile. —**fertility,** n., **fertilize,** v.

fertile eunuch syndrome, a hypogonadotropic hormonal disorder that occurs only in males in which the quantity of testosterone and follicle-stimulating hormone is inadequate for the inducement of spermatogenesis and the development of secondary sexual characteristics.

fertile period, the time in the menstrual cycle during which fertilization may occur. Spermatozoa can survive for 48 to 72 hours; the ovum lives for 24 hours. Thus the fertile period begins 2 to 3 days before ovulation and lasts for 2 to 3 days afterward.

fertility /fərtil'itē/, the ability to reproduce.

Fertility Preservation, a Nursing Interventions Classification defined as providing information, counseling, and treatment that facilitate reproductive health and the ability to conceive.

fertility rate, the number of live births divided by the number of females aged 15 through 44 years of age. It is usually expressed as the number per 1000 women.

fertilization /fur'tiltzā'shən/ [L, *fertilis,* fruitful], the union of male and female gametes to form a zygote from which the embryo develops. The process usually takes place in the outer one third of the fallopian tube of the female when a spermatozoon, carried in the seminal fluid discharged during coitus, comes in contact with and penetrates the ovum.

fertilization membrane, a viscous membrane surrounding the fertilized ovum that prevents penetration of additional spermatozoa.

fertilizin /fərtil'izin/, a glycoprotein found on the plasma membrane of the ovum in various species.

fester, 1. to become superficially inflamed and pus-producing. 2. to become increasingly virulent.

festinant /fes'tinənt/, pertaining to a gait pattern that accelerates involuntarily as a result of a nervous system disorder. The increased rate of walking represents an automatic attempt by the body to overtake a displaced center of gravity.

festinating gait [L, *festinare,* to hasten], a manner of walking in which a person's speed increases in an unconscious effort to "catch up" with a displaced center of gravity. It is a common characteristic of Parkinson's disease.

festoon [Fr, *feston,* scallop], a carving in the base material of a denture that simulates the contours of the natural gingival tissues.

FET, abbreviation for **forced expiratory time.**

fetal /fē'təl/ [L, *fetus,* fruitful], pertaining to the final stage of development of an embryonic mammal. In humans the fetal period extends from the end of the eighth week of intrauterine life until birth.

fetal abortion [L, *fetus*], termination of pregnancy after the twentieth week of gestation but before the fetus has developed enough to live outside the uterus.

fetal advocate, a person who regards the health and well-being of the fetus as a matter of top priority.

fetal age, the age of the conceptus computed from the time elapsed since fertilization.

fetal alcohol syndrome (FAS) [L, *fetus* + Ar, *alkohl,* essence; Gk, *syn,* together, *dromos,* course], a set of congenital psychologic, behavioral, and physical abnormalities that tend to appear in infants whose mothers consumed at least 1 ounce of absolute alcohol per day during pregnancy. It is characterized by typical craniofacial and limb defects, cardiovascular defects, intrauterine growth retardation, and retarded development. The most serious cases have involved infants born to mothers who were chronic alcoholics and drank heavily during pregnancy. Women who drank less reportedly gave birth to infants with less serious malformations, or **fetal alcohol effects (FAEs),** but it is not known whether there is a lower limit to alcohol consumption during pregnancy or a particular period in embryonic life when the offspring is most vulnerable to effects of alcohol.

fetal alveoli, the terminal pulmonary sacs of a fetus, which are filled with fluid before birth.

fetal asphyxia, a condition of hypoxemia, hypercapnia, and respiratory and metabolic acidosis that may occur in the uterus.

fetal attitude, the relationship of the fetal parts to each other. An example is the "military" attitude, in which the fetal head is not flexed and the chin is not on the chest as usual but is held straight up.

fetal bradycardia, an abnormally slow fetal heart rate, usually below 100 beats/min.

fetal circulation, the pathway of blood circulation in the fetus. Oxygenated blood from the placenta travels through the umbilical vein to the heart. The blood enters the right atrium at a pressure sufficient to direct most of the flow across the atrium and through the foramen ovale into the left atrium; thus oxygenated blood is available for circulation through the left ventricle to the head and upper extremities. The blood is returned to the placenta through the umbilical arteries.

fetal death, the intrauterine death of a fetus, or the death of a fetus weighing at least 500 g or after 20 or more weeks of gestation.

fetal distress, a compromised condition of the fetus, usually discovered during labor, characterized by a markedly abnormal rate or rhythm of myocardial contraction.

fetal dose, the estimated amount of radiation received by a fetus during a radiographic examination of a pregnant woman.

fetal heart rate (FHR), the number of heartbeats in the fetus that occur in a given unit of time. The FHR varies in cycles of fetal rest and activity and is affected by many factors, including maternal fever, uterine contractions, maternal-fetal hypotension, and many drugs. The normal FHR is between 110 beats/min and 160 beats/min.

fetal heart sound [L, *fetus,* fruitful; AS, *heorte* + L, *sonus,* sound], the heartbeats of the fetus as detected by auscultation or electronic fetal monitoring. The embryonic heart begins beating at about 14 days of intrauterine life.

fetal hemoglobin, hemoglobin F, the major hemoglobin present in the blood of a fetus and neonate.

fetal hydantoin syndrome (FHS), a complex of birth defects associated with prenatal maternal ingestion of hydantoin derivatives. Symptoms of FHS include microcephaly, hypoplasia or absence of nails on the fingers or toes, abnormal fa cies, mental and physical retardation, and cardiac defects.

fetal lie, the relationship of the long axis of the fetus to the long axis of the mother.

fetal membranes, the structures that protect, support, and nourish the embryo and fetus, including the yolk sac, allantois, amnion, chorion, placenta, and umbilical cord.

fetal mortality, the number of fetal deaths per 1000 births, or per live births.

fetal movements [L, *fetus* + *movere,* to move], muscular motions produced by the fetus in utero beginning around the fifth month of life. The early fetal movements can be felt by the mother.

fetal placenta [L, *fetus* + *placenta,* flat cake], the part of the placenta that is formed from the shaggy chorion frondosum, the villi of which invade the decidua basalis.

fetal position, the relationship of the part of the fetus that presents in the pelvis to four quadrants of the maternal pelvis, identified by initial L (left), R (right), A (anterior), and P (posterior). The presenting part is also identified by initial O (occiput), M (mentum), and S (sacrum). If a fetus presents with the occiput directed to the posterior aspect of the mother's right side, the fetal position is right occiput posterior (ROP).

fetal presentation, the part of the fetus that lies closest to or has entered the true pelvis. Cephalic presentations are vertex, brow, face, and chin. Breech presentations include frank breech, complete breech, incomplete breech, and single or double footling breech. Shoulder presentations are rare.

fetal respiration, the exchange of gases between the blood of the mother and that of the fetus through the placenta.

fetal rotation [L, *fetus* + *rotare,* to rotate], the turning of the head of the fetus as it begins the descent through the birth canal. The fetal head may be rotated by hand or with forceps if needed to guide the body in a proper position for delivery.

fetal stage, (in embryology) the interval from the end of the embryonic stage, at the end of the seventh or eighth week of gestation, to birth, 38 to 42 weeks after the first day of the last menstrual period.

fetal tachycardia, a fetal heart rate that continues at 160 beats/min or more for more than 10 minutes.

fetid /fet'id, fē'tid/ [L, *fetere,* to stink], pertaining to something that has a foul or putrid odor.

fetish [Fr, *fetiche,* artificial], **1.** any object or idea given unreasonable or exces-

sive attention or reverence. **2.** (in psychology) any inanimate object or any body part not of a sexual nature that arouses erotic feelings or fixation. **—fetishism,** *n.*

fetishist /fet'ishist/, a person who believes in or receives erotic gratification from fetishes.

fetochorionic /fē'tōkôr'ē·on'ik/ [L, *fetus,* fruitful; Gk, *chorion,* skin], pertaining to the fetus and the chorion.

fetoglobulins /fē'tōglob'yəlinz/, proteins found in large amounts in fetal blood and normally in very small amounts in adult blood. Th group includes alpha-fetoprotein.

fetography /fētog'rəfē/ [L, *fetus* + Gk, *graphein,* to record], roentgenography of the fetus in utero.

fetology /fētol'əjē/ [L, *fetus* + Gk, *logos,* science], the branch of medicine that is concerned with the fetus in utero, including the diagnosis of abnormalities, congenital anomalies, the prevention of teratogenic influences, and the treatment of certain disorders.

fetometry /fētom'ətrē/ [L, *fetus* + Gk, *metron,* measure], the measurement of the size of the fetus, especially the diameter of the head and circumference of the trunk. A kind of fetometry is **roentgen fetometry.**

fetoplacental /-pləsen'təl/ [L, *fetus* + *placenta,* flat cake], pertaining to the fetus and the placenta.

fetoprotein /-prō'tēn/ [L, *fetus* + Gk, *proteios,* first rank], an antigen that occurs naturally in fetuses and occasionally in adults as the result of certain diseases. Leukemia, hepatoma, sarcoma, and other neoplasms are associated with **beta-fetoprotein** in the blood of adults. An increased amount of **alpha-fetoprotein** in the fetus is diagnostic for neural tube defects.

fetor hepaticus [L, *stench, hepar,* liver], foul-smelling breath associated with severe liver disease.

fetoscope /fē'təskōp'/ [L, *fetus* + Gk, *skopein,* to look], a stethoscope for monitoring the fetal heartbeat through the mother's abdomen.

fetoscopy /fētos'kəpē/, a procedure in which a fetus may be directly observed in utero, using a fetoscope introduced through a small incision in the abdomen under local anesthesia.

fetotoxic /-tok'sik/ [L, *fetus* + Gk, *toxikon,* poison], pertaining to anything that is poisonous to a fetus.

fetus /fē'təs/ [L, fruitful], the unborn offspring of any viviparous animal after it has attained the particular form of the species; more specifically the human being in utero

F

after the embryonic period and the beginning of the development of the major structural features, usually from the eighth week after fertilization until birth. —**fetal, foetal,** *adj.*

fetus amorphus, a shapeless conceptus that has no formed or recognizable parts.

fetus in fetu /infē′tōō/, a fetal anomaly in which a small, imperfectly formed twin, incapable of independent existence, is contained within the body of the normal twin, the autosite.

fetus papyraceus, a twin fetus that has died in utero early in development and has been pressed flat against the uterine wall by the living fetus.

fetus sanguinolentis /sang′gwinəlen′tis/, a darkly colored, partly macerated fetus that has died in utero.

FEV, abbreviation for **forced expiratory volume.**

FEVC, abbreviation for **forced expiratory vital capacity.**

fever [L, *febris*], an abnormal elevation of body temperature above 37° C (98.6° F) caused by disease. Fever results from an imbalance between the elimination and the production of heat. Exercise, anxiety, and dehydration may increase the temperature of healthy people. Infection, neurologic disease, malignancy, pernicious anemia, thromboembolic disease, paroxysmal tachycardia, congestive heart failure, crushing injury, severe trauma, and many drugs may cause the development of fever. Fever has no recognized function in conditions other than infection. It increases metabolic activity by 7% per degree Celsius, requiring a greater intake of food. The course of a fever varies with the cause and condition of the patient and the treatment given.

fever blister, a cold sore caused by herpesvirus I or II. It generally appears around the mouth or nasal mucous membranes following a febrile episode or cold.

fever of unknown origin (FUO), a fever of any duration that proves to be a cause for study and for which there is at least at first no discovery of the cause despite intensive search.

fever treatment, the care and management of a person who has an elevated temperature.

Fever Treatment, a Nursing Interventions Classification defined as management of a patient with hyperpyrexia caused by nonenvironmental factors.

F factor, (in bacterial genetics) an episome present in conjugating male bacteria but absent in females.

FFA, abbreviation for **free fatty acid.**

^{18}F-FDG, symbol for [^{18}F]-2-fluoro-2-deoxy-D-glucose, a sugar analog used in positron emission tomography to determine the local cerebral metabolic rate of glucose as a measure of neural activity in the brain.

FGT cytologic smear, abbreviation for female genital tract cytologic smear, any sample of tissues from the female reproductive tract smeared on a microscope slide for examination.

FHR, abbreviation for **fetal heart rate.**

FHS, abbreviation for **fetal hydantoin syndrome.**

fiber /fī′bər/, **1.** a long, threadlike, acellular structure found in plant and animal tissues. Plant fibers usually consist of structural carbohydrates such as cellulose in cell walls. Animal fibers are composed mainly of the protein collagen, which forms elastic threads of loose connective tissue in skin and other organs. **2.** a skeletal muscle cell. **3.** the axon of a nerve cell.

fiberglass dermatitis, a pruritic papular skin disease produced by mechanical irritation from glass fibers.

fiberoptic bronchoscopy /-op′tik/ [L, *fibra* + Gk, *optikos,* sight], the visual examination of the tracheobronchial tree through a fiberoptic bronchoscope.

fiberoptic duodenoscope, an instrument for visualizing the interior of the duodenum, consisting of an eyepiece, a flexible tube incorporating bundles of coated glass or plastic fibers with special optic properties, and a terminal light.

fiberoptics /-op′tiks/, the technical process by which an internal organ or cavity can be viewed, using glass or plastic fibers to transmit light through a specially designed tube and reflect a magnified image. —**fiberoptic,** *adj.*

fiberscope /fī′bərskōp/ [L, *fibra* + Gk, *skopein,* to look], a flexible fiberoptic instrument designed for the examination of particular organs and cavities of the body and used in bronchoscopy, endoscopy, and gastroscopy.

fibril /fī′bril/ [L, *fibrilla,* small fiber], a small filamentous structure that often is a component of a cell, as in a mitotic spindle.

fibrillation /fī′brilā′shən/ [L, *fibrilla,* small fiber, *atio,* process], involuntary recurrent contraction of a single muscle fiber or of an isolated bundle of nerve fibers. Fibrillation is usually described by the part that is contracting abnormally, such as atrial fibrillation or ventricular fibrillation.

fibrillin /fibri′lin/ [L, *fibrilla,* small fiber], a major component of elastin-associated microfibrils linked to Marfan syndrome by findings of immunohistochemical studies

fibrin /fī′brin/ [L, *fibra,* fiber], a stringy insoluble protein produced by the action of thrombin on fibrinogen in the clotting process. Fibrin is responsible for the semisolid character of a blood clot.

fibrinocellular /fī′brinōsel′yələr/, composed of fibrin and cells, as occurs in some exudates that result from inflammation.

fibrinogen /fībrin′əjən/ [L, *fibra,* fiber; Gk, *genein,* to produce], a plasma protein that is converted into fibrin by thrombin in the presence of calcium ions.

fibrinogenopenia /fī′brinōjen′ōpē′nē·ə/ [L, *fibra* + Gk, *genein,* to produce, *penia,* poverty], a deficiency of fibrinogen in the blood.

fibrinogenous /fī′brinōj′ənəs/ [L, *fibra,* fiber; Gk, *genein,* to produce], pertaining to the characteristics or properties of fibrinogen or the production of fibrin.

fibrinokinase /fī′brinōkī′nās/ [L, *fibra* + Gk, *kinesis,* motion], a nonwater-soluble enzyme in animal tissue that activates plasminogen.

fibrinolysin /fī′brinol′isin/ [L, *fibra* + Gk, *lysein,* to loosen], a proteolytic enzyme that dissolves fibrin. It is formed from plasminogen in the blood plasma.

fibrinolysis /fī′brinol′isis/, the continual process of fibrin decomposition by fibrinolysin that is the normal mechanism for the removal of small fibrin clots. —**fibrinolytic,** *adj.*

fibrinopeptide /fī′hrinōpep′tīd/ [L, *fibra* + Gk, *peptein,* to digest], a product of the action of thrombin on fibrinogen.

fibrinous pericarditis [L, *fibra,* fiber; Gk, *peri,* near, *kardia,* heart, *itis,* inflammation], a condition in which a lymph exudate accumulates on the pericardium and coagulates. The coagulated exudate may acquire a thick buttery appearance.

fibroadenoma /fī·brō·ad′ino′mə/ [L, *fibra* + Gk, *aden,* gland, *oma*], a benign tumor composed of dense epithelial and fibroblastic tissue.

fibroblast /fī′brəblast/ [L, *fibra* + Gk, *blastos,* germ], a flat, elongated undifferentiated cell in the connective tissue that gives rise to various precursor cells such as the chondroblast, collagenoblast, and osteoblast, which form the fibrous, binding, and supporting tissue of the body. —**fibroblastic,** *adj.*

fibroblastoma /-blastōmə/ [L, *fibra* + Gk, *blastos,* germ, *oma*], a tumor derived from a fibroblast, now differentiated as a fibroma or a fibrosarcoma.

fibrocartilage /-kär′tilij/ [L, *fibra* + *cartilago*], cartilage that consists of a dense matrix of white collagenous fibers. —**fibrocartilaginous,** *adj.*

fibrochondritis /-kondrī′tis, an inflammation of fibrocartilage.

fibrochondroma /-kondrō′mə/, a tumor composed of mixed fibrous and cartilaginous tissues.

fibrocyst /fī′brəsist/, **1.** any cystic lesion within a fibrous connective tissue. **2.** a cystic fibroma.

fibrocystic /-sis′tik/, pertaining to a fibrocyst or cystic fibroma.

fibrocystic disease of breast [L, *fibra* + Gk, *kystis* bag], (of the breast) the presence of single or multiple cysts that are palpable in the breasts. The cysts are benign and fairly common, yet must be considered potentially malignant and observed carefully for growth or change.

fibroepithelial papilloma /-ep′ithē′lē·əl/ [L, *fibra* + Gk, *epi,* above, *thele,* nipple; L, *papilla,* nipple; Gk, *oma,* tumor], a benign epithelial tumor containing extensive fibrous tissue.

fibroepithelioma /fī′brō·ep′ithē′lē·ō′mə/ [L, *fibra* + Gk, *epi,* above, *thele,* nipple, *oma,* tumor], a neoplasm consisting of fibrous and epithelial components.

fibrofolliculoma /-folik′yəlō′mə/, a benign tumor derived from the dermal part of a hair follicle.

fibrogliosis /-glī·ō′sis/, the formation of scar tissue in the brain in reaction to a penetrating injury. The scar is produced by fibroblasts and astrocytes.

fibroid /fī′broid/ [L, *fibra* + Gk, *eidos,* form], **1.** having fibers. **2.** *informal.* a fibroma or myoma, particularly of the uterus.

fibroidectomy /fī′broidek′təmē/ [L, *fibra,* fiber; Gk, *eidos,* form, *ektome,* excision], the surgical removal of a fibrous tumor, such as a uterine fibromyoma.

fibrolipoma /fī′brōlipō′mə/, a fibrous tumor that also contains fatty material.

fibroma /fībrō′mə/ [L, *fibra* + Gk, *oma,* tumor], a benign neoplasm consisting largely of fibrous or fully developed connective tissue.

fibroma cavernosum, a tumor that contains large vascular spaces, an excessive amount of fibrous tissue, and blood or lymph vessels.

fibroma cutis, a fibrous tumor of the skin.

fibroma mucinosum, a fibrous tumor in which degenerating mucoid material is present.

fibroma of breast [L, *fibra,* fiber; Gk, *oma,* tumor; AS, *braest*], a connective tissue tumor of the breast. It is usually benign and painless.

fibroma pendulum, a pendulous fibrous tumor of the skin.

fibromatosis /-mətō′sis/ [L, *fibra* + Gk,

oma, tumor, *osis,* condition], a gingival enlargement believed to be hereditary, manifested in the permanent dentition. It is characterized by a firm hyperplastic tissue that covers the surfaces of the teeth.

fibromuscular dysplasia (FMD) /mus'-kyələr/, an arterial disorder sometimes associated with strokes or transient ischemic attacks. The condition is characterized by intraluminal folds of fibrous endothelial tissue. The condition commonly involves the renal arteries and is associated with hypertension.

fibromyalgia, a form of nonarticular rheumatism characterized by musculoskeletal pain, spasm, and stiffness; fatigue; and severe sleep disturbance. Common sites of pain or stiffness can be palpated in the lower back, neck, shoulder region, arms, hands, knees, hips, thighs, legs, and feet.

fibromyomectomy /fī'brōmī'ōmek'təmē/, a surgical procedure for removing a uterine fibroma or other type of fibromyoma.

fibromyositis /fī'brōmī'əsī'tis/ [L, *fibra* + Gk, *mys,* muscle, *itis,* inflammation], any one of a large number of disorders in which the common elements are stiffness and joint or muscle pain accompanied by localized inflammation of the muscle tissues and fibrous connective tissues. Kinds of fibromyositis include **lumbago, pleurodynia,** and **torticollis.**

fibroplasia /-plā'zhə/, the formation of a scar during the fibroblastic repair phase of healing.

fibrosarcoma /-särkō'mə/ [L, *fibra* + Gk, *sarx,* flesh, *oma,* tumor], a sarcoma that contains fibrous connective tissue.

fibrosing alveolitis /fī'brōsing/ [L, *fibra* + *alviolus,* small hollow; Gk, *itis,* inflammation], a severe form of alveolitis characterized by dyspnea and hypoxia. It occurs in advanced rheumatoid arthritis and other autoimmune diseases.

fibrosis /fībrō'sis/ [L, *fibra* + Gk, *osis,* condition], **1.** a proliferation of fibrous connective tissue. **2.** an abnormal condition in which fibrous connective tissue spreads over or replaces normal smooth muscle or other normal organ tissue. Fibrosis is most common in the heart, lung, peritoneum, and kidney.

fibrosis of the lungs [L, *fibra* + Gk, *osis,* condition; AS, *lungen*], the formation of scar tissue in the connective tissue of the lungs as a sequel to any inflammation or irritation caused by tuberculosis, bronchopneumonia, or a pneumoconiosis. Localized fibrosis may be complicated by infarction, abscess, or bronchiectasis.

fibrothorax /-thôr'aks/, fibrosis of the pleural membranes.

fibrous /fī'brəs/ [L, *fibra,* fiber], consisting mainly of fibers or fiber-containing materials, such as fibrous connective tissue.

fibrous astrocyte, a glial cell with long, fibrous processes found in the white matter of the brain and spinal cord.

fibrous capsule, 1. the external layer of an articular capsule. It surrounds the articulation of two adjoining bones. **2.** the external, tough membranous envelope surrounding some visceral organs such as the liver.

fibrous dysplasia, an abnormal condition characterized by the fibrous displacement of the osseous tissue within the bones affected. The distinct kinds of fibrous dysplasia are monostotic fibrous dysplasia, polyostotic fibrous dysplasia, and polyostotic fibrous dysplasia with associated endocrine disorders. The initial signs may be a limp, a pain, or a fracture on the affected side. Pathologic fractures are frequently associated with this process, and angulation deformities may follow.

fibrous goiter, an enlargement of the thyroid gland characterized by hyperplasia of the capsule and connective tissue.

fibrous joint, any one of many immovable joints, such as those of the skull segments, in which a fibrous tissue or sometimes a form of cartilage connects the bones.

fibrous thyroiditis, a disorder characterized by slowly progressive fibrosis of an enlarged thyroid with replacement of normal thyroid tissue by dense fibrous tissue. Symptoms include a choking sensation, dyspnea, dysphagia, and hypothyroidism, but in some patients the gland functions normally.

fibrous tissue, the connective tissue of the body, consisting of closely woven elastic fibers and fluid-filled areolae.

fibrovascular proliferation /-vas'kyələr/, the growth of new blood vessels and fibrous tissues on the surface of the retina and optic nerve in diabetic retinopathy.

fibula /fib'yələ/ [L, buckle], one of the two bones of the lower leg, lateral to and smaller in diameter than the tibia. In proportion to its length it is the most slender of the long bones and presents three borders and three surfaces for attaching various muscles.

fibular /fib'yələr/ [L, *fibula,* clasp], pertaining to the fibula.

Fick's law [Adolf E. Fick], **1.** (in chemistry and physics) an observed law stating that the rate at which one substance diffuses through another is directly proportional to the concentration gradient of the diffusing substance. **2.** (in medicine) an observed law stating that the rate of diffusion across a membrane is directly proportional to the concentration gradient of the substance on the two sides of the membrane and inversely related to the thickness of the membrane.

Fick's principle [Adolf E. Fick, German physiologist, 1829–1901], a method for making indirect measurements, based on the law of conservation of mass. It is used specifically to determine cardiac output, in which the amount of oxygen uptake of each unit of blood as it passes through the lungs is equal to the oxygen concentration difference between arterial and mixed venous blood.

F.I.C.S., abbreviation for *Fellow of the International College of Surgeons.*

fictive kin /fĭk'tĭv/, people who are regarded as being part of a family even though they are not related.

FID, abbreviation for **free induction decay.**

field [AS, *feld*], a defined space, area, or distance. The field of vision represents the total area that can be seen with one fixed eye. The binocular field is the area that can be seen with both eyes.

field fever, a form of leptospirosis caused by *Leptospira grippotyphosa,* which primarily affects agricultural workers. It is characterized by fever, abdominal pain, diarrhea, vomiting, stupor, and conjunctivitis.

field of vision [AS, *feld* + L, *visio,* seeing], the area of space in which objects are visible at the same time when the eye is fixed and the face is turned so as to exclude the limiting effects of the orbital margins and nose.

fiery serpent /fī'ərē/ [AS, *fyre* + L, *serpere,* to creep], an informal term for *Dracunculus medinensis.*

FIGLU, abbreviation for **formiminoglutamic acid.**

FIGO, a classification system for cancers of the uterine cervix established by the French Fédération Internationale de Gynécologie et d'Obstétrique. Tumors are classified by Roman numerals from I to IV, representing a range from precancerous or in situ to highly malignant. Classification subdivisions are represented by letters such as IA, IIB, and so on.

figure-ground relationship /fig'(y)ər/ [L, *figura,* form; AS, *grund* + L, *relatus,* carry back], a perceptual field that is divided into a figure, which is the object of focus, and a diffuse background.

figure-of-eight bandage, a bandage with successive laps crossing over and around

each other to resemble the numeric figure eight.

figure-of-eight suture [L, *sutura*], a suture that begins at the deepest layer on each side of a wound, then crosses over to pass through the superficial layers on the opposite side before being tied.

filament /fĭl'əmənt/ [L, *filare,* to spin], a fine threadlike fiber. Filaments are found in most tissues and cells of the body and serve various morphologic or physiologic functions.

filamentous /fĭl'əmen'təs/, [L, *filare,* to spin], pertaining to something that is threadlike or capable of being drawn out into a threadlike structure.

filariasis /fĭl'ərī'əsis/ [L, *filum,* thread; Gk, *osis,* condition], a disease caused by the presence of filariae or microfilariae in body tissues. Filarial worms are round, long, and threadlike and are common in most tropic and subtropic regions. They tend to infest the lymph glands and channels after entering the body as microscopic larvae through the bite of an insect. The infection is characterized by occlusion of the lymphatic vessels, with swelling and pain of the limb distal to the blockage.

filariform /filer'ifôrm/, pertaining to a structure or organism that is threadlike.

file, **1.** (in dentistry) a tool for scaling or removing plaque from the teeth. **2.** a collection of related data or information, assembled for a specified purpose and stored as a unit.

filial generation /fĭl'ē·əl/ [L, *filius,* son, *generare,* to beget], the offspring produced from a given mating or cross in a genetic sequence.

filiform bougie /fĭl'ifôrm/ [L, *filum,* thread, *forma,* form; Fr, *bougie,* candle], an extremely thin device for passage through a narrow pathway such as a sinus tract.

filiform catheter, a catheter with a slender, threadlike tip that allows the wider part of the instrument to be passed through canals that are constricted or irregular.

filling, a material such as silver amalgam that is inserted into a hole drilled in a tooth to repair a caries.

filling factor [AS, *fyllan,* filling; L, *factor,* a maker], a measure of the geometric relationship of a radiofrequency coil used in magnetic resonance imaging and the body.

filling pressure, the pressure in the left ventricle at the end of diastole.

film [AS, *filmen,* membrane], **1.** a thin sheet or layer of any material, such as a coating of oil on a metal part. **2.** (in photography and radiography) a thin, flexible transparent sheet of cellulose acetate or

polyester plastic material coated with a light-sensitive emulsion, used to record images.

film badge, a photographic film packet, sensitive to ionizing radiation, used for estimating the exposure of personnel working with x-rays and other radioactive sources.

film development, the processing of photographic or x-ray films to manifest the latent image resulting from exposure of the chemically treated gelatin emulsion to a pattern of electromagnetic radiation.

film fault, a defect in a photograph or radiograph, usually caused by a chemical, physical, or electrical error in its production.

film on teeth, a collection of mucinous deposits that adhere to the teeth by means of acquired pellicle. Plaque, the film on teeth, contains microorganisms, desquamated tissue elements, blood cellular elements, and other debris.

film screen mammography, a breast radiographic technique in which a special single-emulsion film and high-detail intensifying screens are used.

filopressure, the temporary compression of a blood vessel by a ligature. The ligature is removed when the blood flow has stopped.

Filovirus, a genus of single-stranded negative-sense ribonucleic acid viruses in the Filoviridae family. The genus includes the Ebola and Marburg viruses.

filter [Fr, *filtrer,* to strain], **1.** a device or material through which a gas or liquid is passed to separate out unwanted matter. **2.** (in radiology) a device added to radiographic equipment that selectively removes low-energy x-rays that have no chance of reaching the film.

filtered back projection, a mathematic technique used in magnetic resonance imaging and computed tomography to create images from a set of multiple projection profiles.

filtration /filtrā'shən/ [Fr, *filtrer,* to strain], the addition of sheets of metal to a beam of x-rays, altering the energy spectrum and thus the imaging characteristics and penetrating ability of the radiation. Filtration is generally provided by aluminum or copper at low to medium energy and by tin, copper, and aluminum for higher energy beams.

filum /fī'ləm/, a threadlike structure.

fimbria /fim'brē·ə/ [L, fringe], any structure that forms a border or edge or that resembles a fringe.

fimbriae tubae /fim'brī·ī/, the branched fingerlike projections at the distal end of each of the fallopian tubes.

fimbria hippocampi, a band of efferent fibers formed by the alveus hippocampi that is continuous with the posterior pillar of the fornix.

fimbrial tubal pregnancy /fim'brē·əl/, a kind of tubal pregnancy in which implantation occurs in the fimbriated distal end of one of the fallopian tubes.

fimbria ovarica, the longest of the fimbriae tubae. It extends from the infundibulum to the ovary.

fimbriated /fim'brē·ā'tid/ [L, *fimbria,* a fringe], having fimbria, or the fringelike structure of the ovaries or the nerve fibers along the border of the hippocampus.

finastride /fin'əstrīd, finas'trīd/, a drug used to treat prostatic hypertrophy by reversing the progressive enlargement of the gland.

finding, 1. an observation made about a particular disease state, usually in relation to physical examination and laboratory tests. **2.** a conclusion drawn from an examination, study, or experiment.

fine motor skills [Fr, *fin,* thin; L, *movere* + ONor, *skilja,* to cut apart], the use of precise coordinated movements in such activities as writing, buttoning, cutting, tracing, or visual tracking.

fine-needle aspiration, a diagnostic technique that uses a very thin needle and gentle suction to obtain tissue samples. The needle is thinner than that used for venipuncture, and the procedure is less painful than drawing of blood.

fineness /fīn'nes/ [Fr, *fin,* thin], (in dentistry) a means of grading alloys in relation to gold content. The fineness of an alloy is designated in parts per thousand of pure gold.

fine tremor [Fr, *fin,* thin; L, *tremor,* to tremble], a vibration that occurs after a voluntary movement or one that results from fatigue in the corresponding muscle group.

finger [AS, *fingar*], any of the digits of the hand. The fingers are composed of three bony phalanges. Some anatomists regard the thumb as a finger.

finger agnosia, a neurologic disorder in which a patient is unable to distinguish between stimuli applied to two different fingers without visual clues.

finger goniometer [AS, *finger* + Gk, *gonia,* angle, *metron,* meter], an instrument for measuring the angle of a finger joint, or of an arm or leg.

finger-nose test [AS, *finger* + *nosu* + L, *testum,* crucible], a test of the coordination of the arms. The patient is asked to draw the tip of the index finger quickly to the nose, first with the eyes open, then with the eyes closed. An inability to per form the test accurately may be an indication of cerebellar disease.

finger phenomenon, a diagnostic test for organic hemiplegia. With the patient's elbow on the table, the examiner grasps the patient's wrist and uses the thumb to put pressure on the radial side of the patient's pisiform bone. If the hemiplegia is organic, the patient's fingers spread fanwise.

fingerprint, an image left on a smooth surface by the pattern of the pad of a distal phalanx. The distinctive pattern of loops and whorls represents the fine ridges marking the skin. Because each individual's fingerprints are unique, a classification system of the patterns is useful in identifying patients.

finger stick, the act of puncturing the tip of the finger to obtain a small sample of capillary blood.

finger sweep, a technique for clearing a mechanical obstruction from the upper airway of an unconscious patient. The rescuer opens the victim's mouth by grasping the lower jaw and tongue between the thumb and fingers. The rescuer then attempts to sweep the foreign object out of the victim's mouth with a finger.

FIO$_2$, 1. abbreviation for **fraction of inspired oxygen.** 2. the percentage of inspired oxygen a patient is receiving, usually expressed as a fraction.

fire ant sting, a potentially lethal venomous injection of piperidine alkaloids by a fire ant. The ant attaches itself to the skin with its mandibles and injects venom through a stinger in the posterior part of its abdomen. The ant injects repeatedly as it rotates its body around the attachment site. All victims experience a local wheal and flare reaction.

Fire-Setting Precautions, a Nursing Interventions Classification defined as prevention of fire-setting behaviors.

first aid [AS, *fyrst* + Fr, *aider*, to help], the immediate care that is given to an injured or ill person before treatment by medically trained personnel. Attention is directed first to the most critical problems: evaluation of the patency of the airway, the presence of bleeding, and the adequacy of cardiac function.

First Aid, a Nursing Interventions Classification defined as providing initial care of a minor injury.

first-dollar coverage, an insurance plan under which the third-party payer assumes liability for covered services as soon as the first dollar of expense for such services is incurred, without requiring the insured to pay a deductible.

first metacarpal bone, the metacarpal bone of the thumb.

first-order change, a change within a system that itself remains unchanged.

first-order kinetics, a chemical reaction in which the rate of decrease in the number of molecules of a substrate is proportional to the concentration of substrate molecules remaining. The rate of metabolism of most drugs follows the rule of first-order kinetics and is independent of the dose.

First Responder, the first emergency care person to arrive at an accident scene. This person is trained to follow standards set up by the United States Department of Transportation (DOT).

first rib, the highest rib of the thoracic cage. It moves about the axis of its neck, raising and lowering the sternum.

first stage of labor [ME, *fyrst* + OFr, *estage* + L, *labor*, work], a period of 8 to 12 hours marked by the onset of regular contractions of the uterus with full dilation of the cervix and the appearance of a small amount of blood-tinged mucus. Danger signs of the first stage include abnormal bleeding, abnormal fetal heart rate, and abnormal fetal presentation and position.

Fishberg concentration test [Arthur M. Fishberg, American physician, 1898–1992] a test of the ability of the kidneys to concentrate urine by measurement of the specific gravity of morning urine samples after overnight deprivation of fluid intake.

fish poisoning, toxic effects caused by ingestion of fish that contain substances that may produce symptoms ranging from nausea and vomiting to respiratory paralysis.

fish tapeworm infection [AS, *fisc*, fish], an infection caused by the tapeworm *Diphyllobothrium latum* that is transmitted to humans when they eat contaminated raw or undercooked freshwater fish.

fission /fish′ən/ [L, *fissio*, splitting], 1. the act or process of splitting or breaking up into parts. 2. a type of asexual reproduction common in bacteria, protozoa, and other simpler forms of life in which the cell divides into two or more equal components, each of which eventually develops into a complete organism. 3. (in physics) the splitting of the nucleus of an atom and subsequent release of energy.

fissiparous /fisip′ərəs/, reproduced by fission.

fissural angioma /fish′ərəl/ [L, *fissura,* cleft], a tumor composed of a cluster of dilated blood vessels found on the lip, face, or neck in an embryonal fissure.

fissure /fish′ər/ [L, *fissura,* cleft], 1. a cleft or a groove on the surface of an organ, often marking its division into parts, such as the lobes of the lung. 2. a crack-

F

like lesion of the skin, such as an anal fissure. **3.** a lineal fault on a bony surface that occurs during the development of a part, such as a fissure in the enamel of a tooth. —**fissured,** *adj.*

fissured tongue /fish´ərd/ [L, *fissura,* cleft; AS, *tunge*], a tongue with deep surface furrows that may radiate outward. It may be inherited as an autosomal-dominant trait.

fissure fracture, any fracture in which a crack extends into the cortex of the bone but not through the entire bone.

fistula /fis´chōōlə, -chələ/, *pl.* **fistulas, fistulae** [L, pipe], an abnormal passage from an internal organ to the body surface or between two internal organs. —**fistulous, fistular, fistulate,** *adj.*

fistulectomy /fis´chəlek´təmē/ [L, *fistula,* pipe; Gk, *ektome,* excision], the surgical removal of a fistula.

fit, 1. *nontechnical.* a paroxysm or seizure. **2.** the sudden onset of an episode of symptoms such as a fit of coughing. **3.** the manner in which one surface is aligned to another, such as the alignment of a denture with the gingiva and jaw.

fitness, a measure of the ability of a person to perform certain tasks.

Fitzgerald factor, a high–molecular weight kininogen that may be required for the interaction of factors XII and XI in the coagulation process.

Fitzpatrick, Joyce J., a nursing theorist who derived her Life Perspective Rhythm Model from Martha Rogers' conceptualization of unitary man. Fitzpatrick believes a central concern of nursing science and the nursing profession is the meaning attributed to life as the basic understanding of human existence. The four major concepts in this model are expressed as nursing, person, health, and environment. The person is viewed as a unified open rhythmic system with temporal patterns, consciousness patterns, and motion and perceptual patterns.

five-day fever, *informal.* trench fever.

five-step nursing process, a nursing process comprising five broad categories of nursing behaviors: assessing, analyzing, planning, implementing, and evaluating.

fixating eye /fik´sāting/ [L, *figere,* to fasten; AS, *eage*], (in strabismus) the normal eye that can be focused.

fixation /fiksā´shən/ [L, *figere,* to fasten, *atio,* process], (in psychoanalysis) an arrest at a particular stage of psychosexual development, such as anal fixation. —**fixate,** *v.,* **fixated,** *adj.*

fixational ocular movements /fiksā´-shənəl/, rotation of the eyes during voluntary fixation on an object.

fixation muscle, a muscle that acts to hold a part of the body in appropriate position.

fixative /fik´sətiv/ [L, *figere,* to fasten], **1.** any substance used to bind, glue, or stabilize. **2.** any substance used to preserve gross or histologic specimens of tissue for later examination.

fixator, a device composed of rods and pins designed to provide stabilization of a body part. The external skeletal apparatus may be attached directly to the bone.

fixed anions /fikst/, anions that are not part of the body's buffer anions.

fixed bridgework, a dental device that incorporates artificial teeth permanently attached to natural teeth or implants in the upper or the lower jaw.

fixed cations, cations that are not part of the body's metabolic buffering system.

fixed-combination drug [L, *figere,* to fasten, *combinare,* to combine; Fr, *drogue*], any of a group of multiple-ingredient preparations that provide concomitant administration of specific amounts of two or more medications.

fixed coupling, a precise distance between a normal and an ectopic beat that is duplicated each time the ectopic beat occurs.

fixed delusion [L, *figere,* to fasten, *deludere,* to deceive], a delusion that is consistent, unaltered, and difficult to interrupt.

fixed dressing, a dressing usually made of gauze impregnated with a hardening agent such as plaster of paris, sodium silicate, starch, or dextrin applied to support or immobilize a part of the body.

fixed-drug eruption, well-defined red to purple lesions that appear at the same sites on the skin and mucous membranes each time a particular drug is used.

fixed fulcrum, a tomographic fulcrum that remains at a fixed height.

fixed idea, 1. a persistent, obsessional thought or notion. **2.** in certain mental disorders, especially obsessive-compulsive disorder, an idea that dominates mental activity and persists despite contrary evidence.

fixed interval (FI) reinforcement, (in psychiatry) reinforcement given after a specific amount of time has elapsed.

fixed macrophage [L, *figere,* to fasten; Gk, *makros,* large, *pagein,* to eat], a nonmotile mononuclear phagocyte in the liver sinuses, spleen, lymph glands, and other tissues.

fixed orthodontic appliance, a prosthetic device cemented to the teeth or attached by adhesive material, for changing the relative positions of dentitions.

fixed pupil [L, *figere,* to fasten, *pupilla,*

little girl], an abnormal condition in which the pupils fail to dilate or contract when stimulated. The cause is commonly adhesions that bind the iris to the lens capsule or interference with the nerve supply of the iris in acute glaucoma.

fixed rate pacemaker [L, *figere,* to fasten, *ratum,* calculate, *passus,* step; ME, *maken*], an artificial electronic cardiac stimulus that delivers impulses to the cardiac muscle at a preset rate, regardless of the heart's independent activity.

fixed ratio (FR) reinforcement, (in psychiatry) reinforcement given after a specific number of responses have occurred.

fixed torticollis [L, *figere,* to fasten, *tortus,* twisted, *collum,* neck], a condition in which neck muscles on one side are so short that the head is held continuously in the same position.

fixer, a chemical product used in processing photographic or x-ray film. Applied after the developing phase, it neutralizes any developer remaining on the film, removes undeveloped silver halides, and hardens the emulsion.

flaccid /flak′sid/ [L, *flaccus,* flabby], weak, soft, and flabby; lacking normal muscle tone, such as flaccid muscles.— **flaccidity, flaccidness,** *n.*

flaccid bladder, a form of neurogenic bladder caused by interruption of the reflex pathways associated with the voiding reflex in the spinal cord.

flaccid paralysis, an abnormal condition characterized by the weakening or the loss of muscle tone.

flagella /flajel′ə/ [L, *flagellum,* whip], typically long, hairlike projections that extend from some acellular organisms and aid in their movement.

flagellant /flaj′ələnt/, a person who receives sexual gratification from the practice of flagellation.

flagellate /flaj′əlāt′, -lit/ [L, *flagellum,* whip], a microorganism that propels itself by waving whiplike filaments or cilia behind its body, such as *Trypanosoma, Leishmania, Trichomonas,* and *Giardia.*

flagellation /flaj′əlā′shən/, **1.** the act of whipping, beating, or flogging. **2.** a type of massage administered by tapping the body with the fingers. **3.** a type of sexual deviation in which a person is erotically gratified by being whipped or by whipping another. **4.** the arrangement of flagella on an organism; exflagellation.

flail chest /flāl/ [ME, *fleyl,* whip; AS, *cest,* box], a thorax in which multiple rib fractures cause instability in part of the chest wall and paradoxic breathing, with the lung underlying the injured area contracting on inspiration and bulging on expiration.

flame photometry [L, *flagrare,* to burn; Gk, *phos,* light, *metron,* measure], measurement of the wavelength of light rays emitted by excited metallic electrons exposed to the heat energy of a flame, used to identify characteristics in clinical specimens of body fluids.

flammable, the property of igniting ad burning easily and rapidly.

flange /flanj/, **1.** the part of a denture base that extends from the cervical ends of the teeth to the border of the denture. **2.** a prosthesis with a lateral vertical extension designed to direct a resected mandible into centric occlusion.

flank, the posterior portion of the body between the ribs and the ilium.

flap, a layer of skin or other tissue surgically separated from deeper structures for transplantation, coverage of an area that has been injured, or examination of deeper tissues.

flap reconstruction, an alternative to skin expansion as a method of breast reconstruction after mastectomy. It involves creation of a skin flap using tissue from another part of the body, such as the back or abdomen.

flap surgery, a type of breast reconstruction that is performed in a single stage, in some cases at the same time as a mastectomy.

flare /fler/, **1.** a red blush on the skin at the periphery of an urticarial lesion seen in immediate hypersensitivity reactions. **2.** an expanding skin flush, spreading from an infective lesion or extending from the principal site of a reaction to an irritant. **3.** the sudden intensification of a disease.

flaring of nostrils, nasal widening during inspiration, a sign of air hunger or respiratory distress.

flash, a sudden or intermittent brief burst of intense heat or light.

flashback, a phenomenon experienced by persons who have taken a hallucinogenic drug and unexpectedly reexperience its effects.

flash burn, a lesion caused by a very brief exposure to an extremely intense source of radiant energy or heat.

flashover phenomenon, an effect of a lightning strike or other intense electric discharge in which the electric current passes over the body instead of through it. The result is a red, featherlike branching pattern on the skin.

flask, **1.** a narrow-neck glass vessel used for heating liquids, distilling chemicals, or culturing fluid media. **2.** a small glass receptacle for holding liquids or powders.

flask closure [L, *vasculum,* small vessel, *claudere,* to close], (in dentistry) the joining of two halves of a flask that encloses and forms a mold for a denture base.

flat affect, the absence or near absence of emotional response to a situation that normally elicits emotion. It is observed in schizophrenia and some depressive disorders.

flat bone [AS, *flet,* floor], any of the bones that provide structural contours of the skeleton. Examples include ribs and bones of the cranium.

flat electroencephalogram, a graphic chart on which no tracings are recorded during electroencephalography, indicating a lack of brain wave activity.

flat spring contraceptive diaphragm, a kind of contraceptive diaphragm in which the flexible metal spring that forms the rim is a thin, light, flat band made of stainless steel.

flatulence /flach′ələns/ [L, *flatus,* a blowing], the presence of an excessive amount of air or gas in the stomach and intestinal tract, causing distension of the organs and in some cases mild to moderate pain.

Flatulence Reduction, a Nursing Interventions Classification defined as prevention of flatus formation and facilitation of passage of excessive gas.

flatulent /flach′ələnt/ [L, *flatus,* a blowing], pertaining to gas or air in the digestive tract.

flatus /flā′təs/ [L, a blowing], air or gas in the intestine that is passed through the rectum.

Flavivirus. a genus of a family of Flaviviridae single-stranded positive-sense ribonucleic acid viruses, including species that cause yellow fever, dengue, and St. Louis encephalitis.

flavone /flā′vōn/ [L, *flavus,* yellow], a colorless crystalline flavonoid derivative and component of bioflavonoid that increases capillary resistance.

flavoprotein, a group of conjugated proteins that make yellow enzymes essential for cellular respiration.

flavoxate hydrochloride /flavok′sāt/, a smooth muscle relaxant prescribed for spastic conditions of the urinary tract.

fl. dr., abbreviation for **fluid dram.**

flea [AS], a wingless, bloodsucking insect of the order Siphonaptera, some species of which transmit arboviruses to humans by acting as host or vector to the organism.

flea bite, a small puncture wound produced by a bloodsucking flea. Certain species of fleas transmit plague, murine typhus, and probably tularemia.

flecainide acetate /flekā′nīd/, an oral antiarrhythmic drug prescribed for the treatment of ventricular arrhythmias.

Fleischner method /flīsh′nər/, [Felix Fleischner, American radiologist, 1893–1969], a technique for producing lordotic x-ray projections of the lungs. The patient is placed in posteroanterior projection position while leaning backward from the waist to a nearly 45-degree posterior inclination.

flesh, the soft, muscular tissues of the body.

Fletcher factor, a prekallikrein blood coagulation substance that interacts with both factor XII and Fitzgerald factor, activating both and accelerating thrombin formation.

FLEX, abbreviation for **Federation Licensing Examination.**

flexion /flek′shən/ [L, *flectere,* to bend], **1.** a movement allowed by certain joints of the skeleton that decreases the angle between two adjoining bones, such as bending the elbow. **2.** (in obstetrics) a resistance to the descent of the fetus through the birth canal that causes the neck to flex so the chin approaches the chest.

flexion jacket, a corset designed to provide spinal immobility.

flexor /flek′sər/ [L, bender], a muscle that flexes a joint.

flexor carpi radialis [L, *flexor,* bender], a slender, superficial muscle of the forearm that lies on the ulnar side of the pronator teres. It functions to flex and to help abduct the hand.

flexor carpi ulnaris, a superficial muscle lying along the ulnar side of the forearm. It functions to flex and adduct the hand.

flexor digitorum superficialis, the largest superficial muscle of the forearm, lying on the ulnar side under the palmaris longus. The muscle flexes the second phalanx of each finger and, by continued action, the hand.

flexor retinaculum of ankle [L, *flexor,* bender, *retinaculum,* halter; AS, *ancleow*], a strong band of fascia from the medial malleolus to the calcaneum, passing over the long flexor tendons and blood vessels and nerves of the posterior tibia.

flexor retinaculum of the hand, the thick fibrous band of antebrachial fascia that wraps the carpal canal surrounding the tendons of flexor muscles of the forearm at the distal ends of the radius and the ulna.

flexor retinaculum of wrist [L, *flexor,* bender, *retinaculum,* halter; AS, *wrist*], a strong ligament across the front of the hollow of the carpus and over the flexor tendons of the fingers and median nerve.

flexor withdrawal reflex, a common cutaneous reflex consisting of a widespread contraction of physiologic flexor muscles and relaxation of physiologic extensor muscles. It is characterized by abrupt withdrawal of a body part in response to painful or injurious stimuli.

flextime /fleks'tīm/ [L, *flectere*, to bend; AS, *tima*], a system of staffing that allows the individualization of work schedules.

flexure /flek'shər/, a normal bend or curve in a body part, such as the colic flexure of the colon or the dorsal flexure of the spine.

flicks, rapid fixation involuntary movements of the eye.

flight into health [AS, *fleogan*, to fly], an abnormal but common reaction to an unpleasant physical sensation or symptom in which the person denies the reality of the feeling or observation, insisting there is nothing wrong.

flight of ideas, (in psychiatry) a continuous stream of talk in which the patient switches rapidly from one topic to another and each subject is incoherent and unrelated to the preceding one.

flight-or-fight reaction [AS, *fleogan*, to fly, *feohtan*, to fight; L, *reagere*, to act again], **1.** (in physiology) the reaction of the body to stress, in which the sympathetic nervous system and the adrenal medulla act to increase the cardiac output, dilate the pupils of the eyes, increase the rate of the heartbeat, constrict the blood vessels of the skin, increase the levels of glucose and fatty acids in the circulation, and induce an alert, aroused mental state. **2.** (in psychiatry) a person's reaction to stress by either fleeing from a situation or remaining and attempting to deal with it.

flight to illness, the effort of the patient to convince the therapist that he or she is too ill to terminate therapy and that continued support is needed.

flip angle, (in magnetic resonance imaging) the amount of rotation of the macroscopic magnetization vector produced by a radiofrequency pulse with respect to the direction of the static magnetic field.

floater [AS, *flotian*, to float], one or more spots that appear to drift in front of the eye, caused by a shadow cast on the retina by vitreous debris. Most floaters are benign and represent remnants of a network of blood vessels that existed prenatally in the vitreous cavity. The sudden onset of several floaters may indicate serious disease.

floating head [AS, *flotian*, to float, *heafod*], unengaged fetal head.

floating kidney, a kidney that is not securely fixed in the normal anatomic location because of congenital malplacement or traumatic injury.

floating patella [AS, *flotian* + L, *patella*, small pan], a patella that has been forced away from the femoral condyle by an effusion into the knee joint.

float nurse, a nurse who is available for assignment to duty on an ad hoc basis, usually to assist in times of unusually heavy work loads or to assume the duties of absent nursing personnel.

flocculant /flok'yōōlənt/, an agent or substance that causes flocculation.

flocculation test /flok'yōōlā'shən/ [L, *floccus,* flock of wool], a serologic test in which a positive result depends on the degree of flocculent precipitation produced in the material being tested.

flocculent /flok'yōōlənt/ [L, *floccus,* flock of wool], clumped or tufted, such as a cloud, or covered with a woolly, fuzzy surface.—**flocculate,** *v.,* **flocculation, floccule,** *n.*

flooding [AS, *flod*], **1.** profuse bleeding from the uterus especially after childbirth or prolonged menses. **2.** a technique used in behavior therapy for the reduction of anxiety associated with various phobias. Exposure to a stimulus that usually provokes anxiety desensitizes a person to that stimulus, thereby reducing fear and anxiety.

floor, the lower inner surface of any cavity or organ.

floppy infant syndrome [ME, *flappe,* slap; L, *infans,* speechless], a general term for juvenile spinal muscular atrophies, including Werdnig-Hoffmann disease and Wohlfart-Kugelberg-Welander disease.

floppy-valve syndrome, a cardiac disorder in which mitral or tricuspid valves slip beyond their point of closure during left ventricular systole.

flora /flôr'ə/, microorganisms that live on or within a body to compete with disease-producing microorganisms and provide a natural immunity against certain infections.

florid /flôr'id/ [L, *floridus,* flower], in human skin complexion or wound appearance, a bright red color.

flossing, the mechanical cleansing of interproximal tooth surfaces, subgingivally and supragingivally, by tape or waxed or unwaxed dental floss.

flotation device /flōtā'shən/ [Fr, *flotter,* to float], a foam mattress with a gellike pad located in its center, designed to protect bony prominences and distribute pressure evenly against the skin's surface.

flotation therapy, a state of semiweightlessness produced by various types of hospital equipment and used in the treatment and prevention of pressure ulcers.

flow, **1.** the movement of a liquid or gas. **2.** copious menstruation but less profuse than flooding.

flowmeter, a device operated by a needle valve in an anesthetic gas machine that measures gases by speed of flow, according to their viscosity and density.

flow sheet, (in a patient record) a graphic summary of several changing factors, especially the patient's vital signs or weight and the treatments and medications given. In labor the flow sheet displays the progress of labor.

flow transducer, a measuring device that calculates volume by dividing flow by time.

flow-volume curve, a graphic representation of the instantaneous volumetric flow rates achieved during a forced expiratory vital capacity maneuver. It is plotted as a function of the lung volume. It may be a maximum expiratory flow-volume curve or a partial expiratory flow-volume curve.

flow-volume loop, a pulmonary function test system in which the patient breathes into an electronic spirometer and performs a forced inspiratory and expiratory vital capacity maneuver while flow and volume are displayed on an oscilloscope screen. The data are displayed graphically as a loop whose shape indicates lung volume and other data through the complete respiratory cycle.

floxuridine /floksyŏŏr'ədēn/, an antineoplastic agent prescribed in the treatment of malignant neoplastic disease of the brain, breast, liver, and gallbladder.

fl. oz., abbreviation for **fluid ounce.**

flu /flōō/, *informal.* **1.** influenza. **2.** any viral infection, especially of the respiratory or intestinal system.

fluctuant /fluk'chōō-ənt/, pertaining to a wavelike motion that is detected when a structure containing a liquid is palpated.

fluctuation /fluk·chōō-ā'shən/ [L, *fluctuare,* to wave], **1.** a wavelike motion of fluid in a body cavity that follows a shaking motion. **2.** a variation in a fixed value or mass.

flucytosine /flōōsī'təsēn/, an antifungal prescribed in the treatment of certain serious fungal infections.

fludarabine, a fluorinated nucleotide analog of the antiviral agent vidarabine. It is prescribed in the treatment of patients with B-cell chronic lymphocytic leukemia.

fluent aphasia /flōō'ənt/ [L, *fluere,* to flow; Gk, *a,* not, *phasis,* speech], form of aphasia in which the patient articulates words easily, although the words may be unintelligible or may not be related to a particular stimulus. Types include **Wernicke's aphasia** and **conduction aphasia.**

fluid /flōō'id/ [L, *fluere,* to flow], **1.** a substance, such as a liquid or gas, that is able to flow and to adjust its shape to that of a container because it is composed of molecules that are able to change positions with respect to each other without separating from the total mass. **2.** a body fluid, either intracellular or extracellular, that is involved in the transport of electrolytes and other vital chemicals to, through, and from tissue cells.

fluid balance, a state of equilibrium in which the amount of fluid consumed equals the amount lost in urine, feces, perspiration, and exhaled water vapor.

fluid dram (fl. dr.), a unit of liquid measure equal to 3.696 milliliters (ml), 60 minims, or ⅛ fluid ounce.

Fluid Management, a Nursing Interventions Classification defined as promotion of fluid balance and prevention of complications resulting from abnormal or undesired fluid levels.

Fluid/Electrolyte Management, a Nursing Interventions Classification defined as regulation and prevention of complications from altered fluid and/or electrolyte levels.

fluidic ventilator /flōō·id'ik/, a device used in respiratory therapy that applies the Coanda effect to the movement of the flow of air or gases.

Fluid Monitoring, a Nursing Interventions Classification defined as collection and analysis of patient data to regulate fluid balance.

fluidotherapy /flōō'idōther'əpē, a modality of dry heat that uses a suspended air stream with the properties of a liquid. It simultaneously performs the functions of applied heat, massage, sensory stimulation, levitation, and pressure oscillations.

fluid ounce (fl. oz.), a measure of liquid volume in the apothecaries' system, which is equal to 8 fluid drams or 29 ml, 480 minims, ½₀ imperial pint, or the volume occupied by 437.5 grains of distilled water at a temperature of 16.7° C.

fluid overload, an excessive accumulation of fluid in the body caused by excessive parenteral infusion or deficiencies in cardiovascular or renal fluid volume regulation.

Fluid Resuscitation, a Nursing Interventions Classification defined as administering prescribed intravenous fluids rapidly.

fluid retention, a failure to excrete excess fluid from the body. Causes may include renal, cardiovascular, or metabolic disorders.

fluid therapy, the regulation of wate

balance in patients with impaired renal, cardiovascular, or metabolic function by careful measurement of fluid intake against daily losses.

fluid volume deficit, a NANDA-accepted nursing diagnosis of the state in which an individual experiences decreased intravascular, interstitial, and/or intracellular fluid. This refers to dehydration, water loss alone without change in sodium. Defining characteristics include decreased urine output, increased urine concentration, sudden weight loss, decreased venous filling, increased hematocrit, decreased skin/tongue turgor, decreased blood pressure, and dry skin/mucous membranes.

fluid volume deficit, risk for, a NANDA-accepted nursing diagnosis of the state in which an individual is at risk of experiencing vascular, cellular, or intracellular dehydration. Risk factors include advanced age; excessive weight; extreme loss of fluid through normal routes, such as diarrhea, or abnormal routes, such as indwelling tubes; lack of intake of fluids, as happens during physical immobility; increased fluid needs, as created by hypermetabolic states; and use of diuretics or other medications affecting the retention and excretion of body fluids.

fluid volume excess, a NANDA-accepted nursing diagnosis of a state in which an individual experiences increased isotonic fluid retention. Defining characteristics include edema, effusion, anasarca, weight gain, shortness of breath, intake greater than output, abnormal breath sounds, rales (crackles), decreased hemoglobin and hematocrit, increased central venous pressure, jugular vein distension, and positive hepatojugular reflex.

fluke /flōōk/, a parasitic flatworm of the class Trematoda, including the genus *Schistosoma.*

flunisolide, an intranasal steroid antiinflammatory agent prescribed in the treatment of seasonal or continuing allergic rhinitis that involves inflammation of the mucous membranes of the nasal passages.

fluocinolone acetonide /flōō´osin´əlōn/, a topical glucocorticoid prescribed for skin inflammation.

fluocinonide /flōō´osin´ənīd/, a synthetic corticosteroid prescribed to reduce skin inflammation.

fluorescence /flŏŏres´əns/ [L, *flux,* a discharge], the emission of light of one wavelength (usually ultraviolet) when exposed to energy of a different, usually shorter wavelength.—**fluoresce,** *v.,* **fluorescent,** *adj.*

fluorescent antibody test (FA test) /flŏŏres´ənt/, a test in which a fluorescent dye is used to stain an antibody for identification of clinical specimens. Fluorescent dyes make the dyed organisms glow visibly when examined under a fluorescent microscope. Kinds of fluorescent antibody tests include the FTA-ABS test.

fluorescent microscopy, examination with a fluorescent microscope equipped with a source of ultraviolet light rays, used to study specimens that have been stained with fluorescent dye.

fluorescent treponemal antibody absorption test (FTA-ABS test), a serologic test for syphilis.

fluoridation /flŏŏr´idā´shən/ [L, *fluere,* to flow], the process of adding fluoride, especially to a public water supply, to reduce tooth decay.

fluoride /flŏŏr´īd/, an anion of fluorine, fluoride compounds are introduced into drinking water or applied directly to the teeth to prevent tooth decay.

fluoride dental treatment [L, *fluere,* to flow, *dens,* tooth; Fr, *traitment*], the direct oral application of fluoride compounds to reduce dental caries.

fluoride poisoning [L, *fluere,* to flow, *potio,* drink], the toxic effects of contact with compounds of fluorine, an intensely poisonous pale yellow gas. Sodium fluoroacetate is a powerful rodent poison. The fluoroacetate compounds inhibit enzymes of the citric acid cycle. Inhalation of hydrogen fluoride can lead to bronchospasm, laryngospasm, and pulmonary edema.

fluorine (F) /flŏŏr´ēn/ /flōō´ərēn/ [L, *fluere,* to flow], an element of the halogen family and the most reactive of the nonmetals. Its atomic number is 9; its atomic mass (weight) is 19.00. Small amounts of sodium fluoride are added to the water supply of many communities to harden tooth enamel and decrease dental caries. Excessive amounts of fluoride can mottle tooth enamel and cause osteosclerosis. Acute fluoride poisoning and death can result from the accidental ingestion of insecticides and rodenticides containing fluoride salts.

fluoroacetic acid /flŏŏr´ō-asē´tik, -aset´ik/, a colorless water-soluble, highly toxic compound that blocks the citric acid cycle, causing convulsions and ventricular fibrillation. It is derived from a South African tree and is used in some potent pesticides.

fluorocarbons /flŏŏr´ōkär´bəns/ [L, *fluere,* to flow, *carbo,* coal], hydrocarbons that contain fluorine. Fluorocarbons are generally colorless, nonflammable gases, but some are liquids at room temperature. The compounds can produce mild upper respiratory tract irritation, and excessive exposure has been cited as a cause of central nervous system depression.

fluorometry /floŏrom'ətrē/ [L, *fluere* + Gk, *metron*, measure], measurement of fluorescence emitted by compounds when exposed to ultraviolet or other intense radiant energy. Fluorometry is used to measure urinary estrogens, triglycerides, catecholamines, and other substances. —**fluorometric**, *adj.*

fluoroscope /floŏr'əskōp'/ [L, *fluere* + Gk, *skopein*, to look], a device used for the immediate projection of a radiographic image on a fluorescent screen for visual examination. —**fluoroscopic**, *adj.*

fluoroscopic compression device /floŏr'-əskop'ik/, any of several objects that can be placed on a specific area of the patient's abdomen to compress the exterior surface during fluoroscopy of the digestive tract.

fluoroscopy /floŏros'kəpē/, a technique in radiology for visually examining a part of the body or the function of an organ with a fluoroscope.

fluorosis /floŏrō'sis/ [L, *fluere* + Gk, *osis*, condition], the condition that results from excessive prolonged ingestion of fluorine. Severe chronic fluorine poisoning leads to osteosclerosis and other pathologic bone and joint changes in adults.

fluorouracil /floŏr'ōyoŏr'əsil/ /floŏ'-ərōyoŏr'əsil/, an antineoplastic prescribed in the treatment of malignant neoplastic disease of the skin and internal organs.

fluoxetine hydrochloride /floŏ·ok'sətēn/, an oral antidepressant that acts by selectively preventing serotonin uptake.

fluoxymesterone /floŏ·ok'simes'tərōn/, an androgenic and anabolic steroid prescribed in the treatment of testosterone deficiency, breast cancer in females, and delayed puberty in males.

fluphenazine hydrochloride /floŏfen'-əzēn/, a phenothiazine tranquilizer prescribed in the treatment of psychotic disorders.

fluprednisolone /floŏ'prednis'əlōn/, a glucocorticoid with antiinflammatory activity and toxicity similar to those of cortisol.

flurandrenolide /floŏ'rəndren'əlīd/, a topical glucocorticoid prescribed for skin inflammation.

flurazepam hydrochloride /floŏraz'əpam/, a benzodiazepine minor tranquilizer prescribed in the treatment of insomnia.

flush [ME, *fluschen*], **1.** a blush or sudden reddening of the face and neck. **2.** a sudden subjective feeling of heat. **3.** a prolonged reddening of the face such as

may be seen with fever, use of certain drugs, or hyperthyroidism. **4.** a sudden rapid flow of water or other liquid.

flush device, apparatus for the accurate transmission of a pressure wave from a catheter to a transducer in an IV line.

flutamide, a hormonal antineoplastic agent prescribed in the treatment of recurrent forms of cancer that respond to hormone therapy, such as cancer of the breast, prostate, or kidney. It acts by preventing sex hormones (that aid cancer growth) from getting to cancerous tissue. It may also help other anticancer drugs to reach cancer cells and stop further cancer growth.

flutter, a rapid vibration or pulsation that may interfere with normal function.

flutter-fibrillation [AS, *fleotan,* to move quickly; L, *fibrilla,* small fiber], a type of atrial fibrillation (involuntary recurrent contraction) in which the irregular fibrillatory line resembles atrial flutter mixed with atrial fibrillatory waves.

fluvoxamine maleate, an antidepressant drug prescribed in the treatment of obsessive-compulsive disorder in adult patients.

flux gain /fluks/, (in radiology) the ratio of the number of light photons at the output phosphor of an image intensifier tube to the number at the input phosphor.

fly [AS, *flyge*], a two-winged insect of the order Diptera, some species of which transmit arboviruses to humans.

fly bites, bites that may be caused by species of deer, horse, or sand flies. Such bites produce a small painful wound with swelling caused by substances in the insect's saliva that are injected beneath the surface of the skin.

Fm, symbol for the element **fermium.**

FMD, abbreviation for **fibromuscular dysplasia.**

FMET, abbreviation for **formylmethionine.**

FMG, abbreviation for **foreign medical graduate.**

FMR-1, the symbol for a gene associated with a mental retardation disorder of the **fragile X syndrome.** The normal function of the gene has not been determined.

FMRI, abbreviation for **functional magnetic resonance imaging.**

FNP, abbreviation for **family nurse practitioner.**

foam bath [AS, *fam* + *baeth*], a bath taken in water containing a saporin substance that covers the surface of the liquid and through which air or oxygen is blown to form the foam.

focal /fō'kəl/ [L, *focus,* hearth], pertaining to a focus.

focal lesion [L, *focus* + *laesio,* hurting], an infection, tumor, or injury that develops at a restricted or circumscribed area of tissue.

focal plane, the plane of tissue that is in focus on a tomogram.

focal point [L, *focus,* hearth, *punctus,* pricked], a point at which rays of light meet when deflected, either by reflection or refraction.

focal seizure [L, *focus,* hearth; OFr, *seisir*], a transitory disturbance in motor, sensory, or autonomic function that results from abnormal neuronal discharges in a localized part of the brain, most frequently motor or sensory areas adjacent to the central sulcus. Focal motor seizures commonly begin as spasmodic movements in the hand, face, or foot and may spread progressively to other muscles to end in a generalized convulsion. Focal seizures may be caused by localized anoxia or a small brain lesion.

focal spot, the area on the anode of an x-ray tube or the target of an accelerator that is struck by electrons and from which the resulting x-rays are emitted. The shape and size of a focal spot influence the resolution of a diagnostic image.

focal symptom [L, *focus,* hearth; Gk, *symptoma,* that which happens], a body function disturbance centered on a specific body system or part.

focal zone, (in ultrasonography) the distance along the beam axis of a focused transducer assembly, from the point where the beam area first becomes equal to four times the focal area to the point beyond the focal surface where the beam area again becomes equal to four times the focal area.

focus /fō'kəs/ [L, hearth], a specific location, as the site of an infection or the point at which an electrochemical impulse originates.

focused activity /fō'kəst/, a therapeutic technique of actively leading the patient to adaptive coping skills and away from maladaptive ones.

focused grid, (in radiography) an x-ray grid that has lead foils placed at an angle so that they all point to a focus at a specific distance.

fogged film fault /fogd/ [Dan, *spray* + AS, *filmen,* membrane; L, *fallere,* to deceive], a defect in a photograph or radiograph, which appears as a foggy image or image area.

fogging [ME, *fogge*], a method of determining refractive error, particularly in cases of astigmatism, by placing excessively convex or concave lenses in front of the eyes. The patient is made artificially myopic by means of the spheres in order to relax all accommodation.

fog nebulizer /neb'yəlī'zer/, (in respiratory care) a device that humidifies by producing large volumes of particles.

foil pellet, a loosely rolled piece of gold foil, used for making various dental restorations, as a permanent tooth cavity filling or tooth crown.

folate /fō'lāt/, **1.** a salt of folic acid. **2.** any of a group of substances found in some foods and in mammalian cells that act as coenzymes and promote the chemical transfer of single carbon units from one molecule to another.

folded cravat sling, a bandage suspended from the neck, usually for supporting a forearm. It is prepared by placing a broad fold of cloth on the chest vertically with one end over the shoulder of the affected arm. The other end hangs in front of the chest, and the lower end is moved up and over the shoulder and arm.

Foley catheter /fō'lē/ [Frederick E. B. Foley, American physician, 1891–1966], a rubber catheter with a balloon tip to be filled with a sterile liquid after it has been placed in the bladder. This kind of catheter is used when continuous drainage of the bladder is desired, such as in surgery.

foliate papillae /fō'lē·āt/, a series of nipplelike processes that occur in folds along the lateral margins and in the front of the palatoglossus muscle of the tongue.

folic acid /fō'lik, fol'ik/, a yellow crystalline water-soluble vitamin of the B complex group essential for cell growth and reproduction. It functions as a coenzyme with vitamins B_{12} and C in the breakdown and use of proteins and in the formation of nucleic acids and heme in hemoglobin. It also increases the appetite and stimulates the production of hydrochloric acid in the digestive tract.

folic acid deficiency anemia, a form of megaloblastic (macrocytic) anemia caused by a lack of folic acid in the diet.

folie /fōlē'/ [Fr, madness], a psychiatric condition in a person who has previously been in good mental health.

folie du doute /dΥdo͞ot'/ [Fr, madness of doubts], an extreme obsessive-compulsive reaction characterized by persistent doubting, vacillation, repetition of a particular act, and pathologic indecisiveness.

folie du pourquoi /dΥpo͞orkwô·ä'/ [Fr, madness of why], a psychopathologic condition characterized by the persistent tendency to ask questions, usually concerning unrelated topics.

folie gemellaire /zhemeler'/ [Fr, madness in twins], a psychotic condition that occurs simultaneously in twins, sometimes in those not living together or closely associated at the time.

folie musculaire /mYskYler′/, severe chorea.

folie raisonnante /rezônäNt′/ [Fr, deliberating reason], a delusional form of any psychosis marked by an apparent logical thought process but lacking common sense.

folinic acid /fōlin′ik/, an active form of folic acid.

folk illnesses /fōk/, health disorders that are attributed to nonscientific causes.

follicle /fol′ikəl/ [L, *folliculus,* small bag], **1.** a pouchlike depression, such as the dental follicles that enclose the teeth before eruption or the hair follicles within the epidermis. **2.** fluid- or colloid-filled ball of cells in some glands such as the thyroid.—**follicular,** *adj.*

follicle-stimulating hormone (FSH), a gonadotropin that stimulates the growth and maturation of graafian follicles in the ovary and promotes spermatogenesis in the male.

follicle stimulating hormone releasing factor (FSH-RF) [L, *folliculus,* small bag, *stimulare,* to incite; Gk, *horaein,* to set in motion; ME, *relesen* + L, *facere,* to do], the gonadotropin-releasing hormone.

follicular adenocarcinoma /fōlik′yələr/, a neoplasm characterized by a follicular arrangement of cells often seen in the thyroid gland. The follicular thyroid carcinoma has a tendency to metastasize distantly to the lungs and bones.

follicular cyst, an odontogenic sac that arises from the epithelium of a tooth bud and dental lamina. The kinds of follicular cysts are dentigerous, primordial, and multilocular.

follicular goiter, an enlargement of the thyroid gland characterized by proliferation of the follicles and epithelial tissue.

follicular phase, the first part of the menstrual cycle, when ovarian follicles mature to prepare for ovulation.

follicular tonsillitis [L, *folliculus,* a small bag, *tonsilla* + Gk, *itis,* inflammation], an inflammation of the tonsils accompanied by a purulent infection of the tonsillar crypts.

follicular vulvitis [L, *folliculus,* a small bag, *vulva,* a wrapper; Gk, *itis,* inflammation], an inflammation of the skin follicles of the vulva.

folliculitis /fōlik′yōōlī′tis/, inflammation of hair follicles, such as in sycosis barbae.

folliculogenesis /fōlik′yəlōjen′əsis/, **1.** the stimulation of follicle development in the ovary by hormones or drugs. **2.** the development of follicles in the ovary, nor-

mally under the influence of the follicle stimulating hormone secreted by the anterior pituitary gland.

folliculosis /fōlik′yōōlōsis/, a condition characterized by the development of a large number of lymph follicles, which may or may not be associated with an infection.

follow-up, an act of renewing contact with sources of information and reviewing data needed to reinforce or evaluate a previous action or report.

fomentation /fō′mentā′shən/ [L, *fomentare,* to apply a poultice], **1.** a topical treatment for pain or inflammation that uses a warm, moist application. **2.** a substance or poultice that is used as a warm, moist application.

fomite /fō′mīt/ [L, *fomes,* tinder], nonliving material such as bed linen that may transmit microorganisms.

Fones' method /fōnz/, [Alfred C. Fones, American dentist, b. 1869], a toothbrushing technique that uses large, sweeping scrubbing circles over occluded teeth, with the toothbrush held at right angles to the tooth surfaces.

fontanel /fon′tənel′/ [Fr, *fontaine,* fountain], a space covered by tough membranes between the bones of an infant's cranium.

fonticulus /fontik′yələs/ [L, little fountain], fontanel or fontanelle.

food [AS, *foda*], **1.** any substance, usually of plant or animal origin, consisting of carbohydrates, proteins, fats, and such supplementary elements as minerals and vitamins, that is ingested or otherwise taken into the body and assimilated to provide energy and to promote the growth, repair, and maintenance essential for sustaining life. **2.** nourishment in solid form, as contrasted with liquid form. **3.** a particular kind of solid nourishment, such as breakfast food or snack food.

food additives, a large variety of substances that are added to foods to prevent spoilage, improve appearance, enhance flavor or texture, or increase nutritional value. Most food additives must be approved by the U. S. Food and Drug Administration to determine whether they can cause cancer, birth defects, or other health problems.

food allergy, a hypersensitive state that results from the ingestion of a specific food antigen. Symptoms of sensitivity to specific foods can include allergic rhinitis, bronchial asthma, urticaria, angioneurotic edema, dermatitis, pruritus, headache, labyrinthitis and conjunctivitis, nausea, vomiting, diarrhea, pylorospasm, colic, spastic constipation, mucous colitis, and perianal eczema. Food allergens are predominantly protein in nature.

Food and Drug Administration (FDA), a U. S. federal agency responsible for the enforcement of federal regulations on the manufacture and distribution of food, drugs, and cosmetics intended to prevent the sale of impure or dangerous substances.

food and drug interactions, adverse health effects of certain combinations of foods and medications. A thiazide diuretic may cause depletion of potassium from body tissues, a vitamin C deficiency may reduce activity of drug-metabolizing enzymes, and isoniazid may interfere with the function of pyridoxine. Monoamine oxidase inhibitors may react with tyramine in certain cheeses, wines, and pickled seafood to produce a life-threatening hypertensive crisis.

food chain [AS, *foda* + *chaine*], an ecologic sequence in which the various organisms within a community subsist on a species lower in the sequence, as the human eats the bird that eats the fish that eats the worm, and so on. Each level within the chain has a fundamental role, and destruction of any one member affects the rest of the chain negatively.

food contaminants /kəntam′inənts/, substances that make food unfit for human consumption. Examples include bacteria, toxic chemicals, carcinogens, teratogens, and radioactive materials. Also regarded as contaminants are basically harmless substances, such as water, that may be added to food to increase its weight.

food exchange list. See **Exchange Lists for Meal Planning.**

food poisoning, any of a large group of toxic processes that result from the ingestion of a food contaminated by toxic substances or by bacteria that contain toxins.

food pyramid, a diagrammatic proportional representation of human nutritional needs devised in 1992 by the U. S. Department of Agriculture to replace the "four food groups" pie chart used since the 1950s. The USDA "Food Guide Pyramid" features a relatively wide base of 6 to 11 servings daily of grains and cereals beneath a layer representing 5 to 9 servings daily of fruits and vegetables. A third tapering level represents 2 to 3 daily servings of meats and 2 to 3 of dairy products. At the peak of the pyramid are fats and sweets, to be eaten sparingly.

food service administrator, a member of a hospital staff who is responsible for the planning and management of the food service system of the facility.

food service department, the section of a hospital or similar health facility that is responsible for food preparation and services to patients and personnel. It also provides nutritional care to patients.

foot [AS, *fot*], the distal extremity of the leg, consisting of the tarsus, the metatarsus, and the phalanges.

foot-and-mouth disease, an acute extremely contagious rhinovirus infection of cloven-hooved animals. It is characterized by the development of ulcers on the skin around the mouth, on the mucous membrane in the mouth, and on the udders. Horses are immune. Uncommonly the virus is transmitted to humans by direct contact with infected animals or their secretions or with contaminated milk. Symptoms and signs in humans include headache, fever, malaise, and vesicles on the tongue, oral mucous membranes, hands, and feet.

footboard, a board or open box placed at the end of a patient's bed and at a level above the top of the mattress to prevent the weight of the top sheet and blankets from resting on the feet. It is situated so that the soles of the feet are positioned firmly against the board with the legs at right angles to it. Its purposes are to help the bedridden patient retain normal posture and prevent footdrop.

Foot Care, a Nursing Interventions Classification defined as cleansing and inspecting the feet for the purposes of relaxation, cleanliness, and healthy skin.

footdrop /fŏŏt′drop/ [AS, *fot* + *dropa*], an abnormal neuromuscular condition of the lower leg and foot, characterized by an inability to dorsiflex, or evert, the foot caused by damage to the common peroneal nerve.

footling breech [AS, *fot* + ME, *brech*], an intrauterine position of the fetus in which one or both feet are folded under the buttocks at the inlet of the maternal pelvis; one foot presents in a single footling breech, both in a double footling breech.

foot-pound, a unit for the measurement of work or energy. One foot-pound is the amount of work required to move 1 pound a distance of 1 foot in the same direction as that of the applied force.

footprinting, a method for determining the location of binding between a protein and a deoxyribonucleic acid (DNA) molecule. The technique involves nuclease digestion of the unbound components of DNA.

foramen /fôrā′mən/, *pl.* **foramina** [L, hole], an opening or aperture in a membranous structure or bone, such as the apical dental foramen and the carotid foramen.

F

foramen magnum, a passage in the occipital bone through which the spinal cord enters the spinal column.

foramen of Monro /monrō'/, a passage between the lateral and third ventricles of the brain.

foramenotomy, surgical removal of small pieces of bone around an intervertebral foramen, allowing more room for the spinal nerve. The procedure usually accompanies a laminectomy.

foramen ovale /ōvā'lē, ōvä'lä/, **1.** an opening in the septum between the right and the left atria in the fetal heart. This opening provides a bypass for blood that would otherwise flow to the fetal lungs. **2.** an oval foramen situated laterally to the foramen rotundum of the sphenoid bone.

foramen rotundum, one of a pair of rounded apertures in the greater wings of the sphenoid bone.

foramen spinosum, a small opening near the posterior angle of the greater wing of the sphenoid bone.

foramen venosum, an aperture in the greater wing of the sphenoid bone, through which a small vein passes from the cavernous sinus.

Forbes-Albright syndrome /fôrbsôl'brīt/ [Anne P. Forbes, American physician, 1911–1992; Fuller Albright, American physician, 1900–1969], an endocrine disease characterized by amenorrhea, prolactinemia, and galactorrhea, caused by an adenoma of the anterior pituitary.

forbidden clone theory [AS, *forbeodan* + Gk, *klon,* a cutting, *theoria,* speculation], a theory, associated with autoimmunity, that certain clone cells that can react against the body persist after birth and can be activated by a viral infection or by some metabolic change.

force [L, *fortis,* strong], **1.** energy applied so that it initiates motion, changes the speed or direction of motion, or alters the size or shape of an object. **2.** a push or pull defined as mass times acceleration.

forced expiratory flow (FEF), the average volumetric flow rate during any stated volume interval while a forced expired vital capacity test is performed. It is usually expressed as a percentage of vital capacity.

forced expiratory time (FET), the time required to exhale a given volume of vital capacity.

forced expiratory volume (FEV), the volume of air that can be forcibly expelled in a fixed period after full inspiration.

forced expired vital capacity (FEVC), a pulmonary function test of the maximal volume of gas that can be forcibly and rapidly exhaled starting from the position of full inspiration.

forced-inhalation abdominal breathing, a respiratory therapy technique in which the patient inhales through the nose with an effort forceful enough to lift small sandbag weights placed on the abdomen.

forceps, *pl.* **forceps** [L, pair of tongs], a pair of any of a large variety and number of surgical instruments, all of which have two handles or sides, each attached to a dull blade. Forceps are used to grasp, handle, compress, pull, or join tissue, equipment, or supplies.

forceps delivery, an obstetric operation in which instruments are used to deliver a baby. It is performed to overcome dystocia, to quickly deliver a baby experiencing fetal distress, or, most often, to shorten normal labor.

forceps rotation, an obstetric operation in which forceps are used to turn a baby's head that is arrested in transverse or posterior position in the birth canal.

forcible inspiration [L, *fortis,* strong, *inspirare*], breathing that is assisted by a mechanical ventilator that forces air into the lungs during inspiration but allows a return to ambient pressure as the patient exhales passively.

Fordyce-Fox disease /fôr'disfoks'/ [G. H. Fox, American dermatologist, 1846–1937; John A. Fordyce, American dermatologist, 1858–1925], an apocrine gland disorder that produces symptoms similar to those of miliaria.

Fordyce's disease [John A. Fordyce], the presence of enlarged oil glands in the mucosal membranes of the lips, cheeks, gums, and genitalia. It is a common condition and may be symptomless.

forearm, the portion of the upper extremity between the elbow and the wrist. It contains two long bones, the radius and ulna.

forefinger, the first, or index, finger.

forefoot, the portion of the foot that includes the metatarsus and toes.

foregut /fôr'gut/ [AS, *fore,* in front, *guttas*], the cephalic portion of the embryonic alimentary canal.

foreign body /fôr'in/ [Fr, *forain,* alien; AS, *bodig*], any object or substance found in an organ or tissue in which it does not belong under normal circumstances, such as a bolus of food in the trachea or a particle of dust in the eye.

foreign body granuloma [OFr, *forain* + AS, *bodig* + L, *granulum,* little grain; Gk, *oma,* tumor], a chronic inflammatory mass of tissue that accumulates around foreign bodies such as gravel, splinters, or bits of sutures.

foreign body in airway, anything found in the airway that is not normally present. Examples include food, coins, small pieces of toys, and bones. Observation is made for changes in breathing pattern, dyspnea, and color (cyanosis). Removal is generally performed with a fiberoptic laryngoscope and forceps, or via bronchoscopy.

foreign body in ear [OFr, *forain* + AS, *bodig* + *eare*], any object found in the ear canal that is not normally part of it, such as a bean, insect, or pebble.

foreign body in esophagus [OFr, *forain* + AS, *bodig* + Gk, *oisophagos,* gullet], anything found in the esophagus that is not normally a part of the tissue.

foreign body in eye [OFr, *forain* + AS, *bodig* + *eage*], anything found in the eye that is not a normal part of the tissue.

foreign body in throat [OFr, *forain* + AS, *bodig* + *throte*], anything found in throat tissue that is not normally present. A common foreign body in the throat is a posteriorly displaced tongue.

foreign body obstruction, a disturbance in normal function or a pathologic condition caused by an object lodged in a body orifice, passage, or organ. Most cases occur in children who suddenly inhale or swallow a foreign object or insert it into a body opening.

foreign medical graduate (FMG), a physician trained in and graduated from a medical school outside the United States and Canada. U. S. citizens graduated from medical schools outside the United States and Canada are also classified as FMGs.

forensic /fôren'sik/ [L, *forum,* public place], pertaining to courts of law.

forensic dentistry, the branch of dentistry that deals with the legal aspects of professional dental practices and treatment.

forensic medicine [L *forum,* public place, *medicinus,* physician], a branch of medicine that deals with the legal aspects of health care.

forensic psychiatry [L, *forum,* public place; Gk, *psyche,* mind, *iatreia,* treatment], a branch of psychiatry concerned with the application of psychiatry to law, including criminal responsibility, guardianship, and competence to stand trial.

foreplay /fôr'plā/, sexual activities, such as kissing and fondling, that precede coitus.

foreskin /for'skin/ [AS, *fore* + *skinn*], a loose fold of skin that covers the end of the penis or clitoris. Its removal constitutes circumcision.

forest yaws /for'ist/ [L, *foris,* outside; Afr, *yaw,* strawberry], a cutaneous form of American leishmaniasis, common in South and Central America, caused by *Leishmania guyanensis.* The disease is chronic, with multiple deep skin ulcers that occasionally spread to the nasal mucosa.

forewaters /fôr'wôtərs/ [AS, *fore* + *waeter*], the part of the amniotic sac that pouches into the cervix in front of the presenting part of the fetus.

forked tongue /fôrkt/ [L, *furca* + AS, *tunge*], a tongue divided by a longitudinal fissure.

formaldehyde /fərmal'dəhīd/, a toxic, colorless foul-smelling gas that is soluble in water and used in that form as a disinfectant, fixative, or preservative.

formalin /fôr'məlin/, a clear solution of formaldehyde in water. A 37% solution is used for fixing and preserving biologic specimens for pathologic and histologic examination.

formation /fôrmā'shən/, a cluster of people who occupy and therefore define a quantum of space.

formative evaluation /fôr'mətiv/, judgments made about effectiveness of nursing interventions as they are implemented.

formboard, equipment used in tactual performance testing. It consists of a board with cutouts of various shapes and sizes and blocks of corresponding geometric characteristics. The subject is tested on ability to fit the blocks into their proper cutout spaces.

forme fruste /fôrm' frYst', fôrm' frōost'/, *pl.* **formes frustes** [Fr, rough form], **1.** an incomplete or atypical form of a disease or a disease that is spontaneously arrested before it has run its usual course. **2.** (in genetics) an inherited disorder in which there is minimal expression of an abnormal trait.

formiminoglutamic acid (FIGLU) /fôr-min'imoglūtam'ik/, a compound formed in the metabolism of histidine, present in urine in elevated levels in folic acid deficiency. Increased excretion of FIGLU may indicate folic acid deficiency.

formula /fôr'm(y)ələ/ [L., *forma,* pattern], a simplified statement, generally using numerals and other symbols, expressing the constituents of a chemical compound, a method for preparing a substance, or a procedure for achieving a desired value or result.—**formulaic,** *adj.*

formulary /fôr'myələ'rē/ [L, *forma,* pattern], a listing of drugs intended to include a large enough range of medications and sufficient information about them to enable health practitioners to prescribe treatment that is medically appropriate. Hospitals maintain formularies that list all drugs commonly stocked in their pharmacy.

formulation /fôr'myəlā'shən/ [L, *forma*, pattern], **1.** a pharmacologic substance prepared according to a formula. **2.** a systematic and precise statement of a problem, a theory, or a method of analysis in research.

formylmethionine (FMET) /fôr'mil-məthī'ənēn/, (in molecular genetics) the first amino acid in a protein sequence.

fornication /fôr'nikā'shən/ [L, *fornix*, arch], (in law) sexual intercourse between two people who are not married to each other. The specific legal definition varies from jurisdiction to jurisdiction.

fornix /fôr'niks/, *pl.* **fornices** /fôr'nisēz/ [L, arch], an archlike structure or space.

fornix cerebri /ser'əbrī/, an archlike body of nerve fibers that lies beneath the corpus callosum of the cranium and serves as the efferent pathway from the hippocampus.

forskolin (FSK), an activator of adenylate cyclase. FSK interacts directly with ion channels, increasing glutamate responses and amplitude and decay time of spontaneous excitatory postsynaptic currents.

fortified milk [L, *fortis*, strong; AS *milc*], pasturized milk enriched with one or more nutrients, usually vitamins A and D, that has been standardized at 400 International units per quart **(fortified vitamin D milk).**

forward chaining, a method of measuring rehabilitation performance: The patient performs the first step independently and the therapist helps the patient perform the rest of the steps. The routine is then repeated with the patient performing the first two steps independently, then the first three steps, and so on.

forward-leaning posture, a respiratory therapy technique intended to reduce or eliminate accessory muscle activity in ambulatory patients with breathing difficulty. It involves walking in a slightly stooped, forward-leaning posture.

fosinopril, an angiotensin-converting enzyme inhibitor prescribed in the treatment of high blood pressure. It acts by blocking enzymes involved in body chemistry that results in constriction of blood vessels, increasing blood pressure and causing sodium and fluids to be retained.

fossa /fos'ə/, *pl.* **fossae** [L, ditch], a hollow or depression, especially on the surface of the end of a bone, such as the olecranon fossa or the coronoid fossa.

Foster bed /fos'tər/, trademark for a special bed used in the care and treatment of severely injured patients, especially those with spinal injuries. It consists of two

Bradford frames mounted on a castered base. The assembly is attached to a rotary bearing mechanism, permitting horizontal turning of the patient without moving the spine.

foundation [L, *fundamentum*], **1.** a charitable organization usually established to allocate private funds to worthy projects or to provide other services. **2.** (in dentistry) any device or material added to a remaining tooth structure to enhance the stability and retention of an overlying cast restoration.

foundation model, a health maintenance organization or other health system that is legally established as a tax-exempt, not-for-profit corporation organized to operate as a charitable institution.

fourchette /fŏŏrshet'/ [Fr, fork], a tense band of mucous membranes at the posterior angle of the vagina that connects the posterior ends of the labia minora.

four-handed dentistry, a technique of chairside operation in which four hands simultaneously perform tasks directly associated with dental work being accomplished in the oral cavity of a patient.

Fourier transform (FT) /fŏŏryā'/ [Jean B.J. Fourier, French mathematician, 1768–1830; L, *transformare*, to change form], (in medical physics) a mathematical procedure that separates out the frequency components of a signal from its amplitudes as a function of time, or vice versa.

Fourier transform imaging, (in medical physics) nuclear magnetic resonance (NMR) imaging techniques in which at least one dimension is phase encoded by applying variable gradient pulses along that dimension before "reading out" the NMR signal with a gradient magnetic field perpendicular to the variable gradient. The Fourier transform is then used to reconstruct an image from the set of encoded NMR signals.

Fournier's gangrene /fŏŏrnyāz'/ [Jean A. Fournier, French syphilographer. 1832–1914], an infective gangrene of the scrotum or vulva caused by an anaerobic hemolytic strain of streptococcus.

four-poster cast, a cast to immobilize the cervical vertebrae. It contains four vertical posts or poles on the anterior and posterior lateral sides of the head and is placed over the shoulders. The head is supported under the chin and occiput, and the posts prevent movement.

four-tailed bandage, a narrow piece of cloth with two ties on each end for wrapping a joint, such as an elbow or knee, or a prominence, such as the nose or chin.

fourth-generation scanner, a computed

fourth stage of labor [ME, *feower,* four; OFr, *estage* + L, *labor,* work], a post-partum period of about 4 hours after the third stage, or delivery of the placenta. Some complications, especially hemorrhage, occur at this time, necessitating careful observation of the mother.

fourth ventricle [ME, *feower,* four; L, *ventriculus,* little belly], a cavity with a diamond-shaped floor in the hindbrain, communicating below with the central canal of the spinal cord and above with the cerebral aqueduct of the midbrain. At the bottom of the ventricle are surfaces of the pons and medulla.

fovea capitis /fō'vē-ə/ [L, *fovea,* pit], **1.** a depression on the proximal surface of the head of the radius where it meets the capitulum of the humerus. **2.** a fovea on the head of the femur, where the ligamentum teres is attached.

fovea centralis, an area at the center of the retina where cone cells are concentrated and there are no rod cells.

Fowler's position /fou'lərz/ [George R. Fowler, American surgeon, 1848–1906], the posture assumed by the patient when the head of the bed is raised 45 to 60 degrees and his or her knees are elevated slightly.

foxglove /foks'glov/, a common name for a plant that is a source of digitalis, *Digitalis purpura.*

Fr, symbol for the element **francium.**

fractional dilation and curettage /frak'-shənəl/, a diagnostic technique in which each section of the uterus is examined and curetted to obtain specimens of the endometrium from all parts of the organ.

fractionation /frak'shənā'shən/ [L, *frangere,* to break], **1.** (in neurology) a mechanism within the neural arch of the vertebrae whereby only a portion of the efferent nerves innervating a muscle reacts to a stimulus, even when the reflex requirement is maximal, so that a reserve of neurons remains to respond to additional stimuli. **2.** (in chemistry) the separation of a substance into its basic constituents, by using such procedures as fractional distillation or crystallization. **3.** (in bacteriology) the process of isolating a pure culture by successive culturing of a small portion of a colony of bacteria. **4.** (in histology) the process of isolating the different components of living cells by centrifugation. **5.** (in radiology) the process of administering a dose of radiation in smaller units over time to minimize tissue damage rather than in a single large dose.

fraction of inspired oxygen (F₁O₂) [L, *frangere,* to break, *inspirare,* to breathe in; Gk, *oxys,* sharp, *genein,* to produce], the proportion of oxygen in the air that is inspired.

fracture /frak'chər/ [L, *frangere,* to break], a traumatic injury to a bone in which the continuity of the bone tissue is broken. A fracture is classified by the bone involved, the part of that bone, and the nature of the break, such as a comminuted fracture of the head of the tibia.

fracture-dislocation, a fracture involving the bony structures of any joint, with associated dislocation of the same joint.

fracture of clavicle [L, *frangere* + *clavicula,* little key], a break in the long bone of the shoulder girdle. It is usually accompanied by pain, swelling, and a protuberance and depression over the site of the injury. The patient usually supports the injured arm at the elbow.

fracture of olecranon [L, *frangere* + Gk, *olekranon,* point of the elbow], a fracture of the bony prominence of the ulna at the elbow joint. Different types of olecranon fractures may occur, depending on the articular surfaces involved and possible displacement of the radius. The triceps, which normally extends the elbow, may become spastic as a result of the injury.

fracture of patella [L, *frangere* + *patella,* small pan], a break in the sesamoid knee cap. The fracture often occurs in automobile accidents in which the knee strikes the dashboard. The damage is complicated by the reflex bracing of the quadriceps femoris muscle that pulls the fragments apart.

fracture of radius [L, *frangere* + *ray*], a fracture and dislocation of the lower end of the radius, usually with backward and radial displacement of the wrist and hand. The fracture commonly occurs when a falling person extends the arm and hand in an effort to cushion the impact.

fracture of skull [L, *frangere* + AS, *skulle,* bowl], a break in the structure of one or more of the cranial bones. A fracture of bones in the vault of the skull is usually a compound fracture and complicated by possible damage to brain tissue, particularly if shards of cranial bones are driven into the brain by the force of the trauma.

fracture threshold, a measure of bone density used in predicting osteoporosis risk factors.

fragile X syndrome /fraj'əl/, a reproductive disorder characterized by a nearly broken X chromosome, which has a tip hanging by a flimsy thread. It is the most common inherited cause of mental retardation. Some healthy individuals may possess fragile X chromosomes without exhibiting symptoms and may transmit the condition to children or grandchildren.

fragmented fracture /frag'mentid/ [L, *frangere,* to break], a fracture that produces multiple bone fragments.

frail elder, an older person (usually above 85 years of age) who has multiple physical or mental disabilities that may interfere with the ability to perform activities of daily living independently.

fraise /frāz/ [Fr, strawberry], a smooth hemispheric or conic burr with cutting edges. It is used for enlarging trephine openings or cutting osteopathic flaps.

frame of reference [AS, *framian,* to help; L, *referre,* to carry back], the personal guidelines of an individual, taken as a whole. An individual frame of reference reflects the person's social status, cultural norms, and concepts.

Franceschetti's syndrome /fran'chesket'ēz/ [Adolphe Franceschetti, Swiss ophthalmologist, 1896–1968], a complete form of mandibulofacial dysostosis.

franchise dentistry /fran'chīz/ [Fr, exemption; L *dens,* tooth], the practice of dentistry under a trade name, which has been purchased from another dentist or dental practice.

Francisella, a genus of nonmotile nonspore-forming pathogenic aerobic bacteria. The organisms cause tularemia in humans.

francium (Fr) /fran'sē·əm/ [France], a metallic element of the alkali metal group. Its atomic number is 87; its atomic mass (weight) is 223.

frank [L, *francus,* forthright], obvious or clinically evident, such as the unequivocal presence of a condition or a disease.

Frank biopsy guide, trademark for a device consisting of a long needle containing a hooked wire used to obtain biopsy samples of breast tissue.

frank breech [L, *francus* + ME, *brec*], an intrauterine position of the fetus in which the buttocks present at the maternal pelvic inlet, the legs are straight up in front of the body, and the feet are at the shoulders.

Frankfort horizontal plane [Frankfurt-am-Main (anthropologic) Agreement, 1882], (in dentistry) a craniometric surface determined by the inferior borders of the bony orbits and the upper margin of the auditory meatus, passing through the two orbitales and the two tragions.

Frankfort-mandibular incisor angle (FMTA), (in dentistry) the precumbency of the mandibular incisor tooth to the Frankfort horizontal plane.

Frank-Starling relationship [Otto Frank, German physiologist, 1865–1944; Ernest

H. Starling, English physiologist, 1866–1927], an index for determining cardiac output, based on the length of the myocardial fibers at the onset of contraction. The force exerted per beat of the heart is directly proportional to the length or degree of stretch of the myocardial fiber.

fraud /frôd/ [L, *fraudare,* to cheat], (in law) the act of intentionally misleading or deceiving another person by any means so as to cause him or her legal injury, usually the loss of something valuable or the surrender of a legal right.

Fraunhofer zone /froun'hōfər/ [Joseph von Fraunhofer, German optician, 1787–1826], (in ultrasonography) the zone farthest from the transducer face.

FRC, abbreviation for **functional residual capacity.**

F.R.C.P., abbreviation for *Fellow of the Royal College of Physicians.*

F.R.C.S., abbreviation for *Fellow of the Royal College of Surgeons.*

freckle [ME, *freken*], a brown or tan macule on the skin that results from exposure to sunlight. There is an inherited tendency to freckling.

free-air chamber [AS, *freo,* free; Gk, *aer,* air; L, *camera,* vault], a device used as a primary standard for calibrating x-ray exposure. It is used in national calibration laboratories throughout the world.

free association, 1. spontaneous consciously unrestricted association of ideas, feelings, or mental images. **2.** spontaneous verbalization of thoughts and emotions that enter the consciousness during psychoanalysis.

free clinic, a clinic or health program, usually located in a neighborhood setting, that provides health care for ambulatory patients at nominal or no cost.

free fatty acid (FFA) [AS, *freo* + *faett* + L, *acidus,* sour], nonesterified fatty acids, released by the hydrolysis of triglycerides within adipose tissue. Free fatty acids can be used as an immediate source of energy by many organs and can be converted by the liver into ketone bodies.

free-floating anxiety, a generalized, persistent, pervasive fear that is not attributable to any specific object, event, or source.

free-form foot orthosis, an orthosis that is molded directly to a patient's foot.

free gingiva, the unattached coronal portion of the gum that encircles a tooth and forms a gingival sulcus or crevice.

free gingival groove, a shallow line or depression on the gum surface at the junction of the free and attached gingivae.

free graft [AS, *freo* + Gk, *graphein,* stylus], a graft completely removed from its original site and replaced at a new site in a single one-stage operation.

free-induction decay (FID), (in magnetic resonance imaging), a signal emitted by a tissue after a radiofrequency pulse has excited the nuclear spins of the tissue at resonance. The decaying oscillation back to the normal state is the signal from which an MR image is made.

free macrophage [AS, *freo* + Gk, *makros,* large, *phagein,* to eat], a motile macrophage derived from a monocyte. It responds to chemotactic stimuli and migrates from blood vessels to tissue spaces.

free nerve ending, a receptor nerve ending that is not enclosed in a capsule.

free radical, a compound with an unpaired electron. It is unstable and reacts readily with other molecules.

free-radical theory of aging, a concept of aging based on the premise that the main causative factor is an imbalance between the production and elimination of free chemical radicals in the body tissues.

free-standing tax-exempt clinic, (in U. S. managed care) an organization that may employ physicians or make arrangements with physicians as independent contractors. It is usually organized as a not-for-profit, tax-exempt corporation. It is the direct provider of health care and holds preferred provider organization and health maintenance organization contracts, bills and collects in its own name, and owns the accounts receivable department.

free thyroxine, the amount of the unbound, active thyroid hormone thyroxine (T_4) circulating in the blood, measured by specific laboratory procedures.

free thyroxine index, the amount of unbound, physiologically active thyroxine (T_4) in serum. This amount is determined by direct assay or, more frequently, calculated on the basis of an in vitro uptake test.

free water clearance, the calculated volume of water that must be added to a given volume of urine to make it isotonic to the plasma.

freeway space [AS, *freo* + *wegan* + L, *spatiaum*], the interocclusal distance or separation between the occlusal surfaces of the teeth when the mandible is in its rest position.

freezing, a sudden inability to initiate or continue repetitive motor activity of patients with Parkinson's disease. The patient may be unable to take the first step in walking or, if walking, may find a real or imagined obstacle that causes the feet to remain in one spot.

freezing point [ME, *fresen,* to be cold; L, *punctus,* pricked], the temperature at which a substance changes from a liquid to a solid state. The freezing point for water is 32° on the **Fahrenheit** scale and 0° on the **Celsius** scale.

Freiberg's infraction [Albert H. Freiberg, American surgeon, 1868–1940; L, *infarcire,* to stuff], an abnormal orthopedic condition characterized by osteochondritis or aseptic necrosis of bone tissue, most commonly affecting the head of the second metatarsal.

Frei's test /frī/ [William S. Frei, German dermatologist, 1885–1943], a test performed to confirm a diagnosis of lymphogranuloma venereum.

Frejka splint /frā'kə/, a corrective device consisting of a pillow that is belted between the legs of a baby born with dislocated hips to maintain abduction and articulation of the head of the femur with the acetabulum.

fremitus /frem'itəs/ [L, a growling], a tremulous vibration of the chest wall that is primarily palpated during physical examination.

French scale (Fr), a method of sizing catheters, tubules, and sounds in which each Fr unit is equivalent to 1.3 mm.

frenectomy /frənek'təmē/ [L, *fraenum,* bridle; Gk, *ektome,* excision], a surgical procedure for excising a frenum or frenulum, such as the excision of the lingual frenum from its attachment into the mucoperiosteal covering of the alveolar process to correct ankyloglossia.

Frenkel's exercises [Heinrich S. Frenkel, Swiss neurologist, 1860–1931], a system of slow repetitious exercises of increasing difficulty developed to treat ataxia in multiple sclerosis and similar disorders.

frenotomy /frənot'əmē/ [L, *fraenum* + Gk, *temnein,* to cut], a surgical procedure for repairing a defective frenum, such as the cutting or lengthening of the lingual frenum to correct ankyloglossia.

frenulum of lips /fren'yələm, a fold of movement-limiting mucous membrane running from the gums to the lips or tongue. The frenulum of the lower lip is called the frenulum labii inferioris; that of the upper lip is the frenulum labii superioris.

frenulum of tongue [L, *fraenum,* bridle; AS, *tunge*], a longitudinal fold of mucous membrane connecting the floor of the mouth to the underside of the tongue in midline. A congenital defect causes an abnormal shortness of the frenulum, causing tongue-tie, which can be surgically corrected.

frenum /frē'nəm/, *pl.* **frenums, frena** [L, *fraenum,* bridle], a restraining portion or structure.

frequency *(F)* /frē'kwənsē/ [L, *frequens,* frequent], **1.** the number of repetitions of any phenomenon within a fixed period, such as the number of heartbeats per minute. **2.** (in biometry) the proportion of the number of persons having a discrete characteristic to the total number of persons being studied. **3.** (in electronics) the number of cycles of a periodic quantity, such as alternating current, that occur in a period of 1 second. Electromagnetic frequencies, formerly expressed in cycles per second (cps), are now expressed in hertz (Hz).

freshening, a step in the process of wound repair in which fibrin, granulation, and early scar tissue are removed in preparation for secondary closure.

fresh frozen plasma [ME, *fresen,* to be cold; Gk, *plassein,* to mold], an unconcentrated form of blood plasma containing all of the clotting factors except platelets. It can be used to supplement red blood cells (RBCs) when whole blood is not available for exchange transfusion or to correct a bleeding problem of unknown cause.

Fresnel zone /freznel'/, [Augustine J. Fresnel, French physicist, 1788–1827], (in ultrasonography) the region nearest the transducer face.

Freud, Sigmund /froid/ [Austrian neurologist, 1856–1939], founder of a complex integrated theory of psychologic causes of mental disorders, some, such as hysteria, with physical symptoms. Among tenets of freudian theory: human beings are motivated by a pleasure principle; receive internal stimulation from a sex instinct and a death instinct; have personality structures that can be divided into ego, superego, and id; and have unconscious, preconscious, and conscious levels of mental activity.

freudian /froi'dē·ən/ [Sigmund Freud], **1.** pertaining to Sigmund Freud; his theories and doctrines, which stress the formative years of childhood as the basis for later psychoneurotic disorders, primarily through the unconscious repression of instinctual drives and sexual desires; and his system of psychoanalysis, based on free association and dream analysis, for treating such disturbances. **2.** anything that is easily interpreted according to the theories of Freud or in psychoanalytic terms. **3.** pertaining to the school of psychiatry based on Freud's teachings. **4.** one who adheres to Freud's school of psychiatry.

freudian fixation [Sigmund Freud], an arrest in psychosexual development characterized by a firm emotional attachment to another person or object.

freudianism /froi'dē·əniz'əm/, the school of psychiatry based on the psychoanalytic theories and psychotherapeutic methods of treating disorders developed by Sigmund Freud and his followers.

freudian slip, (in freudian psychology) a behavioral error in speech or action that is believed to reveal a hidden motive in the unconscious of the perpetrator.

friable /frī'əbəl/ [L, *friare,* to crumble], easily shattered, crumbled, or pulverized.

fricative /frik'ətiv/, a consonant speech sound such as an /f/ or /s/, made by forcing an air stream through a constricted opening.

Fricke dosimeter, a chemical radiation dosimeter that uses the change of concentration of ferric ions in a solution subject to irradiation to quantify the amount of dose delivered to the sample.

friction /frik'shən/ [L, *fricare,* to rub], **1.** the act of rubbing one object against another. **2.** a type of massage in which deeper tissues are stroked or rubbed, usually through strong circular movements of the hand.

frictional force /frik'shənəl/, the force component parallel to the surfaces at the point of contact between two objects. It may be increased or decreased by such factors as moisture on a surface.

friction burn, tissue injury caused by abrasion of the skin.

friction rub, a dry, grating sound heard with a stethoscope during auscultation. It is a normal finding when heard over the liver and splenic areas.

Friedländer's bacillus /frēd'lendərz/ [Carl Friedländer, German pathologist, 1847–1887], a bacterium of the species *Klebsiella pneumoniae,* which is associated with infection of the respiratory tract, especially lobar pneumonia.

Friedländer's pneumonia [Carl Friedländer; Gk, *pneumon,* lung], a form of bronchopneumonia with a high mortality rate, particularly among older patients. The pneumonic patches tend to become confluent, and those who survive may experience pulmonary abscesses and necrosis.

Friedman curve /frēd'mən/ [Emanuel A. Friedman, American obstetrician, b. 1926], a graph depicting the progress of labor, prepared by labor attendants to facilitate detection of dysfunctional labor.

Friedman's test [Maurice H. Friedman, American physiologist, b. 1903], a modification of the Aschheim-Zondek test. A sample of urine from a woman is injected into a mature unmated female rabbit. If, days later, the rabbit ovaries contain fresh corpora lutea or hemorrhaging corpora, the result is positive, indicating that the woman is pregnant.

Friedreich's ataxia /frēd′rīshs/ [Nickolaus Friedreich, German physician, 1825–1882], an abnormal condition characterized by muscular weakness, loss of muscular control, weakness of the lower extremities, and an abnormal gait. The primary pathologic feature is pronounced sclerosis of the posterior columns of the spinal cord with possible involvement of the spinocerebellar tracts and the corticospinal tracts.

Friedreich's sign [Nikolaus Friedreich; L, signum, sign], the diastolic collapse of the jugular veins in adherent pericardium.

Fried's rule, a method of estimating the dose of medicine for a child by multiplying the adult dose by the child's age in months and dividing the product by 150.

frigid /frij′id/ [L, frigidus, cold], **1.** lacking warmth of feeling; unemotional; unimaginative; without passion or ardor and stiff or formal in manner. **2.** (of a woman) unresponsive to sexual advances or stimuli, abnormally indifferent or averse to sexual intercourse, or unable to have an orgasm during sexual intercourse. —**frigidity,** n.

fringe field /frinj/, (in magnetic resonance imaging) the part of a magnetic field that extends away from the confines of the magnet and cannot be used for imaging. It may affect nearby equipment and personnel.

frit /frit, frē/ [Fr, fried], a partially or wholly fused porcelain from which dental porcelain powders are made.

frôlement /frôlmäN′/ [Fr, brushing], **1.** the rustling type of sound often heard on auscultating the chest in diseases of the pericardium. **2.** a kind of massage that uses a light brushing stroke with the hand.

frontal bone /frun′tal/ [L, frons, forehead], a single cranial bone that forms the front of the skull, from above the orbits, posteriorly to a junction with the parietal bones at the coronal suture.

frontal lobe, the largest of five lobes constituting each of the two cerebral hemispheres. It lies beneath the frontal bone; occupies part of the lateral, the medial, and the inferior surfaces of each hemisphere; and extends posteriorly to the central sulcus and inferiorly to the lateral fissure. It is responsible for voluntary control over most skeletal muscles and is associated with the higher mental activities, such as planning, judgment, and conceptualization.

frontal lobe syndrome, behavioral and personality changes usually observed after a neoplastic or traumatic frontal lobe lesion. The patient may become sociopathic, boastful, hypomanic, uninhibited, exhibitionistic, and subject to outbursts of irritability or violence; in other cases the person may become depressed, apathetic, lacking in initiative, negligent about personal appearance, and inclined to perseverate.

frontal plane, any of the vertical planes passing through the body from the head to the feet, perpendicular to the sagittal planes, dividing the body into front and back portions.

frontal pole [L, frons, forehead, polus], the anterior extremity of the frontal lobe of the cerebrum.

frontal section [L, frons, forehead, sectio, a cutting], a section of the head or other body part cut into anterior and posterior portions.

frontal sinus, one of a pair of small cavities in the frontal bone of the skull that communicate with the nasal cavity. Each sinus opens into the anterior part of the middle meatus through the frontonasal duct.

frontal vein, one of a pair of superficial veins of the face, arising in the plexus of the forehead.

frostbite [AS, frost + bitan], traumatic effect of extreme cold on skin and subcutaneous tissues that is first recognized by distinct pallor of exposed skin surfaces, particularly the nose, ears, fingers, and toes. Vasoconstriction and damage to blood vessels impair local circulation and cause anoxia, edema, vesiculation, and necrosis. Gentle warming is appropriate first-aid treatment.

frottage /frôtäzh′/ [Fr, rubbing], sexual gratification obtained by rubbing (especially the genital area) against the clothing of another person, as can occur in a crowd.

frotteur /trôtœr′/ [Fr], a person who obtains sexual gratification by the practice of frottage.

frozen section [ME, fresen + L, sectio], a histologic section of tissue that has been frozen by exposure to dry ice.

frozen section method [AS, freosan, to freeze; L, sectio, a cutting; Gk meta order, hodos path], (in surgical pathology) a method used in preparing a selected portion of tissue for pathologic examination. The tissue is moistened and, fixed or unfixed, is rapidly frozen and cut by a microtome in a cryostat.

F.R.S.C., abbreviation for Fellow of the Royal Society of Canada.

fructokinase /fruk′tōki′nās/, an enzyme that catalyzes the transfer of a high-energy phosphate group from adenosine triphosphate to d-fructose.

fructose /fruk'tōs, frŏŏk'-/, a yellowish-to-white crystalline water-soluble levorotatory ketose monosaccharide that is sweeter than sucrose. It is found in honey and several fruits and combines with glucose to form the disaccharide sucrose.

fructose intolerance [L, *fructus,* fruit, *in* + *tolerare,* to bear], an inherited disorder marked by an absence of enzymes needed to metabolize fructose. Symptoms include sweating, tremors, confusion, and digestive distress, with vomiting, and failure of infants to grow.

fructosemia /frŏŏk'tōsē'mē·ə/ [L, *fructus,* fruit; Gk, *haima,* blood], the presence of fructose in the blood.

fructose test, a laboratory fertility examination of the semen of azoospermic men. Fructose comes primarily from the seminal vesicles. The purpose of the test is to rule out possible ejaculatory duct obstruction or agenesis of seminal vesicles.

fructosuria /frŏŏk'tōsŏŏr'ē·ə/, presence of the sugar fructose in the urine.

frustration /frustrā'shən/, a feeling that results from interference with one's ability to attain a desired goal or satisfaction.

FSH, abbreviation for **follicle-stimulating hormone.**

FSH-RF, abbreviation for **follicle-stimulating hormone releasing factor.**

FSK, abbreviation for **forskolin.**

FT, abbreviation for *fast-twitch.*

FTC, abbreviation for **Federal Trade Commission.**

FTT, abbreviation for **failure to thrive.**

fucosidosis /fyŏŏ'kōsidō'sis/, a hereditary lysosomal storage disorder that results from the absence of the enzyme required to metabolize fucoside moieties. It causes mental retardation, neurologic deterioration, coarse facial features, thickened skin, and hepatosplenomegaly.

fugue /fyŏŏg/ [L, *fuga,* running away], a state of dissociative reaction characterized by amnesia and physical flight from an intolerable situation. During the episode the person appears normal and seems consciously aware of what may be very complex activities and behavior, but afterward he or she has no recollection of the actions or behavior.

fulcrum /fŏŏl'krəm, ful'-/ [L, *fulcire,* to support], **1.** the stable point or the position on which a lever, such as the ulna or the femur, turns. Numerous common body movements, such as raising the arm and walking, are combinations of lever actions involving fulcrums. **2.** (in radiology) an imaginary pivot point about which the x-ray tube and film move.

fulfillment [AS, *fullfyllan,* to make full], a perception of harmony in life that results when an individual has found meaning and acts purposefully.

fulgurate /ful'gyərāt/ [L, *fulgur,* lightning], **1.** pertaining to sudden, intense, sharp pain. **2.** the use of a movable electrode to destroy superficial tissue.

full-arch wire, a wire that is attached to the teeth and extends from the molar region of one side of the mouth to the other.

full bath [AS, *fol* + *baeth*], a bath in which the patient's body is immersed in water up to the neck.

full denture [AS, *fol* + L, *dens,* tooth], a removable dental prosthetic that replaces all of the natural teeth in the maxillary and/or mandibular arch. The denture is completely supported by the mouth tissues.

full-liquid diet, a diet consisting of only liquids and foods that liquefy at body temperature. The diet is prescribed after surgery, in some acute infections of short duration, to treat acute gastrointestinal disorders, and for patients too ill to chew.

full-lung tomography, a technique of producing general tomographic surveys of both lungs to detect possible occult nodules of metastases.

full pulse [AS, *fol* +, *pulsare,* to beat], a large volume pulse with a low pulse pressure.

full-risk HMO, (in U. S. managed care) a health maintenance organization in which the hospital receives capitation (money paid) for all facility and hospital-based physician services. The physician group receives capitation and shares the deficit or surplus of the hospital risk pool.

full term [AS, *fol* + Gk, *terma,* limit], pertaining to the normal period of human gestation, between 38 and 41 weeks.

full-thickness graft, a tissue transplant that includes the full thickness of the skin and subcutaneous layers.

full weight bearing (FWB) [AS, *fol* + *gewiht* + ME, *beren*], (in radiology) a view that shows the response to stresses of a natural posture. Full weight-bearing views of the foot are useful in studying flatfoot or cave foot.

fulminant hepatitis, a rare and frequently fatal form of acute hepatitis B in which the patient's condition rapidly deteriorates, with hepatic encephalopathy, necrosis of the hepatic parenchyma, blood coagulation disorders, renal failure, and coma. The prognosis for adults is generally unfavorable.

fulminating /ful'minā'ting/ [L, *fulminare,* lightening flash], (of a disease or condition) rapid, sudden, severe, such as an infection, fever, or hemorrhage.—**fulminate,** *v.*

fumigate /fyoo′migāt/, to disinfect by exposing an area or object to pesticidal smoke or fumes.

fuming, producing a visible vapor.

function /fungk′shən/ [L, *functio,* performance], **1.** an act, process, or series of processes that serve a purpose. **2.** to perform an activity or to work properly and normally.

functional /fungk′shənəl/ [L, *functio,* performance], **1.** pertaining to a function. **2.** affecting the functions but not the structure of an organism or organ system.

functional age, a combination of the chronologic, physiologic, mental, and emotional ages.

functional analysis, (in psychiatry) a type of therapy that traces the sequence of events involved in producing and maintaining undesirable behavior.

functional antagonism, (in pharmacology) a situation in which two agonists interact with different receptors and produce opposing effects.

functional differentiation, (in embryology) the specialization or diversification that results from the particular function of a cell or tissue.

functional disease, 1. a disease that affects function or performance. **2.** a condition marked by signs or symptoms of an organic disease or disorder although careful examination fails to reveal any evidence of structural or physiologic abnormalities. Headache, impotence, certain heart murmurs, and constipation may be symptoms of functional disease.

functional dyspepsia, a condition characterized by impaired digestion caused by an atonic or a neurologic problem.

functional illness, a physical disorder with no known structural explanation for the symptoms.

functional imaging, (in nuclear medicine) a diagnostic procedure in which a sequence of radiographic or scintillation camera images of the distribution of an administered radioactive tracer delineates one or more physiologic processes in the body.

functional magnetic resonance imaging (fMRI), a radiographic technique for imaging activity of the brain as it experiences virtual reality. In fMRI the examiner takes a rapid succession of scans designed to detect changes in oxygen consumption in the brain, which reflects small changes in blood flow to various regions of the brain and increased activity in certain cells.

functional murmur [L, *functio,* performance], a heart murmur caused by an alteration of function without structural heart disease or damage, as in a murmur related to anemia rather than an organic heart disorder.

functional nursing, an organizational mode for assigning nursing personnel that is task- and activity-oriented, using auxiliary health workers trained in a variety of skills.

functional occlusal harmony, a biting relationship of opposing teeth in all ranges and movements that provides maximum masticatory efficiency without pathogenic force on the supporting oral structures.

functional overlay, an emotional aspect of an organic disease. It is characterized by symptoms that continue long after clinical signs of the disease have ended.

functional pathology [L, *functio,* performance; Gk, *pathos,* disease, *logos,* science], a study of the functional changes that result from structural alterations in tissues.

functional position of the hand, a position for splinting the hand, including the wrist and fingers. The thumb is abducted and in opposition and alignment with the pads of the fingers.

functional progression, a rehabilitative sequence for a musculoskeletal or similar injury. The program usually progresses from immobilization for primary healing through protection of range of motion to endurance and strengthening activities.

functional psychosis, a severe emotional disorder characterized by personality derangement and loss of ability to function in reality, but without evidence that the disorder is related to the physical processes of the brain.

functional residual capacity, the volume of gas in the lungs at the end of a normal tidal volume exhalation. The functional residual capacity is equal to the residual volume plus the expiratory reserve volume.

functional splint [L, *functio,* performance; ME, *splent*], an orthopedic device that allows or assists a patient's movements.

functional visual skills, various normal eye activities such as depth perception, eye aiming and alignment, and oculomotility.

fundal height /fun′dəl/ [L, *fundus,* bottom; AS, *heightho*], the height of the fundus, measured in centimeters from the top of the symphysis pubis to the highest point in the midline at the top of the uterus.

fundal placenta [L, *fundus,* bottom, *placenta,* flat cake], a placenta that is attached to the fundus of the uterus.

fundamentals of nursing /fun′dəmen′təls/, the basic principles and practices of nursing as taught in educational programs for nurses. This phase of training emphasizes

F

the importance of knowledge and understanding of the fundamental needs of humans as well as competence in basic skills of nursing care.

fundiform ligament of penis /fun'difôrm/, a band of elastic fibers surrounding the penis. It extends from the linea alba above the pubic symphysis and attaches to the penile fascia.

fundoplication /fun'dəplikā'shən/ [L, *fundus*, bottom, *plicare*, to fold], a surgical procedure involving making tucks (plication) in the fundus of the stomach around the lower end of the esophagus.

fundus /fun'dəs/, *pl.* **fundi** [L, bottom], the base or the deepest part of an organ; the portion farthest from the mouth of an organ, such as the fundus of the uterus or the fundus of an eye.

fundus microscopy, examination of the base of the interior of the eye using an instrument that combines an ophthalmoscope and a lens with high magnifying power for observing minute structures in the cornea and iris.

fundus of gallbladder, the closed end of the gallbladder, adjacent to the inferior border of the liver.

fundus of stomach, a cul-de-sac of the stomach that lies above the level of the cardiac orifice, where the esophagus joins the stomach.

fundus of urinary bladder, the bottom of the bladder, formed by the convex posterior wall.

fungal abscess, a collection of pus produced by a fungal infection.

fungal infection [L, *fungus,* mushroom, *inficere,* to stain], any fungal condition caused by a fungus. Most fungal infections are superficial and mild, though persistent and difficult to eradicate. Some kinds of fungal infections are **aspergillosis, blastomycosis, candidiasis, coccidioidomycosis,** and **histoplasmosis.**

fungal infection of nail, an infection of the horny cutaneous plates on the dorsal tips of the fingers and toes. The infection is commonly caused by *Trichophyton* organisms.

fungal septicemia [L, *fungus* + Gk, *septikos,* putrid, *haima,* blood], a form of septicemia in which the causative agent is a fungus.

fungemia /funjē'mē·ə/ [L, *fungus* + Gk, *haima,* blood], the presence of fungi in the blood.

fungi /fun'jī/, *sing.* **fungus** /fun'gəs/ [L, *fungus,* mushroom], a general term for a eukaryotic, thallus-forming organism that requires an external carbon source. Fungi lack both chlorophyll and chemolithotrophic systems. They may be saprophytes or

parasites. A simple fungus reproduces by budding; multicellular fungi reproduce by spore formation. They may invade living organisms, including humans, as well as nonliving organic substances.—**fungal, fungous,** *adj.*

fungicide /fun'jisīd/, a drug that kills fungi.—**fungicidal,** *adj.*

fungiform /fun'ji/fôrm/ [L, *funis* + *forma*], shaped like a mushroom.

fungistatic /fun'jēstat'ik/, having an inhibiting effect on the growth of fungi.

funic presentation [L, *funis* + *praesentare,* to show], (in obstetrics) the appearance of the umbilical cord before the main presenting part of the fetus.

funic souffle /fyōō'nik sōō'fəl/ [L, *funis,* cord; Fr, *souffle,* breath], a soft, muffled blowing sound produced by blood rushing through the umbilical vessels and synchronous with the fetal heart sound.

funiculitis /fənik'yəlī'tis/, any abnormal inflammatory condition of a cordlike structure of the body, such as the spinal cord or spermatic cord.

funiculopexy /fənik'yəlōpek'sē/, a surgical procedure for correcting an undescended testicle, in which the spermatic cord is sutured to surrounding tissue.

funiculus /fənik'yələs/ [L, little cord], a division of the white matter of the spinal cord, consisting of fasciculi or fiber tracts.

funis /fyōō'nis, fōō'nis/, a cordlike structure.

funnel chest [L, *fundere,* to pour], a skeletal abnormality of the chest characterized by a depressed sternum. The deformity may not interfere with breathing, but surgical correction is often recommended for cosmetic reasons.

funnel feeding, a technique in which liquids may be given orally to a patient who cannot move the lips or masticate, such as after surgery at the mouth or lips. A rubber tube attached to a funnel is placed in the mouth, usually at one corner, and a liquid is poured slowly through the funnel and tube into the mouth near the back of the tongue.

funny bone, a popular name for a point at the lower end of the humerus where the ulnar nerve crosses the elbow joint near the surface and, if subjected to external pressure, produces in a tingling sensation.

FUO, abbreviation for **fever of unknown origin.**

furazolidone /fōō'rəzol'idōn/, an antiinfective and antiprotozoal prescribed for certain bacterial or protozoal infections of the GI tract.

furcation /fərkā'shən/ [L, *furca,* fork], the region of division of the root portion of a tooth.

furfuraceous desquamation /fur'fərā'sē--əs/ [L, *furfur,* bran, *desquamare,* to scale off], the shedding of epidermis in large scales.

furosemide /fŏōrō'səmīd fyərō'səmid/, a loop diuretic prescribed in the treatment of congestive heart failure, renal failure, and edema.

furrow /fur'ō/ [AS, *furh*], a groove, such as the atrioventricular furrow that separates the atria from the ventricles of the heart.

furuncle /fyŏŏr'ungkəl/ [L, *furunculus,* petty thief], a localized suppurative staphylococcal skin infection originating in a gland or hair follicle and characterized by pain, redness, and swelling. Necrosis deep in the center of the inflamed area forms a core of dead tissue that is spontaneously extruded, eventually resorbed, or surgically removed. —**furunculous,** *adj.*

furunculosis /fyŏŏrung'kyŏōlō'sis/, an acute skin disease characterized by boils or successive crops of boils that are caused by staphylococci or streptococci.

fusiform /fyŏō'sifôrm/ [L, *fusus,* spindle, *forma,* form], a structure that is tapered at both ends.

fusiform aneurysm, a localized dilation of an artery in which the entire circumference of the vessel is distended.

fusiform gyrus [L, *fusus,* spindle, *forma,* form; Gk, *gyros,* turn], a convolution of the cerebral hemispheres that lies below the collateral fissures and joins the occipital and temporal lobes.

fusimotor /fyŏō'zimō'tər/ [L, *fusus* + *motare,* to move about], pertaining to the motor nerve fibers, or gamma efferent fibers, that innervate the intrafusal fibers of the muscle spindle.

fusion /fyŏō'zhən/ [L, *fusio,* outpouring], **1.** the joining into a single entity, as in optic fusion. **2.** the act of uniting two or more bones of a joint. **3.** the surgical join-ing of two or more vertebrae, performed to stabilize a segment of the spinal column after severe trauma, herniation of a disk, or degenerative disease. **4.** (in psychiatry) the tendency of two people who are experiencing an intense emotion to unite.

fusional movement /fyŏō'zhənəl/, a reflex that moves the visual axes to the point of fixation, producing stereoscopic vision.

fusion beat, (in electrocardiography) a P wave or QRS complex resulting from the concurrent activation of the atria or the ventricles by two stimuli in the same chamber.

Fusobacterium, a large cigar-shaped anaerobic bacillus genus with only one species, *Fusobacterium fusiforme,* pathogenic to humans.

fusospirochetal disease /fyŏō'zōspī'rōkē'-təl/ [L, *fusus,* spindle; Gk, *speira,* coil, *chaite,* hair], any infection characterized by ulcerative lesions in which both a fusiform bacillus and a spirochete are found, such as trench mouth or Vincent's angina.

FVIII, (recombinant blood factor VIII), a large glycoprotein containing more than 2300 amino acids, 24 cysteine residues, and 25 potential glycosylation sites. The factor is used to treat blood-clotting disorders, such as **hemophilia A,** in which the factor is deficient or missing.

F wave, a waveform recorded in electroneuromyographic and nerve conduction tests. It appears on supramaximal stimulation of a motor nerve and is caused by antidromic transmission of a stimulus. The F wave is used in studies of motor nerve function in the arms and legs.

f waves, (in cardiology) on an electrocardiogram tracing, wavy deflections at a rate of 400 or more per minute that represent fibrillation.

FWB, abbreviation for **full weight bearing.**

G

g, abbreviation for **gram.**

G1, the start of a cell-division cycle, a phase during which the cell's future can be influenced by various positive and negative signals, such as growth factors. The signals determine whether the cell is allowed beyond a certain checkpoint.

G2, a phase in the cell-division cycle after deoxyribonucleic acid duplication. During the G2 phase mitosis occurs; it results in the formation of identical cells.

Ga, symbol for the element **gallium.**

GA, abbreviation for **general anesthesia.**

GABA, abbreviation for **gamma-aminobutyric acid.**

GAD, abbreviation for **generalized anxiety disorder.**

gadolinium (Gd) /gad'əlin'ē·əm/ [Johan Gadolin, Finnish chemist, 1760–1852], **1.** a rare earth metallic element. Its atomic number is 64; its atomic mass (weight) is 157.25. **2.** (in radiology) a phosphor used to intensify screens.

gag [ME, *gaggen,* to strangle], **1.** a dental device for holding the jaws open during oral surgery or dental restoration. **2.** to retch or attempt to vomit.

gag reflex [ME, *gaggen,* to strangle; L, *reflectere,* to bend back], a normal neural reflex elicited by touching the soft palate or posterior pharynx; the responses are symmetric elevation of the palate, retraction of the tongue, and contraction of the pharyngeal muscles.

gait [ONorse, *geta,* a way], the manner or style of walking, including rhythm, cadence, and speed.

Gait Assessment Rating Scale (GARS), an inventory of 16 abnormal aspects of gait observed by an examiner as a patient walks at a self-selected pace. Each aspect is graded on a scale of 0-1-2-3, with lower numbers indicating less abnormality.

gait determinant, one of a number of the kinetic anatomic factors that govern an individual's locomotion in the process of walking. Some authorities have defined pelvic rotation, pelvic tilt, knee and hip flexion, knee and ankle interaction, and lateral pelvic displacement as the main determinants of gait.

gait disorder, an abnormality in the manner or style of walking, which usually results from neuromuscular, arthritic, or other body changes.

galactocele /gəlak'təsēl'/, a cyst or hydrocele caused by blockage of a mammary gland milk duct.

galactokinase /gəlak'tōkī'nās/ [Gk, *gala,* milk, *kinesis,* movement; Fr, *diastase,* enzyme], an enzyme that functions in the metabolism of glycogen.

galactokinase deficiency, an inherited disorder of carbohydrate metabolism in which the enzyme galactokinase is deficient or absent. As a result, dietary galactose is not metabolized, galactose accumulates in the blood, and cataracts may develop.

galactophorous duct /-môr'fəs/ [Gk, *gala* + *pherein,* to bear; L, *ducere,* to lead], a passage for milk in the lobes of the breast.

galactorrhea /gəlak'tərē'ə/ [Gk, *gala* + *rhoia,* flowing], lactation not associated with childbirth or nursing. The condition is sometimes a symptom of a pituitary gland tumor.

galactosamine, galactose that contains an amine group on the second group.

galactose /gəlak'tōs/ [Gk, *gala* + *glykys,* sweet], a simple sugar found in the dextrorotatory form in lactose (milk sugar), nerve cell membranes, sugar beets, gums, and seaweed and in the levorotatory form in flaxseed mucilage.

galactosemia /gəlak'tōsē'mē·ə/ [Gk, *gala* + *glykys,* sweet, *haima,* blood], an inherited autosomal-recessive disorder of galactose metabolism. It is characterized by a deficiency of the enzyme galactose-1-phosphate uridyl transferase. Shortly after birth an intolerance to milk occurs; it is evidenced by anorexia, nausea, vomiting, and diarrhea and causes failure to thrive.

galactose tolerance test, a test of the ability of the liver to remove galactose from the blood and convert it to glycogen. The test, which is used to estimate impaired liver function, measures the rate of galactose excretion after ingestion or injection of a measured amount of galactose.

galactoside, a glycoside containing galactose.

galactoside permease /gəlak'tōsīd'/, an

enzyme that catalyses the transport of lactose into the cell.

galactosidose, an enzyme that catalyzes the metabolism of galactosides.

galactosis /gal'əktōsis/, lactation; the formation of milk by the lacteal glands.

galactosuria /-sŏŏr'ē-ə/, the presence of galactose in the urine.

galactosyl ceramide lipidosis /gəlak'təsil/ [Gk, *gala* + *glykys,* sweet; L, *cera,* wax, *lipos,* fat, *osis,* condition], a rare, fatal, inherited disorder of lipid metabolism, present at birth. Infants become paralyzed, blind, deaf, and increasingly retarded; eventually they die of bulbar paralysis.

galactosyl transferase, a protein in the head of a sperm that is involved in fertilizing eggs. Antibodies to galactosyl transferase prevent sperm from binding to eggs.

galactozymase /-zī'māz/, an enzyme in milk that is able to hydrolyze starch.

galacturia /gal'əktŏŏr'ē-ə/ [Gk, *gala,* milk, *ouron,* urine], a condition in which the urine has a milky color caused by the abnormal presence of galactose, a monosaccharide, in the urine.

galanin /galan'in, gal'ənin/, a neuropeptide in the small intestine and central and peripheral nervous systems that has a role in bowel motility, pancreas activity, and prolactin and growth hormone release.

Galant reflex /gəlant'/, a normal response in the neonate to move the hips toward the stimulated side when the back is stroked along the spinal cord.

Galeazzi's fracture /gal'ē-at'sēz/ [Riccardo Galeazzi, Italian surgeon, 1866–1952], a fracture of the distal radius accompanied by dislocation of the radioulnar joint.

Galen's vein /gā'lənz/ [Claudius Galen, Greek physician, circa AD 130–200], the large vein formed by the union of the two terminal cerebral veins. It curves around the splenium of the corpus callosum and continues as the straight sinus of the brain.

gallbladder /gôl'blad'ər/ [ME, *gal* + AS, *blaedre*], a pear-shaped excretory sac lodged in a fossa on the visceral surface of the right lobe of the liver. It stores and concentrates bile, which it receives from the liver via the hepatic duct. In an adult it holds about 32 ml of bile. During digestion of fats the gallbladder contracts, ejecting bile through the common bile duct into the duodenum.

gallbladder carcinoma, a malignant neoplasm of the bile reservoir, characterized by anorexia, nausea, vomiting, weight loss, progressively worsening right upper quadrant pain, and eventually jaundice. Tumors of the gallbladder are predominantly adenocarcinomas and are often associated with biliary calculi.

gallium (Ga) /gal'ē·əm/ [L, *Gallia,* Gaul], a metallic element. Its atomic number is 31; its atomic mass (weight) is 69.72. The melting point of gallium is 29.8° C (88.6° F); it will melt if held in the hand. Because of its high boiling point (1983° C; 3602° F), it is used in high-temperature thermometers. Radioisotopes of gallium are used in total body scanning procedures.

gallop /gal'əp/ [Fr, *galop*], a third or fourth heart sound, which at certain heart rates sometimes sounds like the gait of a horse.

gallop rhythm [Fr, *galop* + Gk, *rhythmos*], a cadence resembling that of a galloping horse produced by an abnormal third or fourth heart sound.

galoche chin /gəlosh/ [Fr, *galosh* + AS, *cin*], a narrow protruding or thrusting chin. It is a congenital condition.

galvanic /galvan'ik/ [Luigi Galvani, Italian physician, 1737–1798], pertaining to or involving electricity.

galvanic electric stimulation [Luigi Galvani], the use of a high-voltage electric stimulator to treat muscle spasms, edema of acute injury, myofascial pain, and certain other disorders.

galvanic skin response (GSR) [Luigi Galvani; AS, *scinn* + L, *respondere,* to reply], a reaction to certain stimuli as indicated by a change in the electrical resistance of the skin. The effect is related to subconscious activity of the sweat glands and may result from pleasant as well as unpleasant stimuli. The GSR is used in some polygraph examinations.

galvanometer /gal'vənomətər, gal'vənom'ətər/ [Luigi Galvani], an instrument used to measure the strength and direction of flow of an electric current. Its action depends on the deflection of a magnetic needle in the field produced by current passing through a coil. Galvanometers are used in certain diagnostic instruments, such as electrocardiographs.

Galveston Orientation and Amnesia Test (GOAT), a series of 10 questions asked of a patient to help evaluate posttraumatic amnesia. The test is repeated on a weekly basis and is scored on a scale of 0 to 100.

Gambian trypanosomiasis /gam'bē·ən/, a usually chronic form of African trypanosomiasis, caused by the parasite *Trypanosoma brucei gambiense.*

game knee [ME, *gamen* + AS, *cneow*], a popular term for any injury or condition that interferes with normal function of the knee joint.

gamete /gam'ēt/ [Gk, marriage partner], **1.** a mature male or female germ cell that

G

is capable of functioning in fertilization or conjugation and contains the haploid number of chromosomes of the somatic cell. **2.** the ovum or spermatozoon. —**gametic,** *adj.*

gamete intrafallopian transfer (GIFT), a human fertilization technique in which male and female gametes are injected through a laparoscope into the fimbriated ends of the fallopian tubes.

gametic /gəmat'ik/, pertaining to a reproductive cell such as a spermatozoon or ovum.

gametic chromosome, any of the chromosomes contained in the haploid cell, specifically the spermatozoon or ovum, as contrasted with those in the diploid, or somatic cell.

gametocide /gəmē'tōsīd/ [Gk, *gamete* + L, *caedere,* to kill], any agent that is destructive to gametes or gametocytes, specifically to the malarial gametocytes. —**gametocidal,** *adj.*

gametocyte /gəmē'tōsīt/ [Gk, *gamete* + *kytos,* cell], (in genetics) any cell capable of dividing into or in the process of developing into a gamete, specifically an oocyte or spermatocyte.

gametogenesis /gam'itōjen'əsis/ [Gk, *gamete* + *genein,* to produce], the origin and maturation of gametes, which occurs through the process of meiosis. —**gametogenic, gametogenous,** *adj.*

gametophyte /gəmē'tōfīt/ [Gk, *gamete* + *phyton,* plant], a cell in the reproductive stage when the nuclei are in a haploid condition.

gamma /gam'ə/, Γ, γ, the third letter of the Greek alphabet. It is a symbol for photon, heavy-chain immunoglobulins, or the third component in a series of certain chemical groups.

gamma-aminobutyric acid (GABA), an amino acid with neurotransmitter activity that can be found in the brain, heart, lungs, kidneys, and certain plants.

gamma camera [Gk, *gamma,* third letter of Greek alphabet; L, *camera,* vault], a device that uses the emission of light from a crystal struck by gamma rays to produce an image of the distribution of radioactive material in a body organ. The light is detected by an array of light-sensitive electronic tubes and is converted to electric signals for further processing.

gamma efferent fiber [Gk, *gamma* + L, *efferre,* to carry out, *fibra,* fiber], any of the motor nerve fibers that transmit impulses from the central nervous system to the intrafusal fibers of the muscle spindle.

gamma-glutamyl transpeptidase (GGT), an enzyme that appears in the serum of patients with several types of liver or gall-

bladder disorders, including drug hepatotoxicity, biliary tract obstruction, and alcohol-induced liver disease.

gamma interferon, a small species-specific glycoprotein produced by mitogen-stimulated T cells. It possesses antiviral and immune activity in response to inducing agents.

gamma knife stereotaxic radiosurgery, a method for destroying deep-seated brain tumors with a focused beam of gamma radiation.

gamma radiation [Gk, *gamma* + L, *radiare,* to emit rays], a very high–frequency electromagnetic emission of photons from certain radioactive elements in the course of nuclear transition or from nuclear reactions. Gamma radiation is more penetrating than alpha and beta radiation but has less ionizing power and is not deflected in electric and magnetic fields. The wavelengths of gamma rays emitted by radioactive substances are characteristic of the radioisotopes involved and range from about 4×10^{-10} to 5×10^{-13} m. The depth to which gamma rays penetrate depends on their wavelength and energy. Gamma and other forms of radiation can injure, distort, or destroy body cells and tissue, especially cell nuclei, but controlled radiation is used in the diagnosis and treatment of various diseases. Gamma radiation can penetrate thousands of meters of air and several centimeters of soft tissue and bone.

gamma ray, an electromagnetic radiation of short wavelength emitted by the nucleus of an atom during a nuclear reaction. Composed of high-energy photons, gamma rays lack mass and an electric charge and travel at the speed of light.

gammopathy /gamop'əthē/, an abnormal condition characterized by the presence of markedly increased levels of gamma globulin in the blood. Monoclonal gammopathy is commonly associated with an electrophoretic pattern showing one sharp, homogenous electrophoretic band in the gamma globulin region. This reflects the presence of excessive amounts of one type of immunoglobulin secreted by a single clone of B cells. Polyclonal gammopathy reflects the presence of a diffuse hypergammaglobulinemia in which all immunoglobulin classes are proportionally increased.

gamogenesis /gam'ōjen'əsis/ [Gk, *gamos,* marriage, *genein,* to produce], sexual reproduction through the fusion of gametes. —**gamogenetic,** *adj.*

gamone /gam'ōn/ [Gk, *gamos,* marriage], a chemical substance secreted by the ova and spermatozoa that supposedly attracts the gametes of the opposite sex to facilitate union. Kinds of gamones are **androgamone** and **gynogamone.**

gancyclovir /gansik′lōvir/, an acrylic nucleoside structurally related to acyclovir. It is used to prevent cytomegalovirus disease after allogenic bone marrow transplantation and in persons with acquired immunodeficiency syndrome.

gangliocytoma /gang′glē·ō′sītō′mə/, a tumor involving ganglion cells. These tumors are frequently found in the pituitary gland.

ganglion /gang′glē·on/, *pl.* **ganglia** [Gk, knot], **1.** a knot or knotlike mass. **2.** one of the nerve cell bodies, chiefly collected in groups outside the central nervous system. The two types of ganglia in the body are the sensory ganglia on the dorsal roots of spinal nerves and on the sensory roots of the trigeminal, facial, glossopharyngeal, and vagus nerves and the autonomic ganglia of the sympathetic and parasympathetic systems.

ganglionar neuroma /gang·glē′ənər/ [Gk, *ganglion* + *neuron*, nerve, *oma*, tumor], a tumor composed of a solid mass of ganglia and nerve fibers. Usually found in abdominal tissues, the tumor occurs most commonly in children.

ganglionated, having ganglia.

ganglionated nerve, a nerve of the sympathetic nervous system.

ganglionic blockade /gang′glē·on′ik/, the blocking of nerve impulses at synapses of autonomic ganglia, usually by the administration of ganglionic blocking agents.

ganglionic blocking agent, any one of a group of drugs prescribed to produce controlled hypotension, as required in certain surgical procedures or in emergency management of hypertensive crisis. The drugs act by occupying receptor sites on sympathetic and parasympathetic nerve endings of autonomic ganglia.

ganglionic glioma [Gk, *ganglion* + *glia*, glue, *oma*, tumor], a tumor composed of glial cells and ganglion cells that are nearly mature.

ganglionitis /gang′glē·ənī′tis/, an inflammation of a nerve or lymph ganglion.

ganglioside /gang′glē·əsīd′/, a glycosphingolipid found in the brain and other nervous system tissues. Accumulation of gangliosides caused by an inborn error of metabolism results in gangliosidosis or Tay-Sachs disease.

gang rape, sexual intercourse against the will of the victim by a group of assailants.

gangrene /gang′grēn/ [Gk, *gangraina*, a gnawing sore], necrosis or death of tissue, usually the result of ischemia (loss of blood supply), bacterial invasion, and subsequent putrefaction. The extremities are most often affected. Dry gangrene is a late complication of diabetes mellitus that is already complicated by arteriosclerosis, in which the affected extremity becomes cold, dry, and shriveled and eventually turns black. Moist gangrene may follow a crushing injury or an obstruction of blood flow by an embolism, tight bandages, or a tourniquet. **—gangrenous,** *adj.*

gangrenous appendicitis /gang′grənəs/ [Gk, *gaggraina,* a gnawing sore; L, *appendere,* to hang upon, Gk, *itis,* inflammation], a condition in which the appendix becomes gangrenous because obstruction of its lumen blocks the flow of blood to that body part.

gangrenous vulvitis [Gk, *gaggraina* + L, *vulva,* wrapper; Gk, *itis,* inflammation], the death of tissues in the area of the vulva that results when an inadequate blood supply causes sloughing of cells.

gantry assembly /gan′trē/, (in computed tomography) a subsystem consisting of the x-ray tube, the detector array, the high-voltage generator, the patient support and positioning couch, and the mechanical support for each.

gap [OE, *gapa,* a hole], (in molecular genetics) a short missing segment in one strand of double-stranded deoxyribonucleic acid.

gap phenomenon, (in cardiology) a condition in which a premature stimulus encounters a block where an earlier or later stimulus could be conducted.

Gardner, Mary Sewell, [1871–1961], an American public health nurse who wrote the classic *Public Health Nurse.* She was instrumental in the development of the National Organization for Public Health Nursing and of public health nursing in the American Red Cross.

Gardner-Diamond syndrome, [Frank H Gardner, American physician, b. 1919; Louis K. Diamond, American physician, b. 1902], a condition resulting from autoerythrocyte sensitization, marked by large, painful transient skin discolorations that appear without apparent cause but often accompany emotional upsets, various collagen disorders, and abnormalities of protein metabolism.

Gardnerella vaginalis /gárd′nərel′ə/ [Herman L. Gardner, twentieth-century American bacteriologist; L, *vagina,* sheath], a genus of rod-shaped gram-negative bacteria normally found in the female genital tract. The bacteria may also be a cause of bacterial vaginitis.

Gardnerella vaginalis **vaginitis** [Herman L. Gardner, L, *vagina,* sheath; Gk, *itis,* inflammation], an infection of the female genital tract by bacteria of the *Gardnerella vaginalis* strain, often in combination with various anaerobic bacteria. It is assumed that the infection is sexually transmitted. The bacteria are also found in normal women without symptoms. The infection often produces a gray or yellow discharge with a "fishy" odor that increases after washing the genitalia with alkaline soaps.

Gardner's syndrome [Eldon J. Gardner, American geneticist, b. 1909], familial polyposis of the large bowel, with fibrous dysplasia of the skull, extra teeth, osteomas, fibromas, and epidermal cysts.

Gardner-Wells tongs, braces that are attached to the skull of patients immobilized with cervical injuries.

gargle /gár'gəl/ [Fr, *gargouille,* drainpipe], **1.** to hold and agitate a liquid at the back of the throat by tilting the head backward and forcing air through the solution. **2.** a solution used to rinse the mouth and oropharynx.

GARS, abbreviation for **Gait Assessment Rating Scale.**

Gartner's duct [Hermann T. Gartner, Danish anatomist, 1785–1827], one of two vestigial closed ducts, each parallel to a uterine tube.

gas [Gk, *chaos*], an aeriform fluid that possesses complete molecular mobility and the property of indefinite expansion. A gas has no definite shape, and its volume is determined by its container and by temperature and pressure.

gas bacillus [Gk, *chaos* + L, *bacillum,* small rod], any of several species of bacillus that produce a gas as a by-product of their metabolism. Examples include *Escherichia coli,* which ferments lactose and glucose, and the clostridial species that produce gas gangrene.

gas chromatography, the separation and analysis of different substances according to their different affinities for a standard absorbent. In the process a gaseous mixture of the substances is passed through a glass cylinder containing the absorbent, which may be dampened with a nonvolatile liquid solvent for one or more of the gaseous components.

gas embolism, an occlusion of one or more small blood vessels, especially in the muscles, tendons, and joints, caused by expanding bubbles of gases. Gas emboli can rupture tissue and blood vessels, causing decompression sickness and death. This phenomenon commonly affects deepsea divers who rise too quickly to the surface without adequate decompression.

gaseous /gas'ē-əs, gash'əs/ [Gk, *chaos*], pertaining to or resembling gas.

gas exchange, impaired, a NANDA-accepted nursing diagnosis of the state in which the individual experiences a decreased passage of oxygen and/or carbon dioxide between the alveoli of the lungs and the vascular system. The cause of the condition is an imbalance in ventilatory perfusion. Defining characteristics include confusion, restlessness, irritability, inability to move secretions, hypercapnia, and hypoxia.

gas gangrene, necrosis accompanied by gas bubbles in soft tissue after surgery or trauma. It is caused by anaerobic organisms such as various species of *Clostridium.* Symptoms include pain, swelling, and tenderness of the wound area; moderate fever; tachycardia; and hypotension. A characteristic finding is toxic delirium. If untreated, gas gangrene is rapidly fatal.

gas-scavenging system, the equipment used to prevent waste anesthetic gases from escaping into the atmosphere of the operating room.

gas sterilization [Gk, *chaos,* gas; L, *sterilis,* barren], the use of a gas such as ethylene oxide, C_2H_4O, to sterilize medical equipment.

gas therapy, the use of medical gases in respiratory therapy. Kinds of gas therapy include **carbon dioxide therapy, controlled oxygen therapy, helium therapy,** and **hyperbaric oxygenation.**

gastrectasia /gas'trektā'zhə/ [Gk, *gaster,* stomach, *ektasis,* stretching], an abnormal dilation of the stomach. It may be accompanied by pain, vomiting, rapid pulse, and falling body temperature. Causes can include overeating, obstruction of the pyloric valve, or a hernia.

gastrectomy /gastrek'əmē/, surgical excision of all or, more commonly, part of the stomach. It is performed to remove a chronic peptic ulcer, to stop hemorrhage in a perforating ulcer, or to remove a malignancy. Before surgery a gastrointestinal series is done, and a nasogastric tube is inserted. With the patient under general anesthesia, one half to two thirds of the stomach is removed, including the ulcer and a large area of acid-secreting mucosa.

gastric /gas'trik/ [Gk, *gaster,* stomach], pertaining to the stomach.

gastric analysis, examination of the contents of the stomach, primarily to determine the quantity of acid present and incidentally to ascertain the presence of blood, bile, bacteria, and abnormal cells.

gastric cancer, a malignancy of the stomach with symptoms of gastric cancer are vague epigastric discomfort, dysphagia, anorexia, weight loss, and unexplained iron deficiency anemia. Many cases are asymptomatic in the early stages and metastases may cause the first symptoms.

gastric digestion [Gk, *gaster,* stomach; L, *digere,* to separate], digestion by gastric juice in the stomach.

gastric dyspepsia, pain or discomfort localized in the stomach.

gastric emesis [Gk, *gaster,* stomach, *emesis,* vomiting], vomiting associated with a stomach disorder such as stomach cancer, stomach ulcer, or severe gastritis.

gastric fistula, an abnormal passage into the stomach, communicating most frequently with an opening on the external surface of the abdomen. A gastric fistula may be created surgically to provide tube feeding for patients with severe esophageal disorders.

gastric glands, glands in the stomach mucosa that secrete hydrochloric acid, mucin, and pepsinogen.

gastric inhibitory polypeptide, a gastrointestinal hormone found in the mucosa of the small intestine. Release of the hormone, mediated by the presence of glucose or fatty acids in the duodenum, results in the release of insulin by the pancreas and inhibition of gastric acid secretion.

gastric intubation, a procedure in which a Levin tube or other small-caliber catheter is passed through the nose into the esophagus and stomach. It may also be used for the introduction into the stomach of liquid formulas to provide nutrition for unconscious patients or for premature or sick newborns. Medication or a contrast medium may be instilled for treatment or for radiologic examination.

gastric juice, digestive secretions of the gastric glands in the stomach, consisting chiefly of pepsin, hydrochloric acid, rennin, and mucin. The pH is strongly acid (0.9 to 1.5).

gastric lavage, the washing out of the stomach with sterile water or a saline solution.

gastric motility, the spontaneous peristaltic movements of the stomach that aid in digestion, moving food through the stomach and out through the pyloric sphincter into the duodenum.

gastric mucin [Gk, *gaster,* stomach; L, *mucus*], a viscous secretion of glycoproteins produced from the mucous membrane lining of swine stomachs and formerly used in the treatment of peptic ulcers.

gastric node, a node in one of three groups of lymph glands associated with the abdominal and pelvic viscera supplied by branches of the celiac artery.

gastric resection [Gk, *gaster,* stomach; L,

re + secare, to cut], the surgical removal of part or all of the stomach, usually performed in the treatment of stomach cancer or intractable peptic ulcer.

gastrin /gas′trin/ [Gk, *gaster,* stomach], a polypeptide hormone secreted by the pylorus that stimulates the flow of gastric juice and contributes to the stimulus for bile and pancreatic enzyme secretion.

gastrinoma /gas′trinō′mə/, a tumor found in the pancreas and duodenum.

gastritis /gastrī′tis/, an inflammation of the lining of the stomach that occurs in two forms. Acute gastritis may be caused by severe burns; major surgery; aspirin or other antiinflammatory agents (nonsteroidal antiinflammatory drugs); corticosteroids; drugs; food allergens; or viral, bacterial, or chemical toxins. The symptoms —anorexia, nausea, vomiting, and discomfort after eating—usually abate after the causative agent has been removed. Chronic gastritis is usually a sign of underlying disease such as peptic ulcer, stomach cancer, Zollinger-Ellison syndrome, or pernicious anemia.

gastrocamera /gas′trōkam′ərə/, a small camera that can be lowered into the stomach through the esophagus and retrieved after recording images of the stomach lining.

gastrocnemius /-knē′mē′əs/ [Gk, *gastroknemia,* calf of the leg], the most superficial calf muscle in the posterior part of the leg. It joins the tendon of the soleus as part of the tendo calcaneus.

gastrocnemius gait, an abnormal gait associated with a weakness of the gastrocnemius. It is characterized by the dropping of the pelvis on the affected side at the last moment of the stance phase in the walking cycle, accompanied by lagging or slowness in forward pelvic movement.

gastrocnemius test, a test of the function of the gastrocnemius muscle by ankle plantar flexion while the patient is in a prone position. The examiner places fingers for palpation on the posterior of the calf while the patient pulls the heel upward.

gastrocolic reflex /-kol′ik/ [Gk, *gaster + kolon,* colon; L, *reflectere,* to bend backward], a mass peristaltic movement of the colon that often occurs 15 to 20 minutes after food enters the stomach.

gastrodidymus /-did′iməs/ [Gk, *gaster + didymos,* twin], conjoined, equally developed twins united at the abdominal region.

gastrodisciasis /gas′trōdiskī′əsis/ [Gk, *gaster + diskos,* disk, *eidos,* form, *osis,* condition], an infection of trematodes of the genus *Gastrodiscoides,* which are digestive tract parasites.

gastroduodenal /dōō'ədē'nəl/ [Gk, *gaster* + L, *duodeni,* 12 fingers], pertaining to the stomach and duodenum.

gastroduodenitis /-dōō'ədenī'tis/ [Gk, *gaster,* stomach; L, *duodeni,* 12 fingers; Gk, *itis,* inflammation], inflammation of the stomach and duodenum.

gastroduodenoscopy /-dōō'ədenos'kəpē/, inspection of the stomach and duodenum by means of a gastroscope passed through the oral cavity and esophagus or through an incision in the abdominal wall.

gastroduodenostomy /-dōō'ədenos'təmē/, surgical establishment of a passageway between the stomach and the duodenum.

gastroenteritis /gas'trō·en'tərī'tis/ [Gk, *gaster* + *enteron,* intestine, *itis* inflammation], inflammation of the stomach and intestines accompanying numerous gastrointestinal disorders. Symptoms are anorexia, nausea, vomiting, fever (depending on causative factor), abdominal discomfort, and diarrhea. The condition may be attributed to bacterial enterotoxins, bacterial or viral invasion, chemical toxins, or miscellaneous conditions such as lactose intolerance.

gastroenterologist /gas'trō·en'tərol'əjist/, a physician who specializes in diseases affecting the gastrointestinal tract.

gastroenterology /gas'trō·en'tərol'əjē/ [Gk, *gaster* + *enteron,* intestine, *logos,* science], the study of diseases affecting the gastrointestinal tract, including the stomach, intestines, gallbladder, and bile duct.

gastroenterostomy /gas'trō·en'təros'təmē/ [Gk, *gaster* + *enteron,* intestine, *stoma,* mouth], surgical formation of an artificial opening between the stomach and the small intestine, usually at the jejunum. The operation is performed with a gastrectomy to route food from the remainder of the stomach into the small intestine or alone to treat a perforating ulcer of the duodenum.

gastroesophageal /gas'trō·isof'əjē'əl/ [Gk, *gaster* + *oisophagos,* gullet], pertaining to the stomach and esophagus.

gastroesophageal reflux, a backflow of contents of the stomach into the esophagus that is often the result of incompetence of the lower esophageal sphincter. Gastric juices are acid and therefore produce burning pain in the esophagus.

gastroesophagitis /gas'trō·ēsof'əjī'tis/, inflammation of the stomach and esophagus.

gastrofiberscope /-fī'bərskōp'/, a flexible fiber endoscope for examination of the stomach.

gastrointestinal (GI) /gas'trō·intes'tinəl/ [Gk, *gaster* + L, *intestinum,* intestine], pertaining to the organs of the gastrointestinal tract, from mouth to anus.

gastrointestinal allergy, an immediate reaction of hypersensitivity after the ingestion of certain foods or drugs. Gastrointestinal allergy differs from food allergy, which can affect organ systems other than the digestive system. Characteristic symptoms include itching and swelling of the mouth and oral passages, nausea, vomiting, diarrhea (sometimes containing blood), severe abdominal pain, and, if severe, anaphylactic shock.

gastrointestinal bleeding, any bleeding from the gastrointestinal tract. The most common underlying conditions are peptic ulcer, Mallory-Weiss syndrome, esophageal varices, diverticulosis, ulcerative colitis, and carcinoma of the stomach and colon. Vomiting of bright red blood or passage of coffee ground vomitus indicates upper gastrointestinal bleeding, usually from the esophagus, stomach, or upper duodenum.

gastrointestinal infection, any infection of the digestive tract caused by bacteria, viruses, or parasites. All may have common clinical features of nausea, vomiting, diarrhea, and anorexia.

Gastrointestinal Intubation, a Nursing Interventions Classification defined as insertion of a tube into the gastrointestinal tract.

gastrointestinal obstruction, any obstruction of the passage of intestinal contents, caused by mechanical blockage or failure of motility. Mechanical blockage may be caused by adhesions resulting from surgery or inflammatory bowel disease, an incarcerated hernia, fecal impaction, tumor, intussusception, volvulus, or foreign body ingestion. Failure of motility may follow anesthesia, abdominal surgery, or occlusion of any of the mesenteric arteries to the gut. Symptoms vary with the cause of obstruction but generally include vomiting, abdominal pain, and increasing abdominal distension.

gastrointestinal system assessment, an evaluation of the patient's digestive system and symptoms. Discussion of symptoms is encouraged. The patient is asked whether there is or has been pain or tenderness in the oral cavity, gums, tongue, lips, abdomen, or rectum, and whether there have been instances of dysphagia, belching, heartburn, anorexia, nausea, vomiting, constipation, diarrhea, or painful defecation. Information is elicited about changes in eating; bowel habits; the color, character, and frequency of stool and urine; the use of laxatives or enemas; and the occurrence of fatigue, hemorrhoids, and edema of the extremities. Diagnostic aids include a complete blood count, stool examination, prothrombin time, and determinations of levels of alkaline phosphatase, serum and urine bilirubin, serum glutamic oxaloacetic transaminase, serum glutamic pyruvic transaminase, lactic acid dehydrogenase, blood urea nitrogen, serum lipase, cholinesterase, calcium, albumin, and glucose.

gastrokinetic drugs /-kinet'ik/, chemicals that stimulate salivation, increase lower esophageal sphincter pressure, and improve esophageal clearance in the supine but not in the upright position.

gastromalacia /-məlā'shə/ [Gk, *gaster,* stomach, *malakia,* softness], an abnormal softening of the walls of the stomach.

gastromegaly /-meg'əlē/ [Gk, *gaster* + *megas,* large], an abnormal enlargement of the stomach or abdomen.

gastroparesis /-pərē'sis/, failure of the stomach to empty caused by decreased gastric motility.

gastroplasty /gas'troplas'tē/ [Gk, *gaster* + *plassein,* to mold], any surgery performed to reshape or repair any stomach defect or deformity.

gastroschisis /gastros'kəsis/ [Gk, *gaster* + *schisis,* division], a congenital defect characterized by incomplete closure of the abdominal wall with protrusion of the viscera.

gastroscope /gas'trŏskōp'/ [Gk, *gaster* + *skopein,* to look], a fiberoptic instrument for examining the interior of the stomach. —**gastroscopy,** *n.,* **gastroscopic,** *adj.*

gastroscopy /gastros'kəpē/, the visual inspection of the interior of the stomach by means of a gastroscope inserted through the esophagus, —**gastroscopic,** *adj.*

gastrostomy /gastros'təmē/ [Gk, *gaster* + *stoma,* mouth], surgical creation of an artificial opening into the stomach through the abdominal wall. It is performed to feed a patient who has esophageal cancer or tracheoesophageal fistula, who may be unconscious for a prolonged period, or who is unable to swallow as a result of a cerebrovascular accident, Alzheimer's disease, or another disorder.

gastrostomy feeding, the introduction of a nutrient solution through a tube that has been surgically inserted into the stomach through the abdominal wall.

gastrothoracopagus /gas'trōthôr'əkop'-əgəs/ [Gk, *gaster* + *thorax,* chest, *pagos,* fixture], conjoined twins who are united at the thorax and abdomen.

gastrula /gas'trŏŏlə/ [Gk, *gaster,* stomach], the early embryonic stage formed by the invagination of the blastula. The cup-shaped gastrula consists of an outer layer of ectoderm and an inner layer of mesentoderm that subsequently differentiates into the mesoderm and endoderm.

gastrulation /gas'trəlā'shən/ [Gk, *gaster,* stomach], the development of the gastrula in lower animals and the formation of the three germ layers in the embryo of humans and higher animals.

Gatch bed /gach/ [William D. Gatch, American surgeon, 1878–1961; AS, *bedd*], a bed that has an adjustable joint, allowing the knees to be flexed and the legs supported.

gatekeeper, a health care professional, usually a primary care physician or a nurse, who is the patient's first contact with the health care system and triages the patient's further access to the system.

gatekeeper effect, a contraction of the endothelium mediated by immunoglobulin. It permits components of the blood to gain access to the extravascular space as a result of the increased vascular permeability.

gateway drugs, minor substances of abuse such as inhalants used in general by children or young people before they experiment with marijuana or hard drugs; entry drugs.

gating, (in magnetic resonance imaging) organizing data so that information used to construct an image originates in the same point in the cycle of a repeating motion, such as a heartbeat.

gating mechanism, 1. (in cardiology) the increasing duration of an action potential from the atrioventricular node to a point in the distal Purkinje system, beyond which it decreases. **2.** the opening and closing of cell membrane channels.

Gaucher's disease /gōshaz'/ [Phillipe C.E. Gaucher, French physician, 1854–1918], a rare familial disorder of fat metabolism caused by an enzyme deficiency, characterized by widespread reticulum cell hyperplasia in the liver, spleen, lymph nodes, and bone marrow.

gauntlet bandage /gônt'lit/ [Fr, *gantlet,* small glove, *bande,* strip], a glovelike bandage covering the hand and fingers.

gauss /gôs, gous/ [J.K.F. Gauss, German physicist, 1777–1855], a unit of magnetic field strength. It is equal to 1/10,000 tesla.

gauze /gôz/ [Fr, *gaze*], a transparent fabric of open weave and differing degrees of fineness, most often cotton muslin, used in surgical procedures and for bandages and dressings. It may be sterilized and permeated by an antiseptic or lotion.

gauze sponge [Fr, *gaze* + Gk, *spoggia*],

a piece of folded gauze used during surgery to wipe up bleeding surfaces and thereby help locate any sources of blood loss.

gavage /gávázh'/ [Fr, *gaver*, to gorge], the process of feeding a patient through a nasogastric tube.

gavage feeding of the newborn, a procedure in which a tube passed through the nose or mouth into the stomach is used to feed a newborn with weak sucking, uncoordinated sucking and swallowing, respiratory distress, tachypnea, or repeated apneic spells.

gay [Fr, *gai,* merry], **1.** any person who is homosexual. **2.** pertaining to homosexuality.

gay bowel syndrome, a group of gastrointestinal symptoms that occur commonly in homosexual males. Clinical features include bloating, flatulence, diarrhea, polyps, fissures, and hemorrhoids.

Gay-Lussac's law /gā'ləsaks'/ [Joseph L. Gay-Lussac, French scientist, 1778–1850; L, *legu,* a rule], (in physics) a law stating that the volume of a specific mass of a gas increases as the temperature increases if the pressure remains constant.

Gay Nurses' Alliance (GNA), a national organization of homosexual and lesbian nurses.

gaze /gāz/ [ME, *gazen,* to stare], a state of looking in one direction. A person with normal vision has six basic positions of gaze, each determined by control of different combinations of contractions of extraocular muscles.

gaze paresis, a disturbance of eye conjugate movement in which gaze tends to tonically deviated in the direction of normal gaze.

GB, abbreviation for **gallbladder.**

GBIA, abbreviation for **Guthrie's bacterial inhibition assay.**

g.c., *informal.* abbreviation for **gonococcus.**

G-CSF, abbreviation for **granulocyte colony-stimulating factor.**

Gd, symbol for the element **gadolinium.**

GDM, abbreviation for **gestational diabetes mellitus.**

GDNF, abbreviation for **glial cell line-derived neurotrophic factor.**

Ge, symbol for the element **germanium.**

gegenhalten /gā'gənhál'tən/ [Ger, counterpressure], the involuntary resistance to passive movement of the extremities. The effect may be psychogenic in origin or may be a sign of dementia or cerebral deterioration.

Geiger-Müller (GM) counter /gī'gərmil'-ər/ [Hans Geiger, German physicist, 1882–1945; Walther Müller, twentieth-century German physicist; Fr, *conter,* to tell], an electronic device that indicates the level of radioactivity of any substance by counting the number of subatomic particles, as electrons, emitted by the substance. It cannot identify the type or energy of a particle.

gel /jel/ [L, *gelare,* to congeal], a colloid that is firm although it contains a large amount of liquid, used in many medicines as a demulcent, a vehicle for other drugs, an antacid, or an astringent, depending on the drug from which it is derived.

gelatin buildup /jel'ətən/, an x-ray film artifact that may appear as a sharp area of either increased or reduced density.

gelatin film, absorbable, a hemostatic used to attain hemostasis during surgery, particularly neurologic, thoracic, and ophthalmic procedures.

gelatinous /jəlat'ənəs/ [L, *gelare,* to congeal], pertaining to or resembling a viscous, jellylike substance.

gelatin sponge, an absorbable local hemostatic prescribed to control surgical bleeding and treat pressure ulcers.

gel filtration, a method of separating molecules by size. A solution containing molecules of various sizes is passed through a filter consisting of a porous material, generally a polyacrylamide or polysaccharide.

gemellary /jem'ələr'ē/ [L, *gemellus,* twin], pertaining to twins.

gemellipara /jem'əlip'ərə/ [L, *gemellus* + *parare,* to give birth], a woman who has given birth to twins.

gemellology /jem'əlol'əjē/ [L, *gemellus* + Gk, *logos,* science], the study of twins and the phenomenon of twinning.

gemellus /jəmel'əs/, either of a pair of small muscles arising from the ischium. They rotate the thigh laterally.

gemellus test, a test of the function of the gemellus superior and gemellus inferior in hip external rotation while the patient is seated with the knees flexed. The examiner places one hand on the lateral aspect of the knee to prevent flexion or abduction of the hip while the patient rotates the thigh outward by moving the foot medially.

gemfibrozil /jemfī'brəzil/ an antihyperlipidemic agent prescribed for hyperlipidemia.

gemistocyte /gemis'təsīt/, an astrocyte with an eccentric nucleus and swollen cytoplasm, as seen in areas of nervous tissue affected by edema, demyelination, or infarction.

gemma /jem'ə/, *pl.* **gemmae** [L, bud], a budlike projection produced by lower forms of life during the budding process o asexual reproduction. **2.** any budlike or bulblike structure, such as a taste bud or end bulb. —**gemmaceous,** *adj.*

gemmate /jem′āt/ [L, *gemma + atus,* function], **1.** having buds or gemmae. **2.** to reproduce by budding.

gemmation /jemā′shən/ [L, *gemmare,* to produce buds], the process of cell reproduction by budding.

gemmiferous /jemif′ərəs/ [L, *gemma + fer,* bearing], having buds or gemmae; gemmiparous.

gemmiform /jem′ifôrm′/, resembling a bud or gemma.

gemmipara /jemip′ərə/ [L, *gemma + parare,* to give birth], an animal that produces gemmae or reproduces by budding, such as the hydra. —**gemmiparous,** *adj.*

gemmule /jem′yo͞ol/ [L, *gemmula,* small bud], **1.** the small asexual reproductive structure produced by the parent during budding that eventually develops into an independent organism. **2.** (according to the early theory of pangenesis) any of the submicroscopic particles containing hereditary elements that are produced by each somatic cell of the parent, and are transmitted through the bloodstream to the gametes.

gender /jen′dər/ [L, *genus,* kind], **1.** the classification of the sex of a person into male, female, or ambivalent. **2.** the specific sex of a person.

gender identity, the inner sense of maleness or femaleness.

gender identity disorder, a condition characterized by a persistent feeling of discomfort or inappropriateness concerning one's anatomic sex.

gender role, the expression of a person's gender identity; the image that a person presents to both himself or herself and others, demonstrating maleness or femaleness.

gender testing [L, *genus,* kind, *testum,* crucible], a procedure for validating the sex of an individual by examining a tissue sample, usually obtained from oral mucous membrane cells, for the presence of a Y chromosome.

gene /jēn/ [Gk, *genein,* to produce], the biologic unit of genetic material and inheritance. The gene is now considered to be a particular nucleic acid sequence within a deoxyribonucleic acid molecule that occupies a precise locus on a chromosome and is capable of self-replication by coding for a specific polypeptide chain.

gene amplification [Gk, *genein,* to produce; L, *amplus,* large], a gene duplicating process in which ribonucleic acid molecules are transcribed many times in

certain cells in response to defined signals or environmental stresses.

gene library, (in molecular genetics) a collection of all or part of the genetic information of a species, obtained from cloned fragments.

gene pool [Gk, *genein,* to produce; AS, *pol*] the total number of genetic traits within a person or species population. In a population that reproduces by random sexual selection, the distribution of genetic traits follows a normal bell curve.

gene probe, a device used in molecular biology for locating a particular gene on a chromosome. It involves pairing a short known segment of deoxyribonucleic acid or ribonucleic acid with a matching sequence of bases on a chromosome.

general adaptation syndrome (GAS) [L, *genus,* kind; L, *adaptare,* to fit; Gk, *syn,* together, *dromos,* course], the defense response of the body or the psyche to injury or prolonged stress, as described by Hans Selye (1907–1982). It consists of an initial stage of shock or alarm reaction, followed by a phase of increasing resistance or adaptation, using the various defense mechanisms of the body or mind, and culminates in a state of adjustment and healing or of exhaustion and disintegration.

general anesthesia, the absence of sensation and consciousness as induced by various anesthetic agents, given by inhalation or intravenous injection. The components of general anesthesia are analgesia, amnesia, muscle relaxation, control of vital signs, and unconsciousness. The kind of anesthesia selected and the dose and route by which it is given depend on the indication for anesthesia and the patient's physical status. General anesthesia may be administered only by a physician or a Certified Registered Nurse Anesthetist.

generalization /jen′(ə)rəlīzā′shən/ /jen′-(ə)rəlīzā′shən/ [L, *genus,* kind; Gk, *izein,* to cause], **1.** the reasoning by which a basic conclusion is reached, with application to different items that have a common factor. **2.** the process of reducing or subsuming under a general rule or statement, such as classifying items in general categories. **3.** a principle with general application. **4.** (in occupational therapy) the ability of a patient to apply knowledge and skills learned in therapy to a variety of similar but new situations.

generalized anaphylaxis /jen′(ə)rəlīzd′/, a severe reagin-mediated reaction to an allergen characterized by itching, edema, wheezing respirations, apprehension, cyanosis, dyspnea, pupillary dilation, falling blood pressure, and rapid weak pulse that may quickly produce shock and death.

generalized anxiety disorder (GAD), an anxiety reaction characterized by persistent apprehension. The symptoms range from mild, chronic tenseness with feelings of timidity, fatigue, apprehension, and indecisiveness to more intense states of restlessness and irritability that may lead to aggressive acts. In extreme cases the overwhelming emotional discomfort is accompanied by physical reactions. The symptoms of anxiety may be controlled with medication such as tranquilizers, but psychotherapy is the preferred treatment.

generalized peritonitis [L, *genus,* kind; Gk, *peri,* near, *tenein,* to stretch, *itis,* inflammation], a bacterial infection of the peritoneum secondary to an infection in another organ, as when an appendix ruptures or an ulcer perforates the gastric wall. The symptoms are usually acute and severe.

generally recognized as effective (GRAE), one of the statutory criteria that must be met by a drug before it can be approved as a new drug. Meeting these criteria relieves the manufacturer of the necessity of obtaining premarket approval as required by the Federal Food, Drug, and Cosmetic Act. To be recognized as effective, the drug must be, according to the act, considered safe and effective by "experts qualified by scientific training and experience."

generally recognized as safe (GRAS), a 1958 rule established by the U. S. Food and Drug Administration to identify foods regarded as safe to use because of lack of evidence that they may be harmful.

general paresis [L, *genus,* kind; Gk, paralysis], an organic mental disorder that results from chronic syphilitic infection. It is characterized by degeneration of the cortical neurons; progressive dementia, tremor, and speech disturbances; muscular weakness; and ultimately generalized paralysis.

general practitioner (GP) [L, *genus,* kind; Gk, *praktikos,* practical], a family practice physician.

general relaxation [L, *genus,* kind, *relaxare,* to ease], a slackening of strain or tension of the entire body, but particularly of the muscles.

general symptom [L, *genus* + Gk, *symptoma,* that which happens], a symptom that affects the entire body rather than a specific organ or location.

generation /jen′ərā′shən/ [L, *generare,* to beget], **1.** the act or process of reproduction; procreation. **2.** a group of contemporary individuals, animals, or plants that are the same number of life cycles from a common ancestor. **3.** the period between the birth of one individual or organism and that of its offspring.

generative /jen′ərā′tiv/ [L, *generare,* to beget], pertaining to activity that generates new physical or mental growth, such as creative problem solving.

generic /jəner′ik/ [L, *genus,* kind], **1.** pertaining to a genus. **2.** pertaining to a substance, product, or drug that is not protected by trademark. **3.** pertaining to the name of a kind of drug that is also the description of the drug, such as penicillin or tetracycline.

generic equivalent, a drug product sold under its generic name, identical in chemical composition to one or more others sold under trademark but not necessarily equivalent in therapeutic effect.

generic name, the official established nonproprietary name assigned to a drug. A drug is licensed under its generic name, and all manufacturers of the drug list it by its generic name. However, a drug is usually marketed under trademark chosen by the manufacturer.

generic nursing program, a program that prepares people with no professional nursing experience for entry into the field of nursing.

genesis /jen′əsis/ [Gk, origin], **1.** the origin, generation, or developmental evolution of anything. **2.** the act of producing or procreating.

gene splicing /jēn/, (in molecular genetics) the process by which a segment of deoxyribonucleic acid (DNA) is attached to or inserted into a strand of DNA from another source.

gene therapy, a procedure that involves injection of "healthy genes" into the bloodstream of a patient to cure or treat a hereditary disease or similar illness. Blood is withdrawn from the patient; the white cells are separated and cultured in a laboratory and inserted into modified viruses. Normal genes from a volunteer are inserted into the viruses, which, in turn, transfer the normal gene into the chromosomes of the patient's white cells. The white cells containing the normal genes are finally injected into the patient's bloodstream.

genetic /jənet′ik/ [Gk, *genesis,* origin], **1.** pertaining to reproduction, birth, or origin. **2.** pertaining to genetics or heredity. **3.** pertaining to or produced by a gene; inherited.

genetic affinity, relationship by direct descent.

genetically significant dose (GSD) /jənet′iklē/, an arbitrary measure of the esti mated annual gonadal radiation received by the population gene pool. In the United States the estimated GSD is 20 mrad. The figure is not intended to suggest possible genetic effects of exposure to that level of radiation.

genetic association, a condition in which specific genotypes are associated with other factors, such as specific diseases.

genetic carrier, a person who carries a gene without exhibiting the effects of that gene. Such a gene is usually recessive, but it may also be dominant and latent, with symptoms that do not appear until adulthood.

genetic code, the information carried by the deoxyribonucleic acid molecules that determines the specific amino acids and their arrangement in the polypeptide chain of each protein synthesized by the cell. Any change in the code results in the incorrect arrangement of the amino acids in the protein, causing a mutation.

genetic colonization, the process by which a parasite introduces into its host genetic information that induces the host to synthesize products solely for the use of the parasite.

genetic counseling, the process of determining the occurrence or risk of occurrence of a genetic disorder within a family and of providing appropriate information and advice about the courses of action that are available, whether care of a child already affected, prenatal diagnosis, termination of a pregnancy, sterilization, or artificial insemination is involved.

Genetic Counseling, a Nursing Interventions Classification defined as use of an interactive helping process focusing on the prevention of a genetic disorder or on the ability to cope with a family member who has a genetic disorder.

genetic death, **1.** the failure of an organism to survive as a result of its genetic makeup. **2.** the removal of a gene or genotype from the gene pool of a population or a given familial descent because of sterility, failure of the individual or organism to reproduce, or death before sexual maturity.

genetic drift, the chance fluctuations in gene frequencies within a population. The smaller the population, the greater the tendency for variation within each generation, so that eventually small isolated inbreeding groups become genetically quite different from their ancestors.

genetic engineering, the process of producing recombinant deoxyribonucleic acid (DNA) so that the genotype and phenotype of organisms can be altered and controlled. Enzymes are used to break the DNA molecule into fragments so that genes from another organism can be inserted and the nucleotides can be rearranged in any desired sequence.

genetic equilibrium, the state within a population at which the frequency of genes and genotypes does not change from generation to generation.

genetic homeostasis, the maintenance of genetic variability within a population through adaptation to varied or changing environments and conditions of life as a result of shifts or resistance to shifts in gene frequencies.

genetic isolate, a group of plants, animals, or individuals that are genetically separated by geographic, racial, social, cultural, or other barriers that prevent them from interbreeding with those outside the group.

geneticist /jənet′isist/, one who specializes in the study or application of genetics.

genetic load, the average number of accumulated detrimental genes per individual within a population, including those caused by mutation and selection within a recent generation and those inherited from ancestors.

genetic map, the graphic representation of the linear arrangement of genes on a chromosome and the relative distances between them, as expressed in map or morgan units.

genetic marker, any specific gene that produces a readily recognizable genetic trait that can be used in family and population studies or in linkage analysis.

genetic polymorphism, the recurrence within a population of two or more discontinuous genetic variants of a specific trait in such proportions that they cannot be maintained simply by mutation, such as the sickle cell trait, the Rh factor, and the blood groups.

genetics /jənet′iks/, **1.** the science that studies the principles and mechanics of heredity, specifically the means by which traits are passed from parents to offspring and the causes of the similarities and differences between related organisms. **2.** the total genetic makeup of a particular individual, family, group, or condition.

genetic screening, the process of investigating a specific population of persons for the purpose of detecting the presence of disease, either incipient or overt, such as the generalized screening of all newborns for phenylketonuria.

gene transfer [Gk, *genein,* to produce; L, *transferre,* to bring across], a type of gene therapy in which a gene is transplanted from a donor organism into a recipient organism.

geniculate neuralgia /jənik'yəlāt/ [L, *geniculum,* little knee; Gk, *neuron,* nerve, *algos,* pain], a severe debilitating inflammatory condition of the geniculate ganglion of the facial nerve. It is characterized by pain, loss of the sense of taste, facial paralysis, and a decrease in salivation and lacrimation.

geniohyoideus /jē'nē·ōhī·oi'dē·əs/ [Gk, *genion,* chin, *hyoides,* Y-shaped], one of the four suprahyoid muscles that draw the hyoid bone and the tongue forward.

genitals /jen'itəlz/ [L, *genitalis*], the sex, or reproductive, organs visible on the outside of the body. In the female they include the vulva, mons veneris, labia majora, labia minora, clitoris, and vaginal vestibule. The male genitals include the penis, scrotum, and testicles. —**genital,** *adj.*

genital stage /jen'itəl/ [L, *genitalis* + Fr, *stage,* trial period], (in psychoanalysis) the final period in freudian psychosexual development, beginning with adolescence and continuing through the adult years when the genitals are the predominant source of pleasurable stimulation.

genital wart [L, *genitalis* + AS, *wearte*], a small soft, moist pink or red swelling that becomes pedunculated. The growth may be solitary, or a cauliflower-like group may be present in the same area of the prepuce or vulva. It is caused by a human papilloma virus and is contagious. Atypical genital warts should have biopsy as possible carcinomas because they are associated with cervical cancer.

genitourinary (GU) /jen'itō·yŏŏr'iner'ē/ [L, *genitalis* + Gk, *ouron,* urine], referring to the genital and urinary systems of the body: the organ structures, functions, or both.

genocide /jen'əsīd/, the systematic extermination of a national, ethnic, political, religious, or other population.

genogram /jē'nōgram/, a diagram that depicts family relationships over at least three generations.

genome /jē'nōm/ [Gk, *genein,* to produce], the complete set of genes in the chromosomes of each cell of a specific organism.

genome map, a graphic representation of the locations of genes in a genome. The human genome map, completed in 1996, locates 5264 markers for genes and has led to the discovery of 223 genes linked to more than 200 diseases.

genomic /jēnō'mik/, pertaining to genome.

genotoxic /jē'nōtok'sik/, capable of altering deoxyribonucleic acid, thereby causing cancer or mutation.

genotoxic carcinogens, cancer-causing agents that can alter deoxyribonucleic acid molecules.

genotype /jē'nōtīp'/ [Gk, *genos,* birth, *typos,* mark], **1.** the complete genetic constitution of an organism or group, as determined by the specific combination and location of the genes on the chromosomes. **2.** the alleles situated at one or more sites on homologous chromosomes. The genetic information carried by a pair of alleles determines a specific characteristic or trait. **3.** a group or class of organisms having the same genetic makeup; the type species of a genus. —**genotypic,** *adj.*

gentamicin sulfate /jen'təmī'sin/, an aminoglycoside antibiotic prescribed to relieve the effects of severe infections caused by organisms sensitive to gentamicin.

gentian violet /jen'shən/, an antibacterial antiinfective, antifungal, and anthelmintic. It is prescribed in the treatment of pinworms, superficial infections of the skin, and vaginal infections.

genu /jē'nōō/ [L, knee], the knee or any angular structure resembling the flexed knee.

genupectoral position /je'nōōpek'tərəl/ [L, *genu,* knee, *pectus,* breast, *positio*], knee-chest position. To assume the genupectoral position the person kneels so that the weight of the body is supported by the knees and chest, with the abdomen raised. The head is turned to one side, and the arms are flexed so that the upper part of the body can be supported in part by the elbows.

genu recurvatum [L, *genu,* knee, *recurvare,* to bend back], a backward deformity, hyperextension, at the knee joint.

genus /jē'nəs/, *pl.* **genera** /jen'ərə/ [L, kind], a subdivision of a family of animals or plants. A genus usually is composed of several closely related species. The genus *Homo* has only one species, *Homo sapiens* (humans).

genu valgum [L, *genu,* knee, *valgus,* bent inward], a deformity in which the legs are curved inward so that the knees are close together, knocking as the person walks, with the ankles widely separated.

genu varum [L, knee, *varus,* bent outward], a deformity in which one or both legs are bent outward at the knee.

geographic tongue /jē'əgraf'ik/ [Gk, *ge,* earth, *graphein,* to record; AS, *tunge*], an inflammatory disorder on the dorsal surface of the tongue characterized by numerous and continually changing areas of loss and regrowth of the filiform papillae.

geophagia, the practice of eating clay or dirt. A form of pica, the compulsion is associated with disorders of mineral balance.

geotrichosis /jē′ōtrikō′sis/ [Gk, *ge,* earth, *thrix,* hair, *osis,* condition], a condition associated with the fungus *Geotrichum candidum* that may cause oral, bronchial, pharyngeal, and intestinal disorders. Geotrichosis most commonly occurs in immunosuppressed individuals with diabetes. Geotrichosis has been associated with allergic asthmatic reactions similar to allergic aspergillosis and a type of intestinal disorder characterized by abdominal pain, diarrhea, and rectal bleeding.

geriatric day care /jer′ē·at′rik/ [Gk, *geras,* old age; AS, *daeg* + L, *garrire,* chatter], an ambulatory health care facility for elderly people. It usually offers a broad range of professional and community services to maximize functional independence of the patients.

Geriatric Depression Scale (GDS), a brief depression screening inventory composed of 30 questions that require yes or no answers. The 30-item score of 11 or above indicates depressed individuals.

geriatrician /jer′ē·ətrish′ən/, a physician who has specialized postgraduate education and experience in the medical care of older persons.

geriatric nurse practitioner, a registered nurse with additional education obtained through a master's degree program in nursing or a nondegree-granting certificate program that prepares the nurse to deliver primary health care to elderly adults.

geriatrics /jer′ē·at′riks/, the branch of medicine dealing with the physiologic characteristics of aging and the diagnosis and treatment of diseases affecting the aged.

germ /jurm/ [L, *germen,* sprout], 1. any microorganism, especially one that is pathogenic. 2. a unit of living matter able to develop into a self-sufficient organism such as a seed, spore, or egg. 3. (in embryology) the first stage in development, such as a spermatozoon or other germ cell.

germanium (Ge) /jərmā′nē·əm/ [Germany], a metallic element with some nonmetallic semiconductor properties. Its atomic number is 32; its atomic mass (weight) is 72.61.

germ cell, 1. a sexual reproductive cell in any stage of development, from the primordial embryonic form to the mature gamete. 2. an ovum or spermatozoon or any of their preceding forms. 3. any cell undergoing gametogenesis.

germ-free animal, a laboratory animal raised under sterile conditions, free of exposure to microorganisms.

germicide /jur′misīd/ [L, *germen,* sprout,

caedere, to kill], a drug that kills pathogenic microorganisms. —**germicidal,** *adj.*

germinal /jur′minəl/ [L, *germen,* sprout], pertaining to or characteristic of a germ cell or to the early stages of development.

germinal center [L, *germen,* sprout; Gk, *kentron,* center], an antigen-localizing primary follicle with lymphoid tissue. It reacts to antigens, enlarging and becoming filled with lymphoblasts and macrophages at the center of a ring of small lymphocytes.

germinal epithelium, 1. the epithelial layer covering the genital ridge from which the gonads are derived in early embryonic development. 2. the epithelial covering of the ovary, formerly thought to be the site of the formation of the oogonia.

germinal infection, an infection transmitted to a child by the ovum or sperm of a parent.

germinal stage, (in embryology) the interval of time from fertilization to implantation during which the ovum undergoes cell division several times, travels to the uterus, and, in the form of a blastocyst, begins to implant itself in the endometrium.

germination /jur′minā′shən/ [L, *germen,* sprout], 1. the initial growth and development of an organism from the time of fertilization to the formation of the embryo. 2. the sprouting of a spore or the seed of a plant. —**germinate,** *v.*

germinoma /jur′minō′mə/, a neoplasm of the germinal tissue of the gonads, the mediastinum, or the pineal region.

germ layer, one of the three primordial cell layers formed during gastrulation in the early stages of embryonic development from which the entire range of body tissue is derived.

germ line, genetic material in a cell lineage that is passed down through the gametes before it is modified by somatic recombination or maturation.

germ plasm, 1. the protoplasm of the germ cells containing the basic reproductive and hereditary material; the total of the deoxyribonucleic acid in a specific cell or organism. 2. *nontechnical.* germ cells in any stage of development together with the tissues from which they originated.

germ theory [L, *germen,* sprout; Gk, *theoria,* speculation], the concept that all infectious and contagious diseases are caused by living microorganisms.

geroderma /jer′ədur′mə/ [Gk, *geron,* old man, *derma,* skin], 1. the atrophic skin of aging. 2. skin that is thin and wrinkled as a result of a defective state of nutrition. 3. any condition characterized by skin that is thin and wrinkled, resembling the skin of old age.

gerodontology /jer'ōdontol'əjē/, **1.** the study of the dentition and dental needs of the elderly. **2.** dental geriatrics.

gerontic nursing, nursing care pertaining to an older person, a compromise between geriatric nursing (nursing care primarily for older persons who are ill) and gerontologic nursing (a more holistic view of the nursing care of older persons).

gerontogen /jeron'təjən/, environmental agent that contributes to the aging process by accelerating the onset and/or rate of progression of aging.

Gerontological Society of America (GSA), an organization of scientific and academic professionals interested in studies of the nature of the aging process and the clinical manifestations of disease in the aging organism. GSA members participate with the International Association of Gerontology in periodic seminars at which worldwide research on longevity is presented.

gerontology /jer'əntol'əjē/ [Gk, geras, old age, logos, science], the study of all aspects of the aging process, including the clinical, psychologic, economic, and sociologic issues encountered by older persons and their consequences for both the individual and society.

geropsychiatry /jer'ōsīkī'ətrē/ [Gk, geras, old age, psyche, mind], the study and treatment of psychiatric aspects of aging and mental disorders of elderly people.

Gesell Developmental Assessment [Arnold L. Gesell, American pediatrician and psychologist, 1880–1961], an evaluation program that provides information on gross motor, fine motor, language, personal-social, and cognitive development.

Gestalt /gəshtält'/, pl. **Gestalts, Gestalten** /gəshtäl'tən/ [Ger, form], a single physical, psychologic, or symbolic configuration, pattern, or experience that consists of a number of elements and has an effect as a whole different from that of the sum of its parts.

Gestalt psychology, a school of psychology, originating in Germany, that maintains that a psychologic phenomenon is perceived as a total configuration or pattern, rising from the relationships among its constituent elements, rather than as discrete elements possessing attributes of their own.

Gestalt therapy, a form of psychotherapy that stresses the unity of self-awareness, behavior, and experience.

gestate /jes'tāt/ [L, gestare, to bear], **1.** to carry a developing fetus in the womb. **2.** to grow and develop slowly toward maturity, such as a fetus in the womb.

gestation /jestā'shən/ [L, gestare, to bear], the period from the fertilization of the ovum until birth. Gestation varies with the species; in humans the average duration is 266 days, or approximately 280 days from the onset of the last menstrual period.

gestational age /jestā'shənəl/ [L, gestare + aetas, time of life], the age of a fetus or a newborn, usually expressed in weeks dating from the first day of the mother's last menstrual period.

gestational assessment [L, gestare, to bear, assidere, to sit beside], calculation of the fetal age of the offspring, based on such factors as the menstrual history of the mother, the date when fetal heart sounds are first detected, and the evaluation of ultrasound data. The information is important in planning emergency care in the event of premature birth signs.

gestational diabetes mellitus (GDM), a disorder characterized by an impaired ability to metabolize carbohydrate, usually caused by a deficiency of insulin, occurring in pregnancy. It disappears after delivery of the infant but, in a significant number of cases, returns years later.

gestational psychosis [L, gestare, to bear; Gk, psyche, mind, osis, condition], any mental disorder that can be attributed to a pregnancy.

gestational sac, a pouch containing the fetus in extrauterine gestation.

gestures in physical examination /jes'-chərs/, physical appearance clues in diagnosis, such as a patient's pressing a clenched fist against the sternum as a "body language" message of the pain experienced during a myocardial infarction.

Getman visuomotor theory, a concept that visual perception is based on developmental sequences of physiologic actions in children. The sequence of eight stages begins with innate response systems and advances to cognitive integration of perceptions, abstractions, and higher symbolic activity.

GFR, abbreviation for **glomerular filtration rate.**

GFP, abbreviation for **green fluorescent protein.**

GH, abbreviation for **growth hormone.**

Ghon's complex [Anton Ghon, Czechoslovakian pathologist, 1866–1936], a combination of pleural surface-healed granulomas or scars on the middle lobe of the lung together with hilar lymph node granulomas. The complex is evidence that a primary tuberculosis case has healed.

ghost cells [AS, gast + L, cella, storeroom], red blood cells that have lost their hemoglobin so that only the plasma membranes are observed in microscopic examinations of urine samples. The hemoglobin is destroyed by the presence of urine.

GI, abbreviation for **gastrointestinal.**

giant cell /jī'ənt/ [L, *gigant,* huge, *cella,* storeroom], an abnormally large tissue cell. It often contains more than one nucleus and may appear as a merger of several normal cells.

giant cell carcinoma, a malignant epithelial neoplasm characteristically containing many large anaplastic cells.

giant cell myeloma, a bone tumor of multinucleated giant cells that resembles osteoclasts scattered in a matrix of spindle cells.

giant chromosome, any of the excessively large chromosomes found in insects and lower animals, specifically the lampbrush chromosome and polytene chromosome.

giant follicular lymphoma, a nodular, well-differentiated lymphocytic malignant lymphoma in which nodules distort the normal structure of a lymph node.

giant hypertrophic gastritis, a rare disease characterized by large folds of nodular gastric rugae that may cover the wall of the stomach, causing anorexia, nausea, vomiting, and abdominal distress.

giant peristaltic contraction, a propulsive contraction of the bowel that normally occurs periodically in the distal small intestine and colon. The contractions are 1.5 to 2 times larger than normal in amplitude and 4 to 6 times longer in duration than usual.

Giardia /jē·ár'dē·ə/ [Alfred Giard, French biologist, 1846–1908], a common genus of flagellate protozoans. Many species of *Giardia* normally inhabit the digestive tract and cause inflammation in association with other factors that produce rapid proliferation of the organism.

giardiasis /jē·árdī'əsis/ [Alfred Giard; Gk, *osis,* condition], an inflammatory intestinal condition caused by overgrowth of the protozoan *Giardia lamblia.* The source of infection is usually untreated water contaminated with *G. lamblia* cysts.

gibbus /gib'əs, jib'əs/ [L, hump], **1.** a hump, swelling, or enlargement on a body surface, usually confined to one side. **2.** a convex spinal curvature that may occur after the collapse of a vertebral body as may result from a fracture or tuberculosis of the spine.

Gibson's murmur [George A. Gibson, Scottish physician, 1854–1913], a heart murmur that is heard continuously throughout the cardiac cycle. It waxes at the end of systole and wanes near the end of diastole and is often described as a "machinery-like" murmur.

Gibson walking splint, a kind of Thomas splint that enables a patient to be ambulatory.

Giemsa's stain /gē·em'səz/ [Gustav Giemsa, German chemist, 1867–1948; Fr, *teindre,* to dye], an azure dye used as a stain in the microscopic examination of the blood for certain protozoan parasites, viral inclusion bodies, and rickettsia and, more routinely, in the preparation of a smear for a differential white cell count.

GIFT, abbreviation for **gamete intrafallopian transfer.**

gigantism /jigan'tizəm/, [L, *gigas,* giant], an abnormal condition characterized by excessive size and stature. It is caused most frequently by hypersecretion of growth hormone and occurs to a lesser degree in hypogonadism and in certain genetic disorders.

Gilbert's syndrome [Nicolas A. Gilbert, French physician, 1858–1927], a benign hereditary condition characterized by hyperbilirubinemia and jaundice.

Gilles de la Tourette's syndrome /zhēl'dəlätŏŏrets'/ [George Gilles de la Tourette, French neurologist, 1857–1927], an abnormal condition characterized by facial grimaces, tics, and involuntary arm and shoulder movements. In adolescence the condition worsens; the patient may grunt, snort, and shout involuntarily. Coprolalia often develops.

Gillies' operation /gil'ēz/ [Harold D. Gillies, English surgeon, 1882–1960], a surgical procedure for reducing fractures of the zygoma and zygomatic arch by making an incision in the temporal hairline.

ginger jake paralysis /jin'jərjāk'/, a polyneuropathy that primarily affects motor nerves to the distal parts of the extremities. First observed in Jamaica, it is caused by drinking an alcoholic extract of Jamaican ginger adulterated with a pesticide.

gingiva /jinjī'və/, *pl.* **gingivae** [L, gum], the gum tissues of the mouth, a mucous membrane with supporting fibrous tissue that overlies the crowns of unerupted teeth and encircles the necks of those that have erupted. —**gingival,** *adj.*

gingival abscess, a pocket of pus that arises under the mucosal covering of the gum and spreads to the neck of a tooth.

gingival blanching /jinjī'vəl/ [L, *gingiva* + Fr, *blanchir,* to whiten], the lightening of gum color, usually temporary, caused by stretching of gum tissue and decreased blood supply.

gingival blood supply, the vascular supply to the gum tissue, arising from blood vessels that pass on the gum side of the outer periosteum of bone and anastomose with blood vessels of the periodontal membrane and intra-alveolar blood vessels.

gingival cavity, a cavity that occurs in the third of the clinical crown of the tooth nearest to the gum.

gingival color, the color of healthy or diseased gum tissues. It varies with the thickness and degree of keratinization of the epithelium, blood supply, pigmentation, and alterations produced by medications and gingival and systemic diseases.

gingival consistency, the combination of visual and tactile characteristics of healthy gum tissue.

gingival corium, the most stable connective tissue of the gingiva, which lies between the periosteum and the lamina propria mucosae.

gingival crater, a depression in the gum tissue, especially in the area of the former apex of interdental papilla.

gingival crevice, a normal space located circumferentially around all teeth between the wall of the unattached gum tissue and the enamel and/or cementum surface of the tooth.

gingival discoloration, a change in the normal color of the gum tissue, associated with inflammation, reduced blood supply, abnormal pigmentation, and other problems.

gingival festoon, the distinct rounding and enlargement of the margins of the gum tissue found in early gingival involvement.

gingival hormonal enlargement, the enlargement of the gum tissue associated with hormonal imbalance during pregnancy, puberty, and postmenopausal therapy.

gingival hyperplasia, overgrowth of the gum tissue, often in patients treated with phenytoin for epileptic seizures.

gingival hypertrophy, an overgrowth of gum tissue encircling the teeth. It may be caused by the ingestion of dilantin, a medication prescribed for the treatment of epilepsy.

gingival line [L, *gingiva,* gum, *linea*], the scalloped line formed by the edge of the unattached gum tissue at the margin of the soft tissues beside the teeth.

gingival massage, the rubbing of the gum tissues for cleansing purposes, improvement of tissue tone and blood circulation, and keratinization of the surface epithelium.

gingival mat, the connective tissue of the gum, composed of coarse, broad collagen fibers that attach the gingivae to the teeth and hold the unattached gum close to the teeth.

gingival physiology, the function of the gum tissue as supportive and protective investments of the teeth and subjacent tissues.

gingival position, the level of the gum margin in relation to the teeth.

gingival shrinkage, the reduction in the size of the gum tissue, especially as the result of therapeutic elimination of subgingival deposits and curettage of the soft tissue wall of the gingival pocket.

gingival stippling, a series of small depressions in the surface of healthy gum tissue, producing an appearance that varies from that of smooth, undulated velvet to that of an orange peel.

gingivectomy /jin′jīvek′təmē/ [L, *gingiva* + Gk, *ektome,* excision], surgical removal of infected and diseased gum tissue performed to arrest the progress of periodontal disease.

gingivitis /jin′jivī′tis/ [L, *gingiva* + Gk, *itis,* inflammation], a condition in which the free gingival margins close to the teeth are red, swollen, and bleeding. Generally gingivitis is the result of poor oral hygiene, but it may be a sign of other conditions such as diabetes mellitus.

gingivoplasty /jin′jivōplas′tē/ [L, *gingiva* + Gk, *plassein,* to shape], the surgical contouring of the gum tissues and interdental papillae to restore gingival tissue to more normal form and function.

gingivostomatitis /jin′jivōstō′matī′tis/ [L, *gingiva* + Gk, *stoma,* mouth, *itis,* inflammation], multiple painful ulcers on the gums and mucous membranes of the mouth, the result of a herpesvirus infection.

ginseng /jin′seng/, a folk remedy prepared from the root of any species of the genus *Panax.* It is used by some Asian populations as a heart tonic, aphrodisiac, and stimulant.

Giordano-Giovannetti diet /jôrdā′nōjō′-vənet′ē/, a low-protein, low-fat, high-carbohydrate diet with controlled potassium and sodium intake, used in chronic renal insufficiency and liver failure. Protein is given only in the form of essential amino acids so that the body will use excess blood urea nitrogen to synthesize the nonessential amino acids for the production of tissue protein.

gipoma /gipō′mə/, a pancreatic tumor that causes changes in secretion of gastric inhibitory polypeptide.

girdle /gur′dəl/, any curved or circular structure, such as the hipline formed by the bones and related tissues of the pelvis.

girdle pad, a covering that fits over the iliac crests and sacrum to protect the hip area in contact sports.

Giuliani's sign, a posterior left chest thrill felt between the left scapula and spinal column of mitral insufficiency caused by anterior mitral leaf prolapse.

glabella /gləbəl′ə/ [L, *glabrum,* bald], a flat triangular area of bone between the two superciliary ridges of the forehead. It is sometimes used as a baseline for cephalometric measurements.

glabrous skin /glā′brəs/ [L, *glaber,* smooth; AS, *scinn*], smooth, hairless skin.

glacial acetic acid /glā′shəl/, a clear, colorless liquid or crystalline substance (CH_3COOH) with a pungent odor. It is obtained by the destructive distillation of wood or from acetylene and water or by the oxidation of ethyl alcohol by aerobic bacteria, as in the production of vinegar. Glacial acetic acid is strongly corrosive and potentially flammable, having a low flash point.

gland [L, *glans,* acorn], any one of many organs in the body, comprising specialized cells that secrete or excrete materials not related to their ordinary metabolism. Some glands lubricate; others such as the pituitary gland produce hormones; hematopoietic glands such as the spleen and certain lymph nodes take part in the production of blood components. **Exocrine glands** discharge their secretions into ducts. **Endocrine glands** are ductless and discharge their secretion products directly into the blood or interstitial fluid.

glanders [OFr, *glandres,* neck gland swelling], an infection caused by the bacillus *Pseudomonas mallei,* transmitted to humans from horses and other domestic animals. It is characterized by purulent inflammation of the mucous membranes and development of skin nodules that ulcerate.

glandular epithelium [L, *glandula,* small gland; Gk, *epi,* above, *thele,* nipple], epithelium that contains glandular cells.

glandular tissue [L, *glandula,* small gland; OFr, *tissu*], a group of epithelial secreting cells composing a definitive glandular organ such as the thyroid.

glans /glanz/, *pl.* **glandes** /glan′dēz/ [L, acorn], **1.** a general term for a small rounded mass or a glandlike body. **2.** erectile tissue, as on the ends of the clitoris and the penis.

glans of clitoris [L, *glans* + Gk, *kleitoris*], the erectile tissue at the end of the clitoris. It comprises two corpora cavernosa enclosed in a dense, fibrous membrane and connected to the pubis and ischium.

glans penis, the conical tip of the penis that covers the end of the corpora cavernosa penis and the corpus spongiosum like a cap. The urethral orifice is normally located at the distal tip of the glans penis.

glare, a strong, dazzling light that may cause discomfort to the eye.

Glasgow Coma Scale, a quick, practical standardized system for assessing the degree of conscious impairment in the critically ill and for predicting the duration and ultimate outcome of coma, primarily in patients with head injuries. The system involves three determinants, eye opening, verbal response, and motor response, all of which are evaluated independently according to a rank order that indicates the level of consciousness and degree of dysfunction.

Glasgow Outcome Scale, a functional assessment inventory based on five global categories: death, persistent vegetative state, severe disability, moderate disability, and good recovery. It measures outcome. It has been criticized as lacking sensitivity to functionally significant changes.

glaucoma /glôkō′mə, glou-/ [Gk, cataract], an abnormal condition of elevated pressure within an eye caused by obstruction of the outflow of aqueous humor. Acute (angle-closure, closed-angle, or narrow-angle) glaucoma occurs if the pupil in an eye with a narrow angle between the iris and cornea dilates markedly, causing the folded iris to block the exit of aqueous humor from the anterior chamber. Chronic (open-angle or wide-angle) glaucoma is much more common, often bilateral; it develops slowly and is genetically determined. The obstruction is believed to occur within the Schlemm's canal. —**glaucomatous,** *adj.*

glaucomatocyclitic crisis /glôkom′ə-tōsiklit′ik/, a recurrent rise in intraocular pressure in one eye, resembling acute angle-closure glaucoma and accompanied by signs of uveitis.

glaucomatous halo /glôkom′ətəs/, **1.** an illusion of a circle of brightness surrounding a light, observed by some glaucoma patients. **2.** a yellowish-white ring surrounding the optic disc.

glenohumeral /glē′nōhyo͞o′mərəl/, [Gk, *glene,* joint socket; L, *humerus,* shoulder], pertaining to the glenoid cavity and the humerus at the shoulder joint.

glenohumeral joint, the shoulder joint, formed by the glenoid cavity of the scapula and the head of the humerus.

glenohumeral ligaments [Gk, *glene,* joint socket, *humerus,* shoulder], three thickened bands of connective tissue attached proximally to the anterior margin of the

glenoid cavity and labrum and distally to the lesser tuberosity and neck of the humerus.

glenoid cavity /glē'noid/ [Gk, *glene,* joint socket, *eidos,* form; L, *cavum*], a shallow depression with which the head of the humerus articulates.

glia cells /glī'ə, glē'ə/ [Gk, *glia,* glue; L, *cella,* storeroom], neural cells that have a connective tissue supporting function in the central nervous system. Examples include astrocytes and oligodendroglial cells of ectodermal origin and microglial cells of mesodermal origin.

gliadin /glī'ədin/ [Gk, *glia,* glue], a protein substance that is obtained from wheat and rye. Its solubility in diluted alcohol distinguishes it from another grain protein, glutenin.

glial cell line-derived neurotrophic factor (GDNF) /glī'əl/, a nerve growth drug. It has been used in laboratory animals to reverse the progression of symptoms of Parkinson's disease. GDNF is believed to act as a biologic shield, protecting dopamine nerve cells from damage that normally would destroy them.

gliding [AS, *glidan,* to glide], **1.** one of the four basic movements allowed by the various joints of the skeleton. It is common to all movable joints and allows one surface to move smoothly over an adjacent surface, regardless of shape. **2.** a smooth, continuous movement.

gliding contusion, a brain injury caused by displacement of the gray matter of the cerebral cortex during angular acceleration of the head. Most of the damage occurs at the junction between the gray matter and the white matter. Such contusions are associated with diffuse axonal injuries and acute subdural hematomas.

gliding joint, a synovial joint in which articulation of contiguous bones allows only gliding movements, as in the wrist and the ankle.

gliding zone, an articular cartilage surface area immediately adjacent to a joint space.

glioblastoma multiforme /glī'ōblastō'mə mul'tifôr'mē/ [Gk, *glia,* glue, *blastos,* germ, *oma,* tumor; L, *multus,* many, *forma,* form], a malignant, rapidly growing pulpy or cystic tumor of the cerebrum or the spinal cord. The lesion spreads with pseudopod-like projections.

glioma /glī·ō'mə/ [Gk, *glia* + *oma,* tumor], any of the largest group of primary tumors of the brain, composed of malignant glial cells. Kinds of gliomas are **astrocytoma, ependymoma, glioblastoma multiforme, medulloblastoma,** and **oligodendrogli- oma.**

glioneuroma /glī'ōno͞oro͞o'mə/ [Gk, *glia* + *neuron,* nerve, *oma,* tumor], a neoplasm composed of nerve cells and elements of their supporting connective tissue.

gliosarcoma /glī'ōsärkō'mə/ [Gk, *glia* + *sarx,* flesh, *oma,* tumor], a tumor composed of spindle-shaped cells in the delicate supporting connective tissue of nerve cells.

gliosis /glī·ō'sis/, a proliferation of astrocytes that may appear as a sign of healing after a central nervous system injury.

glipizide /glip'izīd/, an oral antidiabetic drug prescribed as an adjunct to diet and exercise in lowering blood glucose levels of patients with noninsulin-dependent diabetes.

Glisson's capsule /glis'ənz/ [Francis Glisson, English physician, 1597–1677; L, *capsula,* little box], the fibrous tissue sheath around lobules of the liver that carry branches of the hepatic artery, portal vein, and bile duct.

glitter cells [ME, *gliteren,* to shine], white blood cells in which movement of granules is observed in their cytoplasm. They are seen in microscopic examination of urine samples in cases of pyelonephritis.

Gln, abbreviation for **glutamine.**

global aphasia /glō'bəl/ [L, *globus,* ball; Gk, *a* + *phasis,* without speech], a loss of ability to use any form of written or spoken language. The condition involves both sensory and motor nerve tracts. Communication is attempted through gestures or the use of automatic words and phrases.

global price, (in U. S. managed care) an all-inclusive price for services rendered. It may refer to comprehensive physician services alone or include both hospital and physician services, depending on the contractual agreement.

global warming, an ecologic model of world climate changes based on the **greenhouse effect,** exacerbated by burning of fossil fuels, massive deforestation, and conversion of cropland to industrial and other urban uses, all contributing to an increase in the earth's temperature.

globin /glō'bin/ [L, *globus,* ball], a group of four globulin protein molecules that become bound by the iron in heme molecules to form hemoglobin or myoglobin.

globose nucleus, one of four deeply placed cerebellar nuclei located medial to the emboliform nucleus. It receives input from the intermediate zone of the cerebellar cortex, and its axons exit via the superior cerebellar peduncle.

globule /glob'yo͞ol/ [L, *globulus,* small ball], a small spheric mass.

globulin /glob'yōōlin/, one of a broad category of simple proteins classified by solubility, electrophoretic mobility, and size.

globulinuria /-ōōr'ē·ə/ [L, *globulus,* small ball; Gk, *ouron,* urine], the presence of globulin class proteins in the urine.

globus hystericus /glō'bus/ [L, small ball; Gk, *hystera,* womb], a transitory sensation of a lump in the throat that cannot be swallowed or coughed up, often accompanying emotional conflict or acute anxiety.

globus pallidus /pal'idəs/ [L, small ball, pale], the smaller and more medial part of the lentiform nucleus of the brain, separated from the putamen by the lateral medullary lamina.

glomangioma /glōman'jē·ō'mə/ [L, *glomus,* ball of thread; Gk, *angeion,* vessel, *oma*], a benign tumor that develops from a cluster of blood cells in the skin.

glomerular /glōmer'yōōlər/ [L, *glomerulus,* small ball], pertaining to a glomerulus, especially a renal glomerulus.

glomerular disease, any of a group of diseases in which the glomerulus of the kidney is affected. Depending on the particular disease, there may be hyperplasia, atrophy, necrosis, scarring, or deposits in the glomeruli.

glomerular filtration, the renal process whereby fluid in the blood is filtered across the capillaries of the glomerulus and into the urinary space of Bowman's capsule.

glomerular filtration rate (GFR), [L, *glomerulus,* small ball; Fr, *filtre* + L, *ratus*], a kidney function test in which results can be determined from the amount of ultrafiltrate formed by plasma flowing through the glomeruli of the kidney. It may be calculated from insulin and creatinine clearance, serum creatinine, and blood urea nitrogen.

glomerulonephritis /glōmer'yōōlōnəfrī'tis/ [L, *glomerulus,* small ball; Gk, *nephros,* kidney, *itis*], an inflammation of the glomerulus of the kidney, characterized by proteinuria, hematuria, decreased urine production, and edema.

glomerulosclerosis /-sklərō'sis/ [L, *glomerulus,* small ball; Gk, *sklerosis,* a hardening, *osis,* condition], a severe kidney disease in which glomerular function of blood filtration is lost as fibrous scar tissue replaces the glomeruli. The disease commonly follows an infection or arteriosclerosis.

glomerulus /glōmer'yōōləs/, *pl.* **glomeruli** [L, small ball], **1.** a tuft or cluster. **2.** a structure composed of blood vessels or nerve fibers, such as a renal glomerulus.

glomus /glō'məs/, *pl.* **glomera** /glom'ərə/ [L, ball of thread], a small group of arterioles connecting directly to veins and having a rich nerve supply.

glomus cell, 1. an epithelioid cell surrounding a coiled arteriovenous anastomosis of a glomus body. **2.** a modified smooth muscle cell.

glomus tumor, a frequently painful neoplasm involving the arteriovenous anastomoses of the skin.

glossectomy /glosek'təmē/ [Gk, *glossa,* tongue, *ektome,* excision], the surgical removal of all or a part of the tongue.

glossitis /glosī'tis/ [Gk, *glossa,* tongue, *itis*], inflammation of the tongue. Acute glossitis, characterized by swelling, intense pain that may be referred to the ears, salivation, fever, and enlarged regional lymph nodes, may develop during an infectious disease or after a burn, bite, or other injury.

glossodynia /glos'ōdin'ē·ə/ [Gk, *glossa* + *odyne,* pain], pain in the tongue, caused by acute or chronic inflammation, an abscess, an ulcer, or trauma.

glossoepiglottic /glos'ō·ep'iglot'ik/, pertaining to the epiglottis and the tongue.

glossolalia /glos'ōlā'lyə/ [Gk, *glossa* + *lalein,* to babble], speech in an unknown 'language,' as 'speaking in tongues' during a state of religious ecstasy.

glossoncus /glosong'kəs/ [Gk, *glossa* + *onkos,* swelling], a local swelling or general enlargement of the tongue.

glossopathy /glosop'əthē/ [Gk, *glossa* + *pathos,* disease], a pathologic condition of the tongue, such as acute inflammation caused by a burn, bite, injury, or infectious disease; enlargement resulting from congenital lymphangioma; or a disorder produced by mycotic infection, a malignant lesion, or a congenital anomaly.

glossopexy /glos'əpek'sē/ [Gk, *glossa* + *pexis,* fixation], an adhesion of the tongue to the lip.

glossopharyngeal /glos'ōfərin'jē·əl/ [Gk, *glossa* + *pharynx,* throat], pertaining to the tongue and pharynx.

glossopharyngeal breathing (GPB), a technique of forcing air into the lungs with the pharynx and tongue muscles. The technique can be taught to patients whose respiratory muscles are weak.

glossopharyngeal nerve, either of a pair of cranial nerves essential to the sense of taste, sensation in some viscera, and secretion from certain glands.

glossopharyngeal neuralgia, a disorder of unknown origin characterized by recurrent attacks of severe pain in the back of the pharynx, the tonsils, the base of the tongue, and the middle ear.

glossophytia /glos'əfit'ē·ə/ [Gk, *glossa* + *phyton,* plant], a condition of the tongue characterized by a blackish patch on the dorsum on which filiform papillae are greatly elongated and thickened like bristly hairs.

glossoplasty /glos'ōplas'tē/ [Gk, *glossa* + *plassein,* to mold], a surgical procedure or plastic operation on the tongue performed to correct a congenital anomaly, repair an injury, or restore a measure of function after excision of a malignant lesion.

glossoptosis /glos'optō'sis/ [Gk, *glossa* + *ptosis,* falling], the retraction or downward displacement of the tongue.

glossopyrosis /glos'ōpīrō'sis/ [Gk, *glossa* + *pyr,* fire, *osis,* condition], a burning sensation in the tongue caused by chronic inflammation, exposure to extremely hot or spicy food, or psychogenic glossitis.

glossorrhaphy /glosôr'əfē/ [Gk, *glossa* + *rhaphe,* seam], the surgical suturing of a wound in the tongue.

glossotrichia /glos'ətrik'ē·ə/ [Gk, *glossa* + *thrix,* hair], a condition of the tongue characterized by a hairlike appearance of the papillae.

glossy skin [ONorse, *glosa,* smooth and shiny; AS, *scinn*], a shiny skin that is usually secondary to neuritis and may be associated with other integumentary disorders, including alopecia, skin fissuring, and ulceration. It usually begins as an erythematous area on an extremity.

glottis, *pl.* **glottises, glottides** [Gk, opening to larynx], **1.** a slitlike opening between the true vocal cords (plica vocalis). **2.** the phonation apparatus of the larynx, composed of the true vocal cords and the opening between them (rima glottidis). —**glottal, glottic,** *adj.*

gloves, sterile fitted coverings for the hands, usually with a separate sheath for each finger and thumb. Gloves are worn to protect health care personnel from urine, stool, blood, saliva, and drainage from wounds and lesions of patients, but also to protect patients from health care personnel who may have cuts.

glow curve, (in thermoluminescence dosimetry) the graphic representation of the emitted light intensity that increases with the increasing phosphor temperature.

GLP-1, abbreviation for **glucagon-like peptide 1.**

Glu, abbreviation for **glutamic acid.**

glucagon /glōō'kəgon/ [Gk, *glykys,* sweet, *agaein,* to lead], a polypeptide hormone produced by alpha cells in the islets of Langerhans that stimulates the conversion of glycogen to glucose in the liver. Secretion of glucagon is stimulated by hypoglycemia and by the growth hormone of the anterior pituitary.

glucagon-like peptide 1 (GLP-1), an appetite-suppressing substance found in the brain and intestine. In the brain GLP-1 acts as a satiety signal. In the intestine it slows emptying of the stomach and stimulates the release of insulin from the pancreas.

glucagonoma syndrome /glōō'kəgonō'mə/ [Gk, *glykys* + *agaein* + *oma,* tumor], a disease associated with a glucagon-secreting tumor of the islet cells of the pancreas. It is characterized by hyperglycemia, stomatitis, glossitis, anemia, weight loss, and a characteristic rash.

glucocorticoid /glōō'kōkôr'təkoid/ [Gk, *glykys* + L, *cortex,* bark; Gk, *eidos,* form], an adrenocortical steroid hormone that increases glyconeogenesis, exerts an antiinflammatory effect, and influences many body functions. The most important of the three glucocorticoids is cortisol (hydrocortisone); corticosterone is less active, and cortisone is inactive until converted to cortisol. Glucocorticoids promote the release of amino acids from muscle, mobilize fatty acids from fat stores, and increase the ability of skeletal muscles to maintain contractions and avoid fatigue.

gluconeogenesis /glōō'kō·nē'ō·jen'əsis/, the formation of glycogen from fatty acids and proteins rather than from carbohydrates.

glucosan /glōō'kəsan/ [Gk, *glykys,* sweet], any of a large group of anhydrous polysaccharides that on hydrolysis yield a hexose, primarily anhydrides of glucose. The glucosans include cellulose, glycogen, starch, and the dextrins.

glucose /glōō'kōs/ [Gk, *glykys,* sweet], a simple sugar found in certain foods, especially fruits, and a major source of energy present in human and animal body fluids.

glucose electrode, a specialized electric terminal that contains incorporated enzyme for glucose determination.

glucose 1-phosphate, an intermediate compound in carbohydrate metabolism.

glucose 6-phosphate, an intermediate compound in carbohydrate metabolism.

glucose-6-phosphate dehydrogenase (G-6-PD) deficiency, an inherited disorder characterized by red cells partially or completely deficient in glucose-6-phosphate dehydrogenase, an enzyme critical in aerobic glycolysis. The disorder is associated with episodes of acute hemolysis under conditions of stress or in response to certain chemicals or drugs.

glucose tolerance test, a test of the body's ability to metabolize carbohydrates by administering a standard dose of glucose and measuring the blood and urine for glucose level at regular intervals thereafter.

glucosuria /glōō′kōsŏŏr′ē·ə/ [Gk, *glykys* + *ouron*, urine], abnormal presence of glucose in the urine resulting from the ingestion of large amounts of carbohydrate or from a kidney disease such as nephrosis or a metabolic disease such as diabetes mellitus. **—glucosuric,** *adj.*

glucosyl, 1. pertaining to glucose. 2. a glucose radical.

glue sniffing [Gk, *gloios* + ME, *sniffen*], the practice of inhaling the vapors of toluene, a volatile organic compound used as a solvent in certain glues.

glutamate /glōō′təmāt/, a salt of glutamic acid, a major excitatory amino acid of the central nervous system.

glutamic acid (Glu) /glōōtam′ik/ [L, *gluten,* glue, *amine,* ammonia; *acidus,* sour], a nonessential amino acid that occurs widely in a number of proteins. Preparations of glutamic acid are used as aids for digestion.

glutamic acid decarboxylase autoantibody, an antibody found in patients with insulin-dependent diabetes mellitus (IDDM), and in stiff man syndrome, a neurologic condition associated with IDDM. The antibody recognizes glutamic acid decarboxylase, an intracellular enzyme.

glutamic acidemia /glōōtam′ikas′idē′-mē·ə/, an inherited disorder of amino acid metabolism that causes an excessive level of glutamic acid.

glutamic acid hydrochloride, a gastric acidifier prescribed for hypoacidity.

glutamine (Gln) /glōō′təmēn/ [L, *gluten* + *amine,* ammonia], a nonessential amino acid found in the juices of many plants and in many proteins in the body. It functions as an amino donor for many reactions. It is also a nontoxic transport for ammonia.

glutaraldehyde /glōō′täral′dəhīd/, a histologic fixative and sterilant for medical instruments.

glutargin /glōōtär′gin/, arginine glutamate.

glutathione /glōō′təthī′ōn/ [L, *gluten* + Gk, *theione,* sulfur], a tripeptide of glutamic acid, cysteine, and glycine whose deficiency is commonly associated with hemolytic anemia.

gluteal /glōō′tē·əl/ [Gk, *gloutos,* buttocks], pertaining to the buttocks or to the muscles that form the buttocks.

gluteal fold, 1. a fold of the buttock. 2. the horizontal lower margin of the buttock at its junction with the thigh.

gluteal reflex, contraction of the gluteus muscles elicited by stroking the back.

gluteal tuberosity, a ridge on the lateral posterior surface of the femur to which is attached the gluteus maximus.

gluten /glōō′tən/ [L, glue], the insoluble protein constituent of wheat and other grains.

glutethimide /glōōteth′əmīd/, a sedative prescribed in the treatment of anxiety and insomnia.

gluteus /glōōtē′əs/, any of the three muscles that form the buttocks. The gluteus maximus acts to extend the thigh. The gluteus medius acts to abduct and rotate the thigh. The gluteus minimus acts to abduct the thigh.

Gly, abbreviation for **glycine.**

glyburide /glī′bərīd/, an oral antidiabetic drug prescribed as an adjunct to diet and exercise in lowering blood glucose levels of patients with noninsulin-dependent diabetes.

glycate, the product of a nonenzymic reaction between a sugar and a free amino group of a protein.

glycerin /glis′ərin/ [Gk, *glykys,* sweet], a sweet, colorless oily fluid that is a pharmaceutic grade of glycerol. It is used as a moistening agent for chapped skin, as an ingredient of suppositories for constipation, and as a sweetening agent and vehicle for drug preparations.

glycerol /glis′ərôl/ [Gk, *glykys,* sweet], an alcohol that is a component of fats. Glycerol is soluble in ethyl alcohol and water.

glycerol kinase, an enzyme in the liver and kidneys that catalyzes the transfer of a phosphate group from adenosine triphosphate to form adenosine diphosphate and L-glycerol-3-phosphate.

glycine (Gly) /glī′sin/ [Gk, *glykys* + L, *amine,* ammonia], a nonessential amino acid occurring widely as a component of animal and plant proteins.

glycocholic acid /glī′kōkol′ik/ [Gk, *glykys,* sweet; L, *acidus,* sour], a substance in bile, formed by glycine and cholic acid, that aids in digestion and absorption of fats.

glycogen /glī′kəjən/ [Gk, *glykys,* sweet, *genein,* to produce], a polysaccharide that is the major carbohydrate stored in animal cells. It is formed from repeating units of glucose and stored chiefly in the liver and, to a lesser extent, in muscle cells.

glycogenesis /glī′kōjen′əsis/, the synthesis of glycogen from glucose.

glycogenolysis /glī′kōjenol′isis/ [Gk, *glykys* + *genein* + *lysis,* loosening], the breakdown of glycogen to glucose.

glycogen storage disease [Gk, *glykys* + *genein* + L, *instaurare,* to renew, *dis,* opposite of; Fr, *aise,* ease], any of a group of inherited disorders of glycogen metabolism. An enzyme deficiency causes glycogen to accumulate in abnormally large amounts in various parts of the body.

glycogen storage disease, type I. See **von Gierke's disease.**

glycogen storage disease, type Ib, a form of glycogen storage disease in which excessive amounts of glycogen are deposited in the liver and leukocytes.

glycogen storage disease, type II. See **Pompe's disease.**

glycogen storage disease, type III. See **Cori's disease.**

glycogen storage disease, type IV. See **Andersen's disease.**

glycogen storage disease, type V. See **McArdle's disease.**

glycogen storage disease, type VI. See **Hers' disease.**

glycogen storage disease, type VII. See **Tarui's disease.**

glycolipid /glī′kōlip′id/ [Gk, *glykys,* sweet, *lipos,* fat], a compound that consists of a lipid and a carbohydrate, usually galactose, found primarily in the tissue of the nervous system.

glycolysis /glīkol′isis/ [Gk, *glykys* + *lysis,* loosening], a series of enzymatically catalyzed reactions by which glucose and other sugars are broken down to yield lactic acid (anaerobic glycolysis) or pyruvic acid (aerobic glycolysis). The breakdown releases energy in the form of adenosine triphosphate.

glycometabolism /glī′kōmətab′əliz′əm/, the metabolism of sugar in the animal body.

glycopenia /-pē′nē·ə/, **1.** hypoglycemia. **2.** a deficiency of sugar in the blood or tissues.

glycopeptides /-pep′tīdz/, a class of peptides that contain sugars linked with amino acids, as in bacterial cell walls.

glycophorin /-fôr′in/, one of a group of proteins that project through the membrane of red blood cells. The outside end of glycophorins carries antigen of the MNS blood group. The sialic acid component of glycophorins contributes to the negative charge of the outer erythrocyte plasma membrane.

glycoprotein /glī′kōprō′tēn/ [Gk, *glykys,* sweet, *proteios,* first rank], any of the large group of conjugated proteins in which the nonprotein substance is a carbohydrate. These include the mucins, the mucoids, and the chondroproteins.

glycopyrrolate /glī′kōpir′əlāt/, an anticholinergic prescribed as an adjunct to ulcer therapy.

glycoside /glī′kəsīd/ [Gk, *glykys,* sweet], any of several carbohydrates that yield a sugar and a nonsugar on hydrolysis. The plant *Digitalis purpurea* yields a glycoside used in the treatment of heart disease.

glycosphingolipids /glī′kōsfing′gōlip′ids/, compounds formed from carbohydrates and ceramide, a fatty substance, found in tissues of the central nervous system and also in erythrocytes.

glycosuria /glī′kōsŏŏr′ē·ə/ [Gk, *glykys* + *ouron,* urine], abnormal presence of a sugar, especially glucose, in the urine. It is a finding most routinely associated with diabetes mellitus. —**glycosuric,** *adj.*

glycosuric acid /-sŏŏr′ik/ [Gk, *glykys* + *ouron,* urine; L, *acidus,* sour], a compound that is an intermediate product of the metabolism of tyrosine. It forms a melanin-like staining substance in the urine of people who have alkaptonuria.

glycosylated hemoglobin (GHb/Hb A₁c) /glīkō′silā′tid/, a hemoglobin A molecule with a glucose group on the *N*-terminal valine amino acid unit of the beta chain. The glycosylated hemoglobin concentration represents the average blood glucose level over the previous several weeks.

glycyrrhizic acid /glis′iriz′ik/, a sweet compound containing potassium and calcium salts derived from licorice root.

gm, abbreviation for **gram.** The preferred abbreviation is **g.**

GM-CSF, abbreviation for **granulocyte-macrophage colony-stimulating factor.**

GMENAC, abbreviation for **Graduate Medical Education National Advisory Committee.**

GMP, abbreviation for **guanosine monophosphate.**

GM-2, a carbohydrate found in much larger quantities in cancer cells than in normal cells. It is used in some experimental cancer therapy. When it is mixed with bacille Calmette-Guérin and injected into melanoma patients, some patients make antibodies against the cancer cells.

GN, abbreviation for **graduate nurse.**

GNA, abbreviation for **Gay Nurses' Alliance.**

gnathic /nath′ik/ [L, *gnathos,* jaw], pertaining to the jaw or cheek.

gnathion /nā′thē·on/ [L, *gnathos,* jaw], the lowest point in the lower border of the mandible in the median plane. It is a common reference point in the diagnosis and orthodontic treatment of various kinds of malocclusion.

gnathodynamometer /nā'thōdī'nəmom'-ətər/ [Gk, *gnathos* + *dynamis*, force, *metron*, measure], an instrument used for measuring the biting pressure of the jaws of an individual.

gnathodynia /nā'thōdin'ē-ə/ [Gk, *gnathos* + *odyne*, pain], a pain in the jaw, such as that commonly associated with an impacted wisdom tooth.

gnathology /nāthol'əjē/ /nāthol'əjē/ [Gk, *gnathos* + *logos*, science], a field of dental or medical study that deals with the entire masticatory apparatus, including its anatomic, histologic, morphologic, physiologic, pathologic, and therapeutic characteristics.

gnathostatic cast /nā'thōstat'ik/ [Gk, *gnathos* + *statike*, weighing; ME, *casten*], a cast of the teeth trimmed so that its occlusal plane is in its normal oral attitude when the cast is set on a plane surface.

gnathostatics /nā'thōstat'iks/ [Gk, *gnathos* + *statike*, weighing], a technique of orthodontic diagnosis based on an analysis of the relationships between the teeth and certain reference points on the skull.

gnotobiotic /nō'tōbī·ot'ik/, pertaining to an animal or an environment in which all the microorganisms are known.

GnRH, abbreviation for **gonadotropin-releasing hormone.**

goal /gōl/ [ME, *gol,* limit], the purpose toward which an endeavor is directed, such as the outcome of diagnostic, therapeutic, and educational management of a patient's health problem.

goal-oriented movements, voluntary movements that are organized around behavioral goals, environmental context, and task specificity, as distinguished from reflexive movements.

GOAT, abbreviation for **Galveston Orientation and Amnesia Test.**

goblet cell [ME, *gobelet,* small bowl], one of the many specialized epithelial cells that secrete mucus and form glands of the epithelium of the stomach, the intestine, and parts of the respiratory tract.

goiter [L, *guttur,* throat], an enlarged thyroid gland, usually evident as a pronounced swelling in the neck. The enlargement may be associated with hyperthyroidism, hypothyroidism, or normal levels of thyroid function. It may be cystic or fibrous, containing nodules or an increased number of follicles. —**goitrous,** *adj.*

goitrogenic glycoside /goi'trəjen'ik/, a glycoside that may cause hyperthyroidism or a goiter.

gold (Au) [AS, *geolu,* yellow], a yellowish soft metallic element that occurs naturally as a free metal and as the telluride $AuAgTe_4$. Its atomic number is 79; its atomic mass (weight) is 196.97. It is used as a dental restorative material. Gold salts, in which gold is attached to sulfur, are often used in the treatment, or chrysotherapy, of patients with rheumatoid arthritis but cause serious toxicity in about 10% of patients.

gold 198, a radioactive gold antineoplastic prescribed for treatment of cancer of the prostate, cervix, and bladder and for reduction of fluid accumulation secondary to a cancer.

Goldblatt kidney, an abnormal kidney in which constriction of a renal artery leads to ischemia and release of renin, a pressor substance associated with hypertension.

gold compound, a drug containing gold salts, usually administered with other drugs in the treatment of rheumatoid arthritis. Gold is potentially toxic and is administered only under the supervision of a specialist in chrysotherapy.

gold foil, (in dentistry) pure gold that has been rolled and beaten into a very thin sheet. The main types of gold foil are cohesive, semicohesive, and noncohesive.

gold inlay, an intracoronal cast restoration of gold alloy that restores one or more tooth surfaces.

Goldman-Fox knife, a dental surgical instrument with a sharp cutting edge, designed for the incision and contouring of gingival tissue.

gold sodium thiomalate, an antirheumatic prescribed for rheumatoid arthritis.

gold standard, 1. an accepted test that is assumed to be able to determine the true disease state of a patient, regardless of positive or negative test findings or sensitivities or specificities of other diagnostic tests used. **2.** an acknowledged measure of comparison of the superior effectiveness or value of a particular medication or other therapy as compared with that of other drugs or treatments.

golfer's elbow, a popular term for medial epicondylitis associated with repeated use of the wrist flexors.

Golgi apparatus /gôl'jē/ [Camillo Golgi, Italian histologist and Nobel laureate, 1843–1946; L, *ad,* toward, *praeparare,* to prepare], one of many small membranous structures found in most cells, composed of various elements associated with the formation of carbohydrate side chains of glycoproteins, mucopolysaccharides, and other substances.

Golgi-Mazzoni corpuscles /gôl'jēmatsō'-

nē/ [Camillo Golgi; Vittori Mazzoni, Italian physiologist, 1880–1940], a number of thin capsules enveloping terminal nerve fibrils in the subcutaneous tissue of the fingers.

Golgi's cells [Camillo Golgi; L, *cella,* storeroom], **1. Golgi type I neurons,** nerve cells having long axons that leave the local neuropil area of the parent cell body, traverse the white matter, and project to the rest of the nervous system. **2. Golgi type II neurons,** nerve cells with short trajectory axons such as stellate cells of the cerebral and cerebellar cortex. They generally do not enter white matter but remain within the local neuropil in the cerebral and cerebellar cortices and the retina.

Golgi tendon organ [Camillo Golgi], a sensory nerve ending that is sensitive to both tension and excessive passive stretch of a skeletal muscle.

gomphosis /gomfō'sis/, *pl.* **gomphoses** [Gk, *gomphos,* bolt], an articulation by the insertion of a conic process into a socket, such as the insertion of a root of a tooth into an alveolus of the mandible or the maxilla.

gonad /gō'nad/ [Gk, *gone,* seed], a gamete-producing gland such as an ovary or a testis. —**gonadal,** *adj.*

gonadal aplasia /gō'nədəl/, a congenital state in which there is defective development of the germinal tissues of the gonads.

gonadal dose, a measure of the dose of radiation received by the gonads as a result of a radiographic examination. It may vary from less than 1 mrad for a dental or chest radiograph to 225 mrad for a lumbar spine radiograph and 800 mrad for a fetus during pelvimetry.

gonadal dysgenesis, a general designation for a variety of conditions involving anomalies in the development of the gonads, such as Turner's syndrome, hermaphroditism, and gonadal aplasia.

gonadal shield, a specially designed contact or shadow shield used to protect the gonadal area of a patient from the primary radiation beam during radiographic procedures. It is generally used for all patients who are potentially reproductive, including all those less than 40 years of age and older males.

gonadotrophic /gō'nədōtrof'ik/, **1.** pertaining to genitalia. **2.** capable of influencing the gonads. **3.** relating to the state in which the gonads exert influence on the body.

gonadotropin /gō'nədōtrop'in/ [Gk, *gone* + *trophe,* nourishment], a hormonal substance that stimulates the function of the testes and ovaries. The gonadotrophic

follicle-stimulating hormone and luteinizing hormone are produced and secreted by the anterior pituitary gland. In early pregnancy chorionic gonadotropin is produced by the placenta. —**gonadotropic, gonadotrophic,** *adj.*

gonadotropin-releasing hormone (GnRH) [Gk, *gone,* seed, *trope,* a turn; ME, *relesen;* Gk, *hormaein,* to set in motion], a decapeptide hypophysiotropic hormone secreted by the hypothalamus. It stimulates the release of gonadotropin hormone by the anterior pituitary gland. It also stimulates the release of the **luteinizing hormone (LH)** and **follicle-stimulating hormone (FSH)** by the anterior pituitary.

goniometer /gon'ē·om'ətər/, an instrument used to measure angles, particularly range-of-motion angles of a joint.

goniometry /gon'ē·om'ətrē/ [Gk, *gonia,* angle, *metron,* measure], a system for measuring angles during testing for various labyrinthine diseases that affect the sense of balance. —**goniometric,** *adj.*

gonioscope /gō'nē·əskōp'/ [Gk, *gonia* + *skopein,* to look], an optical instrument used to examine the filtration angle of the anterior chamber of the eye.

goniotomy /gōn'ē·ot'əmē/, an operation performed to remove any obstruction to the flow of aqueous humor in the front chamber of the eye. The procedure is commonly done in patients with glaucoma.

gonococcal /gon'əkok'əl/ [Gk, *gone,* seed, *kokkos,* berry], pertaining to or resembling gonococcus.

gonococcal pyomyositis [Gk, *gone,* seed, *kokkos,* berry, *pyon,* pus, *mys,* muscle, *itis,* inflammation], an acute inflammatory condition of a muscle caused by infection with *Neisseria gonorrhoeae,* characterized by abscess formation and pain. It is an unusual form of gonorrhea and must be differentiated from sarcoma.

gonococcal salpingitis [Gk, *gone,* seed, *kokkos,* berry, *salpigx,* tube, *itis,* inflammation], an inflammation of the fallopian tubes caused by a gonococcal infection.

gonococcal urethritis [Gk, *gone,* seed, *kokkos,* berry, *ourethra,* urethra, *itis,* inflammation], an inflammation of the urethra caused by an infection of *Neisseria gonorrhoeae.*

gonococcus /gon'əkok'əs/, *pl.* **gonococci** /gon'əkok'sī/ [Gk, *gone* + *kokkos,* berry], a gram-negative intracellular diplococcus of the species *Neisseria gonorrhoeae,* the cause of gonorrhea.

gonorrhea /gon'ərē'ə/ [Gk, *gone* + *rhoia,* flow], a common sexually transmitted disease that most often affects the genitourinary tract and occasionally the pharynx, conjunctiva, or rectum. Infection results from contact with an infected person or with secretions containing the causative organism *Neisseria gonorrhoeae.* Gonorrheal infections must be reported to local health departments in the United States. Urethritis; dysuria; purulent, greenish-yellow urethral or vaginal discharge; red or edematous urethral meatus; and itching, burning, or pain around the vaginal or urethral orifice are characteristic. The vagina may be massively swollen and red, and the lower abdomen may be tense and very tender. —**gonorrheal, gonorrheic,** *adj.*

gonorrheal /gon'ərē'əl/ [Gk, *gone,* seed, *kokkos*], pertaining to or resembling gonorrhea.

gonorrheal arthritis [Gk, *gone,* seed, *kokkos,* berry, *arthron,* joint, *itis,* inflammation], a blood-borne gonococcal infection of the joints. It may affect one or several joints, may occur as a chronic or acute form, and often leads to joint fusion. Infection may result in pus formation in an affected joint.

gonorrheal conjunctivitis, a severe, destructive form of purulent conjunctivitis caused by the gonococcus *Neisseria gonorrhoeae.* Newborns receive routine prophylaxis of a topical instillation of 1% solution of silver nitrate or an antibiotic ointment; the treatment has largely eradicated the infection in infants.

gonorrheal proctitis [Gk, *gone,* seed, *rhoia,* flow, *proktos,* anus, *itis,* inflammation], an inflammation of the rectum caused by an infection of gonorrhea.

Gonyaulax catanella /gon'ē-ô'laks/, a species of toxin-producing planktonic protozoa ingested by shellfish along the coasts of North America that causes shellfish poisoning.

Goodell's sign /gŏŏdelz'/ [William Goodell, American gynecologist, 1829–1894], softening of the uterine cervix, a probable sign of pregnancy.

good faith and fair dealing, actions taken with the best interests of the patient in mind and without harmful intent.

Goodpasture's syndrome /gŏŏd'pas·chər/ [Ernest W. Goodpasture, American pathologist, 1886–1960], a chronic relapsing pulmonary hemosiderosis, usually associated with glomerulonephritis and characterized by a cough with hemoptysis, dyspnea, anemia, and progressive renal failure.

Goodrich, Annie Warburton (1866–1954), an American nursing educator who was instrumental in advancing nursing from an apprenticeship to a profession. In 1923 she became dean of the newly formed School of Nursing at Yale University, which awarded a degree similar to that awarded in other professions.

Good Samaritan legislation /səmar'itən/ [good Samaritan, from New Testament parable; L, *lex,* law, *lator,* proposer], laws enacted in some states to protect physicians, dentists, nurses, and some other health professionals from liability in rendering emergency medical or dental aid, unless there is proven willful wrong or gross negligence.

Gordon's elementary body [Mervyn H. Gordon, English physician, 1872–1953], a particle found in tissues containing eosinophils; once thought to be the viral cause of Hodgkin's disease.

Gordon's reflex [Alfred Gordon, American neurologist, 1874–1953], **1.** an abnormal variation of Babinski's reflex, elicited by compressing the calf muscles, characterized by dorsiflexion of the great toe and fanning of the other toes. It is evidence of disease of the pyramidal tract. **2.** an abnormal reflex, elicited by compressing the forearm muscles, characterized by flexion of the fingers or of the thumb and index finger. It is seen in diseases of the pyramidal tract.

Gosselin's fracture /gôslaNz'/ [Leon A. Gosselin, French surgeon, 1815–1847], a V-shaped fracture of the distal tibia, extending to the ankle.

GOT, abbreviation for glutamic-oxaloacetic transaminase.

goundou /gŏŏn'dŏŏ/ [West African], a condition characterized by bony exostoses of the nasal and maxillary bones, usually occurring as a late sequela of yaws in people in Africa and Latin America.

gout [L, *gutta,* drop], a disease associated with an inborn error of uric acid metabolism that increases production or interferes with excretion of uric acid. Excess uric acid is converted to sodium urate crystals that precipitate from the blood and become deposited in joints and other tissues. The condition can cause exceedingly painful swelling of a joint, accompanied by chills and fever. The disorder is disabling and, if untreated, can progress to the development of destructive joint changes, such as tophi.

gouty /gou'tē/ [L, *gutta,* drop], pertaining to or resembling the condition of gout.

GP, abbreviation for **general practitioner.**

GPB, abbreviation for **glossopharyngeal breathing.**

gp160, code for a glycoprotein that provides an outer coat for the human immunodeficiency virus. The outer coat, in turn, is composed of **gp120,** which protrudes from the virus surface, and **gp41,** which is embedded in the envelope coat.

GPT, abbreviation for glutamic-pyruvic transaminase.

GPWW, abbreviation for **group practice without walls.**

gr, abbreviation for **grain.**

graafian follicle /grä′fē·ən, -grä′-/ [Reijnier de Graaf, Dutch physician, 1641–1673; L, *folliculus,* small bag] /gräf′/, a mature ovarian vesicle, measuring about 10 to 12 mm in diameter, that ruptures during ovulation to release the ovum. Many primary ovarian follicles, each containing an immature ovum about 35 μm in diameter, are embedded near the surface of the ovary. Under the influence of the follicle-stimulating hormone from the adenohypophysis, one ovarian follicle ripens into a graafian follicle during the proliferative phase of each menstrual cycle. The cavity of the follicle collapses when the ovum is released, and the remaining follicular cells greatly enlarge to become the corpus luteum.

gracile /gras′il/, long, slender, and graceful.

gracilis /gras′ilis/, the most superficial of the five medial femoral muscles. It functions to adduct the thigh and flex the leg and to assist in the medial rotation of the leg after it is flexed.

gradation of activity /gradā′shən/, therapeutic activities that are appropriately paced and modified to demand maximal capacities at any point in progression or regression of the patient's condition.

graded exercise test (GXT), a test given a cardiac patient during rehabilitation to assess prognosis and quantify maximal functional capacity.

gradient /grā′dē·ənt/ [L, *gradus,* step], **1.** the rate of increase or decrease of a measurable phenomenon, such as temperature or pressure. **2.** a visual representation of the rate of change of a measurable phenomenon; a curve.

gradient former, a device for the preparation of linear density gradient medium in a column for gradient electrophoresis.

gradient gel electrophoresis, gel electrophoresis performed in a concentration gradient gel with progressively decreasing pore size.

gradient magnetic field, a magnetic field that changes in strength in a certain given direction. Such fields are used in magnetic resonance imaging (MRI) to select a region for imaging and also to encode the location of MRI signals received from the object being imaged.

gradient plate technique, a method for isolating antibiotic-resistant bacteria mutants by exposing an agar plate containing concentration gradient of antibiotic to an inoculation of bacteria to be tested.

graduated bath /graj′ oo·a′tid/ [L, *gradus,* step; AS, *baeth*], a bath in which the temperature of the water is slowly reduced.

graduated muscular contractions, controlled shortening of muscle units in properly timed and adequate response to a stimulus. The contractions may be induced by the central nervous system or by electrical stimulation.

graduate medical education /graj′ oo·it/, formal medical education pursued after receipt of the doctor of medicine (M.D.) or other professional degree in the medical sciences.

Graduate Medical Education National Advisory Committee (GMENAC), a committee established by order of the Secretary of the Department of Health, Education, and Welfare (now the Department of Health and Human Services) to study the personnel issues in medicine. The committee issued its final report in September 1980. Among its conclusions was that the supply of nurses in expanded roles, including nurse practitioners and nurse midwives, should be increased.

graduate nurse (GN) [L, *gradus,* step, *nutrix,* nurse], a nurse who is a graduate of an accredited school of nursing.

Graduate Record Examination (GRE), an examination administered to graduates of institutions of higher learning. The scores are used as criteria for admission to master's and doctoral programs in many institutions and areas of specialization, including nursing.

GRAE, abbreviation for **generally recognized as effective.**

graft [Gk, *graphion,* stylus], a tissue or an organ taken from a site or a person and inserted into a new site or person, performed to repair a defect in structure. The graft may be temporary, such as an emergency skin transplant for extensive burns, or permanent with the grafted tissue growing to become a part of the body. Skin, bone, cartilage, blood vessel, nerve, muscle, cornea, and whole organs such as the kidney or the heart may be grafted.

graft facilitation, a method for extending the survival of a graft by conditioning the recipient with an immunoglobulin antibody-blocking factor, which inhibits cell-mediated immunity.

graft rejection, the immunologic destruction of transplanted organs or tissues. The rejection may be based on both cell-mediated and antibody-mediated immunity against cells of the graft by a histoin-compatible recipient.

graft-versus-host disease (GVHD), a rejection response of certain grafts, especially of bone marrow. It involves an incompatibility resulting from a deficiency in the immune response of the recipient and is commonly associated with inadequate donor immunosuppressive therapy. Characteristic signs may include skin lesions with edema, erythema, ulceration, scaling, and loss of hair.

Graham's law /grā'əmz/ [Thomas Graham, English chemist, 1805–1869], the law stating that the rate of diffusion of a gas through a liquid (or the alveolar-capillary membrane) is directly proportional to its solubility coefficient and inversely proportional to the square root of its density.

Graham Steell murmur [Graham Steell, British physician, 1851–1942], an early diastolic murmur heard in the second intercostal space to the left of the sternum. It is associated with pulmonary valve regurgitation in pulmonary hypertension.

grain (gr) [L, *granum,* seed], the smallest unit of mass in avoirdupois, troy, and apothecaries' weights, which is the same in all and is equal to 4.79891 mg. The troy and apothecaries' ounces contain 480 grains; the avoirdupois ounce contains 437.5 grains.

gram (g, gm) [L, *gramma,* small weight], a unit of mass in the metric system equal to 1/1000 kilogram, 15.432 grains, and 0.0353 ounce avoirdupois. The preferred abbreviation is *g.*

gram calorie. See **calorie (cal).**

gram-equivalent weight (gEq), an equivalent weight of a substance calculated as the gram mass that contains, replaces, or reacts (directly or indirectly) with the Avogadro number of hydrogen atoms.

gram-molecular weight (gmW), a mass in grams numerically equal to the molecular weight of a substance, or the sum of all the atomic weights in its molecular formula.

gram-negative [Hans C. J. Gram, Danish physician, 1853–1938; L, *negare,* to say no], having the pink color of the counterstain used in Gram's method of staining microorganisms. This property is a primary method of characterizing organisms in microbiology.

gram-positive [Hans C. J. Gram; L, *positivus*], retaining the violet color of the stain used in Gram's method of staining microorganisms. This property is a primary method of characterizing organisms in microbiology.

Gram's stain [Hans C. J. Gram], the method of staining microorganisms using a violet stain followed by an iodine solution; decolorizing with an alcohol or acetone solution; and counterstaining with safranin. The retention of either the violet color of the stain or the pink color of the counterstain serves as a primary means of identifying and classifying bacteria.

gram-variable, gram-positive bacteria that can become gram-negative after culturing.

grandiose /gran'dē·ōs'/ [L, *grandis,* great], pertaining to something or somebody imposing, impressive, magnificent, or, also, pompous and showy.

grand mal seizure. See **tonic-clonic seizure.**

grand multipara /grand/ [L, *grandis,* great, *multus,* many, *parere,* to give birth], a woman who has carried six or more pregnancies to a viable stage.

grand rounds [L, *grandis* + *rotundus,* wheel], a formal conference in which one usually expert person presents a lecture concerning a clinical issue intended to be educational for the listeners. In some settings grand rounds may be formal teaching rounds conducted by an expert at the bedsides of selected patients.

grant [ME, *granten,* to believe a request], an award given to an institution, a project, or an individual, usually consisting of a sum of money. A grant is awarded by a granting agency, the federal government, a foundation, a private business, or an institution to provide financial support for research, service, or training.

granular /gran'yələr/ [L, *granulum,* little grain], **1.** macroscopically resembling or feeling like sand. **2.** microscopically appearing to have a few or many particles within or on its surface, such as a stained granular leukocyte. —**granularity,** *n.*

granular cast [L, *granulum,* little grain; ONorse, *kasta*], a mass of pathologic debris composed of cells filled with protein and fatty granules.

granular induration, fibrosis of an organ, characterized by the formation of localized granular areas, as seen in cirrhosis of the liver.

granulation tissue /gran'yəlā'shən/ [L, *granulum,* little grain], any soft, pink, fleshy projections that form during the healing process in a wound that does not heal by first intention. It consists of many capillaries surrounded by fibrous collagen.

granule /gran'yōōl/ [L, *granulum,* little grain], a particle, grain, or other small dry mass capable of free movement. Unlike powders, granules are usually free flowing because of small surface forces involved.

granulitis /gran'yəlī'tis/ [L, *granulum*, little grain; Gk, *itis*, inflammation], acute miliary tuberculosis.

granulocyte /gran'yŏŏləsīt'/ [L, *granulum* + Gk, *kytos*, cell], a type of leukocyte characterized by the presence of cytoplasmic granules. Kinds of granulocytes are **basophil, eosinophil,** and **neutrophil.**

granulocyte colony-stimulating factor (G-CSF), a glycoprotein secreted by a variety of cells that stimulates the growth of hematopoietic stem cells and their differentiation into granulocytes.

granulocyte-macrophage colony-stimulating factor (GM-CSF), a glycoprotein secreted by macrophages that stimulates the growth of myeloid progenitor cells and their differentiation into granulocytes and macrophages.

granulocyte transfusion, the use of specially prepared leukocytes for the treatment of severe granulocytopenia and for prophylaxis in the prevention of serious infection in patients with leukemia or those receiving cancer chemotherapy.

granulocytopenia /gran'yŏŏlōsī'tōpē'nē·ə/ [L, *granulum* + Gk, *kytos*, cell, *penia*, poverty], an abnormal decrease in the total number of granulocytes in the blood. **—granulocytopenic,** *adj.*

granulocytosis /gran'yŏŏlōsītō'sis/ [L, *granulum* + Gk, *kytos*, cell, *osis*, condition], an abnormal increase in the total number of granulocytes.

granuloma /gran'yŏŏlō'mə/ [L, *granulum* + Gk, *oma*, tumor], a chronic inflammatory lesion characterized by an accumulation of macrophages; epithelioid macrophages, with or without lymphocytes; and giant cells into a discrete granule. Granulomas may resolve spontaneously, remain static, become gangrenous, spread, or act as a focus of infection.

granuloma annulare, a self-limited chronic skin disease of unknown cause that consists of reddish papules and nodules arranged in a ring. It most commonly occurs on the distal parts of the extremities in children. No treatment is necessary.

granuloma gluteale infantum, a skin condition of the neonate characterized by large elevated bluish or brownish-red nodules on the buttocks. It often occurs as a secondary reaction to the application of strong steroid salves over time.

granuloma inguinale, a sexually transmitted disease characterized by ulcers of the skin and subcutaneous tissues of the groin and genitalia. It is caused by infection with *Calymmatobacterium granulo-*

matis, a small gram-negative rod-shaped bacillus.

granulomatosis /gran'yŏŏlōmətō'sis/ [L, *granulum* + Gk, *oma*, tumor, *osis*, condition], a condition or disease characterized by the development of granulomas such as **berylliosis, pulmonary Wegener's granulomatosis,** or **Wegener's granulomatosis.**

granulomatous /gran'yəlom'ətəs/ [L, *granulum*, little grain], pertaining to or resembling granulomas.

granulomatous lipophagia [L, *granulum*, little grain; Gk, *lipos*, fat, *phagein*, to eat], a disease in which enlarged intestinal and mesenteric lymph spaces become filled with fats and fatty acids.

granulopoietin /gran'yŏŏlō'pō·ē'tin/, a glycoprotein secreted by monocytes that controls production of granulocytes by bone marrow.

granulosa cell tumor /gran'yŏŏlō'sə/ [L, *granulum*, little grain], a fleshy ovarian tumor with yellow streaks that originates in cells of the primordial membrana granulosa and may grow to a large size.

granulosa-theca cell tumor, an ovarian tumor composed of granulosa (follicular) cells or theca cells or both.

granulosis /gran'yŏŏlō'sis/, any disorder characterized by an accumulation of granules in an area of body tissue.

graphanesthesia /graf'anəsthē'zhə/, inability to feel writing on the skin, usually caused by a central nervous system lesion.

graphesthesia /graf'esthē'zhə/, ability to feel writing on the skin.

graphing /graf'ing/, the organization of data consisting of two or more variables along horizontal and vertical axes of a graph to show relationships between specific quantities or other specific factors.

GRAS, abbreviation for **generally recognized as safe.**

grasp reflex [ME, *graspen,* grab; L, *reflectere,* to bend back], a pathologic reflex induced by stroking the palm or sole with the result that the fingers or toes flex in a grasping motion. The reflex occurs in diseases of the premotor cortex.

grass-line ligature [AS, *graes* + L, *linea,* thread, *ligare,* to bind], a fine cord composed of the fibers of a grass-cloth plant, used in orthodontics for minor adjustments or movement of the teeth.

Graves' disease /grāvz/ [Robert J. Graves, Irish physician, 1796–1853], a disorder characterized by pronounced hyperthyroidism usually associated with an enlarged thyroid gland and exophthalmos (abnormal protrusion of the eyeball). The origin is unknown, but the disease is familial and may be autoimmune; antibodies to thyroglobulin or to thyroid microsomes are found in more than 60% of patients with the disorder. Typical signs are nervousness, a fine tremor of the hands, weight loss, fatigue, breathlessness, palpitations, increased heat intolerance, increased metabolic rate, and gastrointestinal motility. An enlarged thymus, generalized hyperplasia of the lymph nodes, blurred or double vision, localized edema, atrial arrhythmias, and osteoporosis may occur. In patients with inadequately controlled disease, infection or stress may precipitate a life-threatening thyroid storm.

gravid /grav'id/ [L, *gravidus,* pregnant], pregnant; carrying fertilized eggs or a fetus. —**gravidity, gravidness,** *n.*

gravida /grav'idə/ [L, *gravidus,* pregnant], a woman who is pregnant. The patient may be identified more specifically as **gravida I,** if pregnant for the first time, or **gravida II,** if pregnant a second time.

gravida macromastia, overdevelopment of the breasts during pregnancy.

gravidarum chloasma /grav'ider'əm, grä'vidär/ [L, *gravidus,* pregnant; Gk, *chloazein,* to be green], a pigmentary change in the skin that occurs in some women during pregnancy. It usually occurs as patches of brown or black discoloration.

gravidum gingivitis /grav'idəm/ [L, *gravidus,* pregnant, *gingiva,* gums, *itis,* inflammation], a type of gum inflammation that is associated with plaque formation during pregnancy. It may be associated with hormonal changes.

gravid uterus [L, *gravidus,* pregnant, *uterus,* womb], a pregnant uterus.

gravity /grav'itē/ [L, *gravis,* heavy], the universal effect of the attraction between any body of matter and any planetary body. The force of the attraction depends on the relative masses of the bodies and on the distance between them.

gravity-eliminated plane, a supported position or plane in which the effect of gravity is absorbed or neutralized. In evaluation of muscle strength certain tests are conducted in the gravity-eliminated plane.

gray (Gy), the SI unit of absorbed radiation dose. One gray equals the energy equivalent of 1 joule/kg of matter; 1 Gy equals 100 rad.

gray scale, (in ultrasonography) the property in which intensity information is recorded as changes in the brightness of the gray scale display.

gray scale display, (in ultrasonography) a signal-processing method of selectively amplifying and displaying the level echoes

from soft tissues at the expense of the larger echoes.

gray substance [AS, *graeg* + L, *substantia*], the gray nervous tissue found in the cortex of the cerebrum, cerebellum, and core of the spinal cord. It is predominantly composed of neuron cell bodies and unmyelinated axons. The gray color is produced by cytoplasmic elements seen in all cell bodies and processes not covered by whitish myelin. Nuclei in the gray substance of the spinal cord function as centers for all spinal reflexes.

gray syndrome, a toxic condition in neonates, especially premature infants, caused by a reaction to chloramphenicol. The condition is named for the characteristic ashen-gray cyanosis, which is accompanied by abdominal distension, hypothermia, vomiting, respiratory distress, and vascular collapse. The syndrome is fatal if the drug is continued.

GRE, abbreviation for **Graduate Record Examination.**

great auricular nerve [AS, large; L, *auricula,* little ear, *nervus,* nerve], one of a pair of cutaneous branches of the cervical plexus, arising from the second and third cranial nerves. It is distributed to the skin of the face and that of the mastoid process.

great calorie. See **Calorie (Cal).**

great cardiac vein, one of the five tributaries of the coronary sinus, beginning at the apex of the heart and ascending along the anterior interventricular sulcus to the base of the ventricles. The great cardiac vein drains the blood through its tributaries from the capillaries of the myocardium.

greater omentum [AS, *great,* large; L, *omentum,* entrails], a filmy transparent extension of the peritoneum, draping the transverse colon and coils of the small intestine. It is attached along the greater curvature of the stomach and the first part of the duodenum.

greater sciatic foramen [AS, *great* + Gk, *ischiadikos,* hip joint; L, *foramen,* hole], an opening between the hip bone, sacrum, and sacrotuberous ligament.

greater sciatic notch [AS, *great,* large; Gk, *ischiadikos,* hip joint; OFr, *enochier,* notch], a notch on the posterior border of the hip bone between the posterior inferior iliac spine and the spine of the ischium.

greater trochanter, a large projection of the femur, to which are attached various muscles, including the gluteus medius, gluteus maximus, and obturator internus.

great membrane, the external components of a membrane, such as the layer of

G

carbohydrate molecules on the outer surface.

great saphenous vein, one of a pair of the longest veins in the body, which contains 10 to 20 valves along its course through the leg and the thigh before ending in the femoral vein. It begins in the medial marginal vein of the dorsum of the foot.

great vessels, the large arteries and veins entering and leaving the heart. They include the aorta, the pulmonary arteries and veins, and the superior and inferior venae cavae.

Greenfield filter [L. Greenfield, twentieth-century American surgeon], a filter placed in the inferior vena cava under fluoroscopic guidance. Used in patients who are particularly vulnerable to pulmonary embolism, it prevents venous emboli from entering the pulmonary circulation.

Greenfield's disease [Joseph G. Greenfield, British pathologist, 1884–1958], a disorder of the white matter of the brain tissue, characterized by an accumulation of sphingolipid in both parenchymal and supportive tissues and a diffuse loss of myelination.

green fluorescent protein (GFP), a protein obtained from the jellyfish *Aequorea victoria* that emits a bright green fluorescence when illuminated. GFP is used to monitor gene expression, gene transfer across plasma membranes, and cell-to-surface activity.

greenhouse effect, a theorized change in the earth's climate caused by accumulation of solar heat in the earth's surface and atmosphere. Human activity contributes increasing amounts of the so-called greenhouse gases, such as carbon dioxide, methane, and chlorofluorocarbon, to the atmosphere. Some of the particles and gases in the atmosphere also allow more sunlight to filter through to the earth's surface but reflect back much of the radiant infrared energy that otherwise would escape through the atmosphere back into space.

green soap [AS, *grene* + L, *sapo*], a soft soap made from vegetable oils with sodium or potassium hydroxide in concentrations adjusted to retain glycerol. The soap actually may be any color, depending on the ingredient oils added.

green soap tincture [AS, *grene* + L, *sapo*, soap, *tinctura*, dyeing], an alcoholic solution of green soap with lavender oil added.

greenstick fracture [AS, *grene* + *stician*], an incomplete fracture in which the bone is bent but fractured only on the outer arc of the bend. Children are particularly likely to have greenstick fractures.

green tea, a common dietary source of an anticarcinogen, epigallocatechin.

green tobacco sickness, a nicotine-induced illness of tobacco harvest workers, characterized by headache, dizziness, vomiting, and prostration.

grenz rays [Ger, *Grenze,* boundary; L, *radius,* ray], low-energy x-rays used for treatment of skin conditions.

Greulich-Pyle method /groi′lish-pīl′, grōō′lik-/, a technique for evaluating the bone age of children, using a single frontal radiograph of the left hand and wrist.

Grey Turner's sign, [George Grey Turner, English surgeon, 1877–1951], bruising of the skin of the loin in acute hemorrhagic pancreatitis.

grid [ME, *gredire*, grate], (in radiology) a device used to absorb scattered radiation produced during a radiographic examination. A grid selectively absorbs radiation that is not heading along straight lines from the x-ray source to the film. A **linear grid** is a simple x-ray grid consisting of parallel lead strips.

grid cutoff, (in radiology) an undesirable absorption of primary-beam x-rays by the grid so that useful x-rays are literally cut off from the film.

grief [L, *gravis,* heavy], a nearly universal pattern of physical and emotional responses to bereavement, separation, or loss. The physical components are similar to those of fear, hunger, rage, and pain.

grief reaction, a complex of somatic and psychologic symptoms associated with extreme sorrow or loss, specifically the death of a loved one. Somatic symptoms include feelings of tightness in the throat and chest with choking and shortness of breath, abdominal distress, lack of muscular power, and extreme tiredness and lethargy. Psychologic reactions involve a generalized awareness of mental anguish and discomfort accompanied by feelings of guilt, anger, hostility, extreme restlessness, inability to concentrate, and lack of capacity to initiate and maintain organized patterns of activities.

Grief Work Facilitation, a Nursing Interventions Classification defined as assistance with the resolution of a significant loss.

Grief Work Facilitation: Perinatal Death, a Nursing Interventions Classification defined as assistance with the resolution of a perinatal loss.

grieving, anticipatory, a NANDA-accepted nursing diagnosis of intellectual and emotional responses and behaviors by which individuals (families, communities) work through the process of modifying self-concept based on the perception of potential loss. Defining characteristics include potential loss of significant object; expression of distress at potential loss; denial of potential loss; denial of the significance of the loss; guilt, anger, sorrow; bargaining; alteration in: eating habits, sleep patterns, activity level, libido; altered communication patterns; difficulty taking on new or different roles; resolution of grief before the reality of loss.

grieving, dysfunctional, a NANDA-accepted nursing diagnosis of extended, unsuccessful use of intellectual and emotional responses by which individuals (families, communities) attempt to work through the process of modifying self-concept upon the perception of potential loss. Defining characteristics include repetitive use of ineffectual behaviors associated with attempts to reinvest in relationships; reliving of past experiences with little or no reduction (diminishment) of intensity of grief; prolonged interference with life functioning; onset of exacerbation of somatic or psychosomatic responses; expression of distress at loss; denial of loss; expression of guilt; expression of unresolved issues; anger; sadness; crying; difficulty in expressing loss; alterations: in eating habits, sleep patterns, dream patterns; activity level, libido, concentration, and/or pursuit of tasks; idealization of lost object; reliving of past experiences; interference with life functioning; developmental regression; and labile affect.

grinder's asthma /grĭn′dərz/ [ME, *grinden,* to crush; Gk, panting], a condition characterized by asthmatic symptoms caused by inhalation of fine particles produced by industrial grinding processes.

grinding-in, a clinical corrective grinding of one or more natural or artificial teeth to improve centric and eccentric occlusions.

grip and pinch strength, the measurable ability to exert pressure with the hand and fingers. It is measured by having a patient forcefully squeeze grip or pinch dynamometers, which may express results in either pounds or kilograms of pressure.

gripes /grĭps/ [AS, *gripan,* to grasp], severe and usually spasmodic pain in the abdominal region caused by an intestinal disorder.

griseofulvin /gris′ē-ōful′vin/, an antifungal prescribed in the treatment of certain infections of the skin, hair, and nails.

Griswald brace, an orthosis for the control of vertebral body compression fractures. It is designed with two anterior forces with each equal to one half the posterior force to extend the spine.

grocer's itch [AS, *gican,* itch], a dermatitis caused by contact with mites found in grain, cheese, or dried foods.

groin [ME, *grynde*], each of two areas where the abdomen joins the thighs.

Grönblad-Strandberg's syndrome /grōn′-bladstrand′bərg/ [Ester E. Grönblad, Swedish ophthalmologist, 1898–1942; James V. Strandberg, Swedish dermatologist, 1883–1942], an autosomal-recessive disorder of connective tissue characterized by premature aging and breakdown of the skin, gray or brown streaks on the retina, and hemorrhagic arterial degeneration, including retinal bleeding that causes vision loss. Angina pectoris and hypertension are common; weak pulse, episodic claudication, and fatigue with exertion may affect the extremities.

groove [AS, *grafan,* to dig], a shallow, linear depression in various structures throughout the body, as those that form channels for nerves along the bones, those in bones for the insertion of muscles, and those between certain areas of the brain.

grooved pegboard test, a method for evaluating psychomotor function by measuring how quickly a subject can insert pegs into grooved holes.

gross [OFr, *gros,* large], **1.** macroscopic, as *gross pathology,* from the study of tissue changes without magnification by a microscope. **2.** large or obese.

gross anatomy, the study of the organs or parts of the body large enough to be seen with the naked eye.

Grossman principle, (in tomography) the principle that when the fulcrum or axis of rotation remains at a fixed height, the focal plane level is changed by raising or lowering the table top through this fixed point to the desired height.

gross motor skills [Fr, *gros,* big; L, *movere,* ONorse, *skilja,* to cut apart], the use of large muscle groups that coordinate body movements required for normal living such as walking, running, jumping, throwing, and balance.

gross sensory testing, an evaluation procedure that includes assessment of passive motion sense in the shoulder, elbow, wrist, and fingers and ability to localize touch stimuli to specific fingers.

gross visual skills, the general ability of a person to track a large, bright object side-to-side or up-to-down without jerkiness, nystagmus, or convergence and to discriminate among various basic shapes and colors.

G

ground [AS, *grund*], **1.** (in electricity) a connection between the electric circuit and the ground, which becomes a part of the circuit. **2.** (in psychology) the background of a visual field that can enhance or inhibit the ability of a patient to focus on an object.

ground itch, pruritic papules, urticarial vesiculopustular lesions secondary to penetration of the skin by hookworm larvae. The condition is prevalent in tropic and subtropic climates and may be prevented by wearing shoes and establishing sanitary disposal of feces.

ground state, 1. the lowest energy level of a physical system. **2.** the stable form of an atom or molecule.

group [Fr, *groupe,* cluster], (in research) any set of items or people under study. An **experimental group** is studied to determine the effect of an event, a substance, or a technique. A **control group** serves as a standard or reference for comparison with an experimental group. A control group is similar to the experimental group in number and is identical in specified characteristics such as sex, age, annual income, parity, or other factors.

group dynamics [Fr, *groupe* + Gk, *dynamis,* force], the interactions and relationships that take place among group members, as well as between the group and the rest of society. It includes interdependence of group members, collective problem solving and decision making, and group conformity.

group function, (in dentistry) the simultaneous contacting of opposing teeth in a segment or a unit.

group-model HMO, a health maintenance (HMO) in which a contract is established with multispecialty medical groups for medical services. The HMO is responsible for marketing and developing contracts with enrollees and hospitals. Care is provided at hospitals where the physicians have admitting privileges or at ancillary facilities with which the HMO subcontracts.

group practice, two or more physicians, advanced practice nurses, and/or physician's assistants who work together and share facilities. The physicians may practice different specialties. Physicians who are part of a group often are prohibited from becoming independent contractors and earning money by providing medical care outside the group.

group practice without walls (GPWW), a medical practice formed to share economic risk, expenses, and marketing efforts. Physicians retain separate offices

and finances. Often a central site is established to house administrative services and some or all ancillary services.

group therapy, the application of psychotherapeutic techniques within a group of people (usually 10 or fewer) who experience similar difficulties. Generally a group leader directs the discussion of problems in an attempt to promote individual psychologic growth and favorable personality change. Group therapy has been found to be particularly effective in the treatment of various addictions.

growing fracture [AS, *growan* + L, *fractura,* to break], a fracture, usually linear, in which consecutive radiographic images show a gradual separation of the fracture edges with the passage of time. The cause often is pressure of soft tissues that forces the edges apart.

growing pains, 1. rheumatism-like pains that occur in the muscles and joints of children or adolescents as a result of fatigue, emotional problems, postural defects, and other causes that are not related to growth and that may be symptoms of various disorders. **2.** emotional and psychologic problems experienced during adolescence.

growth [AS, *growan,* to grow], **1.** an increase in the size of an organism or any of its parts, as measured in increments of weight, volume, or linear dimensions, that occurs as a result of hyperplasia or hypertrophy. **2.** the normal progressive anatomic, physiologic development from infancy to adulthood that is the result of gradual and normal processes of accretion and assimilation. In childhood growth is categorized according to the approximate age at which distinctive physical changes usually appear and at which specific developmental tasks are achieved. **3.** any abnormal localized increase of the size or number of cells, as in a tumor or neoplasm. **4.** a proliferation of cells, specifically a bacterial culture or mold.

growth and development, altered, a NANDA-accepted nursing diagnosis of the state in which an individual demonstrates deviations in norms from his or her age group. Defining characteristics include delay or difficulty in performing skills (motor, social, or expressive) typical of the age group; altered physical growth; inability to perform self-care or self-control activities appropriate for the age; flat affect; listlessness; and decreased responses.

growth charts, graphic displays of normal progressive changes in height, weight, and head circumference. They consider the range of growth as expressed in percentiles, or as standard deviation from the mean for average height or weight for age.

growth curve, a graphic display of data showing proliferation of cell numbers in a culture as a function of time.

growth factor, any cytokine, or highly specific protein, that stimulates the division and differentiation of particular types of cells.

growth factor receptor, a membrane-spanning protein that binds with a specific growth factor and transduces a signal that triggers cell division.

growth failure, a lack of normal physical and psychologic development that results from genetic, nutritional, pathologic, or psychosocial factors.

growth hormone (GH), human, a single-chain peptide secreted by the anterior pituitary gland in response to growth hormone–releasing factor (GHRF) from the hypothalamus. GH promotes protein synthesis in all cells, increases fat mobilization and use of fatty acids for energy, and decreases use of carbohydrate. A deficiency of GH causes dwarfism; an excess results in gigantism or acromegaly.

growth hormone–releasing factor (GHRF), somatotropin-releasing factor released by the hypothalamus.

growth retardation, failure of an individual to develop at a normal rate of height and weight for his or her age.

Grünfelder's reflex /grYn'feldərz, grēn'-/, an involuntary dorsiflexion of the great toe with a fanlike spreading of the other toes, caused by continued pressure on the posterior lateral fontanel.

grunting [ME, *grunten*], abnormal short, deep hoarse sounds in exhalation that often accompany severe chest pain. The grunt occurs because the glottis briefly stops the flow of air, halting the movement of the lungs and their surrounding or supporting structures.

GSA, abbreviation for **Gerontological Society of America.**

G-6-PD deficiency, abbreviation for **glucose-6-phosphate dehydrogenase deficiency.**

GSR, abbreviation for **galvanic skin response.**

gt, abbreviation for the Latin word *gutta,* 'a drop.'

GTP, abbreviation for **guanosine triphosphate.**

gtt, abbreviation for the Latin word *guttae,* 'drops.'

GU, abbreviation for **genitourinary.**

guaiac /gwī'ak/, a wood resin, commonly used as a reagent in laboratory tests for the presence of occult blood.

guaiac test, a test, using guaiac as a reagent, performed on feces and urine for detecting occult blood in the intestinal and urinary tracts.

guaifenesin /gwī'əfen'əsin/, glyceryl guaiacolate, a white to slightly gray powder with a bitter taste and faint odor, widely used as an expectorant.

guanabenz acetate /gwan'abenz/, an antihypertensive agent prescribed in the treatment of hypertension.

guanadrel sulfate /gwan'ədril/, an antihypertensive agent prescribed in the treatment of hypertension in patients who do not respond to first-step agents.

guanethidine sulfate /gwaneth'idēn/, an antihypertensive prescribed in the treatment of moderate and severe hypertension.

guanine /gwan'ēn/, a major purine base found in nucleotides and a fundamental constituent of deoxyribonucleic acid and ribonucleic acid. In free or uncombined form it occurs in trace amounts in most cells, usually as a product of the enzymatic hydrolysis of nucleic acids and nucleotides.

guanine deaminase, an enzyme that catalyzes the hydrolysis of guanine to xanthine and ammonia.

guanine deaminase assay, the measurement of an enzyme in the blood that commonly increases in hepatitis and other types of liver disease and mononucleosis.

guanosine /gwan'ōsēn/, a compound derived from a nucleic acid, composed of guanine and a sugar, D-ribose. It is a major molecular component of the nucleotides guanosine monophosphate and triphosphate and of deoxyribonucleic acid and ribonucleic acid.

guanosine monophosphate (GMP), a nucleotide that plays an important role in various metabolic reactions and in the formation of ribonucleic acid from deoxyribonucleic acid templates.

guanosine triphosphate (GTP), a high-energy nucleotide, similar to adenosine triphosphate, that functions in various metabolic reactions, such as the activation of fatty acids and the formation of the peptide bond in protein synthesis.

guaranine /gwərä'nin/, caffeine.

guardian ad litem /ad lī'təm/, (in law) a person who is appointed by a court to prosecute or defend a suit for an infant or an incapacitated person. A guardian ad litem is sometimes appointed when a person's life is in imminent danger and that person refuses treatment.

guardianship, a legal status that places the care and property of an individual in the hands of another person. Implementation of the law varies in different cases and jurisdictions. Some courts have held as legally incompetent mental patients who have jobs and live independently.

Guarnieri's bodies /gōō'ärnyer'ē/ [Giuseppi Guarnieri, Italian physician, 1856–1918], acidophilic inclusion bodies that are formed in the cytoplasm of cells infected with cowpox or vaccinia virus.

Gubbay test of motor proficiency, a screening test for the identification of developmental dyspraxia.

Guedel's signs /gōō'dəlz/ [Arthur E. Guedel, American anesthesiologist, 1883–1956], a system for describing the stages and planes of anesthesia during an operative procedure. These stages are only applicable to ether anesthesia and are difficult to delineate when combination anesthetics are given.

Guérin's fracture /gāraNz'/ [Alphonse F. M. Guérin, French surgeon, 1816–1895], a fracture of the maxilla.

guide dog [ME, *guiden,* to guard; OE, *docga*], a dog trained to aid in the mobility of a blind person. Guide dogs are usually recruited from certain compatible breeds and tested at 13 weeks of age. If qualified, the dog is then specially trained in private hands for 1 year and retested. Most dogs selected for training pass the final test. Guide dogs also may be trained to serve as "ears" for deaf persons.

guided imagery /gī'did/, a therapeutic technique for relieving pain or discomfort in which a patient is encouraged to concentrate on an image that helps relieve pain or discomfort.

guide plane [ME, *guiden,* to guard; L, *planum,* level ground], **1.** a part of an orthodontic appliance that has an established inclined plane for changing the occlusal relation of the maxillary and mandibular teeth and for permitting their movement to normal positions. **2.** a plane that is developed on the occlusal surfaces of occlusion rims for positioning the mandible in centric relation. **3.** two or more vertically parallel surfaces of abutment teeth shaped to direct the path of placement and removal of a partial denture.

guide-shoe marks, a radiographic image artifact caused by pressure of the guide shoes, curved metal lips that guide x-ray film in automatic developing systems.

guidewire /gīd'wī·ər/ [ME, *guiden,* to guard; AS, *wir*], a device used to position an intravenous catheter, endotracheal tube, central venous line, or gastric feeding tube.

guiding, (in occupational therapy) a method in which therapists assist their patients in perceiving the environment by directing movement of their hands and bodies in functional activities.

Guillain-Barré's syndrome /gēyaN'bärā'/ [Georges Guillain, French neurologist, 1876–1951; Jean A. Barré, French neurologist, 1880–1967], an idiopathic peripheral polyneuritis that occurs 1 to 3 weeks after a mild episode of fever associated with a viral infection or with immunization. Symmetric pain and weakness affect the extremities, and paralysis may develop. The neuritis may spread, ascending to the trunk and involving the face, arms, and thoracic muscles.

guilt [AS, *gylt,* delinquency], a feeling caused by tension between the ego and superego when one falls below the standards set for oneself.

Guilt Work Facilitation, a Nursing Interventions Classification defined as helping another to cope with painful feelings of responsibility, actual or perceived.

guilty, (in criminal law) a verdict by the court that to a moral certainty it is beyond reasonable doubt that the defendant committed the crime and is responsible for the offense as charged.

Gulf War syndrome, a group of medical and psychologic complaints, including fatigue, skin rash, memory loss, and headaches experienced by men and women who served in the 1991 Persian Gulf War.

gum, 1. a sticky excretion from certain plants. **2.** a firm layer of flesh covering the inside of the jaws and the base of the teeth.

gumboil [AS, *goma* + *byl*], an abscess of the gingiva and periosteum resulting from injury, infection, or dental decay. The gum is characteristically red, swollen, and tender.

gumma /gum'ə/ [AS, *goma,* gum], **1.** a granuloma, characteristic of tertiary syphilis, varying from 1 mm to 1 cm in diameter. It is usually encapsulated and contains a central necrotic mass surrounded by inflammatory and fibrotic zones of tissue. **2.** a soft granulomatous lesion that sometimes accompanies tuberculosis.

Gunning's splint [Thomas B. Gunning, American dentist, 1813–1889; D, *splinte,* split], a maxillomandibular splint used for supporting the maxilla and the mandible in surgery of the jaws.

gunshot fracture [ME, *gunne* + AS, *sceotan,* to shoot; L, *fractura,* break], a fracture caused by a bullet or similar missile.

gunshot wound, high-velocity penetration of the body by a bullet, commonly marked by a small entrance wound and a larger exit wound. The wound is usually accompanied by damage to blood vessels, bones, and other tissues.

Gunson method, (in radiology) a method of radiographic examination of the pharynx and upper esophagus during swallowing.

Günther's disease /gun'thərz/ [Hans Gunther, German physician, 1884–1956], a rare congenital disorder of porphyrin metabolism that is associated with sunlight-induced skin lesions.

gurgle [Fr, *gargouiller,* to gurgle], an abnormal coarse sound heard during auscultation, especially over large cavities or over a trachea nearly filled with secretions.

gurry /gur'ē/, *slang.* the detritus incident to physical trauma or surgery, including body fluids, secretions, and tissue.

gustation /gustā'shən/ [L, *gustare,* to taste], the sense and act of tasting foods, beverages, or other substances.

gustatory /gus'tətôr'ē/ [L, *gustare,* to taste], pertaining to the act or sense of taste or the organs of taste.

gustatory hallucination [L, *gustare,* to taste, *alucinari,* wandering mind], a false taste sensation of either food or beverage on the mucous membrane lining the empty mouth.

gustatory papilla [L, *gustare,* to taste, *papilla,* nipple], any of the small tissue elevations in the mouth that contain sense organs of taste such as the circumvallate papilla of the tongue.

gut [AS, *guttas*], **1.** intestine. **2.** *informal.* digestive tract. **3.** suture material manufactured from the intestines of sheep.

Guthrie's bacterial inhibition assay (GBIA) /guth'rē/, a screening for phenylketonuria (PKU) used to detect the abnormal presence of phenylalanine metabolites in the blood. A small amount of blood is obtained and placed in a medium with a strain of *Bacillus subtilis,* a bacterium that cannot grow without phenylalanine.

gutta (gt) /gut'ə, gōōt'ä/ [L, drop], one drop, or about 1 minim, of a medication, as eyedrops or eardrops.

guttae (gtt, gtts, GTTS) [L, drops], the plural of **gutta,** more than one drop, as in **guttae pro auribus,** or eardrops, or **guttae ophthalmicae,** or eyedrops.

gutta-percha /gut'əpur'chə/ [Malay, *getah-percha,* latex sap], the coagulated rubbery sap of various tropical trees, used for temporarily sealing the dressings of prepared tooth cavities.

gutta-percha point, any of the fine tapered cylinders of gutta-percha that may be used to fill a root canal.

guttate psoriasis /gut'āt/ [L, *gutta,* drop; Gk, itch], an acute form of psoriasis that consists of teardrop-shaped red scaly patches measuring 3 to 10 mm all over the body.

guttural /gut'ərəl/ [L, *guttur,* throat], pertaining to or belonging to the throat, including low-pitched, raspy voice quality.

Guyon tunnel [Felix J. Guyon, French surgeon, 1831–1920], a fibroosseous tunnel formed in part by the pisohamate ligament of the hand. It contains the ulnar artery and nerve and may be the site of a compression injury.

GVHD, abbreviation for **graft-versus-host disease.**

GVHR, abbreviation for **graft-versus-host reaction.**

Gy, abbreviation for the SI unit **gray.**

GYC agar, a mixture of glucose, yeast extract, and calcium carbonate used for culturing bacteria.

gyn, 1. *informal.* abbreviation for **gynecologist. 2.** abbreviation for **gynecology.**

gynandrous /gīnan'drəs, jī-/ [Gk, *gyne,* woman, *aner,* man], describing a man or a woman who has some of the physical characteristics usually attributed to the other sex, as a female pseudohermaphrodite. —**gynandry,** *n.*

gynecography /gī'nə-, jin'əkog'rəfē/, the radiologic examination of the female pelvic organs by means of intraperitoneal gas insufflation.

gynecoid pelvis /gī'nəkoid, jin'əkoid/ [Gk, *gyne + eidos,* form; L, *pelvis,* basin], a type of pelvis characteristic of the normal female and associated with the smallest incidence of fetopelvic disproportion.

gynecologic examination /gī'nə-, jin'-əkəloj'ik/, pelvic examination.

gynecologic operative procedures [Gk, *gynaikos,* of a woman; L, *operari,* to work, *procedere,* to proceed], surgical intervention on the female reproductive system. Gynecologic and obstetric problems account for one fifth of all female visits to physicians; many require surgical correction. Essential postoperative care demands that the patient be kept warm and quiet. Because of the risk of shock or hemorrhage, the patient should be closely monitored at frequent intervals during the first few hours. Fluids can be given when tolerated. Urine should be collected and measured periodically. Use of elastic stockings and suitable exercise is recommended to reduce the risk of thrombophlebitis.

gynecologist /gī'nəkol'əjist, jī'-, jin'-/, a physician who specializes in the health care of women, including diseases of the reproductive organs and breasts.

gynecology /gī'nəkol'əjē, jī'-, jin'-/ [Gk, *gyne + logos,* science], the study of diseases of the female reproductive organs, including the breasts. Unlike most specialties in medicine, gynecology encompasses surgical and nonsurgical expertise. It is almost always studied and practiced in conjunction with obstetrics. —**gynecologic, gynecological,** *adj.*

gynecomastia /gī′nəkōmas′tē·ə, jī′-, jin′-/ [Gk, *gyne* + *mastos,* breast], an abnormal enlargement of one or both breasts in men. The condition is usually temporary and benign. It may be caused by hormonal imbalance, tumor of the testis or pituitary, use of medication that contains estrogens or steroidal compounds, or failure of the liver to inactivate circulating estrogen, as in alcoholic cirrhosis.

gynephobia /gī′nəfō′bē·ə, jī′-, jin′-/ [Gk, *gyne* + *phobos,* fear], an anxiety disorder characterized by a morbid fear of women or a morbid aversion to the society of women.

gynogamone /gī′nōgam′ōn/ [Gk, *gyne* + *gamos,* marriage], a gamone secreted by the female gamete.

gypsum /jip′səm/, a mineral composed mainly of crushed calcium sulfate hemihydrate. It is used in making plaster of paris surgical casts and impressions for dentures. Gypsum dust has an irritant action on the mucous membranes of the respiratory tract and the conjunctiva.

gyrase /jī′rās/, an enzyme that promotes the unwinding of the closed circular deoxyribonucleic acid helix of bacteria.

gyrus /jī′rəs/, *pl.* **gyri** /jī′rī/ [Gk, *gyro,* circle], one of the winding convolutions of the surface of the brain, separated from each other by sulci (grooves). They are caused by infolding of the cortex.

H

h, **1.** abbreviation for **haustus. 2.** symbol for **hecto-. 3.** abbreviation for **height. 4.** symbol for *hora,* the Latin word for hour. **5.** abbreviation for *horizontal.* **6.** abbreviation for **hyperopia.**

H, 1. symbol for the element **hydrogen. 2.** symbol for **henry.**

²H, formula for **deuterium,** an isotope of hydrogen.

³H, formula for **tritium,** an isotope of hydrogen.

[H⁺], symbol for hydrogen ion molar concentration.

H₀, symbol for **null hypothesis.**

H₁ receptor, a type of histamine receptor on vascular smooth muscle walls through which histamine mediates vasodilation.

H₂ receptor, a type of histamine receptor on various kinds of cells through which histamine mediates bronchial constriction in asthma and gastrointestinal constriction in diarrhea.

H₂O, formula for water.

HAAg, abbreviation for *hepatitis A antigen.*

Haas method, a technique for producing radiographic images of the interior of the skull. The patient rests the head with the forehead and nose on the table so that the beam enters the skull near the base of the occipital bone and emerges 1 inch above the nasion.

habeas corpus /hā′bē·əs kôr′pəs/ [L, you have the body], a right retained by all psychiatric patients that provides for the release of individuals who claim they are being deprived of their liberty and detained illegally. A hearing for this determination takes place in a court of law, where the patient's sanity is at issue.

habilitation /həbil′itā′shən/, the process of supplying a person with the means to develop maximum independence in activities of daily living through training or treatment.

habit [L, *habitus,* condition], **1.** a customary or particular practice, manner, or mode of behavior. **2.** an involuntary pattern of behavior or thought. **3.** the habitual use of drugs or narcotics.

habitat /hab′itat/ [L, *habitare,* to dwell], a natural environment where a species of a plant or animal, including a human being, may live and grow normally.

habit spasm, an involuntary twitching or tic. It usually involves a small muscle group of the face, neck, or shoulders and causes movements such as spasmodic blinking or rapid jerking of the head to the side.

habit tic [L, *habitus,* condition; Fr, *tic*], a brief recurrent movement of a muscle group, such as a blink, grimace, or sudden head turning, that is of psychogenic rather than organic origin.

habit training, the process of teaching a child how to adjust to the demands of the external world by forming certain habits, primarily those related to eating, sleeping, elimination, and dress.

habitual abortion /həbich′ oo̅·əl/ [L, *habituare,* to become used to], spontaneous termination of three successive pregnancies before the twentieth week of gestation.

habitual dislocation [L, *habitus,* condition, *dis* + *locare,* to place], a dislocation that recurs repeatedly after reduction.

habitual hyperthermia, a condition of unknown cause that occurs in young females, characterized by body temperatures of 99° to 100.5° F regularly or intermittently for years, associated with fatigue, malaise, vague aches and pains, insomnia, bowel disturbances, and headaches.

habituation /həbich′ oo̅·ā′shən/ [L, *habituare,* to become used to], **1.** an acquired tolerance gained by repeated exposure to a particular stimulus. **2.** a decline and eventual elimination of a conditioned response by repetition of the conditioned stimulus. **3.** psychologic and emotional dependence on a drug, tobacco, or alcohol that results from the repeated use of the substance but without the addictive, physiologic need to increase dosage.

habitus /hab′itəs/, describing a person's appearance or physique, as an athletic habitus.

HACEK, acronym for *Hemophilus, Actinobacillus, Cardiobacterium, Eikenella,* and *Kingella,* microorganisms associated with infective endocarditis.

hacking cough [AS, *haeccan* + *cohettan*], a short, weak repeating cough, often caused by irritation of the larynx by a postnasal drip.

Haemophilus /hēmof′iləs/ [Gk, *haima,* blood, *philein,* to love], a genus of gram-negative pathogenic bacteria, frequently found in the respiratory tract of humans and other animals. *Haemophilus influenzae,* which causes respiratory tract infections and one form of meningitis, is an example.

Haemophilus influenzae, a small gram-negative nonmotile parasitic bacterium that occurs in two forms, encapsulated and nonencapsulated, and in six types, a, b, c, d, e, and f. Almost all infections are caused by encapsulated type b organisms.

hafnium (Hf) /haf′nē·əm/ [Hafnia, Medieval Latin name of Copenhagen, Denmark], a hard, brittle silver-gray metallic element of the first transition group. Its atomic number is 72; its atomic mass (weight) is 178.49.

Hagedorn needle /hä′gedôrn/ [Werner Hagedorn, German physician, 1831–1894], a flat surgical needle with a cutting edge near its point and a very large eye at the other end.

Haglund's deformity [Sims E. P. Haglund, Swedish orthopedist, 1870–1937], a foot disorder characterized by an enlarged posterior-superior lateral aspect of the calcaneus, often associated with an inverted subtalar joint. It is a common cause of posterior Achilles bursitis.

hair [AS, *haer*], a filament of keratin consisting of a root and a shaft formed in a specialized follicle in the epidermis. There are three stages of hair development: anagen, the active growing stage; catagen, a short interlude between the growth and resting phases; and telogen, the resting (club) stage before shedding. Scalp hair grows at an average rate of 1 mm every 3 days, body and eyebrow hair at a much slower rate.

hair analysis [AS, *haer* + Gk, a loosening], chemical analysis of a hair sample to find possible evidence of exposure to a toxic substance. Molecules of lead compounds and other chemicals are absorbed and stored in hair shafts. Hair analysis is also used to determine possible causes of malnutrition. Samples for analysis are taken from areas close to the scalp to eliminate chances that toxic chemicals found in the hair may have been absorbed from air pollutants.

Hair Care, a Nursing Interventions Classification defined as promotion of neat, clean, attractive hair.

hair follicle [AS, *haer* + L, *folliculus,* a small bag], a tiny tube of epidermal cells originating in the corium layer of the skin and containing the root of a hair shaft.

hairline fracture [AS, *haer* + L, *linea* + *fractura*], a minor fracture that appears on x-ray film as a thin line between two segments of a bone. The segments remain in alignment, and the fracture may not extend completely through the bone. A fatigue hairline fracture may develop without apparent injury and in the absence of trauma.

hair transplantation, a form of dermatologic and plastic surgery performed to correct scalp hair deficiencies caused by hormonal changes, burns, or injuries. The procedure uses existing hair to fill in bald areas. Several sessions are usually required to achieve the level of hair fullness desired by the patient. The sessions consist of grafting the hair-bearing tissue over the bald area directly or using tiny "plugs" of follicles to restore the hairline. It is important that the patient have healthy hair growth on other parts of the head to serve as donor areas and that color, texture, and other aspects of a matching transplant be compatible.

hairy-cell leukemia [AS, *haer* + L, *cella,* storeroom; Gk, *leukos,* white, *haima,* blood], an uncommon neoplasm of blood-forming tissues, characterized by pancytopenia, enlargement of the spleen, and many fine projections on the surface of reticulum cells in the blood and bone marrow. The disease occurs six times more frequently in men than in women and usually appears in the fifth decade with an insidious onset and a variable course marked by anemia, thrombocytopenia, and spontaneous bruising.

hairy leukoplakia, a form of leukoplakia characterized by a white plaque that is markedly folded in appearance or smooth and is often visible on one or both lateral borders of the tongue. It is associated with severe immunodeficiency, occurs in human immunodeficiency virus–infected patients, and is believed to result from the Epstein-Barr virus.

hairy nevus [AS, *haer* + L, *naevus,* birthmark], a mole, usually pigmented, that has hairs growing from it.

hairy tongue, a dark, pigmented overgrowth of the filiform papillae of the tongue that is a benign and frequent side effect of use of some antibiotics.

halazone /hal′əzōn/, a chlorine antiseptic similar to chloramine. It is used for purification of drinking water.

halcinonide /həlsin′ənīd/, a topical glucocorticoid prescribed topically as an antiinflammatory agent.

half-life (t½) [AS, *haelf* + *lif*], **1.** th

time required for a radioactive substance to lose 50% of its activity through decay. Each radionuclide has a unique half-life. **2.** the amount of time required to reduce a drug level to half of its initial value.

half-normal saline, (in respiratory therapy) a solution of 0.45% NaCl used for mucosal hydration. As the fluid tends to evaporate, the saline concentration increases, achieving nearly normal saline concentration in the respiratory tract.

half-sibling, one of two or more children who have one parent in common; a half-brother or half-sister.

half-value layer (HVL), the amount of material required to attenuate a beam of radiation to half of its original level.

halfway house, a specialized treatment facility, usually for psychiatric patients who no longer require complete hospitalization but who need some care and time to adjust to living independently.

halisteresis /həlis'tərē'sis/ [Gk, *hals,* salt, *steresis,* absence of], a theoretic process of bone resorption in which bone salts may be removed by humoral mechanisms and returned to body tissue fluids, leaving behind a decalcified bone matrix.

halitosis /hal'itō'sis/ [L, *halitus,* breath; Gk, *osis,* condition], offensive breath resulting from poor oral hygiene, dental or oral infections, ingestion of certain foods such as garlic or alcohol, use of tobacco, or some systemic diseases such as the odor of acetone in diabetes and ammonia in liver disease.

Hall, Lydia E., a nursing theorist who presented her Care, Core, and Cure Model in "Nursing: What Is It?" in *The Canadian Nurse* (1964). Hall believed nursing functions differently in three overlapping circles that constitute aspects of patients. She labeled the circles *the body* (the care), *the disease* (the cure), and *the person* (the core).

Hallervorden-Spatz's syndrome /hol'-ərfôr'dən shpots/ [Julius Hallervorden, German neurologist, 1882–1965; H. Spatz, German neurologist, 1888–1969], a progressive neurologic disease of children, with symptoms of parkinsonism. It is characterized by rigidity, athetosis, and dementia.

Hallpike test /hôl'pīk/, a method for evaluating the function of the vestibule of the ear in patients with vertigo or hearing loss. The patient's position is quickly changed from sitting to lying down with the neck hyperextended, and then returned to sitting. Nystagmus can then be evaluated.

hallucination /həlōō'sinā'shən/ [L, *alucinari,* to wander in mind], a sensory perception that does not result from an external stimulus and that occurs in the waking state. It can occur in any of the senses and is classified accordingly as auditory, gustatory, olfactory, tactile, or visual. —**hallucinate,** /həlōō'sənāt/ *v.*

Hallucination Management, a Nursing Interventions Classification defined as promoting the safety, comfort, and reality orientation of a patient experiencing hallucinations.

hallucinatory neuralgia /həlōō'sənətôr'ē/, a feeling of localized pain that persists after an episode of severe throbbing pain has subsided.

hallucinogen /həlōō'sənəjen', hal'əsin'-əjən, hal'yəsin'əjən/ [L, *alucinari* + Gk, *genein,* to produce], a substance that causes excitation of the central nervous system, characterized by hallucination, mood change, anxiety, sensory distortion, delusion, and depersonalization; increased pulse, temperature, and blood pressure; and dilation of the pupils.

hallucinogenesis /-jen'əsīs/ [L, *alucinari,* to wander in mind; Gk, *genein,* to produce], a cause or source of hallucinations.

hallucinosis /halōō'sinō'sis/ [L, *alucinari* + Gk, *osis,* condition], a pathologic mental state in which awareness consists primarily or exclusively of hallucinations.

hallux /hal'əks/, *pl.* **halluces** /hal'yōōsēz/ [L, *hallex,* large toe], the great toe.

hallux rigidus, a painful deformity of the great toe, limiting motion at the metatarso-phalangeal joint.

hallux valgus, a deformity in which the great toe is angulated away from the midline of the body toward the other toes; in some cases the great toe rides over or under the other toes.

hallux varus, fixed displacement of the great toe away from the other toes.

halo cast [Gk, *halos,* circular floor; AS, *kasta*], an orthopedic device used to help immobilize the neck and head. It incorporates the trunk, usually with shoulder straps, and an outrigger within the cast to secure pins to a band around the skull.

haloderma /hal'ōdur'mə/, skin changes caused by ingestion or injection of halogen, usually a bromide or an iodide.

halo effect, the beneficial effect of an interview or other encounter, as may occur in the course of a research project or a health care visit. It is the result of indefinable interpersonal factors present in the interaction.

halogen /hal'ōjən/ [Gk, *hals,* salt, *genein,* to produce], any member of the group 17 elements in the periodic table: fluorine, chlorine, bromine, iodine, and astatine.

They are found in sea water as the corresponding halide ion.

halogenated hydrocarbon /hǝloj'ǝnā'tid/ [Gk, *hals,* salt, *genein,* to produce, *hydor,* water; L, *carbo,* coal], a volatile liquid used for general anesthesia, administered in combination with oxygen or with oxygen in combination with nitrous oxide.

halo nevus, a benign melanocyte that appears as a central brown mole surrounded by a circle of depigmented skin. Over a period of months the central nevus becomes flat and loses its pigment, leaving a round white macule. Eventually the halo repigments.

haloperidol /hal'ōper'ǝdôl/, a butyrophenone tranquilizer prescribed in the treatment of psychotic disorders and in the control of Gilles de la Tourette's syndrome.

halothane /hal'ǝthān/, an inhalation anesthetic prescribed for induction and maintenance of general anesthesia.

halothane-related hepatitis, an adverse reaction of some patients to inhalation of halothane, a general anesthetic. The reaction is characterized by hepatitis and a severe fever that develops several days after exposure to the anesthetic.

Halsted's forceps /hal'stedz/ [William S. Halsted, American surgeon, 1852–1922], **1.** a small pointed hemostatic forceps. **2.** a forceps with slender jaws for grasping arteries and other blood vessels.

Halsted's suture [William S. Halsted], the union of two adjoining skin surfaces by a suture placed through the subcuticular fascia.

HALT, abbreviation for **Hypertension and Lipid Trial.**

hamartoma, a new tissue growth resembling a tumor. It results from a defective overgrowth in tissue formation.

hamate bone /ham'āt/ [L, *hamatus,* hooked], a carpal (wrist) bone that rests on the fourth and fifth metacarpal bones and projects a hooklike process, the hamulus, from its palmar surface.

hammer finger [AS, *hamer + finger*], a permanently flexed terminal phalanx caused by an injury to the extensor tendon.

hammer toe /ham'ǝr tō/ [AS, *hamer + ta*], a foot digit permanently flexed at the mid-phalangeal joint, producing a clawlike appearance. The anomaly may be present in more than one digit but is most common in the second toe.

Hampton's hump [Aubrey O. Hampton, American radiologist, 1900–1955], a soft tissue image in a radiograph of the lung that is a manifestation of a pulmonary infarction.

hamstring muscle [AS, *hamm + streng*], any of the group of three muscles at the back of the thigh: medially the semimembranosus and the semitendinosus and laterally the biceps femoris.

hamstring reflex, a normal deep tendon reflex elicited by tapping one of the hamstring tendons behind the knee, causing contraction of the tendon and flexion of the knee.

hamstring tendon, one of the three tendons from the three hamstring muscles in the back of the thigh. The one lateral and the two medial hamstring tendons connect the hamstring muscles to the knee.

hand [AS, *hand*], the part of the upper limb distal to the forearm. It is the most flexible part of the skeleton and has a total of 27 bones, 8 forming the carpus, 5 forming the metacarpus, and 14 forming the phalangeal section.

handblock [AS, *hand* + Fr, *bloc*], a device made of a wood block several inches high with a firm handle that can assist a disabled patient in sitting push-ups, which can enhance transfers or mobility in bed.

hand condenser, (in dentistry) an instrument for compacting amalgams or gold foil using force applied by the operator.

handedness /han'didnes/ [AS, *hand + ness,* condition], voluntary or involuntary preference for use of either the left or right hand. The preference is related to cerebral dominance: left-handedness corresponds to dominance of the right side of the brain, and vice versa.

hand-foot-and-mouth disease, a coxsackie viral infection characterized by the appearance of painful ulcers and vesicles on the mucous membranes of the mouth and on the hands and feet. The disease is highly contagious and mainly affects children, including infants.

handicapped /han'dikapt/ [*hand in cap,* a seventeenth-century game with forfeits], referring to a person who has a congenital or acquired mental or physical defect that interferes with normal functioning of the body system or the ability to be self-sufficient in modern society.

handpiece /hand'pēs/, a device for holding rotary instruments in a dental engine or condensing points in mechanical condensing units.

hanging drop preparation [ME, *hangen,* to hang; AS, *dropa,* to fall; L, *praeparer,* to make ready], a technique used for the examination and identification of certain microorganisms, such as spirochetes or trichomonads. A drop of a fluid mixture is placed on a glass coverslip, which is then inverted carefully and placed over the slide so that the drop is hanging from the slip into the concavity in the slide. Th delicate structures and the method of movement characteristic of the species may then be viewed through the microscope.

hangman's fracture, a fracture of the posterior elements of the cervical vertebrae with dislocation of C2 or C3.

hangnail [AS, *angnaegl,* troublesome nail], a piece of partially disconnected epidermis of the cuticle or nail fold. Tearing the skin fragment causes a red, painful, easily infected sore.

hangover, a popular term for a group of symptoms, including nausea, thirst, fatigue, headache, and irritability, resulting from the use of alcohol and certain drugs.

Hanot's disease /hanōz'/ [Victor C. Hanot, French physician, 1844–1896], primary biliary cirrhosis.

Hansen's bacillus [Gerard H. A. Hansen, Norwegian physician, 1841–1912; L, *bacillum,* a small rod], the acid-fast *Mycobacterium leprae,* which is the cause of leprosy.

HA-1A, a genetically engineered antibody used in the treatment of certain blood infections. The HA-1A antibody attacks the bacterial toxin rather than directly attacking the bacterium. It is relatively free of side effects.

Hantavirus, a genus of viruses in the *Bunyaviridae* family. *Hantavirus* is the cause of several different forms of hemorrhagic fever with renal syndrome. The severity of the illness is determined by the strain isolated through the use of immunofluorescent assay or enzyme-linked immunosorbent assay.

hapadnavirus /hapad'nəvī'rəs/, a virus similar to that of hepatitis B of the Hepadnaviridae family of microorganisms. that proliferates in the nuclei of liver cells and causes a persistent hepatitis B infection.

haploid /hap'loid/ [Gk, *haploos,* single, *eidos,* form], having only one complete set of nonhomologous chromosomes. —**haploidy,** *n.*

haploid nucleus [Gk, *haploos,* single, *eidos,* form; L, *nucleus,* nut], a nucleus possessing only half the normal somatic number of chromosomes. It may occur in a germ cell after reduction division and before fertilization.

Hapsburg lip, an overdeveloped, thick lower lip, which often accompanies the Hapsburg jaw (a jaw that projects forward).

hapten /hap'tən/ [Gk, *haptein,* to grasp], a nonproteinaceous substance that acts as an antigen by combining with particular bonding sites on an antibody.

haptics /hap'tiks/ [Gk, *haptein,* to grasp], the science concerned with studying the sense of touch. —**haptic,** *adj.*

haptoglobin /hap'tōglō'bin/ [Gk, *haptein,* to grasp; L, *globus,* ball], a plasma protein whose only function is to bind free hemoglobin. The quantity of haptoglobin is increased in certain chronic diseases and inflammatory disorders and is decreased or absent in hemolytic anemia.

harborage transmission /här'bərij/, a mode of infection transmission in which the organism does not undergo morphologic and physiologic changes in the vector.

hard chancre [AS, *heard* + Fr, *canker*], a syphilitic chancre or primary lesion that develops at the site of a syphilis infection. The lesion begins as a small red papule that gradually hardens and erodes into an extremely contagious ulcer. A secretion exuded by the sore contains *Treponema pallidum,* the organism that is the causative agent of syphilis in humans.

hard contact lens [AS, *heard* + L, *contingere,* to touch, *lentil*], a polymethylmethacrylate, or rigid gas-permeable, contact lens that retains its form without support, in contrast with a soft contact lens, which readily yields to pressure.

hard data, information about a patient that is obtained by observation and measurement, including laboratory data, as opposed to information collected by interview of the patient or others.

hardening of the arteries, arteriosclerosis.

hard fibroma, a neoplasm composed of fibrous tissue in which few cells are present.

hardness of x-rays, the relative penetrating power of x-rays. In general, the shorter the wavelength, the harder the radiation.

hard palate [AS, *heard,* hard; L, *palatum*], the bony part of the roof of the mouth, continuous posteriorly with the soft palate and bounded anteriorly and laterally by the alveolar arches and the gums.

hard soap, a detergent soap made with olive oil and sodium hydroxide.

hard water [AS, *heard* + *waeter*], water that contains certain cations, particularly calcium and magnesium, that precipitate with soap solutions.

Hardy-Weinberg equilibrium principle /här'dē wīn'bərg/ [G. H. Hardy, English mathematician, 1877–1947; Wilhelm Weinberg, German physician, 1862–1937; L, *aequilibris,* equal weight, *principium,* a beginning], the mathematic relationship between the frequency of genes and the resulting genotypes in populations. In a large interbreeding population characterized by random mating, mendelian inheritance, and the absence of migration, mutation, and selection, the ratio of individuals homozygous for a dominant gene to those heterozygous to those homozygous for a recessive gene is 1:2:1, at which point equilibrium is established; the frequency of genes and genotypes remains relatively unchanged from generation to generation.

harlequin color /här'lək(w)in/ [It, *arlecchino,* goblin; L, *color,* hue], a temporary flushing of the skin on the lower side of the body with pallor on the other side. Commonly seen in normal young infants, it disappears as the child matures.

harlequin fetus, an infant whose skin at birth is completely covered with thick, horny scales that resemble armor and are divided by deep red fissures. The condition is the most severe form of lamellar exfoliation of the newborn.

Harrison's groove [Edward Harrison, English physician, 1776–1838], a deformity of the thorax that develops as a result of the pull of the diaphragm on ribs weakened by rickets or some other calcium deficiency disorder.

Harris tube [Franklin Harris, American surgeon, b. 1895], a tube used for gastric and intestinal decompression. It is a mercury-weighted single-lumen tube that is passed through the nose and carried through the digestive tract by gravity. The location of the tube and its final placement are checked by fluoroscopy.

Hartmann's curet [Arthur Hartmann, German physician, 1849–1931], a curet used for the removal of adenoids.

Hartnup disease [Hartnup, family name of first patients diagnosed in England, 1956], a rare recessive genetic metabolic disorder characterized by pellagra-like skin lesions, transient cerebellar ataxia, and hyperaminoaciduria.

Hashimoto's disease /hä'shimō'tōz/ [Hakaru Hashimoto, Japanese surgeon, 1881–1934], an autoimmune thyroid disorder. It is characterized by the production of antibodies in response to thyroid antigens and the replacement of normal thyroid structures with lymphocytes and lymphoid germinal centers. The thyroid, typically enlarged, pale yellow, and lumpy on the surface, shows dense lymphocytic infiltration, and the remaining thyroid tissue frequently contains small empty follicles.

haustus (h) /hôs'təs/, a draught of medicine.

HAV, abbreviation for *hepatitis A virus.*

Haverhill fever /hā'vəril/ [Haverhill, Massachusetts, disorder first diagnosed, 1925], a febrile disease, caused by infection with *Streptobacillus moniliformis,* transmitted by the bite of a rat. Characteristically the

wound from the bite heals, but within 10 days fever, chills, vomiting, headache, muscle and joint pain, and a rash appear.

haversian canal /havur'shən/ [Clopton Havers, English physician, 1650–1702], one of the many tiny longitudinal canals in bone tissue, averaging about 0.05 mm in diameter. Each contains blood vessels, connective tissue, nerve filaments, and occasionally lymphatic vessels.

haversian canaliculus /kan'əlik'yələs/ [Clopton Havers], any of the many tiny passages radiating from the lacunae of bone tissue to larger haversian canals.

haversian glands [Clopton Havers; L, *glans,* acorn], extrasynovial fat pads that may project into the joint space.

haversian lamella [Clopton Havers; L, *lamella,* a small plate], one of a series of lamellae (circular layers) arranged around the central haversian canal of an osteon, or cylindric unit of bone structure.

haversian system [Clopton Havers], a circular district of bone tissue, consisting of concentric rings of osteocytes and lamellae in the bone around a central blood vessel canal.

Hawthorne effect /hô'thôrn/, a general unintentional, but usually beneficial effect on a person, a group of people, or the function of the system being studied. It is the effect of an encounter, as with an investigator or health care provider, or of a change in a program or facility, as by painting of an office or change in the lighting system.

hay fever [AS, *heawan,* to hew; L, *febris,* fever], *informal.* an acute seasonal allergic rhinitis stimulated by tree, grass, or weed pollen.

Hayflick limits [Leonard Hayflick, American microbiologist, b. 1928; L, *limes,* border], the concept that the life span of living organisms is limited by the number of times that somatic cells will subdivide. On the basis of human cells in cultures, where divisions occur about 50 times, it is estimated the average human life span is limited to around 115 years.

hazard /haz'ərd/ [Fr, *hasard,* chance], a condition or phenomenon that increases the probability of a loss that may result in injury or illness. **—hazardous,** *adj.*

Hb, abbreviation for **hemoglobin.**

HB, abbreviation for **hepatitis B.**

Hb A, abbreviation for **hemoglobin A.**

Hb A$_2$, abbreviation for **hemoglobin A$_2$.**

HBAg, abbreviation for *hepatitis B antigen.*

Hb C, abbreviation for **hemoglobin C.**

HBE, abbreviation for **His bundle electrogram.**

Hb F, abbreviation for **hemoglobin F.**

HBIG, abbreviation for **hepatitis B immune globulin.**

Hb S, abbreviation for **hemoglobin S.**

HBsAG, abbreviation for hepatitis B surface antigen.

Hb S-C, abbreviation for **hemoglobin S-C.**

HBV, abbreviation for *hepatitis B virus.*

HCG, abbreviation for human chorionic gonadotropin.

HCG radioreceptor assay, a urine test to detect pregnancy or missed abortion, performed by measuring human chorionic gonadotropin, a chemical found only in the urine of pregnant women or in tumors that produce HCG.

HCl, formula for **hydrochloric acid** or hydrogen chloride.

HCV. abbreviation for *hepatitis C virus.*

H deflection, (in cardiology) a deviation observed on the His electrogram that represents activation of the bundle of His.

HDI, abbreviation for **high-definition imaging.**

HDL, abbreviation for **high-density lipoprotein.**

HDV, abbreviation for *hepatitis D virus.*

He, symbol for the element **helium.**

head [AS, *heafod*], **1.** the uppermost extremity, containing the brain, special sense organs, mouth, nose, and related structures. Most of the tissues are enclosed within the skull, composed of 22 bones. **2.** a rounded, usually proximal part of some long bones.

headache /hed′āk/ [AS, *heafod* + *acan,* to hurt], a pain in the head from any cause.

head and neck cancer, any malignant neoplasms of the upper aerodigestive tract, facial features, and structures in the neck, which appear as masses, ulcerations, or flat lesions that usually produce early symptoms.

head banging, a form of physical exertion observed during some temper tantrums. It usually occurs near the peak of excitement and may be associated with other physical or muscular movements.

head bobbing, a sign of respiratory distress in an infant. Because neck extensor muscles are not strong enough to stabilize the head, accessory muscle use produces head bobbing.

head box, a clear plastic chamber that fits over a patient's head with an adjustable seal around the neck for mechanical ventilation. Humidified gas enters the chamber, and excess gas is released through an outlet valve. The device may help prevent the need for intubation.

head, eye, ear, nose, and throat (HEENT), a specialty in medicine concerned with the anatomic, physiologic, and pathologic characteristics of the head, eyes, ears, nose, and throat and with diagnosis and treatment of their disorders.

head injury, any traumatic damage to the head resulting from blunt or penetrating trauma of the skull. Blood vessels, nerves, and meninges can be torn; bleeding, edema, and ischemia may result.

head process, a strand of cells that extends forward from the primitive node in the early stages of embryonic development in vertebrates. It is the precursor of the notochord.

heads-up tilt table test (HUTT), a method of evaluating children with neurocardiac syncope. After baseline signs are recorded in the supine position, the patient is tilted to an 80-degree angle for 30 minutes, or until neurocardiac syncope signs appear.

head-tilt, chin-lift airway technique, a method of providing maximum airway opening in an unconscious person. With the victim lying on his or her back, the rescuer pushes down on the victim's forehead with the palm of the hand, tilting the victim's head back. With the other hand, the rescuer lifts the victim's lower jaw near the chin. The technique opens the airway by moving the tongue away from the back of the throat and the epiglottis away from the opening of the trachea. This technique is not recommended if a cervical spine injury is suspected.

head traction [AS, *heafod* + L, *trahere,* to draw], traction that is applied to the head in the treatment of cervical vertebrae injuries.

Heaf test /hēf/ [Frederick R. G. Heaf, English physician, 1894–1973], a tuberculin skin test that uses a multiple puncture technique.

healing [AS, *haelan,* to cure], the act or process in which the normal structural and functional characteristics of health are restored to diseased, dysfunctional, or damaged tissues, organs, or systems of the body.

health [AS, *haelth*], a condition of physical, mental, and social well-being and the absence of disease or other abnormal condition. It is not a static condition; constant change and adaptation to stress result in homeostasis.

health assessment, an evaluation of the health status of an individual by performing a physical examination after obtaining a health history. Various laboratory tests also may be ordered to confirm a clinical impression or to screen for dysfunction.

health behavior, an action taken by a person to maintain, attain, or regain good health and to prevent illness. Health behavior reflects a person's health beliefs. Some common health behaviors are exercising regularly, eating a balanced diet, and obtaining necessary inoculations.

health belief model, a conceptual framework that describes a person's health behavior as an expression of health beliefs. The model was designed to predict a person's health behavior, including the use of health services, and to justify intervention to alter maladaptive health behavior.

health care consumer, any actual or potential recipient of health care, such as a patient in a hospital, a client in a community mental health center, or a member of a prepaid health maintenance organization.

Health Care Financing Administration (HCFA), the branch of the U.S. Department of Health and Human Services responsible for administering the Medicare and Medicaid programs. HCFA sets the coverage policy and payment and other guidelines and directs the activities of government contractors (e.g., carriers and fiscal intermediaries).

health care industry, the complex of preventive, remedial, and therapeutic services provided by hospitals and other institutions, nurses, doctors, dentists, government agencies, voluntary agencies, noninstitutional care facilities, pharmaceutic and medical equipment manufacturers, and health insurance companies.

Health Care Information Exchange, a Nursing Interventions Classification defined as providing patient care information to health professionals in other agencies.

health care provider, any individual who provides health services to health care consumers.

health care proxy [AS, *haelth* + ME, *caru,* sorrow; L, *procuratio,* a deputy], a person designated to make health care decisions for a patient who has become incapacitated.

health care system, the complete network of agencies, facilities, and all providers of health care in a specified geographic area. Nursing services are integral to all levels and patterns of care, and nurses form the largest number of providers in a health care system.

health certificate, a statement signed by a health care provider that attests to the state of health of a person.

health councils, *(Canada)* organizations that plan and allocate health care facilities. Local participants are represented in the District Health Councils, funded by the Ministry of Health.

health culture, a system that attempts to explain and treat sickness and to maintain health. It may be a popular or folk system, or it may be a technical or scientific one.

health economics, a social system that studies the supply and demand of health care resources and the effect of health services on a population.

health education, an educational program directed to the general public that attempts to improve, maintain, and safeguard the health of the community.

Health Education, a Nursing Interventions Classification defined as developing and providing instruction and learning experiences to facilitate voluntary adaptation of behavior conducive to health in individuals, families, groups, or communities.

health hazard [AS, *haelth* + OFr, *hasard*], a danger to health resulting from exposure to environmental pollutants such as asbestos or ionizing radiation or to a life-style influence such as cigarette smoking or chemical abuse.

health history, (in nursing and medicine) a collection of information obtained from the patient and from other sources concerning the patient's physical status and psychologic, social, and sexual function. The history provides a data base on which a plan for management of the diagnosis, treatment, care, and follow-up observation of the patient may be made.

health maintenance, a program or procedure planned to prevent illness, to maintain maximal function, and to promote health.

health maintenance, altered, a NANDA-accepted nursing diagnosis of an inability to identify, manage, or seek help to maintain health. Defining characteristics include a demonstrated lack of knowledge regarding basic health practices or the inability to take responsibility for meeting those needs, the inability to adapt to internal or external environmental change, a lack of financial or other resources or support systems, a history of a lack of health-seeking behavior, or an increased interest in improving health behavior.

health maintenance organization (HMO), a type of group health care practice that provides basic and supplemental health maintenance and treatment services to voluntary enrollees who prepay a fixed periodic fee set without regard to the amount or kind of services received. Some of the first HMOs, Kaiser-Permanente among them, have demonstrated that high quality medical care often can be provided at less expense by such a system than by other health care systems. In addition to diagnostic and treatment services, including hospitalization and surgery, an HMO often offers supplemental services such as dental, mental, and eye care and prescription drugs. Federal financial support for the establishment of HMOs was provided under Title XIII of the 1973 U.S. Public Health Service Act.

health nurse, a community or visiting nurse usually employed by a public health agency and assigned primarily to promote health maintenance and preventive health measures within the community.

health physicist, a health scientist who directs research, training, and management of programs in which patients and health professionals are exposed to potential hazards associated with the use of diagnostic and therapeutic equipment such as radioactive materials.

health physics, the study of the effects of ionizing radiation on the body and the methods for protecting people from the undesirable effects of the radiation.

health policy, 1. a statement of a decision regarding a goal in health care and a plan for achieving that goal. 2. a field of study and practice in which the priorities and values underlying health resource allocation are determined.

Health Policy Monitoring, a Nursing Interventions Classification defined as surveillance and influence of government and organization regulations, rules, and standards that affect nursing systems and practices to ensure high quality care of patients.

health professional, any person who has completed a course of study in a field of health, such as a registered nurse, physical therapist, or physician. The person is usually licensed by a government agency or certified by a professional organization.

health-related services, actions of a health facility other than providing medical care that may contribute directly or indirectly to the physical or mental health and well-being of patients, such as personal or social services.

health resources, all materials, personnel, facilities, funds, and anything else that can be used for providing health care and services.

Health Resources and Services Administration (HRSA), a U.S. federal agency with responsibilities for the distribution of health information. This includes audiovisual materials relating to a wide range of health subjects such as recruitment of minorities into the health professions and the role of women in dentistry.

health risk, a disease precursor associated with a higher than average morbidity or mortality rate.

health risk appraisal, a process of gathering, analyzing, and comparing an individual's characteristics prognostic of health with those of a standard age group.

health screening, a program designed to evaluate the health status and potential of an individual. Health screening may include taking a personal and family health history and performing a physical examination, tests, laboratory tests, or radiologic examination.

Health Screening, a Nursing Interventions Classification defined as detecting health risks or problems by means of history, examination, and other procedures.

health-seeking behaviors, a NANDA-accepted nursing diagnosis of a state in which a client in stable health is actively seeking ways to alter personal health habits and the environment to move toward optimal health. Defining characteristics include an expressed or observed desire to seek a higher level of wellness, unfamiliarity with wellness community resources, lack of knowledge of health promotion behaviors, desire for increased control of health practice, and concern about environmental conditions or health status.

health service area, a geographic region designated under the U.S. National Health Planning and Resources Development Act of 1974, covering such factors as geographic features, political boundaries, population, and health resources, for the effective planning and development of health services.

health supervision, health teaching, counseling, or monitoring of the status of a patient's health other than for physical care.

Health System Guidance, a Nursing Interventions Classification defined as facilitating a patient's location and use of appropriate health services.

health systems agency (HSA), a body established under the terms of the U.S. National Health Planning and Resources Development Act of 1974. Health planning agencies are intended to provide networks of health planning and resource development services in each of several health service areas established by the Act.

health systems plan, a plan in which the long-range goals of a health services area are specified. Health systems plans are prepared by health systems agencies.

healthy, a condition of physical, mental, and social well-being and of absence of disease or another abnormal condition.

hearing [AS, *hieran*], the sense that enables sound to be perceived. It is the major function of the ear.

hearing aid, an electronic device that amplifies sound used by people with impaired hearing. The device consists of a microphone, a battery power supply, an amplifier, and a receiver.

hearing impairment, loss of hearing that adversely affects an individual's ability to communicate.

hearing loss, an inability to perceive the normal range of sounds audible to an individual with normal hearing. **Conductive hearing loss** is a result of damage to the outer or middle ear, whereas **sensorineural hearing loss** results from damage to the cochlea or auditory nerve.

heart [AS, *heorte*], the muscular cone-shaped hollow organ, about the size of a clenched fist, that pumps blood throughout the body and beats normally about 70 times per minute by coordinated nerve impulses and muscular contractions. Enclosed in pericardium, it rests on the diaphragm between the lower borders of the lungs, occupying the middle of the mediastinum. It is covered ventrally by the sternum and the adjoining parts of the third to the sixth costal cartilages. The layers of the heart, starting from the outside, are the epicardium, the myocardium, and the endocardium. The chambers include two ventricles with thick muscular walls, making up the bulk of the organ, and two atria with thin muscular walls. A septum separates the ventricles and extends between the atria (interatrial septum), dividing the heart into the right and left sides.

heartbeat, a complete cycle of cardiac muscle contraction and relaxation.

heart block, an interference with the normal conduction of electrical impulses that control activity of the heart muscle. Heart block usually is further defined as to the location of the block and the type.

heartburn, a painful burning sensation in the esophagus just below the sternum. Heartburn is usually caused by the reflux of gastric contents into the esophagus but may result from gastric hyperacidity or peptic ulcer.

heart disease risk factors [AS, *heorte,* heart; L, *dis* + Fr, *aise,* ease, *risquer,* chance of injury; L, *facere,* to make], hereditary, life-style, and environmental influences that increase one's chance of development of heart disease. Examples include cigarette smoking, high blood pressure, diabetes, obesity, high cholesterol level, lack of routine exercise, and hereditary factors.

heart failure, a condition in which the heart cannot pump enough blood to meet the metabolic requirements of body tissues. Many of the symptoms associated with heart failure are caused by the dysfunction of organs other than the heart, es-

pecially the lungs, kidneys, and liver. Ventricular dysfunction is usually the basic disorder in congestive heart failure; it often triggers compensatory mechanisms that preserve cardiac output but produce symptoms and signs such as dyspnea, orthopnea, rales, and edema. Most kinds of heart disease initially affect the left side of the heart, and clinicians commonly divide associated heart failure into left-sided and right-sided heart failure.

heart-lung machine, an apparatus consisting of a pump and an oxygenator that takes over the functions of the heart and lungs, especially during open heart surgery. The blood is shunted from the venous system through an oxygenator and returned to the arterial circulation.

heart rate, the pulse, calculated by counting the number of QRS complexes or ventricular beats per minute.

heart scan, a radiographic scan of the heart, performed after injecting a radioactive material into a vein. It is used for determining the size, shape, and location of the heart; for diagnosing pericarditis; and for viewing the chambers of the heart.

heart sound, a normal noise produced within the heart during the cardiac cycle that can be heard over the precordium. It may reveal abnormalities in cardiac structure or function. Cardiac auscultation is performed systematically from apex to base of the heart or from base to apex, using a stethoscope to listen, initially with the diaphragm and then with the bell of the instrument. The first heart sound (S_1), a dull, prolonged "lub," occurs with the closure of the mitral and tricuspid valves and marks the onset of ventricular systole. The second heart sound (S_2), a short, sharp "dup," occurs with the closing of the aortic and pulmonic valves at the beginning of ventricular diastole.

heart surgery, any surgical procedure involving the heart, performed to correct acquired or congenital defects, replace diseased valves, open or bypass blocked vessels, or graft a prosthesis or a transplant in place. Two major types of heart surgery are performed: closed and open. The closed technique is done through a small incision, without using the heart-lung machine. In the open technique the heart chambers are open and fully visible, and blood is detoured around the surgical field by the heart-lung machine.

heart transplantation [AS, *hoerte* + L, *transplantare*], the surgical removal of a donor heart and transfer of the organ to a recipient. The procedure usually involves removing a heart from a healthy individual who may have died in an accident or of another cause unrelated to heart disease and using it to replace the severely diseased heart of another person. Most recipients survive for more than 1 year with a transplanted heart, and nearly three fourths of the recipients are able to return to work. Total ischemic time for heart transplantation is less than 6 hours between donor and recipient.

heart valve, one of the four structures within the heart that prevent backflow of blood by opening and closing with each heartbeat. The valves include two semilunar valves, the aortic and pulmonary; the mitral or bicuspid valve; and the tricuspid valve. The valves permit blood flow in only one direction.

heat cramp [AS, *haetu* + *crammian,* to fill], any cramp or painful spasm of the voluntary muscles in the arm, leg, or abdomen caused by depletion in the body of both water and salt. It usually occurs after vigorous physical exertion in an extremely hot environment or under other conditions that cause profuse sweating and depletion of body fluids and electrolytes.

Heat Exposure Treatment, a Nursing Interventions Classification defined as management of a patient overcome by heat as a result of excessive environmental heat exposure.

Heat/Cold Application, a Nursing Interventions Classification defined as stimulation of the skin and underlying tissues with heat or cold for the purpose of decreasing pain, muscle spasms, or inflammation.

heated nebulization, a method of inhalation therapy that uses a heating device with a nebulizer that produces a spray with a higher water content than that of a cold atomizer. The mist may be administered through a mask or in a tent.

heat exhaustion, an abnormal condition characterized by weakness, vertigo, nausea, muscle cramps, and loss of consciousness, caused by depletion of body fluid and electrolytes, which results from exposure to intense heat or inability to acclimatize to heat. Body temperature is near normal; blood pressure may drop but usually returns to normal as the person is placed in a recumbent position; the skin is cool, damp, and pale.

heat hyperpyrexia, a severe and sometimes fatal condition resulting from failure of the temperature regulating capacity of the body, caused by prolonged exposure to sun or to high temperature. Reduction or cessation of sweating is sometimes an early symptom. Body temperature of 105° F or higher, tachycardia, hot and dry skin,

headache, altered mental status, and seizures may occur.

heat labile [L, *labilis,* liable to slip], readily destroyed by heat.

heat-labile antibody, an immunoglobulin that loses its ability to interact with antigens when heated above 56° C.

heat rash, a finely papular or vesicular inflammation of the skin that results from prolonged exposure to heat and high humidity.

heat shock protein (HsP), an intracellular protein that increases in concentration during metabolic stress, such as exposure to heat.

heaves /hēvz/ [AS, *hebban,* to lift], *informal.* vomiting and retching.

heavy chain, a high molecular–weight polypeptide that is part of an immunoglobulin molecule. Different types of heavy chains characterize the various categories of immunoglobulins (Igs) such as IgG and IgA.

heavy chain disease [AS, *heafig* + L, *catena,* chain; *dis,* opposite of; Fr, *aise,* ease], a plasma cell disorder characterized by a proliferation of immunoglobulin heavy chains. Effects tend to vary according to the predominant type of heavy chain. For example, most gamma heavy chain disease patients are elderly men who have symptoms resembling those of malignant lymphoma. Mu heavy chain disease presents symptoms of chronic lymphocytic leukemia.

heavy function, (in dentistry) an increase in the functional activities of the teeth, which enhances occlusal force.

heavy metal, a metallic element with a specific gravity five or more times that of water. The heavy metals are antimony, arsenic, bismuth, cadmium, cerium, chromium, cobalt, copper, gallium, gold, iron, lead, manganese, mercury, nickel, platinum, silver, tellurium, thallium, tin, uranium, vanadium, and zinc. Small amounts of many of these elements are common and necessary in the diet. Large amounts of any of them may cause poisoning.

heavy metal poisoning, poisoning caused by the ingestion, inhalation, or absorption of various toxic heavy metals.

heavy water, water in which the hydrogen component is deuterium (^{2}H), or heavy hydrogen. It has properties different from those of ordinary water. Because of its ability to absorb neutrons, heavy water is used as a moderator in nuclear reactions. Also written as D_2O.

Heberden's node /hē′bərdənz/ [William Heberden, English physician, 1710–1801; L, *nodus,* knot], an abnormal cartilaginous or bony enlargement of a distal interphalangeal joint of a finger, usually occurring in degenerative diseases of the joints.

hebetude /heb′itōōd′/ [L, *hebeo,* to be blunt], a state of dullness or lethargy, characteristic of some forms of schizophrenia.

heel [AS, *hela*], the posterior part of the foot, formed by the largest tarsal bone, the calcaneus.

heel cup, a plastic device designed to help relieve pain of a heel spur or contusion by pushing the fat pad of the heel under the calcaneus to increase the cushioning effect.

heel-knee test [AS, *hela* + *cneow,* knee; L, *testum,* crucible], a method of assessing coordination of movements of the extremities. In the test the patient, lying supine, is asked to touch the knee of one leg with the heel of the other.

heel lift, a form of foot orthosis, usually made of sheets of cork, to correct a dysfunction that may result from anatomic limb length differences or decreased flexibility.

heel puncture [AS, *hela* + L, *punctura*], a method of obtaining a blood sample from a newborn or premature infant by a puncture in the lateral or medial areas of the plantar surface of the heel. Care must be exercised to prevent puncture of the posterior curvature of the heel and to make the puncture as shallow as feasible.

heel-shin test [AS, *hela* + *scinu,* shin; L, *testum,* crucible], a method of assessing coordination of movements of the extremities. In the test the patient, lying supine, is asked to pass the heel of one leg slowly down the shin of the other leg from the knee to the ankle.

HEENT, abbreviation for **head, eye, ear, nose, and throat.**

Hegar's dilators /hā′gərz/ [Alfred Hegar, German gynecologist, 1830–1914], a series of bougies used to dilate the cervical canal.

Hegar's sign [Alfred Hegar; L, *signum,* sign], a softening of the isthmus of the uterine cervix that occurs early in gestation. It is a probable sign of pregnancy.

height (ht) /hīt/ [AS, *hiehtho*], the vertical measurement of a structure, organ, or other object from bottom to top, when it is placed or projected in an upright position.

height of contour, the greatest convexity of a tooth surface, viewed from a predetermined position.

Heimlich maneuver /hīm′lik, -lish/ [H. J. Heimlich, American physician, b. 1920; Fr, *manœuvre,* work done by hand], an emergency procedure for dislodging a bolus of food or other obstruction from the trachea to prevent asphyxiation. The chok-ing person is grasped from behind by the rescuer, whose fist, thumb side in, is placed just below the victim's sternum with the other hand placed firmly over the fist. The rescuer then pulls the fist firmly and abruptly upward into the epigastrium, forcing the obstruction up the trachea. If repeated attempts do not free the airway, an emergency cricothyrotomy may be necessary.

Heimlich sign [H. J. Heimlich; L, *signum*], a universal distress signal that a person is choking and unable to speak, made by grasping the throat with a thumb and index finger, thereby attracting the attention of others nearby.

Heinz bodies /hīnts/ [Robert Heinz, German pathologist, 1865–1924], irregularly shaped bits of altered hemoglobin found in the red blood cells of people who are hypersensitive to certain chemicals such as aniline, phenylhydrazine, and primaquine.

Helen, Sister (Helen Bowden), a nurse who received her education in England and became the first director of the newly formed Bellevue Hospital Training School for Nurses in New York in 1873. Although she had not trained under Florence Nightingale, she set up the Bellevue school according to Nightingale's principles.

helical virus /hel′ikəl/, a virus in which the protein capsid appears in a coiled pattern.

helicopod gait /hel′ikōpod′/ [Gk, *helix,* coil, *pous,* foot], a manner of walking in which the feet describe half-circles. It is associated with some mental disorders.

helium (He) /hē′lē·əm/ [Gk, *helios,* sun], a colorless, odorless gaseous element; the second lightest element. Its atomic number is 2; its atomic mass (weight) is 4.00. Helium is one of the rare or inert gases and does not usually combine with other elements. The main physiologic and medical uses of helium are in respiratory therapy and testing and the prevention of nitrogen narcosis and decompression sickness in hyperbaric environments. A mixture of 80% helium and 20% oxygen is commonly breathed by deep-sea divers to prevent gas emboli and by patients undergoing treatment to clear obstruction of the respiratory tract. Helium is used in pulmonary function testing to calculate the diffusion and residual capacities of the lungs.

helium therapy, the use of helium-oxygen gas mixtures to treat patients with airway obstruction. Because of its low density, helium can negotiate an obstruction more easily.

helix /hē′liks/ [Gk, coil], a coiled, spiral-like formation characteristic of many organic molecules such as deoxyribonucleic acid.

Heller's test, a laboratory test for proteinuria in which urine is layered on nitric acid. Appearance of a ring of precipitated protein at the junction of the fluids is a positive sign.

Hellin's law, a generalized formula for calculating the ratio of multiple births in any population, stating that if twin births occur at the rate of $1:N$, then the rate of triplet births is approximately $1:N^2$, quadruplets $1:N^3$, quintuplets $1:N^4$, and so on, with the exponent of N being one less than the number in the multiple set. The constant N varies greatly with population, although it was originally set at 89 when the law was formulated. In general, twin births occur approximately once in every 80 pregnancies.

HELLP syndrome /help/, acronym for a form of severe preeclampsia, a hypertensive complication of late pregnancy. The letters stand for *h*emolysis, *e*levated *l*iver function, and *l*ow *p*latelet level.

helmet cells, fragmented red blood cells that have been "scooped out" so they resemble helmets. They are found in patients with carcinomatosis, hemolytic anemia, and thrombotic thrombocytopenic purpura. Helmet cells can be seen in blood samples of people with prosthetic heart valves.

helminth /hel′minth/ [Gk, *helmins*, worm], a worm, especially one of the pathogenic parasites of the division Metazoa, including flukes, tapeworms, and roundworms.

helminthemesis /hel′minthem′əsis/ [Gk, *helmins*, worm, *emesis*, vomiting], the vomiting of intestinal worms.

helminthiasis /hel′minthī′əsis/ [Gk, *helmins*, worm, *osis*, condition], a parasitic infestation of the body by helminths that may be cutaneous, visceral, or intestinal. Ascariasis, bilharziasis, filariasis, hookworm, and trichinosis are common forms of the disease.

helminthic /helmin′thik/ [Gk, *helmins*, worm], pertaining to worms.

helminthology /hel′minthol′əjē/, a branch of medicine concerned with parasitic worms.

helper factor, a protein produced by helper T lymphocytes that stimulates proliferation and antibody production by other lymphocytes.

helper T cell, a T lymphocyte that promotes the immune response of other lymphocytes to foreign antigens by releasing soluble proteins called helper factors.

helper virus, a virus that is necessary in a phenotypically mixed infection to mediate the replication of a defective virus. Viruses

that mature by budding through the plasma membrane require the coding of a helper virus.

helplessness /help′ləsnəs/, a feeling of loss of control or ability, usually after repeated failures, with the result that one is unable to make autonomous choices.

Helsinki Accords /helsing′kē/, a declaration signed by the representatives of 35 member nations of the Conference on Security and Cooperation in Europe in Helsinki, Finland, on August 1, 1975. The Helsinki accords grew from the precedent set by the judgments at the Nuremberg tribunals that crimes against humanity are offenses subject to criminal prosecution. The principle and the practice of informed consent in health care grew from this precedent.

helvolic acid /helvol′ik/, an antibiotic, derived from the mold *Aspergillus fumigatus*, formerly used as an amebicide.

hemacytometer /-sītom′ətər/ [Gk, *haima*, blood, *kytos*, cell, *metron*, measure], an apparatus for counting the number of cells in a known volume of blood or other fluid.

hemadsorption /hē′madsôrp′shən, hem′-/ [Gk, *haima*, blood; L, *ad* to, *sorbere*, to swallow], a process in which a substance or an agent, such as certain viruses and bacilli, adheres to the surface of an erythrocyte.

hemagglutination /hē′məgloō′tinā′shən, hem′-/ [Gk, *haima* + L, *agglutinare*, to glue], the coagulation of erythrocytes.

hemagglutination inhibition, 1. the inhibition of virus-induced hemagglutination as a procedure for identifying hemagglutinating viruses. **2.** a method for measuring the concentration of soluble antigens in biologic specimens in which the specimen is incubated first with homologous antibodies and then with antigen-coated erythrocytes.

hemagglutinin [Gk, *haima* + L, *agglutinare*], a type of antibody that agglutinates red blood cells. It is classified according to the source of cells agglutinated as **autologous** (from the same organism), **homologous** (from an organism of the same species), and heterologous (from an organism of a different species).

hemangiectasis, dilation of a blood vessel.

hemangioblast /hēman′jē·ōblast′/, an embryonic mesodermal cell that gives rise to vascular endothelium and bloodforming cells.

hemangioblastoma /hēman′jē·ōblastō′mə/ [Gk, *haima* + *angeion*, vessel, *blastos*, germ, *oma*, tumor], a brain tumor composed of a proliferation of capillaries and

H

of disorganized clusters of capillary cells or angioblasts.

hemangioendothelioma /hēman'jē·ō·en'dōthē'lē·ō'mə/ [Gk, *haima + endon,* inside, *thele,* nipple, *oma,* tumor], a tumor consisting of endothelial cells that grows around an artery or a vein. The tumor rarely becomes malignant.

hemangiofibroma /-fībrō'mə/ [Gk, *haima,* blood; L, *fibra,* fiber; Gk, *oma,* tumor], a tumor that has the characteristics of both a hemangioma and a fibroma.

hemangioma /hēman'jē·ō'mə/ [Gk, *haima + angeion,* small vessel, *oma*], a benign tumor consisting of a mass of blood vessels.

hemapoiesis /hem'əpō·ē'sis/ [Gk, *haima,* blood, *poiein,* to make], the formation of blood cells.

hemarthros /hem'är'thrəs/ [Gk, *haima,* blood, *arthron,* joint], the extravasation of blood into a joint.

hematemesis /hē'mətem'əsis, hem'-/ [Gk, *haima + emesis,* vomiting], vomiting of bright red blood, indicating rapid upper gastrointestinal bleeding, commonly associated with esophageal varices or peptic ulcer.

hematinic /hem'ətin'ik/, a therapeutic agent that produces an increase in the number of erythrocytes and/or hemoglobin concentration in erythrocytes, such as iron or B complex vitamins.

hematinuria /hem'ətinōōr'ē·ə/ [Gk, *haima,* blood, *ouron,* urine], a dark-colored urine resulting from the presence of hematin or hemoglobin.

hematocele /hem'ətōsēl'/, a cystlike accumulation of blood within the tunica vaginalis of the scrotum. It is usually caused by injury.

hematochezia /hem'ətōkē'zhə/ [Gk, *haima + chezo,* feces], the passage of red blood through the rectum. The cause is usually bleeding in the colon or rectum, but it may result from the loss of blood higher in the digestive tract. Cancer, colitis, and ulcers are among causes of hematochezia.

hematocrit /hemat'ōkrit/ [Gk, *haima + krinein,* to separate], a measure of the packed cell volume of red cells, expressed as a percentage of the total blood volume. The normal range is between 43% and 49% in men and between 37% and 43% in women.

hematocyte /hem'ətōsīt/ [Gk, *haima,* blood, *kytos,* cell], a blood cell, particularly a red blood cell.

hematocytoblast /hem'ətōsī'təblast'/ [Gk, *haima,* blood, *kytos,* cell, *blastos,* germ], a large nucleated reticuloendothelial cell

found in bone marrow. It is believed to be a common precursor of various blood elements.

hematogenesis /-jen'əsis/ [Gk, *haima,* blood, *genein,* to produce], pertaining to the formation of blood cells or an increase in the production of blood elements.

hematogenous /hēmatoj'ənəs/ [Gk, *haima + genein,* to produce], originating or transported in the blood.

hematogenous pigment /hem'ətoj'ənəs/ [Gk, *haima,* blood, *genein,* to produce; L, *pingere,* to paint], the red color of erythrocytes caused by the presence of hemoglobin.

hematogenous tuberculosis [Gk, *haima,* blood, *genein,* to produce; L, *tuberculum,* a small swelling; Gk, *osis,* condition], a form of tuberculosis that is blood-borne.

hematoid /hem'ətoid/, bloodlike or resembling blood.

hematologic death syndrome /hemə'tōloj'ik/, a group of clinical signs and symptoms of radiation damage to the blood cells. The condition is characterized by nausea, vomiting, fever, diarrhea, infections, anemia, leukopenia, and hemorrhage. It can result from exposure to a dose of 200 to 1000 rad. The mean survival time for a person with hematologic death syndrome is estimated at between 10 and 60 days.

hematologic effect, (in radiology) the response of blood cells to radiation exposure. In general, all types of blood cells are destroyed by radiation, and the degree of cell depletion increases with increasing dose.

hematologist /hē'mətol'əjist, hem'-/, a medical specialist in the field of blood and blood-forming tissues.

hematology /hē'mətol'əjē, hem'-/ [Gk, *haima + logos,* science], the scientific study of blood and blood-forming tissues. **—hematologic, hematological,** *adj.*

hematoma /hē'mətō'mə, hem'-/ [Gk, *haima + oma,* tumor], a collection of extravasated blood trapped in the tissues of the skin or in an organ, resulting from trauma or incomplete hemostasis after surgery. Initially there is frank bleeding into the space; if the space is limited, pressure slows and eventually stops the flow of blood. The blood clots, serum collects, the clot hardens, and the mass becomes palpable to the examiner and is often painful to the patient.

hematometra /hē'mətōmē'trə/, an accumulation of blood or menstrual fluid in the uterine cavity.

hematometry /hem'ətom'ətrē/, an examination of a blood sample to determine the number, type, and properties of blood cells and platelets and the amount of hemoglobin.

hematomyelia /hē′mətōmē′lē·ə/ [Gk, *haima* + *meylos,* marrow], the appearance of frank blood in the fluid of the spinal cord.

hematoperitoneum /-per′itōnē′əm/ [Gk, *haima,* blood, *peri,* near, *tenein,* to stretch], the effusion of blood into the peritoneal cavity.

hematophagous /hem′ətof′əgəs/, **1.** pertaining to the feeding on blood by insects or other parasites. **2.** the destruction of erythrocytes by phagocytes.

hematopoiesis /hē′mətōpō·ē′sis, hem′-/ [Gk, *haima* + *poiein,* to make], the normal formation and development of blood cells in the bone marrow. In severe anemia and other hematologic disorders, cells may be produced in organs outside the marrow (extramedullary hematopoiesis). —**hematopoietic,** *adj.*

hematopoietic growth factor /-pō·et′ik/, one of a group of proteins, including erythropoietin, interleukin, and colony-stimulating factors, that promote the proliferation of blood cells.

hematopoietic malignancies, diseases such as leukemia that arise as a result of unregulated clonal proliferation of stem cells.

hematopoietic stem cell, an actively dividing cell that is the source of blood cells.

hematopoietic syndrome a group of clinical features associated with effects of radiation on the blood and lymph tissues. It is characterized by nausea and vomiting, anorexia, lethargy, hemolysis and destruction of the bone marrow, and atrophy of the spleen and lymph nodes.

hematopoietic system [Gk, *haima,* blood, *poiein,* to make; L, *systema*], body organs and tissues involved in the formation and functioning of blood elements. It includes the bone marrow and spleen.

hematoporphyrinuria /-pôr′firinŏŏ′ē·ə/, the presence of elevated levels of hematoporphyrin in the urine that results from destruction of lysis of erythrocytes.

hematospermia /-spur′mē·ə/, the presence of blood in the semen. Causes may include vascular congestion, infection involving seminal vesicles, coitus interruptus, sexual abstinence, or frequent coitus.

hematoxylin-eosin /hē′mətok′silin/ [*Haematoxylon campechianum,* logwood; Gk, *eos,* dawn], a stain commonly used to treat tissue sections on microscope slides.

hematuria /hē′mətŏŏr′ē·ə, hem′-/ [Gk, *haima* + *ouron,* urine], abnormal presence of blood in the urine. It is symptom-

atic of many renal diseases and disorders of the genitourinary system. Microscopic examination of the urine, culture and sensitivity of the urine, as well as physical examination of the patient are usually performed. —**hematuric,** *adj.*

heme /hēm/ [Gk, *haima,* blood], the pigmented iron-containing nonprotein part of the hemoglobin molecule. There are four heme groups in a hemoglobin molecule, each consisting of a cyclic structure of four pyrrole residues, called protoporphyrin, and an atom of iron in the center.

hemeralopia /hem′ərəlō′pē·ə/ [Gk, *hemera,* day, *alaos,* blind, *ops,* eye], an abnormal visual condition in which bright light causes blurring of vision. —**hemeralopic,** *adj.*

hemiacephalus /hem′ē·āsef′ələs/ [Gk, *hemi,* half, *a* + *kephale,* without head], a fetus in which the brain and most of the cranium are lacking.

hemiachromatosia /hem′ē·ak′rōmətō′zhə/, a state of being color-blind in only one half of the visual field.

hemialgia /hem′ē·al′jē·ə/, pain that affects one side of the body.

hemiamblyopia /hem′ē·am′blē·ō′pē·ə/ [Gk, *hemi,* half, *amblys,* dull, *ops,* eye], blindness in half of the normal visual field.

hemianalgesia /hem′ē·an′əljē′sē·ə/ [Gk, *hemi,* half, *a* + *algos,* without pain], a loss of feeling or sensitivity to pain affecting half of the body or one side of the body.

hemianesthesia /hem′ē·an′esthē′zhə, hem′ē·nō′pē·ə/ [Gk, *hemi* + *anaisthesia,* absence of feeling], a loss of feeling on one side of the body.

hemiarthroplasty /hem′ē·är′thrəplas′tē/, a surgical procedure for repair of an injured or diseased hip joint. It involves replacing the head of the femur with a prosthesis.

hemiarthrosis /hem′ē·ärthrō′sis/ [Gk, *hemi,* half, *arthron,* joint, *osis,* condition], a false articulation between two bones.

hemiataxia /hem′ē·ətak′sē·ə/, a loss of muscle control affecting one side of the body, usually as a result of a stroke or cerebellar injury.

hemiazygous vein /hem′ē·əzī′gəs/ [Gk, *hemi* + *a* + *zygon,* without yoke], one of the tributaries of the azygous vein of the thorax.

hemiblock, a failure to conduct an impulse down one division of the left bundle branch, such as an anterior superior or posterior inferior hemiblock.

hemic /hem′ik, hē′mik/ pertaining to blood.

hemicellulose /hem′ēsel′yŏŏlōs/ [Gk, *hemi*

+ L, *cellula,* little cell], any of a group of polysaccharides that constitute the chief part of the skeletal substances of the cell walls of plants. They resemble cellulose but are more soluble and more easily extracted and decomposed.

hemicephalia /-sefā'lyə/ [Gk, *hemi* + *kephale,* head], a congenital anomaly characterized by the absence of half of the cerebrum, caused by severe arrest of brain development in the fetus.

hemicephalus [Gk, **hemi,** half, **kephale,** head], a fetus with congenital absence of half of the cerebrum.

hemicrania /-krā'nē-ə/ [Gk, *hemi* + *kranion,* skull], **1.** a headache, usually migraine, that affects only one side of the head. **2.** a congenital anomaly characterized by the absence of half of the skull in the fetus; incomplete anencephaly.

hemicraniectomy /-kran'ē-ek'təmē/ [Gk, *hemi,* half, *kranion,* skull, *ektome,* excision], a surgical procedure in which part or all of one half of the skull is excised and reflected as a preliminary step to certain types of brain operations.

hemidiaphragm /-dī'əfram/, either the left or right functional half of the diaphragm. Although the diaphragm is a single anatomic unit, it is divided by the union of its central tendon and the pericardium into separate leaves. Each hemidiaphragm can function independently.

hemidystrophy /-dis'trəfē/, a condition in which the two sides of the body do not develop equally.

hemiectromelia /hem'ē-ek'trōmē'lyə/ [Gk, *hemi* + *ektosis,* miscarriage, *melos,* limb], a congenital anomaly characterized by the incomplete development of the limbs on one side of the body. **—hemiectromelus,** *n.*

hemiepilepsy /hem'ē-ep'əlepsē/, a form of epilepsy that affects only one side of the body.

hemigastrectomy /-gastrek'təmē/, surgical removal of one half of the body of the stomach.

hemiglossal /-glos'əl/, pertaining to one side of the tongue.

hemignathia /hem'ēnā'thē-ə/ [Gk, *hemi* + *gnathos,* jaw], **1.** a congenital anomaly characterized by incomplete development of the lower jaw on one side of the face. **2.** a condition of having only one jaw. **—hemignathus,** *n.*

hemihyperplasia /-hī'pərplā'zhə/ [Gk, *hemi* + *hyper,* excessive, *plassein,* to form], overdevelopment or excessive growth of half of a specific organ or part or all of the organs and parts on one side of the body.

hemihypertonia /-hī'pərtō'nē-ə/ [Gk, *hemi*

+ *hyper* + *tonikos,* stretching], exaggerated tension in the muscles on one side of the body, causing tonic contraction. In one form of the disorder, tonic spasms may occur occasionally in different muscle groups on one side of the body.

hemihypertrophy /-hīpur'trəfē/ [Gk, *hemi* + *hyper* + *trophe,* nourishment], an unusual enlargement or overgrowth of half of the body or half of a body part.

hemihypoplasia /-hī'pōplā'zhə/ [Gk, *hemi* + *hypo,* under, *plassein,* to form], partial or incomplete development of half of a specific organ or part or all of the organs and parts on one side of the body.

hemikaryon /hem'ēker'ē-on/ [Gk, *hemi* + *karyon,* nut], a cell nucleus that contains the haploid number of chromosomes, or one half of the diploid number, as that of the gametes. **—hemikaryotic,** *adj.*

hemilateral /-lat'ərəl, pertaining to one side.

hemimelia /-mē'lyə/ [Gk, *hemi* + *melos*], a developmental anomaly characterized by the absence or gross shortening of the lower part of one or more of the limbs.

hemiopia /hem'ē-ō'pē-ə/ [Gk, *hemi,* half, *ops,* eye], a condition involving only one eye or half the visual field.

hemipagus /hemip'əgəs/ [Gk, *hemi* + *pagos,* fixture], symmetric twins who are conjoined at the thorax.

hemiparesis /-pərē'sis/ [Gk, *hemi* + *paralyein,* to be palsied], muscular weakness of one half of the body.

hemiparesthesia /-per'esthē'zhə/ [Gk, *hemi,* half, *para,* beside, *aisthesis,* sensation], a numbness or other abnormal or impaired sensation that is experienced on only one side of the body.

hemiplegia /hem'iplē'jə/ [Gk, *hemi* + *plege,* stroke], paralysis of one side of the body. **—hemiplegic,** *adj.*

hemiplegic gait /-plē'jik/ [Gk, *hemi,* half, *plege,* stroke; ONorse, *gata,* a way], a manner of walking in which an affected limb moves in a semicircle with each step.

hemisection /-sek'shən/ [Gk, *hemi,* half; L, *sectare,* to cut], half of a body or other object divided along a longitudinal plane, producing two lateral halves.

hemisomus /hem'isō'məs/ [Gk, *hemi* + *soma,* body], a fetus or individual in whom one side of the body is malformed, defective, or absent.

hemisphere /hem'isfir/ [Gk, *hemi* + *sphaira,* sphere], **1.** one half of a sphere or globe. **2.** the lateral half of the cerebrum or cerebellum. **—hemispherical,** *adj.*

hemiteras /hem'ēter'əs/, *pl.* **hemiterata** [Gk, *hemi* + *teras,* monster], any individual with a congenital malformation that is not so severe or disabling as to be classified as a monstrous or teratic condition. —**hemiteratic,** *adj.*

hemithorax /-thô′aks/, one side of the chest.

hemithyroidectomy /-thī′roidek′təmē/, surgical removal of one lobe of the thyroid gland.

hemivertebra /-vur′tə.brə/, an abnormal condition characterized by the congenital failure of a vertebra to develop completely. It is possibly caused by the complete failure of the growth center of one vertebral body. Usually half of the vertebra involved is completely or partially developed, and the other half is absent.

hemizygote /-zī′gōt/ [Gk, *hemi* + *zygon*, yoke], an individual, organism, or cell that has only one of a pair of genes for a specific characteristic. —**hemizygosity,** *n.,* **hemizygous, hemizygotic,** *adj.*

hemlock, the common name for *Conium maculatum,* a plant indigenous to most of Europe and the source of a poisonous alkaloid, coniine. An extract of the leaves and flowers of conium has been used as a respiratory sedative; its hydrochloride salts have been used as an antispasmodic.

Hemlock Society, a group who provide information about euthanasia.

hemobilinuria /hē′mōbil′inŏŏr′ē·ə/, the presence of the brown pigment urobilin in the blood and urine.

hemochromatosis /hē′mōkrō′mətō′sis, hem′-/ [Gk, *haima,* blood, *chroma,* color, *osis,* condition], a rare disease of iron metabolism, characterized by excess iron deposits throughout the body.

hemoclip, a malleable metal clip used to ligate small blood vessels during surgery and to mark the location of body structures in radiographic procedures.

hemoconcentration /-kon′səntrā′shən/ [Gk, *haima* + L, *cum,* together with, *centrum,* center], an increase in the number of red blood cells resulting from either a decrease in plasma volume or increased production of erythrocytes.

hemocyanin /he′mōsī′ənin/, an oxygen-carrying protein molecule present in certain lower animals, particularly arthropods and mollusks. The molecule is similar to the hemoglobin molecule of human blood but uses copper atoms rather than iron.

hemocytology /-sītol′əjē/ [Gk, *haima,* blood, *kytos,* cell, *logos,* science], the study of the components of blood.

hemodiafiltration /-dī′əfiltrā′shən/, a technique similar to hemofiltration, used to treat uremia by convective transport of the solute rather than by diffusion.

hemodialysis /hē′mōdī·al′isis, hem′-/ [Gk,

haima + *dia,* apart, *lysis,* loosening], a procedure in which impurities or wastes are removed from the blood. It is used in treating renal failure and various toxic conditions. The patient's blood is shunted from the body through a machine for diffusion and ultrafiltration and then returned to the patient's circulation. Hemodialysis requires access to the patient's bloodstream, a mechanism for the transport of the blood to and from the dialyzer, and a dialyzer. Access may be achieved by an external shunt or an arteriovenous fistula. Various dialyzers may be used. The procedure takes from 3 to 8 hours and may be necessary daily in acute conditions or two or three times a week in chronic renal failure.

hemodialysis technician, a registered health professional who has received special training in the operation of hemodialysis equipment and treatment of patients with kidney disorders.

hemodilution /-diloo′shən/ [Gk, *haima,* blood; L, *diluare,* to wash away], a condition in which the concentration of erythrocytes or other blood elements is lowered.

hemodynamics /-dīnam′iks/ [Gk, *haima* + *dynamis,* force], the study of the physical aspects of blood circulation, including cardiac function and peripheral vascular physiologic characteristics.

hemofiltration /-filtrā′shən/, a type of hemodialysis in which there is convective transport of the solute through ultrafiltration across the membrane.

hemoglobin (Hb) /hē′məglō′bən/ [Gk, *haima* + L, *globus,* ball], a complex protein-iron compound in the blood that carries oxygen to the cells from the lungs and carbon dioxide away from the cells to the lungs. Each erythrocyte contains 200 to 300 molecules of hemoglobin, each molecule of hemoglobin contains several molecules of heme, and each molecule of heme can carry one molecule of oxygen. A hemoglobin molecule contains four globin polypeptide chains, designated in adults as the alpha (α), beta (β), gamma (γ), and delta (δ) chains. Hemoglobin releases the carboxyhemoglobin in the lungs for excretion and picks up more oxygen for transport to the cells.

hemoglobin A (Hb A), a normal hemoglobin.

hemoglobin A$_2$ (Hb A$_2$), a normal hemoglobin present in small amounts in adults, characterized by the substitution of δ chains for β chains.

hemoglobin C (Hb C), an abnormal type of hemoglobin characterized by the substitution of lysine for glutamic acid at posi-

H

tion 6 of the β chain of the hemoglobin molecule.

hemoglobin C disease, a genetic blood disorder characterized by a moderate chronic hemolytic anemia and associated with the presence of hemoglobin C.

hemoglobin E disease [Gk, *haima,* blood; L, *globus,* ball; *E;* Gk, *dis,* not; Fr, *aise,* ease], a mild form of anemia caused by a genetic abnormality of the hemoglobin molecule. Worldwide it is the third most common form of hemoglobin disorder, primarily affecting persons in Southeast Asia and black populations.

hemoglobin electrophoresis, a test to identify various abnormal hemoglobins in the blood, including certain genetic disorders such as sickle cell anemia.

hemoglobinemia /hē′mōglō′binē′mē·ə, hem′-/, presence of free hemoglobin in the blood plasma.

hemoglobin F (Hb F), the normal hemoglobin of the fetus. Most Hb F is replaced by hemoglobin A in the first days after birth. Hb F has an increased capacity to carry oxygen and is present in increased amounts in some pathologic conditions.

hemoglobin M disease [Gk, *haima,* blood; L, *globus,* ball; *M;* Gk, *dis,* not; Fr, *aise,* ease], a type of anemia in which part of the hemoglobin contains iron in the Fe(III) state and is unable to combine with oxygen. The patient may experience cyanosis but is able to function because part of the hemoglobin is normal.

hemoglobinometer /-om′ətər/ [Gk, *haima,* blood; L, *globus,* ball; Gk, *metron,* measure], any of several types of instruments designed to measure the percentage of hemoglobin in a blood sample. Some use colorimetric techniques, comparing the color of the blood sample with a standard red color.

hemoglobinopathy /hē′mōglō′binop′əthē, hem′-/ [Gk, *haima* + L, *globus,* ball; Gk, *pathos,* disease], a group of inherited disorders characterized by structural variations of the hemoglobin molecule. An abnormality may occur in the heterozygous or the homozygous form.

hemoglobin oxygen saturation, a quantitative measure of volume of oxygen per volume of blood, depending on the grams of hemoglobin per deciliter of blood.

hemoglobin S (Hb S), an abnormal type of hemoglobin, characterized by the substitution of the amino acid valine for glutamic acid in the β chain of the hemoglobin molecule. It moves more slowly and is much less soluble than hemoglobin A.

hemoglobin saturation, the amount of oxygen combined with hemoglobin in proportion to the amount of oxygen the hemoglobin is capable of carrying.

hemoglobin S-C (Hb S-C) disease, a genetic blood disorder in which two different abnormal alleles, one for hemoglobin S and one for hemoglobin C, are inherited.

hemoglobin_Seattle, an abnormal hemoglobin in which glutamic acid replaces alanine at position 76 of the β chain, decreasing the hemoglobin molecule's affinity for oxygen.

hemoglobinuria /-ŏŏr′ē-ə/ [Gk, *haima* + L, *globus,* ball; Gk, *ouron,* urine], abnormal presence of hemoglobin that is not attached to red blood cells in the urine.

hemoglobinuric /-ŏŏr′ik/ [Gk, *haima,* blood; L, *globus,* ball; Gk, *ouron,* urine], pertaining to the presence of hemoglobin in the urine.

hemogram /hē′məgram/ [Gk, *haima* + *gramma,* record], a written or graphic record of a differential blood count that emphasizes the size, shape, special characteristics, and numbers of the solid components of the blood.

hemolysin /himol′əsin/ [Gk, *haima* + *lysis,* loosening], any one of the numerous substances that lyse or dissolve red blood cells. Hemolysins are produced by bacterial strains, including staphylococci and streptococci. Hemolysins appear to aid the invasive power of bacteria.

hemolysis /himol′isis/ [Gk, *haima* + *lysis,* loosening], the breakdown of red blood cells and the release of hemoglobin that occur normally at the end of the life span of a red cell. Hemolysis may occur in antigen-antibody reactions, metabolic abnormalities of the red cell that significantly shorten red cell life span, and mechanical trauma such as cardiac prosthesis.

hemolytic anemia /-lit′ik/ [Gk, *haima* + *lysis* + *a* + *haima,* without blood], a disorder characterized by chronic premature destruction of red blood cells. Anemia may be minimal or absent, reflecting the ability of the bone marrow to increase production of red blood cells.

hemolytic antibody /hē′məlit′ik/, an antibody capable of dissolving red blood cells in the presence of complement.

hemolytic jaundice, a yellowish discoloration of the skin caused by a breakdown of red blood cells, which causes excessive amounts of bilirubin.

hemolytic uremia syndrome, a rare kidney disorder marked by renal failure, microangiopathic hemolytic anemia, and platelet deficiency.

hemopathology /-pəthol′əjē/, the study of diseases of the blood.

hemoperfusion /-pərfyŏŏ′zhən/, the perfusion of blood through a sorbent device such as activated charcoal or resin beads, rather than through dialysis equipment. Hemoperfusion may be used in treating uremia, liver failure, and certain forms of drug toxicity.

hemopericardium /-per'ikär'dē·əm/ [Gk, *haima* + *peri,* near, *kardia,* heart], an accumulation of blood within the pericardial sac surrounding the heart.

hemoperitoneum /-per'itōnē'əm/ [Gk, *haima* + *peri,* around, *tenein,* to stretch], the presence of extravasated blood in the peritoneal cavity.

hemophil /hē'mōfil/ [Gk, *haima,* blood, *philein,* to love], bacteria of the genus *Haemophilus,* which thrive in culture media containing blood.

hemophilia /hē'mōfē'lyə, hem'-/ [Gk, *haima* + *philein,* to love], a group of hereditary bleeding disorders characterized by a deficiency of one of the factors necessary for coagulation of the blood. The two most common forms of the disorder are hemophilia A and hemophilia B. Greater than usual loss of blood during dental procedures, epistaxis, hematoma, and hemarthrosis are common problems in patients with hemophilia. Severe nonsurgical internal hemorrhage and hematuria are less common. —**hemophiliac,** *n.,* **hemophilic,** *adj.*

hemophilia A, a hereditary blood disorder transmitted as an X-linked recessive trait and caused by a deficiency of coagulation factor VIII. Hemophilia A is considered the classic type of hemophilia.

hemophilia B, a hereditary blood disorder transmitted as an X-linked recessive trait and caused by a deficiency of factor IX.

hemophilia C, a hereditary blood disorder transmitted as an X-linked recessive trait and caused by a deficiency of factor XI.

hemopneumopericardium /hē'mōnoo'-mōper'ikär'dē·əm/ [Gk, *haima,* blood, *pneuma,* air, *kardia,* heart], an accumulation of both blood and air in the pericardium.

hemopneumothorax /hē'mōnoo'mothôr'aks/ [Gk, *haima,* blood, *pneuma,* air, *thorax,* chest], an accumulation of both air and blood in the pleural cavity.

hemopoietic /hē'mōpō·et'ik, hem'-/ [Gk, *haima* + *poiein,* to make], related to the process of formation and development of the various types of blood cells.

hemoptysis /himop'tisis/ [Gk, *haima* + *ptyein,* to spit], coughing up of blood from the respiratory tract. Blood-streaked sputum often is present in minor upper respiratory infections or bronchitis. More

profuse bleeding may indicate *Aspergillus* infection, lung abscess, tuberculosis, or bronchogenic carcinoma.

hemorheology /-rē·ol'əjē/ [Gk, *haima,* blood, *rhoia,* flow, *logos,* science], the study of the effects of blood flow on the cellular components of blood and walls of blood vessels.

hemorrhage /hem'ərij/ [Gk, *haima* + *rhegnynei,* to gush], a loss of a large amount of blood in a short period, either externally or internally. Hemorrhage may be arterial, venous, or capillary. Symptoms of massive hemorrhage are related to hypovolemic shock: rapid, thready pulse; thirst; cold, clammy skin; sighing respirations; dizziness; syncope; pallor; apprehension; restlessness; and hypotension. If bleeding is contained within a cavity or joint, pain will develop as the capsule or cavity is stretched by the rapidly expanding volume of blood. —**hemorrhagic,** *adj.*

hemorrhagic diathesis /-raj'ik/, an inherited predisposition to any of a number of abnormalities characterized by excessive bleeding.

hemorrhagic disease of newborn, a bleeding disorder of neonates that is usually caused by a deficiency of vitamin K.

hemorrhagic fever, a group of viral aerosol infections. Hemorrhagic fever is characterized by fever, chills, headache, malaise, and respiratory or gastrointestinal symptoms, followed by capillary hemorrhages and in severe infection by oliguria, kidney failure, hypotension, and possibly death. Many forms of the disease occur in specific geographic areas.

hemorrhagic gastritis, a form of acute gastritis usually caused by a toxic agent such as alcohol, aspirin or other drugs, or bacterial toxins that irritate the lining of the stomach. Nausea, vomiting, and epigastric distress may persist after the irritant is removed.

hemorrhagic infarct [Gk, *haima,* blood, *rhegnynei,* to gush; L, *infarcire,* to stuff], an area of necrosis that has accumulated so much blood that it resembles a red, swollen bruise.

hemorrhagic jaundice [Gk, *haima,* blood, *rhegnynei,* to gush; Fr, *jaune,* yellow], a form of jaundice that occurs in Weil's syndrome or other forms of **leptospirosis** in which capillary injury and anemia are present.

hemorrhagic measles [Gk, *haima,* blood, *rhegnynei,* to gush; ME, *masalas*], a severe form of measles characterized by bleeding into the skin and mucous membranes.

hemorrhagic pericarditis [Gk, *haima,*

H

blood, *rhegnynei*, to gush, *peri*, near, *kardia*, heart, *itis*, inflammation], an inflammation of the pericardium with a bloody effusion. The condition is frequently caused by tuberculosis or a tumor.

hemorrhagic plague [Gk, *haima*, blood, *rhegnynei*, to gush; L, *plaga*, stroke], a severe form of bubonic plague in which bleeding occurs under the skin.

hemorrhagic pleurisy [Gk, *haima*, blood, *rhegnynei*, to gush, *pleuritis*], an inflammation of the pleura in which effusion of blood into the tissues occurs.

hemorrhagic purpura [Gk, *haima*, blood, *rhegnynei*, to gush; L, *purpura*, purple], a form of purpura associated with thrombocytopenia and prolonged bleeding time.

hemorrhagic shock, a state of physical collapse and prostration associated with the sudden and rapid loss of significant amounts of blood. Severe traumatic injuries often cause such blood losses, which in turn produce low blood pressure in affected individuals.

hemorrhagic urticaria [Gk, *haima*, blood, *rhegnynei*, to gush; L, *urtica*, nettle], a skin eruption characterized by bleeding in the wheals, usually as a complication of another disease such as nephritis. In some cases the bleeding occurs first, and the wheals become superimposed.

hemorrhoid /hem′əroid/ [Gk, *haima* + *rhoia*, flow], a varicosity in the lower rectum or anus caused by congestion in the veins of the hemorrhoidal plexus. Internal hemorrhoids originate above the internal sphincter of the anus. If they become large enough to protrude from the anus, they become constricted and painful. Small internal hemorrhoids may bleed with defecation. External hemorrhoids appear outside the anal sphincter. They are usually not painful, and bleeding does not occur unless a hemorrhoidal vein ruptures or thromboses.

hemorrhoidal /hem′əroi′dəl/ [Gk, *haimorrhois*, a vein that discharges blood], pertaining to or resembling hemorrhoids.

hemorrhoidal tag, an anal skin tag that was originally part of hemorrhoidal tissue.

hemorrhoidectomy /hem′əroidek′təmē/ [Gk, *haimorrhois*, a vein that discharges blood, *ektome*, excision], a surgical procedure performed for excision of a hemorrhoid.

hemosalpinx /hē′mōsal′pinks/ [Gk, *haima*, blood, *salpinx*, tube], a collection of blood in a fallopian tube.

hemosiderin /hē′mōsid′ərin/ [Gk, *haima* + *sideros*, iron], an iron-rich pigment that is a product of red cell hemolysis. Iron is often stored in this form.

hemosiderosis /hē′mōsid′ərō′sis, hem′-/ [Gk, *haima* + *sideros*, iron, *osis*, condition], an increased deposition of iron in a variety of tissues, usually in the form of hemosiderin and usually without tissue damage.

hemostasis /himos′təsis, hē′məstā′sis/ [Gk, *haima* + *stasis*, halting], the termination of bleeding by mechanical or chemical means or by the complex coagulation process of the body, which consists of vasoconstriction, platelet aggregation, and thrombin and fibrin synthesis.

hemostatic /-stat′ik/ [Gk, *haima* + *stasis*, halting], pertaining to a procedure, device, or substance that arrests the flow of blood. Direct pressure, tourniquets, and surgical clamps are mechanical hemostatic measures. Cold applications, including the use of an ice bag on the abdomen to halt uterine bleeding and irrigation of the stomach with an iced solution to check gastric bleeding, are hemostatic. Gelatin sponges, solutions of thrombin, and microfibrillar collagen, which causes the aggregation of platelets and the formation of clots, are used to arrest bleeding in surgical procedures.

hemotherapeutics /ther′əpyoo̅′tiks/, a form of treatment that involves the use of fresh blood plasma or serum.

hemothorax /hē′mōthôr′aks, hem′-/ [Gk, *haima* + *thorax*, chest], an accumulation of blood and fluid in the pleural cavity, between the parietal and visceral pleura, usually the result of trauma. Hemothorax also may be caused by the rupture of small blood vessels that results from inflammation.

hemotroph /hē′mətrof/, the total nutritive substances supplied to the embryo from the maternal circulation after the development of the placenta. —**hemotrophic,** *adj.*

Henderson-Hasselbalch equation [Lawrence J. Henderson, American chemist, 1878–1942; Karl A. Hasselbach, Danish biochemist, 1874–1962], the relationship among pH, the pK_a of a buffer system, and the ratio of the concentrations of the conjugate base and a weak acid.

Henderson, Virginia (1897–1996), a nursing theorist who introduced a holistic approach to the profession in 1966. The method is based on the concepts that the body and mind are inseparable, no two individuals are alike, and the role of nursing is independent of the functions of the physician.

Henle's fissure /hen′lēz/ [Friedrich G. J. Henle, German anatomist, 1809–1885], one of many patches of connective tissue between the muscle fibers of the heart.

Henle's loop, a U-shaped part of the renal tubule.

Henoch-Schönlein purpura /hen'ôkh-shœn'līn/ [Eduard H. Henoch, German physician, 1820–1910; Johannes L. Schönlein, German physician, 1793–1864], a self-limited hypersensitivity vasculitis, chiefly of children. It is characterized by purpuric skin lesions that appear predominantly on the lower abdomen, buttocks, and legs and are usually associated with pain in the knees and ankles. Other joint involvement, gastrointestinal bleeding, and hematuria are also common findings.

henry (H) [Joseph Henry, American physicist, 1797–1878], an International System (SI) unit of electrical inductance equal to 1 volt-second per ampere.

Henry's law [William Henry, English chemist, 1774–1836], (in physics) a law stating that the solubility of a gas in a liquid is proportional to the pressure of the gas if the temperature is constant and if the gas does not chemically react with the liquid.

Henschen method, (in radiology) a technique for positioning a patient's head in a true lateral position to produce a radiographic image of the mastoid and petrous parts of the head.

heparin /hep'ərin/ [Gk, *hepar,* liver], a naturally occurring mucopolysaccharide that acts in the body as an antithrombin factor to prevent intravascular clotting. The substance is produced by basophils and mast cells.

heparin lock flush solution (USP) [Gk, *hepar,* liver; OE, *loc* + ME, *fluschen* + L, *solutus,* dissolved], a sterile solution of heparin sodium, saline solution, and benzyl alcohol that is intended for use in maintaining patency in intravenous equipment. It is not used in anticoagulant therapy.

heparin rebound, the phenomenon of reactivation of heparin effect that occurs from 5 minutes to 5 hours after neutralization with protamine sulfate.

heparin sodium, an anticoagulant prescribed in the treatment and prophylaxis of a variety of thromboembolic disorders.

hepatectomy /hep'ətek'təmē/ [Gk, *hepar,* liver, *ektome,* excision], a surgical procedure performed to remove a part of the liver.

hepatic /hepat'ik/ [Gk, *hepar,* liver], pertaining to the liver.

hepatic adenoma, a rapidly growing tumor of the liver that may become very large and rupture, causing a lethal internal hemorrhage.

hepatic amebiasis, a disorder characterized by enlargement and tenderness of the liver that is often associated with amebic dysentery.

hepatic bile, a "C" form of bile obtained from a duodenal drainage tube after the gallbladder has been emptied.

hepatic coma, a neuropsychiatric manifestation of extensive liver damage caused by chronic or acute liver disease. Either endogenous or exogenous waste toxic to the brain is not neutralized in the liver before being shunted back into the peripheral circulation of the blood, or substances required for cerebral function are not synthesized in the liver. The condition is characterized by variable consciousness, including lethargy, stupor, and coma; tremor of the hands; personality change; memory loss; hyperreflexia; and hyperventilation. Respiratory alkalosis, mania convulsions, and death may occur.

hepatic cord, a mass of cells arranged in irregular radiating columns and plates, spreading outward from the central vein of the hepatic lobule.

hepatic dyspepsia, a digestive difficulty caused by a liver disorder.

hepatic fistula, an abnormal passage from the liver to another organ or body structure.

hepatic insufficiency, a failure or partial failure of normal liver function.

hepatic lobes [Gk, *hepar,* liver, *lobos,* lobes], the large divisions of the liver: caudate, quadrate, left, and right.

hepatic node, a node in one of three groups of lymph glands associated with the abdominal and pelvic viscera supplied by branches of the celiac artery.

hepaticoduodenostomy /hepat'ikōdoo'-ōdənostəmē/, surgical establishment of a passageway between the hepatic duct and the duodenum.

hepaticoenterostomy /həpat'ikō·en'ros'-təmēl, surgical establishment of a passageway between the hepatic duct and the intestine.

hepaticolithotomy /-thiot'əmē/, an incision made in the bile duct for the removal of gallstones.

hepaticolithotripsy /-lith'ətrip'sē/, a surgical procedure in which gallstones in the bile duct are crushed for removal.

hepatic pulse, pulsation of the liver, such as may occur in tricuspid incompetence.

hepatic siderosis [Gk, *hepar,* liver, *sideros,* iron, *osis,* condition], a chronic disease in which hemosiderin, an iron-containing pigment, accumulates in the liver and causes a bronze skin pigmentation.

hepatic vein catheterization, the intro-

H

duction of a long, fine catheter into a hepatic venule for the purpose of recording intrahepatic venous pressure. The catheter is inserted through a vein in the arm.

hepatic veins [Gk, *hepar,* liver; L, *vena*], the three main veins, the right, middle, and left, that drain the blood of the liver into the inferior vena cava.

hepatitis /hep´ətī´tis/ [Gk, *hepar* + *itis,* inflammation], an inflammatory condition of the liver characterized by jaundice, hepatomegaly, anorexia, abdominal and gastric discomfort, abnormal liver function, clay-colored stools, and tea-colored urine. The condition may be caused by bacterial or viral infection, parasitic infestation, alcohol, drugs, toxins, or transfusion of incompatible blood. Severe hepatitis may lead to cirrhosis and chronic liver dysfunction.

hepatitis A, a form of infectious viral hepatitis caused by the hepatitis A virus **(HAV),** characterized by slow onset of signs and symptoms. The virus may be spread by direct contact through fecally contaminated food or water.

hepatitis B, a form of viral hepatitis caused by the hepatitis B virus **(HBV).** The virus is transmitted in contaminated serum in blood transfusion, by sexual contact with an infected person, or by the use of contaminated needles and instruments.

hepatitis B immune globulin (HBIG), a passive immunizing agent prescribed for postexposure prophylaxis against infection by the hepatitis B virus.

hepatitis B vaccine, a vaccine prepared from the blood plasma of asymptomatic human carriers of hepatitis B virus or in yeast cells by recombinant deoxyribonucleic acid technology. A series of three doses is recommended to achieve immunity.

hepatitis B vaccine (recombinant), a genetically engineered vaccine produced in yeast cells by recombinant deoxyribonucleic acid technology.

hepatitis C (non-A, non-B hepatitis, [HCV]), a type of hepatitis transmitted largely by blood transfusion or percutaneous inoculation, as when intravenous drug users share needles. The disease progresses to chronic hepatitis in up to 50% of the patients acutely infected.

hepatitis D (delta hepatitis, [HDV]), a form of hepatitis that occurs only in patients infected with hepatitis B. HDV relies on hepatitis B virus replication and cannot replicate independently. The disease usually develops into a chronic state. It is transmitted sexually and through needle sharing.

hepatitis E (epidemic non-A, non-B hepatitis, [HEV]), a self-limited type of hepatitis that may occur after natural disasters because of fecally contaminated water or food.

hepatization /hep´ətīzā´shən/ [Gk, *hepatizein,* like the liver], transformation of lung tissue into a solid mass resembling the liver. In early pneumococcal pneumonia consolidation and effusion of red blood cells in the alveoli produce **red hepatization.** In later stages of pneumococcal pneumonia, when white blood cells fill the alveoli, the consolidation becomes gray hepatization, or yellow hepatization, when infiltrated by fat deposits.

hepatoblastoma /hep´ətō´blastō´mə/, a cancer of the liver that tends to occur in children. Hepatoblastoma also may be associated with precocious puberty.

hepatocarcinogen /-kärsin´əjən/, an agent that causes carcinoma of the liver.

hepatocele [Gk, *hepar,* liver, *kele,* hernia], a hernia of a part of the liver through the diaphragm or the abdominal wall.

hepatocellular jaundice /-sel´yələr/, jaundice resulting from disease or injury to liver cells.

hepatocholangitis /hep´ətōkō´lanjī´tis/, an inflammation of both the liver and the bile ducts.

hepatocyte /hep´ətōsīt/ [Gk, *hepar* + *kytos,* cell], a parenchymal liver cell that performs all the functions ascribed to the liver.

hepatoduodenal ligament /hep´ətōdoo´-ədē´nəl, -doo-od´inəl/ [Gk, *hepar* + L, *duodeni,* twelve fingers], the part of the lesser omentum between the liver and the duodenum, containing the hepatic artery, the common bile duct, the portal vein, the lymphatics, and the hepatic plexus of nerves.

hepatogastric ligament /hep´ətōgas´trik/ [Gk, *hepar* + *gaster,* stomach], the part of the lesser omentum between the liver and the stomach.

hepatogenous jaundice /hep´ətoj´ənəs/ [Gk, *hepar,* liver, *genein,* to produce; Fr, *jaune,* yellow], a type of jaundice caused by a condition of the liver.

hepatogram /hep´ətōgram´/, **1.** a sphygmographic tracing of the liver pulse. **2.** a radiographic image of the liver.

hepatography /hep´ətog´rəfē/, **1.** the recording of a tracing of the liver pulse. **2.** the radiographic or isotope scintigraphic visualization of the liver.

hepatojugular /hep´ətōjug´yŏŏlər/ [Gk, *hepar,* liver; L, *jugulum,* neck], pertaining to the liver and the jugular vein.

hepatojugular reflux [Gk, *hepar* + L, *jugulum,* neck], an increase in jugular venous pressure when pressure is applied for 30 to 60 seconds over the abdomen, suggestive of right-sided heart failure.

hepatolenticular degeneration /həpat'-ōlentik'yo͞olər/ [Gk, *hepar* + L, *lens,* lentil], an abnormal condition associated with defective copper metabolism in the body, characterized by decreased serum ceruloplasmin and copper levels and increased secretion of urinary copper. In individuals with this condition tissue deposits of copper associated with hepatic cirrhosis, deep marginal pigmentation of the cornea, and extensive degeneration of the central nervous system develop.

hepatolithiasis /lithī'əsis/, the presence of stones in the liver.

hepatologist /hep'ətol'əjist/, a physician who specializes in diseases of the liver.

hepatology /hep'ətol'əjē/, the branch of medicine that is concerned primarily with diseases of the liver.

hepatoma /hep'ətō'mə/ [Gk, *hepar* + *oma,* tumor], a primary malignant tumor of the liver characterized by hepatomegaly, pain, hypoglycemia, weight loss, anorexia, ascites, as well as elevated serum alpha fetoprotein levels, portal hypertension, and jaundice in the plasma.

hepatomegaly /hep'ətōmeg'əlē/ [Gk, *hepar* + *megas,* large], abnormal enlargement of the liver that is usually a sign of disease. Hepatomegaly may be caused by hepatitis or other infection, fatty infiltration as in alcoholism, biliary obstruction, or malignancy.

hepatonecrosis /-nekrō'sis/, **1.** the death of liver cells. **2.** gangrene of the liver.

hepatopancreatic ampulla /-pan'krē-at'ik/ [Gk, *hepar* + *pan,* all, *kreas,* flesh], the dilation formed by the junction of the pancreatic and bile ducts as they open into the lumen of the duodenum.

hepatorenal /hep'ətōrē'nəl/, [Gk, *hepar,* liver; L, *ren,* kidney], pertaining to the liver and kidneys.

hepatorenal syndrome a type of kidney failure characterized by a gradual loss of function without signs of tissue damage.

hepatosplenomegaly /-splē'nōmeg'əlē/ [Gk, *hepar,* liver, *splen* + *megas,* large], enlargement of the spleen and liver.

hepatotoxic /-tok'sik/, potentially destructive of liver cells.

hepatotoxicity /hep'ətōtoksis'itē/ [Gk, *hepar* + *toxikon,* poison], the tendency of an agent, usually a drug or alcohol, to have a destructive effect on the liver.

hepatoxin /-tok'sin/, a poison that damages parenchymal cells of the liver.

heptachlor poisoning /hep'təklôr'/ [Gk, *hepar,* seven, *chloros,* green; L, *potio,* drink], a form of chlorinated organic insecticide poisoning.

herb /(h)urb/ [L, *herba,* grass], **1.** any plant that is used for culinary or medicinal purposes. **2.** a leafy plant without a wooden stem. **3.** a plant with aerial parts that do not persist from one year to the next.

herbalist /hur'bəlist/, **1.** a person who specializes in the study of herbs. **2.** a dealer in medicinal herbs.

herb bath [L, *herba,* grass; AS, *baeth*], a medicinal bath taken in water containing a decoction of aromatic herbs.

herbicide poisoning /hur'bisīd/ [L, *herba,* grass, *caedere,* to kill], a poisoning caused by the ingestion, inhalation, or absorption of a substance intended for use as a weed killer or defoliant. Many of the commonly used agricultural herbicides can produce symptoms ranging from skin irritation to hypotension, liver and kidney damage, and coma or convulsions.

herbivorous /hərbiv'ərəs/ [L, *herba,* grass, *vorare,* to devour], pertaining to feeding on plants or to animals that subsist mostly or entirely on plants.

herb tea, a medicinal beverage prepared by the infusion of a water-soluble extract of leaves, roots, bark, or other parts of an herb. The vegetable matter is commonly macerated and steeped in boiling water, which is strained and served hot.

herd immunity [ME, *heord,* group; L, *immunis,* free from], the level of disease resistance of a community or population.

herd instinct [ME, *heord* + L, *instinctus,* impulse], the basic need of social animals, including humans, for the companionship of peers and a tendency to find compatibility with the behavioral standards of others in the group.

hereditability /həred'itəbil'itē/ [L, *hereditas,* inheritance], the degree to which a specific trait is controlled by inheritance.

hereditary /həred'iter'ē/ [L, *hereditas,* inheritance], pertaining to a characteristic, condition, or disease transmitted from parent to offspring; inborn; inherited.

hereditary angioedema, an inherited autosomal-dominant disorder characterized by the episodic appearance of nonpitting edema involving any part of the body.

hereditary ataxia, one of a group of inherited degenerative diseases of the spinal cord, cerebellum, and often other parts of the nervous system, characterized by tremor, spasm, muscle wasting, skeletal change, and sensory disturbances resulting in impaired motor activity.

hereditary multiple exostoses, a rare familial dyschondroplastic disease in which bony protuberances form on the shafts of the long bones and eventually develop into

H

caps of cartilage covering the ends of the bones.

hereditary oral disease, any abnormal condition characterized by genetic defects of oral and paraoral structures, such as deformed dentition, ankyloglossia, hereditary gingivofibromatosis, or cleft palate.

heredity /həred′itē/ [L, *hereditas,* inheritance], **1.** the process by which particular traits or conditions are genetically transmitted from parents to offspring, causing resemblance of individuals related by descent. **2.** the total genetic constitution of an individual; the sum of the qualities inherited from ancestors and the potentialities of transmitting these qualities to offspring.

Hering-Breuer reflexes /her′ingbroi′ər/ [Heinrich E. Hering, German physiologist, 1866–1948; Joseph Breuer, Austrian physician, 1842–1925], inhibitory and excitatory impulses that maintain the rhythm of respiration and prevent the overdistension of alveoli.

hermaphroditism /hərmaf′rədītiz′əm/ [Gk, *Hermaphrodites,* son of Hermes and Aphrodite], a rare condition in which both testicular and ovarian tissue exist in the same person; the testicular tissue contains seminiferous tubules or spermatozoa, and the ovarian tissue contains follicles or corpora albicantia.

hermetic /hərmet′ik/ [Gk, *Hermes*], from use in alchemy, pertaining to sealing a container to make it airtight.

hernia /hur′nē·ə/ [L, rupture], protrusion of an organ through an abnormal opening in the muscle wall of the cavity that surrounds it. A hernia may be congenital, may result from the failure of structures to close after birth, or acquired later in life as a result of obesity, muscular weakness, surgery, or illness.

hernial /hur′nē·əl/, pertaining to or resembling a hernia.

hernial sac [L, *hernia,* rupture; Gk, *sakkos,* sack], a pouch of peritoneum into which organs or other tissues pass to form a hernia.

herniated /hur′nē·ā′tid/, pertaining to a tear or abnormal bulge of an organ or organ part through a retaining tissue.

herniated disk, a rupture of the fibrocartilage surrounding an intervertebral disk, releasing the nucleus pulposus that cushions the vertebrae above and below. The resultant pressure on spinal nerve roots may cause considerable pain and damage the nerves. The condition most frequently occurs in the lumbar region.

herniation /hur′nē·ā′shən/, a protrusion of a body organ or part of an organ through an abnormal opening in a membrane, muscle, or other tissue.

herniography /hur′nē·og′rəfē/, the radiographic examination of a hernia after it has been injected with a contrast medium.

herniorrhaphy /hur′nē·ôr′əfē/, the surgical repair of a hernia.

herniotomy /hur′nē·ot′əmē/ [L, *hernia* + Gk, *tenein,* to cut], a surgical procedure to reduce a hernia.

heroin /her′ō·in/ [Ger, heroine, originally trademark for diacetylmorphine], a morphinelike drug with no currently acceptable medical use in the United States. Heroin is included in Schedule I of the Controlled Substances Act of 1970. Like other opium alkaloids, it can produce analgesia, respiratory depression, gastrointestinal spasm, and physical dependence. It produces its major effects on the central nervous system and bowel and alters the endocrine and autonomic nervous systems.

herpangina /hur′panjī′nə/ [Gk, *herpein,* to creep; L, *angina,* quinsy], a viral infection, usually of young children, characterized by sore throat, headache, anorexia, and pain in the abdomen, neck, and extremities. Febrile convulsions and vomiting may occur in infants. Papules or vesicles may form in the pharynx and on the tongue, the palate, or the tonsils. The cause is often infection by a strain of coxsackievirus.

herpes genitalis /hur′pēz jen′ital′is/ [Gk, *herpein,* to creep; L, *genitalis,* genitalia], a chronic infection caused by type 2 herpes simplex virus (HSV2), usually transmitted by sexual contact. It causes painful vesicular eruptions on the skin and mucous membranes of the genitalia of males and females. When acquired during pregnancy, HSV2 may be transmitted through the placenta to the fetus and to the newborn by direct contact with infected tissue during birth. It is a precursor of cervical cancer.

herpes gestationis [Gk, *herpein* + L, *gestare,* to bear], a generalized pruritic vesicular or bullous rash that appears in the second or third trimester of pregnancy and disappears several weeks after delivery. The lesions often recur with succeeding pregnancies and are associated with premature birth and increased fetal mortality rate.

herpes menstrualis [Gk, *herpein,* to creep; L, *menstruare*], a form of herpes simplex that tends to erupt during menstrual periods.

herpes simplex [Gk, *herpein* + L, *simplex,* uncomplicated], an infection caused by a herpes simplex virus (HSV), which has an affinity for the skin and nervous system and usually produces small, transient, irritating, and sometimes painful fluid-filled blisters on the skin and mucous membranes. HSV1 (oral herpes, herpes labialis) infections tend to occur in the facial area, particularly around the mouth and nose; HSV2 (herpes genitalis) infections are usually limited to the genital region. The initial symptoms of a herpes simplex infection usually include burning, tingling, or itching sensations about the edges of the lips or nose within 1 or 2 weeks after contact with an infected person. Small vesicles, or fever blisters, filled with fluid erupt and generally are associated with itching, pain, or similar discomfort.

herpes simplex encephalitis, a necrotizing inflammation of the brain that follows an infection with herpes simplex virus (HSV-1). It is a common acute form of encephalitis and similar to other viral encephalitis infections. The mortality rate varies, but even desperately ill patients may recover completely.

herpesvirus /hur′pēzvī′rəs/ [Gk, *herpein* + L, *virus,* poison], any of seven related viruses: herpes simplex viruses 1 and 2, varicella zoster virus, Epstein-Barr virus, cytomegalovirus, HHV6, and HHV7.

herpesvirus simiae encephalomyelitis, a typically fatal infection of the central nervous system by a B form of herpes simplex virus that usually affects simians. Persons most likely to be infected by the monkey virus are veterinarians and animal laboratory workers.

herpes zoster /zos′tər/ [Gk, *herpein* + *zoster,* girdle], an acute infection caused by reactivation of the latent varicella zoster virus (VZV), which mainly affects adults. It is characterized by the development of painful vesicular skin eruptions that follow the underlying route of cranial or spinal nerves inflamed by the virus. Distribution of the pain and vesicular eruptions is usually unilateral, although both sides of the body may be involved. Any sensory nerve may be affected, but the virus in most cases tends to invade the posterior root ganglia associated with thoracic and trigeminal nerves. The pain usually precedes other effects and may mimic that of other disorders such as appendicitis or pleurisy. Evidence indicates that VZV remains latent in the body of a person who has been infected, and a person lacking varicella immunity can acquire chickenpox from a herpes zoster patient.

herpes zoster ophthalmicus, a form of herpes zoster causing pain and skin eruptions along the ophthalmic branch of the fifth cranial nerve. There also may be involvement of the third cranial nerve. The infection frequently leads to corneal ulceration or other ocular complications.

herpes zoster oticus, a herpes zoster infection of the eighth cervical (vestibulocochlear) nerve ganglia and geniculate ganglion, causing severe pain in the external ear structures and pain or paralysis along the facial nerve. The disease also may cause hearing loss and vertigo.

herpetic keratitis /hərpet′ik/ [Gk, *herpein,* to creep, *keras,* horn, *itis,* inflammation], an inflammation of the cornea caused by a herpesvirus.

herpetic neuralgia [Gk, *herpein,* to creep, *neuron,* nerve, *algos,* pain], a form of neuralgia with intractable pain that develops at the site of a previous eruption of herpes zoster.

herpetic sore throat, a herpes inflammation that develops in the region of the pharynx.

herpetic stomatitis [Gk, *herpein,* to creep, *stoma,* mouth, *itis,* inflammation], a form of inflammation of the mouth caused by a herpesvirus infection.

herpetiform /hərpet′ifôrm′/ [Gk, *herpein* + L, *forma,* form], having clusters of vesicles; resembling the skin lesions of some herpesvirus infections.

Hers' disease /herz, hurz/ [H. G. Hers, twentieth-century Belgian physiologist; L, *dis,* opposite of; Fr, *aise,* ease], an uncommon metabolic disorder of glycogen storage. It is characterized by hepatomegaly and an accumulation of abnormally large amounts of glycogen in the liver as a result of its inability to break down glycogen. The condition is inherited as an autosomal-recessive trait.

hertz (Hz) /hurts, herts/ [Heinrich R. Hertz, German physicist, 1857–1894], a unit of measurement of wave frequency equal to 1 cycle per second (cps).

Herxheimer's reaction /herks′hī′mərz/ [Karl Herxheimer, German dermatologist, 1861–1944], an increase in symptoms after administration of a drug. The reaction was originally discovered in penicillin treatment of syphilis, but it has been found to occur with other diseases as well.

Herzog taping protocol, a procedure for immobilizing and balancing a foot with tape after a musculoskeletal injury.

Heschl's gyrus /hesh′əl/ [Richard L. Heschl, Austrian pathologist, 1824–1881; Gk, *gyros,* turn], any of several small gyri that run transversely on the upper surface of the temporal operculum of the insula of the cortex.

hesperidin /hesper′idin/, a crystalline flavone glycoside found in bioflavonoid and present in most citrus fruits, especially in the spongy casing of oranges and lemons.

Hesselbach's hernia /hes'əlbaks, hes'-əbkhs/ [Franz K. Hesselbach, German surgeon, 1759–1816], a protrusion of diverticula through the femoral sheath.

hetastarch /het'əstärch/, a plasma volume extender prescribed as an adjunct in shock and leukophoresis.

heteroallele /het'ərō-əlēl'/ [Gk, *heteros,* different, *alleolon,* of one another], one of a set of genes at a specific locus on homologous chromosomes that differs from the other of the pair, causing a mutation. —**heteroallelic,** *adj.*

heteroantibody /het'ərō-an'tibod'ē/, an antibody that is specific with respect to antigen from a species other than that of the antibody producer.

heteroantigen /he'tərō-an'təjən/, an antigen that originates in a different species and is foreign to the antibody producer.

heteroblastic /het'ərōblas'tik/ [Gk, *heteros* + *blastos,* germ], developing from different germ layers or kinds of tissue rather than from a single type.

heterocellular /-sel'yələr/, (in biology) a structure formed by more than one kind of cell.

heterocephalus /-sef'ələs/ [Gk, *heteros* + *kephale,* head], a malformed fetus that has two heads of unequal size. —**heterocephalous, heterocephalic,** *adj.*

heterochromatin /-krō'mətin/ [Gk, *heteros,* different, *chroma,* color], that part of chromosome material that is inactive in gene expression but may function in controlling metabolic activities, transcription, and cell division. —**heterochromatic,** *adj.*

heterochromatinization /-krō'mətīzā'-shən/, the transformation of genetically active euchromatin into genetically inactive heterochromatin; the inactivation of one of the X chromosomes in the mammalian female during the early stages of embryogenesis.

heterochromosome /-krō'məsōm/, a sex chromosome. —**heterochromosomal,** *adj.*

heterocytotropic antibody /-sī'tətrop'ik/, an immunoglobulin E class antibody that has a greater affinity for antigens when fixed to mast cells of a different species than the one in which the antibody was produced.

heterodidymus /het'ərōdid'iməs/ [Gk, *heteros* + *didymos,* twin], a conjoined twin fetus in which the parasitic elements consist of a head, neck, and thorax attached to the thoracic wall of the autosite.

heteroduplex /-dōō'pleks, -dōō'pleks/ [Gk, *heteros* + L, *duoplicare,* to double], (in molecular genetics) a deoxyribonucleic acid molecule in which the two strands are derived from different individuals, with the result that some pairs or blocks of base pairs may not match.

heteroduplex mapping a method for determining the location of insertions, deletions, and other heterogeneities in the two strands of a deoxyribonucleic acid molecule.

heteroenzyme /het'ərō-en'zim/, a functionally identical enzyme from a different species.

heteroeroticism /het'ərō·irot'isiz'əm/ [Gk, *heteros,* different, *eros,* love], sexual feeling or activity directed toward another individual.

heterofermentation /-fur'məntā'shun/, fermentation that produces major products that are different.

heterogamete /-gam'ēt/ [Gk, *heteros* + *gamete,* spouse], a gamete that differs considerably in size and structure from the one with which it unites, specifically denoting those of higher organisms as opposed to those of lower plants and animals.

heterogamy /het'ərog'əmē/ [Gk, *heteros* + *gamos,* marriage], **1.** sexual reproduction in which there is fusion of dissimilar gametes, usually differing in size and structure. **2.** reproduction by the alternation of sexual and asexual generations; heterogenesis. —**heterogamous,** *adj.*

heterogeneity /-jənē'itē/, **1.** a quality of being dissimilar in kind. **2.** a state of having different characteristics and qualities.

heterogeneous /het'əroj'ənəs/ [Gk, *heteros,* different, *genos,* kind], **1.** consisting of dissimilar elements or parts; unlike; incongruous. **2.** not having a uniform quality throughout. —**heterogeneity,** *adj.*

heterogenesis /-jen'əsis/ [Gk, *heteros* + *genein,* to produce], **1.** reproduction that differs in successive generations, such as the alternation of sexual with asexual reproduction, so that offspring have characteristics different from those of the parents. **2.** asexual generation. **3.** abiogenesis. —**heterogenetic, heterogenic,** *adj.*

heterogenous /het'əroj'ənəs/ [Gk, *heteros* + *genos,* kind], derived or developed from another source or from two different sources.

heterogenous vaccine [Gk, *heteros,* different, *genein,* to produce; L, *vaccinus,* cow], a vaccine made from a source other than the patient's own tissues.

heteroimmunization /-im'yənīzā'shun/, immunization of an individual with antigens from a different species.

heteroinfection /-infek'shən/ [Gk, *heteros,* different; L, *inficere,* to stain], infection by a microorganism originating outside the body.

heterolactic acid fermentation /-lak'tik/, bacterial fermentation that produces a mixture of lactic acid and other products.

heterologous anaphylaxis /het'ərol'əgəs/ [Gk, *heteros,* different, *logos,* relation, *ana,* again, *phylaxis,* protection], a form of passive anaphylaxis that results from the transfer of serum between two animals of different species.

heterologous tumor [Gk, *heteros + logos,* relation], a neoplasm consisting of tissue different from that of its site.

heterometropia /-mətrō'pē·ə/ [Gk, *heteros,* different, *metron,* measure, *ops,* eye], a generally mild visual disorder in which one eye refracts differently from the other, causing slightly different images to be perceived by the right and left eyes.

heteronymous /het'əron'iməs/ [Gk, *heteros,* different, *onyma,* name], **1.** having different names; the opposite of synonymous. **2.** an optical phenomenon in which two images are produced by one object.

heterophil /het'ərofil'/ [Gk, *heteros + philein,* to love], having affinity for something unusual or abnormal, as an antibody that reacts to an antigen other than the one it is expected to challenge.

heterophil antibody test [Gk, *heteros + philein,* to love], a test for the presence of heterophil antibodies in the serum of patients suspected of having infectious mononucleosis, based on an agglutination reaction between heterophil antibodies in a person's serum and heterophil antigen.

heterophilic leukocyte /-fil'ik/ [Gk, *heteros,* different, *philein,* to love, *leukos,* white, *kytos,* cell], a neutrophil of certain animal species that takes an acid stain.

heteroplastic transplantation /-plas'tik/ [Gk, *heteros,* different, *plassein,* to mold; L, *transplantare*], the transfer of tissue from one animal to another of a different species.

heteroploid /het'ərəploid'/ [Gk, *heteros + ploos,* times, *eidos,* form], **1.** pertaining to an individual, organism, strain, or cell that has a variation in the number of whole chromosomes characteristic for the somatic cell of the species. **2.** such an individual, organism, strain, or cell.

heteroploidy /het'ərəploi'dē/, the state or condition of having an abnormal number of chromosomes, either more or less than that characteristic of the somatic cell of the species.

heteropolymer /-pol'imir/ [Gk, *heteros + polys,* many, *meros,* part], a compound formed from subunits that are not all the same, such as a protein composed of various amino acid subunits.

heterosexual /-sek'shəl/ [Gk, *heteros,* different; L, *sexus,* male or female], **1.**

a person whose sexual desire or preference is for people of the opposite sex. **2.** pertaining to sexual desire or preference for people of the opposite sex. **—heterosexuality,** *n.*

heterosexual panic, an acute attack of anxiety that results in the frantic pursuit of heterosexual activity in response to unconscious or latent homosexual impulses.

heterosis /het'ərō'sis/ [Gk, *heteros + osis,* condition], the superiority of first-generation hybrid plants and animals in respect to one or more traits when compared with either of the parent strains or with corresponding inbred strains.

heterotopic ossification /-top'ik/ [Gk, *heteros + topos,* place], a nonmalignant overgrowth of bone, frequently occurring after a fracture, that is sometimes confused with certain bone tumors when visualized on x-ray film.

heterotopic pain, pain that appears in the wrong part of the body, as pain originating in the gallbladder that may be felt in the right shoulder. The phenomenon seems to be caused by projection of sensory neurons from different parts of the body into the same regions of the central nervous system.

heterotopic pregnancy, a pregnancy that is both intrauterine and extrauterine.

heterotopic transplantation [Gk, *heteros,* different, *topos,* place; L, *transplantare*], the transfer of tissue from one part of a body of a donor to another area of the body of a recipient.

heterotransplant /-trans'plant/ [Gk, *hetero,* different; L, *transplantare*], the transfer of tissue from one animal to another of a different species.

heterotypic /het'ərōtip'ik/ [Gk, *heteros + typos,* pattern], pertaining to or characteristic of a type differing from the usual or normal, specifically regarding the first meiotic division of germ cells in gametogenesis as distinguished from the second or mitotic division.

heterotypic chromosomes, any unmatched pair of chromosomes, specifically the sex chromosomes.

heterotypic mitosis, the division of bivalent chromosomes, as occurs in the first meiotic division of germ cells in gametogenesis; a reduction division.

heterozygosis /het'ərōzīgō'sis/ [Gk, *heteros + zygotos,* yoked], **1.** the formation of a zygote by the union of two gametes that have dissimilar pairs of genes. **2.** the production of hybrids through crossbreeding. **—heterozygotic,** *adj.*

heterozygote /-zī'gōt/ [Gk, *heteros,* different, *zygotos,* yoked], an organism whose somatic cells have two different allelomor-

H

phic genes on the same locus of each pair of chromosomes. It can produce two different types of gametes.

heterozygote detection, the use of amniocentesis and other techniques to identify potential inherited X-linked recessive disorders such as Hunter's syndrome or Duchenne's muscular dystrophy.

heterozygous /het′ərəzī′gəs/ [Gk, *heteros* + *zygotos,* yoked], having two different genes at corresponding loci on homologous chromosomes. An individual who is heterozygous for a characteristic has inherited a gene for that characteristic from one parent and the alternative gene from the other parent.

heuristic /hyŏŏris′tik/ [Gk, *heuriskein,* to discover], **1.** serving to stimulate interest for further investigation. **2.** a teaching method in which the student is encouraged to learn through independent research and investigation.

HEV, abbreviation for *hepatitis E virus.*

hexachlorophene /hek′səklôr′əfēn/, a topical antiinfective and detergent used as an antiseptic scrub and as a disinfectant for inanimate objects.

hexafluorenium bromide /-flŏŏrē′nē·əm/, an inhibitor of acetylcholinesterase used as an adjunct to anesthesia to prolong the skeletal muscle relaxation caused by succinylcholine.

hexamethonium /-məthō′nē·əm/, a cholinergic blocking agent used to control bleeding and treat peptic ulcers and hypertension.

hexamethylmelamine /-meth′ilmel′əmēn/, an antineoplastic that is used to treat persistent or recurrent ovarian carcinomas.

hexocyclium methylsulfate /-sī′klē·əm/, an anticholinergic prescribed as an adjunct to ulcer therapy.

hexokinase /hek′səkī′nās/ [Gk, *hex,* six, *glykys,* sweet, *kinein,* to move, *ase,* enzyme], an enzyme present in muscle that catalyzes the transfer of a phosphate group from adenosine triphosphate to d-glucose.

hexose /hek′sōs/ [Gk, *hex,* six, *glykys,* sweet], a monosaccharide that contains six carbon atoms in the molecule. Glucose, maltose, and fructose are the principal hexoses found in nature.

hexylcaine hydrochloride /hek′silkān/, a local anesthetic for use on intact mucous membranes of the respiratory, upper gastrointestinal, and urinary tracts.

hexylresorcinol /hek′ilrəsôr′sənol/, a topical skin anesthetic that is also administered for the treatment of certain types of worm infestations.

Hf, symbol for the element **hafnium.**

HFV, abbreviation for **high-frequency ventilation.**

Hg, symbol for the element **mercury.**

Hgb, abbreviation for **hemoglobin.**

HGE, abbreviation for human granulocytic ehrlichiosis.

HGF, 1. abbreviation for *human growth factor* **2.** abbreviation for *hyperglycemic-glycogenolytic factor.*

HHS, abbreviation for **Department of Health and Human Services.**

HI, abbreviation for **hemagglutination inhibition.**

hiatal hernia, protrusion of a part of the stomach upward through the diaphragm. The major difficulty in symptomatic patients is gastroesophageal reflux, the backflow of the acid contents of the stomach into the esophagus.

hiatus /hī·ā′təs/ [L, *hiare,* to stand open], a usually normal opening in a membrane or other body structure. —**hiatal,** *adj.*

hiatus aorticus [L, *hiare,* to stand open; Gk, *aerein,* to raise], an opening in the diaphragm for the aorta and thoracic duct.

hiatus esophagus [L, *hiare,* to stand open; Gk, *oisophagos,* gullet], the opening in the diaphragm for the esophagus.

hibakusha /hē′bäkōō′shä/ [Japanese], people who were exposed to atomic bomb explosions in Hiroshima and Nagasaki.

Hib disease, an infection caused by *Haemophilus influenzae* type b (Hib), which mainly affects children in the first 5 years of life. It is a leading cause of bacterial meningitis, as well as pneumonia, joint or bone infections, and throat inflammations.

hibernation /hībərnā′shun/, [L, *hibernare,* to winter], a natural physiologic state or process wherein a generalized slowdown in metabolic and body functions produces a somnolescent condition.

hibernoma /hī′bərnō′mə/, *pl.* **hibernomas, hibernomata** [L, *hibernus,* winter; Gk, *oma,* tumor], a benign tumor, usually on the hips or the back, composed of fat cells that are partly or entirely of fetal origin.

hiccup /hik′əp/, a characteristic sound that is produced by the involuntary contraction of the diaphragm, followed by rapid closure of the glottis. Hiccups have various causes, including indigestion, rapid eating, certain types of surgery, and epidemic encephalitis.

hidrosis /hidrō′sis, hī-/ [Gk, *hidros,* sweat], sweat production and secretion. —**hidrotic,** *adj.*

hieralgia /hī′ərəl′jə/, [Gk, *hieron.* sacrum, *algos,* pain], a painful sacrum.

high-altitude edema [ME, *heigh* + L, *altitudo* + Gk, *oidema,* swelling], a form of pulmonary edema that occurs in people who move rapidly to higher altitudes. Fluid accumulates in the lungs as atmospheric pressure decreases.

high-calorie diet, a diet that provides 1000 or more calories a day beyond what is ordinarily recommended. It may be prescribed for nursing mothers, patients with severe weight loss caused by illness, or people with abnormally high metabolic rates or energy requirements.

high-copy number, a large number of repetitive copies of a gene, such as may be produced by cloning.

high-definition imaging (HDI), an ultrasound test technique used in breast cancer diagnosis to determine without biopsy whether a lump is a solid tumor or a relatively harmless fluid-filled cyst.

high-density lipoprotein (HDL) [ME, *heigh,* high; L, *densus,* thick; Gk, *lipos,* fat, *proteios,* first rank], a plasma protein made in the liver and containing about 50% protein (apoprotein) with cholesterol and triglycerides (phospholipid). It may serve to stabilize very low-density lipoprotein and is involved in transporting cholesterol and other lipids to the liver to be disposed.

high-dose tolerance, the absence of an expected immunologic response after repeated injections of large amounts of an antigen.

high enema [ME, *heigh* + Gk, *einienai,* to send in], an enema that is inserted into the colon through a long catheter.

high-energy phosphate compound, a chemical compound containing a high-energy bond between phosphoric acid residues and certain organic substances. When the bond is hydrolyzed, a large amount of energy is released.

highest intercostal vein [ME, *heigh* + L, *inter,* between, *costa,* rib, *vena,* vein], one of a pair of veins that drain the blood from the upper two or three intercostal spaces.

high-flow oxygen delivery system, respiratory care equipment that supplies inspired gases at a consistent preset oxygen concentration.

high forceps, an obstetric operation in which forceps are used to deliver a baby whose head is not engaged in the birth canal. The procedure is considered hazardous and is generally condemned.

high-Fowler's position [ME, *heigh,* high; George R. Fowler, American surgeon, 1848–1906], placement of the patient in a semisitting position by raising the head of the bed more than 20 inches.

high-frequency hearing loss [ME, *heigh* + L, *frequens;* AS, *deaf*], a loss of ability to hear high-frequency sounds. It is most commonly associated with aging and noise exposure. Hearing loss may begin in early adulthood with a loss of hearing to frequencies in the range of 18 to 20 kHz. At about 60 years of age, loss of hearing may begin to affect lower frequencies, in the range of 4 to 8 kHz. Hearing loss caused by noise exposure is often greatest at or near 4 kHz.

high-frequency ventilation (HFV), a technique for providing ventilatory support to patients by operating at a breathing rate of 60 breaths per minute or more. Kinds of high-frequency ventilation include high-frequency jet ventilation (HFJV) and high-frequency oscillation (HFO). HFJV uses a high-pressure gas source that can be regulated to produce short, rapid jets of gas through a small-bore cannula into the airway above the carina. It has a respiratory rate of 100 to 400 cycles per minute. HFO forces small impulses of gas into and out of the airway at frequencies of 400 to 4000 per minute.

high labial arch, a labial arch wire adapted to lie gingival to the anterior tooth crowns, having auxiliary springs that extend downward in contact with the teeth to be moved.

high-level wellness, a concept of optimal health that emphasizes the integration of body, mind, and environment to maximize the function of an individual.

high lithotomy, a suprapubic approach for surgical removal of urinary bladder stones that are not easily removed by ultrasonic crushing.

high-potassium diet, a diet that contains foods rich in potassium, including all leafy green vegetables, brussels sprouts, citrus fruits, bananas, dates, raisins, legumes, meats, and whole grains. It is indicated for any condition that causes loss of extracellular fluid.

high-pressure liquid chromatography, a method of chromatography to separate and quantitate mixtures of substances in a solution.

high-protein diet, a diet that contains large amounts of protein, consisting largely of meats, fish, milk, legumes, and nuts. It may be indicated in protein depletion that results from any cause.

high-residue diet /-rez'idyoo͞ [ME, *heigh* + L, *residuum,* remaining; Gk, *diaita,* way of living], a diet that contains a greater than usual proportion of substances the digestive tract will not metabolize and absorb, such as fiber and other cellulose products.

high-risk infant, any neonate, regardless of birth weight, size, or gestational age, who has a greater than average chance of morbidity or mortality, especially within the first 28 days of life. Risk factors include preconceptual, prenatal, natal, or postnatal conditions or circumstances that interfere with the normal birth process or impede adjustment to extrauterine growth and development.

high-speed handpiece, a rotary cutting instrument that operates at high speeds of up to 450,000 rpm. Modern high-speed handpieces are powered by miniature turbines driven by compressed air.

high-vitamin diet, a dietary regimen that includes a variety of foods that contain therapeutic amounts of all of the vitamins necessary for the metabolic processes of the body. It is often ordered in combination with other therapeutic diets that contain larger than usual amounts of protein or calories, especially when treating severe or chronic infection, malnutrition, or vitamin deficiency.

hilar /hī'lär/ [L, *hilum,* a trifle], pertaining to a hilum.

Hill-Burton Act, a 1946 amendment to the U.S. Public Health Service Act authorizing grants to states for surveying their hospital and public health center needs and for planning and constructing additional facilities.

Hill-Burton programs, a cluster of programs created by U.S. legislation included in the National Health Planning and Resources Development Act of 1974. The programs allow federal monetary assistance for modernization of health facilities, construction of outpatient health centers, construction of inpatient facilities in underserved areas, and conversion of existing health care facilities for the provision of new health services.

hilum /hī'ləm/ /hī'ləs/, *pl.* **hila** [L, *hilum,* a trifle], a depression or pit at that part of an organ where vessels and nerves enter.

hindbrain /hīnd'brān/ [ME, *hind* + AS, *bragen*], the division in the brain of an embryo that eventually becomes the pons, the medulla oblongata, and the cerebellum.

hindgut /hīnd'gut/ [ME, *hind* + AS, *guttas*], the caudal part of the embryonic alimentary canal.

hinge axis, the joint where the mandible meets the skull and the point of rotation of the mandible.

hinge axis-orbital plane, a craniofacial plane that is usually determined by marking three points on the cephalogram of the patient's skull. The hinge axis-orbital plane is a reference plane for the diagnosis of various types of malocclusions and the development of associated prostheses.

hinged knee, an appliance designed to protect and support the knee during activity. It consists of an elastic sleeve with medial and lateral steel or aluminum bars hinged at the axis of the knee joint. The hinged bars are stabilized with straps.

hinge joint [AS, *hangian,* to hang; ME, *jointe,* a connection], a synovial joint providing a connection in which articular surfaces are closely molded together in a manner that permits extensive motion in one plane.

hip-joint disease [AS, *hype* + L, *jungere,* to join; Gk, *dis,* not; Fr, *aise,* ease], any abnormal condition of the hip joint, such as Perthes' disease or congenital dislocation of the hip.

Hippel's disease [Eugen von Hippel, German ophthalmologist, 1867–1939], a familial disease, hereditary hemangioma confined mainly to the retina, first described by Hippel.

hippocampal /hip'ōkam'pəl/ [Gk, *hippokampos,* seahorse], pertaining to the hippocampus.

hippocampal commissure [Gk, *hippokampos,* seahorse; L, *commissura,* a joint], a thin triangular layer of transverse fibers that connects the medial edges of the posterior pillars of the fornix in the brain.

hippocampal fissure, a fissure reaching from the posterior aspect of the corpus callosum to the tip of the temporal lobe.

hippocampal formation [Gk, *hippokampos,* seahorse; L, *formatio*], a part of the rhinencephalon, including the dentate gyrus, longitudinal striae, and hippocampus.

hippocampal gyrus [Gk, *hippokampos,* seahorse, *gyros,* turn], a convolution on the medial side of the temporal lobe of the cerebral cortex.

hippocampus /hip'ōkam'pəs/, *pl.* **hippocampi** [Gk, *hippokampos,* seahorse], a curved convoluted elevation of the floor of the inferior horn of the lateral ventricle of the brain.

Hippocrates /hipok'rətēz/, a Greek physician born about 460 BC on the island of Cos, a center for the worship of Æsculapius. Called the "Father of Medicine," Hippocrates introduced a scientific approach to healing.

Hippocratic oath /hip'əkrat'ik/, an oath, attributed to Hippocrates, that serves as an ethical guide for the medical profession. It is traditionally incorporated into the graduation ceremonies of medical colleges.

hippuric acid [Gk, *hippos,* horse, *ouron,* urine; L, *acidus,* sour], a detoxication product in the urine of some animals. It has been used as a medication in the treatment of arthritic diseases.

hip replacement [AS, *hype*], substitution of an artificial ball and socket joint for the hip joint. Hip replacement is performed to relieve a chronically painful and stiff hip in advanced osteoarthritis, an improperly healed fracture, or degeneration of the joint. Antibiotic therapy is begun before surgery, and the patient is taught to walk with crutches or a walker. During surgery the femoral head, neck, and part of the shaft are removed, and the contours of the socket are smoothed. A prosthesis of a durable, hard metal alloy or stainless steel is shaped to resemble a head of a femur and is attached to the femur. A metal or a plastic acetabulum is implanted.

Hirschberg's reflex /hursh'bərgz/, a diagnostic test for pyramidal tract disease. The test result is regarded as positive if inversion of the foot occurs when the sole is stroked at the base of the great toe.

Hirschfeld-Dunlop file, a kind of periodontal file, used with a pull stroke to remove tooth calculus. Various models with different angulations are available for different tooth surfaces.

Hirschfeld's method [Isador Hirschfeld, American dentist, 1881–1965], a toothbrushing technique in which the bristles are placed against the axial surfaces of the teeth at a slight incisal or occlusal angle and in contact with the teeth and gingivae, then vigorously rotated in very small circles.

Hirschsprung's disease /hirsh'sprŏŏngz/ [Harald Hirschsprung, Danish physician, 1830–1916], the congenital absence of autonomic ganglia in the smooth muscle wall of the colon, which causes poor or absent peristalsis in the involved segment of colon, accumulation of feces, and dilation of the bowel (megacolon). Symptoms include intermittent vomiting, diarrhea, and constipation. The abdomen may become distended to several times its normal size.

hirsutism /hur'sŏŏtiz'əm/ [L, hirsutus, hairy], excessive body hair in a masculine distribution pattern as a result of heredity, hormonal dysfunction, porphyria, or medication. Treatment of the specific cause usually stops growth of more hair. —**hirsute,** adj., **hirsuteness,** n.

hirsutoid papilloma of the penis /hur'-sŏŏtoid/ [L, hirsutus, shaggy; Gk, eidos, form], a condition characterized by clusters of small white papules on the coronal edge of the glans penis.

His, abbreviation for **histidine.**

His bundle electrogram (HBE) [Wilhelm His, Jr., German physician, 1863–1934], (in cardiology) a direct recording of the electrical activity in the bundle of His.

His-Purkinje system /his'pərkin'jē/ [Wilhelm His, Jr.; Johannes E. Purkinje, Czechoslovakian physiologist, 1787–

1869], the conduction system in the cardiac tissues from the bundle of His to the distal Purkinje fibers.

histaminase /histam'inās/, a soft tissue enzyme found in various body tissues. It catalyzes the deamination of histamine and converts histamine into inactive imidazolacetic acid.

histamine /his'təmēn, -min/ [Gk, histos, tissue; L, amine, ammonia], a compound, found in all cells, produced by the breakdown of histidine. It is released in allergic inflammatory reactions and causes dilation of capillaries, decrease in blood pressure, increase in secretion of gastric juice, and constriction of smooth muscles of the bronchi and uterus.

histamine blocking agent, a substance that interferes with stimulation of cells by histamine.

histamine headache, a headache associated with the release of histamine from the body tissues and marked by symptoms of dilated carotid arteries, fluid accumulation under the eyes, tearing or lacrimation, and rhinorrhea (runny nose).

histamine-proved achlorhydria [Gk, histos, tissue, amine + a, not, chlorhydria, hydrochloric acid], the absence of normal hydrochloric acid production by cells in the lining of the stomach as demonstrated by the **histamine test.**

histamine test [Gk, histos, tissue, amine + L, testum, crucible], a test for achylia gastrica, or the lack of hydrochloric acid in the stomach. The stomach is emptied and washed out before subcutaneous injection of 0.1% histamine to stimulate gastric acid secretion. The stomach is aspirated continuously. If no acid is produced, that outcome is considered evidence that the stomach is not producing hydrochloric acid.

histenzyme /histen'zīm/, a renal tissue enzyme that splits hippuric acid into glycine and benzoic acid.

histidine (His) /his'tidēn/ [Gk, histos, tissue], a basic amino acid found in many proteins and a precursor of histamine. It is an essential amino acid in infants.

histidinemia /his'tidinē'mē·ə/, an inherited metabolic disorder caused by an enzyme defect involving l-histidine ammonia lyase and affecting the amino acid histidine. The condition leads to retardation and nervous system disorders.

histioblast /his'tē·, a tissue-forming cell.

histiocytic malignant lymphoma /his'-tē·ōsit'ik/ [Gk, histos + kytos, cell], a lymphoid neoplasm containing undifferentiated primitive cells or differentiated reticulum cells.

histiotypic growth /his'tē·ōtip'ik/ [Gk, his-

H

tos + *typos*, mark], the uncontrolled proliferation of cells, as occurs in bacterial cultures and molds.

histocompatibility /his′tōkəmpat′ibil′itē/ [Gk, *histos*, tissue; L, *compatibilis*, agreeing], a measure of the similarity of the antigens of donor and recipient of transplanted tissue.

histocompatibility antigens [Gk, *histos* + L, *compatibilis*, agreeable], a group of genetically determined antigens on the surface of many cells. They are the cause of most graft rejections.

histocompatibility complex, a group of genes whose products determine the compatibility of tissues or organs transplanted from one individual to another of the same species or from one species to another.

histocompatibility gene [Gk, *histos*, tissue; L, *compatibilis* + *genein*, to produce], the gene that determines histocompatibility of the donor and recipient of transplanted tissue.

histocompatibility locus, a set of positions on a chromosome occupied by a complex of genes that govern several tissue antigens.

histocyte /his′təsīt/ [Gk, *histion*, web, *kytos*, cell], a macrophage of connective tissue that plays a role in the body's immune system.

histogram /his′təgram′/ [Gk, *histos* + *gramma*, record], (in research) a graph showing the values of one or more variables plotted against time or against frequency of occurrence.

histography /histog′rəfē/ [Gk, *histos* + *graphein*, to record], the process of describing or creating visualizations of tissues and cells. —**histographer,** *n.,* **histographic,** *adj.,* **histographically,** *adv.*

histoincompatible /his′tō·in′kəmpat′əbəl/, pertaining to host and donor tissues that have different genotypes and are therefore likely to induce an immune response, leading to rejection of a tissue graft or organ transplant.

histologic [Gk, *histos*, tissue, *logos*, science], pertaining to the study of the microscopic anatomic and physiologic characteristics of tissues and the cells found therein.

histologic technician/technologist, an allied health professional who works in a clinical laboratory preparing sections of body tissue for examination by a pathologist. This process includes preparation of tissue specimens of human and animal origin for diagnostic, research, or teaching purposes. The tissue sections enable the pathologist to diagnose body dysfunction and malignancy.

histologist /histol′əjist/, a medical scientist who specializes in the study of the structure of organ tissues, including the composition of cells and their organization into various body tissues.

histology /histol′əjē/ [Gk, *histos* + *logos*, science], **1.** the science dealing with the microscopic identification of cells and tissue. **2.** the structure of organ tissues, including the composition of cells and their organization into various body tissues. —**histologic, histological,** *adj.*

histolysis [Gk, *histos*, tissue, *lysis*, loosening], breakdown or dissolution of living organic tissue.

histolytic /his′tōlit′ik/, pertaining to or causing the breakdown or dissolution of living organic tissue.

histone /his′tōn/ [Gk, *histos*, tissue], any of a group of strongly basic low–molecular weight proteins that are soluble in water and insoluble in dilute ammonia and combine with nucleic acid to form nucleoproteins. They are found in the cell nucleus.

histopathology /his′tōpəthol′əjē/ [Gk, *histos*, tissue, *pathos*, disease, *logos*, science], the study of diseases involving the tissue cells.

histoplasma agglutinin /-plaz′mə/ [Gk, *histos* + *plasma*, a formation], a specific antibody that interacts with antigens, causing clumping that is associated with fungal lung infections.

Histoplasma capsulatum [Gk, *histos* + *plasma* + L, *capsula*, little box], a dimorphic fungal organism that is a single budding yeast at body temperature and a mold at room temperature. It is the causative organism in histoplasmosis.

histoplasmin test /-plaz′min/, a skin test for diagnosis of an infection caused by *Histoplasma capsulatum* fungus.

histoplasmosis /his′tōplazmō′sis/ [Gk, *histos* + *plasma* + *osis*, condition], an infection caused by inhalation of spores of the fungus *Histoplasma capsulatum.* Primary histoplasmosis is characterized by fever, malaise, cough, and lymphadenopathy. Progressive histoplasmosis, the sometimes fatal disseminated form of the infection, is characterized by ulcerating sores in the mouth and nose; enlargement of the spleen, liver, and lymph nodes; and severe and extensive infiltration of the lungs.

history /his′tərē/ [L, *historia,* inquiry], **1.** a record of past events. **2.** a systematic account of the medical, emotional, and psychosocial occurrences in a patient's life and of factors in the family, ancestors, and environment that may have a bearing on the patient's condition.

history of present illness, an account obtained during the interview with the patient of the onset, duration, and character of the present illness, as well as of any acts or factors that aggravate or ameliorate the symptoms.

histotoxin /-tok′sin/ [Gk, *histos* + *toxikon*, poison], any substance that is poisonous to the body tissues. It is usually generated within the body rather than being introduced externally.

histrionic /his′trē·on′ik/ [L, *histrio*, actor], pertaining to exaggerated facial expressions, speech, or body movements, such as used on the stage.

histrionic paralysis [L, *histrio*, actor; Gk, *paralyein*], a condition such as **Bell's palsy** in which paralysis of facial muscles results in dramatic, excitable behavior.

histrionic personality [L, *histrio*, actor, *persona*, role played], a personality characterized by behavioral patterns and attitudes that are overreactive, emotionally unstable, overly dramatic, and self-centered, exhibited as a means of attracting attention, consciously or unconsciously.

histrionic personality disorder, a disorder characterized by dramatic, reactive, and intensely exaggerated behavior, which is typically self-centered. It results in severe disturbance in interpersonal relationships that can lead to psychosomatic disorders, depression, alcoholism, and drug dependency.

His-Werner disease [Wilhelm His, Jr., German physician, 1863–1934; Heinrich Werner, German physician, 1874–1947; Gk, *dis*, not; Fr, *aise*, ease], trench fever, an acute louse-borne infection that mainly affected soldiers in World War I.

HIV, abbreviation for **human immuno-deficiency virus.**

HIVNET, an international vaccine test network organized to conduct studies of prospective vaccines for human immunodeficiency virus (HIV) infection. It also supports behavioral and other studies of HIV infections.

HLA, abbreviation for **human leukocyte antigen.**

HLA-A, abbreviation for *human leukocyte antigen A.*

HLA-B, abbreviation for *human leukocyte antigen B.*

HLA complex, human leukocyte antigen group A, the major human histocompatibility complex that enables the immune system to differentiate tissues or proteins between "self" and "nonself." It consists of groups of loci on the short arm of chromosome 6. They are identified by numbers and letters, such as HLA-B27. HLA-A, -B, and -C are cell surface antigens that

occur on the surface of all nucleated cells and platelets and are important in tissue transplantation. If donor and recipient HLA antigens do not match, the nonself antigens are recognized and destroyed by killer T cells.

HLA-D, abbreviation for *human leukocyte antigen D.*

HLH, abbreviation for *human luteinizing hormone.*

HMD, abbreviation for *hyaline membrane disease.*

HME, abbreviation for *human monocytic erlichiosis.*

HMG-CoA reductase, a rate-controlling enzyme of cholesterol synthesis.

HMO, abbreviation for **health maintenance organization.**

Ho, symbol for the element **holmium.**

H₂O, symbol for **water.**

hoarseness /hôrs′nəs/, a condition marked by a rough, harsh, grating voice, indicating an inflammation of the throat and larynx.

Hodgkin's disease /hoj′kinz/ [Thomas Hodgkin, English physician, 1798–1866], a malignant disorder characterized by painless, progressive enlargement of lymphoid tissue, usually first evident in cervical lymph nodes; splenomegaly; and the presence of Sternberg-Reed cells, large, atypical macrophages with multiple or hyperlobulated nuclei and prominent nucleoli. Symptoms include anorexia, weight loss, generalized pruritus, low-grade fever, night sweats, anemia, and leukocytosis. There is a threefold increased risk of development of Hodgkin's disease in first-degree relatives, suggesting an unknown genetic mechanism.

Hodgson's disease /hoj′sənz/ [Joseph Hodgson, English physician, 1788–1869; Gk, *dis*, not; Fr, *aise*, ease], an aneurysmal dilation of the aorta.

Hoffmann's reflex [Johann Hoffmann, German neurologist, 1857–1919], an abnormal reflex elicited by sudden forceful flicking of the nail of the index, middle, or ring finger, which causes flexion of the thumb and of the middle and distal phalanges of one of the other fingers.

holandric /holan′drik/ [Gk, *holos*, whole, *aner*, man], **1.** designating genes located on the nonhomologous part of the Y chromosome. **2.** pertaining to traits or conditions transmitted only through the paternal line.

holandric inheritance, the acquisition or expression of traits or conditions only through the paternal line, transmitted by genes carried on the nonhomologous part of the Y chromosome.

hold-relax, a technique of facilitating

neuromuscular sensation and awareness. It is used in treating hypertonicity or motor dysfunction. It is often applied when there is muscle tightness on one side of a joint and when immobility is the result of pain.

holism /hō′lizəm/ [Gk, *holos,* whole], a philosophic concept in which an entity is seen as more than the sum of its parts.

holistic /hōlis′tik/ [Gk, *holos*], pertaining to the whole; considering all factors, as holistic medicine.

holistic counseling, an alternative form of psychotherapy that focuses on the whole person (mind, body, and spirit) and health.

holistic health care, a system of comprehensive or total patient care that considers the physical, emotional, social, economic, and spiritual needs of the person; his or her response to illness; and the effect of the illness on the ability to meet self-care needs. Holistic nursing is the modern nursing practice that expresses this philosophy of care.

Holliday-Segar formula, a method of estimating the daily caloric needs of the average hospital patient under conditions of bed rest, based on the body weight in kilograms of the patient.

hollow cathode lamp [ME, *holg* + Gk, *kata,* down, *hodos,* way, *lampas*], a lamp consisting of a metal cathode and an inert gas.

holmium (Ho) /hōl′mē·əm/ [L, *Holmia,* Stockholm, Sweden], a rare earth metallic element. Its atomic number is 67; its atomic mass (weight) is 164.93.

holoacardius /hol′ō·ākär′dē·əs/ [Gk, *holos* + *kardia,* heart], a separate, grossly defective monozygotic twin fetus.

holoacardius acephalus, a grossly defective separate twin fetus that lacks a heart, a head, and most of the upper part of the body.

holoacardius acormus, a grossly defective, separate twin fetus in which the trunk is malformed and little more than the head is recognizable.

holoacardius amorphus, a malformed separate twin fetus in which there are no recognizable or formed parts.

holoarthritis /-ärthrī′tis/, a form of arthritis that involves all or most of the joints.

holoblastic /hol′əblas′tik/ [Gk, *holos* + *blastos,* germ], pertaining to an ovum that contains little or no yolk and undergoes total cleavage.

holocephalic /hō′lōsifal′ik/ [Gk, *holos* + *kephale,* head], a malformed fetus in which several parts are deficient although the head is complete.

holocrine /hol′əkrēn/ [Gk, *holos,* whole,

krienein, to secrete], pertaining to a gland whose only function is to secrete or whose secretion consists of disintegrated cells of the gland itself.

holocrine secretion [Gk, *holos,* whole, *krienein,* to secrete], a secretion that consists of disintegrated or altered cells of the gland, as in the example of sebaceous glands.

holoendemic /hol′ō·endem′ik/, pertaining to an intensely endemic disease area.

holoenzyme /hol′ō·en′zīm/ [Gk, *holos* + *en,* in, *zymos,* ferment], a complete enzyme-cofactor complex that gives rise to full catalytic activity.

holographic reconstruction /-graf′ik/, a method of producing three-dimensional images with diagnostic ultrasound equipment.

hologynic /hol′ōjin′ik/ [Gk, *holos* + *gyne,* female], **1.** designating genes located on attached X chromosomes. **2.** pertaining to traits or conditions transmitted only through the maternal line.

hologynic inheritance, the acquisition or expression of traits or conditions only through the maternal line, transmitted by genes located on attached X chromosomes. The phenomenon is not known to occur in humans.

holoprosencephaly /hol′ōpros′ensef′əlē/ [Gk, *holos* + *pro,* before, *enkephalos,* brain], a congenital defect characterized by multiple midline facial defects, including cyclopia in severe cases. **—holoprosencephalic, holoprosencephalous,** *adj.*

Holter monitor [Norman J. Holter, American biophysicist, 1914–1983; L, *monere,* to remind], trademark for a device for making prolonged electrocardiograph recordings (usually 24 hours) on a portable tape recorder while the patient conducts normal daily activities.

Holtzman inkblot technique, a modification of the Rorschach test in which many more pictures of inkblots are used, the subject is permitted only one response to each design, and the scoring is predominantly objective rather than subjective.

Homans' sign [John Homans, American surgeon, 1877–1954; L, *signum,* mark], pain in the calf with dorsiflexion of the foot, indicating thrombophlebitis or thrombosis.

home assessment [AS, *ham,* village; L, *assidere,* to sit beside], an examination of the living area of a physically challenged person for the purposes of making recommendations about elimination of safety hazards and suggesting architectural or other modifications that would allow for independent functioning.

home care [AS, *ham,* village; L, *garrire,* to chatter], a health service provided in the patient's place of residence for the purpose of promoting, maintaining, or restoring health or minimizing the effects of illness and disability. Service may include such elements as medical, dental, and nursing care; speech and physical therapy; homemaking services of a home health aide; and provision of transportation.

home health agency, an organization that provides health care in the home. Medicare certification for a home health agency in the United States requires provision of skilled nursing services and at least one additional therapeutic service.

home health nurse, a registered nurse who visits patients in the home. The nurse works primarily in the area of secondary or tertiary care, providing hands-on care and educating the patient and family on care and prevention of future episodes.

homeless person, an individual who has no permanent home, haven, or domicile. Such individuals usually are indigent and depend on charity or public assistance for temporary lodging and medical care.

home maintenance management, impaired, a NANDA-accepted nursing diagnosis of the inability to independently maintain a safe, growth-promoting immediate environment. Defining characteristics include difficulty in maintaining the home, a need for help from the outside in maintaining the home, the existence of debt or a financial crisis. The critical defining characteristics, at least one of which must be present for the diagnosis to be made, are unwashed or unavailable cooking utensils, clothes, or linens; presence of accumulations of dirt, food, waste, and refuse; exhausted or distressed family or household members, and repeated infections and infestations resulting from a lack of hygiene.

homeodynamics /hō′mē·ədīnam′iks/ [Gk, *homoios,* similar, *dynamis,* force], the constantly changing interrelatedness of body components while maintaining an overall equilibrium.

homeomorphous /-môr′fəs/, similar in appearance but different in composition.

Homeopathic Pharmacopoeia of the United States, one of the three official drug compendia specified in the Federal Food, Drug, and Cosmetic Act.

homeopathist /hō′mē·op′əthist/, a physician who practices homeopathy.

homeopathy /hō′mē·op′əthē/ [Gk, *homoios,* similar, *pathos,* disease], a system of therapeutics based on the theory that "like cures like." The theory was advanced in the late eighteenth century by Dr. Samuel Hahnemann, who believed that a large amount of a particular drug may cause symptoms of a disease and moderate dosage may reduce those symptoms; thus some disease symptoms could be treated by very small doses of medicine. —**homeopathic,** *adj.*

homeostasis /hō′mē·əstā′sis/ [Gk, *homoios* + *stasis,* standing still], a relative constancy in the internal environment of the body, naturally maintained by adaptive responses that promote healthy survival. Various sensing, feedback, and control mechanisms function to effect this steady state. Some of the functions controlled by homeostatic mechanisms are heartbeat, hematopoiesis, blood pressure, body temperature, electrolytic balance, respiration, and glandular secretion. —**homeostatic,** *adj.*

homeotherapy /-ther′əpē/, the treatment or prevention of disease by homeopathic methods.

homeotic mutation /hō′mē·ot′ik/, a mutation that causes tissues to alter their normal differentiation pattern, producing integrated structures but in unusual locations.

homeotypic /hō′mē·ōtip′ik/ [Gk, *homoios* + *typos,* mark], pertaining to or characteristic of the regular or usual type, specifically applied to the second meiotic division of germ cells in gametogenesis, as distinguished from the first meiotic division.

homeotypic mitosis, the equational division of chromosomes, as occurs in the second meiotic division of germ cells in gametogenesis.

Home's silver precipitation method, (in dentistry) a technique for depositing silver in enamel and dentin by application of ammoniac silver nitrate solution and its reduction with formalin or eugenol.

homicide /hom′isīd/ [L, *homo,* man, *caedere,* to kill], the death of one human being caused by another. Homicide is usually intentional and often violent.

hominal physiology /hom′inəl/ [L, *hominis,* human; Gk, *physis,* nature, *logos,* science], the study of the specific physical and chemical processes involved in the normal functioning of humans; human physiology.

hominid /hom′inid/ [L, *homo,* man; Gk, *eidos,* form], pertaining to the primate family, Hominidae, which includes humans.

homoblastic /hō′mōblas′tik/ [Gk, *homos* + *blastos,* germ], developing from the same germ layer or a single type of tissue.

homochronous inheritance /hōmok′rənəs/ [Gk, *homos* + *chronos,* time], the ap-

homocysteine /-sis′tēn/, an amino acid containing sulfur and a homolog of cysteine, produced in the demethylation of methionine. It is also an intermediate product in the biosynthesis of cysteine from L-methionine via L-cystathionine in the breakdown of proteins. High levels of homocysteine are associated with an increased risk of collagen cardiovascular disorders.

homocystine /sis′tin/, a disulfide analog of homocysteine produced by the oxidation of homocysteine.

homocystinemia /-sis′tinē′mē·ə/, an amino acid disorder that causes an excess of homocystine in the blood.

homocystinuria /hō′mōsis′tinŏŏr′ē·ə/ [Gk, homos + (cystine); Gk, ouron, urine], a rare biochemical abnormality characterized by the abnormal presence of homocystine, an amino acid, in the blood and urine, which is caused by any of several enzyme deficiencies in the metabolic pathway of methionine to cystine. —**homocystinuric,** adj.

homogenate /hōmoj′ənit/, a tissue that is or has been made homogenous.

homogeneous /hō′mōjē′nē·əs/ [Gk, homos + genos, kind], **1.** consisting of similar elements or parts. **2.** having a uniform quality throughout. —**homogeneity,** adj.

homogenesis /hō′mōjen′əsis/ [Gk, homos + genesis, origin], reproduction by the same process in succeeding generations so that offspring are similar to the parents.

homogenetic /-jenet′ik/, **1.** pertaining to homogenesis. **2.** homogenous, def. 2.

homogenized /hōmoj′ənīzd/ [Gk, homos, same, genein, to produce], the state of having undergone homogenization: having a uniform texture or consistency throughout.

homogenized milk [Gk, homos + genos, kind], pasteurized milk that has been mechanically treated to reduce and emulsify the fat globules so that the cream cannot separate and the protein is more digestible.

homogenous /hōmoj′ənəs/ [Gk, homos + genos, kind], **1.** homogeneous. **2.** having a likeness in form or structure as a result of a common ancestral origin. **3.** homoplasty.

homogeny /hōmoj′ənē/ [Gk, homos + genos, kind], **1.** homogenesis. **2.** a likeness in structure or form that results from a common ancestral origin.

homoiothermic /hom′ē·əthur′mik/ [Gk, homos, same, therme, heat], pertaining to the ability of warm-blooded animals to maintain a relatively stable internal temperature, regardless of the temperature of the environment. This ability is not fully developed in newborn humans.

homolateral /hō′mōlat′ərəl/, pertaining to the same side of the body.

homolateral limb synkinesis, a condition of hemiplegia in which there appears to be a mutual dependency between the affected upper and lower limbs. Efforts at flexion of an upper extremity cause flexion of the lower extremity.

homolog /hom′əlog/ [Gk, homos, same], **1.** any organ corresponding in function, origin, and structure to another organ, as the flippers of a seal that correspond to human hands. **2.** (in chemistry) one of a series of compounds, each formed by an added common element; for example, CO, carbon monoxide, is followed by CO_2, carbon dioxide, with the addition of an oxygen atom. —**homologous,** adj.

homologous [Gk, homos, same, logos, relation], pertaining to corresponding attributes; similar in structure.

homologous anaphylaxis /hōmol′əgəs/ [Gk, homos, same, logos, relation, ana, back, phylaxis, protection], a form of passive anaphylaxis resulting from the transfer of serum between animals of the same species.

homologous chromosomes [Gk, homos, same, chroma color, soma body], any two chromosomes in the diploid complement of the somatic cell that are identical in size, shape, and gene loci. In humans there are 22 pairs of homologous chromosomes and 1 pair of sex chromosomes.

homologous graft [Gk, homos, same, logos, relation, graphein, stylus], a tissue removed from a donor for transplantation to a recipient of the same species.

homologous organs, [Gk, homos, same, logos, relation, organon, instrument], body parts of different species (or sexes) that are structural equivalents, such as the arms of humans and the forelegs of dogs and cats.

homologous tumor, a neoplasm made up of cells resembling those of the tissue in which it is growing.

homonymous /hōmon′iməs/ [Gk, homos, same, onyma, name], having the same name or sound.

homonymous diplopia [Gk, homos, same, onyma, name, diploos, double, opsis, vision], a type of diplopia in which the image observed by the right eye is located to the right of the image observed by the left eye.

homonymous hemianopia [Gk, homos + onyma, name], blindness or defective vi sion in the right or left halves of the visual fields of both eyes.

homophobia /hō'mōfō'bē·ə/ [Gk, *homos,* same, *phobos,* fear], the fear of or prejudice against homosexuals.

homoplastic transplantation [Gk, *homos,* same, *plassein,* to mold; L, *transplantare,* to transplant], the homologous transplantation of tissue from one human to another or from one animal to another of the same species.

homoplasty /hō'məplas'tē/ [Gk, *homos* + *plassein,* to mold], having a likeness in form or structure acquired through similar environmental conditions or parallel evolution rather than resulting from common ancestral origin. —**homoplastic,** *adj.*

homopolymer /hō'mōpol'imir/ [Gk, *homos* + *poly,* many, *meros,* part], a compound formed from subunits that are the same, such as a carbohydrate composed of a series of glucose units.

Homo sapiens /hō'mō sā'pē·əns, sä'pē·ens/ [L, *homo,* human, *sapere,* to know or taste], the scientific term for the genus and species identifying humans.

homosexual /-sek'shəl/ [Gk, *homos* + L, *sexus,* sex, gender], **1.** pertaining to or denoting the same sex. **2.** a person who is sexually attracted to members of the same sex.

homosexual panic, an acute attack of anxiety based on unconscious conflicts concerning gender identity and a fear of being homosexual.

homosexual sexual intercourse [Gk, *homos,* same; L, *sexus,* male or female, *intercursus,* interposition], sexual activity of members of the same sex ranging from feelings and fantasies to kissing and genital, oral, or anal contact.

homotopic pain /hō'mōtop'ik/, pain experienced at the point of injury.

homotype /hō'mōtīp/, any structure or body part, such as a hand or foot, that appears in reversed symmetry with a similar part.

homovanillic acid /hō'mōvənil'ik/, an acid that is produced by normal metabolism of dopamine and may occur at an elevated level in urine in association with tumors of the adrenal gland.

homozygosis /hō'mōzīgō'sis/ [Gk, *homos* + *zygon,* yoke], **1.** the formation of a zygote by the union of two gametes that have one or more pairs of identical genes. **2.** the production of purebred organisms or strains through the process of inbreeding.

homozygote /hō'məzī'gōt/ [Gk, *homos,* same, *zygon,* yoke], an organism whose somatic cells have identical genes on the same locus on one of the chromosome pairs.

homozygous /hō'məzī'gəs/ [Gk, *homos* + *zygon,* yoke], having two identical genes at corresponding loci on homologous chromosomes.

homunculus /hōmung'kyələs/, *pl.* **homunculi** [L, little man], **1.** a dwarf in whom all the body parts are proportionally developed and in which there is no deformity or abnormality. **2.** (in early embryologic theories of development, primarily preformation) a minute and complete human being contained in each of the germ cells that after fertilization grows from the microscopic to normal size. **3.** a small anatomic model of the human form; a manikin. **4.** (in psychiatry) a little man created by the imagination who possesses magical powers.

hook grasp, a type of prehension in which an object is grasped with the fingers alone.

hookworm [AS, *hok* + *wyrm*], nontechnical. a nematode of the genera *Ancylostoma, Necator,* and *Uncinaria.* Most hookworm infections in the Western Hemisphere are caused by the species *Necator americanus.*

hookworm disease [AS, *hok* + *wyrm* + Gk, *dis,* not; Fr, *aise,* ease], a roundworm infestation that may involve either of two important intestinal parasites of humans, *Ancylostoma duodenale* and *Necator americanus.* Both forms of the disease are characterized by abdominal pain and iron deficiency anemia. The worm enters the human body as a larva by penetrating the skin, traveling to the lungs via the circulatory system, and ascending the respiratory tract, where it is swallowed. In the intestinal tract the hookworm attaches its mouth to the mucosa and subsists on the blood of the host

hopelessness [AS, *hopian,* to hope, *laes,* less, *ness,* condition], a NANDA-accepted nursing diagnosis of a state in which an individual sees limited or no alternatives or personal choices available and is unable to mobilize energy on his or her own behalf. Defining characteristics include passivity, decreased verbalization, decreased affect, lack of initiative, decreased response to stimuli, turning away from the speaker, shrugging in response to the speaker, closing eyes, decreased appetite, increased or decreased sleep, and lack of involvement in care.

hordeolum /hôrdē'ələm/ [L, *hordeum,* barley], a furuncle of the margin of the eyelid originating in the sebaceous gland of an eyelash.

horizon /hôrī'zən/ [Gk, *horizein,* to en-

H

circle], a specific stage of human embryonic development determined by the appearance and ultimate formation of certain anatomic characteristics. The classification comprises 23 stages, each lasting 2 to 3 days, beginning with the fertilization of the ovum.

horizontal abdominal position /hôr'izon'təl/, prone position.

horizontal angulation [Gk, *horizein*, to encircle; L, *angularis*, angle], (in dentistry) the measured angle within the occlusal plane at which the primary x-ray beam is directed, relative to a reference in the vertical or sagittal plane.

horizontal fissure of the right lung, a cleft that marks the separation of the upper and middle lobes of the right lung.

horizontal plane [Gk, *horizein*, to encircle; L, *planum*, level ground], **1.** any plane of the erect body parallel to the horizon, dividing the body into upper and lower parts. **2.** a plane passing through a tooth at right angles to its long axis.

horizontal position, a position in which the patient lies on the back with the legs extended.

horizontal pursuit, a visual screening test in which the patient is asked to follow with both eyes a target moving in a horizontal plane while the examiner observes accuracy of alignment and supportive head movements.

horizontal resorption, a pattern of bone reduction in marginal periodontitis whereby the marginal crest of the alveolar bone between adjacent teeth remains level and the bases of the periodontal pockets are supracrestal.

horizontal transmission, the spread of an infectious agent from one person or group to another, usually through contact with contaminated material such as sputum or feces.

horizontal vertigo, a giddiness or feeling of instability experienced while lying down, frequently caused by a labyrinthine disorder.

hormic psychology /hôr'mic/ [Gk, *hormaien*, to begin action], (in psychology) the school that stresses the purposive, goal-oriented nature of human behavior.

hormonal /hôr'mōnəl/ [Gk, *hormaein*, to set in motion], pertaining to or resembling hormones.

hormone /hôr'mōn/ [Gk, *hormaein*, to set in motion], a complex chemical substance produced in one part or organ of the body that initiates or regulates the activity of an organ or a group of cells in another part. Hormones secreted by the endocrine glands are carried through the bloodstream to the target organ.

hormone therapy, the treatment of diseases with hormones obtained from endocrine glands or substances that simulate hormonal effects.

horn, a projection or protuberance on a body structure. Examples include the horn of the hyoid bone and the iliac horn.

Horner's syndrome [Johann F. Horner, Swiss ophthalmologist, 1831–1886], a neurologic condition characterized by miotic pupils, ptosis, and facial anhidrosis, which results from a lesion in the spinal cord, with damage to a cervical nerve.

horse serum [AS, *hors* + L, *serum*, whey], immune serum prepared from the blood of a horse. Because many people are sensitive to horse serum, a skin test for sensitivity is recommended before immunization.

horseshoe fistula /hôrs'shoo͞o/ [AS, *hors* + *scoh*, shoe], an abnormal semicircular passage in the perianal area with both openings on the surface of the skin.

horseshoe kidney, a relatively common congenital anomaly characterized by an isthmus of parenchymal tissue connecting the two kidneys at the lower poles.

hospice /hos'pis/ [L, *hospes*, host], a system of family-centered care designed to assist the terminally ill person to be comfortable and to maintain a satisfactory lifestyle through the phases of dying.

hospital /hos'pitəl/ [L, *hospitium*, guesthouse], a health care facility that provides inpatient beds, continuous nursing services, and an organized medical staff. Diagnosis and treatment are provided to both surgical and medical patients for a variety of diseases and disorders.

hospital clinic, a medical center that furnishes space, supplies, and equipment and contracts with physicians to provide patient services. The hospital bills the patient for technical and professional services dispensed.

hospitalism /hos'pitəliz'əm/, the physical or mental effects of hospitalization or institutionalization on patients, especially infants and children in whom the condition is characterized by social regression, personality disorders, and stunted growth.

host /hōst/ [L, *hospes*], **1.** an organism in which another, usually parasitic organism is nourished and harbored. A primary or **definitive host** is one in which the adult parasite lives and reproduces. A secondary or **intermediate host** is one in which the parasite exists in its nonsexual, larval stage. A **reservoir host** is a primary animal host for organisms that are sometimes parasitic in humans and through which humans may become infected. **2.** the recipient of a transplanted organ or tissue.

host defense mechanisms, a group of

body protective systems, including physical barriers and the immune response, that normally guard against infective organisms.

hostility /hostil′itē/ [L, *hostilis,* hostile], an emotional state characterized by enmity toward others and a desire to harm those at whom the antagonism is directed. The hostility may be expressed passively and actively.

hot bath [AS, *hat* + *baeth*], a bath in which the temperature of the water is gradually raised to about 106° F.

hot compress [AS, *hat* + L, *comprimere,* to press together], a heated pad of damp, thickly folded cloth applied to an area to reduce pain or inflammation.

hot flash, a transient sensation of warmth experienced by some women during or after menopause. Hot flashes result from autonomic vasomotor disturbances that accompany changes in the neurohormonal activity of the ovaries, hypothalamus, and pituitary.

hot line, a means of contacting a trained counselor or specific agency for help with a particular problem, such as a rape hot line or a battered child hot line. The person needing help calls a telephone number and speaks to a counselor, who remains anonymous.

hot spot, 1. (in molecular genetics) a site in a gene sequence at which mutations occur with an unusually high frequency. **2.** (in nuclear medicine) an area on a nuclear medicine image that has an abnormally high amount of detected radiation as the result of increased absorption of radionuclide.

Hounsfield unit /hounz′fēld/, [Godfrey N. Hounsfield, twentieth-century English scientist] (in computed tomography) the numeric information contained in each pixel. It has a relationship to the composition and nature of the tissue imaged.

hourglass uterus [Gk, *hora* + AS, *glaes*], a uterus in which a segment of circular muscle fibers contracts during labor, causing constriction ring dystocia.

housekeeping department, a unit of a hospital staff responsible for cleaning the hospital premises and furnishings, including controlling pathogenic organisms.

housemaid's knee [AS, *hus* + *maeden* + *cneow,* knee], a chronic inflammation of the bursa in front of the kneecap, characterized by redness and swelling. It is caused by prolonged and repetitive pressure of the knee on a hard surface.

house organ, a publication designed for distribution to the employees or members of an institution or business.

house physician [AS, *hus* + Gk, *physikos,*

natural], a physician on call and immediately available in a hospital or other health care facility.

house staff, the interns and residents who are employed at a hospital while receiving additional training after graduation from medical college.

house surgeon, a surgeon on call and immediately available on the premises of a hospital.

housewives' eczema [AS, *hus* + *wif* + Gk, *ekzein,* to boil over], *nontechnical.* contact dermatitis of the hands caused and exacerbated by their frequent immersion in water and by the use of soaps and detergents.

Howell-Jolly bodies /hou′əljol′ē/ [William H. Howell, American physiologist, 1860–1945; Justin M. J. Jolly, French histologist, 1870–1953], spheric and granular inclusions in the erythrocytes observed on microscopic examination of stained blood smears.

HPG, abbreviation for *human pituitary gonadotropin.*

HPL, abbreviation for **human placental lactogen.**

HPV, 1. abbreviation for **human papilloma virus. 2.** abbreviation for **human parvovirus.**

hr, abbreviation for *hour.*

HRIG, abbreviation for *human rabies immune globulin* vaccine.

HRSA, abbreviation for **Health Resources and Services Administration.**

hs, h.s., abbreviation for the Latin *hora somni,* at bedtime.

HSA, abbreviation for **health systems agency.**

HsP, abbreviation for **heat shock protein.**

HSV, abbreviation for *herpes simplex virus.*

HSV1, abbreviation for *herpes simplex virus type 1.*

ht, abbreviation for **height.**

HTLV-I, abbreviation for **human T-cell lymphotropic virus-I.**

HTLV-II, abbreviation for **human T-cell lymphotropic virus-II.**

HTLV-III, abbreviation for **human T-cell lymphotropic virus-III.**

Hubbard tank [Carl P. Hubbard, American engineer, b. 1857; Port, *tanque*], a large whirlpool tank containing warm water in which patients can perform underwater exercise. The patient's trunk and extremities are submerged on a stretcher. The water provides buoyancy and heat for the benefit of weakened or painful muscles or joints with limited active range of motion.

huffing, a type of forced expiration with

an open glottis to replace coughing when pain limits normal coughing.

HUGO /hyo͞o′gō, an acronym for **Human Genome Organization.**

Huhner test /ho͞o′nər/ [Max Huhner, American urologist, 1873–1947], a test for male fertility in which a semen sample aspirated from the vagina within an hour after coitus is examined for spermatozoal activity.

Huhn's gland, an anterior lingual gland embedded in tissues on the inferior surface and near the apex and midline of the tongue.

human /h(y)o͞o′mən/ [L, *humanus*], a member of the genus *Homo* and particularly of the species *H. sapiens.*

human bite [L, *humanus* + AS, *bitan*], a wound caused by the piercing of skin by human teeth. Bacteria are usually present, and serious infection often follows.

human chorionic somatomammotropin (HCS), a hormone produced by the syncytiotrophoblast during pregnancy. It regulates carbohydrate and protein metabolism of the mother.

human diploid cell rabies vaccine (HDCV), an inactivated rabies virus vaccine prepared from rabies virus grown in human diploid cell cultures. Active immunization with HDCV begins on the day of exposure, followed by four or five additional injections.

human ecology, the study of interrelationships between individuals and their environments, as well as among individuals within the environment.

Human Genome Organization (HUGO), an international group established in 1989 to coordinate activities concerned with the human genome project, including the distribution of funding and dissemination of information.

human immunodeficiency virus (HIV-1) /im′yo͞onō′difish′ənsē/ [L, *humanus* + *immunis*, free from, *de*, from, *facere*, to make, *virus*, poison], a retrovirus that causes acquired immunodeficiency syndrome (AIDS). Retroviruses produce the enzyme reverse transcriptase, which allows transcription of the viral genome onto the deoxyribonucleic acid of the host cell. It is transmitted through contact with an infected individual's blood, semen, breast milk, cervical secretions, cerebrospinal fluid, or synovial fluid. HIV infects T-helper cells of the immune system and causes infection with a long incubation period, averaging 10 years. With the immune system destroyed, AIDS develops as opportunistic infections such as **Kaposi's sarcoma,** *Pneumocystis carinii* **pneumonia, candidiasis,** and **tuberculosis** that at-

tack organ systems throughout the body. Aside from the initial antibody tests (enzyme-linked immunosorbent assay and Western blot) that establish the diagnosis for HIV infection, the most important laboratory test for monitoring the level of infection is the CD4 lymphocyte test, which determines the percentage of T lymphocytes that are CD4 positive.

human insulin, a biosynthetic product manufactured from *Escherichia coli* by recombinant deoxyribonucleic acid technology. The advantage of human insulin is that it eliminates allergic reactions that occur with the use of animal insulins.

human investigations committee, a group established in a hospital, school, or university to review research proposals involving human subjects to protect the rights of the people to be studied.

humanism /h(y)o͞o′məniz′əm/, a system of thought pertaining to the interests, needs, and welfare of human beings.

humanistic existential therapy /hyo͞o′mənis′tik/, a kind of psychotherapy that promotes self-awareness and personal growth by stressing current reality and by analyzing and altering specific patterns of response to help a person realize his or her potential.

humanistic nursing model, a conceptual framework in which the nurse-patient relationship is analyzed as a human-to-human event rather than a nurse-to-patient interaction.

humanistic psychology, a branch of psychology that emphasizes a person's struggle to develop and maintain an integrated, harmonious personality as the primary motivational force in human behavior.

human leukocyte antigen (HLA), any one of four significant genetic markers identified as specific loci on chromosome 6: HLA-A, HLA-B, HLA-C, and HLA-D. Each locus has several genetically determined alleles; each of these is associated with certain diseases or conditions.

human natural killer cell, a lymphocyte that is able to lyse tumor and virally infected cells as part of the body's natural defense against malignancy and invasion by pathogens.

human papilloma virus (HPV), a virus that is the cause of common warts of the hands and feet, as well as lesions of the mucous membranes. The virus can be transmitted through sexual contact and is a precursor to cancer of the cervix.

human parvovirus (HPV), a small single-stranded deoxyribonucleic acid virion that has been associated with several diseases, including erythema infectiosum and aplastic crises of chronic hemolytic anemias.

human placental lactogen (HPL), a placental hormone that may be deficient in certain abnormalities of pregnancy.

human prion diseases [L, *humanus* + *proteinaceous infection particle* + Gk, *dis,* not; Fr, *aise,* ease], a group of neurodegenerative diseases that are unique in having both infectious and genetic causes. Examples include **Creutzfeldt-Jakob's disease (CJD)** and Gerstmann-Straussler's syndrome. A homozygous prion protein genotype predisposes individuals to susceptibility to the diseases.

human protein C, an anticoagulant that inactivates coagulation cofactors 5 and 8c and mediates clot lysis by tissue plasminogen activator (t-PA).

human rhinovirus 14, the common cold virus. It has a complex protein coat containing "sticky sites" that help attach the virus to cell receptors in the upper respiratory system.

human T-cell lymphotropic virus-I (HTLV-I), one of several type C oncoviruses with an affinity for helper and inducer T lymphocytes. HTLV-I is a source of T cell leukemia/lymphoma that causes chronic infection and is associated with tropical spastic paraparesis.

human T-cell lymphotropic virus-II (HTLV-II), a type C oncovirus with serologic cross-reactivity with HTLV-I. It has been associated with hairy cell leukemia and various hematologic diseases.

human T-cell lymphotropic virus-III (HTLV-III), a slow-acting virus associated with acquired immunodeficiency virus.

humectant /hyōōmek'tənt/, a substance that promotes retention of moisture.

humerus /hyoo'mərəs/, *pl.* **humeri** [L, *shoulder*] the bone of the upper arm, comprising a body, a head, and a condyle. The nearly hemispheric head articulates with the glenoid cavity of the scapula and has a constriction called the surgical neck, frequently the seat of a fracture. The condyle at the distal end has several depressions into which articulate the radius and ulna. —**humeral,** *adj.*

humidification /hyōōmid'ifikā'shən/ [L, *humiditas,* moist, *facere,* to make], the process of increasing the relative humidity of the atmosphere around a patient through the use of aerosol generators or steam inhalers that exert an antitussive effect. Humidification acts by decreasing the viscosity of bronchial secretions.

humidifier /hyōōmid'ifī'ər/ [L, *humidus,* moist, *facere,* to make], a machine designed to adjust the amount of moisture in

the atmosphere of a room or respiratory device.

humidity /hyōōmid'itē/ [L, *humidus,* moist], pertaining to the level of moisture in the atmosphere, which varies with the temperature. The percentage is usually represented in terms of **relative humidity,** with 100% the point of air saturation, or the level at which the air can absorb no additional water.

humor /hyōō'mər/ [L, *humidus,* moist], any body fluid such as blood or lymph. The term is often used in reference to the **aqueous humor** or the **vitreous humor** of the eye.

humoral immunity /hyōō'mərəl/ [L, *humor,* liquid, *immunis,* freedom], one of the two forms of immunity that respond to antigens such as bacteria and foreign tissue. Humoral immunity is the result of circulating antibodies carried in the immunoglobulins IgA, IgB, and IgM.

humoral response, one of a broad category of hypersensitivity reactions. Humoral responses are mediated by B cell lymphocytes and occur in type I, type II, and type III hypersensitivity reactions.

humpback /hump'bak/ [Du, *homp,* thick slice; AS, *baec*], a colloquial term for **kyphosis,** an abnormal curvature of the cervicothoracic spine.

hunger, a physical sensation usually associated with a craving or desire for food.

hunger contractions, strong contractions of the stomach usually associated with a desire for food.

hunger pain, epigastric cramps often associated with a desire for food.

hung-up reflex, a deep tendon reflex in which, after a stimulus is given and the reflex action takes place, the limb slowly returns to its neutral position.

Hunter's syndrome [Charles Hunter, Canadian physician, 1873–1955; Gk, *syn,* together, *dromos,* course], a hereditary defect in mucopolysaccharide metabolism affecting only males, characterized by dwarfism, kyphosis, gargoylism, and mental retardation.

Huntington's chorea [George S. Huntington, American physician, 1851–1916; Gk, *choreia,* dance], a rare abnormal hereditary condition characterized by chronic progressive chorea and mental deterioration that terminates in dementia. An individual afflicted with the condition usually shows the first signs in the fourth decade of life and dies within 15 years.

Hurler's syndrome [Gertrude Hurler, German physician, 1889–1965], a type of mucopolysaccharidosis, transmitted as an autosomal-recessive trait, that produces severe mental retardation. Characteristic

H

signs of the disease are enlargement of the liver and spleen, often with cardiovascular involvement. Facial characteristics include a low forehead and enlargement of the head, sometimes resulting from hydrocephalus.

Hürthle cell tumor /hirt'lə, hōōrth'lē/ [Karl W. Hürthle, German histologist, 1860–1945], a neoplasm of the thyroid gland composed of large cells with granular eosinophilic cytoplasm (Hürthle cells); it may be benign (Hürthle cell adenoma) or malignant (Hürthle cell carcinoma).

Hutchinson's freckle [Jonathan Hutchinson, English surgeon, 1828–1913], a tan patch on the skin that grows slowly and becomes mottled, dark, thick, and nodular. The lesion is usually seen on one side of the face of an elderly person.

Hutchinson's teeth [Jonathan Hutchinson], a characteristic of congenital syphilis in which the permanent lateral incisor teeth are peg-shaped, widely spaced, and notched at the end with a centrally placed crescent-shaped deformity.

Hutchinson's triad [Jonathan Hutchinson], the interstitial keratitis, notched teeth, and deafness characteristic of congenital syphilis.

Hutchison-type neuroblastoma [Robert G. Hutchison, English pediatrician, 1871–1960; Gk, typos, mark], a neuroblastoma that has metastasized to the cranium.

HUTT, abbreviation for **heads-up tilt table test.**

HVA, abbreviation for **homovanillic acid.**

HV interval /in'tərvəl/, (in cardiology) the conduction time through the His-Purkinje system. It is measured from the onset of the His potential to the onset of ventricular activation as recorded on an electrogram.

HVL, abbreviation for **half-value layer.**

hyaline /hī'əlin/ [Gk, hyalos, glass], pertaining to substances that are clear or glasslike.

hyaline bodies [Gk, hyalos + AS, bodig], **1.** the residue of colloidal degeneration found in some cells. **2.** globules of neurosecretory material found in the posterior lobe of the pituitary. **3.** deposits of homogenous eosinophilic material found in renal tubular epithelium and representing excess protein molecules that cannot be metabolized or transported.

hyaline cartilage [Gk, hyalos, glass; L, cartilago], a type of elastic connective tissue composed of specialized cells in a translucent, pearly blue matrix. Hyaline cartilage thinly covers the articulating ends of bones; connects the ribs to the

sternum; and supports the nose, the trachea, and part of the larynx.

hyaline cast, a transparent cast composed of mucoprotein.

hyaline membrane [Gk, hyalos, glass; L, membrana], a fibrous covering of acinar epithelium in infants caused by a lack of pulmonary surfactant associated with prematurity and low birth weight.

hyaline thrombus, a translucent colorless mass consisting of hemolyzed erythrocytes.

hyalinuria /-ŏŏr'ē·ə/ [Gk, hyalos, glass, ouron, urine], the presence of hyaline casts of protein in the acid pH of urine.

hyaloid /hī'əloid/ [Gk, hyalos, glass, eidos, form], pertaining to or resembling hyaline.

hyaloid artery [Gk, hyalos + eidos, form], an embryonic blood vessel that branches to supply the vitreous body of the eye. It persists in the adult as a narrow passage through the vitreous body from the optic disc to the posterior surface of the crystalline lens.

hyaloid membrane [Gk, hyalos, glass; L, membrana], a surface layer of the vitreous body of the eye, at the interface between the primary and secondary vitreous and at the boundaries of the hyaloid canal.

hyaloplasm /hī'əlōplaz'əm/ [Gk, hyalos + plasma, formation], the part of the cytoplasm that is clear and more fluid than the granular and reticular part.

hyaluronic acid /hī'əlyŏŏron'ik/, a mucopolysaccharide formed by the polymerization of acetylglucosamine and glucuronic acid. Known as the cement substance of tissues, it forms a gel in intercellular spaces.

hyaluronidase /hī'əlyŏŏron'ədās/, an enzyme that hydrolyzes hyaluronic acid. It is prescribed to increase the absorption and dispersion of other parenteral drugs, for hypodermoclysis, and for improvement of resorption of radiopaque agents.

hybrid /hī'brid/ [L, hybrida, offspring], **1.** an offspring produced by mating plants or animals from different species, varieties, or genotypes. **2.** pertaining to such a plant or animal.

hybridization /hī'bridīzā'shən/, **1.** the process of producing hybrids by crossbreeding. **2.** (in molecular genetics) the process of combining single-stranded nucleic acids whose base composition is identical but whose base sequence is different to form stable double-stranded duplex molecules.

hybridoma /hī'bridō'mə/, a hybrid cell formed by the fusion of a myeloma cell and an antibody-producing cell. Hybridomas are used in the production of monoclonal antibodies.

hybrid subtraction, a two-step subtraction method for producing digitalized radiographic images that uses at least four images.

hydantoin /hīdan′tō·in/, any one of a group of anticonvulsant medications, chemically and pharmacologically similar to the barbiturates, that act to limit seizure activity and reduce the spreading of abnormal electrical excitation from the focus of the seizure.

hydatid /hī′dətid/ [Gk, *hydatis,* water drop], a cyst or cystlike structure that usually is filled with fluid, especially the cyst formed around the developing scolex of the dog tapeworm *Echinococcus granulosus.* —**hydatic,** *adj.*

hydatid cyst, a cyst in the liver that contains larvae of the tapeworm *Echinococcus granulosus,* whose eggs are carried from the intestinal tract to the liver via the portal circulation. Patients are generally asymptomatic, except for hepatomegaly and a dull ache over the right upper quadrant of the abdomen.

hydatidiform /hī′dədid′ifôrm/ [Gk, *hydatis,* water drop; L, *forma*], having the appearance or form of a **hydatid.**

hydatid mole, an intrauterine neoplastic mass of grapelike enlarged chorionic villi. Characteristic signs are extreme nausea, uterine bleeding, anemia, hyperthyroidism, an unusually large uterus for the duration of pregnancy, absence of fetal heart sounds, edema, and high blood pressure.

hydatidosis /hī′dətidō′sis/ [Gk, *hydatis* + *osis,* condition], infestation with the tapeworm *Echinococcus granulosus.*

hydradenitis /hī′dradəni′tis/ [Gk, *hydos,* water, *aden,* gland, *itis,* inflammation], an infection or inflammation of the sweat glands.

hydralazine /hīdral′əzēn/, a vasodilator prescribed in the treatment of hypertension.

hydramnios /hīdram′nē·əs/ [Gk, *hydos* + *amnos,* lamb's caul], an abnormal condition of pregnancy characterized by an excess of amniotic fluid. It is associated with maternal disorders, including toxemia of pregnancy and diabetes mellitus.

hydranencephaly /hī′dran′ənsef′əlē/, a neurologic disorder in which the cerebral hemispheres are lacking, although the cerebellum, brainstem, and other central nervous system tissues may be intact. The newborn with hydranencephaly may have normal neurologic functions but does not develop.

hydrate /hī′drāt/ [Gk, *hydor,* water], **1.** a combination of a substance with one or more water molecules. **2.** a molecular association of a substance with water.

hydration /hīdrā′shən/ [Gk, *hydor,* water], a chemical process in which water is taken up (added) without disrupting the rest of the molecule.

hydremic ascites /hīdrem′ik/ [Gk, *hydor* + *haima,* blood, *askos,* bag], an abnormal accumulation of fluid within the peritoneal cavity accompanied by hemodilution, as in protein calorie malnutrition.

hydroa /hīdrō′ə/ [Gk, *hydor* + *oon,* egg], an unusual vesicular and bullous skin condition of childhood that recurs each summer after exposure to sunlight, sometimes accompanied by itching and lichenification.

hydrobilirubin /hī′drōbil′iroo̅′bin/ [Gk, *hydor,* water; L, *bilis,* bile, *ruber,* red], a reddish-brown bile pigment produced by the reduction of bilirubin.

hydrocarbon /-kär′bən/ [Gk, *hydor* + L, *carbo,* charcoal], any of a large group of organic compounds whose molecules are composed of hydrogen and carbon, many of which are derived from petroleum.

hydrocele /hī′drōsēl′/ [Gk, *hydor* + *kele,* hernia], an accumulation of fluid in any saclike cavity or duct, specifically in the tunica vaginalis testis or along the spermatic cord. The condition is caused by inflammation of the epididymis or testis or by lymphatic or venous obstruction in the cord.

hydrocephalic cry /-səfal′ik/, an involuntary loud nighttime cry of a child who has acquired hydrocephalus.

hydrocephalocoele, a hernia consisting of a watery sac of brain tissue protruding through a fissure into the skull.

hydrocephalus /-sef′ələs/ [Gk, *hydor* + *kephale,* head], a pathologic condition characterized by an abnormal accumulation of cerebrospinal fluid, usually under increased pressure, within the cranial vault and subsequent dilation of the ventricles. Interference with the normal flow of cerebrospinal fluid may result from increased secretion of the fluid, obstruction within the ventricular system (noncommunicating or intraventricular hydrocephalus), or defective resorption from the cerebral subarachnoid space (communicating or extraventricular hydrocephalus), caused by developmental anomalies, infection, trauma, or brain tumors.

hydrochloric acid /-klôr′ik/ [Gk, *hydor* + *chloros,* green], an aqueous solution of hydrogen and chlorine. Hydrochloric acid is secreted in the stomach and is a major component of gastric juice.

H

hydrochlorothiazide /-klôr′ōthī′əzīd/, a thiazide diuretic and antihypertensive prescribed in the treatment of hypertension and edema.

hydrocholeretics /-kō′ləret′iks/ [Gk, *hydor* + *chloe,* bile, *eresis,* removal], drugs that stimulate the production of bile with a low specific gravity or with a minimal proportion of solid constituents.

hydrocodone bitartrate /-kō′dōn/, a narcotic antitussive prescribed in the treatment of cough.

hydrocolloid, a gelatinous colloid in which water is the dispersion material. It is used in dentistry as an impression material.

hydrocortisone valerate /-kôr′tisōn/, a topical corticosteroid prescribed for skin inflammation.

hydroflumethiazide /-flōō′methī′əzīd/, a diuretic and antihypertensive prescribed in the treatment of hypertension and edema.

hydrogel, a gel in which water is the dispersion medium.

hydrogen (H) /hī′drəjən/ [Gk, *hydor* + *genein,* to produce], a gaseous univalent element. Its atomic number is 1; its atomic mass (weight) is 1.008. It is the simplest and lightest of the elements and is normally a colorless, odorless, highly inflammable diatomic gas. It occurs in pure form only sparsely in the earth and the atmosphere but is plentiful in the sun and in many other stars. Hydrogen is a component of numerous compounds, many of them produced by the body. As a component of water, hydrogen is crucial in the metabolic interaction of acids, bases, and salts within the body and in the fluid balance necessary for the body to survive.

hydrogenase /hī′drōjənās′/ [Gk, *hydor,* water, *genein,* to produce, *ase,* suffix indicating an enzyme], an enzyme that catalyzes reduction of molecules by combining them with molecular hydrogen.

hydrogen bonding, the attractive force of compounds in which a hydrogen atom covalently linked to an electronegative element such as oxygen, nitrogen, or fluorine has a large degree of positive character relative to the electronegative atom, thereby causing the compound to possess a large dipole.

hydrogen cyanide (HCN), a colorless, toxic, volatile liquid or gas with the aroma of bitter almonds. It occurs naturally in almonds and in the stone pits of peaches, plums, and other fruits. When dissolved in water, it is called hydrocyanic acid, prussic acid.

hydrogen donor, a compound that gives up hydrogen (usually H^+, a proton) to another compound.

hydrogen ion [H^+], a positively charged hydrogen atom.

hydrogen ion [H^+] concentration of blood, a measure of blood pH and its effect on the ability of the hemoglobin molecule to hold oxygen.

hydrogen peroxide, a topical antiinfective prescribed for cleansing of open wounds, as a mouthwash, and for the removal of cerumen from the external ear.

hydrokinetics /-kinet′iks/ [Gk, *hydor,* water, *kinesis,* motion], the study of movement of fluids.

hydrolase /hī′drōlās/, an enzyme that cleaves ester bonds by the addition of water.

hydrolysis /hīdrol′isis/ [Gk, *hydor* + *lysis,* loosening], the chemical alteration or decomposition of a compound with water.

hydrolytic /-lit′ik/ [Gk, *hydor,* water, *lysis,* loosening], pertaining to or having the ability to produce hydrolysis.

hydrolyze /hī′drōlīz/ [Gk, *hydor,* water, *lysis,* loosening], **1.** to cause or bring about hydrolysis. **2.** to cause a substance to split into component parts by the addition of water.

hydrometer /hīdrom′ətər/ [Gk, *hydor* + *metron,* measure], a device that determines the specific gravity or density of a liquid by a comparison of its weight with that of an equal volume of water. A calibrated hollow glass device is placed in the liquid being examined, and the depth to which the device settles in the liquid is noted.

hydromorphone hydrochloride /-môr′-fōn/, a narcotic analgesic used to treat moderate to severe pain.

hydronephrosis /hī′drōnefrō′sis/ [Gk, *hydor* + *nephros,* kidney, *osis,* condition], distension of the pelvis and calyces of the kidney by urine that cannot flow past an obstruction in a ureter. Ureteral obstruction may be caused by a tumor, a calculus lodged in the ureter, inflammation of the prostate gland, or edema caused by a urinary tract infection. The person may experience pain in the flank and in some cases hematuria, pyuria, and hyperpyrexia. —**hydronephrotic,** *adj.*

hydropenia /-pē′nē·ə/, lack of water in the body tissues.

hydropericarditis, inflammation of the pericardium accompanied by excessive accumulation of serous fluid.

hydropericardium, an excessive accumulation of fluid in the pericardium.

hydroperitoneum /-per′itōnē′əm/, an accumulation of fluid in the peritoneum.

hydrophilic /-fil′ik/ [Gk, *hydor* + *philein,*

to love], pertaining to the property of attracting water molecules, possessed by polar radicals or ions.

hydrophobia /-fō'bē-ə/ [Gk, *hydor* + *phobos,* fear], **1.** *nontechnical.* rabies. **2.** a morbid, extreme fear of water.

hydrophobiaphobia, a morbid fear of hydrophobia, with symptoms that may simulate those of rabies.

hydrophobic [Gk, *hydor* + *phobos,* fear], pertaining to the property of repelling water molecules, a quality possessed by nonpolar radicals or molecules that are more soluble in organic solvents than in water.

hydrophone /hī'drəfōn/, a small diameter probe with a piezoelectric element, usually about 0.5 mm in diameter, at one end. When placed in an ultrasound beam, the hydrophone produces an electric signal.

hydropic /hīdrop'ik/ [Gk, *hydrops*], pertaining to the condition of dropsy.

hydrops /hī'drops/ [Gk, dropsy], an abnormal accumulation of clear watery or serous fluid in a body tissue or cavity such as a joint, a graafian follicle, a fallopian tube, the abdomen, the middle ear, or the gallbladder.

hydrops fetalis, massive edema in the fetus or newborn, usually in association with severe erythroblastosis fetalis. Severe anemia and effusions of the pericardial, pleural, and peritoneal spaces also occur.

hydrops gravidarum [Gk, *hydor,* water; L, *gravidus,* pregnant], edema caused by pregnancy.

hydroquinone /hī'drōkwin'ōn/, a dermatologic bleaching agent prescribed to reduce pigmentation of the skin in certain conditions in which an excess of melanin causes hyperpigmentation.

hydrosalpinx /hī'drōsal'pingks/ [Gk, *hydor* + *salpinx,* tube], an abnormal condition of the fallopian tube in which it is cystically enlarged and filled with clear fluid. It is the result of an infection that has previously occluded the tube at both ends.

hydrosis [Gk, *hydor,* water, *osis,* condition], pertaining to the production of sweat.

hydrostatic /-stat'ik/ [Gk, *hydor,* water, *statos,* standing], pertaining to fluids at rest or in equilibrium and the pressure they exert.

hydrostatic pressure, the pressure exerted by a liquid.

hydrostatic dosimetry, the weighing of a person under water to determine the ratio of lean tissue to body fat.

hydrostatics, the study of pressures in liquids at rest or in equilibrium.

hydrotherapy /-ther'əpē/ [Gk, *hydor* + *therapeia,* treatment], the use of water in the treatment of various disorders. Hydrotherapy may include continuous tub baths, wet sheet packs, or shower sprays.

hydrothorax /-thôr'aks/ [Gk, *hydor* + *thorax,* chest], a noninflammatory accumulation of serous fluid in one or both pleural cavities.

hydrotropism /-trō'pizəm/ [Gk, *hydor* + *trope,* turning], the tendency of a cell or organism to turn or move in a certain direction under the influence of a water stimulus.

hydrous /hī'drəs/ [Gk, *hydor,* water], pertaining to a substance or object that contains water or is moist.

hydroxide /hīdrok'sīd/, an ion with the formula OH⁻.

hydroxyamphetamine hydrobromide /hīdrok'se-əmfet'əmēn/, an adrenergic and mydriatic prescribed for dilation of the pupil for ophthalmoscopy and as a diagnostic aid in Horner's syndrome.

hydroxyandrosterone /hīdrok'se·andros'-tərōn/ [Gk *hydor* + *andros,* male, *stereos,* solid], a sex hormone secreted by the testes and adrenal glands.

hydroxyapatite /hīdrok'se·ap'ətīt/, an inorganic compound composed of calcium, phosphate, and hydroxide. It is found in the bones and teeth in a crystallized latticelike form that gives these structures rigidity.

hydroxychloroquine sulfate /-klôr'əkwīn/, an antiprotozoal antirheumatic drug that is also a suppressant of lupus erythematosus and of polymorphous light eruption. It is prescribed in the treatment of malaria and the suppression of acute paroxysmal attacks of the disease; in the treatment of extraintestinal, usually hepatic, amebiasis; and in the reduction of symptoms of lupus erythematosus and rheumatoid arthritis.

17-hydroxycorticosteroid /-kôr'tikos'-təroid/, any steroid hydroxylated at carbon-17 secreted by adrenal glands and measured in the urine in a test for determining adrenal function and diagnosing hypoadrenalism or hyperadrenalism.

11-hydroxyetiocholanolone /hīdrok'se-ē'-tē-ōkolan'əlōn/, a sex hormone secreted by the testes and adrenal glands.

5-hydroxyindoleacetic acid /hīdrok'se·in'-dōlē·əset'ik/, an acid produced by serotonin metabolism, measured in the blood and urine to aid in the diagnosis of certain kinds of tumors. It commonly rises above normal levels in whole blood in association with asthma, diarrhea, rapid heartbeat, and other symptoms and is elevated in the urine of patients with carcinoid syndrome.

hydroxyl (OH) /hīdrok'sil/, a monovalent radical consisting of an oxygen and a hydrogen atom.

hydroxyprogesterone caproate /-prōjes'-tərōn/, a progestational steroid prescribed in the treatment of advanced adenocarcinoma of the uterine corpus, amenorrhea, and abnormal uterine bleeding caused by hormonal imbalance in the absence of organic disease.

hydroxyproline /-prō'lēn/, an amino acid whose level is elevated in the urine in diseases of the bone and certain genetic disorders such as Marfan's syndrome.

hydroxyurea /hīdrok′siyoorē′ə/, an antineoplastic prescribed in the treatment of a variety of neoplasms.

hydroxyzine hydrochloride /hīdrok'-səzēn/, a minor tranquilizer/antihistamine prescribed to relieve anxiety, nervous tension, hyperkinesis, itching, and motion sickness.

hygiene /hī'jēn [Gk, *Hygieia,* the goddess of health], the principles and science of the preservation of health and prevention of disease.

hygienist /hī'jənist, hījē'nist/ [Gk, *Hygieia*], one who practices the principles and laws of **hygiene.**

hygrometer /hīgrom'ətər/ [Gk, *hygros,* moist, *metron,* measure], an instrument that directly measures relative humidity of the atmosphere or the proportion of water in a specific gas or gas mixture, without extracting the moisture.

hygroscopic humidifier /-skop'ik/, a humidifying device attached to the tubing circuit of a mechanical ventilator or anesthesia gas machine to maintain a constant rate of humidity in the trachea.

hymen /hī'mən/ [Gk, membrane], a fold of mucous membrane, skin, and fibrous tissue at the introitus of the vagina. It may be absent, small, thin and pliant, or rarely tough and dense, completely occluding the introitus.

hymenal /hī'mənəl/ [Gk, *hymen,* membrane], pertaining to the hymen.

hymenal tag, normal redundant hymenal tissue protruding from the floor of the vagina during the first weeks after birth.

hymenectomy /hī'mənek'təmē/ [Gk, *hymen,* membrane, *ektome,* excision], the surgical excision of a membrane, particularly the hymen.

Hymenolepis /hī'minol'əpis/ [Gk, *hymen* + *lepis,* rind], a genus of intestinal tapeworms that infest humans, such as *Hymenolepis nana,* the dwarf tapeworm, and *H. diminuta.* Heavy infestation by *H. nana* may cause abdominal pain, bloody stools, and disorders of the nervous system, especially in children. Contaminated food spreads the disease.

hymenotomy /hī'mənot'əmē/ [Gk, *hymen* + *temnein,* to cut], the surgical incision of the hymen.

hyoglossal [Gk, *hyoeides* + *glossa,* tongue], pertaining to the tongue and the horseshoe-shaped hyoid bone at the base of the tongue immediately above the thyroid cartilage.

hyoglossal membrane /-glos'əl/, a widening of the lingual septum connecting the root of the tongue to the hyoid bone.

hyoglossus /-glos'əs/ [Gk, *hyoeides* + *glossa,* tongue], a depressor muscle of the tongue that arises from the hyoid bone.

hyoid /hī'oid/ [Gk, *hyoeides,* upsilon, U-shaped], **1.** the hyoid bone. **2.** pertaining to the hyoid bone.

hyoid arch [Gk, *hyoeides* + L, *arcus,* bow], the second pharyngeal or branchial arch. It is present in typical form in the embryo, but the skeletal elements develop into the stapes and styloid process of the temporal bone of the adult.

hyoid bone /hī'oid/ [Gk, *hyoeides,* upsilon, U-shaped; AS, *ban,* bone], a single U-shaped bone suspended from the styloid processes of the temporal bones. The body of the bone attaches to various muscles such as the hypoglossus and the sternohyoideus.

hyoscyamine /hī'əsī'əmēn/, an anticholinergic prescribed in the treatment of hypermotility of the gastrointestinal and lower urinary tracts.

hypalgesia /hī'paljē'zē·ə/ [Gk, *hypo,* below, *algesis,* pain], the perception of a painful stimulus to a degree that varies significantly from a normal perception of the same stimulus.

hyperacidity /-əsid'itē/ [Gk, *hyper,* excess; L, *acidus,* sour], an excessive amount of acidity, as in the stomach.

hyperactivity /-aktiv'itē/ [Gk, *hyper* + L, *activus,* active], any abnormally increased motor activity or function involving either the entire organism or a particular organ such as the heart or thyroid.

hyperacuity /akyoo'itē/ [Gk, *hyper,* excessive, *akouien,* to hear], excessive sensitivity to sounds.

hyperadenosis /-ad'ənō'sis/ [Gk, *hyper,* excessive, *aden,* gland, *osis,* condition], a condition characterized by enlarged glands.

hyperalbuminemia /albyoo''minē'mē·ə/, an excessive amount of albumin in the blood.

hyperalgia /-al'jə/, extreme sensitivity to pain.

hyperalimentation /-al'iməntā'shən/ [Gk, *hyper* + L, *alimentum,* nourishment], overfeeding or the ingestion or administration of an amount of nutrients that exceeds the demands of the appetite.

hyperalkalinity /-al'kəlin'itē/, a condition of excessive alkalinity.

hyperammonemia /hī'pəram'ōnē'mē·ə/ [Gk, *hyper* + (ammonia), *haima*, blood], abnormally high levels of ammonia in the blood. Untreated, the condition leads to hepatic encephalopathy characterized by asterixis, vomiting, lethargy, coma, and death.

hyperbaric chamber /-ber'ik/ [Gk, *hyper,* excess, *baros,* weight, *kamara,* arched roof], an airtight chamber containing an oxygen atmosphere under high pressure. A patient may be placed in the chamber for the treatment of certain infections, tumors, and cardiovascular diseases in which atmospheric oxygen pressures up to three times normal may have therapeutic value.

hyperbaric oxygenation [Gk, *hyper* + *baros,* weight, *oxys,* sharp, *genein,* to produce], the administration of oxygen at greater than normal atmospheric pressure. The procedure is performed in specially designed chambers that permit the delivery of 100% oxygen at atmospheric pressure that is three times normal. The technique is used to overcome the natural limit of oxygen solubility in blood, which is about 0.3 ml of oxygen per 100 ml of blood. Hyperbaric oxygenation has been used to treat carbon monoxide poisoning, air embolism, smoke inhalation, acute cyanide poisoning, decompression sickness, clostridial myonecrosis, and certain cases of blood loss or anemia in which increased oxygen transport may compensate in part for hemoglobin deficiency.

hyperbaric solution [Gk, *hyper,* excess, *baros,* weight], a type of spinal anesthetic that has a specific gravity greater than that of cerebrospinal fluid so it will settle into the lowest parts of the spinal canal.

hyperbarism /-ber'izəm/, any disorder resulting from exposure to increased ambient pressure, usually caused by sudden exposure to or a significant increase in pressure.

hyperbetalipoproteinemia /hī'pərbā'tə lip'ōprō'tēnē'mē·ə/ [Gk, *hyper* + *beta,* second letter of Greek alphabet, *lipos,* fat, *proteios,* first rank, *haima,* blood], type II hyperlipoproteinemia, a genetic disorder of lipid metabolism in which there are abnormally high levels of serum cholesterol and xanthomas appear on the tendons of the heels, knees, and fingers.

hyperbilirubinemia /hī'pərbil'iroo'binē'-mē·ə/ [Gk, *hyper* + L, *bilis,* bile, *ruber,* red; Gk, *haima,* blood], greater than normal amounts of the bile pigment bilirubin in the blood, often characterized by jaundice, anorexia, and malaise. Hyperbilirubinemia is most often associated with liver disease or biliary obstruction, but it also occurs when there is excessive destruction of red blood cells.

hyperbilirubinemia of the newborn, an excess of bilirubin in the blood of the neonate. It is usually caused by a deficiency of an enzyme that results from physiologic immaturity, or by increased hemolysis, especially that produced by blood group incompatibility, which, in severe cases, can lead to kernicterus.

hypercalcemia /hī'pərkalsē'mē·ə/ [Gk, *hyper* + L, *calx,* lime; Gk, *haima,* blood], greater than normal amounts of calcium in the blood, most often resulting from excessive bone resorption and release of calcium, as occurs in hyperparathyroidism, metastatic tumors of bone, Paget's disease, and osteoporosis. Clinically patients with hypercalcemia are confused and have anorexia, abdominal pain, muscle pain, and weakness. —**hypercalcemic,** *adj.*

hypercalcemic nephropathy /-kalsē'mik/ [Gk, *hyper,* excessive; L, *calx,* lime, *haima,* blood; Gk, *nephros,* kidney, *pathos,* disease], a progressive disorder of kidney function caused by an excessive level of calcium in the blood. The calcium causes cumulative functional and histologic abnormalities that lead to a decreased glomerular filtration rate and kidney failure.

hypercalciuria /hī'pərkal'sēyŏŏr'ē·ə/ [Gk, *hyper* + L, *calx,* lime; Gk, *ouron,* urine], the presence of abnormally great amounts of calcium in the urine, resulting from conditions such as sarcoid, hyperparathyroidism, or certain types of arthritis that are characterized by augmented bone resorption. Concentrated amounts of calcium in the urinary tract may form kidney stones. —**hypercalciuric,** *adj.*

hypercapnia /hī'pərkap'nē·ə/ [Gk, *hyper* + *kapnos,* vapor], greater than normal amounts of carbon dioxide in the blood.

hypercapnic acidosis /-kap'nik/ [Gk, *hyper,* excessive, *kapnos,* vapor; L, *acidus,* sour, *osis,* condition], an excessive acidity in body fluids caused by an increase in carbon dioxide tension in the blood. The condition may be secondary to pulmonary insufficiency; as carbon dioxide accumulates in the blood, its acidity increases.

hyperchloremia /-klôrē'mē·ə/ [Gk, *hyper* + *chloros,* green, *haima,* blood], an excessive level of chloride in the blood that results in acidosis.

hyperchlorhydria /-klôrhid'rē·ə [Gk, *hyper* + *chloros* + *hydor,* water], the ex-

H

cessive secretion of hydrochloric acid by cells lining the stomach.

hypercholesterolemia /-kōles'tərōlē'mē·ə/ [Gk, *hyper* + *chole,* bile, *stereos,* solid, *haima,* blood], a condition in which greater than normal amounts of cholesterol are present in the blood. High levels of cholesterol and other lipids may lead to the development of atherosclerosis.

hyperchromia /-krō'mē·ə/ [Gk, *hyper,* excessive, *chroma,* color], an increase of hemoglobin in the erythrocytes.

hyperchromic /-krō'mik/ [Gk, *hyper* + *chroma,* color], having a greater density of color or pigment.

hyperchylomicronemia /-kī'lōmī'krōnē'-mē·ə/ [Gk, *hyper* + *chylos,* juice, *mikros,* small, *haima,* blood], type I hyperlipoproteinemia, a rare congenital deficiency of an enzyme essential to fat metabolism. Fat accumulates in the blood as chylomicrons. The condition affects children and young adults, in whom xanthomas (fatty deposits) in the skin, hepatomegaly, and abdominal pain develop.

hypercoagulability /-kō·ag'yələbil'itē/ [Gk, *hyper* + L, *coagulare,* to curdle, *habilis,* able], a tendency of the blood to coagulate more rapidly than normal.

hyperdynamic syndrome /-dīnam'ik/ [Gk, *hyper* + *dynamis,* force], a cluster of symptoms that signal the onset of septic shock, often including a shaking chill, rapid rise in temperature, flushing of the skin, galloping pulse, and alternating rise and fall of the blood pressure. This is a medical emergency treated by keeping the patient warm, elevating the legs to assist venous return, usually ordering intravenous fluids and antibiotics, and managing blood pressure.

hyperemesis gravidarum /hī'pərem'isis/ [Gk, *hyper* + *emesis,* vomiting; L, *gravida,* pregnant], an abnormal condition of pregnancy characterized by protracted vomiting, weight loss, and fluid and electrolyte imbalance. If the condition is severe and intractable, brain damage, liver and kidney failure, and death may result. Dry mucous membranes are a sign of dehydration. Other signs include decreased skin elasticity, a rapid pulse, and falling blood pressure. The volume of urine excreted falls. The hematocrit is elevated because of hemoconcentration. Loss of electrolytes in vomitus leads to metabolic acidosis with hypokalemia, hypochloremia, and hyponatremia. Forceful vomiting may cause retinal hemorrhages that impair vision and gastroesophageal tears that bleed, causing hematemesis or melena.

hyperemesis lactentium, a condition of excessive vomiting by infants.

hyperemia /hī'pərē'mē·ə/ [Gk, *hyper* + *haima,* blood], an excess of blood in part of the body, caused by increased blood flow, as in the inflammatory response, local relaxation of arterioles, or obstruction of the outflow of blood from an area. Skin overlying a hyperemic area usually becomes reddened and warm. **—hyperemic,** *adj.*

hyperesthesia /-esthē'zhə/, an extreme sensitivity of one of the body's sense organs such as pain or touch receptors in the skin.

hyperextension /-ikten'shən/ [Gk, *hyper* + L, *extendere,* to stretch out], (of a joint) a position of maximum extension.

hyperextension bed, a bed used in pediatric orthopedics to maintain any correction achieved by suspension of a body part and to increase the range of motion of the hips after an operative muscle release procedure.

hyperextension suspension, an orthopedic procedure used in the postoperative positioning of hip muscles. The procedure uses traction equipment, including metal frames, ropes, and pulleys to relieve the weight of the lower limbs and to position the muscles of the hip properly, without applying traction to the involved lower limbs.

hyperflexia /-flek'shə/ [Gk, *hyper* + L, *flectere,* to bend], the forcible overflexion or bending of a limb.

hyperfunction /-fungk'shən/ [Gk, *hyper* + L, *functio,* performance], increased function of any organ or system.

hypergenesis /-jen'əsis/ [Gk, *hyper* + *genesis,* origin], excessive growth or overdevelopment. The condition may involve the entire body, as in gigantism, or any part, or it may result in the formation of extra parts, such as additional fingers or toes. **—hypergenetic,** *adj.*

hypergenetic teratism /-jənet'ik/ [Gk, *hyper+ genesis* + *teras,* monster], a congenital anomaly in which there is excessive growth of a part, an organ, or the entire body, as in gigantism.

hypergenitalism /-jen'itəliz'əm/, the presence of abnormally large external genitalia. The condition is usually associated with precocious puberty.

hyperglobulinemia /-glob'yəlinē'mē·ə/ [Gk, *hyper,* excessive; L, *globulus,* small globe, *haima,* blood], an excess of globulin in the blood.

hyperglycemia /hī'pərglīsē'mē·ə/ [Gk, *hyper* + *glykys,* sweet, *haima,* blood], a greater than normal amount of glucose in the blood. Most frequently associated with diabetes mellitus, the condition may occur in newborns, after the administration of glucocorticoid hormones, and with an excess infusion of intravenous solutions containing glucose.

hyperglycemic-hyperosmolar nonketotic coma /-glīsē′mik/ [Gk, *hyper* + *glykys* + *hyper* + *osmos,* impulse; L, *non,* not, (ketone); Gk, deep sleep], a diabetic coma in which the level of ketone bodies is normal; caused by hyperosmolarity of extracellular fluid and resulting in dehydration of intracellular fluid, often a consequence of overtreatment with hyperosmolar solutions.

hyperglyceridemia /-glī′səridē′mē·ə/ [Gk, *hyper,* excessive, *glykys* + *haima,* blood], an excess of glycerides, particularly triglycerides, in the blood.

hyperglycogenolysis /-glī′kōjənol′isis/, excessive breaking down of glycogen and its conversion to glucose in animal tissue.

hyperglycosemia /-glī′kəsē′mē·ə/, an excess of sugar in the blood.

hyperglycosuria /-glī′kōsŏŏr′ē·ə/, an excess of sugar in the urine.

hypergonadism /-gō′nədiz′əm/ [Gk, *hyper,* excessive, *gone,* seed], excessive activity of the ovaries or testes.

hyperhidrosis /hī′pərhīdrō′sis, -hidrō′sis/ [Gk, *hyper* + *hidros,* perspiration], excessive perspiration often caused by heat, hyperthyroidism, strong emotion, menopause, or infection.

hyperimmune /-imyōōn′/ [Gk, *hyper* + L, *immunis,* freedom], a characteristic associated with an unusual abundance of antibodies, producing a greater than normal immunity.

hyperimmune plasma, plasma containing extremely high levels of antibodies.

hyperinsulinism /-in′səliniz′əm/ [Gk, *hyper* + L, *insula,* island], an excessive amount of insulin in the body. It may be caused by administration of an insulin dose greater than required.

hyperirritability /-irit′əbil′itē/ [Gk, *hyper,* excessive; L, *irritare,* to tease], excessive excitability or sensitivity, or exaggerated response to a stimulus.

hyperkalemia /hī′pərkəlē′mē·ə/ [Gk, *hyper* + L, *kalium,* potassium; Gk, *haima,* blood], greater than normal amounts of potassium in the blood. This condition is seen frequently in acute renal failure, massive trauma, major burns, and Addison's disease. Early signs are nausea, diarrhea, and muscle weakness.

hyperkeratinization /-ker′ətinīzā′shən/ [Gk, *hyper,* excessive, *keras,* horn], an abnormal horny thickening of the epithelium of the palms and soles.

hyperkeratosis /-ker′ətō′sis/ [Gk, *hyper* +

keras, horn, *osis,* condition], overgrowth of the cornified epithelial layer of the skin.

hyperketonemia /-kē′tōnē′mē·ə/, an abnormally high level of ketone bodies in the blood.

hyperketonuria /-kē′tōnŏŏr′ē·ə/, an abnormally high level of ketone bodies in the urine.

hyperlactation /-laktā′shən/, a condition in which lactation continues beyond the usual period of breast-feeding.

hyperlipemia /-lipē′mē·ə/, an excessive level of blood fats, usually caused by a lipoprotein lipase deficiency or a defect in the conversion of low-density lipoprotein to high-density lipoprotein.

hyperlipidemia /-lip′idē′mē·ə/ [Gk, *hyper* + *lipos,* fat, *haima,* blood], an excess of lipids, including glycolipids, lipoproteins, and phospholipids, in the plasma.

hyperlipidemia type I, a condition of elevated lipid levels in the blood, characterized by an increase in both cholesterol and triglycerides and caused by the presence of chylomicrons. It is inherited as an autosomal-recessive trait with a low risk of atherosclerosis.

hyperlipidemia type IIA, hyperlipidemia type IIB. See **familial hypercholesterolemia.**

hyperlipidemia type III. See **broad beta disease.**

hyperlipidemia type IV, a relatively common form of hyperlipoproteinemia characterized by a slight elevation in cholesterol levels, a moderate elevation of triglyceride levels, and an elevation of the normal triglyceride carrier protein very low-density lipoprotein level. It is sometimes familial and is associated with an increased risk for coronary atherosclerosis.

hyperlipidemia type V, a condition of elevated blood lipid levels, characterized by slightly increased cholesterol level, greatly increased triglyceride level, elevation of the triglyceride carrier protein very low-density lipoprotein level, and chylomicrons. It is a genetically heterogenous disorder.

hyperlipoproteinemia /hī′pərlip′ōprō′-tēnē′mē·ə/ [Gk, *hyper* + *lipos,* fat, *proteios,* first rank, *haima,* blood], any of a large group of inherited and acquired disorders of lipoprotein metabolism. They are characterized by greater than normal amounts of certain protein-bound lipids and other fatty substances in the blood.

hypermagnesemia /hī′pərmag′nisē′mē·ə/ [Gk *hyper* + *magnesia* magnesium, *haima,* blood], a greater than normal amount of magnesium in the plasma, found in people with kidney failure and in those who use large doses of drugs con-

H

taining magnesium, such as antacids. Toxic levels of magnesium cause cardiac arrhythmias and depression of deep tendon reflexes and respiration.

hypermature cataract /-məchŏŏr'/ [Gk, *hyper,* excessive; L, *maturare,* to make ripe; Gk, *katarrhaktes,* portcullis], an opaque lens that has lost water and has become soft and reduced in size.

hypermetabolic state /-met'əbol'ik/, an abnormally increased rate of metabolism, as in a high fever or hyperthyroidism.

hypermetabolism /-mətab'əliz'əm/, increased metabolism, usually accompanied by excessive body heat.

hypermetaplasia /-met'əplā'zhə/, an abnormal increase in the rate of transformation of one kind of tissue into another, as in the development of tumors.

hypermetria /hī'pərmē'trē·ə/ [Gk, *hyper* + *metron,* measure], an abnormal condition, a form of dysmetria, characterized by a dysfunction of the power to control the range of muscular action and causing movements that overreach the intended goal of the affected individual.

hypermnesia /hī'pərm·nē'zhə/, an extraordinarily good state of memory.

hypermobility /-mōbil'itē/ [Gk, *hyper,* excessive; L, *mobilis,* movable], a form of laxity characterized by an abnormally wide range of movement of the joints. The condition is seen in children and may be associated with **Marfan's syndrome** or degenerative joint diseases.

hypermorph /hī'pərmôrf'/ [Gk, *hyper* + *morphe,* form], **1.** a person whose arms and legs are disproportionately long in relation to the trunk and whose sitting height is disproportionate to the standing height. **2.** (in genetics) a mutant gene that shows an increased activity in the expression of a trait.

hypermotility /-motil'itē/, an excessive movement of the involuntary muscles, particularly in the gastrointestinal tract.

hypernatremia /hī'pərnatrē'mē·ə/ [Gk, *hyper* + L, *natrium,* sodium], a greater than normal concentration of sodium in the blood, caused by excessive loss of water and electrolytes that results from polyuria, diarrhea, excessive sweating, or inadequate water intake. People with hypernatremia may become mentally confused, have seizures, and lapse into coma. Care must be taken to restore water balance slowly, because further electrolyte imbalances may occur.

hyperopia /-ō'pē·ə/ [Gk, *hyper* + *ops,* eye], farsightedness, or an inability of the eye to focus on nearby objects. It results from an error of refraction in which rays of light entering the eye are brought into focus behind the retina.

hyperorchidism /-ôr'kidiz'əm/ [Gk, *hyper,* excessive, *orchis,* testis], excessive endocrine activity of the testes.

hyperornithinemia /-ôr'nithinē'mē·ə/, a metabolic disorder involving the amino acid ornithine, which tends to accumulate in the tissues, causing seizures and retardation.

hyperosmia /-oz'mē·ə/, an abnormally increased sensitivity to odors.

hyperosmolarity /-oz'məler'itē/ [Gk, *hyper* + *osmos,* impulse], a state or condition of abnormally increased osmolarity. —**hyperosmolar,** *adj.*

hyperosmotic /-osmot'ik/, pertaining to an increased concentration of osmotically active components.

hyperostosis /-ostō'sis/ [Gk, *hyper,* excessive, *osteon,* bone, *osis,* condition], an overgrowth of bone. It may involve adjacent cartilage or occur as a bone swelling or osteoma.

hyperoxaluria /-ok'səlŏŏr'ē·ə/, an excessive level of oxalic acid or oxalates, primarily calcium oxalate, in the urine. An excess of oxalates may lead to the formation of renal calculi and renal failure.

hyperoxemia /-oksē'mē·ə/ [Gk, *hyper,* excessive, *oxys,* sharp, *haima,* blood], increased oxygen content of the blood.

hyperoxia /-ok'sē·ə/, abnormally high oxygen tension in the blood.

hyperoxygenation /-ok'sijonā'shən/ [Gk, *hyper* + *oxys,* sharp, *genein,* to produce], the use of high concentrations of inspired oxygen before and after endotracheal aspiration.

hyperparathyroidism /-per'əthī'roidiz'-əm/ [Gk, *hyper* + *para,* beside, *thyreos,* shield, *eidos,* form], an abnormal endocrine condition characterized by hyperactivity of any of the four parathyroid glands with excessive secretion of parathyroid hormone, increased resorption of calcium from the skeletal system, and increased absorption of calcium by the kidneys and gastrointestinal system. The condition may be primary, originating in one or more of the parathyroid glands, or secondary, resulting from an abnormal hypocalcemia-producing condition in another part of the body, which causes a compensatory hyperactivity of the parathyroid glands.

hyperperistalis /-per'istal'is/ [Gk, *hyper,* excessive, *peristellein,* to clasp], a state of excessive motility of the waves of alternate contractions and relaxations that propel contents forward through the digestive tract.

hyperphenylalaninemia /hī'pərfen'ilal'-əninē'mē-ə/ [Gk, *hyper* + (phenylalanine), *haima*, blood], an abnormally high concentration of phenylalanine in the blood. This symptom may be the result of one of several defects in the metabolic process of breaking down phenylalanine.

hyperphoria /hī'pərfôr'ē-ə/ [Gk, *hyper* + *pherein*, to bear], the tendency of an eye to deviate upward.

hyperphosphoremia /-fos'fərē'mē-ə/, an abnormally high level of phosphorus compounds in the blood.

hyperpigmentation /-pig'məntā'shən/ [Gk, *hyper* + L, *pigmentum*, paint], darkening of the skin. Causes include heredity, drugs, exposure to the sun, and adrenal insufficiency.

hyperpituitarism /-pityoo'itəriz'əm/ [Gk, *hyper*, excessive; L, *pituita*, phlegm], overactivity of the anterior lobe of the pituitary gland, leading to such conditions as **acromegaly** and **Cushing's disease.**

hyperplasia /hī'pərplā'zhə/ [Gk, *hyper* + *plassein*, to mold], an increase in the number of cells of a body part that results from an increased rate of cellular division.

hyperplastic gingivitis [Gk, *hyper*, excessive, *plassein*, to mold; L, *gingiva*, gum; Gk, *itis*, inflammation], a condition of enlarged and inflamed gum tissue that results from an increase in the number of cells, usually because of dental plaque accumulation.

hyperploid /hī'pərploid/ [Gk, *hyper* + *eidos*, form], **1.** pertaining to an individual, organism, strain, or cell that has one or more chromosomes in excess of the basic haploid number or of an exact multiple of the haploid number characteristic of the species. **2.** such an individual, organism, strain, or cell.

hyperploidy /hī'pərploi'dē/, any increase in chromosome number that involves individual chromosomes rather than entire sets, resulting in more than the normal haploid number characteristic of the species, as in Down's syndrome.

hyperpnea /hī'pərpnē'ə/ [Gk, *hyper* + *pnoe*, blowing], an exaggerated deep, rapid, or labored respiration. It occurs normally with exercise and abnormally with aspirin overdose, pain, fever, hysteria, or any condition in which the supply of oxygen is inadequate, such as cardiac disease and respiratory disease. —**hyperpneic, hyperpnoic,** *adj.*

hyperpolarized helium /-pō'lərizd/, a gas used in magnetic resonance imaging studies of respiratory disorders to produce images of the air spaces in the lungs.

hyperprolactinemia /-prōlak'tinē'mē-ə/ [Gk, *hyper* + L, *pro,* before, *lac,* milk; Gk, *haima,* blood], an excessive amount of prolactin in the blood. The condition is caused by a hypothalamus-pituitary dysfunction. In women it is usually associated with gynecomastia, galactorrhea, and secondary amenorrhea; in men it may be a factor in decreased libido and impotence.

hyperproteinemia /-prō'tēnē'mē-ə/ [Gk, *hyper,* excessive, *proteios,* first rank, *haima,* blood], an abnormally high level of protein elements in the blood.

hyperpyrexia /hī'pərpīrek'sē-ə/ [Gk, *hyper* + *pyressein,* to be feverish], an extremely elevated temperature that sometimes occurs in acute infectious diseases, especially in young children. Malignant hyperpyrexia, characterized by a rapid rise in temperature, tachycardia, tachypnea, sweating, rigidity, and blotchy cyanosis, occasionally occurs in patients undergoing general anesthesia. —**hyperpyretic,** *adj.*

hyperreactivity /-rē'activa'itē/ [Gk, *hyper* + L, *re,* again, *activus,* active], an abnormal condition in which responses to stimuli are exaggerated.

hyperreflection /-riflek'shən/, a compulsion to devote excessive attention to oneself.

hyperreflexia /-riflek'sē-ə/ [Gk, *hyper* + L, *reflectere,* to bend back], increased reflex reactions.

hypersensibility /-sen'səbil'itē/, excessive ability to perceive or feel, as excessive sensibility to pain.

hypersensitivity /-scn'sitiv'itē/ [Gk, *hyper* + L, *sentire,* to feel], an abnormal condition characterized by a cxaggerated response of the immune system to an antigen. —**hypersensitive,** *adj.*

hypersensitivity pneumonitis, an inflammatory form of interstitial pneumonia that results from an immunologic reaction in a hypersensitive person. The reaction may be provoked by a variety of inhaled organic dusts, often those containing fungal spores. A wide variety of symptoms may occur, including asthma, fever, chills, malaise, and muscle aches, which usually develop 4 to 6 hours after exposure.

hypersensitivity reaction, an inappropriate and excessive response of the immune system to a sensitizing antigen. The antigenic stimulant is an allergen. Hypersensitivity reactions are classified by the components of the immune system involved in their mediation. Humoral reactions, mediated by the circulating B lymphocytes, are immediate and of three types: anaphylactic hypersensitivity, cytotoxic hypersensitivity, and immune complex disease. Cellular reactions, mediated by the T

H

lymphocytes, are delayed cell-mediated hypersensitivity reactions.

hypersensitization /-sen'sitīzā'shən/ [Gk, *hyper,* excessive; L, *sentire,* to feel], a state of increased reactivity or sensitivity to a stimulus.

hypersomnia /hī'pərsom'nē-ə/ [Gk, *hyper* + L, *somnus,* sleep], **1.** sleep of excessive depth or abnormal duration, usually caused by psychologic rather than physical factors and characterized by a state of confusion on awakening. **2.** extreme drowsiness, often associated with lethargy. **3.** a condition characterized by periods of deep, long sleep.

hypersplenism /hī'pərsplē'nizəm/ [Gk, *hyper* + *splen,* spleen], a syndrome consisting of splenomegaly and a deficiency of one or more types of blood cells. The numerous causes of this syndrome include portal hypertension, the lymphomas, the hemolytic anemias, malaria, tuberculosis, and various connective tissue and inflammatory diseases. Patients complain of abdominal pain on the left side and often experience fullness after eating very little, because the greatly enlarged spleen is pressing against the stomach.

hypersthenic /hī'pərsthen'ik/, **1.** pertaining to a condition of excessive strength or tonicity of the body or a body part. **2.** pertaining to a body type characterized by massive proportions.

hypersystole, abnormal force or duration of the heart systole.

hypertelorism /hī'pərtel'əriz'əm/ [Gk, *hyper* + *tele,* far, *horizo,* separate], a developmental defect characterized by an abnormally wide space between two organs or parts. A kind of hypertelorism is **ocular hypertelorism.**

hypertension /-ten'shən/ [Gk, *hyper* + L, *tendere,* to stretch], a common, often asymptomatic disorder characterized by elevated blood pressure persistently exceeding 140/90 mm Hg. Essential hypertension, the most common kind, has no single identifiable cause, but the risk of the disorder is increased by obesity, a high serum sodium level, hypercholesterolemia, and a family history of high blood pressure. Known causes of hypertension include adrenal disorders such as aldosteronism, Cushing's syndrome, and pheochromocytoma; thyrotoxicosis; preeclampsia; and chronic glomerulonephritis. People with mild or moderate hypertension may be asymptomatic or may experience suboccipital headaches, especially on rising; tinnitus; lightheadedness; ready fatigability; and palpitations. Malignant hypertension, characterized by a diastolic pressure higher than 120 mm Hg,

severe headaches, blurred vision, and confusion, may result in fatal uremia, myocardial infarction, congestive heart failure, or a cerebrovascular accident.

Hypertension and Lipid Trial (HALT), a study to assess the efficacy and safety of alpha-adrenergic blockers in patients with hypertension.

hypertensive /-ten'siv/ [Gk, *hyper,* excessive; L, *tendere,* to stretch], pertaining to high blood pressure, its cause, or its effects.

hypertensive arteriosclerosis, a form of arteriosclerosis complicated by a buildup of the muscular and elastic tissues of the arterial walls caused by hypertension.

hypertensive crisis [Gk, *hyper* + L, *tendere,* to stretch; Gk, *krisi,* turning point], a sudden severe increase in blood pressure to a level exceeding 200/120 mm Hg, occurring most frequently in individuals who have untreated hypertension and in patients who have stopped taking prescribed antihypertensive medication. Characteristic signs include severe headache, vertigo, diplopia, tinnitus, nosebleed, twitching of muscles, tachycardia or other cardiac arrhythmia, distended neck veins, narrowed pulse pressure, nausea, and vomiting. The patient may be confused, irritable, or stuporous; and the condition may lead to convulsions, coma, myocardial infarction, renal failure, cardiac arrest, or stroke.

hypertensive encephalopathy [Gk, *hyper* + L, *tendere,* to stretch; Gk, *enkephalos,* brain, *pathos,* disease], a set of symptoms, including headache, convulsions, and coma, associated with glomerulonephritis.

hypertensive retinopathy [Gk, *hyper* + L, *tendere,* to stretch, *rete* + *net,* web; Gk, *pathos,* disease], a condition in which retinal changes occur in association with arterial hypertension. The changes may include blood vessel alterations, hemorrhages, exudates, and retinal edema.

hyperthermia, /hī'pərthur'mē-ə/ [Gk, *hyper* + *therme,* heat], **1.** a much higher than normal body temperature induced therapeutically or iatrogenically. **2.** *nontechnical.* malignant hyperthermia.

hyperthermia, a NANDA-accepted nursing diagnosis of a state in which an individual's body temperature is elevated above his or her normal range. Defining characteristics include increase in body temperature, flushed skin, skin warm to the touch, increased respiratory rate, tachycardia, and seizures or convulsions.

hyperthyroidism /-thī'roidiz'əm/ [Gk, *hyper* + *thyreos,* shield, *eidos,* form], a condition characterized by hyperactivity of the thyroid gland. The gland is usually enlarged, secreting greater than normal amounts of thyroid hormones, and the metabolic processes of the body are accelerated. Nervousness, exophthalmos, tremor, constant hunger, weight loss, fatigue, heat intolerance, palpitations, and diarrhea may develop.

hypertonia /-tō'nē-ə/, **1.** abnormally increased muscle tone or strength. The condition is sometimes associated with genetic disorders and may be expressed in arm or leg deformities. **2.** a condition of excessive pressure, such as the intraocular pressure of glaucoma.

hypertonic /hī'pərton'ik/ [Gk, hyper + tonos, stretching], (of a solution) having a greater concentration of solute than another solution, hence exerting more osmotic pressure than that solution, such as a hypertonic saline solution that contains more salt than is found in intracellular and extracellular fluid.

hypertonic bladder [Gk, hyper, excessive, tonos, tone; AS, blaedre], a condition of excessive pressure in the detrusor muscle of the bladder, usually caused by an irritant such as a calculus.

hypertonic contracture, prolonged muscle contraction that results from continuous nerve stimulation in spastic paralysis.

hypertonicity /-tənis'itē/ [Gk, hyper, excessive, tonos, tone], **1.** excessive tone, tension, or activity. **2.** (in ophthalmology) increased intraocular pressure. **3.** excessive tension of the arteries or muscles. **4.** increase in osmotic pressure.

hypertonic saline, a saline solution that contains 1% to 15% sodium chloride (compared with normal saline solution at 0.9%). It is used as a bronchial lavage to stimulate sputum production and to promote coughing.

hypertonic solution, a solution that increases the degree of osmotic pressure on a semipermeable membrane.

hypertonus /-tō'nəs/, an excessive level of skeletal muscle tension or activity.

hypertrophic /-trof'ik/ [Gk, hyper, excessive, trophe, nourishment], pertaining to an increase in size, structure, or function.

hypertrophic cardiomyopathy, an abnormality in the structure and function of heart muscle characterized by gross hypertrophy of the interventricular septum and left ventricular free wall. Ventricular outflow obstruction results in impaired diastolic filling and reduced cardiac output. Signs and symptoms, such as fatigue and syncope, are often associated with exercise when the demand for increased cardiac output cannot be met.

hypertrophic catarrh [Gk, hyper + trophe, nourishment, kata, down, rhoia, flow], a chronic condition characterized by inflammation and discharge from a mucous membrane, accompanied by the thickening of the mucosal and submucosal tissue.

hypertrophic cirrhosis, a stage of cirrhosis characterized by an overgrowth of liver tissue.

hypertrophic gastritis, an inflammatory condition of the stomach characterized by epigastric pain, nausea, vomiting, and distension. It is differentiated from other forms of gastritis by the presence of prominent rugae (folds), enlarged glands, and nodules on the wall of the stomach. This condition often accompanies peptic ulcer, Zollinger-Ellison syndrome, or gastric hypersecretion.

hypertrophic gingivitis [Gk, hyper, excessive; trophe, nourishment], a condition in which the gum tissue becomes enlarged and inflamed, usually because of an underlying systemic disorder.

hypertrophic scarring, scarring caused by excessive formation of new tissue in the healing of a wound. It has the appearance of a hard, tumorlike keloid.

hypertrophy /hīpur'trəfē/ [Gk, hyper + trophe, nourishment], an increase in the size of an organ caused by an increase in the size rather than the number of the cells. —**hypertrophic,** adj.

hypertrophy of heart [Gk, hyper, excessive, trophe, nourishment; AS, heorte], an increase in the size of the heart secondary to enlargement of the heart muscle, but without an increase in the size of the heart chambers.

hyperventilation /-ven'tilā'shən/ [Gk, hyper + ventilare, to fan], a pulmonary ventilation rate that is greater than that metabolically necessary for pulmonary gas exchange. It is the result of an increased frequency of breathing, an increased tidal volume, or a combination of both and causes excessive intake of oxygen and elimination of carbon dioxide. Hypocapnia and respiratory alkalosis then occur, leading to dizziness, faintness, numbness of the fingers and toes, possibly syncope, and psychomotor impairment.

hyperventilation tetany, a nervous disorder characterized by muscle twitches, cramps, or spasms caused by abnormally low blood levels of CO_2 from forced overbreathing.

hyperviscosity /-viskos'itē/ [Gk, hyper, excessive; L, viscosus, sticky], pertaining to an extremely viscous or thick fluid.

hypervitaminosis /-vī'təminō'sis/, an abnormal condition resulting from excessive intake of toxic amounts of one or more vitamins, especially over a long period. Seri-

H

ous effects may result from overdoses of fat-soluble vitamins A, D, E, or K; but adverse reactions are less likely with the water-soluble B and C vitamins.

hypervolemia /-vōlē′mē-ə/ [Gk, *hyper* + L, *volumen,* paper roll; Gk, *haima,* blood], an increase in the amount of intravascular fluid, particularly in the volume of circulating blood or its components.

hypesthesia /hī′pəristhē′zhə/ [Gk, *hypo,* under, *aisthesis,* feeling], a decrease in sensation in response to stimulation of the sensory nerves or body organs or areas they innervate. —**hypesthetic,** *adj.*

hypha /hī′fə/, *pl.* **hyphae** [Gk, *hyphe,* web], the threadlike structure of the mycelium in a fungus.

hyphema /hīfē′mə/ [Gk, *hypo,* under, *haima,* blood], a hemorrhage into the anterior chamber of the eye, usually caused by a blunt injury or trauma. Glaucoma may result from recurrent bleeding.

hypnagogic hallucination /hip′nəgoj′ik/ [Gk, *hypnos,* sleep, *agogos,* leading], a vivid image that occurs in the period between wakefulness and sleep.

hypnagogue /hip′nəgog/ [Gk, *hypnos* + *agogos,* leading], an agent or substance that tends to induce sleep or the feeling of dreamy sleepiness, as occurs before falling asleep. —**hypnagogic,** *adj.*

hypnoanalysis /hip′nə·anal′isis/ [Gk, *hypnos* + *analyein,* to loosen], the use of hypnosis as an adjunct to other techniques in psychoanalysis.

hypnogenic zone /hip′nəjen′ik, a specific area on the body that, when stimulated with pressure, can cause a person to enter a hypnotic state.

hypnosis /hipnō′sis/ [Gk, *hypnos,* sleep], a passive, trancelike state that resembles normal sleep during which perception and memory are altered, resulting in increased responsiveness to suggestion. The condition is usually induced by the monotonous repetition of words and gestures while the subject is completely relaxed.

hypnotherapy /hip′nəther′əpē/ [Gk, *hypnos* + *therapeia,* treatment], the use of hypnosis as an adjunct to other techniques in psychotherapy.

hypnotics /hipnot′iks/ [Gk *hypnos,* sleep], a class of drugs often used as sedatives.

hypnotic sleep /hipnot′ik/ [Gk, *hypnos,* sleep; ME, *slep*], sleep induced by hypnosis through the administration of hypnotic medicines.

hypnotic suggestion [Gk, *hypnos,* sleep; L, *suggerere,* to suggest], a suggestion implanted in the mind of a person under hypnosis.

hypnotic trance, an artificially induced sleeplike state, as in hypnosis.

hypnotism /hip′nətiz′əm/ [Gk, *hypnos,* sleep], the study or practice of inducing hypnosis.

hypnotist /hip′nətist/, one who practices hypnotism.

hypnotize /hip′nətīz/, **1.** to put into a state of hypnosis. **2.** to fascinate, entrance, or control through personal charm.

hypoacidity /hī′pō·əsid′itē/, a deficiency of acid.

hypoactivity /-aktiv′itē/ [Gk, *hypo,* under; L, *activus,* active], any abnormally diminished activity of the body or its organs, such as decreased cardiac output, thyroid secretion, or peristalsis.

hypoacusis /-əkŌŌ′sis/ [Gk, *hypo,* under, *akouein,* to hear], a reduced sensitivity to sounds that may be conductive or sensorineural in nature.

hypoalbuminemia /-albŌŌ′minē′mē-ə/, a condition of abnormally low levels of albumin in the blood.

hypoalimentation /-al′iməntā′shən/ [Gk, *hypo* + L, *alimentum,* nourishment], a condition of insufficient or inadequate nourishment.

hypoallergenic /-al′ərjen′ik/ [Gk, *hypo,* under, *allos,* other, *ergein,* to work], pertaining to a lowered potential for producing an allergic reaction.

hypobarism /-ber′izəm/, air pressure that is significantly less than sea level normal of 760 mm Hg.

hypobetalipoproteinemia /hī′pōbā′təlip′-ōprō′tēnē′mē-ə/ [Gk, *hypo* + *beta,* second letter of Greek alphabet, *lipos,* fat, *proteios,* first rank, *haima,* blood], an inherited disorder in which there are less than normal amounts of beta-lipoprotein in the serum.

hypocalcemia /hī′pōkalsē′mē-ə/ [Gk, *hypo* + L, *calx,* lime; Gk, *haima,* blood], a deficiency of calcium in the serum that may be caused by hypoparathyroidism, vitamin D deficiency, kidney failure, acute pancreatitis, or inadequate amounts of plasma magnesium and protein. Mild hypocalcemia is asymptomatic. Severe hypocalcemia is characterized by cardiac arrhythmias and tetany with hyperparesthesia of the hands, feet, lips, and tongue. —**hypocalcemic,** *adj.*

hypocalcemic tetany /-kalsē′mik/ [Gk, *hypo,* under, *calx,* calcium, *haima,* blood, *tetanos,* convulsive tension], a disease caused by an abnormally low level of calcium in the blood. It is characterized by hyperexcitability of the neuromuscular system. A common cause is a deficiency of parathyroid secretion.

hypocalciuria /-kal′siuŌŌr′ē-ə/ [Gk, *hypo,* under; L, *calx,* lime; Gk, *ouron,* urine], a diminished level of calcium in the urine

hypocapnia /-kap'nē-ə/, an abnormally low arterial carbon dioxide level.

hypochloremia /-klôrē'mē-ə/ [Gk, *hypo* + *chloros*, green, *haima*, blood], a decrease in the chloride level in the blood serum. The condition may result from prolonged gastric suctioning.

hypochloremic alkalosis /-klôrē'mik/, a metabolic disorder resulting from an increase in blood bicarbonate level secondary to loss of chloride from the body.

hypochlorhydria /-klôrhid'rē-ə/ [Gk, *hypo* + *chloros*, green, *hydor*, water], a deficiency of hydrochloric acid in the stomach's gastric juice.

hypochlorite poisoning /-klôr'īt/, toxic effects of ingestion of or skin contact with household or commercial bleaches or similar chlorinated products. Symptoms include pain and inflammation of the mouth and digestive tract, vomiting, and breathing difficulty.

hypochlorous acid /-klôr'əs/ [Gk, *hypo* + *chloros*, green; L, *acidus*, sour], a greenish-yellow liquid derived from an aqueous solution of chlorinated lime.

hypocholesteremia /-kəles'tərē'mē-ə/, an abnormally low level of cholesterol in the blood.

hypochondriac /-kon'drē-ak/ [Gk, *hypo*, under, *chondros*, cartilage], **1.** pertaining to the regions of the upper abdomen beneath the lower ribs. **2.** pertaining to a person who is so preoccupied with matters of ill health that the state of mind itself becomes a disability. —**hypochondriacal** /-kəndrī'əkəl/, *adj.*

hypochondriac region [Gk, *hypo* + *chondros*, cartilage; L, *regio*, direction], the part of the abdomen in the upper zone on both sides of the epigastric region and beneath the cartilages of the lower ribs.

hypochondriasis /hī'pokəndrī'əsis/ [Gk, *hypo* + *chondros*, cartilage, *osis*, condition], a chronic abnormal concern about the health of the body. It is characterized by extreme anxiety, depression, and an unrealistic interpretation of real or imagined physical symptoms as indications of a serious illness or disease despite rational medical evidence that no disorder is present.

hypochondroplasia /-kon'drōplā'zhə/, an inherited form of dwarfism that resembles a mild form of achondroplasia.

hypochromic /hī'pōkrō'mik/ [Gk, *hypo* + *chroma*, color], pertaining to less than normal color. The term usually describes a red blood cell and characterizes anemias associated with decreased synthesis of hemoglobin.

hypochromic anemia, 1. a group of anemias characterized by a decreased concentration of hemoglobin in the red blood cells. **2.** a form of anemia in which the hemoglobin is deficient in proportion to the size of erythrocytes or the individual erythrocyte has the capacity to contain more hemoglobin.

hypocycloidal motion /-sī'kloidəl/, (in tomography) a complex circular pattern of movement of the x-ray tube and film that results in blurring of structures outside the focal plane and elimination of ghost images.

hypodermic /-durmic/ [Gk, *hypo* + *derma*, skin], pertaining to the area below the skin, such as a hypodermic injection.

hypodermic implantation [Gk, *hypo*, under, *derma*, skin; L, *implantare*, to set into], the introduction of a solid medicine under the skin, usually on the chest or abdominal wall, to ensure local action or slow absorption.

hypodermic needle, a short, thin hollow needle that attaches to a syringe for injecting a drug or medication under the skin or into vessels and for withdrawing a fluid such as blood for examination.

hypodermic syringe [Gk, *hypo*, under, *derma,* skin, *syringx,* tube], an instrument designed to direct fluid under the skin into subcutaneous tissue through a fine hollow needle.

hypodermic tablet, a compressed or molded dosage form of a medication that can be dissolved in water for intravenous administration.

hypodermoclysis /hī'pōdərmok'lisis/ [Gk, *hypo* + *derma,* skin, *klysis,* flushing out], the injection of an isotonic or hypotonic solution into subcutaneous tissue to supply a continuous and large amount of fluid, electrolytes, and nutrients. The procedure is used to replace the loss or inadequate intake of water and salt during illness or surgery or after shock or hemorrhage. It is performed only when a patient is unable to take fluids intravenously, orally, or rectally. The rate of absorption into the circulatory system is increased with the addition to the solution of the enzyme hyaluronidase.

hypodipsia /-dip'sē-ə/, a condition in which health is threatened by an abnormally low fluid intake.

hypofibrinogenemia /-fī'brinōjənē'mē-ə/ [Gk, *hypo* + L, *fibra,* fiber; Gk, *genein,* to produce, *haima,* blood], a deficiency of fibrinogen, a blood clotting factor, in the blood. The condition may occur as a complication of abruptio placentae.

hypofunction /-fungk'shən/ [Gk, *hypo*, under; L, *functio,* performance], a diminished or inadequate level of activity of an organ system or its parts.

hypogammaglobulinemia /-gam'əglō'-byəlinē'mē-ə/ [Gk, *hypo* + *gamma*, third letter in Greek alphabet; L, *globus*, small sphere; Gk, *haima*, blood], a less than normal concentration of gamma globulin in the blood, usually the result of increased protein catabolism or loss of protein in the urine. The condition is associated with a decreased resistance to infection.

hypogastric /-gas'trik/ [Gk, *hypo*, under, *gaster*, stomach], pertaining to the hypogastrium, or the lower abdominal region below the umbilical region and between the right and left iliac regions.

hypogastric pain, pain in the lower abdomen.

hypogastric plexus, a complex of nerve fibers in the pelvic area near the termination of the aorta and the beginning of the common iliac artery.

hypogenitalism /-jen'itəliz'əm/ [Gk, *hypo* + L, *genitalis*, fruitful], a condition of retarded sexual development caused by a defect in male or female hormonal production in the testis or ovary.

hypogeusia /-gōō'zē-ə/, reduced taste.

hypoglossal /-glos'əl/ [Gk, *hypo*, under, *glossa*, tongue], pertaining to nerves or other structures under the tongue.

hypoglossal nerve [Gk, *hypo* + *glossa*, tongue], either of a pair of cranial nerves essential for swallowing and moving the tongue.

hypoglossus /-glos'əs/, **1.** a muscle that retracts and pulls down the side of the tongue. **2.** the hypoglossal nerve.

hypoglycemia /hī'pōglīsē'mē-ə/ [Gk, *hypo* + *glykys*, sweet, *haima*, blood], a less than normal amount of glucose in the blood, usually caused by administration of too much insulin, excessive secretion of insulin by the islet cells of the pancreas, or dietary deficiency. The condition may cause weakness, headache, hunger, visual disturbances, ataxia, anxiety, personality changes, and, if untreated, delirium, coma, and death.

hypoglycemic /-glīsē'mik/, [Gk, *hypo*, under, *glykys*, sweet, *haima*, blood], pertaining to or resembling a state of low blood sugar level.

hypoglycemic agent, any of a large heterogeneous group of drugs prescribed to decrease the amount of glucose circulating in the blood. Hypoglycemic agents include insulin, the sulfonylureas, and the biguanides. Insulin in its various forms is given parenterally and acts by increasing the use of carbohydrates and the metabolism of fats and protein. The sulfonylureas act by stimulating the release of endogenous insulin from the pancreas.

hypoglycemic coma [Gk, *hypo*, under, *glykys*, sweet, *koma*, deep sleep], a loss of consciousness that results from abnormally low blood sugar levels.

hypoglycogenolysis /-glī'kōjənol'isis/, a metabolic disorder in which defective splitting of glycogen molecules results in a decreased formation of glucose.

hypogonadism /-gō'nədiz'əm/, a deficiency in the secretory activity of the ovary or testis. The condition may be primary or caused by a gonadal dysfunction involving the Leydig's cells in the male, or it may occur secondary to a hypothalamus-pituitary disorder.

hypoinsulinism /-in'səliniz'əm/ [Gk, *hypo*, under; L, *insula*, island (of Langerhans)], a deficiency of insulin secretion by cells of the pancreas and associated signs and symptoms of diabetes.

hypokalemia /hī'pōkəlē'mē-ə/ [Gk, *hypo* + L, *kalium*, potassium; Gk, *haima*, blood], a condition in which an inadequate amount of potassium, the major intracellular cation, is found in the circulating bloodstream. Hypokalemia is characterized by abnormal electrocardiographic findings, weakness, confusion, mental depression, and flaccid paralysis. The cause may be starvation, treatment of diabetic acidosis, adrenal tumor, or diuretic therapy. —**hypokalemic,** *adj.*

hypokalemic alkalosis /-kalē'mik/, a pathologic condition resulting from the accumulation of base or the loss of acid from the body associated with a low level of serum potassium.

hypokalemic periodic paralysis [Gk, *hypo*, under; L, *kalium*, potassium; Gk, *peri*, near, *hodos*, way, *paralyein*, to be palsied], a state of recurring attacks of muscular weakness associated with low blood levels of potassium.

hypokinesia /-kīnē'zhə/, a condition of abnormally diminished motor activity.

hypokinetic /-kinet'ik/ [Gk, *hypo*, under, *kinesis*, movement], pertaining to diminished power of movement or motor function, which may or may not be accompanied by a mild form of paralysis.

hypolipoproteinemia /hī'pōlip'ōprō'tēnē'mē-ə/ [Gk, *hypo* + *lipos*, fat, *proteios*, first rank, *haima*, blood], a group of defects of lipoprotein metabolism that cause varying complexes of signs. Primary, or hereditary, hypolipoproteinemia factors include abnormal transport of triglycerides in the blood, low levels of high-density lipoproteins, high levels of low-density lipoproteins, and abnormal fat deposits in the body.

hypomagnesemia /hī'pōmag'nisē'mē-ə/, an abnormally low concentration of magnesium in the blood plasma, which causes nausea, vomiting, muscle weakness, tremors, tetany, and lethargy. Mild hypomagnesemia is usually the result of inadequate absorption of magnesium in the kidney or intestine. A more severe form is associated with malabsorption syndrome, protein malnutrition, and parathyroid disease.

hypomania /-mā′nē·ə/ [Gk, *hypo* + *mania*, madness], a mild degree of mania characterized by optimism; excitability; energetic, productive behavior; marked hyperactivity and talkativeness; heightened sexual interest; quick anger and irritability; and a decreased need for sleep. —**hypomaniac**, *n.*, **hypomanic**, *adj.*

hypometria /hī′pōmē′trē·ə/ [Gk, *hypo* + *metron*, measure], an abnormal condition, a form of dysmetria, characterized by a dysfunction of the power to control the range of muscular action, resulting in movements that fall short of the intended goals of the affected individual.

hypomobility /-mōbil′itē/, a lack of normal movement of a joint or body part, as may result from an articular surface dysfunction or from disease or injury that affects a bone or muscle.

hypomorph /hī′pōmôrf/ [Gk, *hypo* + *morphe*, form], **1.** a person whose legs are disproportionately short in relation to the trunk and whose sitting height is greater in proportion than his or her standing height. **2.** (in genetics) a mutant allele that has a reduced effect on the expression of a trait but at a level too low to cause abnormal development.

hypomotility /-motil′ite/ [Gk, *hypo,* under; L, *motare,* to move frequently], a state of diminished motility or loss of power to move about.

hyponatremia /hī′pōnatrē′mē·ə/ [Gk, *hypo* + L, *natrium,* sodium; Gk, *haima,* blood], a lower than normal concentration of sodium in the blood, caused by inadequate excretion of water or by excessive water in the circulating bloodstream. In a severe case the person may experience water intoxication with confusion and lethargy, leading to muscle excitability, convulsions, and coma.

hypoosmolality [Gk, *hypo* + *osmos,* impulse], a state or condition of abnormally reduced osmolality.

hypoparathyroidism /-per′əthī′roidiz′əm/ [Gk, *hypo* + *para,* beside, *thyreos,* shield, *eidos,* form], a condition of insufficient secretion of the parathyroid glands. It can be caused by primary parathyroid dysfunction or by elevated serum calcium level.

hypoperistalsis /-per′istal′sis/ [Gk, *hypo,* under, *peristellein,* to clasp], a state of abnormally slow motility of waves of alternate contraction and relaxation that impel contents forward through the digestive tract.

hypopharyngeal /-fərin′jē·əl/ [Gk, *hypo* + *pharynx,* throat], **1.** pertaining to the hypopharynx. **2.** situated below the pharynx.

hypopharynx /-fer′ingks/, the inferior part of the pharynx, between the epiglottis and the larynx. It corresponds to the height of the epiglottis and is a critical dividing point in separating solids and fluids from air entering the region.

hypophonia /-fō′nē·ə/ [Gk, *hypo,* under, *phone,* voice], a weak or whispered voice.

hypophoria /-fôr′ē·ə/, a type of strabismus in which the patient may not show signs of ocular muscle imbalance until the affected eye is covered, resulting in a downward deviation.

hypophosphatasia /hī′pōfos′fətā′zhə/ [Gk, *hypo* + *phosphoros,* lightbearing], congenital absence of alkaline phosphatase, an enzyme essential to the calcification of bone tissue.

hypophosphatemic rickets /hī′pōfos′-fətē′mik/, a rare familial disorder characterized by impaired resorption of phosphate in the kidneys and poor absorption of calcium in the small intestine, which result in osteomalacia, retarded growth, skeletal deformities, and pain.

hypophyseal /-fizē′əl, -fiz′ē·əl/ [Gk, *hypo,* under, *phyein,* to grow], pertaining to the hypophysis or pituitary body.

hypophyseal hormones, hormones that are associated with body growth and exercise effects, such as luteinizing hormone, which stimulates testosterone production and muscular hypertrophy; growth hormone; and antidiuretic hormone.

hypophyseal portal system, a set of veins that carry blood and regulatory hormones from the hypothalamus to the adenohypophysis.

hypophysectomy /hīpof′əsek′təmē/ [Gk, *hypo* + *phyein,* to grow, *ektome,* excision], surgical removal of the pituitary gland. It may be performed to slow the growth and spread of endocrine-dependent malignant tumors or to excise a pituitary tumor. —**hypophysectomize,** *v.*

hypophyseoprivic /-fiz′ē·ōpriv′ik/ [L, *privus,* deprived], a deficiency of hormone secretions by the pituitary gland (hypophysis). The condition may be caused by functional inactivity or surgical removal of the gland.

hypophysis /hīpof′isis/ [Gk, *hypo,* under, *phyein,* to grow], the pituitary body (gland). The anterior lobe is sometimes identified as the **adenohypophysis, and**

the posterior lobe as the **neurohypophysis.**

hypopigmentation /-pig´məntā´shən/ [Gk, *hypo* + L, *pigmentum*, paint], unusual lack of skin color, as seen in albinism.

hypopituitarism /-pityōō´iteriz´əm/ [Gk, *hypo* + L, *pituita*, phlegm], an abnormal condition caused by diminished activity of the pituitary gland and marked by excessive deposits of fat and persistence or acquisition of adolescent characteristics.

hypoplasia /hī´pōplā´zhə/ [Gk, *hypo* + *plassein*, to mold], incomplete or underdeveloped organ or tissue, usually the result of a decrease in the number of cells. **—hypoplastic,** *adj.*

hypoplastic anemia /-plas´tik/, a broad category of anemias characterized by decreased production of red blood cells.

hypoploid /hī´pəploid/ [Gk, *hypo* + *eidos*, form], **1.** pertaining to an individual, organism, strain, or cell that has fewer than the normal haploid number or an exact multiple of the haploid number of chromosomes characteristic of the species. **2.** such an individual, organism, strain, or cell.

hypoploidy /hī´pōploi´dē/, any decrease in chromosome number that involves individual chromosomes rather than entire sets, so that fewer than the normal haploid number of chromosomes characteristic of the species are present, as in Turner's syndrome.

hypopnea /hīpop´nē·ə, hī´pōnē´ə/ [Gk, *hypo* + *pnoe*, breath], abnormally shallow and slow respiration. In wellconditioned athletes it may be appropriate and is often accompanied by a slow pulse; otherwise it is characteristic of damage to the brainstem. Accompanied by a rapid, weak pulse, it is a grave sign.

hypopotassemia /-pot´əsē´mē·ə/ [Gk, *hypo* + D, *potasschen*, potash; Gk, *haima*, blood], a deficiency of potassium in the blood.

hypoproliferative anemias /-prolif´ər-ətiv´/, a group of anemias caused by inadequate production of erythrocytes. The condition is associated with protein deficiencies, renal disease, and myxedema.

hypoproteinemia /hī´pōprō´tēnē´mē·ə/ [Gk, *hypo* + *proteios*, first rank, *haima*, blood], a disorder characterized by a decrease in the amount of protein in the blood to an abnormally low level, accompanied by edema, nausea, vomiting, diarrhea, and abdominal pain.

hypoprothrombinemia /hī´pōprōthrom´-binē´mē·ə/ [Gk, *hypo* + L, *pro*, before; Gk, *thrombos*, lump, *haima*, blood], an abnormal reduction in the amount of prothrombin (factor II) in the circulating blood, characterized by poor clot formation, longer bleeding time, and possible hemorrhage.

hypopyon /hīpō´pē·on/ [Gk, *hypo* + *pyon*, pus], an accumulation of pus in the anterior chamber of an eye, which appears as a gray fluid between the cornea and the iris. It may occur as a complication of conjunctivitis, herpetic keratitis, or corneal ulcer.

hyporeflexia /-riflek´sē·ə/ [Gk, *hypo* + L, *reflectere*, to bend back], decreased reflex reactions.

hyposalivation /-sal´ivā´shən/ [Gk, *hypo* + L, *saliva*, spittle], a decreased flow of saliva that may be associated with dehydration, radiation therapy of the salivary gland regions, anxiety, use of drugs such as atropine and antihistamines, vitamin deficiency, various forms of parotitis, or various syndromes such as Plummer-Vinson syndrome.

hypostatic /-stat´ik/ [Gk, *hypo* + *stasis*, standing still], pertaining to an accumulation of deposits of substances or congestion in a body area that results from a lack of activity.

hypostatic lung collapse [Gk, *hypo*, under, *stasis*, standing still; AS, *lungen* + L, *collabi*, to fall together], a lung disorder in which the settling or pooling of fluids or suspended solids results in congestion caused by the effects of gravity in a dependent part.

hypostatic pneumonia, a type of pneumonia associated with elderly or debilitated people who remain in the same position for long periods. Gravity tends to accelerate fluid congestion in one area of the lungs, increasing the susceptibility to infection.

hyposthenic /hī´pōsthen´ik/, **1.** pertaining to a lack of strength or muscle tone. **2.** a body type characterized by a slender build.

hypotelorism /hī´pōtel´əriz´əm/ [Gk, *hypo* + *tele*, far, *horizo*, separate], a developmental defect characterized by an abnormally decreased distance between two organs or parts.

hypotension /-ten´shən/ [Gk, *hypo* + L, *tendere*, to stretch], an abnormal condition in which the blood pressure is not adequate for normal perfusion and oxygenation of the tissues. An expanded intravascular space, a decreased intravascular volume, or diminished cardiac output may be the cause.

hypotensive /-ten´siv/ [Gk, *hypo*, under; L, *tendere*, to stretch], pertaining to abnormally low blood pressure.

hypothalamic amenorrhea /-thalam´ik/ [Gk, *hypo* + *thalamos*, chamber], cessation of menses caused by disorders that inhibit the hypothalamus from initiating the cycle of neurohormonal interactions of the brain, pituitary, and ovary necessary for ovulation and subsequent menstruation.

hypothalamic hormones, a group of hormones secreted by the hypothalamus, including vasopressin, oxytocin, and the thyrotropin-releasing and gonadotropin-releasing hormones.

hypothalamic obesity [Gk, *hypo,* under, *thalamos,* chamber; L, *obesitas,* fatness], obesity that is caused by damage or a functional disturbance involving the hypothalamus.

hypothalamic-pituitary-adrenal axis, the combined system of neuroendocrine units that in a negative feedback network regulate the body's hormonal activities.

hypothalamus /hī′pōthal′əməs/ [Gk, *hypo* + *thalamos,* chamber], a part of the diencephalon of the brain, forming the floor and part of the lateral wall of the third ventricle. It activates, controls, and integrates the peripheral autonomic nervous system, endocrine processes, and many somatic functions such as body temperature, sleep, and appetite. **—hypothalamic,** *adj.*

hypothenar eminence /hīpoth′ənär, hī′-pōthē′när/ [Gk, *hypo* + *thenar,* palm], a fleshy pad on the ulnar side of the palm of the hand.

hypothermal /-thur′mə/ [Gk, *hypo,* under, *therme,* heat], **1.** pertaining to a condition in which the body temperature is significantly below normal as a result of external exposure to cold or has been reduced markedly for surgical or therapeutic purposes. **2.** pertaining to temperatures that are tepid to slightly warm.

hypothermia /hī′pōthur′mē·ə/ [Gk *hypo* + *therme,* heat], **1.** an abnormal and dangerous condition in which the temperature of the body is below 95° F (35° C), usually caused by prolonged exposure to cold and/or damp conditions. Respiration is shallow and slow, and the heart rate is faint and slow. The person may appear to be dead. Treatment includes slowly warming the person. Hospitalization is necessary. **2.** the deliberate and controlled reduction of body temperature with cooling mattresses or ice as preparation for some surgical procedures.

hypothermia, a NANDA-accepted nursing diagnosis of the state in which an individual's body temperature is reduced below his or her normal range but not below 96° F (rectal) or 97.5° F (rectal newborn). Defining characteristics include mild shivering, cool skin, moderate pallor, slow

capillary refill, tachycardia, cyanotic nail beds, hypertension, and piloerection.

hypothermia blanket, a covering used to conserve heat in the body of a patient suffering from hypothermia.

hypothermia therapy, the reduction of a patient's body temperature to counteract high prolonged fever caused by an infectious or neurologic disease or less frequently as an adjunct to anesthesia in heart or brain surgery. Hypothermia may be produced by placing crushed ice around the patient, by immersing the body in ice water, by autotransfusing blood after it is circulated through coils submerged in a refrigerant, or most commonly by applying cooling blankets or vinyl pads containing coils through which cold water and alcohol are circulated by a pump.

hypothesis /hīpoth′isis/ [Gk, groundwork], (in research) a statement derived from a theory that predicts the relationship among variables representing concepts, constructs, or events.

hypothrombinemia /-throm′binē′mē·ə/, a deficiency of the clotting factor thrombin in the blood.

hypothyroid /-thī′roid/ [Gk, *hypo,* under, *thyreos,* shield, *eidos,* form], pertaining to or resembling thyroid deficiency.

hypothyroidism /-thī′roidiz′əm/ [Gk, *hypo* + *thyreos,* shield, *eidos,* form], a condition characterized by decreased activity of the thyroid gland. It may be caused by surgical removal of all or part of the gland, overdosage with antithyroid medication, decreased effect of thyroid releasing hormone secreted by the hypothalamus, decreased secretion of thyroid-stimulating hormone by the pituitary gland, or atrophy of the thyroid gland itself. Weight gain, mental and physical lethargy, dryness of the skin, constipation, arthritis, and slowing of the body's metabolic processes may occur. Untreated, hypothyroidism leads to myxedema, coma, and death.

hypotonia /-tō′nē·ə/ [Gk, *hypo,* under, *tonos,* stretching], a condition of diminished tone or tension that may involve any body structure.

hypotonic, [Gk, *hypo,* under, *tonos,* stretching], pertaining to a lower or lessened tone or tension in any body structure, as in paralysis.

hypotonic saline [Gk, *hypo,* under, *tonos,* tone; L, *sal,* salt], a saline solution that is less than isotonic in strength.

hypotonic solution /hī′pōton′ik/ [Gk, *hypo* + *tonikos,* a stretching], a solution having a lower concentration of solute than another solution, hence exerting less osmotic pressure than that solution.

hypoventilation /-ven′tilā′shən/ [Gk, *hypo*

H

+ L, *ventilare,* to fan], an abnormal condition of the respiratory system, characterized by cyanosis, polycythemia, increased arterial carbon dioxide tension, and generalized decreased respiratory function. Hypoventilation may be caused by uneven distribution of inspired air (such as in bronchitis), obesity, neuromuscular or skeletal disease affecting the thorax, decreased response of the respiratory center to carbon dioxide, and reduced functional lung tissue such as in atelectasis, emphysema, and pleural effusion. The results of hypoventilation are hypoxia, hypercapnia, pulmonary hypertension with cor pulmonale, and respiratory acidosis.

hypovolemia /-vōlē'mē-ə/ [Gk, *hypo* + L, *volumen,* whirl; Gk, *haima,* blood], an abnormally low circulating blood volume.

hypovolemic shock /-vōlē·mik/, a state of physical collapse and prostration caused by massive blood loss, circulatory dysfunction, and inadequate tissue perfusion. The common signs include low blood pressure, feeble pulse, clammy skin, tachycardia, rapid breathing, and reduced urinary output. The associated blood losses may stem from gastrointestinal bleeding, internal hemorrhage, external hemorrhage, or excessive reduction of intravascular plasma volume and body fluids. Disorders that may cause hypovolemic shock are dehydration from excessive perspiration, severe diarrhea, protracted vomiting, intestinal obstruction, peritonitis, acute pancreatitis, and severe burns, which deplete body fluids.

hypoxemia /hī'poksē'mē-ə/ [Gk, *hypo* + *oxys,* sharp, *genein,* to produce, *haima,* blood], an abnormal deficiency of oxygen in arterial blood. Symptoms of acute hypoxemia are cyanosis, restlessness, stupor, coma, Cheyne-Stokes respiration, apnea, increase in blood pressure, tachycardia, and an initial increase in cardiac output that later falls, producing hypotension and ventricular fibrillation or asystole. Chronic hypoxemia stimulates red blood cell production by the bone marrow, leading to secondary polycythemia.

hypoxia /hīpok'sē-ə/ [Gk, *hypo* + *oxys,* sharp, *genein,* to produce], inadequate oxygen at the cellular level, characterized by tachycardia, hypertension, peripheral vasoconstriction, dizziness, and mental confusion. The tissues most sensitive to hypoxia are the brain, heart, pulmonary vessels, and liver.

hypoxic drive /-hīpok'sik/, the low arterial oxygen pressure stimulus to respiration that is mediated through the carotid and aortic bodies.

hypsibrachycephaly /hips'ibrakisef'əlē/

[Gk, *hypsi,* high, *brachys,* short, *kephale,* head], the condition of having a skull that is high with a broad forehead. —**hypsibrachycephalic,** *adj., n.*

hysterectomy /his'tərek'təmē/ [Gk, *hystera,* womb, *ektome,* excision], surgical removal of the uterus. It is performed to remove fibroid tumors of the uterus or to treat chronic pelvic inflammatory disease, severe recurrent endometrial hyperplasia, uterine hemorrhage, and precancerous and cancerous conditions of the uterus. Types of hysterectomy are total hysterectomy, in which the uterus and cervix are removed, and radical hysterectomy, in which ovaries, oviducts, lymph nodes, and lymph channels are removed with the uterus and cervix. Menstruation ceases after either type is performed. One or both ovaries and oviducts may be removed at the same time. —**hysterectomize,** *v.*

hysteresis /his'tərē'sis/ [Gk, *hysterein,* to be late], **1.** a lagging or retardation of one of two associated phenomena or a failure to act in unison. **2.** the influence of the previous condition or treatment of the body on its subsequent response to a given force.

hysteria /histir'ē·ə/ [Gk, *hystera,* womb], a general state of tension or excitement in a person or a group, characterized by unmanageable fear and temporary loss of control over the emotions.

hysteric /hister'ik/ [Gk, *hystera,* womb], pertaining to or resembling hysteria.

hysteric amaurosis [Gk, *hystera* + *amauroein,* to darken], monocular or, more rarely, binocular blindness that follows an emotional shock. It may last for hours, days, or months.

hysteric aphonia [Gk, *hystera,* womb, *a,* not, *phone,* voice], an inability to produce vocal sounds, usually psychogenic in nature.

hysteric ataxia [Gk, *hystera,* womb, *ataxia,* without order], a loss of control over voluntary movements in walking or standing. although the involved muscles function normally when the person is lying or sitting.

hysteric chorea [Gk, *hystera,* womb, *choreia,* dance], a condition in which an individual has choreiform movements, usually associated with his or her occupation, although the actions are the result of hysteria rather than true chorea.

hysteric convulsion, a violent involuntary contraction and relaxation of the skeletal muscles marked by spasmodic muscular contractions with no organic cause.

hysteric dyspepsia, difficulty in digestion caused by emotional disturbances.

hysteric paralysis [Gk, *hystera,* womb,

paralyein, to be palsied], a loss of movement or muscular weakness that is caused by hysteria rather than an identifiable organic defect.

hysteric syncope, a temporary loss of consciousness or a fainting spell caused by emotional agitation.

hysteric tremor [Gk, *hystera*, womb; L, *tremere*, to tremble], **1.** a fine, rhythmic shaking in one extremity or of a generalized nature that may be an expression of fear, anxiety, or hysteria. **2.** a coarse irregular shaking that increases with voluntary movements. **3.** a shaking that is transient and caused by exposure to drugs or toxic substances rather than an organic disorder.

hysteric vertigo, a giddiness or loss of stability, often with a sensation of rotation, with no organic cause.

hysterogram /his'tərōgram'/ [Gk, *hystera* + *gramma*, record], the radiographic record of a uterus made after the injection of a contrast medium into the uterine cavity.

hysterography /his'tərog'rəfē/ [Gk, *hystera*, womb; *graphein*, to record], the use of x-ray film and other instruments to make a medical assessment of the condition of the uterus.

hysterolaparotomy /his'tərōlap'ərot'əmē/ [Gk, *hystera* + *lapara*, loin, *temnein*, to cut], abdominal hysterectomy or hysterotomy.

hystero-oophorectomy /-ō'əfərek'təmē/ [Gk, *hystera*, womb, *oophoron*, ovary, *ektome*, excision], the surgical removal of both the uterus and the ovaries.

hysterosalpingogram /his'tərō'salping'-gōgram'/ [Gk, *hystera* + *salpinx*, tube, *gramma*, record], an x-ray film of the uterus and the fallopian tubes using gas or a radiopaque substance introduced through the cervix to allow visualization of the cavity of the uterus and the passageway of the tubes.

hysterosalpingography /his'tərosal'ping-gog'rəfē/, a method of producing radiographic images of the uterus and fallopian tubes as part of the diagnosis of abnormalities in the reproductive tract of a nonpregnant woman.

hysterosalpingo-oophorectomy /-salping'-gō-ō'əfərek'təmē/ [Gk, *hystera* + *salpinx*, tube, *oophoron*, ovary, *ektome*, excision], surgical removal of one or both ovaries and oviducts along with the uterus, performed commonly to treat malignant neoplastic disease of the reproductive tract and chronic endometriosis. To prevent the severe symptoms of sudden menopause in premenopausal women, a part of one ovary is left, unless a malignancy is present.

hysteroscopy /his'təros'kepē/ [Gk, *hystera* + *skopein*, to look], direct visual inspection of the cervical canal and uterine cavity through a hysteroscope. Hysteroscopy is performed to examine the endometrium, to secure a specimen for biopsy, to remove an intrauterine device, or to excise cervical polyps. —**hysteroscope**, *n*., **hysteroscopic**, *adj*.

hysterotome /his'tərotom'/ [Gk, *hystera*, womb, *temnein*, to cut], a surgical knife used for certain procedures involving uterus.

hysterotomy /his'tərot'əmē/ [Gk, *hystera* + *temnein*, to cut], surgical incision of the uterus, performed as a method of abortion in a pregnancy beyond the first trimester of gestation in which a saline injection abortion was incomplete or in which a tubal sterilization is to be done with the abortion.

hysterovaginoenterocele /-vaj'inō·en'-tərōsēl'/ [Gk, *hystera*, womb; L, *vagina*, sheath; Gk, *enteron*, bowel, *kele*, hernia], a hernia involving the uterus, vagina, and intestines.

Hz, abbreviation for **hertz.**

HZV, abbreviation for *herpes zoster virus*.

I

I, 1. symbol for *inspired gas.* **2.** symbol for the element **iodine.**

¹³¹I, symbol for *radioactive iodine, isotopic mass (atomic weight) 131.*

¹³²I, symbol for *radioactive iodine, isotopic mass (atomic weight)132.*

IABC, abbreviation for **intraaortic balloon counterpulsation.**

IABP, abbreviation for **intraaortic balloon pump.**

IADL, abbreviation for **instrumental activities of daily living.**

I.A.D.R., abbreviation for **International Association for Dental Research.**

IAH, abbreviation for **idiopathic diffuse alveolar hemorrhage.**

I and O, abbreviation for *intake and output.*

iatrogenic /ī′atrōjen′ik, yat-/ [Gk, *iatros,* physician, *genein,* to produce], caused by treatment or diagnostic procedures. —**iatrogenesis, iatrogeny,** *n.*

iatrogenic diabetes mellitus, a form of diabetes that develops as an adverse effect of treatment for a different medical problem.

iatrogenic pneumothorax, a condition in which air or gas is present in the pleural cavity as a result of mechanical ventilation, tracheostomy tube placement, or other therapeutic intervention.

iatrology, the science of medicine.

iatropic /ī′atrōp′ik/, [Gk, *iatros,* physician, *trepein,* to turn], describing a need to see a physician.

iatropic stimulus, the symptoms that induce a patient to seek professional health care.

I band [ME, *band,* flat strip], an isotropic band within a striated muscle fiber that appears dark in polarized light but light when stained.

IBC, abbreviation for *iron-binding capacity.*

IBD, abbreviation for **inflammatory bowel disease.**

IBS, abbreviation for **irritable bowel syndrome.**

ibuprofen /ībyōō′prəfin/, a nonsteroidal antiinflammatory agent prescribed in the treatment of rheumatoid arthritis and osteoarthritis, muscle aches, and menstrual cramps.

■ CONTRAINDICATIONS: Renal dysfunction; disorders of the gastrointestinal tract; or known hypersensitivity to this drug, to other nonsteroidal antiinflammatory drugs, or to aspirin prohibits its use.

■ ADVERSE EFFECTS: Among the more serious adverse reactions are gastrointestinal disturbances, gastric or duodenal ulceration, dizziness, skin rash, and tinnitus. Ibuprofen may interact with other drugs.

ibutilide, a drug that controls atrial fibrillation and atrial flutter. It is prescribed in the treatment of heart arrhythmias by converting atrial fibrillation and atrial flutter of recent onset to normal sinus rhythm.

IBW, abbreviation for *ideal body weight.*

IC, abbreviation for **inspiratory capacity.**

ICA, abbreviation for **islet cell antibody.**

ICD, abbreviation for **implantable cardioverter-defibrillator.**

ICD, abbreviation for *International Classification of Diseases.*

ICDA, abbreviation for *International Classification of Diseases Adapted for Use in the United States.*

ice burn, partial-thickness thermal necrosis of the skin caused by prolonged therapy entailing applications of ice.

Iceland disease /īs′land/, a group of symptoms associated with effects of a viral infection of the nervous system, including muscular pain and weakness, depression, and sensory changes.

I cell disease, a form of lysosomal disease characterized by progressive mental deterioration, heart disease, and respiratory failure in the first 10 years of life. A number of lysosomal enzymes are lacking and fibroblasts display numerous coarse inclusions.

ice pack [ME, *is* + *pakke*], a container of crushed ice used to reduce tissue temperature, relieve pain, soothe inflamed tissue, or control bleeding.

ICF, abbreviation for **intermediate care facility.**

ICF/MR, abbreviation for *intermediate care facility for the mentally retarded.*

ICH, abbreviation for **intracerebral hemorrhage.**

ichor /ī′kôr/, a thin watery fluid discharged from a sore.

ichthyoid /ik'thē·oid/ [Gk, *ichthys,* fish, *eidos,* form], pertaining to objects or structures that are fish-shaped or fishlike.

ichthyosis /ĭk'thē-ō'sis/ [Gk, *ichthys* + fish, *osis,* condition], any of several inherited dermatologic conditions in which the skin is dry and hyperkeratotic, resembling fish scales. It usually appears at or shortly after birth and may be part of one of several rare syndromes. —**ichthyotic,** *adj.*

ichthyosis vulgaris [Gk, *ichthys* + *osis* + L, *vulgaris,* common], a hereditary skin disorder characterized by large, dry dark scales that cover the face, neck, scalp, ears, back, and extensor surfaces but not the flexor surfaces of the body.

ICN, abbreviation for **International Council of Nurses.**

ICP, abbreviation for **intracranial pressure.**

I.C.S., abbreviation for **International Congress of Surgeons.**

ICSH, abbreviation for **interstitial cell-stimulating hormone.**

ictal /ik'təl/ [Gk, *ikteros,* jaundice], pertaining to a sudden acute onset, as convulsions of an epileptic seizure.

icteric /ikter'ik/ [Gk, *ikteros,* jaundice], pertaining to or resembling jaundice.

icterogenic /ik'tərōjen'ik/, causing jaundice.

icterus gravis neonatorum /ik'tərəs/ [Gk, *ikteros,* jaundice; L, *gravis,* weight, *neonatus,* newborn], a hemolytic jaundice of the newborn caused by incompatibility between the mother's serum and the infant's red corpuscles.

icterus index [Gk, *ikteros* + L, *index,* pointer], a liver function test in which the blood serum is compared in intensity of color with that of potassium dichromate, where normal values are represented by a numeric range of 3 to 5. When an excessive amount of bilirubin is present and jaundice becomes apparent, the index is usually 15 or higher; subnormal values are associated with various anemias.

icterus neonatorum, a jaundiced condition in a newborn.

ictus /ik'təs/, *pl.* **ictuses, ictus** [L, stroke], **1.** a seizure. **2.** a cerebrovascular accident. —**ictal, ictic,** *adj.*

ICU, abbreviation for **intensive care unit.**

id [L, it], **1.** (in freudian psychoanalysis) the part of the psyche functioning in the unconscious that is the source of instinctive energy, impulses, and drives. **2.** the true unconscious.

ID, abbreviation for *infectious disease.*

IDDM, abbreviation for **insulin-dependent diabetes mellitus.**

idea [Gk, form], any thought, concept, intention, or impression that exists in the mind as a result of awareness, understanding, or other mental activity.

ideal gas law /īdē'əl/ [Gk, *idea,* form, *chaos,* gas; AS, *lagu,* law], the rule that $PV = nRT$, with the product of pressure (P) and volume (V) equal to the product of the number of moles of gas (n), absolute temperature (T), and a gas constant (R).

idealized image /īdē'əlizd/, a self-concept of a person with a compulsive craving for perfection and admiration. It results in unrealistically high and unattainable goals.

idea of influence, an idea held less firmly than a delusion, often seen in paranoid disorders, that external forces or persons are controlling one's thoughts, actions, and feelings.

idea of persecution, an idea held less firmly than a delusion, often seen in paranoid disorders, that one is being threatened, discriminated against, or mistreated by other persons or external forces.

idea of reference, a delusion that the statements or actions of others, usually interpreted as deprecatory, refer to oneself. It is often seen in paranoid disorders.

ideational apraxia /ī'dē·ā'shənəl/ [Gk, *idea,* form, *a* + *prassein,* not to do], a condition in which the conceptual process is lost, often because of a lesion in the submarginal gyrus of the parietal lobe. The individual is unable to formulate a plan of movement and does not know the proper use of an object because of a lack of perception of its purpose. There is no loss of motor movement.

identification /īden'tifikā'shən/ [L, *idem,* the same, *facere,* to make], an unconscious defense mechanism by which a person patterns his or her personality on that of another person, assuming the person's qualities, characteristics, and actions. The process is a normal function of personality development and learning.

identity /īden'titē/, a component of self-concept characterized by one's persisting consciousness of being oneself, separate and distinct from others. **Identity diffusion,** or identity confusion, is a lack of clarity and consistency in one's perception of the self, which produces a high degree of anxiety.

identity crisis [L, *idem,* the same; Gk, *krisis,* turning point], a period of confusion concerning an individual's sense of self and role in society, which occurs most frequently in the transition from one stage of life to the next. It is often expressed by isolation, negativism, extremism, and rebelliousness.

identity disorder of childhood, a mental

disturbance of childhood in which the person is abnormally uncertain and concerned about long-term goals such as career choice or sexual preference.

ideology /ī′de·ol′əjē/ [Gk, *idea*], a scheme of ideas or systematic organization of ideas associated with doctrine and philosophy.

ideomotor apraxia /īde·əmō′tor/ [Gk, *idea* + L, *motare,* to move about; Gk *a* + *prassein,* not to do], the inability to translate an idea into motion, resulting from some interference with the transmission of the appropriate impulses from the brain to the motor centers. There is no loss of the ability to perform an action automatically, such as tying the shoelaces, but the action cannot be performed on request.

ideophobia /-fō′bē·ə/ [Gk, *idea* + *phobos,* fear], an anxiety disorder characterized by the irrational fear or distrust of ideas or reason.

idiogram /id′ē·əgram′/, a diagram or graphic representation of a karyotype, showing the number, relative sizes, and morphologic characteristics of the chromosomes of a species, individual, or cell.

idiojunctional rhythm /-jungk′shənəl/ [Gk, *idios,* own; L, *jungere,* to join; Gk, *rhythmos*], a heart rhythm emanating from the nodo-His region of the atrioventricular junction but without retrograde conduction to the atria.

idiopathic /-path′ik/ [Gk, *idios* + *pathos,* disease], without a known cause.

idiopathic diffuse alveolar hemorrhage (IAH), bleeding into the alveoli of the lungs caused by any of a number of disorders.

idiopathic disease, a disease that develops without an apparent or known cause, although it may have a recognizable pattern of signs and symptoms and may be curable.

idiopathic gangrene [Gk, *idios,* own, *pathos,* disease, *gaggraina*], a gangrenous condition of unknown cause.

idiopathic guttate hypomelanosis /hī′-pōmel′ənō′sis/, a drop-shaped hypopigmented skin lesion of unknown origin.

idiopathic hemosiderosis, the accumulation of intracellular iron containing deposits in the lungs as a result of bleeding in the lungs.

idiopathic hypoventilation, a disorder of unknown cause associated with a deficiency of air to the alveoli of the lungs.

idiopathic midline destructive disease (IMDD), a disorder of unknown cause characterized by ulceration and necrosis of the midline facial tissues and obstruction of the upper airways.

idiopathic necrotizing crescentic glo-

merulonephritis, an autoimmune disorder that causes intracapsular hemorrhage and cellular crescent formation in the renal glomerulus.

idiopathic nephrotic syndrome [Gk, *idios,* own, *pathos,* disease, *nephros,* kidney], a kidney disease of unknown origin characterized by hematuria, albuminuria, edema, and hypertension caused by damage in the glomeruli capillaries.

idiopathic neuralgia [Gk, *idios,* own, *pathos,* disease, *neuron,* nerve, *algos,* pain], a form of neuralgia that occurs without any identifiable structural nerve lesion.

idiopathic pericarditis [Gk, *idios,* own, *pathos,* disease, *peri,* near, *kardia,* heart, *itis,* inflammation], an inflammation of the pericardium of unknown cause.

idiopathic postpartum renal failure, kidney failure that begins 1 day to several weeks after delivery following an uneventful gestation. Symptoms include oliguria or anuria, which progresses to azotemia, with complications of hemolytic anemia or coagulopathy.

idiopathic pulmonary fibrosis [Gk, *idios,* own, *pathos,* disease; L, *pulmoneous,* the lungs, *fibra,* fiber], fibrosis of the lungs that may follow an earlier inflammation or disease such as tuberculosis or pneumoconiosis.

idiopathic pulmonary hemorrhage, bleeding in the lungs without a known cause. It may be a cause of secondary spontaneous pneumothorax.

idiopathic reactive hypoglycemia, a condition of diminished blood sugar level that occurs after the ingestion of carbohydrates and has no known cause.

idiopathic scoliosis, an abnormal condition characterized by a lateral curvature of the spine. The main factors in diagnosing idiopathic scoliosis are the degree, balance, and rotational component of the curvature. The rotational component may contribute to rib cage deformities and impingement on the pulmonary and cardiac systems. Neurologic deficits are commonly associated with severe curvature and vary according to the extent to which the curvature has impinged on the spinal cord. Some signs of such impingement are reflex, sensation, and motor alterations of the lower extremities.

idiopathic steatorrhea [Gk, *idios,* own, *pathos,* disease, *stear,* fat, *rhoia,* flow], excess fat in the stools, particularly as in celiac disease in adults.

idiopathic tetanus [Gk, *idios,* own, *pathos,* disease, *tetanos,* convulsive tension], a tetanus infection of unknown cause.

idiopathic thrombocytopenic purpura (ITP), a deficiency of platelets that results in bleeding into the skin and other organs. Acute ITP is a disease of children that may follow a viral infection, lasts a few weeks to a few months, and usually has no residual effects. Chronic ITP is more common in adolescents and adults, begins more insidiously, and lasts longer. Antibodies to platelets are found in patients with ITP.

idiopathic ventricular tachycardia, a heart rhythm with a consistently excessive rate despite the absence of an apparent organic cause for the abnormality.

idiopathy /id′ē·op′əthē/, any primary disease that arises without an apparent cause. —**idiopathic,** adj.

idiosyncrasy /-sin′krəsē/ [Gk, idios + synkrasis, mixing together], **1.** a physical or behavioral characteristic or manner that is unique to an individual or a group. **2.** an individual's unique hypersensitivity to a particular drug, food, or other substance. —**idiosyncratic,** adj.

idiosyncratic /-sinkrat′ik/ [Gk, idios, own, synkrasis, mixing together], pertaining to personal peculiarities or mannerisms.

idiosyncratic drug [Gk, idios, own, sygkrasis, mixing together; Fr, drogue], an individual sensitivity to effects of a drug caused by inherited or other body constitution factors.

idiotope /id′ē·ətōp′/, an antigenic determinant of an idiotype of the variable regions of an immunoglobulin.

idiotrophic /-trof′ik/, describing an organism capable of choosing its own food.

idiot savant /idē·ō′ savänt′/, an individual with mental retardation who is nonetheless capable of performing certain unusual mental feats, primarily those involving music, puzzle solving, or manipulation of numbers

idiotype /id′ō ətīp′/ [Gk, idios + typos, mark], the part of an immunoglobulin molecule that confers unique character, most often including its binding site.

idioventricular /-ventrik′yələr/ [Gk, idios + L, ventriculus, little belly], originating in a ventricle.

idioventricular rhythm [Gk, idios, own; L, ventriculus, little belly; Gk, rhythmos], an independent cardiac rhythm caused by a repeated discharge of impulses at a rate of <100 beats/min from a focus within a ventricle.

IDL, abbreviation for **intermediate-density lipoprotein.**

IDM, abbreviation for infant of a diabetic mother.

idoxuridine /ī′doksyŏōr′ədēn/, an ophthalmic antiviral prescribed for herpes simplex keratitis.

id reaction, the autosensitization result-

ing from any inflammatory condition that causes pruritus and vesicular lesions. These secondary lesions are caused by circulating antigens and are usually distant from the primary infection.

I:E ratio, (in respiratory therapy) the duration of inspiration to expiration. A range of 1:1.5 to 1:2 for an adult is considered acceptable for mechanical ventilation. Ratio increases to 1:1 or 2:1 or higher may cause hemodynamic complications.

Ig, abbreviation for **immunoglobulin.**

IgA, abbreviation for **immunoglobulin A.**

IgA deficiency, a selective lack of immunoglobulin A, the most common type of immunoglobulin deficiency. Immunoglobulin A is a major protein antibody in the saliva and the mucous membranes of the intestines and the bronchi that protects against bacterial and viral infections. A deficiency of immunoglobulin A is associated with autosomal-dominant or autosomal-recessive inheritance and with autoimmune abnormalities. The IgA deficiency is common in patients with rheumatoid arthritis and in those with systemic lupus erythematosus. Common symptoms are respiratory allergies associated with chronic sinopulmonary infection.

IgD, abbreviation for **immunoglobulin D.**

IgE, abbreviation for **immunoglobulin E.**

IGF, abbreviation for **insulin-like growth factors.**

IgG, abbreviation for **immunoglobulin G.**

IgM, abbreviation for **immunoglobulin M.**

ignipeditis /ig′nēpedī′tēz/ [L, ignis, fire, pes, foot], a burning pain in the soles of the feet caused by peripheral neuritis.

IGT, abbreviation for **impaired glucose tolerance.**

IH, abbreviation for infectious hepatitis.

IL-1, abbreviation for **interleukin-1.**

IL-2, abbreviation for **interleukin-2.**

IL-3, abbreviation for **interleukin-3.**

IL-4, abbreviation for **interleukin-4.**

IL-5, abbreviation for **interleukin-5.**

IL-6, abbreviation for **interleukin-6.**

IL-7, abbreviation for **interleukin-7.**

IL-8, abbreviation for **interleukin-8.**

IL-9, abbreviation for **interleukin-9.**

IL-10, abbreviation for **interleukin-10.**

IL-11, abbreviation for **interleukin-11.**

IL-12, abbreviation for **interleukin-12.**

IL-13, abbreviation for **interleukin-13.**

IL-14, abbreviation for **interleukin-14.**

IL-15, abbreviation for **interleukin-15.**

ILD, abbreviation for **interstitial lung disease;** interstitial lung disorder.

Ile, abbreviation for **isoleucine.**

ileal bypass /il'ē·əl/ [L, *ilium,* intestine; AS, *bi,* near; Fr, *passer*], a surgical procedure for treating obesity by anastomosing the upper part of the small intestine to a part closer to the end of the small intestine, thereby bypassing much of the length of the ileum that normally absorbs nutrients.

ileal conduit [Fr, *conduire,* to guide], a method of urinary diversion through intestinal tract tissue. Ureters are implanted in a section of dissected ileum. This section is sutured closed on one end, and the other end is drawn through the abdominal wall (right lower quadrant) to create a stoma. The patient wears a pouch to collect the urine.

ileectomy /il'ē·ek'təmē/, surgical removal of the ileum.

ileitis /il'ē·ī'tis/ [L, *ileum,* intestine; Gk, *itis*], inflammation of the ileum.

ileoanal anastomosis /il'ē·ō·ā'nəl/, a surgical procedure in which the colon and rectum are removed but the anus and anal sphincter are left intact. An anastomosis is formed between the lower end of the small intestine and the anus.

ileocecal /il'ē·ōsē'kəl/ [L, *ilium,* intestine, *caecus,* blind], pertaining to both the ileum and the cecum and the region where they are joined.

ileocecal syndrome, appendicitis.

ileocecal valve [L, *ileum,* intestine, *caecus,* blind, *valvarum,* folding door], the valve between the ileum of the small intestine and the cecum of the large intestine. It consists of two flaps that project into the lumen of the large intestine, immediately above the vermiform appendix.

ileocolic node /il'ē·ōkol'ik/ [L, *ileum* + Gk, *kolon,* colon; L, *nodus,* knot], a node in one of three groups of superior mesenteric lymph glands, forming a chain of approximately 15 nodes around the ileocolic (mesenteric) artery.

ileocolitis /-kōlī'tis/, an inflammation of the ileum and colon.

ileocystoplasty /-sis'təplas'tē/ [L, *ileum* + Gk, *kystis,* bag, *plassein,* to mold], a surgical procedure in which the bladder is reconstructed by using a segment of the ileum for the bladder wall.

ileocystostomy /-sistos'təmē/ [L, *ilium* + intestines; Gk, *kystis,* bag, *stoma,* mouth], a surgical procedure to form a passage to direct urine through the abdominal wall by using a segment of small intestine as a tube from the bladder.

ileorectal /-rek'təl/, pertaining to the ileum and rectum.

ileosigmoidostomy /-sig'moidos'təmē/, surgical establishment of a passageway between the ileum and the colon.

ileostomate /il'ē·os'təmāt/, a person who has undergone an ileostomy.

ileostomy /il'ē·os'təmē/ [L, *ileum* + Gk, *stoma,* mouth, *temnein,* to cut], surgical formation of an opening of the ileum onto the surface of the abdomen, through which fecal matter is emptied. The operation is performed in advanced or recurrent ulcerative colitis, Crohn's disease, or cancer of the large bowel. Intestinal antibiotics are given to decrease the bacterial count. A nasogastric or intestinal tube is passed. The diseased part of the large bowel is removed in a permanent ileostomy; occasionally the distal and proximal segments of bowel may be reconnected after ulcerated areas have healed. A loop of the proximal ileum is then drawn out onto the abdomen and sutured in place, and a stoma is formed. After surgery the patient wears a disposable bag to collect the semiliquid fecal matter, which begins to drain once peristalsis is restored and the nasogastric tube is removed.

ileum /il'ē·əm/, *pl.* **ilea** [L, intestine], the distal part of the small intestine, extending from the jejunum to the cecum. It ends in the right iliac fossa, opening into the medial side of the large intestine. —**ileac, ileal,** *adj.*

ileus /il'ē·əs/ [L; Gk, *eilein,* to twist], an obstruction of the intestines, such as an adynamic ileus caused by immobility of the bowel or a mechanical ileus in which the intestine is blocked by mechanical means.

iliac circumflex node /il'ē·ak/ [L, *ilium* + flank; *circum,* around, *flectere,* to bend, *nodus,* knot], a node in one of the seven clusters of parietal lymph nodes of the abdomen. This node is one of a group found along the course of the deep iliac circumflex vessels.

iliac crest [L, *ilia,* intestines; ME, *creste*], the upper elevated margins of the ilium.

iliac fascia, the part of the endoabdominal fascia that is attached with the iliacus to the crest of the ilium and passes under the inguinal ligament into the thigh.

iliac horns, accessory bony spurs on the posterior of the ilium, one of the symptoms of nail-patella syndrome.

iliacus /ilī'əkəs/ [L, *ilium,* flank], a flat triangular muscle that covers the inner curved surface of the iliac fossa. It acts to flex and laterally rotate the thigh.

iliofemoral /il'ē·ōfem'ərəl/, pertaining to the ilium and femur.

iliofemoral ligament [L, *ilium* + flank, *femur,* thigh, *ligamentum*], a triangular band of connective tissue attached by its apex to the anterior inferior spine of the ilium and acetabular margin and by its base to the intertrochanteric line of the femur.

iliofemoral thrombosis, a thrombus in the iliofemoral circulation.

ilioinguinal /il′ē-ō-ing′gwinəl/ [L, *ilium* + *inguen,* groin], pertaining to the hip and inguinal regions.

iliolumbar ligament /-lum′bər/ [L, *ilium* + *lumbus,* loin, *ligare,* to bind], one of a pair of ligaments forming part of the connection between the vertebral column and the pelvis. Each iliolumbar ligament attaches to a transverse process of the fifth lumbar vertebra and passes to the base of the sacrum.

iliopectineal line /-pek′tənəl/ [L, *ilium* + *pectus,* breast, *linea*], a bony ridge on the inner surface of the ilium and pubic bones that divides the true and false pelves.

iliopsoas /il′ē-ōsō′əs/ [L, *ilium* + Gk, *psoa,* loin muscle], one of the pair of muscle complexes that flex the thigh and the lumbar vertebral column.

iliopsoas abscess [L, *ilium,* intestine], an abscess, possibly tuberculous in origin, that spreads from the thoracic or lumbar spine to the upper leg muscles.

iliotibial tract /-tib′ē-əl/ [L, *ilium,* flank, *tibia,* shinbone], a band of connective tissue that extends from the iliac crest to the knee and links the gluteus maximus to the tibia.

ilium /il′ē-əm/, *pl.* **ilia** [L, flank], the uppermost of the three bones that make up the innominate bone (hipbone). The ilium forms the superior part of the acetabulum and provides attachment for several muscles, including the obturator internus, the gluteals, the iliacus, and the sartorius. —**iliac,** *adj.*

illegitimate /il′ejit′imit/ [L, *in, legitimatus,* not lawful], **1.** not authorized by law. **2.** born out of wedlock. **3.** abnormal.

illicit /ilis′it/ [L, *illicitus,* unlawful], pertaining to an act that is unlawful or otherwise not permitted.

illiterate /ilit′ərit/, unable to read and write.

illness [ME, unhealthy condition], an abnormal process in which aspects of the social, physical, emotional, or intellectual condition and function of a person are diminished or impaired, compared with that person's previous condition.

illness behavior, the manner in which individuals monitor the structure and functions of their own bodies, interpret symptoms, take remedial action, and make use of health care facilities.

illness experience, the process of being ill, comprising five stages: phase I, experiencing a symptom; phase II, assuming a sick role; phase III, making contact for health care; phase IV, being dependent (a patient); and phase V, recovering or being rehabilitated. Each stage is characterized by certain decisions, behaviors, and end points.

illness prevention, a system of health education programs and activities directed to protecting patients from real or potential health threats, minimizing risk factors, and promoting healthy behavior.

illumination /ilōō′minā′shən/ [L, *illuminare,* to make light], the lighting up of a part of the body or of an object under a microscope for the purpose of examination. —**illuminate,** *v.*

illusion /ilōō′zhən/ [L, *illudere,* to mock], a false interpretation of an external sensory stimulus, usually visual or auditory, such as a mirage in the desert or voices on the wind.

IM, abbreviation for *intramuscular.*

I.M.A., abbreviation for **Industrial Medical Association.**

image /im′ij/ [L, *imago,* likeness], **1.** a representation or visual reproduction of the likeness of someone or something, such as a painting, photograph, or sculpture. **2.** an optic representation of an object, such as that produced by refraction or reflection. **3.** a person or thing that closely resembles another; semblance. **4.** a mental picture, representation, idea, or concept of an objective reality. **5.** (in psychology) a mental representation of something previously perceived and subsequently modified by other experiences.

image acquisition time, the time required to perform a magnetic resonance imaging procedure, comprising only the data acquisition time.

image foreshortening, (in radiology) a type of shape distortion in which the image appears shorter and wider than a non distorted image of the same object. It results from misalignment of the x-ray tube to the patient, of the patient to the film, or of the tube to the film.

image format, (in computed tomography) the manner in which an image is stored, such as on a floppy disk, magnetic tape, or film.

image intensifier, an electronic device used to produce a fluoroscopic image with a low-radiation exposure. A beam of x-rays passing through the patient is converted in a special vacuum tube into a pattern of electrons. The electrons are accelerated and concentrated onto a small fluorescent screen.

image matrix, (in radiology) an arrangement of columns or rows of imaginary cells, or pixels, forming a digital image.

imagery /im'ijrē/ [L, *imago*], (in psychiatry) the formation of mental concepts, figures, ideas; any product of the imagination.

imagination /imaj'inā'shən/ [L, *imaginare*, picture to oneself], **1.** the ability to form, or the act or process of forming, mental images or conscious concepts of things that are not immediately available to the senses. **2.** (in psychology) the ability to reproduce images or ideas stored in the memory by the stimulation or suggestion of associated ideas.

imaging /im'ijing/ [L, *imago*], the formation of a mental picture or representation of someone or something using the imagination.

imago /imā'gō/ [L, likeness], (in analytic psychology) an unconscious, usually idealized mental image of a significant individual, such as one's mother, in a person's early formative years.

imbalance /imbal'əns/ [L, *im*, not, *bilanx*, having two scales], **1.** lack of balance between opposing muscle groups. **2.** abnormal balance of fluid and electrolytes in the body tissues. **3.** unequal distribution of subjects in a population group. **4.** pertaining to a person with mental abilities that are remarkable in one area but deficient in others, as an idiot savant.

imbricate /im'brikāt/ [L, *imbrex*, roofing tile], to build a surface with overlapping layers of material. Surgeons may imbricate with layers of tissue when closing a wound or other opening in a body part. —**imbrication,** *n.*

IMDD, abbreviation for **idiopathic midline destructive disease.**

imiglucerase, an analog of a human enzyme produced by recombinant deoxyribonuclease technology. It is prescribed as enzyme replacement therapy for patients with type I Gaucher disease.

iminoglycinuria /im'inōglī'sinōōr'ē·ə/, a benign familial condition characterized by the abnormal urinary excretion of the amino acids glycine, proline, and hydroxyproline.

imipenem-cilastatin sodium /im'ipē'nəm sil'əstat'in/, a broad-spectrum parenteral antibiotic. It is prescribed for the treatment of infections caused by susceptible organisms in the lower respiratory or urinary tracts, skin, abdomen, reproductive organs, bones, or joints. It is also used in the treatment of endocarditis and septicemia.

imipramine hydrochloride /imip'rəmēn/, a tricyclic antidepressant prescribed in the treatment of mental depression.

immature baby /iməchŏŏr'/ [L, *im*, not, *maturare*, to make ripe], a term sometimes applied to an infant who weighs less than 1134 g (2.5 lb) and who is significantly underdeveloped at birth.

immature cataract [L, *im + maturus*, ripe; Gk, *katarrhaktes*], a cataract at an early stage of development when the lens, partially opaque, absorbs fluid and increases by swelling. Only part of the lens is opaque.

immature erythrocyte [L, *im + maturus*, ripe; Gk, *erythros*, red, *kytos*, cell], any of the intermediate blood cells between the hemocytoblasts and nonnucleated red blood cells. They may be found in the blood circulation after birth of the fetus.

immediate auscultation /imē'dē·it/ [L, *im + medius*, middle, *auscultare*, to listen], a method of examining a patient by placing an ear or stethoscope on the skin directly over the body part being studied.

immediate automatism, a state in which a person acts spontaneously and automatically and later has no recollection of the behavior.

immediate denture [L, *im + medius + dens*, tooth], a removable artificial denture that is placed in the mouth to maintain normal appearance and ability to masticate food. It may be full or partial.

immediate hypersensitivity, an allergic reaction that occurs within minutes after exposure to an allergen.

immediate postoperative fit prosthesis (IPOF), a temporary or preparatory prosthesis such as a pylon.

immediate posttraumatic automatism, a posttraumatic state in which a person acts spontaneously and automatically and later has no recollection of the behavior.

immersion /imur'zhən/ [L, *im + mergere*, to dip], the placing of a body or an object into water or other liquid so that it is completely covered by the liquid. —**immerse,** *v.*

immersion foot, an abnormal condition of the feet characterized by damage to the muscles, nerves, skin, and blood vessels, caused by prolonged exposure to dampness or prolonged immersion in cold water.

Immerslund-Gräsbeck's syndrome, a familial form of megaloblastic anemia and cobalamin deficiency. It is characterized by selective intestinal malabsorption of vitamin B_{11}, uninfluenced by intrinsic factor.

immiscible /imis'əbəl/ [L, *im + miscere*, to mix], not capable of being mixed, such as oil and water.

immobilization /imō'bəlīzā'shən/, **1.** fixation of a body part so that it cannot move during surgery or after setting of a fracture. **2.** prolonged inactivity of an individual.

immobilization test, a procedure for identifying antibodies to motile microorganisms by measuring the ability of the antibodies to restrict the motility of the microorganisms.

immotile cilia syndrome /imō′til/ [L, *im, motilis,* movable, *cilia,* eyelashes; Gk, *syn,* together, *dromos,* course], a condition in which the hairlike processes of epithelial and other cells fail to function normally. As a result, the patient has difficulty in filtering dust and other airborne debris from the respiratory system.

immune /imyo͞on′/ [L, *immunis,* free from], being protected against infective or allergic diseases by a system of antibody molecules and related resistance factors.

immune complex, a multimolecular complex formed when an antibody binds to a specific antigen. The complex is capable of activating complement.

immune complex assay, a laboratory assessment of the amounts of components in multimolecular antigen-antibody complexes. The assay is used in various diagnostic tests for collagen-vascular disorders, glomerulonephritis, vasculitis, hepatitis, and neoplastic diseases.

immune complex hypersensitivity [L, *immunis,* free; *complexus,* embrace; Gk, *hyper,* excess; L, *sentire,* to feel], an immunoglobulin (Ig) G or IgM complement dependent, immediate-acting humoral hypersensitivity to certain soluble antigens.

immune cytolysis, cell destruction mediated by a specific antibody in conjunction with complement.

immune deviation, modification of an immune response to an antigen caused by a previous exposure to the same antigen.

immune elimination, 1. a method for determining antibody response by measuring the rate of removal of labeled antigens from the circulation. 2. an accelerated removal of antigens as a result of their binding to antibodies.

immune exclusion, the prevention of an antigen from entering the body by a specific immune response.

immune gamma globulin, passive immunizing agent obtained from pooled human plasma. It is prescribed for immunization against measles, poliomyelitis, chickenpox, serum hepatitis after transfusion, hepatitis A, agammaglobulinemia, and hypogammaglobulinemia.

immune hemolysis, the destruction of red blood cells caused by the formation of specific antigen-antibody complexes in the presence of complement.

immune human globulin, a sterile solution of globulins that is used as a passive immunizing agent and derived from adult human blood.

immune neutropenia, neutrophil destruction caused by antibodies specific for neutrophil epitopes, as often occurs in autoimmune diseases.

immune proteins [L, *immunis,* free from; Gk, *proteios,* first rank], proteins in the form of antibodies or antitoxins that contribute to the immunity of a host.

immune recognition, the activation of a T or B cell by an antigen.

immune response, a defense function of the body that produces antibodies to destroy invading antigens and malignancies. Important components of the immune system and response are immunoglobulins, lymphocytes, phagocytes, complement, properdin, the migratory inhibitory factor, and interferon. The kinds of immune response are humoral immune response, involving B lymphocytes or B cells, and cell-mediated immune response, involving T lymphocytes or T cells. The B cells and the T cells derive from the hemopoietic stem cells. The receptor sites on the surface membranes of the B cells are the combining sites of immunoglobulin molecules. The classes of immunoglobulins, identified by letter names, are M, G, A, E, and D. Immunoglobulin M (IgM), the antibody that immature B cells synthesize and incorporate in their cytoplasmic membranes, is the predominant antibody produced. The T cells develop in the thymus gland and proliferate with antigen receptors on their surface membranes. They assist in the antigen-antibody reaction of the B cells and control the cell-mediated response.

immune system, a biochemical complex that protects the body against pathogenic organisms and other foreign bodies. The system incorporates the humoral immune response, which produces antibodies to react with specific antigens, and the cell-mediated response, which uses T cells to mobilize tissue macrophages in the presence of a foreign body.

immunity /imyo͞o′nitē/ [L, *immunis,* free], 1. (in civil law) exemption from a duty or an obligation generally required by law, as an exemption from taxation or from penalty for wrongdoing or protection against liability. 2. the quality of being insusceptible to or unaffected by a particular disease or condition. —**immune,** *adj.*

immunization /im′yənīzā′shən/ [L, *immunis,* free], a process by which resistance to an infectious disease is induced or augmented.

Immunization/Vaccination Administration, a Nursing Interventions Classification defined as provision of immunizations for prevention of communicable disease.

immunoabsorbent /im′yənō′absôr′bənt/, a gel or other inert substance used to absorb antibodies from a solution or to purify them.

immunoabsorption /im′yənō′absôrp′shən/, **1.** removal of a specific group of antibodies by antigens. **2.** removal of antigen by interaction with specific antibodies.

immunoadsorbent /im′yənō′adsôr′bənt/, an insoluble preparation of antigens or antibodies used to bind homologous antibodies or antigens and remove them from a mixture of substances.

immunoassay /im′yənō·as′ā/ [L, *immunis* + Fr, *essayer,* to try], a competitive-binding assay in which the binding protein is an antibody.

immunobead /im′yənōbēd/, a tiny, inert plastic sphere coated with antigens or antibody, used for immunoassays, such as the isolation of B cells from T cells.

immunoblastic lymphoma /-blas′tik/, a proliferation of immunoblasts involving the lymph nodes.

immunoblotting /-blot′ing/, a method for identifying antigens. The antigens are allowed to adhere to cellulose sheets where they bond nonspecifically and are identified by staining with labeled antibodies. The method is also used to detect monoclonal proteins.

immunochemistry, the study of the chemical properties of antigens and antibodies, complement, and T cell receptors.

immunochemotherapy /-kem′ōther′əpē/, a combination of biotherapy and chemotherapy.

immunocompetence /-kom′pətəns/, the ability of an immune system to mobilize and deploy its antibodies and other responses to stimulation by an antigen.

immunocompromised /-kom′prəmīzd′/ [L, *immunis,* free from, *compromittere,* to promise mutually], pertaining to an immune response that has been weakened by a disease or an immunosuppressive agent.

immunocompromised host, an individual whose immune response is defective as a result of an immunodeficiency disorder or exposure to immunosuppressive drugs or irradiation.

immunodeficiency disease /-difish′ənsē/, any of a group of health conditions caused by a defect in the immune system and generally characterized by susceptibility to infections and chronic diseases. The diseases are sometimes classified as B cell (antibody) deficiencies, T cell (cellular) deficiencies, combined T and B cell defi-

ciencies, defects of cell movement, and defects of microbicidal activity.

immunodeficient /-difish′ənt/ [L, *immunis* + *de,* from, *facere,* to make], pertaining to an abnormal condition of the immune system in which cellular or humoral immunity is inadequate and resistance to infection is decreased. Kinds of immunodeficient conditions are **hypogammaglobulinemia** and **lymphoid aplasia.**

immunodiagnostic /-dī′əgnos′tik/ [L, *immunis* + Gk, *dia,* through, *gnosis* knowledge], pertaining to or characterizing a diagnosis based on an antigen-antibody reaction.

immunodiffusion /-difyŌŌ′zhən/ [L, *immunis* + *diffundere,* to spread], a technique for the identification and quantification of any of the immunoglobulins. It is based on the presence of a visible precipitate that results from an antigen-antibody combination under certain circumstances. Gel diffusion is a technique that involves evaluation of the precipitin reaction in a clear gel. Electroimmunodiffusion is a gel diffusion to which an electrical field is applied, accelerating the reaction. Double gel diffusion is a technique that permits identification of antibodies in mixed specimens.

immunoelectroadsorption /im′yənō′ilek′trō·adsôrp′shən/, an antibody assay technique in which antigens are adsorbed onto a metal-coated glass slide with an electric current. Serum containing antibodies is then applied to the slide.

immunoelectron microscopy /im′yənō′-ilek′tron/, electron microscopy of specimens labeled with antibodies that have been conjugated with gold. The gold makes the antibody labels electron-dense.

immunoelectrophoresis /-ilek′trōfôrē′sis/ [L, *immunis* + Gk, *elektron,* amber, *pherein,* to bear], a technique that combines electrophoresis and immunodiffusion to separate and allow identification of complex proteins. The proteins in the test serum are spread out in agar and separated by electrophoresis. —**immunoelectrophoretic,** *adj.*

immunoenhancement /im′yənō′enhans′mənt/, the augmentation of immune responsiveness by immunization or other means.

immunoferritin /fer′itin/, an antibody labeled with ferritin used to identify specific antigens in electron microscopy.

immunoferritin technique, a method of labeling antibody molecules with ferritin, an electron-dense material. The ferritin renders the sites of antibody attachment visible in electron microscopy.

immunofixation /-fiksā′shən/, a process

by which antigens in a protein mixture are separated on an electrophoretic gel and identified by the application of labeled antibodies.

immunofluorescence /-floŏres′əns/ [L, *immunis* + *fluere,* to flow], a technique used for the rapid identification of an antigen by exposing it to known antibodies tagged with the fluorescent dye fluorescein and observing the characteristic antigenantibody reaction of precipitation. —**immunofluorescent,** *adj.*

immunogen /imyoo′nəjən/ [L, *immunis* + Gk, *genein,* to produce], any agent or substance capable of provoking an immune response or producing immunity. —**immunogenic,** *adj.*

immunogenetics /-jənet′iks/, a branch of medicine concerned with the role of genetics in tissue transplantation and immunologic response.

immunogenicity /-jənis′itē/, the ability of an antigen to induce a specific immune response.

immunoglobulin /-glob′yəlin/ [L, *immunis* + *globus,* small sphere], any of five structurally and antigenically distinct antibodies present in the serum and external secretions of the body.

immunoglobulin A (IgA), one of the five classes of humoral antibodies produced by the body and one of the most prevalent. It is found in all secretions of the body and is the major antibody in the mucous membrane lining the intestines and in the bronchi, saliva, and tears. IgA combines with a protein in the mucosa and defends body surfaces against invading microorganisms.

immunoglobulin D (IgD), one of the five classes of humoral antibodies produced by the body. It is a specialized protein found in small amounts in serum tissue. The precise function of IgD is not known, but it increases in quantity during allergic reactions to milk, insulin, penicillin, and various toxins.

immunoglobulin E (IgE), one of the five classes of humoral antibodies produced by the body. It is concentrated in the lung, the skin, and the cells of mucous membranes. It provides the primary defense against environmental antigens. IgE reacts with certain antigens to release certain chemical mediators that cause type I hypersensitivity reactions characterized by wheal and flare.

immunoglobulin G (IgG), one of the five classes of humoral antibodies produced by the body. It is a specialized protein synthesized by the body in response to invasions by bacteria, fungi, and viruses.

immunoglobulin M (IgM), one of the

five classes of humoral antibodies produced by the body and the largest in molecular structure. It is the first immunoglobulin the body produces when challenged by antigens and is found in circulating fluids. It is the dominant antibody in ABO incompatibilities.

immunohematology /-hem′ətol′əjē/ [L, *immunis* + Gk, *haima,* blood, *logos,* science], the study of antigen-antibody reactions and their effects on blood.

immunoincompetence /im′yənō′inkom′-pətəns/, an inability to develop an immune reaction.

immunoincompetent /im′yənō′inkom′-pətənt/, an inability to develop an immune response to the challenge of antigens.

immunologic barrier /-loj′ik/, an apparent protection against an immune response afforded by certain areas of the body as demonstrated by the prolonged survival of foreign grafts in those areas.

immunologic disease [L, *immunis,* free from; Gk, *logos,* science; L, *dis* + Fr, *aise,* ease], the signs and symptoms of reactions of antibodies to antigens, as in anaphylaxis.

immunologic granuloma, a small, organized, compact collection of mononuclear phagocytes that develops within 2 or 3 weeks after the introduction of a foreign material, provoking an inflammatory response.

immunologic pregnancy test, a method of detecting pregnancy through an increase in the concentration of human chorionic gonadotropin in the plasma or urine.

immunologic surveillance [L, *immunis,* free from; Gk, *logos,* science; Fr, *surveiller,* to watch over], the theory that the immune system protects human organisms from microorganisms, foreign tissue, and diseases caused by altered cells, especially cancer cells.

immunologic tests [L, *immunis* + *testum,* crucible], tests based on the principles of antigen-antibody reactions.

immunologic theory of aging, a concept based on the premise that because of decline in the function of T cells and B cells, normal cells are unrecognized as such, thereby triggering immune reactions within the individual's own body.

immunologist /im′yənol′əjist/, a specialist in immunology.

immunology /im′yənol′əjē/ [L, *immunis* + Gk, *logos,* science], the study of the reaction of tissues of the immune system of the body to antigenic stimulation.

immunomodulator /-mod′yəlā′tər/ [L, *immunis* + *modulus,* little measure], a substance that acts to alter the immune response by augmenting or reducing the ability of the immune system to produce specifically modified serum antibodies or sensitized cells that recognize and react with the antigen that initiated their production. Corticosteroids, cytotoxic agents, thymosin, and the immunoglobulins are among the immunomodulating substances. —**immunomodulation,** *n.*

immunopathology /-pəthol'əjē/, **1.** the study of disease processes that have an immunologic cause. **2.** injury to tissues and cells induced by antibodies or other products of an immune response.

immunophenotypic analysis /-fē'nōtip'ik/, a method for dividing lymphomas and leukemias into clonal subgroups on the basis of differences in cell surfaces and cytoplasmic antigens.

immunopotency /-pō'tənsē/ [L, *immunis* + *potentia,* power], the ability of an antigen to elicit an immune response.

immunoprecipitation /-prisip'itā'shən/, a procedure used to isolate target molecules with which antibodies react.

immunoproliferative disorder, a condition characterized by the continuous proliferation of a subset of immune cells, such as lymphocytes or plasma cells.

immunoproliferative small intestine disease (IPSID), a disorder characterized by a small, diffuse lesion with cells that have features of plasma cells, histiocytes, and atypical lymphocytes. The disease mainly affects the duodenum and proximal jejunum.

immunoprophylaxis /-prō'filak'sis/, the introduction of active immunization through vaccines or passive immunization through antisera.

immunoradiometric assay /-rā'dē·ōmet'-rik/, a method to measure certain plasma proteins by using radiolabeled antibody.

immunoregulation /-reg'yəlā'shən/, control of immune response functions, by manipulation of suppressor and contrasuppressor lymphocyte circuits.

immunoregulatory hormones /-reg'-yəlatôr'ē/, chemical substances secreted by endocrine glands and lymphocytes that influence activities of the immune system.

immunoselection /-silek'shən/ [L, *immunis* + *seligere,* to select], **1.** the survival of certain cells that results from their lack of surface antigens that would otherwise make them vulnerable to attack and destruction by antibodies of an immune system. **2.** the chance of survival of a fetus that results from the compatibility of its genotype with that of the mother's immune system.

immunosorbent /-sôr'bənt/, a substance containing attached antigens used to re-

move homologous antibodies from a solution.

immunostimulant /-stim'yələnt/, an agent such as bacille Calmette-Guerin vaccine that induces an immune response.

immunosuppression /-səpresh'ən/ [L, *immunis* + *supprimere,* to press down], **1.** the administration of agents that significantly interfere with the ability of the immune system to respond to antigenic stimulation by inhibiting cellular and humoral immunity. Immunosuppression may be deliberate, such as in preparation for bone marrow or other transplantation to prevent rejection by the host of the donor tissue, or incidental, such as often results from chemotherapy for the treatment of cancer. **2.** an abnormal condition of the immune system characterized by markedly inhibited ability to respond to antigenic stimuli. —**immunosuppressed,** *adj.*

immunosuppressive /-səpres'iv/, **1.** pertaining to a substance or procedure that lessens or prevents an immune response. **2.** an immunosuppressive agent, such as immunosuppressive drugs used to prevent homograft rejection.

immunotherapy /-ther'əpē/ [L, *immunis* + Gk, *therapeia,* treatment], the application of immunologic knowledge and techniques to prevent and treat disease. Examples include the use of immunostimulants and immunosuppressants and the transfer of immunocompetent cells and tissues from one person to another. An increasingly important role in immunotherapy is that of cytokines, including interferon, now widely used for its antiviral and antitumor properties. —**immunotherapeutic,** *adj.*

immunotoxin (IT) /-tok'sin/, a plant or animal toxin that is attached to a monoclonal antibody and used to destroy a specific target cell.

impacted /impak'tid/ [L, *impingere,* to drive against], tightly or firmly wedged in a limited amount of space. —**impact,** *v.,* **impaction,** *n.*

impacted fracture, a bone break in which the adjacent fragmented ends of the fractured bone are wedged together.

impacted tooth, a tooth so positioned against another tooth, bone, or soft tissue that its complete and normal eruption is impossible or unlikely.

impaction /impak'shən/, **1.** an obstacle or malposition that prevents a tooth from erupting. **2.** the presence of a large or hard fecal mass in the rectum or colon.

impaired glucose tolerance (IGT) /imperd'/ [L, *impejorare,* to make worse; Gk, *glykys,* sweet; L, *tolerare,* to endure], a condition in which fasting plasma glucose levels are higher than normal but lower than those diagnostic of diabetes mellitus.

impairment [L, *impejorare*, to make worse], any disorder in structure or function resulting from anatomic, physiologic, or psychologic abnormalities that interfere with normal activities.

impedance /impē′dəns/ [L, *impedire*, to entangle], a form of electrical resistance observed in an alternating current that is analogous to the classic electric resistance that occurs in a direct current circuit.

impedance plethysmography, a technique for detecting blood vessel occlusion that determines volumetric changes in the limb by measuring changes in its girth as indicated by changes in the electrical impedance of mercury-containing polymeric silicone (Silastic) tubes in a pressure cuff.

imperative conception /imper′ətiv/ [L, *imperare*, to command], a thought or impression that appears spontaneously in the mind and cannot be eliminated, such as an obsession.

imperforate /impur′fərit/ [L, *im*, not, *perforare*, to pierce], lacking a normal opening in a body organ or passageway.

imperforate anus, any of several congenital developmental malformations of the anorectal part of the gastrointestinal tract. The most common form is anal agenesis, in which the rectal pouch ends blindly above the surface of the perineum. Other forms include anal stenosis, in which the anal aperture is small, and anal membrane atresia, in which the anal membrane covers the aperture, creating an obstruction.

imperforate hymen [L, *im* + *perforare*, to pierce through; Gk, *hymen*, membrane], a hymen that completely encloses the external orifice of the vagina.

impermeable /impur′mē·əbəl/ [L, *im*, not, *permeare*, to pass through]. (of a tissue, membrane, or film) preventing the passage of a substance through it.

impetigo /im′pətī′gō/ [L, *impetus*, an attack], a streptococcal, staphylococcal, or combined infection of the skin beginning as focal erythema and progressing to pruritic vesicles, erosions, and honey-colored crusts. Lesions usually form on the face and spread locally. The disorder is highly contagious through contact with the discharge from the lesions. —**impetiginous** /im′petij′inəs/, *adj.*

impetigo contagiosa [L, *impetus*, attack; *contingere*, to touch], an acute contagious superficial infection of the skin. It is characterized by vesicles that rupture, leaving a purulent exudate that dries into golden crusts.

impetigo herpetiformis [L, *impetus*, at-

tack; Gk, *herpein*, to creep; L, *forma*], a skin disorder that mainly affects pregnant women, beginning as an eruption in the genitofemoral area and spreading to other areas. The eruptions are usually irregular or circular groups of pustules that tend to coalesce.

impingement injection test /impinj′mənt/, an appraisal of shoulder injury in which a reduction of more than half the painful arc of abduction is relieved after injection of 10 ml of lidocaine in the subacromial space.

impingement sign, a painful arc produced by forceful abduction of the internally rotated arm against the acromion in evaluation of a shoulder injury.

impingement syndrome, a progressive condition of shoulder pain and dysfunction, usually caused by repetitive placement of the arm in overhead positions. The disorder is a common sports injury.

implant /im′plant, implant′/ [L, *implantare*, to set into], **1.** (in radiotherapy) an encapsulated radioactive substance embedded in tissue for therapy. For example, seeds containing iodine-125 may be implanted permanently in prostate and chest tumors, and seeds of iridium-192 in ribbons or wire may be embedded temporarily in head and neck cancers. **2.** (in surgery) material inserted or grafted into an organ or structure of the body. The implant may be of tissue such as in a blood vessel graft or of an artificial substance such as in a hip prosthesis, a cardiac pacemaker, or a container of radioactive material.

implantable cardioverter-defibrillator (ICD), a surgically implanted electric device that automatically terminates lethal ventricular arrhythmias by delivering low-energy shocks to the heart, restoring proper rhythm when the heart begins beating rapidly or erratically.

implantation, (in embryology) the process involving the attachment, penetration, and embedding of the blastocyst in the lining of the uterine wall during the early stages of prenatal development.

implantation dermoid cyst, a tumor derived from embryonal tissues, caused by an injury that forces part of the ectoderm into the body.

implantation endometriosis [L, *implantare*, to set into; Gk, *endon*, within, *metra*, womb, *osis*, condition], ectopic endometrial tissue prevalent throughout the peritoneal cavity.

implant denture, an artificial full or partial denture that consists of a subperiosteally or intraperiosteally implanted framework in contact with alveolar bone.

implanted fusion port, a self-sealing silicone septum encased in a metal or plastic case with an attached silicone catheter.

implanted suture [L, *implantare,* to set into, *sutura*], a suture formed by inserting pins on opposite sides of a wound and drawing the edges of the wound together by winding thread tightly around the pins.

implant restoration, a single-tooth implant crown or multiple-tooth implant crown or bridge that replaces a missing tooth or teeth.

implementation /im'pləməntā'shən/ [L, *implere,* to fill], a deliberate action performed to achieve a goal, such as carrying out a plan in caring for a patient.

implementation mechanism, the means by which innovations are transferred from the planners to the units of service.

implementing /im'pləmen'ting/ [L, *implere,* to fill], (in five-step nursing process) a category of nursing behavior in which the actions necessary for accomplishing the health care plan are initiated and completed. Implementing includes performing or assisting in the performance of the patient's activities of daily living, counseling and teaching the patient or the patient's family, giving care to achieve therapeutic goals and to optimize the patient's achievement of health goals, supervising and evaluating the work of staff members, and recording and exchanging information relevant to the patient's continued health care.

implied consent /implīd'/ [L, *implicare,* to involve, *consentire,* to feel], the granting of permission for health care without a formal agreement between the patient and health care provider. An example is an appointment made with a physician by a patient with a physical complaint; it is implied that by making the appointment the patient gives consent to the physician to make a diagnosis and offer treatment.

implosion /implō'zhən/ [L, *im* + *plaudere,* to strike], 1. a bursting inward. 2. a psychiatric treatment for people disabled by phobias and anxiety in which the person is desensitized to anxiety-producing stimuli by repeated intense exposure in imagination or reality, until the stimuli are no longer stressful. —**implode,** *v.*

impotence /im'pətəns/ [L, *im,* not, *potentia,* power], 1. weakness. 2. inability of the adult male to achieve penile erection or less commonly to ejaculate after achieving an erection. Functional impotence has a psychologic basis. Anatomic impotence results from physically defective genitalia. Atonic impotence involves disturbed neuromuscular function. —**impotent,** *adj.*

impregnate /impreg'nāt/ [L, *impregnare,* to

make pregnant], 1. to inseminate and make pregnant; to fertilize. 2. to saturate or mix with another substance. —**impregnable,** *adj.,* **impregnation,** *n.*

impression /impresh'ən/ [L, *imprimere,* to press into], 1. (in dentistry and prosthetic medicine) a mold of a part of the mouth or other part of the body from which a replacement or prosthesis may be formed. 2. (in the medical record) the examiner's diagnosis or assessment of a problem, disease, or condition. 3. a strong sensation or effect on the mind, intellect, or feelings.

impression material [L, *imprimere,* to press into, *materia,* stuff], any substance used for making impressions of teeth and oral structures for the purpose of producing dental restorations.

imprinting [Fr, *empreindre,* to impress], (in ethology) a special type of learning that occurs at critical points during the early stages of development in animals.

imprisonment /impriz'ənment/ [Fr, *emprisonner,* to confine], (in law) the act of confining, detaining, or arresting a person or in any way restraining personal liberty and preventing free exercise of movement.

impulse /im'puls/ [L, *impellere,* to drive], 1. (in psychology) a sudden irresistible, often irrational inclination, urge, desire, or action resulting from a particular feeling or mental state. 2. (in physiology) the electrochemical process involved in neural transmission. —**impulsive,** *adj.*

impulse-control disorder, a behavior in which the individual fails to resist performing a potentially harmful act.

Impulse Control Training, a Nursing Interventions Classification defined as assisting the patient to mediate impulsive behavior through application of problem-solving strategies to social and interpersonal situations.

impulse-conducting system [L, *impellere,* to drive before, *conducere,* to conduct; Gk, *systema*], the Purkinje fibers within the heart muscle that conduct impulses controlling the contractions of the atria and ventricles.

impulsion /impul'shən/ [L, *impellere,* to drive], an abnormal, irrational urge to commit an unlawful or socially unacceptable act.

IMV, abbreviation for **intermittent mandatory ventilation.**

In, symbol for the element **indium.**

inactivated measles virus vaccine /inak'tivā'tid/ [L, *in,* not, *activus* + OE, *masala,* blister; L, *virus,* poison, *vaccinus,* of a cow], a measles vaccine virus that has been treated so that it is no longer capable of replication. It is an alternative to live attenuated measles vaccine, which may be contraindicated for some individuals, such as those who are immunocompromised.

inactivation /inak′tivā′shən/ [L, *in,* not, *activus,* active], a reversible denaturation of a protein.

inactivation of complement [L, *in* + *activus, complere,* to complete], the loss of activity of the enzymatic proteins in blood, achieved by heating the serum to about 122° F (55° C). Inactivation of complement is a step in the process of **complement fixation.**

inactive colon /inak′tiv/ [L, *in,* not, *activus,* active; Gk, *kolon,* colon], hypotonicity of the bowel that results in decreased contractions and propulsive movements and a delay in the normal 12-hour transit time of luminal contents from the cecum to the anus. Colonic inactivity may be caused by acquired or congenital megacolon, anticholinergic drugs, depression, faulty habits of elimination, inadequate fluid intake, lack of exercise, a low-residue or starvation diet, neuroendocrine response to surgical stress, prolonged bed rest, or a neurologic disease such as diabetic visceral neuropathy, multiple sclerosis, parkinsonism, and spinal cord lesions. Normal motility of the colon is frequently compromised by the continued use of laxatives.

inadequate personality /inad′əkwit/ [L, *in,* not, *adaequare,* to equal, *personalis,* of a person], a personality characterized by a lack of physical stamina, emotional immaturity, social instability, poor judgment, reduced motivation, ineptness—especially in interpersonal relationships—and an inability to adapt or react effectively to new or stressful situations.

inanimate /inan′imit/ [L, *in,* not, *animus,* life spirit], not alive; lacking signs of life.

inanition /in′ənish′ən/ [L, *inanis,* empty], **1.** an exhausted condition resulting from lack of food and water or a defect in assimilation; starvation. **2.** a state of lethargy characterized by a loss of vitality or vigor in all aspects of social, moral, and intellectual life.

inanition fever, a temporary mild febrile condition of the newborn in the first few days after birth, usually caused by dehydration.

inborn /in′bôrn/ [L, *in,* within; AS, *beran,* to bear], innate; acquired or occurring during intrauterine life, with reference to both normally inherited traits and developmental or genetically transmitted anomalies.

inborn error of metabolism, one of many abnormal metabolic conditions caused by an inherited defect of a single enzyme or other protein. People with such diseases generally display a large number of physical signs that are characteristic of the genetic trait. Inborn errors of metabolism may be detected in the fetus in utero by the examination of squamous and blood cells obtained by amniocentesis and fetoscopy. Laboratory tests after birth often show higher than normal levels of particular metabolites in the blood and urine, such as phenylpyruvic acid and phenylalanine in phenylketonuria and galactose in galactosemia.

inborn lysosomal disease, one of many inherited disorders of metabolism involving degradative enzymes normally located in lysosomes. The condition leads to storage of abnormal amounts of lysosomal agents.

inbreeding /in′brēding/ [L, *in,* within; AS, *bredan,* to reproduce], the production of offspring by the mating of closely related individuals, organisms, or plants; self-fertilization is the most extreme form, which normally occurs in certain plants and lower animals. The practice provides a greater chance for recessive genes for both desirable and undesirable traits to become homozygous and to be expressed phenotypically.

incandescent [L, *incandescere,* to begin to glow], hot to the point of glowing or emitting intense light rays, as an incandescent light bulb.

incarcerate /inkar′sərāt/ [L, *in,* within, *carcerare,* to imprison], to trap, imprison, or confine, such as a loop of intestine in an inguinal hernia.

incarcerated hernia [L, *in* + *carcerare,* to imprison, *hernia,* rupture], a loop of bowel with ends occluded so that solids cannot pass; the herniated bowel will not return to its normal position without manipulation or surgery.

incentive spirometry /insen′tiv/, a method of encouraging voluntary deep breathing by providing visual feedback about inspiratory volume.

inception /insep′shən/ [L, *incipere,* to begin], the origin or beginning of anything.

incest /in′sest/ [L, *incestum,* defiled], sexual intercourse between members of the same family who are so closely related as to be legally prohibited from marrying by reason of their consanguinity. —**incestuous,** *adj.*

incidence /in′sidəns/ [L, *incidere,* to happen], **1.** the number of times an event occurs. **2.** (in epidemiology) the number of new cases in a particular period.

incidence rate, the rate of new cases of a disease in a specified population over a defined period.

incidental additives /in'siden'təl/ [L, *incidere*, to happen, *additio*, something added], material added to food by the use of pesticides, herbicides, or chemicals used in food processing.

incident report, a document, usually confidential, describing any accident or deviation from policies or orders involving a patient, employee, visitor, or student on the premises of a health care facility.

Incident Reporting, a Nursing Interventions Classification defined as written and verbal reporting of any event in the process of patient care that is inconsistent with desired patient outcomes or routine operations of the health care facility.

incineration /insin'ərā'shən/ [L, *incinerare*, to burn to ashes], the removal or reduction of waste materials by burning.

incipient /insip'ē·ənt/ [L, *incipire*, to commence], coming into existence; at an initial stage; beginning to appear, such as a symptom or disease.

incipient dental caries, a dental condition in which a lesion of tooth decay is initially detectable.

incisal angle /insī'səl/ [L, *incidere*, to cut into, *angulus*, corner], the degree of slope between the axis-orbital plane and the discluding surface of the maxillary incisor teeth.

incisal guide, the part of a dental articulator that maintains the incisal guide angle.

incisal guide pin, a metal rod, attached to the upper member of an articulator, that touches the incisal guide table to maintain the established vertical separation of the upper and lower members of the articulator.

incision /insizh'ən/ [L, *incidere*, to cut into], **1.** a cut produced surgically by a sharp instrument that creates an opening into an organ or space in the body. **2.** the act of making an incision.

incisional hernia /insish'ənəl/ [L, *incidere*, to cut into, *hernia*, rupture], a herniation through a surgical scar.

Incision Site Care, a Nursing Interventions Classification defined as cleansing, monitoring, and promotion of healing in a wound that is closed with sutures, clips, or staples.

incisor /insī'zər/, one of the eight front teeth, four in each dental arch, that first appear as primary teeth during infancy, are replaced by permanent incisors during childhood, and last until old age. The crown of the incisor is chisel shaped and has a sharp cutting edge. The upper incisors are larger and stronger than the lower and are directed obliquely downward and forward.

incisura /in'sisyōō'rə/ [L, *incidere*, to cut into], a notch or indentation on an organ or body part.

inclusion /inklōō'zhən/ [L, *in*, within, *claudere*, to shut], **1.** the act of enclosing or the condition of being enclosed. **2.** a structure within another, such as an inclusion in the cytoplasm of the cells.

inclusion bodies, microscopic objects of various shapes and sizes observed in the nucleus or cytoplasm of blood cells or other tissue cells, depending on the type of disease.

inclusion conjunctivitis, an acute purulent conjunctival infection caused by *Chlamydia* organisms. It occurs in two forms: the infection in infants is characterized by bilateral chemosis, redness, and purulent discharge; the adult variety is unilateral, less severe, and less purulent and is associated with preauricular lymphadenopathy.

inclusion dermoid cyst, a tumor derived from embryonal tissues, caused by the inclusion of foreign tissue when a developmental cleft closes.

inclusiveness principle /inklōō'sivnəs/ [L, *in*, within, *claudere*, to shut, *principium*, a beginning], a rule that response to various objects in the environment is proportional to the amount of stimulus provided by each object.

inclusive rate /inklōō'siv/, a method of calculating inpatient hospital charges in which a fixed amount covers all services, regardless of the number or intensity of services provided.

incoercible /in'kō·ur'sibəl/, pertaining to something that cannot be restrained or willfully terminated, as a siege of hiccups.

incoercible vomiting, vomiting that is intractable or out of control.

incoherent /in'kōhir'ənt/ [L, *in*, not, *cohaere*, to hold together], **1.** disordered; without logical connection; disjointed; lacking orderly continuity or relevance. **2.** unable to express one's thoughts or ideas in an orderly, intelligible manner, usually as a result of emotional stress.

incompatibility /in'kəmpat'ibil'itē/ [L, *in* + *compatibilus*, agreeing], a state of not being able to exist in harmony, as when transfused blood produces adverse effects because the donor and recipient blood groups conflict.

incompatible /in'kəmpat'əbəl/ [L, *in*, not, *compatibilus*, agreeing], unable to coexist. A tissue transplantation may be rejected because recipient and donor antibody factors are incompatible.

incompetence /inkom'pətəns/ [L, *in*, not, *competentia*, capable], lack of ability. Body organs that do not function adequately may be described as incompetent. —**Incompetent,** *adj.*

incompetency /inkomp'ətənsē/, legal status of a person declared to be unable to provide for his or her own needs and protection.

incompetent cervix [L, *in*, not, *competentia,* capable, *cervix,* neck], (in obstetrics) a condition characterized by painless dilation of the cervical os of the uterus before term without labor or contractions of the uterus. Miscarriage or premature delivery may result.

incomplete abortion /in'kəmplēt'/ [L, *in*, not, *complere,* to fill, *ab,* away from, *oriri,* to be born], termination of pregnancy in which the products of conception are not entirely expelled or removed. It often causes hemorrhage that may require surgical evacuation by curettage, oxytocics, and blood replacement.

incomplete dislocation [L, *in* + *complere,* to fill up, *dis* + *locare,* to place], a partial abnormal separation of the articular surfaces of a joint.

incomplete fracture, a bone break in which the crack in the osseous tissue does not completely traverse the width of the affected bone but may angle off in one or more directions.

incomplete hemianopia, loss of only a part of the half of the visual field.

incomplete hernia [L, *in* + *complere,* to fill up, *hernia,* rupture], a hernia that has not yet protruded through a weak spot or opening.

incomplete protein, a food that is deficient in one or more of the nine essential amino acids.

incongruent communication /inkong'-grōō·ənt/, a communication pattern in which the sender gives conflicting messages on verbal and nonverbal levels and the listener does not know which message to accept.

incontinence /inkon'tinəns/ [L, *incontinentia,* inability to retain], the inability to control urination or defecation. Urinary incontinence may be caused by cerebral clouding, infection, lesions in the brain or spinal cord, damage to peripheral nerves of the bladder, or injury to the sphincter or perineal structures, sometimes during childbirth. Stress incontinence precipitated by coughing, straining, or heavy lifting occurs more often in women than in men. Fecal incontinence may result from relaxation of the anal sphincter or central nervous system or spinal cord disorders and may be treated by a program of bowel training. —**incontinent,** *adj.*

incontinence, bowel, a NANDA-accepted nursing diagnosis of a state in which an individual experiences a change in normal bowel habits characterized by involuntary passage of stool. The cause of the condition is neuromuscular or musculoskeletal impairment; depression, severe anxiety, or perceptive or cognitive impairment; multiple life changes; inadequate relaxation; little or no exercise; poor nutrition; work-related tensions; no vacations; unmet expectations; unrealistic perceptions; and inadequate support systems or coping methods. The defining characteristic is an involuntary passage of stool.

incontinence, functional, a NANDA-accepted nursing diagnosis of the state in which an individual experiences an involuntary, unpredictable passage of urine. The critical defining characteristics are the urge to void or bladder contractions sufficiently strong to result in loss of urine before reaching an appropriate receptacle.

incontinence, reflex, a NANDA-accepted nursing diagnosis of the state in which an individual experiences an involuntary loss of urine occurring at somewhat predictable intervals when a specific bladder volume is reached. Defining characteristics include lack of awareness of bladder filling; lack of urge to void or feeling of bladder fullness; or uninhibited bladder contractions/spasms at regular intervals.

incontinence, stress, a NANDA-accepted nursing diagnosis of the state in which an individual experiences a loss of urine of less than 50 ml occurring with increased abdominal pressure, such as experienced during coughing, sneezing, laughing, and lifting. The major defining characteristic is reported or observed dribbling with increased abdominal pressure. Minor characteristics include urinary urgency or urinary frequency (more often than every 2 hours).

incontinence, total, a NANDA-accepted nursing diagnosis of the state in which an individual experiences a continuous and unpredictable loss of urine. Defining characteristics include a constant flow of urine that occurs at unpredictable times without distension or uninhibited bladder contractions or spasms, unsuccessful incontinence refractory treatments, nocturia (urination more than two times per night), lack of perineal or bladder awareness, and unawareness of incontinence.

incontinence, urge, a NANDA-accepted nursing diagnosis of the state in which an individual experiences involuntary passage of urine occurring soon after a strong sense of urgency to void. Defining characteristics are urinary urgency, frequency (voiding more often than every 2 hours), bladder contractions or spasms, nocturia

I

(urination more than two times per night), voiding in small amounts (less than 100 ml) or in large amounts (500 ml), and an inability to reach a toilet on time.

increment /ing'krəmənt/ [L, *incresere*, to grow], **1.** an increase or gain. **2.** the act of growing or increasing. **3.** the amount of an increase or gain in intrauterine pressure as uterine contractions begin in labor. —**incremental**, *adj.*

incremental line /ing'krəmen'təl/, **1.** one of a series of lines showing successive layers deposited in a tissue. **1.** a very fine line of cementum that follows the contours of a tooth.

incremental lines of Ebner [Victor von Ebner, Austrian histologist, 1842–1925], delicate lines seen on ground sections of a tooth, indicating periods of rest between increments of dentin.

incrustation, hardened exudate, scale, or scab.

incubation period /in'kyəbā'shən/ [L, *incubare,* to lie on; Gk, *peri,* around, *hodos,* way], **1.** the time between exposure to a pathogenic organism and the onset of symptoms of a disease. **2.** the time required to induce the development of an embryo in an egg or to induce the development and replication of tissue cells or microorganisms being grown in culture media. **3.** the time allowed for a chemical reaction or process to proceed.

incubator /in'kyəbā'tər/, an apparatus used to provide a controlled environment, especially a particular temperature.

incudectomy /in'kyoōodek'təmē/ [L, *incus,* anvil, *ektome,* excision], surgical removal of the incus, performed to treat conductive hearing loss that results from necrosis of the tip of the incus. Local or general anesthesia is used. The defective incus is excised and replaced with a bone chip graft so that sound vibrations are again transmitted.

incurable /inkyoō'rəbəl/, not responding to medical or surgical treatment.

incus /ing'kəs/, *pl.* **incudes** /inkoō'dēz/ [L, anvil], one of the three ossicles in the middle ear, resembling an anvil. It transmits sound vibrations from the malleus to the stapes.

IND, abbreviation for **investigational new drug.**

indanedione derivative /indan'dē·ōn/, one of a small group of oral anticoagulants designed for long-term therapeutic use in patients who cannot tolerate other oral anticoagulants.

indemnify /indem'nifi/, to protect against loss or injury by compensating for the loss or injury.

indentation /in'dəntā'shən/ [L, *in,* within,

dens, tooth], a notch, pit, or depression in the surface of an object, such as toothmarks on the tongue or skin. —**indent,** *v.*

independence /in'dəpen'dəns/ [L, *in,* not, *de,* from, *pendere,* to hang], **1.** the state or quality of being independent; autonomy; free of the influence, guidance, or control of a person or a group. **2.** a lack of requirement or reliance on another for physical existence or emotional needs. —**independent,** *adj.*

independent assortment [L, *in,* not, *dependere,* to hang from, *ad,* towards, *sortiri,* to cast lots], (in genetics) a basic principle that the members of a pair of genes are randomly distributed in the gametes, independently of the distribution of other pairs of genes.

independent living center, rehabilitation facility in which disabled persons can receive special education and training in the performance of all or most activities of daily living with a particular handicap.

independent practice, (in nursing) the practice of certain aspects of professional nursing that are encompassed by applicable licensure and law and require no supervision or direction from others. Nurses in independent practice may have an office in which they see patients and charge fees for service. In all nursing settings state practice acts define certain aspects of nursing practice that are independent and may define those that must be done only under supervision or direction of another individual, usually a physician.

Independent Practice Association (IPA), a U.S. type of physician alliance in which the physicians own the practice, as opposed to physicians employed by an entity such as a health maintenance organization.

independent variable, (in research) a variable that is manipulated by the researcher and evaluated by its measurable effect on the dependent variable or variables.

indeterminate cleavage /in'ditur'minit/ [L, *in,* not, *determinare,* to fix limits; AS, *cleofan,* to split], mitotic division of the fertilized ovum into blastomeres that have similar developmental potential and, if isolated, can give rise to a complete individual embryo.

index astigmatism [L, *indicare,* to make known, *a + stigma,* point], an astigmatism caused by unequal refractive indices in different parts of the lens.

index case [L, *indicare,* to make known], (in epidemiology) the first case of a disease, as contrasted with subsequent cases.

Index Medicus, an index published monthly by the National Library of Medicine, which lists articles from the medical.

nursing, and allied health literature from throughout the world by subject and by author.

index myopia, a kind of nearsightedness caused by a variation in the index of refraction of the eye media.

Indian Health Service, a bureau of the Department of Health and Human Services for providing public health and medical services to Native Americans in the United States. In Canada the services are provided by the Ministry of Indian Affairs.

indican /in'dikən/ [Gk, *indikon,* indigo], a substance (potassium indoxyl sulfate) produced in the intestine by the decomposition of tryptophan, absorbed by the intestinal wall, and excreted in the urine.

indication /in'dikā'shən/ [L, *indicare,* to make known], a reason to prescribe a medication or perform a treatment. A bacterial infection may be an indication for the prescription of a specific antibiotic; appendicitis is an indication for appendectomy. —**indicate,** *v.*

indicator /in'dikā'tər/, a tape, paper, tablet, or other substance that is used to test for a specific reaction because it changes in a predictable visible way. Some kinds of indicators are **autoclave indicator, dipsticks,** and **litmus paper.**

indicator-dilution method, a method for measuring blood volume. A known amount of a substance that dissolves freely in blood but does not leave the capillaries is injected intravenously. After a few minutes a sample of blood is withdrawn, and the volume of blood in the body is calculated from the concentration of the substance in the sample, the volume of the sample, and the hematocrit.

indifference to pain syndrome /indif'-ərəns/, a congenital lack of pain sensitivity caused by defective development of sensory nerve endings in the skin.

indigence /in'dijəns/ [L, *indigere,* to need], a condition of having insufficient income to pay for adequate medical care without depriving oneself or one's dependents of food, clothing, shelter, or other living essentials.

indigenous /indij'ənəs/ [L, *indigena,* a native], native to or occurring naturally in a specified area or environment, as certain species of bacteria in the human digestive tract.

indigestible /in'dijes'təbəl/ [L, *in,* not, *digerere,* to separate], pertaining to a food substance that cannot be broken down by the digestive tract and converted into an absorbable nutrient.

indinavir, an antiretroviral protease in-

hibitor prescribed in the treatment of human immunodeficiency virus infection.

indirect anaphylaxis [L, *in,* not, *directus,* straight; Gk, *ana,* again, *phylaxis,* protection], an exaggerated reaction of hypersensitivity to a person's own antigen that occurs because the antigen has been altered in some way.

indirect calorimetry, the measurement of the amount of heat generated in an oxidation reaction by determining the intake or consumption of oxygen or by measuring the amount of carbon dioxide or nitrogen released and translating these quantities into a heat equivalent.

indirect Coombs' test a blood antibody screening technique in which a small amount of the recipient's serum is added to the donor's red blood cells. Coombs' serum is then added to the mixture. Visible agglutination indicates that the recipient has antibodies to the donor's red blood cells.

indirect laryngoscopy [L, *in,* not, *directus,* straight; Gk, *larynx* + *skopein,* to view], a method of examining the larynx with a mirror.

indirect nursing care functions, liaison nurse activities used to solve problems with a consultee who is responsible and accountable for implementing and evaluating any recommended changes.

indirect ophthalmoscope, an ophthalmoscope with a biconvex lens that produces a reversed direct image.

indirect provider reimbursement, a method of payment to an agency for health services delivered by providers such as nurses.

indirect restorative method, the technique for fabricating a restoration on a cast of the original, such as the indirect construction of an inlay.

indirect retainer, a part of a removable partial denture that resists movement of a distal extension away from its tissue support by means of lever action opposite the fulcrum line of the direct retention.

indirect transfusion [L, *in* + *directus,* straight, *transfundere,* to pour through], the transfusion of blood to a recipient after the donor blood has been prepared with anticoagulants, defibrinating agents, or other substances, as opposed to direct transfusion of blood from donor to recipient.

indirect vision [L, *in* + *directus,* straight, *visio,* seeing], a visual sensation caused by stimulation of the extramacular part of the retina.

indium (In) [L, *indicum,* indigo], a silvery metallic element with some nonmetallic chemical properties. Its atomic number is 49; its atomic mass (weight) is 114.82.

individual immunity /in'divij'oo·əl/ [L, *individuus,* indivisible, *immunis,* free], a form of natural immunity not shared by most other members of the race and species.

individual-model HMO, a health maintenance organization (HMO) in which individual physicians contract directly and independently with the HMO.

individual psychology, a modified system of psychoanalysis, developed by Alfred Adler, that views maladaptive behavior and personality disorders as resulting from a conflict between the desire to dominate and feelings of inferiority.

indole /in'dōl/, a volatile chemical produced during tryptophan metabolism. It is a component of intestinal gas.

indoleacetic acid /in'dōləsē'tik, -əset'ik/, a major terminal metabolite of tryptophan that is present in very small amounts in normal urine and excreted in elevated quantities by patients with carcinoid tumors.

indolent /in'dələnt/ [L, *in* + *dolere,* to suffer pain], pertaining to an organic disorder that is accompanied by little or no pain.

indomethacin /in'dōmeth'əsin/, a nonsteroidal antiinflammatory agent prescribed in the treatment of arthritis, gout attacks, and certain other inflammatory conditions.

induce /ind(y)oos'/ [L, *inducere,* to lead in], to cause or stimulate the start of an activity, as an enzyme induces a metabolic activity. —**inducer, induction,** *n.*

induced abortion, an intentional termination of pregnancy before the fetus has developed enough to live if born.

induced fever, a deliberate elevation of body temperature by application of heat or by inoculation with a fever-producing organism to kill heat-sensitive pathogens.

induced lethargy, a trancelike state produced during hypnosis.

induced mutation [L, *inducere,* to lead in, *mutare,* to change], a mutation that has been produced by treatment with a physical or chemical agent that affects the deoxyribonucleic acid molecules of a living organism.

induced phagocytosis [L, *inducere,* to lead in; Gk, *phagein,* to eat, *kytos,* cell], the ingestion of microorganisms and other foreign particles by cells of the reticuloendothelial system.

induced psychotic disorder, a severe mental disturbance in which there is a withdrawal from reality, resulting from exposure to a toxic agent such as a drug or hallucinogen.

induced trance, a somnambulistic state resulting from hypnotism.

induced vomiting [L, *inducere,* to lead in; *vomere,* to vomit], vomiting produced by administration of ipecac syrup, soapy water, or handwashing liquid detergent or by insertion of a finger or blunt instrument into the throat. Vomiting may be medically indicated in cases of ingestion of noncaustic poisons but may also be self-induced by patients afflicted with **bulimia.**

inducer /indoo'sər/, (in molecular genetics) a substance, usually a molecular substrate of a specific enzyme, that combines with and deactivates the active repressor produced by the regulator gene.

induction /induk'shən/ [L, *inducere,* to lead in], (in embryology) the process of stimulating and determining morphogenetic differentiation in a developing embryo through the action of chemical substances transmitted from one to another of the embryonic parts.

induction of anesthesia, all parts of the anesthetic process that occur before the desired level of anesthesia is attained.

induction of labor, an obstetric procedure in which labor is initiated artificially by means of amniotomy or administration of oxytocics. It is performed electively or for fetal or maternal indications. Elective induction is carried out for the convenience of the mother or the obstetrician, often to avert the possibility of delivery outside the hospital when labor is judged to be imminent and the mother is expected to have an unusually rapid birth.

induction phase, the period during which a normal cell becomes transformed into a cancerous cell.

inductive approach /induk'tiv/, the analysis of data and examination of practice problems within their own context rather than from a predetermined theoretic basis.

inductor /induk'tər/ [L, *inducere,* to lead in], (in embryology) a tissue or cell that emits a chemical substance that stimulates some morphogenetic effect in the developing embryo.

induration /in'dyərā'shən/ [L, *indurare,* to make hard], hardening of a tissue, particularly the skin, caused by edema, inflammation, or infiltration by a neoplasm. —**indurated,** *adj.*

indurative myocarditis /in'dyərē'tiv/ [L, *indurare,* to make hard; Gk, *mys,* muscle, *kardia,* heart, *itis,* inflammation], a form of myocarditis in which the inflammation leads to a hardening of the muscles of the heart walls.

industrial health [L, *industria,* diligence; ME, *helthe*], the health concerns associated with the workplace, such as exposure to asbestos, mining and milling dusts, metal and acid vapors, lighting, and ergonomic factors.

Industrial Medical Association (I.M.A.), a professional organization whose members are concerned with the identification, prevention, diagnosis, and treatment of disorders associated with technology and industry.

industrial psychology [L, *industria,* diligence], the application of psychologic principles and techniques to the problems of business and industry, including the selection of personnel, the motivation of workers, and the development of training programs.

indwelling catheter /in'dweling/ [L, *in,* within; AS, *dwellan,* to remain], any catheter designed to be left in place for a prolonged period.

inebriant /ine'brē-ənt/ [L, *inebriare,* to make drunk], a substance that induces inebriation or intoxication, as does ethanol.

inebriate /inur'/ /ine'brē-āt/, to make drunk.

inert /inurt'/ [L, *iners,* idle], **1.** not moving or acting, such as inert matter. **2.** (of a chemical substance) not taking part in a chemical reaction. **3.** (of a medical ingredient) not active pharmacologically; serving only as a bulking, binding, or sweetening agent or other excipient in a medication.

inert gas, a chemically inactive gaseous element. The inert gases are argon, helium, krypton, neon, radon, and xenon.

inertia /inur'shə/ [L, idleness], **1.** the tendency of a body at rest to remain at rest unless acted on by an outside force, and the tendency of a body in motion to remain at motion in the direction in which it is moving unless acted on by an outside force. **2.** an abnormal condition characterized by a general inactivity or sluggishness, such as colonic inertia or uterine inertia.

inertial impaction /inur'shəl/, the deposition of large aerosol particles on the walls of an airway conduit. The impaction caused by inertia tends to occur where the airway direction changes.

inevitable abortion /inev'itəbəl/ [L, *inevitabilis,* unavoidable], a condition of pregnancy in which spontaneous termination is imminent and cannot be prevented. It is characterized by bleeding, uterine cramping, dilation of the cervix, and presentation of the conceptus in the cervical os.

in extremis, in the extremity, or at the point of death.

infant /in'fənt/ [L, *infans,* unable to speak],

1. a child who is in the earliest stage of extrauterine life, a time extending from the first month after birth to approximately 12 months of age, when the baby is able to assume an erect posture. **2.** (in law) a person not of full legal age; a minor. **3.** pertaining to infancy; in an early stage of development. —**infantile,** *adj.*

infant behavior, disorganized, a NANDA-accepted nursing diagnosis of an alteration in integration and modulation of the physiologic and behavioral systems of functioning (i.e., the autonomic, motor, state, organizational, self-regulatory, and attentional-interactional systems). Defining characteristics include change from baseline physiologic measures; tremors, startles, and twitches; hyperextension of arms and legs; diffuse/unclear sleep; deficient self-regulatory behaviors; deficient response to visual/auditory stimuli; and yawning and apnea.

infant behavior, disorganized: risk for, a NANDA-accepted nursing diagnosis of a risk for alteration in integration and modulation of the physiologic and behavioral systems of functioning (i.e., autonomic, motor, state, organizational, self-regulatory, and attentional-interactional systems). The risk factors are pain, oral motor problems, environmental overstimulation, lack of containment or boundaries, prematurity, and invasive or painful procedures.

infant behavior, organized: potential for enhanced, a NANDA-accepted nursing diagnosis of a pattern of modulation of the physiologic and behavioral systems of functioning of an infant (i.e., autonomic, motor, state, organizational, self-regulatory, and attentional-interactional systems) that is satisfactory but can be improved, producing higher levels of integration in response to environmental stimuli. The defining characteristics are stable physiologic measures, definite sleep/wake states, use of some self-regulatory behaviors, and response to visual or auditory stimuli.

infant botulism, an intoxication by neurotoxins produced by *Clostridium botulinum* that occurs in children less than 6 months of age. The condition is characterized by severe hypotonicity of all muscles, constipation, lethargy, and feeding difficulties; and it may lead to respiratory insufficiency. The botulism neurotoxin is usually found in the gastrointestinal tract rather than in the blood, indicating that it is probably produced in the gut rather than ingested.

Infant Care, a Nursing Interventions Classification defined as provision of developmentally appropriate family-centered care to the child less than 1 year of age.

infant death, the death of a live-born infant before 1 year of age.

infant feeder, a device for nourishing small or weak babies who cannot suck hard enough to get milk from the breast or a bottle. The feeder resembles a bulb syringe with a long soft nipple on the end.

infant feeding pattern, ineffective, a NANDA-accepted nursing diagnosis of a state in which an infant demonstrates an impaired ability to suck or coordinate the suck-swallow response. The defining characteristics are an inability to initiate or sustain an effective suck and inability to coordinate sucking, swallowing, and breathing.

infanticide /infan′tisīd/ [L, *infans,* unable to speak, *caedere,* to kill], **1.** the killing of an infant or young child. **2.** one who takes the life of an infant or young child. —**infanticidal,** *adj.*

infantile /in′fəntīl/ [L, *infans,* unable to speak], **1.** of, relating to, or characteristic of infants or infancy. **2.** lacking maturity, sophistication, or reasonableness. **3.** affected with infantilism. **4.** being in a very early stage of development.

infantile amnesia, (in psychology) the inability to remember events from early childhood.

infantile arteritis, a disorder in infants and young children characterized by inflammation of many arteries in which atherosclerotic lesions are rarely present.

infantile autism, a pervasive developmental disorder characterized by abnormal emotional, social, and linguistic development in a child. Symptoms include abnormal ways of relating to people, objects, and situations. It may result from organic brain dysfunction, in which case it occurs before 3 years of age.

infantile cerebral ataxic paralysis [L, *infans,* unable to speak, *cerebrum,* the brain; Gk, *ataxia,* without order, *paralyein,* to be palsied], a form of congenital diplegia, characterized by cerebral maldevelopment, ataxia, spasticity of the legs, and possibly mental deficiency.

infantile cirrhosis, a progressive fibrous liver disorder caused by protein malnutrition.

infantile colic [L, *infans,* unable to speak; Gk, *kolikos,* pain in the colon], a descriptive term for a suggested intestinal cause of discomfort in a newborn; specific causes and mechanisms have not been defined. The typical infantile colic patient eats and gains weight but may also appear excessively hungry. Aerophagia caused by

crying may lead to flatulence and abdominal distension.

infantile cortical hyperostosis, a familial disorder characterized in an infant by bony swellings and tenderness in the affected areas. The mandible is most commonly involved.

infantile dwarf, a person whose mental and physical development is greatly retarded as a result of various causes such as genetic or developmental defects.

infantile encephalitis [L, *infans,* unable to speak; Gk, *enkephalos,* brain, *itis,* inflammation], any of a group of brain inflammation conditions affecting infants. The cause may be a direct viral infection or a secondary encephalitis as a complication of measles, chickenpox, rubella, or other diseases.

infantile hemiplegia, paralysis of one side of the body that may occur at birth as a result of a cerebral hemorrhage, in utero as a result of lack of oxygen, or during a febrile illness in infancy.

infantile hydrocele [L, *infans* + Gk, *hydor,* water, *kele,* hernia], an accumulation of fluid in the tunica vaginalis. It may be present at birth or acquired.

infantile scurvy, a nutritional disease caused by an inadequate dietary supply of vitamin C, which most commonly occurs because cow's milk unfortified with vitamin C is the principal food in an infant's diet.

infantile spinal paralysis [L, *infans,* unable to speak, *spina* + Gk, *paralyein,* to be palsied], acute anterior poliomyelitis, a viral infection characterized by nonspecific illnesses, aseptic meningitis, and flaccid weakness of muscle groups.

infantile uterus, a uterus that has failed to attain adult characteristics.

infantilism /infan′tiliz′əm/ [L, *infans,* unable to speak], **1.** a condition in which various anatomic, physiologic, and psychologic characteristics of childhood persist in the adult. **2.** a condition, usually of psychologic rather than organic origin, characterized by speech and voice patterns in an older child or adult that are typical of very young children.

infant mortality, the statistical rate of infant death during the first year after live birth, expressed as the number of such deaths per 1000 live births in a specific geographic area or institution in a given period.

infant of chemically dependent mother, a newborn who shows withdrawal symptoms, usually within the first 24 hours of life, most commonly caused by maternal antepartum dependence on heroin, methadone, diazepam, phenobarbital, or alcohol.

Characteristic symptoms include tremors, irritability, hyperactive reflexes, increased muscle tone, twitching, increased mucus production, nasal congestion, respiratory distress, excessive sweating, elevated temperature, vomiting, diarrhea, and dehydration. The infants cry shrilly, often sneeze, frantically suck their fists but feed poorly, and frequently yawn but have difficulty falling asleep. They are usually pale, are often born with nose and knee abrasions, and are subject to convulsions.

infant stimulation [L, *infans,* unable to speak, *stimulare,* to incite], the testing of sensory inputs for newborns and infants, usually through the performance of tasks involving coordination and manipulation.

infarct /infärkt'/ [L, *infarcire,* to stuff], a localized area of necrosis in a tissue, vessel, organ, or part resulting from tissue anoxia. It is caused by an interruption in the blood supply to the area or, less frequently, by circulatory stasis produced by the occlusion of a vein that ordinarily carries blood away from the area. An infarct may resemble a red swollen bruise because of hemorrhage and an accumulation of blood in the area. Some infarcts are pale and white, caused by a lack of circulation to the area.

infarct extension, a myocardial infarction that has spread beyond the original area, usually as a result of the death of cells in the ischemic margin of the infarct zone.

infarction /infärk'shən/ [L, *infarcire,* to stuff], **1.** the development and formation of an infarct. **2.** an infarct. Kinds of infarction include **myocardial infarction** and **pulmonary infarction.**

infect [L, *inficere,* to stain], to transmit a pathogen that may induce development of an infectious disease in another person.

infected abortion, a spontaneous or induced termination of an immature pregnancy in which the products of conception have become infected, causing fever and requiring antibiotic therapy and evacuation of the uterus.

infection /infek'shən/ [L, *inficere,* to stain], **1.** the invasion of the body by pathogenic microorganisms that reproduce and multiply, causing disease by local cellular injury, secretion of a toxin, or antigen-antibody reaction in the host. **2.** a disease caused by the invasion of the body by pathogenic microorganisms. —**infectious,** *adj.*

infection control, the policies and procedures of a hospital or other health facility to minimize the risk of spreading of nosocomial or community-acquired infections to patients or members of the staff.

Infection Control, a Nursing Interventions Classification defined as minimizing the acquisition and transmission of infectious agents.

infection control committee, a group of hospital health professionals composed of infection control personnel, with medical, nursing, administrative, and occasionally dietary and housekeeping department representatives who plan and supervise infection control activities.

Infection Control: Intraoperative, a Nursing Interventions Classification defined as preventing nosocomial infection in the operating room.

infection control nurse, a registered nurse who is assigned responsibility for surveillance and infection prevention, education, and control activities.

Infection Protection, a Nursing Interventions Classification defined as prevention and early detection of infection in a patient at risk.

infection, risk for, a NANDA-accepted nursing diagnosis of the state in which an individual is at increased risk for being invaded by pathogenic organisms. Risk factors include inadequate primary defenses such as broken skin, decrease in ciliary action, change in pH secretions, and altered peristalsis; inadequate secondary defenses such as decreased hemoglobin, suppressed inflammatory response, and immunosuppression; inadequate acquired immunity; tissue destruction and increased environmental exposure; chronic disease; invasive procedures; malnutrition; pharmaceutic agents; trauma; and rupture of amniotic membranes.

infectious /infek'chəs/, **1.** capable of causing an infection. **2.** caused by an infection.

infectious bulbar paralysis [L, *inficere,* to stain, *bulbus,* swollen root; Gk, *paralyein,* to be palsied], a herpesvirus disease of animals that may cause a mild pruritus when transmitted to humans.

infectious disease [L, *inficere,* to stain, *dis* + Fr, *aise,* ease], any communicable disease, or one that can be transmitted from one human being to another or from animal to human by direct or indirect contact.

infectious granuloma [L, *inficere,* to stain, *granulum,* little grain; Gk, *oma,* tumor], a lumpy lesion of granuloma tissue that may develop in diseases such as tuberculosis, syphilis, and actinomycosis.

infectious isolation [L, *inficere,* to stain; It, *isolare,* to detach], a practice of confining a patient with a particularly virulent disease to an isolated room or other area to reduce the risk of contact and spread of the disease among hospital personnel.

infectious mononucleosis [L, *inficere,* to stain; Gk, *monos,* single; L, *nucleus,* nut; Gk, *osis,* condition], an acute herpesvirus infection caused by the Epstein-Barr virus. It is characterized by fever, sore throat, swollen lymph glands, atypical lymphocytes, splenomegaly, hepatomegaly, abnormal liver function, and bruising.

infectious myringitis, an inflammatory contagious condition of the eardrum caused by viral or bacterial infection. It is characterized by the development of painful vesicles on the drum.

infectious nucleic acid, deoxyribonucleic acid or, more commonly, viral ribonucleic acid that is able to infect the nucleic acid of a cell and to induce the host to produce viruses.

infective endocarditis /infek′tiv/ [L, *inficere,* to stain; Gk, *endon,* within, *kardia,* heart, *itis,* inflammation], a bacterial infection of the innermost lining of the heart. It usually occurs after rheumatic fever or another febrile disease. Subacute bacterial endocarditis may lead to vegetation on the heart valves or ulceration of the valve cusps.

infective tubulointerstitial nephritis [L, *inficere,* to stain; *tubulus,* tubule, *interstitium,* space between], an acute inflammation of the kidneys caused by an infection by *Escherichia coli* or another pyogenic pathogen. The condition is characterized by chills, fever, nausea and vomiting, flank pain, dysuria, proteinuria, and hematuria. The kidney may become enlarged, and parts of the renal cortex may be destroyed.

infectivity /infektiv′itē/ [L, *inficere,* to stain], the ability of a pathogen to spread rapidly from one host to another.

inferior /infir′ē·ər/ [L, *inferus,* lower], **1.** situated below or lower than a given point of reference, as the feet are inferior to the legs. **2.** of poorer quality or value.

inferior alveolar artery, an artery that descends with the inferior alveolar nerve from the first or mandibular part of the maxillary artery to the mandibular foramen.

inferior aperture of minor pelvis, an irregular aperture bounded by the coccyx, the sacrotuberous ligaments, part of the ischium, the sides of the pubic arch, and the pubic symphysis.

inferior aperture of thorax, an irregular opening bounded by the twelfth thoracic vertebra, the eleventh and twelfth ribs, and the edge of the costal cartilages as they meet the sternum.

inferior carotid triangle [L, *inferior,*

lower; Gk, *karos,* heavy sleep; L, *triangulus,* three-cornered], a triangular area bounded by the midline of the neck, the superior belly of the omohyoid muscle above, and the sternocleidomastoid muscle behind.

inferior conjunctival fornix, the space in the fold of conjunctiva created by the reflection of the conjunctiva covering the eyeball and the lining of the lower eyelid.

inferior gastric node, a node in one of two groups of gastric lymph glands, lying between the two layers of the lesser omentum along the pyloric half of the greater curvature of the stomach.

inferiority complex /infir′ē·ôr′itē/, **1.** a personal feeling or sense of being inadequate. It is largely unconscious and influences attitudes and behaviors. **2.** (in psychoanalysis) a complex characterized by striving for unrealistic goals motivated by an unresolved Oedipus complex. **3.** *informal.* a feeling of being inferior.

inferior mesenteric artery, a visceral branch of the abdominal aorta, supplying the left half of the transverse colon, all of the descending and iliac colons, and most of the rectum.

inferior mesenteric node, a node in one of the three groups of visceral lymph glands serving the viscera of the abdomen and the pelvis.

inferior mesenteric vein, the vein in the lower body that returns the blood from the rectum, the sigmoid and descending colons, and part of the transverse colon.

inferior olivary nucleus [L, *inferior,* lower, *oliva,* olive, *nucleus,* nut kernel], a small purse-shaped collection of nerve cells lying posterolateral to the pyramid, just below the level of the pons. It is a source of cerebellar climbing fibers.

inferior orbital fissure, a groove in the inferolateral wall of the orbit that contains the infraorbital and zygomatic nerves and the infraorbital vessels.

inferior phrenic artery, a small visceral branch of the abdominal aorta that arises from the aorta itself, the renal artery, or the celiac artery.

inferior sagittal sinus, one of the six venous channels of the posterior dura mater, draining blood from the brain into the internal jugular vein.

inferior subscapular nerve /subskap′-yŏŏlər/, one of two small nerves on opposite sides of the back that arise from the posterior cord of the brachial plexus.

inferior thyroid vein, one of the few veins that arise in the venous plexus on the thyroid gland and form a plexus ventral to the trachea, under the sternothyroideus muscle.

inferior ulnar collateral artery, one of a pair of branches of the deep brachial arteries, carrying blood to the muscles of the forearm.

inferior vena cava, the large vein that returns deoxygenated blood to the heart from parts of the body below the diaphragm. It is formed by the junction of the two common iliac veins to the right of the fifth lumbar vertebra and ascends along the vertebral column, pierces the diaphragm, and opens into the right atrium of the heart.

inferolateral /in'fərōlat'ərəl/ [L, *inferus,* lower, *latus,* side], pertaining to a location situated below and to the side.

inferomedial /in'fərōmē'dē·əl/ [L, *inferus,* lower, *medius,* middle], pertaining to a location situated below and toward the center.

infertile /infur'təl/ [L, *in,* not, *fertilis,* fruitful], denoting the inability to produce offspring. This condition may be present in one or both sex partners and may be temporary and reversible. The cause may be physical, or it may result from psychologic or emotional problems. The condition is classified as primary, in which pregnancy has never occurred, and secondary, when there have been one or more pregnancies.

infertility /in'furtil'itē/, the condition of being unable to produce offspring.

infest /infest'/, to attack, invade, and subsist on the skin or in the internal organs of a host.

infestation /in'festā'shən/ [L, *infestare,* to attack], the presence of animal parasites in the environment, on the skin, or in the hair of a host.

infiltrate /in'filtrāt, infil'trāt/ [L, *in* + *filtrare,* to strain through], **1.** to perform the process of infiltration. **2.** a substance that seeps through a filter.

infiltration /in'filtrāshən/ [L, *in,* within, *filtare,* to strain through], the process whereby a fluid passes into the tissues, such as when a local anesthetic is administered.

infiltrative disorder /infil'trətiv/, a condition caused by the diffusion or accumulation in cells or tissues of substances not normally found in those cells or tissues.

infirmary /infur'mərē/ [L, *infirmus,* weak], a hospital, originally a part of a monastery, that provides care for sick or infirm persons, particularly indigent patients.

inflammation [L, *inflammare,* to set afire], the protective response of body tissues to irritation or injury. Inflammation may be acute or chronic; its cardinal signs are redness (rubor), heat (calor), swelling (tu-

mor), and pain (dolor), often accompanied by loss of function. Histamine, kinins, and various other substances mediate the inflammatory process.

inflammatory /inflam'ətôr'ē/ [L, *inflammare,* to set afire], pertaining to or resembling inflammation.

inflammatory autobullectomy, a procedure for shrinking a bulla caused by an inflammation in patients with bullous emphysema.

inflammatory dysmenorrhea [L, *inflammare* + Gk, *dys+* + *men,* month, *rhein,* to flow], menstrual pain that accompanies pelvic infection, fibroids, or endometritis.

inflammatory fracture [L, *inflammare,* to set afire, *fractura,* break], a fracture of bone tissue weakened by inflammation.

inflammatory response, a tissue reaction to injury or an antigen. The response may include pain, swelling, itching, redness, heat, loss of function, or a combination of symptoms.

inflammatory scoliosis [L, *inflammare* + Gk, *skoliosis,* curvature], a form of scoliosis caused by muscle spasms associated with acute inflammation.

inflatable splint /inflā'təbəl/ [L, *in,* within, *flare,* to blow; ME, *splente*], a tubular device that is placed around a patient's extremity and inflated with air to maintain rigidity.

influenza /in'flōō·en'zə/ [It, influence], a highly contagious infection of the respiratory tract caused by a myxovirus and transmitted by airborne droplet infection. Symptoms include sore throat, cough, fever, muscular pains, and weakness. The incubation period is brief (from 1 to 3 days), and the onset is usually sudden, with chills, fever, and general malaise. Fever and constitutional symptoms distinguish influenza from the common cold. Three main strains of influenza virus have been recognized: type A, type B, and type C. New strains of the virus emerge at regular intervals and are named according to their geographic origin. Asian flu is a type A influenza. Yearly vaccination with the currently prevalent strain of influenza virus is recommended for elderly or debilitated persons and health care personnel.

influenza-virus vaccine, an active immunizing agent prescribed for immunization against influenza.

informal admission, a type of admission to a psychiatric hospital in which there is no formal or written application and the patient is free to leave at any time.

information systems director [L, *informatio,* idea], a person who directs and administers the data processing facilities of a hospital or other health facility.

informed consent [L, *informare,* to give form, *consentire,* to sense], permission obtained from a patient to perform a specific test or procedure. Informed consent is required before performing most invasive procedures and before admitting a patient to a research study.

infraclavicular fossa /in′frəkləvik′yələr/, a small pocket or indentation just below the clavicle on both sides of the body.

infraction fracture /infrak′shən/ [L, *infractio,* a breaking, *fractura,* break], a pathologic fracture characterized by a small radiolucent line and most commonly associated with a disorder of metabolism.

infradian rhythm /in′frərā′dē·ən/ [L, *infra,* below, *dies,* day; Gk, *rhythmos*], a biorhythm that repeats in patterns more frequent than 24-hour periods.

infrahyoid /in′frəhī′oid/, pertaining to the area below the hyoid bone, particularly the group of muscles attached to it.

inframaxillary, 1. pertaining to the mandible, or lower jaw. 2. lying below the maxilla, or upper jaw.

infranodal block /in′frənō′dəl/ [L, *infra,* below, *nodus,* knot; Fr, *bloc*], a type of atrioventricular (AV) block in which the abnormality is below the AV node, that is, in the bundle of His or in both bundle branches. The condition is often the result of arteriosclerosis, degenerative diseases, a defect in the conduction system, or a tumor. Symptoms include frequent episodes of fainting and a pulse rate of between 20 and 40 beats/min.

infranodal disease, a cardiac disorder involving the electrical conduction system of the heart below the atrioventricular node.

infraorbital /in′frə·ô′bitəl/ [L, *infra,* below, *orbita,* wheeltrack], pertaining to the area beneath the floor of the bony cavity in which the eyeball is located.

infraorbital foramen [L, *infra,* below, *orbita,* wheeltrack, *foramen,* hole], an opening on the anterior aspect of the maxilla. Through it pass the inferior orbital nerves and blood vessels.

infrapatellar fat pad /in′frəpətel′ər/, an area of palpable soft tissue in front of the joint space on either side of the patellar tendon.

infrared radiation /in′frəred′/ [L, *infra* + AS, *read,* red; L, *radiare,* to emit rays], electromagnetic radiation in which the wavelengths are between 10^{-5} m and 10^{-4} m, or longer than those of visible light waves but shorter than those of radio waves. Infrared radiation that strikes the body surface is perceived as heat.

infrared therapy, treatment by exposure to various wavelengths of infrared radiation. Infrared treatment is performed to relieve pain and to stimulate circulation of blood.

infrared thermography, measurement of temperature through the detection of infrared radiation emitted from heated tissue.

infrasonics /in′frəson′iks/, sound frequencies that are below the range of human hearing.

infundibular stalk /in′fundib′yələr/ [L, *infundibulum,* funnel; ME, *stalke*], an elongated funnel-shaped structure that connects the hypothalamus with the pituitary gland.

infundibulum /in′fundib′yələm/ *pl.* **infundibula,** [L, funnel], a funnel-shaped structure or passage, such as the cavity formed by the fimbriae tubae at the distal end of the fallopian tubes.

infusate /infyōō′sāt/, a parenteral fluid slowly introduced into a patient over a specific period.

infusate contamination, nosocomial infections transmitted through intravascular devices such as catheters, cannulas, or needles during surgery or other procedures.

infusion /infyōō′zhən/ [L, *in,* within, *fundere,* to pour], 1. the introduction of a substance such as a fluid, electrolyte, nutrient, or drug, directly into a vein or interstitially by means of gravity flow. 2. the substance introduced into the body by infusion. 3. the steeping of a substance, such as an herb, to extract its medicinal properties. 4. the extract obtained by the steeping process. —**infuse,** *v.*

infusion pump, an apparatus designed to deliver measured amounts of a drug or intravenous (IV) solution through IV injection over time. Some kinds of infusion pumps can be implanted surgically.

ingestion /injes′chən/ [L, *in,* within, *gerere,* to carry], the oral taking of substances into the body. The term is generally applied to both nutrients and medications.

ingrown hair [L, *in,* within; AS, *growen,* to grow, *haer*], a hair that fails to follow the normal follicle channel to the surface, with the free end becoming embedded in the skin.

ingrown toenail, a toenail whose distal lateral margin grows or is pressed into the skin of the toe, causing an inflammatory reaction.

inguinal /ing′gwinəl/ [L, *inguen,* groin], pertaining to the groin.

inguinal canal, the tubular passage through the lower muscular layers of the abdominal wall that contains the spermatic cord in the male and the round ligament in the female. It is a common site for hernias.

inguinal falx, the inferior terminal part of the common aponeurosis of the internal abdominal oblique and the transverse abdominis.

inguinal hernia, a hernia in which a loop of intestine enters the inguinal canal; in a male it sometimes fills the entire scrotal sac.

inguinal node, any of the approximately 18 nodes in the group of lymph glands in the upper femoral triangle of the thigh.

inguinal region, the part of the abdomen surrounding the inguinal canal, in the lower zone on both sides of the pubic region.

inguinal ring, either of the two apertures of the inguinal canal, the internal end opening into the abdominal wall and the external end opening into the aponeurosis of the obliquus externus abdominis above the pubis.

inguinocrural hernia /ing'gwinəlkroo'rəl/ [L, *inguen,* groin, *crus,* thigh, *hernia,* rupture], an inguinal hernia that has turned from the inguinal canal laterally over the groin.

inhalant /inhā'lənt/, a substance introduced into the body by inhalation. It may be a medication or a volatile chemical.

inhalation administration of medication /in'həlā'shən/ [L, *in,* within, *halare,* to breathe], the administration of a drug by inhalation of the vapor released from a fragile ampule packed in a fine mesh that is crushed for immediate administration. The medication is absorbed into the circulation through the mucous membrane of the nasal passages. Vaporized medication is also given by inhalation.

inhalation anesthesia, surgical narcosis achieved by the inhalation of an anesthetic gas or a vapor. Administration of an inhalation anesthetic is usually preceded by intravenous administration of a short-acting hypnotic drug. The procedure may require endotracheal intubation.

inhalation injury, damage to the pulmonary parenchyma caused by inhalation of very hot air, toxic gas, asbestos, or chemical products of plastic manufacture.

inhalation therapy, a treatment in which a substance is introduced into the respiratory tract with inspired air. Oxygen, water, and various drugs may be administered by techniques of inhalation therapy.

inhalation toxicity, a severe neuromuscular disorder with symptoms like those of Parkinson's disease, caused by prolonged inhalation of manganese dust.

inhale /inhāl'/ [L, *in,* within, *halare,* to

breathe], to breathe in or to draw in with the breath. —**inhalation,** *n.*

inhaler [L, *in + halare;* to breathe], a device for administering medications to be inhaled, such as vapors, fine powders, or volatile substances. An inhaler also may be designed to administer anesthetic gases.

inherent /inhir'ənt/ [L, *inhaerere,* to cling to], inborn, innate; natural to an environment.

inherent rate, the frequency of impulse formation attributed to a given pacemaker location.

inheritance /inher'itəns/ [L, *in,* within, *hereditare,* to inherit], **1.** the acquisition or expression of traits or conditions by transmission of genetic material from parents to offspring. **2.** the sum of the genetic qualities or traits transmitted from parents to offspring; the total genetic makeup of the fertilized ovum. —**inherited,** *adj.* **inherit,** *v.*

inherited disorder /inher'itid/, any disease or condition that is genetically determined and involves either a single gene mutation, multifactorial inheritance, or a chromosomal aberration.

inherited trait [L, *in,* within, *hereditare,* to inherit; Fr, *trait,* a draft], a distinguishing quality or characteristic that is transmitted genetically from one generation to the next.

inhibin /inhib'in/, a testicular hormone that inhibits activity of the follicle-stimulating hormone secreted by the anterior pituitary gland.

inhibiting gene /inhib'iting/ [L, *inhibere,* to restrain; Gk, *genein,* to produce], a gene that prevents the expression of another gene.

inhibition /in'hibish'ən/ [L, *inhibere,* to restrain], **1.** (in psychology) the unconscious restraint of a behavioral process, usually resulting from the social or cultural forces of the environment; the condition inducing such restraint. **2.** (in psychoanalysis) the process in which the superego prevents the conscious expression of an unconscious instinctual drive, thought, or urge. **3.** (in physiology) restraining, checking, or arresting the action of an organ or cell or reducing a physiologic activity by antagonistic stimulation. **4.** (in chemistry) the stopping or slowing of the rate of a chemical reaction.

inhibition assay, an immunoassay in which an excess of antigens prevents or inhibits the completion of either the initial or the indicator phase of the reaction.

inhibition of reflexes [L, *inhibere,* to restrain, *reflectere,* to bend back], **1.** the prevention of a reflex action, requiring a series of biochemical mechanisms to restrict the flow of excitatory impulses at presynaptic and postsynaptic points in the system. **2.** a negative reflex effect that may become established during differential conditioning. The negative conditioned reflex represents an inhibition of a conditioned reflex.

inhibitor /inhib'itor/, a drug or other agent that prevents or restricts a certain action.

inhibitory /inhib'itôr'ē/ [L, *inhibere,* to restrain], tending to stop or slow a process, such as a neuron that suppresses the intensity of a nerve impulse.

inhibitory enzyme [L, *inhibere,* to restrain; Gk, *en,* within; *zyme,* ferment], an enzyme that blocks rather than catalyzes a chemical reaction.

inion /in'ē·on/ [Gk], the most prominent point of the back of the head, where the occipital bone protrudes farthest.

initial contact stance stage /inish'əl/ [L, *initium,* beginning, *contigere,* to touch], one of the five stages in the stance phase of walking or gait, specifically associated with the moment when the foot touches the ground or floor and the leg prepares to accept the weight of the body.

initiation codon /inish'ē·ā'shən kō'don/ [L, *initium,* beginning, *caudex,* book], (in molecular genetics) the triplet of nucleotides, usually adenine-uracil-guanine, that code for formylmethionine, the first amino acid in protein sequences.

initiator /inish'ē·ā'tər/, a cocarcinogenic factor that causes a usually irreversible genetic mutation in a normal cell and primes it for uncontrolled growth. Examples include radiation, aflatoxins, urethane, and nitrosamines.

injectable silicone /injek'təbəl/ [L, *in* + *jacere,* to throw, *silex,* silicon], polymeric organic compounds of silicone that are used in plastic surgery. The silicones are injected beneath the skin for cosmetic benefits.

injection /injek'shən/ [L, *in,* within, *jacere,* to throw], **1.** the act of forcing a liquid into the body by means of a needle and syringe. Injections are designated according to the anatomic site involved; the most common are intraarterial, intradermal, intramuscular, intravenous, and subcutaneous. **2.** the substance injected. **3.** redness and swelling observed in the physical examination of a part of the body, caused by dilation of the blood vessels secondary to an inflammatory or infectious process. **—inject,** *v.*

injection cap, a rubber diaphragm covering a plastic cap. It permits needle insertion into a catheter or vial.

injunction /injungk'shən/ [L, *injungere,* to enjoin], a court order that prevents a party from performing a specified act.

injury, risk for /in'jərē/, a NANDA-accepted nursing diagnosis of a state in which an individual is at risk of injury as a result of environmental conditions interacting with the individual's adaptive and defensive resources. The cause of the condition may be somatic (internal) or environmental (external). A somatic risk for injury includes abnormal sensory function, autoimmune condition, malnutrition, hemoglobinopathy or other abnormal hematologic condition, broken skin, developmental abnormality, and psychologic dysfunction. An environmental risk for injury includes lack of immunization; presence of pathogenic microorganisms, chemical pollutants, poisons, alcohol, nicotine, or food additives; modes of transportation; physical aspects of the community, buildings, equipment, or facilities; nosocomial agents; nonavailability of assistance; and various psychologic factors.

injury, perioperative positioning: risk for, a NANDA-accepted nursing diagnosis of a state in which the client is at risk for injury as a result of the environmental conditions found in the perioperative setting. The risk factors are disorientation, immobilization, muscle weakness, sensory or perceptual disturbances resulting from anesthesia, obesity, emaciation, and edema.

injury severity score (ISS), an evaluation system developed to predict the outcomes of traumas, including mortality and length of hospital stay.

inlay splint [L, *in,* within; AS, *lecan,* lay], a casting for fixing or supporting one or more approximating teeth.

inlet [L, *in,* within; ME, *leten*], a passage leading into a cavity, such as the pelvic inlet that marks the brim of the pelvic cavity.

in loco parentis /in lō'kō pəren'tis/ [L, *in* + *locus,* place, *parentis,* parent], the assumption by a person or institution of the parental obligations of caring for a child without adoption.

innate /in'āt, ināt'/ [L, *innatus,* inborn], **1.** existing in or belonging to a person from birth; inborn; hereditary; congenital. **2.** a natural and essential characteristic of something or someone; inherent. **3.** originating in or produced by the intellect or the mind.

inner cell mass [AS, *innera,* within; L, *cella,* storeroom, *massa,* lump], a cluster of cells localized around the animal pole of the blastocyst of placental mammals from which the embryo develops.

innervate /in'ərvāt/ [L, *in* + *nervus*], to supply a body part or organ with nerves or nervous stimuli.

innervation /in'ərvā'shən/ [L, *in,* within, *nervus,* nerve], the distribution or supply of nerve fibers or nerve impulses to a body part.

innocent /in'əsənt/ [L, *innocens,* harmless], benign, innocuous, or functional; not malignant, such as an innocent heart murmur.

innocuous /inok'yōō-əs/ [L, *innocuus,* harmless], pertaining to use of a substance or procedure that causes no ill effects.

innominate /inom'ināt/ [L, *innominatum,* nameless], without a name; unnamed. The term is traditionally applied to certain anatomic structures, often identified by their descriptive name, such as the hipbone.

innominate artery, one of the three arteries branching from the arch of the aorta.

innominate bone, the hipbone. It consists of the ilium, ischium, and pubis and unites with the sacrum and coccyx to form the pelvis.

innominate vein, a large vein on either side of the neck that is formed by the union of the internal jugular and subclavian veins. The two veins drain blood from the head, neck, and upper extremities and unite to form the superior vena cava.

inoculate /inok'yəlāt/ [L, *inoculare,* to graft], to introduce a substance (inoculum) into the body to produce or to increase immunity to the disease or condition associated with the substance.

inoculum /inok'yōōləm/, *pl.* **inocula** [L, *inoculare,* to graft a bud], a substance introduced into the body to cause or to increase immunity to a specific disease or condition. It may be a toxin; a live, attenuated, or killed virus or bacterium; or an immune serum.

inoperable /inop'ərəbəl/ [L, *in* + *operari,* to work], pertaining to a medical condition that would not benefit from surgical intervention or for which the risk outweighs the benefits.

inorganic /in'ôrgan'ik/ [L, *in,* not; Gk, *organikos,* natural], (in chemistry) a chemical compound that does not contain hydrocarbon or other derivatives.

inorganic acid, a compound containing no carbon that is composed of hydrogen and an electronegative element such as chlorine. An example is hydrochloric acid.

inorganic chemistry, the study of the properties and reactions of all chemical elements and compounds other than hydrocarbons or their derivatives.

inorganic dust, dry, finely powdered particles of an inorganic substance, especially dust, which, when inhaled, can cause abnormal conditions of the lungs.

inorganic phosphorus, phosphorus that may be measured in the blood as phosphate ions.

inosine /in'əsēn, -sīn/, a nucleoside, derived from animal tissue, especially intestines. It has been used in the treatment of cardiac disorders and now is under investigation in studies of cancer and virus chemotherapy.

inosiplex /inō'sipleks/, a form of inosine that acts as a stimulator of the immune system. It is currently under investigation for use in cancer therapy and in the treatment of herpesvirus and rhinovirus infections.

inositol /inō'sətōl, inos'-/, an isomer of glucose that occurs widely in plant and animal cells.

inotropic /in'ōtrop'ik/ [Gk, *inos,* fiber, *trope,* turning], pertaining to the force or energy of muscular contractions, particularly those of the heart muscle.

inotropic agent, a substance that influences the force of muscular contractions.

inpatient /in'pāshənt/ [L, *in,* within, *patior,* to suffer], **1.** a patient who has been admitted to a hospital or other health care facility for at least an overnight stay. **2.** pertaining to the treatment or care of such a patient or to a health care facility to which a patient may be admitted for 24-hour care.

inpatient care unit, a unit of a hospital organized for medical and continuous nursing services for a group of inpatients who are usually grouped according to diagnosis or other common characteristics, such as maternity or surgical patients.

input, the information or material that enters a system.

inquest /in'kwest/ [L, *in* + *quaerere,* to seek], a legal inquiry into the cause, manner, and circumstances of a sudden, unexpected, or violent death.

INR, abbreviation for *International Normalized Ratio.*

insane /insān'/ [L, *in,* not, *sanus,* sound], a legal term for unsound, diseased, or deranged mental functioning, particularly pertaining to a person who is unable to provide adequate self-care if there is a need to protect the patient and the public from each other. In the United States the precise definition of this legal term varies from state to state.

insanity, /insan'itē/ [L, *in,* not, *sanus,* sound] *informal.* a term used more in legal and social than in medical terminology. It refers to those mental illnesses that are of such a serious or debilitating nature as to interfere with one's capability of functioning within the legal limits of society and performing the normal activities of daily living.

insatiable /insā′sh(ē)əbəl/ [L, *insatiatus*, not satisfied], pertaining to an appetite for food or other needs that cannot be satisfied.

insect bite [L, *in*, within, *secare*, to cut], the bite of any parasitic or venomous arthropod such as a louse, flea, mite, tick, or arachnid. Many arthropods inject venom that produces poisoning or severe local reaction, saliva that may contain viruses, or substances that produce mild irritation.

insecticide /insek′tisīd/, a chemical agent that kills insects.

insemination /insem′inā′shən/, the injection of semen into the vagina. It may involve an artificial process unrelated to sexual intercourse.

insenescence /in′sines′əns/ [L, *insenescere*, to begin to grow old], **1.** the process of aging. **2.** the state of being chronologically old but retaining the vitality of a young person.

insensible /insen′sibəl/ [L, *in* + *sentire*, to feel], **1.** pertaining to a person who is unconscious for any reason. **2.** pertaining to a person who is apathetic or deprived of normal sense perceptions.

insensible perspiration [L, *in*, not, *sentire*, to feel, *per*, through, *spirare*, to breath], the loss of fluid from the body by evaporation, such as normally occurs during respiration.

insertion /insur′shən/ [L, *inserere*, to introduce], (in anatomy) the place of attachment, such as that of a muscle to the bone it moves.

insertion site, the point in a vein where a needle or catheter is inserted.

in-service education [L, *in*, within, *servus*, a slave, *educare*, to rear], a program of instruction or training that is provided by an agency or institution for its employees.

insidious /insid′ē-əs/ [L, *insidiosus*, cunning], describing a development that is gradual, subtle, or imperceptible.

insight /in′sīt/ [L, *in*, within; AS, *gesihth*, sight], **1.** the capacity of comprehending the true nature of a situation or of penetrating an underlying truth. **2.** an instance of penetrating or comprehending an underlying truth, primarily through intuitive understanding. **3.** (in psychology) a type of self-understanding encompassing both intellectual and emotional awareness of the unconscious nature, origin, and mechanisms of one's attitudes, feelings, and behavior.

insipid /insip′id/ [L, *in* + *sapidus*, savory], dull, tasteless, or lifeless.

in situ /in sī′tōō, sit′ōō/ [L, *in*, within, *si-*

tus, position], **1.** in the natural or usual place. **2.** describing a cancer that has not metastasized or invaded neighboring tissues, such as carcinoma in situ.

insoluble /insol′yəbəl/ [L, *in*, not, *solubilis*, soluble], unable to be dissolved, usually in a specific solvent, such as a substance that is insoluble in water.

insomnia /insom′nē·ə/ [L, *in*, not, *somnus*, sleep], chronic inability to sleep or to remain asleep throughout the night; wakefulness; sleeplessness.

insomniac /insom′nē·ak/, **1.** a person with insomnia. **2.** pertaining to, causing, or associated with insomnia. **3.** characteristic of or occurring during a period of sleeplessness.

inspiration /in′spirā′shən/ [L, *inspirare*, to breathe in], the act of drawing air into the lungs in order to exchange oxygen for carbon dioxide, the end product of tissue metabolism. The major muscle of inspiration is the diaphragm, the contraction of which creates a negative pressure in the chest, causing the normal lungs to expand and air to flow inward. Lungs at maximal inspiration have an average total capacity of 5500 to 6000 ml of air.

inspiratory /inspī′rətôr′ē/ [L, *inspirare*, to breathe in], pertaining to inspiration.

inspiratory capacity (IC), the maximum volume of gas that can be inhaled from the end of a resting exhalation.

inspiratory dyspnea [L, *inspirare*, to breathe in; Gk, *dys*, without, *pnoia*, breath], a form of breathing difficulty caused by an obstruction in the larynx, trachea, or bronchi. The patient attempts to compensate for this deficiency with prolonged deep inspirations.

inspiratory gas flow rate, the amount of gas delivered per minute to a patient's lungs by mechanical ventilation.

inspiratory hold, either of two kinds of modification in an intermittent positive-pressure breathing pressure waveform: (1) a pressure hold, in which a preset pressure is reached and held for a designated period, and (2) a volume hold, in which a predetermined volume is delivered and then held for a designated period.

inspiratory muscle fatigue, weakness or exhaustion of the inspiratory muscles that produces a condition of threatened acute respiratory failure.

inspiratory reserve volume, the maximum volume of gas that can be inhaled beyond a normal resting inspiration.

inspiratory resistance muscle training, exercises that require inhalation against some type of resisting force, such as abdominal breathing practice. The resistance may be provided by a therapist pushing against the ribs or by applying a belt or swathe tightly about the costal margin.

inspiratory waveform, one of several inspiratory flow patterns associated with mechanical ventilation. These include a square wave, a sinusoidal wave, and a descending ramp wave.

inspirometer /in'spirom'ətər/ [L, *inspirare,* to breathe in; Gk, *metron,* measure], an apparatus used to measure the volume, force, and frequency of a patient's inspirations.

inspissate /inspis'āt/ [L, *inspissare,* to thicken], (of a fluid) to thicken or harden through the absorption or evaporation of the liquid part, such as milk in an inspissated milk duct. **—inspissation,** *n.*

instillation /in'stilā'shən/ [L, *instillare,* to drip], **1.** a procedure in which a fluid is slowly introduced into a cavity or passage of the body and allowed to remain for a specific length of time before being drained or withdrawn. **2.** a solution so introduced. **—instill,** *v.*

instinct /in'stingkt/ [L, *instinctus,* impulse], an inborn psychologic representation of a need, such as life instincts of hunger, thirst, and sex, as well as the destructive and aggressive death instincts.

institutionalism syndrome /in'stityoo'-shənəliz'əm/, a condition characterized by apathy, withdrawal, submissiveness, and lack of initiative. The person may resist leaving a hospital, even when the surroundings are barely adequate, because it is familiar and predictable.

institutionalize /in'stityoo'shənəliz'/ [L, *instituere,* to put in place], to place a person in an institution for psychologic or physical treatment or for the protection of the person or society. **—institutionalization,** *n.,* **institutionalized,** *adj.*

institutional licensure /in'stityoo'shənəl/ [L, *instituere,* to put in place, *licere* to be permitted], a proposed procedure in which licensure for almost all health professions would be abandoned and the responsibility for assessing professional competence would fall to the health care facility where the health professional is used.

institutional review board (IRB), a federally approved committee that reviews all research proposals before submission of requests for funding by granting agencies.

instrument /in'strəmənt/ [L, *instrumentum,* tool], a surgical tool or device designed to perform a specific function, such as cutting, dissecting, grasping, holding, retracting, or suturing. Some kinds of instruments arc **clamp, needle holder, retractor,** and **speculum.**

instrumental activities of daily living

(IADL), the activities often performed in the course of a normal day in a person's life.

instrumental labor /in'strəmen'təl/ [L, *instrumentum,* tool, *labor,* work], child delivery in which the use of instruments, such as forceps or perforators, is required.

instrumentation /in'strəməntā'shən/, the use of instruments for treatment and diagnosis.

insufficiency /in'səfish'ənsē/ [L, *in,* not, *sufficere,* to be adequate], inability to perform a necessary function adequately.

insufficient sleep syndrome /in'səfish'ənt/, a neurologic disorder in which individuals persistently fail to obtain enough sleep to support normal wakefulness.

insufflate /in'səflāt insuf'lāt/ [L, *insufflare,* to blow into], to blow a gas or powder into a tube, cavity, or organ to allow visual examination, to remove an obstruction, or to apply medication. **—insufflation,** *n.*

insufflator /in'səflā'tər/ [L, *insufflare,* to blow into], an apparatus used to blow air or gas into a body cavity.

insulation /in'səlā'shən/, a nonconducting substance that offers a barrier to the passage of heat or electricity.

insulin /in'səlin/ [L, *insula,* island], **1.** a naturally occurring hormone secreted by the beta cells of the islets of Langerhans in the pancreas in response to increased levels of glucose in the blood. The hormone acts to regulate the metabolism of glucose and the processes necessary for the intermediary metabolism of fats, carbohydrates, and proteins. Insulin lowers blood glucose level and promotes transport and entry of glucose into the muscle cells and other tissues. **2.** a pharmacologic preparation of the hormone administered in treating diabetes mellitus. The various preparations of insulin available for prescription vary in onset, intensity, and duration of action. They are termed short-acting, intermediate-acting, and long-acting.

insulinase, an enzyme that inactivates insulin.

insulin-dependent diabetes mellitus (IDDM), an inability to metabolize carbohydrate caused by an absolute insulin deficiency, occurring in children and adults. It is characterized by excessive thirst, increased urination, increased desire to eat, loss of weight, diminished strength, and marked irritability. IDDM patients are sensitive to insulin, physical activity, and diet and likely to experience ketoacidosis.

insulinemia /in'səlinēmē·ə/ [L, *insula,* island; Gk, *haima,* blood], an abnormally high level of insulin in the blood.

insulin hypoglycemic test, a postoperative procedure for determining the completeness of vagotomy for peptic ulcer disease.

insulin injection sites, body tissue areas that allow optimal use of subcutaneous injections of insulin. The choice of sites can affect the rate of absorption and peak action times, but repeated use of the same injection site can lead to localized tissue damage, resulting in malabsorption of insulin and misdiagnosis of insulin resistance. These problems are minimized by systematic rotation of injection sites.

insulin kinase, an enzyme, assumed to be present in the liver, that activates insulin.

insulin-like growth factor, a hormone that stimulates protein synthesis and sulfation.

insulin lipodystrophy [L, *insula,* island; Gk, *lipos,* fat; *dys,* bad, *trophe,* nourishment], the loss of local fat deposits in patients with diabetes as a complication of repeated insulin injections into the same area.

insulinogenic /in'səlin'ōjen'ik/ [L, *insula* + Gk, *genein,* to produce], promoting the production and release of insulin by the islets of Langerhans in the pancreas.

insulinoma /in'səlinō'mə/ [L, *insula* + Gk, *oma,* tumor], a tumor of the insulin-secreting cells of the islets of Langerhans. The majority are benign. Surgical resection of the tumor may be possible, thus limiting the development of hypoglycemia.

insulin pump [L, *insula,* island; ME, *pumpe*], a portable, battery-powered instrument that delivers a measured amount of insulin through the abdominal wall. It can be programmed to deliver varied doses of insulin according to the body's needs at the time.

insulin reaction, the adverse effects caused by excessive levels of circulating insulin.

insulin resistance, a complication of diabetes mellitus characterized by a need for more than 200 units of insulin per day to control hyperglycemia and ketosis. The cause is associated with insulin binding by high levels of antibody.

insulin shock, a condition of hypoglycemic shock caused by an overdose of insulin, decreased intake of food, or excessive exercise. It is characterized by sweating, trembling, chilliness, nervousness, irritability, hunger, hallucination, numbness, and pallor. Uncorrected, it progresses to convulsions, coma, and death. Treatment requires an immediate dose of glucose.

insulin tolerance test, a test of the body's ability to use insulin, in which insulin is given and blood glucose is measured at regular intervals.

insulintropin /in'səlintrop'in/ [L, *insula,* island], a naturally occurring hormone produced in the intestines when food is ingested. It causes the release of insulin from the pancreas, which in turn regulates blood sugar levels. It has been administered to type II diabetes patients but is not useful in its present form in the treatment of type I diabetes patients, in whom the pancreas does not secrete insulin.

insulitis /in'səlī'tis/, a lymphocytic infiltration of the pancreatic beta cells in the islets of Langerhans.

Insurance Authorization, a Nursing Interventions Classification defined as assisting the patient and provider to secure payment for health services or equipment from a third party.

intake [L, *in,* within; AS, *tacan,* to take], **1.** the process in which a person is admitted to a clinic or hospital or is signed in for an office visit. The reason for the visit and various identifying data about the patient are noted. **2.** (in nursing) the amount of food or fluid ingested in a given period.

integral dose /in'təgrəl/ [L, *integrare,* to make whole; Gk, *dosis,* giving], (in radiotherapy) the total amount of energy absorbed by a patient or object during exposure to radiation.

Integrated Group Without Walls /in'-təgrā'tid/, a network of physicians who have merged legally but continue to practice individually.

Integrated Health Care Delivery System a managed care system in the United States that includes a hospital organization that provides acute patient care, a multispecialty medical care delivery system, the capability of contracting for any other needed services, and a payer.

Integrated Multispecialty Group, a managed care system similar to a single-specialty medical group, except that various specialties and usually primary care are also provided.

integrated system, **1.** (in managed care) a legal partnership between groups of physicians and hospitals that contract and share risk while working together. **2.** a group of interconnected units that form a functioning computer system.

integrating dose meter /in'təgrā'ting/, (in radiotherapy) an ionization chamber, usually designed to be placed on the patient's skin, with a measuring system for determining the total radiation administered during an exposure.

integration /in'təgrā'shən/ [L, *integrare,* to make whole], **1.** the act or process of unifying or bringing together. **2.** (in psychology) the organization of all elements of the personality into a coordinated functional whole that is in harmony with the environment. —**integrate,** *v.*

integration of self, one of the components of high-level wellness. It is a prerequisite for the achievement of maturity and is characterized by the integration of mind, body, and spirit into one harmoniously functioning unit.

integrin /integ′rin, **1.** a protein that links the outside of a cell with its interior. **2.** a heterodimeric molecule involved in cell-substate and cell-cell adhesion.

integument /integ′yo͞omənt/ [L, *integumentum,* a covering], a covering or skin. —**integumentary,** *adj.*

integumentary system /integ′yəmen′tərē/, the skin and its appendages, hair, nails, and sweat and sebaceous glands.

integumentary system assessment, an evaluation of the general condition of a patient's integument and of factors or abnormalities that may contribute to the presence of a dermatologic disorder. The patient is asked about itching, pain, rashes, blisters, or boils; whether the skin usually is dry, oily, thin, rough, bumpy, or puffy; or whether it feels hot or cold, peels, changes in color, or is marked with dark liver (aging) spots. Observations are made of the intactness, turgor, elasticity, temperature, cleanliness, odor, wetness or dryness, and color of the skin. Cyanosis of the lips, circumoral area, or mucous membranes, earlobes, or nailbeds; jaundice of the sclera; paleness of conjunctivae; and distribution of pigment are noted. Evidence of rashes, edema, needle marks, insect bites, scabies, acne, sclerema, decubiti, uremic frost on the beard or eyebrows, or pressure areas over bony prominences is recorded. The nails are examined for brittleness, lines, a convex ram's horn or concave spoon shape, and the condition of surrounding tissue including clubbing of the fingers and toes. The existence and characteristics of lesions such as maculae, papules, vesicles, pustules, bullae, hives, warts, moles, ulcers, scars, keloids, petechiae, lipomas, crusts of dried exudate, flakes of dead epidermis, excoriations, blackheads, and chancres are noted.

intellect /in′təlekt/ [L, *intellectus,* perception], **1.** the power and ability of the mind for knowing and understanding, as contrasted with feeling or with willing. **2.** a person possessing a great capacity for thought and knowledge. —**intellectual,** *adj., n.*

intellectualization /in′təlek′cho͞o·əlīzā′-shən/ [L, *intellectus* + Gk, *izein,* to cause], **1.** (in psychiatry) a defense mechanism in which reasoning is used as a

means of blocking a confrontation with an unconscious conflict and the emotional stress associated with it. **2.** the overuse of abstract thinking or generalizations to control or minimize painful feelings.

intelligence /intel′ijəns/ [L, *intelligentia,* perception], **1.** the potential ability and capacity to acquire, retain, and apply experience, understanding, knowledge, reasoning, and judgment in coping with new experiences and solving problems. **2.** the manifestation of such ability. See also **intelligence quotient.** —**intelligent,** *adj.*

intelligence quotient (IQ), a numeric expression of a person's intellectual level as measured against the statistical average of his or her age group. On several of the traditional scales it is determined by dividing the mental age, derived through psychologic testing, by the chronologic age and multiplying the result by 100. Average IQ is considered to be 100.

intelligence test, any of a variety of standardized tests designed to determine the mental age of an individual by measuring the relative capacity to absorb information and to solve problems.

intemperance /intem′pərəns/ [L, *in,* not, *temperare,* to moderate], excessive indulgence in eating, drinking, or other lifestyle functions.

intensifying screen /inten′sifi′ing/ [L, *intensus,* tighten, *facere,* to make; ME, *screne*], a device consisting of fluorescent material, which is placed in contact with the film in a radiographic cassette. Radiation interacts with the fluorescent phosphor, releasing light photons. These photons expose the film with greater efficiency than would radiation alone; thus patient exposure can be reduced.

intensive care /inten′siv/ [L, *intensus,* tighten, *garrire,* to chatter], constant complex health care as provided in various acute life-threatening conditions such as multiple trauma, severe burns, or myocardial infarction or after certain kinds of surgery.

intensive care unit (ICU), a hospital unit in which patients requiring close monitoring and intensive care are housed for as long as needed. An ICU contains highly technical and sophisticated monitoring devices and equipment, and the staff in the unit is educated to give critical care as needed.

intention /inten′shən/ [L, *intendere,* to aim], a kind of healing process. Healing by primary intention is the initial union of the edges of a wound, progressing to complete healing without granulation. Healing by secondary intention is wound closure in which the edges are separated, granula-

I

tion tissue develops to fill the gap, and epithelium grows in over the granulations, producing a scar. Healing by **tertiary intention** is wound closure in which granulation tissue fills the gap between the edges of the wound, with epithelium growing over the granulation at a slower rate and producing a larger scar than results from healing from second intention.

intentional additives, substances that are deliberately added in the manufacture of food or pharmaceutical products to improve or maintain flavor, color, texture, or consistency or to enhance or conserve nutritional value.

intention tremor, fine, rhythmic purposeless movements that tend to increase during voluntary movements.

interactional model /-ak′shənəl/ [L, *inter,* between, *agere,* to do], a therapy model that views the family as a communication system comprising interlocking subsystems of family members. Family dysfunction occurs when the rules governing family interaction become vague and ambiguous. The therapeutic goal is to help the family clarify the rules governing their relationships.

interactionist theory /-ak′shənist/, an aging theory that views age-related changes as resulting from the interactions among the individual characteristics of the person, the circumstances in society, and the history of social interaction patterns of the person.

interaction processes, a component of the theory of effective practice. The processes consist of a series of interactions between a nurse and a patient. The series occurs in a sequence of actions and reactions until the patient and the nurse both understand what is wanted and the desired behavior or act is achieved.

interalveolar /-alvē′ələr/ [L, *inter,* between, *alveolus,* little hollow], pertaining to the area between alveoli.

interarticular /-ärtik′yələr/ [L, *inter,* between, *articulus,* joint], pertaining to the areas between two joints or between facing surfaces of a joint.

interarticular fibrocartilage [L, *inter* + *articulus,* joint], one of four kinds of fibrocartilage, consisting of flattened fibrocartilaginous plates between the articular cartilage of the most active joints such as the sternoclavicular, wrist, and knee joints.

intercalary /intur′kələr′ē, in′tərkal′ərē/ [L, *intercalare,* to insert], occurring between two others, such as the absence of the middle part of a bone with the proximal and distal parts present.

intercalate /intur′kəlāt/ [L, *intercalare*],

to insert between adjacent surfaces or structures. —**intercalation,** *n.*

intercapillary glomerulosclerosis /-kap′-iler′ē/ [L, *inter* + *capillaris,* hairlike, *glomerulus,* small ball; Gk, *sklerosis,* a hardening], an abnormal condition characterized by degeneration of the renal glomeruli. It is associated with diabetes and often produces albuminuria, nephrotic edema, hypertension, and renal insufficiency.

intercavernous sinuses /-kav′ərnəs/ [L, *inter,* between, *caverna,* cavity, *sinus,* curve], the cavities through which the cavernous sinuses of the dura mater communicate.

intercellular /-sel′yələr/ [L, *inter* + *cella,* storeroom], pertaining to the area between or among cells.

intercellular bridge, a structure that connects adjacent cells, occurring primarily in the epithelium and other stratified squamous epithelia. It consists of slender strands of cytoplasm that project from the surfaces of adjacent cells.

intercerebral /-ser′əbəl/ [L, *inter,* between, *cerebrum,* brain], pertaining to the area between the left and right cerebral hemispheres.

interclavicular /-kləvik′yələr/ [L, *inter,* between, *clavicula,* little key], pertaining to the area between the clavicles.

interconceptional gynecologic care /-kənsep′shənəl/ [L, *inter* + *concipere,* to take in], health care of a woman during her reproductive years, between pregnancies, and after 6 weeks after delivery. Papanicolaou's test for cervical cancer, breast and pelvic examinations, evaluation of general health, and laboratory determination of glucosuria and proteinuria and of the hematocrit or hemoglobin are common and routine aspects of interconceptional care.

intercondylar fracture /in′tərkon′dilər/ [L, *inter* + Gk, *kondylos,* knuckle], a fracture of the tissue between condyles.

intercostal /-kos′təl/ [L, *inter* + *costa,* rib], pertaining to the space between two ribs.

intercostal bulging, the visible bulging of the soft tissues of the intercostal spaces that occurs when increased expiratory effort is needed to exhale, as in asthma, cystic fibrosis, or obstruction of an airway by a foreign body.

intercostal muscles, the muscles between adjacent ribs. They are designated as external and internal and function as secondary ventilatory muscles.

intercostal neuralgia, pain in the intercostal spaces of the chest wall, involving intercostal nerves.

intercostal node, a node in one of three

groups of thoracic parietal lymph nodes situated near the dorsal parts of the intercostal spaces. The nodes are associated with lymphatic vessels that drain the posterolateral area of the chest.

intercostal space [L, *inter,* between, *costa,* rib, *spatium*], the region between the ribs.

intercourse /in'tərkôrs'/ [L, *intercursus,* running between], *informal.* sexual intercourse between individuals.

intercristal /-kris'təl/ [L, *inter* + *crista,* ridge], pertaining to the space between two crests.

intercurrent disease /-kur'ənt/ [L, *intercurrere,* to run between], a disease that develops in and may alter the course of another disease.

interdental canal /-den'təl/ [L, *inter* + *dens,* tooth], any one of the nutrient channels that pass upward to the teeth through the body of the mandible.

interdental gingiva, the supporting gingival tissues, consisting of prominent horizontal collagen fibers, that normally fill the space between two approximating teeth.

interdental groove, a linear vertical depression on the surface of the interdental papillae, which functions as a sluiceway for the egress of food from the interproximal areas.

interdental spillway, a sluiceway formed by the interproximal contours of adjoining teeth and their investing tissues.

interdigestive migrating motor complex /-dijes'tiv/, a pattern of small bowel cyclic motor activity that follows completion of food digestion and absorption.

interest tests, psychologic tests designed to clarify an individual's vocational potential or to compare an individual's performance with the average scores of a specific population.

interference /-fir'əns/ [L, *inter* + *ferire,* to strike], the effect of a component on the accuracy of measurement of the desired analyte.

interferent /-fir'ənt/ [L, *inter* + *ferire,* to strike], any chemical or physical phenomenon that can interfere with or disrupt a reaction or process.

interferential current therapy /-fərən'-shəl/, a form of electrical stimulation therapy using two or three distinctly different currents that are passed through a tissue from surface electrodes. Parts of each current are canceled by the other, with the result that a different net current is applied to the target tissue.

interferon /-fir'on/ [L, *inter* + *ferire,* to strike], a natural cellular protein formed when cells are exposed to a virus or another foreign particle of nucleic acid. It induces the production of translation inhibitory protein (TIP) in noninfected cells. TIP blocks translation of viral ribonucleic acid, thus giving other cells protection against both the original and other viruses. Interferon is species specific.

interferon alpha-2a, recombinant, a parenteral antineoplastic drug administered in the treatment of hairy-cell leukemia.

interferon alpha-2b, recombinant, a parenteral antineoplastic drug with indications, contraindications, and adverse effects similar to those of **interferon alpha-2a, recombinant.**

interferon beta-1a, an antiviral and immune system regulator. It is prescribed in the treatment of relapsing forms of multiple sclerosis. It can help reduce the number of neurologic attacks and slow the progress toward physical disability.

interferon nomenclature, a system recommended by the International Interferon Nomenclature Committee for identifying interferon compounds. For a specific isolated product, "interferon" is the first word of the name. It is followed by a Greek letter, spelled out; an arabic number; and a lowercase letter appended by a dash, as in the example, *interferon alpha-2a.*

interim rate /in'tərim/ [L, meanwhile, *ratum,* calculate], a method of third-party payment for costs of hospital services in which an amount is paid periodically pending an accounting of actual costs at the end of a designated period.

interiorization /intir'ē-ərīzā'shən/ [L, *interior,* inner; Gk, *izein,* to cause], the merging of reflex and cognitive processes as a response to the environment.

interior mesenteric artery [L, inner; Gk, *mesos* middle, *enteron,* intestine, *arteria,* airpipe], a visceral branch of the abdominal aorta, supplying the left half of the transverse colon, all of the descending and iliac colons, and most of the rectum.

interkinesis /in'tərkinē'sis, -kinē'sis/ [L, *inter* + Gk, *kinein,* to move], the interval between the first and second nuclear divisions in meiosis.

interlace mode /-lās'/, (in radiology) a process whereby a conventional television (TV) camera tube reads off its target assembly so that each of two fields represents repeated adjacent active traces and horizontal retraces of the electron beam across a TV screen.

interleukin /-loo'kin/, one of a large group of cytokines produced mainly by T cells or in some cases by mononuclear phagocytes or other cells. Most interleukins direct other cells to divide and differentiate.

interleukin-1 (IL-1) /-l$\overline{oo}$′kin/, a protein with numerous immune system functions, including activation of resting T cells and endothelial and macrophage cells, mediation of inflammation, and stimulation of synthesis of lymphokines, collagen, and collagenases.

interleukin-2 (IL-2), a protein with various immunologic functions, including the ability to initiate proliferation of activated T cells. IL-2 is used in the laboratory to grow T cell clones with specific helper, cytotoxic, and suppressor functions.

interleukin-3 (IL-3), an immune response protein that supports the growth of pluripotent bone marrow stem cells and is a growth factor for mast cells.

interleukin-4 (IL-4), an immune response protein that is a growth factor for activated B cells, resting T cells, and mast cells.

interleukin-5 (IL-5), an eosinophil differentiation cytokine produced by helper T cells. Its functions are to stimulate B cells and eosinophils and to facilitate the differentiation of B cells that secrete immunoglobulin A.

interleukin-6 (IL-6), a cytokine derived from fibroblasts, macrophages, and tumor cells. It is an antiviral compound also used in the treatment of some types of cancer.

interleukin-7 (IL-7), a cytokine produced by bone marrow stromal cells that causes lymphoid stem cell differentiation into progenitor B and T cells and stimulates cell-mediated killing by T cells and monocytes.

interleukin-8 (IL-8), a cytokine produced by various cell types involved in inflammation that attracts and activates neutrophils.

interleukin-9 (IL-9), a glycoprotein factor that helps induce growth of some T helper cell clones but not cytotoxic T cell clones.

interleukin-10 (IL-10), a protein factor expressed by CD4$^+$ and CD8$^+$ T cells, monocytes, macrophages, and activated B cells. It inhibits cytokine synthesis and suppresses macrophage and natural killer T cell functions.

interleukin-11 (IL-11), a cytokine produced by bone marrow stromal cells. The protein factor induces IL-6-dependent murine plasmacytoma cells to proliferate and plays an important role in early platelet hematopoiesis.

interleukin-12 (IL-12), a protein factor that acts on T cells as a cytotoxic lymphocyte maturation factor. Its source is activated T cells, and its function is to stimulate cell-mediated killing by natural killer cells and lymphocytes.

interleukin-13 (IL-13), a protein factor produced by activated T cells. It inhibits inflammatory cytokine production by lipopolysaccharide in peripheral blood monocytes. It suppresses cell-mediated immune responses and promotes B cell differentiation.

interleukin-14 (IL-14), a protein factor produced by follicular dendritic cells, germinal T cells, and some malignant B cells. It also enhances the proliferation of B cells and induces memory B cell production and maintenance.

interleukin-15 (IL-15), a T cell growth factor that enhances peripheral blood T cell production.

interlobular duct /-lob′yələr/ [L, *inter* + *lobulus*, small lobe], any duct connecting or draining the lobules of a gland.

interlocked twins [L, *inter* + AS, *loc*, a fastening], monozygotic twins so positioned in the uterus that the neck of one becomes entwined with that of the other during presentation so that vaginal delivery is not possible.

intermediary /-mē′dē·er′ē/ [L, *inter* + *mediare*, to divide], a private insurance company or public or private agency selected by health care providers to pay claims under the Medicare program.

intermediary metabolism [L, *inter*, between, *mediary*, to divide; Gk, *metabole*, change], the metabolic processes involved in the synthesis of cellular components between digestion of food and excretion of waste products.

intermediate-acting insulin [L, *inter* + *mediare*, to divide, *activus*, active], a preparation of the antidiabetic principle of beef pancreas or pork pancreas modified by interaction with zinc under specific chemical conditions and having an intermediate range of action.

intermediate care /-mē′dē·it/, a level of medical care for certain chronically ill or disabled individuals in which room and board are provided but skilled nursing care is not.

intermediate care facility (ICF), a health facility that provides medically related services to persons with a variety of physical or emotional conditions requiring institutional facilities but without the degree of care provided by a hospital or skilled nursing facility.

intermediate care unit, a transitional unit for patients from critical care units that provides close monitoring before discharge.

intermediate cuneiform bone, the smallest of the three cuneiform bones of the foot, located between the medial and lateral cuneiform bones.

intermediate-density lipoprotein (IDL), a lipid-protein complex with a density between those of very low–density lipoprotein and low-density lipoprotein. In a type III hyperlipoproteinemic state, the IDL concentration in the blood is elevated.

intermediate host, any animal in which the larval or intermediate stage of a parasite develops. Humans are intermediate hosts for malaria parasites.

intermediate mass, the connecting mass of nervous tissue between two lobes of the diencephalon.

intermenstrual /-men′stro͞o·əl/ [L, *inter* + *menstruum,* menstrual fluid], pertaining to the time between menstrual periods.

intermenstrual fever, the normal slight elevation of temperature that marks ovulation, usually occurring about 14 days before the onset of menses.

intermittent /-mit′ənt/ [L, *inter* + *mittere,* to send], occurring at intervals; alternating between periods of activity and inactivity such as rheumatoid arthritis, which is marked by periods of signs and symptoms followed by periods of remission.

intermittent assisted ventilation (IAV), (in respiratory therapy) a system in which an assisted rate is combined with spontaneous breathing.

intermittent compression, external compression used to control and reduce accumulation of lymph in body tissues. Devices to provide intermittent compression in an on-off timing sequence include inflated pressure sleeves and linear compression pumps. Intermittent compression is also used to decrease acute bleeding.

intermittent explosive disorder, a mental disturbance beginning in childhood and characterized by discrete episodes of violence and aggressive behavior or destruction of property in otherwise normal individuals.

intermittent fever, a fever that recurs in cycles of paroxysms and remissions, such as in malaria.

intermittent hydrosalpinx /hī′drōsal′-pingks/ [L, *inter,* between, *mittere,* to send; Gk, *hydor,* water, *salpinx,* tube], a fluid accumulation in a fallopian tube. The fluid is released periodically through the uterine cavity.

intermittent incontinence [L, *inter,* between, *mittere,* to send, *incontinentia,* inability to retain], urinary incontinence that occurs only when there is pressure on the bladder or exertion of muscular effort.

intermittent mandatory ventilation (IMV), a mode of mechanical ventilation in which the patient is allowed to breathe independently and then, at certain prescribed intervals, a ventilator delivers a breath either under positive pressure or in a measured volume.

intermittent pulse [L, *inter,* between, *mittere,* to send, *pulsare,* to beat], a pulse in which an occasional beat is absent. It tends to occur with second-degree heart block or extrasystole.

intermittent torticollis [L, *inter,* between, *mittere,* to send, *tortus,* twisted, *collum,* neck], intermittent spasms of the neck muscles, drawing the head to one side. The powerful contractions usually occur in the sternocleidomastoid muscle.

intermittent tremor [L, *inter,* between, *mittere,* to send, *tremere,* to tremble], a rhythmic involuntary shaking that occurs intermittently or a tremor that occurs after a voluntary movement is attempted.

intern /in′turn/ [L, *internus,* inward], **1.** a physician in the first postgraduate year, learning medical practice under supervision before beginning a residency program. **2.** any immediate postgraduate trainee in a clinical program. **3.** to work as an intern.

internal /intur′nəl/ [L, *internus,* inward], within or inside. —**internally,** *adv.*

internal abdominal oblique muscle, one of a pair of anterolateral muscles of the abdomen. It functions to compress the abdominal contents and assists in micturition, defecation, emesis, parturition, and forced expiration. Both sides acting together serve to flex the vertebral column.

internal acoustic meatus, an opening in the petrous part of the temporal bone through which the facial, intermediate, and vestibulocochlear nerves and the labyrinthine artery pass.

internal aperture of tympanic canaliculus, the upper opening of the tympanic channel in the temporal bone, leading to the tympanum.

internal bleeding [L, *internus,* inward; AS, *blod*], any hemorrhage from an internal organ or tissue, such as intraperitoneal bleeding into the peritoneal cavity or intestinal bleeding into the bowel.

internal carotid artery, each of two arteries starting at the bifurcation of the common carotid arteries, opposite the cranial border of the thyroid cartilage, through which blood circulates to many structures and organs in the head.

internal carotid plexus, a network of nerves on the internal carotid artery, formed by the internal carotid nerve. The internal carotid plexus supplies sympathetic fibers to the branches of the internal carotid artery, the tympanic plexus, the nerves of the cavernous sinus, and the cranial parasympathetic ganglia through which the fibers pass.

internal cervical os, an internal opening of the uterus that corresponds to the slight constriction or isthmus of that organ about midway in its length. The internal cervical os separates the body of the uterus from the cervix.

internal ear, the complex inner structure of the ear, containing receptors for hearing and balance. The maculae and crystae cells help maintain equilibrium; the organ of Corti cells translate sound vibrations into impulses for the sense of hearing. The auditory receptor cells are innervated by the cochlear nerve.

internal fertilization, the union of gametes within the body of the female after insemination.

internal fistula, an abnormal passage between two internal organs or structures.

internal fixation, any method of holding together the fragments of a fractured bone without the use of appliances external to the skin. After open reduction of the fracture, through an appropriate incision smooth or threaded pins, Kirschner wires, screws, plates attached by screws, or medullary nails may be used to stabilize the fragments.

internal hemorrhage, bleeding into a serous cavity, a hollow viscus, or tissues.

internal hemorrhoid, a fold of mucous membrane at the anorectal junction, caused by edema or dilation of the interior rectal vein.

internal hernia, a protrusion of an intraperitoneal viscus into a recess or compartment within the peritoneal cavity.

internal iliac artery, a division of the common iliac artery, supplying the walls of the pelvis, the pelvic viscera, the genital organs, and part of the medial thigh.

internal iliac node, a node in one of seven groups of parietal lymph nodes serving the abdomen and the pelvis.

internal iliac vein, one of the pair of veins in the lower body that join the external iliac vein to form the two common iliac veins.

internal injury [L, *internus,* inward, *injuria*], any hurt, wound, or damage to the viscera.

internalization /intur'nəlīzā'shən/ [L, *internus* + Gk, *izein,* to cause], the process of adopting within the self, either unconsciously or consciously through learning and socialization, the attitudes, beliefs, values, and standards of another person or more generally of the society or group to which one belongs.

internal jugular vein, one of a pair of veins in the neck. Each vein collects blood from one side of the brain, the face, and the neck, and both unite with the subclavian vein to form the brachiocephalic vein.

internal mammary artery bypass, a surgical procedure to correct a coronary artery obstruction. The internal mammary artery in situ and still attached to the subclavian artery is anastomosed to the coronary artery beyond the obstruction.

internal medicine, the branch of medicine concerned with the study of the physiologic and pathologic characteristics of the internal organs and with the medical diagnosis and treatment of disorders of these organs.

internal os, the internal opening of the cervical canal.

internal pterygoid muscle, one of the four muscles of mastication. It acts to close the jaws.

internal rotation, the turning of a limb toward the midline of the body.

internal secretion [L, *internus,* inward, *secernere,* to separate], a type of secretion in which substances pass directly from a gland into the bloodstream.

internal standard, an element or compound added in a known amount to yield a signal against which an instrument or an analyte to be measured can be calibrated.

internal strangulation [L, *internus,* inward, *strangulare,* to choke], a state of extreme constriction of an organ, such as a loop of intestine trapped in an opening, resulting in an interruption in the blood supply and ischemia.

internal thoracic artery, one of a pair of arteries that arise from the first parts of the subclavian arteries and descend to the margin of the sternum. The artery supplies the pectoral muscles, breasts, pericardium, and abdominal muscles.

internal thoracic vein, one of a pair of veins that accompany the internal thoracic artery, receiving tributaries that correspond to those of the artery.

International Association for Dental Research (IADR), an international organization concerned with research in dentistry and the exchange of information regarding such research.

International Classification of Disease Adapted for Use in the United States (ICDA), a classification system adapted by the U.S. Public Health Service from the parent system developed by the World Health Organization. The system is used in categorizing and indexing hospital records. Each disease is listed as belonging to a major section, such as infectious disease or neoplastic disease, and then further coded into major disease categories.

and subdivisions. The system is updated every 10 years.

International Classification of Diseases (ICD), an official list of categories of diseases, physical and mental, issued by the World Health Organization. It is used primarily for statistical purposes in the classification of morbidity and mortality data.

International Commission on Radiation Protection (ICRP), a nongovernmental organization founded in England in 1928 to provide general guidance on the safe use of radiation sources, including appropriate protective measures and codes of practice for medical radiology. The ICRP was reorganized in 1950 to include effects of nuclear energy.

International Congress of Surgeons (ICS), an international professional organization of surgeons.

International Council of Nurses (ICN), the oldest international health organization. It is a federation of nurses' associations from 112 countries and was one of the first health organizations to develop strict policies of nondiscrimination based on nationality, race, creed, color, politics, sex, or social status. The objectives of the ICN include promotion of national associations of nurses, improvement of standards of nursing and competence of nurses, improvement of the status of nurses within their countries, and provision of an authoritative international voice for nurses.

International Normalized Ratio (INR), a comparative rating of a patient's prothrombin time (PT) ratio, used as a standard for monitoring the effects of warfarin. The INR indicates what the patient's PT ratio would have been if measured by using the primary World Health Organization International Reference reagent.

International Red Cross Society, an international philanthropic organization based in Geneva, Switzerland, concerned primarily with the humane treatment and welfare of the victims of war and calamity and with the neutrality of hospitals and medical personnel in times of war.

International System of Units (SI), an internationally accepted scientific system of expressing length, mass, and time in base units (IU) of meters, kilograms, and seconds, replacing the old centimeter-gram-second system (CGS). The SI system includes as standard measurements the **ampere, kelvin, candela,** and **mole.**

International Unit (IU, I.U.), a unit of measure in the International System of Units.

interneuron /-nŏŏr′on/, a nerve cell whose axon and dendrite lie entirely within the central nervous system (CNS) and whose function is to relay impulses within the CNS.

internist /intur′nist, in′turnist/ [L, *internus,* inward], a physician who specializes in internal medicine.

internship /in′turnship′/, a period of apprenticeship for a medical school graduate who serves in a hospital for a specified period before beginning a professional practice.

internuncial neuron /-nun′sē·əl/ [L, *inter + nuntius,* messenger], a connecting neuron in a neural pathway, usually serving as a link between two other neurons.

interocclusal record /-əklŏŏ′səl/, a record of the positional relation of opposing teeth or jaws to each other, made on the surfaces of occlusal rims or teeth with a plastic material that hardens, such as acrylic resin.

interoceptive /in′tərōsep′tiv/ [L, *internus,* inward, *capere,* to take], pertaining to stimuli originating from within the body that are related to the functioning of the internal organs or the receptors they activate.

interoceptor /-sep′tər/ [L, *internus + capere,* to take], any sensory nerve ending located in cells in the viscera that responds to stimuli originating from within the body in relation to the function of the internal organs, such as digestion, excretion, and blood pressure.

interosseous /-os′ē·əs/ [L, *inter,* between, *os,* bone], pertaining to an area between bones or a structure such as a ligament connecting two bones.

interparoxysmal /-per′əksis′məl/ [L, *inter,* between, *paroxysmos,* irritation], pertaining to something that happens between paroxysms.

interperiosteal fracture /in′tərper′ē·os′-tē·əl/ [L, *inter + Gk, peri,* around, *osteon,* bone], an incomplete fracture in which the periosteum is not disrupted.

interpersonal /-pur′sənəl/ [L, *inter,* between, *personalis*], pertaining to the interactions of individuals.

interpersonal psychiatry [L, *inter + persona,* mask], a theory of psychiatry introduced by Harry Stack Sullivan [1892–1949] that stresses the nature and quality of relationships with significant others as the most critical factor in personality development.

interpersonal therapy, a kind of psychotherapy that views faulty communications, interactions, and interrelationships as basic factors in maladaptive behavior. A kind of interpersonal therapy is **transactional analysis.**

interphase /in'tərfās'/ [L, *inter* + Gk, *phasis*, phase], the metabolic stage in the cell cycle during which the cell is not dividing, the chromosomes are not individually distinguishable, and such biochemical and physiologic activities as deoxyribonucleic acid synthesis occur.

interpleural space /-ploȯr'əl/ [L, *inter*, between; Gk, *pleura*, rib; L, *spatium*], the potential space of the mediastinum between the two pleural linings.

interpolated PVC /intur'pələ'tid/ [L, *interpolare*, to refurbish], a ventricular extrasystole sandwiched between two consecutive sinus-conducted beats.

interpolation /intur'pəlā'shən/, **1.** the transfer of tissues, as in plastic surgery or transplantation. **2.** (in statistics) the introduction of an estimated intermediate value of a variable between known values.

interpubic disk /-pyoo͞o'bik/ [L, *inter* + *os pubis*, pubic bone; Gk, *diskos*, flat plate], the fibrocartilaginous plate connecting the opposed surfaces of the pubic bones at the pubic symphysis.

interpulse interval /-puls/, the time elapsed between successive nerve impulses; the reciprocal of impulse frequency.

interradicular space /-radik'yələr/ [L, *inter* + *radix*, root, *spatium*], the area between the roots of a multirooted tooth, normally occupied by a bony septum and the periodontal membrane.

interrogatories /in'tərog'ətôr'ēz/ [L, *inter* + *rogare*, to ask], (in law) a series of written questions submitted to a witness or other person having information of interest to the court. The answers are transcribed and sworn to under oath.

interrupted suture /in'tərup'tid/ [L, *interrumpere*, to sever, *sutura*], a single suture tied separately, as distinguished from a continuous suture.

intersection syndrome, a condition of pain, crepitus, and a squeaky sensation in the dorsal radial forearm. It occurs most commonly among weight lifters and rowers.

intersex /in'tərseks'/ [L, *inter* + *sexus*, sex, gender], any individual who has anatomic characteristics of both sexes or whose external genitalia are ambiguous or inappropriate for either the normal male or female.

intersexuality /-sek'shoo͞o·al'itē/ [L, *inter* + *sexus*, male or female], the condition in which an individual has both male and female anatomic characteristics to varying degrees or in which the appearance of the external genitalia is ambiguous or differs from that characteristic of the gonadal or genetic sex. **—intersexual,** *adj.*

interspinal ligament /-spī'nəl/ [L, *inter* + *spina*, spine, *ligare*, to bind], one of many thin, narrow membranous ligaments that connect adjoining spinous processes of the vertebrae and extend from the root of each process to the apex.

interspinous /-spī'nəs/ [L, *inter* + *spina*, spine], pertaining to the space between any spinous processes.

interstitial /in'tərstish'əl/ [L, *inter* + *sistere*, to stand], pertaining to the space between cells, as interstitial fluid.

interstitial cell-stimulating hormone (ICSH), the luteinizing hormone that also stimulates the production of testosterone by the Leydig, or interstitial, cells of the testis.

interstitial cystitis, an inflammation of the bladder, believed to be associated with an autoimmune or allergic response. The bladder wall becomes inflamed, ulcerated, and scarred, causing frequent painful urination. Hematuria often occurs.

interstitial emphysema, a form of emphysema in which air or gas escapes into the interstitial tissues of the lung after a penetrating injury or a rupture in an alveolar wall. Since the alveoli must be decompressed, there is danger that the pleura will be torn, causing a pneumothorax.

interstitial fibroid [L, *interstitium,* space between, *fibra,* fiber; Gk, *eidos,* form], a fibrous tumor that develops in the muscular wall of the uterus and tends to grow inward.

interstitial fluid, an extracellular fluid that fills the spaces between most of the cells of the body and provides a substantial part of the liquid environment of the body. Formed by filtration through the blood capillaries, it is drained away as lymph.

interstitial growth, an increase in size by hyperplasia or hypertrophy within the interior of a part or structure that is already formed.

interstitial implantation, (in embryology) the complete embedding of the blastocyst within the endometrium of the uterine wall.

interstitial inflammation [L, *interstitium,* space between, *inflammare,* to set afire], an inflammation in an area of connective tissues.

interstitial keratitis, an uncommon inflammation within the layers of the cornea. The first symptom is a diffuse haziness. Blood vessels may grow into the area and cause permanent opacities. The causes are syphilis, tuberculosis, leprosy and vascular hypersensitivity.

interstitial lung disease, a respiratory disorder characterized by a dry unproduc tive cough and dyspnea on exertion. The patient may have swallowing disorders or joint and muscle pain and a history of industrial exposure to inorganic dusts such as asbestos or silica. Interstitial lung disease may result from viral, bacterial, or other types of infection; uremic pneumonitis; cancer; a congenital or inherited disorder; or circulatory impairment.

interstitial mastitis [L, *interstitium,* space between; Gk, *mastos,* breast], an inflammation of the connective tissue between ducts of the breast.

interstitial nephritis, inflammation of the interstitial tissue of the kidney, including the tubules. Acute interstitial nephritis is an immunologic adverse reaction to certain drugs, often sulfonamide or methicillin. Acute renal failure, fever, rash, and proteinuria are characteristic of this condition. Chronic interstitial nephritis is a syndrome of interstitial inflammation and structural changes, sometimes associated with such conditions as ureteral obstruction, pyelonephritis, exposure of the kidney to a toxin, rejection of a transplant, and certain systemic diseases. Gradually renal failure, nausea, vomiting, weight loss, fatigue, and anemia develop.

interstitial pneumonia, a diffuse chronic inflammation of the lungs beyond the terminal bronchioles, characterized by fibrosis and collagen formation in the alveolar walls and by the presence of large mononuclear cells in the alveolar spaces. The symptoms are progressive dyspnea, clubbing of the fingers, cyanosis, and fever. The disease may result from a hypersensitive reaction to busulfan, chlorambucil, hexamethonium, or methotrexate. Interstitial pneumonia may also be an autoimmune reaction, since it often accompanies celiac disease, rheumatoid arthritis, Sjögren's syndrome, and systemic sclerosis.

interstitial therapy, radiotherapy in which needles or wires that contain radioactive material are implanted directly into tumor areas.

interstitial tissue [L, *interstitium,* space between; OFr, *tissu*], the connective and supporting tissue within and surrounding major functional elements of an organ.

interstitial tubal pregnancy, a kind of tubal pregnancy in which implantation occurs in the proximal interstitial part of one of the fallopian tubes.

interstitium /-stish'ē-əm/, the space between cells in a tissue.

intertransverse ligament /-transvurz'/ [L, *inter* + *transversus,* cross-direction], one of many fibrous bands connecting the transverse processes of vertebrae.

intertrigo /in'tərtrī'gō/ [L, *inter* + *terere,* to scour], an erythematous irritation of opposing skin surfaces caused by friction. Common sites are the axillae, the folds beneath large or pendulous breasts, and the inner aspects of the thighs. —**intertriginous,** *adj.*

intertrochanteric crest /in'tərtrō'kanter'-ik/ [L, *inter* + *trochanter,* runner, *crista,* ridge], one of a pair of ridges along the thigh bones, curving obliquely from the greater to the lesser trochanter.

intertrochanteric fracture, a fracture characterized by a crack in the tissue of the proximal femur between the greater and lesser trochanters.

intertrochanteric line, a line that runs across the anterior surface of the thigh bone from the greater to the lesser trochanter, winding around the medial surface and ending in the linea aspera.

intertuberous diameter /-tōō'bərəs/ [L, *inter* + *tuber,* swelling; Gk, *dia,* across, *metron,* measure], the distance between the ischial tuberosities, a factor used in determining the dimensions, including the narrowest diameter, of the pelvic outlet.

interval /in'tərval/ [L, *intervallum,* space between], a space between things or events, or a break or interruption in an otherwise continuous flow.

interval health history [L, *intervallum,* space between], a kind of health history that notes the general condition of a client during the period between visits and is not limited to facts relevant to a particular condition. The interval health history provides an ongoing account of a person's health, serving to bring the data base up to date.

intervention /in'tərven'shən/ [L, *inter* + *venire,* to come], any act performed to prevent harming of a patient or to improve the mental, emotional, or physical function of a patient. A physiologic process may be monitored or enhanced, or a pathologic process may be arrested or controlled. Independent intervention is any health care activity pertaining to certain aspects of professional practice that are encompassed by applicable licensure and law and require no supervision or direction from others. Interdependent intervention refers to any health care activity carried out by one health care professional in collaboration with another.

interventricular /-ventrik'yələr/ [L, *inter,* between, *ventriculus,* little belly], pertaining to the location between the ventricles, as the septum of the heart.

interventricular septum [L, *inter,* between, *ventriculus,* little belly, *saeptum,* fence], the wall between the ventricles of the heart.

intervertebral /in'tərvur'təbrəl/ [L, *inter* + *vertebra*, back joint], pertaining to the space between any two vertebrae, such as the fibrocartilaginous disks.

intervertebral disk, one of the fibrous disks found between adjacent spinal vertebrae, except the axis and the atlas. The disks vary in size, shape, thickness, and number, depending on the location in the back and on the particular vertebrae they separate.

intervertebral foramen, any of the passages between adjacent vertebrae through which the spinal nerves and vessels pass.

intervertebral ganglion [L, *inter,* between; *vertebra,* back joint; Gk, *ganglion,* knot], the ganglionic enlargement of a spinal nerve root between adjacent vertebrae.

interview /in'tərvyōō/, a communication with a patient initiated for a specific purpose and focused on a specific content area. A problem-seeking interview is an inquiry that focuses on gathering data to identify problems the patient needs to resolve. A problem-solving interview focuses on problems that have been identified by the patient or health care professional.

intervillous space /in'tərvil'əs/ [L, *inter* + *villus,* hair, *spatium*], one of many spaces between the chorionic villi of the endometrium of the gravid uterus, beneath the placenta. The intervillous spaces act as small reservoirs for oxygenated maternal blood.

intestinal /intes'tinəl/ [L, *intestinum*], pertaining to the intestines.

intestinal absorption [L, *intestinum,* intestine, *absorbare* to swallow], the passage of the products of digestion from the lumen of the small intestine into the blood and lymphatic vessels in the wall of the gut. The surface area of the intestine is greatly increased by the presence of fingerlike projections, called *villi,* each of which contains capillaries and a lymphatic vessel, or lacteal.

intestinal angina, chronic vascular insufficiency of the mesentery caused by atherosclerosis and resulting ischemia of the smooth muscle of the small bowel.

intestinal apoplexy, the sudden occlusion of one of the three principal arteries to the intestine by an embolism or a thrombus. This condition leads rapidly to necrosis of intestinal tissue and is often fatal.

intestinal atresia [L, *intestinum* + Gk, *a* + *tresis,* boring], a pathologic obstruction of the continuous lumen of the intestinal tract caused by a defect of development in utero.

intestinal bypass surgery [L, *intestinum* + AS, *bi* + Fr, *passer* + Gk, *cheirourgos*], a surgical procedure to shorten the digestive tract. It is performed so that less intestinal surface will be available to absorb nutrients from the digested food passing through, as in morbid obesity, or to bypass a blocked or diseased part of the intestine. The technique usually involves anastomosing the jejunum to the ileum.

intestinal colic [L, *intestinum* + Gk, *kolikos,* colonic pain], spasmodic pain in intestinal disorders.

intestinal dyspepsia, an abnormal condition characterized by impaired digestion associated with a disorder that originates in the intestines.

intestinal fistula, an abnormal passage from the intestine to an external abdominal opening or stoma, usually created surgically for the exit of feces after removal of a malignant or severely ulcerated segment of the bowel.

intestinal flora [L, *intestinum* + *flos,* flowers], the natural bacterial content of the inside of the digestive tract.

intestinal flu, a viral gastroenteritis, usually caused by infection by an enterovirus. It is characterized by abdominal cramps, diarrhea, nausea, and vomiting.

intestinal fluke [L, *intestinum* + AS, *floc*], any internal parasite of the genera *Fasciolopsis, Heterophyes,* and *Metagonimus* in North America and of other genera in Asia and in tropical countries. They enter the body through the mouth as encysted larvae in aquatic vegetation or freshwater fish. Symptoms of intestinal fluke infestation usually include abdominal pain and obstruction and diarrhea.

intestinal gas [L, *intestinum*], gas in the digestive tract arising from three sources—swallowed air, gas produced by digestive processes, and blood gases diffused into the intestinal lumen. Gases produced in the intestine and diffused from blood are mainly hydrogen (H_2), most of which is a bacterial fermentation product of ingested carbohydrates; carbon dioxide (CO_2); and methane (CH_4).

intestinal juices, the secretions of glands lining the intestine.

intestinal obstruction, any obstruction that results in failure of the contents of the intestine to progress through the lumen of the bowel. The most common cause is a mechanical blockage resulting from adhesions, impacted feces, tumor of the bowel, hernia, intussusception, volvulus, or the strictures of inflammatory bowel disease. Obstruction of the small bowel may cause severe pain, vomiting of fecal matter, dehydration, and eventually a drop in blood pressure. Obstruction of the colon causes less severe pain, marked abdominal distension, and constipation.

intestinal perforation [L, *intestinum* + *perforare,* to pierce], the escape of digestive tract contents into the peritoneal cavity that results from trauma or a disease condition such as a ruptured appendix or perforated ulcer. The condition inevitably leads to peritonitis.

intestinal strangulation, the arrest of blood flow to the bowel, causing edema, cyanosis, and gangrene of the affected loop of bowel. This condition is usually caused by a hernia, intussusception, or volvulus. Early signs of intestinal strangulation resemble those of intestinal obstruction.

intestinal tonsil, one of a group of lymphatic nodules forming a single layer in the mucous membrane of the ileum opposite the mesenteric attachment.

intestinal tract [L, *intestinum* + *tractus*], the segments of the small and large intestines between the pyloric valve and the rectum. It forms part of the digestive tract.

intestinal tubes [L, *intestinum* + *tubus*], the alimentary canal or digestive tract.

intestine /intes'tin/ [L, *intestinum*], the part of the alimentary canal extending from the pyloric opening of the stomach to the anus. It includes the small and large intestines. —**intestinal,** *adj.*

intima /in'timə/, *pl.* **intimae** [L, *intimus,* innermost], the innermost layer of a structure, such as the lining membrane of an artery, vein, lymphatic vessel, or organ. —**intimal,** *adj.*

intimal sclerosis [L, *intimus,* innermost; Gk, *sklerosis,* hardening], a hardening of the innermost layer of a blood vessel.

intolerance /intol'ərəns/ [L, *in,* not, *tolerare,* to bear], a condition characterized by inability to absorb or metabolize a nutrient or medication. Exposure to the substance may cause an adverse reaction, as in lactose intolerance.

intoxicant /intok'sikənt/ [L, *in* + Gk, *toxikon,* poison], any agent that can cause intoxication or poisoning.

intoxication /intok'sikā'shən/ [L, *in,* within; Gk, *toxikon,* poison], **1.** the state of being poisoned by a drug or other toxic substance. **2.** the state of being inebriated as a result of an excessive consumption of alcohol. **3.** a state of mental or emotional hyperexcitability, usually euphoric.

intraabdominal infections /in'trə·abdom'inəl/, diseases caused by organisms, usually bacterial or fungal, situated within the cavity of the abdomen. Treatment depends on the type of infectious organism and the site of the infection.

intraabdominal pressure [L, *intra,* within, *abdomen,* belly], the degree of pressure within the abdominal cavity.

intraaortic balloon pump /in'trə·ā·ôr'tik/ [L, *intra* + *aeirein,* to rise], a counterpulsation device that provides temporary cardiac assist in the management of refractory left ventricular failure that may follow myocardial infarction or occur in preinfarction angina.

intraarterial /in'trə·ärtir'ē·əl/, pertaining to a structure or action inside an artery.

intraarticular /in'trə·ärtik'yələr/ [L, *intra* + *articulus,* joint], within a joint.

intraarticular fracture, a fracture involving the articular surfaces of a joint.

intraarticular injection, the injection of a medication into a joint space, usually to reduce inflammation, such as in bursitis or fibromyositis.

intraarticular ligament, a ligament that forms part of the joints between 16 of the 24 ribs, dividing the joints into two cavities, each containing a synovial membrane.

intraatrial /in'trə·ā'trē·əl/ [L, *intra* + *atrium,* hall], pertaining to the space or substance within an atrium in the heart.

intraatrial block, delayed or abnormal conduction within the atria. It is identified on an electrocardiogram by a prolonged and often notched P wave.

intracanalicular fibroma /-kan'əlik'yələr/ [L, *intra* + *canaliculus,* small channel], a tumor containing glandular epithelium and fibrous tissue, occurring in the breast.

intracanicular papilloma /-kənik'yələr/, a benign warty growth in certain glands, especially the breast.

intracapsular fracture /-kap'syələr/ [L, *intra* + *capsula,* little box], a fracture within the capsule of a joint.

intracardiac /-kar'dē·ak/ [L, *intra,* within; Gk, *kardia,* heart], pertaining to the interior of the heart chambers.

intracardiac lead /lēd/ [L, *intra* + Gk, *kardia,* heart; AS, *laedan,* lead], **1.** an electrocardiographic conductor in which the exploring electrode is placed within one of the cardiac chambers, usually by means of cardiac catheterization. **2.** *informal.* a tracing produced by such a lead on an electrocardiograph.

intracatheter /-kath'ətər/ [L, *intra* + Gk, *katheter,* something lowered], a thin, flexible plastic catheter introduced through a stainless steel needle and threaded into a blood vessel to infuse blood, fluid, or medication.

intracavitary /in'trəkav'itər'ē/ [L, *intra* +

cavum, cave], pertaining to the space within a body cavity.

intracavitary therapy, a kind of radiotherapy in which one or more radioactive sources are placed, usually with the help of an applicator or holding device, within a body cavity to irradiate the walls of the cavity or adjacent tissues.

intracellular /-sel′yələr/ [L, *intra,* within, *cella,* storeroom], pertaining to the interior of a cell.

intracellular fluid (ICF) [L, *intra + cella,* storeroom, *fluere,* to flow], a fluid within cell membranes throughout most of the body, containing dissolved solutes that are essential to electrolytic balance and to healthy metabolism.

intracerebral /-ser′əbrəl/ [L, *intra + cerebrum,* brain], pertaining to the area or substance within the cerebrum.

intracerebral hematoma, a localized collection of blood within the cerebrum, associated with a cerebral laceration resulting from a contusion.

intracerebral hemorrhage (ICH), a type of hemorrhagic stroke in which bleeding directly into the brain occurs. It is most often caused by hypertension and is associated with increased intracranial pressure. ICH usually occurs in the basal ganglia, thalamus, pons, and cerebral and cerebellar white matter.

intracistronic /in′trəsistron′ik/ [L, *intra + cis,* this side, *trans,* across], within a cistron.

intracoronal retainer /-kôr′ənəl/ [L, *intra + corona,* crown], **1.** a retainer in which the prepared tooth cavity and its cast restoration lie largely within the body of the coronal part of a tooth and within the contour of the tooth crown, such as an inlay. **2.** a direct retainer used in the construction of removable partial dentures. It consists of a female part within the coronal segment of the crown of an abutment and a fitted male part attached to the denture proper.

intracostal /-kos′təl/, pertaining to the inner surface of a rib.

intracranial /-krā′nē·əl/ [L, *intra,* within; Gk, *kranion,* skull], pertaining to the area within the cranium (the bony skull).

intracranial aneurysm, any aneurysm of any of the cerebral arteries. Characteristics of the condition include sudden severe headache, stiff neck, nausea, vomiting, and sometimes loss of consciousness.

intracranial hemorrhage [L, *intra,* within; Gk, *kranion,* skull, *haima,* blood], a hemorrhage within the cranium.

intracranial pressure, pressure that occurs within the cranium.

Intracranial Pressure (ICP) Monitoring, a Nursing Interventions Classification defined as measurement and interpretation of patient data to regulate intracranial pressure.

intractable /intrak′təbəl/ [L, *intractabilis,* hard to manage], having no relief, such as a symptom or a disease that is not relieved by the therapeutic measures used.

intractable pain [L, *intractabilis,* hard to manage, *poena,* penalty], pain that is not relieved by ordinary medical, surgical, and nursing measures. The pain is often chronic, persistent, and psychogenic in nature.

intracutaneous /-kyōōtā′nē·əs/ [L, *intra + cutis,* skin], within the skin.

intracystic papilloma /-sis′tik/ [L, *intra + Gk, kystis,* bag], a benign epithelial tumor formed within a cystic adenoma.

intradermal /-dur′məl/ [L, *intra,* within; Gk, *derma,* skin], within the dermis..

intradermal injection, the introduction of a hypodermic needle into the dermis for the purpose of instilling a substance such as a serum or vaccine.

intradermal test [L, *intra + Gk, derma,* skin], a procedure used to identify suspected allergens by subcutaneously injecting the patient with small amounts of extracts of the suspected allergens.

intraductal /-duk′təl/, within a duct.

intraductal carcinoma [L, *intra + ductus,* duct], a neoplasm that occurs most often in the breast.

intraductal papilloma, a small benign epithelial tumor in a milk duct of the breast, occasionally marked by bleeding from the nipple.

intradural lipoma [L, *intra + dura,* hard], a fatty tumor in or beneath the dura mater of the spine or sacrum that tends to infiltrate the dorsal column and roots of spinal nerves, causing pain and dysfunction.

intraepidermal carcinoma /in′trə·ep′-idur′məl/ [L, *intra + Gk, epi,* above, *derma,* skin], a neoplasm of squamous epidermal cells that does not proliferate into the basal area and often occurs in many sites simultaneously.

intraepidermal vesicle, a fluid-filled blisterlike cavity within the epidermis. It is usually less than 1 cm in diameter.

intrafusal muscle fiber /-fyōō′zəl/, the striated muscle fiber within a muscle spindle.

intraluminal /-lōō′minəl/, **1.** within the lumen of any tubular structure or organ. **2.** between or among tubes.

intraluminal coronary artery stent, a device permanently inserted into a coronary artery to maintain patency of the lumen of the blood vessel.

intramammary abscess /-mam′ərē/, a

collection of pus within a mammary gland.

intramenstrual pain /-men'stroo·əl/ [L, *intra*, within, *menstrualis*, monthly, *poena*, penalty], pelvic or lower abdominal pain that occurs about midway between menstrual periods and may be associated with ovulation.

intramural /-myoo'rəl/ [L, *intra*, within, *murus*, wall], pertaining to events or structures within the walls of an organ or body part or cavity.

intramuscular /-mus'kyələr/ [L, *intra*, within, *musculus*], pertaining to the interior of muscle tissue.

intramuscular injection [L, *intra* + *musculus*, muscle], the introduction of a hypodermic needle into a muscle to administer a medication.

intraocular /-ok'yələr/ [L, *intra* + *oculus*, eye], pertaining to structures or substances within the eyeball.

intraocular pressure, the internal pressure of the eye, regulated by resistance to the flow of aqueous humor through the fine sieve of the trabecular meshwork. Contraction or relaxation of the longitudinal muscles of the ciliary body affects the size of the opening in the meshwork.

intraoperative /-op'ərətiv'/ [L, *intra* + *operari*, to work], pertaining to the period during a surgical procedure.

intraoperative hyperthermia [L, *intro* + *operari*, to work], hyperthermia delivered as a therapeutic measure to internal sites that have been exposed by a surgical procedure.

intraoperative ultrasound, a diagnostic technique that uses a portable ultrasound device to scan the spinal cord during spinal surgery. Intraoperative ultrasound can distinguish between syrinxes, or fluid-filled cysts, and neoplastic growths in nervous system tissue.

intraoral orthodontic appliance /in'trə·ôr'əl/ [L, *intra* + *oralis*, mouth], an orthodontic device placed inside the mouth to correct or alleviate malocclusion.

intraosseous /in'trə·os'ē·əs/ [L, *intra*, within, *os*, bone], pertaining to the interior of bone.

intraosseous infusion, the injection of blood, medications, or fluids into bone marrow rather than into a vein. The technique may be performed in emergency treatment of a child when intravenous infusion is not feasible.

intraparietal sulcus /-perī'ətəl/ [L, *intra* + *paries*, wall, *sulcus*, groove], an irregular groove on the convex surface of the parietal lobe that marks the division of the inferior and superior parietal lobules.

intrapartal care /-pär'təl/ [L, *intra* + *partus*, birth], care of a pregnant woman from the onset of labor to the completion of the fourth stage of labor with the expulsion of the placenta.

Intrapartal Care, a Nursing Interventions Classification defined as monitoring and management of stages one and two of the birth process.

Intrapartal Care: High-Risk Delivery, a Nursing Interventions Classification defined as assisting vaginal birth of multiple or malpositioned fetuses.

intrapartal period, the period spanning labor and birth.

intrapartum /-pär'təm/, pertaining to the period of labor and birth.

intrapartum hemorrhage, copious bleeding, usually caused by abruptio placentae or placenta previa during labor.

intraperiosteal fracture /in'trəper'ē·os'-tē·əl/ [L, *intra* + Gk, *peri*, around, *osteon*, bone], a fracture that does not rupture the periosteum.

intrapleural space /-ploor'əl/ [L, *intra*, within; Gk, *pleura*, rib; L, *spatium*], pertaining to the cavity of the pleura.

intrapsychic conflict /-sī'kik/ [L, *intra* + Gk, *psyche*, mind], an emotional clash of opposing impulses within oneself.

intrapulmonary /-pul'məner'ē/ [L, *intra*, within, *pulma*, lung], pertaining to the interior of the lungs.

intrapulmonary shunt [L, *intra* + *pulmoneus*, relating to the lung], (in respiratory therapy) a condition of perfusion without ventilation, expressed as a ratio of QS/QT, with QS reflecting the difference between end capillary oxygen content and mixed venous oxygen content and QT representing cardiac output. The condition may occur in atelectasis, pneumonia, pulmonary edema, and adult respiratory distress syndrome.

intrarenal hemodynamics /-rē'nəl/ [L, *intra* + *ren*, kidney], the pattern of blood flow or distribution in the various parts of the kidney. Normally the renal cortex and outer medulla receive the major part of renal blood flow.

intraspinal hypodermic /-spī'nəl/ [L, *intra*, within, *spina*, spine, *hypo*, under, *derma*, skin], pertaining to the injection of a substance into the spinal canal.

intrathecal /in'trathē'kəl/ [L, *intra* + *theca*, sheath], pertaining to a structure, process, or substance within a sheath, such as within the spinal canal.

intrathecal injection, the introduction of a hypodermic needle into the subarachnoid space for the purpose of instilling a material for diffusion throughout the spinal fluid.

intrathoracic goiter /-thôras′ik/ [L, *intra* + Gk, *thorax*, chest; L, *guttur*, throat], an enlargement of the thyroid gland that protrudes into the thoracic cavity.

intrauterine /in′trayoo̅′tərin/ [L, *intra*, within, *uterus*, womb], pertaining to the inside of the uterus.

intrauterine device (IUD) [L, *intra* + *uterus*, womb; Fr, *devise*], a contraceptive device. It consists of a bent strip of radiopaque plastic with a fine monofilament tail.

intrauterine fracture, a fracture that occurs during fetal life.

intrauterine growth curve, a line on a standardized graph representing the mean weight for gestational age through pregnancy to term.

intrauterine growth retardation, an abnormal process in which the development and maturation of the fetus are impeded or delayed more than two deviations below the mean for gestational age, sex, and ethnicity. It may be caused by genetic factors, maternal disease, or fetal malnutrition that results from placental insufficiency.

intravascular /-vas′kyələr/ [L, *intra* + *vasculum*, little vessel], pertaining to the inside of a blood vessel.

intravascular coagulation test [L, *intra* + *vasculum*, little vessel], a test for detecting internal coagulation of blood.

intravenous (IV) /-vē′nəs/ [L, *intra* + *vena*, vein], pertaining to the inside of a vein, as of a thrombus or an injection, infusion, or catheter.

intravenous bolus, a relatively large dose of medication administered into a vein in a short period, usually within 1 to 30 minutes. The intravenous bolus is commonly used when rapid administration of a medication is needed such as in an emergency; when drugs that cannot be diluted, such as many cancer chemotherapeutic drugs, are administered; and when the therapeutic purpose is to achieve a peak drug level in the bloodstream of the patient.

intravenous catheter [L, *intra*, within, *vena*, vein; Gk, *katheter*, a thing inserted], a catheter that is inserted into a vein for supplying medications or nutrients directly into the bloodstream or for diagnostic purposes such as studying blood pressure.

intravenous cholangiography (IVC), (in diagnostic radiology) a procedure for outlining the major bile ducts. A radiopaque contrast material is injected intravenously, and serial radiographic films are taken.

intravenous controller, any of several devices that automatically deliver intravenous fluid at selectable flow rates. The controller is commonly equipped with a rate selector, drop sensor, and alarm. When the infusion does not flow at the prescribed rate, the drop alarm emits a visual and an audible signal.

intravenous DSA (IV-DSA), a form of digital subtraction angiography in which radiopaque contrast medium is injected into a vein, rather than an artery, to allow visualization of arteries.

intravenous fat emulsion, a preparation of 10% fat administered into a vein to help maintain the weight of an adult patient or the weight and growth of a younger patient. The intravenous fat emulsion is isotonic and may be administered into a peripheral vein, but it is not mixed with other solutions used in parenteral alimentation.

intravenous feeding, the administration of nutrients through a vein or veins.

intravenous infusion, 1. a solution administered into a vein through an infusion set that includes a plastic or glass vacuum bottle or bag containing the solution and tubing connecting the bottle to a catheter or a needle in the patient's vein. 2. the process of administering a solution intravenously.

intravenous infusion filter, any of the numerous devices used in helping to ensure the purity of an intravenous (IV) solution. IV filters strain the solution to remove such contaminants as dissolved impurities (detergents, proteins, and polysaccharides), extraneous salts, microorganisms, particles, precipitates, and undissolved drug powders. Any such contaminants may complicate the IV therapy and patient recovery. Some filters are built into the primary IV tubing; others must be attached.

intravenous infusion technique, the calculations for determining the delivery rate of intravenous fluid for the individual patient and the necessary spiking of the container and priming of the tubing before venipuncture and administration of the fluid.

intravenous injection, a hypodermic injection into a vein for the purpose of instilling a single dose of medication, injecting a contrast medium, or beginning an intravenous infusion of blood, medication, or a fluid solution such as saline or dextrose in water.

Intravenous (IV) Insertion, a Nursing Interventions Classification defined as insertion of a needle into a peripheral vein for the purpose of administering fluids, blood, or medications.

intravenously, through a vein.

intravenous medication [L, *intra*, within, *vena*, vein, *medicare*, medicine], pharmaceutical delivered directly into the bloodstream via a vein.

intravenous peristaltic pump, any one of several devices for administering intravenous (IV) fluids by exerting pressure on the IV tubing rather than on the fluid itself. Most peristaltic pumps operate with normal IV tubing and deliver fluid at a selectable cubic centimeter per hour rate. An alarm sounds when the infusion does not flow at the prescribed rate.

intravenous piston pump, any of several devices that accurately control the infusion of intravenous (IV) fluids by piston action. Most IV piston pumps can be operated by battery, as well as by electric current, and require special tubing. Some models are portable.

intravenous pump, a pump designed to regulate the rate of flow of a fluid administered through an intravenous catheter.

intravenous pyelography (IVP), a technique in radiology for examining the structures and evaluating the function of the urinary system. A contrast medium is injected intravenously, and serial x-ray films are taken as the medium is cleared from the blood by glomerular filtration. The renal calyces, renal pelvis, ureters, and urinary bladder are all visible on the radiographs.

intravenous syringe pump, any one of several devices that automatically compress a syringe plunger at a controlled rate. Such devices are used with disposable syringes that can deliver blood, medications, or nutrients by intravenous, arterial, or subcutaneous routes. They are often used in the treatment of infants and are especially useful in the care of ambulatory patients.

intravenous team, a group of registered nurses and licensed practical nurses with special training who administer intravenous therapy under the direction of a physician.

intravenous therapy, the administration of fluids or drugs, or both, into the general circulation through a venipuncture.

Intravenous (IV) Therapy, a Nursing Interventions Classification defined as administration and monitoring of intravenous fluids and medications.

intraventricular /-ventrik′yələr/ [L, *intra* + *ventriculus,* little belly], pertaining to the space within a ventricle.

intraventricular block, the altered conduction of the cardiac impulse within the ventricles. The block can occur as a right bundle branch block, a left bundle branch block, or a left anterior or posterior fascicular block. The block is identified on an electrocardiogram when the QRS duration is wider than normal.

intraventricular conduction defect, a delay in conduction of a ventricular impulse within the ventricles.

intraventricular pressure [L, *intra,* within, *ventriculus,* little belly], the pressure of the blood within the ventricles of the heart. It varies with the phase of the cardiac cycle.

intrinsic /intrin′sik/ [L, *intrinsecus,* inside], **1.** denoting a natural or inherent part or quality. **2.** originating from or situated within an organ or tissue.

intrinsic asthma, a nonseasonal, nonallergic form of asthma, which usually first occurs later in life than allergic asthma and tends to be chronic and persistent rather than episodic. Precipitating factors include inhalation of irritating pollutants such as dust particles, smoke, aerosols, strong cooking odors, paint fumes, and other volatile substances.

intrinsic factor, a substance secreted by the gastric mucosa that is essential for the intestinal absorption of cyanocobalamin. A deficiency of intrinsic factor causes pernicious anemia.

intrinsic minus hand deformity, an abnormality that results from interruption of the ulnar and median nerves at the wrist. It causes metacarpophalangeal joint hyperextension and interphalangeal joint flexion.

intrinsic muscles, muscles that are entirely within the body part or segment moved by them, as the tongue muscles.

introitus /intrō′itəs/ [L, *intro,* inside, *ire,* to go], an entrance or orifice to a cavity or a hollow tubular structure of the body, such as the vaginal introitus.

introjection /-jek′shən/ [L, *intro* + *jacere,* to throw], an ego defense mechanism whereby an individual unconsciously incorporates into his own ego structure the qualities of another person.

intromission /-mish′ən/, the insertion of one object into another, such as the introduction of the penis into the vagina.

intron /in′tron/ [L, *intra,* within, *regin,* region], (in molecular genetics) a sequence of base pairs in deoxyribonucleic acid that interrupts the continuity of genetic information.

introspection /-spek′shən/ [L, *introspicere,* to look into], **1.** the act of examining one's own thoughts and emotions by concentrating on the inner self. **2.** a tendency to look inward and view the inner self. **—introspective,** *adj.*

introsusception /-susep′shən/ [L, *intro,* inside, *suscipere,* to receive], the telescoping or invagination of one segment of the digestive tract into another segment, usually a lower segment. The process can cause obstruction and strangulation of the bowel.

introversion /-vur'zhən/ [L, *intro* + *vertere,* to turn], **1.** the tendency to direct one's interests, thoughts, and energies inward or toward things concerned with the self. **2.** the state of being totally or primarily concerned with one's own intrapsychic experience.

introvert /in'trəvurt/ [L, *intro* + *vertere,* to turn], **1.** a person whose interests are directed inward and who is shy, withdrawn, emotionally reserved, and self-absorbed. **2.** to turn inward or to direct one's interests and thoughts toward oneself.

introverted personality /-vur'tid/ [L, *intro,* inside, *vertere,* to turn, *personalis*], a personality that is preoccupied with inner thoughts and fantasies rather than with the outer world of people and things.

intubate /in'tyoobāt/ [L, *in,* within, *tubus,* tube], to catheterize or insert a tube into an organ or body part.

intubation [L, *in,* within, *tubus,* tube, *atio,* process], passage of a tube into a body aperture, specifically the insertion of a breathing tube through the mouth or nose into the trachea to ensure a patent airway for the delivery of anesthetic gases and oxygen or both. **Blind intubation** is the insertion of a breathing tube without the use of a laryngoscope.

intussusception /in'təsəsep'shən/ [L, *intus,* within, *suscipere,* to receive], prolapse of one segment of bowel into the lumen of another segment. This kind of intestinal obstruction may involve segments of the small intestine, the colon, or the terminal ileum and cecum. Intussusception occurs most often in infants and small children and is characterized by abdominal pain, vomiting, and presence of bloody mucus in the stool (currant jelly stool).

inulin /in'yoolin/, a fructose-derived substance used as a diagnostic aid in tests of kidney function, specifically glomerular filtration. It is not metabolized or absorbed by the body but is readily filtered through the kidney.

inulin clearance, a test of the rate of filtration of a starch, inulin, in the glomerulus of the kidney. Inulin is given by mouth, and the glomerular filtration rate can be estimated from the time needed for the inulin to appear in the urine.

inunction /inungk'shən/ [L, *in,* within, *ungere,* to smear], **1.** the rubbing of a drug mixed with an oil or fatty substance into the skin, with absorption of the active ingredient. **2.** any compound so applied.

in utero /inyoo'tərō/, inside the uterus.

invagination /invaj'ənā'shən/ [L, *in,* within, *vagina,* sheath], **1.** a condition

in which one part of a structure telescopes into another, as the intestine during peristalsis. If the invagination is extensive or involves a tumor or polyp, it may cause an intestinal obstruction. **2.** surgery for repair of a hernia by replacement of the contents of the hernial sac in the abdominal cavity. —**invaginate,** *v.*

invariable behavior /inver'ē·əbəl/ [L, *in,* not, *variare,* to vary], behavior that results from physiologic response to a stimulus and is not modified by individual experience, such as a reflex.

invasion /invā'zhən/ [L, *in,* within, *vadere,* to go], the process by which malignant cells move through the basement membrane and gain access to blood vessels and lymphatic channels.

invasion of privacy, (in law) the violation of another person's right to be left alone and free of unwarranted publicity and intrusion.

invasive /invā'siv/ [L, *in,* within, *vadere,* to go], characterized by a tendency to spread, infiltrate, and intrude.

invasive carcinoma, a malignant neoplasm composed of epithelial cells that infiltrate and destroy surrounding tissues.

Invasive Hemodynamic Monitoring, a Nursing Interventions Classification defined as measurement and interpretation of invasive hemodynamic parameters to determine cardiovascular function and regulate therapy as appropriate.

invasive procedure [L, *in* + *vadere,* to go, *procedere,* to proceed], a diagnostic or therapeutic technique that requires entry of a body cavity or interruption of normal body functions. Examples include the Papanicolaou's (Pap) test and colonoscopy.

invasive thermometry, measurement of tissue temperature using probes placed directly into the tissue.

inverse anaphylaxis /invurs', in'vurs/, an exaggerated reaction of hypersensitivity induced by an antibody rather than by an antigen.

inverse I:E ratio, an inspiratory/expiratory ratio in which the duration of inspiration is prolonged relative to time allowed for exhalation. This procedure is sometimes instituted to improve oxygenation.

inverse square law, a law stating that the amount of radiation measured is inversely proportional to the square of the distance between the source and the irradiated surface. For example, a person 2 feet from a patient being treated with radium is exposed to four times more radiation than he or she would be exposed to at 4 feet.

inversion /invur'zhən/ [L, *invertere,* to turn over], **1.** an abnormal condition in which an organ is turned inside out, such as a uterine inversion. **2.** a chromosomal defect in which two or more segments of a chromosome break off and become separated. They rejoin the chromosome in the wrong order.

inversion traction, a positional form of traction for the prevention and treatment of back disorders. Special equipment is used to lengthen the spinal column while the patient is in an inverted position.

invert /in'vurt/ [L, *invertere,* to turn over], to turn something upside down or inside out.

invertebrate /invur'təbrit/, designating a category of animals that lack a vertebral column.

invert sugar [L, *invertere,* to turn over; Gk, *sakcharon*], a mixture of glucose and fructose produced by the hydrolysis of sucrose. The process results in an inversion of optical rotation from dextrorotation of sucrose to levorotation of the mixture.

investigational device exemption (IDE) /inves'tigā'shənəl/ [L, *investigare,* to search for], an agreement through which the federal government permits the testing of new medical devices.

investigational new drug (IND), a drug not yet approved for marketing by the Food and Drug Administration and available only for use in experiments to determine its safety and effectiveness.

invisible differentiation /inviz'ibəl/ [L, *in,* not, *visibilis,* visible, *differentia,* difference], (in embryology) a fixed determination for specialization and diversification that exists in embryonic cells but is not yet visibly apparent.

in vitro /invē'trō/ [L, *in,* within, *vitreus,* glassware], (of a biologic reaction) occurring in laboratory apparatus.

in vitro fertilization (IVF), a method of fertilizing human ova outside the body by collecting the mature ova and placing them in a dish with a sample of spermatozoa. After an incubation period of 48 to 72 hours, the fertilized ova are injected into the uterus through the cervix. The procedure takes from 2 to 3 days.

in vitro susceptibility testing, a laboratory trial of the sensitivity of microorganisms, particularly fungi, to potential therapeutic chemicals.

in vivo /invē'vō/ [L, *in,* within, *vivo,* alive], (of a biologic reaction) occurring in a living organism.

in vivo fertilization, a method of fertilization of an ovum within a fallopian tube of a fertile female donor for transplantation into an infertile recipient.

in vivo tracer study, (in nuclear medicine) a diagnostic procedure in which a series of radiograms of an administered radioactive tracer, as it passes through a compartment in the patient's body, demonstrates normal or abnormal structures or processes.

involucrum /in'vəloo'krəm/, *pl.* **involucra** [L, *involvere,* to wrap up], a sheath or coating, such as that encasing a sequestrum of necrotic bone.

involuntary /invol'ənter'ē/ [L, *in,* not, *voluntas,* will], occurring without conscious control or direction.

involuntary patient, a person admitted to a psychiatric facility against his or her will.

involution /in'vəloo'shən/ [L, *involvere,* to wrap up], **1.** a normal process characterized by a decrease in the size of an organ caused by a decrease in the size of its cells, such as postpartum involution of the uterus. **2.** (in embryology) a developmental process in which a group of cells grows over the rim at the border of the organ or part and, rolling inward, rejoins the organ or part to form a tube.

involutional melancholia, a former term for a state of depression that occurs during the climacteric. It is now treated as a form of a major depressive episode.

inward aggression /in'wərd/ [AS, *inweard*], destructive behavior that is directed against oneself.

iodide /ī'ədīd/ [Gk, *ioeides,* violet], an anion of iodine. Sodium and potassium iodide are the salts most commonly used in medicine.

iodinated ^{125}**I serum albumin** /ī'ədinā'tid/, a sterile buffered isotonic solution containing radioiodinated normal human serum adjusted to provide not more than 1 mCi of radioactivity per milliliter in diagnostic tests of blood volume and cardiac output.

iodine (I) /ī'ədīn/ [Gk, *ioeides,* violet], a nonmetallic element of the halogen group. Its atomic number is 53; its atomic mass (weight) is 126.90. Iodine is an essential micronutrient or trace element; almost 80% of the iodine present in the body is in the thyroid gland, mostly in the form of thyroglobulin. Iodine deficiency can result in goiter or cretinism. Iodine is found in seafood, iodized salt, and some dairy products. It is used as a contrast agent for blood vessels in computed tomography scans. Radioisotopes of iodine are used in radioisotope scanning procedures and in palliative treatment of cancer of the thyroid.

iodine poisoning [Gk, *ioeides,* violet; L, *potio,* drink], toxic effects of ingesting iodine. Symptoms include burning pain in the mouth and esophagus, abdominal pain, vomiting, diarrhea, shock, nephritis, laryngeal edema, and circulatory collapse.

iodism /ī'ədiz'əm/ [Gk, *ioeides* + *ismos,* process], a condition produced by excessive amounts of iodine in the body. It is characterized by increased lacrimation and salivation, rhinitis, weakness, and a typical skin eruption.

iodize /ī'ədīz/ [Gk, *ioeides* + *izein,* to cause], to treat or impregnate with iodine or an iodide.

iodized salt [Gk, *ioeides,* violet; AS, *sealt*], table salt to which potassium or sodium iodide has been added to protect against goiter, particularly in regions where soil and drinking water have low iodine content. The iodides are added to achieve a ratio of approximately 100 ppm.

iodochlorhydroxyquin /ī·ō'dōklôr'hī-drok'səkwin/, an antiamebic and topical antiinfective prescribed in the treatment of eczema, athlete's foot, and other fungal infections.

iododerma /ī·ō'dōdur'mə/ [Gk, *ioeides* + *derma,* skin], a skin rash caused by a hypersensitivity to ingested iodides. The lesions may be acneiform, bullous, or fungating.

iodoform /ī·ō'dəfôrm/ [Gk, *ioeides* + (chloroform)], a topical antiinfective used as an antiseptic.

iodophor /ī·ōdəfôr/ [Gk, *ioeides* + *phoros,* bearer], an antiseptic or disinfectant that combines iodine with another agent such as a detergent.

iodopsin /ī'ōdop'sin/ [Gk, *ioeides* + *optikos,* vision], a photosensitive chemical in the cones of the retina that reacts in association with other chemicals and plays a part in color vision. Iodopsin is more stable when exposed to bright light than rhodopsin, which is found in the rods of the retina.

iodoquinol /ī'ōdō·kwinol/, an amebicide prescribed in the treatment of intestinal amebiasis.

iodotherapy /ī·ō'dōther'əpē, a treatment that uses iodine or an iodide.

ion /ī'ən, ī'on/ [Gk, *ienai,* to go], an atom or group of atoms that has acquired an electrical charge through the gain or loss of an electron or electrons.

ion exchange chromatography, the process of separating and analyzing different substances according to their affinities for chemically stable but very reactive synthetic exchangers, which are composed largely of polystyrene and cellulose. Ion exchange chromatography is often used to separate components of nucleic acids and proteins elaborated by various structures throughout the body.

ionic bonding /ī·on'ik/ [Gk, *ienai* + ME, *band,* to bind], an electrostatic force between ions. Ionic compounds do not form true molecules; in aqueous solution they break down into their hydrated constituent ions.

ionic dissociation, a phenomenon whereby ions in ionic compounds in an aqueous solution are freed from their mutual attractions and distribute themselves uniformly throughout the solvent.

ionic strength, the sum of the concentrations of all ions in a solution multiplied by the square of their charge.

ionization /ī'ənīzā'shən/ [Gk, *ienai* + *izein,* to cause], the process in which a neutral atom or molecule gains or loses electrons and thus acquires a negative or positive electrical charge. Ionization can cause cell death or mutation.

ionization chamber, a small cavity filled with air that has the capability of collecting the ionic charge liberated during irradiation.

ionization constant (K), after establishment of ionic equilibrium, the product of the molar concentration of the ions divided by the molar concentration of the nonionized molecules.

ionize /ī'ənīz/ [Gk, *ienai* + *izein,* to cause], to separate or change into ions.

ionized calcium, the ionized, unbound, noncomplexed fraction of serum calcium that is biologically active.

ionizing energy /ī·nī'zing/, the average energy lost by ionizing radiation in producing an ion pair in a gas.

ionizing radiation, high-energy electromagnetic waves (such as x-rays and gamma rays) and particulate rays (such as alpha particles, beta rays, electrons, neutrons, positrons, protons, and heavy nuclei) that dissociate substances in their paths into ions. High-energy x-rays penetrate deeply, most beta particles penetrate only a few millimeters, and alpha particles penetrate only a fraction of a millimeter, but all produce intense ionization along their tracks.

ionizing radiation injury [Gk, *ion,* going; L, *radiare,* to shine, *injuria*], damage or ill effects suffered by exposure to ionizing radiation, including cellular harm resulting from radiation for diagnostic or therapeutic application. The risk of cell death or injury from radiation depends on the type of tissue cells, the stage of cell division at the time of exposure, the intensity and time span of exposure, and the type of radiation administered.

ion-selective electrode, a potentiometric electrode that develops a potential in the presence of one ion (or class of ions) but not in the presence of a similar concentration of other ions.

iontophoresis /ī·on'tōfôrē·sis/ [Gk, *ion,* going, *pherein,* to carry], the introduction of ions of soluble salts into the tissues by direct current.

iontophoretic pilocarpine test [Gk, *ienai* + *pherein,* to carry], a sweat test used in the diagnosis of cystic fibrosis. Pilocarpine iontophoresis is used to stimulate production of sweat, which is absorbed from the forearm in a previously weighed gauze pad. The sweat sample is then analyzed for concentrations of sodium and chloride electrolytes.

ion transfer, a method of transporting chemicals across a membrane, using an electric current as a driving force.

iota /ī·ō'təl/, I, ι, the ninth letter of the Greek alphabet.

IPA, abbreviation for **independent practice association.**

IPA-Model HMO, a health maintenance organization (HMO) that contracts with an independent practice association (IPA) for physician services. The IPA processes and adjudicates claims. The HMO provides enrollees and hospital contracts.

IPA paradigm shift, an independent practice association that takes on the role of the health maintenance organization and contracts with its participating providers, but is neither a payer nor a provider.

Ipecac /ip'əkak/, an emetic prescribed to cause emesis in certain types of poisoning and drug overdose.

IPOF, abbreviation for **immediate postoperative fit prosthesis.**

ipomea /ipəmē'ə/, a resin prepared from the dried root of *Ipomoea orizabensis,* formerly used as a cathartic.

IPPB (intermittent positive-pressure breathing), a form of assisted or controlled respiration produced by a ventilatory apparatus in which compressed gas is delivered under positive pressure into a person's airways until a preset pressure is reached. Passive exhalation is allowed through a valve, and the cycle begins again as the flow of gas is triggered by inhalation.

IPPB unit, a pressure-cycled ventilator for providing a flow of air into the lungs at a predetermined pressure. As the pressure is attained, the flow is stopped, pressure is released, and the patient exhales.

IPPV, abbreviation for *intermittent positive-pressure ventilation.*

IPSID, abbreviation for **immunoproliferative small intestine disease.**

IPSP, abbreviation for *inhibitory postsynaptic potential.*

IQ, abbreviation for **intelligence quotient.**

Ir, symbol for the element **iridium.**

IRB, abbreviation for **institutional review board.**

Ir g, abbreviation for *immune response function gene.* See **immune response.**

iridectomy /ī'ridek'təmē/ [Gk, *iris,* rainbow, *ektome,* excision], surgical removal of part of the iris of the eye. It is performed most often to restore drainage of the aqueous humor in glaucoma or to remove a foreign body or a malignant tumor.

iridemia /ī'ridē'mə/, hemorrhage from the iris.

iridescence /ir'ides'əns/ [L, *iridescere,* to shine like a rainbow], the property of light interference or ability to break up light waves into colors of the spectrum.

iridium (Ir) /irid'ē·əm/ [Gk, *iris,* rainbow], a silvery-bluish metallic element. Its atomic number is 77; its atomic mass (weight) is 192.22.

iridology /ī'ridol'əjē/ [Gk, *iris,* rainbow, *logos,* science], the science that specializes in relations between disease and the shape, color, and other individual characteristics of the iris.

iridopathy /ī'ridop'əthē/, any disease of the iris.

iridoplegia /ī'ridōplē'jə/ [Gk, *iris,* rainbow, *plege,* stroke], a condition of paralysis of the sphincter muscle of the iris or the dilator muscle or both.

iridotomy /ī'ridot'əmē/ [Gk, *iris* + *temnein,* to cut], a surgical incision into the iris of the eye. It is performed to relieve occlusion of the pupil, to enlarge the pupil in cataract extraction, or to treat postoperative glaucoma.

iris /ī'ris/ [Gk, rainbow], an annular contractile disc suspended in aqueous humor between the cornea and the crystalline lens of the eye enclosing a circular pupil. The periphery of the iris is continuous with the ciliary body and is connected to the cornea by the pectinate ligament. The iris divides the space between the lens and the cornea into an anterior and a posterior chamber. Dark pigment cells under the translucent tissue of the iris are variously arranged in different people to produce different colored irises. —**iridic,** *adj.*

iritis /īrī'tis/ [Gk, *iris* + *itis*], an inflammatory condition of the iris of the eye characterized by pain, lacrimation, photophobia, and, if severe, diminished visual acuity. On ophthalmic examination the eye looks cloudy, the iris bulges, and the pupil is contracted.

iron (Fe) /ī'ərn/ [AS, *iren*], a common metallic element essential for the synthesis of hemoglobin. Its atomic number is 26; its atomic mass (weight) is 55.85. It is used as a hematinic in the form of its salts and complexes.

iron deficiency anemia, a microcytic hypochromic anemia caused by inadequate supplies of iron needed to synthesize hemoglobin, characterized by pallor, fatigue, and weakness. Iron deficiency may be the result of an inadequate dietary supply of iron, poor absorption of iron in the digestive system, or chronic bleeding.

iron dextran, an injectable hematinic prescribed in the treatment of iron deficiency anemia that is not responsive to oral iron therapy.

iron metabolism, a series of processes involved in the entry of iron into the body and its absorption, transport, storage, use in the formation of hemoglobin and other iron compounds, and eventual excretion. Iron normally enters through the epithelium of the intestinal mucosa and is oxidized from ferrous to ferric iron in the process. Once in the blood, iron cycles between the plasma and the reticuloendothelial or erythropoietic system. For hemoglobin synthesis plasma iron is delivered to the normoblast, where it remains up to 4 months, in the hemoglobin molecules of a mature red cell. Senescent red cells then deteriorate and break down. The iron is released from the hemoglobin by the reticuloendothelial system to reenter the transport pool for recycling.

iron poisoning [AS, *iren* + L, *potio,* drink], toxic effects of ingesting iron salts, particularly ferrous sulfate and ferrous chloride. Ferrous sulfate tablets, sometimes mistaken for candy, can cause vomiting, collapse, and liver necrosis. Ferrous chloride, a corrosive substance, causes vomiting, diarrhea, and hemorrhage when taken internally. Iron encephalopathy has resulted from excessive use of iron preparations.

iron-rich food, any nutrient containing a relatively large amount of iron. The best source of dietary iron is liver. Oysters, clams, heart, kidney, lean meat, seafood, and iron-fortified foods are other good sources.

iron salt poisoning, poisoning caused by overdose of ferric or ferrous salt, characterized by vomiting, bloody diarrhea, cyanosis, and gastric and intestinal pain.

iron saturation, the capacity of iron to saturate transferrin, measured in the blood to detect iron excess or deficiency.

iron-storage disease, an abnormal accumulation of iron in the parenchyma of many organs, as in hemosiderosis.

iron transport, the process whereby iron is carried from the intestinal mucosa to sites of use and storage. Iron binds with transferrin and shuttles to storage and utilization sites.

irradiation /irā'dē-ā'shən/ [L, *irradiare,* to beam upon], exposure to any form of radiant energy such as heat, light, or x-ray. Radioactive sources of radiant energy such as x-rays or isotopes of iodine or cobalt are used diagnostically to examine internal body structures. Similar sources of radioactivity in larger amounts are used to destroy microorganisms or tissue cells that have become cancerous. Ultraviolet light is also used to identify certain bacteria and toxic molds. —**irradiate,** *v.*

irrational /irash'ənəl/ [L, *irrationalis,* contrary to reason], pertaining to events, conditions, or behavior that may be considered unreasonable.

irreducible /ir'əd(y)oo'sibəl/ [L, *in,* not, *reducere,* to bring back], unable to be returned to the normal position or condition, as an irreducible hernia.

irregular pulse /ireg'yələr/ [L, *in,* not, *regula,* rule, *pulsare,* to beat], a variation in force or rhythm of impulses in an artery caused by cardiac arrhythmia.

irreversible /ir'əvur'sibəl/ [L, *irrevertere,* to not turn back], pertaining to a situation or condition that cannot be reversed.

irreversible shock, a condition in which shock does not respond to available forms of treatment and in which recovery is impossible as a result of massive cellular damage.

irrigate /ir'igāt/ [L, *irrigare,* to supply water], to flush with a fluid, usually with a slow, steady pressure on a syringe plunger. It may be done to cleanse a wound or to clear tubing.

irrigation /ir'igā'shən/, the process of washing out a body cavity or wounded area with a stream of water or other fluid. It is also used to cleanse a tube or drain inserted into the body such as an indwelling catheter. —**irrigate,** *v.*

irrigator /ir'igā'tər/, an apparatus with a flexible tube for flushing or washing out a body cavity.

irritability /ir'itəbil'itē/ [L, *irritare,* to tease], a condition of abnormal excitability or sensitivity.

irritable bladder /ir'itəbəl/ [L, *irritare,* to tease; AS, *blaedre*], a condition characterized by a nearly constant urge to urinate despite the lack of evidence of a cause such as inflammation or a kidney stone.

irritable bowel syndrome (IBS) [L, *irritare,* to tease; OFr, *boel* + Gk, *syn,* together, *dromos,* course], abnormally increased motility of the small and large intestines, generally associated with emotional stress. Most of those affected are young adults, who complain of diarrhea and occasionally pain in the lower abdomen. The pain is usually relieved by passing flatus or stool. In diagnosing irritable bowel syndrome, other more serious conditions such as dysentery, lactose intolerance, and the inflammatory bowel diseases must be ruled out.

irritant /ir'itənt/ [L, *irritare,* to tease], an agent that produces inflammation or irritation.

irritant poison [L, *irritare,* to tease, *potio,* drink], any of a large number of toxic substances in the environment that can cause pain in the digestive tract, diarrhea, vomiting, abdominal cramps, and urinary tract disorders. Some irritant chemicals are industrial gases such as ammonia, chlorine, phosgene, sulfur dioxide, hydrogen sulfide, and nitrogen dioxide, which may leak into the atmosphere.

irritation fibroma /ir'itā'shən/, a localized peripheral tumorlike enlargement of connective tissue caused by prolonged irritation. It commonly develops on the gingivae or the buccal mucosa.

IRV, abbreviation for **inspiratory reserve volume.**

ischemia /iskē'mē-ə/ [Gk, *ischein,* to hold back, *haima,* blood], a decreased supply of oxygenated blood to a body organ or part. The condition is often marked by pain and organ dysfunction, as in ischemic heart disease. —**ischemic,** *adj.*

ischemic heart disease /iskē'mik/, a pathologic condition of the myocardium caused by lack of oxygen in tissue cells.

ischemic lumbago, a pain in the lower back and buttocks caused by vascular insufficiency, as in occlusion of the abdominal aorta.

ischemic necrosis, death of tissue caused by interruption of its blood supply.

ischemic pain, the unpleasant, often excruciating sensation associated with decreased blood flow caused by mechanical obstruction, constricting orthopedic casts, or insufficient blood flow that results from injury or surgical trauma. Ischemic pain caused by occlusive arterial disease is often severe and may not be relieved, even with narcotics. The individual with peripheral vascular disease may experience ischemic pain only while exercising because the metabolic demands for oxygen cannot be met as a result of occluded blood flow.

ischemic paralysis, loss of motor control in a body area caused by an interruption in the blood supply to the area's muscles or nerves.

ischemic pericarditis [Gk, *ischein,* to hold back, *haima,* blood, *peri,* near, *kardia,* heart, *itis,* inflammation], an inflammation of the pericardium caused by interruption of its blood supply during myocardial infarction.

ischemic stroke, a cerebrovascular disorder caused by deprivation of blood flow to an area of the brain, generally as a result of thrombosis, embolism, or reduced blood pressure.

ischial spines /is'kē-əl/ [Gk, *ischion,* hip joint; L, *spina,* thorn], two relatively sharp posterior bony projections into the pelvic outlet from the ischial bones that form the lower border of the pelvis.

ischial tuberosity [Gk, *ischion,* hip joint; L, *tuber,* swelling], a rounded protuberance of the lower part of the ischium. It forms a bony area on which the human body rests when in a sitting position.

ischium /is'kē-əm/, *pl.* **ischia** [L; Gk, *ischion,* hip joint], one of the three parts of the hip bone, which joins the ilium and the pubis to form the acetabulum. The ischium comprises the dorsal part of the hip bone and is divided into the body of the ischium, which forms the posteroinferior two fifths of the acetabulum, and the ramus, which joins the inferior ramus of the pubis.

ISCLT, abbreviation for *International Society of Clinical Laboratory Technologists.*

ISG, abbreviation for *immune serum globulin.*

ISH, abbreviation for **isolated systolic hypertension.**

Ishihara color test /ish'ēhä'rə/ [Shinobu Ishihara, Japanese ophthalmologist, 1879–1963], a test of color vision that uses a series of plates on which are printed round dots in a variety of colors and patterns. People with normal color vision are able to discern specific numbers or patterns on the plates; the inability to pick out a given number or shape is symptomatic of a specific deficiency in color perception.

Islands of Langerhans /lang'gorhanz/ [L, *insula,* island; Paul Langerhans, German pathologist, 1847–1888], clusters of cells within the pancreas that produce insulin, glucagon, and pancreatic polypeptide. They form the endocrine part of the gland, and their hormonal secretions released into the bloodstream are balanced, important regulators of carbohydrate metabolism.

islet cell antibody (ICA) /i'lit/ [OFr, *islette,* little island], an immunoglobulin that reacts with the cytoplasm of all of the

I

cells of the pancreatic islets. These antibodies occur in about 60% to 70% of newly diagnosed insulin-dependent diabetic patients.

islet cell tumor, any tumor of the islands of Langerhans.

isoagglutination /ī'sō·əgeloo'tinā'shən/ [Gk, *sos,* equal; L, *agglutinate,* to glue], the clumping of erythrocytes by agglutinins from the blood of another individual of the same species.

isoagglutinin /ī'sō·əgeloo'tinning/ [Gk, *sos,* equal; L, *agglutinate,* to glue], an antibody that causes agglutination of erythrocytes in other members of the same species that carry an isoagglutinogen on their erythrocytes.

isoagglutinogen /ī'sō·əglootin'əjən/ [Gk, *sos* + L, *agglutinate,* to glue; Gk, *Geenen,* to produce], an antigen that causes the agglutination of erythrocytes in others of the same species that carry a corresponding isoagglutinin in their serum.

isoantibody /ī'sō·an'tibod'ē/ [Gk, *sos* + *anti,* against; AS, *boding,* body], an antibody to isoantigens found in other members of the same species.

isoantigen /ī'sō·an'tijən/ [Gk, *sos* + *anti,* against; AS, *boding,* body; Gk, *Geenen,* to produce], a substance that interacts with isoantibodies in other members of the same species.

isobar /ī'səbär/ [Gk, *sos* + *barrios,* weight], **1.** a line connecting points of equal pressure on a graph. **2.** (in nuclear medicine) one of a group of nuclides having the same total number of neutrons and protons in the nucleus but so proportioned that their atomic numbers have different values.

isobaric /-bär'ik/ [Gk, *sos,* equal, *barrios,* weight], **1.** pertaining to two substances or solutions of the same specific gravity. **2.** pertaining to two isotopes that have the same mass number but different atomic numbers. **3.** having the same barometric pressure.

isobutyl alcohol /ī'sōbyoo'til/ [Gk, *sos* + *butyrin,* butter, *Hyl,* matter; AR, *alcohol,* essence], a clear, colorless liquid that is miscible with ethyl alcohol or ether.

isocapnic /-kap'ink/, pertaining to a steady level of carbon dioxide in the tissues despite changing levels of ventilation.

isocarboxazid /-kärbok'səzid/, a monoamine oxidase inhibitor prescribed in the treatment of mental depression.

isochromosome /-krō'məsōm/, a chromosome with identical arms on each side of the centromere.

isocrotic, (in chromatography) separation

of a mixture using a single solvent or solvent mixture.

isodose chart /ī'sədōs/ [Gk, *sos* + *doss,* giving, *charta,* paper], (in radiotherapy) a graphic representation of the distribution of radiation in a medium; lines are drawn through points receiving equal doses.

isodynamic law /ī'sōdīnam'ik/, the rule that for energy purposes different foods may replace one another in accordance with their caloric values when burned in a calorimeter.

isoeffect lines /ī'sō·ifekt'/, (in radiotherapy) lines on a graph representing doses of radiation that have tumoricidal effects in normal tissues.

isoelectric /ī'sō·ilek'trik/ [Gk, *sos* + *electron,* amber], pertaining to the electric baseline of an electrocardiogram.

isoelectric focusing, the ordering and concentration of substances according to their isoelectric points.

isoelectric period, a period in physiologic activity, such as nerve conduction or muscle contraction, when there is no variation in electric potential.

isoelectric point, the pH at which a molecule containing two or more ionizable groups is electrically neutral. The average number of positive charges equals the average number of negative charges.

isoenzyme /ī'sō·en'zīm/ [Gk, *sos* + *en,* in, *Syme,* ferment], a chemically distinct form of an enzyme. The various forms are distinguishable in analysis of blood samples, which aids in the diagnosis of disease. Isoenzymes that catalyze the same physiologic reaction may also appear in different forms in different animal species.

isoetharine mesylate /ī'sō·eth'ərēn/, a beta-adrenergic bronchodilator prescribed in the treatment of bronchial asthma, bronchitis, and emphysema.

isoexposure lines /ī'sō·ikspō'zhər/, (in radiology) imaginary lines representing positions of equal exposure to radiation in the area around fluoroscopic equipment.

isoflows /ī'sōflōz/, (in respiratory therapy) a measure of early small airway dysfunction in a patient made by comparing forced expiratory flow rates between air and helium at fixed points in time.

isoflurophate /-floo'rōfāt/, a cholinesterase inhibitor prescribed in the treatment of open-angle glaucoma and esotropia.

isogamete /ī'sōgam'ēt/ [Gk, *sos* + *gamete,* wife], a reproductive cell of the same size and structure as the one with which it unites. **—isogametic,** *adj.*

isogamy /īsog'əmē/ [Gk, *sos* + *gamos,* marriage], sexual reproduction in which there is fusion of gametes of the same size and structure, such as in certain algae, fungi, and Protista. —**isogamous,** *adj.*

isogenesis /-jen'əsis/ [Gk, *sos* + *Geenen,* produce], development from a common origin and according to similar processes. —**isogenetic, isogenic,** *adj.*

isograft /ī'səgraft'/ [Gk, *sos* + *graphion,* stylus], surgical transplantation of histocompatible tissue obtained from genetically identical individuals, such as between a patient and his or her identical twin.

isohydric shift [Gk, *sos* + *hydor,* water; AS, *sciftan,* to divide], the series of reactions in red blood cells in which CO_2 is taken up and oxygen is released without the production of excess hydrogen ions.

isoimmunization /ī'so·im'yənīzā'shən/, the development of antibodies against antigens from the same species (isoantigens), such as the development of anti-Rh antibodies in an Rh-negative person.

isokinetic /-kinet'ik/, pertaining to a concentric or eccentric contraction that occurs at a set speed against a force of maximal resistance produced at all points in the range of motion.

isokinetic exercise [Gk, *sos,* equal, *kinesis,* motion; L, *exercere,* to keep at work], a form of exercise in which maximum force is exerted by a muscle at each point throughout the active range of motion as the muscle contracts. The effort of the patient to resist the movement is measured.

isolate /ī'səlāt/ [It, *isolare,* to detach], **1.** to separate a pure chemical substance from contamination by foreign matter. **2.** to derive from any source a pure culture of a microorganism. **3.** to prevent an individual from having contact with the rest of a population.

isolated systolic hypertension (ISH), a type of hypertension in which only the systolic blood pressure is elevated. This condition increases the risk of stroke or heart attack.

isolation /-lā'shən/ [L, *insula,* island], the separation of a seriously ill patient from others to prevent the spread of an infection or to protect the patient from irritating environmental factors.

isolation incubator, an incubator bed regularly maintained for premature or other infants who require isolation.

isolation ward [It, *isolare,* to detach; ME, *warden*], a room or section of a hospital in which certain categories of patients, particularly those infected with acute contagious diseases, can be treated with a minimum of contact with the rest of the patients and hospital personnel.

Isolette, trademark for a self-contained incubator unit that provides a controlled heat, humidity, and oxygen microenvironment for the isolation and care of premature and low–birth weight neonates.

isoleucine (Ile) /ī'səlo͞o'sēn/ [Gk, *sos* + *leukos,* white], an amino acid that occurs in most dietary proteins and is essential for proper growth in infants and for nitrogen balance in adults.

isologous graft /īsol'əgəs/ [Gk, *sos,* equal, *logos,* relation, *graphion,* stylus], a tissue transplant between two individuals who are genetically identical, as identical twins.

isomeric /-mer'ik/ [Gk, *sos,* equal, *meros,* part], pertaining to a chemical phenomenon in which two compounds of the same proportion of elements and molecular mass (weight) may differ in chemical and physical properties. The difference is the result of the arrangement of atoms in the respective molecules, either the connections between the atoms or their arrangements in three-dimensional space.

isomers /ī'səmərz/, molecules that have the same molecular mass (weight) and formula but different structures, resulting in different properties.

isometheptene hydrochloride /-məthep'-tēn/, an antispasmodic and vasoconstrictor drug that is a component in some fixed-combination drugs used to treat migraine.

isometric /ī'səmet'rik/ [Gk, *sos* + *metron,* measure], maintaining the same length or dimension.

isometric contraction [Gk, *sos,* equal, *metron,* measure; L, *contractio,* a drawing together], muscular contraction not accompanied by movement of the joint. The muscle is neither lengthened nor shortened, but tension changes can be measured.

isometric exercise, a form of active exercise that increases muscle tension by applying pressure against stable resistance. This exercise may be accomplished by imposing different muscles in the same individual, such as by making a limb push or pull against an immovable object. There is no joint movement, and the length of the muscle remains unchanged.

isometric growth, an increase in size of different organs or parts of an organism at the same rate.

isoniazid /ī'sənī'əzide/, a tuberculostatic antibacterial prescribed in the treatment of tuberculosis caused by mycobacteria sensitive to the drug.

isoosmotic solution /ī'sō·osmot'ik/ [Gk, *sos,* equal; L, *solutus,* dissolved], a solution with electrolytes that will exert the same osmotic pressure as another solution.

isophane insulin suspension /ī′səfān/ [Gk, *sos* + *phanein*, to show; L, *insula*, island; *suspendere*, to hang up], a modified form of protamine zinc insulin suspension. It is an intermediate-acting insulin that is a stable, commonly prescribed preparation.

isophosphamide /-fos′fəmīd/, an antineoplastic that is a derivative of cyclophosphamide; its use is similar to that of cyclophosphamide.

isopropamide iodide /-prō′pəmīd/, an anticholinergic prescribed as an adjunct to ulcer therapy.

isopropyl alcohol /ī′sōprō′pil/, a clear, colorless bitter aromatic liquid that is miscible with water, ether, chloroform, and ethyl alcohol.

isoproterenol hydrochloride /ī′sōprəter′-ənol/, a beta-adrenergic stimulant used as a bronchodilator and cardiac stimulant.

isosorbide dinitrate /-sôr′bīd/, an antianginal agent prescribed as a coronary vasodilator in the treatment of angina pectoris and congestive heart failure.

isotachophoresis /-tak′ōfôrē′sis/ [Gk, *sos* + *tachos*, speed, *pherein*, to bear], the ordering and concentration of substances of intermediate effective mobilities between an ion of high effective mobility and one of much lower effective mobility, followed by their migration at a uniform speed.

isothermal /-thur′məl/ [Gk, *sos*, equal, *therme*, heat], having the same temperature.

isotones /ī′sətōnz′/, atoms that have the same number of neutrons but different numbers of protons.

isotonic /ī′sətōn′ik/ [Gk, *sos* + *tonikos*, stretching], (of a solution) having the same concentration of solute particles as another solution, hence exerting the same amount of osmotic pressure as that solution.

isotonic exercise, a form of active exercise in which the muscle contracts and causes movement. Throughout the procedure there is no significant change in the resistance, so that the force of the contraction remains constant.

isotonicity law /ī′sətonis′itē/, a law that describes a state of equal osmotic pressure in extracellular body fluids that results from equal concentrations of electrolytes and other solute particles in the fluid.

isotonic solutions [Gk, *sos*, equal, *tonos*, tone, *solutus*, dissolved], solutions exerting equal osmotic pressures.

isotope /ī′sətōp/ [Gk, *sos* + *topos*, place], one of two or more forms of a chemical element having almost identical properties:

they have the same number of protons in the atomic nucleus and the same atomic number, but they differ in the number of their neutrons and atomic mass (weights). Many hundreds of radioactive isotopes are used in diagnostic and therapeutic procedures.

isotopic tracer /ī′sətop′ik/ [Gk, *sos* + *topos*, place; Fr, *tracer*, to track], an isotope or artificial mixture of isotopes of an element incorporated into a sample to permit observation of the course of the element, alone or in combination, through a chemical, physical, or biologic process. The observations may be made by measuring the radioactivity or the abundance of the isotope.

isotretinoin /-trətin′ō·in/, an antiacne agent prescribed for cystic acne.

isotype /ī′sətīp/, an antigenic determinant that occurs in all members of a subclass of an immunoglobulin class. An antigenic determinant that is isotypic in one subclass may appear as an allotypic marker in another class.

isovaleric acid /-vəler′ik/ [Gk, *sos* + L, *valeriana*, herb, *acidus*, sour], a fatty acid with a pungent taste and disagreeable odor that is found in valerian and other plant products, as well as in cheese. It also occurs as a metabolite of the amino acid leucine and is found in the sweat of feet and in urine of patients with smallpox, hepatitis, and typhus.

isovolume pressure-flow curve /-vol′-yəm/, a curve on a graph describing the relationship of driving pressure to the resulting volumetric flow rate in the airways at any given lung inflation.

isovolumic contraction /-vəlōō′mik/ [Gk, *sos* + L, *volumen*, paper roll, *contractio*, drawing together], (in cardiology) an early phase of systole in which the left ventricle is generating enough tension to overcome the resistance of the aortic end-diastolic pressure.

isoxsuprine hydrochloride /īsok′səprēn/, a peripheral vasodilator prescribed for the symptomatic relief of cerebrovascular insufficiency and improvement of circulation in arteriosclerosis, Raynaud's disease, and Buerger's disease.

ISS, abbreviation for **injury severity score.**

isthmus /is′məs/, *pl.* **isthmuses, isthmi** [Gk, *isthmos,* a narrow, connection, passage, or constriction], a narrow connection between two larger bodies or parts, such as the isthmus of the thyroid.

isthmus of thyroid [Gk, *isthmos* + *thyreos* + *eidos,* form], a part of the thyroid gland, anterior to the trachea, which joins the two lateral lobes of the gland.

IT, abbreviation for **immunotoxin.**

itch [AS, *giccan*], **1.** to feel a sensation, usually on the skin, that makes one want to scratch. **2.** a tingling, annoying sensation on an area of the skin that makes one want to scratch it. **3.** the pruritic condition of the skin caused by infestation with the parasitic mite *Sarcoptes scabiei.* —**itchy,** *adj.*

itch mite [AS, *giccan* + *mite*], a tiny eight-legged insect with piercing and sucking mouth parts. At least three genera of itch mites are recognized: *Chorioptes, Notoëdres,* and *Sarcoptes.*

ITP, abbreviation for **idiopathic thrombocytopenic purpura.**

IU, I.U., abbreviation for **International Unit.**

IUD, abbreviation for **intrauterine device.**

IUPC, abbreviation for *intrauterine pressure catheter.*

IV, 1. abbreviation for **intravenous** or **intravenously. 2.** *informal.* equipment consisting of a bottle or bag of fluid, infusion set with tubing, and intravenous catheter, used in intravenous therapy. **3.** intravenous administration of fluids or medication by injection into a vein.

IVAC pump, trademark for a portable intravenous (IV) pump that electronically regulates and monitors the flow of intravenous fluid. It is usually attached to the IV stand.

IVC, abbreviation for **intravenous cholangiography.**

Ivemark syndrome /ĭ′vmärk, ē′vəmr̆k/, a congenital defect in which organs on the left side of the body are a mirror image of their counterparts on the right side.

IVF, abbreviation for **in vitro fertilization.**

IVP, abbreviation for **intravenous pyelography.**

IVT, abbreviation for *intravenous transfusion.*

IV-type traction frame, a metal support that holds traction equipment consisting of two metal uprights, one at each end of the bed, which support an overhead metal bar.

Ivy method [Robert H. Ivy, American surgeon, 1881–1947], a test of bleeding time in which a blood pressure cuff on the upper arm is inflated to 40 mm of mercury and a small wound is made with a scalpel and a template on the volar surface of the arm. Normal adult Ivy bleeding time is from 1 to 9 minutes.

Ixodes /iksō′dēz/ [Gk, sticky], a genus of parasitic hard-shelled ticks associated with the transmission of a variety of arbovirus infections, such as Rocky Mountain spotted fever.

ixodiasis /ik′sō·dī′əsis/, **1.** skin lesions created by the bites of ixodid ticks. **2.** any tick-transmitted disease.

ixodid /iksod′id, iksō′did/, pertaining to hard ticks of the family Ixodidae.

J, abbreviation for **joule.**

Jaccoud's dissociated fever /zháko͞oz´/ [Sigismond Jaccoud, French physician, 1830–1913], a form of meningitic fever accompanied by a paradoxic slow pulse rate.

jacket [Fr, *jaquette*], a supportive or confining therapeutic casing or garment for the torso.

jacket restraint, an orthopedic device used to help immobilize the trunk of a patient in traction and to discourage the patient from sitting up in bed. The jacket restraint is attached to both sides of the bedspring frame by means of buckled webbing straps that are sewn into the side seams of the restraint. The jacket restraint may be used with most kinds of traction.

jackknife position /jak´nīf/, an anatomic position in which the patient is placed on the back in a semisitting position, with the shoulders elevated and the thighs flexed at right angles to the abdomen. Examination and instrumentation of the male urethra are facilitated by this position.

Jackson crib, a removable orthodontic appliance retained in position by crib-shaped wires.

Jackson's sign [John H. Jackson, English neurologist, 1835–1911], (in hemiparesis) an observation that during quiet respiration the movement of the paralyzed side of the chest may be greater than that of the opposite side.

Jacquemier's sign /zhákmē-āz´/ [Jean M. Jacquemier, French obstetrician, 1806–1879], a deepening of the color of the vaginal mucosa just below the urethral orifice. It may sometimes be noted after the fourth week of pregnancy.

jactitation /jak´titā´shən/ [L, *jactare,* show off, display], twitchings or spasms of muscles or muscle groups, as observed in the restless body movements of a patient with a severe fever.

JADA, abbreviation for *Journal of the American Dental Association.*

JAMA /já´má, jam´ə, jā´ā´em´ā´/, abbreviation for *Journal of the American Medical Association.*

jamais vu /zhámāvY´, -vē´, -vo͞o´/ [Fr, never seen], the sensation of being a

stranger when with a person one knows or when in a familiar place.

Janeway lesion /jān´wā/ [Edward G. Janeway, American physician, 1841–1911; L, *laedere,* to injure], a small erythematous or hemorrhagic macule on the palms or soles. It is diagnostic of subacute bacterial endocarditis.

janiceps /jan´əseps/ [L, *Janus,* two-faced Roman god, *caput,* head], a conjoined twin fetus in which the heads are fused, with the faces looking in opposite directions.

Japanese encephalitis, a severe epidemic infection of brain tissue seen in East Asia and the South Pacific, including Australia and New Zealand. It is characterized by shaking chills, paralysis, and weight loss and is caused by a group of B arboviruses transmitted by mosquitoes.

JAPHA /jaf´ə, jā´ā´pē´āch´ā´/, abbreviation for *Journal of the American Public Health Association.*

jar, to shake or jolt.

jar, a cylindric vessel.

jargon (jar.) /jár´gən/ [Fr, **jargonner,** to speak indistinctly], **1.** incoherent speech or gibberish. **2.** a language used by scientists, artists, or others of a professional subculture that is not understood by the general population.

jargon aphasia [Fr, *jargonner* + Gk, *a* + *phasis,* speech], a form of speech in which several words are combined in a single word but in a jumbled manner with incorrect accents or words mixed with neologisms. Although outwardly incomprehensible, the speech may be meaningful when analyzed by a psychotherapist.

Jarisch-Herxheimer reaction /já´-risherks´hīmər/ [Adolph Jarisch, Austrian dermatologist, 1850–1902; Karl Herxheimer, German dermatologist, 1861–1944], an acute febrile reaction that may follow therapy for syphilis. It is often accompanied by headache and myalgia and is more common in patients with early syphilis.

Jarotzky's treatment /jərot´skēz/ [Alexander Jarotsky, Russian physician, b. 1866], therapy of gastric ulcer using a bland diet consisting of egg whites, fresh butter, bread, milk, and noodles.

Jarvik-7 [Robert K. Jarvik, American cardiologist, b. 1946], an artificial heart designed by R. K. Jarvik for use in humans. The Jarvik-7 was an early model that depended on air pressure to drive the ventricles.

jaundice /jôn′dis, ján′dis/ [Fr, *jaune*, yellow], a yellow discoloration of the skin, mucous membranes, and sclerae of the eyes, caused by greater than normal amounts of bilirubin in the blood. Persons with jaundice may experience nausea, vomiting, and abdominal pain and may pass dark urine and clay-colored stools. Jaundice is a symptom of many disorders, including liver diseases, biliary obstruction, and the hemolytic anemias. Physiologic jaundice commonly develops in newborns and disappears after a few days. —**jaundiced,** *adj.*

jaw [AS, *ceowan*, to chew], a common term used to describe the maxillae and the mandible and the soft tissue that covers these structures.

jaw reflex, an abnormal reflex elicited by tapping the chin with a rubber hammer while the mouth is half open and the jaw muscles are relaxed. A quick snapping shut of the jaw implies damage to the area of cerebral cortex governing motor activity of the fifth cranial nerve.

jaw relation, any relation of the mandible to the maxilla.

jaw-winking, an involuntary facial movement phenomenon in which the eyelid droops, usually on one side of the face, when the jaw is closed but raises when the jaw is opened or when the jaw is moved from side to side.

JCAHO, abbreviation for **Joint Commission on Accreditation of Health Care Organizations.**

J chain, the part of the immunoglobulin M(IgM) molecule that may hold the structure together, thus "joining chain."

J/deg, abbreviation for *joules per degree.*

Jefferson fracture, a fracture characterized by bursting of the ring of the atlas.

jejunal feeding tube, a hollow tube inserted into the jejunum through the abdominal wall for administration of liquefied foods.

jejunectomy /jij′ōōnek′təmē/, the surgical removal of all or part of the jejunum.

jejunocolostomy /jijōō′nōkələs′təmē/, the surgical creation of an anastomosis between the jejunum and colon.

jejunostomy /jijōō′ōnos′təmē/, a surgical procedure to create an artificial opening to the jejunum through the abdominal wall. It may be a permanent or a temporary opening.

jejunotomy /jij′ōōnot′əmē/, a surgical incision in the jejunum.

jejunum /jijōō′nəm/, *pl.* **jejuna** [L, *jejunus,* empty], the intermediate or middle of the three parts of the small intestine, connecting proximally with the duodenum and distally with the ileum. —**jejunal,** *adj.*

jelly, a semisolid nonliquid colloidal solution.

jellyfish sting [L, *gelare,* to congeal; AS, *fisc + stingan*], a wound caused by skin contact with a jellyfish, a sea animal with a gelatinous body and tentacles containing stinging structures. In most cases a tender, red welt develops on the affected skin. In some cases, depending on the sensitivity of the person and the species of jellyfish, severe localized pain and nausea, weakness, excessive lacrimation, nasal discharge, muscle spasm, perspiration, and dyspnea may occur.

Jendrassik's maneuver /yendrá′shiks/ [Ernst Jendrassik, Hungarian physician, 1858–1921; Fr, *manoeuvre,* action], (in neurology) a diagnostic procedure in which the patient hooks the flexed fingers of the two hands together and forcibly tries to pull them apart. While this tension is being exerted, the lower extremity reflexes, particularly the patellar reflex, are tested.

jerk, 1. a sudden abrupt motion such as a thrust, yank, push, or pull. **2.** a quick muscular contraction induced when a tendon over a bone is tapped.

jerk nystagmus, a slow drift of the eyes in one direction, followed by a rapid recovery movement in the other direction.

jerks, a form of choromania, or morbid desire to make rhythmic movements, sometimes associated with emotional fervor.

jet humidifier, a humidifier that increases the surface area for exposure of water to gas by breaking the water into small aerosol droplets. Gas issuing from the unit has a maximum amount of water vapor and a minimum of liquid water particles.

jet lag [L, *jacere,* to throw; Scand, *lagga,* to fall behind], a condition characterized by fatigue, insomnia, and sluggish body functions caused by disruption of the normal circadian rhythm resulting from rapid travel across several time zones.

jet nebulizer [L, *nebula,* mist], a humidifier that uses the Bernoulli effect to convert a source of liquid into a fine mist of aerosol particles.

Jeune's syndrome /zhœnz, zhōōnz/ [Mathis Jeune, French pediatrician, b. 1910], a form of lethal short-limbed dwarfism characterized by constriction of the upper thorax and occasionally by polydactylism.

It is inherited as an autosomal-recessive trait.

jimson weed /jim′sən/, a common name for *Datura stramonium,* a poisonous plant with large, trumpet-shaped flowers. Its chief components are the anticholinergics hyoscyamine and scopolamine.

jitters, 1. irregularities in ultrasound echo locations caused by mechanical or electronic disturbances. **2.** a very uneasy, nervous feeling.

J/kg, abbreviation for *joules per kilogram.*

Jobst garment, trademark for a type of pressure wrap applied to control hypertrophic scar formation.

JOD. abbreviation for *juvenile-onset diabetes.*

Jod-Basedow phenomenon /jod′bá′zədō′/ [Ger, *Jod,* iodine; Karl A. von Basedow, German physician, 1799–1854], thyrotoxicosis occurring when dietary iodine is given to a patient with endemic goiter in an area of environmental iodine deficiency. It is presumed that iodine deficiency protects some patients with endemic goiter from development of thyrotoxicosis.

Joffroy's reflex /zhôfrô-äz′, jof′roiz/ [Alexis Joffroy, French physician, 1844–1908], a reflex contraction of the gluteus muscles produced when firm pressure is applied to the buttocks of patients with spastic paralysis or the lower limbs.

Joffroy's sign [Alexis Joffroy], **1.** an upward direction of a patient's gaze, caused by the absence of facial muscle contraction in ophthalmic goiter. **2.** an inability to perform simple mathematic exercises such as addition or multiplication, caused by an organic brain disease.

jogger's heel [ME, *joggen,* to shake; AS, *hela,* heel], a painful condition, common among joggers and distance runners. It is characterized by bruising, bursitis, fasciitis, or calcaneal spurs that result from repetitive and forceful strikes of the heel on the ground.

Johnson, Dorothy E., a nursing theorist who developed a Behavioral Systems Model presented in *Conceptual Models for Nursing Practice* (Riehl and Roy, eds., 1973). Johnson's theory addresses two major components: the patient and nursing. The patient is a behavioral system with seven interrelated subsystems. Each subsystem has structural and functional requirements. Johnson considered that problems in nursing are caused by disturbances in the structure or functions of the subsystems or the system. Her behavioral systems theory provides a conceptual framework for nursing education, practice, and research.

Johnson's method, (in dentistry) a technique for filling root canals, in which gutta-percha cones are dissolved in a chloroform-rosin solution in the root canal to form a plastic mass.

joint [L, *jungere,* to join], any one of the connections between bones. Each is classified according to structure and movability as fibrous, cartilaginous, or synovial. Fibrous joints are immovable, cartilaginous joints are slightly movable, and synovial joints are freely movable. Typical immovable joints are those connecting most of the bones of the skull with a sutural ligament. Typical slightly movable joints are those connecting the vertebrae and the pubic bones.

joint and several liability, (in law) a condition in which several persons share the liability for a plaintiff's injury and may be found liable individually or as a group.

joint appointment, 1. a faculty appointment to two institutions within a university or system, as to the schools of nursing and medicine of the same university. **2.** (in academic nursing) the appointment of a member of the faculty of a university to a clinical service of an associated service institution.

joint capsule [L, *jungere,* to join, *capsula,* little box], a fibrous connective tissue envelope surrounding a joint.

joint chondroma, a cartilaginous mass that develops in the synovial membrane of a joint.

Joint Commission on Accreditation of Health Care Organizations (JCAHO), a private nongovernmental agency that establishes guidelines for the operation of hospitals and other health care facilities, conducts accreditation programs and surveys, and encourages the attainment of high standards of institutional medical care in the United States.

joint conference committee, a hospital organization composed of the governing board, administration, and medical staff representatives whose purpose is to facilitate communication between the groups.

joint fracture, a fracture of the articular surfaces of the bony structures of a joint.

joint instability, an abnormal increase in joint mobility.

joint mouse, a small movable calculus in or near a joint, usually a knee.

joint planning, the development by two or more health care providers of a strategic plan to serve the health care needs of an area while sharing clinical or administrative services or data but not assets.

joint practice, 1. the practice of one or more physicians, nurses, and other health professionals, usually private, who work as a team, sharing responsibility for a group of patients. **2.** (in inpatient nursing) the practice of making joint decisions about patient care by committees of the physicians and nurses working on a division.

joint protection, the use of orthotics with therapeutic exercise to prevent damage or deformity of a joint during rehabilitation to restore power and range of motion.

Jones criteria /jōnz/, a standardized set of guidelines for the diagnosis of rheumatic fever, as recommended by the American Heart Association.

joule /jōōl/ [James P. Joule, English physicist, 1818–1889], a unit of energy or work in the meter-kilogram-second system. It is equivalent to 10^7 ergs or 1 watt second.

J-pouch, a fecal reservoir formed surgically by folding over the lower end of the ileum in an ileoanal anastomosis.

JRA, abbreviation for **juvenile rheumatoid arthritis.**

Judd method, (in radiology) a technique for positioning a patient for radiographic examination of the atlas and odontoid process.

judgment /juj′mənt/ [L, judicare, to judge], **1.** (in law) the final decision of the court regarding the case before it. **2.** the reason given by the court for its decision; an opinion. **3.** an award, penalty, or other sentence of law given by the court. **4.** (in psychiatry) the ability to recognize the relationships of ideas and to form correct conclusions from those data as well as from those acquired from experience.

judgment call, slang. a decision based on experience, especially a judgment that resolves a serious problem in which the data are inconclusive or equivocal.

jugal /jōō′gəl/ [L, jugum, yoke], pertaining to structures attached or yoked, as the zygomatic bone.

jugular /jug′yələr/ [L, jugulum, neck], **1.** pertaining to or involving the neck. **2.** informal. the jugular vein.

jugular foramen [L, jugulum, neck, foramen, hole], one of a pair of openings between the lateral part of the occipital bone and the petrous part of the temporal bones in the skull.

jugular fossa, a deep depression adjacent to the interior surface of the petrosa of the temporal bone of the skull.

jugular process, a part of the occipital bone that projects laterally from the squamous part. On its anterior border a deep notch forms the posterior and medial boundary of the jugular foramen.

jugular pulse, a pulsation in the jugular vein caused by conditions that inhibit diastolic filling of the right side of the heart.

jugular venous pressure (JVP), blood pressure in the **jugular vein,** which reflects the volume and pressure of venous blood. With elevated JVP the neck veins may be distended as high as the angle of the jaw.

jugum /jōō′gəm/ [L, yoke], a ridge or furrow joining to structures.

juice /jōōs/ [L, jus, broth], any fluid secreted by the tissues of animals or plants. In humans it usually refers to the secretions of the digestive glands.

jumentous /jōōmen′təs/ [L, jumentum, beast of burden], having a strong animal odor, especially that of a horse. The term is used to describe the odor of urine during certain disease conditions.

jumping gene, (in molecular genetics) a unit of genetic information associated with a segment of deoxyribonucleic acid that can move from one position in the genome to another.

junction /jungk′shən/ [L, jungere, to join], an interface or meeting place for tissues or structures.

junctional bigeminy /jungk′shənəl/ [L, jungere, to join, bis, twice, geminus, twin], cardiac arrhythmia in which each sinus beat is precisely linked to a junctional beat.

junctional epithelium [L, jungere, to join; Gk, epi + thele, nipple], an area of epithelial soft tissue surrounding the abutment post of a tooth.

junctional extrasystole [L, jungere, to join, extra, beyond; Gk, systole, contraction], a premature beat that usually arises from the nodal-His region, the primary junctional pacing site, but may also arise from within the bundle of His.

junctional rhythm, a cardiac rhythm usually originating in the nodal-His region. It may be a normal escape rhythm (rate less than 60 beats/min) or an active focus (rate 60 beats/min or more.)

junctional tachycardia, a nonparoxysmal (gradual onset) cardiac rhythm emanating from the nodal-His region with a rate faster than the inherent rate of the atrioventricular junction (a rate of more than 60 beats/min).

junction lines, (in radiology) vertical lines that appear in the mediastinum on a posterior-anterior (P-A) projection radiographic image.

junction nevus [L, jungere, to join, naevus, birthmark], a hairless flat or slightly raised brown skin blemish arising from pigment cells at the epidermal-dermal junction. Malignant change may be signaled by increase in size, hardness or darkening, bleeding, or appearance of satellite discoloration around the nevus.

juncture, a joint or union of two parts.

juniper tar /joo′nipər/ [L, *juniperus* + AS, *teoru*], a dark, oily liquid obtained by the destructive distillation of the wood of *Juniperus oxycedrus* trees. It is used as an antiseptic stimulant in ointments for skin disorders such as psoriasis and eczema.

jurisprudence /joo′risproo′dəns/ [L, *jus*, law, *prudentia*, knowledge], the science and philosophy of law. **Medical jurisprudence** relates to the interfacing of medicine with criminal and civil law.

justice [L, *justus*, sufficient], a principle of fair and equal treatment for all, with due reward and honor.

juvenile /joo′vənəl, -vənīl/ [L, *juvenus*, youthful], **1.** a young person; youth; child; youngster. **2.** pertaining to, characteristic of, or suitable for a young person; youthful. **3.** physiologically underdeveloped or immature. **4.** denoting psychologic or intellectual immaturity; childish.

juvenile alveolar rhabdomyosarcoma, a rapidly growing tumor of striated muscle occurring in children and adolescents, chiefly in the extremities. The prognosis is grave.

juvenile delinquency, persistent antisocial, illegal, or criminal behavior by children or adolescents to the degree that it cannot be controlled or corrected by the parents, it endangers others in the community, and it becomes the concern of a law enforcement agency.

juvenile delinquent, a person who performs illegal acts and who has not reached an age at which treatment as an adult can be accorded under the laws of the community having jurisdiction.

juvenile glaucoma [L, *juvenis,* young man; Gk, *glaukcos,* bluish-gray], increased intraocular tension in a young adult caused by developing structural defects that restrict the outflow of fluid.

juvenile laryngeal respiratory papillomatosis, multiple squamous cell tumors that develop in the larynx, usually in young children. The growths are transmitted by a papilloma virus and may be acquired from the mother.

juvenile myoclonic syndrome, a condition in which myoclonic seizures begin to appear around the time of puberty.

juvenile periodontitis, an abnormal condition that may affect the dental alveoli, especially in the anterior and first molar regions of children and adolescents. It is characterized by severe pocketing and bone loss.

juvenile rheumatoid arthritis (JRA), a form of rheumatoid arthritis, usually affecting the larger joints of children less than 16 years of age and often accompanied by systemic manifestations. As bone growth in children is dependent on the epiphyseal plates of the distal epiphyses, skeletal development may be impaired if these structures are damaged.

juvenile spinal muscular atrophy, a disorder beginning in childhood in which progressive degeneration of anterior horn and medullary nerve cells leads to skeletal muscle wasting. The condition usually begins in the legs and pelvis.

juvenile xanthogranuloma, a skin disorder characterized by groups of yellow, red, or brown papules or nodules on the extensor surfaces of the arms and legs, and in some cases on the eyeball, meninges, and testes. The lesions typically appear in infancy or early childhood and usually disappear in a few years.

juxtaarticular /juk′stə·ártik′yələr/ [L, *juxta,* near, *articulus,* joint], pertaining to a location near a joint.

juxtacrine /juks′təkrin/, describing a hormonal relationship in which the secretory cell is adjacent to an effector cell.

juxtaglomerular /-glōmer′ələr/ [L, *juxta,* near, *glomerulus,* small ball], pertaining to an area between the afferent and efferent arterioles of the kidney glomerulus.

juxtaglomerular apparatus, a collection of cells located beside each renal glomerulus. It is involved in the secretion of renin in response to blood pressure changes and is important in autoregulation of certain kidney functions.

juxtaglomerular cells [L, *juxta,* near, *glomerulus,* small ball, *cella,* storeroom], smooth muscle cells lining the glomerular end of the afferent arterioles in the kidney that are in opposition to the macula densa region of the early distal tubule. These cells synthesize and store renin.

juxtamedullary /-med′əler′ē/, near the border of a medulla.

juxtaposition /-pəzish′ən/, the placement of objects side by side or end to end.

JVP, abbreviation for **jugular venous pressure.**

K

k, abbreviation for **kilo,** 1000, or 10^3.

K, 1. symbol for **ionization constant. 2.** symbol for **Kelvin scale. 3.** symbol for the element **potassium** (kalium). **4.** abbreviation for kilobyte. **5.** symbol in electronics for 1024 (2^{10}). **6.** abbreviation for **katal.**

K_m, symbol for *Michaelis-Menten constant.*

kA, abbreviation for *kiloampere.*

Kahn test [Reuben L. Kahn, American bacteriologist, b. 1887], **1.** one of the older serologic tests for syphilis. The appearance of a white precipitate in a serum sample allowed to stand overnight in a mixture with a sensitized antigen is regarded as a positive reaction. **2.** a test for the presence of cancer by measuring the proportion of albumin A in a blood sample.

kainate /kī'nāt/, a non-NMDA (*N*-methyl-D-aspartate) receptor agonist. The natural mineral is used as a fertilizer.

kala-azar /ká'lə-ȧ·zár'/ [Hindi, *kala,* black; Assamese, *azar,* fever], a disease caused by the protozoan *Leishmania donovani,* transmitted to humans, particularly to children, by the bite of the sand fly. Kala-azar occurs primarily in Asia, parts of Africa, several South and Central American countries, and the Mediterranean region. The liver and spleen are the main sites of infection; signs and symptoms include anemia, hepatomegaly, splenomegaly, irregular fever, and emaciation.

kalak /kal'ak/, a pustular skin disease observed among Eskimos.

kalemia /kəlē'mē·ə/, the presence of potassium in the blood.

kalium (K) /kā'lē·əm/ [Ar, *quali,* potash], potassium.

kaliuresis /kal'iyoorē'sis/, the excretion of potassium in the urine.

kallikrein-kinin system /kalik'rē·in-/, a proposed hormonal system that functions within the kidney, with the enzyme kallikrein in the renal cortex mediating production of bradykinin, which acts as a vasodilator peptide.

Kallmann's syndrome [Franz J. Kallman, American psychiatrist, 1897–1965], a condition characterized by the absence of the sense of smell. It is caused by agenesis of the olfactory bulbs and secondary hypogonadism related to a decrease of luteinizing hormone–releasing hormone.

kanamycin /kan'əmī'sin/, an antibacterial substance derived from *Streptomyces kanamyceticus.*

kanamycin sulfate, an aminoglycoside antibiotic prescribed in the treatment of certain severe infections and those resistant to other antibiotics.

Kangaroo Care, a Nursing Interventions Classification defined as promoting closeness between parent and physiologically stable preterm infant by preparing the parent and providing the environment for skin-to-skin contact.

Kanner's syndrome [Leo Kanner, Austrian-born American child psychiatrist, b. 1894], a form of infantile psychosis with an onset in the first 30 months of life. It is characterized by infantile autism.

kaolin /kā'əlin/ [Chin, *kao-ling,* high ridge], an adsorbent used internally to treat diarrhea, often in combination with pectin. Kaolin in an ointment base is also used topically as an absorbent and a protective emollient.

kaolinosis /kā'əlinō'sis/, a form of pneumoconiosis acquired by inhaling clay dust (kaolin).

Kaposi's disease /kap'əsēz/ [Moritz K. Kaposi, Austrian dermatologist, 1837–1902; L, *dis* + Fr, *aise,* ease], a rare inherited skin disorder that begins in childhood and involves mainly exposed skin areas. Exposure to sunlight results in erythema and vesiculation, followed by increased pigmentation and telangiectasia, skin ulcers, warts, and malignant epitheliomas.

Kaposi's sarcoma (KS, ks) [Moritz K. Kaposi], a malignant, multifocal neoplasm of reticuloendothelial cells that begins as soft brownish or purple papules on the feet and slowly spreads in the skin, metastasizing to the lymph nodes and viscera. It occurs most often in men and is associated with diabetes, malignant lymphoma, acquired immunodeficiency syndrome, or other disorders.

kappa /kap'ə/, K, κ, the tenth letter of the Greek alphabet, used to denote: (in chemistry) the tenth carbon atom in a chain; a type of killer particle present in certain strains of *Paramecium;* and a visual axis angle.

kappa (κ) light chain, one of two kinds of smaller peptide chains present in an immunoglobulin molecule.

karaya powder /kár′áyá/ [Hindi, *karayal,* resin; L, *pulvis,* dust], a dried form of *Sterculia urens* or other species of *Sterculia,* used as a bulk cathartic. Methylcellulose has largely replaced this drug in modern use. Externally it is used as a drying agent for stage I and stage II pressure ulcers.

Kardex, trademark for a card-filing system that allows quick reference to the particular needs of each patient for certain aspects of nursing care.

Kartagener's syndrome /kártag′ənərz/, an inherited disorder characterized by bronchiectasis, chronic paranasal sinusitis, and transposed viscera, usually dextrocardia.

karyocyte /ker′ē·əsīt′/ [Gk, *karyon,* nut, *kytos,* cell], a normoblast, or developing red blood cell with a nucleus condensed into a homogenous staining body. It is normally found in the red bone marrow.

karyogamy /ker′ē·og′əmē/ [Gk, *karyon,* nut, *gamos,* marriage], the fusion of cell nuclei, as in conjugation and zygosis. —**karyogamic,** *adj.*

karyogenesis /ker′ē·ōjen′əsis/ [Gk, *karyon* + *genein,* to produce], the formation and development of the nucleus of a cell. —**karyogenetic,** *adj.*

karyokinesis /ker′ē·ōkinē′sis, -kīnē′sis/ [Gk, *karyon* + *kinesis,* motion], the division of the nucleus and equal distribution of nuclear material during mitosis and meiosis. —**karyokinetic,** *adj.*

karyoklasis /ker′ē·ok′ləsis/ [Gk, *karyon* + *klasis,* breaking], **1.** the disintegration of the cell nucleus or nuclear membrane. **2.** the interruption of mitosis. —**karyoklastic, karyoclastic,** *adj.*

karyology /ker′ē·ol′əjē/ [Gk, *karyon* + *logos,* science], the branch of cytology that concentrates on the study of the cell nucleus, especially the structure and function of the chromosomes. —**karyologic, karyological,** *adj.,* **karyologist,** *n.*

karyolymph /ker′ē·əlimf′/ [Gk, *karyon* + *lympha,* water], the clear, usually nonstaining, fluid substance of the nucleus. It consists primarily of proteinaceous, colloidal material in which the nucleolus, chromatin, linin, and various submicroscopic particles are dispersed. —**karyolymphatic,** *adj.*

karyolysis /ker′ē·ol′isis/ [Gk, *karyon* + *lysis,* loosening], the dissolution of the cell nucleus. It occurs normally, both as a form

of necrobiosis and during the generation of new cells through mitosis and meiosis.

karyolytic /ker′ē·əlit′ik/, **1.** pertaining to karyolysis. **2.** that which causes the destruction of the cell nucleus.

karyomegaly /ker′ē·ōmeg′əlē/ [Gk, *karyon,* nut, *megas,* large], an increase in the nuclear size of tissue cells.

karyomere /ker′ē·əmir′/ [Gk, *karyon* + *meros,* part], **1.** a saclike structure containing an unequal part of the nuclear material after atypical mitosis. **2.** a segment of the chromosome.

karyometry /ker′ē·om′ətrē/, the measurement of the nucleus of a cell. —**karyometric,** *adj.*

karyomit /ker′ē·əmit′/ [Gk, *karyon* + *mitos,* thread], **1.** a single chromatin fibril of the network within the nucleus of a cell. **2.** a chromosome.

karyomitome /ker′ē·om′itōm/ [Gk, *karyon* + *mitos,* thread], the fibrillar chromatin network within the nucleus of a cell.

karyomorphism /-môr′fizəm/ [Gk, *karyon* + *morphe,* form], the shape or form of a cell nucleus, especially that of the leukocyte. —**karyomorphic,** *adj.*

karyon /ker′ē·on/ [Gk, nut], the nucleus of a cell. —**karyontic,** *adj.*

karyophage /ker′ē·ōfāj′/ [Gk, *karyon* + *phagein,* to eat], an intracellular protozoan parasite that destroys the nucleus of the cell it infects. —**karyophagic, karyophagous,** *adj.*

karyopyknosis /-piknō′sis/ [Gk, *karyon* + *pyknos,* thick], the state of a cell in which the nucleus has shrunk and the chromatin has condensed into solid masses. —**karyopyknotic,** *adj.*

karyorrhexis /-rek′sis/ [Gk, *karyon* + *rhexis,* rupture], the fragmentation of chromatin and distribution of it throughout the cytoplasm as a result of nuclear disintegration. —**karyorrhectic,** *adj.*

karyosome /ker′ē·əsōm′/ [Gk, *karyon* + *soma,* body], a dense irregular mass of chromatin filaments in the cell nucleus.

karyospheric /-sfer′ikəl/ [Gk, *karyon* + *sphaira,* ball], **1.** pertaining to a nucleus that is spheric in shape. **2.** such a nucleus.

karyostasis /ker′ē·os′təsis/ [Gk, *karyon* + *stasis,* standing], the resting stage of the nucleus between cell division. —**karyostatic,** *adj.*

karyotheca /-thē′kə/ [Gk, *karyon* + *theke,* sheath], the membrane that encloses a cell nucleus. —**karyothecal,** *adj.*

karyotype /ker′ē·ətīp′/ [Gk, *karyon* + *typos,* mark], **1.** the total morphologic characteristics of the somatic chromosome complement of an individual or species, described in terms of number, form, size, and arrangement within the nucleus, as determined by a microphotograph taken during the metaphase stage of mitosis. **2.** a diagrammatic representation of the chromosome complement of an individual or species, arranged in pairs in descending order of size and according to the position of the centromere. —**karyotypic,** *adj.*

Kasabach method /kas'əbak/, (in radiology) a technique for positioning a patient for radiographic examination of the odontoid process.

Kashin-Bek disease [Nikolai I. Kashin, Russian orthopedist, 1825–1872; E. V. Bek; L, *dis* + Fr, *aise,* ease], a form of osteoarthrosis afflicting mainly children living in China, Korea, and eastern Siberia. It is believed to be caused by eating foods made with wheat contaminated by a fungus, *Fusarium sporotrichiella.*

kat, abbreviation for **katal.**

katadidymus /kat'ədid'əməs/ [Gk, *kata,* down, *didymos,* twin], conjoined twins united in the lower part of the body and separated at the top.

katal (K, kat) /kat'al/ [Gk, *kata,* down], an enzyme unit in moles per second.

Kayser-Fleischer ring /kī'zərflī'shər/ [Bernhard Kayser, German ophthalmologist, 1869–1954; Bruno Fleischer, German ophthalmologist, 1874–1904], a gray-green to red-gold pigmented ring at the outer margin of the cornea, pathognomonic of hepatolenticular degeneration, a rare progressive disease caused by a defect in copper metabolism and transmitted as an autosomal-recessive trait.

Kazanjian's operation /kasan'jē·ənz/ [Varaztad J. Kazanjian, Armenian-born maxillofacial surgeon in U.S., 1879–1974], a surgical procedure for extending the vestibular sulcus to improve the prosthetic foundation of edentulous ridges.

kbp, abbreviation for **kilobase pair.**

kcal, abbreviation for **kilocalorie.**

kCi, abbreviation for **kiloCurie.**

KE, abbreviation for **kinetic energy.**

keel, (in prosthetics) a device in a stored-energy foot prosthesis that bends the foot upward when weight is applied to the toe.

kefir /kef'ər/ [Russ, fermented milk], a slightly effervescent, acidulous beverage prepared from the milk of cows, sheep, or goats through fermentation by kefir grains, which contain yeasts and lactobacilli. It is an important source of the bacteria necessary in the gastrointestinal tract to synthesize vitamin K.

Keith-Wagener-Barker classification system [Norman M. Keith, Canadian physician, b. 1885; Henry P. Wagener, American physician, b. 1890; N. W. Barker, twentieth-century American physician], a method of classifying the degree of hy-pertension in a patient on the basis of retinal changes. The stages are group 1, identified by constriction of the retinal arterioles; group 2, constriction and sclerosis of the retinal arterioles; group 3, characterized by hemorrhages and exudates in addition to group 2 conditions; and group 4, papilledema of the retinal arterioles.

Kellgren's syndrome /kel'grinz/ [Henry Kellgren, Swedish physician, b. 1827], a form of osteoarthritis affecting the proximal and distal interphalangeal joints, the first metatarsophalangeal and carpometacarpal joints, the knees, and the spine.

Kelly clamp [Howard A. Kelly, American gynecologist, 1858–1943; AS, *clam,* to fasten], a curved hemostat without teeth, used primarily in gynecologic procedures for grasping vascular tissue.

Kelly's pad, a horseshoe-shaped inflatable rubber drainage pad used in a bed or on the operating table.

keloid /kē'loid/ [Gk, *kelis,* spot, *eidos,* form], an overgrowth of collagenous scar tissue at the site of a wound of the skin. The new tissue is elevated, rounded, and firm. —**keloidal, cheloidal,** *adj.*

keloid acne [Gk, *kelis,* spot, *eidos* + *form* + *akme,* point], pyoderma in and around the pilosebaceous structures, resulting in keloid scarring. Blacks are highly susceptible.

keloidosis /kē'loidō'sis/ [Gk, *kelis* + *eidos* + *osis,* condition], habitual or multiple formation of keloids.

keloid scar [Gk, *kelis,* spot, *eidos,* form, *eschara,* scab], an overgrowth of tissue in a scar at the site of skin injury, particularly a wound or a surgical incision. The amount of tissue growth is in excess of that necessary to repair the wound and is partially caused by an accumulation of collagen at the site.

kelp [ME, *culp*], **1.** any of the brown seaweed species of *Laminaria* found on the Atlantic coast of Europe. **2.** the ashes of *Laminaria* seaweed burned in a process of extracting iodine and potassium salts.

Kelvin scale (K) [Lord Kelvin (William Thomson), British physicist, 1824–1907], an absolute temperature scale calculated in Celsius units from the point at which molecular activity apparently ceases, −273.15° C. To convert Celsius degrees to Kelvin, add 273.15.

Kennedy classification [Edward Kennedy, American dentist, b. 1883], a method of classifying edentulous conditions and partial dentures, based on the position of the spaces of the missing teeth in relation to the remaining teeth.

kenophobia /kē'nōfō'bē·ə/ [Gk, *kenos,*

empty, *phobos,* fear], the morbid fear of large and open spaces; agoraphobia.

Kent bundle [Albert F. S. Kent, English physiologist, 1863–1958; AS, *byndel,* to bind], an accessory pathway between an atrium and a ventricle outside of the conduction system. This congenital anomaly causes Wolff-Parkinson-White's syndrome.

kerasin /ker′əsin/ [L, *cera,* wax], a cerebroside, found in brain tissue, that consists of a fatty acid, galactose, and sphingosine.

keratectomy /ker′ətek′təmē/ [Gk, *keras,* horn, *ektome,* excision], surgical removal of a part of the cornea performed to excise a small, superficial lesion that does not warrant a corneal graft. Corneal epithelium grows rapidly, filling a small surgical area in about 60 hours.

keratic /kərat′ik/ [Gk, *keras,* horn; L, *icus,* like], 1. pertaining to keratin. 2. pertaining to the cornea.

keratic precipitate, a group of inflammatory cells deposited on the endothelial surface of the cornea after trauma or inflammation, sometimes obscuring vision.

keratin /ker′ətin/ [Gk, *keras,* horn], a fibrous sulfur-containing protein that is the primary component of the epidermis, hair, nails, enamel of the teeth, and horny tissue of animals.

keratin cyst, an epithelial cyst containing keratin.

keratinization /-īzā′shən/ [Gk, *keras* + L, *izein,* to cause], a process by which epithelial cells lose their moisture and are replaced by horny tissue.

keratinize /ker′ətinīz/, to make or become horny tissue.

keratinocyte /kerat′inōsīt′/ [Gk, *keras* + *kytos,* cell], an epidermal cell that synthesizes keratin and other proteins and sterols. These cells constitute 95% of the epidermis, being formed from undifferentiated, or basal, cells at the dermal-epidermal junction.

keratinophilic /kerat′inōfil′ik/, describing a type of fungi that uses keratin as a substrate.

keratitis /ker′ətī′tis/, any inflammation of the cornea. **—keratic,** *adj.*

keratoacanthoma /ker′ətō·ak′antho′mə/ [Gk, *keras* + *akantha,* thorn, *oma,* tumor], a benign, rapidly growing, flesh-colored papule or nodule of the skin with a central plug of keratin. The lesion is most common on the face or the back of the hands and arms.

keratocele /ker′ətōsēl/, a hernia of Descemet's membrane through an ulcer in the outer layers of the cornea.

keratoconjunctivitis /ker′ətokᵊnjungk′-tivī′tis/ [Gk, *keras* + L, *conjunctivus,* connecting; Gk, *itis,* inflammation], inflammation of the cornea and conjunctiva.

keratoconjunctivitis sicca, dryness of the cornea caused by a deficiency of tear secretion in which the corneal surface appears dull and rough and the eye feels gritty and irritated. The condition may be associated with erythema multiforme, Sjögren's syndrome, trachoma, and vitamin A deficiency.

keratoconus /ker′ətōkō′nəs/ [Gk, *keras* + *konos,* cone], a noninflammatory protrusion of the central part of the cornea. It is more common in females and may cause marked astigmatism.

keratocyst /ker′ətōsist/, a thin-walled odontogenic cyst lined by keratinizing epithelium.

keratoderma blennorrhagica /-dur′mə/, the development of hyperkeratotic skin lesions of the palms, soles, and nails. The condition tends to occur in some patients with Reiter's syndrome.

keratodermatitis /-dur′mətī′tis/, an inflammation and proliferation of the cells of the horny layer of the skin.

keratoectasia /ker′ətō·ektäzhə/, a forward bulging or protrusion of the cornea.

keratoepithelioplasty /-ep′ithē′lē·əplas′-tē/, a surgical procedure for the repair of corneal epithelial defects. The defective cornea is removed and replaced with small pieces of donor cornea, which proliferate and replace the original tissue.

keratogenesis /-jen′əsis/, the formation of horny tissue caused by the growth of keratin-producing cells.

keratogenic /jen′ik/, pertaining to an agent that induces a growth of horny tissue.

keratogenous /ker′ətoj′ənəs, pertaining to development of the horny layer of the skin or its growth.

keratoglobus /-glō′bəs/, a congenital anomaly characterized by distension of the eyeball or the anterior segment of the eye.

keratohyalin /-hī′əlin/ [Gk, *keras* + *hyalos,* glass], a substance in the granules found in keratinocytes of the epidermis.

keratoid /ker′ətoid/ [Gk, *keras,* horn, *eidos,* form], resembling horny or corneal tissue.

keratoiritis /ker′ətō·īrī′tis/, an inflammation of the cornea in association with iritis.

keratolysis /ker′ətol′əsis/ [Gk, *keras* + *lysis,* loosening], the loosening and shedding of the outer layer of the skin, which may occur normally by exfoliation or as a congenital condition in which the skin is shed at periodic intervals. **—keratolytic,** *adj.*

keratoma /ker′ətō′mə/, a hard, thick, epidermal growth caused by hypertrophy of the horny layer of the skin. See also **callus.**

keratomalacia /-məlā′shə/ [Gk, *keras* + *malakia*, softness], a condition characterized by xerosis and ulceration of the cornea, resulting from severe vitamin A deficiency. Early symptoms include night blindness; photophobia; swelling and redness of the eyelids; and drying, roughness, pain, and wrinkling of the conjunctiva. In advanced deficiency Bitot's spots appear; the cornea becomes dull, lusterless, and hazy; and without adequate therapy it eventually softens and perforates, resulting in blindness.

keratomycosis /-mīkō′sis/, a fungal disease of the cornea.

keratopathy /ker′ətop′əthē/ [Gk, *keras* + *pathos*, disease], any noninflammatory disease of the cornea.

keratophakia /-fā′kē·ə/, the surgical implantation of donor cornea to the anterior cornea to modify a refractive error.

keratoplasty /ker′ətōplas′tē/ [Gk, *keras* + *plassein*, to mold], an ophthalmologic surgical procedure in which an opaque part of the cornea is excised.

keratosis /ker′ətō′sis/ [Gk, *keras* + *osis*, condition], any skin lesion in which there is overgrowth and thickening of the cornified epithelium. —**keratotic,** *adj.*

keratosis follicularis, a group of several skin disorders characterized by keratotic papules that coalesce to form brown or black crusted, wartlike patches.

kerion /kir′ē·on/ [Gk, honeycomb], an inflamed, boggy granuloma that develops as an immune reaction to a superficial fungus infection, generally in association with *Tinea capitis* of the scalp.

Kerley lines /kur′lē/ [Peter J. Kerley, English radiologist, b. 1900], (in radiology) lines resembling interstitial infiltrate that appear on chest x ray images and are associated with certain disease conditions. They are several centimeters in length and may be oriented in many directions. Kerley lines may occur with congestive heart failure and pleural lymphatic engorgement.

KERMA, abbreviation for *kinetic energy released in material,* a quantity that describes the transfer of energy from a photon to a medium as the ratio of energy transferred per unit mass at each point of interaction.

kernicterus /kərnik′tərəs/ [Ger, *Kern,* kernel; Gk, *ikteros,* jaundice], an abnormal toxic accumulation of bilirubin in central nervous system tissues caused by hyperbilirubinemia.

Kernig's sign /ker′niks/ [Vladimir M. Kernig, Russian physician, 1840–1917],

a diagnostic sign for meningitis marked by a loss of the ability of a supine patient to completely straighten the leg when it is fully flexed at the knee and hip.

kerosene poisoning /ker′əsēn/ [Gk, *keros,* wax; L, *potio,* drink], a toxic condition caused by the ingestion of kerosene or the inhalation of its fumes. Symptoms after ingestion include drowsiness, fever, a rapid heartbeat, tremors, and severe pneumonitis if the fluid is aspirated. Vomiting is not induced.

ketamine hydrochloride /kē′təmēn/, a nonbarbiturate general anesthetic administered parenterally to achieve dissociative anesthesia. Ketamine hydrochloride is a potent somatic analgesic and is particularly useful for brief, minor surgical procedures and for the induction of inhalation anesthesia.

ketoacidosis /-as′idō′sis/ [Gk, *keton,* form of acetone; L, *acidus,* sour, *osis,* condition], acidosis accompanied by an accumulation of ketones in the body, resulting from extensive breakdown of fats because of faulty carbohydrate metabolism. It occurs primarily as a complication of diabetes mellitus and is characterized by a fruity odor of acetone on the breath, mental confusion, dyspnea, nausea, vomiting, dehydration, weight loss, and, if untreated, coma. Emergency treatment includes the administration of insulin and intravenous fluids and the evaluation and correction of electrolyte imbalance. —**ketoacidotic,** *adj.*

ketoaciduria /-as′idŏŏr′ē·ə/ [Gk, *keton* + L, *acidus,* sour; Gk, *ouron,* urine], presence in the urine of excessive amounts of ketone bodies, occurring as a result of uncontrolled diabetes mellitus, starvation, or any other metabolic condition in which fats are rapidly catabolized. **ketoaciduric,** *adj.*

11-ketoandrosterone /-andros′tərōn/, a sex hormone secreted by the testes and adrenal glands that may be measured in the urine to assess hormonal and adrenal functions.

ketoconazole /kō′nəzōl/, an antifungal agent prescribed for the treatment of candidiasis, coccidioidomycosis, histoplasmosis, and other fungal diseases.

11-ketoetiocholanolone /kē′tō·ē′tē·ō-kəlan′əlōn/, a sex hormone secreted by the testes and adrenal glands that may be measured in the urine to assess hormonal and adrenal functions.

ketogenesis /-jen′əsis/ [Fr, *acetone* + Gk, *genein,* to produce], the formation or production of ketone bodies.

ketogenic amino acid /-jen′ik/, an amino

K

acid whose carbon skeleton serves as a precursor for ketone bodies.

ketogenic diet /-jen′ik/, a diet high in fats and low in carbohydrates.

ketone /kē′tōn/ [Fr, *acetone*], an organic chemical compound characterized by having in its structure a carbonyl, or keto, group, =CO, attached to two alkyl groups. It is produced by oxidation of secondary alcohols.

ketone alcohol, [Gk, *keton* + Ar, *alkohl*, essence], an alcohol containing the ketone group.

ketone bodies, the normal metabolic products, beta-hydroxybutyric acid and aminoacetic acid, from which acetone may arise spontaneously. The two acids are products of lipid pyruvate metabolism, via acetyl-CoA in the liver, and are oxidized by the muscles.

ketone group, the chemical carbonyl group with attached hydrocarbons.

ketonemia /kē′tōnē′mē·ə/, the presence of ketones, mainly acetone, in the blood. It is characterized by the fruity breath odor of ketoacidosis.

ketoprofen /-prō′fən/, a nonsteroidal antiinflammatory drug with analgesic and antipyretic actions. It is prescribed for the treatment of rheumatoid and osteoarthritis and related conditions.

ketose /kē′tōs/ [Gk, *keton* + *glykys,* sweet], the chemical form of a monosaccharide in which the carbonyl group is a ketone.

ketosis /kitō′sis/ [Gk, *keton* + *glykys,* sweet, *osis,* condition], the abnormal accumulation of ketones in the body as a result of excessive breakdown of fats caused by a deficiency or inadequate use of carbohydrates. Fatty acids are metabolized instead, and the end products, ketones, begin to accumulate. This condition is seen in starvation, occasionally in pregnancy if the intake of protein and carbohydrates is inadequate, and most frequently in diabetes mellitus. It is characterized by ketonuria, loss of potassium in the urine, and a fruity odor of acetone on the breath. —**ketotic,** *adj.*

17-ketosteroid /-stir′oid/ /kētō′stəroid/, any of the adrenal cortical hormones, or ketosteroids, that has a ketone group attached to its seventeenth carbon atom. They are commonly measured in the blood and urine to aid the diagnoses of Addison's disease; Cushing's syndrome; stress; and endocrine problems associated with precocious puberty, feminization in men, and excessive hair growth.

ketotic /kētot′ik/ [Fr, *acetone*], **1.** pertaining to the presence of ketone in the body. **2.** denoting the presence of a carbonyl group in a chemical compound.

keV, an abbreviation for *kiloelectron volts,* an energy unit equivalent to 1000 electron volts.

key points of control, areas of the body that can be handled by a therapist in a specific manner to change an abnormal pattern, to reduce spasticity throughout the body, and to guide the patient's active movements. The key points are the shoulder and pelvic girdles.

key ridge, the lowest point of the zygomaticomaxillary ridge.

kg, abbreviation for **kilogram.**

kG, abbreviation for *kilogauss.*

kg cal, abbreviation for *kilogram calorie.*

kHz, abbreviation for *kilohertz.*

kidney [ME, *kidnere*], one of a pair of bean-shaped urinary organs in the dorsal part of the abdomen; one is located on each side of the vertebral column between the twelfth thoracic and third lumbar vertebrae. In most individuals the right kidney is slightly lower than the left. Each kidney is about 11 cm long, 6 cm wide, and 2.5 cm thick. The kidneys filter the blood and eliminate wastes in the urine through a complex filtration network and resorption system comprising more than 2 million nephrons. The nephrons are composed of glomeruli and renal tubules that filter blood under high pressure, removing urea, salts, and other soluble wastes from blood plasma and returning the purified filtrate to the blood. More than 1183 L of blood pass through the kidneys every day.

kidney cancer, a malignant neoplasm of the renal parenchyma or renal pelvis. Factors associated with an increased incidence of disease are exposure to aromatic hydrocarbons or tobacco smoke and the use of drugs containing phenacetin. The characteristic symptoms include hematuria, flank pain, fever, and a palpable mass.

kidney disease, any one of a large group of conditions, including infectious, inflammatory, obstructive, vascular, and neoplastic disorders of the kidney. Characteristics of kidney disease are hematuria, persistent proteinuria, pyuria, edema, dysuria, and pain in the flank. Specific symptoms vary with the type of disorder. For example, hematuria with severe, colicky pain suggests obstruction by a kidney stone; hematuria without pain may indicate renal carcinoma; proteinuria is generally a sign of disease in the glomerulus, or filtration unit, of the kidney; pyuria indicates infectious disease; and edema is characteristic of the nephrotic syndrome.

Kielland's rotation /kē′land/ [Christian Kielland, Norwegian obstetrician, 1871–1941], an obstetric operation in which Kielland's forceps are used in turning the head of the fetus from an occiput posterior or occiput transverse position to an occiput anterior position.

Kiesselbach's plexus /kē′səlbákhs′, -báks′/ [Wilhelm Kiesselbach, German laryngologist, 1839–1902], a convergence of small fragile arteries and veins located superficially on the anterosuperior part of the nasal septum.

killed vaccine [ME, *killen* + L, *vaccinus,* of a cow], a vaccine prepared from dead microorganisms. Killed vaccines are generally used to produce immunization from organisms that are too virulent to be used in the living attenuated state. The immune system reacts to the presence of the pathogen in the same manner, whether the organism is live or dead. However, when possible, immunity produced by a live, attenuated vaccine is usually more effective.

killer cell, a small lymphocyte without B or T cell markers. It is the effector cell of antibody-dependent cell-mediated cytotoxicity, recognizes antibodies on target cells, and lyses those cells through a cell-cell interaction that does not require complement.

killer T cells, antigen-stimulated T lymphocytes or cytotoxic T cells that attack foreign antigens directly and destroy cells that bear those antigens.

killer yeast, strains of yeast cells that contain killer plasmid, a toxic protein that destroys other yeast strains.

kilobase (kb), a length of nucleic acid equal to 1000 bases or nucleotides.

kilobase pair (kbp), a length of double-stranded deoxyribonucleic acid or double-stranded ribonucleic acid equal to 1000 purine or pyrimidine base pairs.

kilocalorie (kcal) /-kəl′ərē/ [Gk, *chilioi,* thousand; L, *calor,* heat], a unit of heat equal to 1000 small calories (cal) or 4186 joules

kilogram (kg) /-gram/ /kil′əgram/ [Gk, *chilioi,* thousand; Fr, *gramme*], a unit for the measurement of mass in the metric system. One kilogram is equal to 1000 grams or to 2.2046 pounds avoirdupois.

kilohertz (kHz) /-hurts/ [Gk, *chilioi,* thousand; *hertz,* Heinrich R. Hertz, German physicist, 1857–1894], unit of frequency equal to 1000 (10^3) hertz.

kiloliter (kl) /lē′tər/ [Gk, *chilioi,* thousand; Fr, *litre*], unit of volume equivalent to 1057 quarts, 1000 liters.

kilometer (km) /-mē′tər/ [Gk, *chilioi,* thousand, *metron*], measure equivalent to 1000 meters (about 0.62 miles).

kilovolt (kv) /-volt/ [Gk, *chilioi,* thousand; volt, Count Alessandro Volta, Italian scientist, 1745–1827], measure of electrical potential, 1000 volts.

kilovolt peak (kVp), a measure of the maximum electrical potential in kilovolts across an x-ray tube.

kinanesthesia /kin′anesthē′zhə/, **1.** an inability to perceive the movement or position of one's body parts. The condition is observed as a sign of ataxia. **2.** loss of movement sense.

kinase /kī′nās/ [Gk, *kinesis,* motion; *ase,* enzyme], **1.** an enzyme that catalyzes the transfer of a phosphate group or another high-energy molecular group to an acceptor molecule. **2.** an enzyme that activates a preenzyme (zymogen).

kind firmness, (in psychology) a direct, clear, and confident approach to a patient in which rules and regulations are calmly cited in response to infractions and requests.

kindred /kin′drid/, a group of genetically related individuals.

kinematic face-bow /kin′əmat′ik/, an adjustable caliper-like device used for precisely locating the axis of rotation of a mandible through the sagittal plane.

kinematics /kin′əmat′iks, kī-′/ [Gk, *kinema,* motion], (in physiology) the geometry of the motion of the body without regard to the forces acting to produce the motion. The most common types of motions studied in kinematics are flexion, extension, adduction, abduction, internal rotation, and external rotation. Kinematics is especially important in orthopedics, rehabilitation medicine, and physical therapy.

kinesia /kīnē′zhə/ [Gk, *kinein,* to move], any feeling of nausea caused by the sensation of motion, as in sea sickness or car sickness.

kinesic behavior /kīnē′sik/, nonverbal cues of communication that function to achieve and maintain bonds of attachments between people.

kinesics /kīnē′siks/ [Gk, *kinesis,* motion], the study of body position, posture, movement, and facial expression in relation to communication.

kinesiologic electromyography /kinē′-sē·oloj′ik/, the study of muscle activity involved in body movements.

kinesiology /-ol′əjē/ [Gk, *kinesis* + *logos,* science], the scientific study of muscular activity and the anatomy, physiology, and mechanics of the movement of body parts.

kinesiotherapist, a health professional who uses exercise and movement to rehabilitate patients and who is commonly employed in government hospitals. Kinesiotherapists do not use physical agents.

kinesiotherapy, a specialized area of medicine in which exercise and movement are used as the primary form of rehabilita-

K

tion; typically used in the treatment of amputees.

kinesis /kīnē'sis, kinē'sis/, physical movement or force, particularly when induced by a stimulus.

kinesthesia /kin'esthē'zhə/ [Gk, *kinesis,* motion, *aisthesis,* feeling], the perception of one's own body parts, weight, and movement.

kinesthetic memory /kin'esthet'ik/, the recollection of movement, weight, resistance, and position of the body or parts of the body.

kinesthetic sense [Gk, *kinesis,* motion; L, *sentire,* to feel], an ability to be aware of muscular movement and position. By providing information through receptors about muscles, tendons, joints, and other body parts, the kinesthetic sense helps control and coordinate activities such as walking and talking.

kinetic analysis /kinet'ik/, analysis in which the change of the monitored parameter with time is related to concentration, such as change of absorbance per minute, to determine the rate of a reaction.

kinetic energy (KE) [Gk, *kinesis,* motion, *energeia*], the energy possessed by an object by virtue of its motion. It is expressed by the formula $E = 1/2mv^2$, where *m* represents the mass of the object and *v* is its velocity.

kinetic hallucination [Gk, *kinesis,* motion; L, *allucinari,* wandering mind], a false perception of body movement.

kinetic proofreading, 1. a molecular activity in which an enzyme distinguishes correct substrates. 2. a mechanism that permits a ribosome to make correct codon-anticodon interactions.

kinetic reflex [Gk, *kinesis,* motion; L, *reflectere,* to bend back], a postural response resulting from stimulation of the vestibular apparatus.

kinetics /kinet'iks/ [Gk, *kinesis* + L, *icus,* like], (in physiology) the study of the forces that produce, arrest, or modify the motions of the body. Newton's laws are applicable to the forces produced by muscles of the body that act on joints. The reaction forces of the muscles contribute to the equilibrium and the motion of the body.

kinetoplasm /kīet'ōplaz'əm/, the most highly contractile part of a cell.

kinetotherapeutic bath /kinet'ōthur'-əpyo͞o'tik/ [Gk, *kinesis* + *therapeutike,* medical practice; AS, *baeth*], a bath in which underwater exercises are performed to strengthen weak or partially paralyzed muscles.

King, Imogene, a nursing theorist who introduced her theory of goal attainment in her book, *Toward a Theory of Nursing* (1971). King's conceptual framework specifies three interacting systems: personal system, interpersonal system, and social system. King defined nursing as a process of human interactions between nurse and clients who communicate to set goals and then agree to meet the goals.

kin group, family members who are related genetically or by marriage.

kinin /kī'nin/, any of a group of polypeptides with varying physiologic activity such as contraction of visceral smooth muscle, vascular permeability, and vasodilation.

kinky hair disease [Du, *kink,* short twist; AS, *haer* + L, *dis* + Fr, *aise,* ease], an inherited condition characterized by short, sparse, poorly pigmented hair with shafts that are twisted and broken. Other mental and physical disorders are usually associated with the disease.

kinship model family group, a family unit comprising the biologic parents and their offspring. It is like a nuclear family but more closely tied to an extended family.

Kirkland knife [Olin Kirkland, American periodontist, 1876–1969; AS, *cnif*], a surgical knife with a heart-shaped blade that is sharp on all edges; it is used for a primary gingivectomy incision.

Kirklin staging system, a system for determining the prognosis of colon cancer, based on the extent to which the tumor has penetrated the bowel area.

Kirschner's wire /kursh'nərz/ [Martin Kirschner, German surgeon, 1879–1942; AS, *wir*], a threaded or smooth metallic wire available in three diameters and 22.86 cm long. The wire is used in internal fixation of fractures or for skeletal traction.

Kite method, (in radiology) a technique for positioning the leg of a patient with congenital clubfoot for radiographic examination.

kiting /kī'ting/, *informal.* the improper and illegal practice of altering a drug prescription to indicate that more of a drug was prescribed than was actually ordered by the physician.

KJ, abbreviation for *knee jerk.*

kl, abbreviation for **kiloliter.**

Klebsiella /kleb'zē·el'ə/ [Theodore A. E. Klebs, German bacteriologist, 1834–1913], a genus of diplococcal bacteria that appear as small, plump rods with rounded ends. Several respiratory diseases, including bronchitis, sinusitis, and some forms of pneumonia, are caused by infection by species of *Klebsiella.*

Klebsiella pneumoniae [Theodore A. E. Klebs; Gk, *pneumon,* lung], a species of bacteria found in soil, water, cereal grains, and the intestinal tract of humans and other animals. It is associated with several pathologic conditions, including pneumonia.

Klebs-Loeffler bacillus /klebz'lef'lər/ [Theodore A. E. Klebs; Friederich A. J. Loeffler, German bacteriologist, 1852–1915; L, *bacillum,* small rod], *Corynebacterium diphtheriae.*

Kleine-Levin's syndrome /klīn'lev'in/ [Willi Kleine, twentieth-century German psychiatrist; Max Levin, Russian-born American neurologist, b. 1901], a disorder of unknown cause often associated with psychotic conditions that is characterized by episodic sleep, abnormal hunger, and hyperactivity.

kleptolagnia /klep'tōlag'nē·ə/ [Gk, *kleptein,* to steal; *lagneia,* lust], sexual excitement or gratification produced by stealing.

kleptomania /-mā'nē·ə/ [Gk, *kleptein,* to steal; *mania,* madness], an anxiety disorder characterized by an abnormal, uncontrollable, and recurrent urge to steal. The objects are taken not for their monetary value, immediate need, or utility but because of a symbolic meaning usually associated with some unconscious emotional conflict; they are usually given away, returned surreptitiously, or kept and hidden. —**kleptomaniac,** *n.*

Klinefelter's syndrome /klīn'feltərz/ [Harry F. Klinefelter, American physician, b. 1912], a condition of gonadal defects appearing in males after puberty, with an extra X chromosome in at least one cell line. Characteristics are small firm testes, long legs, gynecomastia, poor social adaptation, subnormal intelligence, chronic pulmonary disease, and varicose veins. The severity of the abnormalities increases with greater numbers of X chromosomes.

Klippel-Feil's syndrome /klipel'fel', klip'-əlfil'/ [Maurice Klippel, French neurologist, 1858–1942; Andre Feil, French neurologist, b. 1884], a condition of short neck and limited neck movements because of congenital fusion of the cervical vertebrae or reduction in the number of cervical vertebrae.

Kloehn cervical extraoral orthodontic appliance, a cervical extraoral traction appliance for correcting or improving malocclusion.

Klumpke's palsy /klŏŏmp'kēz/ [Augusta

Dejerine-Klumpke, French neurologist, 1859–1927], atrophic paralysis of the forearm. It is present at birth and involves the seventh and eighth cervical nerves and the first thoracic nerve. The condition may be accompanied by Horner's syndrome, ptosis, and miosis because of involvement of sympathetic nerves.

km, abbreviation for **kilometer.**

kneading /nē'ding/ [AS, *cnedan*], a grasping, rolling, and pressing movement, as is used in massaging the muscles.

knee /nē/ [AS, *cneow*], a joint complex that connects the thigh with the lower leg. It consists of three condyloid joints, 12 ligaments, 13 bursae, and the patella.

knee-ankle interaction, one of the five major kinetic determinants of gait, which helps to minimize the displacement of the body's center of gravity during the walking cycle. The knee and the foot work simultaneously to lower the body's center of gravity. When the heel of the foot is in contact with the ground, the foot is dorsiflexed, and the knee is fully extended so that the associated limb is at its maximum length with the center of gravity at its lower point.

knee-elbow position [AS, *cneow* + *elboga*], a position in which a patient being examined rests on the knees and elbows with the head supported on the hands.

knee-hip flexion, one of the five major kinetic determinants of gait, which allows the passage of body weight over the supporting extremity during the walking cycle. Knee-hip flexion occurs during the stance and swing phases of the cycle. The knee first locks into extension as the heel of the weight-bearing limb strikes the ground and is unlocked by final flexion and initiation of the swing phase in the walking cycle. Hip flexion is synchronized with these movements, which help to minimize the vertical displacement of the body's center of gravity in the act of walking.

knee joint, the complex, hinged joint at the knee, regarded as three articulations in one, comprising condyloid joints connecting the femur and the tibia and a partly arthrodial joint connecting the patella and the femur. The knee joint and its ligaments permit flexion, extension, and, in certain positions, medial and lateral rotation. It is a common site for sprain and dislocation.

knee replacement, the surgical insertion of a hinged prosthesis performed to relieve pain and restore motion to a knee severely affected by osteoarthritis, rheumatoid arthritis, or trauma.

K

knee sling, a leg support in sling form used under the knee for Russell traction.

knife needle /nīf/ [AS, *cnif* + *Neal*], a slender surgical knife with a needle point, used in the discission of a cataract and other ophthalmic procedures such as goniotomy and goniopuncture.

Knoop hardness test /nōōp/ [Frederick Knoop, twentieth-century American metallurgist], a method of measuring surface hardness by resistance to the penetration of an indenting tool made of diamond.

knot /not/ [AS, *cnotta*], (in surgery) the interlacing of the ends of a ligature or suture so that they remain in place without slipping or becoming detached. The ends of the suture are passed twice around each other before being pulled taut to make a simple surgeon's knot.

knowledge deficit /nol'ij/, a NANDA-accepted nursing diagnosis of an absence or deficiency of cognitive information related to specific topics. The nature of the knowledge is to be specified. The defining characteristics are verbalization of the problem; inaccurate follow-through of instruction; inaccurate performance of test; and inappropriate or exaggerated behaviors, e.g., hysterical, hostile, agitated, apathetic.

Kocher's forceps /kō'kərz/ [Emil T. Kocher, Swiss surgeon, 1841–1917], a kind of surgical forceps that has notched jaws, interlocking teeth, and thick curved or straight powerful handles.

Koch's bacillus /kōks/ [Robert Koch, German bacteriologist, 1843–1910; L, *bacillum*, small rod], the *Mycobacterium tuberculosis* microorganism.

Koch's phenomenon [Robert Koch; Gk, *phainomenon*, anything seen], a tuberculin reaction that occurs when a culture of tubercle bacilli is injected into subjects already infected with the disease. In humans a positive tuberculin reaction indicates sensitization resulting from a tuberculosis infection.

Koch's postulates [Robert Koch; L, *postulare*, to demand], the prerequisites for experimentally establishing that a specific microorganism causes a particular disease. The conditions are the following: (1) the microorganism must be observed in all cases of the disease; (2) the microorganism must be isolated and grown in pure culture; (3) microorganisms from the pure culture, when inoculated into a susceptible animal, must reproduce the disease; (4) and the microorganism must be observed in and recovered from the experimentally diseased animal.

Koebner phenomenon /kōb'nər/ [Heinrich

Koebner, Polish dermatologist, 1838–1904; Gk, *phainomenon*, something observed], the development of isomorphic lesions at the site of an injury occurring in psoriasis, lichen nitidus, lichen planus, and verruca plana.

KOH, chemical formula for **potassium hydroxide.**

koilonychia /koi'lōnik'ē-ə/ [Gk, *koilos*, hollow, *onyx*, nail], spoon nails; a condition in which nails are thin and concave from side to side.

Kopan's needle /kō'pənz/, a long biopsy needle used to locate the position of a breast tumor on x-ray film.

Koplik's spots /kop'liks/ [Henry Koplik, American pediatrician, 1858–1927], small red spots with bluish-white centers on the lingual and buccal mucosa, characteristic of measles. The rash of measles usually erupts a day or two after the appearance of Koplik's spots.

Korányi's sign /kôr'ənyēz/ [Friedrich von Korányi, Hungarian physician, 1828–1913; L, *signum*], a paravertebral area of dullness found posteriorly on the side opposite a pleural effusion.

Korotkoff sounds /kôrot'kôf/ [Nickolai Korotkoff, Russian physician, 1874–1920], sounds heard during the taking of blood pressure using a sphygmomanometer and stethoscope. As air is released from the cuff, pressure on the brachial artery is reduced, and the blood is heard pulsing through the vessel.

Korsakoff's psychosis /kôr'səkôfs/ [Sergei S. Korsakoff, Russian psychiatrist, 1854–1900], a form of amnesia often seen in chronic alcoholics that is characterized by a loss of short-term memory and an inability to learn new skills. The person is usually disoriented, may present with delirium and hallucinations, and confabulates to conceal the condition.

kosher [Heb, *kasher*, fit or proper], pertaining to the preparation and serving of foods according to Jewish dietary laws. Inherently kosher foods include common fruits, vegetables, and cereals, as well as tea and coffee. Foods that are not kosher include pork, birds of prey, and seafood that lacks fins and scales such as lobster and eels. Most poultry and meat products, excluding pork, are kosher if properly processed.

Kr, symbol for the element **krypton.**

Kraske position /kras'kə/ [Paul Kraske, Swiss surgeon, 1851–1930], an anatomic position in which the patient is prone, with hips flexed and elevated, head and feet down. The position is used for renal surgery.

kraurosis /krôrō′sis/ [Gk, *krauros,* dry, *osis,* condition], a thickening and shriveling of the skin.

kraurosis vulvae, a skin disease of aged women characterized by dryness, itching, and atrophy of the external genitalia.

Krause's corpuscles [Wilhelm J. F. Krause, German anatomist, 1833–1910; L, *corpusculum,* little body], any of a number of sensory end organs in the conjunctiva of the eye; mucous membranes of the lips and tongue; epineurium of nerve trunks, the penis, and the clitoris; and synovial membranes of certain joints. Krause's corpuscles are tiny cylindric oval bodies. They contain a soft, semifluid core in which the axon terminates either in a bulbous extremity or in a coiled mass.

Krukenberg's tumor /kroo′kənbərgz/ [Friedrich E. Krukenberg, German pathologist, 1871–1946], a neoplasm of the ovary that is a metastasis of a gastrointestinal malignancy, usually stomach cancer.

KS, ks, abbreviation for **Kaposi's sarcoma.**

KUB, abbreviation for *kidney, ureter, and bladder;* a term used in a radiographic examination to determine the location, size, shape, and malformation of the kidneys, ureters, and bladder.

Kuchendorf method /koo′kəndôrf/ (in radiology) a technique for positioning a patient for radiography of the patella.

Kufs' disease /koofs/ [H. Kufs, German psychiatrist, 1871–1955; L, *dis* + Fr, *aise,* ease], an adult form of hereditary cerebral sphingolipidosis (amaurotic familial idiocy), characterized by cerebromacular degeneration, hypertonicity, and progressive spastic paralysis.

Kümmell's disease /kim′əlz/ [Hermann Kümmell, German surgeon, 1852–1937; L, *dis* + Fr, *aise,* ease], a set of symptoms that develop after a compression fracture of the vertebrae with spinal injury. They include spinal pain, intercostal neuralgia, kyphosis, and weakness in the legs.

Küntscher nail /koon′chər, kin′chər/ [Gerhard Küntscher, German surgeon, 1902–1972; AS, *naegel*], a stainless steel nail used in orthopedic surgery for the fixation of fractures of the long bones, especially the femur.

Kupffer's cells /koop′fərz/ [Karl W. von Kupffer, German anatomist, 1829–1902], specialized cells of the reticuloendothelial system lining the sinusoids of the liver. Kupffer's cells filter bacteria and other small foreign proteins out of the blood.

kuru /koo′roo/ [New Guinea, trembling], a slow, progressive, fatal infection of the central nervous system seen only in natives of the New Guinea highlands. Incidence of the disease has declined with the decline of cannibalism.

Kussmaul breathing /koos′moul/ [Adolf Kussmaul, German physician, 1822–1902; AS, *braeth*], abnormally deep, very rapid sighing respirations characteristic of diabetic ketoacidosis.

Kussmaul's coma [Adolf Kussmaul; Gk, *koma,* deep sleep], a diabetic coma characterized by acidosis and deep breathing or extreme hyperpnea.

Kussmaul's sign [Adolf Kussmaul; L, *signum,* mark], **1.** a paradoxic rise in venous pressure with distension of the jugular veins during inspiration, as seen in constrictive pericarditis or mediastinal tumor. **2.** conditions of convulsions and coma associated with a gastrointestinal disorder caused by absorption of a toxic substance.

kv, abbreviation for **kilovolt.**

Kveim reaction [Morton A. Kveim, Norwegian physician, b. 1892; L, *re,* again, *agere,* to act], a reaction used in a diagnostic test for sarcoidosis, based on an intradermal injection of antigen derived from a lymph node known to be sarcoid.

kvp, abbreviation for **kilovolt peak.**

kvp test cassette, (in radiology) a light-proof box containing a copper filter, a series of stepwedges, and an optical attenuator, used to test the accuracy of kVp settings for peak electrical potential across an x-ray tube.

kwashiorkor /kwä′shē·ôr′kôr/ [Afr], a malnutrition disease, primarily of children, caused by severe protein deficiency that usually occurs when the child is weaned from the breast. Eventually the following symptoms occur: retarded growth, changes in skin and hair pigmentation, diarrhea, loss of appetite, nervous irritability, lethargy, edema, anemia, fatty degeneration of the liver, necrosis, dermatoses, and fibrosis, often accompanied by infection and multivitamin deficiencies.

Kyasanur Forest disease, an arbovirus infection transmitted by the bite of a tick that is harbored by shrews and other forest animals in western tropical India. Characteristics of the infection include fever, headache, muscle ache, cough, abdominal and eye pain, and photophobia.

kymography /kēmog′rəfē/ [Gk, *kyma,* wave, *graphein,* to record], a technique for graphically recording motions of body organs, as of the heart and the blood vessels.

kyphos /kī′fəs/ [Gk, *kyphos,* hunchbacked],

K

the hump in the thoracic vertebral column that is associated with kyphosis.

kyphoscoliosis /kī'fōskō'lē·ō'sis/ [Gk, *kyphos*, hunchbacked, *skolios* curved, *osis*, condition], an abnormal condition characterized by an anteroposterior and a lateral curvature of the spine. **—kyphoscoliotic,** *adj.*

kyphosis /kīfō'sis/ [Gk, *kyphos*, hunchbacked], an abnormal condition of the vertebral column, characterized by increased convexity in the curvature of the thoracic spine as viewed from the side. It may be caused by rickets or tuberculosis of the spine. **—kyphotic,** *adj.*

L

L, **1.** symbol for *kinetic potential.* **2.** abbreviation for *Lactobacillus.* **3.** abbreviation for **lambert. 4.** abbreviation for *Latin.* **5.** symbol for **liter. 6.** abbreviation for **lung.**

La, symbol for the element **lanthanum.**

LA, abbreviation for **left atrium.**

L&A, abbreviation for *reaction of the pupil to light accommodation.*

lab, abbreviation for **laboratory.**

label [ME, band], **1.** a substance with a special affinity for an organ, tissue, cell, or microorganism in which it may become deposited and fixed. **2.** the process of depositing and fixing a substance in an organ, tissue, cell, or microorganism. **3.** an atom or molecule attached to either a ligand or binding protein and capable of generating a signal for monitoring in the binding reaction. **4.** the process of attaching a radio isotope to a compound for the purpose of tracing it during a physiologic action in the body.

labeled compound, a chemical substance in which part of the molecules are labeled with a radionuclide or isotope so that observations of the radioactivity or isotopic composition make it possible to follow the compound or its fragments through physical, chemical, or biologic processes.

labeling, **1.** the providing of information on a drug, food, device, or cosmetic to the purchaser or user. Regulations for labeling are provided by the Food and Drug Administration. **2.** the assignment of a word or term to a form of behavior. **3.** the act of classifying a patient according to a diagnostic category. Labeling can be misleading because not all patients conform to defined characteristics of standard diagnostic categories.

la belle indifference /lä bel eNdifäräNs'/ [Fr, nice indifference], an air of unconcern displayed by some patients toward their physical symptoms. It is believed the physical symptoms may relieve anxiety.

labetalol hydrochloride /ləbet'əlol/, an antihypertensive drug with beta and alpha blocking properties. It is prescribed for the treatment of hypertension.

labia /lā'bē·ə/ *sing.* **labium** [L, lip], **1.** the lips; the fleshy liplike edges of an organ or tissue. **2.** the folds of skin at the opening of the vagina.

labial bar /lā'bē·əl/, a major connector that is installed labially or buccally to the dental arch and joins bilateral parts of a mandibular removable partial denture.

labial flange, the part of a denture that occupies the outer vestibule of the mouth.

labial glands [L, *labium,* lip, *glans,* acorn], small mucous or serous glands embedded in the lips.

labial notch, a depression in the denture border that accommodates the labial frenum.

labia majora /majôr'ə/, *sing.* **labium majus** /mā'jəs/, two long lips of skin, one on each side of the vaginal orifice outside the labia minora. They extend from the anterior labial commissure to the posterior labial commissure and form the lateral boundaries of the pudendal cleft.

labia minora /minôr'ə/, *sing.* **labium minus** /mē'nəs/, two folds of skin between the labia majora, extending from the clitoris backward on both sides of the vaginal orifice, ending between it and the labia majora.

labile /lā'bil/ [L, *labilis,* slipping], **1.** unstable; characterized by a tendency to change or be altered or modified. **2.** (in psychiatry) characterized by rapidly shifting or changing emotions, as in bipolar disorder and certain types of schizophrenia; emotionally unstable. —**lability,** *n.*

labiodental /lā'bē·ōden'təl/ [L, *labium,* lip, *dens,* tooth], **1.** pertaining to the labial, or cheek, surfaces of the 12 anterior teeth. **2.** (in speech therapy), sounds of speech that require a special coordination of teeth and lips.

labiolingual fixed orthodontic appliance /lā'bē·ōling'gwəl/ [L, *labium,* lip, *lingua,* tongue], an orthodontic appliance for correcting or improving malocclusion, characterized by anchorage to the maxillary and mandibular first permanent molars and by labial and lingual arches.

labor [L, work], the time and the processes that occur during parturition from the beginning of cervical dilation to the delivery of the placenta.

laboratory (lab) /lab'(ə)rətôr'e/ [L, *laborare,* to labor], **1.** a facility, room, build-

657

ing, or part of a building in which scientific research, experimentation, testing, or other investigative activities are carried out. **2.** pertaining to a laboratory.

Laboratory Data Interpretation, a Nursing Interventions Classification defined as critical analysis of patient laboratory data in order to assist with clinical decision-making.

laboratory diagnosis, a diagnosis arrived at after study of secretions, excretions, or tissue through chemical, microscopic, or bacteriologic means or by biopsy.

laboratory error, any error made by the personnel in a clinical laboratory in performing a test, interpreting data, or reporting or recording the results.

laboratory medicine, the branch of medicine in which specimens of tissue, fluid, or other body substance are examined outside of the person, usually in the laboratory. Some fields of laboratory medicine are chemistry, cytology, hematology, histology, and pathology.

laboratory test, a procedure, usually conducted in a laboratory, that is intended to detect, identify, or quantify one or more significant substances, evaluate organ functions, or establish the nature of a condition or disease.

labor coach, a person who assists a woman in labor and delivery by closely attending to her emotional needs and encouraging her to use properly the breathing patterns, concentration techniques, body positions, and massage techniques that were taught in a program of psychophysical preparation for childbirth. The task of a labor coach is to decrease or eliminate the use of analgesia or anesthesia.

labored breathing, abnormal respiration characterized by evidence of increased effort, including use of the accessory muscles of respiration of the chest wall, stridor, grunting, or nasal flaring.

Labor Induction, a Nursing Interventions Classification defined as initiation or augmentation of labor by mechanical or pharmacologic methods.

labor pains [L, *labor,* work, *poena,* penalty], pain associated with contraction of the uterus in labor.

Labor Suppression, a Nursing Interventions Classification defined as controlling uterine contractions prior to 37 weeks of gestation to prevent preterm birth.

labyrinthectomy /lab′ərinthk′təmē/, the surgical excision of the aural labyrinth.

labyrinthine /lab′ərin′thīn/ [Gk, *labyrinthos,* maze], pertaining to or resembling a labyrinth or maze, such as the structure of the inner ear.

labyrinthine righting, one of the five basic neuromuscular reactions involved in a change of body positions. The change stimulates cells in the semicircular canals of the inner ear, causing neck muscles to respond by automatically adjusting the head to the new position.

labyrinthitis /lab′ərinthī′tis/ [Gk, *labyrinthos,* maze, *itis*], inflammation of the labyrinthine canals of the inner ear, resulting in vertigo.

laceration /las′ərā′shən/ [L, *lacerare,* to tear], **1.** the act of tearing or slashing. **2.** a torn, jagged wound. —**lacerate,** *v.,* **lacerated,** *adj.*

laceration of cervix [L, *lacerare,* to tear, *cervix,* neck], a wound or irregular tear of the cervix uteri during childbirth.

laceration of the perineum [L, *lacerare,* to tear; Gk, *perineos*], a wound or irregular tear of the perineal tissues during childbirth.

lacrimal /lak′riməl/ [L, *lacrima,* tear], pertaining to tears.

lacrimal apparatus, a network of structures of the eye that secrete tears and drain them from the surface of the eyeball. These parts include the lacrimal glands, lacrimal ducts, lacrimal canals, lacrimal sacs, and nasolacrimal ducts.

lacrimal bone, one of the smallest and most fragile bones of the face, located at the anterior part of the medial wall of the orbit. It unites with the maxilla to form the groove for the lacrimal sac.

lacrimal caruncle, the small, reddish, fleshy protuberance that fills the triangular space between the medial margins of the upper and lower eyelids.

lacrimal duct, one of a pair of channels through which tears pass from the lacrimal lake to the lacrimal sac of each eye.

lacrimal fold [L, *lacrima,* tear; AS, *fealdan*], a valvelike fold of mucous membrane at the lower part of the nasolacrimal duct.

lacrimal gland, one of a pair of glands situated superior and lateral to the eye bulb in the lacrimal fossa of the frontal bone. The watery secretion from the gland consists of the tears, slightly alkaline and saline, that moisten the conjunctiva.

lacrimal papilla, the small conic elevation on the medial margin of each eyelid, supporting an apex pierced by the punctum lacrimale through which tears emerge to moisten the conjunctiva.

lacrimal reflex [L, *lacrima,* tear, *reflectere,* to bend back], a release of tears in response to stimulation or irritation of the corneal conjunctiva.

lacrimal sac, the dilated end of each of the two nasolacrimal ducts. The lacrimal sacs fill with tears secreted by the lacrimal glands and conveyed through the lacrimal ducts.

lacrimation /lak'rimā'shən/, **1.** the normal continuous secretion of tears by the lacrimal glands. **2.** an excessive amount of tear production, as in crying or weeping.

lacrimator /lak'rimā'tər/, an agent that stimulates the secretion of tears.

lacrimotomy /lak'rimot'əmē/, a surgical incision in the lacrimal gland.

lactalbumin /lak'təlbyoo'min/ [L, *lac*, milk, *albus*, white], a simple, highly nutritious protein found in milk. It is similar to serum albumin.

lactam /lak'təm/, a cyclic amide created by the elimination of a molecule of water from aminocarboxylic acid.

lactase /lak'tās/ [L, *lac* + Fr, *diastase*, enzyme], an enzyme that catalyzes the hydrolysis of lactose to glucose and galactose.

lactase deficiency, an inherited abnormality in which the amount of the digestive enzyme lactase is deficient, resulting in the inability to digest lactose, except for the bacterial breakdown of lactose in the large intestine.

lactate /lak'tāt/, an anion of lactic acid.

lactate dehydrogenase (LDH), an enzyme that is found in the cytoplasm of almost all body tissues, where its main function is to catalyze the oxidation of L-lactate to pyruvate. It is assayed as a measure of anaerobic carbohydrate metabolism and as one of several serum indicators of myocardial infarction and muscular dystrophies.

lactation /laktā'shən/ [L, *lac*, milk, *atio*, process], the process of synthesis and secretion of milk from the breasts in the nourishment of an infant or child.

Lactation Counseling, a Nursing Interventions Classification defined as use of an interactive helping process to assist in maintenance of successful breastfeeding.

Lactation Suppression, a Nursing Interventions Classification defined as facilitating the cessation of milk production and minimizing breast engorgement after giving birth.

lacteal /lak'tē-əl/, pertaining to milk.

lacteal fistula, an abnormal passage opening into a lacteal duct.

lacteal vessel, one of the many central lymphatic capillaries in the villi of the small intestine. They open into the lymphatic vessels in the submucosa. The capillary is filled with milky-white chyle caused by the absorption of fat from the lumen (chylomicrons).

lactic /lak'tik/ [L, *lac* + *icus*, like], referring to milk and milk products.

lactic acid, a three-carbon organic acid produced by anaerobic respiration. There are three forms: L-lactic acid in muscle and blood is a product of glucose and glycogen metabolism; D-lactic acid is produced by the fermentation of dextrose by a species of micrococcus; DL-lactic acid is a racemic mixture found in the stomach, in sour milk, and in certain other foods prepared by bacterial fermentation.

lactic acid fermentation, 1. the production of lactic acid from sugars by various bacteria. **2.** the souring of milk.

lactic acidosis, a disorder characterized by an accumulation of lactic acid in the blood, resulting in a lowered pH in muscle and serum. The condition occurs most commonly in tissue hypoxia.

lactiferous /laktif'ərəs/ [L, *lac* + *ferre*, to carry], pertaining to a structure that produces or conveys milk, such as the tubules of the breasts.

lactiferous duct, one of many channels that carry milk from the lobes of each breast to the nipple.

lactiferous glands [L, *lac*, milk, *ferre*, to carry, *glans*, acorn], glands that secrete or convey milk such as mammary glands.

Lactobacillus /lak'tōbəsil'əs/ [L, *lac* + *bacillum*, small rod], any one of a group of nonpathogenic gram-positive rod-shaped bacteria that produce lactic acid from carbohydrates.

Lactobacillus acidophilus [L, *lac*, milk, *bacillum*, small rod, *acidus*, sour; Gk, *philein*, to love], a bacterium found in milk and dairy products, feces of bottlefed babies and adults, saliva, and carious teeth. The strain is used to manufacture a fermented milk product.

Lactobacillus bulgaricus, a genus of bacteria used in the production of yogurt.

lactoferrin /lak'tō-fer'in/, an iron-binding protein present in neurophil granules.

lactogen /lak'təjən/ [L, *lac* + Gk, *genein*, to produce], a drug or other substance that enhances the production and secretion of milk. – **lactogenic,** *adj.*

lacto-ovo-vegetarian /lak'tō-ōv'ōvej'əter'-ē-ən/, one whose diet consists primarily of foods of vegetable origin but also includes some animal products such as eggs *(ovo),* milk, and cheese *(lacto)* but no meat, fish, or poultry.

lactoperoxidase /-pərok'sidās/, an enzyme found in milk and saliva. It is believed to inhibit a number of microorganisms, functioning in a nonspecific immunity role.

lactose /lak'tos/ [L, *lac* + Gk, *glykys*, sweet], a disaccharide found in the milk

L

of all mammals. On hydrolysis, lactose yields the monosaccharides glucose and galactose.

lactose intolerance, a sensitivity disorder resulting in the inability to digest lactose because of a deficiency of or defect in the enzyme lactase. Symptoms of the disorder are bloating, flatus, nausea, diarrhea, and abdominal cramps.

lactosuria /lak′təsŏŏr′ē·ə/ [L. *lac* + Gk, *glykys,* sweet, *ouron,* urine], the presence of lactose in the urine, a condition that may occur in late pregnancy or during lactation.

lactotherapy /-ther′əpē/ [L, *lac,* milk; Gk, *therapeia,* treatment], any treatment that depends on a diet consisting exclusively or almost exclusively of milk.

lactotoxin /-tok′sin/, any toxic base occurring in milk as a result of decomposition of its proteins.

lacto-vegetarian /-vej′əter′ē·ən/, one whose diet consists of milk and milk products *(lacto)* in addition to foods of vegetable origin but does not include eggs, meat, fish, or poultry.

lactulose /lak′tyəlōs/, a nonabsorbable synthetic disaccharide, 4-0-[β]-D-galactopyranosyl-D-fructose, $C_{12}H_{22}O_{11}$. It is hydrolyzed in the colon by bacteria primarily to lactic acid.

lacuna /ləkyŏŏ′nə/, *pl.* **lacunae** [L, pit], **1.** a small cavity within a structure, especially bony tissue. **2.** a gap, as in the field of vision.

lacunar /lakyŏŏ′nər/ [L, *lacuna,* pit], pertaining to or characterized by the presence of pits, depressions, hollows, or spaces.

lacunar state, a pseudobulbar disorder characterized by the appearance of small, smooth-walled cavities in the brain tissue. The condition usually follows a series of small strokes, particularly in older adults with arterial hypertension and arteriosclerosis.

lacus lacrimalis /lā′kəs lak′rimā′ləs/ [L, *lacus,* lake, *lacrimalis,* tears], a triangular space separating the medial ends of the upper and lower eyelids.

LAD, **1.** abbreviation for *left anterior descending.* **2.** abbreviation for **leukocyte adhesion deficiency.**

LADME /lad′mē/, an abbreviation for the time course of drug distribution, representing the terms *liberation, absorption distribution, metabolism,* and *elimination.*

Laënnec's catarrh /lā′əneks′/ [René T. H. Laënnec, French physician, 1781–1826; Gk, *kata,* down, *rhoia,* flow], a form of bronchial asthma characterized by the discharge of small, viscous, beadlike bodies of sputum. These bodies, **Laënnec's pearls,** are formed in the bronchioles and

appear in the asthmatic person's expectorated bronchial secretions.

Laënnec's cirrhosis [René T. H. Laënnec; Gk, *kirrhos,* yellow, *osis,* condition], a fibrotic form of cirrhosis precipitated by alcohol abuse.

laetrile /lā′ətril/, a substance composed primarily of amygdalin, a cyanogenic glycoside derived from apricot pits. Laetrile has been offered as a cancer medication despite clinical studies by the National Cancer Institute that failed to show benefits from its use.

laf, abbreviation for **laminar air flow.**

lagophthalmos /lag′əfthal′məs/ [Gk, *lagos,* hare, *ophthalmos,* eye], an abnormal condition in which an eye may not be fully closed because of a neurologic or muscular disorder.

lag phase [Dan, *lakke,* go slowly; Gk, *phasis,* appearance], a time span during which bacteria injected into a fresh medium have not begun to multiply, although they may enlarge.

laity /lā′itē/ [Gk, *laikos,* of the people], a nonprofessional segment of the population, as viewed from the perspective of a member of a particular profession. A clergyman may regard a physician as a member of the laity and vice versa.

LAK, abbreviation for **lymphokine-activated killer cells.**

laked blood /lākt/ [Fr, *laque,* a deep red color], blood that is clear, red, and homogenous because of hemolysis of the red blood cells, as may occur in poisoning and severe extensive burns.

La Leche League International /lä lech′ā/ [Sp, *la leche,* the milk], an organization that promotes and provides education about breastfeeding.

laliatry [Gk, *lalia,* speech, *iatreia,* treatment], the study of speech disorders and their treatment.

lallation /lalā′shən/ [L, *lallare,* to babble], **1.** babbling, repetitive, unintelligible utterances, such as the babbling of an infant and the mumbled speech of schizophrenics, alcoholics, and the severely mentally retarded. **2.** a speech disorder characterized by a defective pronunciation of words containing the sound /l/ or by the use of the sound /l/ in place of the sound /r/.

lallognosis [Gk, *lalia,* speech, *gnosis,* knowing], the science of understanding speech.

lalophobia /lal′ōfō′bē·ə/ [Gk, *lalia,* speech, *phobos,* fear], a morbid dread of talking caused by fear and anxiety that one will stammer or stutter.

lamarckism /ləmär′kizəm/ [Jean B. P. de Lamarck, French naturalist, 1744–1829; Gk, *ismos,* practice], the theory postulated that organic evolution results from structural changes in plants and animals caused by adaptation to environmental conditions and that these acquired characteristics are transmitted to offspring. — **lamarckian,** *adj., n.*

Lamaze method /ləmäz'/ [Fernand Lamaze, French obstetrician, 1890–1957], a method of psychophysical preparation for childbirth developed in the 1950s. It requires classes, practice at home, and coaching during labor and delivery, often by a trained coach called a 'monitrice.' The classes, given during pregnancy, teach the physiology of pregnancy and childbirth, exercises to develop strength in the abdominal muscles and control of isolated muscles of the vagina and perineum, and techniques of breathing and relaxation to promote control and relaxation during labor. The kind and rate of breathing change with the advancing stages of labor.

lambda /lam'də/, **1.** Λ, λ, the eleventh letter of the Greek alphabet. **2.** a posterior fontanel of the skull marking the point where the sagittal and lambdoidal sutures meet.

lambdacism /lam'dəsiz'əm/ [Gk, *lambda* + *ismos,* practice], a speech disorder characterized by a defective pronunciation of words containing the sound /l/, by the excessive use of the sound, or by the substitution of the sound /r/ for /l/.

lambda (λ) light chain, one of two kinds of smaller polypeptide chains present in an immunoglobulin molecule.

lambdoid /lam'doid/, having the shape of the Greek letter lambda.

lambdoidal suture /lamdoi'dəl/, the interdigitating connection between the occipital bone and the parietal bones of the skull.

lambert (L) /lam'bert, lam'bərt/ [J. H. Lambert, German physicist, 1728–1777], a unit of luminance or brightness of a perfectly diffusing surface, whether emitting or reflecting, equal to a total luminous flux of one lumen per square centimeter.

lamella /ləmel'ə/, *pl.* **lamellae** [L, small plate], **1.** a thin leaf or plate, as of bone. **2.** a medicated disk, prepared from glycerin and an alkaloid, for insertion under the eyelid, where it dissolves and is absorbed.

lamellar /ləmel'ər/ [L, *lamella,* small plate], pertaining to or characterized by lamella.

lamellar exfoliation of the newborn [L, *lamella* + *ex,* without, *folium,* leaf; AS, *niwe,* new, *boren,* born], a congenital skin disorder transmitted as an autosomal-recessive trait in which a parchmentlike scaly membrane that covers the infant peels off within 24 hours of birth.

lameness /lām'nəs/ [ME, *lama,* to break], a condition of diminished function, particularly because of a foot or leg injury. The term may also be applied to a stiff or painful back that makes walking difficult.

lamina /lam'inə/, *pl.,* **laminae** [L, thin plate], any thin, flat layer of membrane or other bulkier tissue. It may be structureless or part of a structure, as the laminae of the vertebral arch.

lamina densa, a layer of epithelial basal lamina that appears dark in electron micrographs.

lamina dura, 1. a sheet of compact alveolar bone that lies adjacent to the periodontal membrane, the lining of the tooth socket. **2.** a radiographic term to identify the radiopaque lining of the tooth socket (alveolus)

lamina lucida, a layer of epithelial basal lamina that appears light or clear in electron micrographs.

lamin antibody /lam'in/, a type of immunoglobulin found in the serum of some patients with autoimmune diseases, including systemic lupus erythematosus.

lamina propria, a layer of connective tissue that lies just under the epithelium of the mucous membrane.

laminar air flow (laf) /lam'iner/ [L, *lamina,* plate; Gk, *aer;* AS, *flowan*], a system of circulating filtered air in parallel flow planes in hospitals or other health care facilities. The system reduces the risk of bacterial contamination or exposure to chemical pollutants in surgical theaters, food preparation areas, hospital pharmacies, and laboratories.

laminaria /lam'iner'ē·ə/ [L, *lamina,* plate], a type of seaweed that swells on absorption of water.

laminaria tent, a cone of dried seaweed that swells as it absorbs water and therefore is used to dilate the cervix nontraumatically in preparation for induced abortion or induced labor.

laminated thrombus /lam'inā'tid/, a thrombus composed of an aggregation of blood platelets, fibrin, clotting factors, and cellular elements arranged in layers, apparently formed at different times.

laminectomy /lam'inek'təmē/ [L, *lamina* + Gk, *ektome,* excision], surgical removal of the bony arches of one or more vertebrae. It is performed to relieve compression of the spinal cord caused by a bone displaced in an injury or as the result of degeneration of a disk, or to reach and remove a displaced intervertebral disk. Spinal fusion may be necessary for stabil-

L

ity of the spine if several laminae are removed. —**laminectomize,** *v.*

laminin /lam′inin/, any of several large glycoproteins consisting of three polypeptide subunits and found in basement membranes.

laminotomy /-ot′əmē/, the surgical division of the lamina of a vertebral arch. Also called **rachiotomy.**

laminotrigine, an anticonvulsant drug prescribed as adjunctive therapy in the treatment of partial seizures in epilepsy patients over the age of 16.

lampbrush chromosome [Gk, *lampas,* torch; AS, *bryst,* bristle], an excessively large type of chromosome found in the oocytes of many lower animals. It has a hairy, brushlike appearance.

lamprophonia [Gk, *lampros,* clear, *phone,* sound], an unusually clear and distinct sound.

lance [L, *lancea,* spear], to incise a furuncle or an abscess to release accumulated pus.

Lancefield's classification [Rebecca C. Lancefield, American bacteriologist, 1895–1981], a serologic classification of streptococci based on their antigenic characteristics. The bacteria are divided into 13 groups by the identification of their pathologic action.

lancet /lan′sit/ [L, *lancea,* lance], a short pointed blade used to obtain a drop of blood for a capillary sample.

lancinating /lan′sinā′ting/ [L, *lancea,* lance], sharply cutting or tearing, such as lancinating pain.

Landau reflex /lan′dou/, a normal response of infants when held in a horizontal prone position to maintain a convex arc with the head raised and the legs slightly flexed.

landmark position [AS, *land* + *meark,* mark; L, *positio*], the correct placement of the hands on the chest in cardiopulmonary resuscitation.

Landsteiner's classification /land′stī′nərz/ [Karl Landsteiner, American pathologist and Nobel laureate, 1868–1943], the classification of blood groups A, B, AB, and O on the basis of the presence or absence of the two agglutinogens A and B on the erythrocytes in human blood.

Langerhans' cells /lung′ərhuns, lang′ərhans/, [Paul Langerhans, German pathologist, 1847–1888], a stellate dendritic cell found mostly in the stratum spinosum of the epidermis.

language /lang′gwij/ [L, *lingua,* tongue], a defined set of characters that, when used alone or in combination, form a meaningful set of words and symbols that are used for communication.

language disorder, a partial or complete disruption in the ability to understand and produce the conventional symbols or words that comprise one's native language.

lanolin /lan′əlin/ [L, *lana,* wool, *oleum,* oil], a fatlike substance from the wool of sheep. It contains about 25% water as a water-in-oil emulsion and is used as an ointment base and an emollient for the skin.

lanthanum (La) /lan′thənəm/ [Gk, *lanthanein,* to escape notice], a rare earth metallic element. Its atomic number is 57; its atomic mass (weight) is 138.91.

lanuginous /lənōō′jinəs/ [L, *lanugo,* down], pertaining to lanugo.

lanugo /lanyōō′gō/ [L, down], **1.** the soft, downy hair covering a normal fetus beginning in the fifth month of gestation and almost entirely shed by the ninth month. **2.** the fine, soft hair covering all parts of the body except palms, soles, and areas where other types of hair are normally found.

lanulous /lan′yōōləs/ [L, *lana,* wool, *osus,* filled with], downy or covered with short, fine wooly hair, such as the skin of a fetus.

LAP, abbreviation for **leukocyte alkaline phosphatase.**

lap, 1. abbreviation for **laparotomy. 2.** abbreviation for *left atrial pressure.*

laparectomy /lap′ərek′təmē/, the surgical excision of tissue from the wall of the abdomen, usually performed to correct a problem of abdominal muscle laxity.

laparoenterostomy /lap′ərō·en′təros′təmē/ [Gk, *lapara,* loin, *enteron,* bowel, *stoma,* mouth], the surgical installation of a tube through an external opening in the abdomen to drain the bowel. A similar procedure may be used to supply nutrients to a patient with an upper digestive tract obstruction.

laparoenterotomy /lap′ərō·en′tərot′əmē/ [Gk, *laparo,* loin, *enteron,* bowel, *tennein,* to cut], a surgical incision in the intestine through the abdominal wall.

laparohysterectomy /-his′tərek′təmē/ [Gk, *lapara,* loin, *hystera,* womb, *ektome,* excision], a hysterectomy performed by making an excision through the abdominal wall.

laparohystero-oophorectomy /-his′tərō-/, the surgical removal of the uterus and ovaries through a small incision in the abdominal wall.

laparohysterosalpingo-oophorectomy /-his′tərō′salping′gō-/, the surgical removal of the uterus, ovaries, and fallopian tubes through a small incision in the abdominal wall.

laparomyitis /-mī-ī′tis/, an inflammation of the abdominal or lumbar muscles.

laparosalpingo-oophorectomy /-salping′-gō-/, the surgical removal of the ovaries and fallopian tubes through a small incision in the abdominal wall.

laparoscope /lap′ərəskōp′/ [Gk, *lapara*, loin, *skopein*, to look], a type of endoscope consisting of an illuminated tube with an optical system. It is inserted through the abdominal wall for examining the peritoneal cavity. —**laparoscopic**, *adj.,* **laparoscopy**, *n.*

laparoscopic-assisted vaginal hysteroscopy /-skop′ik/, a procedure for viewing the inner surface of the uterus with a specially designed endoscope inserted through the cervix. Before insertion the uterus is inflated with carbon dioxide or a glucose solution administered through the cervix.

laparoscopic laser cholecystectomy, the surgical removal of the gallbladder through an incision in the abdominal wall, using a laser with the guidance and illumination of a laparoscope.

laparoscopic sterilization /-skop′ik/ [Gk, *lapara*, loin, *skopein*, to view; L, *sterilis*, barren], the process of rendering a woman incapable of reproduction by inserting a specialized endoscope through a small incision in the abdominal wall. Sterilization may be performed through the incision with clips to occlude the fallopian tubes or by electrocoagulation and severance.

laparoscopy /lap′əros′kəpē/, the examination of the abdominal cavity with a laparoscope through one or more small incisions in the abdominal wall, usually at the umbilicus.

laparotomy (lap) /lap′ərot′əmē/ [Gk, *lapara* + *temnein*, to cut], any surgical incision into the peritoneal cavity, usually performed under general or regional anesthesia, often on an exploratory basis. Some kinds of laparotomy are **appendectomy, cholecystectomy,** and **colostomy.** —**laparotomize**, *v.*

lap-board [ME, *lappa* + *bord,* plank], a flat board placed over the lap to serve as a temporary desk or table.

lapis /lap′is/ [L, stone], any substance that does not easily volatilize, as lapis dentalis, or tooth tartar.

Laplace's law /läpläs′/ [Pierre S. de Laplace, French physicist, 1749–1827], a principle of physics that the tension on the wall of a sphere is the product of the pressure times the radius of the chamber and the tension is inversely related to the thickness of the wall.

large for gestational age (LGA) infant, an infant whose fetal growth was accelerated and whose size and weight at birth fall above the ninetieth percentile of appropriate for gestational age infants, whether delivered prematurely, at term, or later than term. Factors other than genetic influences that cause accelerated intrauterine growth include maternal diabetes mellitus and Beckwith's syndrome.

large intestine [L, *largus,* abundant, *intestinum*], the part of the digestive tract comprising the cecum; appendix; ascending, transverse, descending, and sigmoid colons; and rectum.

lariat structure /ler′ē-ət/, a ring of intron segments that have been spliced out of a messenger ribonucleic acid molecule by enzymes. Some introns form a long tail attached to the ring, giving the structure the appearance of a microscopic cowboy lariat.

Larmor frequency [Joseph Larmor, Irish physicist, 1857–1942], the frequency of the precession of a charged particle when its motion comes under the influence of an applied magnetic field and a central force.

larva /lär′və/ [L, specter], the early immature form of an animal, which undergoes metamorphosis to an adult form.

larval /lär′vəl/, pertaining to an organism in the preadult stage of a larva.

laryngeal /lerin′jē-əl/ [Gk, *larynx*], pertaining to the larynx.

laryngeal cancer [Gk, *larynx* + L, *cancer,* crab], a malignant neoplastic disease characterized by a tumor arising from the epithelium of the structures of the larynx. Chronic alcoholism and heavy use of tobacco increase the risk of developing the cancer. Persistent hoarseness is usually the first sign; advanced lesions may cause a sore throat, dyspnea, dysphagia, and cervical adenopathy.

laryngeal catheterization, the insertion of a catheter into the larynx for the purpose of removing secretions or introducing gases.

laryngeal polyp [Gk, *larynx* + *poly,* many, *pous,* foot], a polyp on the vocal cords that causes hoarseness as a result of vocal abuse or smoking.

laryngeal reflex [Gk, *larynx* + L, *reflectere,* to bend back], a cough reflex caused by irritation of the fauces and larynx.

laryngeal vertigo [Gk, *larynx* + L, *vertere,* to turn], a short episode of dizziness or unconsciousness following a paroxysmal attack of coughing or laryngeal spasm.

laryngectomy /ler′injek′təmē/ [Gk, *larynx* + *ektome,* excision], surgical removal of the larynx performed to treat cancer of the larynx. —**laryngectomize**, *v.*

L

laryngismus /ler′injiz′məs/ [Gk, *laryngismos,* whooping], spasm of the larynx. Laryngismus stridulus, a condition characterized by sudden laryngeal spasm with a crowing sound on inspiration and the possible development of cyanosis, occurs in inflammation of the larynx.

laryngitis /ler′injī′tis/ [Gk, *larynx + itis*], inflammation of the mucous membrane lining the larynx, accompanied by edema of the vocal cords with hoarseness or loss of voice, occurring as an acute disorder caused by a cold, by irritating fumes, by sudden temperature changes, or as a chronic condition resulting from excessive use of the voice, heavy smoking, or exposure to irritating fumes. In acute laryngitis there may be a cough, and the throat usually feels scratchy and painful.

laryngocele /ləring′gōsēl′/, an abnormal air-containing cavity connected to the laryngeal ventricle. It is caused by an evagination of the mucous membrane of the ventricle and may displace and enlarge the false vocal cord, resulting in hoarseness and airway obstruction. Because a laryngocele is also a potential reservoir of infection, it is usually excised.

laryngologist /ler′ing·gol′əjist/, a physician who specializes in the diagnosis and treatment of disorders of the larynx.

laryngology /ler′ing·gol′əjē/, [Gk, *larynx + logos,* science], the branch of medicine that specializes in the causes and treatments of disorders of the larynx.

laryngopharyngeal /-ferin′jē·əl/. pertaining to the larynx and pharynx.

laryngopharyngitis /ləring′gōfer′injī′tis/ [Gk, *larynx + pharynx,* throat, *itis*], inflammation of the larynx and pharynx.

laryngopharyngography /lering′gōfer′ingog′rəfē/ [Gk, *larynx + pharynx + graphein,* to record], the radiographic examination of the larynx and pharynx.

laryngopharynx /lering′gōfer′ingks/ [Gk, *larynx + pharynx,* throat], one of the three regions of the throat, extending from the hyoid bone to the esophagus.

laryngoscope /ləring′gəskōp/, an endoscope for examining the larynx.

laryngoscopic /-skop′ik/ [Gk, *larynx + skopein,* to view], pertaining to the use of a laryngoscope.

laryngoscopy /ler′ing·gos′kəpē/ [Gk, *larynx + skopein,* to view], the use of a laryngoscope to view the larynx.

laryngospasm /ləring′gōspaz′əm/ [Gk, *larynx + spasmos,* spasm], a spasmodic closure of the larynx.

laryngotomy /ler′ing·got′əmē/ [Gk, *larynx + temnein,* to cut], a surgical incision into the larynx through the cricovocal membrane. It is usually an emergency pro-

cedure that is performed when a standard tracheotomy cannot be done.

laryngotracheitis /-trā′kē·ī′tis/, an inflammation of the larynx and trachea.

laryngotracheobronchitis (LTB) /lering′-gōtrā′kē·ō′brongkī′tis/ [Gk, *larynx + L, tractus,* trachea; Gk, *bronchos,* windpipe, *itis*], an inflammation of the major respiratory passages, usually causing hoarseness, nonproductive cough, and dyspnea.

laryngotracheotomy /-trā′kē·ot′əmē/, a surgical incision into the larynx and trachea.

larynx /ler′ingks/ [Gk], the organ of voice that is part of the air passage connecting the pharynx with the trachea. The larynx forms the caudal part of the anterior wall of the pharynx and is lined with mucous membrane that is continuous with that of the pharynx and trachea. It is composed of three single cartilages and three paired cartilages, all connected together by ligaments and moved by various muscles. —**laryngeal,** *adj.*

LAS, abbreviation for **lymphadenopathy syndrome.**

laser /lā′zər/, acronym for *light amplification by stimulated emission of radiation,* a source of intense monochromatic radiation of the visible, ultraviolet, or infrared parts of the spectrum. Lasers are used in surgery to divide or cause adhesions or to destroy or fix tissue in place.

laser angioplasty, the opening of an occluded artery with laser energy delivered to the site through a fiberoptic probe.

laser bronchoscopy, bronchoscopy that is performed with the aid of a carbon dioxide laser beam directed through fiberoptic equipment in the diagnosis and treatment of bronchial disorders.

laser iridotomy, a procedure for the treatment of closed-angle glaucoma in which the patient has intermittent periods of increased intraocular pressure. The angle-closure mechanism is controlled by creating an opening in the iris. Specific techniques vary with the type of laser used.

laser pain management, the use of lasers to relieve pain. This treatment has been applied effectively to specific acupuncture points where there is no anatomic dysfunction at the base of the pain.

Laser Precautions, a Nursing Interventions Classification defined as limiting the risk of injury to the patient related to use of a laser.

laser trabeculoplasty, an application of laser energy in the treatment of primary open-angle glaucoma. The procedure may be recommended when intraocular pressure increases despite administration of topical agents. Laser trabeculoplasty creates a fistula between the anterior chamber and the subconjunctival space of the eye, bypassing an obstruction to aqueous outflow. The eye is anesthetized with a topical anesthetic. A potential complication is a temporary increase in intraocular pressure, which is treated with drugs. The procedure is usually not effective with additional application, and most patients continue to require antiglaucoma medications.

Lassa fever /lä′sə/ [Lassa, Nigeria; L, *febris*, fever],   a highly contagious disease caused by a virulent arenavirus. It is characterized by fever, pharyngitis, dysphagia, and ecchymoses. Pleural effusion, edema and renal involvement, mental disorientation, confusion, and death from cardiac failure often ensue.

last sacraments [ME, *laste* + L, *sacramentum*, solemn oath],   a religious ceremony performed by a member of the clergy in behalf of a person about to die.

latchkey children,   minors who are often at home alone because their parents are at work.

latency period /lā′tənsē/ [L, *latere*, to be concealed; Gk, *peri* + *hodos*, way],   **1.** the period between contact with a pathogen and development of symptoms. **2.** the time between stimulus and response. **3.** a period between early childhood and puberty when there is little overt interest in the opposite sex.

latency stage [L, *latere*, to be concealed; Fr, *estage*, stage],   (in psychoanalysis) a period in psychosexual development occurring between early childhood and puberty when sexual motivation and expression are repressed or transferred, through sublimation, to the feelings and behavioral patterns expected as typical of the age.

latent /lā′tənt/ [L, *latere*, to be concealed],   dormant; existing as a potential; for example, tuberculosis may be latent for extended periods of time and become active under certain conditions.

latent energy [L, *latere*, to be concealed; Gk, *energeia*],   the energy contained in an object as a result of its position in space, its internal structure, and stresses imposed on it.

latent heat [L, *latere*, to be concealed; AS, *haetu*],   the heat absorbed by a substance when it changes from a solid to a liquid or from a liquid to a gas without an accompanying rise in temperature.

latent image,   (in radiology) an invisible image produced in the x-ray film emulsion by x-rays or visible light that can be converted to a visible image by development.

latent learning [L, *latere*, to be concealed; ME, *lernen*],   learning acquired unintentionally. It may remain in the subconscious, or be latent, until a need for the knowledge arises.

latent malaria [L, *latere*, to be concealed; It, *mal* + *aria*, bad air],   a continuing infection without clinical symptoms, resulting from a balance established between the parasite and the body's immune system.

latent period,   (in radiology) an interval of seeming inactivity between the time of exposure to an injurious dose of radiation and the response.

latent phase,   the early stage of labor that is characterized by irregular, infrequent, and mild contractions and little or no dilation of the cervix or descent of the fetus.

latent syphilis [L, *latere*, to be concealed; Gk, *syn*, together, *philein*, to love],   a stage of syphilis infection in which no clinical symptoms appear but serologic tests indicate the presence of the syphilis spirochete.

latent tetany [L, *latere*, to be concealed; Gk, *tetanos*, convulsive tension],   a form of tetany that is elicited only by mechanical or electrical stimuli.

late-phase hypersensitivity reaction,   an inflammatory response in IgE allergic diseases. It begins 2 to 4 hours after exposure to an antigen, peaks at 6 to 12 hours, and disappears after 24 hours.

lateral /lat′ərəl/ [L, *latus*, side],   **1.** pertaining to the side. **2.** away from the midsagittal plane. **3.** farther from the midsagittal plane. **4.** to the right or left of the midsagittal plane.

lateral aortic node,   a lumbar lymph node in any of three clusters of nodes serving the pelvis and abdomen.

lateral aperture of the fourth ventricle,   an opening between the end of each lateral recess of the fourth ventricle and the subarachnoid space.

lateral cerebral sulcus,   a deep cleft marking the division of the temporal from the frontal and parietal lobes of brain.

lateral condensation method,   a technique for filling and sealing tooth root canals. A preselected gutta-percha cone is sealed into the apex of the root; other cones are forced laterally with a spreader until the canal is filled.

lateral cuneiform bone,   one of the three cuneiform bones of the foot. It is located in the center of the front row of tarsal bones.

lateral decentering,   (in radiology) an error in positioning of a focused grid, resulting in partial grid cutoff over the entire film. The error may also be a result of improperly positioning the tube head rather than the grid.

lateral geniculate body, one of two elevations of the lateral posterior thalamus receiving visual impulses from the retina via the optic nerves and tracts and relaying the impulses to the calcarine (visual) cortex.

lateral humeral epicondylitis, inflammation of the tissue at the lower end of the humerus at the elbow joint, caused by the repetitive flexing of the wrist against resistance. It may result from athletic activity or manual manipulation of tools or other equipment.

lateral incisal guide angle, (in dentistry) the inclination of the incisal guide in the frontal plane.

lateralization /lat'ərəl·īzā'shən/, the tendency for certain processes to be more highly developed on one side of the brain than the other, such as development of spatial and musical thoughts in the right hemisphere and verbal and logical processes in the left hemisphere in most persons.

lateral lobes of thyroid gland [L, *latus,* side; Gk, *lobos* + *thyreos,* shield; L, *glans,* acorn], the left and right lobes of a highly vascular thyroid gland situated in front of the neck. The two conical lobes lying on either side of and attached to the larynx are connected by a narrow isthmus.

lateral nystagmus [L, *latus,* side; Gk, *nystagmos,* nodding], an involuntary jerky movement in which the eyes move from side to side.

lateral pectoral nerve, one of a pair of branches from the brachial plexus that, with the medial pectoral nerve, supplies the pectoral muscles.

lateral pelvic displacement, one of the five major kinetic determinants of gait. It helps to synchronize the rhythmic movements of walking and is produced by the horizontal shift of the pelvis or relative hip abduction.

lateral pinch, a grasp in which the thumb is opposed to the middle phalanx of the index finger.

lateral projection, (in radiology) a position of a patient between the x-ray tube and the film cassette so the beam will travel from the left to the right side of the body, or vice versa.

lateral recumbent position, the posture assumed by the patient lying on the left side with the right thigh and knee drawn up.

lateral region, the part of the abdomen in the middle zone on both sides of the umbilical region.

lateral resolution, (in ultrasonography) the resolution of objects in a plane perpendicular to the axis of the beam. It is a measure of the ability of the system to detect closely separated objects such as adjacent blood vessels.

lateral rocking, a sideways rocking of the body used to move the body forward or backward when normal muscle action is not possible. The technique is used by some handicapped patients to move the body to or from the edge of a chair or to a different sitting position on a bed.

lateral rotation, a turning away from the midline of the body.

lateral sinus [L, *latus,* side, *sinus,* hollow], one of the transverse bilateral sinuses of the dura mater that lie along the attached margin of the tentorium cerebelli. They receive the superior sagittal and straight sinuses and drain into the internal jugular veins.

lateral spinal curvature [L, *latus,* side, *spina,* backbone, *curvatura,* bend], a bending or abnormal curve of the vertebral column to the right or left side.

lateral umbilical fold, a fold in the peritoneum produced by a slight protrusion of the inferior epigastric artery and the interfoveolar ligament.

lateral ventricle [L, *latus,* side, *ventriculus,* little belly], a cavity in each cerebral hemisphere that communicates with the third ventricle through the interventricular foramen.

late rickets [Gk, *rhachis,* backbone], a form of rickets in which bone changes because of a kidney defect that results in a vitamin D or calcium deficiency. The disorder tends to affect older children.

lateroduction /lat'ərōduk'shən/, **1.** muscular action in movement to one side or the other. **2.** a turning away from the midline.

laterognathism /lat'ərōnath'izəm/, an asymmetric mandible resulting from irregular growth and development, fractures, tumors, or soft tissue atrophy or hypertrophy.

laterotorsion /-tôr'shən/, displacement of the uterus to one side.

lateroversion /-vur'zhən/, the act of turning over or being deflected from one side to the other.

latex /lā'teks/ [L, liquid], an emulsion or fluidlike sap produced in special cells or vessels of certain plants. Latex contains resins, proteins, and other substances and is a source of rubber. It can cause allergic reactions in some individuals.

latex fixation test [L, *latex,* fluid, *figere,* to fasten], a serologic test used in the diagnosis of rheumatoid arthritis in which antigen-coated latex particles agglutinate with rheumatoid factors in a slide specimen of serum or synovial fluid.

Latex Precautions, a Nursing Interventions Classification defined as reducing the risk of a systemic reaction to latex.

Lathrop, Rose Hawthorne (1851–1926), an American nurse who was a daughter of Nathaniel Hawthorne. She established a home in New York for incurable cancer patients, mostly those who were poor and not accepted in hospitals because of the nature of their disease. She founded the order of sisters called Servants of Relief for Incurable Cancer. The order founded hospitals wherever there was sufficient need and offered quality care to their patients.

latissimus dorsi /latis'iməs dôr'sī/ [L, widest, *dorsum,* the back], one of a pair of large triangular muscles on the thoracic and lumbar areas of the back. The latissimus dorsi extends, adducts, and rotates the arm medially, draws the shoulder back and down, and, with the pectoralis major, draws the body up when climbing.

latitude [L, *latitudio,* breadth], the ability of an x-ray imaging system to produce acceptable images over a range of exposures. If a system has wide latitude, it is possible to image parts of the body that vary in thickness or density with only one exposure.

LATS, abbreviation for **long-acting thyroid stimulator.**

LATS-P, abbreviation for **long-acting thyroid stimulator protector.**

lattice formation [OFr, *lattis,* geometric design], a three-dimensional cross-linked structure formed by the reaction of multivalent antigens with antibodies.

Lauenstein method, (in radiology) a technique for positioning a patient to x-ray the hip joint with emphasis on the relationship of the femur to the acetabulum. The knee of the affected leg is flexed, and the thigh drawn up to a near right angle.

laughing gas /laf'ing/, *informal.* nitrous oxide, a side effect of which is laughter or giggling when administered in less than anesthetizing amounts.

Laurence-Moon-Bardet-Biedl's syndrome /lôr'əns mōōn' bärdā' bē'dəl/ [John Z. Laurence, English ophthalmologist, 1829–1870; Robert C. Moon, American ophthalmologist, 1844–1933; Georges Bardet, French physician, b. 1885; Artur Biedl, Czechoslovakian physician, 1869–1933], a hereditary condition characterized by obesity, hypogenitalism, mental deficiency, polydactylism, and retinitis pigmentosa.

lavage /ləväzh'/ [Fr, washing], **1.** the process of washing out an organ, usually the bladder, bowel, paranasal sinuses, or stomach for therapeutic purposes. **2.** to perform a lavage.

law [AS, *lagu*], **1.** (in a field of study) a rule, standard, or principle that states a fact or a relationship between factors, such as Dalton's law regarding partial pressures of gas. **2.** a rule, principle, or regulation established and promulgated by a government to protect or restrict the people affected.

Law method, (in radiology) any of several techniques for positioning a patient for x-ray examination of the facial bones, sinuses, and relationship of the teeth to the jaw bones.

law of definite composition, (in chemistry) a law stating that a given compound is always made of the same elements present in the same proportion.

law of dominance, formerly considered as a separate principle of Mendel's laws of inheritance, but in modern genetics it is incorporated as part of the first mendelian law, the law of segregation.

law of initial value, the physiologic and psychologic principle that states that, with a given intensity of stimulation, the degree of change produced tends to be greater when the initial value of that variable is low; or the higher the initial level of functioning, the smaller is the change that can be produced.

law of universal gravitation, (in physics) the law stating that the force with which bodies are attracted to each other is directly proportional to the masses of the objects and inversely proportional to the square of the distance by which they are separated.

lawrencium (Lr) /lôren'sē·əm/ [Ernest O. Lawrence, American physicist, 1901–1958], a synthetic transuranic metallic element. Its atomic number is 103; its atomic mass (weight) is 257.

lax, 1. abbreviation for **laxative. 2.** a condition of relaxation or looseness.

laxative (lax) /lak'sətiv/ [L, *laxare,* to loosen], **1.** pertaining to a substance that causes evacuation of the bowel by a mild action. **2.** a laxative agent that promotes bowel evacuation by increasing the bulk of the feces, softening the stool, or lubricating the intestinal wall.

laxative regimen, a diet that ensures an adequate intake of high-fiber bulk foods, including fruits and vegetables, to avoid chronic constipation. The regimen is supplemented with fluids and physical exercise.

lay referral system, an illness referral system through which a person passes from the first recognition of an abnormality to an announcement to the family, to

L

members of the community, to traditional or culturally recognized healers, and then to the regular medical system that includes nurses and physicians. Depending on the culture and the medical care available, some steps may be omitted.

lazy leukocyte syndrome, an immunodeficiency disease of children characterized by recurrent stomatitis, gingivitis, otitis media, and low-grade fever with severe neutropenia.

lb [L, *libra*], abbreviation for **pound.**

lb ap, abbreviation for *apothecary pound.*

lb avdp, abbreviation for *avoirdupois pound.*

LBBB, abbreviation for *left bundle branch block.*

lbd, abbreviation for *lower back disorder.*

lbf, abbreviation for *pound-force.*

lbf/ft², abbreviation for *pound-force per square foot.*

lbf/in², abbreviation for *pound-force per square inch.*

lbm, abbreviation for **lean body mass.**

lbp, 1. abbreviation for **low back pain. 2.** abbreviation for *low blood pressure.*

L-carnitine /elkär′nitēn/, an oral drug for carnitine deficiency prescribed for the treatment of primary systemic carnitine deficiency.

LCAT, abbreviation for **lecithin-cholesterol acetyltransferase.**

LCBF abbreviation for **local cerebral blood flow.**

LCMRG abbreviation for **local cerebral metabolic rate of glucose utilization.**

LD, abbreviation for **lethal dose.**

LD₅₀, symbol for **median lethal dose.**

LDH, abbreviation for **lactate dehydrogenase.**

LDL, abbreviation for **low-density lipoprotein.**

le, abbreviation for *left eye.*

LE, abbreviation for *lupus erythematosus.*

leaching /lē′ching/, removal of the soluble contents of a substance by running water or another liquid through it, leaving the insoluble part behind.

lead (Pb) /led/ [ME, *leed*], a common soft blue-gray metallic element. Its atomic number is 82; its atomic mass (weight) is 207.19. In its metallic form lead is used as a protective shielding against x-rays. Lead is poisonous, a characteristic that has led to a reduction in the use of lead compounds as pigments for paints and inks. Normal concentrations in whole blood are 0 to 5 µg/dl.

lead /lēd/ [AS, *laedan*, to lead], an electrical connection attached to the body to record electrical activity, especially of the heart or brain.

lead apron /led/ [AS, *led* + Fr, *napperon*], a protective shield of lead and rubber that may be worn by a patient, radiologic technologist or radiologist, or both during exposure to x-rays or other diagnostic radiation. It is intended to guard against excessive exposure of the genitalia and other vital body organs to ionizing radiation.

lead-containing eye glasses /led/, a radiographic shielding device for personnel who are exposed to radiation. The glasses reduce exposure to the lens of the eye.

lead encephalopathy /led/ [AS, *led* + Gk, *enkephalos*, brain, *pathos*, disease], a condition of brain structure and function as a result of lead poisoning, including exposure to tetraethyl lead. Children are commonly afflicted after eating chips of lead-based paints. The untreated disorder is characterized by delirium, convulsions, mania, cortical blindness, and coma.

lead equivalent /led/, (in radiology) the thickness of lead required to achieve the same shielding effect against radiation, under specified conditions, as that provided by a given material.

leadership [AS, *leadan*, to lead, *scieppan*, to shape], the ability to influence others to the attainment of goals.

lead pipe fracture /led/, a fracture that compresses the bony tissue at the point of impact and creates a linear fracture on the opposite side of the bone involved.

lead-pipe rigidity /led/, a state of stiffness and inflexibility that remains uniform throughout the range of passive movement. It is associated with diseases of the basal ganglia.

lead poisoning /led/, a toxic condition caused by the ingestion or inhalation of lead or lead compounds. Many children have developed the condition as a result of eating flaked lead paint. Poisoning also occurs from the ingestion of water from lead pipes and lead salts in certain foods and wines, the use of pewter or earthenware glazed with a lead glaze, and the use of leaded gasoline. Inhalation of lead fumes is common in industry. The acute form of intoxication is characterized by a burning sensation in the mouth and esophagus, colic, constipation or diarrhea, mental disturbances, and paralysis of the extremities, followed in severe cases by convulsions and muscular collapse. Chronic lead poisoning, which is characterized by extreme irritability, anorexia, and anemia, may progress to the acute form.

lead shielding /led/, the use of aprons and other devices containing lead as protective measures against radiation. A layer of lead

1 mm in thickness should attenuate 99% of x-rays of 50 kVp and 94% of x-rays of 100 kVp.

leakage radiation /lē′kij/ [ONorse, *leka,* to drip; L, *radiare,* to emit rays], radiation, exclusive of the primary beam, that is emitted through the housing of equipment used in radiation therapy and radiography.

lean body mass (lbm) [ME, *lenen,* slender; AS, *bodig* + ME, *massa,* lump], the combination of cell solids, extracellular and intracellular water, and mineral mass of the body.

learned helplessness /lurnd/, a behavioral state and personality trait of a person who believes that he or she is ineffectual, responses are futile, and control over reinforcers in the environment has been lost.

learning [AS, *leornian,* to learn], **1.** the act or process of acquiring knowledge or some skill by means of study, practice, or experience. **2.** knowledge, wisdom, or a skill acquired through systematic study or instruction. **3.** (in psychology) the modification of behavior through practice, experience, or training.

learning curve, a graphic presentation of the effects of a specified method of teaching or training on the ability of a subject to learn, as shown by improved performance in a particular task.

learning disability, an abnormal condition often affecting children of normal or above-average intelligence, characterized by difficulty in learning such fundamental procedures as reading, writing, and numeric calculation.

learning-disabled adult, a nonspecific difficulty in the learning process, commonly resulting from developmental lag rather than brain damage or demonstrable illness.

learning environment, the sum of the internal and external circumstances and influences surrounding and affecting a person's learning.

Learning Facilitation, a Nursing Interventions Classification defined as promoting the ability to process and comprehend information.

Learning Readiness Enhancement, a Nursing Interventions Classification defined as improving the ability and willingness to receive information.

learning theory [AS, *leornian,* to learn; Gk, *theoria,* speculation], a group of concepts and principles that attempts to explain the learning process. One concept, Guthrie's contiguous conditioning premise, postulates that each response becomes permanently linked with stimuli present at the time so that contiguity rather than reinforcement is a part of the learning process.

Leber's congenital amaurosis /lā′bərz/ [Theodor von Leber, German ophthalmologist, 1840–1917; L, *congenitus,* born with; Gk, *amauroein,* to darken], a rare kind of blindness or severely impaired vision caused by a defect transmitted as an autosomal-recessive trait and occurring at birth or shortly thereafter. The eyes appear normal externally, but pupillary constriction to light is sluggish or absent, and retinal pigment is degenerated.

Leboyer method of delivery /ləboiyā′/ [Frederick LeBoyer, French obstetrician, b. 1918], a psychophysical approach to delivery with the goal of minimizing the trauma of birth by gently and pleasantly introducing the newborn to life outside the womb. It has four aspects: a gentle controlled delivery in a quiet dimly lit room, avoidance of pulling on the head, avoidance of overstimulation of the infant's sensorium, and encouragement of maternal-infant bonding.

LE cell (lupus erythematosus cell), a neutrophil that has phagocytosed the nucleus of another leukocyte that has already been altered by interacting with the LE factor in the bloodstream.

lecithin /les′ithin/ [Gk, *lekithos,* yolk], any of a group of phospholipids common in plants and animals. They are essential for fat metabolism and are used in the processing of foods, pharmaceutical products, cosmetics, and inks.

lecithin-cholesterol acetyltransferase (LCAT) deficiency, an autosomal-recessive disorder characterized by an accumulation of unesterified cholesterol in the tissues, corneal opacity, hemolytic anemia, proteinuria, renal insufficiency, and premature atherosclerosis.

lecithin/sphingomyelin ratio, the ratio of two components of amniotic fluid, used for predicting fetal lung maturity. The normal ratio in amniotic fluid is 2:1 or greater when fetal lungs are mature.

lecithoblast /les′ithəblast′/, an embryonic cell, the primitive entoderm of a two-layered blastodisc.

lecithroprotein /les′ithəprō′tēn/, a compound formed by a combination of lecithin and a protein.

lectin /lek′tin/, a protein substance occurring in seeds and other parts of certain plants that binds with glycoproteins and glycolipids on the surface of animal cells, causing agglutination.

Leech Therapy, a Nursing Interventions Classification defined as application of medicinal leeches to help drain replanted or transplanted tissue engorged with venous blood.

Lee-Davidsohn test, a heterophil antibody test for infectious mononucleosis using horse red blood cells.

Lee-White method [Roger I. Lee, American physician, b. 1881; Paul D. White, American physician, 1886–1973; Gk, *meta,* beyond, *hodos,* way], a method of determining the length of time required for a clot to form in a test tube of venous blood.

left atrium (LA), the uppermost chamber on the left side of the heart. It receives blood from the pulmonary veins.

left brachiocephalic vein [ME, *left,* weak; Gk, *brachys,* short, *kephale,* head], a vessel that starts in the root of the neck at the junction of the internal jugular and the subclavian veins on the left side and runs obliquely across the thorax to join the right brachiocephalic vein and form the superior vena cava.

left common carotid artery, the longer of the two common carotid arteries, arising from the aortic arch and having cervical and thoracic parts.

left coronary artery, one of a pair of branches from the ascending aorta, arising in the left posterior aortic sinus, dividing into the left interventricular artery and the circumflex branch, and supplying both ventricles and the left atrium.

left-handedness /left'han'didnes/, a natural tendency by some persons to favor the use of the left hand in performing certain tasks.

left-heart failure, an abnormal cardiac condition characterized by the impairment of the left side of the heart and elevated pressure and congestion in the pulmonary veins and capillaries. Left-heart failure may be related to right-heart failure, because both sides of the heart are part of a circuit and the impairment of one side will eventually affect the other.

left hepatic duct, the duct that drains the bile from the left lobe of the liver into the common bile duct.

left lateral recumbent position [ME, *left* + L, *latus,* side, *recumbere,* to lie down, *positio*], a position in which the patient lies on the left side with the upper knee and thigh drawn upward.

left pulmonary artery, the shorter and smaller of two arteries conveying venous blood from the heart to the lungs, rising from the pulmonary trunk, and connecting to the left lung.

left subclavian artery, an artery, divided into three parts, that arises from the aortic arch to supply the vertebral column, spinal cord, ear, and brain.

left-to-right shunt, **1.** a diversion of blood from the left side of the heart to the right, such as through a septal defect. **2.** a diversion of blood from the systemic to the pulmonary circulation, such as from a patent ductus arteriosus.

left ventricle (LV), the thick-walled chamber of the heart that pumps blood through the aorta and the systemic arteries, the capillaries, and back through the veins to the right atrium. It has walls about three times thicker than those of the right ventricle and contains a mitral valve with two flaps that controls the flow of blood from the left atrium.

left ventricular assist device (LVAD), a mechanical pump that temporarily and artificially aids the natural pumping action of the left ventricle.

left ventricular failure, heart failure in which the left ventricle fails to contract forcefully enough to maintain a normal cardiac output and peripheral perfusion. Pulmonary congestion and edema develop from back pressure of accumulated blood in the left ventricle. Signs include breathlessness, pallor, sweating, and peripheral vasoconstriction. The heart is usually enlarged.

legacy /leg'əsē/ [L, *legatum,* bequest], something that is handed down from the past or intended to be bestowed on future generations.

legal [L, *lex,* law], actions or conditions that are permitted or authorized by law.

legal blindness [L, *lex,* law; ME, *blend,* sightless], a state of visual acuity in which no better than 20/200 is measured in the better eye with corrective lenses or a visual field of not more than 20 degrees is obtained.

leg cylinder cast [ONor, *leggr* + Gk, *kylindros* + ONorse, *kasta*], an orthopedic device of plaster of paris or fiberglass used to immobilize the leg in treating fractures from the ankle to the upper thigh.

Legg-Calvé-Perthes' disease [Arthur T. Legg, American surgeon, 1874–1939; Jacque Calvé, French orthopedist, 1875–1954; Georg C. Perthes, German surgeon, 1869–1927], osteochondrosis of the head of the femur in children. It is characterized initially by epiphyseal necrosis or degeneration, followed by regeneration or recalcification.

Legionella pneumonia /lē'jənel'ə/ [American Legion; Gk, *pneumon,* lung], a form of pneumonia caused by a gram-negative bacillus identified as *Legionella pneumophila.* It was discovered after an outbreak of the disease among veterans attending a 1976 convention of the American Legion.

Legionella pneumophila /noomof'ələ/,

a small gram-negative rod-shaped bacterium that is the causative agent in **Legionnaires' disease.**

Legionnaires' disease /lē'jənerz'/ [American Legion], an acute bacterial pneumonia caused by infection with *Legionella pneumophila.* It is characterized by an influenza-like illness, followed within a week by high fever, chills, muscle aches, and headache. The symptoms may progress to dry cough, pleurisy, and sometimes diarrhea. Usually the disease is self-limited, but mortality has been 15% to 20% in a few localized epidemics. Contaminated air conditioning cooling towers and stagnant water supplies, including water vaporizers and water sonicators, may be a source of organisms.

legume /leg'yoom/ [L, *legumen,* pulse], any of the members of the Fabales order of dicotyledenous plants, including dried peas, beans, and lentils.

Leiner's disease /lī'nərz/, [Karl Leiner, Austrian pediatrician, 1871–1930], an infant condition of generalized dermatitis, with scaling and erythematosus, as well as seborrheic dermatitis of the scalp.

Leininger, Madeleine, a nursing theorist who is credited with the foundation of transcultural nursing and the resultant nursing research, education, and practice in this subfield of nursing. The most complete account of transcultural care theory is found in her book *Care: The Essence of Nursing and Health* (1984). Some of the major concepts are care, caring, culture, cultural values, and cultural variations. A basic tenet of Leininger's theory is that human beings are inseparable from their cultural background and social structure.

leiomyofibroma /lī'ōmī'ōfībrō'mə/ [Gk, *leios,* smooth, *mys,* muscle; L, *fibra,* fiber; Gk, *oma,* tumor], a tumor consisting of smooth muscle cells and fibrous connective tissue, commonly occurring in the uterus in middle-aged women.

leiomyoma /lī'ōmī·ō'mə/, a benign smooth-muscle tumor occurring most commonly in the uterus, stomach, esophagus, or small intestine.

leiomyoma cutis, a neoplasm of the smooth muscles of the skin. The lesion is characterized by many small, tender red nodules.

leiomyoma uteri, a benign neoplasm of the smooth muscle of the uterus. The tumor is characteristically firm, well circumscribed, round, and gray-white.

leiomyosarcoma /-särkō'mə/ [Gk, *leios,* smooth, *mys,* muscle, *sarx,* flesh, *oma,* tumor], a sarcoma that contains large spindle cells of unstriated muscle.

Leishman-Donovan body /lēsh'məndon'-

əvən/ [William B. Leishman, English pathologist, 1865–1926; Charles Donovan, Irish physician, 1863–1951], the resting stage of an intracellular nonflagellated protozoan parasite *(Leishmania donovani)* that causes kala-azar, or visceral leishmaniasis, as it appears in infected tissue specimens.

Leishmania /lēshmā'nē·ə/ [William B. Leishman], a genus of protozoan parasites. These organisms are transmitted to humans by any of several species of sand flies.

leishmaniasis /lēsh'mənī'əsis/ [William B. Leishman], infection with any species of protozoan of the genus *Leishmania.* The diseases caused by these organisms may be cutaneous or visceral. A typical infection may begin with a cutaneous sore and progress to ulceration of the mouth, palate, and nose. Some cases are accompanied by a febrile illness. There are three major types of leishmaniasis: **visceral leishmaniasis** or **kala-azar, cutaneous leishmaniasis** or **oriental sore,** and **American leishmaniasis. —leishmanial,** *adj.*

lemniscal system /lemnis'kəl/ [Gk, *lemniskos,* fillet, *systema*], a part of the somatosensory network of large-diameter myelinated A fibers. It includes the dorsal columns and the neospinothalamic tract extending from the spinal cord to the thalamus and cortex.

lemniscus /lemnis'kəs/ [Gk, *lemniskos,* fillet], a band or tract of central nervous system fibers, particularly the ascending axons of secondary sensory neurons leading to the thalamus.

Lenègré's disease /lenāgrā/, [Jean Lenègré, twentieth century French cardiologist], sclerodegeneration of the conduction system of the heart that eventually results in complete heart block.

length of stay (LOS), the period of time a patient remains in a hospital or other health care facility as an inpatient.

Lennox-Gastaut's syndrome /len'oks-gästo'/, [William G. Lennox, American neurologist, 1884–1960; Henri Gastaut, French biologist, b. 1914], a condition in which a variety of generalized seizures, such as tonic, tonic-clonic, akinetic, and myoclonic, begin to appear in the first 5 years of life.

lens [L, lentil], **1.** a curved transparent piece of plastic or glass that is shaped, molded, or ground to refract light in a specific way, as in eyeglasses, microscopes, or cameras. **2.** *informal,* the crystalline lens of the eye. **—lenticular,** *adj.*

lens capsule, the clear thin elastic capsule that surrounds the lens of the eye.

lens implant, an artifical lens that is usually implanted at the time of cataract extraction but may also be used for patients with extreme myopia, diplopia, ocular albinism, and certain other abnormalities.

lenticonus /len'tikō'nəs/, an abnormal spheric or conic protrusion on the lens of the eye. It is a congenital defect found in Alport's syndrome.

lenticular nucleus /lentik'yələr/ [L, *lentil,* lens, *nucleus,* nut], biconvex basal ganglia of the cerebrum, composed of lateral putamen and medial globus pallidus tissue as part of the corpus striatum.

lentiform /len'tifôrm/ [L, *lens* + *forma*], pertaining to or resembling a lentil shape, such as the lens of the eye.

lentigo /lentī'gō/, *pl.* **lentigines** /lentij'ənēz/ [L, freckle], a tan or brown macule on the skin brought on by sun exposure, usually in a middle-aged or older person. It is benign.

lentigo maligna melanoma, a neoplasm developing from Hutchinson's freckle on the face or other exposed surfaces of the skin in elderly patients. It is asymptomatic, flat, and tan or brown, with irregular darker spots and frequent hypopigmentation. It is one of the major clinical types of melanoma.

lentivirus /len'tivī'rəs/, a member of a subfamily of retroviruses that includes human immunodeficiency virus. Lentiviruses are usually slow viruses, with long incubation periods that may delay the onset of symptoms until several years after exposure.

Leopold's maneuver [Christian G. Leopold, German physician, 1846–1911], a series of four steps used in palpating the abdomen of a pregnant woman to determine position and presentation of the fetus.

leper /lep'ər/ [Gk, *lepis,* scaly], an outdated term for a person afflicted with leprosy (Hansen's disease).

LE prep, abbreviation for **lupus erythematosus preparation.**

lepromin test /leprō'min/, a skin sensitivity test used to distinguish between the lepromatous and tuberculoid forms of leprosy. The test consists of an intradermal injection of lepromin, which is prepared from heat-sterilized *Mycobacterium leprae.*

leprosarium /lep'rōser'ē·əm/ [Gk, *lepra,* leprosy, sanitarium], a hospital for persons who have Hansen's disease.

leprosy /lep'rəsē/ [Gk, *lepra*], a chronic communicable disease caused by *Mycobacterium leprae* that may take either of two forms, depending on the degree of immunity of the host. Tuberculoid leprosy, seen in those with high resistance, pre-

sents as thickening of cutaneous nerves and anesthetic, saucer-shaped skin lesions. Lepromatous leprosy, seen in those with little resistance, involves many body systems, with widespread plaques and nodules in the skin, iritis, keratitis, destruction of nasal cartilage and bone, testicular atrophy, peripheral edema, and involvement of the reticuloendothelial system. Blindness may result. —**lepromatous, leprotic, leprous,** *adj.*

leptin /lep'tin/ [Gk, thin], a human gene associated with obesity. The gene transmits instructions for the production of a large protein receptor that relays signals to the brain to stop eating, eat less, or burn calories faster.

leptocytosis /lep'tōsītō'sis/ [Gk, *leptos,* thin, *kytos,* cell, *osis,* condition], a hematologic condition in which target cells are present in the blood. Thalassemia, some forms of liver disease, and absence of the spleen are associated with leptocytosis.

leptomeninges /lep'tōminin'jēz/ [Gk, *leptos* + *meninx,* membrane], the arachnoid membrane and the pia mater, two of the three layers covering the brain and spinal cord.

leptomeningitis /-men'inji'tis/, an inflammation of the arachnoid and pia mater layers of the meninges.

leptonema /lep'tənē'mə/ [Gk, *leptos* + *nema,* thread], the threadlike chromosome formation in the leptotene stage in the first meiotic prophase of gametogenesis before the beginning of synapsis.

Leptospira /-spī'rə/ [Gk, *leptos* + *speira,* coil], a genus of the family Treponemataceae, order Spirochaetales; tightly coiled microorganisms having spirals with hooked ends. The spirochete is pathogenic to humans and may cause hepatitis, jaundice, skin hemorrhages, fever, renal failure, mental status changes, and muscular illness.

Leptospira agglutinin, an agglutinin found in the blood of patients with leptospirosis.

leptospirosis /lep'tōspīrō'sis/ [Gk, *leptos* + *speira* + *osis,* condition], an acute infectious disease caused by several serotypes of the spirochete *Leptospira interrogans,* transmitted in the urine of wild or domestic animals, especially rats and dogs. Human infections arise directly from contact with an infected animal's urine or tissues or indirectly from contact with contaminated water or soil. Clinical symptoms may include hepatitis, jaundice, hemorrhage into the skin, fever, chills, renal failure, meningitis with mental status changes, and muscular pain. The most serious form of the disease is called **Weil's disease.**

leptotene /lep′tətēn/ [Gk, *leptos* + *tainia,* ribbon], the initial stage in the first meiotic prophase in gametogenesis in which the chromosomes become visible as single thin filaments.

Leriche's syndrome /lərēshs′/ [Rene Leriche, French surgeon, 1879–1955], a vascular disorder marked by gradual occlusion of the terminal aorta; intermittent claudication in the buttocks, thighs, or calves; absence of pulsation in femoral arteries; pallor and coldness of the legs; gangrene of the toes; and, in men, impotence.

lesbian /lez′bē-ən/ [Gk, island of Lesbos, home of Sappho], 1. a female homosexual. 2. pertaining to the sexual preference or desire of one woman for another. —**lesbianism,** *n.*

Lesch-Nyhan's syndrome /lesh′nī′han/ [Michael Lesch, American pediatrician, b. 1939; William L. Nyhan, Jr., American pediatrician, b. 1926], a hereditary disorder of purine metabolism, characterized by mental retardation, self-mutilation of the fingers and lips by biting, impaired renal function, and abnormal physical development.

Leser-Trélat sign /lā′zər-trālä′/, [Edmund Leser, German surgeon, 1828–1916; Ulysse Trélat, French surgeon, 1828–1890], a condition of malignant cells present in the skin. It is characterized by the sudden onset of seborrheic keratoses with pruritus or enlargement of preexisting keratosis in older adults.

lesion /lē′zhen/ [L, *laesus,* an injury], 1. a wound, injury, or pathologic change in body tissue. 2. any visible, local abnormality of the tissues of the skin, such as a wound, sore, rash, or boil. A lesion may be described as benign, cancerous, gross, occult, or primary.

lesser occipital nerve [AS, *losian,* to lose; L, *occiput,* back of the head, *nervus,* nerve], one of a pair of cutaneous branches of the cervical plexus, arising from the second cervical nerve and ascending along the side of the head behind the ear to supply the skin. It communicates with the posterior auricular branch of the facial nerve.

lesser omentum [AS, *losian,* to lose; L, *omentum,* entrails], a membranous extension of the peritoneum from the peritoneal layers covering the ventral and dorsal surfaces of the stomach and the first part of the duodenum.

lesser sciatic notch [AS, *losian,* to lose; Gk, *ischiadikos,* hip joint; OFr, *enochier*], a notch on the posterior border of the ischium of the hip bone. It is smooth, is

coated with cartilage, and has several ridges corresponding to subdivisions of the obturator internus tendon.

lesser trochanter, one of a pair of conic projections at on the shaft of the femur, just below the neck. It is the site of insertion of the psoas major muscle.

let-down, a sensation in the breasts of lactating women that often occurs as the milk flows into the ducts. It may occur when the infant begins to suck or when the mother hears the baby cry or even thinks of nursing the child.

lethal /lē′thəl/, deadly, capable of causing death.

lethal dose (LD), the amount of toxin that produces death in all members of a species population within a specified period of time.

lethal equivalent [L, *letum,* death, *aequus,* equal, *valere,* to be strong], any recessive gene carried in the heterozygous state that, if homozygous, would be lethal and result in the death of the individual or organism.

lethal gene, any gene that produces a phenotypic effect that causes the death of the organism at some stage of development from conception of the egg to adulthood. The gene may be dominant, incompletely dominant, or recessive.

lethality /lēthal′itē/, the probability that a person threatening suicide will succeed, based on the method described, the specificity of the plan, and the availability of the means.

lethargy /leth′ərjē/ [Gk, *lethargos,* forgetful], the state or quality of dullness, prolonged sleepiness, sluggishness, or serious drowsiness. —**lethargic,** *adj.*

Letterer-Siwe's syndrome /let′ərərzē′və/ [Erich Letterer, German pathologist, b. 1895; Sture A. Siwe, Swedish physician, 1897–1966], any of a group of malignant neoplastic diseases of unknown origin, characterized by histiocytic elements.

leucine (Leu) /lōō′sēn/ [Gk, *leukos,* white], a white crystalline amino acid essential for optimal growth in infants and nitrogen equilibrium in adults. It cannot be synthesized by the body and is obtained by the hydrolysis of food protein during pancreatic enzyme digestion.

leucinosis /lōō′sinō′sis/ [Gk, *leukos* + *osis,* condition], a condition in which the pathways for the degradation of leucine are blocked and large amounts of the amino acid accumulate in body tissue.

leucovorin calcium /lōō′kəvôr′in/, an antianemic prescribed in the treatment of an overdose of a folic acid antagonist and certain cases of megaloblastic anemia.

leukapheresis /lōō′kəfərē′sis/ [Gk, *leukos*

L

+ *aphairesis*, removal], a process by which blood is withdrawn from a vein, white blood cells are selectively removed, and the remaining blood is reinfused in the donor.

leukemia /lookē'mē·ə/ [Gk, *leukos* + *haima*, blood], a broad term given to a group of malignant diseases characterized by diffuse replacement of bone marrow with proliferating leukocyte precursors; abnormal numbers and forms of immature white cells in circulation; and infiltration of lymph nodes, spleen, and liver. The origin of leukemia is not clear, but it may result from genetic predisposition plus exposure to ionizing radiation, benzene, or other chemicals that are toxic to bone marrow. Classification has become increasingly complex, sophisticated, and essential since identification of the subtype has therapeutic and prognostic implications. Leukemia is classified according to the predominant proliferating cells. Acute leukemia usually has a sudden onset and rapidly progresses from early signs such as fatigue, pallor, weight loss, and easy bruising to fever, hemorrhages, extreme weakness, bone or joint pain, and repeated infections. Chronic leukemia develops slowly, and signs similar to those of the acute forms of the disease may not appear for years. —**leukemic,** *adj.*

leukemia cutis, a condition of the skin in which yellow-brown, red, or purple nodular lesions form localized or general diffuse infiltrations.

leukemia inhibitory factor (LIF), a cytokine named for its ability to suppress the spontaneous proliferation of lymphoid stem cells.

leukemogenesis /lookē'mōjen'əsis/, the onset, development, or progression of leukemia.

leukemoid /lookē'moid/, resembling leukemia.

leukemoid reaction [Gk, *leukos* + *eidos*, form; L, *re*, again, *agere*, to act], a clinical syndrome resembling leukemia in which the white blood cell count is elevated in response to an allergy, inflammatory disease, infection, poison, hemorrhage, burn, or severe physical stress.

leukoagglutinin /loo'kō·aglōo'tinin/, an antibody that causes white blood cells to adhere to each other.

leukoblast /loo'kəblast/ [Gk, *leukos*, white, *blastos*, germ], an immature leukocyte, or white blood cell.

leukocyte /loo'kəsīt/ [Gk, *leukos* + *kytos*, cell], a white blood cell, one of the formed elements of the circulating blood system. Five types of leukocytes are classified by the presence or absence of

granules in the cytoplasm of the cell. The agranulocytes are **lymphocytes** and **monocytes**. The granulocytes are **neutrophils, basophils,** and **eosinophils.** —**leukocytic,** *adj.*

leukocyte adhesion deficiency (LAD), an autosomal inherited disorder caused by a defective integrin molecule (CD18) that is important for cellular adhesion. This defect causes neutrophils to be immotile and unable to phagocytose.

leukocyte alkaline phosphatase (LAP), an enzyme present in lymphocytes that is elevated in various diseases such as cirrhosis and polycythemia and in certain infections. It may be measured in the blood to detect these disorders.

leukocytoclastic vasculitis /loo'kəsī'-təklas'tik/, an allergic inflammation of blood vessels, characterized by deposits of fragmented cells, nuclear dust, necrotic debris, and fibrin staining in the vessels.

leukocytogenesis /-jen'əsis/, the origin and development of leukocytes.

leukocytosis /loo'kōsītō'sis/ [Gk, *leukos* + *kytos*, cell, *osis*, condition], an abnormal increase in the number of circulating white blood cells. An increase often accompanies bacterial, but not usually viral, infections. The normal range is 5000 to 10,000 white cells per cubic millimeter of blood. Kinds of leukocytosis include basophilia, **eosinophilia,** and **neutrophilia.**

leukocyturia /loo'kəsītōōr'ē·ə/, the presence of white blood cells in the urine.

leukoderma /lookōdur'mə/ [Gk, *leukos* + *derma*, skin], localized loss of skin pigment caused by several specific causes.

leukodystrophy /-dis'trəfē/ [Gk, *leukos,* white, *dys* + *trophe,* nourishment], a disease of the white matter of the brain, characterized by demyelination.

leukoerythroblastic anemia /loo'kō·-erith'rōblas'tik/ [Gk, *leukos* + *erythros,* red, *blastos*, germ, *a* + *haima*, not blood], an abnormal condition in which large numbers of immature white and red blood cells are present. It is characteristic of some anemias that occur as a result of the replacement of normal bone marrow with malignant tumor.

leukonychia /loo'kōnik'ē·ə/ [Gk, *leukos* + *onyx*, nail], a benign condition in which white patches appear under the nails. Trauma, infection, and many disorders can cause white spots or streaks on nails.

leukopenia /loo'kōpē'nē·ə/ [Gk, *leukos* + *penes*, poor], an abnormal decrease in the number of white blood cells to fewer than 5000 cells per cubic millimeter. The condition may be caused by an adverse drug reaction, radiation poisoning, or pathologic conditions. One or all kinds of white blood cells may be affected. The two most common forms of leukopenia are neutrophilic leukopenia and lymphocytic leukopenia. —**leukopenic,** *adj.*

leukophoresis /lōō'kōfərē'sis/ [Gk, *leukos* + *phoresis,* being transmitted], a laboratory procedure in which white blood cells are separated by electrophoresis for identification and an evaluation of the types of cells and their proportions.

leukoplakia /lōō'kōplā'kē-ə/ [Gk, *leukos* + *plakos,* plate], a precancerous, slowly developing change in a mucous membrane characterized by thickened, white, firmly attached patches that are slightly raised and sharply circumscribed.

leukoplakic vulvitis /-plā'kik/ [Gk, *leukos,* white, *plakos,* plate, *vulva* + *itis,* inflammation], a condition in which the skin of the vulva becomes thick and white, develops bleeding fissures, and later becomes atrophic. The condition may progress to cancer.

leukopoiesis /lōō'kōpō-ē'sis/ [Gk, *leukos* + *poiein,* to make], the process by which white blood cells form and develop. Neutrophils, basophils, and eosinophils are produced in myeloid tissue in the bone marrow. Lymphocytes and monocytes are normally derived from hemocytoblasts in lymphoid tissue, but a few develop in the marrow. —**leukopoietic,** *adj.*

leukorrhea /lōō'kōrē'ə/ [Gk, *leukos* + *rhoia,* flow], a white discharge from the vagina. Normally, vaginal discharge occurs in regular variations in amount and consistency during the course of the menstrual cycle. A greater than usual amount is normal in pregnancy, and a decrease is to be expected after delivery, during lactation, and after menopause.

leukotoxin /loo'kətok'sin/ [Gk, *leukos* + *toxikon,* poison], a substance that can in activate or destroy leukocytes. —**leukotoxic,** *adj.*

leukotrienes /-trī'ēnz/, a class of biologically active compounds that occur naturally in leukocytes and produce allergic and inflammatory reactions similar to those of histamine. They are thought to play a role in the development of allergic and autoallergic disease such as asthma and rheumatoid arthritis.

leukovirus /-vī'rus/ [Gk, *leukos,* white; L, *virus,* poison], any of a group of ribonucleic acid viruses that cause disease in animals.

leuprolide acetate /lōō'prōlīd/, a parenteral antineoplastic drug prescribed for the palliative treatment of advanced prostatic cancer.

levamisole, a drug used as an anthelmintic agent against a wide variety of nematodes.

levator /livā'tər/, *pl.* **levatores** /lev'ətôr'ēz/ [L, *levare,* to lift up], **1.** a muscle that raises a structure of the body, as the levator ani raises parts of the pelvic diaphragm. **2.** a surgical instrument used to lift depressed bony fragments in fractures of the skull and other bones.

levator ani, one of a pair of muscles of the pelvic diaphragm that stretches across the bottom of the pelvic cavity like a hammock, supporting the pelvic organs. It functions to support and slightly raise the pelvic floor. The pubococcygeus draws the anus toward the pubis and constricts it.

levator palpebrae superioris, one of the three muscles of the eyelid, also considered an extrinsic muscle of the eye. It is innervated by the oculomotor nerve. It raises the upper eyelid and is the antagonist of the orbicularis oculi.

levator scapulae, a muscle of the dorsal and lateral aspects of the neck. It acts to raise the scapula and pull it toward the midline.

LeVeen shunt [Harry H. Leveen, American surgeon, b. 1914], a tube that is surgically implanted to connect the peritoneal cavity and the superior vena cava to drain an accumulation of fluid in the peritoneal cavity. It is used in cirrhosis of the liver, right-sided heart failure, or abdominal cancer.

level of activities [OFr, *livel* + L, *activus*], pertaining to the hierarchy of nervous system activity that determines the level responsible for certain functions while also being controlled by a higher level above it, as in the sequence of events in a reflex action.

level of consciousness (LOC) [OFr, *livel* + L, *conscire,* to be aware of], a degree of cognitive function involving arousal mechanisms of the reticular formation of the brain. Impaired LOC may be expressed in obtundation or reduced alertness, stupor, syncope, or unresponsiveness.

level of inquiry [OFr, *livel* + *inquirere,* to ask about], (in nursing research) one of the levels in a rank-ordered system of classification and organization of the questions to be answered in a research study.

levels of care, a classification of health care service levels by the kind of care given, the number of people served, and the people providing the care.

lever /lē'vər, lev'ər/ [L, *levare,* to lift up], (in physiology) any one of the numerous bones and associated joints of the body that act together as a lever so that force applied to one end of the bone to lift a weight at another point tends to rotate the bone in the direction opposite from that of the applied force.

Levine, Myra Estrin, a nursing theorist who developed a framework for nursing practice with the formulation of four conservation principles: energy, structural integrity, personal integrity, and social integrity. The first edition of her book using the conservation principles, *Introduction to Clinical Nursing,* was published in 1969. Levine's emphasis on the ill person in the health care setting reflects the history of health care in the 1960s. Levine's model stresses nursing interventions and interactions based on the scientific background of these principles.

Levin tube /lev'in/ [Abraham L. Levin, American physician, 1880–1940], a plastic catheter introduced through the nose and used in gastric intubation for gastric decompression or gavage feeding.

levitation /lev'itā'shən/ [L, *levitas,* lightness, *atus,* process], (in psychiatry) a hallucinatory sensation of floating or rising in the air. **—levitate,** *v.*

levobunolol hydrochloride /-bun'əlol/, a topical ophthalmic beta-adrenergic blocker drug for glaucoma. It is prescribed for the treatment of chronic open-angle glaucoma and ocular hypertension.

levocardia /-kär'dē-ə/, a congenital anomaly in which the viscera are transposed to the opposite side of the body, except for the heart, which is in its normal position.

levodopa /lē'vōdō'pə/, an antiparkinsonian prescribed in the treatment of Parkinson's disease, juvenile forms of Huntington's disease, and chronic manganese poisoning.

levopropoxyphene napsylate /-prōpək'-sifēn/, an antitussive prescribed for cough.

levorphanol tartrate /lē'vôrfā'nol/, a narcotic analgesic prescribed for pain and preoperative analgesia.

levothyroxine sodium /-thī'rəksēn/, a thyroid hormone prescribed in the treatment of hypothyroidism.

levotorsion /-tôr'shən/, the rotation to the left of the upper pole of the cornea of one or both eyes.

Lev's disease [Maurice Lev, American pathologist, b. 1908], fibrosis or calcification of the conduction system of the heart that results in varying degrees of heart block in patients with normal myocardium and coronary arteries.

Lewis Blood Group System, a blood-group system based on antigens present in soluble forms in blood and secretions. The antigens are adsorbed from the plasma onto the red cell membrane. The expressed Lewis phenotype is based on whether the patient is a secretor or nonsecretor of the Lewis gene product. The system was named for a Mrs. Lewis, an English patient in whom these antibodies were discovered in 1946.

lewisite /lōo'isīt/ [Winford L. Lewis, American chemist, 1878–1943], 2-chlorovinyl arsine; a poisonous blister gas, used in World War I, that causes irritation of the lungs, dyspnea, damage to the tissues of the respiratory tract, tears, and pain.

Lewy bodies /lā'wē, lōo'ē [Frederick H. Lewy, German neurologist, 1885–1950], concentric spheres found inside vacuoles in midbrain and brainstem neurons in patients with idiopathic parkinsonism, Alzheimer's disease, and other neurodegenerative conditions.

Leyden-Möbius muscular dystrophy /lī'-dən-m'bē-əs, -mē'bē-əs/, a form of limb-girdle muscular dystrophy that begins in the pelvic girdle.

Leydig cells /lī'dig/ [Franz von Leydig, German anatomist, 1821–1908], cells of the interstitial tissue of the testes that secrete testosterone.

Leydig cell tumor, a generally benign neoplasm of interstitial cells of a testis that may cause gynecomastia in adults and precocious sexual development if the lesion occurs before puberty.

LF, abbreviation for *low frequency.*

LFA, abbreviation for *left frontoanterior fetal position.*

LFP, abbreviation for *left frontoposterior fetal position.*

LFT, abbreviation for **liver function test.**

LGA, abbreviation for *large for gestational age.*

LGV, abbreviation for **lymphogranuloma venereum.**

LH, abbreviation for **luteinizing hormone.**

Lhermitte's sign /ler'mits/ [Jacques J. Lhermitte, French neurologist, 1877–1959], sudden, transient, electric-like shocks spreading down the body when the head is flexed forward, occurring chiefly in multiple sclerosis but also in compression disorders of the cervical spinal cord.

LHRH, abbreviation for **luteinizing hormone-releasing hormone.**

Li, symbol for the element **lithium.**

liability /lī'əbil'itē/ [L, *ligare,* to bind], **1.** something one is obligated to do or an obligation required to be fulfilled by law, usually financial in nature. **2.** the amount of money required to fulfill a financial obligation.

liaison nursing /lē-ā'zən/, an arrangement with clinical specialists in psychiatric nursing whereby nurses and health professionals in other disciplines obtain consultation services in medical-surgical, parent-child, and geriatric settings.

libel /lī′bəl/ [L, *libellus,* little book], a false accusation written, printed, or typewritten or presented in a picture or a sign that is made with malicious intent to defame the reputation of a person who is living or the memory of a person who is dead, resulting in public embarrassment, contempt, ridicule, or hatred.

liberation /lib′ərā′shən/ [L, *liber,* free], the process of drug release from the dosage form.

libidinous /libid′inəs/ [L, *libidinosus,* lustful], **1.** pertaining to or belonging to the libido. **2.** having or characterized by sexual desire. —**libidinize,** *v.*

libido /libē′dō, libī′dō/, **1.** the psychic energy or instinctual drive associated with sexual energy, pleasure, or creativity. **2.** (in psychoanalysis) the instinctual drives of the id. **3.** lustful desire or striving.

Libman-Sacks endocarditis /lib′mənsaks′/ [Emanuel Libman, American physician, 1872–1946; Benjamin Sacks, American physician, 1896–1939], an abnormal condition and the most common manifestation of lupus erythematosus, characterized by verrucous lesions that develop near the heart valves but rarely affect valvular action.

lice, *sing.* **louse** [AS, *lus*], any of the small wingless insect order of Anoplura. Lice are ectoparasites of birds and mammals and may spend their entire life cycle on a single host, attaching eggs to the hair shafts or feathers. They transfer to humans by direct contact. Three forms that infect humans are the **head louse,** *Pediculus humanus capitis;* the **body louse,** *Pediculus humanus corporis;* and the **crab louse,** *Phthirus pubis.*

license, an agency-or government-granted permission issued to a health-care professional to engage in a given occupation on finding that the applicant has attained the degree of competency necessary to ensure that the public health, safety, and welfare are reasonably well-protected.

licensed practical nurse (LPN) /lī′sənst/ [L, *licere,* to be allowed; Gk, *praktikos,* fit for action; L, *nutrix,* nurse], *U.S.* a person trained in basic nursing techniques and direct patient care who practices under the supervision of a registered nurse. The course of training usually lasts 1 year. In Canada an LPN is called a certified nursing assistant.

licensed psychologist, a person who has earned a PhD in psychology from an ac-

credited graduate school and who has completed 2 to 3 years of postgraduate training with special emphasis on the diagnosis and treatment of psychologic disorders.

licensure /lī′sənshŏŏr/ [L, *licere,* to be allowed], the granting of permission by a competent authority (usually a government agency) to an organization or individual to engage in a practice or activity that would otherwise be illegal. Kinds of licensure include the issuing of licenses for general hospitals or nursing homes, for health professionals such as physicians, and for the production or distribution of biologic products.

lichen amyloidosis /lī′kən/, a common form of amyloidosis. The condition is characterized by symmetric distribution over the skin of translucent yellowish-brown dome-shaped pruritic papules.

lichenification /līken′ifikā′shən/ [Gk, *leichen,* lichen, *facere,* to make], thickening and hardening of the skin, often resulting from the irritation caused by repeated scratching of a pruritic lesion. —**lichenified,** *adj.*

lichen nitidus [Gk, *leichen* + L, *nitidus,* bright], a rare skin disorder characterized by numerous flat, glistening, pale, discrete papules measuring 2 to 3 mm in diameter.

lichenoid eczema /lī′kənoid/, a chronic inflammatory cutaneous condition characterized by skin thickening and accentuated skin lesions.

lichen planus, a nonmalignant, chronic, pruritic skin disease of unknown cause that is characterized by small flat purplish papules or plaques with fine gray lines on the surface.

lichen sclerosis et atrophicus, a chronic skin disease characterized by white flat papules and black hard follicular plugs. In advanced cases the papules tend to coalesce into large white patches of thin pruritic skin.

lichen simplex chronicus, a form of dermatitis characterized by a patch of pruritic confluent papules.

licorice /lik′ərish, -ris/ [Gk, *glykys,* sweet, *rhiza,* root], a dried root of gummy texture from the leguminous plant *Glycyrrhiza glabra.* It has a sweet, astringent taste and is used as a flavoring agent in medicines, especially in cough syrups and laxatives. It may cause an elevation of blood pressure.

lidocaine hydrochloride /lī′dəkān/, a local anesthetic agent prescribed as a local anesthetic for topical administration to skin or mucous membranes. It is used parenterally as an antiarrhythmic agent.

L

lie [AS, *licgan,* position], the relationship between the long axis of the fetus and the long axis of the mother. In a longitudinal lie the fetus is lying lengthwise, or vertically, in the uterus, whereas in a transverse lie the fetus is lying crosswise, or horizontally.

Lieberkühn's glands /lē'bərkēnz/ [Johann N. Lieberkühn, German anatomist, 1711–1756; L, *glans,* acorn], tubular glands between the bases of the villi of the small intestine and on the surface of the epithelium of the large intestine.

lie detector [AS, *leogan,* untruth; L, *detegere,* to uncover], an electronic device or instrument used to detect lying or anxiety in regard to specific questions. A commonly used lie detector is the polygraph recorder that senses and records pulse, respiratory rate, blood pressure, and perspiration.

lienal vein /lī'ənəl, lē-ē'nəl/ [L, *lien,* spleen, *vena*], a large vein of the lower body that unites with the superior mesenteric vein to form the portal vein. It returns blood from the spleen.

lienography /lē'ənog'rəfē/, the radiographic examination of the spleen after it has been injected with a contrast medium.

LIF, abbreviation for **leukemia inhibitory factor.**

life [AS, *lif*], the energy that enables organisms to grow, reproduce, absorb and use nutrients, evolve, and in some organisms achieve mobility, express consciousness, and demonstrate a voluntary use of the senses.

life costs [AS, *lif* + L, *constare,* constant], the mortality, morbidity, and suffering associated with a given disease or medical procedure.

life cycle, 1. the interval of time covered during the sequence of events from conception and birth, through growth and maturity, to natural death. **2.** the series of stages from any stage of one generation to the same stage of the next generation.

life expectancy, the probable number of years a person will live after a given age, as determined by mortality in a specific geographic area. It may be individually qualified by the person's condition or race, sex, age, or other demographic factors.

life extension [AS, *lif,* life; L, *extenere,* to stretch out], the process of extending the life span of an individual or population by intervention that promotes better use of preventive medicine and use of established diagnostic and therapeutic facilities.

life island, a plastic bubble enclosing a bed, used to provide a germ-free environment for patients with a specific kind of immune deficit.

life review, 1. (in psychiatry) a progressive return to consciousness of past experiences. **2.** reminiscences that occur in old age as a consequence of the realization of the inevitability of death.

lifesaving measure, any independent, interdependent, or dependent nursing intervention that is implemented when a patient's physical or psychologic status is threatened.

life science, the study of the laws and properties of living matter.

life space, a term introduced by American psychologist Kurt Lewin to describe simultaneous influences that may affect individual behavior. The totality of the influences make up the life space.

life span, the length of life of an individual or the average length of life in a population or species.

life-style–induced health problems, diseases with natural histories that include conscious exposure to certain health-compromising or risk factors.

life support [AS, *lif,* life; L, *supportare,* to bring up to], the use of any therapeutic technique or device to maintain life functions.

lifetime reserve [AS, *lif* + *tid,* time; L, *re,* again, *servare,* to keep], a lifetime total of days of inpatient hospitalization benefits that may be drawn on by a patient who has exhausted the maximum benefits allowed under Medicare for a single spell of illness.

Li-Fraumeni cancer syndrome /lē'-frômen'ē/, [Frederick P. Li; Joseph F. Fraumeni, Jr.; twentieth-century American epidemiologists], a type of familial breast carcinoma affecting young women and associated with soft-tissue sarcomas and other cancers in close relatives.

lift assessment [AS, *lyft,* loft; L, *assidere,* to sit beside], the selection of the most appropriate lift method to use when moving a patient, as from the bed to a chair.

ligament /lig'əmənt/ [L, *ligare,* to bind], **1.** one of many predominantly white, shiny, flexible bands of fibrous tissue binding joints together and connecting various bones and cartilages. **2.** a layer of serous membrane with little or no tensile strength, extending from one visceral organ to another, such as the ligaments of the peritoneum. **—ligamentous,** *adj.*

ligamenta flava [L, *ligare* + *flavus,* yellow], the bands of yellow elastic tissue connecting the laminae of adjacent vertebrae from the axis to the first segment of the sacrum.

ligamental tear /lig'əmen'təl/ [L, *ligare,* to bind; AS, *teran,* to destroy], a complete or partial tear of a ligamentous structure connecting and surrounding the bones of a joint, caused by an injury to the joint, as by a sudden twisting motion or a forceful blow. Ligamental tears may occur at any joint but are most common in the knees.

ligament of the neck of the rib, one of five ligaments of each costotransverse joint, consisting of short, strong fibers passing from the neck of the rib to the transverse process of the adjacent vertebra.

ligament of the tubercle of the rib, one of the five ligaments of each costotransverse joint, comprising a short thick fasciculus passing obliquely from the transverse process of a vertebra to the tubercle of the associated rib.

ligamentum nuchae /lig′əmen′təm/, the fibrous membrane that reaches from the external occipital protuberance and median nuchal line to the spinous process of the seventh vertebra.

ligand /lig′ənd, lī′gənd/ [L, *ligare*, to bind], **1.** a molecule, ion, or group bound to the central atom of a chemical compound, such as the oxygen molecule in hemoglobin, which is bound to the central iron atom. **2.** an organic molecule attached to a specific site on a cell surface or to a tracer element.

ligases /lī′gāsəz/ [L, *ligare* + Fr, *diastase*, enzyme], a group of enzymes that catalyze the formation of a bond between substrate molecules coupled with the breakdown of a pyrophosphate bond in adenosine triphosphate or a similar donor molecule.

ligation /līgā′shən/ [L, *ligare*, to bind], the procedure of tying off a blood vessel or duct with a suture or wire ligature. It may be performed to stop or prevent bleeding during surgery, to stop spontaneous or traumatic hemorrhage, to prevent passage of material through a duct as in tubal ligation, or to treat varicosities. —**ligate,** *v.*

ligature /lig′əchər/ [L, *ligare*, to bind], **1.** a suture. **2.** a wire, as used in orthodontia.

ligature needle, a long, thin curved needle used for passing a suture underneath an artery for ligation of the vessel.

ligature wire [L, *ligare*, to bind; AS, *wir*], a soft thin wire used in dental procedures, particularly to connect brackets or attachments in orthodontic appliances.

light [AS, *leoht*], **1.** electromagnetic radiation of the wavelength and frequency that stimulate visual receptor cells in the retina to produce nerve impulses that are perceived as vision. **2.** electromagnetic radiation with wavelengths shorter than ultraviolet light and longer than infrared

light, the range of visible light generally in the range of 400 to 800 nm.

light-adapted eye [AS, *leoht* + L, *adaptatio* + AS, *eage*], an eye that has been exposed to bright light long enough for chemical and physiologic changes to take place, such as bleaching of the rhodopsin or visual purple. The loss of cone sensitivity to light may require increased light intensity to obtain the same degree of visual acuity.

light bath, the exposure of the patient's uncovered skin to the sun or to actinic light rays from an artificial source for therapeutic purposes.

light chain, a subunit of an immunoglobulin molecule composed of a polypeptide chain of about 22,000 daltons, or atomic mass units.

light chain deficiency, an alteration in the kappa or lambda light chains of immunoglobulins that is associated with immunodeficiency diseases such as megaloblastic anemia and diarrhea.

light chain disease, a type of multiple myeloma in which plasma cell tumors produce only monoclonal light chain proteins. Persons with light chain disease may develop lytic bone lesions, hypercalcemia, impaired kidney function, and amyloidosis.

lightening /līt′əning/ [AS, *leoht*, light], a subjective sensation reported by many women late in pregnancy as the fetus settles lower in the true pelvis, leaving more space in the upper abdomen.

light film fault [AS, *leoht*, light, *filmen*, membrane; L, *fallere*, to deceive], a defect in a radiograph or developed photographic film that appears as a barely distinct and inadequate image.

light-headedness, a condition of feeling giddy, faint, delirious, or slightly dizzy.

light microscope [AS, *leoht* + Gk, *mikros*, small, *skopein*, to view], a microscope that uses visible light to view objects too small for the naked eye to see.

light reflex, the mechanism by which the pupil of the eye constricts in response to direct or consensual stimulation with light.

light scatter, light dispersion in any direction by suspended particles in a solution. The degree of scattering depends on the size and shape of the particles.

light therapy [AS, *leoht* + Gk, *therapeia*, treatment], exposure of the body to electromagnetic waves of the infrared, ultraviolet, or visible spectrum for therapeutic purposes. In the winter months light therapy may be used to treat depressive disorders.

light-touch palpations [AS, *leoht* + Fr, *toucher* + L, *palpare*, to touch gently],

L

a method of examination by gently depressing the abdomen 1 to 2 cm to outline the size and position of abdominal organs.

ligneous /lig′nē-əs/ [L, *ligum,* wood], woody or resembling wood in texture or other characteristics.

lignin /lig′nin/ [L, *lignum,* wood], a polysaccharide that with cellulose and hemicellulose forms the chief part of the skeletal substances of the cell walls of plants.

lilliputian hallucination /lil′ipyōo′shən/ [Lilliput, mythic island in Swift's *Gulliver's Travels*], a hallucination in which things seem smaller than they actually are.

limb /lim/ [AS, *lim*], **1.** an appendage or extremity of the body, such as an arm or leg. **2.** a branch of an internal organ, such as a loop of a nephron.

limb-girdle muscular dystrophy [AS, *lim,* limb, *gyrdel*], a form of muscular dystrophy transmitted as an autosomal-recessive trait. The characteristic weakness and degeneration of the muscles begins in the shoulder girdle or the pelvic girdle. The condition is progressive, regardless of the area in which it is first manifest.

limbic /lim′bik/ [L, *limbus,* edge], pertaining to something that is marginal or at a junction between structures.

limbic lobe [L, *limbus,* edge; Gk, *lobos,* lobe], the marginal section of the cerebral hemispheres on the medial aspects. It forms a ring of neural tissue around the hypothalamus and some nuclei.

limbic system [L, *limbus,* edge], a group of structures within the rhinencephalon of the brain that are associated with various emotions and feelings such as anger, fear, sexual arousal, pleasure, and sadness. The structures of the limbic system include the cingulate gyrus, the isthmus, the hippocampal gyrus, the uncus, and the amygdala. The structures connect with various other parts of the brain.

limb lead /lēd/ [AS, *lim,* limb, *laeden,* lead], (in electrocardiography) an electrode that is attached to an arm or a leg.

limbus /lim′bəs/, an edge or border, such as the corneal limbus at the edge of the cornea bordering the sclera.

lime [AS, *lim*], **1.** any of several oxides and hydroxides of calcium. **2.** a citrus fruit yielding a juice with a high ascorbic acid content. Lime juice was one of the first effective agents to be used in the treatment of scurvy.

limitation of motion /lim′itā′shən/ [L, *limes,* limit], the restriction of or reduction to a normal range of motion of a body part caused by disease or injury.

limited fluctuation method of dosing [L, *limes,* limit, *fluctuare,* to wave], a method of drug administration in which the dose is not allowed to rise or fall beyond specified maximum and minimum limits.

limiting charge, the maximum amount that can be charged in the United States for the services of a physician who does not accept the restrictions on fees established by Medicare laws.

limiting resolution, (in computed tomography) the spatial frequency at a modulation transfer function equal to 0.1. The absolute object size that can be resolved by a scanner is equal to the reciprocal of the spatial frequency.

limit of stability, the greatest distance in any direction a person can lean away from a midline vertical position without falling, stepping, or reaching for support.

Limit Setting, a Nursing Interventions Classification defined as establishing the parameters of desirable and acceptable patient behavior.

limp [ME, not firm], an abnormal pattern of ambulation in which the two phases of gait are markedly asymmetric.

LINAC, abbreviation for **linear accelerator.**

lincomycin hydrochloride /lin′kəmī′sin/, an antibiotic prescribed in the treatment of certain infections.

lindane /lin′dān/, gamma-benzene hexachloride prescribed in the treatment of pediculosis and scabies.

Lindbergh pump [Charles A. Lindbergh, American technician, 1902–1974; ME, *pumpe*], a pump used to preserve an organ of the body by perfusing its tissues with oxygen and other essential nutrients, usually during the transport of an organ from a donor to a recipient.

line [L, *linea*], **1.** a connection between two points. **2.** a stripe, streak, or narrow ridge, often imaginary, that serves to connect reference points or to separate various parts of the body, as the hairline or nipple line. **3.** a black absorption line in a continuous spectrum passing through a medium. **4.** an accretion line in the enamel of a tooth marking successive layers of calcification. **5.** a catheter or wire that may be inserted in a vein, as an intravenous line. **6.** the base line of an electrocardiogram when neither positive nor negative potentials are recorded. **7.** line of sight.

linea [L, *line*], a line defining anatomic features.

linea alba /lin′ē-ə/ [L, *linea,* line, *albus,* white], the part of the anterior abdominal aponeurosis in the middle line of the abdomen, representing the fusion of three aponeuroses into a single tendinous band extending from the xiphoid process to the symphysis pubis. It contains the umbilicus.

linea albicantes, lines, white to pink or gray, that occur on the abdomen, buttocks, breasts, and thighs and are caused by the stretching of the skin and weakening or rupturing of the underlying elastic tissue.

linea arcuata, the curved tendinous band in the sheath of the rectus abdominis below the umbilicus. It inserts into the linea alba.

linea aspera, the posterior crest of the femur (thigh bone) that extends proximally into three ridges to which are attached various muscles, including the gluteus maximus, pectineus, and iliacus.

linea nigra, a dark line appearing longitudinally on the abdomen of a pregnant woman during the latter 24 weeks of term. It usually extends from the symphysis pubis midline to the umbilicus.

linear /lin′ē·ər/ [L, *linea,* line], pertaining to a line or lines, particularly straight lines.

linear accelerator (LINAC) [L, *linea,* line, *accelerare,* to quicken], an apparatus for accelerating charged subatomic particles used in radiotherapy, physics research, and the production of radionuclides.

linear array, (in radiology) a contiguous sequence of identical discrete detectors, either gas-filled ionization chambers or solid-state semiconductors, used with a fan beam x-ray generator. The detectors read off once for each x-ray pulse. The resulting electronic signal is converted to a digital number and stored in a computer memory.

linear energy transfer (LET), (in radiology) the rate at which energy is transferred from ionizing radiation to soft tissue. It is expressed in terms of kiloelectron volts per micrometer of track length in soft tissue.

linear flow velocity, the velocity of a particle carried in a moving stream, usually measured in centimeters per second.

linear fracture, a fracture that extends parallel to the long axis of a bone but does not displace the bone tissue.

linear IgA bullous disease, a condition characterized by linear deposits of IgA binding to the area of the lamina lucida. Tense bullae are frequent, and the vesicles are likely to occur on the face, thighs, feet, and flexures. The disease tends to affect women more than men.

linearity /lin′ē·er′itē/, (in radiology) the ability to obtain the same exposure for the same milliampere-seconds (mAs), regardless of mA and exposure time used.

linear regression, a statistical procedure in which a straight line is established through a data set that best represents a relationship between two subsets or two methods.

linear scan, (in ultrasonography) the motion of the transducer at a constant speed along a straight line at right angles to the beam.

linear staining, the use of fluorescein-labeled goat or rabbit antiimmunoglobulins to produce smooth-staining patterns for study by immunofluorescence microscopy.

linear tomography, tomography that produces a blurring pattern with linear, or unidirectional, motion. The pattern is caused by elongation of structures outside the focal plane.

linea semilunaris, the slightly curved line on the ventral abdominal wall, approximately parallel to the median line and lying about halfway between the median line and the side of the body. It marks the lateral border of the rectus abdominis and is visible as a shallow groove when that muscle is tensed.

linea terminalis, a hypothetical line dividing the upper, or false, pelvis, from the lower, or true, pelvis.

line compensator, an electrical device that monitors electric power for medical devices such as x-ray equipment and makes adjustments for voltage fluctuations.

line of demarcation [L, *linea* + *de* + *marcare,* to mark], a line that indicates a change in the condition of tissues, such as the boundary between gangrenous and healthy tissues.

line of gravity, an imaginary line that extends from the center of gravity to the base of support.

line pair (lp), (in computed tomography and radiography) a factor in determining spatial frequency. It consists of a bar, or line, and its adjacent equal width interspace, forming a pair. As line pairs per centimeter increase, the fidelity of the line pair image decreases.

Lineweaver-Burk transformation /lī′-nwe′vərburk′/ [Hans Lineweaver, American chemist, b. 1907; Dean Burk, American scientist, 1904–1988; L, *transformare,* to change shape], a method of converting experimental data from studies of enzyme activity so that they can be displayed on a linear plot.

lingual /ling′gwəl/ [L, *lingua,* tongue], pertaining to or resembling the tongue.

lingual artery [L, *lingua,* tongue], one of a pair of arteries that arises from the external carotid arteries and supplies the tongue and surrounding muscles.

lingual bar, a major connector that is in-

L

stalled on the tongue side of the dental arch and joins bilateral parts of a mandibular removable partial denture.

lingual crib, an orthodontic appliance consisting of a wire frame suspended behind the maxillary incisor teeth. It is used for obstructing undesirable thumb and tongue habits that can produce malocclusions.

lingual flange, the part of a mandibular denture that occupies the space adjacent to the residual ridge and next to the tongue.

lingual gingiva [L, *lingua*, tongue, *gingiva*, gum], the gingival tissue covering the teeth on the surfaces facing the tongue.

lingual goiter, a tumor at the back of the tongue formed by an enlargement of the primordial thyrolingual duct.

lingualis leukoplakia [L, *lingua*, tongue; Gk, *leukos*, white, *plako*, plate], a chronic inflammatory lesion characterized by smooth thick white patches on the surface of the tongue, generally attributed to excessive use of alcohol and tobacco. The lesions may be a precursor of epithelioma.

lingual pain, a pain in the tongue, which may be caused by biting the tongue, heavy metal poisoning, Vincent's stomatitis, or infiltration of the lingual muscles by a neoplasm.

lingual rest, a metallic extension onto the tongue side of an anterior tooth to provide support or indirect retention for a removable partial denture.

lingual thyroid, residual thyroid tissue at the base of the tongue that failed to descend into the neck during embryologic development.

lingual tonsil, a mass of lymphoid follicles near the root of the tongue.

lingula /ling′gyələ/ [L, small tongue], any anatomic structure that resembles a tongue.

lingula of the lung [L, *lingula*, small tongue; AS, *lungen*], a tonguelike projection from the costal surface of the upper lobe of the left lung.

lingulectomy /ling′fyəlek′təmē/, a surgical excision of the tongue-shaped lingula part of the left upper lobe of the lung.

liniment /lin′imənt/ [L, *linere*, to smear], a preparation, usually containing an alcoholic, oily, or soapy vehicle, that is rubbed on the skin as a counterirritant.

linin /li′nin/ [Gk, *linon*, flax], the faintly staining threads seen in the nuclei of cells, with granules of chromatin attached to the threads.

linitis /linī′tis/ [Gk, *linon*, flax, *itis*, inflammation], inflammation of cellular tissue of the stomach as in linitis plastica, seen frequently in adenocarcinoma of the stomach.

linitis plastica, a diffuse fibrosis and thickening of the wall of the stomach, resulting in a rigid, inelastic organ. The layer of connective tissue of the stomach becomes fibrotic and thick, and the stomach wall becomes shrunken and rigid. Causes of this condition include infiltrating undifferentiated carcinoma, syphilis, and Crohn's disease involving the stomach.

linkage /ling′kij/ [Gk, *linke*, connection], **1.** (in genetics) the location of two or more genes on the same chromosome so that they do not segregate independently during meiosis but tend to be transmitted together as a unit. The closer the loci of the genes, the more likely they are to be inherited as a group and associated with a specific trait. **2.** (in psychology) the association between a stimulus and the response it elicits. **3.** (in chemistry) the bond between two atoms or radicals in a chemical compound.

linkage disequilibrium, a nonrandom association of two genes on the same chromosome.

linkage group, (in genetics) a group of genes located on the same chromosome that tends to be inherited as a unit.

linked genes [Me, *linke* + Gk, *genein*, to produce], genes that are located on the same chromosome and whose position is close enough so that they tend to be transmitted as a linkage group.

linker [ME, *linke*, connection], (in molecular genetics) a small segment of synthetic deoxyribonucleic acid (DNA) having a place on its surface that can be ligated to DNA fragments in cloning.

linoleic acid /lin′əlē′ik/ [Gk, *linon*, flax, *oleum*, oil], a colorless to straw-colored essential fatty acid with two unsaturated bonds, occurring in linseed and safflower oils.

linolenic acid /lin′ōlen′ik/ [Gk, *linon*, flax, *oleum*, oil], an unsaturated fatty acid essential for normal human nutrition. It occurs in glycerides of linseed and other vegetable oils.

liothyronine sodium /lī′ōthī′rənēn/, a synthetic thyroid hormone prescribed in the treatment of primary hypothyroidism, myxedema, simple goiter, cretinism, and secondary hypothyroidism.

liotrix /lī′ətriks/, a uniform mixture of the thyroid hormones T_3 and T_4. It is prescribed in the treatment of hypothyroid conditions.

lip [AS, *lippa*], **1.** either the upper or lower fleshy structure surrounding the opening of the oral cavity. **2.** any rimlike structure bordering a cavity or groove; labium.

LIP, abbreviation for **lymphocytic interstitial pneumonia.**

lipase /lī′pās, lip′ās/ [Gk, *lipos*, fat; Fr, *diastase*, enzyme], any of several enzymes produced by the organs of the digestive system that catalyze the breakdown of lipids through the hydrolysis of the linkages between fatty acids and glycerol in triglycerides and phospholipids.

lipectomy /lipek′təmē/ [Gk, *lipos* + *ektome*, excision], an excision of subcutaneous fat, as from the abdominal wall.

lipedema /lip′ədē′mə/, a condition in which fat deposits accumulate in the lower extremities from the hips to the ankles, accompanied by symptoms of tenderness in the affected areas.

lipemia /lipē′mē·ə/ [Gk, *lipos* + *haima*, blood], a condition in which increased amounts of lipids are present in the blood, a normal occurrence after eating.

lipid /lip′id, lī′pid/ [Gk, *lipos*, fat, *eidos*, form], any of the free fatty acid fractions in the blood. They are stored in the body and serve as an energy reserve, but are elevated in various diseases such as atherosclerosis. Kinds of lipids are **cholesterol, fatty acids, neutral fat, phospholipids,** and **triglycerides.**

lipidosis /lip′idō′sis/ [Gk, *lipos* + *osis,* condition], a general term that includes several rare familial disorders of fat metabolism. The chief characteristic of these disorders is the accumulation of abnormal levels of certain lipids in the body. Kinds of lipidoses are **Gaucher's disease, Krabbe's disease, Niemann-Pick's disease,** and **Tay-Sachs' disease.**

lipid pneumonia, an inflammation of the spongy tissue of the lung caused by inhalation of oil droplets into the alveoli.

lipiduria /lip′idŏŏr′ē·ə/, the presence of lipids (fatty bodies) in the urine.

lipoatrophic diabetes /lip′ō·atrof′ik/, an inherited disease characterized by insulin-resistant diabetes mellitus, loss of body fat, acanthosis nigricans, and hypertrophied musculature. It is associated with a disorder of the hypothalamus resulting in excessive blood levels of growth hormone and adrenocorticotropic-releasing hormones.

lipoatrophy /lip′ō·at′rəfē/, a breakdown of subcutaneous fat at the site of an insulin injection. It usually occurs after several injections at the same site.

lipochrome /lip′əkrōm/ [Gk, *lipos* + *chroma*, color], any of the naturally occurring pigments that contain a lipid and give a yellow color to fats, such as carotene.

lipodystrophia progressiva /-distrō′fē·ə/ [Gk, *lipos* + *dys,* bad, *trophe,* nourishment; L, *progredior,* to go forth], an abnormal accumulation of fat around the buttocks and thighs and a progressive, symmetric disappearance of subcutaneous fat from areas above the pelvis and on the face.

lipodystrophy /lip′ōdis′trəfē/ [Gk, *lipos* + *dys,* bad, *trophe,* nourishment], any abnormality in the metabolism or deposition of fats.

lip of hip fracture, a fracture of the posterior lip of the acetabulum, often associated with displacement of the hip.

lipofuscin /lip′əfus′in/, a class of fatty pigments consisting mostly of oxidized fats that are found in abundance in the cells of adults.

lipogenesis /-jen′əsis/ [Gk, *lipos,* fat, *genein,* to produce], the production and accumulation of fat.

lipogranuloma /lip′ōgran′yŏŏlō′mə/ [Gk, *lipos* + L, *granulum,* little grain; Gk, *oma,* tumor], a nodule of necrotic, fatty tissue associated with granulomatous inflammation or a foreign-body reaction around a deposit of injected material containing an oily substance.

lipohypertrophy /lip′ōhīpur′trəfē/, a build-up of subcutaneous fat tissue at the site of an insulin injection.

lipoic acid /lipō′ik/, a bacterial growth factor found in liver and yeast.

lipoid /lip′oid/, any substance that resembles a lipid.

lipolysis /lipol′isis/, the breakdown or destruction of fats.

lipolytic /-lit′ik/ [Gk, *lipos,* fat, *lysis,* loosening], the chemical breakdown of fat.

lipolytic digestion /lip′əlit′ik/, a phase of food digestion in which fat molecules are split into glycerol and fatty acids.

lipoma /lipō′mə/ [Gk, *lipos* + *oma,* tumor], a benign tumor consisting of mature fat cells. —**lipomatous,** *adj.*

lipoma annulare colli, a diffuse, symmetric accumulation of fat around the neck, not a true lipoma.

lipoma arborescens, a fatty tumor of a joint, characterized by a treelike distribution of fat cells.

lipoma capsulare, a benign neoplasm characterized by the abnormal presence of fat cells in the capsule of an organ.

lipoma fibrosum, a fatty tumor containing masses of fibrous tissue.

lipomatosis /lip′ōmatō′sis/ [Gk, *lipos* + *oma,* tumor, *osis,* condition], a disorder characterized by abnormal tumorlike accumulations of fat in body tissues.

lipomatosis dolorosa, a disorder characterized by the abnormal accumulation of painful or tender fat deposits.

lipomatosis gigantea, a condition characterized by massive deposits of fat.

lipomatous myxoma, a tumor containing fatty tissue that arises in connective tissue.

lipomatous nephritis, a rare condition in which the renal nephrons are replaced by fatty tissue. Kidney failure may result.

lipometabolism /-metab'əliz'əm/ [Gk, *lipos,* fat, *metabole,* change], the chemical processes involved in building up or breaking down fat molecules.

lipomyoma /-mī·ō'mə/ [Gk, *lipos,* fat; *mys,* muscle, *oma,* tumor], a tumor that combines characteristics of a lipoma and myoma.

lipomyxoma /lip'ōmiksō'mə/ [Gk, *lipos* + *myxa,* mucus, *oma,* tumor], a myxoma that contains fat cells.

lipophilia /-fil'yə/ [Gk, *lipos,* fat, *philein,* to love], a tendency to attract or absorb fat.

lipoprotein /lip'ōprō'tēn/ [Gk, *lipos* + *proteios,* first rank], a conjugated protein in which lipids form an integral part of the molecule. They are synthesized primarily in the liver; contain varying amounts of triglycerides, cholesterol, phospholipids, and protein; and are classified according to their composition and density. Kinds of lipoproteins are **chylomicrons, high-density lipoproteins, low-density lipoproteins,** and **very low–density lipoproteins.**

lipoprotein lipase (LPL), an enzyme that plays a key role in breaking down chylomicrons and very low–density lipoprotein particles, releasing their fatty acids and other lipids for entry into tissue cells.

liposarcoma /lip'ōsárkō'mə/ [Gk, *lipos* + *sarx,* flesh, *oma,* tumor], a malignant growth of primitive fat cells.

liposoluble /-sol'yəbəl/ [Gk, *lipos,* fat; L, *solubilis*], fat soluble.

liposome /lip'əsōm/ [Gk, *lipos,* fat, *soma,* body], a multilayered spheric particle of a lipid in an aqueous medium in a cell.

liposuction /-suk'shən/, a technique for removing adipose tissue with a suction pump device. It is used primarily to remove or reduce localized areas of fat around the abdomen, breasts, legs, face, and upper arms where the skin is contractile enough to redrape in a normal manner.

lip reading, a former name for **speech reading.**

liquefaction /lik'wəfak'shən/ [L, *liquere,* to flow, *facere,* to make], the process in which a solid or a gas is made liquid.

liquifactive degeneration /lik'wəfak'tiv/, dissolution of tissues due to hydrolytic enzymes released by leukocytes and tissue cells. It occurs in the skin of patients with lupus erythematosus.

liquid /lik'wid/ [L, *liquere,* to flow], a state of matter, intermediate between solid and gas, in which the molecules move freely among themselves and the substance flows freely with little application of force and assumes the shape of the vessel in which it is contained.

liquid diet, a diet consisting of foods that can be served in liquid or strained form plus custard, ice cream, pudding, tapioca, and soft-cooked eggs. It is prescribed in acute infections, in acute inflammatory conditions of the gastrointestinal tract, and for patients unable to consume soft or semifluid foods, usually after surgery.

liquid glucose, a thick, syrupy odorless and colorless or yellowish liquid obtained by the incomplete hydrolysis of starch, primarily consisting of dextrose with dextrins, maltose, and water.

liquid scintillation counter, a device for measuring radioactivity, usually beta particles, emitted from a sample dispersed in a liquid scintillation cocktail.

liquor /lik'ər/, any fluid or liquid, such as liquor amnii, the amniotic fluid.

Lisfranc's fracture /lisfrangks'/ [Jacque Lisfranc, French surgeon, 1790–1847], a fracture dislocation of the foot in which one or all of the proximal metatarsals are displaced.

lisping, the defective pronunciation of one or more of the sibilant consonant sounds, usually /s/ and /z/.

Listeria monocytogenes /lister'ē·ə, mon'-ōsītoj'inēz/ [Joseph Lister; Gk, *mono,* single, *kytos,* cell, *genein,* to produce], a common species of gram-positive, motile bacillus that causes listeriosis.

Lister, Joseph [Scottish surgeon, 1827–1912], introduced the use of antiseptic surgery in London hospitals in 1867. Lister operations were performed under a spray of diluted carbolic acid, instruments were dipped in carbolic acid, and wounds were dressed with gauze similarly treated.

listeriosis /listir'ē·ō'sis/ [Joseph Lister; Gk, *osis,* condition], an infectious disease caused by a genus of gram-positive motile bacteria that are nonsporulating. It is transmitted by direct contact from infected animals to humans; through ingesting contaminated meat and dairy products; by inhalation of dust; or by contact with mud, sewage, or soil contaminated with the organism. The disorder is characterized by circulatory collapse, shock, endocarditis, hepatosplenomegaly, and a dark red rash over the trunk and legs. Fever, bacteremia, malaise, and lethargy are commonly seen.

Liston's forceps [Robert Liston, Scottish surgeon, 1794–1847], a kind of bone-cutting forceps.

liter (L) /lē'tər/ [Fr], a derived unit of volume equivalent to 1.057 quarts and defined as the volume occupied by a mass of 1 kg of water at standard temperature and pressure.

lithiasis /lithī'əsis/ [Gk, *lithos,* stone, *osis,* condition], the formation of calculi in the hollow organs or ducts of the body. Calculi are formed of mineral salts and may irritate, inflame, or obstruct the organ in which they form or lodge. Lithiasis occurs most commonly in the gallbladder, kidney, and lower urinary tract. Lithiasis may be asymptomatic, but more often the condition is extremely painful.

lithium (Li) /lith'ē·əm/ [Gk, *lithos,* stone], a silver-white alkali metal occurring in various compounds such as petalite and spodumene. Its atomic number is 3; its atomic mass (weight) is 6.94. Lithium is the lightest known metal. Its salts are used in the treatment of manias.

lithium carbonate, an antimanic agent prescribed in the treatment of manic episodes of manic-depressive disorder.

lithium fluoride (LiF), a compound commonly used for thermoluminescent dosimetry.

lithogenesis /lith'əjen'əsis/ [Gk, *lithos,* stone, *genein,* to produce], the origin of the formation of a calculus.

lithopedion /lith'əpē'dē·ən/ [Gk, *lithos* + *paidion,* child], a fetus that has died in utero and has become calcified or ossified.

lithoscope /lith'əskōp'/, a device used to inspect calculi in the bladder.

lithotomy /lithot'əmē/ [Gk, *lithos* + *temnein,* to cut], the surgical excision of a calculus, especially one from the urinary tract.

lithotomy forceps, a forceps for the extraction of a calculus, usually from the urinary tract.

lithotomy position, the posture assumed by the patient lying supine, with the hips and knees flexed and the thighs abducted and rotated externally.

lithotripsy /lith'ətrip'sē/ [Gk, *lithos,* stone, *tribein,* to wear away], a procedure for eliminating a calculus in the renal pelvis, ureter, bladder, or gallbladder. It may be crushed surgically or by using a noninvasive method such as a pulsed dye laser. The fragments may then be expelled or washed out.

lithotrite /lith'ətrīt/ [Gk, *lithos* + L, *terere,* to rub], an instrument for crushing a stone in the urinary bladder. **—lithotrity,** *n.*

litigant /lit'əgənt/ [L, *litigare,* to go to law], (in law) a party to a lawsuit.

litigate /lit'əgāt/, (in law) to carry on a suit or to contest.

litigious paranoia [L, *litigare,* to go to law; Gk, *paranous,* madness], a form of paranoia in which the person seeks legal proof or justification for systematized delusions.

litmus paper /lit'məs/ [ONorse, *litmosi,* coloring herb; L, *papyrus,* paper], absorbent paper coated with litmus, a blue dye, that is used to determine pH. Acid substances or solutions turn blue litmus to red. Alkaline substances or solutions do not cause a color change in blue litmus.

litter [Fr, *lit,* bed], a stretcher.

live attenuated measles virus vaccine /əten''yōō·ā'tid/, a vaccine prepared from live strains of measles virus that have been cultured under conditions that cause them to lose their virulence without losing their ability to induce immunity. The vaccine is not recommended for pregnant women or others who may have certain medical conditions that tend to diminish immunity.

live attenuated vaccine, a vaccine prepared from live microorganisms or functional viruses whose disease-producing ability has been weakened but whose immunogenic properties have not.

live birth [AS, *libben,* to be alive; ONorse, *byrth*], the birth of an infant, irrespective of the duration of gestation, that exhibits any sign of life such as respiration, heartbeat, umbilical pulsation, or movement of voluntary muscles.

livedo /livē'dō/ [L, *liveo,* bluish spot], a blue or reddish mottling of the skin that worsens in cold weather and is probably caused by arteriolar spasm.

livedo reticularis, a disorder accentuated by exposure to cold and presenting with a characteristic reddish-blue mottling with a typical 'fishnet' appearance. The condition involves the entire leg and, less often, the arms.

live measles and mumps virus vaccine, a vaccine prepared from live strains of measles and mumps viruses. The vaccine is commonly combined with live rubella viruses such as **MMR vaccine** and administered to normal infants at the age of 15 months.

live oral poliovirus vaccine, a vaccine prepared from three strains (trivalent) of live polioviruses. Primary immunization with the vaccine usually begins at the age of 2 months.

liver [AS, *lifer*], the largest gland of the body and one of its most complex organs. More than 500 of its functions have been identified. It is divided into four lobes, contains as many as 100,000 lobules, and is served by two distinct blood supplies. The hepatic artery conveys oxygenated blood to the liver, and the hepatic portal

L

vein conveys nutrient-filled blood from the stomach and the intestines. Some of the major functions performed by the liver are the production of bile by hepatic cells; the secretion of glucose, proteins, vitamins, fats, and most of the other compounds used by the body; the processing of hemoglobin for vital use of its iron content; and the conversion of poisonous ammonia to urea.

liver biopsy, a diagnostic procedure in which a special needle is introduced into the liver under local anesthesia to obtain a specimen for pathologic examination.

liver cancer, a malignant neoplastic disease of the liver, occurring most frequently as a metastasis from another malignancy. Risk factors include hemochromatosis, hepatitis, schistosomiasis, exposure to vinyl chloride or arsenic, and possibly nutritional deficiencies. Alcoholism may be a predisposing factor, but nonalcoholic cirrhosis is a greater risk than alcoholic cirrhosis. Aflatoxins in moldy grain and peanuts appear to be linked to high rates of hepatocellular carcinoma. Characteristics of liver cancer are abdominal bloating, anorexia, weakness, dull upper abdominal pain, ascites, mild jaundice, and a tender enlarged liver; in some cases tumor nodules are palpable on the liver surface.

liver disease, any one of a group of disorders of the liver. Characteristics of liver disease are jaundice, anorexia, hepatomegaly, ascites, and impaired consciousness.

liver failure [AS, *lifer* + L, *fallere,* to deceive], a condition in which the liver fails to fulfill its function or is unable to meet the demands made on it. Anorexia, fatigue, and weakness are common symptoms of liver cell failure, whereas jaundice indicates a biliary obstruction and fever may accompany viral or alcoholic liver diseases.

liver fluke [AS, *lifer* + *floc*], a parasitic trematode belonging to the class Trematoda with six genera that may infest the liver. The most important species affecting humans in industrialized countries is *Clonorchis sinensis,* which is usually acquired by eating freshwater fish containing the encysted larvae. Infestations are most likely to result from ingestion of raw, dried, salted, or pickled freshwater fish and can be prevented by thorough cooking of such fish.

liver function test (LFT), one of several tests used to evaluate various functions of the liver—for example, metabolism, storage, filtration, and excretion. Kinds of liver function tests include **alkaline phos-** phatase, **Bromsulphalein test,** prothrombin time, serum bilirubin, and serum glutamic pyruvic transaminase.

liver scan, a noninvasive technique of visualizing the size, shape, and consistency of the liver by the intravenous injection of a radioactively labeled compound that is readily taken up and trapped in the Kupffer cells of the liver.

liver spot, *nontechnical.* a senile lentigo or actinic keratosis.

liver transplantation, a treatment for end-stage hepatic dysfunction in which a donor liver is matched in size and blood group to the recipient. The transplanted organ may be introduced as an auxiliary liver or as a total replacement. The procedure requires five anastomoses and many units of blood. Because of a shortage of child-size livers, pediatric transplants often are performed with a segment of an adult liver.

livid /liv′id/ [L, *lividus,* bluish], pertaining to an injury that is congested and has a bluish discoloration.

lividity /livid′itē/ [L, *lividus,* bluish], a tissue condition of being red or blue because of venous congestion, as in a contusion.

living will [AS, *libben* + *willa,* wish], **1.** an advance declaration by a patient adjudged to be hopelessly and terminally ill that the person does not want to be connected to life support equipment. The document, signed and witnessed, may generally serve as a "Living Will," depending on current state laws. **2.** a written agreement between a patient and a physician to withhold heroic measures if the patient's condition is found to be irreversible.

livor mortis /lī′vər/, a purple discoloration of the skin in some dependent body areas following death as a result of blood cell destruction.

lizard /liz′ərd/ [L, *lacerta*], a scaly-skinned reptile with a long body and tail and two pairs of legs. The large Gila monster and the beaded lizard are the only North American lizards known to be venomous. The symptoms of their bites and the recommended treatment are similar to those of the bites from poisonous snakes.

LLE, abbreviation for *left lower extremity.*

LLQ, abbreviation for *left lower quadrant of abdomen.*

LMA, abbreviation for *left mentoanterior fetal position.*

L.M.D., abbreviation for *local medical doctor,* used by house staff or others to distinguish a patient's primary physician from university faculty, attending specialist physicians, or house staff.

LMP, **1.** abbreviation for *last menstrual period.* **2.** abbreviation for *left mentoposterior fetal position.*

LMT, abbreviation for *left mentotransverse fetal position.*

LOA, abbreviation for *left occipitoanterior fetal position.*

load, a departure from normal body values for parameters such as water content, salt concentration, and heat. A positive load indicates a higher-than-normal value, whereas a negative load indicates a below-normal value.

loading, **1.** the administration of a substance in sufficient quantity to test a patient's ability to metabolize or absorb it. **2.** the exertion of force on a muscle or ligament to increase its strength.

loading response stance stage [AS, *lad,* support; L, *responsum,* reply], one of the five stages of the stance phase of walking or gait, specifically associated with the moment when the leg reacts to and accepts the weight of the body.

loads [AS, *lad,* support], *slang.* a fixed combination of a sedative hypnotic (glutethimide) and a major narcotic analgesic (codeine). The medications are taken orally by drug abusers for a euphoric effect reported to be similar to that produced by heroin.

Loa loa /lō′álō′á/, a parasitic worm of western and central Africa that causes loiasis.

lobar bronchus /lō′bár [Gk, *lobos,* lobe, *bronchos,* windpipe], a bronchus extending from a primary bronchus to a segmental bronchus into one of the lobes of the right or left lung.

lobar pneumonia, a severe infection of one or more of the five major lobes of the lungs that, if untreated, eventually results in consolidation of lung tissue. The disease is characterized by fever, chills, cough, rusty sputum, rapid shallow breathing, cyanosis, nausea, vomiting, and pleurisy. *Streptococcus pneumoniae* is the usual cause. Complications include lung abscess, atelectasis, empyema, pericarditis, and pleural effusion.

lobate /lō′bāt/, organized in lobes or rounded divisions.

lobe /lōb/ [Gk, *lobos*], **1.** a roundish projection of any structure. **2.** a part of any organ, demarcated by sulci, fissures, or connective tissue, as the lobes of the brain, liver, and lungs. —**lobar, lobular,** *adj.*

lobectomy /lōbek′təmē/ [Gk, *lobos* + *ek-tome,* excision], the surgical excision of a lobe of a lung. It is performed to remove a malignant tumor and to treat uncon-

trolled bronchiectasis, trauma with hemorrhage, or intractable tuberculosis. —**lobectomize,** *v.*

lobe of ear [Gk, *lobos,* lobe; AS, *eare*], the lower part of the auricle that contains no cartilage.

lobotomy /lōbot′əmē/ [Gk, *lobos* + *temnein,* to cut], a neurosurgical procedure in which the nerve fibers in the bundle of white matter in the frontal lobe of the brain are severed to interrupt the transmission of various affective responses. Severe intractable depression and pain are among the indications for the operation. It is seldom performed, because it has many unpredictable and undesirable effects.

lobular carcinoma /lob′yələr/ [Gk, *lobos* + *karkinos,* crab, *oma,* tumor], a neoplasm that often forms a diffuse mass and accounts for a small percentage of breast tumors.

lobule /lob′yo͞ol/, a small lobe, such as the soft lower pendulous part of the external ear. —**lobular,** *adj.*

LOC abbreviation for **level of consciousness.**

local [L, *locus,* place], **1.** pertaining to a small circumscribed area of the body. **2.** pertaining to a treatment or drug applied locally. **3.** *informal.* a local anesthetic.

local adaptation syndrome (LAS), the localized response of a tissue, organ, or system that occurs as a reaction to stress.

local anaphylaxis [L, *locus,* place; Gk, *ana* + *phylaxis*], a condition in which injections of an antigen result in local swellings and localized necrosis of the skin and subcutaneous tissues.

local anesthesia, the administration of a local anesthetic agent into tissues to induce the absence of sensation in a small area of the body. Brief surgical or dental procedures are the most common indications for local anesthesia. The anesthetic may be applied topically to the surface of the skin or membrane or injected subcutaneously or through an intradermal weal.

local anesthetic, a substance used to prevent the transmission of impulses through nerves to eliminate sensation, specifically pain, in a defined area of the body. Drugs available for local anesthesia are classified as members of the ester or the amide family.

local cerebral blood flow (LCBF), (in positron emission tomography) the parametric image of blood flow through the brain. It is expressed in milliliters of blood flow per minute.

local cerebral metabolic rate of glucose utilization (LCMRG), (in positron emission tomography) a parametric image of the brain expressed in milligrams of glucose utilization per minute per 100 g of brain tissue.

local control, the arrest of cancer growth at the site of origin.

local hypothermia, the heating of a local area of tissue to therapeutic temperatures.

local immunity, an immunity of a particular organ, tissue, or anatomic site mediated by localized antibodies or lymphoid cells.

local infection [L, *locus,* place, *inficere,* to stain], an infection involving bacteria that invade the body at a specific point and remain there, multiplying, until eliminated.

localization /lō'kəlīzā'shən/ [L, *locus,* place], **1.** the designation of a particular site for a lesion or organ function. **2.** the determination of the site of a biologic function. **3.** the assignment of a position to an object detected by radiography.

localization film [L, *locus,* place; Gk, *izein,* to cause; AS, *filmen,* membrane], (in radiotherapy) a diagnostic film taken to confirm a treatment effect or to view the position of an intracavitary or interstitial implant, especially for the purpose of computing the dose delivered.

localizer image, (in computed tomography) an image used to localize a specific body part.

local lesion [L, *locus,* place, *laesio,* hurting], a lesion of the central nervous system characterized by distinctive local symptoms.

local osteolytic hypercalcemia (LOH), a syndrome of malignancy-associated hypercalcemia resulting from the action of locally acting osteolytic factors released in conjunction with tumor deposits adjacent to bone.

local paralysis, a loss of motor control that is confined to a single muscle, muscle group, or part of the body.

local reaction [L, *locus,* place , *re + agere,* to act], a reaction to treatment that occurs at the site where it was administered.

locant /lōkənt/, a number or letter code that locates the position of an atom, radical, or compound in the structure of a more complex molecule.

location [L, *locus,* place, *atus,* process], a specific place in the memory of a computer where a unit of information is stored.

lochia /lō'kē·ə/ [Gk, *lochos,* childbirth], the discharge that flows from the vagina after childbirth. During the first 2 to 4 days after delivery, the lochia is red or brownish red (called lochia rubra); is made up of blood, endometrial decidua, fetal lanugo, vernix, and sometimes meconium; and has a fleshy odor. About the third day the amount of blood diminishes; the placental

site exudes serous material, erythrocytes, lymph, cervical mucus, and microorganisms from the superficial layer called lochia serosa. During the next 10 to 14 days bacteria appear in large numbers, along with mucinous decidual material and epithelial cells, causing the lochia to appear whitish yellow (lochia alba). This may continue for 3 to 6 weeks into the postpartum period. **—lochial,** *adj.*

locked-in syndrome [ME, *loc* + Gk, *syn,* together, *dromos,* course], a paralytic condition in which a person may be conscious and alert but unable to communicate except by eye movements or blinking (e.g., pseudocoma). Bilateral destruction of the medulla oblongata or pons has rendered the individual unable to speak or move any of the limbs.

locked knee [AS, *loc* + *cneow*], a condition in which the knee cannot be fully extended, often caused by longitudinal splitting of the medial meniscus.

locking point [AS, *loc,* lock; L, *punctum,* puncture], a point on the body at which light pressure can be applied to help a weak or debilitated patient maintain a desired posture or position. A basic locking point is the body's center of gravity, at the level of the second sacral vertebra, where mild pressure can assist a patient in standing or walking erect.

locomotion [L, *locus,* place, *motio,* movement], movement or the ability to move from one place or position to another.

locomotor [L, *locus* + *motio*], pertaining to locomotion.

loculate /lok'yo͞olāt/ [L, *loculus,* little place], divided into small spaces or cavities.

loculation /lok'yəlā'shən/, the presence of numerous small spaces or cavities.

loculus /lok'yo͞oləs/ [L, little place], a small chamber, pocket, or cavity, such as the interior of a polyp.

locum tenens /lō'kəm ten'ənz/ [L, *locus,* place, *tenere,* to hold], a temporary substitute for a physician who is away from the practice.

locus, *pl.* **loci** /lō'sī, lō'kē/ [L, place], a specific place or position, such as the locus of a particular gene on a chromosome.

locus ceruleus [L, *locus,* place, *caeruleus,* sky-blue], a deeply pigmented group of several thousand neurons in the floor of the fourth ventricle. It is part of a major norepinephrine pathway of the central nervous system.

locus of control [L, *locus,* place; Fr, *controle*], a center of responsibility for one's behavior. Individuals with an **internal locus of control** believe they can control events related to their life, whereas those with an **external locus of control** tend to believe that real power resides in forces outside themselves and determines their life.

locus of infection, a site in the body where an infection originates.

Löffler's syndrome /lef′lərz/ [Wilhelm Löffler, Swiss physician, 1887–1972], a benign, idiopathic disorder marked by episodes of pulmonary eosinophilia, transient opacities in the lungs, anorexia, breathlessness, fever, and weight loss.

logotherapy /log′ōther′əpē/ [Gk, *logos,* word, *therapeia,* treatment], a treatment modality based on the application of humanistic and existential psychology to assist a patient in finding meaning and purpose in life and unique life experiences.

log roll [ME, *logge* + L, *roto,* turn around], a maneuver used to turn a reclining patient from one side to the other or completely over without flexing the spinal column. The arms of the patient are folded across the chest, and the legs extended. A draw sheet under the patient is manipulated by attending nursing personnel to facilitate the procedure.

LOH, abbreviation for **local osteolytic hypercalcemia.**

loiasis /lō·ī′əsis/, a form of filariasis caused by the worm *Loa loa.* The worms may migrate in subcutaneous tissue, producing localized inflammation known as Calabar swellings. The disease is acquired through the bite of an infected African deer fly.

loin [ME, *loyn,* flank], a part of the body on each side of the spinal column between the false ribs and the hip bones.

lomustine /lōmus′tēn/, an antineoplastic alkylating agent prescribed in the treatment of a variety of malignant neoplastic diseases.

loneliness, risk for, a NANDA-accepted nursing diagnosis of a subjective state in which an individual is at risk of experiencing vague dysphonia. The risk factors are affectional deprivation, physical isolation, cathectic deprivation, and social isolation.

long-acting drug [AS, *lang* + L, *agere,* to do; Fr, *drogue,* drug], a pharmacologic agent with a prolonged effect because of a formulation resulting in the slow release of the active principle or the continued absorption of small amounts of the dosage of the drug over an extended period.

long-acting insulin, a preparation of insulin (of beef or pork pancreas) modified by an interaction with zinc under specific chemical conditions and supplied as a suspension with a prolonged action. An injection of the preparation takes effect within 8 hours, reaches a peak of action in 16 to 24 hours, and has a duration of action of more than 36 hours.

long-acting thyroid stimulator (LATS), an immunoglobulin, probably an autoantibody, that exerts a prolonged stimulatory effect on the thyroid gland, causing rapid growth of the gland and excess activity of thyroid function, resulting in hyperthyroidism.

long-acting thyroid stimulator protector (LATS-P), an antibody that inhibits the neutralization of long-acting thyroid stimulator and is found in the serum of persons with Graves' disease.

long-arm cast [As, *lang* + *earm,* arm; ONorse, *kasta*], an orthopedic cast applied to immobilize the upper extremities from the hand to the upper arm.

long bones, the bones that contribute to the height or length of an extremity, particularly the bones of the legs and arms.

longevity /lonjev′itē/ [L, *longus,* long, *aveum,* age], the number of years an average person of a particular age is expected to continue living. It is determined by statistical tables based on mortality rates of various population groups.

longitudinal /lon′jətoo′dənəl/ [L, *longitudo,* length], **1.** pertaining to a measurement in the direction of the long axis of an object, body, or organ, such as the longitudinal arch of the foot. **2.** pertaining to a scientific study that is conducted over a long period of time.

longitudinal diffusion, the diffusion of solute molecules in the direction of flow of the mobile phase.

longitudinal dissociation, (in cardiology) the insulation of parallel pathways of impulses from each other, usually in the atrioventricular junction.

longitudinal fissure [L, *longitudo,* length, *fissura,* cleft], the largest and deepest groove between the medial surfaces of the cerebral hemispheres.

longitudinal presentation [L, *longitudo,* length, *praesentare,* to show], the normal presentation of a fetus, with the long axis of the infant body parallel to that of the mother.

longitudinal sound waves, pressure waves formed by the oscillation of particles or molecules parallel to the axis of wave propagation. The compression and expansion of such longitudinal waves at high frequencies is the principle on which ultrasonography is based.

long-leg cast, an orthopedic cast applied to immobilize the leg from the toes to the upper thigh.

long-leg cast with walker, an orthopedic cast applied to immobilize the lower extremities from the toes to the upper thigh

L

in treating certain leg fractures. This type of cast is the same as the long-leg cast but incorporates a rubber walker, allowing the patient to walk while the leg is encased in the cast.

long QT syndrome, an inherited cardiac disorder characterized by prolongation of the Q-T interval. The disorder is associated with ventricular tachycardia, cardiac arrhythmias, syncope, and sudden death.

long-scale contrast, (in radiography) a high-kilovolt image containing a wide range and great number of shades of gray with little difference in the adjacent tones.

long-term care (LTC), the provision of medical, social, and personal care services on a recurring or continuing basis to persons with chronic physical or mental disorders.

long-term memory, the ability to recall sensations, events, ideas, and other information for long periods of time without apparent effort.

long thoracic nerve, one of a pair of supraclavicular branches from the roots of the brachial plexus.

long-thoracic nerve injury, damage to the nerve (C5-7) that innervates the serratus muscle, which anchors the apex of the scapula to the posterior of the rib cage.

long tract signs, neurologic signs such as clonus, muscle spasticity, or bladder involvement that usually indicate a lesion in the middle or upper parts of the spinal cord or in the brain.

loop [ME, *loupe*], *informal.* intrauterine device.

loop colostomy [ME, *loupe* + Gk, *kolon,* colon, *stoma,* mouth], a type of temporary colostomy performed as part of the surgical treatment for repair of some colon diseases. The procedure involves bringing an intact segment of colon anterior to the repair through an abdominal incision and suturing it onto the abdomen. A loop is formed and held in position by placing a piece of glass rod between the segment and the abdomen.

loop excision, the surgical removal of dysplastic tissue cells with a small wire loop.

loop of Henle /hen'lē/ [ME, *loupe;* Friedrich G. J. Henle, German anatomist, 1809–1885], the U-shaped part of a renal tubule, consisting of a thin descending limb and a thick ascending limb.

loose association [ME, *lous,* not fastened], (in psychiatry) a disturbance of thinking in which the association of ideas and thought patterns becomes so vague, fragmented, diffuse, and unfocused as to lack any logical sequences or relationship to any preceding concepts or themes.

loose body, a fragment of solid tissue in a body cavity or joint. A kind of loose body is a **joint mouse.**

loose fibrous tissue [ME, *lous,* not fastened], a constrictive, pliable fibrous connective tissue consisting of interwoven elastic and collagenous fibers, interspersed with fluid-filled areolae.

loose-pack joint position, a point in the range of motion at which articulating surfaces are the least congruent and the supporting structures are the most lax.

Looser's zones /lō'zərz/ [Emil Looser, Swiss physician, 1877–1936], transverse translucent bands, sometimes symmetric, seen radiographically in the cortex of bones affected with osteomalacia or certain other deficiency diseases.

LOP, abbreviation for *left occipitoposterior fetal position.*

loperamide hydrochloride /lōper'əmīd/, an antiperistaltic prescribed in the treatment of diarrhea.

lorazepam /lōrā'zəpam/, a benzodiazepine tranquilizer prescribed in the treatment of anxiety, nervous tension, and insomnia.

lordoscoliosis /lôr'dōskō'lē·ō'sis/ [Gk, *lordos,* bent, *skoliosis,* curvature], a combination of lordosis and scoliosis.

lordosis /lôrdō'sis/ [Gk, *lordos,* bent forward, *osis,* condition], an abnormal anterior concavity of the lumbar part of the back.

lordotic pelvis /lôrdot'ik/ [Gk, *lordos,* bent forward; L, *pelvis,* basin], a deformed pelvis that bends forward in the lumbar region and is associated with lordosis.

LOS, abbreviation for *length of stay.*

loss of consortium [ME, *lossen,* to lose; L, *consortionis,* companionship], (in law) a claim for damages sought in recompense for the loss of conjugal relations, including society, affection, and assistance, as well as impairment or loss of sexual relations.

LOT, abbreviation for *left occipitotransverse fetal position.*

lotion [L, *lotio,* a washing], a liquid preparation applied externally to protect the skin or to treat a dermatologic disorder.

loupe /lōōp/ [Fr, magnifying glass], a magnifying lens mounted in a frame worn on the head, as used to examine the eyes.

louse bite, a minute puncture wound produced by a louse that may transmit typhus, trench fever, and relapsing fever. Secondary infection may result from scratching the affected area.

low back pain (LBP) [ME, *low* + AS, *baec* + L, *poena,* penalty], local or referred pain at the base of the spine caused by a sprain, a strain, osteoarthritis, ankylosing spondylitis, a neoplasm, or a prolapsed intervertebral disk. Low back pain is a common complaint and is often associated with poor posture, obesity, sagging abdominal muscles, sitting for prolonged periods of time, or improper body mechanics. Pain may be localized and static; it may be accompanied by muscle weakness or spasms; or it may radiate down the back of one or both legs, as in sciatica. Pain may be initiated or increased by coughing, sneezing, rising from a seated position, lifting, stretching, bending, or turning. To guard against the pain, the person may decrease the range of motion of the spine. If an intervertebral disk is prolapsed, deep pressure over the interspace generally causes pain, and flexion of the hip elicits sciatic pain when the knee is extended but not when the knee is flexed (Lasègue's sign).

low–birth weight (LBW) infant, an infant whose weight at birth is less than 2500 g, regardless of gestational age.

low-calcium diet, a diet that restricts the use of calcium and eliminates most of the dairy foods, all breads made with milk or dry skimmed milk, and deep-green leafy vegetables. It is prescribed for patients who form renal calculi.

low-caloric diet, a diet that is prescribed to limit the intake of calories, usually to cause a reduction in body weight. Such diets may be designated as 800 calorie, 1000 calorie, or other specific numbers of calories.

low cervical cesarean section, a method for surgically delivering a baby through a transverse incision in the thin supracervical part of the lower uterine segment, behind the bladder and the bladder flap. This incision bleeds less during surgery and heals with a stronger scar than the higher vertical scar of the classic cesarean section.

low-cholesterol diet, a diet that restricts foods containing animal fats and saturated fatty acids. It concentrates on poultry, fish, vegetables, fruits, low-fat cottage cheese, and polyunsaturated fats.

low-density lipoprotein (LDL), a plasma protein containing relatively more cholesterol and triglycerides than protein. It is derived in part, if not completely, from the intravascular breakdown of the very low-density lipoproteins.

low-density lipoprotein (LDL) receptor disorder, an inherited autosomal-dominant trait characterized by an abnormality in clearance of low-density lipoprotein.

low-dose tolerance, a temporary and incomplete immunosuppression induced by the administration of subimmunogenic doses of soluble antigen. The tolerance is achieved in the neonatal period, when lymphoid cells have not matured enough to activate a response.

lower extremity suspension [ME, *low* + L, *extremitas* + *suspendere,* to hang], an orthopedic procedure used in the treatment of bone fractures and the correction of orthopedic abnormalities of the lower limbs. The procedure uses traction equipment, including metal frames, ropes, and pulleys, to relieve the weight of the involved lower limb rather than to exert traction pull.

lower level discriminator (LLD), (in nuclear medicine) a radiation energy-sensitive device used to discriminate against all radionuclide pulses whose heights are below the accepted level.

lower motor neuron paralysis, an injury to or lesion that damages the cell bodies or axons, or both, of the lower motor neurons, which are located in the anterior horn cells of the spinal cord and the spinal and peripheral nerves. If complete transection of the spinal cord occurs, voluntary muscle control is totally lost. In partial transection function is altered in varying degrees, depending on the areas innervated by the nerves involved.

lower respiratory tract, one of the two divisions of the respiratory system. The lower respiratory tract includes the left and right bronchi and the alveoli where the exchange of oxygen and carbon dioxide occurs during the respiratory cycle. The bronchi divide into smaller bronchioles in the lungs, the bronchioles into alveolar ducts, the ducts into alveolar sacs, and the sacs into alveoli.

Lowe's syndrome [Charles U. Lowe, American pediatrician, b. 1921], a sex-linked condition in males characterized by progressive mental deterioration, renal tubular dysfunction, and cortical cataracts with or without glaucoma.

low-fat diet [ME, *low;* AS, *faett;* Gk, *diaita,* life-style], a diet containing limited amounts of fat and consisting chiefly of easily digestible foods of high carbohydrate content. It includes all vegetables, lean meats, fish, fowl, pasta, cereals, and whole wheat or enriched bread.

low-fat milk, milk containing 1% to 2% fat, making it an intermediate in fat content between whole and skimmed milk.

low-flow oxygen delivery system, respiratory care equipment that does not supply all the inspired gases. The patient inhales some room air along with the delivered oxygen.

low forceps [ME, *low* + L, *forceps,* pair of

tongs], an obstetric operation in which forceps are used to deliver a baby whose head is on the pelvic floor.

low-grade fever, an oral temperature that is above 98.6°F (37°C) but lower than 100.4°F for 24 hours.

low-grade infection [ME, *lah* + L, *gradus,* degree, *inficere,* to stain], a subacute or chronic infection with mild fever and no pus production.

low-molecular weight heparin, a drug used to prevent potentially fatal blood clots in patients undergoing surgery or other patients at risk for blood clots. It has been used to prevent deep vein thrombosis in patients undergoing hip and knee replacements.

Lown-Ganong-Levine's syndrome (LGL) /loun'gənong'ləvēn'/ [Bernard Lown, American physician, b. 1921; William F. Ganong, American physiologist, b. 1924; S. A. Levine, American physician, 1891–1966], a disorder of the atrioventricular (AV) conduction system marked by ventricular preexcitation. Part or all of the AV nodal connection is bypassed by an abnormal AV connection from the atrial muscle to the bundle of His.

low-power field, the low magnification field of vision under a light microscope.

low-protein diet [ME, *lah* low; Gk, *proteios,* first rank, *diaita,* way of living], a diet proportionally low in protein, usually designed for persons who must restrict protein intake because of a metabolic abnormality associated with kidney failure or a liver disease.

low-purine diet, a diet for gout patients who suffer from a painful accumulation of salts of uric acid in the joints. Purine-rich foods are primary sources of uric acid.

low-residue diet, a diet that will leave a minimal residue in the lower intestinal tract after digestion and absorption. It consists of tender meats, poultry, fish, eggs, white bread, pasta, simple desserts, clear soups, tea, and coffee. Because it is lacking in calcium, iron, and vitamins, it should be used only for a limited time or with nutrient supplementation.

low-sodium diet, a diet that restricts the use of sodium chloride plus other compounds containing sodium such as baking powder or soda, monosodium glutamate, sodium citrate, sodium propionate, and sodium sulfate. The degree of sodium restriction depends on the severity of the condition.

loxapine /lok'səpēn/, a tranquilizer prescribed in the treatment of schizophrenia.

LPL abbreviation for **lipoprotein lipase.**

lpm, abbreviation for *liters per minute.*

LPN, abbreviation for **licensed practical nurse.**

LPO, abbreviation for *left posterior oblique fetal position.*

LPS Act, a California law named for sponsors of the legislation (Lanterman, Petris, and Short) that provides for the protection and treatment of persons judged to be 'gravely disabled' and thus unable to provide food, clothing, or shelter for themselves. The legislation was designed to safeguard the constitutional rights of persons threatened with involuntary commitment on the basis of a psychiatric diagnosis. Some other states have similar laws.

Lr, symbol for the element **lawrencium.**

LSD, abbreviation for *lysergic acid diethylamide.*

L/S ratio, the lecithin/sphingomyelin ratio, used in a test for fetal lung maturity.

LTB, abbreviation for **laryngotracheobronchitis.** See **croup.**

LTC, abbreviation for **long-term care.**

LTH, abbreviation for *luteotropic hormone.*

L-Trp, abbreviation for *L-tryptophan.* See **tryptophan.**

Lu, symbol for the element **lutetium.**

lubb-dupp, (in auscultation) an imitation of the two basic sounds heard in the cardiac cycle. Lubb represents the first sound and is made by closure of the mitral and tricuspid valves. It is lower in pitch and lasts slightly longer than the second sound, dupp, which is made by closure of the aortic valve.

lubricant /lōō'brikənt/ [L, *lubricans,* making slippery], a fluid, ointment, or other agent capable of diminishing friction and making a surface slippery.

lubricating enema /lōō'brəkā'ting/ [L, *lubricans,* making slippery; Gk, *enienai*], an enema used to lubricate the anal canal after surgery for hemorrhoids or to prevent fecal impaction. The enema solution may be made with warm olive oil.

lucid /lōō'sid/ [L, *lucidus,* clear], clear, rational, and able to be understood.

lucid interval, a period of relative mental clarity between periods of irrationality, especially in organic mental disorders such as delirium and dementia.

lucidity /lōōsid'itē/ [L, *lucidus,* clear], pertaining to clarity of mind, perception, or intelligibility.

lucid lethargy, a mental state characterized by a loss of will; hence an inability to act, even though the person is conscious and intellectual function is normal.

lucifugal /lōōsif'yəgəl/, repelled by bright light.

Lucio's leprosy phenomenon [R. Lucio, Mexican physician, 1819–1866], an acute form of diffuse lepromatous infection of the skin, characterized by intensely red, tender plaques, particularly on the legs.

lucipetal /loosip′ətəl/, attracted to bright light.

Ludwig's angina /lood′vigz/ [Wilhelm F. von Ludwig, German surgeon, 1790–1865; L, *angina,* quinsy], a severe form of cellulitis in the region of the submandibular gland. Inflammatory edema may distort the floor of the mouth and make swallowing difficult.

LUE, abbreviation for *left upper extremity.*

Luer-Lok syringe /loo′ərlōk′/, a glass or plastic syringe for injection having a simple screw lock mechanism that securely holds the needle in place.

Lugol's solution [Jean G. A. Lugol, French physician, 1786–1851; L, *solutus,* unbound], an aqueous solution of iodine (5%) and potassium iodide (10%).

Lukes-Collins classification [L. J. Lukes; R. D. Collins, twentieth-century American pathologists], a system of identifying non-Hodgkin's lymphomas according to B cell, T cell, true, and unclassifiable types. B cell types include lymphocytic, plasmacytic, follicular cell lymphomas, and B cell-derived immunoblastic lymphoma. T cell types include T cell–derived immunoblastic lymphoma and convoluted cell lymphoma. True types are of histiocytic origin.

lukewarm bath [ME, *luke* + AS, *wearm, baeth*], a bath in which the temperature of the water is between 90° and 96° F.

LUL, abbreviation for *left upper lobe* of lung.

lumbago /lumbā′gō/ [L, *lumbus,* loin], pain in the lumbar region caused by a muscle strain, rheumatoid arthritis, osteoarthritis, or a herniated intravertebral disk. Ischemic lumbago, characterized by pain in the lower back and buttocks, is caused by vascular insufficiency, as in terminal aortic occlusion.

lumbar /lum′bər, lum′bár/ [L, *lumbus,* loin], pertaining to the part of the body between the thorax and the pelvis.

lumbar nerves, the five pairs of spinal nerves rising in the lumbar region of the vertebral column. They become increasingly large the more caudal their origin and pass laterally and downward under the cover of the psoas major or between its fasciculi and form part of the lumbar plexus.

lumbar node, a node in one of the seven groups of parietal lymph nodes serving the abdomen and the pelvis.

lumbar plexus, a network of nerves formed by the ventral anterior primary divisions of the first three and the greater part of the fourth lumbar nerves. It is located on the inside of the posterior abdominal wall, either dorsal to the psoas major or among its fibers and ventral to the transverse processes of the lumbar vertebrae.

lumbar puncture (LP), the introduction of a hollow needle and stylet into the subarachnoid space of the lumbar part of the spinal canal. With the use of strict aseptic technique, it is performed in various therapeutic and diagnostic procedures. Diagnostic indications include measuring of cerebrospinal fluid (CSF) pressure; obtaining CSF for laboratory analysis; evaluating the canal for the pressure of a tumor; and injecting air, oxygen, or a radiopaque substance for radiographic visualization of the structures of the nervous system of spinal canal and meninges and brain. Therapeutic indications for lumbar puncture include removing blood or pus from the subarachnoid space, injecting sera or drugs, withdrawing CSF to reduce intracranial pressure, introducing a local anesthetic to induce spinal anesthesia, and placing a small amount of the patient's blood in the subarachnoid space to form a clot to patch a rent or hole in the dura to prevent leak of CSF into the epidural space.

lumbar rib, a rudimentary rib that articulates with the transverse process of the first lumbar vertebra.

lumbar subarachnoid peritoneostomy, a surgical procedure for draining cerebrospinal fluid in hydrocephalus, usually in the newborn. A lumbar laminectomy is performed, and then a polyethylene tube is passed from the subarachnoid space around the flank and into the peritoneum.

lumbar subarachnoid ureterostomy, a surgical procedure for draining excess cerebrospinal fluid through the ureter to the bladder in hydrocephalus, usually in the newborn. A lumbar laminectomy and a left nephrectomy are performed, after which a polyethylene tube is passed from the lumbar subarachnoid space through the paraspinal muscles and into the free ureter.

lumbar veins, four pairs of veins that collect blood by dorsal tributaries from the loins and abdominal tributaries from the walls of the abdomen.

lumbar vertebra, one of the five largest segments of the movable part of the vertebral column, distinguished by the absence of a foramen in the transverse process and by vertebral bodies without facets. The body of each lumbar vertebra is flattened or slightly concave superiorly and inferiorly and is deeply constricted ventrally at the sides.

lumbocostal /lum'bōkos'təl/, pertaining to the lumbar region and ribs.

lumbosacral /lum'bōsā'krəl/ [L, *lumbus,* loin, *sacrum,* sacred], pertaining to the lumbar vertebrae and the sacrum.

lumbosacral plexus [L, *lumbus,* loin, *sacrum,* sacred, *plexus,* braided], the combination of all the ventral anterior primary divisions of the lumbar, sacral, and coccygeal nerves. The lumbar and sacral plexuses supply the lower limb. The sacral nerves also supply the perineum through the pudendal plexus and the coccygeal area through the coccygeal plexus.

lumbrical plus deformity /lum'brikəl/, a complication of rheumatoid arthritis in which the lumbricals (muscles in the hands and feet) become contracted, with a resultant action of extension rather than flexion.

lumen /lōō'mən/, *pl.* **lumina, lumens** [L, light], **1.** a tubular cavity or the channel within any organ or structure of the body. **2.** a unit of luminous flux that equals the flux emitted in a unit solid angle by a point source of one candle intensity. —**lumenal, luminal,** *adj.*

luminescence /lōō'mines'əns/ [L, *lumen,* light, *escens,* beginning], **1.** the emission of light by a material after excitation by some stimulus. **2.** (in radiology) the emission of light by intensifying screen phosphors after x-ray interaction.

luminiferous /lōō'minif'ərəs/ [L, *lumen,* light, *ferre,* to bear], pertaining to a medium that will transmit light.

luminophore /lōōmin'əfôr/, **1.** an organic compound or chemical grouping that emits light. **2.** a substance that emits light when illuminated.

lumpectomy /lumpek'təmē/ [ME, *lump,* mass, *ektome,* excision], surgical excision of a tumor without removing large amounts of surrounding tissue.

lunar month /lōō'nər/ [L, *luna,* moon; AS, *monath,* month], a period of 4 weeks or 28 days, approximately the time required for the moon to revolve about the earth.

lunate bone /lōō'nāt/ [L, *luna,* moon; AS, *ban*], the carpal bone in the center of the proximal row of carpal bones between the scaphoid and triangular bones.

Lundh test, a pancreatic function test in which the pancreas is stimulated by oral intake of a formula diet and lipase values are measured in aspirate from the duodenum.

lung (L) [AS, *lungen*], one of a pair of light, spongy organs in the thorax, constituting the main component of the respiratory system. The two highly elastic lungs

are the main mechanisms in the body for inhaling (inspiring) air from which oxygen is extracted for the arterial blood system and for exhaling carbon dioxide dispersed from the venous system. The right lung is divided into three lobes; the left lung, two lobes. Each lung is composed of an external serous coat, a subserous layer of areolar tissue, and the parenchyma. The serous coat comprises the thin, visceral pleura. The subserous areolar tissue contains many elastic fibers and invests the entire surface of the organ. The parenchyma is composed of secondary lobules divided into primary lobules, each of which consists of blood vessels, lymphatics, nerves, and an alveolar duct connecting with air spaces.

lung abscess [AS, *lungen* + L, *abscedere,* to go away], a complication of an inflammation and infection of the lung, often caused by aspiration of infected material from the mouth.

lung cancer, a pulmonary malignancy attributable in the majority of cases to cigarette smoking. Other predisposing factors are exposure to acronitrile, arsenic, asbestos, beryllium, chloromethyl ether, chromium, coal products, ionizing radiation, iron oxide, mustard gas, nickel, petroleum, uranium, and vinyl chloride. Lung cancer develops most often in scarred or chronically diseased lungs. It is usually far advanced when detected, because metastases may precede detection of the primary lesion in the lung. Symptoms of lung cancer include persistent cough, dyspnea, purulent or blood-streaked sputum, chest pain, and repeated attacks of bronchitis or pneumonia. Epidermoid cancers and adenocarcinomas each account for approximately 30% of lung tumors, about 25% are small or oat cell carcinomas, and 15% are large-cell anaplastic cancers.

lung capacities, lung volumes that consist of two or more of the four primary nonoverlapping volumes. Functional residual capacity is the sum of residual volume and expiratory reserve volume. Inspiratory capacity is the sum of the tidal volume and inspiratory reserve volume. Total lung capacity, at the end of maximal inspiration, is the sum of functional residual capacity and inspiratory capacity.

lung compliance, a measure of the ease of expansion by the lungs and thorax. It is determined by pulmonary volume and elasticity, with a high degree of compliance indicating a loss of elastic recoil of the lungs, as in old age or emphysema. Decreased compliance of the lungs occurs in conditions when greater pressure is needed for changes of volume, as in atelectasis, edema, fibrosis, pneumonia, or absence of surfactant.

lung fluke [AS, *lungen,* lung, *floc*], a parasitic flatworm of the genus and species *Paragonimus westermani* found throughout Africa, the Orient, and Latin America, but rarely in North America. It may enter the body as encysted larvae in crabs and crayfish. Symptoms of infestation include peribronchiolar distress and hemoptysis.

lung scan, a radiographic examination of a lung and its function.

lung surfactant, a detergent-like agent that reduces the surface tension of the liquid film covering the lining of the pulmonary alveoli.

lung transplantation, the transfer of an entire pulmonary organ system to a new site. The procedure may be performed as a combined cardiopulmonary transplantation.

lunula /loon'yələ/, *pl.* **lunulae** [L, *luna,* moon], a semilunar structure, such as the crescent-shaped pale area at the base of the nail of a finger or toe.

lupoid. resembling **lupus.**

lupoid hepatitis. an autoimmune form of hepatitis with the histologic appearance of chronic active hepatitis. Many patients show lupoid cells in the blood without systemic lupus erythematosus.

lupus /loo'pəs/ [L, wolf], *nontechnical.* lupus erythematosus. **—lupoid,** *adj.*

lupus anticoagulant, an antibody specific for phospholipoproteins or phospholipid components of coagulation factors found in patients with lupus erythematosus.

lupus band test, a direct immunofluorescent method of visualizing a band of immunoglobulins and complement at the dermal-epidermal junction of involved skin in patients with lupus erythematosus.

lupus erythematosus preparation (LE prep), a laboratory test for lupus erythematosus in which normal neutrophils are incubated with a specimen of the patient's serum, resulting in the appearance of large spheric phagocytized inclusions within the neutrophils if the patient has lupus erythematosus.

lupus pernio, a cutaneous form of sarcoidosis characterized by smooth, shiny plaques on the face, fingers, and toes, clinically resembling frostbite.

lupus vulgaris, a rare cutaneous form of tuberculosis in which areas of the skin become ulcerated and heal slowly, leaving deeply scarred tissue. The disease is not related to lupus erythematosus.

LUQ, abbreviation for *left upper quadrant of abdomen.*

lusus naturae /loo'səs/ [L, *lusus,* sport, *natura,* nature], a congenital anomaly; teratism.

luteal /loo'tē-əl/, pertaining to the corpus luteum or its functions or effects.

luteal hormone [L, *luteus,* yellow; Gk, *hormaein,* to set in motion], a hormone produced by the **corpus luteum.**

luteal phase deficiency, female infertility caused by inadequate secretion of progesterone during the luteal phase of the menstrual cycle.

lutein /loo'tē-in/ [L, *luteus,* yellow], a yellow-red crystalline carotenoid pigment found in plants with carotenes and chlorophylls and also in animal fats, egg yolk, the corpus luteum, or any lipochrome.

luteinization /loo'tē-in'īzā'shən/ [L, *luteus,* yellow], the formation of the corpus luteum from an ovarian follicle that had recently discharged an ovum. The process involves the hypertrophy of the follicular lutein cells and the development of blood vessels and connective tissue at the site.

luteinizing hormone (LH) /loo'tē-inī'zing/ [L, *luteus,* yellow; Gk, *izein,* to cause, *hormein,* to begin activity], a glycoprotein hormone produced by the anterior pituitary gland. It stimulates the secretion of sex hormones by the ovary and the testes and is involved in the maturation of spermatozoa and ova. In men it induces the secretion of testosterone by the interstitial cells of the testes. In females, LH, working together with follicle-stimulating hormone, stimulates the growing follicle in the ovary to secrete estrogen.

luteinizing hormone-releasing hormone (LHRH), a neurohormone of the hypothalamus that stimulates and regulates the pituitary gland's release of the luteinizing hormone.

luteoma /loo'tē-ō'mə/ [L, *luteus* + Gk, *oma,* tumor], **1.** a granulosa or theca cell tumor whose cells resemble those of the corpus luteum. **2.** a unilateral or bilateral nodular hyperplasia of ovarian lutein cells, occasionally developing during the last trimester of pregnancy.

lutetium (Lu) /lootē'shē-əm/ [L, *Lutetia,* Paris], a rare earth metallic element. Its atomic number is 71; and its atomic mass (weight) is 174.97.

lux (lx), a unit of illumination equivalent to one lumen per square meter of surface when measured at right angles to the direction of the light.

luxated joint /luk'sātid/, a condition of complete dislocation, with no contact between articular surfaces of the joint.

luxation /luksā'shən/ [L, *luxare,* to dislocate], dislocation.

LV, abbreviation for **left ventricle.**

LVAD, abbreviation for **left ventricular assist device.**

LVN, abbreviation for *licensed vocational nurse.*

LWD, abbreviation for *living with disease.*

lx, abbreviation for **lux.**

lyases /līˈāsez/ [Gk, *lyein,* to loosen; Fr, *disastase,* enzyme], a group of enzymes that reversibly split carbon bonds with carbon, nitrogen, or oxygen without hydrolysis or oxygen reduction reactions.

lycopene /līˈkəpēn/ [Gk, *lykopersikon,* tomato], a red, crystalline unsaturated hydrocarbon that is the carotenoid pigment in tomatoes and various berries and fruits. It is considered the primary substance from which all natural carotenoid pigments are derived.

lycopenemia /līˈkōpēnēˈmē·ə/, a condition characterized by a high concentration of the carotenoid pigment lycopene in the blood, the result of ingesting large amounts of tomato products and other lycopene-rich fruits. Lycopenemia patients may develop a yellowish skin coloring.

lye poisoning /lī/ [AS, *leah,* lye; L, *potio,* drink], toxic effects of ingesting caustic soda or sodium hydroxide (NaOH), a powerful alkali. If the chemical has a pH above 11.5, the chemical burn damage to the mouth and throat is usually irreversible. An alkali burn can be more serious than an acid burn because an acid is usually neutralized by the tissues it contacts.

lying-in [AS, *licgan,* lying; L, *in*], **1.** designating the time before, during, and after childbirth. **2.** designating a hospital that provides care for women in childbirth and the puerperium. **3.** the condition of being in confinement, or childbed.

Lyme disease /līm/, an acute recurrent inflammatory infection transmitted by a tickborne spirochete, *Borrelia burgdorferi.* The condition was originally described in the community of Lyme, Connecticut. The disease is spread by two species of deer ticks, *Ixodes dammini* and *I. pacificus.* An early sign of an infection is the appearance of a red macule at the site of the bite. The bite site may expand to form concentric circles in a 'bull's eye' pattern. Knees, other large joints, and temporomandibular joints are most commonly involved, with local inflammation and swelling. Chills, fever, headache, malaise, and erythema chronicum migrans, an expanding annular, erythematous skin eruption, often precede the joint manifestations. Occasionally cardiac conduction abnormalities, aseptic meningitis, and Bell's palsy are associated conditions.

lymph /limf/ [L, *lympha,* water], a thin watery fluid originating in organs and tissues of the body that circulates through the lymphatic vessels and is filtered by the lymph nodes. Lymph enters the bloodstream at the junction of the internal jugular and subclavian veins. Lymph contains chyle, erythrocytes, and leukocytes, most of which are lymphocytes.

lymphadenitis /limfadˈinīˈtis, limˈfəd-/ [L, *lympha* + Gk, *aden,* gland, *itis,* inflammation], an inflammatory condition of the lymph nodes, usually the result of systemic neoplastic disease, bacterial infection, or other inflammatory condition. The nodes may be enlarged, hard, smooth or irregular, and red and may feel hot.

lymphadenopathy /limfadˈinopˈəthē/, any disorder characterized by a localized or generalized enlargement of the lymph nodes or lymph vessels.

lymphadenopathy syndrome (LAS), a persistent generalized swelling of the lymph nodes. It is often a part of the acquired immunodeficiency syndrome–related complex.

lymphangiectasia /limfanˈjē·ektāˈzhə/ [L, *lympha* + Gk, *angeion,* vessel, *ektasis,* stretching], dilation of the smaller lymphatic vessels. It usually results from obstruction in the larger vessels.

lymphangiogram /limfanˈjē·əgram′/ [L, *lympha,* water; Gk, *angeion,* vessel, *gramma,* record], a radiographic visualization of a part of the lymphatic system.

lymphangiography /-jē·ogˈrəfē/ [L, *lympha* + Gk, *angeion,* vessel, *graphein,* to record], the x-ray examination of lymph glands and lymphatic vessels after an injection of contrast medium.

lymphangioma /limfanˈjē·ōˈmə/ [L, *lympha* + Gk, *angeion,* vessel, *oma,* tumor], a benign yellowish-tan tumor on the skin, composed of a mass of dilated lymph vessels.

lymphangioma cavernosum, a tumor formed by dilated lymphatic vessels and filled with lymph mixed with coagulated blood.

lymphangioma circumscriptum, a benign skin lesion that develops from superficial hypertrophic lymph vessels.

lymphangioma simplex, a growth formed by moderately dilated lymph vessels in a circumscribed area on the skin.

lymphangiosarcoma /limfanˈjē·ōˈsárkōˈmə/ [L, *lympha,* water; Gk, *angeion,* vessel, *sarx,* flesh, *oma,* tumor], a tumor arising from the lymphatic vessels.

lymphangitis /limˈfanjīˈtis/ [L, *lympha* + Gk, *angeion,* vessel, *itis*], an inflammation of one or more lymphatic vessels, usually resulting from an acute streptococcal infection of one of the extremities. It is characterized by fine red streaks extending from the infected area to the axilla or groin and by fever, chills, headache, and myalgia. The infection may spread to the bloodstream.

lymphatic /limfat′ik/ [L, *lympha* + *icus,* form], **1.** pertaining to the lymphatic system of the body, consisting of a vast network of tubes transporting lymph. **2.** any of the vessels associated with the lymphatic network.

lymphatic capillary plexus, one of the numerous networks of lymphatic capillaries that collect lymph from the intercellular fluid and constitute the beginning of the lymphatic system. The lymphatic vessels arise from the capillary plexuses, which vary in size and number in different regions and organs of the body.

lymphatic organ [L, *lympha,* water; Gk, *organon,* instrument], any body structure composed of lymphatic tissue, such as the thymus, spleen, tonsils, and lymph nodes.

lymphatic system, a vast, complex network of capillaries, thin vessels, valves, ducts, nodes, and organs that helps to protect and maintain the internal fluid environment of the entire body by producing, filtering, and conveying lymph and producing various blood cells. The lymphatic network also transports fats, proteins, and other substances to the blood system and restores 60% of the fluid that filters out of the blood capillaries into interstitial spaces during normal metabolism. Small semilunar valves throughout the lymphatic network help to control the flow of lymph and, at the junction with the venous system, prevent venous blood from flowing into the lymphatic vessels. The lymph collected throughout the body drains into the blood through two ducts situated in the neck. Various body dynamics such as respiratory pressure changes, muscular contractions, and movements of organs surrounding lymphatic vessels combine to pump the lymph through the lymphatic system. The system also includes specialized lymphatic organs such as the tonsils, the thymus, and the spleen.

lymphatic vasculitis, a condition of blood vessel necrosis in which the vessels acquire fibrinoid deposits and are infiltrated by lymphocytes.

lymphatic vessels [L, *lympha,* water, *vascellum,* little vase], fine transparent valved channels distributed through most tissues. They are often distinguished by their beaded appearance, which is caused by an irregular lumen. The collecting branches form two systems, one generally running with the superficial veins and the

other below the deep fascia and including the intestinal lacteals. They drain through a thoracic duct and a right lymphatic duct into the venous system near the base of the neck.

lymphedema /lim′fidē′mə/ [L, *lympha* + Gk, *oidema,* swelling], a primary or secondary condition characterized by the accumulation of lymph in soft tissue and the resultant swelling caused by inflammation, obstruction, or removal of lymph channels. Congenital lymphedema (Milroy's disease) is a hereditary disorder characterized by chronic lymphatic obstruction. Lymphedema praecox occurs in adolescence, chiefly in females, and causes puffiness and swelling of the lower limbs. Secondary lymphedema may follow surgical removal of lymph channels in mastectomy, obstruction of lymph drainage caused by malignant tumors, or the infestation of lymph vessels with adult filarial parasites. —**lymphedematous, lymphedematose,** *adj.*

lymph node [L, *lympha* + *nodus,* knot], one of the many small oval structures that filter the lymph and fight infection and in which lymphocytes, monocytes, and plasma cells are formed. The lymph nodes are of different sizes, some as small as pinheads, others as large as lima beans. Each node is enclosed in a capsule; is composed of a lighter-colored cortical part and a darker medullary part; and consists of closely packed lymphocytes, reticular connective tissue laced by trabeculae, and three kinds of sinuses: subcapsular, cortical, and medullary. Lymph flows into the node through afferent lymphatic vessels. Most lymph nodes are clustered in areas such as the mouth, the neck, the lower arm, the axilla, and the groin.

lymph nodule [L, *lympha,* water, *nodulus,* small knot] any of the small densely packed spheric nodes or aggregations of lymph cells embedded in the reticular meshwork of the lymphatic system, mainly in the tonsils, spleen, and thymus.

lymphoblast /lim′fəblast′/, a large, immature cell that develops into a lymphocyte after an antigenic or mitogenic challenge.

lymphocele /lim′fəsēl/, a cystic mass that contains lymph from injured lymph vessels.

lymphocyte /lim′fəsīt/ [L, *lympha* + Gk, *kytos,* cell], small agranulocytic leukocytes originating from fetal stem cells and developing in the bone marrow. Lymphocytes normally comprise 25% of the total white blood cell count but increase in number in response to infection. Two forms occur: B cells and T cells. Both reproduce mitotically, each of the clones displaying identical antibodies on their surface membranes. When an immature B cell is exposed to a specific antigen, the cell is activated, traveling to the spleen or to the lymph nodes, differentiating, and rapidly producing **plasma cells and memory cells.** T cells are lymphocytes that have circulated through the thymus gland and have differentiated to become thymocytes.

lymphocyte activation, the stimulation of lymphocytes by antigens or mitogens, rendering them metabolically active and causing them to differentiate into immune effector cells.

lymphocyte transformation, an in vitro immunity test process in which a patient's lymphocytes are placed in a culture with an antigen. The rate of transformation, in terms of proliferation and enlargement of T memory cells, is measured by the uptake of radioactive thymidine by the lymphocytes, indicating protein synthesis.

lymphocytic choriomeningitis /lim'fəsit'-ik/ [L, *lympha* + Gk, *kytos,* cell, *chorion,* skin, *meninx,* membrane, *itis,* inflammation], an arenavirus infection of the meninges and the cerebrospinal fluid. It is caused by the lymphocytic choriomeningitis virus and characterized by fever, headache, and stiff neck.

lymphocytic hypophysitis, the massive infiltration of the pituitary gland by lymphocytes and plasma cells, with destruction of the normal parenchyma.

lymphocytic interstitial pneumonia (LIP), a diffuse respiratory disorder characterized by fibrosis and accumulation of lymphocytes in the lungs. It is commonly associated with lymphoma.

lymphocytopenia /lim'fōsī'təpē'nē·ə/ [L, *lympha* + Gk, *kytos,* cell, *penes,* poor], a decreased number of lymphocytes in the peripheral circulation, occurring as a primary hematologic disorder or in association with nutritional deficiency, malignancy, or infectious mononucleosis.

lymphocytosis /lim'fōsītō'sis/, a proliferation of lymphocytes, as occurs in certain chronic diseases and during convalescence from acute infections.

lymphocytotoxic antibody /lim'fōsītətok'-sik/, an antibody that induces the cell-killing activity of killer lymphocytes on combining with a certain antigen.

lymphoepithelioma /lim'fō·ep'ithē'lē·ō'-mə/ [L, *lympha* + Gk, *epi,* above, *thele,* nipple, *oma,* tumor], a poorly differentiated neoplasm developing from the epithelium overlying lymphoid tissue in the nasopharynx.

lymphogenesis /jen'əsis/, the formation of lymph.

lymphogranulomatosis /-gran'yəlō'mətō'-sis/ [L, *lympha,* water, *granulum,* small grain + Gk, *oma,* tumor, *osis,* condition], an infectious granuloma of the lymphatic system. The term is used to identify several inflammatory, granulomatous or sarcomatous disorders, such as **Hodgkin's disease, sarcoidosis,** and **lymphadenoma.**

lymphogranuloma venereum (LGV) /-gran'yəlō'mə/ [L, *lympha* + *granulum,* small grain; Gk, *oma,* tumor; L, *Venus,* goddess of love], a sexually transmitted disease caused by a strain of the bacterium *Chlamydia trachomatis.* It is characterized by ulcerative genital lesions, marked swelling of the lymph nodes in the groin, headache, fever, and malaise. Ulcerations of the rectal wall occur less commonly.

lymphoid /lim'foid/ [L, *lympha,* water; Gk, *eidos,* form], pertaining to lymph or lymphatics.

lymphoid interstitial pneumonia (LIP), a form of pneumonia that involves the lower lobes with extensive alveolar infiltration by mature lymphocytes, plasma cells, and histiocytes. It is associated with human immunodeficiency virus, dysproteinemia, and Sjögren's syndrome.

lymphoid tissue [L, *lympha,* water; Gk, *eidos,* form; OFr, *tissu*], tissue that consists of lymphocytes on a framework of reticular cells and fibers, as the tonsils and adenoids.

lymphokine /lim'fōkīn/ [L, *lympha* + Gk, *kinesis,* motion], one of the chemical factors produced and released by T lymphocytes that attract macrophages to the site of infection or inflammation and prepare them for attack. Kinds of lymphokines include **chemotactic factor, lymphotoxin, migration inhibiting factor,** and **mitogenic factor.**

lymphokine-activated killer (LAK) cells, nonspecific cytotoxic cells that are generated in the presence of interleukin-2 and the absence of antigen.

lympholysis /limfol'əsis/ [L, *lympha* + Gk, *lysein,* to loosen], cellular destruction of lymphocytes, especially of certain lymphocytes in the process of an immune response. **—lympholytic,** *adj.*

lymphoma /limfō'mə/ [L, *lympha* + Gk, *oma,* tumor], a type of neoplasm of lymphoid tissue that originates in the reticuloendothelial and lymphatic systems. It is usually malignant but in rare cases may be benign. Two main kinds of lymphomas are Hodgkin's disease and non-Hodgkin's lymphoma. The various lymphomas differ in degree of cellular differentiation and content, but the manifestations are similar in all types. Characteristically the appearance of a painless enlarged lymph node or nodes is followed by weakness, fever, weight loss, and anemia. With widespread involvement of lymphoid tissue, the spleen and liver usually enlarge; and gastrointestinal disturbances, malabsorption, and bone lesions frequently develop. — **lymphomatoid,** *adj.*

lymphoma staging, a system for classifying lymphomas according to the extent of the disease for the purpose of treatment and prognosis. Stage I is characterized by the involvement of a single lymph node region or one extralymphatic organ or site. Stage II is characterized by the involvement of two or more lymph node regions on the same side of the diaphragm or a localized involvement of an extralymphatic organ or site plus one or more node regions on the same side of the diaphragm. In stage III lymph nodes on both sides of the diaphragm are affected, and there may be involvement of the spleen or localized involvement of an extralymphatic organ or site. Stage IV is typified by diffuse or disseminated involvement of one or more extralymphatic organs or sites with or without associated lymph node involvement.

lymphomatoid granulomatosis /limfō'-mətoid/, a condition of unknown cause in which lymphocytes and plasma cells infiltrate the blood vessels, producing an angiocentric lesion.

lymphopoiesis /-pō-ē'sis/ [L, *lympha,* water; Gk, *poien,* to make], the formation of lymphocytes. —**lymphopoietic** /-pō·et'ik/, *adj.*

lymphoproliferative /-prōlif'ərətiv', -prō-lif'ərətiv/ [L, *lympha,* water, *prolles,* offspring, *ferre,* to bear], pertaining to the proliferation of lymphoid tissue.

lymphoproliferative syndrome (HTLV-1), induced a group of malignant neoplasms associated with infections by human T cell leukemia-lymphoma virus. The neoplasms arise from the clonal proliferation of lymphoid cells.

lymphoreticular malignancy /-retik'-yələr/, a disease of the lymphoreticular system commonly associated with cell-mediated immune deficiencies in which patients have a scarcity of normal white blood cells.

lymphoreticulosis /-retik'yəlō'sis/ [L, *lympha* + *reticulum,* little net; Gk, *osis,* condition], subacute granulomatous inflammation of lymphoid tissue with proliferation of reticuloendothelial cells, occurring most commonly as the result of a cat scratch. The disorder is characterized

by the formation of an ulcerated papule at the site of the scratch, fever, and tender lymphadenopathy, sometimes progressing to suppuration.

lymphorrhagia, an escape of lymph from a damaged vessel.

lymphorrhoid /limfôr'oid/, a dilated lymph vessel.

lymphosarcoma cell leukemia /-sárkō'mə/ [L, *lympha* + Gk, *sarx,* flesh, *oma,* tumor], a malignancy of blood-forming tissues characterized by many lymphosarcoma cells in the peripheral circulation that tend to infiltrate surrounding tissues.

lymphoscintigraphy /-sintig'rəfē/, a diagnostic technique using scintillation scanning of technetium-99m antimony trisulfide colloid in a noninvasive test for primary and secondary lymphedema. The radiopharmaceutical is injected subcutaneously in the interdigital space of the hands and feet.

lymphotrophy /limfot'rəfē/, the nourishment of cells by lymph, particularly in areas lacking adequate blood vessels.

lymph sinuses [L, *lympha,* water, *sinus,* hollow], continuous small endothelial-lined spaces just below the capsule of the lymph node. The sinuses slow the flow of lymph through the nodes.

Lyon hypothesis /lī'ən/ [Mary L. Lyon, English geneticist, b. 1925], (in genetics) a hypothesis stating that only one of the two X chromosomes in a female is functional, the other having become inactive early in development.

lyonization /lī'ənīzā'shən/ [Mary L. Lyon; Gk, *izein,* to cause], the process of random inactivation of one of the X chromosomes in the female gamete to compensate for the presence of the double X gene complement.

Lyon's ring [Mary L. Lyon], a type of congenital uropathy in females in which submeatal or distal urethral stenosis causes enuresis, dysuria, and recurring infections.

lyophilic /lī'ōfil'ik/ [Gk, *lyein,* to dissolve, *philein,* to love], pertaining to substances having an affinity for stability, in solution. Lyophilic substances are used to stabilize colloids.

lyophilize, to freeze-dry a substance under vacuum conditions.

lypressin /līpres'in/, an antidiuretic and vasoconstrictor prescribed in diabetes insipidus to decrease urinary water loss.

Lys, abbreviation for **lysine.**

lysate /lī'sāt/, a product of dissolution of matter by lysis, as in the destruction of proteins by hydrolysis.

lysemia /līsē'mē·ə/, the disintegration of

red blood cells, accompanied by the release of hemoglobin in the plasma.

lysergide /līsur'jīd/, a psychotomimetic, semisynthetic derivative of ergot that acts at multiple sites in the central nervous system from the cortex to the spinal cord. The drug may cause pupillary dilation, increased blood pressure, hyperreflexia, tremor, muscle weakness, piloerection, and increased body temperature. Larger doses also produce dizziness, drowsiness, paresthesia, euphoria or dysphoria, and synesthesias; colors may be heard, sounds may be visualized, and time is felt to pass slowly.

Lysholm method, (in radiology) any of several techniques for positioning a patient for x-ray examination of the cranial base, the mastoid and petrous regions of the temporal bone, and the optic foramen and orbital fissure.

lysin /lī'sin/, a specific complement-fixing antibody that initiates the lysis of cells.

lysine (Lys) /lī'sēn, lī'sin/, an essential amino acid needed for proper growth in infants and for maintenance of nitrogen balance in adults.

lysine intolerance, a congenital disorder resulting in the inability to use the essential amino acid lysine because of an enzyme deficiency or defect.

lysinemia /lī'sinē'mē·ə/, a condition caused by an inborn error of metabolism and resulting in the inability to use the essential amino acid lysine because of an enzyme defect or deficiency. It is characterized by muscle weakness and mental retardation.

lysine monohydrochloride, a salt of the amino acid lysine, used as a dietary supplement to increase the use of vegetable proteins such as corn, rice, and wheat.

lysinogen /līsin'əjən/, an antigen that

stimulates the production of a specific lysin.

lysinurea /lī'sinŏŏr'ē·ə/, the presence of lysine in the urine.

lysis /lī'sis/ [Gk, lysein, to loosen], **1.** destruction or dissolution of a cell or molecule through the action of a specific agent. Cell lysis is frequently caused by a lysin. **2.** gradual diminution in the symptoms of a disease. Compare **crisis.**

lysis of adhesions, surgery performed to free adhesions of tissues.

lysogenesis /lī'səjen'əsis/ [Gk, lysein, loosening, genein, to produce], the formation of lysins, or antibodies that cause partial or complete dissolution of the target cell.

lysokinase /lī'sōkī'nās/, an activating agent (enzyme) for the production of plasmin.

lysosome /lī'səsōm/ [Gk, lysein + soma, body], a cytoplasmic, membrane-bound particle that contains hydrolytic enzymes that function in intracellular digestive processes. If the hydrolytic enzymes are released into the cytoplasm, they cause self-digestion of the cell so that lysosomes may play an important role in certain self-destructive diseases characterized by the wasting of tissue such as muscular dystrophy.

lysotype /lī'sətīp/, a bacterial species type determined by its reaction to certain phages.

lysozyme /lī'səzīm/ [Gk, lysein + en, within, zyme, ferment], an enzyme with antiseptic actions that destroys some foreign organisms. It is found in granulocytic and monocytic blood cells and is normally present in saliva, sweat, breast milk, and tears.

lytes /līts/, an informal abbreviation of electrolytes, especially the levels of potassium, sodium, phosphorus, magnesium, and calcium in the blood, as determined by laboratory testing.

m, 1. abbreviation **meter.** 2. abbreviation for **milli-.**

M, 1. abbreviation for *mega.* 2. abbreviation for **molar.** 3. abbreviation for *metastasis* in the tumor, node, metastasis (TNM) system for staging malignant neoplastic disease.

ma, MA, abbreviation for **milliampere.**

MA, abbreviation for **mental age.**

M.A., abbreviation for *Master of Arts* degree.

MAA, abbreviation for **methacrylic acid.**

Maass, Clara [an American nurse, (1876–1901)], After training and working at the Newark German Hospital, which has since been renamed for her, she volunteered for military service at the outbreak of the Spanish-American War. After working at army camps where soldiers were dying of yellow fever, she volunteered to go to Havana to participate in the experiments being done to determine the cause of the disease. She was bitten by a mosquito and died 10 days later of yellow fever. She was one of the first nurses to be inducted into the Hall of Fame of the American Nurses Association.

Mab, abbreviation for **monoclonal antibodies.**

mabp, abbreviation for *mean arterial blood pressure.*

MAC, 1. abbreviation for **membrane attack complex.** 2. abbreviation for **microcystic adnexal carcinoma.** 3. abbreviation for **midupper arm circumference.** 4. abbreviation for **minimum alveolar concentration.**

MAC AWAKE, the dose of an inhalation anesthetic at which a patient is capable of responding to a verbal command.

mace /mās/, the oil-containing red fibrous wrapping of the nutmeg kernel. Dried and ground, it is used as an aromatic spice and flavoring.

Mace, trademark for a chemical lacrimator. The name is an acronym formed by letters in *m*ethyl*c*hloroform-2-chloro*ace*tophenone, which is dispersed from a pressurized container to immobilize an attacker.

macerate /mas'ərāt/ [L, *macerare*, to soften], to soften something solid by soaking. —**maceration**, *n.*

maceration /-ā'shən/, the softening and breaking down of skin resulting from prolonged exposure to moisture.

machinery murmur /məshēn'ərē/ [L, *machina* + *murmur*, humming], a continuous murmur heard throughout systole and diastole, with systolic accentuation. It is audible to the left of the sternum in patients with a ductus arteriosus condition.

machismo /mächis'mō/, (in psychology) a concept of the male that includes both desirable traits of courage and fearlessness and the dysfunctional behaviors of heavy drinking, seduction of women, and abusive spouse behavior.

Macleod, John J. [Scottish physiologist, 1876–1935], co-winner, with Sir Frederick G. Banting, of the 1923 Nobel prize for medicine and physiology, for their discovery of insulin.

macrencephaly /mak'rənsef'əlē/ [Gk, *makros*, large, *enkephalos*, brain], a congenital anomaly characterized by abnormal largeness of the brain. —**macrencephalic**, *adj.*

macroadenoma /-ad'ənō'mə/, a glandular tumor more than 10 mm in diameter.

macroamylase /-am'ilās/, a form of serum amylase in which the enzyme is bound to a globulin. Because the resulting complex is too large for renal clearance, plasma amylase levels are increased.

macroamylasemia /mak'rō·am'ilāsē'-mē·ə/, the presence of macroamylase in the blood.

macrobiosis /-bī·ō'sis/ [Gk, *makros*, long, *bios*, life], a long life.

macrobiotic diet /-bī·ot'ik/, a restrictive dietary regimen consisting of grains and unprocessed foods.

macroblepharia /mak'rōblifer'ē·ə/ [Gk, *makros* + *blepharon*, eyelid], the condition of having abnormally large eyelids.

macrocephaly /mak'rōsef'əlē/ [Gk, *makros* + *kephale*, head], a congenital anomaly characterized by abnormal largeness of the head and brain in relation to the rest of the body, resulting in some degree of mental and growth retardation. The head is more than two standard deviations above the average circumference size for age, sex, race, and period of gestation, with excessively wide fontanelles; the facial features are usually normal. There is symmetric overgrowth at the head without increased intracranial pressure, as differentiated from hydrocephalus. —**macrocephalic, macrocephalous,** *adj.,* **macrocephalus,** *n.*

macrocyte /mak′rəsīt/ [Gk, *makros* + *kytos,* cell], an abnormally large mature erythrocyte usually exceeding 9 μm in diameter that is commonly seen in megaloblastic anemias.

macrocytic /mak′rōsit′ik/ [Gk, *makros* + *kytos* + L, *icus,* form], (of a cell) larger than normal, such as the erythrocytes in macrocytic anemia.

macrocytic anemia, a disorder of the blood characterized by impaired erythropoiesis and the presence of large red blood cells in the circulation.

macrocytosis /mak′rōsītō′sis/ [Gk, *makros* + *kytos* + *osis,* condition], an abnormal proliferation of macrocytes in the peripheral blood.

macrodrip /mak′rōdrip/ [Gk, *makros* + AS, *drypan,* to fall in drops], (in intravenous therapy) an apparatus that is used to deliver measured amounts of intravenous solutions at specific flow rates based on the size of drops of the solution. The size of the drops is controlled by the fixed diameter of a plastic delivery tube.

macroelement, a chemical element required in relatively large quantities for the normal physiologic processes of the body. Macroelements include carbon, hydrogen, oxygen, nitrogen, potassium, sodium, calcium, chloride, magnesium, phosphorus, and sulfur.

macrogamete /-gam′ēt/ [Gk, *makros* + *gamete,* spouse], a large nonmotile female gamete of certain thallophytes and sporozoa, specifically the malarial parasite *Plasmodium.*

macrogametocyte /-gamē′təsīt/ [Gk, *makros* + *gamete* + *kytos,* cell], an enlarged merozoite that undergoes meiosis to form the mature female gamete during the sexual phase of the life cycle of certain thallophytes and sporozoa, specifically the malarial parasite *Plasmodium.*

macrogenitosomia /mak′rōjen′itōsō′mē·ə/ [Gk, *makros* + L, *genitalis,* genitalia; Gk, *soma,* body], a congenital condition in which the genitalia are abnormal because of an excess of androgen during fetal development. It is characterized in boys by enlarged external genitalia and in girls by pseudohermaphroditism.

macroglobulin /-glob′yəlin/, a globular serum protein with a molecular mass

above 1 kDa, such as the proteinase inhibitor alpha₂-macroglobulin.

macroglobulinemia /mak′rōglob′yŏŏlinē′-mē·ə/ [Gk, *makros* + L, *globulus,* small ball; Gk, *haima,* blood], a form of monoclonal gammopathy in which immunoglobulin (IgM) is overproduced by the clones of a plasma B cell in response to an antigenic signal.

macroglossia /mak′rōglos′ē·ə/ [Gk, *makros* + *glossa,* tongue], an excessively large tongue. It is seen in certain syndromes of congenital defects, including Down's syndrome.

macrognathia /mak′rōnā′thē·ə/ [Gk, *makros* + *gnathos,* jaw], an abnormally large growth of the jaw. —**macrognathic,** *adj.*

macrolide /ma′krōlīd/, any of a group of antibiotics produced by actinomycetes. They include erythromycin and troleandomycin. Macrolides are generally used against gram-positive bacteria and in patients allergic to penicillins.

macromolecule /-mol′əkyōōl/ [Gk, *makros* + L, *moles,* mass], a molecule of colloidal size, such as a protein, nucleic acid, or polysaccharide.

macronodular adrenal disease /-nod′-yələr/, a form of Cushing's syndrome characterized by massively enlarged adrenal glands.

macronucleus /-nōō′klē·əs/ [Gk, *makros* + L, *nucleus,* nut], **1.** a large nucleus. **2.** (in protozoa) the larger of two nuclei in each cell; it governs cell metabolism and growth.

macronutrient /-nōō′triənt/ [Gk, *makros* + L, *nutriens,* food that nourishes], nutrient required in the greatest amounts: carbohydrate, protein, fat or lipid, and water.

macrophage /mak′rəfāj/ [Gk, *makros* + *phagein,* to eat], any phagocytic cell of the reticuloendothelial system, including specialized Kupffer's cells in the liver and spleen and histocyte in loose connective tissue.

macrophage activating factor (MAF) [Gk. *makros,* large, *phagein,* to eat; L, *activus,* active, *facere,* to make], a lymphokine released from a sensitized leukocyte that induces changes in the appearance and function of macrophages as needed to make them active against certain antigens.

macrophage colony-stimulating factor (M-CSF), a glycoprotein growth factor that induces committed bone marrow stem cells to differentiate and mature into mononuclear phagocytes.

macrophage migration inhibiting factor [Gk, *makros,* large; *phagein,* to eat; L, *migrare,* to wander, *inhibere,* to restrain,

ere, to make], a lymphokine pro-
.ced by leukocytes that immobilizes
.acrophages after contact with an an-
.gen.

macroprolactinoma /-prōlak'tinō'mə/,
a pituitary tumor more than 10 mm in diameter that secretes serum prolactin levels
greater than 200 ng/ml.

macropsia /makrop'sē·ə/ [Gk, *makros,*
large, *opsis,* vision], a visual abnormality in which objects appear larger than
they actually are.

macroreentry /mak'rōrē·en'trē/ [Gk, *makros* + L, *re,* again; Fr, *entree,* entry], (in
cardiology) a relatively large reentry circuit. An example is a reentry circuit that
uses one bundle branch for anterograde
conduction and another for retrograde
conduction to produce the highly malignant bundle branch reentry ventricular
tachycardia.

macroscopic /-skop'ik/ [Gk, *makros,* large,
skopein, to view], large enough to be examined with the naked eye.

macroshock, shock from an electric current of 1 milliampere (mA) or greater.
Currents from 1 to 15 mA produce a tingling sensation and some muscle contraction, those from 15 to 100 mA can cause
a painful shock, those from 100 to 200
mA can cause cardiac fibrillation or respiratory arrest, and those above 200 mA
may produce rapid burning and destruction of tissue.

macrosis /makrō'sis/ [Gk, *makros,* large,
osis, condition], an increase in the size
or volume of an object.

macrotear /-ter, a significant damage to
soft tissues caused by acute trauma.

macula /mak'yələ/, *pl,* **maculae** [L, spot],
a small pigmented area of a spot that appears separate or different from the surrounding tissue.

macula albida [L, *macula,* spot, *albidare,*
to make white], small white areas in the
serous membranes of the pericardium or in
the peritoneum or pleura.

macula atrophica, a condition of cutaneous atrophy characterized by the appearance of small glistening white spots on
the skin.

macula densa [L, *macula,* spot, *densus,*
thick], a thickening in the wall of a distal
tubule of the kidney nephron at a point
where it is in contact with the afferent glomerulus. It may be part of a negative-
feedback system for sodium.

macula folliculi, a spot on the wall of an
ovary where a mature follicle will rupture
to release an ovum.

macula lutea, an oval yellow spot at the
optical "center" of the retina 2 mm from
the optic nerve. It contains a pit, no blood

vessels, and the fovea centralis. Central
high-acuity vision occurs when an image
is focused directly on the fovea centralis
of the macula lutea.

macular degeneration /mak'yələr/ [L,
macula, spot, *degenerare,* to deviate],
a progressive deterioration of the maculae
of the retina and choroid of the eye. The
condition is an effect of several diseases,
such as **retinitis pigmentosa.**

macular dystrophy, any of a variety of
eye disorders that damage the central part
of the retina. Several of the disorders are
related to gene mutations that affect older
adults.

macular rash [L, *macula,* spot; OFr,
rasche], a skin eruption in which the
lesions are flat and less than 1 cm in diameter.

macula solaris [L, *macula,* spot, *solaris,*
sun], a freckle.

macule /mak'yōōl/ [L, *macula,* spot], **1.**
a small flat blemish or discoloration that is
level with the skin surface. **2.** a gray scar
on the cornea that is visible without magnification. —**macular,** *adj.*

maculopapular rash /mak'yələpap'yələr/
[L, *macula,* spot, *papula,* pimple; OFr, *rasche*], a skin eruption characterized by
distinctive macules or papules.

maculopathy /mak'yəlop'əthē/ [L, *macula,*
spot; Gk, *pathos,* disease], a form of
macular degeneration primarily involving
the macula lutea.

MAD, abbreviation for **multiple autoimmune disorder.**

Madura foot /maj'ŏŏr'e/ [Madura, India;
AS, *fot,* foot], a progressive destructive
tropical fungal infection of the foot.

MAF, abbreviation for **macrophage activating factor.**

mafenide acetate /maf'ənīd/, a topical
antiinfective prescribed in the treatment of
burns.

Maffucci's syndrome, enchondromatosis
associated with multiple cavernous (cutaneous or visceral) hemangiomas.

magaldrate /mag'əldrāte/, an antacid
containing a combination of magnesium
and aluminum compounds. It is prescribed
in the treatment of hypersensitivity and
stomach upset associated with heartburn,
sour stomach, or acid indigestion.

magical thinking /maj'ikəl/, (in psychology) a belief that merely thinking about an
event in the external world can cause it to
occur. It is regarded as a form of regression to an early phase of development.

magic-bullet approach [Gk, *magikos,* sor-
cerer; Fr, *boulette,* small ball; L, *ad,* toward, *prope,* near], **1.** a therapeutic or
diagnostic method that makes use of a specific relationship between a drug and a dis-

M

ease or organ. **2.** (in clinical medicine) the administration of a specific drug to cure or ameliorate a given disease or condition. **3.** (in traditional diagnostic radiology) the administration of a specific dye to facilitate the radiographic visualization of a given organ. **4.** (in nuclear medicine) the administration of a specific radionuclide tagged to an appropriate carrier to provide a scintillation camera image of a given organ or structure.

Magill forceps, an intubation forceps used to guide a tracheal tube into the larynx.

magnesemia /mag′nəsē′mē·ə/, the presence of magnesium in the blood.

magnesium (Mg) /magnē′sē·əm, magnē′-zhəm/ [magnesia, lodestone], a silver-white mineral element. Its atomic number is 12; its atomic mass (weight) is 24.32. Magnesium is the second most abundant cation of the intracellular fluids in the body. It is essential for many enzyme activities. It also is important to neurochemical transmissions and muscular excitability. Excess magnesium (hypermagnesemia) in the body can slow the heartbeat and also cause vasodilation by direct effects on the blood vessels and by ganglionic blockade.

magnesium sulfate, a salt of magnesium prescribed parenterally to prevent seizures, especially in preeclampsia, and orally to treat constipation and heartburn and to correct magnesium deficiency.

magnetic field /magnet′ik/ [Gk, magnesia, lodestone; AS, feld], the region around any magnet in which its effects can be detected.

magnetic lines of force [Gk, magnesia, lodestone; L, linea, line, fortis, strong], theoretic lines of magnetism that surround a magnet or fill a magnetic field. The presence of the magnetic force along the imaginary lines can be demonstrated by inserting a sensitive material such as iron filings into the lines of magnetic effect.

magnetic moment [Gk, magnesia, lodestone, momentum, movement], a measure of the net magnetic field produced by an elementary particle or an atomic nucleus spinning about its own axis. It is the basis for magnetic resonance imaging.

magnetic permeability, the ratio of the magnetism induced in a body to the strength of the magnetic field of induction.

magnetic resonance (MR), 1. a phenomenon in which the atomic nuclei of certain materials placed in a strong static magnetic field absorb radio waves supplied by a transmitter at particular frequencies. **2.** spectra emitted by phosphorus in body tissues as measured and imaged on phosphorus nuclear magn[etic] resonance instruments.

magnetic resonance imaging (MRI) [G[k,] magnesia, lodestone, resonare, to soun[d] again, imago, image], medical imaging that uses radiofrequency radiation as its source of energy.

magnetic susceptibility, a measure of the ability of a substance to become magnetized.

magnetization /mag′nətīzā′shən/ [Gk, magnesia, lodestone; Gk, izein, to cause], the magnetic polarization of a material produced by a magnetic field (magnetic moment per unit volume).

magnetron /mag′nətron/ [Gk, magnesia, lodestone, trum, device], a source of microwave energy used in medical linear accelerators to accelerate electrons to the therapeutic energies.

magnification /mag′nifikā′shən/, (in psychology) cognitive distortion in which the effects of one's behavior are magnified.

magnification factor, (in radiology) the image size divided by the object size.

MAHA, abbreviation for **microangiopathic hemolytic anemia.**

Mahaim fibers [I. Mahaim, twentieth century French physician], conductive tracts in cardiac tissue running between the atrioventricular node and His bundle and the muscle of the ventricular septum. They conduct early excitation impulses.

Mahoney, Mary Eliza [the first black American nurse, (1845–1926)], Mahoney was active in furthering intergroup relationships and improving the role of the black nurse in the community. A medal in her name, established after her death, is given to a black nurse in recognition of an outstanding contribution to the nursing profession.

mainstreaming /mān′strēming/ [OE, maegan, strength; ME, strem], **1.** the system of educating children with disabilities in regular classrooms, with special assistance as needed. **2.** the return of persons recovering from mental illness to the community.

maintenance dose /mān′tənəns/ [Fr, maintenir, to uphold; Gk, dosis, giving], the amount of drug required to keep a desired mean steady-state concentration in the tissues.

Majocchi's granuloma /mäjok′ēz/ [Domenico Majocchi, Italian dermatologist, 1849–1929; L, granulum, small grain; Gk, oma, tumor], a rare type of tinea corporis that mainly affects the lower legs. It is caused by the fungus Trichophyton, which infects the hairs of the affected site and raises spongy granulomas.

major connector, a metal plate or bar

…ed for joining the components of one …de of a removable partial denture to …hose on the opposite side of the dental arch.

major depressive disorder, a major disorder of mood characterized by a persistent dysphoric mood, anxiety, irritability, fear, brooding, appetite and sleep disturbances, weight loss, psychomotor agitation or retardation, decreased energy, feelings of worthlessness or guilt, difficulty in concentrating or thinking, possible delusions and hallucinations, and thoughts of death or suicide. The disorder, which occurs in children, adolescents, and adults, may develop over a period of days, weeks, or months; episodes may occur in clusters or singly; separated by several years of normality. Treatment includes use of antidepressants and electroconvulsive therapy, followed by long-term psychotherapy.

major histocompatibility antigen, one of a group of antigens encoded by genes of the histocompatibility complex on chromosomes.

major histocompatibility complex (MHC) [L, *magnus,* great; Gk, *histos,* tissue; L, *compatibilis,* agreement, *complexus,* embrace], a group of proteins on the outer membrane of a cell that help identify self and nonself cells. MHC class I proteins normally help the immune system discriminate between healthy body cells and those that may be precancerous or infected by viruses. MHC class II molecules normally recognize foreign proteins and resemble the GP 120 protein on the outer membranes of human immunodeficiency virus, leading confused antibodies to attack the body's own T helper cells. Individuals with type I diabetes have lower than normal levels of MHC class I proteins, a susceptibility marker; their immune system fails to recognize their own beta cells.

major hysteria [ME, *maiour,* great; Gk, *hystera,* womb], an episode of psychogenic illness affecting a large group of individuals at the same time. An example is the witchcraft trials of the seventeenth century.

major medical insurance, insurance coverage designed to offset the costs of prolonged or catastrophic illness and injury.

major surgery, a surgical procedure that is extensive and/or life-threatening. It can be and often is done under other than general anesthesia.

making weight, (in sports medicine) the practice of rapid weight loss based on the belief that training at a heavier body weight, then dropping weight shortly before competition, gives an athlete an advantage.

mal /mal, mäl/ [L, *malus,* bad], an illness or disease, such as grand mal or petit mal epilepsy.

malabsorption /mal'əbsôrp'shən/ [L, *malus + absorbere,* to swallow], impaired absorption of nutrients from the gastrointestinal tract. It occurs in celiac disease, sprue, dysentery, diarrhea, inflammatory bowel disease, and other disorders.

malabsorption syndrome, a complex of symptoms resulting from disorders in the intestinal absorption of nutrients, characterized by anorexia, weight loss, abdominal bloating, muscle cramps, bone pain, and steatorrhea. Anemia, weakness, and fatigue occur because iron, folic acid, and vitamin B_{12} are not absorbed in sufficient amounts.

malacia /məlā'shə/ [Gk, *malakia,* softness], **1.** a morbid softening or sponginess in any part or tissue of the body. **2.** a craving for spicy foods such as mustard, hot peppers, or pickles. —**malacic,** *adj.*

maladaptation /mal'adəptā'shən/ [L, *malus + adaptatio*], faulty intrapersonal adjustment to stress or change. It may involve a failure to make necessary changes in the desires, values, needs, and attitudes or an inability to make necessary adjustments in the external world.

maladjusted /mal'adjus'tid/ [L, *malus,* bad, *adjuxtare,* to bring together], appearing unable to maintain effective relationships needed to fit into the environment and showing irritability, depression, and other psychogenic influences.

malady /mal'ədē/ [ME, *maladie,* sick], a disease or illness.

malaise /malāz'/ [Fr, discomfort], a vague uneasy feeling of body weakness, distress, or discomfort, often marking the onset of and persisting throughout a disease.

malalignment /mal'əlīn'mənt/ [L, *malus + ad,* to, *linea,* line], a failure of parts of the body to align normally, such as the teeth in the dental arch.

malar /mā'lər/ [L, *mala,* cheek], pertaining to the cheek or the cheekbone.

malaria /məler'ē·ə/ [It, *mal,* bad, *aria,* air], a severe infectious illness caused by one or more of at least four species of the protozoan genus *Plasmodium.* The disease is transmitted from human to human by a bite from an infected *Anopheles* mosquito. Malarial infection can also be spread by blood transfusion from an infected patient or by the use of an infected hypodermic needle. Malaria is characterized by chills, fever, anemia, an enlarged spleen, and a tendency to recurrence. *Plasmodium* parasites penetrate the erythrocytes of the hu-

M

man host, where they mature, reproduce, and burst out periodically. Malarial paroxysms occur at regular intervals, coinciding with the development of a new generation of parasites in the body. —**malarial,** *adj.*

malarial parasite /məler'ē·əl/ [It, *mal aria,* bad air; Gk, *parasitos,* guest], one of four known species of *Plasmodium* that may be injected into the human bloodstream by an anopheline mosquito to begin the cycle of malarial disease.

Malassezia /mal'əsē'zē·ə/ [Louis C. Malassez, French physiologist, 1842–1910], a genus of fungi. *Malassezia furfur* causes tinea versicolor. *M. ovalis* is a nonpathogenic organism found in sebaceous areas.

malathion poisoning /malā'thē·on, məl'-əthī'on/, a toxic condition caused by the ingestion or absorption through the skin of malathion, an organophosphorus insecticide. Symptoms include vomiting, nausea, abdominal cramps, headache, dizziness, weakness, confusion, convulsions, and respiratory difficulties.

male [L, *mas*], **1.** pertaining to the sex that produces sperm cells and fertilizes the female egg to beget children; masculine. **2.** a male person.

male catheterization, the passage of a catheter through the male urethra for the purpose of draining the urinary bladder. The male patient is placed in a supine position with the legs extended. The catheter is inserted 17.5 to 22.5 cm, or until urine flows. Sterile technique is important throughout the procedure to prevent the introduction of infectious organisms into the bladder.

male menopause [L, *mas,* male, *men,* month; Gk, *pauein,* to cease], a late middle-age psychogenic condition affecting some men, who experience anxiety over diminished potency, increased fatigue, thinning and graying hair, and other signs of aging.

male pattern alopecia [L, *mas,* male; ME, *patron* + Gk, *alopex,* fox mange], a common form of baldness in males, beginning at the front and spreading gradually until a fringe remains around the back and temples. Individual differences are determined by heredity, androgenic stimulation, and aging.

male reproductive system assessment, an evaluation of the condition of the patient's genitalia, reproductive history, and past and present genitourinary infections and disorders. A careful, understanding evaluation of the male patient's reproductive system helps to establish the diagnosis and plan the treatment and aids in allaying the patient's anxiety. The assessment also serves as a public health measure by encouraging the reporting of a sexually transmitted disease to the patient's contacts and proper authorities.

male sexual dysfunction, impaired or inadequate ability of a man to carry on his sex life to his own satisfaction. Symptoms, often psychologic in origin, include difficulties in starting and maintaining an erection, premature ejaculation, inability to ejaculate, and even loss of desire.

male sterility [L, *mas* + *sterilis,* barren], the inability of a man to produce sperm. Causes may include environmental factors such as exposure to heat or radiation, undescended testes, varicocele, prolonged fever, endocrine disorders, and abuse of alcohol or marijuana.

malfeasance /malfē'zəns/ [Fr, *malfaire,* to do evil], performance of an unlawful, wrongful act.

malformation /mal'fôrmā'shən/ [L, *malus,* bad, *forma,* shape], an anomalous structure in the body.

malfunction /mal'fungk'shən/ [L, *malus,* bad, *functio,* performance], **1.** the inability to function normally. **2.** not to function normally.

Malgaigne's fracture of pelvis /malgā'-nyəz/ [Joseph F. Malgaigne, French surgeon, 1806–1865], trauma involving multiple pelvic fractures, including fracture of the wing of the ilium or sacrum and fracture of the ipsilateral pubic rami, with associated upper displacement of the hemipelvis.

malicious prosecution /məlish'əs/ [L, *malitia,* wickedness, *prosequi,* to pursue], (in law) a suit begun in malice and pursued without sufficient cause.

malign /məlīn'/ [ME, *malignen,* deceptive], to show ill will or maliciousness; to act viciously; to harm.

malignant /məlig'nənt/ [L, *malignus,* bad disposition], **1.** tending to become worse and to cause death. **2.** (describing a cancer) anaplastic, invasive, and metastatic. —**malignancy,** *n.*

malignant atrophic papulosis, a form of cutaneous lymphocytic vasculitis. The skin disease shows erythematous papules with characteristic porcelain-white centers and elevated borders. The early signs are followed by perforated intestinal ulcers, leading to peritonitis, occluded arterioles, and progressive neurologic disability.

malignant dysentery [L, *malignus,* bad disposition; Gk, *dys,* bad, *enteron,* bowel], a potentially fatal form of dysentery in which symptoms are severe.

malignant endocarditis [L, *malignus,* bad disposition; Gk, *endon,* within, *kardia,* heart, *itis,* inflammation], a bacterial infection of the innermost layer of the heart but primarily affecting the valves after they have already been damaged by rheumatic fever or another disease. The valve cusps may be perforated or ulcerated. The patient usually experiences fever and sweating, emboli, and possibly septicemia.

malignant granuloma [L, *malignus,* bad disposition, *granulum,* little grain, *oma,* tumor], a malignant lymphoma, such as Hodgkin's disease, or a lymphosarcoma.

malignant hepatoma, a primary liver cancer.

malignant hypertension, the most lethal form of hypertension. It is a fulminating condition, characterized by severely elevated blood pressure that commonly damages the intima of small vessels, brain, retina, heart, and kidneys.

malignant hyperthermia (MH), a metabolic disease characterized by often fatal hyperthermia with rigidity of the skeletal muscles occurring in affected people exposed to certain anesthetic agents, particularly the inhalation anesthetics and succinylcholine.

Malignant Hyperthermia Precautions, a Nursing Interventions Classification defined as prevention or reduction of hypermetabolic response to pharmacologic agents used during surgery.

malignant mesenchymoma, a sarcoma that contains mesenchymal elements.

malignant neoplasm, a tumor that tends to grow, invade, and metastasize. It usually has an irregular shape and is composed of poorly differentiated cells. If untreated, it may result in death.

malignant transformation, the changes that a normal cell undergoes as it becomes a cancerous cell.

malignant tumor, a neoplasm that characteristically invades surrounding tissue, metastasizes to distant sites, and contains anaplastic cells. A malignant tumor may cause death if treatment does not intervene.

malingering /məling'gəring/ [Fr, *malingre,* puny, weak], a willful and deliberate feigning of the symptoms of a disease or injury to gain some consciously desired end. —**malinger,** *v.,* **malingerer,** *n.*

malleable /mal'ē-əbəl/ [L, *malleare,* to beat], able to be pressed, hammered, or otherwise forced into a shape without breaking.

malleolus /məlē'ələs/, *pl.* **malleoli** [L, little hammer], a rounded bony process, such as the protuberance on each side of the ankle.

mallet deformity [ME, *maillet,* maul], a flexion abnormality of the distal joint of a finger or toe. It may be caused by severe

damage such as rupture of the terminal tendon.

mallet fracture, avulsion fracture of the dorsal base of a distal phalanx of the hand or foot, involving the associated extensor apparatus and causing dropped flexion of the distal segment.

malleus /mal'ē-əs/, *pl.* **mallei** [L, hammer], one of the three ossicles in the middle ear, resembling a hammer, with a head, neck, and three processes. It is connected to the tympanic membrane and transmits sound vibrations to the incus.

Mallory body /mal'ərē/ [Frank B. Mallory, American pathologist, 1862–1941; AS, *bodig,* body], an eosinophilic cytoplasmic inclusion, alcoholic hyalin, found in the liver cells. It is typically, but not always, associated with acute alcoholic liver injury.

Mallory-Weiss' syndrome [G. Kenneth Mallory, American pathologist, b. 1926; Soma Weiss, American physician, 1899–1942], a condition characterized by massive bleeding after a tear in the mucous membrane at the junction of the esophagus and the stomach. The laceration is usually caused by protracted vomiting, most commonly in alcoholics or in people whose pylorus is obstructed.

malnutrition /mal'nootrish'ən/ [L, *malus,* bad, *nutrire,* to nourish], any disorder of nutrition. It may result from an unbalanced, insufficient, or excessive diet or from impaired absorption, assimilation, or use of foods.

malocclusion /mal'əkloo'zhən/ [L, *malus* + *occludere,* to shut up], abnormal contact of the teeth of the upper jaw with the teeth of the lower jaw.

malonic acid /məlo'nik/, a white, crystalline, highly toxic substance used as an intermediate compound in the production of barbiturates.

malpighian body /malpig'ē-ən/ [Marcello Malpighi, Italian physician, 1628–1694; AS, *bodig,* body], **1.** the renal corpuscle, which includes a glomerulus with Bowman's capsule. **2.** lymphoid tissue surrounding the arteries of the spleen.

malpighian corpuscle [Marcello Malpighi; L, *corpusculum,* little body], one of a number of small, round, deep-red bodies in the cortex of the kidney, each communicating with a renal tubule. The corpuscles are part of a filtering system through which nonprotein components of blood plasma enter the tubules for urinary excretion.

malposition /mal'pəzish'ən/, a placement of a body part that is dislodged, wrong, or faulty, such as in an untreated fracture.

malpractice /malprak'tis/ [L, *malus* + Gk,

M

praktikos, practical], (in law) professional negligence that is the proximate cause of injury or harm to a patient, resulting from a lack of professional knowledge, experience, or skill that can be expected in others in the profession or from a failure to exercise reasonable care or judgment in the application of professional knowledge, experience, or skill.

malpresentation /malpres′əntā′shən/ [L, *malus,* bad, *praesentare,* to show], an abnormal position of the fetus in the birth canal.

malrotation /mal′rōtā′shən/, **1.** any abnormal rotation of an organ or body part, such as the vertebral column or a tooth. **2.** a failure of the intestinal tract or other viscera to undergo normal rotation during embryonic development.

malt /môlt/ [[AS, *mealt*], a preparation obtained from germinated grain, such as barley, that contains partially degraded starch and protein with nutritive and digestive properties.

malunion /malyo͞o′nyən/ [L, *malus* + *unus,* one], an imperfect union of previously fragmented bone or other tissue.

mamillary body /mam′iler′ē/ [L, *mammilla,* nipple; AS, *bodig,* body], either of the two small round masses of gray matter in the hypothalamus located close to one another in the interpeduncular space.

mammary /mam′ərē/ [L, *mamma,* breast], pertaining to the breast.

mammary glands [L, *mamma,* breast, *glans,* acorn], lactiferous glands within the breasts. Glandular tissue forms a radius of lobes containing alveoli, each lobe having a system of ducts for the passage of milk from the alveoli to the nipple. The central part of the breast is filled with glandular tissue.

mammogram /mam′əgram/ [L, *mamma* + Gk, *gramma,* record], an x-ray film of the soft tissues of the breast.

mammography /mamog′rəfē/, radiography of the soft tissues of the breast to allow identification of various benign and malignant neoplastic processes.

mammoplasty /mam′əplas′tē/ [L, *mamma* + Gk, *plassein,* to mold], plastic reshaping of the breasts, performed to reduce or lift large or sagging breasts, to enlarge small breasts, or to reconstruct a breast after removal of a tumor.

mammothermography /mam′ōthərmog′-rəfē/ [L, *mamma* + Gk, *therme,* heat, *graphein,* to record], a diagnostic procedure in which thermography is used for examining the breast to detect abnormal growths.

managed care, a health care system in which there is administrative control over

primary health care services in a medical group practice. Redundant facilities and services are eliminated, and costs are reduced.

managed care organization (MCO), an organization that combines the functions of health insurance, delivery of care, and administration. Examples include the independent practice association, third-party administrator, management service organization, and physician-hospital organization.

management of therapeutic regimen, community: ineffective, a NANDA-accepted nursing diagnosis of a pattern of regulating and integrating into community processes programs for treatment of illness and sequelae of illness that are unsatisfactory for meeting health-related goals. The defining characteristics are deficits in persons and programs to be accountable for illness care of aggregates; deficits in advocates for aggregates; deficits in community activities for secondary and tertiary prevention; illness symptoms above the norm expected for the number and type of population; number of health care resources insufficient for the incidence or prevalence of illness(es); and unexpected acceleration of illness.

management of therapeutic regimen, families: ineffective, a NANDA-accepted nursing diagnosis of a pattern of regulating and integrating into family processes a program for treatment of illness and the sequelae of illness that are unsatisfactory for meeting specific health goals. Defining characteristics include inappropriate family activities for meeting the goals of a treatment or prevention program; acceleration (expected or unexpected) of illness symptoms of a family member; lack of attention to illness and its sequelae; verbalized desire to manage the treatment of illness and prevention of the sequelae; verbalized difficulty with regulation/integration of one or more effects or prevention of complications; and verbalizing that the family did not take action to reduce risk factors for progression of illness and sequelae.

management of therapeutic regimen, individual: effective, a NANDA-accepted nursing diagnosis of a pattern of regulating and integrating into daily living a program for treatment of illness and its sequelae that is satisfactory for meeting specific health goals. The defining characteristics are appropriate choices of daily activities for meeting the goals of a treatment or prevention program; illness symptoms within a normal range of expectation; verbalized desire to manage the atment of illness and prevention of sequelae; and verbalized intent to reduce risk factors for progression of illness and sequelae.

management of therapeutic regimen, individual: ineffective, a NANDA-accepted nursing diagnosis of a pattern of regulating and integrating into daily living a program for treatment of illness and the sequelae of illness that is unsatisfactory for meeting specific health goals. Defining characteristics include choices of daily living ineffective for meeting the goals of a treatment or prevention program; acceleration of illness symptoms, verbalized desire to manage the treatment and prevention of sequelae, verbalized difficulty with regulation/integration of one or more prescribed regimens for treatment of illness and its effects or prevention of complications, verbalization that intimates that the patient would not attempt to include treatment regimens in daily routines, and verbalization that intimates that the patient would not attempt to reduce risk factors for progression of illness and sequelae.

management service organization (MSO), an entity that under contract provides services such as a facility, equipment, staffing, contract negotiation, administration, and marketing. Services may be provided to solo practitioners or groups.

mandible /man′dibəl/ [L, *mandere,* to chew], a large bone constituting the lower jaw. It contains the lower teeth and consists of a horizontal part, a body, and two perpendicular rami that join the body at almost right angles. The body of the mandible is curved, somewhat resembling a horseshoe, and has two surfaces and two borders. —**mandibular,** *adj.*

mandibular arch /mandib′yələr/ [L, *mandere,* to chew, *arcus,* bow], the first visceral arch from which the lower jawbone develops.

mandibular block, (in dentistry) a regional anesthesia of the lower jaw produced by injection of a local analgesic near the third division of the trigeminal nerve.

mandibular canal [L, *mandere* + *canalis,* channel], (in dentistry) a passage or channel that extends from the mandibular foramen on the medial surface of the ramus of the mandible to the mental foramen. It holds blood vessels and a part of the mandibular branch of cranial nerve II (trigeminal).

mandibular notch, a depression in the inferior border of the mandible, anterior to the attachments of the masseter muscle,

where the external facial muscles cross the lower border of the mandible.

mandibular process [L, *mandere,* to chew, *processus*], **1.** the upper alveolar part of the mandible. **2.** the projection of the upper posterior part of the ramus of the mandible bearing the condyle.

mandibular ramus [L, *mandere,* to chew, *ramus,* branch], a broad quadrilateral part of the mandible projecting upward from the posterior end of the body behind the lower teeth. It has two surfaces, four borders, and two processes.

mandibular reflex [L, *mandere,* to chew, *reflectere,* to bend back], a reflex contraction of the masseter muscle after a downward tap on the point of the jaw while the mouth is open.

mandibular sling, the connection between the mandible and the maxilla, formed by the masseter and the pterygoideus at the angle of the mandible.

mandibular spine, a protuberance on the mandibular ramus to which the sphenomandibular ligament is attached.

mandibulofacial dysostosis /mandib′-yəlofā′shəl/ [L, *mandere* + *facies,* face; Gk, *dys,* bad, *osteon,* bone], an abnormal hereditary condition characterized by an antimongoloid slant of the palpebral fissures, coloboma of the lower lid, micrognathia and hypoplasia of the zygomatic arches, and microtia.

mandrel /man′drəl/ [Fr, *mandrin,* boring tool], the shaft of an object, which is inserted into a handpiece or lathe and supports the object while it is rotating.

maneuver /mənoo̅o̅′vər/ [Fr, *manœuvre,* action], **1.** an adroit or skillful manipulation or procedure. **2.** (in obstetrics) a manipulation of the fetus performed to aid in delivery.

manganese (Mn) /mang′gənēs/ [L, *manganesium,* associated with magnesium], a metallic element found in trace amounts in tissues of the body, where it aids in the functions of various enzymes. Its atomic number is 25; its atomic mass (weight) is 54.938.

manganese nodules, small nodes produced by microbial reduction of manganese oxides.

mania /mā′nē·ə/ [Gk, madness], a mood characterized by an unstable expansive emotional state; extreme excitement; excessive elation; hyperactivity; agitation; overtalkativeness; flight of ideas; increased psychomotor activity; fleeting attention; and sometimes violent, destructive, and self-destructive behavior.

manipulation /mənip′yələ′shən/ [L, *manipulare,* to work with the hands], the skillful use of the hands in therapeutic or diagnostic procedures, such as palpation, reduction of a dislocation, turning a fetus, or various treatments in physical therapy and osteopathy.

mannitol /man′itol/, a poorly metabolized sugar used as an osmotic diuretic and in kidney function tests. It is prescribed to promote diuresis, to decrease intraocular and intracranial pressure, to promote the excretion of poisons and other toxic wastes, and to evaluate renal function.

manometer /mənom′ətər/ [Gk, *manos*, thin, *metron*, measure], a device for measuring the pressure of a fluid, consisting of a tube marked with a scale and containing a relatively incompressible fluid, such as mercury. The level of the fluid in the tube varies with the pressure of the fluid being measured. Kinds of manometers are aneroid manometer and **sphygmomanometer.**

manometry /mənom′ətrē/ [Gk, *manos*, thin, *metron*, measure], **1.** the science of pressure movements of liquids or gases. **2.** a technique for measuring changes in the pressure of a gas or liquid that result from a biologic or chemical action.

Mansonella ozzardi /man′sənel′ə/, a parasitic worm that is indigenous to Latin America and the Caribbean islands. It is a relatively benign nematode that infects humans. The larvae live in the bloodstream, and adult worms are found in the visceral mesenteries.

Mantoux test /mantoo′/ [Charles Mantoux, French physician, 1877–1947], a tuberculin skin test that consists of intradermal injection of a purified protein derivative of the tubercle bacillus. A hardened, raised red area of 8 to 10 mm that appears 24 to 72 hours after injection is a positive reaction.

manual rotation /man′yoo·əl/ [L, *manualis*, hand, *rotare*, to turn], an obstetric maneuver in which a baby's head is turned by hand from a transverse to an anteroposterior position in the birth canal to facilitate delivery.

manubriosternal articulation /mənoo′-brē·ōstur′nəl/ [L, *manubrium*, handle; Gk, *sternum*, chest; L, *articularis*, joints], the fibrocartilaginous connection between the manubrium and the body of the sternum.

manubrium /mənoo′brē·əm/ [L, handle], the most anterior of the three bones of the sternum, presenting a broad quadrangular shape that narrows caudally at its articulation with the superior end of the body of the sternum. —**manubrial,** *adj.*

manudynamometer /man′oodīnə′mom′-ətər/ [L, *manus*, hand; Gk, *dynamis*, force,

metron, measure], a device for measuring the force or extent of thrust.

many-tailed bandage [AS, *manig, man taegel,* tail; Fr, *bande,* strip], **1.** a broad evenly shaped bandage with both ends split into strips of equal size and number. As the bandage is placed on the abdomen, chest, or limb, the ends may be overlapped and secured. **2.** an irregularly shaped bandage with torn or cut ends that are secured together.

MAO, abbreviation for **monoamine oxidase.**

MAOI, abbreviation for **monoamine oxidase inhibitor.**

MAP, 1. abbreviation for *medical aid post.* **2.** abbreviation for **mean arterial pressure.**

maple bark disease [AS, *mapul* + ONorse, *bark* + L, *dis,* opposite of; Fr, *aise,* ease], a hypersensitivity pneumonitis caused by exposure to the mold *Cryptostroma corticale,* found in the bark of maple trees. In the susceptible person the condition may be acute, accompanied by fever, cough, dyspnea, and vomiting, or chronic, characterized by fatigue, weight loss, dyspnea on exertion, and a productive cough.

maple syrup urine disease [AS, *mapul* + Ar, *sharab* + Gk, *ouron,* urine], an inherited metabolic disorder in which an enzyme necessary for the breakdown of the amino acids valine, leucine, and isoleucine is lacking. The disease is usually diagnosed in infancy; it is recognized by the characteristic maple syrup odor of the urine and by hyperreflexia.

mapping [L, *mappa,* napkin], (in genetics) the process of locating the relative position of genes on a chromosome through the analysis of genetic recombination.

maprotiline hydrochloride /maprō′tilēn/, an antidepressant similar to the tricyclics. It is prescribed for the treatment of depression.

map unit [L, *mappa,* napkin, *unus,* one], (in genetics) an arbitrary unit of measure used to designate the distance between genes on a chromosome. It is calculated from the percentage of recombinations that occur between specific genes so that 1% of crossing over represents one unit on a genetic map.

marasmic kwashiorkor /məraz′mik/ [Gk, *marasmos,* a wasting; Afr], a malnutrition disease, primarily of children, resulting from the deficiency of both calories and protein. The condition is characterized by severe tissue wasting, dehydration, loss of subcutaneous fat, lethargy, and growth retardation.

marasmoid /mərāz'moid/, resembling marasmus.

marasmus /məraz'məs/ [Gk, *marasmos,* a wasting], a condition of extreme malnutrition and emaciation, occurring chiefly in young children. It is characterized by progressive wasting of subcutaneous tissue and muscle. Marasmus results from a lack of adequate calories and proteins and is seen in children with failure to thrive and individuals in a state of starvation.

marathon encounter group /mer'əthon/ [Marathon, Greece; L, *in,* in, *contra,* against; Fr, *groupe*], an intensive group experience that accelerates self-awareness and promotes personal growth and behavioral change through the continuous interaction of group members for a period ranging from 16 to more than 40 hours.

Marburg virus disease /mär'bȯrg/, a severe febrile disease characterized by rash, hepatitis, pancreatitis, and severe gastrointestinal hemorrhages. The disease is transmitted by the Marburg virus, a member of the Filoviridae family, which also includes the Ebola virus. An epidemic in Marburg, Germany in 1967 was apparently contracted from infected imported African green monkeys. The disease may be transmitted to hospital personnel by improper handling of contaminated needles or from hemorrhagic lesions of patients.

march foot [Fr, *marcher,* to walk; AS, *fot*], an abnormal condition of the foot caused by excessive use, such as in a long march. The forefoot is swollen and painful, and one or more of the metatarsal bones may be broken.

march hemoglobinuria, a rare abnormal condition, characterized by the presence of hemoglobin in the urine, that occurs after strenuous physical exertion or prolonged exercise such as marching or distance running.

Marchiafava-Micheli's disease /mär'-kyəfä'vəmikä'lē/ [Ettore Marchiafava, Italian physician, 1847–1935; F. Micheli, Italian physician, 1872–1929], a rare disorder of unknown origin characterized by episodic hemoglobinuria, which occurs usually, but not always, at night.

Marchi's method /mär'kēz/ [Vittoria Marchi, Italian physician, 1851–1908], a laboratory staining procedure for demonstrating degenerated nerve fibers.

Marcus Gunn pupil sign [Robert Marcus Gunn, English ophthalmologist, 1850–1909], paradoxic dilation of the pupils in an ophthalmologic examination in response to afferent visual stimuli. In a dark room a beam of light is moved from one eye to the other. Normal miosis is caused by the consensual pupil reaction when the normal eye is illuminated; but, as the light is moved to the opposite, abnormal eye, the direct reaction to light is weaker than the consensual reaction; hence both pupils dilate.

Marfan's syndrome /märfäNz'/ [Bernard-Jean A. Marfan, French pediatrician, 1858–1942], a hereditary condition characterized by elongation of the bones, often with associated abnormalities of the eyes and the cardiovascular system. It causes major pathologic musculoskeletal disturbances such as muscular underdevelopment, ligamentous laxity, joint hypermobility, and bone elongation. Pathologic alterations of the cardiovascular system appear to produce fragmentation of the elastic fibers in the media of the aorta, which may lead to aneurysm. Ocular changes include a variety of disorders, including dislocation of the lens. The extremities of individuals with Marfan's syndrome are very long and spiderlike, with greatly extended hands, feet, and fingers.

marginal gingiva /mär'jənəl/ [L, *margo,* margin, *gingiva,* gum], the uppermost part of the free gingiva that overlaps the neck and base of the crown of the tooth.

marginal gyrus [L, *margo,* margin; Gk, *gyros,* turn], the superior frontal convolution on the surface of the cerebral hemispheres.

marginal peptic ulcer [L, *margo,* margin; Gk, *peptein,* to digest; L, *ulcus,* ulcer], an ulcer that develops after surgery at the surgical anastomosis of the stomach and jejunum.

marginal placenta previa, placenta previa in which the placenta is implanted in the lower uterine segment, with its margin touching or spreading to some degree over the internal os of the uterine cervix. During labor, as the cervix dilates, bleeding may occur from the separation of the edge of the placenta from the uterus beneath it.

marginal ridge, an elevation of enamel that forms the proximal boundary of the occlusal surface of a tooth.

marginal sinus [L, *margo* + *sinus,* hollow], a sinus that may encircle the placenta.

marginal sinus rupture, a detachment of the placenta from the implantation site. It may be complete, partial, or marginal in abruptio placentae.

Marie's hypertrophy [Pierre Marie, French neurologist, 1853–1940; Gk, *hyper,* excess, *trophe,* nourishment], chronic enlargement of the joints caused by periostitis.

M

Marin Amat's syndrome [Manuel Marin Amat, Spanish ophthalmologist, b. 1879] an involuntary facial movement phenomenon in which the eyes close when the mouth opens or when the jaws move in mastication. The effect results from a facial nerve paralysis.

marital rape [L, *rapere,* to seize], forcible sexual intercourse by a man with his wife.

mark [AS, *mearc*], any nevus or birthmark.

markers [AS, *mearc*], body language movements that serve as indicators and punctuation marks in interpersonal communication.

Marseilles fever /märsälz', märsä/ [Marseilles, France; L, *febris,* fever], a disease endemic around the Mediterranean, in Africa, in the Crimea, and in India, caused by *Rickettsia conorii* transmitted by the brown dog tick *(Rhipicephalus sanguineus).* Characteristic symptoms are chills, fever, an ulcer covered with a black crust at the site of the tick bite, and a rash appearing on the second to fourth day.

Marshall-Marchetti operation [Victor F. Marshall, American urologist, b. 1913; Andrew A. Marchetti, American obstetrician, 1901–1970], a surgical procedure performed to correct stress incontinence. The vesicourethropexy involves a retropubic incision and suturing of the urethra, vesicle neck, and bladder to the posterior surface of the pubic bone.

marsupialize /märsoo'pē·əlīz/ [L, *marsupium,* pouch; Gk, *izein,* to cause], to form a pouch surgically to treat a cyst when simple removal would not be effective, such as in a pancreatic or a pilonidal cyst.

masculine /mas'kyəlin/ [L, *masculinus,* male], having the characteristics of a male.

masculinization /mas'kyəlin'īzā'shən/ [L, *masculinus* + Gk, *izein,* to cause], the normal development or induction of male sex characteristics. —**masculinize,** *v.*

MASER /mā'sər/, acronym for *microwave amplification by stimulated emission of radiation.*

MASH /mash/, acronym for *mobile army surgical hospital.*

mask [Fr, *masque*], **1.** to obscure, as in symptomatic treatment that may conceal the development of a disease. **2.** to cover, as does a skin-toned cosmetic that may hide a pigmented nevus. **3.** a cover worn over the nose and mouth to prevent inhalation of toxic or irritating materials, to control delivery of oxygen or anesthetic gas, or (by medical personnel) to shield a patient during aseptic procedures from pathogenic organisms normally exhaled from the respiratory tract.

masked residue, the amino acid part of a peptide that is not accessible for activity after a condensation reaction.

mask image, (in digital fluoroscopy) a radiographic image made immediately after contrast material has been injected but before it reaches the anatomic site being examined. The initial mask image is then subtracted electronically from a series of additional images. The technique has the effect of enhancing the image of the tissues being studied.

masking, **1.** the covering or concealing of a disorder by a second condition. An example is a person's beginning a weight-loss diet while an undiagnosed wasting disease such as cancer has developed. **2.** the unconscious display of a personality trait that conceals a behavioral aberration.

masking agent, a cosmetic preparation for covering nevi, surgical scars, and other blemishes.

masklike facies [Fr, *masque* + L, *facies,* face], an immobile expressionless face with staring eyes and slightly open mouth. It is sometimes associated with parkinsonism.

Maslow's hierarchy of needs /mas'lōz/ [Abraham H. Maslow, American psychiatrist, 1908–1970; Gk, *hierarches,* position of authority; AS, *nied,* obligation], (in psychology) a hierarchic categorization of the basic needs of humans. The most basic needs on the scale are the physiologic or biologic such as the need for air, food, or water. Of second priority are the safety needs. The subsequent order of needs in the hierarchic progression are the need to belong, to love, and to be loved; the need for self-esteem; and ultimately the need for self-actualization.

masochism /mas'ōkiz'əm/ [Leopold von Sacher-Masoch, Austrian author, 1836–1895], pleasure or gratification derived from receiving physical, mental, or emotional abuse. —**masochistic,** *adj.*

masochist /mas'ōkist/ [Leopold von Sacher-Masoch], a person who derives pleasure or gratification from masochistic acts or abuse.

mass [L, *massa*], **1.** the physical property of matter that gives it weight and inertia. **2.** (in pharmacology) a mixture from which pills are formed. **3.** an aggregate of cells clumped together, such as a tumor.

mass action law, **1.** the mathematic description of reversible reactions that attain equilibrium, generally regarded as applicable to competitive assay. **2.** the rate of a chemical reaction that is proportional to the active masses of the resulting substances.

massage /məsäzh, məsäj'/ [Fr, *masser,* to stroke], the manipulation of the soft tissue of the body through stroking, rubbing, kneading, or tapping to increase circulation, improve muscle tone, and relax the patient. The procedure is performed either with the bare hands or through some mechanical means such as a vibrator.

masseter /mase'tər/ [Gk, one who chews], the thick rectangular muscle in the cheek that functions to close the jaw. It is one of the four muscles of mastication.

mass fragment [L, *massa,* lump, *frangere,* to shatter], a degraded part of a molecule containing one or more charges.

massive lung collapse, a condition in which an entire lung or one of its lobes becomes airless, frequently as a result of an obstruction in a bronchus.

mass number (A), the sum of the number of protons and neutrons in the nucleus of an atom or isotope.

mass reflex, an abnormal condition, seen in patients with transection of the spinal cord, characterized by a widespread nerve discharge. Stimulation below the level of the lesion results in flexor muscle spasms, incontinence of urine and feces, priapism, hypertension, and profuse sweating. A mass reflex may be triggered by scratching or other painful stimulus to the skin, overdistension of the bladder or intestines, cold weather, prolonged sitting, or emotional stress.

mass spectrometer, an analytic instrument for identifying a substance by sorting a stream of charged particles (ions) according to their mass.

mass spectrometry, (in chemistry) a technique for the analysis of a substance in which the constituents are identified by mass and fragmentation pattern and quantified using a mass spectrometer.

mass spectrum, a characteristic pattern obtained from a mass spectrometer.

mass transfer, the movement of mass from one phase to another.

mastalgia /mastal'jə/ [Gk, *mastos,* breast, *algos,* pain], pain in the breast caused by congestion or "caking" during lactation, an infection, or fibrocystic disease, especially during or before menstruation, or in advanced cancer. **—mastalgic,** *adj.*

mast cell [Ger, *Mast,* fattening; L, *cella,* storeroom], a constituent of connective tissue containing large basophilic granules that contain heparin, serotonin, bradykinin, and histamine.

mast cell leukemia, a malignant neoplasm of leukocytes characterized by connective tissue mast cells in circulating blood.

mast cell tumor [Ger, *Mastzelle,* food cell; L, *tumor*], a connective tissue tumor composed of mast cells.

mastectomy /mastek'təmē/ [Gk, *mastos,* breast, *ektome,* excision], the surgical removal of one or both breasts, most commonly performed to remove a malignant tumor. In a simple mastectomy only breast tissue is removed. In a radical mastectomy some of the muscles of the chest are removed with the breast, together with all lymph nodes in the axilla. In a modified radical mastectomy the large muscles of the chest that move the arm are preserved. **—mastectomize,** *v.*

master problem list, a list of a patient's problems that serves as an index to his or her record. Each problem, the date when it was first noted, the treatment, and the outcome are added to the list as each becomes known.

master's degree program in nursing, a postgraduate program in a school of nursing, based in a university setting, that grants the degree Master of Science in Nursing to successful candidates. Nurses with this degree function in leadership roles in clinical nursing, as consultants in various settings, in faculty positions in schools of nursing, and as nurse practitioners in the various specialties.

mastery /mas'tərē/ [L, *magister,* chief], command or control of a situation.

mastication /mas'tikā'shən/ [L, *masticare,* to chew], chewing, tearing, or grinding food with the teeth while it becomes mixed with saliva.

masticatory movement /mas'tikətôr'ē/, motion of the lower jaw in chewing.

masticatory system [L, *masticare,* to chew; Gk, *systema*], the combination of organs, structures, and nerves involved in chewing. It includes but is not limited to the jaws, the teeth and their supporting structures, the mandibular and maxillary musculature, the mandible, the maxillae, the temporomandibular joints, the tongue, the lips, the cheeks, the oral mucosa, the blood supply, and the cranial nerves.

mastitis /mastī'tis/ [Gk, *mastos,* breast, *itis,* inflammation], an inflammatory condition of the breast, usually caused by streptococcal or staphylococcal infection. Acute mastitis, most common in the first 2 months of lactation, is characterized by pain, swelling, redness, axillary lymphadenopathy, fever, and malaise. **Chronic tuberculous mastitis** is rare; when it occurs, it represents extension of tuberculosis from the lungs and ribs beneath the breast.

M

mastocarcinoma /mas′təkär′sinō′mə/, carcinoma of the mammary gland.

mastocytoma /mas′təsītō′mə/, a tumor that contains mast cells.

mastocytosis /mas′təsītō′sis/ [Ger, *Mast,* fattening; Gk, *kytos,* cell, *osis,* condition], local or systemic overproduction of mast cells, which in rare instances may infiltrate liver, spleen, bones, the gastrointestinal system, and skin.

mastoid /mas′toid/ [Gk, *mastos,* breast, *eidos,* form], **1.** pertaining to the mastoid process of the temporal bone. **2.** breast-shaped.

mastoid cells [Gk, *mastos,* breast, *eidos,* form; L, *cella,* storeroom], air cells in the mastoid process of the temporal bone.

mastoidectomy /mas′toidek′təmē/ [Gk, *mastos* + *eidos,* form, *ektome,* excision], surgical excision of a part of the mastoid part of the temporal bone. It is performed to treat chronic suppurative otitis media or mastoiditis when systemic antibiotics are ineffective. In a simple mastoidectomy with the patient under general anesthesia, infected bone cells are removed, and the eardrum is incised to drain the middle ear.

mastoid fontanel, a posterolateral fontanel that is usually not palpable.

mastoiditis /mas′toidī′tis/ [Gk, *mastos* + *eidos,* form, *itis,* inflammation], an infection of one of the mastoid bones, usually an extension of a middle ear infection. It is characterized by earache, fever, headache, and malaise. Residual hearing loss may follow the infection.

mastoid process, the conic projection of the caudal, posterior part of the temporal bone, serving as the attachment for various muscles, including the sternocleidomastoideus, splenius capitis, and longissimus capitis.

mastopathy /mastop′əthē/, any disease of the breast.

mastopexy, a reconstructive procedure in cosmetic surgery to lift the breasts.

masturbation /mas′tərbā′shən/ [L, *masturbari,* to masturbate], sexual activity in which the penis or clitoris is stimulated, usually to orgasm, by means other than coitus. **—masturbate,** *v,* **masturbatic, masturbatory,** *adj.*

materia /mətir′ē·ə/, matter or material.

material fact /mətir′ē·əl/ [L, *materia,* matter, *factum*], (in law) a fact that establishes or refutes an element essential to the complaint, charge, or defense.

materia medica, 1. the study of drugs and other substances used in medicine: their origins, preparation, uses, and effects. **2.** a substance or a drug used in medical treatment.

maternal /mətur′nəl/ [L, *maternus,* moth-

erhood], **1.** inherited, derived, or received from a mother. **2.** motherly in behavior. **3.** related through the mother's side of the family, such as a maternal grandfather.

maternal and child health (MCH) services, various facilities and programs organized for the purpose of providing medical and social services for mothers and children. Medical services include prenatal and postnatal services, family planning care, and pediatric care in infancy.

maternal antibody, an antibody transmitted from mother to fetus via the placenta. Such antibodies can confer immunity to the fetus and the newborn for up to 6 months after birth.

maternal death, the death of a woman during the childbearing cycle.

maternal deprivation syndrome [L, *maternus,* motherhood, *deprivare,* to deprive; Gk, *syn,* together, *dromos,* course], a condition characterized by developmental retardation that occurs as a result of physical or emotional deprivation. It is seen primarily in infants. Typical symptoms include lack of physical growth, with weight below the third percentile for age and size; malnutrition; pronounced withdrawal; silence; apathy; irritability; and a characteristic posture and body language, featuring unnatural stiffness and rigidity with a slow response reaction to others.

maternal immunity, an immunity acquired by a fetus through the passage of maternal antibodies via the placenta.

maternal-infant bonding, the complex process of attachment of a mother to her newborn. In the first minutes and hours after birth, a sensitive period occurs during which the baby and the mother become intimately involved with each other through behaviors and stimuli that are complementary and that provoke further interactions. The mother touches the baby and holds it en face to achieve eye-to-eye contact. The infant looks back eye to eye. The mother and the baby move in turn to the voice and sounds of the other, a process known as entrainment. The infant's movements constitute a response to the mother's voice, and she is encouraged to continue the process.

maternal inheritance, the transmission of traits or conditions controlled by cytoplasmic factors within the ovum that are not self-replicating and are determined by genes within the nucleus.

maternal mortality, 1. the death of a woman as a result of childbearing. **2.** the number of maternal deaths per 100,000 live births.

maternal placenta [L, *maternus,* motherhood, *placenta,* flat cake], the part of the placenta that develops from the decidua basalis of the uterus and is usually shed along with the fetal elements.

maternal serum alpha-fetoprotein (MSAFP) test, a test of a pregnant woman's blood designed to indicate an increased risk for fetal open neural tube defects such as spina bifida. It may also indicate an increased risk for Down's syndrome.

maternity (mat., matern.) /mətur′nitē/ [L, *maternus,* motherhood], motherhood, the character and quality of a mother.

maternity cycle [L, *maternus,* motherhood; Gk, *kyklos,* circle], the antepartal, intrapartal, and postpartal periods of pregnancy and the puerperium, from conception to 6 weeks after birth.

maternity nursing, nursing care of women and their families during pregnancy, during parturition, and through the first days of the puerperium.

mat gold [Fr, *mat,* dull; AS, *geolu,* yellow], a noncohesive form of pure gold.

mating /mā′ting/ [D, *mate,* companion], the pairing of individuals of the opposite sex, primarily for purposes of reproduction.

mat. med., abbreviation for **materia medica.**

matrifocal family /mat′rifō′kəl/ [L, *mater,* mother, *focus,* hearth, *familia,* household], a family unit composed of a mother and her children. Biologic fathers may have a temporary place in the family during the first years of the children's lives, but they maintain a more permanent position in their own original families.

matrix /mā′triks, mat′riks/ [L, womb], **1.** an intercellular substance **2.** a basic substance from which a specific organ or kind of tissue develops. **3.** a form used in shaping a tooth surface in dental procedures. **4.** (in analytic chemistry) material of no interest in an analysis that may have an effect on the analysis.

matrix retainer, a mechanical device used to secure the ends of a matrix band around a tooth and help compact a restoration into a prepared tooth cavity.

matroclinous inheritance /mātrō′klinəs/ [L, *mater,* mother; Gk, *kleinin,* to incline], a form of heredity in which the traits of the offspring have been transmitted from the mother.

matter [L, *materia*], **1.** anything that has mass and occupies space. **2.** any substance not otherwise identified as to its constituents, such as gray matter, pus, or serum exuding from a wound.

maturation /mach′ərā′shən/ [L, *maturare,* to ripen], **1.** the process or condition of attaining complete development. In humans it is the unfolding of full physical, emotional, and intellectual capacities that enable a person to function at a higher level of competency and adaptability within the environment. **2.** the final stages in the meiotic formation of germ cells in which the number of chromosomes in each cell is reduced to the haploid number characteristic of the species. **3.** suppuration. —**maturate,** *v.*

maturational crisis /mach′ərā′shənəl/, a transitional or developmental period within a person's life, such as puberty, when psychologic equilibrium is upset.

mature /məchŏŏr′/ [L, *maturus,* ripe], **1.** to become fully developed; to ripen. **2.** fully developed or ripened.

maturity (mat.) /məchŏŏ′ritē/ [L, *maturus,* ripe], **1.** a state of complete growth or development, usually designated as the period of life between adolescence and old age. **2.** the stage at which an organism is capable of reproduction.

max, 1. abbreviation for *maxima.* **2.** abbreviation for *maximum.*

maxilla /maksil′ə/, *pl.* **maxillae** [L, *mala,* jaw], one of a pair of large bones (often referred to as one bone) that form the upper jaw, consisting of a pyramidal body and four processes: the zygomatic, frontal, alveolar, and palatine.

maxillary /mak′sələr′ē/ [L, *maxilla,* upper jaw], pertaining to the upper jawbone.

maxillary arch [L, *maxilla,* upper jaw, *arcus,* bow], the curved bony ridge of the upper jawbone, in the shape of a horseshoe, including the dentition and supporting structures.

maxillary artery [L, *maxilla,* upper jaw; Gk, *arteria,* airpipe], either of two larger terminal branches of the external carotid arteries that rise from the neck of the mandible near the parotid gland and divide into three branches, supplying the deep structures of the face.

maxillary process [L, *maxilla,* upperjaw, *processus*], **1.** the alveolar process of the upper jaw that contains the tooth sockets. **2.** the frontal process that extends upward to articulate with the frontal and nasal bones. **3.** the palatine process that helps form the hard palate. **4.** the zygomatic process or anterior surface that articulates with the zygomatic bone.

maxillary sinus, one of a pair of large air cells forming a pyramidal cavity in the body of the maxilla.

maxillary tuberosity, a rounded eminence on the posterior surface of the body of the maxilla, behind the root of the third molar.

maxillary vein, one of a pair of deep

M

veins of the face, accompanying the maxillary artery. Each maxillary vein is a tributary of the internal and external jugular veins.

maxillodental /mak'silōden'təl/, pertaining to or affecting the upper jaw and teeth.

maxillofacial /mak'silōfā'shəl/ [L, *maxilla,* upper jaw, *facies,* face], pertaining to the maxilla and face.

maxillofacial prosthesis [L, *maxilla,* upper jaw, *facies* face], a prosthetic replacement for part, or all, of the upper jaw, nose, or cheek. It is applied when surgical repair alone is inadequate.

maxillofacial syndrome, a congenital defect of fetal ossification characterized by anteroposterior shortening of the maxilla and various other anomalies, including mandibular prognathism, slanting of the eyes, and malformation of the auricles.

maxillofacial trauma, injury to the jaw and face. Fractures requiring reconstructive surgery tend to occur most frequently in auto accidents and short falls.

maxillolacrimal suture /-lak'riməl/, a line of union between the anterior border of the lacrimal bone and the frontal process of the maxilla.

maxillomandibular /maksil'ōmandib'-yōōlər/, pertaining to the upper and lower jaws.

maxillomandibular fixation [L, *maxilla,* upper jaw, *mandere,* to chew, *figere,* to fasten], stabilization of fractures of the face or jaw by temporarily connecting the maxilla and mandible by wires, elastic bands, or metal splints.

maximal diastolic membrane potential, (in cardiology) the greatest degree of negative transmembrane potential achieved by a cell during repolarization.

maximal expiratory flow rate (MEFR), the rate of the most rapid flow of gas from the lungs during a forced vital capacity maneuver.

maximal expiratory pressure (MEP), the greatest force of exhalation achieved by a person after a full inhalation.

maximal midexpiratory flow rate (MMFR), the average volumetric rate of gas flow during the middle half (in terms of volume) of a forced expiratory vital capacity maneuver.

maximal treadmill test (MTT), an exercise stress test in which subjects increase their heart rate during exercise to 80% to 90% of the maximal rate, which is estimated from each subject's age and sex.

maximal voluntary ventilation (MVV), the maximal volume of gas that a person can ventilate by voluntary effort per unit of time breathing as quickly and deeply as possible.

maximum breathing capacity (MBC) /mak'siməl/ [L, *maximus,* greatest; AS, *braeth* + L, *capacitas*], the amount of gas exchanged per minute with maximal rate and depth of respiration.

maximum inspiratory pressure (MIP) /mak'səməm/ [L, *maximus,* greatest, *inspirare,* to breathe in, *premere,* to press], the maximum pressure within the alveoli of the lungs that occurs during a maximum inspiratory effort.

maximum oxygen uptake, the greatest amount of oxygen that can be transported from the lungs to the working muscle tissue.

maximum permissible dose (MPD), the largest amount of ionizing radiation a person may receive according to radiation protection guidelines for persons working with radioactive materials or x-rays. It is 5 rem per year or a lifetime accumulation of 1 rem times the age of the person.

maximum voluntary isometric contraction (MVIC), the peak rotary force produced by a muscular contraction.

Mayer's reflex /mā'ərz/ [Karl Mayer, Austrian neurologist, 1862–1932], a normal reflex elicited by grasping the ring finger and flexing it at the metacarpophalangeal joint of a person whose hand is relaxed with thumb abducted. The normal responses are adduction and apposition of the thumb.

May-Hegglin anomaly, a rare autosomal-dominant inherited blood cell disorder characterized by thrombocytopenia and granulocytes with blue-colored ribonucleic acid containing cytopathic inclusions, similar to Döhle's bodies.

mazindol /mā'zindōl/, an anorexiant prescribed to decrease the appetite in the treatment of exogenous obesity.

mb, mbar, abbreviation for *millibar.*

M.B., abbreviation for *Bachelor of Medicine.*

MBC, abbreviation for **maximum breathing capacity.**

MBD, M.B.D., abbreviation for *minimal brain dysfunction.*

mbp, abbreviation for *mean blood pressure.*

mbt, abbreviation for *mean body temperature.*

mc, abbreviation for *millicycle.*

mC, abbreviation for **millicoulomb.**

Mc, abbreviation for *megacycle.*

MC, 1. abbreviation for *medical certificate.* 2. abbreviation for *Medical Corps.*

McArdle's disease /məkär'dəlz/ [Brian McArdle, English neurologist, b. 1911], an inherited metabolic disease marked by an absence of myophosphorylase B and abnormally large amounts of glycogen in

...eletal muscle. It is milder than other glycogen storage diseases.

MCAT, abbreviation for **Medical College Aptitude Test.**

McBurney's incision /makbur'nēz/ [Charles McBurney, American surgeon, 1845–1913], a surgical wound that begins 2 to 5 cm above the anterior superior iliac spine and runs parallel to the external oblique muscle of the abdomen. This procedure is used for an appendectomy.

McBurney's point [Charles McBurney; L, *pungere*, to puncture], a site of extreme sensitivity in acute appendicitis, situated in the normal area of the appendix about 2 inches from the right anterosuperior spine of the ilium, on a line between that spine and the umbilicus.

McBurney's sign [Charles McBurney], a reaction of the patient indicating severe pain and extreme tenderness when McBurney's point is palpated. Such a reaction indicates appendicitis.

McCall's festoon /məkôlz'/, (in dentistry) a rimlike enlargement of the gingival margin that may be associated with occlusal trauma.

mcg, abbreviation for **microgram.**

M.Ch., abbreviation for *Master of Surgery.*

MCH, 1. abbreviation for **maternal and child health services. 2.** abbreviation for **mean corpuscular hemoglobin.**

MCHC, abbreviation for **mean corpuscular hemoglobin concentration.**

mCi-hr, abbreviation for *millicurie hour.*

McManus, R. Louise [American nurse, b. 1885], the individual who established the first national testing service for the nursing profession.

McMurray's sign /makmur'ēz/ [Thomas P. McMurray, English surgeon, 1887–1949], an audible click heard when rotating the tibia on the femur, indicating injury to meniscal structures.

MCO, abbreviation for **managed care organization.**

M component, an abnormal immunoglobulin that appears in large numbers in patients with macroglobulinemia, heavy chain disease, and multiple myeloma.

MCP, abbreviation for **metacarpophalangeal joint dislocation.**

M-CSF, abbreviation for **macrophage colony-stimulating factor.**

MCTD, abbreviation for **mixed connective tissue disease.**

MCV, abbreviation for **mean corpuscular volume.**

Md, symbol for the element **mendelevium.**

MD, abbreviation for **muscular dystrophy.**

M.D., abbreviation for *Doctor of Medicine.*

MDA, abbreviation for *Muscular Dystrophy Association.*

MDI, abbreviation for **metered dose inhaler.**

MDR, abbreviation for **minimum daily requirement.**

M.D.V., abbreviation for *Doctor of Veterinary Medicine.*

Me, abbreviation for the methyl radical CH_3-.

MEA, abbreviation for **multiple endocrine adenomatosis.**

Meals on Wheels, a program designed to deliver hot meals to elderly, physically disabled, or other people who lack the resources to provide nutritionally adequate warm meals for themselves on a daily basis.

mean [ME, *mene,* in the middle], occupying a position midway between two extremes of a set of values or data. The arithmetic mean is a value that is derived by dividing the total of a set of values by the number of items in the set. The geometric mean is a value between the first and last of a set of values organized in a geometric progression.

mean arterial pressure (MAP), the arithmetic mean of the blood pressure in the arterial part of the circulation.

mean corpuscular hemoglobin (MCH), an estimate of the amount of hemoglobin in an average erythrocyte, derived from the ratio between the amount of hemoglobin and the number of erythrocytes present.

mean corpuscular hemoglobin concentration (MCHC), an estimation of the concentration of hemoglobin in grams per 100 ml of packed red blood cells, derived from the ratio of the hemoglobin to the hematocrit.

mean corpuscular volume (MCV), an evaluation of the average volume of each red cell, derived from the ratio of the volume of packed red cells (the hematocrit) to the total number of red blood cells.

mean marrow dose (MMD), an arbitrary measure of the estimated average annual somatic radiation received by the population of the United States. The figure is 77 mrad and represents a weighted average for people exposed to radiation and those not exposed during the period. It is expressed in terms of bone marrow because irradiation of that tissue is assumed to be a cause of leukemia.

measles /mē'zəlz/ [ME, *meseles,* skin spots], an acute, highly contagious viral disease involving the respiratory tract and characterized by a spreading maculopapu-

M

lar cutaneous rash. It occurs primarily in young children who have not been immunized and in teenagers or young adults who are inadequately immunized. Measles is caused by a paramyxovirus and is transmitted by direct contact with droplets spread from the nose, throat, and mouth of infected people. It is characterized by fever, malaise, coryza, cough, conjunctivitis, photophobia, anorexia, and the pathognomonic Koplik's spots, which appear 1 to 2 days before onset of the rash. Pharyngitis and inflammation of the laryngeal and tracheobronchial mucosa develop, and the temperature may rise to 103° or 104° F. Within 3 to 5 days the fever subsides and the lesions flatten and begin to fade, causing a fine desquamation, especially over heavily affected areas.

measles and rubella virus vaccine live, an active immunizing agent prescribed for immunization against measles and rubella.

measles, mumps, and rubella virus vaccine live (MMR), an active immunizing agent prescribed for simultaneous immunization against measles, mumps, and rubella.

measurement /mezh′ərment/ [L, *mensura*], the determination, expressed numerically, of the extent or quantity of a substance, energy, or time.

measure of central tendency, (in descriptive statistics) an indication of the middle point of distribution for a particular group. Measures include the mean average score, the median or middle score of distribution, and the mode, the most frequently occurring measure.

measure of variability, (in descriptive statistics) a mathematic determination of how much the performance of the group as a whole deviates from the mean or median. The most frequently used measure of variability is the standard deviation.

meatorrhaphy /mē′ətôr′əfē/ [L, *meatus*, channel; Gk, *rhaphe*, suture], the suturing of the cut end of the urethra to the glans penis after surgery to enlarge the urethral meatus.

meatoscopy /mē′ətos′kəpē/ [L, *meatus* + Gk, *skopein*, to look], the visual examination of any meatus, especially the urethra, usually performed with the aid of a speculum.

meatus /mē·ā′təs/, *pl.* **meatuses** [L, channel], an opening or tunnel through any part of the body, such as the external acoustic meatus that leads from the external ear to the tympanic membrane.

mebendazole /məben′dəzōl/, an anthelmintic prescribed in treatment of pinworm, whipworm, roundworm, and hookworm infestations.

MEC, abbreviation for *minimum effecti* concentration, or the minimum inhibitor concentration that allows a drug to be ac tive. The drug is effective at any level above this threshold value.

mecamylamine hydrochloride /mek′-əmil′əmēn/, a ganglionic blocking agent prescribed in the management of hypertensive cardiac disease.

mechanical advantage [Gk, *mechane*, machine; L, *abante*, superior position], (in physiology) the ratio of the output force developed by the muscles to the input force applied to the body structures that the muscles move.

mechanical condenser, a device that delivers automatically controlled impacts for condensing restorative material in the filling of tooth cavities.

mechanical dead airspace [Gk, *mechane* + AS, *dead* + Gk, *aer* + L, *spatium*], the volume of air that fills the breathing circuits of a mechanical ventilator. The mechanical dead space may be increased if necessary to control hypocapnia and respiratory alkalosis.

mechanical heart-lung, a device connected to the circulatory system to maintain oxygenated blood flow during surgery that requires interruption of normal heart-lung functions.

mechanical restraint [Gk, *mechane* + L, *restringere*, to confine], a straitjacket, chair, bed, or other device used to enforce confinement of a patient.

Mechanical Ventilation, a Nursing Interventions Classification defined as use of an artificial device to assist a patient to breathe.

Mechanical Ventilatory Weaning, a Nursing Interventions Classification defined as assisting the patient to breathe without the aid of a mechanical ventilator.

mechanism /mek′əniz′əm/, **1.** an instrument or process by which something is done, results, or comes into being. **2.** a machine or machinelike system. **3.** a stimulus-response system. **4.** a habit or drive.

mechanism of injury, the circumstance in which an injury occurs: for example, caused by sudden deceleration, wounded by a projectile, crushed by a heavy object.

mechanoreceptor /mek′ənō′risep′tər/ [Gk, *mechane*, machine; L, *recipere*, to receive], any sensory nerve ending that responds to mechanical stimuli, such as touch, pressure, sound, and muscular contractions.

mechlorethamine hydrochloride /mek′-lôreth′əmēn/, an antineoplastic alkylating agent prescribed in the treatment of variety of neoplasms.

Meckel's diverticulum [Johann F. Meckel, German anatomist, 1781–1833], an anomalous sac protruding from the wall of the ileum. It is congenital, resulting from the incomplete closure of the yolk stalk.

meclizine hydrochloride /mek'lizēn/, an antihistamine prescribed in the prevention and treatment of motion sickness.

meclofenamate sodium /mek'lōfen'əmāt/, a nonsteroidal antiinflammatory agent prescribed in the treatment of rheumatoid arthritis and osteoarthritis.

meconium /mikō'nē-əm/ [Gk, *mekon,* poppy], a material that collects in the intestines of a fetus and forms the first stools of a newborn. It is thick and sticky, usually greenish to black, and composed of secretions of the intestinal glands, some amniotic fluid, and intrauterine debris such as bile pigments, fatty acids, epithelial cells, mucus, lanugo, and blood.

meconium aspiration, the inhalation of meconium by the fetus or newborn. It can block the air passages and cause failure of the lungs to expand or other pulmonary dysfunction.

meconium ileus, obstruction of the small intestine in the newborn caused by impaction of thick, dry, tenacious meconium, usually at or near the ileocecal valve. Symptoms include abdominal distension, vomiting, failure to pass meconium within the first 24 to 48 hours after birth, and rapid dehydration with associated electrolyte imbalance.

meconium plug syndrome, obstruction of the large intestine in the newborn caused by thick, rubbery meconium that may fill the entire colon and part of the terminal ileum. Symptoms include failure to pass meconium within the first 24 to 48 hours after birth, abdominal distension, and vomiting if complete intestinal blockage occurs.

med, 1. abbreviation for *medical.* **2.** abbreviation for *medicine.* **3.** abbreviation for *minimum effective dose.*

MED, 1. abbreviation for *minimal effective dose.* **2.** abbreviation for *minimal erythema dose.*

medcard /med'kärd/, (in nursing) a small card listing the name, dose, and schedule of administration of each patient's medications, used in dispensing drugs to each patient.

medevac, abbreviation for *medical evacuation.*

MEDEX /med'eks/, **1.** an educational program accredited by the American Medical Association for training military personnel with medical experience to become physician's assistants. **2.** a physician's assistant who has gained medical experience during military service and further training in a physician's assistant program.

medial /mē'dē-əl/ [L, *medius,* middle], **1.** pertaining to, situated in, or oriented toward the midline of the body. **2.** pertaining to the tunica media, the middle layer of a blood vessel wall.

medial antebrachial cutaneous nerve, a nerve of the arm that arises from the medial cord of the brachial plexus, medial to the axillary artery.

medial brachial cutaneous nerve, a nerve of the arm arising from the medial cord of the brachial plexus and distributed to the medial side of the arm.

medial cuneiform bone, the largest of three cuneiform bones of the foot, situated on the medial side of the tarsus, between the scaphoid bone and the first metatarsal. It serves as the attachment for various ligaments.

medial geniculate body, one of a pair of areas on the posterior dorsal thalamus, relaying auditory impulses from the lateral lemniscus to the auditory cortex.

medialis /mē'dē-ā'lis/ [L, *medius,* middle], pertaining to the middle or to the median plane.

medial malleolus, the rounded process of the tibia forming the internal surface of the ankle joint.

medial pectoral nerve, a branch of the brachial plexus that, with the lateral pectoral nerve, supplies the pectoral muscles.

medial rotation, a turning toward the midline of the body.

median /mē'dē-ən/ [L, *medius,* middle], (in statistics) the number representing the middle value of the scores in a sample. In an odd number of scores arrayed in ascending order, it is the middle score; in an even number of scores so arrayed, it is the average of the two central scores.

median antebrachial vein /an'tēbrā'kē-əl/, one of the superficial veins of the upper limb, which drains the venous plexus on the palmar surface of the hand.

median aperture of fourth ventricle, an opening between the roof of the fourth ventricle and the subarachnoid space.

median atlantoaxial joint, one of three points of articulation of the atlas and the axis. It allows rotation of the axis and the skull, the extent of rotation limited by the alar ligaments.

median basilic vein, one of the superficial veins of the upper limb, often formed as one of two branches from the median cubital vein. It is commonly used for venipuncture, phlebotomy, or intravenous infusion.

median effective dose (ED$_{50}$), the dose

M

of a drug that may be expected to cause a specific intensity of effect in half of the patients to whom it is given.

median jaw relation, (in dentistry) any jaw relation that exists when the mandible is in the median sagittal plane.

median lethal dose (MLD, LD$_{50}$), 1. (in radiotherapy) the amount of radiation that kills 50% of the individuals in a large group of animals or organisms within a specified period. 2. (in toxicology) the amount of a substance sufficient to kill one half of the population of test subjects.

median nerve, one of the terminal branches of the brachial plexus, which extends along the radial parts of the forearm and the hand and supplies various muscles and the skin of these parts.

median palatine suture, the line of junction between the horizontal parts of the palatine bones that extends from both sides of the skull to form the posterior part of the hard palate.

median plane, a vertical plane that divides the body into right and left halves and passes approximately through the sagittal suture of the skull.

median rhomboid glossitis, a red depressed, diamond-shaped area on the dorsum of the tongue, frequently irritated by alcohol, hot drinks, or spicy foods.

median sternotomy, a chest surgery technique in which an incision is made from the suprasternal notch to below the xiphoid process. The sternum is then opened with a saw. Closure requires reunion of the sternum with stainless steel sutures.

median toxic dose (TD$_{50}$), the dosage that may be expected to cause a toxic effect in half of the patients to whom it is given.

mediastinal /mē′dē·əstī′nəl/ [L, *mediastinus,* midway], pertaining to a median septum or space between two parts of the body.

mediastinitis, an inflammation of the mediastinum.

mediastinoscopy /mē′dē·as′tinos′kəpē/ [L, *mediastinus,* midway; Gk, *skopein,* to view], an examination of the mediastinum through an incision in the suprasternum, using an endoscope with light and lenses.

mediastinum /mē′dē·əstī′nəm/, *pl.* **mediastina** [L, *mediastinus,* midway], a part of the thoracic cavity in the middle of the thorax, between the pleural sacs containing the two lungs. It extends from the sternum to the vertebral column and contains all the thoracic viscera except the lungs. It is enclosed in a thick extension of the thoracic subserous fascia. —**mediastinal,** *adj.*

mediate /mē′dē·āt/ [L, *medio,* in the middle], 1. to cause a change, as in stimulation by a hormone. 2. to settle a dispute, as in collective bargaining. 3. situated between two places, things, parts, or terms. 4. (in psychology) an event that follows one process or event and precedes another. —**mediating,** *adj.,* **mediator,** *n.*

mediated transport, the movement of a solute across a membrane with the assistance of a transport agent, such as a protein, that aids entry of specific substances into a cell.

medic, abbreviation for **paramedic.**

Medicaid /med′ikād/, a U.S. federally funded state-operated program of medical assistance to people with low incomes, authorized by Title XIX of the Social Security Act. Under broad federal guidelines the individual states determine benefits, eligibility, rates of payment, and methods of administration.

Medicaid mill, *informal.* a health program or facility that solely or primarily serves people eligible for Medicaid. Such facilities are found mainly in depressed areas where few other health services are available.

medical antishock trousers (MAST) [L, *ante,* opposed; Fr, *choc* + Gael, *triubhas,* trews], a garment designed to produce pressure on the lower part of the body, thereby preventing the pooling of blood in the legs and abdomen. The trousers are used to combat shock, stabilize fractures, promote hemostasis, increase peripheral vascular resistance, and permit autotransfusion of small amounts of blood.

medical assistant /med′ikəl/ [L, *medicare,* to heal; *assistere,* to stand by], a person who, under the direction of a physician, performs various routine administrative and nontechnical clinical tasks in a hospital, clinic, or similar facility.

medical care, the provision by a physician of services related to the maintenance of health, prevention of illness, and treatment of illness or injury.

medical care plan [L, *medicare,* to heal; OE, *caru,* sorrow, *planus,* floor], a long-range program of professional medical guidance designed to meet specific health objectives.

medical center, 1. a health care facility. 2. a hospital, especially one staffed and equipped to care for many patients and for a large number of diseases and dysfunctions, using sophisticated technology.

Medical College Aptitude Test (MCAT), an examination taken by persons applying to medical school; the score attained is an important criterion for acceptance.

medical consultation, a procedure whereby, on request by one physician, another physician reviews a patient's medical history, examines the patient, and makes recommendations as to care and treatment. The medical consultant often is a specialist with expertise in a particular field of medicine.

medical corpsman /kōr′man/ [L, *medicare,* to heal, *corpus,* body], **1.** a member of a military medical unit. **2.** a paramedic.

medical decision level, the concentration of analyte, or body fluid sample being analyzed, at which some medical action is indicated for proper patient care.

medical diagnosis [L, *medicare* + Gk, *dia,* through, *gnosis,* knowledge], the determination of the cause of a patient's illness or suffering by the combined use of physical examination, patient interview, laboratory tests, review of the patient's medical records, knowledge of the cause of observed signs and symptoms, and differential elimination of similar possible causes.

medical diathermy [L, *medicare* + *dia,* through, *therme,* heat], the application of high-frequency electrical currents to generate therapeutic heat in diseased tissues.

medical directive, a general term for documents that provide direction on the type of care a person desires.

medical director, a physician who is usually employed by a hospital to serve in a medical and administrative capacity as head of the organized medical staff.

medical emergency kit, a package of drugs and devices that may be used to deal with life-threatening medical situations. The kit may include positive-pressure ventilation equipment, an oxygen tank, nitroglycerin spray or tablets, ammonia inhalants, tourniquets, a sugar source, a bronchial asthma inhaler or injectable corticosteroids or antihistamines, and drugs that can reverse the effects of common substance abuse.

medical engineering, a field of study of biomedical engineering and technologic concepts applied to develop equipment and instruments required in health care delivery.

Medic Alert, a nonprofit U.S. organization that maintains a huge database of information about individuals who are taking one or more medications for a chronic disorder. The database also includes emergency telephone numbers for physicians treating the patients and provides bracelets or pendants to alert paramedics, interns, or other emergency medical personnel of the

medical condition and prescription drugs taken by the patient, who may be unconscious or confused after an accident or episode of illness.

medical ethics [L, *medicare* + Gk, *ethikos*], the moral conduct and principles that govern members of the medical profession.

medical futility, 1. a judgment that further medical treatment of a patient would have no useful result. **2.** a medical treatment, the success of which is possible, but reasoning and experience suggest is highly improbable.

medical illustrator, an artist qualified by special training in preparing illustrations of organs, tissues, and medical phenomena in normal and abnormal states.

medical indigency /in′dijen′sē/, the lack of financial reserves adequate to pay for medical care, especially that of a person or family able to manage other basic living expenses.

medical jurisprudence [L, *medicare* + *jus,* law, *prudentia,* knowledge], the interaction of medicine with civil and criminal law.

medical laboratory technician, a person who, under the supervision of a medical technologist or physician, performs microscopic and bacteriologic tests of human blood, tissue, and fluids for diagnostic and research purposes.

medical model, the traditional approach to the diagnosis and treatment of illness in which the physician focuses on the defect, or dysfunction, within the patient. The medical history, physical examination, and diagnostic tests provide the basis for the identification and treatment of a specific illness.

medical outcomes study, an evaluation of comparable medical care approaches and their relative prognoses.

medical pathology [L, *medicare* + Gk, *pathos,* disease, *logos,* science], the study of diseases not readily treated by surgical procedures.

medical record [L, *medicare* + ME, *recorden,* to report], that part of a client's health record that is made by physicians and is a written or transcribed history of various illnesses or injuries requiring medical care; inoculations; allergies; treatments; prognosis; and frequently health information about parents, siblings, occupation, and military service. The record may be reviewed by a physician in diagnosing the condition.

medical record administrator, a person who maintains records of patients' medical histories, diagnoses, treatment, and

M

outcome in a condition that meets medical, administrative, legal, ethical, regulatory, and institutional requirements.

medical record technician, a health professional responsible for maintaining components of health information systems consistent with the medical, administrative, ethical, legal, accreditation, and regulatory requirements of the health care delivery system.

medical secretary, a person who prepares and maintains medical records and performs related secretarial duties.

medical snatch bag, *informal.* a light, compact, waterproof, and shockproof container of emergency medical equipment for advanced prehospital care. It should provide all that is required to control an obstructed airway, provide artificial ventilation, arrest hemorrhage from a peripheral site, and establish an intravenous access for transfusion.

medical staff, physicians and dentists who are approved and given privileges to provide health care to patients in a hospital or other health care facility.

medical staff, courtesy, physicians and dentists who meet certain qualifications of the medical staff of a hospital but who admit patients only occasionally or act as consultants. They are ineligible to participate in medical staff activities.

medical staff, honorary, physicians and dentists, usually retired, who are recognized by the hospital medical staff for their noteworthy contributions but who may not admit patients to the hospital or participate in medical staff activities.

medical-surgical nursing, the nursing care of adult patients whose conditions or disorders are treated pharmacologically or surgically.

medical technologist, a person who, under the direction of a pathologist or other physician or medical scientist, performs specialized chemical, microscopic, and bacteriologic tests of blood, tissue, and fluids. A certified medical technologist is one who has successfully completed an examination by the Board of Registry of the American Society of Clinical Pathologists or a similar professional body.

medical transcriptionist, a health professional who prepares a written record of patient data dictated by a physician. A certified medical transcriptionist is one who has met the qualifying standards of the American Association of Medical Transcription.

medical waste, any discarded biologic product such as blood or tissue removed from operating rooms, morgues, laboratories, or other medical facilities. The term

may also be applied to bedding, bandages, syringes, and similar materials that have been used in treating patients and to animal carcasses or body parts used in research.

Medical Women's International Association (M.W.I.A.), an international professional organization of women physicians.

medicamentosus /med′ikəmen′tōsəs/ [L, *medicamentum,* drug], pertaining to a drug, particularly to an adverse reaction attributed to a medication.

Medicare /med′iker/, **1.** a U.S. federally funded national health insurance program for people over 65 years of age. The program is administered in two parts. Part A provides basic protection against costs of medical, surgical, and psychiatric hospital care. Part B is a voluntary medical insurance program financed in part from federal funds and in part from premiums contributed by people enrolled in the program. Medicare was authorized by Title XVIII of the Social Security Act of 1965. **2.** (in Canada) Medicare is the name of the national health insurance program.

medicate /med′ikāt/ [L, *medicare,* to heal], to treat an illness by administering drugs.

medicated bougie /med′ikātid/ [L, *medicare,* to heal; Fr, candle], a bougie containing a medicated agent.

medicated enema, a medication administered via an enema. It is usually used before surgery with patients scheduled for bowel surgery.

medicated tub bath, a therapeutic bath in which medication is dispersed in water, usually in the treatment of dermatologic disorders.

medication /med′ikā′shən/ [L, *medicare,* to heal], **1.** a drug or other substance that is used as a medicine. **2.** the administration of a medicine.

Medication Administration, a Nursing Interventions Classification defined as preparing, giving, and evaluating the effectiveness of prescription and nonprescription drugs.

Medication Administration: Enteral, a Nursing Interventions Classification defined as delivering medications through an intestinal tube.

Medication Administration: Interpleural, a Nursing Interventions Classification defined as administration of medication through an interpleural catheter for reduction of pain.

Medication Administration: Intraosseous, a Nursing Interventions Classification defined as insertion of a needle through the bone cortex into the medullary cavity for the purpose of short-term emergency administration of fluid, blood, or medication.

Medication Administration: Oral, a Nursing Interventions Classification defined as preparing and giving medications by mouth and monitoring patient responsiveness.

Medication Administration: Parenteral, a Nursing Interventions Classification defined as preparing and giving medications via the intravenous, intramuscular, intradermal, and/or subcutaneous route.

Medication Administration: Topical, a Nursing Interventions Classification defined as preparing and applying medications to the skin and mucous membranes.

Medical Administration: Ventricular Reservoir, a Nursing Interventions Classification defined as administration and monitoring of medication through an indwelling catheter into the lateral ventricle.

medication error, any incorrect or wrongful administration of a medication, such as a mistake in dosage or route of administration, failure to prescribe or administer the correct drug or formulation for a particular disease or condition, use of outdated drugs, failure to observe the correct time for administration of the drug, or lack of awareness of adverse effects of certain drug combinations.

Medication Management, a Nursing Interventions Classification defined as facilitation of safe and effective use of prescription and over-the-counter drugs.

medication order, a written order by a physician, dentist, or other designated health professional for a medication to be dispensed by a hospital pharmacy for administration to an inpatient.

Medication Prescribing, a Nursing Interventions Classification defined as prescribing medication for a health problem.

medicinal restraint /mədis'ənəl/ [L, *medicina,* art of healing, *restringere,* to confine], the use of psychotropics, hypnotics, or anxiolytics to control a potentially violent patient.

medicinal treatment, therapy of disorders based chiefly on the use of appropriate pharmacologic agents.

medicine [L, *medicina,* art of healing], **1.** a drug or a remedy for illness. **2.** the art and science of the diagnosis, treatment, and prevention of disease and the maintenance of good health. **3.** the art or technique of treating disease without surgery. Two major divisions of medicine are academic medicine and clinical medicine. —**medical,** *adj.*

medicolegal /med'ikōlē'gəl/ [L, *medicina,* art of healing, *lex,* law], pertaining to both medicine and law. Medicolegal considerations, decisions, definitions, and policies provide the framework for informed consent, professional liability, and many other aspects of current practice in the health care field.

meditation /med'itā'shən/ [L, *meditari,* to consider], a state of consciousness in which the individual eliminates environmental stimuli from awareness so that the mind has a single focus, producing a state of relaxation and relief from stress.

Meditation, a Nursing Interventions Classification defined as altering the patient's level of awareness by focusing specifically on an image or thought.

meditation therapy, a method of achieving relaxation and consciousness expansion by focusing on a mantra or a key word, sound, or image while eliminating outside stimuli from one's awareness.

medium, /mē'dē·əm/, *pl.* **media** [L, *medius,* middle], a substance through which something moves or through which it acts. A **contrast medium** is a substance that has a density different from that of body tissues, permitting visual comparison of structures when used with imaging techniques such as x-ray film. A culture medium is a substance that provides a nutritional environment for the growth of microorganisms or cells. A dispersion medium is the substance in which a colloid is dispersed. A **refractory medium** is the transparent tissues and fluid of the eye that refract light.

medium-chain triglyceride (MCT), a glycerine ester combined with an acid, distinguished from other triglycerides by having 8 to 10 carbon atoms. MCTs in foods are usually high in calories and easily digested.

MEDLARS /med'lärs/, abbreviation for *Medical Literature Analysis and Retrieval System,* a computerized literature retrieval service of the National Library of Medicine in Bethesda, Maryland.

MEDLINE /med'līn/, a U.S. National Library of Medicine computer data base that covers approximately 600,000 references to biomedical journal articles published currently and in the 2 preceding years. The files duplicate the contents of the monthly and annual volumes of the *Unabridged Index Medicus,* also published by the National Library of Medicine.

MedRC, abbreviation for *medical reserve corps.*

medroxyprogesterone acetate /medrok'-sēprōjes'tərōn/, a progestin prescribed in the treatment of menstrual disorders caused by hormone imbalance.

medrysone /med'risōn/, a glucocorticoid

M

that decreases the infiltration of leukocytes at the site of inflammation.

Med.Sc.D., abbreviation for *Doctor of Medical Science.*

Med Tech, abbreviation for *medical technician.*

medulla /mədul′ə/, *pl.* **medullas, medullae** [L, marrow], **1.** the most internal part of a structure or organ, such as the renal medulla. **2.** *informal.* medulla oblongata.

medulla oblongata, a bulbous continuation of the spinal cord just above the foramen magnum and separated from the pons by a horizontal groove. It is one of three parts of the brainstem and contains the cardiac, vasomotor, and respiratory centers of the brain.

medulla of the kidney [L, *medulla,* marrow; ME, *kidenei*], a part of the parenchyma of the kidney, beneath the cortex, including the renal pyramids and columns. An inner layer contains the papillae, and the outer part contains the thick ascending limbs of the loop of Henle.

medullary /med′əler′ē, mədul′erē, med′-yəler′ē/ [L, *medulla,* marrow], **1.** pertaining to the medulla of the brain. **2.** pertaining to the bone marrow. **3.** pertaining to the spinal cord.

medullary carcinoma, a soft malignant neoplasm of the epithelium containing little or no fibrous tissue.

medullary cystic disease, a chronic familial disease of the kidney, characterized by the slow onset of uremia. The disease appears in young children or adolescents who pass large volumes of dilute urine with greater than normal amounts of sodium.

medullary sponge kidney, a congenital defect of the kidney, leading to cystic dilation of the collecting tubules. People with this defect often develop a kidney stone or an infection of the kidney caused by urinary stasis.

medullated /med′yəlā′tid/ [L, *medulla,* marrow], enclosed by a marrowlike substance, such as the myelin sheath of a nerve fiber.

medulloblastoma /mədul′ōblastō′mə/ [L, *medulla* + Gk, *blastos,* germ, *oma,* tumor], a poorly differentiated malignant neoplasm composed of tightly packed cells of spongioblastic and neuroblastic lineage. The tumor usually arises in the cerebellum, is extremely radiosensitive, and grows rapidly.

mefenamic acid /mef′ənam′ik/, a nonsteroidal antiinflammatory agent and analgesic prescribed in the treatment of mild to moderate pain.

mefloquine /mef′ləkēn/, an antimalarial for the prophylaxis and treatment of chloroquine-resistant falciparum and vivax malaria.

MEFR, abbreviation for **maximal expiratory flow rate.**

megacolon /meg′əkōlən/ [Gk, *megas* + *kolon,* colon], abnormal massive dilation of the colon that may be congenital, toxic, or acquired. Congenital megacolon (Hirschsprung's disease) is caused by the absence of autonomic ganglia in the smooth muscle wall of the colon. Toxic megacolon is a grave complication of ulcerative colitis and may cause perforation of the colon, septicemia, and death. Acquired megacolon is the result of a chronic refusal to defecate, which usually occurs in children who are psychotic or mentally retarded. The colon becomes dilated by an accumulation of impacted feces.

megadose /meg′ədōs/, a dose that greatly exceeds the amount usually prescribed or recommended.

megadyne /meg′ədīn/, a unit of force equal to one million dynes.

megaesophagus /meg′ə·isof′əgəs/ [Gk, *megas* + *oisophagos,* gullet], abnormal dilation of the lower segments of the esophagus caused by distension resulting from the failure of the cardiac sphincter to relax and allow the passage of food into the stomach.

megahertz (MHz) /meg′əhurts/ [Gk, *megas,* large, *hertz,* a number of cycles per second], a unit of frequency equal to a million cycles per second.

megakaryocyte /meg′əker′ē·əsīt′/ /meg′-əker′ē·əsīt′/ [Gk, *megas,* large, *karyon,* nut, *kytos,* cell], an extremely large bone marrow cell having a nucleus with many lobes. Megakaryocytes are essential for the production and proliferation of platelets in the marrow and are normally not present in the circulating blood. —**megakaryocytic,** *adj.*

megakaryocytic leukemia /meg′əker′-ē·ōsit′ik/ [Gk, *megas* + *karyon,* nut, *kytos,* cell], a rare malignancy of blood-forming tissue in which megakaryocytes proliferate in the bone marrow and circulate in the blood in large numbers.

megalencephaly /meg′əlensef′əlē/ [Gk, *megas* + *enkephalos,* brain], a condition characterized by pathologic parenchymal overgrowth of the brain. In some cases generalized cerebral hyperplasia is associated with mental retardation or a brain disorder, such as epilepsy. —**megalencephalic, megalencephalous,** *adj.*

megaloblast /meg′əlōblast′/ [Gk, *megas* + *blastos,* germ], an abnormally large nucleated immature erythrocyte that develops in large numbers in the bone marrow and is plentiful in the circulation in anemias associated with deficiency of vitamin B_{12}, folic acid, or intrinsic factor. —**megaloblastic,** adj.

megaloblastic anemia /-blas′tik/, a hematologic disorder characterized by the production and peripheral proliferation of immature large dysfunctional erythrocytes. Megaloblasts are usually associated with severe pernicious anemia or folic acid deficiency anemia.

megalocystis /meg′əlōsis′tis/ [Gk, megas + kystis, bag], an abnormal condition primarily affecting girls, characterized by an enlarged and thin-walled bladder.

megalocyte /meg′əlōsīt/, an extremely large erythrocyte.

megalomania /meg′əlōmā′nē·ə/ [Gk, megas + mania, madness], an abnormal mental state characterized by delusions of grandeur in which one believes oneself to be a person of great importance, power, fame, or wealth.

megaloureter /meg′əlōyŏŏrē′tər/ [Gk, megas + oureter, ureter], an abnormal condition characterized by marked dilation of one or both ureters, resulting from dysfunctional peristaltic action of the smooth muscle in the ureters.

megavitamin therapy /-vī′təmin/, a type of treatment that involves the administration of large doses of certain vitamins and minerals.

megestrol acetate /məjes′trōl/, an antineoplastic progestational agent prescribed to treat endometrial cancer and more commonly to palliate advanced endometrial and breast cancer.

meibomian gland /mēbō′mē·ən/ [Heinrich Meibom, German physician, 1638–1700], one of several sebaceous glands that secrete sebum from their ducts on the posterior margin of each eyelid. The glands are embedded in the tarsal plate of each eyelid.

Meigs′ syndrome /megz/ [Joe V. Meigs, American gynecologist, 1892–1963], ascites and hydrothorax associated with a fibroma of the ovaries or other pelvic tumor.

meiocyte /mī′əsīt/ [Gk, meiosis, becoming smaller, kytos, cell], any cell undergoing meiosis.

meiogenic /mī′əjen′ik/ [Gk, meiosis + genein, to produce], producing or causing meiosis.

meiosis /mī-ō′sis/ [Gk, becoming smaller], the division of a sex cell as it matures into two, then four haploid cells; the nucleus of each receives one half of the number of chromosomes present in the somatic cells of the species. —**meiotic** /mī-ot′ik/, adj.

Meissner′s corpuscle /mīs′nərz/ [Georg Meissner, German anatomist, 1829–1905;

L, corpusculum, little body], any one of a number of small, special pressure-sensitive sensory end organs with a connective tissue capsule and tiny stacked plates in the corium of the hand and foot, the front of the forearm, the skin of the lips, the mucous membrane of the tongue, the palpebral conjunctiva, and the skin of the mammary papilla.

Meissner′s plexus /mīs′nərz/, [Georg Meissner; L, plaited], small aggregations of ganglion cells located in the submucosa of the intestine.

mel [L, honey], a mixture of invert sugars and polysaccharides produced from the nectar of flowers by enzymes secreted by the honeybee, Apis mellifica.

melancholia /mel′angkō′lē·ə/ [Gk, melas, black, chole, bile], a severe form of depression.

melaniferous /mel′ənif′ərəs/ [Gk, melas, black; L, ferre, to bear], pertaining to a black pigment.

melanin /mel′ənin/ [Gk, melas, black], a black or dark brown pigment that occurs naturally in the hair, skin, and iris and choroid of the eye.

melanism /mel′əniz′əm/ [Gk, melas, black], an abnormal deposit of dark brown to black melanin pigment in the skin, hair, and other tissues.

melanoameloblastoma /mel′ənō·am′-əlōblastō′mə/, a benign neoplasm appearing as a blue-black lesion on the anterior maxilla of infants. The growth is of neuroectodermal origin and consists of small round undifferentiated tumor cells and larger melanin-producing cells.

melanoblast /mel′ənōblast′/ [Gk, melas, black, blastos, germ], an epithelial tissue cell containing black granules. It develops into a melanocyte.

melanoblastoma /mel′ənō·blastō′mə/, a tumor of poorly differentiated melanin-producing cells.

melanocarcinoma /-kär′sinō′mə/, a malignant melanoma.

melanocyte /mel′ənōsīt′, məlen′ōsīt/ [Gk, melas + kytos, cell], a body cell capable of producing melanin. Melanocytes are distributed throughout the basal cell layer of the epidermis and form melanin pigment from tyrosine, an amino acid.

melanocyte-stimulating hormone (MSH), a polypeptide hormone, secreted by the anterior pituitary gland, that controls the intensity of pigmentation in pigmented cells.

melanocytic nevus /-sit′ik/, a congenital pigmented lesion of the skin caused by a disorder involving melanocytes.

melanoderma /mel′ənōdur′mə/ [Gk, melas + derma, skin], any abnormal darkening

M

of the skin caused by increased deposits of melanin or the salts of iron or silver.

melanoma /mel′ənō′mə/ [Gk, *melas* + *oma,* tumor], any of a group of malignant neoplasms that originate in the skin and are composed of melanocytes. A melanocytic nevus may be acquired or congenital. The congenital melanocytic nevus is regarded as more likely to develop into a malignant melanoma, primarily because of its larger size. Smaller melanomas tend to develop from a pigmented nevus over several months or years. They may be sporadic and occur most commonly in fair-skinned people having light-colored eyes. A previous sunburn increases a person's risk. Any black or brown spot having an irregular border; pigment appearing to radiate beyond that border; a red, black, and blue coloration observable on close examination; or a nodular surface is suggestive of melanoma and is usually excised for biopsy. Melanomas may metastasize and are among the most malignant of all skin cancers. Prognosis depends on the kind of melanoma; its size, depth of invasion, and location; and the age and condition of the patient.

melanomatosis /-mətō′sis/, **1.** a condition characterized by many widespread melanoma lesions. **2.** the development of melanomas throughout the body.

melanosis coli /mel′ənō′sis/, an abnormal condition in which the mucous membrane of the colon is pigmented with melanin.

melanosome /mel′ənōsōm′/, the oval pigment granules within melanocytes that synthesize melanin.

melanotic carcinoma /mel′ənot′ik/, a malignant pigmented skin cancer.

melanuria /mel′ənŏŏr′ē·ə/, urine that has a dark color caused by the presence of melanin or other pigments.

melasma gravidarum /məlaz′mə/ [Gk, *melas,* black; L, *gravida,* pregnant], a dark pigment or discoloration that may appear on the skin of pregnant women.

melatonin /mel′ətō′nin/ [Gk, *melas* + *tonikos,* stretching], the only hormone secreted into the bloodstream by the pineal gland. The hormone appears to inhibit numerous endocrine functions, including the gonadotropic hormones, and to decrease skin pigmentation. When injected, exogenous melatonin causes drowsiness.

melena /məlē′nə/ [Gk, *melas,* black], abnormal black tarry stool that has a distinctive odor and contains digested blood. It usually results from bleeding in the upper gastrointestinal tract and is often a sign of peptic ulcer or small bowel disease.

melena neonatorum [Gk, *melas,* black, *neos,* new; L, *natus,* born], the passage of dark tarry stools by a newborn. The cause is usually the alteration of blood pigment associated with hemorrhage. Normal meconium stools are greenish to black.

melioidosis /mel′ē·oidō′sis/ [Gk, *melis,* distemper, *eidos,* form, *osis,* condition], an infection caused by the gram-negative bacillus *Malleomyces pseudomallei.* Acute melioidosis is fulminant and usually characterized by pneumonia, empyema, lung abscess, septicemia, and liver or spleen involvement. Chronic melioidosis is associated with osteomyelitis, multiple abscesses of the internal organs, and development of fistulas from the abscesses. The disease is acquired by direct contact with infected animals.

melon-seed body /mel′ən/, a small fibrous loose body in a joint or tendon sheath.

melphalan /mel′fəlan/, an antineoplastic alkylating agent prescribed in the treatment of malignant neoplastic diseases, including multiple myeloma.

melting, 1. the liquefaction effect of heat. **2.** the thermal denaturation of double-stranded deoxyribonucleic acid into two component strands.

melting point (mp) [AS, *meltan* + L, *punctus,* pricked], a characteristic temperature at which the solid and liquid forms of a substance are in equilibrium. The mp of ice is 32° F, or 0° C, at one atmosphere pressure.

membrana tectoria /membrā′nə/ [L, *membrana,* thin skin, *tectorium,* a covering], **1.** the broad, strong ligament covering the dens and helping to connect the axis to the occipital bone of the skull. **2.** a spiral membrane projecting from the vestibular lip of the cochlea over the organ of Corti.

membrane /mem′brān/ [L, *membrana,* thin skin], a thin layer of tissue composed of epithelial cells and connective tissue that covers a surface, lines a cavity, or divides a space in the body.

membrane attack complex (MAC), a cluster of complement components that creates a pore in the membrane of a cell, leading to its lysis.

membrane conductance, (in cardiology) the degree of permeability of a cellular membrane to certain ions.

membrane diffusion coefficient, a component of total pulmonary diffusing capacity. It includes qualitative and quantitative characteristics of the functioning alveolar-capillary membrane.

membrane potential [L, *membrana* + *potentia*], the difference in electrical polar-

ization or charge between two sides of a membrane or cell wall.

membrane responsiveness, (in cardiology) the relationship between the membrane potential at the time of stimulation and the maximal rate of depolarization of the action potential.

membranoproliferative glomerulonephritis (MPGN) /mem'brənō'prōlif'-ərotiv'/, a chronic form of glomerulonephritis, characterized by mesangial cell proliferation, irregular thickening of glomerular capillary walls, thickening of the mesangial matrix, and low serum levels of complement.

membranous /mem'brənəs/ [L, *membrana*], resembling or consisting of a membrane.

membranous dysmenorrhea [L, *membrana* + Gk, *dys*, bad, *men*, month, *rhein*, to flow], a form of spasmodic pain associated with menstruation, in which a cast of the uterine cavity is passed.

membranous labyrinth [L, *membrana* + *labyrinthos*, a maze], a network of three fluid-filled membranous semicircular ducts suspended within the bony semicircular canals of the inner ear, associated with the sense of balance.

membranous pharyngitis [L, *membrana* + Gk, *pharynx*, throat], a diphtheric inflammation of the pharynx with the formation of a false membrane in the throat.

memory /mem'ərē/ [L, *memoria*], **1.** the mental faculty or power that enables one to retain and to recall, through unconscious associative processes; previously experienced sensations, impressions, ideas, concepts; and all information that has been consciously learned. **2.** the reservoir of all past experiences and knowledge that may be recollected or recalled at will. **3.** the recollection of a past event, idea, sensation, or previously learned knowledge.

memory image, a sensation, impression, or sense perception as it is recalled in the memory

memory, impaired, a NANDA-accepted nursing diagnosis of the state in which an individual experiences the inability to remember or recall bits of information or behavioral skills. Impaired memory may be attributed to pathophysiologic or situational causes that may either be temporary or permanent. Defining characteristics include observed or reported experiences of forgetting; inability to determine whether a behavior was performed; inability to learn or retain new skills or information; inability to perform a previously learned skill; inability to recall factual information; inability to recall recent or past

events; and forgetting to perform a behavior at a scheduled time.

Memory Training, a Nursing Interventions Classification defined as facilitation of memory.

MEN, abbreviation for **multiple endocrine neoplasia.**

menadiol sodium diphosphate /men'ədī'-ol/, a water-soluble analog of vitamin K.

menadione, menaphthone /men'ədī'ōn/, a synthetic form of vitamin K_3. A water-soluble injectable form of the product is menadiol sodium diphosphate.

menarche /menär'kē/ [Gk, *men*, month, *archaios*, from the beginning], the first menstruation and the commencement of cyclic menstrual function. It usually occurs between 9 and 17 years of age.

mendelevium (Md) /men'dəlē'vē·əm/ [Dimitri I. Mendeleyev, Russian chemist, 1834–1907], a synthetic element in the actinide group. Its atomic number is 101. The atomic mass (weight) of its most stable isotope is 256. It is the ninth transuranic element.

mendelism /men'dəliz'əm/ [Gregor J. Mendel, Austrian geneticist, 1822–1884], the concept of inheritance derived from the application of Mendel's laws. —**mendelian,** *adj.*

Mendel's laws [Gregor J. Mendel], the basic principles of inheritance based on the breeding experiments of garden peas. These are usually stated as two laws, commonly called the law of segregation and the law of independent assortment. According to the first, each characteristic of a species is represented in the somatic cells by a pair of units, now known as genes, which separate during meiosis so that each gamete receives only one gene for each trait. According to the second law, members of a gene pair on different chromosomes segregate independently from other pairs during meiosis so that the gametes show all possible combinations of factors.

Mendelson's syndrome [Curtis L. Mendelson, American obstetrician, b. 1913], a respiratory condition caused by the chemical pneumonia resulting from the aspiration of acid gastric contents into the lungs. It usually occurs when an inebriated person vomits or when a person is stuporous from anesthesia or unconscious, such as during a seizure.

Ménière's disease /mānē·erz'/ [Prosper Ménière, French physician, 1799–1862], a chronic disease of the inner ear characterized by recurrent episodes of vertigo; progressive sensorineural hearing loss, which may be bilateral; and tinnitus. The cause is unknown, although occasionally the condition follows middle ear infection or head trauma. There also may be associated nausea, vomiting, and profuse sweating. Attacks last from a few minutes to several hours.

meninges /minin'jēz/, *sing.* **meninx** /mē'ningks, men'-/ [Gk, *meninx,* membrane], the three membranes enclosing the brain and spinal cord, comprising the dura mater, the pia mater, and the arachnoid membrane. —**meningeal,** *adj.*

meningioma /minin'jē·ō'mə/ [Gk, *meninx,* membrane, *oma,* tumor], a mesenchymal fibroblastic tumor of the membranes enveloping the brain and spinal cord. The tumors may be nodular, plaquelike, or diffuse lesions that invade the skull, causing bone erosion and compression of brain tissue.

meningism /minin'jizəm/ [Gk, *menigx* + *ismos,* process], an abnormal condition characterized by irritation of the brain and spinal cord and by symptoms that mimic those of meningitis. In meningism, however, there is no actual inflammation of the meninges.

meningismus /men'injis'məs/ [Gk, *menigx,* membrane], a condition in which the patient shows signs of meningitis but examination reveals no pathologic changes in the meninges. The condition is associated with cases of pneumonia in small children.

meningitis /min'injī'tis/, *pl.* **meningitides** [Gk, *menigx* + *itis,* inflammation], any infection or inflammation of the membranes covering the brain and spinal cord. It is usually purulent and involves the fluid in the subarachnoid space. The most common causes in adults are bacterial infection with *Streptococcus pneumoniae, Neisseria meningitidis,* or *Haemophilus influenzae.* Aseptic meningitis may be caused by nonbacterial agents. Meningitis is characterized by severe headache, stiffness of the neck, irritability, malaise, and restlessness. Nausea, vomiting, delirium, and complete disorientation may develop quickly. Temperature, pulse rate, and respirations are increased.

meningocele /mining'gōsēl'/ [Gk, *menigx* + *kele,* hernia], a saclike protrusion of either the cerebral or spinal meninges through a congenital defect in the skull or the vertebral column. It forms a hernial cyst that is filled with cerebrospinal fluid but does not contain neural tissue. The anomaly is designated a cranial meningocele or spinal meningocele, depending on the site of the defect.

meningococcal polysaccharide vaccine /-kok'əl/, either of two active immunizing agents against group A and group C meningococcal organisms. It is prescribed for immunization against meningococcal meningitis.

meningococcemia /mining'gōkoksē'mē·ə/ [Gk, *menigx* + *kokkos,* berry, *haima,* blood], a disease caused by *Neisseria meningitidis* in the bloodstream. Onset is sudden, with chills, pain in the muscles and joints, headache, petechiae, sore throat, and severe prostration. Tachycardia is present, respirations and pulse rate are increased, and fever is intermittent.

meningococcus /mining'gōkok'əs/, *pl.,* **meningococci** /-kok'sī/ [Gk, *menigx* + *kokkos,* berry], a bacterium of the genus *Neisseria meningitidis,* a nonmotile gram-negative diplococcus, frequently found in the nasopharynx of asymptomatic carriers, that may cause septicemia or epidemic cerebrospinal meningitis. —**meningococcal,** *adj.*

meningoencephalitis /-ensef'əlī'tis/ [Gk, *menigx,* membrane, *enkephalos,* brain, *itis,* inflammation], an inflammation of both the brain and the meninges, usually caused by a bacterial infection.

meningoencephalocele /mining'gō·ensef'-əlōsēl'/ [Gk, *menigx* + *enkephalos,* brain, *kele,* hernia], a saclike cyst containing brain tissue, cerebrospinal fluid, and meninges that protrudes through a congenital defect in the skull.

meningoencephalomyelitis /mining'gō-ensef'əlōmī'əlī'tis/, a combined inflammation of the brain, spinal cord, and meninges.

meningoencephalopathy /mining'gō·ensef'əlōp'əthē/, a noninflammatory disease of the brain and its membranes.

meningomyelitis /-mī'əlī'tis/ [Gk, *menigx,* membrane, *myelos,* marrow, *itis,* inflammation], an inflammation of the spinal cord and its surrounding membranes.

meningovascular neurosyphilis /-vas'-kyələr/ [Gk, *menigx,* membrane; L, *vasculum,* little vessel; Gk, *neuron,* nerve, *syn,* together, *philein,* to love], a neurosyphilis inflammation of the supporting and nutrient tissues of the central nervous system.

meniscectomy /men'isek'təmē/ [Gk, *meniskos,* crescent, *ektome,* excision], surgical excision of one of the crescent-shaped cartilages of the knee joint. It is performed when a torn cartilage results in chronic pain and in instability or locking of the joint.

meniscus /minis'kəs/, *pl.* **menisci** [Gk, *meniskos,* crescent], **1.** the interface between a liquid and air. **2.** a lens with both convex and concave aspects. **3.** a curved, fibrous cartilage in the knees and other joints.

Menkes' kinky hair syndrome /men'kēz/

[John H. Menkes, American neurologist, b. 1928; D, *kinke*, tight twist; AS, *haer*], a familial disorder affecting the normal absorption of copper from the intestine, characterized by the growth of sparse, kinky hair. Infants with the syndrome suffer cerebral degeneration, retarded growth, and early death.

menometrorrhagia /men'ōmet'rōrā'jē·ə/ [L, *men,* month; Gk, *metra,* womb, *rhegnyai,* to burst forth], excessive menstrual and uterine bleeding other than that caused by menstruation.

menopause /men'əpôz/ [L, *men,* month; Gk, *pausis,* to cease], strictly, the cessation of menses, but commonly referring to the period of the female climacteric. Menses stop naturally with the decline of cyclic hormonal production and function between 35 and 60 years of age but may stop earlier in life as a result of illness or surgical removal of the uterus or both ovaries. As the production of ovarian estrogen and pituitary gonadotropins decreases, ovulation and menstruation become less frequent and eventually stop. Fluctuations in the circulating levels of these hormones occur as the levels decline. Hot flashes are a common symptom of the menopause. Occasionally heavy irregular bleeding occurs at this time, usually associated with myomata (fibroids) or other uterine pathologic condition.

menorrhagia /men'ərā'jē·ə/ [L, *men* + *rhegnyai,* to burst forth], abnormally heavy or long menstrual periods. Menorrhagia occurs occasionally during the reproductive years of most women's lives. If the condition becomes chronic, anemia from recurrent excessive blood loss may result. Abnormal bleeding after menopause always warrants investigation to rule out malignancy. —**menorrhagic,** *adj.*

menorrhea /men'ōrē'ə/ [L, *men* + Gk, *rhoia,* flow], the normal discharge of blood and tissue from the uterus.

menostasis /minos'təsis/ [L, *men* + Gk, *stasis,* stand still], an abnormal condition in which the products of menstruation cannot escape the uterus or vagina because of stenosis, an occlusion of the cervix or the introitus of the vagina. —**menostatic,** *adj.*

menotropins /men'ōtrop'inz/ [L, *men* + Gk, *trepein,* to turn], a preparation of gonadotropic hormones from the urine of postmenopausal women. It is prescribed with chorionic gonadotropin to induce ovulation.

menoxenia /men'oksē'nē·ə/ [L, *men* + Gk, *xenos,* strange], any abnormality relating to menstruation.

menses /men'sēz/ [L, *men,* month], the normal flow of blood and decidua that occurs during menstruation. The first day of the flow of the menses is the first day of the menstrual cycle.

menstrual age [L, *menstrualis,* monthly, *aetas,* lifetime], the age of an embryo or fetus as calculated from the first day of the last menstrual period.

menstrual colic [L, *menstrualis,* monthly; Gk, *kolikos,* colon pain], a form of dysmenorrhea characterized by abdominal pain during or immediately before menstruation.

menstrual cramps, low abdominal pain that may range from a colicky feeling to a constant dull ache. The pain may radiate to the lower back and legs. Menstrual cramps are often associated with the beginning of menses.

menstrual cycle, the recurring cycle of change in the endometrium during which the decidual layer of the endometrium is shed, then regrows, proliferates, is maintained for several days, and sheds again at menstruation. The average length of the cycle, from the first day of bleeding of one cycle to the first of another, is 28 days. The duration and character vary greatly among women. Menstrual cycles begin at menarche and end with menopause. The uterine phases of the cycle are the **proliferative phase, secretory phase,** and **menstrual phase.**

menstrual period [L, *menstrualis,* monthly; Gk, *peri* + *hodos,* way], the periodic discharge of blood and cellular debris from the uterus.

menstrual phase, the final of the three phases of the menstrual cycle, the one in which menstruation occurs. The necrotic mucosa of the endometrium is shed, leaving the stratum basale; bleeding, primarily from the spiral arteries, occurs. For convenience, the days of the menstrual cycle are counted from the first day of the menstrual phase.

menstrual sponge, a small natural sponge or a piece of a synthetic sponge to which a loop of string is attached. It is inserted into the vagina to absorb the menstrual flow and is removed by pulling the string. Menstrual sponges are not commonly used.

menstruation /men'strōō·ā'shən/ [L, *menstruare,* to menstruate], the periodic discharge through the vagina of a bloody secretion containing tissue debris from the shedding of the endometrium from the nonpregnant uterus. The average duration of menstruation is 4 to 5 days, and it recurs at approximately 28-day intervals throughout the reproductive life of nonpregnant women. —**menstruate,** *v.*

M

mental /men′təl/ [L, *mens,* mind], **1.** relating to, or characteristic of the mind or psyche. **2.** existing in the mind; performed or accomplished by the mind. **3.** relating to, or characterized by a disorder of the mind.

mental [L, *mentum,* chin], pertaining to the chin.

mental age (MA), the age level at which one functions intellectually, as determined by standardized psychologic and intelligence tests and expressed as the age at which that level is average.

mental disorder, any disturbance of emotional equilibrium, as manifested in maladaptive behavior and impaired functioning, caused by genetic, physical, chemical, biologic, psychologic, or social and cultural factors.

mental foramen [L, *mentum,* chin], an opening on the lateral part of the body of the mandible, inferior to the second premolar, through which the mental nerve and blood vessels pass.

mental handicap, any mental defect or characteristic resulting from a congenital abnormality, traumatic injury, or disease that impairs normal intellectual functioning and prevents a person from participating normally in activities appropriate for a particular age group.

mental health, a relative state of mind in which a person who is healthy is able to cope with and adjust to the recurrent stresses of everyday living in an acceptable way.

Mental Health Association (MHA), a voluntary nonprofessional agency dedicated to the improvement of mental health facilities and services in community clinics and hospitals, the recruitment and training of volunteers, and the promotion of mental health legislation.

mental health consultation, any interaction between two or more health care professionals related to a specific issue.

mental health service, any one of a group of government, professional, or lay organizations operating at a community, state, national, or international level to aid in the prevention and treatment of mental disorders.

mental hygiene, the study concerned with the development of healthy mental and emotional habits, attitudes, and behavior and with the prevention of mental illness.

mental image, any concept or sensation produced in the mind through memory or imagination.

mentality /mental′itē/ [L, *mens,* mind], **1.** the functional power and capacity of the mind. **2.** intellectual character.

mental retardation, a disorder characterized by subaverage general intellectual function, with deficits or impairments in the ability to learn and to adapt socially. The cause may be genetic, biologic, psychosocial, or sociocultural.

mental ridge [L, *mentum,* chin; AS, *hyrcg*], (in dentistry) a dense elevation that extends from the symphysis to the premolar area on the anterolateral aspect of the body of the mandible.

mental status, the degree of competence shown by a person in intellectual, emotional, psychologic, and personality functioning as measured by psychologic testing with reference to a statistical norm.

mental status examination, a diagnostic procedure for determining the mental status of a person. The trained interviewer poses certain questions in a carefully standardized manner and evaluates the verbal responses and behavioral reactions.

mental tubercle [L, *mentum,* chin], one of a bilateral pair of prominences on the lower border of the body of the mandible.

mentation /mentā′shən/ [L, *mens,* mind, *atus,* process], any mental activity, including conscious and unconscious processes.

menthol /men′thol/ [L, *menta,* mint], a topical antipruritic with a cooling effect that relieves itching. It is an ingredient in many topical creams and ointments.

mentholated camphor /men′thəlā′tid/, a mixture of equal parts of camphor and menthol, used as a local counterirritant.

menton /men′ton/ [L, *mentum,* chin], the most inferior point on the chin in the lateral view of a cephalogram. It is a cephalometric landmark.

mentor /men′tər/ [Gk, *Mentor,* mythic educator], an older, trusted adviser or counselor who offers helpful guidance to younger colleagues.

mentum /men′təm/ [L, chin], **1.** the chin, especially of the fetus. **2.** a fetal reference point in designating the position of the fetus with respect to the maternal pelvis.

MEP, 1. abbreviation for **maximal expiratory pressure. 2.** abbreviation for *mean effective pressure.*

mepenzolate bromide /mepen′zəlāt/, an anticholinergic agent prescribed in the treatment of gastrointestinal hypermotility and as an adjunct in treating peptic ulcer.

meperidine hydrochloride /meper′idēn/, a narcotic analgesic used to treat moderate to severe pain and to relieve pain and allay anxiety before surgery.

mephenesin /mifen′isin/, a curare-like skeletal muscle relaxant sometimes prescribed in the relief of muscle spasm.

mephenytoin /mifen′ətō′in/, an anticonvulsant prescribed for the control of seizures in epilepsy when less toxic medications have not been effective.

mephobarbital /mef'ōbär'bitol/, an anticonvulsant and sedative prescribed in the treatment of anxiety, nervous tension, insomnia, and epilepsy.

meprednisone /mepred'nisōn/, an oral glucocorticoid prescribed in the treatment of several inflammatory conditions.

meprobamate /miprō'bəmāt/, a sedative prescribed in treatment of anxiety and tension and as a muscle relaxant.

mEq, abbreviation for **milliequivalent.**

mEq/L, abbreviation for **milliequivalent per liter.**

meralgia /miral'jə/ [Gk, *meros,* thigh, *algos,* pain], the presence of pain in the thigh.

meralgia paresthetica /per'esthet'ikə/, a condition characterized by pain, paresthesia, and numbness on the lateral surface of the thigh in the region supplied by the lateral femoral cutaneous nerve. The cause of the condition is ischemia of the nerve caused by its entrapped position in the inguinal ligament.

mercaptopurine /mərkap'təpyoo̅'rēn/, an antineoplastic and immunosuppressive prescribed in the treatment of malignant neoplastic diseases, including acute lymphocytic leukemia.

Mercer, Ramona, T., a nursing theorist who developed the Maternal Role Attainment model presented in her book *First-Time Motherhood: Experiences from Teens to Forties* (1986). Maternal role attainment is an interactional and developmental process. It occurs over a period during which the mother becomes attached to her infant, acquires competence in the caregiving tasks, and expresses pleasure and gratification in her role. The focus of Mercer's work went beyond the concept of the "traditional" mother to encompass a variety of mothering roles.

mercurial /mərkyoor'ē-əl/, **1.** pertaining to mercury, particularly a medicine containing the element mercury. **2.** an adverse effect associated with the administration of a mercurial medication, such as a mercurial tremor caused by mercury poisoning.

mercurial diuretic, any one of several diuretic agents that contain mercury in an organic chemical form. The principal use for the drugs is in treating edema of cardiac origin, ascites associated with cirrhosis, or oliguria in the nephrotic stage of glomerulonephritis. Because of the toxicity of these drugs, current practice usually recommends their replacement with more convenient and less toxic diuretics.

mercury (Hg) /mur'kyərē/ [L, *Mercurius,* mythic messenger of the gods], a metallic element. Its atomic number is 80; its atomic mass (weight) is 200.59. It is the only common metal that is liquid at room temperature. Mercury is used in dental amalgams, thermometers, barometers, and other measuring instruments. It forms many poisonous compounds.

mercury poisoning, a toxic condition caused by the ingestion or inhalation of mercury or a mercury compound. The chronic form, resulting from inhalation of the vapors or dust of mercurial compounds or from repeated ingestion of very small amounts, is characterized by irritability, excessive saliva, loosened teeth, gum disorders, slurred speech, tremors, and staggering. Symptoms of acute mercury poisoning appear in a few minutes to a half hour and include a metallic taste in the mouth, thirst, nausea, vomiting, severe abdominal pain, bloody diarrhea, and renal failure that may result in death.

mercury thermometer [L, *Mercurius,* mythic messenger of the gods; Gk, *therme,* heat, *metron,* measure], a thermometer in which the expandable indicator is mercury.

merergasia /mer'ərgā'zhə/ [Gk, *meros,* part, *ergein,* to work], a mild mental incapacity characterized by some emotional instability and some anxiety. —**merergastic,** *adj.*

merisis /mer'isis/ [Gk, *merizein,* to divide into parts], an increase in size as a result of cell division and the addition of new material rather than of cell expansion.

Merkel cell carcinoma /mer'kəl, mur'kəl/ [Friedrich S. Merkel, German anatomist and physiologist, 1845–1919], a rapidly growing malignant skin tumor that tends to occur on sun-exposed surfaces of older Caucasian individuals.

meroblastic /mer'əblas'tik/ [Gk, *meros* + *blastos,* germ], pertaining to or characterizing an ovum that contains a large amount of yolk and in which cleavage is restricted to a part of the cytoplasm.

merocrine secretion /mer'əkrin/ [Gk, *meros,* part, *krinein,* to separate; L, *secernere,* to separate], a secretion in which the secreting cell remains intact while producing and releasing the secretory product.

meromelia /mer'əmē'lyə/ [Gk, *meros* + *melos,* limb], a general designation for the congenital absence of any part of a limb. It is used in reference to such conditions as adactyly, hemimelia, or phocomelia.

merozoite /mer'əzō'īt/ [Gk, *meros* + *zoon,* animal], an organism produced from segmentation of a schizont during the asexual reproductive phase of the life cycle of a sporozoon, specifically the malarial parasite *Plasmodium.*

merozygote /mer′əzī′gōt/, an incomplete zygote that contains only part of the genetic material of one of the parents. It occurs in bacterial genetics.

Merrifield's knife, a surgical knife with a long, narrow triangular blade set into a shank, used for gingivectomy incisions.

mesangial /mesan′jē·əl/, pertaining to the mesangium.

mesangium /mesan′jē·əm/, a cellular network in the renal glomerulus that helps support the capillary loops.

mescaline /mes′kəlēn, -lin/ [Mex, *mezcal*], a psychoactive poisonous alkaloid derived from a colorless alkaline oil in the flowering heads of the cactus *Lophophora williamsii.* Closely related chemically to epinephrine, mescaline causes heart palpitations, diaphoresis, pupillary dilation, and anxiety.

mescalism /mes′kəliz′əm/ [Mex, *mezcal*], a type of chemical dependence on the effects of mescal, an intoxicant spirit obtained from a species of cactus.

mesencephalon /mes′ensef′əlon/ [Gk, *mesos,* middle, *enkephalos,* brain], one of the three parts of the brainstem, lying just below the cerebrum and just above the pons. It consists primarily of white substance with some gray substance around the cerebral aqueduct. —**mesencephalic** /mes′ensifal′ik/, *adj.*

mesenchymal chondrosarcoma /meseng′kəməl/ [Gk, *mesos,* middle, *enchyma,* infusion, *chondros,* cartilage, *sarx,* flesh, *oma,* tumor], a malignant cartilaginous tumor that develops in many sites.

mesenchyme /mes′engkīm/ [Gk, *mesos* + *enchyma,* infusion], a diffuse network of tissue derived from the embryonic mesoderm. It consists of stellate cells embedded in gelatinous ground substance with reticular fibers.

mesenchymoma /mes′engkimō′mə/ [Gk, *mesos* + *enchyma,* infusion, *oma,* tumor], a mixed mesenchymal neoplasm composed of two or more cellular elements that are not usually associated and fibrous tissue.

mesenteric node [Gk, *mesos* + *enteron,* intestine; L, *nodus,* knot], a node in one of three groups of superior mesenteric lymph glands serving parts of the intestine.

mesentery proper /mez′ənter′ē/ [Gk, *mesos* + *enteron,* intestine; L, *propius,* more suitable], a broad fan-shaped fold of peritoneum suspending the jejunum and the ileum from the dorsal wall of the abdomen. The root of the mesentery proper is

connected to certain structures ventral to the vertebral column. The intestinal border of the mesentery proper separates to enclose the intestine. The cranial part of the mesentery suspends the small intestine and various nerves and arteries.

MESH /mesh/, an acronym derived from *Medical Subject Headings,* the list of medical terms used by the U.S. National Library of Medicine (NLM) for its computerized system of storage and retrieval of published medical reports.

mesh graft, a partial or split-thickness skin graft that has had multiple slits cut into it. The slits allow the graft to be stretched to several times its original size for coverage of a larger area on the recipient.

mesiobucco-occlusal /mē′zē·ōbuk′ō·ok-loo′zəl/ [Gk, *mesos,* middle; L, *bucca,* cheek; L, *occludere,* to close up], pertaining to the angle formed by the mesial, buccal, and occlusal surfaces of a tooth.

mesiocclusion /mē′zē·okloo′zhən/ [Gk, *mesos* + L, *occludere,* to close up], an occlusal relationship in which the lower teeth are positioned mesially to the upper teeth.

mesiodens /mē′zē·ədenz/ [Gk, *mesos* + L, *dens,* tooth], a supernumerary erupted or unerupted tooth that develops between two maxillary central incisors.

mesiolinguo-occlusal, pertaining to the angle formed by the mesial, lingual, and occlusal surfaces of a tooth.

mesioversion /mē′zē·ōvur′zhən/ [Gk, *mesos* + L, *vertere,* to turn], **1.** a condition in which one or more teeth are closer than normal to the midline. **2.** a condition in which the maxilla or mandible is positioned more anteriorly than normal.

mesmerism /mez′məriz′əm/ [Franz A. Mesmer, Austrian physician, 1734–1815], a practice of hypnotism introduced by Mesmer, who believed human health was affected by "celestial magnetic forces." Mesmer was regarded as a fraud by the medical profession, but his work led to serious studies of the health effects of the power of suggestion.

mesocolic node /mes′ōkol′ik/ [Gk, *mesos* + *kolon,* colon; L, *nodus,* knot], a node in one of three groups of superior mesenteric lymph glands, proliferating between the layers of the transverse mesocolon, close to the transverse colon.

mesocolopexy /mes′ōkō′ləpek′sē/ [Gk, *mesos* + *kolon,* colon, *pexis,* fixation], suspension or fixation of the mesocolon.

mesoderm /mes′ōdurm/ [Gk, *mesos* + *derma,* skin], (in embryology) the middle of the three cell layers of the developing embryo. It lies between the ectoderm and the endoderm. Bone, connective tissue, muscle, blood, vascular and lymphatic tissue, and the pleurae of the pericardium and peritoneum are all derived from the mesoderm.

mesoduodenum /-dōō'ədē'nəm/ [Gk, *mesos,* middle; L, *duodeni,* 12 fingers long], a fold of tissue that joins the duodenum to the wall of the abdomen of the fetus. The membrane sometimes persists in later life as the duodenal mesentery.

mesogastric /-gas'trik/ [Gk, *mesos,* middle, *gaster,* belly], pertaining to the mesogastrium, a mesentery of the embryonic stomach.

mesomere /mez'əmir/ [Gk, *mesos,* middle, *meros,* part], a row of mesodermal cells between the mesothelium and epimere of the embryo. It develops into the renal tubules.

mesomorph /mes'əmôrf'/ [Gk, *mesos* + *morphe,* form], a person whose physique is characterized by a predominance of muscle, bone, and connective tissue, structures that develop from the mesodermal layer of the embryo.

mesonephric duct /-nef'rik/ [Gk, *mesos* + *nephros,* kidney; L, *ducere,* to lead], (in embryology) a duct that in the male gives rise to the ducts of the reproductive system (ductus epididymidis, ductus deferens, seminal vesicle, ejaculatory duct). In the female it persists vestigially as **Gartner's duct.**

mesonephric tubule, any of the embryonic renal tubules composing the mesonephros. They function as excretory structures during the early embryonic development of humans and other mammals but are later incorporated into the reproductive system. In males the tubules give rise to the efferent and aberrant ductules of the testes, the appendix epididymis, and the paradidymis; in females the epoophoron, paroöphoron, and vesicular appendices.

mesonephros /-nef'rəs/, *pl.* **mesonephroi, mesonephra** [Gk, *mesos* + *nephros,* kidney], the second type of excretory organ to develop in the vertebrate embryo. It consists of a series of twisting tubules that arise from the nephrogenic cord caudal to the pronephros and that at one end form the glomerulus and at the other connect with the excretory mesonephric duct. —**mesonephric, mesonephroid,** *adj.*

mesoridazine /mez'ərid'əzēn/, a phenothiazine tranquilizer prescribed in the treatment of psychotic disorders, behavioral problems in mental retardation, and alcoholism.

mesosalpinx /mes'ōsal'pingks/ [Gk, *mesos* + *salpinx,* tube], the superior, free border of the broad ligament in which the uterine tubes lie.

mesothelial /mez'ōthē'lē·əl/, pertaining to the mesothelium cell layer.

mesothelioma /mes'ōthē'lē·ō'mə/ [Gk, *mesos* + *epi,* above, *thele,* nipple, *oma,* tumor], a rare malignant tumor of the mesothelium of the pleura or peritoneum, associated with exposure to asbestos.

mesothelium /mes'ōthē'lē·əm/ [Gk, *mesos* + *epi,* above, *thele,* nipple], a layer of cells that line the body cavities of the embryo and continue as a layer of squamous epithelial cells covering the serous membranes of the adult.

messenger RNA (mRNA) /mes'ənjər/ [ME, *messangere,* message bearer; *RNA,* ribonucleic acid], (in molecular genetics) an RNA fraction that carries information from deoxyribonucleic acid to the protein-synthesizing ribosomes of cells.

mestranol /mes'trənōl/, an estrogen prescribed in fixed-combination drugs with a progestin as an oral contraceptive.

Met, abbreviation for the amino acid **methionine.**

MET, abbreviation for **metabolic equivalent of task.**

meta-analysis, a systematic method of evaluating statistical data based on results of several independent studies of the same problem.

metabiosis /met'əbī·ō'sis/, **1.** a condition in which the growth and metabolism of one organism alters the environment to allow the growth of another organism. **2.** the parasitic dependence of the existence of one organism on that of another.

metabolic /met'əbol'ik/ [Gk, *metabole,* change], pertaining to **metabolism.**

metabolic acidosis, acidosis in which excess acid is added to the body fluids or bicarbonate is lost from them. In starvation and in uncontrolled diabetes mellitus, glucose is not present or is not available for oxidation for cellular nutrition. The plasma bicarbonate of the body is used up in neutralizing the ketones that result from the breakdown of body fat for energy that occurs to compensate for the lack of glucose. Metabolic acidosis also occurs when oxidation takes place without adequate oxygen, as in heart failure or shock. Severe diarrhea, renal failure, and lactic acidosis also may result.

metabolic alkalosis, an abnormal condition characterized by the significant loss of acid in the body or by increased levels of base bicarbonate. The reduction of acid may be caused by excessive vomiting, insufficient replacement of electrolytes, hyperadrenocorticism, and Cushing's disease. An increase in base bicarbonate may

M

be caused by various problems such as the ingestion of excessive bicarbonate of soda and other antacids during the treatment of peptic ulcers and the administration of excessive intravenous fluids containing high concentrations of bicarbonate. Signs and symptoms of metabolic alkalosis may include apnea, headache, lethargy, muscle cramps, hyperactive reflexes, tetany, shallow and slow respirations, irritability, nausea, vomiting, and atrial tachycardia.

metabolic balance [Gk, *metabole,* change; L, *bilanx,* having two scale trays], an equilibrium between the intake of nutrients and their eventual loss through absorption or excretion. In a positive balance the intake of a nutrient exceeds its loss; in a negative balance a nutrient is used or excreted faster than it is consumed in the diet.

metabolic body size, an estimate of the active tissue mass of a person, calculated by the body weight in kilograms to the 0.75 power.

metabolic cirrhosis, cirrhosis of the liver associated with a metabolic disorder such as Wilson's disease.

metabolic component, the bicarbonate component of plasma.

metabolic disorder, any pathophysiologic dysfunction that results in a loss of metabolic control of homeostasis in the body.

metabolic equivalent of task (MET), a unit of measurement of heat production by the body. One MET is equal to 50 kilogram calories (kcal) per hour per square meter of body surface of a resting individual.

metabolic failure, the severe and usually rapid failure of mental and physical functions, resulting in death.

metabolic pathway, a series of consecutive biochemical reactions or steps through which digested food is transformed into basic nutrients such as amino acids, free fatty acids, and simple carbohydrates.

metabolic rate, the amount of energy liberated or expended in a given unit of time. Energy is stored in the body in energy-rich phosphate compounds (adenosine triphosphate, adenosine monophosphate, and adenosine diphosphate) and in proteins, fats, and complex carbohydrates.

metabolic waste products [Gk, *metabole,* change; L, *vastare,* to destroy, *producere,* to produce], the products of metabolic activity after oxygen and nutrients have been supplied to a cell. These mainly include water and carbon dioxide, along with sodium chloride and soluble nitrog-

enous salts, which are excreted in urine, feces, and exhaled air.

metabolism /mətab′əliz′əm/ [Gk, *metabole,* change, *ismos,* process], the aggregate of all chemical processes that take place in living organisms, resulting in growth, generation of energy, elimination of wastes, and other body functions as they relate to the distribution of nutrients in the blood after digestion. Metabolism takes place in two steps: anabolism, the constructive phase, in which smaller molecules (such as amino acids) are converted to larger molecules (such as proteins); and catabolism, the destructive phase, in which larger molecules (such as glycogen) are converted to smaller molecules (such as pyruvic acid). The metabolic rate is customarily expressed (in calories) as the heat liberated in the course of metabolism.

metabolite /mitab′əlīt/ [Gk, *metabole,* change], a substance produced by metabolic action or necessary for a metabolic process. An essential metabolite is one required for a vital metabolic process.

metabolize /mətab′əlīz/ [Gk, *metabole,* change], to undergo metabolism, the breaking down of carbohydrates, proteins, and fats into smaller units; reorganizing those units as tissue building blocks or as energy sources; and eliminating waste products of the processes.

metacarpal phalanx /-kär′pəl/ [Gk, *meta* + *karpos,* wrist, *phalanx,* line of soldiers], the hands and fingers, particularly phalanges that articulate with carpal bones.

metacarpophalangeal /-kar′pōfəlan′jē·əl/ [Gk, *meta,* beyond, *karpos,* wrist, *phalanx,* line of soldiers], pertaining to the metacarpal bones of the hand and the phalanges of fingers, as in metacarpophalangeal joints.

metacarpophalangeal (MCP) joint dislocation [Gk, *meta* + *karpos* + *phalanx* + L, *jungere,* to join, *dis* + *locare,* to place], the dislocation of a finger at the junction with the metacarpal bone, usually with damage to tendons and other structures.

metacarpus /met′əkär′pəs/ [Gk, *meta,* beyond, *karpos,* wrist], the middle part of the hand, consisting of five slender bones numbered from the thumb side, metacarpals I through V. Each metacarpal consists of a body and two extremities. **—metacarpal,** *adj., n.*

metacentric /met′əsen′trik/ [Gk, *meta* + *kentron,* center], pertaining to a chromosome in which the centromere is located near the center so that the arms of the chromatids are of approximately equal length.

metachromasia /-krōmā′zhē·ə/ [Gk, *meta,*

beyond, *chroma,* color], a tissue staining phenomenon in which cells being examined acquire a color other than that of the dye used. Cartilage cells, for example, may appear red after being stained with a blue dye. The cause is an interaction between the dye molecules and the acidic radicals of the tissue cells.

metachromatic lipids /-krōmat'ik/ [Gk, *meta,* beyond, *chroma,* color, *lipos,* fat], lipid molecules that accumulate in the central nervous system, peripheral nerves, and internal organs of infants who inherit a lipidosis disorder.

metachromatic stain [Gk, *meta* + *chroma,* color; OFr, *desteindre,* to dye], a basic dye, such as toluidine, that can stain substances a different color than that of the stain.

metacommunication /-kəmyoo̅'nikā'shən/ [Gk, *meta* + L, *communicare,* to inform], communication that indicates how verbal information should be interpreted. It may support or contradict verbal communication.

metagenesis /met'əjen'əsis/ [Gk, *meta* + *genein,* to produce], the regular alternation of sexual with asexual methods of reproduction within the same species. —**metagenetic, metagenic,** *adj.*

metal [Gk, *metallon,* a mine], any element that conducts heat and electricity, is malleable and ductile, and forms positively charged ions (cations).

metal fume fever, an occupational disorder caused by the inhalation of fumes of metallic oxides and characterized by symptoms similar to those of influenza.

metallesthesia /met'əlesthē'zhə/ [Gk, *metallon,* a mine, *aisthesia,* perception], an ability to identify a metal through the sense of touch.

metalloprotein /mətal'ōprō'tēn/, a protein that contains one or more metal ions.

metallurgy /met'əlur'jē/ [Gk, *metallon,* a mine, *ergein,* to work], the theoretic and applied sciences of the nature and uses of metals.

metamorphopsia /met'əmôrfop'sē·ə/ [Gk, *meta* + *morphe,* form, *opsis,* sight], a defect in vision in which objects are seen as distorted in shape, which results from disease of the retina or imperfection of the media.

metamorphosis /met'əmôr'fəsis/ [Gk, *meta* + *morphe,* form], a change in shape or structure, especially a change from one stage of development to another, such as the transition from the larval to the adult stage.

metamyelocyte /met'əmī'əlōsīt'/ [Gk, *meta* + *myelos,* marrow, *kytos,* cell], a stage in the development of the granulo-

cyte series of leukocytes, between the myelocyte stage and the mature granulocyte.

metanephrine /met'ənef'rin/, one of the two principal urinary metabolites of epinephrine and norepinephrine in the urine; the other is vanillylmandelic acid.

metanephrogenic /met'ənef'rəjen'ik/ [Gk, *meta* + *nephros,* kidney, *genein,* to produce], capable of forming the metanephros, or fetal kidney.

metanephros /-nef'rəs/, *pl.* **metanephroi, metanephra** [Gk, *meta* + *nephros,* kidney], the third, and permanent, excretory organ to develop in the vertebrate embryo. It consists of a complex structure of secretory and collecting tubules that develop into the kidney.

metaphase /met'əfāz/ [Gk, *meta* + *phasis,* appearance], the second of the four stages of nuclear division in mitosis and in each of the two divisions of meiosis, during which the chromosomes become arranged in the equatorial plane of the spindle to form the equatorial plate, with the centromeres attached to the spindle fibers in preparation for separation.

metaphyseal dysostosis /mətaf'izē'əl, met'əfiz'ē·əl/ [Gk, *meta* + *phyein,* to grow, *dys,* bad, *osteon,* bone], an abnormal condition that affects the skeletal system and is characterized by a disturbance of the mineralization of the metaphyseal area of the bones, resulting in dwarfism. Metaphyseal dysostosis is classified as the Gansen, Schmidt, or Spahar-Hartmann type or cartilage-hair hypoplasia. The Gansen type is characterized by metaphyseal alterations similar to those of achondroplasia but not involving the skull or the epiphyses of the long bones. The Schmidt type of metaphyseal dysostosis is characterized by developmental changes from the weight bearing age to approximately 5 years of age. The Spahar-Hartmann type is characterized by skeletal changes and severe genu varum. Cartilage-hair hypoplasia is characterized by severe dwarfism and hair that is sparse, short, and brittle.

metaphyseal dysplasia, an abnormal condition characterized by disordered modeling of the cylindric bones.

metaphysis /mətaf'əsis/ [Gk, *meta* + *phyein,* to grow], a region of a growing long bone in which diaphysis and epiphysis converge.

metaplasia /met'əplā'zhə/, the reversible conversion of normal tissue cells into another, less differentiated cell type in response to chronic stress or injury.

metaproterenol sulfate /met'əprōter'inôl/, a beta-adrenergic bronchodilator prescribed in the treatment of bronchial asthma.

M

metaraminol bitartrate /met'äram'inol/, an adrenergic vasopressor prescribed in the treatment of hypotension and shock.

metarubricyte /-rōō'brisīt/ [Gk, *meta* + L, *ruber*, red, *kytos*, cell], a red blood cell possessing a nucleus. Such cells, also known as normoblasts, are not normally found in circulating blood.

metastasis /mətas'təsis/, *pl.* **metastases** [Gk, *meta* + *stasis*, standing], **1.** the process by which tumor cells spread to distant parts of the body. Because malignant tumors have no enclosing capsule, cells may escape, become emboli, and be transported by the lymphatic circulation or the bloodstream to implant in lymph nodes and other organs far from the primary tumor. **2.** a tumor that develops away from the site of origin. —**metastatic,** *adj.*, **metastasize (metas)** /mətas'təsīz/, *v.*

metastatic abscess /-stat'ik/ [Gk, *meta,* beyond, *stasis*, standing; L, *abscedere,* to go away], any secondary abscess that develops at a point distant from an original infection; the infectious particles are transported to other locations in the bloodstream.

metastatic calcification [Gk, *meta* + *stasis,* standing; L, *calx,* lime, *facere,* to make], the pathologic process whereby calcium salts accumulate in previously healthy tissues.

metastatic endometriosis [Gk, *meta,* beyond, *stasis,* standing, *endon,* within, *metra,* womb, *osis,* condition], extraperitoneal lesions that resemble metastases from a carcinoma.

metastatic survey [Gk, *meta,* beyond, *stasis,* standing; OFr, *surveoir,* to examine], a method of monitoring the spread of a cancer by taking a series of periodic x-ray films.

metatarsal /met'ətär'səl/ [Gk, *meta* + *tarsos,* flat surface], **1.** pertaining to the metatarsus of the foot. **2.** any one of the five bones making up the metatarsus.

metatarsalgia /met'ətärsal'jə/ [Gk, *meta* + *tarsos* + *algos,* pain], a painful condition around the metatarsal bones caused by an abnormality of the foot or recalcification of degenerated heads of metatarsal bones.

metatarsal phalanx /-tär'səl/ [Gk, *meta* + *tarsos,* flat surface, *phalanx,* line of soldiers], any one of the bones of the foot and toes.

metatarsal stress fracture, a break or rupture of a metatarsal bone, resulting from prolonged running or walking. The condition is often difficult to diagnose with x-ray films.

metatarsus /-tär'səs/ [Gk, *meta* + *tarsos,* flat surface], a part of the foot, consisting of five bones numbered I to V from the

medial side. Each bone has a long, slender body; a wedge-shaped proximal end; a convex distal end; and flattened, grooved sides for the attachment of ligaments. —**metatarsal,** *adj.*

metatarsus valgus, a congenital deformity of the foot in which the forepart rotates outward away from the midline of the body and the heel remains straight.

metatarsus varus, a congenital deformity of the foot in which the forepart rotates inward toward the midline of the body and the heel remains straight.

metathalamus /met'əthal'əməs/ [Gk, *meta* + *thalamos,* chamber], one of five parts of the diencephalon. The medial geniculate body acts as a relay station for nerve impulses between the inferior brachium and the auditory cortex. The lateral geniculate body is a superficial oval bulge at the posterior end of the thalamus, which accommodates the terminal ends of the fibers of the optic tract. Relay cells project to the visual cortex. —**metathalamic,** *adj.*

metaxalone /metak'səlōn/, a skeletal muscle relaxant prescribed as an adjunct in the treatment of acute skeletal muscle spasm.

metazoa /-zō'ə/ [Gk, *meta* + *zoon,* animal], a category of multicellular motile heterotrophic animals whose cells have become differentiated into tissues and organs, particularly those possessing a digestive tract.

Metchnikoff's theory /mech'nikofs/ [Elie Metchnikoff, Russian-French biologist, 1845–1916; Gk, *theoria,* speculation], the theory that living cells ingest microorganisms. The theory proved correct, as seen in the process of phagocytosis and the ingestion of injurious microbes by leukocytes.

meteorism [Gk, *meteorizein,* to hold up], accumulation of gas in the abdomen or the intestine, usually with distension.

meteorotropism /mē'tē·ərətrō'pizəm/ [Gk, *meteors,* high in the air, *trope,* turning], a reaction to meteorologic influences shown by various biologic occurrences such as sudden death, attacks of arthritis, and angina. —**meteorotropic,** *adj.*

meter (m) /mē'tər/ [Gk, *metron,* measure], a metric unit of length equal to 39.37 inches.

metered dose inhaler (MDI) /mē'tərd/, a device designed to deliver a measured dose of an inhalation drug. It usually consists of a canister of aerosol spray, mist, or fine powder that releases a specific dose each time it is pushed against a dispensing valve. It is intended to reduce the risk of overmedication by the person.

metformin hydrochloride, an oral antidiabetic agent prescribed in the treatment of type II (noninsulin-dependent) diabetes mellitus in adults.

methacholine challenge /meth'əkō'lēn/, a method of measuring airway activity by an inhalation challenge test. It consists of inhaling a saline aerosol as a control, followed by increasing concentrations of methacholine chloride, a cholinergic drug. It is used to confirm the diagnosis of asthma when symptoms are present.

methacrylic acid /meth'əkril'ik/, an organic acid obtained from Roman chamomile oil. The methyl ester of methacrylic acid is used in medical and dental products. A copolymer is used in tablet coatings.

methacycline hydrochloride /meth'əsī'-klēn/, a tetracycline antibiotic prescribed in the treatment of infections.

methadone /meth'ədōn/, a synthetic narcotic analgesic prescribed for relief of severe pain, for treatment in detoxification, and in treatment programs for opiate-addicted patients.

methamphetamine hydrochloride /meth'-amfet'əmēn/, a central nervous system stimulant prescribed in the treatment of narcolepsy and hyperkinesis and the reduction of the appetite in exogenous obesity.

methandriol /methan'drē·ol/, an anabolic hormone used as adjunctive therapy in senile and postmenopausal osteoporosis.

methane (CH₄) /meth'ān/, a simple hydrocarbon in the form of colorless gas, produced by the decomposition of organic matter.

methanol /meth'ənol/, a clear, colorless, toxic liquid distillate of wood miscible with water, other alcohols, and ether. It is widely used as a solvent and in the production of formaldehyde.

methanol poisoning, a toxic effect of ingestion, inhalation, or absorption through the skin of methanol (methyl alcohol, wood alcohol) that may impair the central nervous system; cause severe acidosis, blindness, and shock; and result in death.

methaqualone /methak'wəlōn/, a sedative-hypnotic prescribed in the treatment of anxiety and insomnia.

metharbital /methär'bital/, an anticonvulsant prescribed in the treatment of epilepsy.

methazolamide /meth'əzō'ləmīd/, a carbonic anhydrase inhibitor prescribed in the treatment of glaucoma.

methdilazine /methdil'əzēn/, a phenothiazine antihistamine prescribed to relieve itching.

methemoglobin /met'hēməglō'bin, met-he'məglō'bin/, a form of hemoglobin in which the iron component has been oxidized from the ferrous to the ferric state. Methemoglobin cannot carry oxygen.

methemoglobinemia /-ē'mē·ə/, the presence of methemoglobin in the blood.

methemoglobinuria /-ōōr'ē·ə/ [Gk, meta, beyond, haima, blood; L, globus, ball; Gk, ouron, urine], the presence of methemoglobin in the urine.

methenamine /methē'nəmēn/, a urinary antibacterial prescribed in the treatment of urinary tract infections.

methimazole /məthim'əzōl/, an orally administered antithyroid drug prescribed in the treatment of hyperthyroidism.

methionine (Met) /methī'ənēn/, an essential amino acid needed for proper growth in infants and for maintenance of nitrogen balance in adults. It is a source for methyl groups and sulfur in the body.

methocarbamol /meth'əkär'bəmol/, a skeletal muscle relaxant prescribed in the treatment of skeletal muscle spasm.

method /meth'əd/ [Gk, meta, beyond, hodos, way], a technique or procedure for producing a desired effect, such as a surgical procedure, a laboratory test, or a diagnostic technique.

methodology /meth'ədol'əjē/ [Gk, meta + hodos + logos, science], 1. a system of principles or methods of procedure in any discipline, such as education, research, diagnosis, or treatment. 2. the section of a research proposal in which the methods to be used are described. —methodologic, adj.

methohexital sodium /meth'ōhek'sitōl/, an intravenous barbiturate used for the induction of anesthesia in short surgical procedures as a supplement to other anesthetics.

methotrexate /meth'ōtrek'sāt/, an antineoplastic antimetabolite prescribed in the treatment of severe psoriasis and a variety of malignant neoplastic diseases.

methoxamine hydrochloride /methok'-səmēn/, an adrenergic that acts as a vasoconstrictor. It is prescribed for use during anesthesia for maintaining blood pressure and in the treatment of paroxysmal supraventricular tachycardia.

methoxsalen /methok'sələn/, a pigmentation agent used topically for enhancement of pigmentation or for repigmentation in vitiligo.

methscopolamine bromide /meth'skōpō'-ləmēn/, an anticholinergic prescribed in the treatment of hypermotility of the gastrointestinal tract and as an adjunct in treatment of peptic ulcer.

methsuximide /methsuk'simīd/, an anticonvulsant prescribed in the treatment of refractory petit mal epilepsy.

methyclothiazide /məthī'klōthī'əzīd/ /meth'əeklōthī'əzīd/, a diuretic and antihypertensive prescribed in the treatment of hypertension and edema.

methyl (Me) /meth'il/, the chemical radical -CH₃.

methylate /meth'ilāt/ [Gk, *methy,* wine, *hyle,* matter], **1.** a compound of methyl and a base. **2.** to add a methyl group, -CH₃, to a chemical compound.

methylation /-lā'shən/ [Gk, *methy,* wine, *hyle,* matter], **1.** the introduction of a methyl group, -CH₃, to a chemical compound. **2.** the addition of methyl alcohol and naphtha to ethanol to produce denatured alcohol.

methylbenzethonium chloride /ben'-zəthō'nē·əm/, a topical antiinfective prescribed for the prevention and treatment of diaper rash and other dermatoses.

methyldopa /-dō'pə/, an antihypertensive prescribed for the reduction of high blood pressure.

methylene blue /meth'əlēn/, a bluish-green crystalline substance used as a histologic stain and as a laboratory indicator. It is also used in the treatment of cyanide poisoning and methemoglobinemia.

methylergonovine maleate /-ərgon'əvēn/, a synthetic ergot alkaloid prescribed as an oxytocic to prevent or to treat postpartum uterine atony, hemorrhage, or subinvolution.

methylphenidate hydrochloride /-fen'i-dāt/, a central nervous system stimulant prescribed in the treatment of attention deficit disorder in children and narcolepsy in adults.

methylprednisolone /-prednis'əlōn/, a glucocorticoid prescribed in the treatment of inflammatory conditions, including rheumatic fever and rheumatoid arthritis.

methyltestosterone /meth'iltəstos'tərōn/, an androgen prescribed in the treatment of testosterone deficiency, osteoporosis, and female breast cancer and in stimulation of growth, weight gain, and red blood cell production.

methyprylon /meth'əprī'lon/, a sedative and hypnotic prescribed in the treatment of insomnia.

methysergide maleate /meth'isur'jīd/, a vasoconstrictor prescribed for relief of migraine headache.

metoclopramide hydrochloride /met'-əklō'prəmīd/, a gastrointestinal stimulant prescribed to stimulate motility of and increase the tone of gastric contractions of the upper gastrointestinal tract and to prevent emesis.

metocurine iodide /met'əkyoo'rēn/, a potent neuromuscular blocking agent. It is given to produce flaccid paralysis as an adjunct to anesthesia, to reduce muscle spasm in tetanus, and to assist controlled ventilation.

metolazone /mətō'ləzōn/, a diuretic and antihypertensive prescribed for the treatment of edema and high blood pressure.

"me-too" drug, *informal.* a drug product that is similar, identical, or closely related to a drug for which a manufacturer has obtained a new drug application. On the assumption that the new drug has been recognized as safe and effective, clinical trials required of the original manufacturer are not required of the new supplier, but information regarding the manufacture, bioavailability, and labeling of the product is required.

metopic /mətō'pik/, pertaining to the forehead.

metoprolol tartrate /metop'rəlol/, an antiadrenergic (beta-receptor) prescribed in the treatment of hypertension.

metralgia /mətral'jə/ [Gk, *metra,* womb, *algos,* pain], tenderness or pain in the uterus.

metric /met'rik/, pertaining to a system of measurement that uses the meter as a basis.

metric equivalent [Gk, *metron,* measure; L, *aequus,* equal, *valare,* to be strong], any value in metric units of measurement that equals the same value in English units, for example, 2.54 cm equals 1 inch, and 1 L equals 1.0567 quarts.

metric system, a decimal system of measurement based on the meter (39.37 inches) as the unit of length, on the gram (15.432 grains) as the unit of weight or mass, and, as a derived unit, on the liter (0.908 U.S. dry quart or 1.0567 U.S. liquid quart) as the unit of volume.

metritis /mətrī'tis/ [Gk, *metra,* womb, *itis,* inflammation], inflammation of the walls of the uterus. Kinds of metritis are **endometritis** and **parametritis.**

metrocarcinoma /met'rōkär'sinō'mə/ [Gk, *metra,* womb, *karkinos,* crab, *oma,* tumor], a cancer of the uterus.

metronidazole /met'rənī'dəzōl/, an antimicrobial prescribed in the treatment of amebiasis, trichomoniasis, and certain bacterial infections.

metronoscope /mətron'əskōp/, **1.** a device that exposes a small amount of reading matter to the eyes for brief preset periods. It is used in testing and in aiding individuals to increase reading speed. **2.** an apparatus that exercises the eyes rhythmically to improve binocular coordination.

metroplasty /mē'trəplas'tē/ [Gk, *metra,* womb], reconstructive surgery on the uterus.

metrorrhagia /met'rōrā'jē·ə/ [Gk, *metra,* womb, *rhegnynai,* to burst forth], uterine bleeding other than that caused by menstruation. It may be caused by uterine lesions and may be a sign of a urogenital malignancy.

metyrapone /metir'əpōn/, a diagnostic test drug. It is used to test hypothalamic and pituitary function.

metyrosine /mətir'əsēn/, an antihypertensive prescribed in the treatment of pheochromocytoma.

mev, MeV, abbreviation for *million electron volts,* the equivalent of 3.82×10^{-14} small calories, or 1.6×10^{-6} ergs.

mevalonate kinase /məval'ənāt/, an enzyme in the liver and in yeast. It catalyzes the transfer of a phosphate group from adenosine triphosphate to produce adenosine diphosphate and 5-phosphomevalonate.

Mexican typhus [Gk, *typhos,* fever], a form of epidemic typhus carried by lice in Mexico.

mexiletine hydrochloride /mek'silē'tin/, an oral antiarrhythmic drug prescribed for the treatment of symptomatic ventricular arrhythmias.

Meynet's node /mānāz'/, any of the numerous nodules that may develop within the capsules surrounding joints and in tendons affected by rheumatic diseases, especially in children.

mezlocillin sodium /mezlos'ilin/, a semisynthetic penicillin antibiotic prescribed for lower respiratory tract, intraabdominal, urinary tract, gynecologic, and skin infections and bacterial septicemia caused by susceptible strains of multiple microorganisms.

mɪ̄Γ, abbreviation for *millifarad.*

mF, symbol for *microfarad.*

MFCC, abbreviation for *Marriage, Family, and Child Counselor.*

MFD, abreviation for *minimum fatal dose.*

mg, abbreviation for **milligram.**

μg, symbol for **microgram,** unit of mass equal to one millionth of a gram.

Mg, symbol for the element **magnesium.**

MH, 1. abbreviation for **malignant hyperthermia. 2.** abbreviation for **mental health.**

MHA, abbreviation for **Mental Health Association.**

MHC, abbreviation for **major histocompatibility complex.**

MHD, abbreviation for **minimum hemolytic dose.**

mho, symbol for **siemens.**

MHz, abbreviation for **megahertz.**

MI, abbreviation for **myocardial infarction.**

miasma /mī·az'mə/ [Gk, *miainein,* defilement], an unwholesome, polluted atmosphere or environment, such as a marsh or swamp containing rotting organic matter.

MIC, abbreviation for **minimal inhibitory concentration.**

mica /mī'kə/, an aluminum silicate mineral that occurs in thin laminated scales.

micatosis /mī'kətō'sis/, a form of pneumoconiosis caused by inhalation of mica particles.

micellar chromatography /mīsel'ər/, a method of monitoring minute quantities of drugs in whole body fluids by using micellar or colloidal compounds to keep proteins in solution. The technique eliminates the need to remove proteins that usually interfere with chromatographic analysis of blood serum, urine, or saliva.

Michaelis-Menten kinetics [Leonor Michaelis, American biochemist, 1875–1949; Maud L. Menten, Canadian physician in U.S. practice, 1879–1960], a method of transforming drug plasma levels into a linear relationship using the parameters of drug concentration and a constant, K_m, which is a measure of enzyme-substrate affinity.

miconazole nitrate /mīkon'əzōl/, an antifungal used topically to treat certain fungal infections of the skin and vagina and parenterally to treat systemic fungal infections.

micrencephalon /mī'krənsef'əlon/, an abnormally small brain. —**micrencephalic,** *adj., n.*

microabscess /mīkrō·ab'ses/ [Gk, *mikros,* small; L, *abscedere,* to go away], a very small abscess.

microadenoma /mī'krō·ad'ənō'mə/, a pituitary adenoma less than 10 mm in diameter.

microaerophile /mī'krō·er'ōfil/ [Gk, *mikros,* small, *aer,* air, *philein,* to love], a microorganism that requires free oxygen for growth but at a lower concentration than that contained in the atmosphere. —**microaerophilic,** *adj.*

microaerotonometer /mī'krō·er'ətonom'ətər/ [Gk, *mikros* + *aer,* air, *tonos,* tension, *metron,* measure], instrument for measuring the volume of gases in blood or other fluids.

microaggregate recipient set /mi'krō·ag'rəgāt/ [Gk, *mikros* + L, *ad,* to, *gregare,* to collect, *recipere,* to receive; AS, *settan*], a device composed of plastic components for the intravenous delivery of large volumes of stored whole blood or of packed blood cells.

microalbuminuria /mī'krō·al'binōōr'ē·ə/, the urinary excretion of small amounts of albumin, below the detection level of rou-

M

tine dipstick analysis. The condition is an early indicator of altered glomerular permeability in diabetes.

microampere /mī'krō·am'pir/, one millionth of an ampere.

microanalysis /mī'krō·anal'isis/, **1.** analysis of minute quantities of material. **2.** identification of substances by examination under a microscope.

microaneurysm /mi'krō·an'yəriz'əm/ [Gk, *mikros* + *aneurysma*, a widening], a microscopic aneurysm characteristic of thrombotic purpura.

microangiopathic hemolytic anemia (MAHA) /mī'krō·anjē·əpath'ik/, a disorder in which narrowing or obstruction of small blood vessels results in distortion and fragmentation of erythrocytes, hemolysis, and anemia.

microangiopathy /mī'krō·an'jē·op'əthē/ [Gk, *mikros* + *angeion*, vessel, *pathos*, disease], a disease of the small blood vessels. Examples are diabetic microangiopathy, in which the basement membrane of capillaries thickens, and thrombotic microangiopathy, in which thrombi form in the arterioles and the capillaries.

microbe /mī'krōb/, a microorganism. —**microbial**, *adj.*

microbial ecology /mīkrō'bē·əl/, a branch of biology that deals with the interaction of microorganisms with their environment.

microbial pesticides, pathogenic microorganisms that are toxic to a particular bacterium, insect, or other pest.

microbicide /mīkrō'bisīd/ [Gk, *mikros*, small, *bios*, life; L, *cadere*, to kill], any drug, chemical, or other agent that can kill microorganisms.

microbiologic assay /-bī·əloj'ik/, **1.** the use of microorganisms for measuring the activity of organic compounds. **2.** the calculation of the purity of nutritional factors by measuring the growth of certain bacteria.

microbiology /mī'krōbī·ol'əjē/ [Gk, *mikros* + *bios*, life, *logos*, science], the branch of biology concerned with the study of microorganisms, including algae, bacteria, viruses, Protista, fungi, and rickettsiae.

microbiology technologist, a medical technologist who specializes in the identification of bacteria and other microorganisms found in patient tissues and other specimens.

microblast /mī'krōblast'/ [Gk, *mikros*, small, *blastos*, germ], a very small immature red blood cell.

microbrachia /mī'krōbrā'kē·ə/ [Gk, *mikros* + *brachion*, arm], a developmental defect characterized by abnormal smallness of the arms. —**microbrachius**, *n.*

microcarrier /-ker'ē·ər/, microscopic bead or sphere that increases the surface area in a tissue culture for the attachment and yield of anchorage-dependent cells.

microcephaly /mī'krōsef'əlē/ [Gk, *mikros* + *kephale*, head], a congenital anomaly characterized by abnormal smallness of the head in relation to the rest of the body and by underdevelopment of the brain, resulting in some degree of mental retardation. The head is more than two standard deviations below the average circumference size for age, sex, race, and period of gestation. The facial features are generally normal. —**microcephalic, microcephalous,** *adj.*, **microcephalic, microcephalus,** *n.*

microcheiria /mī'krōkī'rē·ə/ [Gk, *mikros* + *cheir*, hand], a developmental defect characterized by abnormal smallness of the hands. The condition is usually associated with other congenital malformations or with bone and muscle disorders.

microcide /mī'krəsīd/, an antimicrobial flavoprotein enzyme. It has antibacterial activity only in the presence of glucose and oxygen as it reduces the oxygen to hydrogen peroxide.

microcirculation /-sur'kyəlē'shən/, the flow of blood throughout the system of smaller vessels of the body, particularly the capillaries.

microcurie (μCi, μc) /mī'krōkyŏŏr'ē/ [Gk, *mikros* + *curie*, Marie Curie], a unit of radiation equal to one millionth (10^{-6}) of a curie.

microcystic adnexal carcinoma (MAC), a form of adnexal tumor that often appears on the face as a yellow, indurated plaque with ill-defined margins.

microcyte /mī'krəsīt/ [Gk, *mikros* + *kytos*, cell], an abnormally small erythrocyte, often occurring in iron deficiency anemias.

microcythemia /-thē'mē·ə/ [Gk, *mikros*, small, *kytos*, cell, *haima*, blood], an excessive amount of microcytes in the blood.

microcytic /mī'krōsit'ik/ [Gk, *mikros* + *kytos*, cell], (of a cell) pertaining to a smaller-than-normal cell.

microcytic anemia, a hematologic disorder characterized by abnormally small erythrocytes, usually associated with chronic blood loss or a nutritional anemia such as iron deficiency anemia.

microcytosis /mī'krōsītō'sis/ [Gk, *mikros* + *kytos* + *osis*, condition], a hematologic condition characterized by erythrocytes that are smaller than normal. Microcytosis is found in iron deficiency anemia. —**microcytic**, *adj.*

microdactyly /mī'krōdak'təlē/ [Gk, *mikros* + *dactylos*, finger], a developmental defect characterized by abnormal smallness of the fingers and toes. The condition is usually associated with bone and muscle disorders.

microdrepanocytic /mī′krōdrep′ənōsit′ik/ [Gk, *mikros* + *drepane,* sickle, *kytos,* cell], pertaining to a blood disorder marked by the presence of both microcytes and drepanocytes, such as occurs in sickle cell-thalassemia.

microdrip /mī′krōdrip′/, (in intravenous therapy) an apparatus for delivering relatively small measured amounts of intravenous solutions at specific flow rates. A microdrip is usually used to deliver small volumes of solution over a long time.

microelectrode /mī′krō·ilek′trōd/, an electrode with a very small tip for use in brain studies. The device can be inserted without membrane damage into nervous tissue to record the bioelectrical activity of a simple neuron.

microencapsulation /mī′krō·enkap′syəlā′shən/ [Gk, *mikros* + *en,* in; L, *capsula,* little box], a laboratory technique used in the bioassay of hormones in which certain antibodies are encapsulated with a perforated membrane. The antibodies cannot escape through the tiny perforations, but hormones that bind with the antibodies may enter the structure to bind with them.

microencephaly /mī′krō·ensef′əlē/ [Gk, *mikros,* small, *egkephalos,* brain], the condition of being born with an abnormally small brain.

microequivalent /mī′krō·ikwiv′ələnt/, one millionth of an equivalent, the amount of a substance that corresponds to its equivalent mass in micrograms.

microfarad (μF) /mī′krōfer′əd/ [Gk, *mikros* + *farad,* Michael Faraday], a unit of capacitance that equals one millionth of a farad.

microfiche /mī′krōfēsh′/ [Gk, *mikros* + Fr, *fiche,* peg], a sheet of microfilm that contains several separate photographic reproductions. The sheet is a convenient size for filing and enables large amounts of data to be stored in a relatively small space.

microfilament /-fil′əmənt/, any of the submicroscopic cellular filaments, such as the tonofibrils, found in the cytoplasm of most cells, that function primarily as a supportive system.

microfilaria /mī′krōfiler′ē·ə/, pl. **microfilariae** [Gk, *mikros* + L, *filum,* thread], the prelarval form of any filarial worm.

microfilm /mī′krəfilm/, a strip of 16 mm or 35 mm film that contains photographic reproductions of pages of books, documents, or other library or medical records

in greatly reduced size. The film is viewed through a machine that enlarges the photographic images to normal reading size.

microgamete /-gam′ēt/, the small motile male gamete of certain thallophytes and sporozoa, specifically the malarial parasite *Plasmodium.* It corresponds to the sperm of the higher animals.

microgametocyte /-gamē′təsīt/ [Gk, *mikros* + *gamete,* spouse, *kytos,* cell], an enlarged merozoite that undergoes meiosis to form the mature male gamete during the sexual phase of the life cycle of certain thallophytes and sporozoa.

microgenitalia /-jen′itā′lē·ə/, a condition characterized by abnormally small external genitalia.

microglia /mīkrog′lē·ə/ [Gk, *mikros* + *glia,* glue], small migratory interstitial cells that form part of the central nervous system. Microglia serve as phagocytes that collect waste products of the nerve tissue of the body.

micrognathia /mī′krōnā′thē·ə/ [Gk, *mikros* + *gnathos,* jaw], underdevelopment of the jaw, especially the mandible. **—micrognathic,** *adj.*

microgram (μg), /mī′krəgram/, a unit of measurement of mass equal to one millionth (10^{-6}) of a gram.

microgyria /mī′krōjī′rē·ə/ [Gk, *mikros* + *gyros,* turn], a developmental defect of the brain in which the convolutions are abnormally small, resulting in structural malformation of the cortex. The condition is usually associated with mental retardation and physical defects.

microgyrus /mī′krōjī′rəs/, pl. **microgyri,** an underdeveloped, malformed convolution of the brain.

microhm /mī′krōm/ [Gk, *mikros* + *ohm,* George Ohm], a unit of electrical resistance equal to one millionth of an ohm.

microinjection /mī′krō·injek′shən/, the injection of tiny amounts of a substance into a cell, using micromanipulation instruments.

microinjector /mī′krō·injek′tər/, an instrument that delivers tiny amounts of a substance into a cell.

microinvasive carcinoma /mī′krō·invā′siv/ [Gk, *mikros* + L, *in,* within, *vadere,* to go], a squamous epithelial neoplasm that has penetrated the basement membrane, the first stage in invasive cancer.

microlevel interventions /-lev′əl/, health-generating changes performed at the individual level, such as in conditioning or stimulus control therapies.

microliter (μl) /mī′krəlē′tər/, a unit of liquid volume equal to one millionth of a liter.

M

microlith /mī′krəlith/ [Gk, *mikros* + *lithos*, stone], a small rounded mass of mineral matter or calcified stone.

micromanipulation /-mənip′yəlā′shən/, surgical displacement or dissection of very small tissues, using either miniature instruments or mechanical devices that translate large motions into smaller movements.

micromanipulator /-mənip′yəlā′tər/, a guidance accessory to a microscope that performs displacement or dissection of very small tissues.

micromelic dwarf /-mē′lik/ [Gk, *mikros* + *melos*, limb], a dwarf whose limbs are abnormally short.

micrometer (μ, mu) /mīkrom′ətər/, 1. an instrument used for measuring small angles or distances on objects being observed through a microscope or telescope. 2. /mī′krōmē′tər/, a unit of measurement, commonly referred to as a *micron*, that equals one thousandth (10^{-3}) of a millimeter.

micromyeloblastic leukemia /mī′krōmī′-əlōblas′tik/ [Gk, *mikros* + *myelos*, marrow, *blastos*, germ], a malignant neoplasm of blood-forming tissues, characterized by the proliferation of small myeloblasts distinguishable from lymphocytes only by special staining techniques and microscopic examination.

micron (μ, mu) /mī′kron/ [Gk, *mikros*, small], 1. a metric unit of length equal to one millionth of a meter; micrometer (def. 2). 2. (in physical chemistry) a colloidal particle with a diameter between 0.2 and 10 μg.

microneurography /-nyo͝orog′rəfē/, the recording of impulse conduction in individual nerve fibers by means of a microelectrode. The technique is used in studies of the relationship between body mass and the sympathetic nervous system.

micronodular /-nod′yələr/, characterized by the presence of very small nodules.

micronodular adrenal disease, a rare form of Cushing's syndrome caused by multiple bilateral small, pigmented autonomous adrenocorticotropic hormone–independent) cortisol-secreting adenomas.

micronucleus /-no͞o′klē·əs/, 1. a small or minute nucleus. 2. (in protozoa) the smaller of two nuclei in each cell; it functions in sexual reproduction as opposed to the macronucleus, which governs cell metabolism and growth.

micronutrient /-no͞otrē·ənt/, any dietary element essential only in minute amounts for the normal physiologic processes of the body.

microorganism /-ôr′gəniz′əm/ [Gk, *mikros* + *organon*, instrument], any tiny, usu-ally microscopic entity capable of carrying on living processes. Kinds of microorganisms include **bacteria, fungi, protozoa,** and **viruses.**

microphage /mī′krəfāj/ [Gk, *mikros* + *phagein*, to eat], a neutrophil capable of ingesting small things such as bacteria. —**microphagic,** *adj.*

microphallus /-fal′əs/ [Gk, *mikros* + *phallos*, penis], an abnormally small penis.

microphthalmos /mī′krəfthal′məs/ [Gk, *mikros* + *ophthalmos*, eye], a developmental anomaly characterized by abnormal smallness of one or both eyes. When the condition occurs in the absence of other ocular defects, it is called pure microphthalmos or nanophthalmos. —**microphthalmic,** *adj.*

micropodia /-pō′dē·ə/ [Gk, *mikros* + *pous*, foot], a developmental anomaly characterized by abnormal smallness of the feet. The condition is often associated with other congenital malformations or with bone and skeletal disorders.

microprolactinoma /-prōlak′tinō′mə/, a prolactin-secreting pituitary tumor less than 10 mM in diameter.

microprosopus /mī′krōprō′səpəs, -prəsō′-pəs/ [Gk, *mikros* + *prosopon*, face], a fetus having an abnormally small or underdeveloped face.

micropsia /mīkrop′sē·ə/ [Gk, *mikros* + *opsis*, sight], a condition of vision in which a person perceives objects as smaller than they really are. —**microptic,** *adj.*

microreentry /-rē·en′trē/ [Gk, *mikros* + L, *re*, again; Fr, *entree*, entry], (in cardiology) pertaining to abnormal transmission of electrical impulses and involving a very small circuit, within Purkinje fibers or myocardial tissue.

microscope /mī′krəskōp′/ [Gk, *mikros*, small, *skopein*, to view], an instrument with lenses for viewing very small objects. An electron microscope uses a beam of electrons instead of visible light.

microscopic /mī′krəskop′ik/ [Gk, *mikros* + *skopein*, to look], 1. pertaining to a microscope. 2. very small; visible only when magnified and illuminated by a microscope.

microscopic anatomy, the study of the microscopic structure of the tissues and cells. Kinds of microscopic anatomy are **cytology** and **histology.**

microscopy /mīkros′kəpē/ [Gk, *mikros* + *skopein*, to look], a technique for observing minute materials using a microscope. Kinds of microscopy include **dark-field microscopy, electron microscopy,** and **immunofluorescent microscopy.**

microshock /mī′krəshok/, 1. shock from

an electric current of less than 1 milliampere. It may not be felt. **2.** the passage of current directly into the cardiac tissue.

microsomal enzymes /-sō'məl/, a group of enzymes associated with a certain particulate fraction of liver homogenate that plays a role in the metabolism of many drugs.

microsome /mī'krəsōm/, a fragment of endoplasmic reticulum associated with ribosomes, found in cells that have been homogenized and ultracentrifuged.

microsomia /-sō'mē·ə/ [Gk, *mikros* + *soma,* body], the condition of having an abnormally small and underdeveloped yet otherwise perfectly formed body with normal proportionate relationships of the various parts.

microspheres /mī'krəsfirs'/, **1.** centrosomes. **2.** microscopic globules of radiolabeled material.

microspherocytosis /-sfir'əsītō'sis/, a hemolytic disorder characterized by the presence in the blood of an excess number of tiny spherocytes, erythrocytes whose diameter is less than normal but whose thickness is increased.

Microsporum /-spôr'əm/ [Gk, *mikros* + *sporos,* seed], a genus of dermatophytes of the family Moniliaceae. One species is *M. audouinii,* which causes epidemic tinea capitis in children.

microstomia /-stō'mē·ə/ [Gk, *mikros,* small, *stoma,* mouth], the condition of having an abnormally small mouth.

microsurgery /-sur'jərē/ [Gk, *mikros,* small, *cheirourgos,* surgery], surgery that involves dissection and manipulation of minute tissue structures under a microscope.

microtear /mī'krāter/, minor damage to soft tissue.

microthermy /-thur'mē/ [Gk, *mikros* + *therme,* heat], the use of heat generated by radio wave conversion in physical therapy.

microtome /mī'krətōm/ [Gk, *mikros* + *temnein,* to cut], a device that cuts specimens of tissue prepared in paraffin blocks into extremely thin slices for microscopic study by a surgical pathologist.

microtrauma /-trô'mə/, a very slight injury or lesion.

microtubule, a hollow cylindric structure that occurs widely within plant and animal cells. Microtubules increase in number during cell division.

microvascular /-vas'kyələr/, pertaining to the part of the circulatory system that is composed of the capillary network.

microvilli /-vil'ī/ [Gk, *mikros,* small; L, *villus,* shaggy hair], tiny hairlike folds in the plasma membrane that extend from the

surface of many absorptive or secretory cells.

microwave interstitial system /mī'-krəwāv/ [Gk, *mikros* + AS, *wafian,* wave], a microwave-generated hyperthermia system that creates a heat field in certain accessible tumors beneath the skin. The treatment can be monitored on a video terminal that shows location of the tumor and heat applicators.

microwaves, electromagnetic radiation in the frequency range of 300 to 2450 Mhz.

microwave thermography, measurement of temperature through the detection of microwave radiation emitted from heated tissue.

micturition reflex /mik'chərish'ən/ [L, *micturire,* to urinate, *reflectere,* to bend back], a normal reaction to a rise in pressure within the bladder, resulting in contraction of the bladder wall and relaxation of the urethral sphincter. Voluntary inhibition normally prevents incontinence; urination follows withdrawal of the inhibition.

micturition syncope [L, *micturire,* to urinate; Gk, *syn,* together, *koptein,* to cut], a temporary loss of consciousness that tends to affect some adult males after arising from a reclining posture to urinate in an upright posture. The effect is caused by a brief interruption of blood flow to the brain and is often associated with the use of alcohol, which contributes to vasodilation.

MICU, abbreviation for *medical intensive care unit.*

MID, abbreviation for **minimal infecting dose.**

midarm muscle circumference, a calculation made by subtracting the triceps skin fold from the midupper arm circumference measurement.

midaxillary line /midak'siler'ē/, an imaginary vertical line that passes midway between the anterior and posterior axillary folds.

midazolam hydrochloride /midaz'əlam/, a parenteral central nervous system depressant. It is prescribed for preoperative sedation and impairment of memory of preoperative events, and for conscious sedation before short diagnostic or endoscopic procedures.

midbody, 1. the middle of the body, or the midregion of the trunk. **2.** a mass of granules that appears in the middle of the spindle during mitotic anaphase.

midclavicular line /mid'kləvik'yōōlər/ [AS, *midd* + L, *clavicula,* little key, *linea,* line], (in anatomy) an imaginary line that extends downward over the trunk from the midpoint of the clavicle, dividing

M

each side of the anterior chest into two parts.

middle adult [AS, *middel* + L, *adultus,* grown up], an individual in the transitional age span between young adult and elderly, approximately 45 to 65 years of age.

middle cardiac vein, one of the five tributaries of the coronary sinus that drain blood from the capillary bed of the myocardium. It receives tributaries from both ventricles and ends in the right extremity of the coronary sinus.

middle ear, the tympanic cavity with the auditory ossicles contained in an irregular space in the temporal bone. It is separated from the external ear by the tympanic membrane and from the inner ear by the oval window. The auditory (pharyngotympanic or eustachian) tube carries air from the posterior nasopharynx into the middle ear.

middle lobe syndrome, localized atelectasis of the middle lobe of the right lung, characterized by chronic infection, cough, dyspnea, wheezing, and obstructive pneumonitis. Asymptomatic obstruction of the bronchus may occur. The condition is caused by enlargement of the surrounding cuff of lymphatic glands.

middle mediastinum, the widest part of the mediastinum, containing the heart, ascending aorta, lower half of the superior vena cava, pulmonary trunk, and phrenic nerves.

middle sacral artery, a small visceral branch of the abdominal aorta, descending to the fourth and fifth lumbar vertebrae, the sacrum, and the coccyx.

middle suprarenal artery, one of a pair of small visceral branches of the abdominal aorta, arising opposite the superior mesenteric artery and supplying the suprarenal gland.

middle temporal artery, one of the branches of the superficial temporal artery on each side of the head.

middle temporal gyrus [AS, *middel* + L, *tempus,* time; Gk, *gyros,* turn], the middle of three gyri of the temporal area of the surface of the brain. It runs horizontally between the inferior and superior temporal sulci of the temporal lobe.

middle umbilical fold, the fold of peritoneum over the urachal remnant within the abdomen.

mid forceps [AS, *midd* + L, *forceps,* pair of tongs], an obstetric operation in which forceps are applied to the baby's head when it has reached the midplane of the mother's pelvis. An episiotomy is usually performed, and local, regional, or inhalation anesthesia is provided. In some cases such as severe fetal distress, mid forceps may be the most rapid and safest means of delivery.

midgut [AS, *midd* + *guttas*], the middle part of the embryonic alimentary canal. It is connected to the yolk sac during early prenatal development and eventually gives rise to some of the small intestine and part of the large intestine.

midlife transition, a period between early adulthood and middle adulthood that occurs between 40 and 45 years of age.

midline /mid′līn/ [AS, *midd* + L, *linea,* line], an imaginary line that divides the body into right and left halves.

midoccipital /mid′oksip′itəl/, pertaining to the center of the occiput.

midparental height /-pəren′təl/, the average height of both parents at 25 to 45 years of age.

midposition /mid′pəzish′ən/, the end-expiratory or end-tidal level or position of the lung-chest system under any given condition, defining the patient's functional residual capacity.

midstance /mid′stanz/ [AS, *midd* + L, *stare,* to stand], one of the five stages in the stance phase of walking, or gait, directly associated with the period of single-leg support of body weight or the period during which the body advances over the stationary foot.

midsternum /midstur′nəm/ [AS, *midd* + Gk, *sternon,* chest], the body of the breast bone (sternum).

midstream catch urine specimen [AS, *midd* + *stream* + L, *captere,* to capture], a urine specimen collected during the middle of a flow of urine, after the urinary opening has been carefully cleaned.

midupper arm circumference (MAC), a measurement of the circumference of the arm at a midpoint between the tip of the acromial process of the scapula and the olecranon process of the ulna.

midwife [AS, *midd* + *wif*], **1.** (in traditional use) a (female) person who assists women in childbirth. **2.** (according to the International Confederation of Midwives, World Health Organization, and Federation of International Gynecologists and Obstetricians) "a person who, having been regularly admitted to a midwifery educational program fully recognized in the country in which it is located, has successfully completed the prescribed course of studies in midwifery and has acquired the requisite qualifications to be registered and/or legally licensed to practice midwifery." **3.** a lay midwife. **4.** a nurse midwife or Certified Nurse Midwife.

midwifery /mid′wĭf(ə)rē/ [AS, *midd* + *wif*], the employment of a person who is qualified by special training and experience to assist a woman in childbirth.

MIF, abbreviation for *macrophage inhibition factor.*

mifepristone /mif'əpris'tōn/,   a drug that induces abortion if taken within the first 7 weeks of pregnancy. Two days after taking the drug to end the pregnancy, the woman must take a second drug to cause strong uterine contractions that expel the fetus. If the drug regimen fails to terminate the pregnancy, the woman must arrange for a surgical abortion to complete the process.

migraine /mī'grān/ [Gk, *hemi,* half, *kranion,* skull],   a recurring vascular headache characterized by a prodromal aura, unilateral onset, and severe pain, photophobia, and autonomic disturbances during the acute phase, which may last for hours or days. The head pain is related to dilation of extracranial blood vessels, which may be the result of chemical changes that cause spasms of intracranial vessels. Attacks often occur during a period of relaxation after physical or psychic stress. An impending attack may be heralded by visual disturbances, such as flashing lights or wavy lines, or by a strange taste or odor, numbness, tingling, vertigo, tinnitus, or a feeling that part of the body is distorted in size or shape. The acute phase may be accompanied by nausea, vomiting, chills, polyuria, sweating, facial edema, irritability, and extreme fatigue.

migrainous cranial neuralgia /mī'grānəs, mīgrā'nəs/ [Gk, *hemi,* half, *kranion,* skull; L, *osus,* having],   a variant of migraine, characterized by closely spaced episodes of excruciating throbbing unilateral headaches often accompanied by dilation of temporal blood vessels, flushing, sweating, lacrimation, nasal congestion or rhinorrhea, ptosis, and facial edema. Repeated episodes usually occur in clusters within a few days or weeks and may be followed by a relatively long remission period.

migrating phlebitis /mī'grāting/ [L, *migrare,* to wander; Gk, *phleps,* vein, *itis,* inflammation],   a form of phlebitis characterized by inflammation in one part of a vein and, after remission, in another part of the vein.

migration /mīgrā'shən/ [L, *migrare,* to wander],   the passage of the ovum from the ovary into a fallopian tube and then into the uterus.

migratory polyarthritis /mī'grətôr'ē/, arthritis progressively affecting a number of joints and finally settling in one or more, which occurs in persons with gonorrhea and develops a few days to a few weeks after the onset of gonorrheal urethritis. The patient usually has a moderate fever. Large joints are most affected; after the swelling subsides, the overlying skin may peel.

migratory thrombophlebitis, a condition in which multiple thromboses appear in both superficial and deep veins. It may be associated with malignancy, especially carcinoma of the pancreas, often preceding other evidence of cancer by several months.

Mikulicz's syndrome /mik'yōōlich'ēz/ [Johann von Miculicz-Radecki, Polish surgeon, 1850–1905],   a bilateral enlargement of the salivary and lacrimal glands. It is found in a variety of diseases, including leukemia, tuberculosis, and sarcoidosis.

mild [AS, *milde,* soft],   gentle, subtle, or of low in intensity.

mildew /mil'dyōō/,   any of numerous species of saprophytic fungal growths with visible mycelium.

milia neonatorum [L, *milium,* millet; Gk, *neo,* new; L, *natus,* born],   a nonpathologic dermatologic condition characterized by minute epidermal cysts consisting of keratinous debris that occur on the face and occasionally on the trunk of the newborn.

miliaria /mil'ē·er'ē·ə/ [L, *milium,* millet],   minute vesicles and papules, often with surrounding erythema, caused by occlusion of sweat ducts during times of exposure to heat and high humidity.

miliary /mil'ē·er'ē/ [L, *milium,* millet],   describing a condition marked by the appearance of very small lesions the size of millet seeds, such as miliary tuberculosis, which is characterized by tiny tubercles throughout the body.

miliary carcinosis,   a condition characterized by numerous cancerous nodules resembling miliary tubercles.

miliary fever [L, *milium,* millet; L, *febris*],   an inflammatory skin eruption caused by sweat retention. Sweat trapped in the dermis or epidermis causes irritation.

miliary tuberculosis,   extensive dissemination by the bloodstream of tubercle bacilli. In children it is associated with high fever, night sweats, and often meningitis, pleural effusions, or peritonitis. A similar illness may occur in adults but with a less abrupt onset and occasionally with weeks or months of nonspecific symptoms such as weight loss, weakness, and low-grade fever. Multiple small opacities resembling millet seeds may be evident on chest x-ray films.

milieu /milyœ, milyōō'/, *pl.* **milieus, milieux** [Fr, middle],   the environment, surroundings, or setting.

M

milieu extérieur /eksterē·œr'/, the external or physical surroundings of an organism, including the social environment, especially the home, school, and recreational facilities, which play a dominant role in personality development.

milieu intérieur /aNterē·œr'/, the basic concept in physiology that multicellular organisms exist in an aqueous internal environment composed of the blood, lymph, and interstitial fluid that bathes all cells and provides a medium for the elementary exchange of nutrients and waste material. All fundamental processes necessary for the maintenance and life of the tissue elements depend on the stability and balance of this environment.

milieu therapy, a type of psychotherapy in which the total environment is used in treating mental and behavioral disorders. It is primarily conducted in a hospital or other institutional setting, where the entire facility acts as a therapeutic community.

Milieu Therapy, a Nursing Interventions Classification defined as use of people, resources, and events in the patient's immediate environment to promote optimal psychosocial functioning.

military attitude, (in obstetrics) a fetal position in which the fetal head is not flexed and the chin is held straight up.

milium /mil'ē·əm/, *pl.* **milia** [L, millet], a minute white cyst of the epidermis caused by obstruction of hair follicles and eccrine sweat glands. One variety is seen in newborns and disappears within a few weeks. Another type is found primarily on the faces of middle-aged women.

milk [AS, *meoluc*], a liquid secreted by the mammary glands or udders of mammalian animals that suckle their young. Milk is a basic food containing carbohydrate (in the form of lactose); protein (mainly casein, with small amounts of lactalbumin and lactoglobulin); suspended fat; the minerals calcium and phosphorus; and the vitamins A, riboflavin, niacin, thiamin, and, when the milk is fortified, D. It is a valuable nutrient for adults and a nearly complete food for infants, especially breast milk.

milk-alkali syndrome, a condition of alkalosis caused by the excessive ingestion of milk, antacid medications containing calcium, or other sources of absorbable alkaline substances. The condition results in hypercalcemia, hypocalciuria, and calcium deposits in the kidneys and other tissues.

milk baby, an infant with iron deficiency anemia caused by ingestion of excessive amounts of milk and delayed or inadequate addition of iron-rich foods to the diet.

milk bath, a bath taken in milk for cosmetic or emollient reasons.

milk ejection reflex, a normal reflex in a lactating woman elicited by tactile stimulation of the nipple, resulting in release of milk from the glands of the breast.

milker's nodule, a smooth brownish-red papilloma of the fingers or palm that begins as a macule and progresses through a vesicular stage to become a nodule. The disease is acquired from pustular lesions on the udder of a cow infected with poxvirus.

milk fever, *nontechnical.* postpartum fever that begins with the onset of lactation. It was formerly considered a normal reaction to lactation. Maternal oral temperature during the puerperium does not normally exceed 100.4° F; continued high readings may indicate infection.

milk globule, a spheric droplet of fat in milk that tends to separate out as cream.

milking, a procedure used to express the contents of a duct or tube, to test for tenderness, or to obtain a specimen for study. The examiner compresses the structure with a finger and moves the finger firmly along the duct or tube to its opening.

Milkman's syndrome [Louis A. Milkman, American radiologist, 1895–1951], a form of osteomalacia characterized by multiple bilateral symmetric absorption stripes, indicating pseudofractures, in hypocalcified long bones and the pelvis and scapula.

milk of magnesia, a laxative and antacid containing magnesium hydroxide. It is prescribed to relieve constipation and acid indigestion.

milk therapy, a nutritional treatment used in the therapy of Curling's ulcer in patients who have been severely burned. Cool homogenized milk is administered in doses of 1 to 2 ounces every hour through a nasogastric tube. After instillation the tube is clamped for 5 minutes and then unclamped. Milk remaining in the stomach is allowed to flow into a basin.

Miller-Abbott tube [Thomas G. Miller, American physician, 1886–1981; William O. Abbott, American physician, 1902–1943], a long small-caliber double-lumen catheter used in intestinal intubation for decompression. One lumen ends in a perforated metal tip, and the other in a collapsible balloon. These tubes are radiopaque and can therefore be seen on a radiogram.

milliampere (mA) /-am'pir/ [L, *mille,* thousand; Andre Ampere], a unit of electric current that is one thousandth of an ampere.

milliampere seconds (mAs), the product obtained by multiplying the electric quantity in milliamperes by the time in seconds.

millicoulomb (mC) /-kōō′lōm/ [L, *mille,* thousand; Charles A. de Coulomb], a unit of electric charge that is one thousandth of a coulomb.

millicurie (mCi, mc) /-kōōr′ē/ [L, *mille,* thousand; Marie Curie], a unit of radioactivity equal to one thousandth of a curie, or 3.70×10^{-7} disintegrations per second.

milliequivalent (mEq) /-ikwiv′ələnt/ [L, *mille + aequus,* equal, *valere,* to be strong], **1.** the number of grams of solute dissolved in 1 ml of a normal solution. **2.** one thousandth of a gram equivalent.

milliequivalent per liter (mEq/L), one thousandth of 1 gram of a specific substance dissolved in 1 L of plasma.

milligram (mg) /-gram/ [L, *mille* + Fr, *gramme,* small weight], a metric unit of weight equal to one thousandth (10^{-3}) of a gram.

milliliter (ml) /-lē′tər/ [L, *mille* + Fr, *litre,* a measure], a metric unit of volume that is one thousandth (10^{-3}) of a liter.

millimeter (mm) /-mē′tər/, a metric unit of length equal to one thousandth (10^{-3}) of a meter.

millimole (mmol, mM) /-mōl/ [L, *mille + moles,* mass], a unit of metric measurement that is equal to one thousandth (10^{-3}) of a mole.

milliosmol /mil′ē·oz′mōl/, one thousandth of an osmole. —**milliosmolar,** *adj.*

millipede /mil′ipēd′/ [L, *mille + pes,* foot], a many-legged wormlike arthropod. Certain species squirt irritating fluids that may cause dermatitis.

millirad (mrad) /-rad/, one thousandth (10^{-3}) of a rad, a unit of measurement of absorbed dose of ionizing radiation.

millirem (mrem), one thousandth (10^{-3}) of a rem. See also **rem.**

milliroentgen (mR, mr) /mil′irent′gən, -jən/ [L, *mille,* thousand; Wilhelm K. Roentgen], a unit of radiation that is equal to one thousandth (10^{-3}) of a roentgen.

millisecond (msec) /-sek′ənd/ [L, *mille,* thousand; ME, *seconde,* small part], one thousandth of a second.

millivolt (mV, mv) /-vōlt/ [L, *mille,* thousand; Alessandro Volta], a unit of electromotive force equal to one thousandth of a volt.

Milwaukee brace /milwô′kē/ [Milwaukee, Wisconsin; OFr *bracier* to embrace], an orthotic device that helps immobilize the torso and neck of a patient in the treatment or correction of scoliosis, lordosis, or kyphosis. It is usually constructed of strong but light metal and fiberglass supports lined with rubber to protect against abrasion.

mimicry /mim′ikrē/ [Gk, *mimetikos,* imitation], **1.** the effort of one species or organism to resemble another to obtain an offensive or defensive advantage. **2.** an autonomic nervous system phenomenon in which facial expressions may be the unwilled and largely unconscious expression of feelings and ideas.

mimic spasm /mim′ik/ [Gk, *mimetikos,* imitative, *spasmos,* spasm], involuntary stereotyped movements of a small group of muscles such as of the face. The spasm is usually psychogenic and may be aggravated by stress or anxiety but is generally controllable.

min, 1. abbreviation for **minim. 2.** abbreviation for *minute.*

Minamata disease /min′əmä′tə/, a severe degenerative neurologic disorder caused by the ingestion of seed grain heated with alkyl compounds of mercury or of seafood taken from waters polluted with industrial wastes contaminated by soluble mercuric salts. The term is derived from a tragedy involving Japanese who ate seafood from Minamata Bay.

mind [AS, *gemynd*], **1.** the part of the brain that is the seat of mental activity and that enables one to know, reason, understand, remember, think, feel, react to, and adapt to surroundings and all external and internal stimuli. **2.** the totality of all conscious and unconscious processes of the individual that influence and direct mental and physical behavior. **3.** the faculty of the intellect or understanding, in contrast to emotion and will.

mineral /min′ərəl/ [L, *minera,* mine], **1.** an inorganic substance occurring naturally in the earth's crust, having a characteristic chemical composition and (usually) crystalline structure. **2.** (in nutrition) a mineral usually referred to by the name of a metal, nonmetal, radical, or phosphate rather than by the name of the compound of which it is a part. Minerals play a vital role in regulating many body functions.

mineral deficiency, the inability to use one or more of the mineral elements essential in human nutrition because of a genetic defect, malabsorption dysfunction, or lack of that mineral in the diet. The symptoms and manifestations vary, depending on the specific function or functions of the element in promoting growth and maintaining health.

M

mineralization /-ĭzā'shən/ [L, *minera* + Gk, *izein*, to cause], the addition of any mineral to the body.

mineralocorticoid /min'əral'ōkôr'tikoid/ [L, *minera* + *cortex*, bark; Gk, *eidos*, form], a hormone secreted by the adrenal cortex that maintains normal blood volume, promotes sodium and water retention, and increases urinary excretion of potassium and hydrogen ions. Aldosterone, the most potent mineralocorticoid with regard to electrolyte balance, and corticosterone, a glucocorticoid and a mineralocorticoid, act on the distal tubules of the kidneys to enhance the resorption of sodium into the plasma.

mineral oil, a laxative, stool softener, emollient, and pharmaceutic aid used as a solvent. It is prescribed to prevent constipation, to treat mild constipation, to prepare the bowel for surgery or examination, and to act as a solvent for various preparations.

miner's elbow [L, *minera* + AS, *elboga*], an inflammation of the olecranon bursa, caused by resting the weight of the body on the elbow, as in some coal mining activities. The condition is sometimes seen in schoolchildren who lean on their elbows.

Minerva cast /minur'və/ [L, *Minerva*, Roman goddess of wisdom; ONorse, *kasta*], an orthopedic cast applied to the trunk and head, with spaces cut out for the face area and the ears. The section encasing the trunk extends to the sternum and the distal rib border anteriorly and across the distal rib border posteriorly. The cast is used for immobilizing the head and part of the trunk in the treatment of torticollis, cervical and thoracic injuries, and cervical spinal infections.

minim (min) /min'im/ [L, *minimum,* smallest], a measurement of volume in the apothecaries' system, originally one drop (of water). Sixty minims equals 1 fluid dram. One minim equals 0.06 ml.

minimal bactericidal concentration, the lowest concentration of drug that results in a 99.9% reduction in the initial bacterial density.

minimal care unit /min'iməl/ [L, *minimum,* smallest], a unit for the treatment of inpatients who are ambulatory and able to meet many of their own daily living needs but require minimal nursing care.

minimal change disease, a kidney disorder characterized by subtle changes in renal function, including albuminuria and presence of lipid droplets in the proximal tubules. It mainly affects small children but also occurs in adults with idiopathic nephrotic syndrome.

minimal infecting dose, the smallest amount of infective material that produces infection.

minimal inhibitory concentration (MIC), the lowest concentration of an antibiotic medication in the blood that is effective against an infection, determined by injecting infected venous blood into a culture medium containing various concentrations of a proposed antibiotic.

minimal occlusive volume (MOV), the volume of endotracheal or tracheostomy tube cuff inflation that is sufficient to obliterate an air leak during the inspiratory phase of ventilation.

Mini-Mental State Examination (MMS), a brief psychologic test designed to differentiate among dementia, psychosis, and affective disorders. It may include ability to identify common objects such as a pencil and a watch, to write a sentence, to spell simple words backward, and to demonstrate orientation by identifying the day, month, and year, as well as town and country.

minimization /min'imīzā'shən/ [L, *minimum,* smallest; Gk, *izein,* to cause], (in psychology) cognitive distortion in which the effects of one's behavior are underestimated.

minimum alveolar concentration (MAC) /min'iməm/, the smallest amount of a gas detected and measured in the alveoli of the lungs.

minimum daily requirement (MDR) [L, *minimum* + OE, *daeglie* + L, *requirere,* to seek], the daily human requirement of nutrients for health and as needed for prevention of a deficiency disease. The figures, established by the U.S. Food and Drug Administration, are generally extrapolated from experimental animal studies and include an added margin for safety.

minimum dose [L, *minimum,* smallest; Gk, *dosis,* giving], the smallest amount of a drug or other substance needed to produce a desired or specified effect. Because of individual variations in drug response, the minimal dose for one person may be either excessive or insufficient for another patient.

minimum hemagglutinating dose, the smallest amount of hemagglutinating agent that causes a complete hemagglutinating reaction in a standard volume of red blood cells.

minimum hemolytic dose (MHD), the smallest amount of a reagent that produces complete lysis of a specified amount of red blood cells.

minimum lethal dose (MLD) [L, *minimum,* smallest, *lethum,* death; Gk, *dosis,* giving], the smallest dose of a drug, relative to body weight, that will kill an experimental animal. The MLD may vary with the species of animal tested.

miniprotein /min′iprō′tēn/, a protein that has been reduced to half its natural size without loss of its ability to function. A miniprotein may consist of about 30 amino acid molecules and retain the normal activity of the natural protein.

Minnesota Multiphasic Personality Inventory (MMPI), a commonly used psychologic test that includes 550 statements for interpretation by the subject, used clinically for evaluating personality and detecting various disorders.

minocycline hydrochloride /min′əsī′klēn/, a tetracycline antibiotic active against bacteria, rickettsia, and other organisms. It is prescribed in the treatment of infections.

minor /mī′nər/ [L, smaller], (in law) a person not of legal age; a person beneath the age of majority.

minor connector, (in dentistry) a device that links the major connector or base of a removable partial denture to other denture units, such as rests and direct and indirect retainers.

minor hysteria [Gk, hystera, womb], a mild disorder that may be expressed in emotional outbursts, repressed anxieties, or conversion of unconscious conflicts into physical symptoms.

minor surgery, surgical procedure for minor problems or injuries that are not considered life-threatening or hazardous.

Minot-Murphy diet [George R. Minot, American physician, 1885–1950; William P. Murphy, American physician, b. 1892], a dietary regimen developed in the 1930s for the treatment of pernicious anemia with large amounts of raw or slightly cooked liver or crude extracts of fresh calf liver.

minoxidil /mīnok′sidil/, a vasodilator prescribed in the treatment of severe refractory hypertension and as a topical solution for the treatment of androgenic alopecia.

minute ventilation /min′it/ [L, minus, very small], the total ventilation per minute, the product of tidal volume and respiratory rate, as measured by expired gas collection for a period of 1 to 3 minutes.

miosis /mī·ō′sis/ [Gk, meiosis, becoming less], **1.** contraction of the sphincter muscle of the iris, causing the pupil to become smaller. **2.** an abnormal condition characterized by excessive constriction of the sphincter muscle of the iris, resulting in very small, pinpoint pupils.

miotic /mē·ot′ik/, **1.** pertaining to miosis. **2.** causing constriction of the pupil of the eye. **3.** any substance or pharmaceutic that causes constriction of the pupil of the eye. Such agents are used in the treatment of glaucoma.

MIP, abbreviation for **maximum inspiratory pressure.**

miracidium /mir′əsid′ē·əm/, pl. **miracidia** [Gk, meirakidion, youthfulness], the ciliated larva of a parasitic trematode that hatches from an egg and can survive only by further developing within a host snail.

mirage /miräzh′/ [L, mirari, to look at], an optical illusion caused by the refraction of light through air layers of different temperatures, such as the illusionary sheets of water that appear to shimmer over stretches of hot sand and pavement.

mirror image /mir′ər/ [L, mirare, to look at, imago], **1.** an image formed by a reflection in a plane mirror. **2.** a kind of reversed asymmetry of characteristics often found in sets of monozygotic twins. **3.** chemical molecules with the same composition but with asymmetric arrangement of the atoms.

mirror speech [L, mirari, to look at; AS, spaec, speech], an abnormal manner of speaking characterized by the reversal of the order of syllables in a word.

miscible /mis′ibəl/ [L, miscere, to mix], able to be mixed or blended with another substance.

misdemeanor /mis′dəmē′nər/ [AS, missan, to miss; ME, demenen, conduct], (in criminal law) an offense that is considered less serious than a felony and carries a lesser penalty, usually a fine or imprisonment for less than 1 year.

misfeasance /misfē′zəns/ [AS, missan, to miss; L, facere, to make], an improper performance of a lawful act, especially in a way that may cause damage or injury.

misogamy /misog′əmē/ [Gk, misein, to hate, gamos, marriage], an aversion to marriage. —**misogamic, misogamous,** adj., **misogamist,** n.

misogyny /misoj′inē/ [Gk, misein, to hate, gyne, women], an aversion to women. —**misogynist,** n., **misogynistic,** adj.

misopedia /mis′ōpē′dē·ə/ [Gk, misein + pais, children], an aversion to children. —**misopedic,** adj., **misopedist,** n.

missed abortion [OE, missan, to be lacking; L, ab, away from, oriri, to be born], a condition in which a dead immature embryo or fetus is not expelled from the uterus for 2 months or more. The uterus diminishes in size, and symptoms of pregnancy abate; maternal infection and blood clotting disorders may follow.

missed period [OE, missan, to be lacking; Gk, peri + hodos, way], an unexplained interruption in the menstrual cycle.

M

missile fracture [L, *mittere,* to throw], a penetration fracture caused by a projectile such as a bullet or a piece of shrapnel.

mistura /misty͞oo′rə/ [L, mixture], any of a number of mixtures of drugs, usually containing suspensions of insoluble substances intended for internal use. An example is **mistura cretae pro infantibus,** a mixture of chalk, tragacanth, chloroform water, and other ingredients formulated for the treatment of gastrointestinal disorders in infants.

mite /mīt/ [AS], a minute arachnid with a flat, almost transparent body and four pairs of legs. Many species of these relatives of ticks and spiders are parasitic, including the chigger and *Sarcoptes scabiei,* which cause localized pruritus and inflammation.

mitleiden /mit′līdən/ [Ger, *mit,* with, *leiden,* to suffer], psychosomatic symptoms sometimes experienced by expectant fathers.

mitochondrion /mī′tōkon′drē·on/, *pl.* **mitochondria** [Gk, *mitos,* thread, *chondros,* cartilage], a small rodlike, threadlike, or granular organelle within the cytoplasm that functions in cellular metabolism and respiration and occurs in varying numbers in all living cells except bacteria, viruses, blue-green algae, and mature erythrocytes. Mitochondria provide the principal source of cellular energy through oxidative phosphorylation and adenosine triphosphate synthesis. They also contain the enzymes involved with electron transport and the citric and fatty acid cycles. —**mitochondrial,** *adj.*

mitogen /mī′təjən, mit′-/ [Gk, *mitos* + *genein,* to produce], an agent that triggers mitosis. —**mitogenic,** *adj.*

mitogenesia /mī′tōjənē′zhə/ [Gk, *mitos* + *genein,* to produce], the production by or formation resulting from mitosis.

mitogenesis /mī′tōjen′əsis/, the induction of mitosis in a cell. —**mitogenetic,** *adj.*

mitogenetic radiation /-jənet′ik/, the force or specific energy that is supposedly given off by cells undergoing division.

mitogenic factor /-jen′ik/, a lymphokine that is released from activated T lymphocytes and stimulates the production of normal unsensitized lymphocytes.

mitome /mī′tōm/, the reticular network sometimes observed within the cytoplasm and nucleoplasm of fixed cells.

mitomycin /mī′təmī′sin/, an antineoplastic antibiotic prescribed in the treatment of malignant neoplastic diseases.

mitosis /mītō′sis, mit-/ [Gk, *mitos,* thread], a type of cell division that occurs in somatic cells and results in the formation of two genetically identical daughter cells containing the diploid number of chromosomes characteristic of the species. Mitosis is the process by which the body produces new cells for both growth and repair of injured tissue. —**mitotic,** *adj.*

mitotane /mī′totān/, an antineoplastic that destroys normal and neoplastic adrenal cortical cells. It is prescribed in the treatment of carcinoma of the adrenal cortex.

mitotic figure [Gk, *mitos* + L, *figura,* form], any chromosome or chromosome aggregation during any of the stages of mitosis.

mitotic index, the number of cells per unit (usually 1000) undergoing mitosis during a given time. The ratio is used primarily as an estimation of the rate of tissue growth.

mitoxantrone, a synthetic antineoplastic anthracenedione for intravenous use. It is prescribed in combination with other approved drugs in the initial treatment of acute lymphocytic leukemia in adults.

mitral /mī′trəl/ [L, *mitra,* turban], **1.** pertaining to the mitral valve of the heart. **2.** shaped like a miter.

mitral atresia, a congenital absence of the mitral valve associated with transposition of the great vessels or hypoplastic left heart syndrome.

mitral commissurotomy [L, *mitra,* turban, *commissura,* joining together; Gk, *temnein,* to cut], a closed-heart surgical procedure in which the mitral valve is divided at the junction of its cusps for the treatment of mitral stenosis.

mitral gradient, the difference in pressure in the left atrium and left ventricle during diastole.

mitral murmur [L, *mitra,* turban, *murmur,* humming], a heart murmur caused by a defective mitral valve.

mitral regurgitation, a backflow of blood from the left ventricle into the left atrium in systole across a diseased valve. The condition may result from congenital valve abnormalities, rheumatic fever, mitral valve prolapse, endocardial fibroelastosis, dilation of the left ventricle as a result of severe anemia, myocarditis, or myocardiopathy. Symptoms include dyspnea, fatigue, intolerance of exercise, and heart palpitations. Congestive heart failure may ultimately occur.

mitral valve, a bicuspid valve situated between the left atrium and the left ventricle; the only valve with two, rather than three, cusps. The mitral valve allows blood to flow from the left atrium into the left ventricle but prevents blood from flowing back into the atrium. Ventricular contraction in systole forces the blood against the valve, closing the two cusps and ensuring the flow of blood from the ventricle into the aorta.

mitral valve prolapse (MVP), protrusion of one or both cusps of the mitral valve back into the left atrium during ventricular systole.

mitral valve stenosis, an obstructive lesion in the mitral valve caused by adhesions on the leaflets of the valve, usually the result of recurrent episodes of rheumatic endocarditis or age-related calcification of the valve leaflets. Hypertrophy of the left atrium develops and may be followed by right-sided heart failure and pulmonary edema (cor pulmonale).

mittelschmerz /mit'əlshmerts/ [Ger, *Mitte,* middle, *Schmerz,* pain], abdominal pain in the region of an ovary during ovulation, which usually occurs midway through the menstrual cycle. Present in many women, mittelschmerz is useful for identifying ovulation, thus pinpointing the fertile period of the cycle.

Mittendorf's dot, an eye anomaly characterized by the presence of a small, dense, floating opacity behind the posterior lens capsule. It is a remnant of the hyaloid artery that was present in the eye during embryonic development. The object usually does not affect vision.

mixed cell malignant lymphoma [L, *miscere,* to mix], a lymphoid neoplasm containing lymphocytes and histiocytes (macrophages).

mixed cell sarcoma, a tumor consisting of two or more cellular elements, excluding fibrous tissue.

mixed connective tissue disease (MCTD), a systemic disease characterized by the combined symptoms of various collagen diseases such as synovitis, polymyositis, scleroderma, and systemic lupus erythematosus.

mixed culture [L, *miscere,* to mix, *colere,* to cultivate], a laboratory culture that contains two or more different strains of organisms.

mixed dentition, a phase of dentition during which some of the teeth are permanent and some are deciduous.

mixed glioma, a tumor, composed of glial cells, that contains more than one kind of cell; the most common being nonneural cells of ectodermal origin.

mixed infection, an infection by several microorganisms, as in some abscesses, pneumonia, and infections of wounds. Numerous combinations of bacteria, viruses, and fungi may be involved.

mixed leukemia, a malignancy of blood-forming tissues characterized by the proliferation of more than one predominant cell line.

mixed lymphocyte culture (MLC) reaction, an assay of the function of the T cell lymphocytes. It is used primarily for histocompatibility testing before grafting.

mixed neoplasm [L, *miscere,* to mix; Gk, *neos,* new + *plasma,* something formed], a tumor or growth involving two germinal layers of tissue.

mixed nerve [L, *miscere,* to mix, *nervus*], a nerve that contains both sensory and motor fibers.

mixed sleep apnea, a condition marked by signs and symptoms of both central sleep apnea and obstructive sleep apnea. It often begins as central sleep apnea and is followed by development of the obstructive form.

mixed tumor, a growth composed of more than one kind of neoplastic tissue.

mixed vaccine, an immunizing preparation that protects against more than one kind of pathogen, such as the diphtheria, tetanus, and pertussis or measles, mumps, and rubella vaccine.

mixed venous blood, blood that is composed of the venous blood from the heart and all systemic tissues in proportion to their venous returns. In the absence of abnormalities, mixed venous blood is present in the main pulmonary artery.

mixture /miks'chər/ [L, *miscere,* to mix], **1.** a substance composed of ingredients that are not chemically combined and do not necessarily occur in a fixed proportion. **2.** (in pharmacology) a liquid containing one or more medications in suspension. The proportions of the ingredients are specific to each mixture.

ml, abbreviation for **milliliter.**

MLC, abbreviation for *mixed lymphocyte culture.*

MLD, abbreviation for **minimum lethal dose.**

mm, abbreviation for **millimeter.**

mM, abbreviation for **millimole.**

MMFR, abbreviation for **maximal mid-expiratory flow rate.**

M-mode, abbreviation for *motion mode,* a variation of B-mode ultrasound scanning. It is used in echocardiography.

mmol, abbreviation for **millimole.**

MMPI, abbreviation for **Minnesota Multiphasic Personality Inventory.**

MMR, abbreviation for **measles, mumps, and rubella virus vaccine live.**

MMWR, abbreviation for *Morbidity and Mortality Weekly Report.*

Mn, symbol for the element **manganese.**

mnemonics [Gk, *mnemonikos*], a system of memory training that links a new concept or image with one already established in the memory, such as associating the numbers of a combination lock with a birthday or telephone number.

MNL, abbreviation for **mononuclear leukocyte.**

Mo, symbol for the element **molybdenum.**

mobile arm support /mō'bəl, mōbēl'/, a forearm support device that enables people with upper extremity disabilities to fulfill some activities of daily living, as by helping to move the hand into position for self-feeding. It may also be used as a training device. The orthotic device may be mounted on a wheelchair.

mobile unit, (in radiology) an easily transportable radiography unit designed for use outside the radiology department.

mobility /mōbil'itē/ [L, *mobilis,* movable], the velocity a particle or ion attains for a given applied voltage and a relative measure of how quickly an ion may move in an electric field.

mobility, impaired physical, a NANDA-accepted nursing diagnosis of a state in which an individual experiences a limitation of ability for independent physical movement. Defining characteristics include an inability to achieve a functional level of mobility in the environment, a reluctance to move, a limited range of motion of the limbs or extremities, a decrease in the strength or control of the musculoskeletal system, an abnormal or impaired ability to coordinate movements, or any of a large number of imposed restrictions on movement such as medically required bed rest or traction.

mobilization lipase /mō'bilizā'shən/, an enzyme that catalyzes the release of fatty acids from adipose tissues.

Mobitz I heart block /mō'bits/ [Woldemar Mobitz, German physician, b. 1889; AS, *hoerte,* heart; Fr, *bloc,* block], second-degree or partial atrioventricular block in which the PR interval increases progressively until the propagation of an atrial impulse to the ventricles does not occur.

Mobitz II heart block, second-degree or partial atrioventricular block, characterized by the sudden nonconduction of an atrial impulse and a periodic dropped beat without prior or subsequent lengthening of the PR interval. This kind of block usually results from bilateral impaired conduction in the bundle branches. It may be caused by anterior myocardial infarction, myocarditis, drug toxicity, electrolyte disturbances, rheumatoid nodules, and various degenerative diseases.

Möbius' syndrome /mē'bē·əs/ [Paul J. Möbius, German neurologist, 1853–1902], a rare developmental disorder characterized by congenital bilateral facial palsy usually associated with oculomotor or other neurologic dysfunctions, speech disorders, and various anomalies of the extremities.

modality /mōdal'itē/, **1.** the method of application of a therapeutic agent or regimen. **2.** a sensory entity, such as the sense of vision or taste.

mode /mōd/ [L, *modus,* measure], a value or term in a set of data that occurs more frequently than other values or terms.

model /mod'əl/ [L, *modulus,* small measure], (in nursing research) a symbolic representation of the interrelations exhibited by a phenomenon within a system or a process. The model is presented as a conceptual framework or a theory that explains a phenomenon and allows predictions to be made about a patient or a process.

Model HMO Act, a comprehensive health maintenance organization (HMO) statute adopted by several states. It requires that enrollees be entitled to receive copies of individual and group contracts and documented evidence of coverage describing the essential services and features of the HMO.

modeling /mod'əling/, a technique used in behavior therapy in which a person learns a desired response by observing and imitating the behavior.

Modeling and Role Modeling, a theory developed by the nursing theorists Helen C. Erickson, Evelyn M. Tomlin, and Mary Ann P. Swain. Their book, *Modeling and Role Modeling: A Theory and Paradigm for Nursing,* was published in 1983. From a synthesis of multiple concepts related to basic needs, developmental tasks, object attachment, and adaptive coping potential, they developed their highly abstract role-modeling theory. Role modeling is the nursing intervention, or nurturance, that requires unconditional acceptance. Role modeling provides a framework for understanding the way clients structure their world. Erickson, Tomlin, and Swain view nursing as a self-care model based on the client's perception of the world and adaptations to stressors.

moderator band /mod'ərā'tər/ [L, *moderari,* to restrain; AS, *bindan,* to bind], a thick bundle of muscle in the central part of the right ventricle of the heart.

modesty, propriety of dress, speech, and conduct in relations between patients and health care personnel, including draping and covering of the patient to the greatest extent possible, depending on the type of care or examination.

modification /mod'ifikā'shən/, **1.** a process whereby a substance is changed from one form to another. **2.** a change in an organism that is acquired or learned but does not involve inheritance.

modified jaw thrust /mod'ifīd/, an upper airway control maneuver to maintain an open airway of an unconscious person in cases of potential spinal injury. In such persons in-line stabilization of the head and neck can be obtained primarily by forward jaw thrust with minimum head extension.

modified milk [L, *modus*, measure, *facere*, to make], cow's milk in which the protein content has been reduced and the fat content increased to correspond to the composition of breast milk.

modified radical mastectomy, a surgical procedure in which a breast is completely removed with the underlying pectoralis minor and some of the adjacent lymph nodes. The pectoralis major is not excised.

modifying gene /mod'ifī'ing/b [L, *modus*, measure; Gk, *genein*, to produce], a gene that alters or influences the expression function of another gene, including the suppression or reduction of the usual function of the modified gene.

modulation /mod'yəlā'shən/, an alteration in the magnitude or any variation in the duration of an electrical current. Modulation, which affects physiologic responses to various waveforms, may be continuous, interrupted, pulsed, or surging.

modulation transfer function (MTF) [L, *modulus*, small measure; L, *transferre*, to carry, *functio*, performance], a quantitative measure of the ability of an imaging system to reproduce patterns that vary in spatial frequency.

Moeller's glossitis /mel'əz/ [Julius O. L. Moeller, German surgeon, 1819–1887], a form of chronic glossitis, characterized by burning or pain in the tongue and increased sensitivity to hot or spicy foods.

moexipril, an angiotensin-converting enzyme inhibitor prescribed in the treatment of high blood pressure.

mohel /mō'əl, mōhāl'/, an ordained Jewish circumciser.

moiety /moi'itē/ [L, *medietas*, middle], a part of a molecule that exhibits a particular set of chemical and pharmacologic characteristics.

moist crackle [OFr, *moiste*, fresh; ME, *krakelen*], an abnormal breathing sound heard on auscultation when air bubbles through fluid or secretions in the bronchi or trachea.

moist heat [OFr, *moiste* + AS, *haetu*], the use of hot water, towels soaked in hot water, or hot water vapors to reduce in-

flammation and pain, stimulate circulation, and/or relieve symptoms as directed by a physician. Hot towels should be wrung out to remove surplus moisture and should not be too hot to be held in the hands of the person applying moist heat.

molality /mōlal'itē/ [L, *moles*, mass], the number of moles of solute per kilogram of water or other solvent; it refers to the weight of the solvent.

molar /mō'lər/ [L, *moles*, mass], **1.** any one of the 12 molar teeth, 6 in each dental arch, 3 located posterior to the premolar teeth. **2. (M)** pertaining to the gram molecular weight of a substance.

molarity /mōler'itē/ [L, *moles*, mass], the number of moles of solute per liter of solution; it refers to the volume of the solution.

molar pregnancy, pregnancy in which a hydatid mole develops from the trophoblastic tissue of the early embryonic stage of development. The signs of pregnancy are all exaggerated: the uterus grows more rapidly than is normal, morning sickness is often severe and constant, blood pressure is likely to be elevated, and blood levels of chorionic gonadotropins are extremely high.

molar solution, a solution that contains one mole of solute per liter of solution.

mold, **1.** a fungus. **2.** a growth of fungi.

mold, a hollow form for casting or shaping an object, as a prosthesis.

molding /mōl'ding/ [ME, *moulde*, shaping], the natural process by which a baby's head is shaped during labor as it is squeezed into and through the birth passage by the forces of labor. The head often becomes quite elongated, and the bones of the skull may be caused to overlap slightly at the suture lines. Most of the changes caused by molding resolve themselves during the first few days of life.

mole [L, mass], *informal,* **1** a pigmented nevus. **2.** (in obstetrics) a hydatid form mole.

mole [L, *molecula*, small mass], the standard unit used to measure the amount of a substance. A mole of a substance is the amount containing the same number of elementary particles (atoms, electrons, ions, molecules, or other particles) as there are atoms in 12 g of carbon 12. —**molar,** *adj.*

molecular biology /məlek'yələr/ [L, *molecula*, small mass; Gk, *bios*, life, *logos*, science], the study of biology from the viewpoint of the physical and chemical interactions of molecules involved in life functions.

molecular genetics [L, *molecula*, small mass; Gk, *genesis*, origin], the branch of genetics that focuses on the chemical

M

structure and the functions, replication, and mutations of the molecules involved in the transmission of genetic information, such as deoxyribonucleic acid and ribonucleic acid.

molecular mass, the mass of a molecule in daltons, derived by addition of the sum of the component atomic masses. Its dimensionless equivalent is molecular weight. The term **relative molecular mass (M_r)** is preferable to **molecular weight.**

molecular mimicry, an antigenic similarity between unrelated macromolecules, believed to play a role in the pathogenesis of rheumatic fever and other diseases.

molecular pathology [L, *molecula*, small mass; Gk, *pathos*, disease, *logos*, science], the branch of the science of disease that is concerned with the health effects of specific molecules.

molecular sieve, 1. a crystalline chemical separation device with molecular size pores that adsorbs small but not large molecules. 2. a crosslinked polymer that forms a porous sieve used as a supporting medium for chromatographic separation of mixtures of solutes.

molecular stutter, a gene defect in which the three-nucleotide code for an amino acid is repeated, missing, or jumbled, causing the gene either to fail to make a specific protein or to make a protein that does not function properly. In Huntington's disease, for example, the code for glutamine may be repeated 40 or 50 times in a row in the mutant gene.

molecular taxonomy, the classification of organisms in appropriate categories on the basis of the distribution and composition of chemical substances in them.

molecular weight (mol wt), the weight of a molecule of a substance as compared with the weight of an atom of carbon-12. It is equal to the sum of the weights of its constituent atoms and is dimensionless. The term **relative molecular mass (M_r)** is preferable.

molecule /mol'əkyōōl/ [L, *molecula*, small mass], the smallest unit that exhibits the properties of an element or compound. A molecule is composed of two or more atoms that are covalently bonded.

mole percent, a percentage calculation expressed in terms of moles of a substance in a mixture or solution rather than in terms of molecular mass.

mole volume, the volume occupied by one mole of a substance, which may be a solid, liquid, or gas. It is numerically equal to the molecular mass divided by the density.

molindone hydrochloride /mol'indōn/,

an antipsychotic agent prescribed in the treatment of schizophrenia.

molluscum /məlus'kəm/ [L, *molluscus*, soft], any skin disease having soft, rounded masses or nodules.

molluscum contagiosum, a disease of the skin and mucous membranes caused by a poxvirus. It is characterized by scattered flesh-toned white papules. Palms of the hands and soles of the feet are not affected. The disease most frequently occurs in children and in adults with an impaired immune response. It is transmitted from person to person by direct or indirect contact.

Moloney test [Paul J. Moloney, Canadian physician, 1870–1939], a skin test for sensitivity to diphtheria toxoid.

mol wt, abbreviation for **molecular weight.**

molybdenum (Mo) /məlib'dənəm/ [Gk, *molybdos*, lead], a grayish metallic element. Its atomic number is 42; its atomic mass (weight) is 95.94. Molybdenum is poisonous if ingested in large quantities.

molybdenum 99, the radionuclide that is the parent of technetium 99 and as such is present as a generator in most nuclear medicine departments.

monad /mon'ad, mō'nəd/, 1. a unicellular free-living organism. 2. a univalent element or radical. 3. a haploid set of chromosomes in a spermatid or ootid.

monarthritis /mon'ärthrī'tis/ [Gk, *monos*, single, *arthron*, joint, *itis*, inflammation], arthritis affecting only one joint.

monarticular /mon'ärtik'yələr/ [Gk, *monos*, single; L, *articulus*, joint], pertaining to only one joint.

monaural /monôr'əl/ [Gk, *monos*, single; L, *auris*, ear], pertaining to one ear.

Mönckeberg's arteriosclerosis /meng'-kəbərgz/ [Johann G. Mönckeberg, German pathologist, 1877–1925], a form of arteriosclerosis in which extensive calcium deposits are found in the media of the artery with little obstruction of the lumen.

Mongolian spot /mong·gōlē·ən/ [*Mongol,* Asian ethnic group; ME, *spotte,* stain], a benign bluish-black macule, between 2 and 8 cm, occurring over the sacrum and on the buttocks of some newborns. It usually disappears during early childhood.

moniliform /mōnil'ifôrm/, resembling a string of beads.

monitor /mon'ətər/ [L, *monere,* to warn], 1. to observe and evaluate a function of the body closely and constantly. 2. a mechanical device that provides a visual or audible signal or a graphic record of a particular function, such as a cardiac monitor or a fetal monitor.

monitrice /mon'itris'/ [Fr, female instructor], a labor coach, usually a registered nurse, who is specially trained in the Lamaze method of childbirth. The coach provides emotional support and leads the mother through labor and delivery.

monkey pox, an epidemic human disease caused by exposure to a monkey pox virus with symptoms resembling those of smallpox. The virus is related antigenically to smallpox and vaccinia organisms.

mono, abbreviation for **mononucleosis.**

monoamine /mon'ō·am'in/, an amine containing one amine group.

monoamine oxidase (MAO), an enzyme that catalyzes the oxidation of amines.

monoamine oxidase (MAO) inhibitor, any of a chemically heterogeneous group of drugs used primarily in the treatment of depression. These drugs also exert an antianxiety effect, especially anxiety associated with phobia. The effects of the drugs vary greatly from patient to patient, and their specific actions leading to clinical benefits are poorly understood. Among the most common adverse effects are drowsiness, dry mouth, orthostatic hypotension, and constipation. MAO inhibitors interact with many drugs and with foods containing large amounts of the amino acid tyramine. Ingestion of these foods by a person taking a MAO inhibitor is likely to cause a severe hypertensive episode associated with headache, palpitations, and nausea.

monobasic acid /mon'ōbā'sik/, an acid with only one replaceable hydrogen atom such as hydrochloric acid.

monobenzone /-ben'zōn/, a depigmenting agent prescribed in the treatment of abnormal skin pigmentation, such as in disseminated vitiligo. It is not to be used for more trivial conditions such as freckles.

monoblast /mon'əblast/ [Gk, monos, single, blastos, germ], an immature monocyte. Increased production of monoblasts in the marrow and the presence of these forms in the peripheral circulation occur in certain leukemias. **—monoblastic,** adj.

monoblastic leukemia, /-blas'tik/ a malignancy of blood-forming organs, characterized by the proliferation of monoblasts and monocytes.

monochromatic /-krōmat'ik/, **1.** pertaining to a single color or a single wavelength of light. **2.** describing a person who is totally color blind. **3.** pertaining to a substance that has only one color or stains with only one color.

monochromaticity /-krō'mətis'itē/, the specificity of light in a single defined wavelength. If the specificity is in the visible light spectrum, it is only one color.

monochrotic pulse /-krot'ik/ [Gk, monos, single, krotein, to strike; L, pulsare, to beat], a pulse characterized by a single wave.

monoclonal /mon'əklō'nəl/ [Gk, monos + klon, twig], pertaining to or designating a group of identical cells or organisms derived from a single cell.

monoclonal antibody (MOAB) [Gk, monos, single, klon, twig; Gk, anti + AS, bodig, body], an antibody produced in a laboratory to isolate and clone individual B lymphocytes, resulting in the production of a pure (monoclonal) antibody.

monocular diplopia /monok'yələr/ [Gk, monos, single, oculus, eye; Gk, diploos, double, opsis, vision], a condition in which a double image is perceived with one eye. The cause is a disorder in the refracting medium of the eye, such as a cataract, or partial dislocation of the lens. In rare cases more than two images may be seen with one eye.

monocular strabismus [Gk, monos, single; L, oculus, eye; Gk, strabismos], a squint that is confined to one particular eye.

monocular vision [Gk, monos, single; L, oculus, eye, visio, seeing], a condition of seeing with only one eye.

monocutaneous candidiasis, a cellular immunodeficiency disorder associated with fungal (Candida) infections of the skin, mucous membranes, nails, and hair.

monocyte /mon'əsīt/ [Gk, monos + kytos, cell], a large mononuclear leukocyte with an ovoid or kidney-shaped nucleus, containing chromatin material with a lacy pattern and gray-blue cytoplasm filled with fine, reddish azurophilic granules.

monocytic leukemia /mon'əsit'ik/, a malignancy of blood-forming tissues in which the predominant cells are monocytes. The disease has an erratic course characterized by malaise, fatigue, fever, anorexia, weight loss, splenomegaly, bleeding gums, dermal petechiae, anemia, and lack of responsiveness to therapy. There are two forms: **Schilling's leukemia,** in which most of the cells are monocytes that probably arise from the reticuloendothelial system, and the more common **Naegeli's leukemia,** in which a large number of the cells resemble myeloblasts.

monocytopenia /-sī'təpē'nē·ə/, an abnormally low level of monocytes in the peripheral blood, that is, less than 200/mm^3.

monocytosis /mon'ōsītō'sis/, an increased proportion of monocytes in the circulation.

monodactylism /-dak'tiliz'əm/ [Gk, monos, single, daktylos, finger or toe], a congenital defect in which the person is

M

born with only one finger on the hand or one toe on the foot.

monoethanolamine /mon′ō·eth′ənol′-əmēn/, an amino alcohol formed by the decarboxylation of serine. It is a component of certain cephalins and phospholipids and is used as a surfactant in pharmaceutical products.

monofactorial inheritance /-faktôr′ē·əl/ [Gk, *monos* + L, *factare,* to make], the acquisition or expression of a trait or condition that depends on the transmission of a single specific gene.

monogamy /mənog′əmē/, **1.** the practice of being married to no more than one person at a time. **2.** (in biology) the habit of pairing with only one mate.

monohybrid /-hī′brid/ [Gk, *monos* + L, *hybrida,* mixed offspring], pertaining to or describing an individual, organism, or strain that is heterozygous for only one specific trait or for the single trait or gene locus under consideration.

monohybrid cross, the mating of two individuals, organisms, or strains that have different gene pairs for only one specific trait or in which only one particular characteristic or gene locus is being followed.

monohydric alcohol /-hī′drik/, an alcohol containing one hydroxyl group.

monoiodotyrosine /mon′ō·ī·ō′dōtī′rəsin/, an iodinated amino acid involved in the synthesis of thyroxine (T_4) and triiodothyronine (T_3).

monokaryotic /-ker′ē·ot′ik/, having a single nucleus.

monolayer /-lā′ər/, a sheet of cells one cell thick such as may be formed on the surface of a culture vessel.

monomer /mon′əmər/ [Gk, *monos* + *meros,* part], a molecule that repeats itself to form a polymer, such as a molecule of fibrin monomer that polymerizes to form fibrin in the blood-clotting process. —**monomeric,** *adj.*

monomolecular elimination reaction /-məlek′yələr/, a first-order chemical kinetic reaction in which only one molecule is involved in the slow step reaction.

monomphalus /mənomf′fələs/ [Gk, *monos* + *omphalos,* navel], conjoined twins that are united at the umbilicus.

mononeuropathy /-nŏŏrop′əthē/ [Gk, *monos* + *neuron,* nerve, *pathos,* disease], any disease or disorder that affects a single nerve trunk. Some common causes of disorders involving single nerve trunks are electric shock, radiation, and fractured bones that may compress or lacerate nerve fibers. Casts and tourniquets that are too tight may also damage a nerve by compression or by ischemia.

mononeuropathy multiplex, a periph-

eral nerve disorder characterized by numbness, pain, and weakness in several areas of the body. The symptoms may develop suddenly in the region supplied by one peripheral nerve and days later in the region of another nerve.

mononuclear /-nyŏŏ′klē·ər/ [Gk, *monos,* single; L, *nucleus,* nut kernel], pertaining to one nucleus, such as a monocyte.

mononuclear leukocyte (MNL), a white blood cell, including lymphocytes and monocytes, with a single round or oval nucleus.

mononucleosis (mono) /mon′ōnŏŏ′klē·ō′-sis/ [Gk, *monos,* single; L, *nucleus,* nut kernel; Gk, *osis,* condition], an abnormal increase in the number of mononuclear leukocytes in the blood.

monooctanoin /mon′ō·ok′tənō′in/, a gallstone-dissolving agent used to dissolve cholesterol gallstones.

monophagia /-fā′jə/, the practice of eating only one kind of food.

monophasic /-fā′sik/, having one phase, part, aspect, or stage.

monoploid /mon′əploid/, haploid.

monopus /mon′əpəs/ [Gk, *monos* + *pous,* foot], a fetus or individual with the congenital absence of a foot or leg.

monorchid /monôr′kid/, a male who has monorchism.

monorchism /mon′ôrkiz′əm/ [Gk, *monos* + *orchis,* testicle, *ismos,* state], a condition in which only one testicle has descended into the scrotum. —**monorchidic,** *adj.*

monosaccharide /-sak′ərīd/ [Gk, *monos* + *sakcharon,* sugar], a simple basic carbohydrate consisting of a single basic unit with the general formula $C_n(H_2O)_n$, with n ranging from 3 to 8.

monosodium glutamate (MSG) /-sō′dē·-əm/, a food flavor enhancer derived from naturally occurring salt of glutamic acid and a cause of **Chinese restaurant syndrome.** It is also used in the treatment of encephalopathies associated with liver disorders.

monosodium urate monohydrate, a uric acid salt deposited as crystals in and around joints in gout patients.

monosome /mon′əsōm/ [Gk, *monos* + *soma,* body], **1.** an unpaired X or Y sex chromosome. **2.** the single, unpaired chromosome in monosomy.

monosomy /mon′əsō′mē/ [Gk, *monos* + *soma,* body], a chromosomal aberration characterized by the absence of one chromosome from the normal diploid complement. —**monosomic,** *adj.*

monospecific /-spəsif′ik/ [Gk, *monos* + L, *species,* form, *facere,* to make], an antibody that reacts with only one type of antigen.

monosynaptic reflex /-sinap'tik/ [Gk, *monos*, single, *synaptein*, to join; L, *reflectere*, to bend back], a reflex requiring only one afferent and one efferent neuron.

monotropy /mənot'rəpē/ [Gk, *monos* + *trepein*, to turn], a phenomenon in which a mother appears to be able to bond with only one infant at a time. When one twin is taken home from the hospital earlier than the other, the mother often reports that she does not feel that the baby discharged later is hers. —**monotropic,** *adj.*

monovalent /-vā'lənt/, **1.** describing an atom or radical having the valence or combining power of one hydrogen atom. **2.** describing a serum antibody capable of combining with only one antigen or complement.

monovulatory /mənō'vyələtôr'ē/ [Gk, *monos* + L, *ovulum*, small egg, *orius*, characterized by], routinely releasing one ovum during each ovarian cycle.

monozygotic (MZ) /-zīgō'tik/ [Gk, *monos* + *zygon*, yoke], pertaining to or developed from a single fertilized ovum, or zygote, such as occurs in identical twins. —**monozygosity,** *n.*, **monozygous,** *adj.*

monozygotic twins, two offspring born of the same pregnancy and developed from a single fertilized ovum that splits into equal halves during an early cleavage phase in embryonic development, giving rise to separate fetuses. Such twins are always of the same sex, have the same genetic constitution, possess identical blood groups, and closely resemble each other in physical, psychologic, and mental characteristics.

mons /mons/ [L, mountain], a mound or slight elevation.

Monson curve [George S. Monson, American dentist, 1869–1933; L, *curvus*, a bend], the curve of occlusion in which each tooth cusp and incisal edge conform to a segment of the surface of a sphere 8 inches (20 cm) in diameter, with its center in the region of the glabella.

monster [L, *monstrum*], a fetus that is grossly malformed and usually nonviable.

monstrosity /monstros'itē/, **1.** the state or condition of having severe congenital defects. **2.** anything that deviates greatly from the normal; a monster or teras.

mons veneris /ven'əris/ [L, *mons,* mountain; *venus,* love], a pad of fatty tissue and thick skin that overlies the symphysis pubis in the woman.

Monteggia's fracture /montej'əz/ [Giovanni B. Monteggia, Italian physician, 1762–1815], fracture of the ulna, associated with radial dislocation or rupture of the annular ligament and resulting in the angulation or overriding of ulnar fragments.

Montenegro test /mon'tənā'grō/, a test used in the diagnosis of cutaneous leishmaniasis, in which killed *Leishmania* antigens are injected intradermally. A positive reaction is indicated by the appearance of a palpable nodule in 48 to 72 hours.

Montercaux fracture /mont'ərkō'/, a fracture of the neck of the fibula associated with the diastasis of ankle mortise.

Montgomery straps /mont·gom'ərē/, bands of adhesive tape featuring a lace-up design, which is used to secure dressings that must be changed frequently.

Montgomery's tubercle [William F. Montgomery, Irish gynecologist, 1797–1859; L, *tuber,* swelling], one of several sebaceous glands on the areolae of the breasts. The sebaceous material that is secreted from the ducts of the glands to the skin of each areola serves to lubricate and protect the breast from infection and trauma during breastfeeding.

mood, a prolonged subjective emotional state that influences one's whole personality and perception of the world. Examples include sadness, elation, and anger.

mood-congruent psychotic features /-kon'gro͞o·ənt/ [AS, *mod,* mind; L, *congruere,* to come together], the characteristics of a psychosis in which the content of hallucinations or delusions is consistent with an elevated, expansive mood or with a depression.

mood disorder [AS, *mod,* mind; L, *dis* + *ordo,* rank], a variety of conditions characterized by a disturbance in mood as the main feature. If mild and occasional, the feelings may be normal. If more severe, they may be a sign of a major depressive disorder or dysthymic reaction or symptomatic of a bipolar disorder. Other mood disorders may be caused by a general medical condition.

Mood Management, a Nursing Interventions Classification defined as providing for safety and stabilization of a patient who is experiencing dysfunctional mood.

mood swing, an oscillation between periods of feelings of well-being and depression. Occasional "blue" periods are not regarded as abnormal.

moon face [AS, *mona,* moon; L, *facies,* face], a condition characterized by a rounded, puffy face. It occurs in people treated with large doses of corticosteroids, such as those with chronic asthma, rheumatoid arthritis, or acute childhood leukemia. The features return to normal when the medication is stopped.

M

Moore's fracture [Edward M. Moore, American surgeon, 1814–1902], a fracture of the distal radius with associated dislocation of the ulnar head, which causes the styloid process to be secured under the annular ligaments of the wrist.

MOPP /mop/, abbreviation for a combination drug regimen used in the treatment of cancer, containing three antineoplastics, Mustargen (mechlorethamine), Oncovin (vincristine sulfate), and Matulane (procarbazine hydrochloride), as well as prednisone (a glucocorticoid). MOPP is prescribed in the treatment of Hodgkin's disease.

Moraxella, a genus of the Neisseriaceae family of gram-negative nonmotile cocci. They are found as pathogens and parasites on the mucous membranes of warm-blooded animals.

Moraxella catarrhalis, a species of aerobic nonmotile bacteria found in both the normal and the diseased nasopharynx. It is a cause of otitis media and respiratory diseases.

Moraxella lacunata, a species of nonmotile cocci that causes corneal infections and subacute conjunctivitis or angular conjunctivitis in humans.

morbid [L, *morbidus,* diseased], pertaining to a pathologic or diseased condition, either physical or mental.

morbidity /môrbid'itē/ [L, *morbidus,* diseased], **1.** an illness or an abnormal condition or quality. **2.** (in statistics) the rate at which an illness or abnormality occurs, calculated by dividing the number of people who are affected within a group by the entire number of people in that group. **3.** the rate at which an illness occurs in a particular area or population.

Morbidity and Mortality Weekly Report (MMWR), a weekly epidemiologic report on the incidence of communicable diseases and deaths in 120 urban areas of the United States. It is published by the Centers for Disease Control and Prevention in Atlanta, Georgia.

morbidity rate [L, *morbidus,* diseased, *ratum,* calculation], the number of cases of a particular disease occurring in a single year per a specified population unit, as x cases per 1000. It also may be calculated on the basis of age groups, sex, occupation, or other population unit.

morbidity statistics [L, *morbidus,* diseased, *status,* condition], a branch of statistics that is concerned with the disease rate of a population or geographic region.

morbid obesity [L, *morbidus,* diseased, *obesitas,* fatness], an excess of body fat that threatens necessary body functions such as respiration.

morbilliform /môrbil'ifôrm/ [L, *morbilli,* little disease, *forma,* form], describing a skin condition that resembles the erythematous maculopapular rash of measles.

mordant /môr'dənt/, a substance capable of deepening the reaction of a biologic specimen to a stain. The chief mordants are alum, aniline, oil, and phenol.

Morgagni's globule /môrgan'yēz/ [Giovanni B. Morgagni, Italian anatomist, 1682–1771], a minute opaque sphere that may form from fluid coagulation between the eye lens and its capsule, especially in cataract.

Morgagni's tubercle [Giovanni B. Morgagni], one of several small soft nodules on the surface of each of the areolas in women. The tubercles are produced by large sebaceous glands just below the surface of the areolae.

morgan /môr'gən/ [Thomas H. Morgan, American biologist, 1866–1945], (in genetics) a unit of measure used in mapping the relative distances between genes on a chromosome.

morgue /môrg/ [Fr, mortuary], a unit of a hospital with facilities for the storage and autopsy of the dead.

moribund /môr'ibund/ [L, *moribundus,* dying], near death or in the act of dying.

Morita therapy /môrē'tä/ [Shomei Morita, twentieth-century Japanese physician], an alternative therapy that has as its focus the symptoms of the patient. Its goal is character building, which enables the patient to live responsibly and constructively, even if the symptoms persist.

morning after pill [AS, *morgen* + *aefter* + *pilian,* to peel], *informal.* a large dose of an estrogen given orally, over a short period, to a woman within 24 to 72 hours after sexual intercourse to prevent conception, most commonly in an emergency such as rape or incest.

morning dip, a significant decline in respiratory function observed in some asthmatic people during the early morning hours.

morning ptosis, a temporary paralysis of the upper eyelid on awakening from sleep.

morning stiffness [OE, *morgen* + *stif*], a period of muscular stiffness after awakening in the morning, a common complaint of patients with arthritis or similar musculoskeletal disorders.

Moro reflex /môr'ō/ [Ernst Moro, German pediatrician, 1874–1951], a normal mass reflex in a young infant (up to 3 to 4 months of age) elicited by a sudden loud noise, such as by striking the table next to the child or raising the head slightly and allowing it to drop. A normal response consists of flexion of the legs, an

embracing posture of the arms, and usually a brief cry.

morphea /môr'fē·ə/ [Gk, *morphe,* form], a skin disease consisting of patches of yellowish or ivory-colored hard, dry, smooth skin.

morphine /môt'fēn/ [Gk, *Morpheus,* god of sleep], a white crystalline alkaloid derived from the opium poppy, *Papaver somniferum,* the source of its principal pharmacologic activity. Morphine acts on the central nervous system to produce both depression and euphoric stimulation. It depresses the motor cortex but stimulates the spinal cord. Even in small amounts morphine depresses the respiratory system. It has a marked analgesic effect, and its principal therapeutic value is pain relief. Morphine rarely provides total relief of pain, but in most cases it reduces the level of suffering. It stimulates the third cranial nerve, resulting in pupillary constriction. Repeated use leads to physical dependence.

morphine poisoning, adverse effect of injection or ingestion of opioid narcotics, marked by symptoms of pinpoint pupils, drowsiness, and shallow respiration. Emergency treatment includes gastric lavage, charcoal, and respiratory support.

morphine sulfate, a narcotic analgesic prescribed to reduce pain.

morphine tartrate, a white crystalline powder used in injections of morphine. It is more soluble in water than morphine itself and is used in various parenteral preparations.

morphinism /môr'finiz'əm/, a pathologic state caused by morphine addiction.

morphogenesis /môr'fəjen'əsis/ [Gk, *morphe* + *genein,* to produce], the development and differentiation of the structures and form of an organism, specifically the changes that occur in the cells and tissue during embryonic development.

morphogens /môr'fəjens/, **1.** soluble substances that control the embryonic differentiation of cells and tissues. **2.** substances secreted by one group of cells that cause specific changes in the growth and differentiation of a different group.

morphogenetic /-jənet'ik/, (in embryology) pertaining to a substance or hormone that acts as an evocator in differentiation.

morphology /môrfol'əjē/ [Gk, *morphe* + *logos,* science], the study of the physical shape and size of a specimen, plant, or animal. **—morphologic** /môr'fəloj'-ik/, *adj.*

morphometry /môfom'ətrē/, the measurement of the structures and parts of organisms.

Morquio's disease /môrkē'ōz/ [Luis

Morquio, Uruguayan physician, 1867–1935], a familial form of mucopolysaccharidosis that results in abnormal musculoskeletal development in childhood. Dwarfism, hunchback, enlarged sternum, and knock-knees may occur.

mortal [L, *mortalis,* perishable], **1.** liable to die. **2.** causing death.

mortality [L, *mortalis,* perishable], **1.** the condition of being subject to death. **2.** the death rate, which reflects the number of deaths per unit of population in any specific region, age group, disease, or other classification, usually expressed as deaths per 1000, 10,000, or 100,000.

mortar /môr'tər/ [L, *mortarium*], a cup-shaped vessel in which materials are ground or crushed by a pestle in the preparation of drugs.

mortinatality /môr'tinātal'itē/ [L, *mors,* death, *natus,* birth], the stillbirth rate. It is calculated by multiplying the number of stillbirths by 1000 and dividing by the total number of births per year.

mortise joint /môr'tis/ [ME, *mortays,* fixed in, *jungere,* to join], the articulatio talocruralis joint of the ankle.

Morton's disease [Thomas G. Morton, American surgeon, 1835–1903; L, *dis* + Fr, *aise,* ease], a form of foot neuralgia caused by a falling metatarsal arch and pressure on the digital branches of the lateral plantar nerve.

Morton's plantar neuralgia [Thomas G. Morton; L, *planta,* foot sole; Gk, *neuron,* nerve, *algos,* pain], a severe throbbing pain that affects the anastomotic nerve branch between the medial and lateral plantar nerves.

Morton's syndrome [Dudley J. Morton, American orthopedist, 1884–1960; Gk, *syn,* together, *dromos,* course], a congenital foreshortening of the first metatarsal segment, causing pain and deformity of the front part of the foot.

mortuary /mô'chəwer'ē/ [L, *mortuarium,* tomb], a building where the bodies of deceased persons are held for identification, postmortem examination, and preparation for burial or cremation.

morula /tuôr'ələ/, *pl.* **morulas, morulae** [L, *morulus,* blackberry], a solid, spheric mass of cells resulting from the cleavage of the fertilized ovum in the early stages of embryonic development. **—morular,** *adj.*

Morvan's disease, a form of syringomyelia with tissue changes in the extremities, such as a paresthesia of the forearms and hands and progressive painless ulceration of the fingertips.

mosaic /mōzā'ik/ [L, *Musa,* goddess of the arts], **1.** (in genetics) an individual or

M

organism that developed from a single zygote but that has two or more kinds of genetically different cell populations. Such a condition results from a mutation, crossing over, or, more commonly in humans, nondisjunction of the chromosomes during early embryogenesis, which causes a variation in the number of chromosomes in the cells. **2.** (in embryology) a fertilized ovum that undergoes determinate cleavage.

mosaic bone, bone tissue appearing to be made up of many tiny pieces cemented together, as seen on microscopic examination of a x-ray film of the affected bone. It is characteristic of Paget's disease of the bone.

mosaic development, a kind of embryonic development occurring in the blastocyst. The fertilized ovum undergoes determinate cleavage, developing according to a precise, unalterable plan in which each blastomere has a characteristic position and limited developmental potency and is a precursor of a specific part of the embryo.

mosaicism /mōzā'isiz'əm/ [L, *Musa,* goddess of the arts], (in genetics) a condition in which an individual or an organism that develops from a single zygote has two or more cell populations that differ in genetic constitution.

mosaic wart, a group of contiguous plantar warts.

mosquito bite /məskē'tō/ [L, *musca,* a fly; AS, *bitan,* to bite], a bite of a blood-sucking arthropod of the subfamily Culicidae that may result in a systemic allergic reaction in a hypersensitive person, an infection, or, most often, a pruritic wheal.

mosquito forceps, a small hemostatic forceps.

Mössbauer spectrometer /mes'bou·ər, ms'bou·ər/ [Rudolf L. Mössbauer, German physicist, b. 1929], an instrument that can detect small changes between an atomic nucleus and its environment, such as caused by alterations in temperature, pressure, or chemical state.

most probable number, a statistical value representing the viable bacterial population in a sample through the use of dilution and multiple tube inoculations.

mother fixation [AS, *modor,* mother; L, *figere,* to fasten], an arrest in psychosexual development characterized by an abnormally persistent, close, and often paralyzing emotional attachment to one's mother.

motile /mō'til/ [L, *motare,* to move often], capable of spontaneous but unconscious or involuntary movement. **—motility,** *n.*

motilin /mōtil'in/, a peptide hormone se-

creted by enterochromaffin cells of the intestinal tract. It stimulates gastrointestinal motility and pepsin secretion.

motion sickness /mō'shən/ [L, *motio,* movement; AS, *seoc,* sick, OE, *nes,* condition], a condition caused by erratic or rhythmic motions in any combination of directions, such as in a boat or a car. Severe cases are characterized by nausea, vomiting, vertigo, and headache; mild cases by headache and general discomfort.

motivation /mō'tivā'shən/ [L, *movere,* to move], conscious or unconscious needs, interests, rewards, or other incentives that arouse, channel, or maintain a particular behavior.

motivational conflict /mō'tivā'shənəl/ [L, *motus,* cause of motion, *alis,* relating to, *confluere,* to come together], a conflict resulting from the arousal of two or more motives that direct behavior toward incompatible goals. Kinds of motivational conflict include **approach-approach conflict, approach-avoidance conflict,** and **avoidance-avoidance conflict.**

motoneuron /mō'tōnŏŏr'on/ [L, *movere,* to move; Gk, *neuron,* nerve], a motor neuron. Its function is to produce muscle contractions.

motor [L, *motare,* to move about], **1.** pertaining to motion, the body apparatus involved in movement, or the brain functions that direct purposeful activities. **2.** pertaining to a muscle, nerve, or brain center that produces or subserves motion.

motor aphasia, the inability to utter remembered words, caused by a cerebral lesion in the inferior frontal gyrus (Broca's motor speech area) of the left hemisphere. The condition most commonly is the result of a stroke. The patient knows what to say but cannot articulate the words.

motor apraxia, the inability to carry out planned movements or to handle small objects, although cognizant of the proper use of the object. The condition results from a lesion in the premotor frontal cortex on the opposite side of the affected limb.

motor area, a part of the cerebral cortex that includes the precentral gyrus and the posterior part of the frontal gyri and that causes the contraction of the voluntary muscles on stimulation with electrodes. Normal voluntary activity requires associations between the motor area and other parts of the cortex; removal of the motor area from one cerebral hemisphere causes paralysis of voluntary muscles, especially of the opposite side of the body.

motor ataxia, an inability to perform coordinated movements.

motor coordination, the harmonious functioning of body parts that involve movement, including gross motor movement, fine motor movement, and motor planning.

motor depressant [L, *motare,* to move about, *deprimere,* to press down], a drug or agent that reduces the normal functioning level of motor neurons, mainly in voluntary muscles.

motor end plate, a large special synaptic contact between motor axons and each skeletal muscle fiber. Each muscle fiber forms one end plate.

motor fiber, one of the fibers (axons) in the cranial and spinal nerves that transmit impulses to and cause contraction of muscle fibers.

motor hallucination [L, *motare,* to move about, *alucinari,* wandering mind], the subjective experience of movement when there is no movement.

motor image, a visual concept of one's bodily movements, real or imagined.

motor nerve, an efferent nerve that conveys impulses to motor end plates or another terminal and is mainly responsible for stimulating muscles and glands.

motor neuron, one of various efferent nerve cells that transmit nerve impulses from the brain or from the spinal cord to muscular or glandular tissue.

motor neuron disease [L, *motare,* to move about, *neuron,* nerve; L, *dis* + Fr, *aise,* ease], any disease of a motor neuron, with degeneration of anterior horn cells, motor cranial nerve nuclei, and pyramidal tracts. An example is **amyotrophic lateral sclerosis (ALS).**

motor neuron paralysis, an injury to the spinal cord that causes damage to the motor neurons and results in various degrees of functional impairment, depending on the site of the lesion.

motor nucleus [L, *motare,* to move about, *nucleus,* nut kernel], the nucleus of a motor nerve or a collection of motor neurons.

motor pathway [L, *motare,* to move about; AS, *paeth*], the route of motor nerve impulses, from the central neuron to a muscle or gland.

motor planning, the ability to plan and execute skilled nonhabitual tasks.

motor point, 1. a point at which a motor nerve enters a muscle. **2.** any point on the skin over a muscle at which electrical stimulation (via electrode) causes contraction of the muscle.

motor protein, protein that moves along a surface, propelled by the energy of adenosine triphosphate hydrolysis.

motor root [L, *motare,* to move about; AS, *rot*], the proximal end of a motor nerve at its attachment to the spinal cord.

motor seizure, a transitory disturbance in brain function caused by abnormal neuronal discharges that arise initially in a localized motor area of the cerebral cortex. The manifestations depend on the site of the abnormal electrical activity, such as tonic contractures of the thumb caused by excessive discharges in the motor area of the cortex controlling the first digit.

motor sense, the feeling or perception enabling a person to accomplish a purposeful movement, presumably achieved by evoking a sensory engram or memory of the pattern for that specific movement.

motor speech areas [L, *motare,* to move about; AS, *spaec* + L, *area,* vacant place], the regions of the cerebral hemispheres that are associated with motor control of speech. For right-handed people the sites are generally located in the left hemisphere. Patients with specific language defects often are found to have lesions in the left hemisphere.

motor tract [L, *motare,* to move about, *tractus*], an efferent nerve pathway that conveys impulses controlling movement.

motor unit, a functional structure consisting of a motor neuron and the muscle fibers it innervates.

motor unit recruitment, the bringing into activity of additional motor neurons, thereby causing greater activity in response to increased tension developed in a muscle. As more units are recruited and as the frequency of discharge increases, muscle tension increases. The pattern of motor unit recruitment varies, depending on the inherent properties of specific motor neurons.

mottle [ME, *motley,* mixed colors], an effect observed in radiologic imaging when the dose of radiation used is reduced to a level where individual quantum effects can be seen.

mourning /mőr'ning/ [AS, *murnan,* to mourn], a response to the loss of a loved object. It is through mourning that grief is resolved.

mouse-tooth forceps, a kind of dressing forceps that has one or more fine sharp points on the tip of each blade. The tips turn in, and the delicate teeth interlock.

mouth [AS, *muth*], **1.** the nearly oval oral cavity at the superior, anterior end of the digestive tube, bounded anteriorly by the lips and containing the tongue and the teeth. It consists of the vestibule and the mouth cavity proper. The vestibule, situated in front of the teeth, is bounded externally by the lips and the cheeks, internally by the gums and the teeth. The mouth cavity proper is bounded by the alveolar arches and the teeth, communicates with

M

the pharynx, and is roofed by the hard and soft palates. The tongue forms the greater part of the floor of the cavity. **2.** an orifice.

mouth guard, a soft plastic intraoral appliance that covers all the occlusal surfaces and the palate. It is worn in contact sports to limit damage to tissues of the mouth, lips, and other oral surfaces.

mouth rinse /mouth'rins/, a solution for cleaning or treating the oral mucosa and controlling dental caries. A typical mouth rinse may contain sodium fluoride, glycerine, alcohol, detergents, and other ingredients.

mouthstick /mouth'wôsh/, a device that is manipulated with the mouth and can be used to type, push buttons, turn pages, operate power wheelchairs, or modify environmental control units and other equipment. It is commonly used by high level (C4 and up) quadriplegics or others.

mouth-to-mouth resuscitation, a procedure in artificial resuscitation, performed most often with cardiac massage. The victim's nose is sealed by pinching the nostrils closed, the head is extended, and air is breathed by the rescuer through the mouth into the lungs.

mouth-to-nose resuscitation, a procedure in artificial resuscitation in which the mouth of the victim is covered and held closed and air is breathed through the victim's nose.

mouthwash /mouth'wôsh/, a medicated liquid used for cleaning the oral cavity and treating mucous membranes of the mouth. Many over-the-counter mouthwashes contain alcohol, which may contribute to surface softening and increased wear of dental resins and composite materials.

MOV, abbreviation for **minimal occlusive volume.**

movement decomposition [L, *movere,* to go, *de,* away, *componere,* to assemble], a distortion in voluntary movement in which motion occurs in a distinct sequence of isolated steps rather than in a normal smooth, flowing pattern.

moving grid, (in radiography) an x-ray grid that is continuously moved or oscillated throughout the exposure of a radiographic film.

moxibustion /mok'səbus'chən/ [Jpn, *moe kusa,* burning herb; L, *comburere,* to burn up], a method of producing analgesia or altering the function of a body system achieved by igniting moxa, wormwood, or another combustible, slow-burning substance and holding it as near the point on the skin as possible without causing pain or burning. It is also sometimes used in conjunction with acupuncture.

moyamoya disease /moi'əmoi'ə/, a cerebral vascular disorder in which the main cerebral arteries at the base of the brain are replaced by a fine network of vessels. It tends mainly to affect Japanese children and young adults and is characterized by convulsions, hemiplegia, mental retardation, and subarachnoid hemorrhage. Patients who survive into adulthood are susceptible to massive intracerebral hemorrhage caused by rupture of the fragile network of new vessels. Few patients live beyond 30 years of age.

MPD, M.P.D., abbreviation for **maximum permissible dose.**

MPGN, abbreviation for **membranoproliferative glomerulonephritis.**

M.P.H., abbreviation for *Master of Public Health.*

MPL + PRED, an anticancer drug combination of melphalan and prednisone.

MPO, abbreviation for **myeloperoxidase.**

MPS, abbreviation for **mucopolysaccharidosis.**

MPS I, abbreviation for *mucopolysaccharidosis I.*

MPS II, abbreviation for *mucopolysaccharidosis II.*

MPS IV, abbreviation for *mucopolysaccharidosis IV.*

MQF, abbreviation for *mobile quarantine facility.*

mr, mR, abbreviation for **milliroentgen.**

M$_r$, symbol for *relative molecular mass.*

mrad, abbreviation for **millirad.**

mrem, abbreviation for **millirem.**

MRI, abbreviation for **magnetic resonance imaging.**

mRNA, abbreviation for **messenger RNA.**

MRSA, methicillin-resistant *Staphylococcus aureus.*

MS, abbreviation for **multiple sclerosis.**

M.S., **1.** abbreviation for *Master of Science.* **2.** abbreviation for *Master of Surgery.*

MSAFP test. abbreviation for **maternal serum alpha-fetoprotein (MSAFP) test.**

msec, abbreviation for **millisecond.**

MSG, abbreviation for **monosodium glutamate.**

MSH, abbreviation for **melanocyte-stimulating hormone.**

MSLT, abbreviation for **multiple sleep latency test.**

MSN, abbreviation for *Master of Science in Nursing.*

MSO, abbreviation for **management service organization.**

M.T., abbreviation for **medical technologist.**

MTT, abbreviation for **maximal treadmill test.**

MTX + MP + CTX, an anticancer drug combination of methotrexate, mercaptopurine, and cyclophosphamide.

mu, /my$\overline{oo}$, m$\overline{oo}$/, **1.** μ, the twelfth letter of the Greek alphabet. **2.** symbol for **micrometer, micron.**

Much's granules /m$\overline{oo}$ks, m$\overline{oo}$khs/ [Hans C. Much, German physician, 1880–1932], granules and rods, found in tuberculosis sputum, that stain with Gram's stain but not by the usual methods for acid-fast bacilli.

mucilage /m(y)$\overline{oo}$'səlij/, **1.** a sticky mixture of carbohydrates produced by plant cell activity. **2.** a thick aqueous solution of a gum used for suspending insoluble substances and for increasing viscosity.

mucin /my$\overline{oo}$'sin/ [L, *mucus,* slime], a mucopolysaccharide, the chief ingredient in mucus. Mucin is present in most glands that secrete mucus and is the lubricant protecting body surfaces from friction or erosion.

mucinoid /my$\overline{oo}$'sinoid/ [L, *mucus* + Gk, *eidos,* form], resembling mucin.

mucinous carcinoma, an epithelial neoplasm characterized by a sticky gelatinous consistency caused by copious mucin secretion.

mucocutaneous /my$\overline{oo}$'k$\overline{oo}$ky$\overline{oo}$tā'nē·əs/ [L, *mucus* + *cutis,* skin, *osus,* having], pertaining to the mucous membrane and the skin.

mucocutaneous lymph node syndrome (MLNS), an acute febrile illness, primarily of young children, characterized by inflamed mucous membranes of the mouth; "strawberry tongue"; cervical lymphadenopathy; polymorphous rash on the trunk; and edema, erythema, and desquamation of the skin on the extremities. Other commonly associated findings include arthralgia, diarrhea, otitis, pneumonia, photophobia, meningitis, and electro cardiographic changes.

mucoepidermoid carcinoma /my$\overline{oo}$'kō·ep'idur'moid/ [L, *mucus* + Gk, *epi,* above, *derma,* skin, *eidos,* form], a malignant neoplasm of glandular tissues, especially the ducts of the salivary glands. The tumor contains mucinous and epidermoid squamous cells.

mucogingival junction /my$\overline{oo}$'kōjinjī'vəl/ [L, *mucus* + *gingiva,* gum, *jungere,* to join], the scalloped linear area of the gums that separates the gingiva from the alveolar mucosa.

mucoid /my$\overline{oo}$'koid/ [L, *mucus* + Gk, *eidos,* form], **1.** resembling mucus. **2.** a group of glycoproteins, including colloid and ovomucoid, similar to the mucins, primarily differing in solubility.

mucoid cyst [L, *mucus* + Gk, *eidos,* form,

kytis, bag], a cyst formed by an overgrowth of a mucus gland or by the spread of mucus into the interstitial tissues.

mucolipidosis /my$\overline{oo}$'kōlip'idō'sis/, any of a group of metabolic disorders characterized by an accumulation of mucopolysaccharides and lipids in the tissues, but without an excess of mucopolysaccharides in the urine.

mucolytic /my$\overline{oo}$'kəlit'ik/ [L, *mucus* + Gk, *lysis,* loosening], **1.** exerting a destructive effect on the mucus. **2.** any agent that dissolves or destroys the mucus.

mucomembranous /my$\overline{oo}$'kəmem'brənəs/ [L, *mucus* + *membrana,* thin skin, *osus,* having], pertaining to a mucous membrane, such as that of the small intestine or the bladder.

mucopolysaccharidase /my$\overline{oo}$'kōpol'ē-sak'əridās/, an enzyme that breaks down molecules of polysaccharides.

mucopolysaccharide /my$\overline{oo}$'kōpol'ē-sak'ərīd/ [L, *mucus* + Gk, *polys,* many, *sakcharon,* sugar], a polysaccharide containing hexosamine and sometimes occurring with protein, such as mucins.

mucopolysaccharidosis (MPS) /my$\overline{oo}$'-kōpol'ēsak'əridō'sis/, *pl.* **mucopolysaccharidoses** [L, *mucus* + *polys,* many, *sakcharon,* sugar, *osis,* condition], one of a group of genetic disorders characterized by greater than normal accumulations of mucopolysaccharides in the tissues, with other symptoms specific to each type. The disorders are numbered MPS I through MPS VII, and each type has a specific eponym. All types are characterized by pronounced skeletal deformity (especially of the face), mental and physical retardation, and decreased life expectancy. Kinds of mucopolysaccharidosis include **Hunter's syndrome (MPS II), Hurler's syndrome (MPS I),** and **Morquio's disease (MPS IV).**

mucoprotein /my$\overline{oo}$·kōprō'tēn, tē·in/ [L, *mucus* + Gk, *proteios,* first rank], a compound present in all connective and supporting tissue that contains polysaccharides combined with protein and is relatively resistant to denaturation.

mucopurulent /my$\overline{oo}$'kōpyŏ̄r'yələnt/ [L, *mucus* + *purulentus,* pus], characteristic of a combination of mucus and pus.

mucosa /my$\overline{oo}$kō'sə/, *pl.* **mucosae,** mucous membrane. **—mucosal,** *adj.*

mucosal immune system /my$\overline{oo}$kō'səl/, the lymphoid tissues of the mucosal surfaces lining the gastrointestinal, respiratory, and urogenital tracts.

mucositis /my$\overline{oo}$'kōsī'tis/, any inflammation of a mucous membrane, such as the lining of the mouth and throat.

mucous membrane /my$\overline{oo}$'kəs/ [L, *mucus*

M

+ *membrana,* thin skin], any one of four major kinds of thin sheets of tissue that cover or line various parts of the body. Mucous membrane lines cavities or canals of the body that open to the outside, such as the linings of the mouth, the digestive tube, the respiratory passages, and the genitourinary tract. It consists of a surface layer of epithelial tissue covering a deeper layer of connective tissue and protects the underlying structure, secretes mucus, and absorbs water, salts, and other solutes.

mucous plug, (in obstetrics) a collection of thick mucus in the uterine cervix that is often expelled at the onset of dilation of the cervix, just before labor begins or in its early hours.

mucus /myōo'kəs/ [L, slime], the viscous, slippery secretions of mucous membranes and glands, containing mucin, white blood cells, water, inorganic salts, and exfoliated cells. —**mucoid,** *adj.,* **mucous** /myōo'kəs/, *adj.*

mucus trap suction apparatus, a catheter containing a trap to prevent mucus from being aspirated from the nasopharynx and trachea of a newborn from entering the mouth of the person operating the device. Mucus traps are also found in adult respiratory equipment.

mud bath, the application of warm mud to the body for therapeutic purposes.

MUGA, abbreviation for *multinucleated gated angiography.*

mulibrey nanism /mul'ibrī/, a rare genetic disorder, transmitted as an autosomal-recessive trait, characterized by dwarfism, constrictive pericarditis, muscular hypotonia, anomalies of the skull and face, and characteristic yellow dots in the ocular fundus. The name of the condition is an acronym composed of the first two letters of the anatomic sites of the principal defects: *mu*scle, *li*ver, *br*ain, and *ey*es.

müllerian duct /miler'ē·ən, mYl-/ [Johannes P. Müller, German physiologist, 1801–1858], one of a pair of embryonic ducts that become the fallopian tubes, uterus, and vagina in females and that atrophy in males.

Müller's law /mil'ərz/ [Johannes P. Müller], the principle that each type of sensory nerve cell normally responds to only one specific stimulus and gives rise to one sensation. A cell may be excited artificially by other forms of stimuli, but the sensation evoked will be the same.

Müller's maneuver [Johannes P. Müller], an inspiratory effort against a closed airway or glottis. The effort decreases intrapulmonary and intrathoracic pressures and expands pulmonary gas.

multicellular /-sel'yələr/, **1.** consisting

of more than one cell. **2.** containing many cavities.

multicomponent virus /-kəmpō'nənt/, a virus that occurs in two or more different particles; each particle contains only one part of the viral genome.

Multidisciplinary Care Conference, a Nursing Interventions Classification defined as planning and evaluating patient care with health professionals from other disciplines.

multidisciplinary health care team /-dis'ipliner'ē/, a group of health care workers who are members of different disciplines, each providing specific services to the patient.

multidrug resistance, the resistance of tumor cells to more than one chemotherapeutic agent.

multifactorial /-faktôr'ē·əl/ [L, *multus,* many, *facere,* to make], pertaining to or characteristic of any condition or disease resulting from the interaction of many factors, specifically the interaction of several genes, usually polygenes, with or without the involvement of environmental factors. Many disorders are considered to be multifactorial.

multifactorial inheritance, the tendency to develop a physical appearance, disease, or condition that is a condition of many genetic and environmental factors such as stature and blood pressure.

multifocal /-fō'kəl/ [L, *multus* + *focus,* hearth], characterized by more than two ectopic foci that pace the heart; may be atrial or ventricular.

multiform /mul'tifôrm/ [L, *multus,* many, *forma*], an organ, tissue, or other object that may appear in more than one shape.

multigenerational model /-jen'ərā'shənəl/, a model of family therapy that focuses on reciprocal role relationships over a period and thus takes a longitudinal approach. The family is viewed as an emotional system in which patterns of interacting and coping can be passed down from one generation to the next and can cause stress to the family members onto whom they are projected.

multigenerational transmission process, the repetition of relationship patterns, including divorce, suicide, and alcoholism, associated with emotional dysfunction that can be traced through several generations of the same family.

multigravida /mul'tigrav'idə/ [L, *multus* + *gravidare,* to impregnate], a woman who has been pregnant more than once.

multihospital system /-hos'pitəl/, a group of two or more hospitals owned, sponsored, or managed by a central organization.

multiinfarct dementia /-infärkt'/ [L, *multus* + *infarcire,* to stuff, *de,* away, *mens,* mind], a form of organic brain disease characterized by the rapid deterioration of intellectual functioning, caused by vascular disease. Symptoms include emotional lability; disturbances in memory, abstract thinking, judgment, and impulse control; and focal neurologic impairment such as gait abnormalities, pseudobulbar palsy, and paresthesia.

multilocular cyst /-lok'yələr/ [L, *multus* + *loculus,* little place; Gk, *kystis,* bag], one of three kinds of follicular cyst, containing many spaces and not associated with a tooth.

multipara /multip'ərə/, *pl.* **multiparae** [L *multus* + *parere,* to bear], a woman who has delivered more than one viable infant.

multiparity /-per'itē/ [L, *multus,* many, *parere,* to give birth], the status of a mother of more than one child.

multiparous /multip'ərous/ [L, *multus,* many, *parere,* to give birth], having given birth to more than one child.

multipenniform /-pen'ifôrm/ [L, *multus* + *penna,* feather, *forma*], (of a body structure) having a shape resembling a pattern of many feathers.

multiphase generator /-fāz'/, (in radiology) a generator that operates on more than single-phase power. It usually has three phases, which greatly increase the number of x-rays produced per unit time.

multiphasic screening /-fā'sik/ [L, *multus* + *phasis,* appearance; ME, *scren*], a technique of screening populations for diseases that combines a battery of screening tests. The technique serves to identify any of several diseases being screened for in a population.

multiple autoimmune disorder (MAD) /mul'tip͡əl/, a condition in which a patient exhibits symptoms of at least two of a group of diseases, including Addison's disease, autoimmune thyroid disease, mucocutaneous candidiasis, hypoparathyroiditis, and insulin-dependent diabetes.

multiple endocrine adenomatosis (MEA), a condition characterized by functioning tumors in more than one endocrine gland. The disorder is commonly associated with Zollinger-Ellison's syndrome and may involve the pituitary, pancreas, and parathyroid glands. It is also seen in multiple endocrine neoplasia type I.

multiple endocrine neoplasia (MEN), a hereditary hormonal disorder that occurs in an autosomal-dominant pattern. The endocrine neoplasms may be expressed as hyperplasia, adenoma, or carcinoma and may develop synchronously or metachronously.

multiple family therapy [L, *multus* + *plica,* fold], psychotherapy in which four or five families meet weekly to confront and deal with problems or issues that they have in common.

multiple fission, cell division in which the nucleus first divides into several equal parts and then the cytoplasm divides into as many cells as there are nuclei.

multiple fracture, 1. a fracture extending several fracture lines in one bone. **2.** the fracture of several bones at one time or from the same injury.

multiple lipomatosis, a rare inherited disorder characterized by discrete localized subcutaneous deposits of fat in the tissues of the body.

multiple mononeuropathy, an abnormal condition characterized by dysfunction of several individual nerve trunks. It may be caused by various diseases such as diabetes mellitus and some inflammatory immunologic conditions.

multiple mucosal neuroma syndrome, a condition of multiple submucosal neuromas or neurofibromas of the lips, tongue, and eyelids. The disease affects young persons and may be associated with tumors of the thyroid or adrenal medulla or with subcutaneous neurofibromatosis.

multiple myeloma, a malignant neoplasm of the bone marrow. The tumor, composed of plasma cells, disrupts normal bone marrow functions, destroys osseous tissue, especially in flat bones; and causes pain, fractures, hypercalcemia, and skeletal deformities.

multiple peripheral neuritis, acute or subacute disseminated inflammation or degeneration of symmetrically distributed peripheral nerves, characterized initially by numbness, tingling in the extremities, hot and cold sensations, and slight fever, progressing to pain, weakness, diminished reflexes, and in some cases flaccid paralysis. The disorder may be caused by toxic substances such as antimony, arsenic, carbon monoxide, copper, lead, and mercury.

multiple personality, a fragmentation of the personality characterized by the presence of two or more distinct subpersonalities.

multiple pregnancy, a pregnancy in which there is more than one fetus in the uterus at the same time.

multiple sclerosis (MS) [L, *multus* + *plica,* fold; Gk, *sklerosis,* hardening], a progressive disease characterized by disseminated demyelination of nerve fibers of the brain and spinal cord. The first signs are paresthesias, or abnormal sensations in the extremities or on one side of the face. Other early signs are muscle weakness,

M

vertigo, and visual disturbances. Later in the course of disease there may be extreme emotional lability, ataxia, abnormal reflexes, and difficulty in urinating.

multiple sleep latency test (MSLT), a test of the propensity to fall asleep. The subject is given five 20-minute nap opportunities at 2-hour intervals. The mean latency to sleep onset and the stages of sleep that occur are determined from polygraph records.

multiple transfusion syndrome [L, *multus,* many, *plica,* fold, *transfundere,* to pour through; Gk, *syn,* together, *dromos,* course], a hemorrhagic reaction to massive transfusions of platelet-poor stored blood. Other clotting factors seldom contribute to the condition.

multipolar mitosis /-pō′lər/ [L, *multus* + *polus,* pole], cell division in which the spindle has three or more poles and results in the formation of a corresponding number of daughter cells.

multisource drug /mul′tisôrs/ [L, *multus* + OFr, *sourse,* origin], a pharmaceutical that can be purchased under any of several trademarks from different manufacturers or distributors.

multispecificity /-spes′ifis′itē/, the ability of an immunoglobulin to bind with more than one type of antigen.

multisynaptic /-sinap′tik/ [L, *multus* + Gk, *synaptein,* to join], pertaining to a nervous process or system of nerve cells requiring a series of synapses.

multivalent /mul′tivā′lənt/ [L, *multus* + *valere,* to be strong], **1.** (in chemistry) denoting the capacity of an element to combine with three or more univalent atoms. **2.** (in immunology) able to act against more than one strain of organism.

multivalent vaccine [L, *multus,* many, *valere,* value, *vaccinus,* cow], a vaccine prepared from several antigenic types within a species.

mummification /mum′ifikā′shən/ [Per, *mum,* wax; L, *facere,* to make], a dried-up state, such as occurs in dry gangrene or a dead fetus in utero.

mummified fetus /mum′ifīd/, a fetus that has died in utero and has shriveled and dried.

mumps [D, *mompen,* to sulk], an acute viral disease, characterized by a swelling of the parotid glands, caused by a paramyxovirus. It is most likely to affect children between 5 and 15 years of age, but it may occur at any age. In adulthood the infection may be severe. The mumps paramyxovirus lives in the saliva of the affected individual and is transmitted in droplets or by direct contact. Symptoms include anorexia, headache, malaise, and

low-grade fever. These signs are commonly followed by earache, parotid gland swelling, and a temperature of 101° to 104° F (38.3° to 40° C). The patient also experiences pain when drinking acidic liquids or when chewing. The prognosis in mumps is good, but the disease sometimes involves complications, such as arthritis, pancreatitis, myocarditis, oophoritis, and nephritis. About one half of the men with mumps-induced orchitis suffer some atrophy of the testicles, but because the condition is usually unilateral, sterility rarely results.

mumps orchitis, an inflammatory disorder of the testis characterized by swelling with fever, malaise, and acute parotitis. It usually occurs in postpubertal men with a recent history of mumps and may result in testicular atrophy.

mumps virus vaccine live, an active immunizing agent prescribed for immunization against mumps.

Münchausen's syndrome /mun′chousənz/ [Baron von Münchausen, German adventurer and confabulator, 1720–1797], an unusual condition characterized by habitual pleas for treatment and hospitalization for a symptomatic but imaginary acute illness. The affected person may logically and convincingly present the symptoms and history of a real disease.

Münchausen's syndrome by proxy [Baron von Münchausen], a variation of Münchausen's syndrome in which the parent persistently fabricates or induces illness in a child with the intent of keeping in contact with hospitals and physicians. The child may endure dozens of surgeries and hospitalizations for illness induced by the parent; nearly 9% of the children die as a result. The mother or father poses as being a good parent by "saving" the child from medical catastrophe, and the child serves as a manipulative object.

mural /myoo̅′rəl/ [L, *murus,* wall], something that is found on or against the wall of a cavity.

mural thrombus [L, *murus,* wall], a thrombus that originates in the wall of a cavity, particularly on a diseased patch of endocardium.

muriatic acid /moo̅′rē·at′ik/ [L, *muria,* brine, *acidus,* sour], hydrochloric acid.

murine typhus /myoo̅′rēn/ [L, *mus,* mouse; Gk, *typhos,* stupor], an acute arbovirus infection caused by *Rickettsia typhi* and transmitted by the bite of an infected flea. The disease is similar to epidemic typhus but less severe. It is characterized by headache, chills, fever, myalgia, and rash.

murmur /mur'mər/ [L, a humming], a gentle blowing, fluttering, or humming sound, such as a heart murmur.

muromonab-CD3 /myoo'rəmon'ab/, a parenteral immunosuppressant drug for kidney transplant rejection. It is used in the control of acute renal transplant rejection.

Murphy's sign, a test for gallbladder disease in which the patient is asked to inhale while the examiner's fingers are hooked under the liver border at the bottom of the rib cage. The inspiration causes the gallbladder to descend onto the fingers, producing pain if the gallbladder is inflamed.

muscarine /mus'kərēn/ [L, musca, fly], a choline-related alkaloid present in the poisonous mushroom Amanita muscaria. It is similar pharmacologically to acetylcholine, although it is not used in therapeutics.

muscarinic /mus'kərin'ik/ [L, musca, fly], stimulating the postganglionic parasympathetic receptor.

muscle /mus'əl/ [L, musculus], a kind of tissue composed of fibers or cells that are able to contract, causing movement of body parts and organs. Muscle fibers are richly vascular, excitable, conductive, and elastic. There are two basic kinds, striated muscle and smooth muscle. Striated muscle, which composes all skeletal muscles except the myocardium, is long and voluntary; it responds very quickly to stimulation and is paralyzed by interruption of its innervation. Smooth muscle, which composes all visceral muscles, is short and involuntary; it reacts slowly to all stimuli and does not entirely lose its tone if innervation is interrupted. The myocardium is sometimes classified as a third (cardiac) kind of muscle, but it is basically a striated muscle that does not contract as quickly as the striated muscle of the rest of the body.

muscle albumin, albumin present in muscle.

muscle biopsy [L, musculus + Gk, bios, life, opsis, view], an examination of surgically removed muscle tissue for diagnosis.

muscle bridge, a band of myocardial tissue over one or more of the large epicardial coronary vessels. It may cause constriction of the artery during systole.

muscle cramp, a sudden intermittent pain in almost any part of the body. It may involve involuntary contractions of variable duration and be accompanied by spasms. Cramps may develop in striated muscle as a result of exertion; high temperature; and excessive loss of sodium, potassium, and magnesium through perspiration. Cramps

can also be associated with arthritic conditions and exposure to cold.

muscle excitability /eksī'təbil'itē/, the ability of a muscle fiber to respond rapidly to a stimulating agent.

muscle guarding, a protective response in muscle that results from pain or fear of movement. The condition may be treated through induced relaxation of the muscle by using biofeedback to reduce electromyographic activity.

muscle receptor, a sensory organ that responds to muscle stretch or tension, including muscle spindles and tendon organs.

muscle reeducation, the use of physical therapeutic exercises to restore muscle tone and strength after an injury or disease.

muscle relaxant, a chemotherapeutic agent that reduces the contractility of muscle fibers. Curare derivatives and succinylcholine compete with acetylcholine and block neural transmission at the myoneural junction. These drugs are used during anesthesia, in the management of patients undergoing mechanical ventilation, and in shock therapy to reduce muscle contractions in pharmacologically or electrically induced seizures.

muscle-setting exercise, a method of maintaining muscle strength and tonality by alternately contracting and relaxing a skeletal muscle or any group of muscles without moving the associated body part.

muscles of mastication, a group of muscles, all innervated by the mandibular division of the trigeminal nerve, responsible for movement of the jaws during the process of chewing. The four muscles of mastication are the masseter, pterygoideus lateralis, pterygoideus medialis, and temporalis.

muscles of ventilation [L, musculus + respirare, to breathe], muscles that provide inspiration, partly by increasing the volume of the chest cavity so that air is drawn into the lungs, including the diaphragm and external intercostal muscles. They are aided during forced breathing by the scalenus muscles, levatores costarum, sternocleidomastoid, pectoralis major, platysma myoides, and serratus superior posterior. Muscles of forced expiration include the external and internal oblique, rectus abdominis, and transverse abdominis.

muscle spindle [L, musculus + AS, spinel], a specialized proprioceptive sensory organ composed of a bundle of fine striated intrafusal muscle fibers innervated by gamma nerve fibers. Their nuclei are gathered together near the center of each fiber to form a nuclear sac, which is surrounded in turn by sensory, annulospiral nerve endings, all enclosed in a fibrous sheath.

muscle testing, a method of evaluating the contractile unit, including the muscle, tendons, and associated tissues, of a moving part of the body by neurologic or resistance testing. The tests may include shortened, middle, and lengthened range-of-motion ability; isokinetic measurement of muscle strength, power, and endurance; and functional tests, such as jogging or specific agility drills, as well as radiography, arthroscopy, electromyography, and other medical tests.

muscle tone, a normal state of balanced muscle tension.

muscular /mus'kyələr/ [L, *musculus*], **1.** pertaining to a muscle. **2.** characteristic of well-developed musculature.

muscular atrophy, a condition of motor unit dysfunction, usually the result of a loss of efferent innervation.

muscular branch of the deep brachial artery, one of several similar branches of the deep brachial artery, supplying certain arm muscles such as the coracobrachialis, biceps brachii, and brachialis.

muscular dystrophy (MD) [L, *musculus* + Gk, *dys,* bad, *trophe,* nourishment], a group of genetically transmitted diseases characterized by progressive atrophy of symmetric groups of skeletal muscles without evidence of involvement or degeneration of neural tissue. In all forms of muscular dystrophy an insidious loss of strength with increasing disability and deformity occurs, although each type differs in the groups of muscles affected, the age of onset, the rate of progression, and the mode of genetic inheritance. The main types of the disease are pseudohypertrophic (Duchenne type) muscular dystrophy, limb-girdle muscular dystrophy, and facioscapulohumeral (Landouzy-Déjérine) muscular dystrophy. Rarer forms include Becker's muscular dystrophy, distal muscular dystrophy, ocular myopathy, and myotonic muscular dystrophy.

muscular fatigue, a refractory condition in which the contractile tissue of a muscle loses its response to stimulation as a result of overactivity. It is usually a period after stimulation during which the muscle is unresponsive to an immediate second stimulus.

muscular incompetence [L, *musculus* + *incompetens*], a failure of a cardiac valve to close properly caused by incompetence of the papillary muscles of the heart.

muscular sarcoidosis, sarcoidosis of the skeletal muscles characterized by interstitial inflammation, fibrosis, atrophy, and damage of the muscle fibers as sarcoid tubercles form within and replace normal muscle cells.

muscular system, all of the muscles of the body, including the smooth, cardiac, and striated muscles, considered as an interrelated structural group.

muscular tension [L, *musculus* + *tendere,* to stretch], strain that results from muscular contractions. Internal tension is caused by cross-bridge activity between the actin and myosin filaments within the muscle fiber. The force generated by these contractile elements is transmitted to the bones via tendons and connective tissue. The bones move and produce external tension.

muscular tone [L, *musculus* + Gk, *tonos,* stretching], a normal degree of tension in muscles at rest.

muscular tremor [L, *musculus* + *tremor,* shaking], minute regular involuntary contraction of individual muscle fasciculi. If the tremors are mild and occasional, the cause may be physiologic. Profuse, persistent, or recurrent widespread muscular twitching often indicates a motor neuron disorder.

musculature /mus'kyəlā'chər/, the arrangement and condition of the muscles.

musculocutaneous nerve /mus'kyəlōky-ōōlōyōōtā'nē-əs/ [L, *musculus* + *cutis,* skin, *osus,* having], one of the terminal branches of the brachial plexus. It is formed on each side by division of the lateral cord of the plexus into two branches. Various branches and filaments supply different structures, such as the biceps, the brachialis, the humerus, and the skin of the forearm.

musculoskeletal /mus'kyōōlōskel'ətəl/ [L, *musculus* + Gk, *skeletos,* dried up], pertaining to the muscles and skeleton.

musculoskeletal system, all of the muscles, bones, joints, and related structures such as the tendons and connective tissue that function in the movement of body parts and organs.

musculoskeletal system assessment, an evaluation of the condition and functioning of the patient's muscles, joints, and bones and of factors that may contribute to abnormalities in these body structures. Health care providers conduct the interview to obtain subjective data, make the necessary observations of the patient, and assemble the information on concurrent and previous disorders, the family history, the patient's social and medication background, and the results of laboratory studies and diagnostic procedures.

mush bite, a procedure used in making simultaneous tooth impressions for the construction of study models or full or partial dentures. The patient draws his or her upper and lower jaws together into a block of softened wax, thus indicating the spatial relationship between the maxilla and mandible.

mushroom [ME, *mucheron*], the fruiting body of the fungus of the class Basidomycetes, especially edible members of the order Agaricales, commonly known as field mushrooms or meadow mushrooms. Mushrooms are composed largely of water and are of limited nutritional value.

mushroom poisoning, a toxic condition caused by the ingestion of certain mushrooms, particularly two species of the genus *Amanita.* Muscarine in *Amanita muscaria* produces intoxication in a few minutes to 2 hours. Symptoms include lacrimation, salivation, sweating, vomiting, labored breathing, abdominal cramps, diarrhea, and in severe cases convulsions, coma, and circulatory failure. More deadly but slower-acting phalloidin in *A. phalloides* and *A. verna* causes similar symptoms, as well as liver damage, renal failure, and death in 30% to 50% of the cases.

music therapy [Gk, *mousike,* music, *therapeia,* treatment], a form of adjunctive psychotherapy in which music is used as a means of recreation and communication, especially with autistic children, and as a means to elevate the mood of depressed and psychotic patients.

Music Therapy, a Nursing Interventions Classification defined as using music to help achieve a specific change in behavior or feeling.

mustard gas /mus'tärd/, a poisonous gas used in chemical warfare during World War I. It causes corrosive destruction of the skin and mucous membranes, often resulting in permanent respiratory damage and death.

mustard plaster [L, *mustum* + Gk, *emplastron*], a mustard medication in a fabric base that can be placed close to the skin for a time as a counterirritant in the form of a poultice.

mutacism /myoo'təsiz'əm/, mimmation, or the incorrect use of /m/ sounds.

mutagen /myoo'təjən/ [L, *mutare,* to change, *genein,* to produce], any chemical or physical environmental agent that induces a genetic mutation or increases the mutation rate. —**mutagenic,** *adj.,* **mutagenicity,** *n.*

mutagenesis /myoo'təjen'əsis/, the induction or occurrence of a genetic mutation.

mutant /myoo'tənt/ [L, *mutare,* to change], **1.** any individual or organism with genetic material that has undergone mutation. **2.** relating to or produced by mutation.

mutant gene, any gene that has undergone a change, such as the loss, gain, or exchange of genetic material, that affects the normal transmission and expression of a trait.

mutase /myoo'tās/, any enzyme that catalyzes the shifting of a chemical group or radical from one position to another within the same molecule or occasionally from one molecule to another.

mutation /myoota'shən/ [L, *mutare,* to change], an unusual change in genetic material occurring spontaneously or by induction. The alteration changes the original expression of the gene. Genes are stable units, but when a mutation occurs, it often is transmitted to later generations. —**mutate,** *v.,* **mutational,** *adj.*

mutein /myoo'tē·in, m(y)oo'tēn/, a protein molecule that results from a mutation.

mutism /myoo'tizəm/ [L, *mutus,* mute], the inability to speak because of a physical defect or emotional problem.

muton /myoo'ton/, (in molecular genetics) the smallest deoxyribonucleic acid segment whose alteration can result in a mutation.

Mutual Goal Setting, a Nursing Interventions Classification defined as collaborating with a patient to identify and prioritize care goals, then developing a plan for achieving those goals through the construction and use of goal attainment scaling.

mutually exclusive categories /myoo'-choo·əlē/, categories on a research instrument that are sufficiently precise to allow each subject, factor, or variable to be classified uniquely.

mutual support group, a type of group in which members organize to solve their own problems. It is led by the group members themselves who share a common goal and use their own strengths to gain control over their lives.

mv, mV, abbreviation for **millivolt.**

MVIC, abbreviation for **maximum voluntary isometric contraction.**

mVO$_2$, symbol for *myocardial oxygen consumption.*

MVV, abbreviation for *maximal voluntary ventilation.*

M.W.I.A., abbreviation for **Medical Women's International Association.**

MX gene, a human gene that helps the body resist viral infections. When exposed to interferon, the MX gene inhibits the production of viral protein and nucleic

M

acid necessary for the proliferation of new viral particles.

myalgia /mī·al′jə/ [Gk, *mys,* muscle, *algos,* pain], diffuse muscle pain, usually accompanied by malaise.

myalgic asthenia /mī·al′jik/ [Gk, *mys* + *algos,* pain, *a* + *sthenos,* without strength], a condition characterized by a general feeling of fatigue and muscular pain, often resulting from or associated with psychologic stress.

myasthenia /mī′əsthē′nē·ə/ [Gk, *mys* + *a* + *sthenos,* without strength], a condition characterized by an abnormal weakness of a muscle or a group of muscles that may be the result of a systemic myoneural disturbance, such as in myasthenia gravis or myasthenia laryngis, which involves the vocal cord tensor muscles. —**myasthenic,** *adj.*

myasthenia gravis, an abnormal condition characterized by chronic fatigability and muscle weakness, especially in the face and throat, as a result of a defect in the conduction of nerve impulses at the myoneural junction. The onset of symptoms is usually gradual, with ptosis of the upper eyelids, diplopia, and weakness of the facial muscles. The weakness may then extend to other muscles innervated by the cranial nerves, particularly the respiratory muscles. Muscular exertion aggravates the symptoms.

myasthenia gravis crisis, acute exacerbation of the muscular weakness characterizing the disease, triggered by infection, surgery, emotional stress, or an overdose or insufficiency of anticholinesterase medication. Typical signs and symptoms include respiratory distress progressing to periods of apnea, extreme fatigue, increased muscular weakness, dysphagia, dysarthria, and fever. The patient may be anxious, restless, irritable, and unable to move the jaws or to raise one or both eyelids.

myasthenic crisis /mī′asthen′ik/, an acute episode of muscular weakness.

mycelium /mīsē′lē·əm/, *pl.* **mycelia** [Gk, *mykes,* fungus, *helos,* nail], a mass of interwoven, branched, threadlike filaments that makes up most fungi.

mycetismus /mī′sitiz′məs/, mushroom poisoning.

mycetoma /mī′sətō′mə/ [Gk, *mykes* + *oma,* tumor], a severe fungal infection involving skin, subcutaneous tissue, fascia, and bone.

mycobacteria /mī′kōbaktir′ē·ə/ [Gk, *mykes* + *bakterion,* small rod], acid-fast microorganisms belonging to the genus *Mycobacterium.* —**mycobacterial,** *adj.*

mycobacteriosis /mī′kōbak′tirē·ō′sis/ [Gk, *mykes* + *bakterion* + *osis,* condition], a tuberculosis-like disease caused by mycobacteria other than *Mycobacterium tuberculosis.*

Mycobacterium /mī′kōbaktir′ē·əm/ [Gk, *mykes* + *bakterion,* small rod], a genus of rod-shaped acid-fast bacteria having two significant pathogenic species: *Mycobacterium leprae,* which causes leprosy, and *M. tuberculosis,* which causes tuberculosis.

Mycobacterium bovis, a species of bacteria that causes tuberculosis in cattle and other animals. It is transmitted to humans by drinking of raw milk contaminated by the microorganism.

Mycobacterium kansasii, a species of slow-growing photochromogenic bacteria that causes tuberculosis-like pulmonary infection in humans. It affects the joints, gonads, spinal fluid, lymph nodes, and viscera.

Mycobacterium marinum, a species of bacteria that causes a form of tuberculosis in cold-blooded animals, including saltwater fish. The bacterium is also found in swimming pools and aquariums and is associated with skin lesions in humans.

mycology /mīkol′əjē/ [Gk, *mykes* + *logos,* science], the study of fungi and fungoid diseases. —**mycologic, mycological,** *adj.,* **mycologist,** *n.*

mycophenolic acid /mī′kōfinō′lik/, a bacteriostatic and fungistatic crystalline antibiotic obtained from *Penicillium brevi compactum* and related species.

Mycoplasma /mī′kōplaz′mə/ [Gk, *mykes* + *plassein,* to mold], a genus of ultramicroscopic organisms lacking rigid cell walls and considered to be the smallest free-living organisms. Some are saprophytes, some are parasites, and many are pathogens.

mycoplasma pneumonia, a contagious disease of children and young adults caused by *Mycoplasma pneumoniae.* It is characterized by symptoms of an upper respiratory infection, dry cough, and fever. Harsh or diminished breath sounds are frequently heard.

mycosis /mīkō′sis/ [Gk, *mykes* + *osis,* condition], any disease caused by a fungus. Some kinds of mycoses are **athlete's foot, candidiasis,** and **coccidioidomycosis.** —**mycotic,** *adj.*

mycosis fungoides /fung·goi′dēz/, a rare chronic lymphomatous skin malignancy resembling eczema or a cutaneous tumor that is followed by microabscesses in the epidermis and lesions simulating those of Hodgkin's disease in lymph nodes and viscera.

mycotic /mīkot'ik/ [Gk, *mykes,* fungus], pertaining to a disease caused by a fungus.

mycotic aneurysm, a localized dilation in the wall of a blood vessel caused by the growth of a fungus. It usually occurs as a complication of bacterial endocarditis.

mycotic granuloma of the larynx /mīkot'ik/, a chronic throat condition characterized by white patches on an otherwise bright red mucous membrane. In the southwestern United States it is associated with histoplasmosis of the larynx. It may also be caused by candidiasis as a complication of chemotherapy or an altered immune state.

mycotoxicosis /mī'kōtok'sikō'sis/ [Gk, *mykes + toxikon,* poison, *osis,* condition], a systemic poisoning caused by toxins produced by fungal organisms.

mycotoxins /mī'kōtok'sins, poisons produced by fungi that are harmful to other organisms.

mydriasis /midrī'əsis/ [Gk, *mydros,* hot mass], **1.** dilation of the pupil of the eye caused by contraction of the dilator muscle of the iris, a muscular sheath that radiates outward like the spokes of a wheel from the center of the iris around the pupil. **2.** an abnormal condition characterized by contraction of the dilator muscle, resulting in widely dilated pupils. —**mydriatic** /mid'rē·at'ik/, *adj.*

mydriatic and cycloplegic agent [Gk, *mydros + kyklos,* circle, *plege,* stroke], any one of several ophthalmic pharmaceutic preparations that dilate the pupil and paralyze the ocular muscles of accommodation. Mydriatics stimulate the sympathetic nerve fibers or block parasympathetic nerve fibers of the eye, temporarily paralyzing the iris sphincter muscle. Cycloplegics temporarily paralyze accommodation while relaxing the ciliary muscle. These drugs are used in diagnostic and refractive examination of the eye, before and after various procedures in eye surgery, in some tests for glaucoma, and in the treatment of anterior uveitis and certain kinds of glaucoma.

myelacephalus /mī'ələsef'ələs/ [Gk, *myelos,* marrow, *a + kephale,* without head], a fetal monster, usually a separate monozygotic twin, whose form and parts are barely recognizable; a slightly differentiated amorphous mass. —**myelacephalous,** *adj.*

myelatelia /mī'ələtē'lē·ə/ [Gk, *myelos + atelia,* unfinished], any developmental defect involving the spinal cord.

myelauxe /mī'əlôk'sē/ [Gk, *myelos + auxe,* increasing], a developmental anomaly characterized by hypertrophy of the spinal cord.

myelencephalon /mī'əlensef'əlon/, the lower part of the embryonic hindbrain, from which the medulla oblongata develops.

myelin /mī'əlin/ [Gk, *myelos,* marrow], a substance constituting the sheaths of various nerve fibers throughout the body. It is largely composed of phospholipids and protein, which gives the fibers a white, creamy color. —**myelinic,** *adj.*

myelinated /mī'əlinā'tid/, (of a nerve) having a myelin sheath.

myelination /mī'əlinā'shən/ [Gk, *myelos + L, atio,* process], the process of furnishing or taking on myelin.

myelin globule, a fatlike droplet found in some sputum.

myelinic /mī'əlin'ik/ [Gk, *myelos + L, icus,* form of], pertaining to myelin.

myelinic neuroma, a neuroma neoplasm composed of myelinated nerve fibers.

myelinization /mī'əlin'izā'shən/ [Gk, *myelos + izein,* to cause], development of the myelin sheath around a nerve fiber.

myelinolysis /mī'əlinol'isis/ [Gk, *myelos + lysein,* to loosen], a pathologic process that dissolves the myelin sheaths around certain nerve fibers, such as those of the pons in alcoholic and undernourished people who are afflicted with central pontine myelinolysis.

myelin sheath, a segmented fatty lamination composed of myelin that wraps the axons of many nerves in the body. The usual thickness of the myelin sheath is between 200 and 800 μm. Various diseases such as multiple sclerosis can destroy myelin wrappings.

myelitis /mī'əlī'tis/, an abnormal condition characterized by inflammation of the spinal cord with associated motor or sensory dysfunction. Some kinds of myelitis are **acute transverse myelitis, leukomyelitis,** and **poliomyelitis.** —**myelitic,** *adj.*

myeloblast /mī'əlōblast'/ [Gk, *myelos + blastos,* germ], one of the earliest precursors of the granulocytic leukocytes. The cytoplasm appears light blue, scanty, and nongranular when seen in a stained blood smear through a microscope. —**myeloblastic,** *adj.*

myeloblastic leukemia /-blas'tik/, a malignant neoplasm of blood-forming tissues, characterized by many myeloblasts in the circulating blood and tissues.

myeloblastomatosis /mī'əlōblas'tōmətō'sis/ [Gk, *myelos + blastos + oma,* tumor, *osis,* condition], abnormal localized clusters of myeloblasts in the peripheral circulation.

myeloblastosis /mī'əloblastō'sis/ [Gk, *myelos + blastos + osis,* condition], an excess of myeloblasts in the blood.

M

myelocele /mī'əlōsēl'/ [Gk, *myelos* + *kele,* hernia], a saclike protrusion of the spinal cord through a congenital defect in the vertebral column.

myeloclast /mī'əlōclast'/ [Gk, *myelos* + *klastos,* broken], a cell that breaks down the myelin sheaths of nerves.

myelocyst /mī'əlōsist'/ [Gk, *myelos* + *kystis,* cyst], any benign cyst formed from the rudimentary medullary canals that give rise to the vertebral canal during embryonic development.

myelocystocele /mī'əlōsis'təsēl'/ [Gk, *myelos* + *kystis* + *kele,* hernia], a protrusion of a cystic tumor containing spinal cord substance through a defect in the vertebral column.

myelocystomeningocele /mī'əlōsis'tōməning'gōsēl/ [Gk, *myelos* + *kystis* + *menix,* membrane, *kele,* hernia], a protrusion of a cystic tumor containing both spinal cord substance and meninges through a defect in the vertebral column.

myelocyte /mī'əlōsīt'/ [Gk, *myelos* + *kytos,* cell], the first of the maturation stages of the granulocytic leukocytes normally found in the bone marrow. Granules are seen in the cytoplasm. The nuclear material of the myelocyte is denser than that of the myeloblast but lacks a definable membrane. The cell is flat and contains increasing numbers of granules as maturation progresses. —**myelocytic,** *adj.*

myelocythemia /mī'əlōsīthē'mē·ə/ [Gk, *myelos* + *kytos* + *haima,* blood], an excessive presence of myelocytes in the circulating blood, such as in myelocytic leukemia.

myelocytic leukemia /mī'əlōsit'ik/, a disorder characterized by the unregulated and excessive production of leukocytes.

myelocytoma /mī'əlō'sītō'mə/ [Gk, *myelos* + *kytos,* cell, *oma,* tumor], a localized cluster of myelocytes in the peripheral vasculature, which may occur in myelocytic leukemia.

myelodiastasis /mī'əlōdī·as'təsis/ [Gk, *myelos* + *diastasis,* separation], disintegration and necrosis of the spinal cord.

myelodysplasia /mī'əkōdisplā'zhə/ [Gk, *myelos* + *dys,* bad, *plassis,* formation], a general designation for the defective development of any part of the spinal cord.

myelofibrosis /mī'əlōfībrō'sis/. the replacement of bone marrow with fibrous tissue. The condition may be associated with anemia, thrombocytopenia, myeloid metaplasia, new bone formation, polycythemia vera, and other abnormalities.

myelogenesis /-jen'əsis/ [Gk, *myelos* + *genein,* to produce], **1.** the formation and differentiation of the nervous system, in particular of the brain and spinal cord,

during prenatal development. **2.** the development of the myelin sheath around the nerve fiber.

myelogenous /mī'əloj'ənəs/, pertaining to the cells produced in bone marrow or to the tissue from which such cells originate.

myelogeny /mī'əloj'ənē/ [Gk, *myelos* + *genein,* to produce], the formation and differentiation of the myelin sheaths of nerve fibers during the prenatal and postnatal development of the central nervous system.

myelogram /mī'əlōgram'/, **1.** an x-ray film taken after the injection of a radiopaque medium into the subarachnoid space to demonstrate any distortions of the spinal cord, spinal nerve roots, and subarachnoid space. **2.** a graphic representation of a count of the different kinds of cells in a stained preparation of bone marrow.

myelography /mī'əlog'rəfē/ [Gk, *myelos* + *graphein,* to record], a radiographic process by which the spinal cord and the spinal subarachnoid space are viewed and photographed after the introduction of a contrast medium. —**myelographic,** *adj.*

myeloid /mī'əloid/ [Gk, *myelos* + *eidos,* form], **1.** pertaining to the bone marrow. **2.** pertaining to the spinal cord. **3.** pertaining to myelocytic forms that do not necessarily originate in the bone marrow.

myeloid metaplasia, a disorder in which bone marrow tissue develops in abnormal sites. Characteristics of the condition are anemia, splenomegaly, immature blood cells in the circulation, and hematopoiesis in the liver and spleen.

myeloidosis /mī'əloidō'sis/ [Gk, *myelos* + *eidos,* form, *osis,* condition], an abnormal condition characterized by general hyperplasia of the myeloid tissue.

myeloma /mī'əlō'mə/ [Gk, *myelos* + *oma,* tumor], an osteolytic neoplasm consisting of a profusion of cells typical of the bone marrow that may develop in many sites and cause extensive destruction of the bone. Intense pain and spontaneous fractures are common.

myeloma kidney disease, a kidney disorder often characterized by irreversible renal failure.

myelomalacia /mī'əlōmələ'shə/ [Gk, *myelos* + *malakia,* softening], an abnormal softening of the spinal cord, caused primarily by inadequate blood supply.

myelomeningocele /mī'əlō'məning'gōsēl/ [Gk, *myelos* + *menix,* membrane, *kele,* hernia], a developmental defect of the central nervous system in which a hernial sac containing a part of the spinal cord, its meninges, and cerebrospinal fluid protrudes through a congenital cleft in the vertebral column. The condition is caused primarily by failure of the neural tube to close during embryonic development, although in some instances it may result from the reopening of the tube as a result of an abnormal increase in cerebrospinal fluid pressure.

myelomere /mī′əlōmir′/ [Gk, *myelos* + *meros,* part], any of the embryonic segments of the brain or spinal cord during prenatal development.

myelopathy /mī′əlop′əthē/, **1.** any disease of the spinal cord. **2.** any disease of the myelopoietic tissues.

myeloperoxidase (MPO) /mī′əlōpərok′-sidās/, a peroxidase enzyme phagocytic cells occurring in that can oxidize halide ions, producing a bactericidal effect.

myeloperoxidase deficiency, an autosomal-recessive inherited disorder in which there is a lack of myeloperoxidase in the primary granules of neutrophils, causing delayed intracellular killing of fungi and bacteria by neutrophils.

myelophthisic anemia /mī′əlofthiz′ik/ [Gk, *myelos* + *phthisis,* wasting], a disorder characterized by anemia and the appearance of immature granulocytes and nucleated erythroid elements in the peripheral blood.

myelopoiesis /mī′əlō′pō·ē′sis/ [Gk, *myelos* + *poiein,* to form], the formation and development of the bone marrow or the cells that originate from it. —**myelopoietic,** /-pō·et′ik/ *adj.*

myeloproliferative disorders /mī′əlō-prōlif′ərətiv′/, a group of conditions characterized by proliferation of myeloid tissue, such as polycythemia vera or chronic myelogenous leukemia.

myeloradiculodysplasia /mī′əlō′rədik′-yəlodis′plā′zhə/ [Gk, *myelos* + L, *radiculus,* small root, Gk, *dys,* bad, *plassein,* to form], any developmental abnormality of the spinal cord and spinal nerve roots.

myeloschisis /mī′əlos′kəsis/ [Gk, *myelos* + *schisis,* cleft], a developmental defect characterized by a cleft spinal cord that results from the failure of the neural plate to fuse and form a complete neural tube.

myelosuppression /-səpresh′ən/, the inhibition of the process of production of blood cells and platelets in the bone marrow.

myenteric plexus /mī′enter′ik/ [Gk, *mys,* muscle, *enteron,* bowel; L, *plexus,* plaited], a group of autonomic nerve fibers and ganglion cells in the muscular coat of the intestine.

myesthesia /mī′esthē′zhə/, perception of any sensation in a muscle, such as touch, direction, proprioception, contraction, relaxation, or extension.

myiasis /mī′yəsis/ [Gk, *myia,* fly, *osis,* condition], infection or infestation of the body by the larvae of flies, usually through a wound or an ulcer, but rarely through intact skin.

mylohyoideus /mī′lōhī·oi′dē·əs/ [Gk, *myle,* mill, *hyoeides,* upsilon, U-shaped], one of a pair of flat triangular muscles that form the floor of the cavity of the mouth. It acts to raise the hyoid bone and the tongue.

myocardial infarction (MI) /mī′ōkär′-dē·əl/ [Gk, *mys,* muscle, *kardia,* heart; L, *infarcire,* to stuff], necrosis of a part of cardiac muscle caused by obstruction in a coronary artery through either atherosclerosis or a thrombus or a spasm. The onset of MI is characterized by a crushing, viselike chest pain that may radiate to the left arm, neck, or epigastrium and sometimes stimulates the sensation of acute indigestion or a gallbladder attack. The patient usually becomes ashen, clammy, short of breath, faint, and anxious and often feels that death is imminent. Typical signs are tachycardia, a barely perceptible pulse, low blood pressure, and mildly elevated temperature, cardiac arrhythmia, and electrocardiographic evidence of elevation of the ST segment and Q wave. Potential complications in MI are pulmonary or systemic embolism, pulmonary edema, shock, ventricular tachycardia, ventricular fibrillation, and cardiac arrest.

myocardial insufficiency, inadequate functioning of the heart muscle.

myocardial ischemia, a condition of insufficient blood flow to the heart muscle via the coronary arteries, often resulting in chest pain (angina).

myocardial perfusion, the flow of blood to the heart muscle. In diagnostic imaging thallium 201 or other substances are injected into the blood to reveal areas of myocardial ischemia.

myocardiograph /mī′ōkär′dē·əgraf′/, a tracing device for recording the activity of heart muscle.

myocardiopathy /mī′ōkär′dē·op′əthē/ [Gk, *mys,* muscle, *kardia,* heart, *pathos,* disease], any disease of the myocardium causing enlargement.

myocarditis /mī′ōkärdī′tis/ [Gk, *mys* + *kardia* + *itis,* inflammation], an inflammatory condition of the myocardium. It may be caused by viral, bacterial, or fungal infection; serum sickness; rheumatic fever; or a chemical agent or may be a complication of a collagen disease. Myocarditis most frequently occurs in an acute viral form and is self-limited, but it may lead to acute heart failure.

M

myocardium /mī'ōkär'dē·əm/ [Gk, *mys,* muscle, *kardia,* heart], a thick contractile middle layer of uniquely constructed and arranged muscle cells that forms the bulk of the heart wall. The myocardium contains a minimum of other tissue, except blood vessels, and is covered interiorly by the endocardium. The contractile tissue of the myocardium is composed of fibers with the characteristic crossstriations of muscular tissue. The fibers are about one third as large in diameter as those of skeletal muscle and contain more sarcoplasm. They branch frequently and are interconnected to form a network that is continuous, except where the bundles and the laminae are attached at their origins and insertions into the fibrous trigone of the heart. Most of the myocardial fibers function to contract the heart. —**myocardial,** *adj.*

myoclonus /mī'ōklō'nəs/ [Gk, *mys* + *klonos,* contraction], a spasm of a muscle or a group of muscles. —**myoclonic,** *adj.*

myocyte /mī'əsīt/, a muscle cell.

myodiastasis /mī'ōdī·as'təsis/ [Gk, *mys* + *diastasis,* separation], an abnormal condition in which there is separation of muscle bundles.

myoedema /mī'ō·idē'mə/, muscle edema.

myoelectrical, pertaining to the electrical property of a muscle.

myofascial /mī·ōfā'shəl/, pertaining to a muscle and its fascia.

myofascial pain, jaw muscle distress associated with chewing or exercise of the masticatory muscles.

myofascial release, a group of massage techniques used to relieve soft tissue from the abnormal grip of tight fascia.

myofibril /-fī'bril/ [Gk, *mys* + L, *fibrilla,* small fiber], a slender striated strand within skeletal and cardiac muscle fibers and composed of bundles of myofilaments.

myogelosis /mī'ōjəlō'sis/ [Gk, *mys* + L, *gelare,* to freeze; Gk, *osis*], a condition in which there are hardened areas or nodules within muscles, especially the gluteal muscles.

myogenic /mī'ōjen'ik/ [Gk, *mys* + *genesis,* origin], pertaining to muscles, particularly cardiac and smooth muscles, that do not require nerves to initiate and maintain contractions.

myoglobin /mī'ōglō'bin/ [Gk, *mys* + L, *globus,* ball], a ferrous globin complex consisting of one heme molecule containing one iron molecule attached to a single globin chain. Myoglobin is responsible for the red color of muscle and for its ability to store oxygen.

myoglobinuria /-glō'binōōr'ē·ə/ [Gk, *mys* + L, *globus* + Gk, *ouron,* urine], the presence of myoglobin, a respiratory pigment of muscle tissue, in the urine.

myoglobinuric renal failure /-glob'-inōōr'ik/, a kidney disease in which large amounts of filtered myoglobin coalesce in the tubules, obstructing nephronal flow and producing epithelial cell injury.

myoma /mī-ō'mə/ [Gk, *mys* + *oma,* tumor], a common benign fibroid tumor of the uterine muscle. Menorrhagia, backache, constipation, dysmenorrhea, dyspareunia, and other symptoms develop in proportion to the size, location, and rate of growth of the tumor.

myomectomy /mī'ōmek'təmē/, the surgical removal of muscle tissue.

myometritis /mī'ōmətrī'tis/, an inflammation or infection of the myometrium of the uterus.

myometrium /mī'ōmē'trē·əm/, *pl.* **myometria** [Gk, *mys* + *metra,* womb], the muscular layer of the wall of the uterus. The smooth muscle fibers of the myometrium course around the uterus horizontally, vertically, and diagonally.

myonecrosis /mī'ōnekrō'sis/ [Gk, *mys* + *necrosis,* death], the death of muscle fibers. Progressive or clostridial myonecrosis is caused by the anaerobic bacteria of the genus *Clostridium.* Seen in deep wound infections, progressive myonecrosis is accompanied by pain, tenderness, a brown serous exudate, and a rapid accumulation of gas within the tissue of the muscle.

myoneural /mī'ōnōōr'əl/ [Gk, *mys* + *neuron,* nerve], pertaining to a muscle fiber and its associated neuron, especially to nerve endings in muscles.

myopathy /mī-op'əthē/ [Gk, *mys* + *pathos,* disease], an abnormal condition of skeletal muscle characterized by muscle weakness, wasting, and histologic changes within muscle tissue, as seen in any of the muscular dystrophies. A myopathy is distinct from a muscle disorder caused by nerve dysfunction. —**myopathic,** *adj.*

myope /mī'ōp/, an individual who is nearsighted or afflicted with myopia.

myopia /mī-ō'pē·ə/ [Gk, *myops,* nearsighted], a condition of nearsightedness caused by the elongation of the eyeball or by an error in refraction so that parallel rays are focused in front of the retina. —**myopic,** *adj.*

myorrhaphy /mī·ôr'əfē/ [Gk, *mys* + *rhaphe,* suture], suturing of a wound in a muscle.

myorrhexis /mī'ərek'sis/ [Gk, *mys* + *rhexis,* rupture], tearing of any muscle. —**myorrhectic,** *adj.*

myosarcoma /mī'ōsärkō'mə/ [Gk, *mys* +

sarx, flesh, *oma,* tumor], a malignant tumor of muscular tissue.

myosin /mī′əsin/ [Gk, *mys* + *in,* within], a cardiac and skeletal muscle protein that makes up close to one half of the proteins that occur in muscle tissue. The interaction of myosin and actin is essential for muscle contraction.

myositis /mī′əsī′tis/, inflammation of muscle tissue, usually of voluntary muscle. Causes of myositis include infection, trauma, and infestation by parasites.

myositis fibrosa, an uncommon inflammation of the muscles, characterized by abnormal formation of connective tissue.

myositis ossificans /əsif′əkanz/, a rare inherited disease in which muscle tissue is replaced by bone. It begins in childhood, with stiffness in the neck and back, and progresses to rigidity of the spine, trunk, and limbs.

myositis purulenta, any bacterial infection of muscle tissue. This condition may result in the formation of an abscess or multiple abscesses.

myositis trichinosa /trik′ənō′sə/, inflammation of the muscles resulting from infection by the parasite *Trichinella spiralis.*

myostasis /mī′ōstā′sis/ [Gk, *mys* + *stasis,* standing], an abnormal condition of weakened muscle in which there is a relatively fixed length of muscle fibers in the relaxed state. —**myostatic,** *adj.*

myostroma /mī′əstrō′mə/ [Gk, *mys* + *stroma,* covering], the framework of muscle tissue.

myotenotomy /-tenot′əmē/ [Gk, *mys* + *tenon,* tendon, *temnein,* to cut], surgical division of the whole or part of a muscle by cutting through its main tendon.

myotherapy /-ther′əpē/ a technique of corrective muscle exercises involving pressure on fingers and joints to relieve pain or spasms.

myotome /mī′ətōm/ [Gk, *mys* + *temnein,* to cut], **1.** the muscle plate of an embryonic somite that develops into a voluntary muscle. **2.** a group of muscles innervated by a single spinal segment. **3.** an instrument for cutting or dissecting a muscle.

myotomic muscle /-tom′ik/, any of the numerous muscles of the trunk of the body, derived from the myotomes and divided into the deep muscles of the back and the thoracoabdominal muscles.

myotomy /mī-ot′əmē/ [Gk, *mys* + *temnein,* to cut], the cutting of a muscle, performed to gain access to underlying tissues or to relieve constriction in a sphincter, such as in severe esophagitis or pyloric stenosis.

myotonia /mī′ətō′nē·ə/ [Gk, *mys* + *tonos,* tone], any condition in which a muscle or a group of muscles does not readily relax after contracting. —**myotonic,** *adj.*

myotonia congenita /konjen′itə/, a rare mild and nonprogressive form of myotonic myopathy evident early in life. The only effects of the disorder are hypertrophy and stiffness of the muscles.

myotonic muscular dystrophy /-ton′ik/, a severe form of muscular dystrophy marked by ptosis, facial weakness, and dysarthria. Weakness of the hands and feet precedes that in the shoulders and hips. Myotonia of the hands is usually present.

myotonic myopathy, any of a group of disorders characterized by increased skeletal muscle tone and decreased relaxation of muscle after contraction.

myringectomy /mir′injek′təmē/ [L, *myringa,* eardrum; Gk, *ektome,* excision], excision of the tympanic membrane.

myringitis /mir′inji′tis/ [L, *myringa* + Gk, *itis*], inflammation or infection of the tympanic membrane.

myringomycosis /miring′gōmīkō′sis/ [L, *myringa* + Gk, *mykes,* fungus, *osis,* condition], a fungal infection of the tympanic membrane.

myringoplasty /miring′gōplas′tē/ [L, *myringa* + Gk, *plassein,* to mold], surgical repair of perforations of the eardrum with a tissue graft, performed to correct hearing loss. The openings in the eardrum are enlarged, and the grafting material is sutured over them.

myringotomy /mir′ing·got′əmē/ [L, *myringa* + Gk, *temnein,* to cut], surgical incision of the eardrum, performed to relieve pressure and release pus or fluid from the middle ear. Antibiotics are given before surgery and continued afterward. The drum is incised, and fluid is gently suctioned from the middle ear. Eardrops may be instilled, or tubes may be inserted to improve drainage.

mysophobia /mē′sə-/ [Gk, *mysos,* anything disgusting, *phobos,* fear], an anxiety disorder characterized by an overreaction to the slightest uncleanliness, or an irrational fear of dirt, contamination, or defilement. —**mysophobic, misophobic,** *adj.*

myxedema /mik′sədē′mə/ [Gk, *myxa,* mucus, *oidema,* swelling], the most severe form of hypothyroidism. It is characterized by swelling of the hand, face, feet, and periorbital tissues. At this stage the disease may lead to coma and death.

myxofibroma /mik′sōfībrō′mə/ [Gk, *myxa* + L, *fibra,* fiber; Gk, *oma,* tumor], a fibrous tumor that contains myxomatous tissue.

myxoma /miksō′mə/ [Gk, *myxa* + *oma,* tumor], a neoplasm of the connective tissue, characteristically composed of stellate

M

cells in a loose mucoid matrix crossed by delicate reticulum fibers. These tumors may grow to enormous size and may occur under the skin but are also found in bones, the genitourinary tract, and the retroperitoneal area. —**myxomatous,** *adj.*

myxopoiesis /mik′sōpō·ē′sis/ [Gk, *myxa* + *poiein,* to make], the production of mucus.

myxosarcoma   /mik′sōsärkō′mə/   [Gk, *myxa* + *sarx,* flesh, *oma,* tumor],   a sarcoma that contains some myxomatous tissue.

myxovirus /mik′sōvī′rəs/ [Gk, *myxa* + L, *virus,* poison], any of a group of medium-size ribonucleic acid viruses that are further divided into orthomyxoviruses and paramyxoviruses. Some kinds of myxoviruses are the viruses that cause influenza, mumps, and parainfluenza.

MZ,   abbreviation for **monozygotic.**

n, 2n, 3n, 4n, symbols for the haploid, diploid, triploid, and tetraploid number of chromosomes in a cell, organism, strain, or individual.

N, 1. symbol for the element **nitrogen.** 2. abbreviation for **normal.** 3. abbreviation for *node* in the TNM system for staging malignant neoplastic disease. See also **cancer staging.** 4. symbol for **Avogadro's number.** 5. symbol for **magnetic flux.**

N/1, symbol for **normal solution.**

nA, abbreviation for *nanoampere,* one billionth of an ampere.

Na, chemical symbol for the element **sodium.**

nabothian cyst /nabō'thē·ən/ [Martin Naboth, German physician, 1675–1721; Gk, *kystis,* bag], a cyst formed in a nabothian gland of the uterine cervix. The cyst, which is pearly white and firm, seldom results in adverse or pathologic effects.

nabothian gland [Martin Naboth; L, *glans,* acorn], one of many small, mucussecreting glands of the uterine cervix.

NAD. abbreviation for *no appreciable disease.*

NADH, abbreviation for *nicotine adenine dinucleotide, reduced.*

nadir /nā'dər/, the lowest point, such as the blood count after it has been depressed by chemotherapy.

nadolol /nad'ənol/, a beta-adrenergic blocking agent prescribed for long-term management of angina pectoris, for hypertension, and after myocardial infarction.

NADPH oxidase defect, a disorder in patients with chronic granulomatosis disease. It is caused by a defect in an enzyme (nicotinamide adenine dinucleotide phosphate oxidase) that catalyzes the conversion of oxygen to superoxide anions and hydrogen peroxide in phagocytes. As a result of this defect, the phagocytes are unable to destroy invading microorganisms.

nafcillin sodium /nafsil'in/, an antibacterial prescribed in the treatment of infections caused by penicillinase-producing staphylococci.

Naffziger sign /naf'zigər/, [Howard C. Naffziger, American surgeon, 1884–1961] a diagnostic sign for sciatica or a herniated nucleus pulposus. Nerve root irritation is produced by the examiner through external jugular venous compression.

Naffziger's syndrome [Howard C. Naffziger], a condition of scalene muscle spasms secondary to intervertebral disk disease, cervical rib disease, or other disorder. The spasms result in pressure on the major nerve plexus of the arm; and the patient experiences pain in the neck, shoulder, arm, and hand.

Nägele's rule /nā'gələz/ [Franz K. Nägele, German obstetrician, 1778–1851; L, *regula,* model], a method for calculating the estimated date of delivery based on a mean length of gestation. Three months are subtracted from the first day of the last normal menstrual period, and 1 year plus 7 days are added to that date.

Nager's acrofacial dysostosis /nā'gərz/ [Felix R. Nager, Swiss physician, 1877–1959; Gk, *akron,* extremity; L, *facies,* face; Gk, *dys,* bad, *osteon,* bone, *osis,* condition], an abnormal congenital condition characterized by limb deformities such as radioulnar synostosis, hypoplasia, and the absence of the radius or of the thumbs.

Nahrungs-Einheit-Milch (nem) /nä'-rŏŏngz īn'hīt milsh, milkh/ [Ger, *Nahrung,* food, *Einheit,* unit, *Milch,* milk], a nutritional unit in Pirquet's system of feeding that is equivalent to 1 g of breast milk.

nail [AS, *naegel*], **1.** a flattened elastic structure with a horny texture at the end of a finger or a toe. Each nail is composed of a root, body, and free edge at the distal extremity. The root fastens the nail to the finger or the toe by fitting into a groove in the skin and is closely molded to the surface of the dermis. The nail matrix beneath the body and the root projects longitudinal vascular ridges. The matrix firmly attaches the body of the nail to the underlying connective tissue. The whitish lunula near the root contains irregularly arranged papillae that are less firmly attached to the connective tissue than the rest of the matrix. The cuticle is attached to the surface of the nail just ahead of the root. **2.** any of various metallic nails used in orthopedics to fasten together bones or pieces of bone.

777

nailbed [AS, *naegle*, nail, *bedd*, bed], the corium beneath the nail. It appears through the clear nail as a series of longitudinal ridges.

nail biting, the habit of excessive biting and chewing one's fingernails and periungual skin, sometimes leading to cutaneous injury. The condition is commonly associated with body manipulations of anxious children. It is also considered a form of motor discharges of inner tension.

Nail Care, a Nursing Interventions Classification defined as promotion of clean, neat, attractive nails and prevention of skin lesions related to improper care of nails.

nail fold, a fold of skin supporting the nail at its base.

nail groove [AS, *naegle* + D, *groeve*, groove], a shallow depression between the nail bed and the nail wall.

nail plate, the hard part of the dorsum of the fingers and thumb, a rigid outer covering that extends about 8 mm under the nail fold and arises from the nail bed.

nail plate avulsion, a temporary partial or complete removal of the nail plate without disrupting the underlying matrix cells.

Nalebuff arthrodesis, an arthrodesis of the wrist in which fusion includes the use of a Steinmann pin.

nalidixic acid /nal′idik′sik/, an antibacterial prescribed in the treatment of certain urinary tract infections.

naloxone hydrochloride /nal′əksōn/, a narcotic antagonist prescribed for reversal of narcotic depression or acute narcotic intoxication.

naltrexone hydrochloride /naltrek′sōn/, an oral opioid antagonist prescribed to block the effects of opioid analgesics, including heroin, morphine, and methadone in patients recovering from addiction.

Namaqualand hip dysplasia, an autosomal-dominant genetic defect found in black children. It is characterized by a growth failure in the femoral epiphysis, resulting in pain and early degenerative arthritis of the hip.

NAMI, abbreviation for **National Alliance for the Mentally Ill.**

NANB, abbreviation for *non-A, non-B hepatitis.*

NANDA, abbreviation for **North American Nursing Diagnosis Association.**

nandrolone decanoate /nan′drəlōn/, an androgen prescribed in the treatment of testosterone deficiency, osteoporosis, and female breast cancer, as well as to stimulate growth, weight gain, and the production of red cells.

nandrolone phenpropionate, an anabolic steroid with androgenic properties. It is prescribed in the treatment of osteoporosis, in certain anemias, in metastatic breast cancers of women, and for protein-sparing effects in many situations.

nanism /nā′nizəm, nan′-/ [Gk, *nanos,* dwarf], an abnormal smallness or under-development of the body; dwarfism.

nanocephaly /nā′nōsef′əlē, nan′-/ [Gk, *nanos* + *kephale,* head], a developmental defect characterized by abnormal smallness of the head. —**nanocephalous,** *adj.,* **nanocephalus,** *n.*

nanocormia /nā′nōkôr′mē·ə/ [Gk, *nanos* + *kormos,* trunk], abnormal disproportionate smallness of the trunk of the body in comparison with the head and limbs. —**nanocormus,** *n.*

nanocurie (nc, nCi) /nan′əkyŏŏr′ē/ [Gk, *nanos,* dwarf; Marie and Pierre Curie], a unit of radiation equal to one billionth of a curie.

nanogram (ng) /nan′əgram/ [Gk, *nanos* + Fr, *gramme,* small weight], one billionth (10^{-9}) of a gram.

nanomelia /nā′nōmē′lyə, nan′-/ [Gk, *nanos* + *melos,* limb], a developmental defect characterized by abnormally small limbs in comparison with the size of the head and trunk. —**nanomelous,** *adj.,* **nanomelus,** *n.*

nanometer (nm) /nan′əmē′tər/ [Gk, *nanos* + *metron,* measure], a unit of length equal to one billionth of a meter.

nanophthalmos /nā′nofthal′məs, nan′-/ [Gk, *nanos* + *ophthalmos,* eye], the condition in which one or both eyes are abnormally small, although other ocular defects are not present.

nanosecond (ns) /nan′əsek′ənd/ [Gk, *nanos,* dwarf; L, *secundus,* second], one billionth (10^{-9}) of a second.

nanosomus /nā′nōsō′məs/ [Gk, *nanos* + *soma,* body], a person of very short stature; a dwarf.

nanukayami /nä′nŏŏkäyä′mē/ [Jpn], an acute, infectious disease caused by one of the serotypes of the spirochete *Leptospira* that is indigenous to Japan.

nanus /nā′nəs/, **1.** a dwarf. **2.** a pygmy. —**nanoid** /nā′noid/, *adj.*

napalm /nā′päm/, abbreviation for *napthenate palmitate,* a form of jellied gasoline used in warfare.

napalm burn [AS, *baernan,* burn], a thermal burn caused by contact with flaming **napalm.**

nape [ME], the back of the neck.

naphazoline hydrochloride /nəfaz′əlēn/, an adrenergic vasoconstrictor prescribed in the treatment of nasal congestion and as an ophthalmic vasoconstrictor.

naphthalene poisoning /naf′thəlēn/ [Gk, *naptha,* flammable liquid; L, *potio,* drink], a toxic condition caused by the ingestion of naphthalene or paradichlorobenzene that may cause nausea, vomiting, headache, abdominal pain, spasm, and convulsions. Naphthalene and paradichlorobenzene are common ingredients in mothballs and moth crystals.

naphthol camphor /naf′thol/, a syrupy mixture of two parts of camphor and one part betanaphthol, used externally as an antiseptic.

napkin ring tumor [ME, *nappekin,* tablecloth, *hring,* band; L, *tumor,* swelling], a tumor that encircles a tubular structure of the body, usually impairing its function and constricting its lumen to some degree.

NAP-NAP, abbreviation for **National Association of Pediatric Nurse Associates/Practitioners.**

NAPNES, abbreviation for **National Association for Practical Nurse Education and Services.**

napping [ME, *nappen,* to doze], periods of sleep, usually during the day, which may last from 15 to 60 minutes without attaining the level of deep sleep.

naproxen /naprok′sən/, a nonsteroidal antiinflammatory agent prescribed for the relief of inflammatory symptoms of arthritis.

NAPT, abbreviation for *National Association of Physical Therapists.*

narc, abbreviation for **narcotic.**

narcissism /när′sisiz′əm/ [Gk, *Narcissus,* mythic youth in love with himself], **1.** an abnormal interest in oneself, especially in one's own body and sexual characteristics; self-love. **2.** (in psychoanalysis) sexual self-interest that is a normal characteristic of the phallic stage of psychosexual development, occurring as the infantile ego acquires a libido.

narcissistic personality /när′sisis′tik/, a disposition characterized by behavior and attitudes that indicate an abnormal love of the self.

narcissistic personality disorder, a psychiatric diagnosis characterized by an exaggerated sense of self-importance and uniqueness, an abnormal need for attention and admiration, preoccupation with grandiose fantasies concerning the self, and disturbances in interpersonal relationships, usually involving the exploitation of others and a lack of empathy.

narcoanalysis /-ənal′isis/, an interview conducted while the patient is deeply sedated with medication so that inhibitions are reduced and responses will be more truthful.

narcohypnosis /-hipnō′sis/ [Gk, *narke,* stupor, *hypnos,* sleep], hypnosis induced with the aid of a narcotic drug such as sodium amobarbital or sodium pentothal.

narcolepsy /när′kəlep′sē/ [Gk, *narke,* stupor, *lambanein,* to seize], a syndrome characterized by sudden sleep attacks, cataplexy, sleep paralysis, and visual or auditory hallucinations at the onset of sleep. Persons with narcolepsy experience an uncontrollable desire to sleep, sometimes many times in one day. Episodes may last from a few minutes to several hours. Momentary loss of muscle tone occurs during waking hours (cataplexy) or while the person is asleep.

narcoleptic /när′kəlep′tik/, **1.** pertaining to a condition or substance that causes an uncontrollable desire for sleep. **2.** a narcoleptic drug. **3.** a person suffering from narcolepsy.

Narcon, abbreviation for *Narcotics Anonymous.*

narcosis /närkō′sis/ [Gk, *narkosis,* numbness], a state of insensibility or stupor caused by narcotic drugs.

narcotic (narc) /narkot′ik [Gk, *narkotikos,* benumbing], **1.** pertaining to a substance that produces insensibility or stupor. **2.** a narcotic drug. Narcotic analgesics, derived from opium or produced synthetically, alter perception of pain; induce euphoria, mood changes, mental clouding, and deep sleep; depress respiration and the cough reflex; constrict the pupils; and cause smooth muscle spasm, decreased peristalsis, emesis, and nausea. Repeated use of narcotics may result in physical and psychologic dependence.

narcotic addict, a person who is psychologically and physically dependent on narcotic drugs, a condition in which the drug is present in the body in amounts great enough to be toxic or sufficient to alter behavior.

narcotic antagonist, a drug that is used primarily in the treatment of narcotic-induced respiratory depression. The narcotic antagonists nalorphine, levallorphan, and naloxone are usually administered parenterally.

narcotic poisoning [Gk, *narkotikos,* stupor; L, *potio,* drink], the toxic effects of a narcotic drug that depresses the brain centers, causing unconsciousness or coma. Narcotic drugs are generally derived from opium, but other drugs, including alcohol, can produce similar effects.

narcotize /när′kətiz/, to subject to the influence of narcotics.

nares /ner′ēz/, *sing.* **naris,** the pairs of anterior and posterior openings to the nasal cavity that allow the passage of air to the pharynx and ultimately the lungs during respiration.

nasal (nas) /nā'zəl/ [L, *nasus,* nose], pertaining to the nose and nasal cavity. —**nasally,** *adv.*

nasal airway, a flexible, curved piece of rubber or plastic, with one wide, trumpet-like end and one narrow end that can be inserted through the nose into the pharynx.

nasal balloon tamponade. a procedure for the control of posterior epistaxis in which a nasal balloon is inserted into the nasal cavity and filled with saline solution. Alternatively, a Foley catheter can be placed through the nostril and used in the same manner.

nasal cannula, a device for delivering oxygen by way of two small tubes that are inserted into the nares.

nasal cartilage [L, *nasus,* nose, *cartilago*], a flat plate of cartilage in the lower anterior part of the nasal septum.

nasal cavity, one of a pair of cavities that open on the face through the pear-shaped anterior nares and communicate posteriorly with the pharynx.

nasal decongestant, a drug that provides temporary relief of nasal symptoms in acute and chronic rhinitis and sinusitis. Most are over-the-counter products compounded with a small amount of vasoconstrictor such as ephedrine or phenylephrine.

nasal drip, a method of slowly infusing liquid into a dehydrated infant by means of a catheter inserted through the nose down the esophagus.

nasal fossa, one of the pair of approximately equal chambers of the nasal cavity that are separated by the nasal septum and open externally through the nares and internally into the nasopharynx through the internal nares. Each fossa is divided into an olfactory region, consisting of the superior nasal concha and part of the septum, and a respiratory region, constituting the rest of the chamber.

nasal glioma, a neoplasm characterized by the ectopic growth of neural tissue in the nasal cavity.

nasal instillation of medication, the instillation of a medicated solution into the nostrils by drops from a dropper or by an atomized spray from a squeeze bottle. Drops are instilled in each nostril as the patient's neck is comfortably hyperextended with the head tilted back over the edge of the bed. The patient's mouth should remain open during the procedure, and the head should stay in the tilted back position for several minutes. Nasal spray is administered to the patient in a sitting position.

nasalis /nāzal'is/ [L, *nasus,* nose], one of the three muscles of the nose, divided into a transverse part and an alar part. The transverse part serves to depress the cartilaginous part of the nose and to draw the alar toward the septum. The alar part serves to dilate the nostril.

nasal obstruction [L, *nasus,* nose, *obstruere*], a narrowing of the nasal cavity, thereby reducing the breathing capacity, caused by an irregular septum, nasal polyps, foreign bodies, or enlarged turbinates. Sinusitis is a common complication of the condition.

nasal polyp, a rounded, elongated bit of pulpy, dependent mucosa that projects into the nasal cavity.

nasal septum, the partition dividing the nostrils. It is composed of bone and cartilage covered by mucous membrane.

nasal sinus, any one of the numerous cavities in various bones of the skull, lined with ciliated mucous membrane continuous with that of the nasal cavity. The nasal sinuses are divided into frontal sinuses, ethmoidal air cells, sphenoidal sinuses, and maxillary sinus.

nascent /nas'ənt, nā'sənt/ [L, *nasci,* to be born], **1.** just born; beginning to exist; incipient. **2.** (in chemistry) pertaining to any substance liberated during a chemical reaction, which, because of its uncombined state, is more reactive.

nascent oxygen, oxygen that has just been liberated from a chemical compound.

nasion /nā'zē·on/ [L, *nasus,* nose], **1.** the anthropometric reference point at the front of the skull where the midsagittal plane intersects a horizontal line tangential to the highest points in the superior palpebral sulci. **2.** the depression at the root of the nose that indicates the junction of the intranasal and the frontonasal sutures.

nasogastric feeding /nā'zōgas'trik/ [L, *nasus,* nose; Gk, *gaster,* stomach; AS, *faedan,* to feed], the process of introducing nutrients in a liquid form directly into the stomach via a nasogastric tube.

nasogastric intubation, the placement of a nasogastric tube through the nose into the stomach to relieve gastric distension by removing gas, gastric secretions, or food; to instill medication, food, or fluids; or to obtain a specimen for laboratory analysis. After surgery and in any condition in which the person is able to digest food but not eat it, the tube may be introduced and left in place for tube feeding until the ability to eat normally is restored.

nasogastric suction, the removal by suction of solids, fluids, or gases from the gastrointestinal tract through a tube inserted into the stomach or intestines via the nasal cavity.

nasogastric tube, any tube passed into the stomach through the nose.

nasojejunal tube /nā′zōjijŏŏ′nəl/, a mercury-weighted tube inserted through the nose to allow natural peristaltic movement from the pylorus into the jejunum.

nasolabial [L, *nasus,* nose, *labium,* lip], pertaining to the nose and lip.

nasolabial reflex /nā′zōlā′bē·əl/ [L, *nasus,* nose, *labium,* lip], a sudden backward movement of the head, arching of the back, and extension and stretching of the limbs that occur in infants in response to a light touch to the tip of the nose with an upward sweeping motion.

nasolacrimal /nā′zōlak′riməl/ [L, *nasus + lacrima,* tears], pertaining to the nasal cavity and associated lacrimal ducts.

nasolacrimal duct, a channel that carries tears from the lacrimal sac to the nasal cavity.

nasolacrimal groove [L, *nasus,* nose, *lacrima,* tear; D, *groeve,* a shallow depression], a groove on the nasal surface of the upper jaw.

nasomandibular fixation /nā′zōmandib′yŏŏlər/ [L, *nasus + mandere,* to chew, *figere,* to fasten], a type of maxillomandibular fixation to stabilize fractures of the jaw by using maxillomandibular splints connected to a wire through a hole drilled in the anterior nasal spine of the maxillary bone.

nasomental reflex /-men′təl/ [L, *nasus,* nose, *mentum,* chin, *reflectere,* to bend back], a reflex elicited by tapping the side of the nose, thereby causing contraction of the mentalis muscle with elevation of the lower lip and wrinkling of the skin of the chin.

nasopharyngeal /nā′zōferin′jē·əl/, pertaining to the cavity of the nose and the nasal parts of the pharynx.

nasopharyngeal angiofibroma [L, *nasus + Gk, pharynx,* throat], a benign tumor of the nasopharynx, consisting of fibrous connective tissue with many vascular spaces. Typical signs are nasal and eustachian tube obstruction, adenoidal speech, and dysphagia.

nasopharyngeal cancer, a malignant neoplastic disease of the nasopharynx. Depending on the site of a nasopharyngeal tumor, there may be nasal obstruction, otitis media, hearing loss, sensory or motor nerve damage, bony destruction of the skull, or deep cervical lymphadenopathy. Squamous cell and undifferentiated carcinomas are the most common lesions.

nasopharyngography /-fer′ingog′rəfē/ [L, *nasus + Gk, pharynx,* throat, *graphein,* to record], radiographic imaging and examination of the nasopharynx.

nasopharyngoscopy /nā′zōfer′ing·gos′-kəpē/ [L, *nasus + Gk, pharynx,* throat, *skopein,* to look], a technique in physical examination in which the nose and throat are visually examined using a laryngoscope, a fiberoptic device, a flashlight, and a dilator for the nares. **—nasopharyngoscopic,** *adj.*

nasopharynx /nā′zōfer′ingks/ [L, *nasus + Gk, pharynx,* throat], the uppermost of the three regions of the throat (pharynx), situated behind the nasal cavity and extending from the posterior nares to the level of the soft palate. On the posterior wall of the nasopharynx, opposite the posterior nares, are the pharyngeal tonsils. **—nasopharyngeal,** *adj.*

nasotracheal tube /-trā′kē·əl/ [L, *nasus + Gk, tracheia,* rough artery; L, *tubus*], a catheter inserted into the trachea through the nasal cavity and the pharynx. It is commonly attached to a mechanical ventilator or a resuscitator bag to administer oxygen.

natal /nā′təl/, **1.** [L, *natus*] pertaining to birth. **2.** [L *nates*] pertaining to the nates, or buttocks.

nates /nā′tēz/, *sing.* natis [L, buttocks], the fleshy hillocks at the lower posterior part of the torso comprising fat and the gluteal muscles.

National Alliance for the Mentally Ill (NAMI), a national organization for family members of psychotic patients.

National Association for Practical Nurse Education and Services (NAPNES), an organization concerned with the education of practical nurses and with the services provided by licensed practical nurses in the United States.

National Association of Pediatric Nurse Associates/Practitioners (NAP-NAP), an organization of nurses who are prepared by training or experience to give primary care to pediatric patients in the United States. NAP-NAP works in conjunction with the American Academy of Pediatrics.

National Bureau of Standards (NBS), a federal agency in the Department of Commerce that sets accurate measurement standards for commerce, industry, and science in the United States. The NBS compares and coordinates its standards with those of other countries.

National Committee for Quality Assurance (NCQA), a U.S. independent nonprofit accrediting body for managed health care organizations. Its focus is on improving quality of care in the managed care industry by assessing compliance of health plans to NCQA-developed standards for quality improvement, utilization management, credentialing processes, member rights and responsibilities, preventive services, and record management.

National Council Licensure Examination (NCLEX), a comprehensive integrated examination, developed and administered by the National Council of State Boards of Nursing, designed to test basic competency for nursing practice. The NCLEX-RN test plan has three components, including nursing behaviors grouped under nursing process categories, the process of decision making that defines the role of nursing, and levels of cognitive ability.

National Eye Institute (NEI), one of several institutes of the National Institutes of Health. NEI was established in 1968 to support research in the normal functioning of the human eye and visual system, the pathology of visual disorders, and the rehabilitation of the visually handicapped.

National Formulary (N.F.), a publication containing the official standards for the preparation of various pharmaceutics not listed in the *United States Pharmacopoeia.* It is revised every 5 years.

national health insurance, a health insurance program that is financed by taxes and administered by the government to provide comprehensive health care that is accessible to all citizens of that nation.

National Health Planning and Resources Development Act of 1974, U.S congressional legislation (PL 93-641) that established a nationwide network of health systems agencies. The act provides for the coordination and direction of national health policy through state and regional regulatory agencies.

National Health Service Corps (NHSC), a program of the U.S. Public Health Service (USPHS) in which health care personnel are placed in areas that are underserved. The Corps was established by the Emergency Health Personnel Act of 1970. Nurses, physicians, and dentists serve in rural and urban areas, usually as employees of local health care agencies.

National Institute of Child Health and Human Development (NICHHD), a branch of the National Institutes of Health that is concerned with all aspects of the growth, development, and health of the children of the United States.

National Institute of Mental Health (NIMH), a branch of the (U.S.) National Institutes of Health within the Alcohol, Drug Abuse, and Mental Health Administration. It is responsible for federal research and education programs dealing with mental health.

National Institute on Aging (NIA), a branch of the (U.S.) National Institutes of Health established in 1974. The NIA supports biomedical, social, and behavioral research and education related to aging.

National Institutes of Health (NIH), an agency within the U.S. Public Health Service made up of several institutions and constituent divisions, including the Bureau of Health Manpower Education, the National Library of Medicine, the National Cancer Institute, and several research institutes and divisions.

National League for Nursing (NLN), an organization concerned with the improvement of nursing education and nursing service and the provision of health care in the United States. Among its many activities are accreditation of nursing programs, preadmission and achievement tests for nursing students, and compilation of statistic data on nursing personnel and trends in health care delivery.

National Male Nurses Association (NMNA), an organization that promotes the interests and practice of male nurses in the United States.

National Marrow Donor Program (NMDP), a coordinating center for bone marrow transplants, providing links with national and international registries of prospective volunteer donors of HLA-compatible bone tissue.

National Organization of Victims Assistance, a private nonprofit organization in the United States of victims and witness assistance practitioners, criminal justice professionals, researchers, former victims, and others committed to the recognition of victims' rights.

National Society of Critical Care Nurses of Canada (NSCCN), an organization of Canadian critical care nurses, established originally in 1975 as the Toronto Chapter of the American Association of Critical-Care Nurses. The group became an independent Canadian organization in 1983.

National Student Nurses Association (NSNA), an organization of students in the field of nursing in the United States. Among its purposes are the improvement of nursing education to improve health care, aid in the development of the nursing student, and encourage optimal achievement in the professional role of the nurse and the health care of people.

natremia /nātrē'mē·ə/, [L, *natrium,* sodium; Gk, *haima,* blood], the presence of sodium in the blood.

natriuresis /nā'trēyŏŏrē'sis/ [L, *natrium,* sodium; Gk, *ouresis,* urination], the excretion of greater than normal amounts of sodium in the urine. The condition may result from the administration of natriuretic diuretic drugs or from various metabolic or endocrine disorders.

natriuretic /nā′trēyŏŏret′ik/, **1.** pertaining to the process of natriuresis. **2.** a substance that inhibits the resorption of sodium ions from the glomerular filtrate in the kidneys, thus allowing more sodium to be excreted with the urine.

natural antibody /nach′(ə)rəl/ [L, *natura,* nature; Gk, *anti* + AS, *bodig,* body], an antibody that is present in serum in the absence of an apparent specific antigen contact.

natural childbirth [L, *natura,* nature; AS, *cild,* child; ME, *bwith,* birth], labor and parturition accomplished by a mother with little or no medical intervention. Prerequisites include normal gestation, an adequate birth canal, strong maternal motivation, physical and emotional preparation, and constant and intensive support of the mother during labor and birth.

natural dentition, the entire array of natural teeth in the dental arches at any given time, consisting of deciduous or permanent teeth or a mixture of the two.

natural family planning method, any of several methods of conception control that does not rely on a medication or a physical device for effectiveness in avoiding pregnancy. Some of the methods are also used to pinpoint the time of ovulation to increase the chance of fertilization when artificial insemination or extraction of an oocyte for in vitro fertilization is to be performed. Kinds of natural family planning include **basal body temperature method of family planning, calendar method of family planning, ovulation method of family planning,** and **symptothermal method of family planning.**

natural foods, foods that have been grown, processed, packaged, and stored without the use of chemical additives.

natural immunity, a usually inherent, nonspecific form of immunity to a specific disease.

naturalistic illness /nach′ərəlis′tik/, an illness thought to be caused by impersonal factors such as the Hispanic model of hot and cold forces.

natural killer (NK) cell [L, *natura* + ME, *kullen,* to kill, *cella,* storeroom], a lymphocyte that is capable of binding to and killing virus-infected and some tumor cells by releasing cytotoxins. It is found in the bone marrow and spleen.

natural law, a doctrine that holds there is a natural moral order or natural moral law inherent in the structure of the universe.

natural network, (in psychiatric nursing) a patient's natural contacts in the community, including church and social groups, friends, family, and occupation that support the person's function outside the hospital environment.

natural pacemaker, any cardiac pacing site in the heart tissues, as opposed to an artificial pacemaker.

natural radiation, radioactivity that emanates from the soil and rocks or particles and rays that reach the earth from cosmic sources, such as actinic radiation from the sun.

natural selection, the natural evolutionary processes by which those organisms best suited for adaptation to the environment tend to survive and propagate the species, whereas those unfit are eliminated.

nature versus nurture /nur′chər/, a name given to a long-standing controversy as to the relative influences of genetics versus the environment in the development of personality. Nature is represented by instincts, and genetic factors and nurture by social influences.

naturopath /nach′ərōpath′/ a person who practices naturopathy.

naturopathy /nach′ərop′əthē/ [L, *natura* + Gk, *pathos,* disease], a system of therapeutics based on natural foods, light, warmth, massage, fresh air, regular exercise, and the avoidance of medications. Advocates believe that illness can be healed by the natural processes of the body.

Nauheim bath /nou′hīm/ [Nauheim, Germany; AS, *baeth,* bath], a bath taken in water through which carbon dioxide is bubbled, followed by systematic exercises, used in the treatment of cardiac conditions.

nausea /nô′zē·ə, nô′zhə/ [Gk, *nausia,* seasickness], a sensation accompanying the urge but not always leading to vomiting. Common causes are seasickness and other motion sicknesses, early pregnancy, intense pain, emotional stress, gallbladder disease, food poisoning, and various enteroviruses. —**nauseate,** *v.,* **nauseous,** *adj.*

nausea and vomiting of pregnancy, a common condition of early pregnancy, characterized by recurrent or persistent nausea, often in the morning, that may result in vomiting, weight loss, anorexia, general weakness, and malaise. The causes of the condition are poorly understood. It usually does not begin before the sixth week after the last menstrual period and ends by the twelfth to the fourteenth week of pregnancy.

nauseous /nô′shəs, nô′zē·əs/ [Gk, *nausia,* seasickness], pertaining to feelings of nausea or reaction to things that may stimulate nausea.

navicular /navik′yələr/, boat-shaped; sunken.

navicular pads, tarsal supports for flat feet. They are inserted directly under the arch of the foot.

n.b., abbreviation for the Latin *nota bene,* 'note well.'

Nb, symbol for the element **niobium.**

NBNA, abbreviation for *National Black Nurses Association.*

NBRC, abbreviation for *National Board for Respiratory Care.*

NBS standard, (in nuclear medicine) a radioactive source standardized or certified or both by the National Bureau of Standards.

nc, nCi, abbreviation for **nanocurie.**

NCI, abbreviation for the *National Cancer Institute.*

NCLEX-RN, abbreviation for **National Council Licensure Examination.**

NCQA, abbreviation for **National Committee for Quality Assurance.**

Nd, symbol for the element **neodymium.**

N.D., abbreviation for *Doctor of Naturopathy.*

NDA, abbreviation for *National Dental Association.*

NE, abbreviation for **niacin equivalent.**

Ne, symbol for the element **neon.**

Neal-Robertson litter, a modified spine board for transporting trauma patients with spinal injuries.

near-death experience [ME, *nere* + *deth* + L, *experientia,* trial], the subjective observations of people either who have been close to clinical death or who may have recovered after having been declared dead. Many claim to have witnessed similar episodes of passing through a tunnel toward a bright light and encountering people who had preceded them in death.

near drowning [ME, *nere,* almost, *drounen,* to drown], a pathologic state in which the victim has survived exposure to circumstances that usually cause drowning. Cardiopulmonary resuscitation is performed immediately; hospitalization is always indicated.

nearest neighbor analysis, (in molecular genetics) a biochemical method used to estimate the frequency with which pairs of bases are located next to one another.

nebula /neb′yələ/, *pl.* **nebulae** [L, cloud], **1.** a slight corneal opacity or scar that seldom obstructs vision and that can be seen only by oblique illumination. **2.** a murkiness in the urine. **3.** an oily concoction that is applied with an atomizer.

nebulization /neb′yəlīzā′shən/ [L, *nebula,* cloud; Gk, *izein,* to cause], a method of administering a drug by spraying it into the respiratory passages of the patient.

nebulize /neb′yəlīz/, to vaporize or disperse a liquid in a fine spray.

nebulizer /neb′yəlī′zər/, a device for producing a fine spray. Intranasal medications are often administered by a nebulizer.

NEC, abbreviation for **necrotizing enterocolitis.**

Necator /nekā′tər/ [L, *necare,* to kill], a genus of nematode that is an intestinal parasite and causes hookworm disease.

necatoriasis /nek′ətərī′əsis/ [L, *necare,* to kill; Gk, *osis,* condition], hookworm disease, specifically that caused by *Necator americanus,* the most common North American hookworm. The larvae live in the soil and reach the human digestive tract through contaminated food and water or through the skin of the feet and legs. Symptoms include diarrhea, nausea, abdominal pain, and anemia in the more severe cases.

neck [AS, *hnecca*], a constricted section, such as the part of the body that connects the head with the trunk. Other such constrictions are the neck of the humerus and the neck of the uterus.

neck dissection, surgical removal of the cervical lymph nodes, performed to prevent the spread of malignant tumors of the head and neck.

neck of femur [AS, *hnecca* + L, *femur,* thigh], the part of the long bone of the thigh between the head and the greater and lesser trochanters.

neck righting reflex, 1. an involuntary response in newborns in which turning the head to one side while the infant is supine causes rotation of the shoulders and trunk in the same direction. The reflex enables the child to roll over from the supine to prone position. **2.** any tonic reflex associated with the neck that maintains body orientation in relation to the head.

neck ring, a metal ring at the neck of a cervicothoracolumbosacral orthosis. It opens posteriorly for ease in putting on or removing the orthosis and is an attachment for a throat mold and occiput pads.

neck shaft angle, an angle created by the intersection of a line drawn through the femoral shaft and a line through the femoral head and neck.

necrobiosis /nek′rōbī·ō′sis/, **1.** the death of a small area of cells in a large area of living tissue. **2.** the normal death of tissue cells as a result of changes associated with development, aging, atrophy, or degeneration.

necrobiosis lipoidica /nek′rōbī·ō′sis lipoi′dikə/ [Gk, *nekros,* dead, *bios,* life, *lipos,* fat, *eidos,* form], a skin disease characterized by thin, shiny, yellow-to-red plaques on the shins or forearms. Telangiectases, crusting, and ulceration of these plaques may occur.

necrobiotic /bī·ot′ik/, pertaining to necrobiosis.

necrobiotic granulomas, granulomas that share some of the characteristics of both immunologic and nonimmunologic collections of mononuclear phagocytes. Relatively acellular areas of the skin become necrobiotic, and the collagen assumes a homogenous, amorphous appearance.

necrogenic /nek′rōjen′ik/ [Gk, *nekros,* dead, *genein,* to produce], **1.** capable of causing death, as of cells or tissue. **2.** originating or caused by infected dead matter.

necrology (necrol) /nekrol′əjē/ [Gk, *nekros,* dead, *logos,* science], the study of the causes of death, including the compilation and interpretation of mortality statistics.

necrolysis /nekrol′isis/ [Gk, *nekros* + *lysis,* loosening], disintegration or exfoliation of dead tissue. **—necrolytic,** *adj.*

necrophilia /nek′rōfil′yə/ [Gk, *nekros* + *philein,* to love], **1.** a morbid liking for being with dead bodies. **2.** a morbid desire to have sexual contact with a dead body, usually of men to perform a sexual act with a dead woman. **—necrophile, necrophiliac,** *n.*

necrophobia [Gk, *nekros,* death, *phobos,* fear], a morbid fear of death and dead bodies.

necrosis /nekrō′sis/ [Gk, *nekros* + *osis,* condition], localized tissue death that occurs in groups of cells in response to disease or injury. In **coagulation necrosis,** blood clots block the flow of blood, causing tissue ischemia distal to the clot; in **gangrenous necrosis,** ischemia combined with bacterial action causes putrefaction to set in.

necrotaxis /nek′rōtak′sis/, the attraction of leukocytes to dead or dying cells.

necrotic /nekrot′ik/, pertaining to the death of tissue in response to disease or injury.

necrotic arachnidism, tissue destruction caused by spider venom.

necrotizing /nek′rōtī′zing/ [Gk, *nekros,* death], causing the death of tissues or organisms.

necrotizing enteritis [Gk, *nekros* + *izein,* to cause, *enteron,* intestine, *itis*], acute inflammation of the small and large intestine by the bacterium *Clostridium perfringens,* characterized by severe abdominal pain, bloody diarrhea, and vomiting.

necrotizing enterocolitis (NEC), an acute inflammatory bowel disorder that occurs primarily in preterm or low–birth weight neonates. It is characterized by ischemic necrosis of the gastrointestinal (GI) mucosa that may lead to perforation and peritonitis. The cause of the disorder is unknown, although it appears to be a defect in host defenses with infection resulting from normal GI flora rather than from invading organisms.

necrotizing vasculitis, an inflammatory condition of blood vessels, characterized by necrosis, fibrosis, and proliferation of the inner layer of the vascular wall. Some cases result in occlusion and infarction. Necrotizing vasculitis may occur in rheumatoid arthritis and is common in systemic lupus erythematosus, periarteritis nodosa, and progressive systemic sclerosis.

needle bath [AS, *naedl,* needle], a shower in which fine jets of water are sprayed over the body.

needle biopsy, the removal of a segment of living tissue for microscopic examination by inserting a hollow needle through the skin or the external surface of an organ or tumor and rotating it within the underlying cellular layers.

needle filter, a device, usually made of plastic, used for filtering medications that are drawn into a syringe before administration.

needle holder, a surgical forceps used to hold and pass a suturing needle through tissue.

needlestick injuries, accidental skin punctures resulting from contact with hypodermic syringe needles. The contact may occur accidentally during efforts to inject a patient or as a result of carelessly touching discarded medical waste. Such injuries can be dangerous, particularly if the needle has been used in treatment of a patient with a severe blood-borne infection such as human immunodeficiency virus. To prevent injuries, used needles are not capped or broken and are disposed of in a rigid puncture-resistant container located near the site of use.

NEEP, abbreviation for **negative end-expiratory pressure.**

Neer and Horowitz classification system, a method of classifying proximal humeral fractures in children based on the degree of separation of the epiphysis from the shaft.

Neer classification system, a method of classifying femoral supracondylar and intercondylar fractures. The system ranges from *type I* for minimal displacement through *type IIA* and *IIB* to *type III* for conjoined supracondylar and shaft fractures. The Neer system is also applied to humeral head and neck fractures.

nefazodone hydrochloride, an antidepressant drug prescribed in the treatment of mental depression in adults.

negative (neg) /neg′ətiv/ [L, *negare,* to deny persistently], **1.** (of a laboratory test) indicating that a substance or a reaction is not present. **2.** (of a sign) indicating on physical examination that a finding is not present, often meaning that there is no pathologic change. **3.** (of a substance) tending to carry or carrying a negative chemical charge.

negative anxiety, (in psychology) an emotional and psychologic condition in which anxiety prevents a person's normal functioning and interrupts the person's ability to perform the usual activities of daily living.

negative catalysis, a decrease in the rate of any chemical reaction caused by a substance that is not consumed and not affected by the reaction.

negative electrode [L, *negare,* to deny; Gk, *elektron,* amber, *hodos,* way], a cathode, or the negative pole of an electric current or of a battery or dry cell.

negative end-expiratory pressure (NEEP), a technique to counterbalance the increase in mean intrathoracic pressure caused by intermittent positive-pressure breathing in an effort to return negative intrathoracic pressure for venous return to the right atrium.

negative feedback, 1. (in physiology) a decrease in function in response to a stimulus; for example, the secretion of follicle-stimulating hormone decreases even as the amount of circulating estrogen increases. **2.** *informal.* a critical, derogatory, or otherwise negative response from one person to what another person has communicated.

negative identity, the assumption of a persona that is at odds with the accepted values and expectations of society.

negative pathognomonic symptom [L, *negare,* to deny; Gk, *pathos,* disease. *gnomen,* index, *symptoma,* that which happens], any symptom that is not usually found in a specific condition and that, if present, would not be compatible with the diagnosis.

negative pi meson (pion), a form of electromagnetic radiation emitted from a proton linear accelerator.

negative pi meson (pion) radiotherapy, a form of radiotherapy using a negative pi meson (pion) beam emitted by a proton linear accelerator. In the treatment of certain tumors, negative pi meson particles are beamed at the tumor; the atomic nuclei of malignant cells take in the radioactive particles and explode, scattering intensely radioactive subatomic particles through the adjacent malignant tissue.

negative pressure, less than ambient atmospheric pressure, such as in a vacuum, at an altitude above sea level, or in a hypobaric chamber.

negative punishment, a form of behavior modification in which the removal of something after an operant (behavior) decreases the probability of the operant's recurrence.

negative reinforcer, (in psychology) a stimulus that, when presented immediately after occurrence of a particular behavior, decreases the rate of occurrence of the behavior.

negative relationship, (in research) an inverse relationship between two variables; as one variable increases, the other decreases.

negative staining, a technique in which an electron-dense substance is mixed with a specimen, resulting in an electron microscopic image in which the specimen appears translucent against an opaque or dark background.

negativism /neg′ətiviz′əm/ [L, *negare,* to deny persistently], a behavioral attitude characterized by opposition, resistance, the refusal to cooperate with even the most reasonable request, and the tendency to act in a contrary manner.

negatron /neg′ətron/, an electron or beta particle with a single negative charge.

neglect /nəglekt′/, a condition that occurs when a parent or guardian fails to provide minimal physical and emotional care for a child or other dependent person.

negligence /neg′lijəns/ [L, *negligentia,* carelessness], (in law) the commission of an act that a prudent person would not have done or the omission of a duty that a prudent person would have fulfilled, resulting in injury or harm to another person.

negligence per se, (in law) a finding of negligence rendered in judgment of a professional action or inaction in violation of a statute or so at odds with common sense that beyond any doubt no prudent person would have been guilty of it.

Negri bodies /nā′grē/ [Adelchi Negri, Italian physician, 1876–1912; AS, *bodig*], intracytoplasmic inclusion bodies found in the brain and central nervous system cells of rabies victims.

NEI, abbreviation for **National Eye Institute.**

Neisseria /nīser′ē·ə/ [Albert L. S. Neisser, Polish dermatologist, 1855–1916], a genus of aerobic to facultatively anaerobic bacteria of the family Neisseriaceae. The gram-negative cocci, which appear in pairs with adjacent sides flattened, are among the normal flora of genitourinary and upper respiratory tracts. Pathogenic species include gonococcus and meningococcus forms.

Neisseriaceae /nī′serē·as′ī-ē/ [Albert L. S. Neisser], a family of four genera of gram-negative aerobic cocci and rod-shaped bacteria occurring singly or in pairs, chains, or clusters. The genera are *Actinobacter, Kingella, Moraxella,* and *Neisseria.*

Neisseria gonorrhoeae [Albert L. S. Neisser; Gk, *gone,* seed, *rhoia,* flow], a gram-negative, nonmotile diplococcal bacterium usually seen microscopically as flattened pairs within the cytoplasm of neutrophils. It is the causative organism of gonorrhea.

Neisseria sicca [Albert L. S. Neisser], a species of dry or slimy white-to-yellow bacteria normally found in the human nasopharynx and in saliva and sputum.

NEJM, abbreviation for *New England Journal of Medicine.*

Nélaton's dislocation /nālätôNz′/ [Auguste Nélaton, French surgeon, 1807–1873], a dislocation of the ankle in which the distal ends of the tibia and fibula are separated and the talus is forced upward between the tibia and fibula.

Nelson's syndrome [Donald H. Nelson, American physician, b. 1925], an endocrine disorder that may follow adrenalectomy for Cushing's disease. It is characterized by a marked increase in the secretion of adrenocorticotropic hormone and melanocyte-stimulating hormone by the pituitary gland.

nem, abbreviation for **Nahrungs-Einheit-Milch.**

nematocides /nəmat′əsīdz/ [Gk, *nema, thread, eidos, form,* L, *caedere,* to kill], chemical pesticides that are used to kill nematode worms.

nematocyst /nem′ətōsist′/ [Gk, *nema,* thread, *eidos,* form, *kystis,* bag], a barbed threadlike process on the surface of coelenterates and attached to a poison sac. The stinger, found on the Portuguese man-of-war and other types of jellyfish, can be ejected into the skin of a human or animal, causing painful and potentially fatal injury.

nematode /nem′ətōd/ [Gk, *nema + eidos,* form], a multicellular, parasitic animal of the phylum Nematoda. All roundworms belong to the phylum.

nematodiasis /nem′ətōdī′əsis/ [Gk, *nema,* thread, *eidos,* form, *osis,* condition], an infestation of nematode worms.

neoadjuvant therapy /nē′ō·ad′jəvənt/, a preliminary cancer treatment, such as chemotherapy or radiation, that usually precedes another phase of treatment.

neoantigen /-an′tijən/ [Gk, *neos,* new, *anti,* against, *genein,* to produce], a new specific antigen that develops in a tumor cell.

neobehaviorism /-bihā′vē·əriz′əm/ [Gk, *neos* + ME, *behaven,* behavior], a school of psychology based on the general principles of behaviorism but broader and more flexible in concept. It stresses experimental research and laboratory analyses in the study of overt behavior and in various subjective phenomena that cannot be directly observed and measured.

neobehaviorist /-ist/, a disciple of the school of neobehaviorism.

neoblastic /-blas′tik/ [Gk, *neos + blastos,* germ], pertaining to a new tissue or development within a new tissue.

neocerebellum /-ser′əbel′əm/, those parts of the cerebellum that receive input via the corticopontocerebellar pathway.

neocortex /-kôr′teks/ [Gk, *neos,* new; L, *cortex,* bark], the most recently evolved part of the brain. In humans the neocortex includes all of the cerebral cortex except for the hippocampal and piriform areas.

neodymium (Nd) /-din′ē·əm/ [Gk, *neos + didymos,* twin], a rare earth element. Its atomic number is 60; its atomic weight (mass) is 144.27.

neogenesis /-jen′əsis/, a process of new tissue formation.

neoglottis /-glot′is/, a vibrating structure that replaces the glottis in alaryngeal speech, such as after a laryngectomy.

neologism /nē·ol′əjiz′əm/ [Gk, *neos + logos,* word], **1.** a word or term newly coined or used with a new meaning. **2.** (in psychiatry) a word coined by a psychotic or delirious patient that is meaningful only to the patient.

neomycin sulfate /-mī′shn/, an aminoglycoside antibiotic prescribed in the treatment of infections of the intestine, in hepatic coma, and topically in the treatment of skin infections.

neon (Ne) /nē′on/ [Gk, *neos,* new], a colorless, odorless gaseous element and one of the inert gases. Its atomic number is 10; its atomic weight (mass) is 20.18. Neon has no compounds and occurs in the atmosphere in the ratio of about 18 parts per million.

neonatal /-nā′təl/ [Gk, *neos* + L, *natus,* born], the period of time covering the first 28 days after birth.

neonatal abstinence syndrome, a behavioral pattern of irritability, tremulousness, and inconsolability exhibited in newborns exposed to heroin and methadone. Follow-

N

ing treatment during the neonatal period, the abnormal signs usually resolve. In some infants hypertonicity has persisted for 6 months.

Neonatal Behavioral Assessment Scale (NBAS), a scale for evaluating and assessing an infant's alertness, motor maturity, irritability, consolability, and interaction with people. It consists of a series of 27 reaction tests, including response to inanimate objects, pinprick, light, and sound of a rattle or bell.

neonatal breathing, respiration in newborns that begins when pulmonary fluid in the lungs is expelled by mechanic compression of the thorax during delivery and resorption from the alveoli into the bloodstream and lymphatics. As air enters the lungs, the chest and lungs recoil to a resting position, but forceful inspirations are necessary to keep the lungs inflated.

neonatal death, the death of a live-born infant during the first 28 days after birth. Early neonatal death is usually considered to be one that occurs during the first 7 days.

neonatal developmental profile, an evaluation of the developmental status of a newborn based on three examinations: a gestational age inventory, a neurologic examination, and a Neonatal Behavioral Assessment score.

neonatal intensive care unit (NICU), a hospital unit containing a variety of sophisticated mechanic devices and special equipment for the management and care of premature and seriously ill newborns.

neonatal mortality, the statistic rate of infant death during the first 28 days after live birth, expressed as the number of such deaths per 1000 live births in a specific geographic area or institution in a given time.

neonatal period, the interval from birth to 28 days of age. It represents the time of the greatest risk to the infant.

neonatal pustular melanosis, a transient skin condition of the neonate characterized by vesicles present at birth that become pustular. The lesions contain neutrophils rather than eosinophils.

neonatal thermoregulation, the regulation of the body temperature of a newborn, which may be affected by evaporation, conduction, radiation, and convection. The infant is kept covered and protected from any means of heat loss. Because the surface area of the newborn's head is proportionately large when compared with the body, heat loss from the head may be great; therefore a cap or fold of blanket is placed around the head.

neonatal unit, a unit of a hospital that

provides care and treatment of newborns through the age of 28 days, and longer if necessary.

neonatal vital signs monitor, equipment in a specialized neonatal intensive care unit that measures mean blood pressure and mean heart rate from a plastic blood pressure cuff, with values digitally displayed on a monitor.

neonate /nē′ənāt/, an infant from birth to 28 days of age.

neonatology /nē′ōnātol′əjē/ [Gk, *neos* + L, *natus,* born; Gk, *logos,* science], the branch of medicine that concentrates on the care of the neonate and specializes in the diagnosis and treatment of the disorders of the newborn. **—neonatologic, neonatological,** *adj.,* **neonatologist,** *n.*

neonatorum encephalitis /-nātôr′əm/ [Gk, *neos,* new; L, *natus,* born; Gk, *enkephalos,* brain, *itis,* inflammation], a brain inflammation that develops in the first 4 weeks of life.

neoplasia /nē′ōplā′zhə/ [Gk, *neos* + *plassein,* to mold], the new and abnormal development of cells that may be benign or malignant. **—neoplastic** /-plas′tik/, *adj.*

neoplasm /nē′ōplaz′əm/ [Gk, *neos* + *plasma,* formation], any abnormal growth of new tissue, benign or malignant. **—neoplastic,** *adj.*

neoplastic /nē′ōplas′tik/ [Gk, *neos,* new, *plassein,* to mold], pertaining to **neoplasty.**

neoplastic fracture, a fracture resulting from a weakness in bone tissue caused by neoplasm or a malignant growth.

neoplastic pericarditis [Gk, *neos,* new, *plasma,* something formed, *peri,* around, *kardia,* heart, *itis,* inflammation], a pericardial inflammation, usually secondary to a malignant tumor within the area.

neoplastic transformation, conversion of a tissue with a normal growth pattern into a malignant tumor.

neoplasty /nē′ōplas′tē/ [Gk, *neos,* new, *plassein,* to mold], a plastic surgery procedure to restore a part or add a new part.

neostigmine bromide /nē′ōstig′mēn/, a cholinergic prescribed in the treatment of myasthenia gravis.

neostriatum /-strī·ā′təm/ the most recently evolved part of the corpus striatum, consisting of the caudate nucleus and putamen. The neostriatum receives input from the entire cerebral cortex and other brain areas and provides output to the basal nuclei.

neoteny /nē·ot′ənē/ [Gk, *neos,* new, *teinein,* to stretch], the attainment of sexual maturity during the larval stage of development such as in certain amphibians.

nephelometer /nef′əlom′ətər/ [Gk, *neph-*

ele, cloud, *metron,* measure], a photometric apparatus used to determine the concentration of solids suspended in a liquid or a gas, such as may be used to determine the number of bacteria in a specimen.

nephelometry /nef′əlom′ətrē/, a technique of determining the concentration of solids suspended in a liquid or gas by use of a nephelometer. **—nephelometric, nephelometrical,** *adj.*

nephrectomy /-ek′təmē/ [Gk, *nephros,* kidney, *ektome,* excision], the surgical removal of a kidney, performed to remove a tumor or otherwise diseased kidney.

nephritic /nəfrit′ik/ [Gk, *nephros,* kidney, *itis,* inflammation], pertaining to an inflammation of the kidney.

nephritic factor, a protein found in the serum of patients with membranoproliferative glomerulonephritis. It activates alternative complement pathways.

nephritic gingivitis [Gk, *nephros* + L, *icus,* like, *gingiva,* gum; Gk, *itis,* inflammation], an inflammatory stomatitis and gingivitis associated with kidney function failure, accompanied by pain, ammoniac odor, and increased salivation.

nephritic syndrome, a group of signs and symptoms of a urinary tract disorder, including hematuria, hypertension, and renal failure.

nephritis /nəfrī′tis/ [Gk, *nephros* + *itis,* inflammation], any one of a large group of diseases of the kidney characterized by inflammation and abnormal function.

nephroangiosclerosis /nef′rō·an′jē·ō′sklerō′sis/ [Gk, *nephros* + *angeion,* vessel, *skleros,* hard, *osis,* condition], necrosis of the renal arterioles, associated with hypertension. Early signs of the condition are headaches, blurring of vision, and a diastolic blood pressure greater than 120 mm Hg. Examination of the retina reveals hemorrhages, vascular exudates, and papilledema. The heart is usually enlarged, especially the left ventricle. Proteins and red blood cells are found in the urine.

nephrocalcinosis /nef′rōkal′sinō′sis/ [Gk, *nephros* + L, *calx,* lime; Gk, *osis,* condition], an abnormal condition of the kidneys in which deposits of calcium form in the parenchyma at the site of previous inflammation or degenerative change.

nephrocystitis /-sistī′tis/, an inflammation involving both the kidney and the urinary bladder.

nephrocystosis /sistō′sis/, the formation of cysts in the kidney.

nephrogenic /nef′rōjen′ik/ [Gk, *nephros* + *genein,* to produce], **1.** generating kidney tissue. **2.** originating in the change.

nephrogenic ascites, the abnormal presence of fluid in the peritoneal cavity of patients undergoing hemodialysis for renal failure. The cause of this type of ascites is unknown.

nephrogenic cord, either of the paired longitudinal ridges of tissue that lie along the dorsal surface of the coelom in the early developing vertebrate embryo. It gives rise to the structures making up the embryonic urogenital system.

nephrogenic diabetes insipidus, an abnormal condition in which the kidneys do not concentrate the urine, resulting in polyuria, polydipsia, and very dilute urine.

nephrogenous /nəfroj′ənəs/, pertaining to the formation and development of the kidneys.

nephrography /nəfrog′rəfē/, radiographic imaging of the kidney.

nephrohypertrophy /-hīpur′trəfē/ [Gk, *nephros,* kidney, *hyper,* excessive, *trophe,* nourishment], enlargement of the kidney.

nephrolith /nef′rəlith/ [Gk, *nephros* + *lithos,* stone], a calculus formed in a kidney. **—nephrolithic,** *adj.*

nephrolithiasis /nef′rōlithī′əsis/, a disorder characterized by the presence of calculi in the kidney.

nephrolithotomy /lithot′əmē/, the surgical removal of renal calculi.

nephrology /nəfrol′əjē/ [Gk, *nephros* + *logos,* science], the study of the anatomy, physiology, and pathology of the kidney. **—nephrologic, nephrological,** *adj.*

nephrolytic /-lit′ik/ [Gk, *nephros* + *lysis,* loosening], pertaining to the destruction of the structure and function of a kidney.

nephron /nef′ron/ [Gk, *nephros,* kidney], a structural and functional unit of the kidney, resembling a microscopic funnel with a long stem and two convoluted tubular sections. Each kidney contains about 1.25 million nephrons, each consisting of the renal corpuscle, the loop of Henle, and the renal tubules. Juxtamedullary nephrons have loops of Henle, whereas cortical nephrons do not. Each renal corpuscle consists of the glomerulus of renal capillaries enclosed within Bowman's capsule.

nephronia /nəfrō′nē·ə/, an inflammation of intrarenal connective tissue that occurs in a small percentage of patients with urinary tract infections.

nephroparalysis /-pəral′isis/ [Gk, *nephros,* kidney, *paralyein,* to be palsied], a paralysis of the kidney resulting in a cessation of its functions.

nephropathy /nefrop′əthē/ [Gk, *nephros* + *pathos,* disease], any disorder of the kidney, including inflammatory, degenerative, and sclerotic conditions.

nephropexy /nef'rəpek'sē/ [Gk, *nephros* + *pexis*, fixation], a surgical operation to fixate a floating or ptotic kidney.

nephroptosis /nef'rəptō'sis/ [Gk, *nephros* + *ptosis*, falling], a downward displacement or dropping of a kidney.

nephrorrhaphy /nəfrôr'əfē/ [Gk, *nephros* + *rhaphe*, suture], an operation that sutures a floating kidney in place.

nephroscope /nef'rəskōp'/ [Gk, *nephros* + *skopein*, to look], a fiberoptic instrument that is used specifically for the disintegration and removal of renal calculi. An ultrasonic probe emitting high-frequency sound waves breaks up the calculi, which are removed by suction through the scope.

nephrostoma /-stō'mə/ [Gk, *nephros* + *stoma*, mouth], the funnel-shaped ciliated opening of the excretory tubules into the coelom of the early developing vertebrate embryo. —**nephrostomic,** *adj.*

nephrostomy /nəfros'təmē/, a surgical procedure in which a flank incision is made so that a catheter can be inserted into the kidney pelvis for the purpose of drainage.

nephrotic syndrome /nəfrot'ik/ [Gk, *nephros* + L, *icus*, like], an abnormal condition of the kidney characterized by marked proteinuria, hypoalbuminemia, and edema. It occurs in glomerular disease and thrombosis of a renal vein and as a complication of many systemic diseases, diabetes mellitus, amyloidosis, systemic lupus erythematosus, and multiple myeloma. —**nephrotic,** *adj.*

nephrotome /nef'rətom/ [Gk, *nephros* + *tome*, section], a zone of segmented mesodermal tissue in the developing vertebrate embryo. It is the primordial tissue for the urogenital system and gives rise to the nephrogenic cord.

nephrotomography /-təmog'rəfē/ [Gk, *nephros* + *tome*, section, *graphein*, to record], sectional radiographic examination of the kidneys.

nephrotomy /nəfrot'əmē/ [Gk, *nephros* + *temnein*, to cut], a surgical procedure in which an incision is made in the kidney.

nephrotoxic /-tok'sik/ [Gk, *nephros* + *toxikon*, poison], toxic or destructive to a kidney.

nephrotoxin /-tok'sin/, a toxin with specific destructive properties for the kidneys.

nephroureterolithiasis /nef'rōyoo'rétərōlithī'əsis/, the presence of calculi in the kidneys and ureters.

neptunium (Np) /nept(y)ōō'nē-əm/ [planet Neptune], a transuranic, metallic element. Its atomic number is 93; its atomic weight (mass) is 237.

Nernst equation [Hermann W. Nernst, German physicist, 1864–1941; L, *ae-*

quare, to make equal], (in cardiology) an expression of the relationship between the electrical potential across a membrane and the concentration ratio between permeable ions on either side of the membrane.

nerve /nurv/ [L, *nervus*], one or more bundles of impulse-carrying fibers that connect the brain and spinal cord with other parts of the body. Nerves transmit afferent impulses from receptor organs toward the brain, spinal cord, and efferent impulses peripherally to the effector organs. Each nerve consists of an epineurium enclosing fasciculi of nerve fibers, each fasciculus surrounded by its own sheath of connective tissue.

nerve accommodation, the ability of nerve tissue to adjust to a constant source and intensity of stimulation so that some change in either intensity or duration of the stimulus is necessary to elicit a response beyond the initial reaction.

nerve cable graft, a multistrand free nerve graft, taken from elsewhere in the body, to bridge a large gap in one of the main nerves in the forearm.

nerve compression, a pathologic event that causes harmful pressure on one or more nerve trunks, resulting in nerve damage and muscle weakness or atrophy. Any nerve that passes over a rigid prominence is vulnerable, and the degree of damage depends on the magnitude and duration of the compressive force.

nerve conduction test, an electrodiagnostic test of the integrity of the peripheral nerves. It involves placing an electrical stimulator over a nerve and measuring the time required for an impulse to travel over a measured segment of the nerve. The test is used in the diagnosis of nerve entrapment syndrome and polyneuropathies.

nerve entrapment, an abnormal condition and type of mononeuropathy, characterized by nerve damage and muscle weakness or atrophy. The peripheral nerve trunks are especially vulnerable to entrapment in which repeated compression results in significant impairment. Nerves that pass over rigid prominences or through narrow bony and fascial canals are particularly prone to entrapment. The common signs of this disorder are pain and muscular weakness. One of the most common types of entrapment is **carpal tunnel syndrome.**

nerve excitability [L, *nervus,* nerve, *excitare,* to rouse], the readiness of a nerve cell to respond to a stimulus.

nerve fiber, a slender process, the axon of a neuron. Each fiber is classified as myelinated or unmyelinated. Myelinated fibers are further designated as A or B fibers; C fibers are unmyelinated. The A fibers are somatic. B fibers are more finely myelinated than A fibers. They are both afferent and efferent and are mainly associated with visceral innervation. The unmyelinated C fibers are efferent postganglionic autonomic fibers and afferent fibers that conduct impulses of prolonged, burning pain sensation from the viscera and periphery.

nerve graft, the transplantation of all or part of a nerve. The procedure may be performed in cases in which the gap in a severed nerve is too large to be repaired by suture alone. The graft provides a pathway that encourages the regrowth of severed axons from the central stump of the damaged nerve. Donor material may consist of heterografts, homografts, or autografts.

nerve growth factor (NGF), a protein resembling insulin whose hormonelike action affects differentiation, growth, and maintenance of neurons.

nerve plexus [L, *nervus,* nerve, *plexus,* plaited], an interwoven network of nerves, such as the lumbar plexus formed by the anterior primary branch of the upper four lumbar nerves.

nerve root impingement, the abnormal protrusion of body tissue into the space occupied by a spinal nerve root. Causes may include disk herniation, tissue prolapse, and inflammation.

nerve sheath [L, *nervus,* nerve; AS, *scaeth*], any of several types of coatings or coverings for nerve fibers and nerve tracts. Kinds of nerve sheaths include **endoneurial, medullary, myelin, neurilemma,** and **notochordal.**

nervous emesis [L, *nervus* + Gk, *emesis,* vomiting], vomiting that is functional and psychogenic. The condition is most common among young women and is regarded as a psychologic representation of a desire to reject something.

nervous prostration [L, *nervus* + *prosternere,* to throw down], a condition of irritable weakness and depression, which may be psychogenic or the result of a severe prolonged illness or exhausting experience.

nervous system [L, *nervus,* nerve; Gk, *system*], the extensive, intricate network of structures that activates, coordinates, and controls all the functions of the body. It is divided into the central nervous system, composed of the brain and spinal cord, and the peripheral nervous system, which includes the cranial nerves and the spinal nerves. These morphologic subdivisions combine and communicate to innervate the somatic and visceral parts of the body with the afferent and efferent nerve fibers.

Afferent fibers carry sensory impulses to the central nervous system; efferent fibers carry motor impulses from the central nervous system to the muscles and other organs. The somatic fibers are associated with the bones, muscles, and skin. The visceral fibers are associated with the internal organs, blood vessels, and mucous membranes.

nervous tachypnea [L, *nervus* + Gk, *tachys,* rapid, *pnoia,* breath], a neurotic symptom characterized by quick shallow breathing.

nested nails, in orthopedic surgery, a pair of nails placed side by side in the medullary canal of long bones.

net charge, the arithmetic sum of positive and negative charges.

net protein utilization (NPU), a measure of protein quality that is based on the percentage of ingested nitrogen that is retained by the body. Because NPU does not take into account differences in the digestibility of proteins, it gives a poorly digested but good-quality protein a false low value.

net radiation, the arithmetic difference between solar radiation received and outgoing terrestrial radiation.

nettle rash [AS, *netele,* nettle; Fr, *rasche,* scurf], a fine, urticarial eruption resulting from skin contact with stinging nettle, a common weed with leaves containing histamine. It is characterized by stinging and itching that lasts from a few minutes to several hours.

Network Design Group, a Medicare-specific oversight group that maintains a log of enrollee complaints related to service and quality of care issues reported to the U.S. Health Care Financing Administration. It participates in investigation of complaints.

networking, 1. the process of developing and using an interaction format with professional colleagues and agencies. 2. (in psychiatric nursing) the process of developing a set of agencies and professional personnel who are able to create a system of communication and support for psychiatric patients, usually those recently discharged from inpatient psychiatric facilities. 3. a network of supportive contacts or services such as the Women's Health Network.

network-model HMO, a managed care system analogous to the group-model health maintenance organization (HMO), but services are provided at multiple sites by multiple groups so a wider geographic area is served. Physicians treat HMO and private patients.

net wt, abbreviation for *net weight.*

Neufeld nail /nyo͞of'əld/ [Alonzo J. Neufeld, American surgeon, b. 1906], an orthopedic nail with a V-shaped tip and shank used for fixating an intertrochanteric fracture. The nail is driven into the neck of the femur until it reaches a round metal plate screwed onto the side of the femur.

Neufeld roller traction, a traction device for a fractured femur, consisting of a cast for the calf and thigh hinged at the knee and suspended by a line to the anterior midthigh looped around a pulley and to a spring attached to the anterior midleg.

Neuman, Betty, a nursing theorist who developed the Neuman Systems Model, first published in 1972. Her model is influenced by Gestalt theory, which states that the homeostatic process is the process by which an organism maintains its equilibrium. Major concepts include total persons approach, holism, open system, lines of resistance and lines of defense, degree of reaction, interventions, levels of prevention, and reconstitution. A spiritual variable was added to her model later and created-environment was added to the typology.

neural /no͞or'əl/ [Gk, neuron, nerve], pertaining to nerve cells and their processes.

neural cell-adhesion molecules, an immunoglobulin that functions as a molecular recognition molecule.

neural crest, the ectodermally derived cells along the outer surface of each side of the neural tube in the early stages of embryonic development.

neural ectoderm, the part of the embryonic ectoderm that develops into the neural tube.

neural fold, either of the paired longitudinal elevations resulting from the invagination of the neural plate in the early developing embryo. The folds unite to enclose the neural groove and form the neural tube.

neuralgia /no͞oral'jə/ [Gk, neuron + algos, pain], an abnormal condition characterized by severe stabbing pain, caused by a variety of disorders affecting the nervous system. —**neuralgic,** adj.

neuralgic amyotrophy /no͞oral'jik/, a brachial plexus disorder characterized by sudden pain and muscle weakness in the upper limbs and possible muscular wasting or atrophy. The cause is unknown.

neural groove, the longitudinal depression that occurs between the neural folds during the invagination of the neural plate to form the neural tube in the early stages of embryonic development.

neural plate, a thick layer of ectodermal tissue that lies along the central longitudinal axis of the early developing embryo and gives rise to the neural tube and subsequently to the brain, spinal cord, and other tissues of the central nervous system.

neural tube, the longitudinal tube lying along the central axis of the early developing embryo that gives rise to the brain, spinal cord, and other neural tissue of the central nervous system.

neural tube defect (NTD), any of a group of congenital malformations involving defects in the skull and spinal column that are caused primarily by the failure of the neural tube to close during embryonic development. In some instances the cleft results from an abnormal increase in cerebrospinal fluid pressure on the closed neural tube during the first trimester of development. The defect may occur at any point along the neural axis or extend the entire length of the spinal column.

neural tube formation, the various processes and stages involved in the embryonic development of the neural tube, which subsequently differentiates into the brain, the spinal cord, and other neural tissue of the central nervous system.

neuraminidase, an enzyme that catalyzes the cleavage of N-acetyl neuraminic acid from mucopolysaccharides. A hereditary deficiency of the enzyme causes sialidosis.

neurapraxia /no͞or'əprak'sē·ə/, the interruption of nerve conduction without loss of continuity of the axon.

neurasthenia /no͞or'əsthē'nē·ə/ [Gk, neuron + a + sthenos, without strength], **1.** an abnormal condition characterized by nervous exhaustion and a vague functional fatigue that often follows depression. **2.** (in psychiatry) a stage in the recovery from a schizophrenic experience, during which the patient is listless and apparently unable to cope with routine activities and relationships. —**neurasthenic,** adj.

neurasthenic /-əsthē'nik/ [Gk, neuron, nerve, asthenia, disability], pertaining to a disorder characterized by excessive fatigue, insomnia, weakness, anxiety, and mental and physical irritability.

neurectomy /no͞oek'təmē/ [Gk, neuron, nerve, ektome, excision], the surgical excision of a nerve segment.

neurenteric canal /no͞or'ənter'ik/ [Gk, neuron + enteron, intestine; L, canalis, channel], a tubular passage between the posterior part of the neural tube and the archenteron in the early embryonic development of lower animals.

neurilemma /no͞or'əlem'ə/ [Gk, neuron + lemma, sheath], a layer of cells composed of one or more Schwann cells that forms the segmented myelin sheaths of

peripheral nerve fibers. It is necessary for regeneration of peripheral nerves when they have been severed. —**neurilemmal, neurilemmatic, neurilemmatous,** *adj.*

neurinoma /noŏr'ino'mə/ [Gk, *neuron* + *oma,* tumor], **1.** a tumor of the nerve sheath. It is usually benign but may undergo malignant change. A kind of neurinoma is **acoustic neuroma. 2.** a neuroma.

neuritic plaque /noŏrit'ik/, an extracellular deposit consisting of beta-amyloid protein mixed with branches of dying nerve cells in the brain of a patient with Alzheimer's disease.

neuritis /noŏrī'tis/, *pl.* **neuritides** [Gk, *neuron* + *itis,* inflammation], an abnormal condition characterized by inflammation of a nerve. Some of the signs of this condition are neuralgia, hypesthesia, anesthesia, paralysis, muscular atrophy, and defective reflexes.

neuroaminodase spikes /noŏr'ō·amē'-nədās/, projections from surfaces of influenza viruses containing neuraminidase that are involved in the release of viruses from infected cells.

neuroanatomy /noŏr'ō·ənat'əmē/, the branch of biology that is concerned with the structure of the nervous system.

neuroarthropathy /-ärthrop'əthē/ [Gk, *neuron* + *arthron,* joint, *pathos,* disease], a condition in which a disease of a joint is secondary to a disease of the nervous system.

neurobiology /-bī'ol'əje/, a branch of biology that is concerned with the anatomy and physiology of the nervous system.

neuroblast /noŏr'əblast/ [Gk, *neuron* + *blastos,* germ], any embryonic cell that develops into a functional neuron; an immature nerve cell. —**neuroblastic,** *adj.*

neuroblastoma /noŏr'ōblastō'mə/ [Gk, *neuron* + *blastos,* germ, *oma,* tumor], a highly malignant tumor composed of primitive ectodermal cells derived from the neural plate during embryonic life. The tumor may originate in any part of the sympathetic nervous system but is most common in the adrenal medulla. Neuroblastomas metastasize early and widely to lymph nodes, liver, lungs, and bone. Symptoms may include an abdominal mass, respiratory distress, and anemia. Hormonally active adrenal lesions may cause irritability, flushing, sweating, hypertension, and tachycardia.

neurobrucellosis /-broō'səlo'sis/, a serious complication of a brucellosis infection that affects the nervous system and may cause meningitis, stroke, cranial nerve lesions, or mycotic aneurysms. The condition may require treatment with drugs that cross the blood-brain barrier.

neurocentral /-sen'trəl/ [Gk, *neuron* + *kentron,* center], pertaining to the centrum and the developing vertebrae in the early stages of embryology.

neurocentrum /-sen'trəm/ [Gk, *neuron* + L, *centrum,* center], the embryonic mesodermal tissue that subsequently gives rise to the vertebrae.

neuro check [Gk, *neuron* + ME, *chek,* stop], *nontechnical.* a brief neurologic assessment. The level of consciousness is evaluated as alert and oriented, lethargic, stuporous, or comatose. The movements of the extremities are determined to be voluntary or involuntary. The pupils of the eyes are observed for equality of dilation, reactivity to light, and ability to accommodate.

neurochemistry /-kem'istrē/, a branch of neurology that is concerned with the biochemistry of the nervous system.

neurocirculatory asthenia /-sur'kyələtô-r'ē/ [Gk, *neuron* + L, *circulare,* to go around; Gk, *a* + *sthenos,* without strength], a psychosomatic disorder characterized by nervous and circulatory irregularities, including dyspnea, palpitation, giddiness, vertigo, tremor, precordial pain, and increased susceptibility to fatigue.

neurocoele /noŏr'əsēl/ [Gk, *neuron* + *koilos,* hollow], a system of cavities in the central nervous system of humans and other vertebrate animals. It consists of the ventricles of the brain and the central canal of the spinal cord.

neurocytolysin /-sītol'isin/, a toxic substance in snake venom that destroys nerve cell membranes.

neurocytolysis /sītol'isis/, the destruction of nerve cells.

neurocytoma /noŏr'ōsītō'mə/ [Gk, *neuron* + *kytos,* cell, *oma,* tumor], a tumor composed of undifferentiated nerve cells that are usually ganglionic.

neurodermatitis /-dur'mətī'tis/ [Gk, *neuron* + *derma,* skin, *itis,* inflammation], a nonspecific, pruritic skin disorder seen in anxious, nervous individuals. Excoriations and lichenification are found on easily accessible, exposed areas of the body such as the forearms and forehead.

neurodevelopmental adaptation /-dəvel'-əpmen'təl/, a type of therapy that emphasizes the inhibition/integration of primitive postural patterns and promotes the development of normal postural reactions and achievement of normal tone. The therapy is used in the treatment of children with cerebral palsy.

neuroectoderm /noŏr'ō·ek'tədurm/ [Gk, *neuron* + *ektos,* outside, *derma,* skin], the part of the embryonic ectoderm that gives rise to the central and peripheral nervous systems, including some glial cells. —**neuroectodermal,** *adj.*

neuroendocrine /nŏŏr′ō·en′dəkrin/ [Gk, *neuron,* nerve, *endon,* within, *krinein,* to secrete], pertaining to or resembling the effects produced by endocrine glands strongly linked with the nervous system.

neuroepithelioma /nŏŏr′ō·ep′ithē′lē·ō′mə/ [Gk, *neuron* + *epi,* upon, *thele,* nipple, *oma,* tumor], an uncommon neoplasm of neuroepithelium in a sensory nerve.

neurofibril /-fī′bril/, a threadlike structure found in the cytoplasm of a neuron.

neurofibrillary tangles /-fī′briler′ē/, an intracellular clump of neurofibrils made of insoluble protein in the brain of a patient with Alzheimer's disease.

neurofibroma /nŏŏr′ōfībrō′mə/ [Gk, *neuron* + L, *fibra,* fiber; Gk, *oma,* tumor], a fibrous tumor of nerve tissue resulting from the abnormal proliferation of Schwann cells. Multiple growths in the peripheral nervous system are often associated with abnormalities in other tissues.

neurofibromatosis /nŏŏr′ōfī′brōmətō′sis/ [Gk, *neuron* + *fibra,* fiber; Gk, *oma,* tumor, *osis,* condition], a congenital condition transmitted as an autosomal-dominant trait, characterized by numerous neurofibromas of the nerves and skin; café-au-lait spots on the skin; and developmental anomalies of the muscles, bones, and viscera.

neurogen /nŏŏr′əjən/ [Gk, *neuron* + *genein,* to produce], a substance within the early developing embryo that stimulates the primary organizer to initiate the formation of the neural plate, which gives rise to the primary axis of the body.

neurogenesis /-jen′əsis/ [Gk, *neuron* + *genesis,* origin], the development of the tissue of the nervous system. —**neurogenetic,** *adj.*

neurogenic /-jen′ik/ [Gk, *neuron* + *genesis,* origin], **1.** pertaining to the formation of nervous tissue. **2.** the stimulation of nervous energy. **3.** originating in the nervous system.

neurogenic arthropathy, an abnormal condition associated with neural damage, characterized by the gradual and usually painless degeneration of a joint.

neurogenic bladder, dysfunction of the urinary bladder caused by a lesion of the nervous system. Treatment is aimed at enabling the bladder to empty completely and regularly, preventing infection, controlling incontinence, and preserving kidney function.

neurogenic fracture, a fracture associated with the destruction of the nerve supply to a specific bone.

neurogenic hoarseness, a sign of unilateral vocal cord paralysis. It is asymptomatic, but there may be excessive air escape during speech as a result of incomplete closure of the glottis. Extra effort is required to generate enough air flow to make speech sounds. Untreated, there is a danger of aspiration pneumonia.

neurogenic impotence, penile erectile dysfunction caused by neurologic disorders. The disorders may involve the parasympathetic sacral spinal cord or the peripheral efferent autonomic fibers to the penis.

neurogenic shock, a form of shock that results from peripheral vascular dilation.

neuroglia /nŏŏrog′lē·ə/ [Gk, *neuron* + *glia,* glue], the supporting or connective tissue cells of the central nervous system. Kinds of neuroglia include **astrocytes, oligodendroglia, microglia,** and **ependyma cells.** —**neuroglial,** *adj.*

neurography /nŏŏrog′rəfē/, **1.** the study of the action potentials of the nerves. **2.** a technique for visualization of peripheral nerve activity by graphic representation of data obtained by media contrast radiographics or by electric recording.

neurohormone /nŏŏr′əhôr′mōn/, a hormone produced in neurosecretory cells such as those of the hypothalamus and released into the bloodstream, the cerebrospinal fluid, or intercellular spaces of the nervous system. The product may or may not be a true systemic hormone such as epinephrine. When the hormone is not a true hormone, it may be a cell product that induces the release of a tropic hormone, which in turn stimulates an endocrine gland to release a systemic hormone.

neurohypophyseal hormone /-hī′pōfiz′ē·əl/ [Gk, *neuron* + *hypo,* under, *phyein,* to grow], a hormone secreted by the posterior pituitary gland. Kinds of neurohypophyseal hormones are **oxytocin** and **vasopressin.**

neurohypophysis /-hīpof′isis/ [Gk, *neuron* + *hypo,* under, *phyein,* to grow], the posterior lobe of the pituitary gland that is the release point of antidiuretic hormone (ADH), vasopressin, and oxytocin. Nervous stimulation from the hypothalamus controls the release of the substances into the blood. The neurohypophysis releases ADH when stimulated by the hypothalamus by an increase in the osmotic pressure of extracellular fluid in the body. The neurohypophysis releases oxytocin under appropriate stimulation from the hypothalamus.

neuroimmunology /nŏŏr′ō·im′yŏŏnol′əjē/ [Gk, *neuron* + L, *immunis,* freedom; Gk, *logos,* science], the study of relationships between the immune and nervous systems, such as autoimmune activity in neurologic diseases.

neurol, abbreviation for **neurology.**

neurolepsis /-lep'sis/ [Gk, *neuron* + *lepsis,* seizure], an altered state of consciousness, as induced by a neuroleptic agent, characterized by quiescence, reduced motor activity, decreased anxiety, and indifference to the surroundings. Sleep may occur, but usually the person can be aroused and can respond to commands.

neurolepsy /nŏŏr'əlep'sē/, a mental state characterized by the blocking of autonomic reflexes, as in hypnosis or antipsychotic drug-induced disorders.

neuroleptanalgesia /-lept'anəljē'zē·ə/ [Gk, *neuron* + *lepsis,* seizure, *a* + *algos,* without pain], a form of analgesia achieved by the concurrent administration of a neuroleptic and an analgesic. Anxiety, motor activity, and sensitivity to painful stimuli are reduced; the person is quiet and indifferent to the environment and surroundings. Sleep may or may not occur, but the patient is not unconscious and is able to respond to commands.

neuroleptanesthesia /-lept'anəsthē'zhə/ [Gk, *neuron* + *lepsis,* seizure, *anaisthesia,* lack of feeling], a form of anesthesia achieved by the administration of a neuroleptic agent, a narcotic analgesic, and nitrous oxide with oxygen. Induction of anesthesia is slow, but consciousness returns quickly after the inhalation of nitrous oxide is stopped.

neuroleptic /-lep'tik/ [Gk, *neuron* + *lepsis,* seizure], pertaining to neurolepsis.

neuroleptic drug, a substance that produces a sedating or tranquilizing effect, such as the butyrophenone derivative, droperidol, and the phenothiazines.

neuroleptic malignant syndrome [Gk *neuron,* nerve, *lepsis,* seizure; L, *malignus,* bad disposition; Gk, *syn,* together, *dromos,* course], a complication of psychotherapy with neuroleptic drugs given in therapeutic doses. It is characterized by hypertonicity, pallor, dyskinesia, hyperthermia, incontinence, unstable blood pressure, and pulmonary congestion.

neurolinguistic programing /-ling·gwis'-tik/, a communication approach based on a conceptualization of levels of experience within the person and levels of the self. It involves both verbal and nonverbal messages, sensory experience, and awareness or perception through behavior patterns that can be observed and perceived.

neurologic assessment /-loj'ik/ [Gk, *neuron* + *logos,* science; L, *icus,* like, *adsidere,* to approximate], an evaluation of the patient's neurologic status and symp-

toms. If alert and oriented, the patient is asked about instances of weakness, numbness, headaches, pain, tremors, nervousness, irritability, or drowsiness. Information is elicited regarding loss of memory, periods of confusion, hallucinations, and episodes of loss of consciousness. The patient's general appearance, facial expression, attention span, responses to verbal and painful stimuli, emotional status, coordination, balance, cognition, and ability to follow commands are noted. If the patient is disoriented, stuporous, or comatose, demonstrated signs of these states are recorded.

neurologic examination, a systematic examination of the nervous system, including an assessment of mental status, the function of each of the cranial nerves, sensory and neuromuscular function, the reflexes, and proprioception and other cerebellar functions.

Neurologic Monitoring, a Nursing Interventions Classification defined as collection and analysis of patient data to prevent or minimize neurologic complications.

neurologist /nŏŏrol'əjist/, a physician who specializes in the nervous system and its disorders.

neurology (neurol.) /nŏŏrol'əjē/ [Gk, *neuron* + *logos,* science], the field of medicine that deals with the nervous system and its disorders. **—neurologic, neurological,** *adj.* **neurologist,** *n.*

neuroma /nŏŏrō'mə/ [Gk, *neuron* + *oma,* tumor], a benign neoplasm composed chiefly of neurons and nerve fibers, usually arising from a nerve tissue. Pain radiating from the lesion to the periphery of the affected nerve is usually intermittent but may become continuous and severe.

neuroma cutis, a neoplasm in the skin that contains nerve tissue and may be extremely sensitive to painful stimuli.

neuromatosis /nŏŏr'ōmətō'sis/ [Gk, *neuron* + *oma,* tumor, *osis,* condition], a neoplastic disease characterized by numerous neuromas.

neuromechanism /-mek'əniz'əm/, a neurologic system whose components work together to produce a central nervous system function.

neuromodulator, a substance that alters nerve impulse transmission.

neuromotor /nŏŏr'ōmō'tər/ [Gk, *neuron,* nerve; L, *mover,* to move], pertaining to both the nerves and muscles or to nerve impulses transmitted to muscles.

neuromuscular /nŏŏr'ōmus'kyŏŏlər/ [Gk, *neuron* + L, *musculus,* muscle], pertaining to the nerves and muscles.

neuromuscular blockade, the inhibition of a muscular contraction activated by the nervous system, possibly resulting in muscle weakness or paralysis.

neuromuscular blocking agent, a chemical substance that interferes locally with the transmission or reception of impulses from motor nerves to skeletal muscles. Nondepolarizing agents such as metocurine, pancuronium, and tubocurarine competitively block the transmitter action of acetylcholine at the postjunctional membrane. Depolarizing blocking agents such as succinylcholine chloride compete with acetylcholine for cholinergic receptors of the motor end plate. Neuromuscular blocking agents are used to induce muscle relaxation in anesthesia, endotracheal intubation, and electroshock therapy and as adjuncts in the treatment of tetanus, encephalitis, and poliomyelitis.

neuromuscular electrical stimulator (NMES), equipment designed to aid in improving or modulating muscular activation. The equipment may be a portable unit for home treatment of a patient needing muscle stimulation over a long period of time or a large clinical model capable of setting a wider variety of waveforms and modulations of the stimulus. The NMES generates pulses or impulses that produce controlled muscle contractions similar to those that occur physiologically. Unless nerve degeneration has occurred, muscles that are weak or paralyzed because of central nervous system involvement should contract when NMES is applied. The procedure may first be tested on an uninvolved muscle on the same or another extremity to establish a normal response.

neuromuscular junction, the area of contact between the ends of a large myelinated nerve fiber and a fiber of skeletal muscle.

neuromuscular spindle, any one of a number of small bundles of delicate muscular fibers, enclosed by a capsule, in which sensory nerve fibers terminate. The nerve fibers end as naked axons encircling the intrafusal fibers with flattened expansions or ovoid disks.

neuromyal transmission /-mī'əl/ [Gk, *neuron* + *mys,* muscle; L, *transmittere,* to transmit], the passage of excitation from a motor neuron to a muscle fiber at the myoneural junction.

neuromyelitis /nŏŏr'ōmī'əlī'tis/ [Gk, *neuron* + *myelos,* marrow, *itis,* inflammation], an abnormal condition characterized by inflammation of the spinal cord and peripheral nerves.

neuron /nŏŏr'on/ [Gk, nerve], the basic nerve cell of the nervous system, containing a nucleus within a cell body and extending one or more processes. Neurons can be classified according to the direction in which they conduct impulses or according to the number of processes they extend. Sensory neurons transmit nerve impulses toward the spinal cord and the brain. Motor neurons transmit nerve impulses from the brain and spinal cord to the muscles and glandular tissue. Multipolar neurons, bipolar neurons, and unipolar neurons are classified according to the number of processes they extend to the different kinds of neurons.

neuronal /nŏŏr'ənəl, nŏŏrō'nəl/ [Gk, *neuron,* nerve], pertaining to or resembling a neuron.

neuronal antibody, an antibody found in the cerebrospinal fluid of most systemic lupus erythematosus (SLE) patients with neuropsychiatric manifestations and in some SLE patients without such manifestations.

neuronal sprouting, the growth of axons or dendrites from a damaged neuron or from an intact neuron that projects to an area denervated by damage to other neurons.

neuronitis /nŏŏr'ənī'tis/ [Gk, *neuron* + *itis,* inflammation], inflammation of a nerve or a nerve cell, especially the cells and the roots of the spinal nerves.

neuroparalysis /-pəral'isis/, loss of muscle power as a result of a disorder involving the part of the nervous system affecting the muscle.

neuropathic joint disease /-path'ik/ [Gk, *neuron* + *pathos,* disease], a chronic progressive degenerative disease of one or more joints, characterized by swelling, joint instability, hemorrhage, heat, and atrophic and hypertrophic changes in the bone. The disease is the result of an underlying neurologic disorder, such as tabes dorsalis from syphilis, diabetic neuropathy, leprosy, or congenital absence or depression of pain sensation.

neuropathic pain syndrome, a condition of autonomic hyperactivity that results in sharp, stinging, or stabbing pain. The disorder is usually noninflammatory but may result in the destruction of peripheral nerve tissue. It may also be accompanied by changes in skin color, temperature, and edema.

neuropathy /nŏŏrop'əthē/ [Gk, *neuron* + *pathos,* disease], inflammation or degeneration of the peripheral nerves, such as that associated with lead poisoning. **neuropathic,** *adj.*

neuropeptide Y (NPY), a natural substance that signals the brain to begin eating. Leptin, a hormone that induces the brain to lose weight, reduces the output of

NPY from the hypothalamus, a major production center.

neurophysin /-fiz'is/, one of a group of proteins released from the posterior pituitary gland at the same time as the hormone vasopressin or oxytocin. It is cleared from a larger protein of which vasopressin or oxytocin is a part.

neuroplasty /nŏŏr'əplas'tē/ [Gk, *neuron,* nerve, *plassein,* to mold], plastic surgery to repair a nerve.

neuroplegia /nŏŏr'ōplē'jē·ə/ [Gk, *neuron* + *plege,* stroke], nerve paralysis caused by disease, injury, or the effect of neuroleptic drugs, administered to achieve **neuroleptanalgesia** or **neuroleptanesthesia.**

neuropore /nŏŏr'opôr/ [Gk, *neuron* + *poros,* pore], the opening at each end of the neural tube during early embryonic development.

neuropraxia /-prak'sē·ə/ [Gk, *neuron,* nerve, *prassein,* to do], a condition in which a nerve remains in place after a severe injury, although it no longer transmits impulses.

neuropsychiatrist /-sīkī'ətrist/, a physician who deals with the relationship between neural processes and psychiatric disorders.

neuropsychiatry /-sīkī'ətrē/, a branch of medicine that deals with problems of psychiatry as it relates to the neurophysiology of brain functions.

neuroradiography /-rā'dē·og'rəfē/, radiography of the tissues of the nervous system.

neuroradiology /-rā'dē·ol'əjē/, the branch of radiology concerned with diagnosing diseases of the central nervous system.

neurorrhaphy /nŏŏrôr'əfē/ [Gk, *neuron, nerve, rhaphe,* suture], a surgical procedure to suture a severed nerve.

neurosarcoidosis /-sär'koidō'sis/, a granulomatous disease that may involve any part of the nervous system but most commonly affects the cranial and spinal nerves. Cranial nerve involvement may result in facial paralysis, whereas spinal nerve involvement may manifest as mononeuritis multiplex. If the central nervous system is affected, the vasculature of the brain may be damaged, resulting in stroke.

neurosarcoma /-särkō'mə/ [Gk, *neuron* + *sarx,* flesh, *oma,* tumor], a malignant neoplasm composed of nerve, connective, and vascular tissues.

neuroscience /nŏŏr'ōsī'əns/ [Gk, *neuron,* nerve; L, *scientia*], the study of neurology and related subjects, including neuroanatomy, neurophysiology, neuropharmacology, and neurosurgery.

neurosis [Gk, *neuron,* nerve, *osis.* condition], *informal;* an emotional disturbance other than psychosis.

neuroskeleton /-skel'ətən/ [Gk, *neuron,* nerve, *skeletos,* dried up], the parts of the skeleton that surround or otherwise protect the nervous system, particularly the skull and vertebrae.

neurosurgery /-sur'jərē/ [Gk, *neuron* + *cheirourgos,* surgeon], any surgery involving the brain, spinal cord, or peripheral nerves. Brain surgery is performed to treat a wound, remove a tumor or foreign body, relieve pressure in intracranial hemorrhage, excise an abscess, treat parkinsonism, or relieve pain. Kinds of brain surgery include craniotomy, lobotomy, and hypophysectomy. Surgery of the spine is performed to correct a defect, remove a tumor, repair a ruptured intervertebral disk, or relieve pain. Kinds of spinal surgery include fusion and laminectomy. Surgery on the peripheral nerves is performed to remove a tumor, relieve pain, or reconnect a severed nerve. One kind of nerve surgery is **sympathectomy.**

neurosyphilis /-sif'ilis/ [Gk, *neuron* + *sys,* hog, *philein,* to love], infection of the central nervous system by *Treponema pallidum,* the causative agent of syphilis, which may invade the meninges and cerebrovascular system. **—neurosyphilitic,** *adj.*

neurotendinous /-ten'dinəs/ [Gk, *neuron,* nerve; L, *tendo,* tendon], pertaining to both nerves and tendons.

neurotendinous spindle [Gk, *neuron* + L, *tendo,* tendon; AS, *spinel,* spindle], a capsule containing enlarged tendon fibers, found chiefly near the junctions of tendons and muscles.

neurotensin /-ten'sin/, a peptide neurotransmitter found in various parts of the brain. It is involved in vasodilation, hypotension, and pain perception.

neurotensinoma /-ten'sinō'mə/, a neuroendocrine tumor of the gastrointestinal tract. Its major secreted product is neurotensin. The tumor originates in nonbeta islet cells but, unlike other neuroendocrine tumors, it has no distinguishing clinical features.

neurotic [Gk, *neuron* + *osis,* condition; L, *icus,* like], **1.** pertaining to neurosis or a neurotic disorder. **2.** pertaining to the nerves. **3.** one who is afflicted with a neurosis. **4.** *informal.* an emotionally unstable person.

neurotic personality [Gk, *neuron,* nerve, *osis,* condition; L, *personalis,* of a person], a disposition characterized by traits and tendencies that increase the likelihood of a specific neurotic behavior. For example, the orderly, cautious, meticulous person may be prone to development of an obsessive-compulsive disorder.

neurotmesis /noŏr'ōtmē'sis/ [Gk, *neuron* + *tmesis,* cutting apart], a peripheral nerve injury in which the nerve is completely disrupted by laceration or traction.

neurotologic /noŏr'ōtōloj'ik/, pertaining to the study of the elements of the ear as they relate to the brain and nervous system.

neurotology /noŏr'ōtol'əjē/, a branch of otology concerned with those parts of the nervous system related to the ear, especially the inner ear and associated brainstem structures.

neurotomy /noŏrot'əmē/, the surgical division of a nerve or nerves.

neurotoxic /noŏr'ōtok'sik/, having a poisonous effect on nerves and nerve cells, such as when ingested lead degenerates peripheral nerves.

neurotoxicity /-toksis'itē/ [Gk, *neuron,* nerve, *toxikon,* poison], the ability of a drug or other agent to destroy or damage nervous tissue.

neurotoxin /noŏr'ōtok'sin/ [Gk, *neuron* + *toxikon,* poison], a toxin that acts directly on the tissues of the central nervous system, traveling along the axis cylinders of the motor nerves to the brain. The toxin may be secreted in the venom of certain snakes, or it may be present on the spines of a shell or in the flesh of fish or shellfish; it may be produced by certain bacteria or by the cellular disintegration of certain bacteria.

neurotransmitter /-transmit'ər/ [Gk, *neuron* + L, *transmittere,* to transmit], any one of numerous chemicals that modify or result in the transmission of nerve impulses between synapses. Neurotransmitters are released from synaptic knobs into synaptic clefts and bridge the gap between presynaptic and postsynaptic neurons. When a nerve impulse reaches a synaptic knob, thousands of neurotransmitter molecules squirt into the synaptic cleft and bind to specific receptors. This flow allows an associated diffusion of potassium and sodium ions that causes an action potential.

neurotripsy /-trip'sē/, the surgical crushing of a nerve.

neurotrophic /trof'ik/, nourishing nerve cells.

neurotropic viruses /-trop'ik/ [Gk, *neuron,* nerve, *tropein,* to turn, *virus,* poison], viruses with an unexplained attraction to nerve tissue. The predilection also applies to certain toxic chemicals.

neurotropism /noŏrot'rəpiz'əm/ [Gk, *neuron,* nerve, *trepein,* to turn], **1.** the tendency for certain microorganisms, poisons, and nutrients to be attracted to nervous tissue. **2.** the tendency of basic dyes to be attracted to nervous tissue.

neurula /noŏr'ələ/, *pl.* **neurulas, neurulae** [Gk, *neuron,* nerve], an early embryo during the period of neurulation when the nervous system tissue begins to differentiate. The embryo at this level of growth represents a third stage in embryonic development.

neurulation /-ā'shən/ [Gk, *neuron* + L, *atus,* process], the development of the neural plate and the processes involved with its subsequent closure to form the neural tube during the early stages of embryonic development.

neutral /n(y)oō'trəl/ [L, *neutralis,* neuter], the state exactly between two opposing values, qualities, or properties; for example, in electricity a neutral state is one in which there is neither a positive nor a negative charge; in chemistry a neutral state is one in which a substance is neither acid nor alkaline.

neutralization /-īzā'shən/ [L, *neutralis* + Gk, *izein,* to cause], the interaction between an acid and a base that produces a solution that is neither acidic nor basic. The usual products of neutralization are a salt and water.

neutral rotation, the position of a limb that is turned neither toward nor away from the body's midline. When a person is supine and the leg is neutrally rotated, the toes should point straight up.

neutral thermal environment, an environment created by any method or apparatus to maintain the normal body temperature to minimize oxygen consumption and caloric expenditure, such as in an incubator for a premature infant.

neutron /n(y)oō'tron/ [L, *neuter,* neither; Gk, *elektron,* amber], (in physics) an elementary particle that is a constituent of the nuclei of all elements except the ^1H form of hydrogen. It has no electric charge and is approximately the same size as a proton.

neutron activation analysis, the analysis of elements in a specimen, performed by exposing it to neutron irradiation to convert many elements to a radioactive form in which they can be identified by measuring their emissions of radiation.

neutropenia /noō'trōpē'nē·ə/ [L, *neuter,* neither; Gk, *penia,* poverty], an abnormal decrease in the number of neutrophils in the blood. The decrease may be relative or absolute. Neutropenia is associated with acute leukemia, infection, rheumatoid arthritis, vitamin B_{12} deficiency, and chronic splenomegaly.

neutrophil /noo'trəfil/ [L, *neuter* + Gk, *philein,* to love], a polymorphonuclear, granular leukocyte that stains easily with neutral dyes. The nucleus contains three to five lobes connected by slender threads of chromatin. The cytoplasm contains fine, inconspicuous granules. Neutrophils are the circulating white blood cells essential for phagocytosis and proteolysis by which bacteria, cellular debris, and solid particles are removed and destroyed.

neutrophilia /-fil'yə/, an elevated number of neutrophils in the blood, a common cause of leukocytosis.

Neviaser procedure, the surgical transfer of a coracoacromial ligament to the clavicle for acromioclavicular separation.

nevirapine, an antiretroviral nonnucleoside analog prescribed in the treatment of human immunodeficiency virus infection.

nevoid basal cell carcinoma syndrome /nē'void/, an inherited form of premalignant skin lesion. It is an autosomal-dominant trait, but the cause is unknown. It is associated with other abnormalities of the skin or bone, the nervous system, the eyes, and the reproductive system. It affects persons under the age of 20 and is accompanied by palmar pits, mandibular cysts, bifid ribs, and other birth defects.

nevoid neuroma [L, *naevus,* birthmark; Gk, *eidos,* form], a tumor of nerve tissue that contains numerous small blood vessels.

nevus /nē'vəs/ [L, *naevus,* birthmark], a pigmented congenital skin blemish that is usually benign but may become cancerous. Any change in color, size, or texture or any bleeding or itching of a nevus merits investigation.

nevus flammeus /flam'ē·əs/, a flat capillary hemangioma that is present at birth and that varies in color from pale red to deep reddish purple. These lesions most often occur on the face. The depth of the color depends on whether the superficial, middle, or deep dermal vessels are involved.

nevus sebaceus of Jadassohn, a congenital skin neoplasm with several cutaneous tissue elements. The most common location is the scalp, face, or neck. It may appear as a yellow or tan waxy patch of alopecia at birth. During puberty the lesion becomes raised, thick, and verrucous. It is usually treated with local excision. Untreated, the lesion may remain benign or become a malignant growth in later life.

New Ballard Score, a system of newborn assessment of gestational maturation. It provides a valid estimation of postnatal maturation for preterm infants with gestational ages greater than 20 weeks and covers a dozen categories, including posture, arm recoil, popliteal angle, skin, plantar surface, and genitals.

newborn [AS, *niwe,* new, *boren,* to bear], **1.** recently born. **2.** a recently born infant; a neonate.

Newborn Care, a Nursing Interventions Classification defined as management of neonate during the transition to extra-uterine life and subsequent period of stabilization.

newborn intrapartal care, care of the newborn in the delivery area during the time after birth before the mother and infant are transferred to the postpartum unit. The nasopharynx and mouth may be suctioned to remove excess mucus as the head is born. Depending on the preference and condition of the mother and the policies of the maternity service, the baby may then be placed on the mother's abdomen and covered with a warm, dry blanket or taken by the nurse to an infant warmer. Apgar scores are assigned at 1 and 5 minutes of age; less commonly another is assigned at 10 minutes of age. The baby is handled gently and quietly and may be put to breast if the mother wishes; bright lights are often avoided, and maternal contact is encouraged.

Newborn Monitoring, a Nursing Interventions Classification defined as measurement and interpretation of physiologic status of the neonate the first 24 hours after delivery.

new drug, a drug for which the Food and Drug Administration requires premarketing approval. A new drug is generally regarded as one for which safety and effectiveness have not yet been demonstrated for its prescribed use.

New England Journal of Medicine *(NEJM),* a weekly professional medical journal that publishes findings of medical research and articles about controversial political and ethical issues in the practice of medicine.

new growth, a neoplasm or tumor.

Newington orthosis, a bilateral orthosis similar to the **Toronto orthosis,** except that flat bars are used and no joints are incorporated.

Newman, Margaret A., a nursing theorist who contributed to the study of nursing theories and models by defining three approaches to the discovery of nursing theory: "borrowing" theories from related disciplines, analyzing nursing practice situations in search of conceptual relationships, and creating new conceptual systems from which theories can be derived.

newton /n(y)oo'tən/ [Isaac Newton, English scientist, 1642–1727], a unit of force in the SI system that would impart an acceleration to 1 kilogram of mass of 1 meter per second per second.

new tuberculin [ME, *newe* + L, *tuber,* swelling], an extract of the tubercle bacillus from which all soluble material has been removed and glycerin added.

Nezelof's syndrome /nez′əlofs/ [Christian Nezelof, French physician, b. 1922], an abnormal condition characterized by absent T cell function, deficient B cell function, fairly normal immunoglobulin levels, and little or no specific antibody production. Nezelof's syndrome causes progressively severe, recurrent, and eventually fatal infections. Signs that often appear in infants or in children up to 4 years of age include recurrent pneumonia, otitis media, chronic fungal infections, upper respiratory tract infections, diarrhea, and hepatosplenomegaly. The disease may enlarge the lymph nodes and the tonsils. These structures may be totally absent in infants with the disease. Involved patients may develop a tendency toward malignancy. Infection may cause sepsis, which is the usual cause of death.

nF, abbreviation for *nanofarad,* one billionth of a farad.

N.F., abbreviation for *National Formulary.*

NF1, a gene associated with neurofibromatosis. The gene is normally part of a family that helps regulate the timing of cell divisions. It may become defective, leading to neurofibromatosis expression, when an itinerant sequence of a deoxyribonucleic acid molecule becomes wedged in the NF1 gene.

ng, abbreviation for **nanogram.**

NGF, abbreviation for **nerve growth factor.**

NG tube, abbreviation for **nasogastric tube.**

NGU, abbreviation for **nongonococcal urethritis.**

NHSC, abbreviation for **National Health Service Corps.**

Ni, symbol for the element **nickel.**

NIA, abbreviation for **National Institute on Aging.**

niacin /nī′əsin/, a white, crystalline water-soluble vitamin of the B complex, usually occurring in various plant and animal tissues as nicotinamide. It functions as a coenzyme necessary for the breakdown and use of all major nutrients and is essential for a healthy skin, normal functioning of the gastrointestinal tract, maintenance of the nervous system, and synthesis of the sex hormones. It also may be effective in improving circulation and reducing high blood cholesterol levels. Symptoms of de-

ficiency include muscular weakness, general fatigue, loss of appetite, various skin eruptions, halitosis, stomatitis, insomnia, irritability, nausea, vomiting, recurring headaches, tender gums, tension, and depression. Severe deficiency results in pellagra.

niacinamide, /nī′əsin′əmīd/ a B complex vitamin. It is closely related to niacin but has no vasodilating action.

niacin equivalent (NE), units used to express niacin content of food. It represents preformed niacin plus tryptophan equivalents (60 mg tryptophan = 1 mg niacin).

NIB, abbreviation for *National Institute for the Blind.*

NIC, abbreviation for **Nursing Interventions Classification.**

nicardipine /nikär·dipin/, a calcium channel blocker and vasodilator. It is prescribed as an antihypertensive and antianginal agent.

N.I.C.H.H.D., abbreviation for **National Institute of Child Health and Human Development.**

Nicholas procedure, a surgical procedure for repairing severe ligamentous injuries to the knee. It involves five procedures: a medial meniscectomy, a medial collateral ligament repair, a vastus medialis advancement, semitendinosus advancement, and a pes anserinus transfer.

nick [ME, *nyke,* notch], (in molecular genetics) a fissure or split in a single strand of deoxyribonucleic acid that can be made with the enzyme deoxyribonuclease or with ethidium bromide.

nickel (Ni) [Ger, *Kupfernickel,* copper demon], a silver-white metallic element. Its atomic number is 28; its atomic mass (weight) is 58.71. Many people are allergic to nickel.

nickel dermatitis, an allergic contact dermatitis caused by the metal nickel. Exposure comes usually from jewelry, wristwatches, metal clasps, and coins. Sweating increases the degree of rash.

nick translation, a method of labeling deoxyribonucleic acid (DNA) in the laboratory by using the enzyme DNA polymerase.

niclosamide /niklō′səmīd/, an anthelmintic prescribed in the treatment of beef and fish tapeworm infestations.

Nicola procedure, the surgical transfer of the long head of the biceps tendon through the humeral head for chronic anterior shoulder dislocation.

nicotine /nik′ətēn/ [Jean Nicot Villemain, French ambassador to Portugal, 1530–1600], a colorless, rapidly acting toxic substance in tobacco that is one of the major contributors to the ill effects of smoking. It is used as an insecticide in agriculture and as a parasiticide in veterinary medicine. Ingestion of large amounts causes salivation, nausea, vomiting, diarrhea, headache, vertigo, slowing of the heartbeat, and in acute cases paralysis of respiratory muscles.

nicotine nasal spray, a product approved by the U.S. Food and Drug Administration for aiding tobacco smoking cessation in adults. One dose of the nasal spray administers 1 mg of nicotine directly into the nasal membranes. Because of the risk of becoming dependent on the nasal spray, it is recommended that patients not use it for more than 6 months.

nicotine poisoning, poisoning from intake of nicotine. Nicotine poisoning is characterized by stimulation of the central and autonomic nervous systems, followed by depression of these systems. In fatal cases death occurs from respiratory failure.

nicotine polacrilex /pōlak′rileks/, a chewing gum (nicotine resin complex) source of nicotine as an adjunct for smoking cessation. It may be prescribed as an aid for patients who are trying to quit cigarette smoking.

nicotine replacement therapy, the use of chewing gum and skin patches as a substitute for tobacco smoke sources to satisfy nicotine cravings.

nicotine withdrawal syndrome, physiologic and psychologic effects of tobacco dependence that make it difficult for addicted smokers to cease use of the alkaloid. Withdrawal symptoms may be diminished by substituting nicotine chewing gum and transdermal nicotine skin patches for cigarettes.

nicotinyl alcohol /nik′ətē′nil/, an alcohol used as a vasodilator in the form of its tartrate salt in the treatment of peripheral vascular disease, vascular spasm, varicose ulcers, decubital ulcers, chilblains, Ménière's disease, and vertigo.

NICU, abbreviation for **neonatal intensive care unit.**

NID, abbreviation for *National Institute for the Deaf.*

NIDA, abbreviation for *National Institute on Drug Abuse.*

nidation /nīdā′shən/ [L, *nidus,* nest], the process by which an embryo burrows into the endometrium of the uterus.

NIDDM, abbreviation for **noninsulin-dependent diabetes mellitus.**

nidus /nī′dəs/ [L, nest], a point or origin, focus, or nucleus of a disease process.

Niebauer prosthesis /nē′bou·ər/, a Silastic prosthesis for interphalangeal and thumb joint replacement.

Niemann-Pick's disease /nē′monpik′/ [Albert Niemann, German pediatrician, 1880–1921; Ludwig Pick, German pediatrician, 1868–1935], an inherited disorder of lipid metabolism in which there are accumulations of sphingomyelin in the bone marrow, spleen, and lymph nodes. The disease is characterized by enlargement of liver and spleen, anemia, lymphadenopathy, and progressive mental and physical deterioration.

nifedipine /nifed′ipēn/, a calcium channel blocker prescribed for the treatment of vasospastic and effort-associated angina and hypertension.

Nightingale, Florence (1820–1910), considered the founder of modern nursing. After limited formal training in nursing in Germany and Paris, she became superintendent in 1853 of a hospital in London. Her success in reorganizing the hospital led the British government to request that she head a mission to the Crimea, where Britain was fighting a war with Russia. After her return to England in 1856, she wrote *Notes on Hospitals* and *Notes on Nursing* and founded a training school for nurses at St. Thomas' Hospital. The graduates became matrons of the most important hospitals in Great Britain, thus raising the standards of nursing around the world. Although she was, by then, bedridden much of the time, she carried on her work on the sanitary reform of India, conducted a study of midwifery, helped establish visiting nurse services, and worked for the reform of the poor laws in which she proposed separate institutions for the sick, the insane, the incurable, and children. After Longfellow wrote *Santa Filomena,* she became known as "The Lady with The Lamp"; the Nightingale Pledge, named after her, embodies her ideals and has inspired thousands of young graduating nurses.

Nightingale ward, a kind of hospital ward designed by Florence Nightingale that revolutionized hospital design. The number of beds allowed in a ward of given size was limited to permit the circulation of air and for general cleanliness and the comfort of patients. Three sides of the ward were windowed to admit light and fresh air.

nightingalism /nī′ting·gā′lizəm/, an ideology emphasizing self-sacrifice on the part of a nurse whose primary concern is the welfare of the patient, with minimum personal attention to the needs of the nurse.

nightmare /nīt′mer/ [AS, *niht,* night, *mara,* incubus], a dream occurring during rapid eye movement sleep that arouses feelings

N

of intense inescapable fear, terror, distress, or extreme anxiety and that usually awakens the sleeper.

night splint, any splint or similar device used only at night.

nightstick fracture, an undisplaced fracture of the ulnar shaft caused by a direct blow.

night sweat [AS, *niht* + *swaetan*], sweating that occurs with a nocturnal fever, as in a wasting disease like pulmonary tuberculosis.

night terrors [AS, *niht* + L, *terrour*], a form of dissociated sleep, usually in children, in which there may be repeated episodes of abrupt awakening from sleep with signs of panic and anxiety. The subject may have only fragmentary dream images of a threatening nature.

night vision [AS, *niht,* night; L, *visio,* seeing], a capacity to see dimly lit objects. It stems from a chemophysical phenomenon associated with the retinal rods. The rods contain the highly light-sensitive chemical rhodopsin, or visual purple, which is essential for the conduction of optic impulses in subdued light. Night vision is sharpest at the periphery of the retina because of the concentration of rods.

nightwalking [AS, *niht* + ME, *walken*], a disorder occurring during nonrapid eye movement sleep in which the subject usually sits up in bed briefly, then gets up and walks around, opening doors, eating, and so on, and eventually returns to bed. The person has no memory of the event the next day.

NIH, abbreviation for **National Institutes of Health.**

nihilistic delusion /nī′hilis′tik/ [L, *nihil,* nothing; *icus,* form of, *deludere,* to deceive], a persistent denial of the existence of particular things or of everything, including oneself, as seen in various forms of schizophrenia.

nikethamide /nīketh′əmīd/, a central nervous system stimulant prescribed as an analeptic in the treatment of depression of the central nervous and respiratory systems.

Nikolsky's sign /nikol′skēz/ [Petr V. Nikolsky, Russian dermatologist, 1858–1940], easy separation of the stratum corneum layer of the epidermis from the basal cell layer by rubbing apparently normal skin areas; found in pemphigus and a few other bullous diseases.

NIMH, abbreviation for **National Institute of Mental Health.**

niobium (Nb) /nī-ō′bē-əm/ [Gk, *Niobe,* mythic daughter of Tantalus and Amphion], a silver-gray metallic element.

Its atomic number is 41; its atomic mass (weight) is 92.906.

nipple [ME, *neb,* beak], a small cylindric, pigmented structure that projects just below the center of each breast. The tip of the nipple has about 20 tiny openings to the lactiferous ducts. The skin of the nipple is surrounded by the lighter pigmented skin of the areola. The depth of pigmentation of the nipple and areola in nulliparas varies from rosy pink to brown, depending on the complexion of the individual.

nipple cancer, an inflammatory malignant neoplasm of the nipple and areola that is usually associated with carcinoma in deeper breast structures. It represents only a small percentage of breast cancers.

nipple discharge, spontaneous exudation of material from the nipple. It may be normal, such as colostrum in pregnancy, or it may be a sign of endocrinologic, neoplastic, or infectious disease.

nipple shield, a device to protect the nipples of a lactating woman. The shield is usually made of soft latex, is 4 or 5 cm wide, and has a tab on one side with which the mother may hold it. The baby nurses from an opening at the center of the shield. It is most often used to allow sore or cracked nipples to heal while maintaining lactation.

niridazole /nirid′əzōl/, an antischistosomal. In the United States it is available from the Centers for Disease Control and Prevention.

Nirschl procedure /nur′shəl/, a surgical procedure for chronic epicondylitis. It involves excision of a hypercapsular tendon segment of the extensor carpi radialis brevis and decortication of the anterolateral condyle.

nirvanic state /nirvä′nik, nirvan′ik/, (in Buddhist meditation) a state in which mental processes cease, often leading to a radical alteration of the personality.

NIS, abbreviation for *Nursing Information System.*

Nissl body /nis′əl/ [Franz Nissl, German neurologist, 1860–1919], any one of the large granular structures in the cytoplasm of nerve cells that stains with basic dyes and contains ribonucleoprotein.

nisoldipine, a calcium channel blocker prescribed in the treatment of hypertension by dilating the arterioles and decreasing peripheral vascular resistance.

nit, the egg of a parasitic insect, particularly a louse. It may be found attached to human or animal hair or to clothing fiber.

nitr, 1. abbreviation for **nitrocellulose.** 2. abbreviation for **nitroglycerin.**

nitrate /nī′trāt/, [Gk, *nitron* soda], **1.** the ion NO_3^-. **2.** a salt of nitric acid.

nitric acid /nī′trik/ [Gk, *nitron,* soda; L, *acidus,* sour], a colorless, highly corrosive liquid that may give off suffocating brown fumes of nitrogen dioxide on exposure to air. Traces of nitric acid are found in rain water during a thunderstorm. Commercially prepared nitric acid is a powerful oxidizing agent used in the manufacture of drugs and occasionally as a cauterizing agent for the removal of warts.

nitric oxide (NO), a colorless free-radical gas commonly found in tissues of humans and other mammals. Nitric oxide participates in many biologic functions such as neurotransmission, vasodilation, cytotoxicity of macrophages, lipid lowering therapy, and inhibition of platelet aggregation. When NO is administered by inhalation, it acts as an endothelium-derived relaxing factor that attenuates the pulmonary vasoconstriction produced by short-term hypoxia. NO deprivation may lead to high blood pressure and the formation of atherosclerotic plaque. On contact with air, NO is quickly converted to the very poisonous nitrogen dioxide (NO_2). Adverse effects of excessive NO exposure include irritation of the eyes, nose, and throat; drowsiness; and loss of consciousness.

nitrite /nī′trīt/ [Gk, *nitron,* soda], an ester or salt of nitrous acid used as a vasodilator and antispasmodic. Among the most widely used nitrites in medicine are amyl, ethyl, potassium, and sodium nitrite.

nitritoid reaction /nī′tritoid/, a group of adverse effects, including hypotension, flushing, lightheadedness, and fainting, produced by administration of arsenicals or gold. The reaction is similar to that caused by administration of nitrites.

nitrobenzene poisoning /-ben′zēn/, a toxic condition caused by the absorption into the body of nitrobenzene, a pale yellow, oily liquid used in the manufacture of aniline, shoe dyes, soap, perfume, and artificial flavors. Nitrobenzene, especially its vapors, is extremely toxic. Exposure in industry is usually by inhalation of the fumes or by absorption through the skin. Symptoms of acute poisoning include headache, drowsiness, nausea, ataxia, cyanosis, and, in extreme cases, respiratory failure.

nitrocellulose (nitr) /-sel′yəlōs/, a mixture of nitrate esters of cellulose made by treating cotton with nitric and sulfuric acids. Solutions in a mixture of ether and alcohol are used as "plastic skin" under the name of **collodion.**

nitrofuran /-fyo͞o′ran/, one of a group of synthetic antimicrobials used to treat infections caused by protozoa or by certain gram-positive or gram-negative bacteria.

nitrofurantoin /nī′trōfyo͞oran′tō·in, -fyo͞o′-rəntō′in/, a urinary antibacterial prescribed in the treatment of certain urinary tract infections.

nitrofurazone /fyo͞o′rəzōn/, a topical antibacterial prescribed in the prophylaxis and treatment of infections in second-and third-degree burns and of the skin and mucous membranes.

nitrogen (N) /nī′trəjən/ [Gk, *nitron,* soda, *genein,* to produce], a gaseous nonmetallic element. Its atomic number is 7; its atomic mass (weight) is 14.008. Nitrogen constitutes approximately 78% of the atmosphere and is a component of all proteins and a major component of most organic substances. Compounds of nitrogen are essential constituents of all living organisms, especially the proteins and the nucleic acids.

nitrogen balance, the relationship between the nitrogen taken into the body, usually as food, and that excreted from the body in urine and feces. Most of the body's nitrogen is incorporated into protein. Positive nitrogen balance, which occurs when the intake of nitrogen is greater than its excretion, implies tissue formation and growth. Negative nitrogen balance, which occurs when more nitrogen is excreted than is taken in, indicates wasting or destruction of tissue.

nitrogen cycle [Gk, *nitron,* soda, *genein,* to produce, *kyklos,* circle], the circulation of nitrogen through natural processes in either of two ways: from the soil to plants and animals that excrete nitrogen products back into the soil or by bacterial fixation of atmospheric nitrogen through plants and animals that decay and release the element back into the atmosphere.

nitrogen dioxide (NO_2), a brownish irritating gas that can be released from silage and the reaction of nitric acid with metals. It may produce symptoms of pulmonary damage in workers who perform ensilage tasks. Organic nitrates or polyol esters of nitric acid such as nitroglycerin, as well as organic nitrites or esters of nitric acid such as amyl nitrite, are effective vasodilators often used in relieving angina.

nitrogen fixation, the process by which free nitrogen in the atmosphere is converted by biologic or chemical means to ammonia and to other forms usable by plants and animals. Biologic nitrogen fixation is the more important process and is accomplished by microorganisms in the soil.

N

nitrogen narcosis, a condition of depressed central nervous system functions through high partial pressure of nitrogen.

nitrogen washout curve, a graphic curve obtained by plotting the concentration of nitrogen in expired alveolar gas during oxygen breathing as a function of time. As a person begins to inhale pure oxygen after breathing ambient air, the nitrogen concentration decreases so that after 4 minutes healthy subjects have a nitrogen concentration in expired alveolar gas of less than 2%.

nitroglycerin (nitr) /-glis′ərin/, a coronary vasodilator prescribed for the prevention or relief of angina pectoris.

nitroglycerin tablets, tablets of glyceryl trinitrate, a volatile ester prepared by the action of nitric and sulfuric acids on glycerol. It is prescribed for the relief of heart symptoms.

nitromersol, /-mur′sol/ an organic mercurial antiseptic that is not a highly effective germicide, sometimes used for the disinfecting of surgical instruments and as an antiseptic on the skin and mucous membranes.

nitrosamines /nīt′rəsam′ēn/, potentially carcinogenic compounds produced by reactions of nitrites with amines or amides normally present in the body. Nitrites are produced by bacteria in saliva and in the intestine from nitrates normally present in vegetables and in nitrate-treated fish, poultry, and meats.

nitrosourea /nītrō′sōyŏŏrē′ə/, one of a group of alkylating drugs used as an antineoplastic drug in the chemotherapy of brain tumors, multiple myeloma, Hodgkin's disease, adenocarcinomas, hepatomas, chronic leukemias, lymphomas, myelomas, and cancers of the breast and ovaries.

nitrous acid (HNO₂), a weak acid and clinical laboratory reagent formed by the action of strong acids on inorganic nitrites. In water it changes into nitric oxide and nitric acid.

nitrous oxide (N₂O, NOx) /nī′trəs/, a colorless, sweet-tasting gas used as an anesthetic in dentistry, surgery, and childbirth. Nitrous oxide alone does not provide enough anesthesia for surgery, for which it is supplemented with other anesthetic agents.

NLN, abbreviation for **National League for Nursing.**

nm, abbreviation for **nanometer.**

N-m, abbreviation for *newton meter.*

N/m², abbreviation for *newton per square meter.*

NMDP, abbreviation for **National Marrow Donor Program.**

NMDS, abbreviation for **nursing minimum data set.**

NMES, 1. abbreviation for *neuromuscular electrical stimulation.* **2.** abbreviation for **neuromuscular electrical stimulator.**

NMNA, abbreviation for **National Male Nurses Association.**

NMR, 1. abbreviation for *nuclear magnetic resonance.* **2.** abbreviation for *nuclear magnetic resonance spectroscopy.*

NNRTI, abbreviation for **nonnucleoside reverse transcriptase inhibitors.**

No, symbol for the element **nobelium.**

NO, abbreviation for **nitric oxide.**

N₂O, symbol for **nitrous oxide.**

nobelium (No) /nōbel′ē-əm/ [Alfred Nobel Institute, Stockholm, Sweden], a synthetic, transuranic metallic element. Its atomic number is 102. The atomic mass (weight) of its most stable isotope is 259.

NOC, abbreviation for **Nursing Outcomes Classification.**

Nocardia /nōkär′dē-ə/ [Edmund I. E. Nocard, French veterinarian, 1850–1903], a genus of gram-positive aerobic bacteria, some species of which are pathogenic, such as *Nocardia asteroides.*

nocardiosis /nōkär′dē-ō′sis/ [Edmund I. E. Nocard; Gk, *osis,* condition], infection with *Nocardia asteroides,* an aerobic gram-positive species of actinomycetes. It is characterized by pneumonia, often with cavitation, and by chronic abscesses in the brain and subcutaneous tissues. The organism enters via the respiratory tract and spreads by the bloodstream, especially in Cushing's syndrome.

nociceptive /nō′sēsep′tiv/ [L, *nocere,* to injure, *capere,* to receive], pertaining to a neural receptor for painful stimuli.

nociceptive reflex [L, *nocere,* to injure, *capere,* to receive, *reflectere,* to bend back], a reflex caused by a painful stimulus.

nociceptive stimulus [L, *nocere,* to injure, *capere,* to receive, *stimulus,* goad], a painful, sometimes detrimental or injurious, stimulus.

nociceptor /nō′sēsep′tər/, a somatic and visceral free nerve ending of thinly myelinated and unmyelinated fibers. It usually reacts to tissue injury but also may be excited by endogenous chemical substances.

no code [AS, *na,* not; L, *caudex,* book], a note written in the patient record and signed by a qualified, usually senior or attending physician, instructing the staff of the institution not to attempt to resuscitate a particular patient in the event of cardiac or respiratory failure. This instruction is usually given only when a patient is so gravely ill that death is imminent and inevitable.

noct., abbreviation for the Latin word, *nocte,* meaning 'at night.'

nocturia /noktōōr′ē·ə/ [L, *nocturnus,* by night; Gk, *ouron,* urine], urination, particularly excessive urination at night. Although it may be a symptom of renal disease, it may occur in the absence of disease in people who drink excessive amounts of fluids, particularly alcohol or coffee, before bedtime or in people with prostatic disease.

nocturnal /noktur′nəl/ [L, *nocturnus,* by night], **1.** pertaining to or occurring during the night. **2.** describing an individual or animal that is active at night and sleeps during the day.

nocturnal emission, involuntary emission of semen during sleep, usually in association with an erotic dream.

nocturnal enuresis [L, *nocturnus,* by night; Gk, *enourein*], involuntary urination while asleep at night.

nocturnal myoclonus, a sleep disorder that usually affects older adults and is marked by thrashing or kicking movements. The condition may be exacerbated by the use of tricyclic depressants used to induce sleep.

nocturnal penile tumescence (NPT) [L, *nocturnus,* by night, *penile,* pertaining to the penis, *tumescere,* to begin to swell], a normal condition of penile erection that occurs during sleep throughout most of the lifetime of a male. The occurrence of NPT is important in the diagnosis of impotence, because it indicates that impotence may be psychogenic.

nodal event /nō′dəl/, an occurrence that may cause anxiety, such as birth, death, divorce, marriage, or a child leaving home.

node /nōd/ [L, *nodus,* knot], **1.** a small rounded mass. **2.** a lymph node.

nodular /nod′yələr/ [L, *nodus,* knot], (of a structure or mass) small, firm, and knotty.

nodular circumscribed lipomatosis, a condition in which circumscribed, encapsulated lipomas are distributed around the neck symmetrically, randomly, or like a collar. The adipose deposits may be painful and tender.

nodular cutaneous angiitis, an inflammatory condition of small arteries that is accompanied by skin lesions.

nodular fasciitis, an inflammation of the fascia that results in the formation of nodules.

nodular goiter [L, *nodus,* knot; Gk, *guttur,* throat], an enlarged goiter that contains nodules.

nodular melanoma, a melanoma that is uniformly pigmented, usually bluish-black and nodular and sometimes surrounded by

an irregular halo of pale, unpigmented skin. The lesion is always raised and may be dome-shaped or polypoid.

nodule /nod′yōōl/ [L, *nodulus,* small knot], **1.** a small node. **2.** a small node-like structure.

noise-induced hearing loss, a gradual loss of hearing caused by exposure to loud noise over an extended period of time. The hearing loss is sensorineural in nature and greatest in the higher frequencies. Although an early hearing loss may be temporary, it becomes permanent with increased exposure to noise.

noise pollution, an unwanted noise level in the environment, causing discomfort and possibly threatening health.

nok, abbreviation for *next of kin.*

noma /nō′mə/ [Gk, *nome,* distribution], an acute, necrotizing ulcerative process involving mucous membranes of the mouth or genitalia. There is rapid spreading and painless destruction of bone and soft tissue accompanied by a putrid odor. Healing eventually occurs but often with disfiguring defects.

nomenclature /nō′mənklā′chər, nōmen′-/ [L, *nomen,* name, *clamare* to call], a consistent, systematic method of naming used in a scientific discipline to denote classifications and to avoid ambiguities in names, such as binomial nomenclature in biology and chemical nomenclature in chemistry.

Nomina Anatomica, the book of official international nomenclature for anatomy as designated by the International Congress of Anatomists.

nominal aphasia /nom′inəl/ [L, *nomen* + Gk, *a* + *phasis,* without speech], a type of speech defect in which the person uses incorrect names in identifying objects. Minor episodes may be due to anxiety, fatigue, or senility; severe cases can indicate a focal lesion on the left side of the brain.

nomogram /nom′əgram, nō′mə-/ [Gk, *nomos,* law, *gramma,* a record], **1.** a graphic representation, by any of various systems, of a numeric relationship. **2.** a graph on which a number of variables is plotted so that the value of a dependent variable can be read on the appropriate line when the values of the other variables are given.

nonabsorbable surgical sutures /-əbsôr′-bəbəl/ [L, *non,* not, *absorbere* + Gk, *cheirourgos,* surgeon; L, *sutura*], sutures of silk, nylon, steel, or other materials that resist absorption. They are used mainly in deep tissues, where it is important for them to remain in place.

nonadaptive immunity /-adap′tiv/, an

N

immune response that persists after repeated exposure to the same antigen.

nonadherent cell /-ədhir'ənt/, a cell such as a lymphocyte that will not adhere to a smooth surface of laboratory equipment.

nonadherent dressing [L, *non* + *adhesio*, sticking to; OFr, *dresser*, to arrange], a dressing designed specifically not to stick to the dried secretions of a wound.

nonadhesive skin traction /-ədhē'siv/ [L, *non*, not, *adhesio*, sticking to], one of two kinds of skin traction in which the therapeutic pull of traction weights is applied over the body structure involved with foam-backed traction straps that do not stick to the skin. The straps decrease the patient's vulnerability to skin breakdown by spreading the traction pull over a wide area of skin surface.

nonbacterial thrombotic endocarditis /-baktir'ē-əl/ [L, *non* + *bakerion*, small rod], one of the three main types of endocarditis, characterized by various kinds of lesions affecting the heart valves. Some studies indicate that this disease may be the first step in the development of bacterial endocarditis and that the lesions involved cause peripheral arterial embolisms, resulting in death.

noncellulose polysaccharides /-sel'yəlōs/, food substances such as hemicellulose, pectins, gums, mucilages, and algal products that absorb water and swell to a larger bulk. They slow emptying of food from the stomach, bind bile acids, provide fermentation material for the colon, and prevent spastic colon pressure.

noncompetitive inhibition /-kəmpet'itiv/, (in pharmacology) a form of inhibition in which a substance occupies a receptor and cannot be displaced from the receptor by increasing the number of other molecules through the principle of mass action.

noncompliance /-kəmplī'əns/ [L, *non* + *complere*, to complete], a NANDA-accepted nursing diagnosis of an informed decision on the part of the client not to adhere to a therapeutic suggestion. The nature of the noncompliance is to be specified, such as 'noncompliance: medications.' The critical defining characteristic, which must be present for the diagnosis to be made, is an observation of the client's failure to adhere to a recommendation or a statement by the client or knowledgeable other person that the recommendations are not being followed.

non compos mentis /non' kom'pos men'tis/ [L, not of sound mind], a legal term applied to a person declared to be mentally incompetent.

nondirective therapy /-direk'tiv/ [L, *non* + *digere*, to direct], a psychotherapeutic approach in which the psychotherapist refrains from giving advice or interpretation as the client is helped to identify conflicts and to clarify and understand feelings and values.

nondisjunction /-disjungk'chən/ [L, *non* + *disjungere*, to disjoint], failure of homologous pairs of chromosomes to separate during the first meiotic division or of the two chromatids of a chromosome to split during anaphase of mitosis or the second meiotic division. The result is an abnormal number of chromosomes in the daughter cells.

nonessential amino acid /-esen'shəl/, any of 11 amino acids that are not essential to the diet because the body can synthesize their molecules from other amino acids.

nonfeasance /nonfē'zəns/ [L, *non* + *facere*, to do], a failure to perform a task, duty, or undertaking that one has agreed to perform or that one had a legal duty to perform.

nongonococcal urethritis (NGU) /-gon'-əkok'əl/ [L, *non* + Gk, *gone*, seed, *kokkos*, berry], an infectious condition of the urethra in males that is characterized by mild dysuria and a scanty to moderate amount of penile discharge. The discharge may be white or clear, thin or mucoid, or, less often, purulent. The infection is often caused by the obligate intracellular parasite *Chlamydia trachomatis*.

nonheme iron /non'hēm/, one of two forms of dietary iron. It is less efficiently absorbed than heme iron. All plant food sources and 60% of animal food sources contain nonheme iron.

nonhemolytic jaundice /-hē'məlit'ik/ [L, *non* + Gk, *haima*, blood, *lysein*, to loosen; Fr, *jaune*, yellow], a form of jaundice that is caused by a liver disease rather than the destruction of red blood cells.

non-Hodgkin's lymphoma (NHL) /-hoj'-kənz/, any of a heterogenous group of malignant tumors involving lymphoid tissue. NHLs differ in their histologic, immunologic, and clinical characteristics, and as to their prognosis with therapy.

nonigravida /nō'nigrav'idə/ [L, *nonus*, nine, *gravida*, pregnant], indicating a woman pregnant for the ninth time.

noninfective valvular mass /-infek'tiv/, a growth or swelling on one of the heart valves associated with autoimmune diseases or with cardiac or extracardiac malignancies. Such masses are frequently asymptomatic and are discovered only at autopsy.

noninflammatory diarrhea /-inflam'ə-tôr'ē/, a profuse watery diarrhea without fever or vomiting that begins 6 to 24 hours after ingesting food contaminated by bacterial toxins produced by either *Clostridium perfringens* or *Bacillus cereus.* The food poisoning usually involves raw meat or other proteinaceous foods exposed to warm temperatures for several hours.

noninsulin-dependent diabetes mellitus (NIDDM), a type of diabetes mellitus in which patients are not insulin-dependent or ketosis prone, although they may use insulin for correction of symptomatic or persistent hyperglycemia and they can develop ketosis under special circumstances such as infection or stress. Onset is usually after 40 years of age but can occur at any age. Two subclasses are the presence or absence of obesity. About 60% to 90% are obese; in these patients glucose tolerance is often improved by weight loss. Hyperinsulinemia and insulin resistance characterize some patients.

noninvasive /-invā′siv/ [L, *non* + *in,* into, *vadere,* to go], pertaining to a diagnostic or therapeutic technique that does not require the skin to be broken or a cavity or organ of the body to be entered, such as obtaining a blood pressure reading by auscultation with a stethoscope and sphygmomanometer.

nonionic /-ī·on′ik/, pertaining to compounds without a net negative or positive charge.

nonionizing radiation /-ī′əni′zing/ [L, *non* + Gk, *ion,* going, *izein,* to cause], radiation for which the mechanism of action in tissue does not directly ionize atomic or molecular systems through a single interaction.

nonipara /nōnip′ərə/ [L, *nonus,* nine, *parere,* to bear], a woman who has given birth to nine offspring.

nonmyelinated nerve fiber /-mī′əlinā′tid/ [L, *non* + Gk, *myelos,* marrow, L, *nervus* nerve, *fibra,* fiber], a nerve fiber that lacks the fatty myelin insulating sheath. Such fibers form the gray matter of the nervous system, as distinguished from the white matter of myelinated fibers.

nonnucleoside reverse transcriptase inhibitors (NNRTI), a class of antiviral drugs that inhibit human immunodeficiency virus replication by interfering with the reverse transcriptase enzyme essential for viral replication. These drugs have a different mechanism of action and a distinct side effect profile from other agents. An example of an NNRTI drug is nevirapine.

Nonnutritive Sucking, a Nursing Interventions Classification defined as provision of sucking opportunities for an infant who is gavage fed or who can receive nothing by mouth.

nonnutritive sweetener /-nōo′tritiv/, a chemical additive such as saccharin, aspartame, or acesulfame that gives a sweet taste to foods without contributing significant calories. The sugar substitute is either not metabolized or so intensely sweet that the calorie count is negligible.

nonossifying fibroma /-os′ifī′ing/, a bone anomaly found in children as a sharply circumscribed, eccentrically located lesion in the metaphysis of long bones. A microscopic examination reveals whorl patterns of spindle cells, fibrous tissue, numerous xanthoma cells, and occasional giant cells.

nonosteogenic fibroma /non′ostē·əjen′ik/, a common bone lesion characterized by degeneration and proliferation of the medullary and cortical tissue near the ends of the diaphyses of the large long bones of the lower extremities.

nonpalpable testis /pal′pəbəl/, a testis that cannot be felt and may be intraabdominal or absent.

nonparametric test of significance /-per′əmet′rik/ [L, *non* + Gk, *para,* beside, *metron,* measure], (in statistics) one of several tests that use a qualitative approach to analyze rank order data and incidence data that cannot be assumed to have a normal distribution. Kinds of nonparametric tests of significance include **chi-square, Spearman's rho.**

nonparous /-per′əs/ [L, *non, parere,* to bear], indicating a woman who has never given birth to a child.

nonpenetrating wound /-pen′ətrā′ting/ [L, *non,* not, *penetrare,* to penetrate; AS, *wund*], a wound that does not break the surface of the skin.

nonpermissive host /-pərmis′iv/, an animal or cell that resists the successful replication of an infectious agent.

nonpolar /-pō′lər/ [L, *non* + *polus,* pole], pertaining to molecules that have a hydrophobic affinity, are "water hating." Nonpolar substances tend to dissolve in nonpolar solvents.

nonpolar solvent, a liquid solvent without significant concentration of charged groups. Liquid hydrocarbons are common examples.

nonproductive cough /-prəduk′tiv/ [L, *non* + *producere,* to produce], a sudden, noisy expulsion of air from the lungs that may be caused by irritation or inflammation and does not remove sputum from the respiratory tract. Intratracheal suctioning may be necessary when secretions cause severe respiratory difficulty and coughing is unproductive.

nonproprietary name /-prəprī′əter′ē/ [L, *non* + *proprietas,* owner, *nomen,* name],

N

the chemical or generic name of a drug or device, as distinguished from a brand name or trademark. A nonproprietary name may be indicated by the letters *USAN,* for United States Adopted Names.

nonprotein nitrogen (NPN) /-prō'tēn/ [L, *non* + Gk, *proteios,* first rank, *nitron,* soda, *genein,* to produce], the nitrogen in the blood that is not a constituent of protein, such as the nitrogen associated with urea, uric acid, creatine, and polypeptides.

nonresponse bias, (in epidemiology) errors that may develop when a part of those selected and identified as study subjects cannot or will not participate in the study. The bias may occur when the group of nonrespondents differs systematically from respondents with respect to exposure or disease status. To minimize this bias, a high participation rate is necessary, or a survey is made of nonresponders to determine whether or how they might differ with regard to the risk of disease or exposure.

nonreversible inhibitor /-rivur'səlǝl/ [L, *non* + *revertere,* to turn back, *inhibere,* to restrain], an effector substance that binds permanently to an active site of an enzyme, inhibiting the normal catalytic activity of the enzyme.

nonsecretor /-sǝkrē'tǝr/ [L, *non* + *secernere,* to separate], a person who does not secrete ABO blood group substances in mucous secretions of the saliva or gastric juice. The condition is genetically determined.

nonseg., abbreviation for *nonsegmented.*

nonseminomatous testicular tumors /-sem'inom'ǝtǝs/, any of a variety of histologic types of testicular carcinoma, including embryonal cell carcinoma, teratocarcinoma, and tumors with mixed elements. Treatment for most cases depends on the stage of the cancer at the time of diagnosis.

nonshivering thermogenesis /-shiv'ǝring/, a natural method by which newborns can produce body heat by increasing their metabolic rate.

nonsmall-cell carcinoma of lung, a major category of histologic types of lung carcinomas, including adenocarcinoma of the lung, large-cell carcinoma, and squamous cell carcinoma. Treatment depends on the stage of development of the cancer at the time of initial presentation. The treatment of choice for otherwise physically fit patients with early stages of disease is resection.

nonspecific binding (NSB) /-spǝsif'ik/, in ligand binding assay, the part of a tracer used in a competitive-binding assay that is found in the bound fraction, independent of the binding reaction.

nonspecific immunosuppression, a therapy, including the use of immunosuppressive drugs and high doses of radiation, that blunts or abolishes the response of the immune system to all antigens.

nonspecific urethritis (NSU) [L, *non,* not, *species,* form], inflammation of the urethra not known to be caused by a specific organism. Onset of symptoms is often related to sexual intercourse. Its acute phase is seldom seen in women, but its chronic phase is a common urologic difficulty among them. The condition is noted by urethral discharge in men and by reddening of the urethral mucosa in women.

nonspecific vaginitis [L, *non,* not, *species,* form, *facere,* to make, *vagina,* sheath; Gk, *itis,* inflammation], a term formerly used for any vaginal inflammation for which no specific pathogen could be identified.

nonsteroidal antiinflammatory drug (NSAID) /-stir'oidǝl/, any of a group of drugs having antipyretic, analgesic, and antiinflammatory effects. They counteract or reduce inflammation by inhibiting prostaglandin synthesis. NSAIDs may be indicated in the treatment of mild-to-moderate pain, rheumatoid arthritis, osteoarthritis, ankylosing spondylosis, gouty arthritis, fever, nonrheumatic inflammation, and dysmenorrhea. Examples include aspirin, ibuprofen, ketoprofen, and indomethacin.

nonstress test (NST) /non'stres/, an evaluation of the fetal heart rate response to natural contractile activity or to an increase in fetal activity.

nonsuppurative osteomyelitis /-sup'yǝrā'-tiv/, tuberculosis of the bone.

nonthrombocytopenic purpura /-throm'-bōsī'tǝpē'ik/, a disorder characterized by purplish or reddish skin areas. The condition does not involve a decrease in the number of platelets.

nontoxic /-tok'sik/, not poisonous.

nontropical sprue /-trop'ikǝl/ [L, *non,* not; Gk, *tropikos,* of the solstice; D, *sprouw*], a malabsorption syndrome resulting from an inborn inability to digest foods that contain gluten.

nonulcerative blepharitis /-ul'sǝrǝtiv'/ [L, *non* + *ilcus,* ulcer; Gk, *blepharon,* eyelid, *itis,* inflammation], a form of blepharitis characterized by greasy scales on the margins of the eyelids around the lashes and hyperemia and thickening of the skin. Nonulcerative blepharitis is often associated with seborrhea of the scalp, eyebrows, and the skin behind the ears.

nonunion /-yōō'nyǝn/, pertaining to a fractured bone that fails to heal properly.

nonverbal communication /-vur'bǝl/,

the transmission of a message without the use of words. It may involve any or all of the five senses.

nonviable /vī'əbəl/ [L, *non* + *vita*, life], unable to exist independently after birth.

nonvital pulp [L, *non*, not, *vita*, life, *pulpa*, flesh], dead dental pulp caused by a disease or trauma that interferes with the blood supply.

Noonan's syndrome /nōō'nənz/ [Jacqueline A. Noonan, American cardiologist, b. 1928], a hypergonadotropic disorder of unknown cause occurring only in males and characterized by short stature, low-set ears, webbing of the neck, and cubitus valgus. Testicular function may be normal, but fertility is often decreased. The number and morphology of the chromosomes are normal.

nootropic /nōətrop'ik/, a chemical designed to increase brain metabolism.

norepinephrine /nôr'epinef'rin/, an adrenergic hormone that acts to increase blood pressure by vasoconstriction but does not affect cardiac output. It is synthesized naturally by the adrenal medulla. It is available also as a drug, levarterenol, which is used to maintain the blood pressure in acute hypotension secondary to trauma, heart disease, or vascular collapse.

norepinephrine bitartrate, an adrenergic vasoconstrictor prescribed in the treatment of cardiac arrest and in certain acute hypotensive states.

no response (NR), the condition for which the maximum decrease in treated tumor volume is less than 50%.

norethindrone /nôreth'indrōn/, a progestin prescribed in the treatment of abnormal uterine bleeding and endometriosis and which is a component in oral contraceptive medications.

norethindrone acetate and ethinyl estradiol, an oral contraceptive prescribed for contraception, endometriosis, and hypermenorrhea.

norfloxacin /nôrflok'səsin/, an oral antibacterial drug prescribed for the treatment of urinary tract infections.

norgestrel /nôrjes'trəl/, a progestin prescribed alone or in combination with estrogen as a contraceptive.

norm [L, *norma*, rule], **1.** a measure of a phenomenon generally accepted as the ideal standard performance against which other measures of the phenomenon may be measured. **2.** abbreviation for **normal.**

norma basalis /nôr'mə bəsā'lis/ [L, rule; Gk, *basis,* foundation], the inferior surface of the base of the skull with the mandible removed, formed by the palatine bones, the vomer, the pterygoid processes, and parts of the sphenoid and temporal bones.

normal (N) /nôr'məl/ [L, *norma*, rule], **1.** describing a standard, average, or typical example of a set of objects or values. **2.** describing a chemical solution in which 1 L contains 1 g of a substance or the equivalent in replaceable hydrogen ions. **3.** people in a nondiseased population. **4.** a gaussian distribution.

normal dental function, the correct and healthy action of opposing teeth during mastication.

normal distribution, (in statistics) a theoretic distribution frequency of variable data usually represented graphically by a bell-shaped curve that reaches a peak about the mean.

normal human plasma [L, *norma*, rule, *humanus* + Gk, *plassein*, to mold], sterile, disease-free human blood prepared from a pooled donor supply.

normal human serum albumin, an isotonic preparation of pooled human serum albumin for treating hypoproteinemia, hypovolemia, and threatened or existing shock.

Normalization Promotion, a Nursing Interventions Classification defined as assisting parents and other family members of children with chronic illnesses or disabilities in providing normal life experiences for their children and families.

normal last shoes, special orthopedic shoes for infants and children constructed with a normal sole, as opposed to a reverse or straight last shoe.

normal phase, a chromatographic mode in which the mobile phase is less polar than the stationary phase.

normal pressure hydrocephalus [L, *norma*, rule, *premere*, to press; Gk, *hydor*, water, *kephale*, head], a condition in which there is dilation of the ventricles without an increase in intracranial pressure. Classic signs and symptoms are gait disturbance, memory/cognitive problems, and urinary incontinence.

normal saline solution [L, *norma*, rule, *sal* + *solutus*, dissolved], a 0.9% w/v (weight of solute per volume of solution) sterile solution of sodium chloride in water that is isotonic with blood and injectable intravenously.

normal sinus rhythm (NSR) [L, *norma*, rule, *sinus*, hollow; Gk, *rhythmos*], the normal heartbeat produced when the pacemaker is in the sinoatrial node and the heart rate is between 60 to 100 beats/min.

normal solution [L, *norma*, rule, *solutus*, dissolved], a solution that contains the gram-equivalent weight of a reagent per liter. It is denoted by the symbols N/l or N.

N

normal strain, a quantity described by the quotient of the change of length of a line and its original length.

normal stress, (in physics) a quantity described by the quotient of distributed force and area when the force is perpendicular to the area.

normal temperature [L, *norma,* rule, *temperatura*], for a normal person at rest, the normal oral clinical temperature is given as 98.6° F or 37° C, but actual "normal" temperatures may range a fraction of a degree or increments of a whole degree higher or lower because of effects of sleep, exercise, eating, sleeping, metabolism, and the ambient temperature. Rectal temperature also averages a fraction of a degree higher than oral temperatures, and axillary readings are usually lower than oral temperatures.

normoblast /nôr'məblast/ [L, *norma* + Gk, *blastos,* germ], a nucleated precursor cell in the bone marrow of the adult circulating erythrocyte. After the extrusion of the nucleus of the normoblast, the young erythrocyte becomes known as a reticulocyte and enters the circulating blood. **—normoblastic,** *adj.*

normochromic /nôr'məkrō'mik/ [L, *norma* + Gk, *chroma,* color], pertaining to a blood cell having normal color caused by the presence of an adequate amount of hemoglobin.

normocyte /nôr'məsīt/ [L, *norma* + Gk, *kytos,* cell], an ordinary, normal, adult red blood cell of average size having a diameter of 7 μ. **—normocytic,** *adj.*

normoglycemic /-glīsē'mik/, pertaining to a normal blood glucose level.

normotensive /-ten'siv/, pertaining to the condition of having normal blood pressure. **—normotension,** *n.*

normoventilation /-ven'tilā'shən/, the alveolar ventilation rate that produces an alveolar carbon dioxide pressure of about 40 mm Hg at any metabolic rate.

normoxia /nôrmok'sē-ə/, an ambient oxygen pressure of about 150 (plus or minus 10) torr, or the partial pressure of oxygen in atmospheric air at sea level.

Norplant System, trademark for a method of implanting capsules of a contraceptive drug, levonorgestrel, beneath the skin of the upper arm of a woman. With the woman under local anesthesia, a set of six capsules, each 2.4 mm in diameter and 34 mm long, is inserted in a fan-shaped pattern through an incision about 10 cm above the elbow crease. The highly progestational drug diffuses through the walls of the capsules. The contraceptive effect can be interrupted by removing the capsules.

North American blastomycosis, an infection caused by inhaling the fungus *Blastomyces dermatitidis.* It may resemble bacterial pneumonia. Painless, well-demarcated, verrucous or ulcerated skin lesions occur on the face and hands. The disease may progress to involve bones and the brain; many viscera are infected in fatal cases.

North American Nursing Diagnosis Association (NANDA), a professional organization of registered nurses created in 1982. The purpose of the organization is "to develop, refine, and promote a taxonomy of nursing diagnostic terminology of general use to the professional."

North Asian tick-borne rickettsiosis, an infection, acquired in the Eastern Hemisphere, caused by *Rickettsia sibirica,* transmitted by ticks. It resembles Rocky Mountain spotted fever. Usual findings include a generalized maculopapular rash involving palms and soles, fever, and lymph node enlargement.

Northern blot test, an electrophoretic test for identifying the presence or absence of particular mRNA molecules and nucleic acid hybridization.

nortriptyline hydrochloride /nôrtrip'-tilēn/, a tricyclic antidepressant prescribed in the treatment of mental depression.

Norwalk agent [Norwalk, Ohio, site where first identified], a strain of virus that produces gastroenteritis symptoms. The infection is transmitted from one person to another and is involved in 40% of the nonbacterial diarrhea cases in children and adults.

Norwegian scabies [Norway; L, *scabere,* to scratch], a severe infestation of human skin by an itch mite *(Sarcoptes scabiei).* The condition is associated with intense itching, crusting and scaling of the skin, and insect egg burrows that appear as discolored lines in the affected skin areas.

nose [AS, *nosu*], the structure that protrudes from the anterior part of the face and serves as a passageway for air to and from the lungs. The nose filters the air, warming, moistening, and chemically examining it for impurities that might irritate the mucous lining of the respiratory tract. The nose also contains receptor cells for smell, and it aids the faculty of speech. The external part, which protrudes from the face, is considerably smaller than the internal part, which lies over the roof of the mouth. The hollow interior part is separated into a right and left cavity by a septum. Each cavity is divided into the superior, middle, and inferior meati by the projection of nasal conchae. The external part of the nose is perforated by two nostrils (anterior nares), and the internal part by two posterior nares.

nosebleed [AS, *nosu* + ME, *blod*, blood], abnormal hemorrhage from the nose. Emergency responses to nosebleed include seating the patient upright with the head thrust forward to prevent swallowing of blood. Pressure with both thumbs directly under the nostril and above the lips may block the main artery supplying blood to the nose. Alternatively, pressure with both forefingers on each side of the nose often slows bleeding by blocking the main arteries and their branches. Continued bleeding may require the insertion of absorbent material within the nostril. Cold compresses on the nose, lips, and back of the head may help control hemorrhage.

NOSIE, abbreviation for **nurses' observation scale for inpatient evaluation.**

nosocomial /nos'əkō'mē·əl/ [Gk, *nosokomeian*, hospital], pertaining to a hospital.

nosocomial infection, an infection acquired at least 72 hours after hospitalization, often caused by *Candida albicans, Escherichia coli,* hepatitis viruses, herpes zoster virus, *Pseudomonas,* or *Staphylococcus.*

nosology /nōsol'əjē/ [Gk, *nosos*, disease, *logos*, science], the science of classifying diseases.

notch [Fr, *noche*], an indentation or a depression in a bone or other organ, such as the auricular notch or the cardiac notch.

nothing by mouth (NPO), [L, *nil per os,* nothing by mouth], a patient care instruction advising that the patient is prohibited from ingesting food, beverage, or medicine. It is usually posted above the bed of a patient who is about to undergo surgery or special diagnostic procedures requiring that the digestive tract be empty.

no-threshold curve, a linear dose-response curve that assumes there is no detectable threshold below which there is no harm. As applied in nuclear medicine, there is no identifiable concentration of radiation below which no response curve occurs.

notifiable [L, *nota*, mark, *facere*, to make], pertaining to certain conditions, diseases, and events that must, by law, be reported to a governmental agency, such as birth, death, smallpox, certain other communicable diseases, and certain violations of public health regulations.

notochord /nō'tōkôrd/ [Gk, *noton*, back, *chorde*, cord], an elongated strip of mesodermal tissue that originates from the primitive node and extends along the dorsal surface of the developing embryo. The structure is replaced by vertebrae, although a remnant of it remains as part of the nucleus pulposus of the intervertebral disks. —**notochordal,** *adj.*

notochordal canal /nō'tōkôr'dəl/ [Gk, *noton* + *chorde*, cord; L, *canalis*, channel], a tubular passage that extends from the primitive pit into the head process during the early stages of embryonic development in mammals.

notogenesis /nō'tōjen'əsis/ [Gk, *noton* + *genein*, to produce], the formation of the notochord. —**notogenetic,** *adj.*

notomelus /nətom'ələs/ [Gk, *noton* + *melos*, limb], a congenital malformation in which one or more accessory limbs are attached to the back.

nourish /nur'ish/ [L, *nutrire*, to suckle], to furnish or supply the essential foods or nutrients for maintaining life.

nourishment /nur'ishmənt/, **1.** the act or process of nourishing or being nourished. **2.** any substance that nourishes and supports the life and growth of living organisms.

NOx, abbreviation for **nitrous oxide,** or any mixture of oxides of nitrogen.

noxious /nok'shəs/ [L, *noxius*, harm], harmful, injurious, or detrimental to health.

Noyes test /noiz/, an orthopedic knee test performed with the knee extended and the thigh relaxed. There is anterolateral tibial subluxation. The knee is gradually flexed, with reduction of the subluxation occurring at about 30 degrees of flexion.

Np, symbol for the element **neptunium.**

NP, abbreviation for **nurse practitioner.**

NPN, abbreviation for **nonprotein nitrogen.**

NPO, abbreviation for **nothing by mouth.**

N-propyl alcohol /en'prō'pil/, a clear, colorless liquid used as a solvent for resins.

NPT, abbreviation for **nocturnal penile tumescence.**

NPU, abbreviation for **net protein utilization.**

NPY, abbreviation for **neuropeptide Y.**

NR, 1. abbreviation for **no response. 2.** abbreviation for *nodal rhythm.*

NREM, abbreviation for *nonrapid eye movement.* See **sleep.**

NRTI, abbreviation for **nucleoside reverse transcriptase inhibitors.**

NSAID, abbreviation for **nonsteroidal antiinflammatory drug.**

NSB, abbreviation for **nonspecific binding.**

NSCCN, abbreviation for **National Society of Critical Care Nurses of Canada.**

n-s/m², abbreviation for *newton second per square meter.*

NSNA, abbreviation for **National Student Nurses Association.**

NSR, abbreviation for **normal sinus rhythm.**

NSU, abbreviation for **nonspecific urethritis.**

ntp, abbreviation for *normal temperature and pressure.*

nu /n(y)oo̅/, N, ν, the thirteenth letter of the Greek alphabet.

nuc, abbreviation for *nuclear.*

nucha /noo̅'kə/, *pl.* **nuchae** [Fr, *nuque,* nape], the nape, or back of the neck. **—nuchal,** *adj.*

nuchal cord /noo̅'kəl/ [Fr, *nuque,* nape; Gk, *chorde*], an abnormal but common condition in which the umbilical cord is wrapped around the neck of the fetus in utero or of the baby as it is being born. It is usually possible to slip the loop or loops of cord gently over the child's head.

nuchal ligament, a large midline posterior ligament in the neck from the base of the skull to the seventh cervical vertebra.

nuchal rigidity, a resistance to flexion of the neck, a condition seen in patients with meningitis.

nuchocephalic reflex /noo̅'kəsefal'ik/, a test for diffuse cerebral dysfunction, such as in senility. When the shoulders are turned to the left or the right, the head fails to turn in the same direction within ½ second.

nuclear family /n(y)oo̅'kle·ər/ [L, *nucleus,* nut kernel, *familia,* household], a family unit consisting of the biologic parents and their offspring.

nuclear isomer, one of two or more nuclides with the same number of neutrons and protons in the nucleus (the same atomic number, or Z, and the same atomic mass, or A) but existing in different energy states.

nuclear medicine, a medical discipline that uses radioactive isotopes in the diagnosis and treatment of disease. The major fields of nuclear medicine are physiologic function studies, radionuclide imaging, and therapeutic techniques.

nuclear medicine technologist, an allied health professional who specializes in the nuclear properties of radioactive and stable nuclides to make diagnostic evaluations of the anatomic or physiologic conditions of the body and to provide therapy with unsealed radioactive tissues.

nuclear problem, (in psychology) an underlying reason for an individual's reaction to a precipitating event.

nuclear radiology, the branch of radiology that uses radioactive materials in diagnosis and treatment of health disorders.

nuclear scanning, a diagnostic technique that uses an injected, ingested, or inhaled radioactive material and a scanning device for determining the size, shape, location, and function of various body parts.

nuclear spin, an intrinsic form of angular momentum possessed by atomic nuclei containing an odd number of nucleons (protons or neutrons).

nuclear transplantation, the transfer of the nucleus of one cell into the cytoplasm of another.

nucleic acid /noo̅kle'ik/ [L, *nucleus* + *acidus,* sour], a polymeric compound of high molecular weight composed of nucleotides, each consisting of a purine or pyrimidine base, a ribose or deoxyribose sugar, and a phosphate group. Nucleic acids are involved in energy storage and release and in the determination and transmission of genetic characteristics. Kinds of nucleic acid are **deoxyribonucleic acid** and **ribonucleic acid.**

nucleocapsid /noo̅'kle·ōkap'sid/ [L, *nucleus* + *capsa,* box], a viral enclosure consisting of a capsid or protein coat that encloses nucleic acid.

nucleochylema /noo̅'kle·ō'kəli̅'mə/ [L, *nucleus* + Gk, *chylos,* juice, *haima,* blood], the ground substance of the nucleus, as distinguished from that of the cytoplasm.

nucleocytoplasmic /noo̅'kle·ōsi̅'tōplas'mik/ [L, *nucleus* + Gk, *kytos,* cell, *plasma,* something formed], of or relating to the nucleus and cytoplasm of a cell.

nucleocytoplasmic ratio, the ratio of the volume of a nucleus of a cell to the volume of the cytoplasm. The proportion is usually constant for a specific cell type, and an increase is indicative of malignant neoplasms.

nucleohistone /noo̅'kle·ōhis'tōn/ [L, *nucleus* + Gk, *histos,* tissue], a complex nucleoprotein that consists of deoxyribonucleic acid and a histone protein. It is the basic constituent of the chromatin in the cell nucleus.

nucleolar organizer /noo̅kle'ələr/ [L, *nucleolus,* little nut kernel; Gk, *organon,* instrument, *izein,* to cause], a part of the nucleus of the cell, thought to consist of heterochromatin, that is responsible for the formation of the nucleolus.

nucleolus /noo̅kle'ələs/, *pl.* **nucleoli** [L, little nut kernel], any one of the small, dense structures composed largely of ribonucleic acid and situated within the cytoplasm of cells. Nucleoli are essential in the formation of ribosomes that synthesize cell proteins.

nucleon /n(y)ōō′klē·on/, a collective term applied to protons and neutrons within the nucleus.

nucleophilic /-fil′ik/, pertaining to some molecules, particularly nucleic acids and proteins, having electrons that can be shared and thus form bonds with alkylating agents.

nucleoplasm /nōō′klē·əplaz′əm/ [L, *nucleus* + Gk, *plasma*, something formed], the protoplasm of the nucleus as contrasted with that of the cell. —**nucleoplasmic**, *adj.*

nucleoplasmin, an acidic protein found in the nucleus that binds to histone and participates in nucleosome assembly.

nucleoprotein /-prō′tēn/ [L, *nucleus* + Gk, *proteios,* first rank], a molecule in which protein is combined with nucleic acid in a cell nucleus.

nucleoside /nōō′klē·əsīd′/, a component of a nucleotide that consists of a nitrogenous base linked to a pentose sugar.

nucleoside monophosphate kinase, a liver enzyme that catalyzes the transfer of a phosphate group from adenosine triphosphate, producing adenosine diphosphate and a nucleoside diphosphate.

nucleoside reverse transcriptase inhibitors (NRTI), a class of antiretroviral drugs that mimic one or more of the components of human immunodeficiency deoxyribonucleic acid (DNA) or ribonucleic acid, interrupting the viral replication process. The drugs (nucleoside analogs) work by blocking the reverse transcriptase enzyme essential for viral replication. Inserting a nucleoside analog into the new viral DNA strand at a specific point terminates the viral chain, halting the replication process before it is completed. Examples of nucleoside analogs include zidovudine (AZT), didanosine (ddI), zalcitabine (ddC), stavudine (d4T) and lamivudine (3TC).

nucleosome /nōō′klē·əsōm/ [L, *nucleus* + Gk, *soma,* body], any one of the repeating nucleoprotein units consisting of histones forming a complex with deoxyribonucleic acid that appear as the beadlike structures at distinct intervals along the chromosome.

5-nucleotidase /nōō′klē·ot′idās/, a non-lipid enzyme, elevated in some liver disorders and cancer of the pancreas. It is measured in the blood to distinguish between certain liver and bone diseases. This enzyme is widely distributed throughout the body but is found in high concentrations in the liver and pancreas.

nucleotide /nōō′klē·ətīd′/, any one of the compounds into which nucleic acid is split by the action of nuclease. A nucleotide consists of a phosphate group, a pentose sugar, and a nitrogenous base. Chains of such structures form deoxyribonucleic acid and/or ribonucleic acid molecules essential for life.

nucleus /n(y)ōō′klē·əs/ [L, nut kernel], **1.** the central controlling body within a living cell, usually a spheric unit enclosed in a membrane and containing genetic codes for maintaining life systems of the organism and for issuing commands for growth and reproduction. **2.** a group of nerve cells of the central nervous system having a common function, such as supporting the sense of hearing or smell. **3.** the center of an atom about which electrons rotate. **4.** the central element in an organic chemical compound or class of compounds. —**nuclear,** *adj.*

nucleus pulposus, the central part of each intervertebral disk, consisting of a pulpy elastic substance that loses some of its resiliency with age.

nuclide /nōō′klīd/ [L, *nucleus,* nut kernel], a species of atom characterized by the constitution of its nucleus, in particular by the number of protons and neutrons.

nudge control, a prosthetic device with a mechanical unit that can be pressed by the chin to lock or unlock one or more joints of the apparatus.

NUG, abbreviation for *necrotizing ulcerative gingivitis.*

Nuhn's gland /noonz/ [Anton Nuhn, German anatomist, 1814–1889], an anterior lingual gland in tissues on the inferior surface and near the apex and midline of the tongue.

nuke, a slang term for nucleoside analog.

null cell [L, *nullus,* not one, *cella,* storeroom], a lymphocyte that develops in the bone marrow and lacks the characteristic surface markers of the B and T lymphocytes (surface immunoglobulin or the pan-T antigen). Null cells represent a small proportion of the lymphocyte population. Stimulated by the presence of antibody, null cells can attack certain cellular targets directly. They kill tumor or viral-infected cells, although not with the specificity of cytotoxic T cells.

null hypothesis (H_0), (in research) a hypothesis that predicts that an observed difference is caused by chance alone and not by systematic observation.

nulligravida /nul′igrav′ədə/ a woman who has never been pregnant.

nullipara /nulip′ərə/, *pl.* **nulliparae** [L, *nullus,* not one, *parere,* to bear], a woman who has not given birth to a viable infant. The designation "para 0" indicates nulliparity.

nulliparity /nul'iper'itē/ [L, *nullus,* none, *parere,* to bear], the status of a woman who has never borne a child.

nulliparous /nulip'ərəs/ [L, *nullus,* none, *parere,* to bear], never having given birth.

num, abbreviation for *number.*

numbness /num'nəs/ [ME, *nomen,* loss of feeling], a partial or total lack of sensation in a body part, resulting from any factor that interrupts the transmission of impulses from the sensory nerve fibers.

numerical taxonomy, a system of classifying organisms based on the overall similarities of the measurable phenotypic characters they share. The system is used to classify strains of bacteria, as well as to separate closely related species of plants and animals.

numeric pain scale /n(y)ōōmer'ik/, a pain assessment system in which patients are asked to rate their pain on a scale from 1 to 10, with 10 representing the worst pain they have experienced or could imagine.

nummular dermatitis /num'yələr/ [L, *nummuli,* petty cash; Gk, *derma,* skin, *itis,* inflammation], a skin disease characterized by coin-shaped, vesicular, or scaling eczema-like lesions on the forearms and front of the calves.

Nuremberg tribunal [Nuremberg, Germany; L, *tribunus,* platform for administration of justice], an international tribunal planned and implemented by the United Nations War Crimes Commission to detect, apprehend, try, and punish people accused of war crimes, establishing the **Nuremberg code.** The principle and practice of informed consent was reinforced by the precedent set in the trials in which Nazi physicians were declared guilty of crimes against humanity in performing experiments on human beings who were not volunteers and did not consent.

nurse [L, *nutrix*], **1.** a person educated and licensed in the practice of nursing; one who is concerned with 'the diagnosis and treatment of human responses to actual or potential health problems' (American Nurses Association). The practice of the nurse includes data collection, diagnosis, planning, treatment, and evaluation within the framework of the nurse's singular concern with the patient's response to the problem, rather than to the problem itself. The concerns of the nurse are thus broader and less discrete and circumscribed than the traditional concerns of medicine. The nurse may be a generalist or a specialist and, as a professional, is ethically and legally accountable for the nursing activities performed and for the actions of others to whom the nurse has delegated responsibility. **2.** to provide nursing care.

nurse anesthetist, a registered nurse qualified by advanced training in an accredited program in the specialty of nurse anesthesia to manage the care of the patient during the administration of anesthesia in selected surgical situations.

nurse cell, a cell that transfers nutrients to an oocyte via a cytoplasmic bridge.

nurse-client interaction, any process in which a nurse and a client exchange or share information, verbally or nonverbally. It is fundamental to communication and is an essential component of the nursing assessment.

nurse-client relationship, a therapeutic relationship between a nurse and a client built on a series of interactions and developing over time. It is time-limited and goal-oriented and has three phases. During the first phase, the phase of establishment, the nurse establishes the structure, purpose, timing, and context of the relationship and expresses an interest in discussing this initial structure with the client. During the middle, developmental, phase of the relationship, the nurse and the client get to know each other better and test the structure of the relationship to be able to trust one another. The last phase, termination, ideally occurs when the goals of the relationship have been accomplished, when both the client and the nurse feel a sense of resolution and satisfaction.

nurse clinician, a nurse who is prepared to identify and diagnose problems of clients by using increased knowledge and skills gained through advanced study in a specific area of nursing practice.

nurse coordinator, a registered nurse who coordinates and manages the activities of nursing personnel engaged in specific nursing services, such as obstetrics or surgery, for two or more patient care units.

Nurse Corps, the branch within each of the armed services comprising the nurses within that service, such as the Army Nurse Corps. In each of the armed services, the members of the Nurse Corps have the rank, title, responsibilities, and status of commissioned officer.

nurse educator, a registered nurse whose primary area of interest, competence, and professional practice is the education of nurses at university level. Minimum education required is Master of Science in Nursing.

nurse midwife, a registered nurse qualified by advanced training in obstetric and neonatal care and certified by the American College of Nurse Midwives. The nurse midwife manages the perinatal care of women having a normal pregnancy, labor, and childbirth.

nurse practice act, a statute enacted by the legislature of any of the states or by the appropriate officers of the districts or possessions. The act delineates the legal scope of the practice of nursing within the geographic boundaries of the jurisdiction.

nurse practitioner (NP), a registered nurse who has advanced education in nursing and clinical experience in a specialized area of nursing practice. The NP collaborates with other health care providers to deliver primary care to patients with common acute or stable chronic medical conditions in ambulatory care settings. Some NPs also function in specialty, tertiary, or long-term care settings. NPs may offer a variety of services such as complete physical examinations, health assessments, and patient education.

nursery diarrhea /nur′sərē/ [L, *nutrix,* nurse; Gk, *dia,* through, *rhein,* to flow], diarrhea of the newborn. In nurseries outbreaks of diarrhea caused by *Escherichia coli, Salmonella,* echoviruses, or adenoviruses are potentially life-threatening to the infant. The most serious aspect of the disease is fluid loss, leading to dehydration and electrolyte imbalance.

nurse's aide, a person who is employed to carry out basic nonspecialized tasks in the care of a patient, such as bathing and feeding, making beds, and transporting patients, under the supervision and direction of a registered nurse.

nurses' observation scale for inpatient evaluation (NOSIE), a systematic, objective behavioral rating scale that is applied by nurses to patient behavior.

nurses' registry, an employment agency or listing service for nurses who wish to work in a specific area of nursing, usually for a short period of time or on a per diem basis.

nurses' station, an area in a clinic, unit, or ward in a health care facility that serves as the administrative center for nursing care for a particular group of patients. It is usually centrally located and may be staffed by a ward secretary or clerk who assists with paperwork, telephone, and other communication. Before going on duty, nurses usually meet there to receive daily assignments, to review the patients' charts, and to update the files.

nursing, 1. the practice in which a nurse assists "the individual, sick or well, in the performance of those activities contributing to health or its recovery (or to a peaceful death) that he would perform unaided if he had the necessary strength, will or

knowledge. And to do this in such a way as to help him gain independence as rapidly as possible." (Virginia Henderson) **2.** "the diagnosis and treatment of human responses to actual or potential health problems," (American Nurses Association). There are four principal characteristics that further define nursing care: the phenomena that concern nurses; the use of theories to observe the need for nursing intervention and to plan nursing action; the nursing action taken; and an evaluation of the effects of the actions relative to the phenomena. **3.** the professional practice of a nurse. **4.** the process of acting as a nurse, of providing care that encourages and promotes the health of the person being served.

nursing assessment, an identification by a nurse of the needs, preferences, and abilities of a patient. Assessment follows an interview with and observation of a patient by the nurse and considers the symptoms and signs of the condition, the patient's verbal and nonverbal communication, medical and social history, and any other information available. Among the physical aspects assessed are vital signs, skin color and condition, motor and sensory nerve function, nutrition, rest, sleep, activity, elimination, and consciousness.

nursing assistant, *Canada.* a person trained in basic nursing techniques and direct patient care who practices under the supervision of a registered nurse.

nursing audit, a thorough investigation designed to identify, examine, or verify the performance of certain specified aspects of nursing care using established criteria. A concurrent nursing audit is performed during ongoing nursing care. A retrospective nursing audit is performed after discharge from the care facility, using the patient's record. Often a nursing audit and a medical audit are performed collaboratively, resulting in a joint audit.

nursing care plan, a plan based on a nursing assessment and a nursing diagnosis carried out by a nurse. It has four essential components: identification of the nursing care problems and statement of the nursing approach to solve those problems; statement of the expected benefit to the patient; statement of the specific actions by the nurse that reflect the nursing approach and achieve the goals specified; and evaluation of the patient's response to nursing care and readjustment of that care as required.

nursing diagnosis, a statement of a health problem or of a potential problem in the client's health status that a nurse is licensed and competent to treat. Four steps are required in the formulation of a nursing diagnosis. A data base is established by collecting information from all available sources, including interviews with the client and the client's family, a review of any existing records of the client's health, observation of the client's response to any alterations in health status, a physical assessment, and a conference or consultation with others concerned in the client's care. The data base is continually updated. The second step includes analysis of the client's responses to the problems, healthy or unhealthy, and classification of those responses as psychologic, physiologic, spiritual, or sociologic. The third step is the organization of the data so that a tentative diagnostic statement can be made that summarizes the pattern of problems discovered. The last step is confirmation of the sufficiency and accuracy of the data base by evaluation of the appropriateness of the diagnosis to nursing intervention and by the assurance that, given the same information, most other qualified practitioners would arrive at the same nursing diagnosis. In use, each diagnostic category has three parts: the term that concisely describes the problem, the probable cause of the problem, and the defining characteristics of the problem. A number of nursing diagnoses have been identified and are listed as accepted by the North American Nursing Diagnosis Association (NANDA), and they are updated and refined at periodic meetings of the group.

nursing differential, an allowance added to payments to hospitals for services rendered Medicaid patients in recognition of the cost of providing nursing services to such patients that is greater than the cost to the general patient population.

nursing director, a nurse whose function is the administrative and clinical leadership of the nursing service of a division of a health care facility, such as a nursing supervisor of maternal and infant care nurses.

nursing ethics [L, *nutrix,* nurse; Gk, *ethikos,* character], the values or moral principles governing relationships between the nurse and patient, the patient's family, other members of the health professions, and the general public.

nursing goal, a general goal of nursing involving activities that are desirable but difficult to measure, such as self-care, good nutrition, and relaxation.

nursing health history, data collected about a patient's level of wellness, changes in life patterns, sociocultural role, and mental and emotional reactions to illness.

nursing intervention, any act by a nurse that implements the nursing care plan or any specific objective of that plan, such as turning a comatose patient to avoid the development of decubitus ulcers or teaching injection technique to a patient with diabetes before discharge from the hospital. The patient may require intervention in the form of support, limitation, medication, or treatment for the current condition or to prevent the development of further stress.

nursing intervention model, (in nursing research) a conceptual framework used to determine appropriate nursing interventions. The model is a holistic representation of the client and the health care system. The goal is to learn what nursing interventions would be most effective for the particular problem within the particular health care system.

Nursing Interventions Classification (NIC), a comprehensive, standardized system to classify treatments performed by nurses. It is a clinical tool developed by a research team at the University of Iowa that describes and defines the knowledge base for nursing curricula and practice. There are at present more than 400 nursing interventions that describe the treatments nurses perform. Each intervention has been labeled, defined, and given a list of appropriate activities. The full range of activities that nurses perform on behalf of patients are included, both independent and collaborative interventions, and both direct and indirect care. A taxonomy is provided to help the nurse find what is most relevant to her or his practice area. NIC interventions have been linked to NANDA diagnoses. It is considered part of the clinical decision making of the nurse to decide and document the nursing diagnoses, desired outcomes, interventions used, and outcomes achieved. The NIC system provides the language to document interventions.

nursing minimum data set (NMDS), a minimum set of items of information with uniform definitions and categories concerning the specific dimension of nursing, which meets the information needs of multiple data users in the health care system. It is the first attempt to standardize the collection of essential nursing data.

nursing objective, a specific aim planned by a nurse to decrease a person's stress, to improve the ability to adapt, or both. A nursing objective may be physical, emotional, social, or cultural and may involve the person's family, friends, and other patients. It is the purpose of any specific nursing order or nursing intervention.

nursing observation, an objective, holistic evaluation made by a nurse of the various aspects of a client's condition. It includes the person's general appearance, emotional affect, nutritional status, habits, and preferences, as well as body temperature, skin condition, and any obvious abnormal processes.

nursing orders, specific instructions for implementing the nursing care plan, including the patient's preferences, timing of activities, details of health education necessary for the particular patient, role of the family, and plans for care after discharge. Nursing orders must be signed by the professional nurse who writes them.

Nursing Outcomes Classification (NOC), a comprehensive, standardized system to classify outcomes of nursing interventions. It is a clinical tool developed by a research team at the University of Iowa that describes and defines the knowledge base for nursing curricula and practice. At present, NOC includes 190 nursing outcomes for use for individual patients or individual family caregivers in the home.

nursing process, the process that serves as an organizational framework for the practice of nursing. It encompasses all of the steps taken by the nurse in caring for a patient: assessment, nursing diagnosis, planning, implementation, and evaluation. The rationale for each step is founded in nursing theory.

nursing process model, a conceptual framework in which the nurse-patient relationship is the basis of the nursing process. The nursing process is represented as dynamic and interpersonal, the nurse and the patient being affected by each other's behavior and by the environment around them. Each successful two-way communication is termed a "transaction" and can be analyzed to discover the factors that promote transactions.

nursing research, a detailed systematic study of a problem in the field of nursing. Nursing research is practice-or discipline-oriented and is essential for the continued development of the scientific base of professional nursing practice.

Nursing Research, a bimonthly refereed journal containing papers and other materials concerning nursing research. The goal of the journal is to stimulate research in nursing and disseminate research findings.

nursing rounds, chart rounds, walking rounds, teaching rounds, or grand rounds that are held specifically for nurses and that focus on nursing care problems.

nursing specialty, a nurse's selected professional field of practice, such as surgical, pediatric, obstetric, or psychiatric nursing.

nursing theorist, a person who develops integrated concepts or frameworks of nursing roles, functions, objectives, and activities and their relationships to clients and the roles of other health professionals.

nursing theory, an organized framework of concepts and purposes designed to guide the practice of nursing.

nursology /nursol′əjē/ [L, *nutrix,* nurse; Gk, *logos,* science], a conceptual framework for the study and practice of nursing. Nursology is intended to provide a model for nursing methods and research. The nurse and the patient have the opportunity to grow, and the science of nursing may emerge from the 'angular' investigations and syntheses.

nurture /nur′chər/, to feed, rear, foster, or care for, such as in the nourishment, care, and training of growing children.

nutation /nōōtā′shən/ [L, *nutare,* to nod], the act of nodding, especially involuntary nodding as occurs in some neurologic disorders.

nutmeg poisoning, a toxic effect of ingesting the dried kernels of the seeds of nutmeg *(Myristica fragrans)* or its volatile oils. The oils contain terpenes and myristicin, which have stimulant and carminative effects. A dose of one to three kernels may produce convulsions for up to 60 hours.

nutrient /nōō′trē-ənt/ [L, *nutriens,* food that nourishes], a chemical substance that provides nourishment and affects the nutritive and metabolic processes of the body.

nutrient artery of the humerus, one of a pair of branches of the deep brachial arteries, arising near the middle of the arm and entering the nutrient canal of the humerus.

nutrient density, the ratio obtained by dividing a food's contribution to the needs for a nutrient by its contribution to calorie needs. When the contribution to nutrient needs exceeds the contribution to calorie needs, the food is considered to have a favorable nutrient density for the nutrient concerned.

nutrient enema [L, *nutriens* + Gk, *enema,* injection], the introduction of saline or glucose into the body via the rectum.

nutrient supplements, vitamins and other nutrients that may not be necessary for healthy adults with an adequate intake of proper nutrients but that may be needed for elderly adults or persons in a debilitated state.

nutriment /nōō′trimənt/ [L, *nutriens,* food that nourishes], any substance that nourishes and aids the growth and development of the body.

nutrition /n(y)ōōtrish′ən/ [L, *nutriens*],

1. nourishment. **2.** the sum of the processes involved in the taking in of nutrients and their assimilation and use for proper body functioning and maintenance of health. **3.** the study of food and drink as related to the growth and maintenance of living organisms.

nutritional /n(y)o͞otrish'ənəl/ [L, *nutrire*, to nourish], pertaining to the quality of food or eating behavior that provides nourishment through assimilation of food to tissues.

nutritional anemia [L, *nutrire*, to nourish; Gk, *a* + *haima*, without blood], a disorder characterized by the inadequate production of hemoglobin or erythrocytes caused by a nutritional deficiency of iron, folic acid, or vitamin B_{12}, or other nutritional disorders.

nutritional care, the substances, procedures, and setting involved in ensuring the proper intake and assimilation of nutriments, especially for the hospitalized patient. Patients who are unable to feed themselves are assisted, and abnormal intake of food is recorded and reported. Supplemental nourishment when indicated and fluids are offered between meals.

Nutritional Counseling, a Nursing Interventions Classification defined as use of an interactive helping process focusing on the need for diet modification.

Nutritional Monitoring, a Nursing Interventions Classification defined as collection and analysis of patient data to prevent or minimize malnourishment.

nutritional science, a body of science that relates to the processes involved in nutrition.

nutrition, altered: less than body requirements, a NANDA-accepted nursing diagnosis of a state in which an individual experiences an intake of nutrients insufficient to meet metabolic needs. Defining characteristics may include loss of weight with adequate food intake, reported intake of less food than is recommended, evidence or report of a lack of food, lack of interest in food, aversion to eating, alteration in the taste of food, feelings of fullness immediately after eating small quantities, abdominal pain with no other explanation, sores in the mouth, diarrhea or steatorrhea, pallor, weakness, and loss of hair.

nutrition, altered: more than body requirements, a NANDA-accepted nursing diagnosis of a state in which an individual is experiencing an intake of nutrients that exceeds metabolic needs. The critical defining characteristics, one of which must be present for the diagnosis to be made, include weight of 20% greater than the ideal for the height and body build of the client and triceps skin fold measurement greater than 15 mm in men and 25 mm in women.

nutrition, altered: risk for more than body requirements, a NANDA-accepted nursing diagnosis of a state in which an individual is at risk of experiencing an intake of nutrients that exceeds metabolic needs. Risk factors include hereditary predisposition; excessive energy intake during late gestational life, early infancy, and adolescence; frequent, closely spaced pregnancies; dysfunctional psychologic conditioning in relationship to food; membership in a lower socioeconomic group; reported or observed obesity in one or both parents; rapid transition across growth percentiles in infants or children; reported use of solid food as a major food source before 5 months of age; observed use of food as reward or comfort measure; reported or observed higher baseline weight at the beginning of each pregnancy; and dysfunctional eating patterns, including pairing food with other activities, concentrating food intake at the end of the day, eating in response to external cues (e.g., time of day or social situation), and eating in response to internal cues other than hunger (e.g., anxiety).

nutrition base, a person's normal nutritional requirements before modification to accommodate a specific condition.

nutritionist /n(y)o͞otrish'ənist/ [L, *nutrire*, to nourish], a professional who has completed academic degrees of BS, MS, EdD, or PhD in foods and nutrition.

Nutrition Management, a Nursing Interventions Classification defined as assisting with or providing a balanced dietary intake of foods and fluids.

Nutrition Therapy, a Nursing Interventions Classification defined as administration of food and fluids to support metabolic processes of a patient who is malnourished or at high risk for becoming malnourished.

Nutting, Mary Adelaide (1858–1947), a Canadian-born American nursing educator and reformer. At Teachers College, Columbia University, she created and developed the Department of Nursing and Health and became the first professor of nursing in the world. With Lavinia Dock she wrote *History of Nursing,* a classic in nursing literature.

nux vomica /nuks' vom'ikə/ [L, *nux*, nut, *vomere*, to vomit], the dried ripe seeds of a small Asian tree, *Strychnos nux-vomica,* a source of the alkaloids strychnine and brucine. The seeds are powdered, and the strychnine content reduced to a little more than 1% by the addition of lactose for use as a bitter tonic and nerve stimulant.

nvm, abbreviation for *nonvolatile matter.*

NVMA, abbreviation for *National Veterinary Medical Association.*

nyctalopia /nik'təlō'pē·ə/ [Gk, *nyx,* night, *alaos,* obscure, *ops,* eye], poor vision at night or in dim light resulting from decreased synthesis of rhodopsin, vitamin A deficiency, retinal degeneration, or a congenital defect. —**nyctalopic,** *adj.*

nyctophobia /nik'tō-/ [Gk, *nyx* + *phobos,* fear], an anxiety reaction characterized by an obsessive, irrational fear of darkness.

nylidrin hydrochloride /nil'idrin/, a peripheral vasodilator prescribed in the treatment of peripheral vascular disease and circulatory disturbances of the inner ear.

nymphomania /nim'fəmā'nē·ə/ [Gk, *nymphe,* maiden, *mania,* madness], a psychosexual disorder of women characterized by an insatiable desire for sexual satisfaction, often resulting from an unconscious conflict concerning personal adequacy.

nymphomaniac /-mā'nē·ak/, **1.** a person with or displaying characteristics of an individual possessing an insatiable desire for sexual satisfaction. **2.** pertaining to or exhibiting nymphomania. —**nymphomaniacal** /nim'fəmənī'əkəl/, *adj.*

nystagmus /nīstag'məs/ [Gk, *nystagmos,* nodding], involuntary, rhythmic movements of the eyes; the oscillations may be horizontal, vertical, rotary, or mixed. Jerking nystagmus is characterized by faster movements in one direction than in the opposite direction. Pendular nystagmus has oscillations that are approximately equal in rate in both directions. Labyrinthine vestibular nystagmus, most frequently rotary, is usually accompanied by vertigo and nausea. Vertical nystagmus is considered pathognomonic of disease of the tegmentum of the brainstem. Seesaw nystagmus, in which one eye moves up and the other down, may be observed in bilateral hemianopia. —**nystagmic,** *adj.*

nystatin /nis'tətin/, an antifungal antibiotic prescribed in the treatment of fungal infections of the gastrointestinal tract, vagina, and skin.

N

O

o, symbol for *ohm*.

O, symbol for the element **oxygen**.

O$_2$, symbol for *oxygen molecule*.

OASDHI, abbreviation for **Old Age, Survivors, Disability and Health Insurance Program.**

oat cell carcinoma [AS, *ate*, oat; L, *cella*, storeroom; Gk, *karkinos*, crab, *oma*, tumor], a malignant, usually bronchogenic epithelial neoplasm consisting of small, tightly packed round, oval, or spindle-shaped epithelial cells that stain darkly and contain neurosecretory granules and little or no cytoplasm. Tumors produced by these cells do not form bulky masses but usually spread along submucosal lymphatics. Many malignant tumors of the lung are of this type.

oatmeal bath, a colloid treatment for pruritus and other skin disorders. The procedure may consist of covering the patient with a layer of muslin containing oatmeal and pouring warm water over the fabric. The bath has a soothing effect. In a variation of the therapy, starch is substituted for oatmeal.

OAWO, abbreviation for **opening abductory wedge osteotomy.**

ob., abreviation for the Latin word *obit*, 'died.'

OB, *informal.*, **1.** abbreviation for **obstetrician. 2.** abbreviation for **obstetrics.**

obduction /əbduk′shən/ [L, *obductio*, a covering], a forensic medical autopsy.

Ober and Barr procedure, a surgical method of treating weak biceps muscles by transfer of the brachioradialis.

Ober procedure, a method for treatment of paralyzed clubfeet by transfer of the posterior tibial tendon to the third cuneiform or metatarsal.

Obersteiner-Redlich zone /ō′bərshtī′-rad′-lish, ō′bərstē′nər-red′lik/ [H. Obersteiner, Austrian neurologist, 1847–1942; Emil Redlich, Austrian neurologist, 1866–1930], a thin line of demarcation between fibers of the peripheral nervous system and the spinal cord or brainstem. It is produced by a basal lamina separating the Schwann cells and collagen of the peripheral nervous system from the neuroglia of the central nervous system.

Ober test, [Frank R. Ober, American surgeon, 1861–1925], an examination for tight tensor fascia lata. The patient lies on one side with the hip and knee flexed on the surface and the opposite hip extended while the knee is flexed. Inability to place the knee being tested on the table surface indicates a tight fascia lata.

obese /ōbēs′/ [L, *obesus*, swollen], pertaining to a corpulent or excessively heavy individual. Generally a person is regarded as medically obese if he or she is 20% above desirable body weight for the person's age, sex, height, and body build. Because the 'average' human body is approximately 25% fat, the proportion may be doubled for a medically defined obese person.

obesity /ōbē′sitē/ [L, *obesitas*, fatness], an abnormal increase in the proportion of fat cells, mainly in the viscera and subcutaneous tissues of the body. Obesity may be exogenous or endogenous. Hyperplastic obesity is caused by an increase in the number of fat cells in the increased adipose tissue mass. Hypertrophic obesity results from an increase in the size of the fat cells in the increased adipose tissue mass.

obex /ō′beks/, a small triangular membrane formed at the caudal angle of the rhomboid fossa or fourth ventricle.

obfuscation /ob′fəskā′shən/ [L, *obfuscare*, to darken], the act of making something confused, clouded, or obscure.

OBG, abbreviation for *obstetrics and gynecology.*

OB-Gyn, *informal.* abbreviation for *obstetrics and gynecology.*

object /ob′jəkt/, (in psychology) something through which an instinct can achieve its goal. In psychoanalytic terms, a person other than self.

object blindness, an inability to recognize objects or analyze spatial relationships. The condition is associated with lesions of the right cerebral hemisphere in right-handed patients.

objective /əbjek′tiv/ [L, *objectare*, to set against], **1.** a goal. **2.** pertaining to a phenomenon or clinical finding that is observed; not subjective. An objective finding is often described in health care as a sign, as distinguished from a symptom, which is a subjective finding.

objective data collection, the process in which data relating to the client's problem are obtained by an observer through direct physical examination, including observation, palpation, and auscultation, and by laboratory analyses and radiologic and other studies.

objective lens, (in radiology) a lens that accepts light from the output phosphor of an image-intensifier tube and converts it into a parallel beam for recording the image on film.

objective sign [L, *objectum,* something cast before, *signum,* sign], a clinical observation that can be seen, heard, measured, or otherwise recorded by an examining physician, nurse, or other health care provider.

objective symptom [L, *objectum,* something cast before; Gk, *symptoma,* that which happens], a symptom accompanied by signs that tend to confirm the patient's physical complaint and enable the examining physician, nurse, or other health care provider to deduce the cause.

objective tinnitus, a noise produced in the ear that can be heard by another person, particularly someone using a stethoscope.

object permanence, a capacity to perceive that something exists even when it is not seen.

object relations, emotional bond between one person and another, as contrasted with interest in and love for the self.

obligate /ob′ligit, -gāt/ [L, *obligare,* to bind], characterized by the ability to survive only in a particular set of environmental conditions, such as an obligate parasite.

obligate aerobe, an organism that cannot grow in the absence of oxygen.

obligate anaerobe, an organism that cannot grow in the presence of oxygen, such as *Clostridium tetani, C. botulinum,* and *C. perfringens.*

obligatory water loss /əblig′ətôr′ē/, the volume of water required for daily urinary excretion of metabolic waste products. This amount of water loss is necessary to maintain normal health.

oblique /əblēk′/ [L, *obliquus,* slanted], a slanting direction or any variation from the perpendicular or the horizontal.

oblique bandage, a circular bandage applied spirally in slanting turns, usually to a limb.

oblique fiber, (in dentistry) any of the collagenous filaments that are bundled together obliquely in the periodontal ligament.

oblique fissure of the lung, 1. the groove marking the division of the lower

and middle lobes in the right lung. **2.** the groove marking the division of the upper and the lower lobes in the left lung.

oblique fracture, a slanted fracture of the shaft on the long axis of a bone.

oblique presentation [L, *obliquus,* slanted, *praesentare,* to show], a presentation in which the long axis of the fetus is oblique to the long axis of the mother.

obliquity of pelvis /əblik′witē/ [L, *obliquus,* aslant], an abnormal tilt of the pelvis with respect to the spinal column.

obliteration /əblit′ərā′shən/ [L, *obliterare,* to efface], the removal or loss of function of a body part by surgery, disease, or degeneration.

obliterative phlebitis /əblit′ərətiv′/ [L, *obliterare,* to efface; Gk, *phleps,* vein, *itis,* inflammation], a form of phlebitis in which the inflammation results in permanent closure of the vessel.

OBS, abbreviation for *organic brain syndrome.*

observation [L, *observare,* to watch], **1.** the act of watching carefully and attentively. **2.** a report of what is seen or noticed, such as a nursing observation.

observation hip, a condition in which a patient experiences a limp, pain, and limited hip motion. Causes may include toxic synovitis, infection, or avascular necrosis.

obsession [L, *obsidere,* to haunt], a persistent thought or idea with which the mind is continually and involuntarily preoccupied and which cannot be expunged by logic or reasoning.

obsessive-compulsive /əbses′iv/ [L, *obsidere,* to haunt, *compellere,* to impel], **1.** characterized by or relating to the tendency to perform repetitive acts or rituals or think repetitive thoughts, usually as a means of releasing tension or relieving anxiety. **2.** describing a person who has an obsessive-compulsive disorder.

obsessive-compulsive disorder an anxiety disposition characterized by recurrent and persistent thoughts, ideas, and feelings of obsessions or compulsions sufficiently severe to cause marked distress, consume considerable time, or significantly interfere with the patient's occupational, social, or interpersonal functioning.

obsolescence /ob′səles′əns/ [L, *obsolescere,* to decay], **1.** to fall into disuse because of age or loss of function. **2.** a state of being useless.

obstetric /əbstet′rik/ [L, *obstetrix,* midwife], pertaining to pregnancy, childbirth.

obstetric anesthesia [L, *obstetrix,* midwife; Gk, *anaisthesia,* lack of feeling], any of various procedures used to provide anesthesia for childbirth. It includes local

O

anesthesia for episiotomy or episiotomy repair; regional anesthesia for labor or delivery, such as by paracervical block or pudendal block; or, for a wider block, epidural, spinal, caudal, or saddle block. Anesthesia for cesarean section may be achieved with an epidural or spinal block or by general anesthesia.

obstetric forceps, forceps used to assist delivery of the fetal head. They vary in weight, length, shape, and mechanism of action, but all consist of a pair of instruments comprising a handle, a shank, and a blade. The several styles of forceps are designed to assist in various clinical situations. The station of the fetus in the pelvis, the position of the head in relation to the pelvis, the size of the fetus, and the preference of the operator all affect the choice of forceps.

obstetrician /ob′stətrish′ən/, a physician who specializes in the branch of medicine concerned with pregnancy and childbirth.

obstetrics /əbstet′riks/ [L, *obstetrix*, midwife], the branch of medicine concerned with pregnancy and childbirth, including the study of the physiologic and pathologic function of the female reproductive tract and the care of the mother and fetus throughout pregnancy, childbirth, and the immediate postpartum period. **—obstetric, obstetrical,** *adj.*

obstipation /ob′stipā′shən/ [L, *obstipare,* to press], 1. a condition of extreme and persistent constipation caused by obstruction in the intestinal or eliminatory system. 2. a process of blocking. **—obstipant,** *n.,* **obstipate,** *v.*

obstruction /əbstruk′shən/ [L, *obstruere,* to build against], 1. something that blocks or clogs. 2. the act of blocking or preventing passage. 3. the condition of being obstructed or clogged. **—obstruct,** *v.,* **obstructive,** *adj.*

obstructive airways disease /əbstruk′tiv/, a classification of respiratory disease characterized by decreased airway size and increased airway secretions. It includes chronic bronchitis, abnormalities of the bronchi, and emphysema.

obstructive anuria [L, *obstruere,* to build against; Gk, *a + ouron,* without urine], an almost complete absence of urination caused by blockage of the urinary tract.

obstructive biliary cirrhosis [L, *obstruere,* to build against, *bilis,* bile; Gk, *kirrhos,* yellow, *osis,* condition], a form of secondary cirrhosis in which a stricture develops in the bile ducts. The condition may develop after cholecystectomy, gallstones, or a tumor.

obstructive constipation [L, *obstruere,* to build against, *constipare,* to crowd together], a condition in which feces are retained in the bowel because of a blockage in the lumen.

obstructive sleep apnea, a form of sleep apnea involving a physical obstruction in the upper airways. The condition is usually marked by recurrent sleep interruptions, choking and gasping spells on awakening, and drowsiness caused by loss of normal sleep.

obstructive uropathy, any pathologic condition that blocks the flow of urine. The condition may lead to impairment of kidney function and an increased risk of urinary infection.

obtund /obtund′/ [L, *obtundere,* to blunt], 1. to deaden pain. 2. to render insensitive to unpleasant or painful stimuli by reducing the level of consciousness, such as by anesthesia or a strong narcotic analgesic. **—obtundation, obtundity,** *n.,* **obtunded, obtundent,** *adj.*

obtundation /ob′tundā′shən/ [L, *obtundere,* to blunt, *atus,* process], the use of an agent that soothes and reduces irritation or pain by blocking sensibility at some level of the central nervous system, such as in the use of narcotics to control pain.

obturation /ob′t(y)ərā′shən/ [L, *obturare,* to stop up], an obstruction of an opening, such as an intestinal blockage.

obturator /ob′tərā′tər, ob′tyərā′tər/ [L, *obturare,* to close], 1. a device used to block a passage or canal or to fill in a space, such as a prosthesis implanted to bridge the gap in the roof of the mouth in a cleft palate. 2. *nontechnical.* an obturator muscle or membrane. 3. (in radiology) a device that is placed into a large-bore cannula during insertion to prevent potential blockage by residual tissues.

obturator externus, the flat, triangular muscle covering the outer surface of the anterior wall of the pelvis. It functions to rotate the thigh laterally.

obturator foramen, a large opening on each side of the lower part of the hip bone, formed posteriorly by the ischium, superiorly by the ilium, and anteriorly by the pubis.

obturator internus, a muscle that covers a large area of the inferior aspect of the lesser pelvis, where it surrounds the obturator foramen. It functions to rotate the thigh laterally and to extend and abduct the thigh when it is flexed.

obturator membrane, a tough fibrous membrane that covers the obturator foramen of each side of the pelvis.

obturator muscles [L, *obturare,* to close, *musculus*], a pair of thigh muscles, the external and internal obturators. The external obturator flexes and rotates the thigh laterally, and the internal obturator abducts and rotates the thigh laterally.

obturator sign [L, *obturare,* to close, *signus,* sign], a sign of appendicitis. The internal rotation of the right leg with the leg flexed to 90 degrees at the hip and knee and a resultant tightening of the internal obturator muscle may cause abdominal discomfort, for example, in appendicitis.

obv, abbreviation for *obverse.*

O.C., abbreviation for **oral contraceptive.**

occ, abbreviation for **occipital.**

occipital /oksip′itəl/, **1.** pertaining to the occiput. **2.** situated near the occipital bone, such as the occipital lobe of the brain.

occipital artery, one of a pair of tortuous branches from the external carotid arteries that divides into six branches and supplies parts of the head and scalp.

occipital bone, the cuplike bone at the back of the skull, marked by a large opening, the foramen magnum, that communicates with the vertebral canal. The occipital bone articulates with the two parietal bones, the two temporal bones, the sphenoid, and the atlas.

occipital condyle syndrome, a condition characterized by a stiff neck and severe localized occipital pain that intensifies with neck flexion. It is associated with unilateral involvement of the twelfth nerve, dysarthria, and dysphagia.

occipitalization /oksip′itəl′īzā′shən/, a process of bony ankylosis of the atlas with the occipital bone.

occipital lobe, one of the five lobes of each cerebral hemisphere, occupying a relatively small pyramidal part of the occipital pole. The occipital lobe lies beneath the occipital bone and presents medial, lateral, and inferior surfaces.

occipital sinus, the smallest of the cranial sinuses and one of six posterior superior venous channels associated with the dura mater.

occipitobregmatic /oksip′itōbregmat′ik/ [L, *occiput,* back of the head; Gk, *bregma,* front of the head], pertaining to the occiput and the bregma.

occipitofrontal /oksip′itōfrun′təl/ [L, *occiput + frons,* forehead], pertaining to the occiput and the frontal bone of the skull.

occipitofrontalis /oksip′itōfrəntal′is/, one of a pair of thin, broad muscles covering the top of the skull, consisting of an occipital belly and a frontal belly connected by an extensive aponeurosis. It is the muscle that draws the scalp and raises the eyebrows.

occiput /ok′sipət/, *pl.* **occiputs, occipita** /oksip′itə′/, the back part of the head.

occluded /əkloo̅′did/ [L, *occludere,* to close up], closed, plugged, or obstructed.

occlusal /əkloo̅′səl/ [L, *occludere,* to close up], pertaining to a closure, such as the contact between the teeth of the upper and lower jaws.

occlusal adjustment, (in dentistry) the intentional mechanical grinding of the biting surfaces of teeth to improve the contact of or relationship between opposing tooth surfaces, their supporting structures, the muscles of mastication, and the temporomandibular joints.

occlusal contouring, the modification by grinding of irregularities of occlusal tooth forms, such as uneven marginal ridges and extruded or malpositioned teeth.

occlusal form, the shape of the occluding surfaces of a tooth, a row of teeth, or any dentition.

occlusal harmony, a combination of healthy and nondisruptive occlusal relationships between the teeth and their supporting structures, the associated neuromuscular mechanisms, and the temporomandibular joints.

occlusal plane [L, *occludere,* to close up, *planum,* level ground], a plane passing through the occlusal surfaces of the teeth. It represents the mean of the curvature of the occlusal or biting surface.

occlusal radiograph, an intraoral radiograph made with the film placed on the occlusal surfaces of one of the arches.

occlusal recontouring, the reshaping of an occlusal surface of a natural or artificial tooth.

occlusal relationship, the relationship of the mandibular teeth to the maxillary teeth when in a defined occlusal contact position.

occlusal rest, a support that is part of a removable partial denture and that is placed on the occlusal surface of a posterior tooth.

occlusal rest angle, (in dentistry) the angle formed by the occlusal rest with the upright minor connector.

occlusal spillway, a natural groove that crosses a cusp ridge or a marginal ridge of a tooth.

occlusal surface [L, *occludere,* to close up, *superficies,* surface], the surfaces of teeth in one arch that make contact or near contact with the corresponding surfaces of the teeth in the opposing arch. It describes the biting surfaces of posterior teeth.

occlusal trauma, injury to a tooth and surrounding structures caused by malocclusive stresses, including trauma, temporomandibular joint dysfunction, and bruxism.

occlusion /əkloo'zhən/ [L, *occludere,* to close up], **1.** (in anatomy) a blockage in a canal, vessel, or passage of the body. **2.** (in dentistry) any contact between the incising or masticating surfaces of the maxillary and mandibular teeth. —**occlude,** *v.,* **occlusive,** *adj.*

occlusion rim, an artificial dental structure with occluding surfaces attached to temporary or permanent denture bases, used for recording the relation of the maxilla to the mandible and for positioning the teeth.

occlusive /əcloo'siv/, pertaining to something that effects an occlusion or closure, such as an occlusive dressing.

occlusive dressing, a dressing that prevents air from reaching a wound or lesion and that retains moisture, heat, body fluids, and medication. It may consist of a sheet of thin plastic affixed with transparent tape.

occult /əkult'/ [L, *occultare,* to hide], hidden or difficult to observe directly, such as occult prolapse of the umbilical cord or occult blood.

occult blood, blood that is not apparent grossly appears from a nonspecific source, with obscure signs and symptoms. It may be detected by means of a chemical test or by microscopic or spectroscopic examination.

occult blood test [L, *occultare,* to hide; AS, *blod* + L, *testum,* crucible], a test for the presence of microscopic amounts of blood in the feces secondary to bleeding in the digestive tract.

occult carcinoma, a small carcinoma that does not cause overt symptoms. The carcinoma may remain localized, be discovered only incidentally at autopsy after death resulting from another cause, or metastasize and be discovered as a result of metastatic disease.

occult ectopic ACTH syndrome, a medical condition that mimics the clinical and biochemical picture of Cushing's disease. The cause is usually a tumor that secretes adrenocorticotropic hormone in the lungs, thymus, pancreas, adrenal medulla, or thyroid gland.

occult fracture, a fracture that cannot be initially detected by radiographic examination but may be evident radiographically weeks later. The break is most likely to occur in the area of the ribs, tibia, metatarsals, or navicula.

occupancy /ok'yəpənse'/ [L, *occupare,* to take possession of], the ratio of average daily hospital census to the average number of beds maintained during the reporting period.

occupancy factor (T), the level of occupancy of an area adjacent to a source of radiation, used to determine the amount of shielding required in the walls. T is rated as full, for an office or laboratory next to an x-ray facility; partial, for corridors and restrooms; and occasional, for stairways, elevators, closets, and outside areas.

occupational accident /ok'yəpā'shənəl/ [L, *occupare,* to take possession of, *accidere,* to happen], an injury to an employee that occurs in the workplace. Occupational accidents account for over 95% of occupational disabilities.

occupational asthma, an abnormal condition of the respiratory system resulting from exposure in the workplace to allergenic or other irritating substances. The condition is most common among people working with detergents, Western red cedar, cotton, flax, hemp, grain, flour, and stone.

occupational deafness, a loss of hearing resulting from noise levels in the workplace.

occupational dermatoses, skin disorders associated with exposure to toxic chemicals or other agents in the workplace. An estimated 80% of cases of contact dermatitis are the result of exposure to chemical irritants. Common agents of contact dermatitis in the workplace are glass fibers, cutting fluids, chemical stains, and polyhalogenated aromatic compounds such as phenol, naphthalene, and aniline herbicides intermediates. Factors influencing development of dermatoses include skin thickness, skin permeability, anatomic site, concentration of chemical, surface area of exposure, and type of substance in which the toxic chemical may be dissolved or mixed.

occupational disability, a condition in which a worker is unable to perform the functions required to complete a job satisfactorily because of an occupational disease or an occupational accident.

occupational disease, a disease that results from a particular employment, usually from the effects of long-term exposure to specific substances or continuous or repetitive physical acts.

occupational health, the ability of a worker to function at an optimum level of well-being at a worksite as reflected in terms of productivity, work attendance, disability compensation claims, and employment longevity.

occupational history, a part of the health history in which questions are asked about the person's occupation, source of income, effects of the work on worker's health or the worker's health on the job, the duration of the job, and to what degree the occupation satisfies the person.

occupational lung disease, any of a group of abnormal conditions of the lungs caused by the inhalation of dusts, fumes, gases, or vapors in an environment where a person works.

occupational medicine, a field of preventive medicine concerned with the medical problems and practices relating to occupations and especially to the health of workers in various industries.

occupational performance tasks, activities that can be used to measure the potential ability or actual proficiency in the handling of certain objects and use of skills related to a given occupation.

occupational socialization, the adaptation of an individual to a given set of job-related behaviors, particularly the expected behavior that accompanies a specific job.

occupational stress, a disorder associated with a job or work. The anxiety may be expressed in the form of extreme tension and anxiety and the development of physical symptoms such as headache or cramps.

occupational therapist (OT), an allied health professional who practices occupational therapy and who must be licensed, registered, certified, or otherwise regulated by law. The OT is concerned with the evaluation, diagnosis, and/or treatment of people of all ages whose ability to cope with activities of daily living is impaired by physical injury, illness, emotional disorder, congenital or developmental disability, or aging. Services include the design, fabrication, and application of orthoses; guidance in the selection and use of adaptive equipment; therapeutic activities to enhance functional performance; prevocational evaluation and training; and consultation concerning the adaptation of physical environment for the handicapped.

occupational therapy (OT), a health rehabilitation profession designed to help people of all ages with physical, developmental, social, or emotional deficits regain and build skills that are important for health and well-being.

occupational therapy aide, a person who, under the supervision of an occupational therapist or assistant, performs clerical and related tasks necessary for the implementation of occupational therapy programs.

occurrence policy /əkur'əns/ [L, *occurere,* to run, *politica,* pertaining to the state], a professional liability insurance policy that covers the holder during the period an alleged act of malpractice occurred. Oc-

currence policies are said to have a 'long tail,' because the statute of limitations on malpractice allegations is unlimited.

ochronosis /ō'krənō'sis/ [Gk, *ochros,* yellow, *osis*], an inherited error of protein metabolism characterized by an accumulation of homogentisic acid, resulting in degenerative arthritis and brown-black pigment deposited in connective tissue and cartilage.

OCN, abbreviation for *Oncology Certified Nurse.*

OCT, abbreviation for **oxytocin challenge test.**

octan /ok'tan/, occurring at 7-day intervals, or every eighth day.

octigravida [L, *octo,* eight, *gravidare,* to impregnate], pertaining to a woman who is pregnant for the eighth time.

ocul., abbreviation for the Latin word *oculis,* pertaining to the eyes.'

ocular /ok'yələr/ [L, *oculus,* eye], **1.** pertaining to the eye. **2.** an eyepiece of an optic instrument.

ocular dysmetria, a visual disorder in which the eyes are unable to fix the gaze on an object or follow a moving object with accuracy.

ocular herpes [L, *oculus,* eye; Gk, *herpein,* to creep], a herpesvirus infection of the eye.

ocular hypertelorism, a developmental defect involving the frontal region of the cranium, characterized by an abnormally widened bridge of the nose and increased distance between the eyes.

ocular hypertension, a condition of intraocular pressure that is higher than normal but that has not resulted in a constricted visual field.

ocular hypotelorism, a developmental defect involving the frontal region of the cranium, characterized by an abnormal narrowing of the bridge of the nose and decreased distance between the eyes, with resulting convergent strabismus.

ocular myopathy, slowly progressive weakness of ocular muscles, characterized by decreased mobility of the eye and drooping of the upper lid. The disorder may be unilateral or bilateral and may be caused by damage to the oculomotor nerve, an intracranial tumor, or a neuromuscular disease.

ocular refraction [L, *oculus,* eye, *refringere,* to break apart], the refraction of the eye.

oculocephalic reflex /ok'yəlō'səfal'ik/ [L, *oculus* + Gk, *kephale,* head; L, *reflectere,* to bend backward], a test of the integrity of brainstem function. When the patient's head is quickly moved to one side and then to the other, the eyes will normally

O

lag behind the head movement and then slowly assume the midline position. Failure of the eyes to either lag properly or revert back to the midline indicates a lesion on the ipsilateral side at the brainstem level.

oculoglandular syndrome /ok'yəlōglan'dyələr/, a unilateral granulomatous form of conjunctivitis. It is associated with a visibly enlarged and tender ipsilateral lymph node and a history of cat-scratch disease.

oculogyric crisis /ok'yəlōjī'rik/ [L, *oculus* + *gyrare,* to turn around], a paroxysm in which the eyes are held in a fixed position, usually up and sideways, for minutes or several hours, often occurring in postencephalitic patients with signs of parkinsonism.

oculomotor /-mō'tər/ [L, *oculus,* eye, *motor,* mover], pertaining to movements of the eyeballs.

oculomotor nerve [L, *oculus* + *motor,* mover], one of a pair of cranial nerves essential for eye movements, supplying certain extrinsic and intrinsic eye muscles.

oculomotor nucleus [L, *oculus,* eye, *motor,* mover, *nucleus,* nut kernel], a nucleus of a third cranial nerve arising in the midbrain.

OD, *(informal).* abbreviation for overdose.

O.D., **1.** abbreviation for *oculus dexter,* a Latin phrase meaning 'right eye.' **2.** abbreviation for *Doctor of Optometry.*

odaxetic /ō'dakset'ik/ [Gk, *odaxein,* a biting pain], causing a tactile sensation such as itching or biting.

OD'd /ōdēd'/ *slang.* overdosed, usually referring to a person who has suffered adverse effects from an excessively large dose of a drug of abuse.

Oddi's sphincter [Ruggero Oddi, Italian surgeon, 1864–1913; Gk, *sphigein,* to bind], a band of circular muscle fibers around the lower part of the common bile duct and pancreatic duct, near the common duct junction with the duodenum.

odontalgia /ō'dontal'jə/ [Gk, *odous,* tooth, *algos,* pain], a toothache.

odontectomy /ōdontek'təmē/ [Gk, *odous,* tooth, *ektome,* cut out], the extraction of a tooth by removal of the bone from around the roots before force is applied.

odontiasis /ō'dontī'əsis/, the process of teething.

odontitis /ō'dontī'tis/ [Gk, *odous* + *itis,* inflammation], abnormal enlargement of a tooth pulp, usually resulting from an inflammation of the odontoblasts (cells responsible for dentin formation) rather than of the mature, or erupted, tooth. It may be caused by infection, tumor, or trauma.

odontoblast /ōdon'təblast'/ [Gk, *odous,* tooth, *blastos,* germ], one of the connective tissue cells of the periphery of the dental pulp that develops into the primary and secondary dentin of a tooth.

odontodysplasia /-displā'zhə/ [Gk, *odous* + *dys,* bad, *plasis,* forming], an abnormality in the development of the teeth, characterized by deficient formation of enamel and dentin.

odontogenesis /-jen'əsis/ [Gk, *odous,* tooth, *genein,* to produce], the origin and formation of developing teeth.

odontogenic /ōdon'tōjen'ik/ [Gk, *odous* + *genein,* to produce], **1.** pertaining to the generation of teeth. **2.** developing in tissues that produce teeth.

odontogenic cyst -jen'ik/, any of a variety of lesions of mouth tissues, including the relatively common dentigerous cyst, which is associated with the crown of an unerupted third molar or maxillary cuspid. Other types are ameloblastic fibroma, odontogenic myxoma, and odontoma.

odontogenic fibroma, a benign neoplasm of the jaw derived from the embryonic part of the tooth germ, dental follicle, or dental papilla or from the periodontal membrane.

odontogenic fibrosarcoma, a malignant neoplasm of the jaw that develops in a mesenchymal component of a tooth or tooth germ.

odontogenic myxoma, a rare tumor of the jaw that may develop from the mesenchyme of the tooth germ.

odontoid process [Gk, *odous* + *eidos,* form; L, *processus*], the toothlike projection that rises perpendicularly from the upper surface of the body of the second cervical vertebra (axis), which serves as a pivot point for the rotation of the atlas (first cervical vertebra), enabling the head to turn.

odontology /ō'dontol'əjē/ [Gk, *odous* + *logos,* science], the scientific study of the anatomy and physiology of the teeth and of the surrounding structures of the oral cavity.

odontoma /ō'donto'mə/ [Gk, *odous* + *oma,* tumor], an anomaly of the mouth that resembles a hard tumor, such as dens in dente, enamel pearl, and complex or composite odontoma.

odor /ō'dər/ [L, a smell], a scent or smell. The sense of smell is activated when airborne molecules stimulate receptors of the first cranial nerve.

odoriferous /ō'dərif'ərəs/ [L, *odor,* smell, *ferre,* to bear], pertaining to something that produces a smell, particularly one that is strong or offensive.

odorous /ō'dərəs/ [L, *odor,* smell], pertaining to something that has an odor, smell, or fragrance.

ODTS, abbreviation for **organic dust toxic syndrome.**

odynacusis [Gk, *odyne,* pain, *akouein,* to hear], a painful sensitivity to noise.

odynophagia /od'inōfā'jə/ [Gk, *odyne,* pain, *phagein,* to swallow], a severe sensation of burning, squeezing pain while swallowing caused by irritation of the mucosa or a muscular disorder of the esophagus such as gastroesophageal reflux, bacterial or fungal infection, tumor, achalasia, or chemical irritation.

Oedipus complex /ed'ipəs, ē'dəpəs/ [Gk, *Oedipus,* mythic king who slew his father and married his mother], **1.** (in psychoanalysis) a child's desire for a sexual relationship with the parent of the opposite sex, usually with strong negative feelings for the parent of the same sex. **2.** a son's desire for a sexual relationship with his mother.

OEM, abbreviation for *optical electron microscope.*

OER, abbreviation for **oxygen enhancement ratio.**

o/f, symbol for *oxidation/fermentation.*

off-center grid, (in radiology) a focused grid that is perpendicular to the central-axis x-ray beam but shifted laterally, resulting in a cutoff across the entire grid.

off-cycle time, (in managed care) a time during which open enrollment in a health plan is usually not permitted.

off-focus radiation, (in radiology) x-rays produced by stray electrons that interact at positions on the anode at points other than the focal spot.

Office of the Inspector General (OIG) of the United States, an agency within the U.S. Department of Health and Human Services that enforces Medicare regulations and investigates and prosecutes charges of Medicare fraud and abuse.

off-level grid, (in radiology) a grid that is not perpendicular to the central-axis x-ray beam. The cause is often a malpositioned x-ray tube rather than an improperly positioned grid.

ofloxacin /oflak'səsin/, an antibiotic of the carboxyfluoroquinolone type.

Ogden classification system, a system of categories for 17 different kinds of epiphyseal fractures.

Ogden plate, a long metal plate with slots designed to accept encircling bands. It is used for fixing long bone fractures associated with preexisting intramedullary devices such as rods or the stem of a prosthesis.

Ogsten line, a line drawn from the adduction tubercle to the intercondylar notch,

used as a guide for transection of the condyle in osteotomy for knock-knee.

o.h., abbreviation for the Latin term *omni hora,* 'hourly.'

OH, symbol for **hydroxyl.**

OHD, abbreviation for *organic heart disease.*

OHF, abbreviation for **Omsk hemorrhagic fever.**

ohm [Georg S. Ohm, German physicist, 1787–1854], a unit of measurement of electrical resistance. One ohm is the resistance of a conductor in which an electrical potential of 1 volt produces a current of 1 ampere.

Ohm's law [Georg S. Ohm], the principle that the strength or intensity of an unvarying electric current is directly proportional to the electromotive force and inversely proportional to the resistance of the circuit.

OIG, abbreviation for **Office of the Inspector General of the United States.**

oil [L, *oleum*], any of a large number of greasy liquid substances not miscible in water. Oil may be fixed or volatile and is derived from animal, vegetable, or mineral matter.

oil retention enema, an enema containing about 200 to 250 ml of an oil-based solution given to soften a fecal mass.

ointment [L, *unguentum,* a salve], a semisolid, externally applied preparation, usually containing a drug. Various ointments are used as local analgesic, anesthetic, antiinfective, astringent, depigmenting, irritant, and keratolytic agents.

O.L., abbreviation for the Latin term *oculus laevus,* 'left eye.'

Old Age, Survivors, Disability and Health Insurance Program (OASDHI), a benefit program, administered by the U.S. Social Security Administration, that provides cash benefits to workers who are retired or disabled, their dependents, and survivors. This part of the program is commonly referred to as Social Security. The program also provides health insurance benefits for people over 65 and disabled people under 65. This part of the program is commonly referred to as Medicare.

Older Americans Act Amendment of 1987, U.S. federal legislation authorizing support of Title III nutrition services for state and county programs on aging. The services include both congregate and home-delivered meals, with related nutrition education.

old dislocation, a dislocation in which inflammatory changes have occurred.

old tuberculin [ME, *ald* + L, *tubercle*], the original formula for an extract of the

O

tubercle bacillus used in the treatment of tuberculosis by Koch.

oleandrism /ō´lē·an´drizəm/, a toxic effect of ingesting or inhaling the cardiac glycoside contained in the roots, bark, flowers, and seeds of oleander *(Nerium oleander),* an evergreen ornamental shrub. Symptoms range from nausea and vomiting to bradycardia and cardiac arrest.

olecranon /ōlek´rənon/ [Gk, *olekranon,* tip of the elbow], a proximal projection of the ulna that forms the point of the elbow and fits into the olecranon fossa of the humerus when the forearm is extended.

olecranon bursa, the bursa of the elbow.

olecranon fossa, the depression in the posterior surface of the humerus that receives the olecranon of the ulna when the forearm is extended.

olefin /ō´ləfin/ [L, *oleum,* oil, *facere,* to make], any of a group of unsaturated aliphatic hydrocarbons containing one or more double bonds in the carbon chain.

oleic acid /ōlē´ik/ [L, *oleum,* oil, *acidus,* sour], a colorless, liquid, monounsaturated fatty acid occurring in almost all natural fats.

oleovitamin /ō´lē·ōvī´təmin/, a preparation of fish-liver oil or edible vegetable oil that contains one or more of the fat-soluble vitamins or their derivatives.

oleovitamin A, an oily preparation, usually fish-liver oil or fish-liver oil diluted with an edible vegetable oil, containing the natural or synthetic form of vitamin A.

Olestra /ōles´trə/, trademark for a synthetic fat substitute derived from sucrose and eight acids of vegetable oils. Olestra adds no calories or fats to the food into which it is incorporated. Because the molecules of Olestra are larger and more tightly packed than those of ordinary fats, they cannot be broken down by digestive enzymes and cannot enter the bloodstream. Adverse effects reported include cramping and loose stools in some people and inhibition of absorption of some vitamins.

olfaction /olfak´shən/ [L, *olfacere,* to smell], **1.** the act of smelling. **2.** the sense of smell.

olfactory /olfak´tərē/, pertaining to the sense of smell. **—olfaction,** *n.*

olfactory bulb [L, *olfactus,* sense of smell, *bulbus,* swollen root], the area of the forebrain where the olfactory nerves terminate and the olfactory tracts arise.

olfactory center [L, *olfactus,* sense of smell; Gk, *kentron*], the part of the brain responsible for the subjective appreciation of odors, a complex group of neurons located near the junction of the temporal and parietal lobes.

olfactory cortex [L, *olfactus,* sense of smell, *cortex,* bark], the part of the cerebral cortex, including the pyriform lobe and the hippocampus formation, that is concerned with the sense of smell.

olfactory foramen, one of several openings in the cribriform plate of the ethmoid bone.

olfactory hallucination [L, *olfactus,* sense of smell, *alucinari,* to wander mentally], a condition in which an individual has false perceptions of odors, which are usually repugnant or offensive. The hallucinations are sometimes associated with guilt feelings.

olfactory lobe [L, *olfactus,* sense of smell; Gk, *lobos,* lobe], a structure involved in the sense of smell in lower animals. Vestiges of the tissue are found in the cerebral hemispheres of humans.

olfactory nerve, one of a pair of nerves associated with the sense of smell. The area in which the olfactory nerves arise is situated in the most superior part of the mucous membrane that covers the superior nasal concha. The olfactory sensory endings are modified epithelial cells, and the least specialized of the special senses. The olfactory nerves connect with the olfactory bulb and the olfactory tract, which are components of the part of the brain associated with the sense of smell.

olfactory organ [L, *olfactus,* sense of smell], the apparatus in the mucous membrane of the nose responsible for the sense of smell. It includes the sensory nerve endings and the olfactory bulb of the brain.

olfactory receptors [L, *olfactus,* sense of smell, *recipere,* to receive], bipolar nerve cells located in the nasal epithelium. Axons of the cells become receptors of the olfactory nerve.

oligemia /ol´ijē´mēə/ [Gk, *oligos,* little, *haima,* blood], a condition of hypovolemia or reduced circulating intravascular volume.

oligoclonal banding /ol´igōklō´nəl/, a process by which cerebrospinal fluid IgG is distributed, after electrophoresis, in discrete bands. Approximately 90% of multiple sclerosis patients show oligoclonal banding.

oligodactyly /ol´igōdak´tilē/ [Gk, *oligos* + *dactylos,* finger], a congenital anomaly characterized by the absence of one or more of the fingers or toes. **—oligodactylic,** *adj.*

oligodendrocyte /ol´igōden´drəsīt/ [Gk, *oligos* + *dendron,* tree, *kytos,* cell], a type of neuroglial cell with dendritic projections that coil around axons of neural cells.

oligodendroglia /ol'igōdendrog'lē·ə/, central nervous system cells that produce myelin.

oligodendroglioma /ol'igōden'drōglī·ō'mə/ [Gk, *oligos* + *dendron,* tree, *glia,* glue, *oma,* tumor], an uncommon brain tumor composed of nonneural ectodermal cells that form part of the supporting connective tissue around nerve cells.

oligodontia /ol'igōdon'shə/ [Gk, *oligos* + *odous,* tooth], a genetically determined dental defect characterized by the development of fewer than the normal number of teeth.

oligogenic /ol'igōjen'ik/ [Gk, *oligos* + *genein,* to produce], pertaining to hereditary characteristics produced by one or only a few genes.

oligohydramnios /-hidram'nē·əs/ [Gk, *oligos* + *hydor,* water, *amnion,* fetal membrane], an abnormally small amount or absence of amniotic fluid.

oligomeganephronia /ol'igōmeg'ənefrō'nē·ə/ [Gk, *oligos* + *megas,* large, *nephros,* kidney], a type of congenital renal hypoplasia associated with chronic renal failure in children. The condition is characterized by a decreased number of functioning nephrons. —**oligomeganephronic,** *adj.*

oligomenorrhea /-men'ôrē'ə/ [Gk, *oligos* + L, *men,* month, *rhoia,* flow], abnormally light or a reduction in menstruation. —**oligomenorrheic,** *adj.*

oligonucleotide /-nōō'klē·ətīd'/, a compound formed by linking a small number of nucleotides.

oligopeptide /-pep'tīd/, a peptide composed of fewer than 20 amino acids.

oligosaccharide /-sak'ərīd/, a compound formed by a small number of monosaccharide units.

oligospermia /ol'igōspur'mē·ə/ [Gk, *oligos* + *sperma,* seed], insufficient spermatozoa in the semen.

oligotroph /ol'igətrof'/, an organism that can survive in a nutrient-poor environment.

oliguria /ol'igyōōr'ē·ə/ [Gk, *oligos* + *ouron,* urine], a diminished capacity to form and pass urine, less than 500 ml in every 24 hours, so that the end products of metabolism cannot be excreted efficiently. —**oliguric,** *adj.*

olisthetic /ōlisthet'ik/, pertaining to olisthy, or bone slippage.

olisthy /ōlis'thē/ [Gk, *olisthanein,* to slip], the slippage of a bone from its normal anatomic site, as in the example of a 'slipped disk.'

olivary body /ol'iver'ē/ [L, *oliva* + AS, *bodig*], an olivary nucleus, part of an aggregate of small densely packed nerve cells, on the medulla oblongata.

olivopontocerebellar /ol'ivōpon'tōsur'-ibel'ər/ [L, *oliva,* olive, *pons,* bridge, *cerebellum,* small brain], pertaining to the olivae, the middle peduncles, and the cerebellum.

olivopontocerebellar atrophy (OPCA) /ol'ivōpon'tōsur'əbel'ər/, a group of hereditary ataxias characterized by mixed clinical features of pure cerebellar ataxia, dementia, Parkinson-like symptoms, spasticity, choreoathetosis, retinal degeneration, myelopathy, and peripheral neuropathy. Various forms of OPCA are transmitted by autosomal-dominant or auto-somal-recessive inheritance.

Ollier's dyschondroplasia /ol'ē·āz'/ [Louis X. E. L. Ollier, French surgeon, 1830–1900; Gk, *dys,* bad, *chondros,* cartilage, *plasis,* formation], a rare disorder of bone development in which the epiphyseal tissue responsible for growth spreads through the bones, causing abnormal irregular growth and eventually deformity.

o.m., abbreviation for the Latin term *omni mane,* 'every morning.'

omalgia /ōmal'jə/ [Gk, *omos,* shoulder, *algos,* pain], pain in the shoulder.

omarthritis /ō'märthrī'tis/, inflammation of the shoulder joint.

ombudsman /om'bədzmən/ [ONorse, *umbothsmathr,* commission man], a person who investigates and mediates patients' problems and complaints in relation to a hospital's services.

omega /ōmē'gə, ōmā'gə, om'əgə/, Ω, ω, the 24th letter of the Greek alphabet.

omega-oxidation, a metabolic pathway of fatty acid oxidation involving the carbon atom farthest removed from the original carboxyl group.

omega-3 fatty acid, a fatty acid with a double bond located at the third carbon atom away from the omega (methyl) end of the molecule. Certain omega-3 fatty acids appear to have protective functions in preventing the formation of blood clots and reducing the risk of coronary heart disease.

omental /ōmen'təl/ [L, *omentum,* membrane of the bowels], pertaining to the omentum.

omental bursa, a cavity in the peritoneum behind the stomach, the lesser omentum, and the lower border of the liver and in front of the pancreas and duodenum.

omentectomy /ō'mentek'təmē/, the surgical excision of a part of the omentum.

omentum /ōmen'təm/, *pl.* **omenta, omentums** [L, fat-skin], an extension of the peritoneum that enfolds one or more organs adjacent to the stomach. —**omental,** *adj.*

omicron /ōm'ikron/, O, o, the 15th letter of the Greek alphabet.

omission /ōmish'ən/ [L, *omittere*, to neglect], (in law) intentional or unintentional neglect to fulfill a duty required by law.

omnifocal lens /om'nēfō'kəl/ [L, *omnis*, all, *focus*, hearth, *lentil*], an eyeglass lens designed for both near and far vision with the reading part in a variable curve.

omnipotence /omnip'ətəns/, (in psychology) an infantile perception that the outside world is part of the organism and within it, which leads to a primitive feeling of all-powerfulness.

omnivorous /omniv'ərəs/ [L, *omnis*, all, *vorare*, to devour], eating both plants and animal flesh.

omn. noct., abbreviation for the Latin term *omni nocte,* 'every night.'

omn. quad. hor., abbreviation for the Latin term *omni quadrante hora,* 'every quarter of an hour.'

omophagia /om'ōfā'jē·ə/ [Gk, *omos*, raw, *phagein*, to eat], the eating of raw foods, particularly raw meat or fish.

omphalic /omfal'ik/ [Gk, *omphalos*, navel], pertaining to the umbilicus.

omphalitis /om'fəlī'tis/, an inflammation of the umbilical stump marked by redness, swelling, and purulent exudate in severe cases.

omphalocele /om'fəlōsēl'/ [Gk, *omphalos* + *kele*, hernia], congenital herniation of intraabdominal viscera through a defect in the abdominal wall around the umbilicus.

omphalogenesis /-jen'əsis/ [Gk, *omphalos* + *genesis*, origin], the formation of the umbilicus or yolk sac during embryonic development. —**omphalogenetic,** *adj.*

omphalosite /om'falōsīt/ [Gk, *omphalos* + *sitos*, food], the underdeveloped parasitic member of unequal conjoined twins united by the vessels of the umbilical cord.

OMS, abbreviation for *Organisation Mondiale de la Santè.*

Omsk hemorrhagic fever (OHF) /ômsk/, an acute infection seen in regions of the former U.S.S.R., caused by an arbovirus transmitted by the bite of an infected tick or by handling infected muskrats. It is characterized by fever, headache, epistaxis, gastrointestinal and uterine bleeding, and other hemorrhagic manifestations.

o.n., abbreviation for the Latin term *omni nocte,* 'every night.'

onanism. coitus interruptus; withdrawal of the penis just before ejaculation during sexual intercourse.

onchocerciasis /ong'kōsərkī'əsis/ [Gk, *onkos*, swelling, *kerkos*, tail, *osis*, condition], a form of filariasis common in Central and South America and Africa, characterized by subcutaneous nodules, pruritic rash, and eye lesions. It is transmitted by the bites of black flies that deposit *Onchocerca volvulus* microfilariae under the skin.

oncofetal protein /-fē'təl/ [Gk, *onkos* + L, *fetus*, pregnant; Gk, *proteios*, first rank], a protein normally produced by fetal tissue and also by cancerous tissues in adult life.

oncogene /ong'kōjēn/ [Gk, *onkos* + *genein*, to produce], a potentially cancer-inducing gene. Under normal conditions such genes play a role in the growth and proliferation of cells, but, when altered in some way by a cancer-causing agent such as radiation, a carcinogenic chemical, or an oncogenic virus, they may cause the cell to be transformed to a malignant state.

oncogenesis /ong'kōjen'əsis/ [Gk, *onkos* + *genesis*, origin], the process initiating and promoting the development of a neoplasm through the action of biologic, chemical, or physical agents.

oncogenic /ong'kōjen'ik/ [Gk, *onkos*, swelling, *genein*, to produce], pertaining to the origin and development of tumors or cancer.

oncogenic virus, any one of over 100 viruses able to cause the development of a malignant neoplastic disease.

oncogenous osteomalacia /ongkoj'ənəs/, a bone disorder caused by mesenchymal tumors. Patients with tumor-induced osteomalacia may have normal-to-low serum calcium levels, low serum phosphorus level, and elevated serum alkaline phosphatase level.

oncologic emergencies /ong'kōloj'ik/, tumor-related disorders that require emergency medical or surgical care. An example is superior vena cava syndrome, in which an expanding tumor mass compresses the thin-walled vena cava, causing obstruction in the venous blood flow from the upper part of the body. Other examples include hypercalcemia, cerebral herniation syndrome, and spinal cord compression.

oncologist /ongkol'əjist/, a physician who specializes in the study and treatment of neoplastic diseases, particularly cancer.

oncology /ongkol'əjē/ [Gk, *onkos*, swelling, *logos*, science], **1.** the branch of medicine concerned with the study of malignancy. **2.** the study of cancerous growths.

Oncology Nursing Society (ONS), an organization of nurses interested or specializing in cancer patient nursing.

oncolysis /ongkol'isis/, **1.** the destruction or disposal of neoplastic cells. **2.** the reduction of a swelling or mass.

oncolytic /ong′kōlit′ik/, pertaining to the destruction of tumor cells.

oncotic /ongkot′ik/ [Gk, *onkos,* a swelling], pertaining to or resulting from the presence of a swelling.

oncotic pressure [Gk, *ogkos,* a swelling; L, *premere,* to press], the osmotic pressure of a colloid in solution, such as when there is a higher concentration of protein in the plasma on one side of a cell membrane than in the neighboring interstitial fluid.

oncotic pressure gradient, the pressure difference between the osmotic pressure of blood and that of tissue fluid or lymph. It is an important force in maintaining fluid balance between the vascular space and the interstitium.

Oncovirinae /ong′kōvir′inē/, a subfamily of ribonucleic acid viruses, including types A, B, C, and D genera of oncoviruses. They are classified on the basis of morphology and type of host.

oncovirus /ong′kōvī′rəs/ [Gk, *onkos* + L, *virus,* poison], a member of a family of viruses associated with leukemia and sarcoma in animals and possibly in humans.

Ondine's curse /ondēnz′/ [L, *Undine,* mythic water nymph; ME, *curs,* invocation], apnea caused by loss of automatic control of respiration. The term refers to a syndrome in patients with decreased sensitivity to retained carbon dioxide. A defect in central chemoreceptor responsiveness to carbon dioxide leaves the patient with hypercapnia and hypoxemia, although fully able to breathe voluntarily.

one-and-a-half spica cast, an orthopedic cast used for immobilizing the trunk of the body cranially to the nipple line, one leg caudally as far as the toes and the other leg caudally as far as the knee.

one gene/one enzyme, a general rule that each gene in a chromosome controls the synthesis of one enzyme. The original rule has been redefined as the one cistron/one polypeptide concept to accommodate posttranslational cleavage to yield multiple peptides, alternate splicing, and alternative promotor sequences.

one gene/one polypeptide, a principle that each gene in a chromosome determines a particular polypeptide. An exception allows many genes to specify only functional ribonucleic acid.

one-to-one care, a method of organizing nursing services in an inpatient care unit by which one registered nurse assumes responsibility for all nursing care provided one patient for the duration of one shift.

one-to-one relationship, a mutually defined, collaborative goal-directed client-therapist relationship for the purpose of psychotherapy.

onlay [AS, *ana,* up, *licagan,* to lie], **1.** a cast type of metal restoration retained by friction and mechanical forces in a prepared tooth for restoring one or more cusps and adjoining occlusal surfaces of a tooth. **2.** an occlusal rest part of a removable partial denture, extended to cover the entire occlusal surface of a tooth.

onlay graft, a bone graft in which the transplanted tissue is laid directly onto the surface of the recipient bone.

on/off phenomenon, a periodic loss of the efficacy of levodopa in the treatment of Parkinson's disease, without obvious relationship to the timing of levodopa administration.

ONS, abbreviation for **Oncology Nursing Society.**

onset of action, the time required after administration of a drug for a response to be observed.

ontogenetic /on′tōjənet′ik/, **1.** of, relating to, or acquired during ontogeny. **2.** an association based on visible morphologic characteristics and not necessarily indicative of a natural evolutionary relationship.

ontogeny /ontoj′ənē/ [Gk, *ontos,* being, *genein,* to produce], the life history of one organism from a single-celled ovum to the time of birth, including all phases of differentiation and growth.

onychia /ōnik′ē·ə/ [Gk, *onyx,* nail], inflammation of the nail bed.

onychodystrophy [Gk, *onyx,* nail, *dys,* bad, *trophe,* nourishment], a condition of malformed or discolored fingernails or toenails.

onychogryphosis /on′ikōgrifō′sis/ [Gk, *onyx* + *gryphein,* to curve, *osis,* condition], thickened, curved, clawlike overgrowth of fingernails or toenails.

onycholysis /on′ikol′isis/ [Gk, *onyx* + *lysein,* to loosen], separation of a nail from its bed, beginning at the free margin, associated with psoriasis, dermatitis of the hand, fungal infection, *Pseudomonas* infection, and many other conditions.

onychomycosis /on′ikō′mīkō′sis/ [Gk, *onyx* + *mykes,* fungus, *osis,* condition], any fungus infection of the nails.

onychosis [Gk, *onyx,* nail, *osis,* condition], a condition of atrophy or dystrophy of the nails, usually caused by a dermatosis such as a fungal infection.

onychotillomania /on′ikōtil′əmā′nē·ə/ [Gk, *onyx,* nail, *tillein,* to pluck, *mania,* madness], a nervous habit of picking at the nails.

onychotomy /on′ikot′əmē/, a surgical incision into a nail bed.

oob, abbreviation for *out of bed.*

oobe, abbreviation for **out-of-body experience.**

ooblast /ō'əblast/ [Gk, *oon*, egg, *blastos*, germ], the female germ cell from which the mature ovum is developed.

oocyesis /ō'əsī-ē'sis/ [Gk, *oon* + *kyesis*, pregnancy], an ectopic ovarian pregnancy.

oocyst /ō'əsist/ [Gk, *oon* + *kystis*, bag], a stage in the development of any sporozoan in which after fertilization a zygote is produced that develops about itself an enclosing cyst wall.

oocyte /ō'əsīt/ [Gk, *oon* + *kytos*, cell], a primordial or incompletely developed ovum.

oocytin /ō'əsī'tin/, the substance in a spermatozoon that stimulates the formation of the fertilization membrane after penetration of an ovum.

oogamy /ō·og'əmē/ [Gk, *oon* + *gamos*, marriage], **1.** sexual reproduction by the fertilization of a large nonmotile female gamete by a smaller, actively motile male gamete, such as occurs in certain algae and the malarial parasite *Plasmodium.* **2.** heterogamy. **—oogamous,** *adj.*

oogenesis /ō'əjen'əsis/ [Gk, *oon* + *genesis*, origin], the process of the growth and maturation of the female gametes, or ova. **—oogenetic,** *adj.*

oogonium /ō'əgō'nē·əm/, *pl.* **oogonia** [Gk, *oon* + *gonos*, offspring], the precursor cell from which an oocyte develops in the fetus during intrauterine life.

ookinesis /ō'əkinē'sis/ [Gk, *oon* + *kinesis*, movement], the mitotic phenomena occurring in the nucleus of the egg cell during maturation and fertilization. **—ookinetic,** *adj.*

ookinete /ō'əkinēt'/ [Gk, *oon* + *kinein*, to move], the motile elongated zygote that is formed by the fertilization of the macrogamete during the sexual reproductive phase of the life cycle of a sporozoan, specifically the malarial parasite *Plasmodium.*

oophoralgia /ō'əfôral'jə/ [Gk, *oophoron*, ovary, *algos*, pain], a pain in an ovary.

oophorectomy /ō'əfərek'təmē/ [Gk, *oophoron*, ovary, *ektome*, excision], the surgical removal of one or both ovaries. It is performed to remove a cyst or tumor, excise an abscess, treat endometriosis, or in breast cancer to remove the source of estrogen, which stimulates some kinds of cancer. If both ovaries are removed, sterility results, and menopause is abruptly induced; in premenopausal women one ovary or a part of one ovary may be left intact unless a malignancy is present. The operation routinely accompanies a hysterectomy in menopausal or postmenopausal women.

oophoritis /ō'əferī'tis/, an inflammatory condition of one or both ovaries, usually occurring with salpingitis or another infection.

oophorosalpingectomy /ō'əfôr'əsal'pinjek'təmē/ [Gk, *oophoron* + *salpinx*, tube, *ektome*, excision], the surgical removal of one or both ovaries and the corresponding fallopian tubes, performed to remove a cyst or tumor, excise an abscess, or treat the condition of endometriosis. In a bilateral procedure the patient becomes sterile, and menopause is induced.

oophorosalpingitis /ō'əfôr'əsal'pinjī'tis/ [Gk, *oophoron*, ovary, *salpigx*, tube, *itis*, inflammation], an inflammation involving both the ovary and the fallopian tube.

ooplasm /ō'əplaz'əm/[Gk, *oon* + *plasma*, something formed], the cytoplasm of the egg, or ovum, including the yolk in lower animals.

oosperm /ō'əspurm/ [Gk, *oon* + *sperma*, seed], a fertilized ovum; the cell resulting from the union of the pronuclei of the spermatozoon and the ovum after fertilization; a zygote.

ootid /ō'ətid/ [Gk, *ootidion*, small egg], the mature ovum after penetration by the spermatozoon and completion of the second meiotic division but before the fusion of the pronuclei to form the zygote.

OP, 1. abbreviation for *operative procedure.* **2.** abbreviation for **outpatient.**

opacity /ōpas'itē/ [L, *opacitus*, shadiness], pertaining to an opaque quality of a substance or object, such as cataract opacity.

opaque /ōpāk'/ [L, *opacus*, obscure], **1.** pertaining to a substance or surface that neither transmits nor allows the passage of light. **2.** neither transparent nor translucent.

OPD, abbreviation for *Outpatient Department.*

open amputation [AS, *offan*, open; L, *amputare*, to cut away], a kind of amputation in which a straight, guillotine cut is made without skin flaps. Open amputation is performed if an infection is probable, developing, or recurrent.

open bite, an abnormal dental condition in which the anterior teeth do not occlude in any mandibular position.

open-chain exercise, exercise in which the distal aspect of the extremity is free in space and not in contact with the ground.

open charting, a system of medical record keeping in which the patient has access to his or her chart.

open circuit, an electrical circuit in which current flow ceases.

open-circuit breathing system, a type of breathing system used in cardiopulmonary therapy in which rebreathing does not occur. Gas is inspired through a breathing branch that is connected to a gas source or open to the ambient atmosphere and then expired into a collecting reservoir or vented back into the atmosphere.

open dislocation, a dislocation in which the skin is broken.

open-drop anesthesia, the oldest and simplest anesthetic technique. A volatile liquid anesthetic agent is dripped onto a porous cloth or mask held over the patient's face.

open-enrollment period, a time during which individuals can enroll in a health care plan.

open fracture grading system, a system of five categories of open fractures, ranging from a less than 1-cm clean wound that communicates to the fracture site to an open fracture requiring repair of arteries.

opening abductory wedge osteotomy (OAWO), a procedure for treating a bunion deformity. It involves the use of a bone graft to open the wedge and bring the first metatarsal closer to the second.

opening pressure, the amount of pressure measured in a manometer after insertion of a spinal needle into the subarachnoid space.

opening wedge osteotomy, a bunion deformity treatment with a proximal cut in the metatarsal and reduction of the deformity. It is performed with or without tendon transfers.

open medical staff, (in managed care) the opening of hospital medical staff membership to all physicians in the community who meet membership and clinical privilege requirements.

open operation, a surgical procedure that provides a full view of the structures or organs involved through membranous or cutaneous incisions.

open-panel HMO, a health maintenance organization (HMO) in which physicians treat both HMO and private patients.

open PHO, a physician-hospital organization in which all physicians on the hospital medical staff can participate.

open pneumothorax [AS, *open* + Gk, *pneuma,* air, *thorax,* chest], the presence of air or gas in the chest as a result of an open wound in the chest wall.

open reduction [AS, *open* + L, *reducere,* to lead back], a surgical procedure for reducing a fracture or dislocation by exposing the skeletal parts involved.

open system, a system that interacts with its environment.

open-wedge osteotomy, a straight cut made across a bone, creating angulation, leaving an open wedge-shaped gap.

open wound [AS, *open* + *wund*], a wound that disrupts the integrity of the skin.

operable /op′ərəbəl/ [L, *operare,* to work], amenable to surgical intervention, as a disease or injury may be.

operant /op′ərənt/ [L, *operare,* to work], any act or response occurring without an identifiable stimulus. The result of the act or response determines whether or not it is repeated.

operant conditioning, a form of learning used in behavior therapy in which the person undergoing therapy is rewarded for the correct response and punished for the incorrect response.

operant level, the frequency or form of a performance under baseline conditions before any systematic conditioning procedures are introduced.

operating microscope /op′ərā′ting/ [L, *operare* + Gk, *mikros,* small, *skopein,* to look], a binocular microscope used in delicate surgery, especially surgery of the eye or ear. The standing type of operating microscope has a motorized zoom system operated by a foot pedal that quickly changes the magnification. The operating microscope that attaches to a surgeon's head has interchangeable lenses for different magnifications.

operating room (OR, O.R.), **1.** a room in a health care facility in which surgical procedures requiring anesthesia are performed. **2.** *informal.* a suite of rooms or an area in a health care facility in which patients are prepared for surgery and undergo surgical procedures.

operating telescope, a magnifying lens that gives low magnification and a wide field of vision.

operation /op′ərā′shən/, any surgical procedure, such as an appendectomy or a hysterectomy.

operationalization of behavior /op′ərā′-shənəl′īzāshən/, (in psychology) the stating of a patient's complaints or problems in specific, observable behavioral terms.

operative cholangiography /op′ərətiv′/ [L, *operare* + Gk, *chole,* bile, *angeion,* vessel, *graphein,* to record], (in diagnostic radiology) a procedure for outlining the major bile ducts. It is performed during surgery by injecting a radiopaque contrast material directly into these ducts.

operator gene /op′ərā′tər/ [L, *operare* + Gk, *genein,* to produce], (in molecular genetics) a genetic unit that regulates the transcription of structural genes in its operon.

operculum /ōpur′kyōōləm/, *pl.* **opercula, operculums** [L, *lid*], a lid or covering,

O

such as the mucous plug that blocks the cervix of the gravid uterus. —**opercular,** *adj.*

operon /op'əron/ [L, *operare,* to work], (in molecular biology) a segment of deoxyribonucleic acid consisting of an operator gene and one or more structural genes with related functions controlled by the operator gene in conjunction with a regulator gene.

ophth, abbreviation for **ophthalmology.**

ophthalmia /ofthal'mē·ə/ [Gk, *ophthalmos,* eye], severe inflammation of the conjunctiva or the deeper parts of the eye.

ophthalmia neonatorum /nē'ōnətôr'əm/, a purulent conjunctivitis and keratitis of the newborn resulting from exposure of the eyes to chemical, chlamydial, bacterial, or viral agents. Chemical conjunctivitis usually occurs as a result of the instillation of silver nitrate in the eyes of a newborn to prevent a gonococcal infection.

ophthalmic /ofthal'mik/, [Gk, *ophthalmos,* eye], pertaining to the eye.

ophthalmic administration of medication /ofthal'mik/, the administration of a drug by instillation of a cream, an ointment, or a liquid drop preparation in the conjunctival sac. The medication is instilled into the eye or eyes as directed. For administration the patient is positioned comfortably, lying back on a bed or examining table or sitting up with the neck hyperextended. The cul-de-sac of the conjunctival sac is exposed by gentle traction on the tissue just below the lower eyelid. The medication is placed into the sac as the patient is instructed to look away from the point of instillation. The dispenser is not allowed to touch the eye, and the medication is not placed directly on the cornea. The eyelid is slowly released, and the patient is asked to roll the eye around a few times to spread the medication over the entire surface of the eye.

ophthalmic medical technician and technologist, an allied health professional who assists ophthalmologists by collecting data and administering treatment ordered by the ophthalmologist. These specialists are qualified to take medical histories; administer diagnostic tests; make anatomic and functional ocular measurements; test ocular functions, including visual acuity, visual fields, and sensorimotor functions; administer topical ophthalmic medications; and instruct the patient in home care and the use of contact lenses.

ophthalmic nerve [Gk, *ophthalmos,* eye; L, *nervus,* nerve], the first division of the trigeminal nerve (CN V), supplying the eyeball through the nasociliary branch.

Branches also innervate the forehead, scalp, lacrimal gland, and dura mater.

ophthalmic solution, a sterile preparation free of foreign particles for installation of a medication into the eye.

ophthalmitis /of'thalmī'tis/ [Gk, *ophthalmos,* eye, *itis,* inflammation], an inflammation of the eye.

ophthalmodynamometer /-din'əmom'ətər/ [Gk, *ophthalmos,* eye, *dynamis,* force, *metron,* measure], an instrument for measuring pressure on the sclera while the fundus is studied with an ophthalmoscope. It may be used to measure blood pressures in the ophthalmic artery.

ophthalmodynia /-din'ē·ə/ [Gk, *ophthalmos,* eye, *odyne,* pain], a pain in the eye.

ophthalmologist /of'thalmol'əjist/, a physician who specializes in ophthalmology.

ophthalmology (ophth) /of'thalmol'əjē/ [Gk, *ophthalmos* + *logos,* science], the branch of medicine concerned with the study of the physiology, anatomy, and pathology of the eye and the diagnosis and treatment of disorders of the eye. —**ophthalmologic, ophthalmological,** *adj.*

ophthalmoplasty /ofthal'mōplas'tē/ [Gk, *ophthalmos,* eye, *plassein,* to mold], plastic surgery of the eye or the area around the eye.

ophthalmoplegia /ofthal'məplē'jē·ə/ [Gk, *ophthalmos* + *plege,* stroke], an abnormal condition characterized by paralysis of the motor nerves of the eye. Bilateral ophthalmoplegia of rapid onset is associated with acute myasthenia gravis, acute thiamin deficiency, botulism, and acute inflammatory cranial polyneuropathy. These diseases are potentially very destructive and require prompt attention.

ophthalmoscope /ofthal'məskōp/ [Gk, *ophthalmos* + *skopein,* to look], a device for examining the interior of the eye. It includes a light, a mirror with a single aperture through which the examiner views, and a dial holding several lenses of varying strengths. The lenses are selected to allow clear visualization of the structures of the eye at any depth.

ophthalmoscopy /of'thalmos'kəpē/, the technique of using an ophthalmoscope to examine the eye.

ophthalmospasm /ofthal'mōspaz'əm/ [Gk, *ophthalmos,* eye, *spasmos*], a sudden involuntary contraction of the eyeball.

opiate /ō'pē·it/ [Gk, *opion,* poppy juice], **1.** a narcotic drug that contains opium, derivatives of opium, or any of several semisynthetic or synthetic drugs with opium-like activity. **2.** *informal.* any soporific or narcotic drug. **3.** pertaining to a substance that causes sleep or relief of pain. Morphine and related opiates may produce unwanted side effects such as nausea, vomiting, dizziness, and constipation.

opiate poisoning [Gk, *opion*, poppy juice; L, *potio*, drink], toxic effects of a potent narcotic, including depression of the brain centers, causing unconsciousness. Acute intoxication is characterized by euphoria, flushing, and itching, followed by reduced rate of respiration, hypotension, lowered body temperature, and abnormally slow heart beat. Withdrawal is marked by effects generally the opposite of opiate poisoning, depending on the size of the dose and the duration of dependence.

opiate receptor [Gk, *opion*, poppy juice; L, *recipere*, to receive], any of a group of cells in the brain that bind to opiate drugs such as morphine. Some along the aqueduct of Sylvius and the center median have been identified as receptors associated with response to pain; others have been found in the striatum.

opinion /əpin'yən/ [L, *opinari*, to suppose], **1.** (in law) a statement by the court, usually in writing, of the reasoning behind its decision or judgment in a particular case. **2.** a statement prepared for a client by an attorney that represents the attorney's understanding of the law as it pertains to a legal question posed by the client.

opioid /ō'pē-oid/ [Gk, *opionm*, poppy juice, *eidos*, form], pertaining to natural and synthetic chemicals that have opium-like effects, although they are not derived from opium. Examples include endorphins or enkephalins produced by body tissues or synthetic methadone.

opisthorchiasis /ō'pisthôrkī'əsis/ [Gk, *opisthen*, behind, *orchis*, testicle, *osis*, condition], infection with one of the species of *Opisthorchis* liver flukes commonly found in the Philippines, India, Thailand, and Laos.

opisthotonos /ō'pisthot'ənəs/ [Gk, *opisthios*, posterior, *tonos*, straining], a prolonged severe spasm of the muscles causing the back to arch acutely, the head to bend back on the neck, the heels to bend back on the legs, and the arms and hands to flex rigidly at the joints.

opium /ō'pē·əm/ [Gk, *opion*, poppy juice], a milky exudate from the unripe capsules of *Papaver somniferum* and *Papaver album* yielding 9.5% or more of anhydrous morphine. It is a narcotic analgesic, a hypnotic, and an astringent. Opium contains several alkaloids, including codeine, morphine, and papaverine.

opium alkaloid, one of several alkaloids isolated from the milky exudate of the unripe seed pods of *Papaver somniferum,* a species of poppy indigenous to the Near East. Three of the alkaloids, codeine, papaverine, and morphine, are used clinically for the relief of pain, but their use entails the risk of physical or psychologic dependence. Morphine is the standard against which the analgesic effect of newer drugs for relief of pain is measured. The opium alkaloids and their semisynthetic derivatives, including heroin, act on the central nervous system, producing analgesia, change in mood, drowsiness, and mental slowness.

opium tincture, an analgesic and antidiarrheal prescribed in the treatment of intestinal hyperactivity, cramping, and diarrhea.

Oppenheim reflex /op'ənhīm/ [Herman Oppenheim, German neurologist, 1858–1919], a variation of Babinski's reflex, elicited by firmly stroking downward on the anterior and medial surfaces of the tibia, characterized by extension of the great toe and fanning of other toes. It is a sign of pyramidal tract disease.

opportunistic infection [L, *opportunus,* convenient, *icus,* form], **1.** an infection caused by normally nonpathogenic organisms in a host whose resistance has been decreased by disorders such as diabetes mellitus, human immunodeficiency virus infection, or cancer; a surgical procedure such as a cerebrospinal fluid shunt or a cardiac or urinary tract catheterization; or immunosuppressive drugs. Long-term use of antibiotics or other drugs also may affect the immune system. **2.** an unusual infection with a common pathogen such as cellulitis, meningitis, or otitis media.

opportunistic pathogen, an organism that exists harmlessly as part of the normal human body environment and does not become a health threat until the body's immune system fails.

opposition [L, *opponere,* to oppose], the relation between the thumb and the other digits of the hand for the purpose of grasping objects between the thumb and fingers.

opscan, abbreviation for *optical scanning.*

opsin, a protein that combines with retinal to form rhodopsin, or visual purple, in the rod photoreceptor cells of the retina.

opsonin /op'sənin/ [Gk, *opsonein,* to supply food], an antibody or complement split product that, on attaching to foreign material, microorganisms, or other antigens, enhances phagocytosis of that substance by leukocytes and other macrophages. —**opsonize,** *v.*

opsonization /op'sənizā'shən/ [Gk, *opsonein* + *izein,* to cause], the process by which opsonins render bacteria more susceptible to phagocytosis by leukocytes.

optic [Gk, *optikos,* sight], pertaining to the eyes or to sight.

optical activity, the rotation of the plane of polarized light clockwise or counterclockwise. Substances that rotate the plane of polarized light to the right are dextrorotatory; those that rotate the plane to the left are levorotatory.

optical brightener, a compound that absorbs ultraviolet light and emits visible light.

optical illusion [Gk, *optikos,* sight; L, *illudere,* to mock], a false visual image derived from a misinterpretation of sensory stimuli caused by physical or psychologic factors or both. A common optical illusion is the appearance of railroad tracks merging in the distance.

optical righting reflex [Gk, *optikos,* sight; AS, *riht* + L, *reflectere,* to bend back], a reflex that restores normal posture and head position with the help of visual clues.

optic atrophy /op'tik/, wasting of the optic disc resulting from degeneration of fibers of the optic nerve and optic tract. Optic atrophy may be caused by a congenital defect, inflammation, occlusion of the central retinal artery or internal carotid artery, alcohol, arsenic, lead, tobacco, or other toxic substances. Degeneration of the disc may accompany arteriosclerosis, diabetes, glaucoma, hydrocephalus, pernicious anemia, and various neurologic disorders.

optic chiasm [Gk, *optikos,* sight, *chiasma,* crossed lines], a point near the thalamus and hypothalamus where parts of each optic nerve cross over.

optic coupling, a method of attaching the crystal window of a scintillator to the window of a photomultiplier tube so there is a minimum loss of light transmitted from the scintillator to the interior of the photomultiplier tube.

optic cup, a two-layered embryonic cavity that develops in early pregnancy. The cells of the optic cup differentiate to form the retina that first develops its layers of rods and cones in the central part of the cup.

optic density, a number describing the blackening of an x-ray film in any specified location.

optic disc, the small blind spot on the surface of the retina, located to the nasal side of the macula. It is the only part of the retina that is insensitive to light.

optic foramen [Gk, *optikos,* sight, *foramen,* hole], an aperture in the root of the lesser wing of the sphenoid bone transmitting the optic nerve.

optic glioma, a slow-growing tumor on the optic nerve or in the chiasm. The tumor is composed of glial cells. Symptoms may include loss of vision, secondary strabismus, exophthalmos, and ocular paralysis.

optician /optish'ən/ [Gk, *optikos,* sight], a person who grinds and fits eyeglasses and contact lenses by prescription. To become an optician, a person must graduate from high school and complete a 4-or 5-year apprenticeship. In some states licensure is required.

optic nerve, one of a pair of cranial nerves that transmit visual impulses. It consists mainly of coarse myelinated fibers that arise in the retinal ganglionic layer, traverse the thalamus, and connect with the visual cortex. The visual cortex functions in the perception of light, shade, and objects. The optic nerve fibers correspond to a tract of fibers within the brain.

optic neuritis [Gk, *optikos,* sight, *neuron,* nerve, *itis,* inflammation], inflammation, degeneration, or demyelinization of an optic nerve caused by a wide variety of diseases. Loss of vision is the cardinal symptom.

optic neuropathy [Gk, *optikos,* sight, *neuron,* nerve, *pathos,* disease], a disease, generally noninflammatory, of the eye, characterized by dysfunction or destruction of the optic nerve tissues. Causes may include an interruption in the blood supply, compression by a tumor or aneurysm, a nutritional deficiency, and toxic effects of a chemical. The disorder, which can lead to blindness, usually affects only one eye.

optic radiation [Gk, *optikos,* sight; L, *radiare,* to shine], a system of fibers from the lateral geniculate body of the thalamus that pass through the sublenticular part of the internal capsule to the striate area.

optic righting, one of the five basic neuromuscular reactions that enable a person to change body positions. It involves a reflex that automatically orients the head to a new optical or visual fixation point, depending on the body position change.

optics /op'tiks/ [Gk, *optikos,* sight], **1.** (in physics) a field of study that deals with the electromagnetic radiation of wavelengths shorter than radio waves but longer than x-rays. **2.** (in physiology) a field of study that deals with vision and the process by which the functions of the eye and the brain are integrated in the perception of shapes, patterns, movements, spatial relationships, and color.

optic stalk, one of a pair of slender embryonic structures that become the optic nerve.

optic system assessment, an evaluation of the patient's eyes, vision, and current and past disorders or injuries that may be responsible for abnormalities in the individual's optic system. A careful assessment of the patient's eyes and vision and of certain aspects of the medical, family, and social history is a significant aid in establishing the diagnosis of an optic system disorder.

optic thermometer, a temperature-measuring device in which the properties of transmission and reflection of visible light are temperature dependent, the detection of which can be related to tissue temperature.

optic tract [Gk, *optikos*, sight; L, *tractus*], a flat band of nerve fibers running backward and laterally around each cerebral peduncle from the optic chiasma to the lateral geniculate body.

optic vesicle, an early embryonic outgrowth from the ventrolateral wall of the forebrain. Its cells develop into the retina and optic nerve of the eye.

optional water loss /op'shənəl/, a volume of average daily water loss, in addition to obligatory water loss, depending on physical activities, climate, and other factors.

optokinetic /op'tōkinet'ik/ [Gk, *optikos*, sight, *kinesis*, motion], pertaining to movement of the eyeballs in response to the movement of objects across the visual field, such as in optokinetic nystagmus.

optometrist /optom'ətrist/ [Gk, *optikos*, sight, *metron*, measure], a person who practices optometry. An optometrist is awarded the degree of Doctor of Optometry (O.D.) after completion of at least 3 years of college followed by 4 years in an approved college of optometry. A state examination and license are also required.

optometry /optom'ətrē/ [Gk, *optikos*, sight, *metron*, measure], the practice of primary eye care, including testing the eyes for visual acuity, diagnosing and managing eye health, prescribing corrective spectacle or contact lenses, and recommending eye exercises.

OPV, abbreviation for **oral poliovirus vaccine.**

OR, O.R., abbreviation for **operating room.**

oral /ôr'əl/ [L, *oralis*, mouth], pertaining to the mouth.

oral administration of medication, the administration of a tablet, a capsule, an elixir, or a solution or other liquid form of medication by mouth. Oral administration of medication includes **buccal administration of medication** and **sublingual administration of medication.**

oral airway, a curved tubular device of rubber, plastic, or metal placed in the oropharynx during general anesthesia and other situations in which the level of consciousness is impaired. Its purpose is to maintain free passage of air and keep the tongue from obstructing the trachea.

oral and maxillofacial surgery [L, *oralis*, mouth; Gk, *cheirourgos*, surgeon], a branch of dentistry that is concerned primarily with surgery on the teeth, jaws, and surrounding soft tissues.

oral cancer, a malignant neoplasm on the lip or in the mouth that occurs at an average age of 60 with a frequency eight times higher in men than in women. Predisposing factors are alcoholism, heavy use of tobacco, poor oral hygiene, ill-fitting dentures, syphilis, Plummer-Vinson's syndrome, betel nut chewing, and in lip cancer pipe smoking and overexposure to sun and wind. Premalignant leukoplakia or erythroplasia or a painless nonhealing ulcer may be the first sign of oral cancer; localized pain usually occurs later, but lymph nodes may be involved early in the course. Almost all oral tumors are epidermoid carcinomas; adenocarcinomas occur occasionally, whereas sarcomas and metastatic lesions from other sites are rare.

oral cavity [L, *oralis*, mouth, *cavum*, cavity], the space within the mouth, containing the tongue and teeth.

oral character, (in psychoanalysis) a kind of personality that exhibits patterns of behavior originating in the oral and first phase of infancy. This personality is characterized by optimism, self-confidence, and carefree generosity reflecting the pleasurable aspects of the stage; or pessimism, futility, anxiety, and sadism as manifestations of frustrations or conflicts occurring during the period.

oral contraceptive, oral hormone medication for contraception. The two major hormones used are progestin and a combination of progestin and estrogen. The hormones act by inhibiting the productivity of gonadotropin-releasing hormone by the hypothalamus, and therefore the pituitary does not secrete gonadotropins to stimulate ovulation. This results in the endometrium of the uterus being thin and the cervical mucus being thick, thus preventing the penetration of sperm.

oral decongestant, a drug such as pseudoephedrine and phenylpropanolamine prescribed for the relief of nasal congestion. Oral decongestants do not appear to cause nasal swelling after long periods of use. They are commonly combined with antihistamines for the treatment of allergic rhinitis.

oral dosage, the administration of a medicine by mouth.

oral eroticism, (in psychoanalysis) libidi-

O

nal fixation at or regression to the oral stage of psychosexual development, often reflected in such personality traits as passivity, insecurity, and oversensitivity.

oral examination [L, *oralis,* mouth, *examinatio,* to weigh], a clinical, visual, and tactile inspection and investigation of the hard and soft structures of the oral cavity for purposes of assessment and diagnosis, planning, treatment, and evaluation.

Oral Health Maintenance, a **Nursing Interventions Classification** defined as maintenance and promotion of oral hygiene and dental health for the patient at risk for developing oral or dental lesions.

Oral Health Promotion, a **Nursing Interventions Classification** defined as promotion of oral hygiene and dental care for a patient with normal oral and dental health.

Oral Health Restoration, a **Nursing Interventions Classification** defined as promotion of healing for a patient who has an oral mucosa or dental lesion.

oral hygiene, the condition or practice of maintaining the tissues and structures of the mouth. Oral hygiene includes brushing the teeth to remove food particles, bacteria, and plaque; massaging the gums with a toothbrush, dental floss, or water irrigator to stimulate circulation and remove foreign matter; and cleansing dentures and ensuring their proper fit to prevent irritation.

oral hypoglycemic agent, an oral antidiabetic agent commonly used in the treatment of adult diabetes. Oral hypoglycemic agents are not prescribed as a substitute for diet and exercise but rather as adjunctive therapy. The available drugs include first-and second-generation sulfonylureas such as tolazamide and glyburide and antihyperglycemics such as biguanide metformin. They are effective but differ in their mechanism of action. Sulfonylureas stimulate pancreatic insulin secretion, whereas metformin suppresses excess glucose production by the liver.

oral mucosa, the mucous membrane of the cavity of the mouth, including the gums.

oral mucous membrane, altered, a NANDA-accepted nursing diagnosis of a state in which an individual experiences disruptions in the tissue layers of the oral cavity. Defining characteristics include oral pain or discomfort, coated tongue, xerostomia (dry mouth), stomatitis, oral lesions or ulcers, lack of or decreased salivation, leukoplakia, edema, hyperemia, oral plaque, desquamation, vesicles, hemorrhagic gingivitis, carious teeth, and halitosis.

oral poliovirus vaccine (OPV), an attenuated preparation of live poliovirus that confers immunity to poliomyelitis. It is routinely prescribed for immunization against poliomyelitis.

oral prophylaxis [L, *oralis,* mouth; Gk, *prophylax,* advance guard], the science and practice of preventing the onset of diseases of the teeth and adjoining mouth tissues. It involves removing plaque, materia alba, food debris, stains, and calculus from the anatomic crowns and roots with hand scaling ultrasonic scaling instruments and hand and electric polishers.

oral rehydration solutions (ORS) [L, *oralis,* mouth, *re + hydor,* water, *solutus,* dissolved], solutions of electrolytes and glucose used in oral rehydration therapy. The recommended electrolytes include NaCl, KCl, and trisodium citrate.

oral rehydration therapy (ORT), the adjustment of water, glucose, and electrolyte balance in a dehydrated patient by giving fluids with measured amounts of essential ingredients by mouth.

oral sadism, (in psychoanalysis) a sadistic form of oral eroticism manifested by such behavior as biting, chewing, and other aggressive impulses associated with eating habits.

oral stage, (in psychoanalysis) according to Freud, the initial stage of psychosexual development occurring in the first 12 to 18 months of life when the feeding experience and other oral activities are the predominant source of pleasurable stimulation.

oral temperature [L, *oralis,* mouth, *temperatura*], the body temperature as recorded by a clinical thermometer placed in the mouth. It is normally around 99° F (37° C), but it may vary within a fraction of a degree, depending on the individual and such factors as time of day, sleep, and exercise and whether measured before or after a meal.

oral tolerance therapy, a treatment in which a patient ingests a foreign protein in an attempt to develop tolerance to the same protein when it is introduced as an antigen. In addition to inhibiting allergic reactions, the therapy may suppress immune responses in general.

orb /ôrb/ [L, *orbis,* circle], describing something spheric or globelike.

orbicular /ôbik′yələr/ [L, *orbiculus,* little circle], pertaining to something round.

orbicular bone [L, *orbiculus,* little circle; AS, *ban*], a knob on the end of the long process of the incus that articulates with the stapes.

orbicularis ciliaris /ôrbik′yōōlär′is/ [L, *orbiculus,* little circle; *cilium,* eyelash], one of the two zones of the ciliary body of the eye, extending from the ora serrata of the retina to the ciliary processes at the margin of the iris.

orbicularis oculi, the muscular body of the eyelid encircling the eye and comprising the palpebral, orbital, and lacrimal muscles. The palpebral muscle functions to close the eyelid gently; the orbital muscle functions to close it more energetically, such as in winking.

orbicularis oris, the muscle surrounding the mouth. It consists partly of fibers derived from other facial muscles such as the buccinator that are inserted into the lips and partly of fibers proper to the lips. It serves to close and purse the lips.

orbicularis pupillary reflex, a normal phenomenon elicited by forceful closure of the eyelids or attempting to close them while they are held apart, resulting first in constriction and then dilation of the pupil.

orbit /ôr′bit/ [L, *orbita,* wheel track], one of a pair of bony, conical cavities in the skull that accommodate the eyeballs and associated structures, such as the eye muscles, nerves, and blood vessels. **—orbital,** *adj.*

orbital aperture /ôr′bitəl/, an opening in the cranium to the orbit of the eye.

orbital fat, a semifluid adipose cushion that lines the bony orbit supporting the eye. Selective loss of fatty tissue caused by hormonal imbalances may produce "bulging" of the eye. Traumatic loss of the fat causes a sunken appearance of the eye.

orbital fissure [L, *orbita,* wheel track, *fissura,* cleft], the space between the floor and lateral wall of the orbit, serving as a conduit for nerves and blood vessels.

orbital myositis, an inflammation of the external ocular muscles. The process, which is generally autoimmune, may be associated with pain, forward displacement of the eyeball, and paralysis of the ocular muscles.

orbital pseudotumor, a specific inflammatory reaction of the orbital tissues of the eye, characterized by exophthalmos and edematous congestion of the eyelids.

orbitography /ôr′bitog′rəfē/, the use of radiology to study the bony cavity containing the eye.

orbitomeatal line /ôr′bitō′mē·ā′təl/ [L, *orbita,* wheel track, *meatus,* passage], a positioning line used in radiography of the skull that passes through the outer canthus of the eye and the center of the external auditory meatus.

Orbivirus /ôr′bivī′rəs/ [L, *orbis,* ring], a genus of the Reoviridae family of viruses that contain double-stranded ribonucleic acid. They are characterized by an outer layer of rings of capsomeres. Insects are hosts for orbiviruses. Colorado tick fever and African horse sickness are among infections caused by species of these viruses.

orchidectomy /ôr′kidek′təmē/ [Gk, *orchis,* testis, *ektome,* excision], a surgical procedure to remove one or both testes. It may be indicated for serious disease or injury to the testis or to control cancer of the prostate by removing a source of androgenic hormones.

orchiopexy /ôr′kē·ōpek′sē/ [Gk, *orchis* + *pexis,* fixation], an operation to mobilize an undescended testis, bring it into the scrotum, and attach it so that it will not retract.

orchioplasty /ôr′kē·ōplas′tē/ [Gk, *orchis,* testis, *plassein,* to mold], a surgical procedure involving a testis.

orchitis /ôrkī′tis/ [Gk, *orchis* + *itis,* inflammation], inflammation of one or both of the testes, characterized by swelling and pain. The condition is often caused by mumps, syphilis, or tuberculosis. **—orchitic,** *adj.*

ordered pairs [L, *ordo,* series, *par,* equal], pertaining to graph coordinates in which the first number of the pair represents a distance along the x (horizontal) axis and the second number is plotted along the y (vertical) axis.

orderly /ôr′dərlē/, **1.** an attendant who assists in the care of hospital patients. **2.** in order; with regular arrangements, method, or system.

order of procedure, the sequence in which the required steps are taken to complete an operation, such as preparation of the patient and cavity and restoration of a tooth.

Order Transcription, a Nursing Interventions Classification defined as transferring information from order sheets to the nursing patient care planning and documentation system.

Orem, Dorthea E., author of the Self-Care Nursing Model, a nursing theory introduced in 1959. The Orem theory describes the role of the nurse in helping a person experiencing inabilities in self-care. The goal of the Orem system is to meet the patient's self-care demands until the family is capable of providing care. The process is divided into three categories: universal, which consists of self-care to meet physiologic and psychosocial needs; developmental, the self-care required when one goes through developmental stages; and health deviation, the self-care required when one has a deviation from a healthy status.

orexigenic /ôrek′sijen′ik/ [Gk, *orexis,* longing, *genein,* to produce], a substance that increases or stimulates the appetite.

oreximania /ôrek′simā′nē·ə/ [Gk, *orexis* + *mania,* madness], a condition characterized by a greatly increased appetite and excessive eating resulting from an unrealistic or exaggerated fear of becoming thin.

orexis /ôrek′sis/ [Gk, longing], **1.** desire, appetite. **2.** the aspect of the mind involving feeling and striving as contrasted with the intellectual aspect.

orf [AS], a contagious viral skin disease acquired from infected sheep and goats, characterized by painless vesicles that may progress to red, weeping nodules and finally to crusting and healing.

organ [Gk, *organon,* instrument], a structural part of a system of the body that is composed of tissues and cells that enable it to perform a particular function, such as the liver, spleen, digestive organs, reproductive organs, or organs of special sense.

organ albumin, albumin characteristic of a particular organ.

organelle /ôrgənel′/ [Gk, *organon,* instrument], **1.** any one of various macromolecular structures bound within most cells, such as the mitochondria, the Golgi apparatus, the endoplastic reticulum, the lysosomes, and the centrioles. **2.** any one of the tiny structures of protozoa associated with locomotion, metabolism, and other processes.

organic /ôrgan′ik/ [Gk, *organikos*], **1.** any chemical compound containing carbon. **2.** pertaining to an organ.

organic chemistry, the branch of chemistry concerned with the composition, properties, and reactions of chemical compounds containing carbon.

organic disease [Gk, *organikos* + L, *dis* + Fr, *aise,* ease], any disease associated with detectable or observable changes in one or more body organs.

organic dust, dried particles of plants, animals, fungi, or bacteria that are fine enough to be windborne.

organic dust toxic syndrome (ODTS), any nonallergic noninfectious respiratory illness caused by inhalation of organic dust from moldy silage, hay, or other agricultural products. Symptoms include shaking chills or sweats, cough or shortness of breath, headache, anorexia, and myalgia.

organic evolution, the theory that all existing forms of animal and plant life have descended with modification from previous simpler forms or from a single cell; the origin and perpetuation of species.

organic foods, foods that have been produced and processed without the use of

commercial chemicals such as fertilizers or pesticides or synthetic substances that enhance color or flavor.

organic headache, a headache caused by any of a wide variety of intracranial disorders, including sinus or ear infections, brain tumors, and subdural hematomas.

organic mental disorders (OMD), a DSM-IV class of psychiatric disorders characterized by progressive deterioration of the mental processes and caused by permanent brain damage or temporary brain dysfunction.

organic murmur, an abnormal cardiac sound caused by a congenital or acquired heart disease.

organic psychosis [Gk, *organikos* + *psyche,* mind, *osis,* condition], a condition characterized by a loss of contact with reality caused by an alteration in brain tissue function.

organic vertigo [Gk, *organikos* + L, *vertigo,* dizziness], vertigo that is associated with a central nervous system disorder such as cerebellar lesions or tabes dorsalis.

organification /ôrgan′ifikā′shən/, a process in the thyroid gland whereby iodide is oxidized and incorporated into tyrosyl residues (tyrosine) of thyroglobulin. Organification is catalyzed by the enzyme thyroid peroxidase.

organism /ôr′gəniz′əm/ [Gk, *organon,* instrument], an individual living animal or plant able to carry on life functions through mutually dependent systems and organs.

organization center /ôr′gənīzā′shən/ [Gk, *organon* + *izein,* to cause], a focal point within the developing embryo from which the organism grows and differentiates.

organizer /ôr′gənī′zər/ [Gk, *organon* + *izein,* to cause], (in embryology) any part of the embryo that induces morphologic differentiation in some other part. Kinds of organizers include **nucleolar organizer, primary organizer.**

organocarbamate insecticide poisoning /-kär′bəmāt/, an adverse reaction to pesticides derived from esters of carbonic acid. Some of those insecticides are formulated in methyl alcohol, acquiring its added toxicity. The effects are similar to those of organophosphate insecticides, but the toxicity is less, and the duration of effects is shorter. The organocarbamate insecticides rarely produce overt central nervous system effects.

organochlorine insecticide poisoning /-klôr′ēn/, an adverse reaction to DDT-like pesticides such as chlordane and methoxychlor. Symptoms include central nervous system disorders, convulsions, increased myocardial irritability, and depressed respiration. Emergency treatment includes decontamination of the gastrointestinal tract without inducing emesis and administration of anticonvulsants.

organ of Corti [Gk, *organon;* Alfonso Corti, Italian anatomist, 1822–1888], the true organ of hearing, a spiral structure within the cochlea containing hair cells that are stimulated by sound vibrations. The hair cells convert the vibrations into nerve impulses that are transmitted by the cochlear part of the vestibulocochlear nerve to the brain.

organogenesis /-jen′əsis/ [Gk, *organon* + *genesis,* origin], (in embryology) the formation and differentiation of organs and organ systems during embryonic development. In humans the period extends from approximately the end of the second week through the eighth week of gestation. —**organogenetic,** *adj.*

organoid /ôr′gənoid/ [Gk, *organon* + *eidos,* form], **1.** resembling an organ. **2.** any structure that resembles an organ in appearance or function, specifically an abnormal tumor mass.

organoid neoplasm, a growth that resembles a body organ.

organomegaly /-meg′əlē/ [Gk, *organon,* instrument, *megas,* large], abnormal enlargement of an organ, particularly an organ of the abdominal cavity.

organophosphate insecticide poisoning /-fos′fāt/, an adverse reaction to organophosphate pesticides such as malathion, chlorothion, and nerve gas agents. Symptoms include nausea, vomiting, abdominal cramping, headache, blurred vision, and excessive salivation. Emergency treatment includes removal of clothing and washing the skin, emptying the stomach, correcting dehydration, and supporting respiration.

organophosphates /-fos′fāts/, a class of anticholinesterase chemicals used in certain pesticides and medications. They act by causing irreversible inhibition of cholinesterase.

organotherapy /-ther′əpē/ [Gk, *organon* + *therapeia,* treatment], the treatment of disease by administering animal endocrine glands or their extracts. Whole glands are no longer implanted, but substances derived from animal organs are widely used. —**organotherapeutic,** *adj.*

organotypic growth /ôr′gənōtip′ik/ [Gk, *organon* + *typos,* mark], the controlled reproduction of cells, such as occurs in the normal growth of tissues and organs.

Organ Procurement, a **Nursing Interventions Classification** defined as guiding families through the donation process to ensure timely retrieval of vital organs and tissue for transplant.

organ specificity, a substance or activity that is identified with a specific organ. The term is commonly applied to enzymes that function in particular organ systems.

orgasm /ôr′gasəm/ [Gk, *orgein,* to be lustful], the sexual climax, a series of strong involuntary contractions of the muscles of the genitalia, accompanied by ejaculation of semen, experienced as exceedingly pleasurable, set off by sexual excitation of critical intensity. —**orgasmic,** *adj.*

orgasmic maturity /ôrgas′mik/, the physiologic maturity of the reproductive system that enables the individual to complete the adult sexual response cycle.

orgasmic platform [Gk, *orgein* + Fr, *plate-forme,* a flat form], congestion of the lower vagina during sexual intercourse.

orient /ôr′ē·ənt/ [L, *oriens,* rising sun], **1.** to make someone aware of new surroundings, including people and their roles; the layout of a facility; and its routines, rules, and services. **2.** to help a person become aware of a situation or simply of reality, such as when a patient recovers from anesthesia. —**orientation,** *n.,* **oriented,** *adj.*

oriental sore /ôr′ē·en′təl/ [L, *oriens* + AS, *sar,* painful], a dermatologic disease caused by the parasite *Leishmania tropica,* transmitted to humans by the bite of the sand fly. This form of leishmaniasis, characterized by ulcerative lesions, causes no systemic symptoms, but the sores are susceptible to secondary infections.

orientation /ôr′ē·əntā′shən/ [L, *oriens* + *itio,* process], **1.** (in molecular genetics) the insertion of a fragment of genetic material into a vector so that the placement of the fragment is in the same direction as the genetic map of the vector (the n orientation) or in the opposite direction (the u orientation). **2.** (in psychiatry) the awareness of one's physical environment with regard to time, place, and the identity of other people.

orifice /ôr′ifis/ [L, *orificium,* opening], the entrance or outlet of any body cavity. —**orificial,** *adj.*

ori gene /ôr′ē/, (in molecular genetics) the site or region in which deoxyribonucleic acid replication starts.

origin /ôr′ijin/ [L, *origo,* source], the more fixed or most proximal end of a muscle attachment.

Orlando (Pelletier), Ida Jean, a nursing theorist who first described her nursing process theory in *The Dynamic Nurse-Patient Relationship* (1972). Her theory stresses the reciprocal relationship be-

O

tween the nurse and patient. She used the nursing process to meet the patient's need and thus alleviate distress. Three elements—patient behavior, nurse reaction, and nursing actions—comprise a nursing situation. Her contribution as a theorist has advanced nursing from personal and automatic responses to disciplined and professional practice responses.

ornithine /ôr′nithēn/, an amino acid, not a constituent of proteins, that is produced as an important intermediate substance in the urea cycle.

ornithine carbamoyl transferase, an enzyme in the blood that increases in patients with liver and other diseases. Its normal concentrations in serum are 8 to 20 mIU/ml.

Ornithodoros /ôr′nithod′ərəs/ [Gk, *ornis,* bird, *doros,* leather bag], a genus of ticks, some species of which are vectors for the spirochetes of relapsing fevers.

orofacial /ôr′ōfā′shəl/ [L, *oris,* mouth, *facies,* face], pertaining to the mouth and face.

oropharyngeal dysphasia /ôr′ōfərin′jē·əl/, a difficulty in initiating a swallow, caused by a neuromuscular disorder of the hypopharynx.

oropharynx /ôr′ōfer′ingks/ [L, *oris,* mouth; Gk, *pharynx,* throat], one of the three anatomic divisions of the pharynx. It extends behind the mouth from the soft palate above to the level of the hyoid bone below and contains the palatine and lingual tonsils. —**oropharyngeal,** *adj.*

orotic acid, a pyrimidine synthesized in the cell from carboxyl phosphate and aspartic acid via condensation, dehydration, and oxidation.

orotic aciduria /ōrot′ik/, a rare autosomal-recessive inherited disorder of pyrimidine metabolism. It includes signs and symptoms of macrocytic hypochromic anemia with megaloblastic changes in bone marrow, leukopenia, retarded growth, and urinary excretion of large amounts of orotic acid.

orphan disease, any rare health disorder for which no treatment has been developed.

orphan drug /ôr′fən/ [Gk, *orphanos,* without parents; ME, *drogge*], any pharmaceutical product that may be available to physicians and patients in countries other than the United States but that has not been 'adopted' by a domestic pharmaceutical manufacturer or distributor.

orphan virus [Gk, *orphanos,* without parents; L, *virus,* poison], a virus that has been isolated and identified, although it has not been associated with any particular disease.

orphenadrine citrate /ôrfen′ədrēn/, a skeletal muscle relaxant with anticholinergic and antihistaminic activity. It is prescribed in the treatment of severe muscle strain.

orphenadrine hydrochloride, an anticholinergic and antihistaminic agent prescribed in the treatment of parkinsonism.

ORS, abbreviation for **oral rehydration solutions.**

ORT, abbreviation for **oral rehydration therapy.**

ortho, abbreviation for *orthopedic.*

orthoclase ceramic feldspar /ôr′thəklās/ [Gk, *orthos,* straight, *klassis,* breaking, *keramikos,* pottery], a plentiful clay in the solid crust of the earth, used as a filler and to give body to fused dental porcelain.

orthodontic appliance /-don′tik/ [Gk, *orthos* + *odous,* tooth], any device used to modify tooth position.

orthodontic band, a thin metal ring, usually made of stainless steel, fitted over a tooth and bonded or cemented to it, for securing orthodontic attachments to a tooth.

orthodontics and dentofacial orthopedics /ôr′thədon′tiks/ [Gk, *orthos* + *odous,* tooth], the specialty of dentistry concerned with the diagnosis and treatment of malocclusion and irregularities of the teeth.

orthodontist /-don′tist/, a practitioner of the branch of dentistry that is concerned with the diagnosis, prevention, and correction of malocclusion of the teeth.

orthodromic conduction /ôr′thədrom′ik/ [Gk, *orthos* + *dromos,* course; L, *conducere,* to connect], the conduction of a neural impulse in the normal direction, from a synaptic junction or a receptor forward along an axon to its termination with depolarization.

orthogenesis /ôr′thəjen′əsis/ [Gk, *orthos* + *genesis,* origin], the theory that evolution is controlled by intrinsic factors within the organism and progresses according to a predetermined course rather than in several directions as a result of natural selection and other environmental factors. —**orthogenetic,** *adj.*

orthogenic /-jen′ik/ [Gk, *orthos* + *genein,* to produce], **1.** pertaining to orthogenesis; orthogenetic. **2.** pertaining to the treatment and rehabilitation of children who are mentally or emotionally disturbed.

orthogenic evolution, change within an animal or plant induced solely by an intrinsic factor, independent of any environmental elements.

orthokinetic cuff /-kinet′ik/ [Gk, *orthos,* straight, *kinesis,* movement; ME, *cuffe*], an elastic covering for a muscle to provide tactile stimulation that will induce contraction and at the same time restrict contraction of an opposing muscle.

orthokinetics /-kinet′iks/ [Gk, *orthos,* straight, *kinesis,* movement], **1.** therapy for hypertrophic osteoarthritis in which an effort is made to change muscular action from one group to another set to protect a joint. **2.** a therapy for spasticity that uses an orthotic device to enable contraction of one muscle while inhibiting its antagonist. **3.** the effect of gravity on the brownian movement as manifested by the movement of particles in the same direction in sedimentation.

orthologous genes /ôrthol′əgəs/, gene loci in different species that are similar in their nucleotide sequences, suggesting they originated from a common ancestral gene.

orthomyxovirus /ôr′thəmik′sōvī′rəs/ [Gk, *orthos* + *mykes,* fungus; L, *virus,* poison], a member of a family of viruses that includes several organisms responsible for human influenza infection.

orthopantogram /ôr′thəpan′təgram/ [Gk, *orthos* + *pan,* all, *gramma,* record], an x-ray film that is taken extraorally and shows a panoramic view of the entire dentition, alveolar bone, and other adjacent structures on a single film.

orthopedic nurse /-pē′dik/ [Gk, *orthos* + *pais,* child], a nurse whose primary area of interest, competence, and professional practice is in orthopedic nursing.

orthopedic oxford, a hard leather shoe with a leather or rubber sole, sometimes with a steel shank between the floor of the shoe and the sole, and with firmly constructed sides that support the foot in an upright position. The shoe is constructed uniformly so that assistive devices can be added.

orthopedics / pū′diks/ [Gk, *orthos,* straight, *pais,* child], a branch of health care that is concerned with the prevention and correction of disorders of the locomotor system of the body, including the skeleton, muscles, joints, and related tissues.

orthopedic surgery [Gk, *orthos,* straight, *pais,* child, *cheirourgia,* surgery], the branch of medicine that is concerned with the treatment of the musculoskeletal system mainly by manipulative and operative methods.

orthopedic traction, a procedure in which a patient is maintained in a device attached by ropes and pulleys to weights that exert a pulling force on an extremity or body part while countertraction is maintained. Traction is applied most often to reduce and immobilize fractures, but it also is used to overcome muscle spasm,

stretch adhesions, correct certain deformities, and help release arthritic contractures. The healthy young adult or adolescent in traction for the treatment of a fracture usually has an uneventful recovery, but diligent attention and nursing care are necessary to avoid the formation of pressure ulcers, infection, constipation, kidney stones, and other sequelae of immobility.

orthopedist /-pēdist/, a physician who specializes in orthopedics.

orthophosphate /-fos′fāt/, a salt of orthophosphoric acid, used in the treatment of kidney disease patients with the complication of hypophosphatemia resulting from a renal phosphate leak.

orthopnea /ôrthop′nē-ə/ [Gk, *orthos* + *pnoia,* breath]], an abnormal condition in which a person must sit or stand to breathe deeply or comfortably. It occurs in many disorders of the cardiac and respiratory systems, such as asthma, pulmonary edema, emphysema, pneumonia, and angina pectoris. —**orthopneic,** *adj.*

orthopneic position /ôr′thopnē′ik/ [Gk, *orthos,* straight, *pnoia,* breath; L, *positio*], a body position that enables a patient to breathe comfortably. Usually it is one in which the patient is sitting up and bent forward with the arms supported on a table or chair arms.

orthopsychiatry /-sīkī′ətrē/ [Gk, *orthos* + *psyche,* mind, *iatreia,* treatment], the branch of psychiatry that specializes in correcting incipient and borderline mental and behavioral disorders, especially in children, and in developing preventive techniques to promote mental health and emotional growth and development.

orthoptic /ôrthop′tik/ [Gk, *orthos* + *ops,* eye], **1.** pertaining to normal binocular vision. **2.** pertaining to a procedure or technique for correcting the visual axes of eyes improperly coordinated for binocular vision.

orthoptic examination, an ophthalmoscopic examination of the binocular function of the eyes. A stereoscopic instrument presents a slightly different picture to each eye. The examiner notes the degree to which the pictures are combined by the normal process of fusion. If the person has diplopia, separate pictures are seen. If the person has suppression amblyopia, only one picture is seen.

orthoptic training [Gk, *orthos,* straight; *ops,* eye; ME, *trainen*], a type of therapy for correction of squint or other ocular muscle disorders by the use of eye exercises.

orthoptist /ôrthop′tist/ [Gk, *orthos* + *ops,* eye], a person qualified by postsecondary training and successful completion of an examination by the American Orthoptist Council who, under the supervision of an ophthalmologist, tests eye muscles and teaches exercise programs designed to correct eye coordination defects.

orthoscopy /ôrthos'kəpē/ [Gk, *orthos,* straight, *skopein,* to view], the use of an **orthoscope** /ôr'thəskōp'/ for examining the fundus of the eye.

orthosis /ôrthō'sis/ [Gk, *orthos,* straight], a force system designed to control, correct, or compensate for a bone deformity, deforming forces, or forces absent from the body. Orthosis often involves the use of special braces. **—orthotic** /ôrthot'ik/, *adj., n.*

orthostasis /-stā'sis/, maintenance of an upright standing posture. In some medical tests a patient may need to maintain orthostasis for a long period to stimulate a rise in aldosterone concentration.

orthostatic /-stat'ik/ [Gk, *orthos* + *statikos,* standing], pertaining to an erect or standing position.

orthostatic hypotension, abnormally low blood pressure occurring when an individual assumes the standing posture.

orthostatic proteinuria, presence of protein in the urine of some people, especially teenagers who have been standing for a long period. It disappears when they recline and is of no pathologic significance.

orthotic /ôrthot'ik/ [Gk, *orthos,* straight], pertaining to **orthosis.**

orthotics /ôrthot'iks/ [Gk, *orthos,* straight], the design and use of external appliances to support a paralyzed muscle, promote a specific motion, or correct musculoskeletal deformities.

orthotist /ôr'thətist/ [Gk, *orthos,* straight], a person who designs, fabricates, and fits braces or other orthopedic appliances prescribed by physicians. A certified orthotist is one who successfully completed the examination of the American Orthotist and Prosthetic Association.

orthotonos /ôrthot'ənəs/ [Gk, *orthos* + *tonos,* tension], a straight, rigid posture of the body caused by a tetanic spasm, resulting from strychnine poisoning or tetanus infection. The neck and all other parts of the body are in a position of extension but not as severely as in opisthotonos.

orthotopic liver transplantation [Gk, *ortho,* straight, *topos,* place], a graft of liver tissue occurring at its natural place or on the proper part of the body.

orthovoltage /-vōl'tij/ [Gk, *orthos,* straight; Count Alessandro Volta], the voltage range of 100 to 350 kiloelectron volts (KeV) supplied by some x-ray generators used for radiation therapy. They have been replaced in many hospitals and other health facilities by equipment that operates in the megavolt range.

Ortolani sign /ôr'təlä'nē/, [Marius Ortolani, twentieth-century Italian surgeon], an audible click heard in a test for a congenital dislocated hip. It is noted in infancy when the hip slips into or out of the socket.

Ortolani's test [Marius Ortolani; L, *testum,* crucible], a procedure used to evaluate the stability of the hip joints in newborns and infants. The baby is placed on his back, and the hips and knees are flexed at right angles and abducted until the lateral aspects of the knees are touching the table. Internal and external rotation are attempted, and symmetry of mobility is evaluated. A click or a popping sensation (Ortolani's sign) may be felt if the joint is unstable.

Os, symbol for the element **osmium.**

OS, abbreviation for *oculus sinister,* a Latin phrase meaning 'left eye.'

Osborne and Cotterill procedure, a surgical method of correcting a chronic dislocated elbow by the use of capsular reefing, the folding in or overlapping of soft tissue by surgical suture to make the structure tighter.

Osborn wave, an abnormal, upward deflection in the electrocardiogram (ECG) occurring at the junction of the QRS complex and the ST segment. It is often found in ECGs of patients with moderate hypothermia and becomes more pronounced as body temperature declines.

osc, 1. abbreviation for **oscillator.** 2. abbreviation for **oscilloscope.**

oscheitis /os'kē-ī'tis/, an inflammation of the scrotum.

oscillation /os'ilā'shən/ [L, *oscillare,* to swing], 1. a back and forth motion. 2. vibration or the effects of a mechanical or electric vibrator.

oscillator (osc) /os'ilā'tər/ [L, *oscillare,* to swing], an electric or other device that produces oscillations, vibrations, or fluctuations, such as an alternating electric current generator.

oscillopsia /os'silop'sē·ə/, abnormal jerky eye movements associated with multiple sclerosis. They create a subjective sensation that the environment is oscillating.

oscilloscope (osc) /osil'əskōp/ [L, *oscillare,* to swing; Gk, *skopein,* to look], an instrument that displays a visual representation of electrical variations on the fluorescent screen of a cathode ray tube. The graphic representation is produced by a beam of electrons on the screen.

Osgood osteotomy /oz'gŏŏd/, a surgical procedure for correction of malrotation of a femur.

Osgood-Schlatter's disease /-shlat′ər/ [Robert B. Osgood, American surgeon, 1873–1956; Carl Schlatter, Swiss surgeon, 1864–1934], inflammation or partial separation of the tibial tubercle caused by chronic irritation, usually as a result of overuse of the quadriceps muscle. The condition is seen primarily in muscular, athletic adolescent boys and is characterized by swelling and tenderness over the tibial tubercle that increase with exercise or any activity that extends the leg.

OSHA /ō′shä/, abbreviation for *Occupational Safety and Health Administration.*

Osler's nodes /ōs′lərz/ [William Osler, American-British physician, 1849–1919], tender, reddish or purplish subcutaneous nodules on the soft tissue on the ends of fingers or toes, seen in subacute bacterial endocarditis and usually lasting only 1 or 2 days. The nodes represent bacterial embolisms from the infected heart valve.

Osler-Weber-Rendu's syndrome /ōs′- lərweb′ərandoo′/ [William Osler; Frederick P. Weber, British physician, 1863–1962; Henri J. L. M. Rendu, French physician, 1844–1902], a vascular anomaly, inherited as an autosomal-dominant trait, characterized by hemorrhagic telangiectasia of skin and mucosa. Small red-to-violet lesions are found on the lips, oral and nasal mucosa, tongue, and tips of fingers and toes. The thin dilated vessels may bleed spontaneously or as a result of only minor trauma, and this condition becomes progressively severe.

osm, **1.** abbreviation for **osmosis.** **2.** abbreviation for **osmotic.**

osmethesia /os′məthē′zhə/ [Gk, *osme,* odor, *aisthesis,* feeling], the ability to perceive and distinguish odors; the sense of smell.

osmium (Os) /oz′mē·əm/ [Gk, *osme,* odor], a hard, grayish, pungent-smelling metallic element. Its atomic number is 76; its atomic weight (mass) is 190.2. Used to produce alloys of extreme hardness, it is highly toxic.

osmoceptors /-sep′tərz/ [Gk, *osme* + L, *recipere,* to receive], receptors in the hypothalamus that respond to osmotic pressure, thereby regulating production of the antidiuretic hormone.

osmolal gap /ozmōl′əl/, a difference between the observed and calculated osmolalities in serum analysis. The calculated osmolar values include sodium concentration multiplied by 2, plus glucose and blood urea nitrogen.

osmolality /oz′mōlal′itē/, the osmotic pressure of a solution expressed in osmols or milliosmols per kilogram of water.

osmolal solution, the solute concentra- tion expressed in the number of osmoles per kilogram of solvent.

osmolar /osmō′lər/, pertaining to the os- motic characteristics of a solution of one or more molecular substances, ionic substances, or both, expressed in osmols or milliosmols.

osmolarity /oz′mōler′itē/, the osmotic pressure of a solution expressed in osmols or milliosmols per liter of the solution.

osmolar solution, the solute concentration expressed in the number of osmoles per liter of solution.

osmole /os′mōl/ [Gk, *osmos,* impulse, *osis,* condition + mole, (molecule)], the quantity of a substance in solution in the form of molecules, ions, or both (usually expressed in grams) that has the same osmotic pressure as one mole of an ideal nonelectrolyte. —**osmolal,** *adj.*

osmology /ozmol′əjē/ [Gk, *osme,* odor, *osmos,* impulse, *logos,* science], **1.** the science of the sense of smell and the production and composition of odors. **2.** the branch of science that is concerned with osmosis.

osmometry /ozmom′ətrē/ [Gk, *osmos,* impulse, *metron,* measure], the field of study that deals with the phenomenon of osmosis and the measurement of osmotic forces. —**osmometric,** *adj.*

Osmone-Clarke procedure, a therapy for talipes valgus. It involves soft tissue release of the medial and lateral foot with peroneus brevis tendon transfer.

osmoreceptor /-risep′tər/ [Gk, *osmos,* impulse; L, *recipere,* to receive], **1.** a neuron in the hypothalamus that is sensitive to the relative fluid/solute concentration in the blood plasma and regulates the secretion of antidiuretic hormone. **2.** a receptor of smell stimuli.

osmoreceptor cell, a cell that recognizes changes in extracellular fluid osmolality.

osmoregulation /-reg′yəlā′shən/ [Gk, *osmos,* impulse; L, *regula,* rule], the act of influencing or controlling the speed and extent of osmosis.

osmosis (osm) /ozmō′sis, os-/ [Gk, *osmos,* impulse, *osis,* condition], the movement of a pure solvent such as water through a differentially permeable membrane from a solution that has a lower solute concentration to one that has a higher solute concentration. Movement across the membrane continues until the concentrations of the solutions equalize. —**osmotic (osm)** /ozmot′ik/, *adj.*

osmotic diarrhea, a form of diarrhea associated with water retention in the bowel resulting from an accumulation of nonabsorbable water-soluble solutes. An excessive intake of hexitols, sorbitol, and man-

O

nitol (used as sugar substitutes in candies, chewing gum, and dietetic foods) can result in slow absorption and rapid small intestine motility, leading to osmotic diarrhea.

osmotic diuresis, diuresis resulting from the presence of certain nonabsorbable substances in tubules of the kidney, such as mannitol, urea, or glucose.

osmotic fragility, a sensitivity to changes in osmotic pressure characteristic of red blood cells. Exposed to a hypotonic concentration of sodium in solution, red cells take in increasing quantities of water, swell until the capacity of the cell membrane is exceeded, and burst. Exposed to a hypertonic concentration of sodium in a solution, red cells give up intracellular fluid, shrink, and break up.

osmotic pressure, 1. the pressure exerted on a differentially permeable membrane separating a solution from a solvent, the membrane being impermeable to the solutes in the solution and permeable only to the solvent. **2.** the pressure exerted on a differentially permeable membrane by a solution containing one or more solutes that cannot penetrate the membrane, which is permeable only by the solvent surrounding it.

osmotic transfection, a method of inserting foreign deoxyribonucleic acid (DNA) molecules into cells by putting cells into a dilute solution that causes them to rupture. The cell membranes quickly repair themselves. During the rupture period the alien DNA is added to the fluid and absorbed into the cell nuclei.

osphresis /osfrē′sis/ [Gk, smell], olfaction; the sense of smell.

osseous /os′ē·əs/ [L, os, bone], bony; consisting of or resembling bone.

osseous labyrinth [L, os, bone; Gk, labyrinthos, maze], the bony part of the internal ear, composed of three cavities: the vestibule, the semicircular canals, and the cochlea, transmitting sound vibrations from the middle ear to the eighth cranial nerve. All three cavities contain perilymph, in which a membranous labyrinth is suspended.

ossicle /os′ikəl/ [L, ossiculum, little bone], a small bone such as the malleus, the incus, or the stapes, which is an ossicle of the middle ear. —**ossicular,** adj.

ossiferous /osif′ərəs/ [L, os, bone, ferre, to bear], pertaining to the formation of bone or bone tissue.

ossification /os′ifikā′shən/ [L, os + facere, to make], the development of bone. Intramembranous ossification is that preceded by membrane, such as in the process initially forming the roof and sides of

the skull. Intracartilaginous endochondral ossification is that preceded by rods of cartilage, such as that forming the bones of the limbs.

ossify /os′ifī/ [L, os, bone, facere, to make], to develop into bone.

ossifying fibroma /os′ifī′ing/ [L, os + facere, to make], a slow-growing, benign neoplasm, occurring most often in the jaws, especially the mandible. The tumor is composed of bone that develops within fibrous connective tissue.

ostealgia /os′tē·al′jə/ [Gk, osteon, bone, algos, pain], any pain that is associated with an abnormal condition within a bone, such as osteomyelitis. —**ostealgic,** adj.

osteitis /os′tē·ī′tis/ [Gk, osteon + itis, inflammation], an inflammation of bone caused by infection, degeneration, or trauma. Symptoms include swelling, tenderness, dull aching pain, and redness in the skin over the affected bone.

osteitis fibrosa cystica, an inflammatory degenerative condition in which normal bone is replaced by cysts and fibrous tissue. It is usually associated with hyperparathyroidism.

ostemia /ostē′mē·ə/, an abnormal congestion of blood in a bone.

ostempyesis /os′təmpī·ē′sis/, an accumulation of pus within a bone.

osteo /os′tē·ō/, **1.** abbreviation for **osteopath. 2.** abbreviation for **osteopathy.**

osteoanagenesis /os′tē·ō·an′əjen′əsis/ [Gk, osteon + ana, again, genesis, origin], the regeneration or formation of bone tissue.

osteoaneurysm /-an′yəriz′əm/, an aneurysm within a bone.

osteoarthritis /os′tē·ō′ärthrī′tis/ [Gk, osteon + arthron, joint, itis, inflammation], a noninflammatory form of arthritis in which one or many joints undergo degenerative changes, including subchondral bony sclerosis, loss of articular cartilage, and proliferation of bone spurs (osteophytes) and cartilage in the joint. Inflammation of the synovial membrane of the joint is common late in the disease. The most common form of arthritis, its cause is unknown but may include chemical, mechanical, genetic, metabolic, and endocrine factors. Emotional stress often aggravates the condition. The condition usually begins with pain after exercise or use of the joint. Stiffness, tenderness to the touch, crepitus, and enlargement develop; deformity, subluxation, and synovial effusion may eventually occur. Involvement of the hip, knee, or spine causes more disability than osteoarthritis of other areas.

osteoarthropathy /-ärthrop′əthē/ [Gk, os-

teon + *arthron,* joint, *pathos,* disease], a disorder affecting bones and joints.

osteoarthrosis /-arthrō′sis/, a condition of chronic arthritis, usually mechanical, without inflammation.

osteoarticular /-artik′yələr/, pertaining to or affecting bones and joints.

osteoarticular brucellosis, a form of brucellosis that affects mainly the weight-bearing joints.

osteoarticular graft, a transplant of bone tissue that contains an articular surface.

osteoblast /os′tē-əblast′/ [Gk, *osteon* + *blastos, germ],* a cell that originates in the embryonic mesenchyme and, during the early development of the skeleton, differentiates from a fibroblast to function in the formation of bone tissue. —**osteoblastic,** *adj.*

osteoblastoma /-blastō′mə/, a small benign, fairly vascular tumor of poorly formed bone and fibrous tissue, occurring most frequently in the vertebrae, femur, tibia, or bones of the upper extremities in children and young adults. The tumor may cause pain, erosion, and resorption of native bone.

osteocachexia /-kəkek′sē-ə/, a chronic disease that results in wasting of the bone, usually caused by malnutrition.

osteocalcin /-kal′sin/, a protein found in the extracellular matrix of bone and dentin. It is involved in regulating mineralization in the bones and teeth.

osteocarcinoma /-kär′sinō′mə/ [Gk, *osteon,* bone, *karkinos,* crab, *oma,* tumor], cancer of the bone.

osteochondral graft /-kon′drəl/, a transplant of tissue composed of both bone and cartilage.

osteochondritis /-kəndrī′tis/ [Gk, *osteon,* bone, *chondros,* cartilage, *itis,* inflammation], a disease of the epiphyses, or bone-forming centers of the skeleton, beginning with necrosis and fragmentation of the tissue, and followed by repair and regeneration.

osteochondritis dissecans [Gk, *osteon,* bone, *chondros,* cartilage; L., *dissecare,* to cut apart], a joint disorder in which a piece of cartilage and neighboring bone tissue become detached from the articular surface.

osteochondrofibroma /-kon′drōfibrō′mə/, a tumor containing tissues of osteoma, chondroma, and fibroma.

osteochondroma /os′tē-ōkondrō′mə/ [Gk, *osteon* + *chondros,* cartilage, *oma,* tumor], a benign tumor composed of bone and cartilage.

osteochondromatosis /-kon′drōmətō′sis/, the transformation of synovial villi into bone and cartilage masses, causing loose bodies in the joints. It usually develops in joints affected by injury or degenerative disease.

osteochondropathy /kəndrop′əthē/, a condition affecting both bone and cartilage and characterized by abnormal enchondral ossification.

osteochondrosarcoma /-kon′drōsärkō′mə/ [Gk, *osteon,* bone, *chondros,* cartilage, *karkinos,* crab, *oma,* tumor], a cancer of the bone and cartilage.

osteochondrosis /-kondrō′sis/ [Gk, *osteon* + *chondros,* cartilage, *osis,* condition], a disease affecting the ossification centers of bone in children. It is initially characterized by degeneration and necrosis, followed by regeneration and recalcification.

osteochondrosis dissecans /dis′əkənz/, the formation of a separate center of bone and cartilage on an epiphyseal surface. The stray fragment may remain in place, be absorbed, or break off and become a loose body.

osteoclasia /-klā′zhə/ [Gk, *osteon* + *klasis,* breaking], **1.** the destruction and absorption of bony tissue by osteoclasts, such as during growth or the healing of fractures. **2.** the degeneration of bone through disease.

osteoclasis /os′tē-ōk′ləsis/, the intentional surgical fracture of a bone to correct a deformity. —**osteoclastic,** *adj.*

osteoclast /os′tē-ōklast′/ [Gk, *osteon* + *klasis,* breaking], **1.** a large type of multinucleated bone cell that functions in the development and periods of growth or repair, such as the breakdown and resorption of osseous tissue. During bone healing of fractures, or during certain disease processes, osteoclasts excavate passages through the surrounding tissue by enzymatic action. **2.** a surgical instrument used in the fracturing or refracturing of bones for therapeutic purposes, such as correction of a deformity.

osteoclast activating factor, a lymphokine that promotes the resorption of bone.

osteoclastic /-klas′tik/, **1.** pertaining to or of the nature of osteoclasts. **2.** destructive to bone.

osteoclastoma /os′tē-ōklastō′mə/ [Gk, *osteon* + *klasis,* breaking, *oma,* tumor], a giant cell tumor of the bone that occurs most frequently at the end of a long bone and appears as a mass surrounded by a thin shell of new periosteal bone. The lesion may be malignant and may cause local pain, loss of function, weakness, and pathologic fracture.

osteocope /os′tē-əkōp/, a painful syphilitic bone disease.

osteocystoma /-sistō′mə/, a cystic tumor in a bone.

O

osteocyte /os'tē·əsīt/ [Gk, *osteon* + *kytos,* cell], a bone cell; a mature osteoblast that has become embedded in the bone matrix. It occupies a small cavity and sends out protoplasmic projections that anastomose with those of other osteocytes to form a system of minute canals within the bone matrix. —**osteocytic,** *adj.*

osteodensitometer /den'sitom'ətər/ [Gk, *osteon,* bone; L, *densus,* thick; Gk, *metron,* measure], an apparatus for measuring the density of bone tissue.

osteodentin /-den'tin/, dentin that resembles bone. It is found chiefly in fish and other animals, but also occurs occasionally in humans when odontoblasts are entrapped by rapidly developing secondary dentin.

osteodermia /-dur'mēə/, a condition in which skeletal changes have occurred in the skin, such as a bony tumor of the skin.

osteodiastasis /-dī·as'təsis/, an abnormal separation of bones.

osteodynia /-din'ē·ə/, bone pain.

osteodystrophy /dis'trəfē/ [Gk, *osteon* + *dys,* bad, *trophe,* nourishment], any generalized defect in bone development, usually associated with disturbances in calcium and phosphorus metabolism and renal insufficiency, such as in renal osteodystrophy.

osteoenchondroma /os'tē·ō·en'kəndrō'mə/, a benign bone and cartilage tumor within a bone.

osteofibrochondrosarcoma /-fī'brōkon'drōsärkō'mə/, a malignant tumor containing bone, cartilage, and fibrous tissues.

osteofibroma /-fībrō'mə/ [Gk, *osteon,* bone; L, *fibra,* fiber; Gk, *oma,* tumor], a tumor composed of both bony and fibrous tissues.

osteogenesis /-jen'əsis/ [Gk, *osteon* + *genesis,* origin], the origin and development of bone tissue. —**osteogenetic, osteogenic,** *adj.*

osteogenesis imperfecta, a genetic disorder involving defective development of the connective tissue. It is characterized by abnormally brittle and fragile bones that are easily fractured by the slightest trauma. In its most severe form, the disease may be apparent at birth, when it is known as osteogenesis imperfecta congenita. The newborn has multiple fractures that have occurred in utero and is usually severely deformed because of imperfect formation and mineralization of bone. If the disease has a later onset, it is called osteogenesis imperfecta tarda and usually runs a milder course. Symptoms generally appear when the child begins to walk, but they become less severe with age, and the

tendency to fracture decreases and often disappears after puberty.

osteogenic, composed of or originating from any tissue involved in the development, growth, or repair of bone.

osteohalisteresis /-hal'istərē'sis/, a condition of soft bones caused by a loss or deficiency of mineral elements.

osteoid /os'tē·oid/ [Gk, *osteon* + *eidos,* form], pertaining to or resembling bone.

osteolipochondroma /-līp'ōkəndrō'mə/, a cartilage tumor with bone and fat elements.

osteolipoma /-līpō'mə/, a fatty tumor containing bone elements.

osteology /os'tē·ol'əgē/ [Gk, *osteon,* bone, *logos,* science], the branch of medicine concerned with the development and diseases of bone tissue.

osteolysis /os'tē·ol'isis/ [Gk, *osteon* + *lysis,* loosening], the degeneration and dissolution of bone caused by disease, infection, or ischemia. The condition commonly affects the terminal bones of the hands and feet. —**osteolytic,** *adj.*

osteolytic hypercalcemia /-lit'ik/, a malignancy associated with excess calcium in the blood. It may be caused by either widespread skeletal metastases or extensive bone marrow involvement by a primary hematologic tumor.

osteoma /os'tē·ō'mə/, a tumor of bone tissue.

osteomalacia /-məlā'shə/ [Gk, *osteon* + *malakia,* softening], an abnormal condition of the lamellar bone, characterized by a loss of calcification of the matrix resulting in softening of the bone and accompanied by weakness, fracture, pain, anorexia, and weight loss. The condition is the result of an inadequate amount of phosphorus and calcium available in the blood for mineralization of the bones. This deficiency may be caused by a diet lacking these minerals or vitamin D; a lack of exposure to sunlight, hence an inability to synthesize vitamin D; or a metabolic disorder causing malabsorption.

osteomesopyknosis /-mez'ōpiknō'sis/, a genetic disorder transmitted as an autosomal trait, characterized by osteosclerosis of the axial spine, pelvis, and proximal areas of long bones.

osteomyelitis /-mī·əlī'tis/ [Gk, *osteon* + *myelos,* marrow, *itis,* inflammation], local or generalized infection of bone and bone marrow. It is usually caused by bacteria introduced by trauma or surgery, by direct extension from a nearby infection, or via the bloodstream. Staphylococci are the most common causative agents. The long bones in children and the vertebrae in adults are the most common sites of infection as a result of hematogenous spread. Persistent, severe, and increasing bone pain; tenderness; guarding on movement; regional muscle spasm; and fever suggest this diagnosis. —**osteomyelitic,** *adj.*

osteomyelodysplasia /os'tē-ōmī'əlō'displā'zhə/ [Gk, *osteon,* bone, *myelos,* marrow, *dys* + *plasis,* forming], a loss of bone tissue through absorption of minerals. The condition is usually associated with leukopenia and sometimes with fever. It may result from an excess of parathyroid hormone.

osteon /os'tē·on/ [Gk, bone], the basic structural unit of compact bone, consisting of the haversian canal and its concentric rings of 4 to 20 lamellae.

osteonal bone /os'tē·ō'nəl/, a microscopic description of bone tissue seen in mature adults. It is composed of tiny chalky tubes with an arteriole running down the middle and circular laminations of bone concentric with an artery.

osteonecrosis /os'tē·ō'nəkrō'sis/ [Gk, *osteon* + *nekros,* dead, *osis* condition], the destruction and death of bone tissue, such as from ischemia, infection, malignant neoplastic disease, or trauma. —**osteonecrotic,** *adj.*

osteopath (osteo) /os'tē·ōpath'/, a physician who specializes in osteopathy.

osteopathology /pathol'əjē/ [Gk, *osteon,* bone, *pathos,* disease, *logos,* science], the study of bone diseases.

osteopathy (osteo) /os'tē·op'əthē/ [Gk, *osteon* + *pathos,* disease], a therapeutic approach to the practice of medicine that uses all the usual forms of medical diagnosis and therapy, including drugs, surgery, and radiation, but that places greater emphasis on the influence of the relationship between the organs and the musculoskeletal system than traditional medicine does. Osteopathic physicians recognize and correct structural problems using manipulation. The process is important in both the diagnosis and treatment of health problems. —**osteopathic,** *adj.*

osteopenia /-pē'nē·ə/ [Gk, *osteon* + *penes,* poverty], a condition of subnormally mineralized bone, usually the result of a failure of the rate of bone matrix synthesis to compensate for the rate of bone lysis.

osteoperiosteal graft /-per'ē·os'tē·əl/, a bone graft that includes the periosteal membrane covering the bone.

osteopetrosis /os'tē·ōpētrō'sis/ [Gk, *osteon* + *petra,* stone, *osis,* condition], an inherited disorder characterized by a generalized increase in bone density, probably caused by faulty bone resorption resulting from a deficiency of osteoclasts. In its most severe form there is obliteration of

the bone marrow cavity, causing severe anemia; marked deformities of the skull; and compression of the cranial nerves, which may result in deafness and blindness and lead to an early death. A milder, benign form is characterized by short stature, fragile bones that fracture easily, and a tendency to develop osteomyelitis. —**osteopetrotic,** *adj.*

osteophlebitis /-fləbī'tis/, an inflammation of the veins that are a part of the vascular system of bones.

osteophyte /os'tē·əfīt/, a bony outgrowth, usually found around the joint area.

osteoplastica /-plas'tikə/, a form of bone inflammation associated with cystic fibrosis.

osteoplasty /o'stē·əplastē/ [Gk, *osteon,* bone, *plassein,* to form], plastic surgery performed on bone tissue.

osteopoikilosis /os'tē·ōpoi'kilō'sis/ [Gk, *osteon* + *poikilos,* mottled, *osis,* condition], an inherited condition of the bones, characterized by multiple areas of dense calcification throughout the osseous tissue, producing a mottled appearance on x-ray examination. It is a benign condition, usually without symptoms, and of unknown cause. —**osteopoikilotic,** *adj.*

osteoporosis /os'tē·ōpərō'sis/ [Gk, *osteon* + *poros,* passage, *osis,* condition], a disorder characterized by abnormal loss of bone density. It occurs most frequently in postmenopausal women, sedentary or immobilized individuals, and patients on long-term steroid therapy. The disorder may cause pain, especially in the lower back, pathologic fractures, loss of stature, and various deformities. Osteoporosis may be without a known cause or secondary to other disorders such as thyrotoxicosis or the bone demineralization caused by hyperparathyroidism.

osteoporosis of disuse [Gk, *osteon,* bone, *poros,* passage, *osis,* condition; L, *dis,* not; ME, *usen,* to act], a thinning of the bone mass that occurs in sedentary people or patients confined to bed for a long period.

osteoporotic /-pərot'ik/ [Gk, *osteon,* bone, *poros,* passage, *osis,* condition], pertaining to osteoporosis.

osteosarcoma /os'tē·ō'särkō'mə/ [Gk, *osteon* + *sarx,* flesh, *oma*], a malignant tumor of the bone, composed of anaplastic cells derived from mesenchyme.

osteosclerosis /os'tē·ōsklerō'sis/ [Gk, *osteon* + *skleros,* hard, *osis,* condition], an abnormal increase in the density of bone tissue. The condition occurs in a variety of disease states; is commonly associated with ischemia, chronic infection, and tumor formation; and may be caused by faulty bone resorption as a result of

O

some abnormality involving the osteoclasts. —**osteosclerotic,** *adj.*

osteosuture /-soo'chər/, the surgical repair of a fractured bone by wiring or suturing the fragments together.

osteosynovitis /-sin'ōvī'tis/ [Gk, *osteon,* bone; Gk, *syn,* together; L, *ovum,* egg; Gk, *itis,* inflammation], an inflammation of the synovial membrane of a joint and the surrounding bone tissue.

osteosynthesis /-sin'thəsis/, the surgical fixation of a bone using any internal mechanical means. It is usually performed in the treatment of fractures.

osteotabes /-tā'bēz/, a condition usually affecting infants in which bone marrow cells are destroyed and the marrow disappears.

osteotelangiectasia /-telan'jē-əktā'zhə/, a sarcoma of the bone characterized by dilated capillaries.

osteothrombophlebitis /-throm'bōfləbī'-tis/, an inflammation through intact bone by progressive thrombophlebitis of small venules.

osteothrombosis /-thrəmbō'sis/, a blockage of the blood vessels in the bone tissue.

osteotome /os'tē-ətōm'/ [Gk, *osteon* + *temnein,* to cut], a surgical instrument for cutting through bone.

osteotomy /os'tē-ot'əmē/ [Gk, *osteon* + *temnein,* to cut], the sawing or cutting of a bone. Kinds of osteotomy include block osteotomy, in which a section of bone is excised; cuneiform osteotomy to remove a bone wedge; and displacement osteotomy, in which a bone is redesigned surgically to alter the alignment or weight-bearing stress areas.

osteotripsy /-trip'sē/, a method of treating callosities or any percutaneous reduction of a bony prominence.

ostomate /os'təmāt/ [L, *ostium,* mouth], a person who has undergone an ostomy.

ostomy /os'təmē/ [L, *ostium,* mouth], *informal.* a surgical procedure in which an opening is made to allow the passage of urine from the bladder or of intestinal contents from the bowel to an incision or stoma surgically created in the wall of the abdomen. An ostomy procedure may be performed to correct an anatomic defect, relieve an obstruction, or permit treatment of a severe infection or injury of the urinary or intestinal tract. Each procedure is named for the anatomic location of the ostomy, such as a colostomy, ureterostomy, cecostomy, or cystostomy.

ostomy care, the management and support of a patient with a surgical opening created in the bladder, ileum, or colon for the temporary or permanent passage of urine or feces, necessitated by carcinoma,

intestinal obstruction, trauma, or severe ulceration distal to the site of the incision. In most cases the opening is covered with a temporary disposable bag in the operating room. The ability of the patient to adjust to the ostomy procedures and equipment is greatly affected by the nursing care received in the days after surgery. A positive patient, matter-of-fact approach, sensitive emotional support, and thorough teaching of self-care measures are essential aspects of ostomy nursing care.

Ostomy Care, a Nursing Interventions Classification defined as maintenance of elimination through a stoma and care of surrounding tissue.

ostomy irrigation, a procedure for cleansing, stimulating, and regulating evacuation of an artificially created orifice. Fluids used in irrigation include tap water and saline or medicated solutions. Loop and double-barrel colostomies require a sequential irrigation of the proximal loop, distal loop, and rectum to prevent the accumulation of discharge.

os trigonum /os'trigō'nəm/, a small foot bone just posterior to the talus. It is sometimes confused with a fracture of the posterior tubercle of the talus.

OT, 1. abbreviation for **occupational therapist. 2.** abbreviation for **occupational therapy.**

otalgia /ōtal'jə/, a pain in the ear.

OTC, abbreviation for **over the counter.**

Othello syndrome /ōthel'ō/ [Othello, jealous Shakespearean character], a psychopathologic condition characterized by suspicion of a spouse's infidelity and morbid jealousy. This condition may be accompanied by rage and violence and is frequently associated with paranoia.

otic /ō'tik, ot'ik/ [Gk, *ous,* ear], pertaining to the ear.

otics /ō'tiks, ot'iks/, a group of drugs used locally to treat inflammation of the external ear canal or to remove excess cerumen.

otic vertigo, a sensation of rotation motion caused by an inner ear disease. Its subcategories are Ménière's disease, inner ear dysfunction, fistula or other pressure sensitivity, unilateral paresis, and benign paroxysmal positional vertigo.

otitic /ōtit'ik/ [Gk, *ous,* ear], pertaining to otitis.

otitis /ōtī'tis/ [Gk, *ous* + *itis,* inflammation], inflammation or infection of the ear.

otitis externa, inflammation or infection of the external canal or the auricle of the external ear. Major causes are allergy, bacteria, fungi, viruses, and trauma. Allergy to nickel or chromium in earrings and to chemicals in hair sprays, cosmetics, hearing aids, and medications, particularly sulfonamides and neomycin, is common. *Staphylococcus aureus, Pseudomonas aeruginosa,* and *Streptococcus pyogenes* are common bacterial causes. Herpes simplex and herpes zoster viruses are frequently implicated. Eczema, psoriasis, and seborrheic dermatitis also may affect the external ear.

otitis mastoidea [Gk, *ous,* ear, *itis,* inflammation, *mastos,* breast, *eidos,* form], an inflammation of the middle ear associated with a mastoid infection.

otitis media, inflammation or infection of the middle ear. It is common in early childhood. Acute otitis media is most often caused by *Haemophilus influenzae* or *Streptococcus pneumoniae.* Chronic otitis media is usually caused by gram-negative bacteria such as *Proteus, Klebsiella,* and *Pseudomonas.* Allergy, *Mycoplasma,* and several viruses also may be causative factors. Otitis media is often preceded by an upper respiratory infection. Organisms gain entry to the middle ear through the eustachian tube. The small diameter and horizontal orientation of the tube in infants predisposes them to infection. Obstruction of the eustachian tube and accumulation of exudate may increase pressure within the middle ear, forcing infection into the mastoid bone or rupturing the tympanic membrane. Symptoms of acute otitis media include a sense of fullness in the ear, diminished hearing, pain, and fever. Usually only one ear is affected. Squamous epithelium may grow in the middle ear through a rupture in the tympanic membrane; development of a cholesteatoma and hearing loss may occur if repeated infections cause an opening to persist. Pneumococcal otitis media may spread to the meninges. Chronic otitis media may result in hearing loss and delays in speech development.

otitis sclerotica [Gk, *ous,* ear, *itis,* inflammation, *sclerosis,* hardening], a sclerosing type of inflammation of the middle ear.

otoacoustic emissions, sounds emitted by the ear. These sounds are used to evaluate the integrity of the ear and to screen hearing in newborns.

otocephalus /ō′tōsef′ələs/, a fetus with otocephaly.

otocephaly /ō′tōsef′əlē/ [Gk, *ous* + *kephale,* head], a congenital malformation characterized by the absence of the lower jaw, defective formation of the mouth, and union or close approximation of the ears on the front of the neck. —**otocephalic, otocephalous,** *adj.*

otocranial debris, otoliths that have been

dislodged by trauma and may move about in the semicircular canals when the head changes position.

otolaryngologist /-ler′ing·gol′əjist/ [Gk, *ous* + *larynx* + *logos,* science], a physician who specializes in the diagnosis and treatment of diseases and injuries of the ears, nose, and throat.

otolaryngology /-ler′ing·gol′əjē/ [Gk, *ous* + *larynx* + *logos,* science], a branch of medicine dealing with the diagnosis and treatment of diseases and disorders of the ears, nose, throat, and adjacent structures of the head and neck.

otolith /ō′təlith/ [Gk, *ous,* ear, *lithos,* stone], **1.** a calculus in the middle ear. **2.** any of the crystals of calcium carbonate attached to the hair cells of the inner ear as gravity orientation receptors.

otolith righting reflex [Gk, *ous* + *lithos,* stone], an involuntary response in newborns in which tilting of the body when the infant is in an erect position causes the head to return to the upright position.

otologist /ōtol′əjist/, a physician trained in the diagnosis and treatment of diseases and other disorders of the ear.

otology /ōtol′əjē/ [Gk, *ous* + *logos,* science], the study of the ear, including the diagnosis and treatment of its diseases and disorders.

otomycosis /ō′tōmīkō′sis/, a lesion of the external ear caused by a fungus infection.

otoplasty /ō′təplas′tē/ [Gk, *ous* + *plassein,* to mold], a common procedure in reconstructive plastic surgery in which, for cosmetic reasons, some of the cartilage in the ears is removed to bring the auricle and pinna closer to the head.

otopyosis, a pus-producing inflammation of the ear, occurring either in the tympanic cavity or the external auditory meatus.

otorrhea /ō′tərē′ə/ [Gk, *ous* + *rhoia,* flow], any discharge from the external ear. Otorrhea may be serous, sanguinous, or purulent or contain cerebrospinal fluid. —**otorrheal, otorrheic, otorrhetic,** *adj.*

otosclerosis /ō′tōsklərō′sis/ [Gk, *ous* + *skleros,* hard, *osis,* condition], a hereditary condition of unknown cause in which irregular ossification occurs in the ossicles of the middle ear, especially of the stapes, causing hearing loss. The condition may worsen during pregnancy.

otoscope /ō′təskōp′/ [Gk, *ous* + *skopein,* to look], an instrument used to examine the external ear, the eardrum, and, through the eardrum, the ossicles of the middle ear. It consists of a light, a magnifying lens, a speculum, and sometimes a device for insufflation.

otoscopy /ōtos′kəpē/ [Gk, *ous,* ear, *skopein,* to view], an inspection of the tympanic

O

membrane and other parts of the outer ear with an otoscope.

ototoxic /ō'tōtok'sik/ [Gk, *ous* + *toxikon*, poison], (of a substance) having a harmful effect on the eighth cranial nerve or the organs of hearing and balance. Common ototoxic drugs include the aminoglycoside antibiotics, aspirin, furosemide, and quinine.

OTR, abbreviation for *occupational therapist, registered.*

Otto pelvis /ot'ō/ [Adolph W. Otto, German surgeon, 1786–1845], a type of hip dislocation in which there is a gradual central displacement of the femur. The cause is unknown.

OU, abbreviation for *oculus uterque,* a Latin phrase meaning 'each eye.'

oubain /wäbā'in/, a crystalline glycoside derived from the seeds of *Strophanthus gratus* and the wood of *Acocanthera oubaio.* It is similar in pharmaceutic action to strophanthin-K and the digitalis glycosides. It is also used as an arrow poison in Africa.

Ouchterlony double diffusion [Orjan T. G. Ouchterlony, Swedish bacteriologist, b. 1914], a form of gel diffusion technique in which antigen and antibody in separate cells are allowed to diffuse toward each other.

ounce (oz) /ouns/ [L, *uncia,* one twelfth], a unit of weight equal to $\frac{1}{16}$ of a pound avoirdupois or 28.349 grams.

outbreeding [AS, *ut,* out, *bredan,* to breed], the production of offspring by the mating of unrelated individuals, organisms, or plants, which can lead to superior hybrid traits or strains.

outcome [AS, *ut* + *couman,* to come], the condition of a client at the end of therapy or a disease process, including the degree of wellness and the need for continuing care, medication, support, counseling, or education.

outcome criteria, standards that focus on observable or measurable results of nursing and other health service activities.

outcome data, information collected to evaluate the capacity of a client to function at a level described in the outcome statement of a nursing care plan or in standards for client care.

outcome measure, a measure of the quality of medical care, the standard against which the end result of the intervention is assessed.

outlet [AS, *ut* + *laetan,* to permit], an opening through which something can exit, such as the pelvic outlet.

outlet contracture, an abnormally small pelvic outlet. It may be anteroposterior or transverse and is of significance in childbirth because it may impede or prevent passage of a baby through the birth canal.

outlier, 1. (in managed care) a case in which costs exceed the allowable amount for the specific diagnosis or treatment. The outlier amount is typically specified in advance in the contract between the provider and payer. 2. (in research) an observation that differs from all others, suggesting that a gross error has occurred in sampling, measurement, or analysis.

outline form [AS, *ut* + *lin,* thread], the shape of the cavosurface of a prepared tooth cavity, before restoring the tooth surface or surfaces.

out-of-body experience, a sensation that the mind has separated temporarily from the body. The feeling tends to occur when the patient is asleep, in a trance, or unconscious as during surgery. The person visualizes his or her body as an impersonal observer might. In some cases the person visualizes objects or persons who are beyond the range of normal senses. Occasionally a patient near death learns after awakening that he or she has ben declared clinically dead during the moments of the experience.

out of phase, pertaining to a series of events or actions that are not synchronous with a previously established periodic process or phenomenon. An oscillation or periodic process that runs in an opposite direction or pattern is sometimes described as 180 degrees out of phase.

out-of-plan services, services given to a patient by a provider outside the managed care system. The patient may be responsible for a larger co-payment than if the services were received within the plan.

outpatient (OP), [AS, *ut* + L, *patientia,* endurance], 1. a patient, not hospitalized, who is being treated in an office, clinic, or other ambulatory care facility. 2. pertaining to a health care facility for patients who are not hospitalized or to the treatment or care of such a patient.

output [AS, *ut* + *putian,* to put], 1. the total of any and all measurable liquids lost from the body, including urine, vomitus, diarrhea; drainage from wounds and fistulas; and those removed by suction equipment. The output is recorded as a means of monitoring a patient's fluid and electrolyte balance. 2. the end product of a system.

output amplifier, an apparatus used to increase the amplitude of the voltage output of a generator and control it at a specific level.

outreach program, a system of delivery of services to geropsychiatric clients, particularly mentally ill older adults in rural environments. They are considered most at risk because mental health and social services are usually not readily available. Outreach programs can diagnose and treat homebound clients with physical limitations or major psychiatric illnesses who are socially isolated.

ova and parasites test /ō′va/, a microscopic examination of feces for detecting parasites, such as amebas or worms and their ova, which are indicators of parasitic disorders.

ovalocytes /ō′vəlōsīts′/ [L, *ovalis*, egg-shaped; Gk, *kytos*, cell], oblong or oval-shaped red blood cells with pale centers that are found occasionally in patients with hemolytic anemias, thalassemias, and hereditary elliptocytosis. A genetic factor may be responsible for the presence of the abnormal blood cells.

oval window /ō′vəl/ [L, *ovum;* ME, *win-doge*], an oval-shaped aperture in the wall of the middle ear, leading to the inner ear. The footplate of the stapes vibrates in the oval window, transmitting sound waves to the cochlea.

ovarian /ōver′ē-ən/ [L, *ovum*, egg], pertaining to the ovary.

ovarian artery, a slender branch of the abdominal aorta, arising caudal to the renal arteries, and supplying an ovary.

ovarian carcinoma, a malignant neoplasm of the ovaries rarely detected in the early stage and usually far advanced when diagnosed. It occurs frequently in the fifth decade of life. Risk factors of the disease are infertility, nulliparity or low parity, delayed childbearing, repeated spontaneous abortion, endometriosis, group A blood type, previous irradiation of pelvic organs, and exposure to chemical carcinogens such as asbestos and talc. After an insidious onset and asymptomatic period, the tumor may become evident as a palpable abdominal or pelvic mass accompanied by irregular or excessive menses or post-menopausal bleeding. In advanced cases the patient may have ascites, edema of the legs, and pain in the abdomen and the backs of the legs. Characteristic of the disease as it advances are abdominal swelling and discomfort, abnormal vaginal bleeding, weight loss, dysuria or abnormal frequency of urination, constipation, and a palpable ovarian mass, especially in post-menopausal women. Most ovarian carcinomas are papillary or serous, followed in frequency by mucinous, endometrial, and undifferentiated cancers. In many cases the cancer spreads over the surface of the peritoneum, and, early in the course of the lesion, tumor cells invade the lymphatic vessels under the diaphragm and the paraaortic nodes. Many kinds of tumors may arise in the ovary.

ovarian cyst, a globular sac filled with fluid or semisolid material that develops in or on the ovary. It may be transient and physiologic or pathologic. Kinds of ovarian cysts include **chocolate cyst,** corpus luteum cyst, and **dermoid cyst.**

ovarian follicle [L, *ovum* + *folliculus,* small bag], a cavity or recess in an ovary containing a liquor that divides the follicular cells into layers and surrounds an ovum.

ovarian pregnancy, a rare type of ectopic pregnancy in which the conceptus is implanted within the ovary.

ovarian varicocele, a varicose swelling of the veins of the uterine broad ligament.

ovarian vein, one of a pair of veins that emerge from convoluted plexuses in the broad ligament near the ovaries and the uterine tubes. The veins from each plexus ascend and unite to form single veins. The right ovarian vein opens into the inferior vena cava, and the left ovarian vein into the renal vein.

ovariocele /ōver′ē-əsēl/, a hernia of an ovary or protrusion of an ovary through the vaginal wall.

ovariocentesis /ōver′ē-ōsentē′sis/, surgical puncture of an ovary or an ovarian cyst.

ovariohysterectomy /-his′tərek′təmē/, the surgical removal of the uterus and ovaries.

ovary /ō′vərē/ [L, *ovum*, egg], one of the pair of female gonads found on each side of the lower abdomen, beside the uterus, in a fold of the broad ligament. At ovulation, an egg is expelled from a follicle on the surface of the ovary under the stimulation of the gonadotrophic hormones, follicle-stimulating hormone (FSH), and luteinizing hormone (LH). The remainder of the follicle (corpus luteum) secretes the hormones estrogen and progesterone, which regulate the menstrual cycle by a negative-feedback system in which an increase in estrogen decreases the secretion of FSH by the pituitary gland and an increase in progesterone decreases the secretion of LH. Each ovary is normally firm and smooth and resembles an almond in size and shape. The ovaries generally are homologous to the testes.

overbite /ō′vərbīt/ [AS, *ofer,* over, *bitan,* to bite], vertical overlapping of lower teeth by upper teeth, usually measured perpendicularly to the occlusal plane.

overclosure /-klō′zhər/ [AS, *ofer* + L, *claudere,* to close], an abnormal condition in which the mandible rises beyond the point of normal occlusal contact, caused by the drifting of teeth, loss of occlusal vertical dimension, change in tooth shapes through grinding, or loss of teeth.

overcompensation /-kom'pənsā'shən/ [AS, *ofer* + L, *compensare*, to weigh together], an exaggerated attempt to overcome a real or imagined physical or psychologic deficit. The attempt may be conscious or unconscious.

overdenture /-den'cher/ [AS, *ofer* + L, *dens*, tooth], a complete or partial removable denture supported by retained roots or teeth to provide improved support, stability, and tactile and proprioceptive sensation and to reduce ridge resorption.

overdose (OD) /-dōs/, an excessive use of a drug, resulting in adverse reactions ranging from mania or hysteria to coma or death.

overdrive suppression /-drīv/ [AS, *ofer* + *drifan*, to drive], the inhibitory effect of a faster cardiac pacemaker on a slower one.

overeruption /-irup'shən/, the projection of a tooth beyond the normal occlusal plane.

overflow /-flō/ [AS, *ofer* + *flowan*], the flooding or excessive discharge of a fluid such as urine, saliva, or bile.

overflow incontinence [AS, *ofer* + *flowan* + L, *incontinentia*, inability to retain], an overflow of urine from a distended paralyzed bladder.

overgrafting /graf'ting/, placing an additional transplant over a previously healed tissue graft. It is sometimes performed to strengthen a split-thickness graft or to replace epithelium that may have been lost.

overgrowth [AS, *ofer* + ME, *growen*], an excessive growth, usually applied to organ or tissue development.

overhang /-hang/ [AS, *ofer* + *hangian*, to *hang*], an excess of dental filling material that projects beyond the margin of the associated tooth cavity preparation.

overhydration /-hīdrā'shən/, an excess of water in the body.

overinclusiveness /-inkloo'sivnəs/ [AS, *ofer* + L, *includere*, to include], a type of association disorder observed in some schizophrenia patients. The individual is unable to think in a precise manner because of an inability to keep irrelevant elements outside perceptual boundaries.

overjet /-jet/ [AS, *ofer* + Fr, *jeter*, to throw], a horizontal projection of upper teeth beyond the lower teeth, usually measured parallel to the occlusal plane.

overlap /lap'/, to extend over and cover part of an existing surface or structure.

overlay /o'vərlā/, to add to an existing condition or structure.

overlearning /-lur'ning/, the practice of an ability that continues beyond the point where performance meets a specified standard.

overload /-lōd/, **1.** a burden greater than the capacity of the system designed to move or process it. **2.** (in physiology) any factor or influence that stresses the body beyond its natural limits and may impair its health.

overnutrition /-nootrish'ən/, a condition of excess nutrient and energy intake over time. Overnutrition may be regarded as a form of malnutrition when it leads to morbid obesity.

overoxygenation /-ok'sijənā'shən/ [AS, *ofer* + Gk, *oxys*, sharp, *genein*, to produce; L, *atio*, process], an abnormal condition in which the oxygen concentration in the blood and other tissues of the body is greater than normal and the carbon dioxide concentration is less than normal. The condition is characterized by a fall in blood pressure, decreased vital capacity, fatigue, errors in judgment, paresthesia of the hands and feet, anorexia, nausea and vomiting, and hyperemia.

overresponse /rispons'/, an abnormally strong reaction to a stimulus.

overriding /-rīding/ [AS, *ofer* + *ridan*], the overlapping or telescoping of body parts, such as when one fragment of a fractured bone rests on another.

overripe cataract /-rīp/ [AS, *ofer* + OE, *reap*], a cataract in which a completely opaque lens solidifies and shrinks.

oversensing /-sen'sing/, the sensation of stimuli, such as magnetism or static electricity, that are not normally detected by the sense organs.

overshoot, 1. /ō'vərshoot'/ to go beyond or exceed a target or goal. **2.** /ō'vərshoot/ an upper part of a structure that extends beyond the lower part.

over the counter (OTC), (of a drug) available to the consumer without a prescription.

overtone, 1. any tone produced by voice or a musical instrument that is of a higher frequency than the lowest or fundamental tone of a sound. **2.** a harmonic.

overweight /-wāt/ [AS, *ofer* + *gewiht*, weight], more than normal in body weight after adjustment for height, body build, and age, or 10% to 20% above the person's 'desirable' body weight.

overwintering /win'təring/, persistence of seasonal infectious agents beyond their normal period of activity, particularly warm weather pathogen vectors that remain operative into the winter months.

ovicidal /ō'visī'dəl/, causing destruction of an ovum.

ovicide /ō′visīd/, an agent that destroys ova.

oviferous /ōvif′ərəs/ [L, *ovum*, egg, *ferre*, to bear], bearing or capable of producing ova (egg cells).

oviparous /ōvip′ərəs/ [L, *ovum* + *parere*, to bring forth], giving birth to young by laying eggs.

oviposition /ō′vipəsish′ən/ [L, *ovum* + *ponere*, to place], the act of laying or depositing eggs by the female member of oviparous animals.

ovipositor /ō′vipos′itər/ [L, *ovum* + *ponere*, to place], a specialized organ, found primarily in insects, for depositing eggs on plants or in the soil. It may be modified into a sting as in worker bees and wasps.

ovocenter /ō′vəsen′tər/ [L, *ovum* + *centrum*, center], the centrosome of a fertilized ovum.

ovoflavin /ō′vəflā′vin/ [L, *ovum* + *flavus*, yellow], a riboflavin derived from the yolk of eggs.

ovoglobulin /ō′vəglob′yŏŏlin/ [L, *ovum* + *globulus*, small sphere], a globulin protein derived from the white of eggs.

ovoid /ō′void/, egg-shaped.

ovoid arch [L, *ovum* + Gk, *eidos*, form; L, *arcus*, bow], a dental arch that curves smoothly from the molars on one side to those on the opposite side to form half an oval.

ovomucin /ō′vəmyoo′sin/ [L, *ovum* + *mucus*, slime], a glycoprotein derived from the white of an egg.

ovomucoid /ō′vəmyoo′koid/ [L, *ovum* + *mucus*, slime; Gk, *eidos*, form], pertaining to a glycoprotein, similar to mucin, derived from the white of an egg.

ovotestis /ō′vətes′tis/ [L, *ovum* + *testis*, testicle], a gonad that contains both ovarian and testicular tissue; a hermaphroditic gonad, —**ovotesticular,** *adj.*

ovoviviparous /ō′vəvivip′ərəs/ [L, *ovum* + *vivus*, living, *parere*, to bring forth], bearing young in eggs that are hatched within the body, such as some reptiles and fishes.

ovucyclic /ov′yəlōsī′klik/, pertaining to recurrent events associated with the ovulatory cycle.

ovucyclic porphyria, episodes of acute abnormalities of porphyrin metabolism that tend to recur in the premenstrual period.

ovulation /ov′yəlā′shən/ [L, *ovum* + *atio*, process], expulsion of an ovum from the ovary on spontaneous rupture of a mature follicle as a result of cyclic ovarian and pituitary endocrine function. It usually occurs on or about the eleventh to the fourteenth day before the next menstrual period and may cause brief, sharp lower abdominal pain on the side of the ovulating ovary. —**ovulate** /ov′yə′lāt/, *v.*

ovulation method of family planning, a natural method of family planning that uses observation of changes in the character and quantity of cervical mucus to determine the time of ovulation during the menstrual cycle. Because pregnancy occurs with fertilization of an ovum extruded from the ovary at ovulation, the method is used to increase or decrease the woman's chance of becoming pregnant by causing or avoiding insemination by spontaneous or artificial means during the fertile period associated with ovulation. The cyclic changes in gonadotropic hormones, especially estrogen, cause changes in the quantity and character of cervical mucus. Daily close monitoring of the mucus is necessary even after several cycles because the length of the 'safe' and 'unsafe' periods and the time of ovulation vary from cycle to cycle, as they do from woman to woman.

ovulatory /ov′yələtôr′ē/ [L, *ovum*], pertaining to ovulation.

ovum /ō′vəm/, *pl.* **ova** [L, egg], **1.** an egg. **2.** the secondary oocyte (female germ cell) extruded from the ovary at ovulation.

owl-eye cell, an enlarged cell infected by cytomegalovirus and containing large inclusion bodies. Owl-eye cells are found mainly in the renal epithelium.

Owren's disease [Paul A. Owren, Norwegian hematologist, b. 1905], a rare congenital bleeding disorder caused by a deficiency of coagulation factor V.

oxacillin sodium /ok′səsil′in/, a penicillinase-resistant penicillin antibiotic prescribed in the treatment of severe infections caused by penicillinase-producing staphylococci.

oxalate /ok′səlāt/, an anion of oxalic acid.

oxalated blood /ok′səlā′tid/, blood to which a soluble ester of oxalic acid has been added to prevent coagulation.

oxalemia /ok′səlē′mē·ə/, elevated levels of oxalates in the blood.

oxalic acid /oksal′ik/, a member of a family of dibasic acids found in many common plants, such as buckwheat, wood sorrel, and rhubarb. It is an important reagent and is used in bleaching and drying. Poisonous if ingested, oxalic acid is used in veterinary medicine as a hemostatic. In dietary intake of foods containing oxalic acid, the substance binds with calcium and is sometimes found in renal calculi and urine of patients with hyperoxaluria.

oxalosis /ok′səlō′sis/, a condition in which calcium oxalate crystals accumulate in the kidneys, heart, and other organs and urinary excretion of oxalate increases. Oxalosis-inducing agents include oxalic acid, methoxyflurane, ethylene glycol, and ascorbic acid.

oxaluric acid /ok'səlo͞or'ik/, a compound derived from uric acid or from parabanic acid, which occurs in normal urine.

oxamniquine /oksam'nəkwēn/, an antischistosomal prescribed in the treatment of infection caused by *Schistosoma mansoni.*

oxandrolone /oksan'drəlōn/, an androgen prescribed in the treatment of testosterone deficiency, osteoporosis, and female breast cancer and for the stimulation of growth, weight gain, and red blood cell production.

oxazepam /oksā'zəpam/, a benzodiazepine tranquilizer prescribed to relieve anxiety and nervous tension.

oxidant /ok'sidənt/ [Gk, *oxys,* sharp], an oxidizing agent.

oxidase /ok'sidās/ [Gk, *oxys,* sharp], an enzyme that induces biologic oxidation by activating the oxygen in molecules containing the element, such as hydrogen peroxide.

oxidation /ok'sidā'shən/ [Gk, *oxys,* sharp, *genein,* to produce, *atio,* process], **1.** any process in which the oxygen content of a compound is increased. **2.** any reaction in which the positive valence of a compound or a radical is increased because of a loss of electrons. **—oxidize,** *v.*

oxidation-reduction reaction, a chemical change in which electrons are removed (oxidation) from an atom, ion, or molecule, accompanied by a simultaneous transfer of electrons (reduction) to another.

oxidative phosphorylation, an ATP-generating process in which oxygen serves as the final electron acceptor. The process occurs in mitochondria and is the major source of adenosine triphosphate generation in aerobic organisms.

oxidative water /ok'sidā'tiv/ [Gk, *oxys,* sharp, *genein,* to produce, *atus,* process], water produced by the oxidation of molecules of food substances, such as the conversion of glucose to water and carbon dioxide.

oxide /ok'sīd/, **1.** a compound of oxygen and another element or radical. **2.** a dianion of oxygen.

oxidize /ok'sidīz/ [Gk, *oxys,* sharp, *genein,* to produce, *izein,* to cause], (of an element or compound) to combine or cause to combine with oxygen, to remove hydrogen, or to increase the valence of an element through the loss of electrons. **—oxidation,** *n.,* **oxidizing,** *adj.*

oxidizing agent, a compound that readily gives up oxygen or attracts hydrogen or electrons from another compound. In chemical reactions an oxidizing agent acts as an acceptor of electrons, thereby increasing the valence of an element.

oxidoreductase /ok'sidō'riduk'tās/, an enzyme that catalyzes a reaction in which one substance is oxidized while another is reduced. An example is alcohol dehydrogenase.

oximeter /oksim'ətər/, any of several devices used to measure oxyhemoglobin in the blood.

oxtriphylline /oks'trəfil'ēn/, a bronchodilator prescribed in the treatment of bronchial asthma, bronchitis, and emphysema.

oxyacoia, an abnormal hearing acuity. Increased sensitivity to sound is sometimes associated with paralysis of the stapedius muscle.

oxybutynin chloride /ok'sibōō'tinin/, an anticholinergic prescribed in the treatment of neurogenic bladder.

oxycalorimeter /ok'sēkal'ôrim'ətər/, an apparatus that measures the heat of combustion of organic materials in terms of oxygen consumed. Each liter of oxygen is roughly equivalent to 5 kilocalories,

oxycellulose /ok'sēsel'yəlōs/, **1.** cellulose that has been oxidized so that all or most of the glucose residues have been converted to glucuronic acid residues for use as an absorbent in chromatography. **2.** cellulose that has been partially oxidized for use as a local hemostatic.

oxycephaly /ok'sisef'əlē/ [Gk, *oxys* + *kephale,* head], a congenital malformation of the skull in which premature closure of the coronal and sagittal sutures results in accelerated upward growth of the head, giving it a long, narrow appearance with the top pointed or conic. **—oxycephalus,** *n.,* **oxycephalous,** *adj.*

oxycodone hydrochloride /ok'sikōdōn/, a narcotic analgesic used to treat moderate-to-severe pain.

oxygen (O) /ok'səjən/ [Gk, *oxys,* sharp, *genein,* to produce], a tasteless, odorless, colorless gas essential for human respiration. Its atomic weight (mass) is 15.9994; its atomic number is 8. In anesthesia, oxygen functions as a carrier gas for the delivery of anesthetic agents to the tissues of the body. In respiratory therapy oxygen is administered to increase the amount circulating in the blood. Overdose of oxygen can cause irreversible toxicity in people with pulmonary abnormalities, especially when complicated by chronic carbon dioxide retention. Prolonged administration of high concentrations of oxygen may cause irreversible damage to infants' eyes.

oxygenation /ok'səjənā'shən/, the process of combining or treating with oxygen. —**oxygenate**, *v.*

oxygen capacity of blood, the maximum amount of oxygen that can be made to combine chemically with hemoglobin in a unit of blood, excluding physically dissolved oxygen.

oxygen concentration in blood, the concentration of oxygen in a blood sample, including both oxygen combined with hemoglobin and oxygen physically dissolved in blood.

oxygen consumption, the amount of oxygen in milliliters per minute that the body requires for normal aerobic metabolism; normally about 250 ml/min.

oxygen cost of breathing, the rate at which the respiratory muscles consume oxygen as they ventilate the lungs.

oxygen debt, the quantity of oxygen that the lungs take up during recovery from a period of exercise or apnea that is in excess of the quantity needed for resting metabolism during the preexercise period.

oxygen enhancement ratio (OER), a measure of tumor sensitivity to the presence or absence of oxygen, expressed as the ratio of radiation dose required to produce a given effect with no oxygen present to the dose required to produce the same effect in 1 atmosphere of air.

oxygen half-saturation pressure of hemoglobin, the oxygen pressure necessary for 50% saturation of hemoglobin at body temperature and at pH 7.4 or 40 mm Hg of carbon dioxide pressure. The value is commonly used as a measure of the affinity between oxygen and hemoglobin.

oxygen hood, a device placed over the head of neonatal patients to deliver high concentrations of oxygen.

oxygen mask, a device used to administer oxygen. It is shaped to fit snugly over the mouth and nose and may be secured in place with a strap or held with the hand. The mask has inspiratory and expiratory valves, allowing oxygen to be inhaled or pumped into the respiratory tract and carbon dioxide to be exhaled into the environment.

oxygen radicals [Gk, *oxys,* sharp; L, *radix,* root], a substituent group of chemical elements rich in oxygen but incapable of prolonged existence in a free state. Oxygen radicals are used in some types of therapy.

oxygen saturation, the fraction of a total hemoglobin in the form of SaO_2 at a defined PO_2.

oxygen store, the total quantity of oxygen normally stored in the various body compartments, including the lungs, arterial and venous blood, and tissues. In a 70-kg human, blood contains about 800 ml of oxygen as oxyhemoglobin, muscles contain about 150 ml as oxymyoglobin, alveolar gas contains a few hundred milliliters, and about 50 ml is dissolved in the tissues.

oxygen tension, the force with which oxygen molecules that are physically dissolved in blood are constantly trying to escape, expressed as partial pressure (PO_2). The tension at any instant is related to the amount of oxygen physically dissolved in plasma; the larger amount carried in chemical combination with hemoglobin serves as a reservoir that releases oxygen molecules to physical solution when the tension decreases and stores additional molecules of the gas when the tension increases.

oxygen tent [Gk, *oxys,* sharp; ME, *tente*], a canopy that encloses the head and neck of a patient and contains a high oxygen tension.

oxygen therapy, any procedure in which oxygen is administered to a patient to relieve hypoxia. Although there are several kinds of hypoxia, all result in hypoxemia. Oxygen administration may relieve hypotension, cardiac arrhythmias, tachypnea, headache, disorientation, nausea, and agitation characteristic of hypoxia, as well as restore the ability of the cells of the body to carry on normal metabolic function.

Oxygen Therapy, a Nursing Interventions Classification defined as administration of oxygen and monitoring of its effectiveness.

oxygen tolerance, an increased capacity to withstand the toxic effects of hyperoxia as a result of any adaptive change occurring within an organism.

oxygen toxicity, a condition of oxygen overdosage that can result in pathologic tissue changes, such as retinopathy of prematurity or bronchopulmonary dysplasia.

oxygen transport, the process by which oxygen is absorbed in the lungs by the hemoglobin in circulating deoxygenated red cells and carried to the peripheral tissues. The process is made possible because hemoglobin has the ability to combine with oxygen present at a high concentration, such as in the lungs, and to release this oxygen when the concentration is low, such as in the peripheral tissues.

oxygen uptake, the amount of oxygen an organism removes from the environment, including the amount the lungs remove from the ambient atmosphere, the amount the blood removes from the alveolar gas in the lungs, or the rate at which an organ or tissue removes oxygen from the blood perfusing it.

oxyhemoglobin /ok'sēhē'məglō'bin, -hem'-/ [Gk, *oxys* + *genein*, to produce, *haima*, blood; L, *globus*, ball], the product of combining hemoglobin with oxygen. The loosely bound complex dissociates easily when the concentration of oxygen is low.

oxyhemoglobin dissociation curve, a graphic expression of the affinity between oxygen and hemoglobin, or the amount of oxygen chemically bound at equilibrium to the hemoglobin in blood as a function of oxygen pressure. To define the curve completely, it should also include the pH, temperature, and carbon dioxide pressure.

oxyhemoglobin saturation, the amount of oxygen actually combined with hemoglobin, expressed as a percentage of the oxygen capacity of that hemoglobin.

oxymesterone /ok'sēmes'tərōn/, an androgen and anabolic steroid involved in tissue building.

oxymetazoline hydrochloride /ok'sēmət-az'əlēn/, a decongestant prescribed in the treatment of nasal congestion.

oxymetholone /ok'sēmeth'əlōn/, an androgen prescribed in the treatment of testosterone deficiency, osteoporosis, and female breast cancer and to stimulate growth, weight gain, and red blood cell production.

oxymorphone hydrochloride /ok'sēmôr'-fōn/, a narcotic analgesic prescribed to reduce moderate-to-severe pain, as a preoperative medication, and to support anesthesia.

oxyntic cell, a hydrochloric-acid producing cell of the stomach.

oxyopia /ok'sē-ō'pē-ə/ [Gk, *oxys* + *opsis* vision], unusual acuteness of vision. A person with normal (20/20) vision when standing 20 feet from the standard Snellen eye chart can read the seventh line of letters, each of which is an eighth of an inch high; an individual with oxyopia can read smaller letters at that distance.

oxyphil cell /ok'səfil/, a cell of the parathyroid glands that takes up acidic stains and has a dark nucleus and fine, granular cytoplasm. Such cells occur singly or in small groups and increase in number with age.

oxytalan /ok'sētal'ən, oksit'ələn/, a type of connective tissue fiber particular to periodontal membrane.

oxytetracycline /ok'sētet'rəsī'klēn/, a tetracycline antibiotic prescribed in the treatment of bacterial and rickettsial infections.

oxytetracycline calcium, a tetracycline antibiotic.

oxytocia /ok'sētō'shə/, rapid childbirth.

oxytocic /ok'sitō'sik/ [Gk, *oxys* + *tokos*,

birth], **1.** pertaining to a substance that is similar to the hormone oxytocin. **2.** any one of numerous drugs that stimulate the smooth muscle of the uterus to contract. Oxytocic agents commonly used include oxytocin, certain prostaglandins, and the ergot alkaloids. These drugs are used to induce or augment labor, control postpartum hemorrhage, correct postpartum uterine atony, produce uterine contractions after cesarean section or other uterine surgery, and induce therapeutic abortion. These drugs are used with extreme caution in parturients with severe hypotension and hypertension, partial placenta previa, cephalopelvic disproportion, or grand multiparity.

oxytocin /ok'sitō'sin/, an oxytocic prescribed to stimulate contractions in inducing or augmenting labor and to contract the uterus to control postpartum bleeding.

oxytocin challenge test, a stress test for the assessment of intrauterine function of the fetus and the placenta. It is performed to evaluate the ability of the fetus to tolerate continuation of pregnancy or the anticipated stress of labor and delivery. A dilute intravenous infusion of oxytocin is begun, regulated by an infusion pump. The uterine activity is monitored with a tocodynamometer, and the fetal heart rate is monitored with an ultrasonic sensor as the uterus is stimulated to contract by the oxytocin. Decelerations of the fetal heart rate in certain repeating patterns may indicate fetal distress.

oxyuricide /ok'sē-ŏŏ'risīd/, an agent that destroys oxyur pinworms, or nematodes.

oz [L, *uncia*], abbreviation for **ounce.**

oz ap [L, *uncia*], abbreviation for *apothecary ounce,* a unit of weight equal to 31.1035 grams.

ozena /ōzē'nə/ [Gk, *ozein*, to have an odor], a condition of the nose characterized by atrophy of the nasal chonchae and mucous membranes. Symptoms include crusting of nasal secretions, discharge, and, especially, a very offensive odor. Ozena may follow chronic inflammation of the nasal mucosa.

ozone [Gk, *ozein*, to have an odor], a form of oxygen consisting of three atoms. Ozone is formed when oxygen is present in an electric discharge, as might occur in a lightning storm. Ozone is used as a bleaching, cleaning, and oxidizing agent and has a faint, chlorinelike odor.

ozone hole, a seasonal depletion of the steady-state ozone concentration in the stratosphere, particularly over Antarctica.

ozone shield, the layer of ozone that hangs in the atmosphere from 20 to 40 miles above the surface of the earth and protects the earth from excessive ultraviolet radiation.

ozone sickness, an abnormal condition caused by the inhalation of ozone that may seep into jet aircraft at altitudes over 40,000 feet. It is characterized by headaches, chest pains, itchy eyes, and sleepiness. Exactly why and how ozone causes this condition is not known. It is more prevalent early in the year and occurs more often over the Pacific Ocean.

oz t [L, *uncia*], abbreviation for *troy ounce,* a unit of weight equal to 31.103 grams.

O

P, 1. symbol for the element **phosphorus. 2.** symbol for *gas partial pressure.* See **partial pressure. 3.** symbol for *after* or *post.*

p17, symbol for a protein that lines the interior of the human immunodeficiency virus envelope.

p24, symbol for a protein that surrounds the ribonucleic acid and reverse transcriptase of the virus in human immunodeficiency virus.

P, 1. (in genetics) symbol for *first parental generation.* **2.** symbol for *first pulmonic sound.*

P$_2$, symbol for *second pulmonic sound.*

P$_{50}$, the partial pressure of oxygen at which hemoglobin is half saturated with bound oxygen.

p-, symbol for **para-.**

pA, abbreviation for *picoampere.*

Pa, 1. symbol for *pascal.* **2.** symbol for the element **protactinium.**

PA, 1. abbreviation for **physician's assistant. 2.** abbreviation for **pulmonary artery.**

P-A, p-a, abbreviation for **posteroanterior.**

P&A, 1. abbreviation for *percussion and auscultation.* See **p and a. 2.** abbreviation for *posterior and anterior.*

PABA, abbreviation for **paraaminobenzoic acid,** a topical sunscreen.

pabulin /pab′yəlin/ [L, *pabulum,* food], products of fat and protein digestion found in the blood after a meal.

pabulum /pab′yələm/ [L, food], any substance that is food or nutrient.

pac, abbreviation for *phenacetin-aspirin-caffeine.*

PAC, abbreviation for **premature atrial complex.**

PA catheter, intravenous catheter that is inserted through a large vein, such as the subclavian, into the pulmonary artery.

pacchionian foramen /pak′ē·ō′nē·ən/ [Antonio Paccioni, Italian anatomist, 1665–1720], an opening in the center of the diaphragm of sella through which the infundibulum passes.

PACE /pās/, acronym for **Program of All-Inclusive Care of the Elderly.**

PACE II, an interdisciplinary assessment and planning system that focuses on evaluation of the physical health of nursing home residents. It includes checklists of defined (diagnosed) conditions, abnormal laboratory or other findings, risk factors, and other impairments and disabilities.

pacemaker [L, *passus,* step; AS, *macian,* to make], **1.** the sinoatrial node composed of specialized nervous tissue located at the junction of the superior vena cava and the right atrium. It initiates the contractions of the atria, which transmit the impulse on to the atrioventricular (AV) node, thereby initiating the contraction of the ventricles. An ectopic or idioventricular pacemaker, originating in the atria, AV node, or ventricle, may cause contractions in cases of abnormal heart functions. **2.** an electric apparatus used in most cases to increase the heart rate in severe bradycardia by electrically stimulating the heart muscle. A pacemaker may be permanent or temporary, emit the stimulus at a constant and fixed rate, or fire only on demand, when the heart does not spontaneously contract at a minimum rate.

pacemaker installation fluoroscopy, the fluoroscopic monitoring of the insertion of an artificial pacemaker, used as an aid for correct installation of the device.

pachyblepharon /-blef′əron/ [Gk, *pachy,* thick], a thickening of the tarsal border of the eyelid.

pachycephalic /-səfal′ik/, pertaining to an abnormal thickening of the skull.

pachycephaly /pak′ēsef′əlē/ [Gk, *pachy,* thick, *kephale,* head], an abnormal thickness of the skull, as in acromegaly. —**pachycephalic, pachycephalous,** *adj.*

pachycheilia /-kī′fē·ə/, an abnormal thickening or swelling of the lips.

pachycholia /-kō′lē·ə/, thickness of the bile.

pachychromatic /-krōmat′ik/, characterized by coarse chromatin filaments.

pachychymia /-kī′mē·ə/, thickness of the chyme.

pachydactyly /pak′ēdak′tilē/ [Gk, *pachy* + *daktylos,* finger], an abnormal thickening of the fingers or the toes. —**pachydactylic, pachydactylous,** *adj.*

pachyderma /-dur′mə/, an overgrowth or

thickening of the skin and subcutaneous tissues.

pachyderma alba /-dur′mə/ [Gk, *pachy* + *derma*, skin; L, *albus*, white], an abnormal state of the buccal mucosa in which the appearance is suggestive of whitened elephant hide.

pachyderma laryngis, an overgrowth of epithelium over the vocal cords.

pachydermatous /-dur′mətəs/, pertaining to a condition of pachyderma.

pachyderma vesicae, a potentially malignant condition of white plaques in the mucous membrane at the base of the bladder.

pachydermoperiostosis /dur′moper′ē·ostō′sis/, a syndrome characterized by a thickening and folding of the facial skin, clubbing of the fingers, and new bone formation over the ends of the long bones.

pachyglossia /-glos′ē·ə/, an abnormal thickening of the tongue.

pachygnathous /-gnoth′əs/, pertaining to an abnormal thickening of the jaw.

pachygyria /-jī′rē·ə/, a broadening and flattening of the gyri of the brain.

pachyleptomeningitis /-lep′təmin′injī′tis/, an inflammation of all the membranes of the brain and spinal cord.

pachylosis /lō′sis/, a condition of rough, dry, and thickened skin.

pachymenia /-mē′nē·ə/, an abnormal thickness of the skin or other membranes.

pachymenic /-mē′mik/, pertaining to pachymenia.

pachymeningitis /-min′injī′tis/, an inflammation of the dura mater.

pachymeningopathy /-mining′gōpath′ē/, an abnormality other than inflammation involving the dura mater.

pachymeninx, *pl.* **pachymeninges** /-mē′-niks/ [Gk, *pachys*, thick, *meninx*, membrame], the dura mater.

pachymeter /pakim′ətər/ [Gk, *pachy* + *metron*, measure], an instrument used to measure thickness, especially of a thin structure, such as a membrane or a tissue.

pachynema /pak′inē′mə/ [Gk, *pachy* + *nema*, thread], the postsynaptic tetradic chromosome formation that occurs in the pachytene stage of the first meiotic prophase of gametogenesis.

pachynsis /pakin′sis/, any thickening of tissues having a pathologic cause.

pachyonychia /pak′ē·ōnik′ē·ə/, an abnormal thickness of the finger or toe nails.

pachyonychia congenita [Gk, *pachy* + *onyx*, nail; L, *congenitus*, born with], a congenital deformity characterized by abnormal thickening and raising of the nails on the fingers and toes and hyperkeratosis of the palms of the hands and the soles of the feet.

pachyotia /pak′ē·ō′shə/, an abnormal thickness of the auricle of the ears.

pachypelviperitonitis /-pel′vēper′itəni′tis/, pelvic peritonitis associated with a thickening of the tissues.

pachyperitonitis /-per′itənī′tis/, an inflammation and abnormal thickening of the tissues of the peritoneum.

pachypleuritis /-plŏŏrī′tis/, an inflammation and thickening of the pleural membranes.

pachysalpingoovaritis /-salping′gō·ō′ver-ī′tis/, an inflammation and thickening of the tissues of the ovaries and fallopian tubes.

pachysomia /-sō′mē·ə/ [Gk, *pachys*, thick, *soma*, body], an abnormal thickening of the soft tissues of the body.

pachytene /pak′itēn/ [Gk, *pachy* + *tainia*, ribbon], the third stage in the first meiotic prophase of gametogenesis in which the paired homologous chromosomes form tetrads. The bivalent pairs become short and thick and intertwine so that four chromatids are visible.

pachyvaginalitis /-vaj′inəlī′tis, an inflammation and thickening of the tunica vaginalis testis.

pachyvaginitis /-vaj′inī′tis/, an inflammation and thickening of the walls of the vagina.

pacifier /pas′ifī′ər/ [L, *pacificare*, to bring peace], **1.** an agent that soothes or comforts. **2.** a nipple-shaped object used by infants and children for sucking.

pacing [L, *passus*, step], the act of electrically stimulating the heart, a normal property of the sinus node; the artificial electrical stimulation of a heart rhythm.

pacing wire [L, *passus*, step; AS, *wir*], the electrical connection between a pulse generator and a pacing electrode.

Pacini's corpuscles /pasē′nez/ [Filippo Pacini, Italian anatomist, 1812–1883; L, *corpusculum*, little body], special sensory end organs resembling tiny white bulbs. Each is attached to the end of a single nerve fiber in the subcutaneous, submucous, and subserous connective tissue of many parts of the body, especially the palm of the hand, the sole of the foot, genital organs, joints, and pancreas. They are pressure sensitive and in cross section resemble an onion.

pacinitis /pas′inī′tis/, an inflammation of the pacinian corpuscles.

pack [ME, *pakke*, bundle], **1.** a treatment in which the entire body or a part of it is wrapped in wet or dry towels or in ice for various therapeutic purposes, as with cold packs for reducing high temperatures and swellings or for inducing hypothermia during certain surgical procedures, espe-

P

cially heart surgery and organ transplantation. **2.** a tampon. **3.** the act of applying a dressing or dental cement to a surgical wound. **4.** a surgical dressing to cover a wound or to fill the cavity left from extraction of a tooth, especially a wisdom tooth.

package insert, a leaflet that, by order of the Food and Drug Administration (FDA), must be placed inside the package of every prescription drug. In it the manufacturer is required to describe the drug, to state its generic name, and to give the applicable indications, contraindications, warnings, precautions, adverse effects, form, dosage, and administration.

packed cells [ME, *pakke,* bundle; L, *cella,* storeroom], a preparation of blood cells separated from liquid plasma, often administered in severe anemia to restore adequate levels of hemoglobin and red cells without overloading the vascular system with excess fluids.

packed cell volume (PCV) [ME, *pakke* + L, *cella,* storeroom, *volumen,* paper roll], a measured quantity of blood to which an anticoagulant has been added and the cells of which have been pressed together by the force of being centrifuged at 2000 rpm.

packer, an instrument for tamponing or introducing a pack of gauze into a wound.

packing [ME, *pakke*], **1.** material used to fill a wound or cavity. **2.** the act of inserting material into a wound or cavity.

PaCO₂, abbreviation for **partial pressure of carbon dioxide in arterial blood.**

pad [D, *paden,* cushion], **1.** a mass of soft material used to cushion shock, prevent wear, or absorb moisture, such as the abdominal pads used to absorb discharges from abdominal wounds. **2.** (in anatomy) a mass of fat that cushions various structures, such as the infrapatellar pad lying below the patella.

PAD, abbreviation for **peripheral arterial disease.**

p.ae. [L, *partes* + *aequales*], symbol for *equal parts.*

pagetoid /paj′ətoid/, a health condition similar to that of Paget's disease.

Paget's disease /paj′əts/ [James Paget, English surgeon, 1814–1899], a common nonmetabolic disease of bone of unknown cause, usually affecting middle-aged and elderly people, characterized by excessive bone destruction and unorganized bone repair. Most cases are asymptomatic or mild; however, bone pain may be the first symptom. Bowed tibias (saber shins), kyphosis, and frequent fractures are caused by the soft, abnormal bone in this condition. Enlargement of the head, headaches, and warmth over involved ar-

eas caused by increased vascularity are additional features. Complications include fractures, kidney stones if the patient is immobilized, heart failure, deafness or blindness caused by pressure from bony overgrowth, and osteosarcoma.

pagophagia /pā′gōfā′jē·ə/ [Gk, *pagos,* frost, *phagein,* to eat], an abnormal condition characterized by a craving to eat enormous quantities of ice. It is associated with a lack of the nutrient iron. —**pagophagic, pagophagous,** *adj.*

PAHA, abbreviation for **paraaminohippuric acid.**

PAHA sodium clearance test, a procedure formerly used for detecting kidney damage or certain muscle diseases that used the sodium salt of paraaminohippuric acid to determine the rate at which the kidneys removed this salt from the blood and urine.

PAHO, abbreviation for *Pan American Health Organization.*

pain [L, *poena,* punishment], an unpleasant sensation caused by noxious stimulation of the sensory nerve endings. It is a subjective feeling and an individual response to the cause. Pain is a cardinal symptom of inflammation and is valuable in the diagnosis of many disorders and conditions. It may be mild or severe, chronic or acute, lancinating, burning, dull or sharp, precisely or poorly localized, or referred.

pain, a NANDA-accepted nursing diagnosis of an unpleasant sensory and emotional experience arising from actual or potential tissue damage or described in terms of such damage (International Association for the Study of Pain); sudden or slow onset of any intensity from mild to severe with an anticipated or predictable end and a duration of less than 6 months. Major defining characteristics are verbal or coded report, observed evidence; antalgic position; protective behavior; guarding behavior; antalgic gestures; facial mask; sleep disturbance (eyes lackluster, "hecohe look," fixed or scattered movement, grimace). Minor defining characteristics are self-focus; narrowed focus (altered time perception, impaired thought process, reduced interaction with people and environment); distraction behavior (pacing, seeking out of other people and/or activities, repetitive activities); autonomic alteration in muscle tone (may span from listless to rigid); autonomic responses (diaphoresis, blood pressure, respiration, pulse change, pupillary dilation); expressive behavior (restlessness, moaning, crying, vigilance, irritability, sighing); and changes in appetite and eating.

pain and suffering, (in law) an element in a claim for damages that allows recovery for the mental and physical pain, suffering, distress, and trauma that an individual has endured as a result of injury.

pain assessment, an evaluation of the reported pain and the factors that alleviate or exacerbate it, used as an aid in the diagnosis and the treatment of disease and trauma. Responses to pain vary widely among individuals, depending on many different physical and psychologic factors, such as specific diseases and injuries and the health, pain threshold, fear, anxiety, and cultural background of the individual involved, as well as the way the person expresses pain experiences. Dramatic relief of intense or chronic pain is often difficult to accomplish, but the patient can be helped to learn to handle pain effectively and to function fairly normally.

pain, chronic, a NANDA-accepted nursing diagnosis of an unpleasant sensory and emotional experience arising from actual or potential tissue damage or described in terms of such damage (International Association for the Study of Pain); sudden or slow onset of any intensity from mild to severe; constant or recurring without an anticipated or predictable end; and a duration of greater than 6 months. Defining characteristics include a verbal or coded report or observed evidence of protective behavior; guarding behavior; facial mask; irritability; self-focusing; restlessness; depression, atrophy of the involved muscle group; changes in sleep pattern; weight changes; fatigue; fear of reinjury; reduced interaction with people; altered ability to continue previous activities; sympathetic mediated responses (temperature, cold, changes of body position, hypersensitivity); and anorexia.

pain intervention, the relief of the painful sensations experienced in suffering the physiologic and psychologic effects of disease and trauma. The most common method of pain intervention is the administration of narcotics, such as morphine. Comprehensive pain intervention uses methods and procedures that incorporate both psychologic and physical measures. Methods of pain intervention for acute pain are different from those for chronic pain. Acute pain, occurring in the first 24 to 48 hours after surgery, is often difficult to relieve, and narcotics seldom alleviate it completely. The type of pain intervention usually depends on the description of the pain by the individual experiencing it. Mild pain may best be relieved by comfort measures and the distraction afforded by television, visitors, reading, and other pas-

sive activities. Moderate pain may best be relieved by a combination of comfort measures and drugs. Cognitive dissonance, often used to dampen moderate pain, encourages the patient to reflect on pleasant experiences and describe them to health care personnel. Intervention to relieve severe pain often includes the administration of narcotics, purposeful interaction between the patient and attending hospital personnel, reduction of environmental stimuli, increased comfort measures, and "waking imagined analgesia," in which the patient is encouraged to concentrate on and become distracted by former pleasant experiences. In the alleviation of all types of pain, dampening or decreasing stimuli that create pain is the chief goal. Pain intervention seeks to reduce the effects of other factors that compound pain, such as fatigue and anxiety. Sensory restriction may increase pain, because it blocks otherwise effective distraction; overstimulation may cause fatigue and anxiety, thus increasing pain. Pain intervention by the use of drugs includes the administration of mild nonnarcotic analgesics and of much more potent and potentially addictive opioids such as morphine. Opioid analgesics administered for the relief of pain, cough, or diarrhea provide only symptomatic treatment and are used cautiously in the care of patients with acute or chronic diseases. The risk of development of psychologic and physical dependency on any drug is always present, especially with opioids. In usual doses opioids relieve suffering by altering the emotional component of the painful experience and by effecting analgesia. Many drugs are appropriate substitutes for the potent opioids morphine and codeine. Some nonnarcotic drugs such as aspirin, indomethacin, ibuprofen or naproxen also have antiinflammatory and antipyretic activity. Pain intervention in the treatment of terminal illnesses uses numerous drugs that relieve pain and produce euphoria and tranquillity in patients who would otherwise suffer greatly. Other techniques include acupuncture; hypnosis; behavior modification, in which treatment consists of reducing medication and gradually increasing mobility through exercise and any other appropriate modality; biofeedback; and transcutaneous electrical nerve stimulation.

Pain Management, a Nursing Interventions Classification defined as alleviation of pain or reduction in pain to a level of comfort that is acceptable to the patient.

pain pathway, the network that communicates unpleasant sensations and the perceptions of noxious stimuli throughout the body in association with physical disease and trauma involving tissue damage. The gate control theory of pain is an attempt to explain the role of the nervous system in the pain response. It states that pain signals that reach the nervous system excite a group of small neurons that form a "pain pool." When the total activity of these neurons reaches a minimum level, a theoretic gate opens up and allows the pain signals to proceed to higher brain centers. The areas in which the gates operate are considered to be in the spinal cord dorsal horn and the brainstem. The pattern theory holds that the intensity of a stimulus evokes a specific pattern, which is interpreted by the brain as pain. This perception is the result of the intensity and frequency of stimulation of a nonspecific end organ. Some authorities believe that bradykinin and histamine, two chemical substances produced by the body, cause pain. Recently discovered pain killers produced naturally by the body are the enkephalins and the endorphins. The immediate reaction to pain is transmitted over the reflex arc by sensory fibers in the dorsal horn of the spinal cord and by synapsing motor neurons in the anterior horn. This anatomic pattern of sensory and motor neurons allows the individual to move quickly at the touch of some harmful stimulus, such as extreme heat or cold.

pain receptor, any one of the many free nerve endings throughout the body that warn of potentially harmful changes in the environment, such as excessive pressure or temperature. The free nerve endings constituting most of the pain receptors are located chiefly in the epidermis and in the epithelial covering of certain mucous membranes. They also appear in the stratified squamous epithelium of the cornea, in the root sheaths and in the papillae of the hairs, and around the bodies of sudoriferous glands. The terminal ends of pain receptors consist of unmyelinated nerve fibers that often anastomose into small knobs between the epithelial cells. Referred pain results only from stimulation of pain receptors located in deep structures such as the viscera, the joints, and the skeletal muscles and never from pain receptors in the skin.

paint [Fr, *peindre*], **1.** to apply a medicated solution to the skin, usually over a wide area. **2.** a medicated solution that is applied in this way. Kinds of paint include **antiseptics, germicides,** and **sporicides.**

pain threshold, the point at which a stimulus, usually one associated with pressure or temperature, activates pain recep-

tors and produces a sensation of pain. Individuals with low pain thresholds experience pain much sooner and faster than those with higher thresholds; individuals' reactions to stimulation of pain receptors vary.

pair, 1. two corresponding items similar in form and function. **2.** one object composed of two joined interdependent parts.

PAL, abbreviation for *posterior axillary line.*

palatable /pal'ətəbəl/ [L, *palatum,* palate], pleasant to the taste, as food may be.

palatal /pal'ətəl/ [L, *palatum,* palate], **1.** pertaining to the palate. **2.** pertaining to the lingual surface of a maxillary tooth.

palate /pal'it/ [L, *palatum*], a structure that forms the roof of the mouth. It is divided into the hard palate and the soft palate. —**palatal, palatine** /pal'ətīn/, *adj.*

palatine /pal'ətin/ [L, *palatum,* palate], pertaining to or belonging to the palate.

palatine arch [L, *palatum* + *arcus,* bow], the vault-shaped muscular structure forming the soft palate between the mouth and the nasopharynx. An opening in the arch connects the mouth with the oropharynx; the uvula is suspended from the middle of the posterior border of the arch.

palatine bone, one of a pair of bones of the skull, forming the posterior part of the hard palate, part of the nasal cavity, and the floor of the orbit of the eye.

palatine ridge, any one of the four to six transverse ridges on the anterior surface of the hard palate.

palatine suture, any one of a number of thin wavy lines marking the joining of the palatine processes that form the hard palate.

palatine tonsil, one of a pair of almond-shaped masses of lymphoid tissue between the palatoglossal and the palatopharyngeal arches on each side of the fauces. They are covered with mucous membrane and contain numerous lymph follicles and various crypts.

palatine uvula, an elongated process that hangs from the middle of the back edge of the soft palate.

palatitis, an inflammation of the hard palate.

palatoglossal /-glos'əl/ [L, *palatum,* palate; Gk, *glossa,* tongue], pertaining to both the palate and the tongue.

palatoglossus /-glos'əs/, a muscle with an origin in the oral surface of the soft palate and an insertion at the side of the tongue. It forms the anterior pillar of the tonsillar fossa and acts to raise the back of the tongue.

palatognathous /pal'ətog'nəthəs/, pertaining to a cleft palate.

palatograph /pal'ətōgraf/, a device that records the movement of the palate while the person is speaking.

palatomaxillary /-mak'siler'ē/ [L, *palatum* + *maxilla,* jaw], pertaining to the palate and the maxilla.

palatonasal /-nā'zəl/ [L, *palatum* + *nasus,* nose], pertaining to the palate and the nose.

palatopharyngeal /-ferin'jē·əl/, pertaining to the palate and pharynx.

palatopharyngeus /-ferin'jē·əs/, a muscle with an origin at the back of the soft palate and an insertion on the posterior border of the thyroid cartilage and the wall of the pharynx. It acts to raise the pharynx.

palatopharyngoplasty /-fering'gōplas'tē/, the surgical excision of palatal and oropharyngeal tissues. The procedure may be performed to treat cases of snoring or sleep apnea thought to be caused by obstructions in the nose or pharynx.

palatoplasty /pal'ətōplas'tē, plastic surgery of the palate.

palatoplegia /-plē'jē·ə/, paralysis of the soft palate.

palatorrhaphy /pal'ətôr'əfē/, the surgical repair of a cleft palate.

palatosalpingeus /-salpin'jē·əs/, the tensor muscle of the soft palate. It arises from the scaphoid fossa of the sphenoid bone.

palatoschisis /pal'ətos'kisis/, a cleft palate.

pale infarct [L, *pallidus,* pallid, *infarcire,* to stuff], a wedge of dead tissue that is white because of an absence of blood and causes an obstruction in an artery.

paleocerebellum /pal'ē·ōser'əbel'əm/, the phylogenetically oldest part of the cerebellum, including the vermis, which connects the cerebellar hemispheres and the flocculus, or lobule, on the posterior lobe.

paleocortex /kôr'ucks/, the phylogenetically oldest part of the cerebral cortex, particularly the olfactory bulb.

paleogenetic /-jənet'ik/ [Gk, *palaios,* long ago, *genesis,* origin], **1.** a trait or structure of an organism or species that originated in a previous generation. **2.** relating to the development of such a trait or structure.

paleokinetic /-kinet'ik/, pertaining to primitive mechanisms of reflexes and other automatic muscular movements.

paleopathology /-pathol'əjē/, the science of disease in ancient eras based on the condition of remains of mummies, skeletons, and other archaeologic findings.

palikinesia /pal'ikinē'zhə., a condition in which involuntary movements are constantly repeated.

palilalia /pal'ilā'lyə/ [Gk, *palin,* again, *la-*

lein, to babble], an abnormal condition characterized by the increasingly rapid repetition of the same word or phrase, usually at the end of a sentence.

palindrome /pal'indrōm'/ [Gk, *palin* + *dromos,* course], (in molecular genetics) a segment of deoxyribonucleic acid in which identical, or almost identical, sequences of bases run in opposite directions.

palindromia /pal'indrō'mē·ə/, the recurrence of a disease.

palingenesis /pal'injen'əsis/ [Gk, *palin* + *genesis,* origin], **1.** the regeneration of a lost part. **2.** the hereditary transmission of ancestral structural characteristics. —**palingenetic, palingenic,** *adj.*

palladium (Pd) /pəlā'dē·əm/ [Gk, *Pallas, Athena,* mythic goddess and protector of Troy], a hard, silvery metallic element. Its atomic number is 46; its atomic mass (weight) is 106.42. Highly resistant to tarnish and corrosion, palladium is used in high-grade surgical instruments and in dental inlays, bridgework, and orthodontic appliances.

pallanesthesia /pal'anesthē'zhə/, a condition characterized by an inability to sense vibrations.

pallesthesia /pal'esthē'zhə [Gk, *pallein,* to quiver], hypersensitivity to vibration, particularly that caused by a tuning fork placed on a bony prominence.

palliate /pal'ē·āt/ [L, *palliare,* to cloak], to soothe or relieve. —**palliation,** *n.,* **palliative,** *adj.*

palliative treatment /pal'ē·ətiv'/ [L, *palliare,* to cloak, *tractare,* to handle], therapy designed to relieve or reduce intensity of uncomfortable symptoms but not to produce a cure. Some kinds of palliative treatment are the use of narcotics to relieve pain in a patient with advanced cancer, the creation of a colostomy to bypass an inoperable obstructing lesion of the bowel, and the debridement of necrotic tissue in a patient with metastatic malignancy.

pallid /pal'id/ [L, *pallidus,* pale], lacking color.

pallidectomy /pal'idek'təmē/ [L, *pallidus,* pale; Gk *exome,* cutting out], the destruction of all or part of the globus pallidus by chemicals or freezing in the treatment of Parkinson's disease.

pallidoamygdalotomy, /pal'idō·amig'dəlot'əmē/, the surgical production of lesions in the globus pallidus and amygdaloid nuclei.

pallidotomy /pal'idot'əmē/, the surgical production of lesions in the globus pallidus for the treatment of extrapyramidal disorders.

pallor /pal′ər/ [L, paleness], an unnatural paleness or absence of color in the skin.

palm /päm/ [L, *palma*], the anterior surface of the hand, beyond the wrist to the base of the fingers. —**palmar,** *adj.*

palm and sole system of identification, a method of identifying individuals by the patterns of ridges in the skin of the palms of the hands and soles of the feet. Like fingerprints, the patterns are helpful in identification of infants and others.

palmar /pal′mər/ [L, *palma*], pertaining to the palm.

palmar aponeurosis [L, *palma* + Gk, *apo,* from, *neuron,* nerve], a sheet of fascia under the skin of the palm and surrounding the muscles.

palmar crease, a normal groove across the palm of the hand.

palmar erythema, an inflammatory redness of the palms of the hands.

palmar grasp reflex [L, *palma,* palm; ONorse, *grapa,* grab], a flexion of the fingers caused by stimulation of the palm of the hand. The reflex is present at birth and usually disappears by 6 months of age.

palmaris longus /pəlmer′is/, a long, slender, superficial fusiform muscle of the forearm, lying on the medial side of the flexor carpi radialis that functions to flex the hand.

palmar metacarpal artery, any one of several arteries arising from the deep palmar arch, supplying the fingers.

palmar pinch, a thumbless grasp in which the tips of the other fingers are pressed against the palm of the hand.

palmar reflex, a reflex that curls the fingers when the palm of the hand is tickled.

palmature /pal′məchər/ [L, *palma*], an abnormal condition in which the fingers are webbed.

Palmer notation, a system for identifying and referring to teeth by either a consecutive alphabetical notation or within each quadrant by lowercase letters.

palmitic acid /palmit′ik/ [L, *palma*], a saturated fatty acid that commonly occurs in animal and vegetable fats and oils. It is used in the manufacture of soaps and candles.

palmitin, /pal′mitin/ a triglyceride consisting of palmitic acid present in palm oil and other vegetable and animal fats.

palmomental reflex /pal′məmen′təl/ [L, *palma* + *mentum,* chin, *reflectere,* to bend back], an abnormal neurologic sign, elicited by scratching the palm of the hand at the base of the thumb, characterized by contraction of the muscles of the chin and corner of the mouth on the same side of the body as the stimulus.

palmoscopy /palmos′kəpē/, detection of the pulse or heartbeat.

palpable /pal′pəbəl/ [L, *palpare,* to touch gently], perceivable by touch.

palpate /pal′pāt/, to use the hands or fingers to examine.

palpation /palpā′shən/ [L, *palpare,* to touch gently], a technique used in physical examination in which the examiner feels the texture, size, consistency, and location of certain body parts with the hands.

palpatory percussion /pal′pətôr′ē/ [L, *palpare,* to touch gently; *percutere,* to strike hard], a technique in physical examination in which the vibrations produced by percussion are evaluated by using light pressure of the flat of the examiner's hand.

palpebral fissure /pal′pəbrəl/ [L, *palpebra,* eyelid, *fissura,* cleft], the opening between the margins of the upper and lower eyelids.

palpebra superior /pal′pəbrə/, *pl.* **palpebrae superiores,** the upper eyelid, larger and more movable than the lower eyelid and furnished with an elevator muscle.

palpebrate /pal′pəbrāt/, **1.** to wink or blink. **2.** having eyelids.

palpitate /pal′pitāt/ [L, *palpitare,* to flutter], to pulsate rapidly, as in the unusually fast beating of the heart under various conditions of stress and in certain heart problems.

palpitation /pal′pitā′shən/ [L, *palpitare,* to flutter], a pounding or racing of the heart. It is associated with normal emotional responses or with heart disorders.

PALS, abbreviation for **pediatric advanced life support.**

palsy /pôl′zē/ [Gk, *para,* beyond, *lysis,* loosening], an abnormal condition characterized by paralysis.

Paltauf's nanism /päl′toufs/ [Arnold Paltauf, Czechoslovakian physician, 1860–1893; Gk, *nanos,* dwarf], dwarfism associated with excessive production or growth of lymphoid tissue.

pampiniform /pampin′ifôrm/, having the shape of a tendril.

pampiniform plexus [L, *pampinus,* vine tendril, *plexus,* plaited], a network of veins in the spermatic cord that drains the testes into the testicular vein in the lower abdomen.

panacea /pan′əsē′ə/ [Gk, *pan,* all, *akeia,* remedy], **1.** a universal remedy. **2.** an ancient name for an herb or a liquid potion with healing properties.

panacinar emphysema /panas′ənər/ [Gk, *pan* + L, *acinus,* grape; Gk, *en* + *physema,* a blowing], a form of emphysema that affects all lung areas by causing dilation and atrophy of the alveoli and by destroying the vascular bed of the lung.

panagglutinable /pan'əglōō'tinəbəl/, pertaining to red blood cells that are agglutinable by the sera of all blood groups of the same species.

panagglutinin /pan'əglōō'tinin/, an antibody that causes clumping (agglutination) of red blood cells of all blood groups of a species.

panangitis /panan'jē-ītis/, an inflammation that affects all layers of a blood vessel.

panarteritis /-är'tərī'tis/ [Gk, pan, all, arteria, artery, itis inflammation], an inflammation that involves all the tissue layers of an artery.

panarthritis /-ärthrī'tis/ [Gk, pan + arthron joint], an abnormal condition characterized by the inflammation of many joints of the body. —**panarthritic,** adj.

panatrophy /panat'rəfē/, **1.** a general atrophy of all parts of a body or structure. **2.** a rare disorder associated with atrophy of cutaneous and subcutaneous tissue. It is characterized by prominence of underlying body structures as all levels of skin and subcutaneous tissue are reduced in thickness.

panbronchiolitis, a chronic inflammation and obstruction of the bronchioles caused by the accumulation of foam cells. It usually leads to bronchiectasis.

pancake kidney /pan'kāk/ [ME, panne, pan, kuka, cake, kidnere], a congenital anomaly in which the left and right kidneys are fused into a single mass in the pelvis. The fused kidney has two collecting systems and two ureters.

pancarditis /-kärdī'tis/ [Gk, pan + kardia, heart, itis, inflammation], an abnormal condition characterized by inflammation of the entire heart, including the endocardium, myocardium, and pericardium.

Pancoast's syndrome /pan'cōsts/ [Henry K. Pancoast, American radiologist, 1875–1939], **1.** a combination of signs associated with a tumor in the apex of the lung. The signs include neuritic pain in the arm, atrophy of the muscles of the arm and the hand, and Horner's syndrome. **2.** an abnormal condition caused by osteolysis in the posterior part of one or more ribs, sometimes involving associated vertebrae.

pancolectomy /-kōlek'təmē/ [Gk, pan + kolon, colon, ektome, excision], the excision of the entire colon, necessitating an ileostomy.

pancreas /pan'krē-əs/ [Gk, pan, all, kreas, flesh], an elongated grayish pink nodular gland that stretches transversely across the posterior abdominal wall in the epigastric and hypochondriac regions of the body and secretes various substances such as digestive enzymes, insulin, and glucagon. A compound, mixed gland composed of exocrine and endocrine tissue; it contains a main duct that runs the length of the organ, draining smaller ducts and emptying into the duodenum.

pancreas scan, a radiographic scan of the pancreas after the intravenous injection of a radioactive contrast medium, used for detecting various abnormalities, such as tumors, cysts, and infections.

pancreatalgia /pan'krē-ətal'jə/, pain in or near the pancreas.

pancreatectomy /pan'krē-ətek'təmē/ [Gk, pan + kreas + ektome, excision], the surgical removal of all or part of the pancreas, performed to excise a cyst or tumor, treat pancreatitis, or repair trauma. A frequent complication is the formation of a fistula in the pancreatic bile duct, allowing digestive enzymes to contact adjacent tissues.

pancreatemphraxis /pan'krē-at'emfrak'sis/, hypertrophy or congestion of the pancreas caused by an obstruction in the pancreatic duct.

pancreatic /pan'krē-at'ik/ [Gk, pan, all, kreas, flesh], pertaining to the pancreas.

pancreatic abscess, an infection characterized by a collection of pus in or around the pancreas.

pancreatic cancer [Gk, pan + kreas + L, cancer, crab], a malignant neoplastic disease of the pancreas, characterized by anorexia, flatulence, weakness, dramatic weight loss, epigastric or back pain, jaundice, pruritus, a palpable abdominal mass, recent onset of diabetes, and clay-colored stools if the pancreatic and biliary ducts are obstructed. About 90% of pancreatic tumors are adenocarcinomas; two thirds are in the head of the pancreas. Radiotherapy or chemotherapy may offer temporary palliation, but cancer of the pancreas has a poor prognosis. People who smoke more than 10 to 20 cigarettes a day, who have diabetes mellitus, or who have been exposed to polychlorinated biphenyl compounds are at increased risk of development of pancreatic cancer.

pancreatic diabetes [Gk, pan, all, kreas, flesh, diabainein, to pass through], diabetes mellitus caused by a deficiency of insulin production by the islet cells of the pancreas.

pancreatic digestion, the action of pancreatic enzymes in the process of breaking down food into its constituents.

pancreatic diverticulum, one of a pair of membranous pouches arising from the em-

P

bryonic duodenum. These two diverticula later form the pancreas and its ducts.

pancreatic dornase, an enzyme from beef pancreas that has been used as a mucolytic for upper respiratory infections and cystic fibrosis.

pancreatic duct, the primary secretory channel of the pancreas.

pancreatic enzyme, any one of the enzymes secreted by the pancreas in the process of digestion. The most important are trypsin, chymotrypsin, steapsin, and amylopsin.

pancreatic hormone, any one of several chemical compounds secreted by the pancreas, associated with the regulation of cellular metabolism. Major hormones secreted by the pancreas are insulin, glucagon, and pancreatic polypeptide.

pancreatic insufficiency, a condition characterized by inadequate production and secretion of pancreatic hormones or enzymes. It usually occurs secondary to a disease process destructive of pancreatic tissue. Nutritional malabsorption, anorexia, poorly localized upper abdominal or epigastric pain, malaise, and severe weight loss often occur. Alcohol-induced pancreatitis is the most common form of the condition.

pancreatic juice, the fluid secretion of the pancreas, produced by the stimulation of food in the duodenum. It contains water, protein, inorganic salts, and enzymes. The juice is essential in breaking down proteins into their amino acid components, in reducing dietary fats to glycerol and fatty acids, and in converting starch to simple sugars.

pancreaticoduodenal /pan′krē·at′ikōdōō′-ədē′nəl/, pertaining to the pancreas and duodenum.

pancreaticolienal node /pan′krē·at′ikō′lī·ē′nəl/ [Gk, *pan* + *kreas* + L, *lien,* spleen, *nodus,* knot], a node in one of three groups of lymph glands associated with branches of the abdominal and pelvic viscera that are supplied by branches of the celiac artery.

pancreatin /pan′krē·ətin′, -krē·ā′tin/, a concentrate of pancreatic enzymes from swine or beef cattle. It is prescribed as an aid to digestion to replace endogenous pancreatic enzymes in cystic fibrosis and after pancreatectomy.

pancreatitis /pan′krē·ətī′tis/ [Gk, *pan* + *kreas* + *itis,* inflammation], an inflammatory condition of the pancreas that may be acute or chronic. **Acute pancreatitis** is generally the result of damage to the biliary tract, as by alcohol, trauma, infectious disease, or certain drugs. It is characterized by severe abdominal pain (generally epigastric or upper left) radiating to the back, fever, anorexia, nausea, and vomiting. There may be jaundice if the common bile duct is obstructed. The causes of **chronic pancreatitis** are similar to those of the acute form. When the cause is alcohol abuse, there may be calcification and scarring of the smaller pancreatic ducts. Abdominal pain, nausea, and vomiting occur, as well as steatorrhea and creatorrhea, caused by the diminished output of pancreatic enzymes. Pancreatic insulin production may be diminished, and diabetes mellitus develops in some patients.

pancreatoduodenectomy /-dōō′ədənek′tə-mē/ [Gk, *pan* + *kreas* + L, *duodeni,* twelve fingers; Gk, *ektome,* excision], a surgical procedure in which the head of the pancreas and the loop of duodenum that surrounds it are excised.

pancreatoduodenostomy, a surgical procedure to establish a fistula or duct from the pancreas into the duodenum.

pancreatogastrostomy /-gastros′təmē/, the surgical establishment of a fistula or duct from the pancreas to the stomach.

pancreatogenic /-jen′ik/, originating in the pancreas.

pancreatography /pan′krē·atog′rəfē/ [Gk, *pan* + *kreas* + *graphein,* to record], visualization of the pancreas or its ducts by injection of x-rays and contrast media into the ducts at surgery or via an endoscope, or by ultrasonography, computed tomography, or radionuclide imaging.

pancreatojejunostomy /-jij′ōōnos′təmē/, the surgical establishment of a fistula or duct from the pancreas to the jejunum.

pancreatolith /-krē·at′əlith/, a stone or calculus in the pancreas.

pancreatolithiasis /-lithī′ə/, the presence of calculi in the pancreas or pancreatic duct.

pancreatolithotomy /lithot′əmē/, the surgical removal of pancreatic calculi.

pancreatolysis /pan′krē·atol′isis/, destruction of the pancreas by pancreatic enzymes.

pancreatomegaly /-meg′əlē/, an abnormal enlargement of the pancreas.

pancreatopathy /pan′krē·atop′əthē/, any disease of the pancreas.

pancreatotomy /pan′krē·ətot′əmē/, a surgical incision in the pancreas.

pancreatropic /pan′krē·ətrop′ik/, exerting an influence on the pancreas.

pancuronium bromide /-kyərō′nē·əm/, a skeletal muscle relaxant prescribed as an adjunct to anesthesia and mechanical ventilation.

pancytopenia /pan′sītōpē′nē·ə/ [Gk, *pan* + *kytos,* cell, *penia,* poverty], marked reduction in the number of red blood cells, white blood cells, and platelets. —**pancytopenic**, *adj.*

p and a, abbreviation for *percussion and auscultation,* as noted in the patient's chart after physical examination of the chest.

pandemia /-dē'mē-ə/ [Gk, *pan,* all, *demos,* people], a disease epidemic that affects all or most of a population group.

pandemic /-dē'mik/ [Gk, *pan* + *demos,* people], (of a disease) occurring throughout the population of a country, a people, or the world.

pandiastolic /-dī'əstol'ik/ [Gk, *pan* + *dia,* through, *stellein,* to set], pertaining to the complete diastole.

Pandy's reaction [Kakman Pandy, Hungarian neurologist, b. 1868], a test for the presence of proteins in spinal fluid. One drop of spinal fluid is added to 1 ml of a carbolic acid solution. If proteins are present, a cloudy precipitate is formed.

panencephalitis /pan'ənsef'əlī'tis/ [Gk, *pan* + *enkephale,* brain, *itis*], inflammation of the entire brain characterized by an insidious onset, a progressive course with deterioration of motor and mental functions, and evidence of a viral cause. Subacute sclerosing panencephalitis is an uncommon childhood disease thought to be caused by a "slow" latent measles virus after recovery from a previous infection. The disease results in ataxia, myoclonus, atrophy, cortical blindness, and mental deterioration.

panendoscope /-en'dəskōp'/ [Gk, *pan* + *endon,* within, *skopein,* to look], a cystoscope that allows a wide view of the bladder and urethra with a special lens system of the interior.

panesthesia /-esthē'zhə/ [Gk, *pan* + *aisthesis,* feeling], the total of all sensations experienced by an individual at one time.

pang, a sudden severe but temporary pain.

pangenesis /-jen'əsis/ [Gk, *pan* + *genesis,* origin], a darwinian theory that each cell and particle of a parent reproduces itself in progeny.

panhidrosis, perspiration over the entire body.

panhypopituitarism /panhī'pōpitoō'-itəriz'əm/ [Gk, *pan* + *hypo,* under, *pituita,* phlegm], generalized insufficiency of pituitary hormones, resulting from damage to or deficiency of the gland. **Prepubertal panhypopituitarism,** a rare disorder usually associated with a suprasellar cyst or craniopharyngioma, is characterized by dwarfism with normal body proportions, subnormal sexual development, and insufficient thyroid and adrenal function. Diabetes insipidus is frequently present;

bitemporal hemianopia or complete blindness may occur; skin is often yellow and wrinkled, but mentality is usually unimpaired. Postpubertal panhypopituitarism may be caused by postpartum pituitary necrosis, resulting from thrombosis of pituitary circulation during or after delivery. Characteristic signs of the disorder are failure to lactate, amenorrhea, weakness, cold intolerance, lethargy, and loss of libido and of axillary and pubic hair. There may be bradycardia or hypotension, and progression of the disorder leads to premature wrinkling of the skin and atrophy of the thyroid and adrenal glands.

panhysterectomy /pan'histərek'təmē/ [Gk, *pan* + *hystera,* uterus, *ektome,* excision], complete surgical removal of the uterus and cervix.

panic /pan'ik/, an intense, sudden, and overwhelming fear or feeling of anxiety that produces terror and immediate physiologic changes that result in paralyzed immobility or senseless, hysteric behavior.

panic attack [Gk, *panikos,* of the god Pan; Fr, *attaquer*], an episode of acute anxiety that occurs unpredictably with feelings of intense apprehension or terror, accompanied by dyspnea, dizziness, sweating, trembling, and chest pain or palpitations. The attack may last several minutes and may occur again in certain situations.

panivorous /paniv'ərəs/ [L, *panis,* bread, *vorare,* to devour], pertaining to the practice of subsisting exclusively on bread. —**panivore,** *n.*

panmyelosis /panmī'əlō'sis/, a pathologic condition characterized by a proliferation of bone marrow cells of all types.

Panner's disease, a rare form of osteochondrosis in which abnormal bony growth occurs in the capitulum of the humerus.

panniculitis /pənik'yəli'tis/ [L, *panniculus,* piece of cloth; Gk, *itis,* inflammation], a chronic inflammation of subcutaneous fat in which the skin becomes hardened, particularly over the abdomen and thorax. Small subcutaneous masses of hard tissue are found in the affected areas.

panniculus /pənik'yələs/, *pl.* **panniculi** [L, small garment], a membranous layer, the many sheets of fascia covering various structures in the body.

pannus /pan'əs/ [L, cloth], an abnormal condition of the cornea, which has become vascularized and infiltrated with granular tissue just beneath the surface. Pannus may develop in the inflammatory stage of trachoma or after a detached retina, glaucoma, iridocyclitis, or other degenerative eye disorder.

P

panography /pənog′rəfē/, a method of tomography that visualizes bodies' curved surfaces at any depth. In dentistry this is accomplished by simultaneous radiography of the maxillary and mandibular dental arches and the associated structures by using two axes of rotation to record these structures.

panophthalmitis /pan′ofthalmī′tis/ [Gk, *pan* + *ophthalmos,* eye, *itis*], an inflammation of the entire eye, usually caused by virulent pyogenic organisms, such as strains of meningococci, pneumococci, streptococci, anthrax bacilli, and clostridia. Initial symptoms are pain, fever, headache, drowsiness, edema, and swelling. As the infection progresses, the iris appears muddy and gray, the aqueous humor becomes turbid, and precipitates form on the posterior surface of the cornea.

panoptic /panop′tik/ [Gk, *pan,* all, *opsis,* vision], pertaining to the enhanced visual effect produced by stains applied to microscopic specimens.

panoramic radiograph /pan′ôram′ik/ [Gk, *pan* + *horama,* view; L, *radiare,* to emit rays; Gk, *graphein,* to record], a method of tomography for visualization of curved body surfaces such as the upper and lower jaws on a single film.

panotitis /pan′ōtī′tis/, a general inflammation of the ear, including the middle ear.

panphobia /-fō′bē-ə/ [Gk, *pan* + *phobos,* fear], an anxiety disorder characterized by an irrational fear of everything. — **panophobic,** *adj.*

panplegia /panplē′jē-ə/, paralysis of all four extremities.

pansclerosis /pan′sklirō′sis/, a general hardening of a tissue or body part.

pansystolic /-sistol′ik/, pertaining to the entire systole.

pantalgia /pantal′jə/, pain that affects all parts of the body.

pantanencephaly /pantan′ensef′əlē/, a congenital absence of all or nearly all brain tissue.

panthenol /pan′thənôl/, **1.** an alcohol converted in the body to pantothenic acid, a vitamin in the B complex. **2.** a viscous liquid derived from pantothenic acid, a member of the vitamin B_{12} group.

panting [Fr, *panteler,* to gasp], a ventilatory pattern characterized by rapid, shallow breathing with small tidal volume. Panting usually moves gas back and forth in the anatomic dead space at a high flow rate, which evaporates water, removes heat with little or no increase in alveolar ventilation rate, and prevents hypocapnia.

pantograph /pan′təgraf′/, **1.** a jointed device for copying a plane figure to any desired scale. **2.** a device that incorporates a pair of face bows fixed to the jaws, used for inscribing centrically related points and arcs leading to the points on segments relatable to the three craniofacial planes.

pantomograph /pantom′əgraf/, a radiographic apparatus that permits visualization of curved body surfaces. In dentistry it is used to produce tomographic views of maxillary and mandibular dental arches.

pantomography /-mog′əfē/ [Gk, *pan* + *graphein,* to record], panoramic radiography for obtaining simultaneous radiographs of the maxillary and mandibular dental arches and related structures.

pantoscopic /pan′təskop′ik/, pertaining to bifocal eyeglasses designed for both reading and distance viewing: the bottom half for close vision and the top half for far vision.

pantothenic acid /pan′təthen′ik/, a member of the vitamin B complex. It is widely distributed in plant and animal tissues and may be an important element in human nutrition.

PaO₂, symbol for **partial pressure of oxygen in arterial blood.**

PAO₂, symbol for *partial pressure of alveolar oxygen.*

pap, any soft, soggy food.

papain /pəpā′ēn/, an enzyme from the fruit of *Carica papaya,* the tropic melon tree. It has been prescribed for enzymatic debridement of wounds and promotion of healing.

Papanicolaou test /pap′ənikəlou′/ [George N. Papanicolaou, Greek physician in U.S. practice, 1883–1962], a simple smear method of examining stained exfoliative cells. It is used most commonly to detect cancers of the cervix, but it may be used for tissue specimens from any organ. A smear, the Papanicolaou (Pap) smear, is usually obtained during a routine pelvic examination annually beginning at 18 years of age. The technique permits early diagnosis of cancer and has contributed to a lower death rate from cervical cancer. The findings are usually reported descriptively and grouped into the following classes: class I, only normal cells seen; class II, atypical cells consistent with inflammation; class III, mild dysplasia; class IV, severe dysplasia, suspicious cells; class V, carcinoma cells seen.

papaverine hydrochloride /papav′ərēn/, a smooth muscle relaxant prescribed in the treatment of cardiovascular or visceral spasms.

papaya /pəpī′ə/, the fruit of the tropical *Carica papaya* (pawpaw) tree and the source of the proteolytic enzyme papain used in blood group serologic evaluation. Papain is also used to prevent adhesions.

paper, a material produced in sheets, usually from wood pulp or other cellulose products. It can be adapted for many purposes, such as litmus paper for testing acidity, filter paper, and articulating carbon paper used to record points of contact between teeth of the upper and lower jaws.

paper chromatography [Gk, *papyrus,* papyrus], the separation of a mixture into its components by filtering it through a strip of special paper.

paper radioimmunosorbent test (PRIST), a technique for determining total immunoglobulin E levels in patients with type I hypersensitivity reactions.

papilla /pəpil'ə/, *pl.* **papillae** [L, nipple], **1.** a small nipple-shaped projection, such as the conoid papillae of the tongue and the papillae of the corium that extend from collagen fibers, the capillary blood vessels, and sometimes the nerves of the dermis. **2.** the optic papilla, a round white disc in the fundus oculi, which corresponds to the entrance of the optic nerve.

papillary /pap'əlerē/ [L, *papilla,* nipple], pertaining to a papilla.

papillary adenocarcinoma, a malignant neoplasm characterized by small papillae of vascular connective tissue covered by neoplastic epithelium that projects into follicles, glands, or cysts. The tumor is most common in the ovaries and thyroid gland.

papillary adenocystoma lymphomatosum, an unusual tumor, consisting of epithelial and lymphoid tissues, that develops in the area of the parotid and submaxillary glands.

papillary adenoma, a benign epithelial tumor in which the membrane lining the glandular tissue forms papillary processes that project into the alveoli or grow out of a cavity's surface.

papillary carcinoma, a malignant neoplasm characterized by fingerlike projections.

papillary duct, any one of the thousands of straight collecting renal tubules that descend through the medulla of the kidney and join with others to form the common ducts opening into the renal papillae.

papillary muscle, any one of the rounded or conical muscular projections attached to the chordae tendineae in the ventricles of the heart. The papillary muscles vary in number; the two main muscles are the anterior papillary muscle and the posterior papillary muscle. The papillary muscles are associated with the atrioventricular valves that they help open and close.

papillate /pap'ilit/, marked by papillae or nipplelike prominences.

papilledema /pap'ilədē'mə/ [L, *papilla* + Gk, *oidema,* swelling], swelling of the optic disc, visible on ophthalmoscopic examination of the fundus of the eye, caused by increase in intracranial pressure. The meningeal sheaths that surround the optic nerves from the optic disc are continuous with the meninges of the brain; therefore increased intracranial pressure is transmitted forward from the brain to the optic disc in the eye to cause swelling.

papilliform /pəpil'ifôrm/, shaped like a papilla.

papillitis /pap'ilī'tis/ [L, *papilla* + Gk, *itis,* inflammation], **1.** inflammation of a papilla, such as the lacrimal papilla. **2.** inflammation of the optic disc.

papilloadenocystoma /pap'ilō·ad'ənō'sistō'mə/, a benign epithelial tumor in which the lining develops in numerous small folds.

papillocarcinoma [L, *papilla,* nipple; Gk, *oma,* tumor, *karkinos,* crab, *oma,* tumor], a malignant tumor in which there are papillary outgrowths.

papilloma /pap'ilō'mə/ [L, *papilla* + Gk, *oma,* tumor], a benign epithelial neoplasm characterized by a branching or lobular tumor.

papillomatosis /pap'ilōmətō'sis/ [L, *papilla* + Gk, *oma,* tumor, *osis,* condition], an abnormal condition characterized by widespread development of nipplelike growths.

papillomavirus /pap'ilō'məvī'rəs/ [L, *papilla* + Gk, *oma,* tumor; L, *virus,* poison], the virus that causes warts in humans.

papilloretinitis /pap'ilōret'inī'tis/ [L, *papilla* + *rete,* net; Gk, *itis,* inflammation], an inflammatory occlusion of a retinal vein.

papovavirus /pap'əvəvī'rəs/ [(acronym) *pa*pilloma, *po*lyoma, *va*cuolating, *virus*], one of a group of small deoxyribonucleic acid viruses, some of which may be potentially cancer-producing. The human wart is caused by a kind of papovavirus, but it very rarely undergoes malignant transformation. Kinds of papovaviruses are papilloma papovavirus, polyoma papovavirus, and SV-40 papovavirus.

Pappenheimer bodies [A. M. Pappenheimer, U.S. pathologist, 1878–1955], phagosomes containing iron granules, found in red blood cells in certain disorders, including sickle cell disease and hemolytic anemia. They may contribute to spurious platelet counts by electro-optical counters.

pappus /pap′əs/ [Gk, *pappos,* down], the first growth of beard, characterized by downy hairs.

papula /pap′yələ/, a small superficial elevation of the skin.

papular /pap′yələr/ [L, *papula,* pimple], pertaining to or resembling a papule.

papular scaling disease [L, *papula,* pimple; AS, *scealu*], any of a group of skin disorders characterized by discrete raised dry, scaling lesions. Some kinds of papular scaling diseases are **lichen planus, pityriasis rosea,** and **psoriasis.**

papulation /pap′yəlā′shən/ [L, *papula,* pimple, *atus,* process], the development of papules.

papule /pap′yool/ [L, *papula,* pimple], a small, solid, raised skin lesion less than 1 cm in diameter, such as the lesions of lichen planus and nonpustular acne. —**papular,** *adj.*

papuloerythematous /pap′yəlō·er′ithem′ətəs/, pertaining to an eruption of papules on an erythematous surface.

papulopustular /pap′yəlōpus′tyələr/, pertaining to a skin eruption of both pustules and papules.

papulosis /pap′yəlō′sis/, a widespread occurrence of papules over the body.

papulosquamous /pap′yəlōskwä′məs/ [L, *papula,* pimple + *squama,* scale], pertaining to a skin eruption that is both papular and scaly.

papulovesicular /pap′yəlō′vesik′yələr/, pertaining to a skin rash characterized by both papules and vesicles.

papyraceous /pap′irā′shəs/ [Gk, *papyros,* paper], having a paperlike quality.

Paquelin's cautery /pak′əlinz/ [Claude A. Paquelin, French physician, b. 1836; Gk, *kauterion,* branding iron], a cauterizing device consisting of a platinum loop through which a heated hydrocarbon is passed.

par, a pair, specifically a pair of cranial nerves, such as the par nonum, or ninth pair.

PAR, abbreviation for **pulmonary arteriolar resistance.**

para [L, *parere,* to bear], a woman who has produced an infant, regardless of whether the child was alive or stillborn. The term is used with numerals to indicate the number of pregnancies carried to more than 20 weeks' gestation, such as para 2, indicating two pregnancies, regardless of the number of offspring produced in a single pregnancy.

paraactinomycosis /per′ə·ak′tinō′mīkō′sis/, a chronic pulmonary infection similar to actinomycosis. The infection is caused by bacteria of the genus *Nocardia.*

paraaminobenzoic acid (PABA) /per′ə-- amē′nōbenzō′ik/, a substance often associated with the vitamin B complex, found in cereals, eggs, milk, and meat and present in detectable amounts in blood, urine, spinal fluid, and sweat. It is widely used as a sunscreen that forms a partial chemical conjugation with constituents of the horny layer and that resists removal by water and sweat. PABA is a sulfonamide antagonist and may be an effective agent for the treatment of scleroderma, dermatomyositis, and pemphigus.

paraaminohippuric acid (PAHA, PHA) /per′ə·amē′-nōhipŏŏr′ik/, the N-acetic acid of paraaminobenzoic acid. Its sodium salt is used for measuring effective renal plasma flow and determining kidney function.

paraaminosalicylic acid (PAS, PASA) /per′ə·amē′-nōsal′isil′ik/, a bacteriostatic agent prescribed for the treatment of pulmonary and extrapulmonary tuberculosis.

paraballism /per′əbôl′izəm/ [Gk, *ballismos,* jumping about], involuntary jerking movements of the legs.

parabiosis /-bī·ō′sis/, the fusion of two eggs or embryos, resulting in conjoined twins.

parabiotic syndrome /-bī·ot′ik/ [Gk, *para,* beside, *bios,* life, *syn,* together, *dromos,* course], a blood transfer condition that can occur between identical twin fetuses as a result of placental vascular anastomoses. One twin may become anemic, and the other plethoric.

parabolic /-bol′ik/, (in ultrasonics) pertaining to flow conditions in blood vessels. Under parabolic flow, blood cells in the middle of the vessels move the fastest, with a gradual decrease in flow velocity for points farther away from the center.

paracanthoma /-kənthō′mə/, a tumor that develops from the abnormal overgrowth of the prickle cell layer of the skin.

paracelsian method /-sel′sē·ən/ [Philippus Aureolus Paracelsus, Swiss alchemist and physician, 1493–1541], the use of chemical agents such as sulfur, iron, lead, and arsenic in the treatment of disease.

paracenesthesia /-sen′esthē′zhə/, any abnormality in the general sense of well-being.

paracentesis /per′əsentē′sis/ [Gk, *para* + *kentesis,* puncturing], a procedure in which fluid is withdrawn from a cavity in the body. An incision is made in the skin; and a hollow trocar, cannula, or catheter is passed through the incision into the cavity to allow outflow of fluid into a collecting device. Paracentesis is most commonly performed to remove excessive accumulations of ascitic fluid from the abdomen.

paracentesis thoracis [Gk, *para* + *kentesis*, puncturing, *thorax*, chest], the aspiration of fluid or air or both through a needle inserted into the pleural cavity.

paracentral /-sen'trəl/ [Gk, *para* + *kentron*], close to a center or a central part.

paracervical /-sur'vikəl/ [Gk, *para* + L, *cervix*, neck], pertaining to the area adjacent to the cervix.

paracervical block, a form of regional anesthesia in which a local anesthetic is injected into the area on each side of the uterine cervix that contains the plexus of nerves innervating the uterine cervix. Paracervical block is not the anesthesia of choice for labor and delivery caused by the high incidence of fetal harm but is an option during abortion and other gynecologic procedures.

paracervix /-sur'viks/, the connective tissue of the pelvic floor, extending from the uterine cervix.

paracholera /-kol'ərə/, an infectious disease with symptoms similar to those of cholera but not caused by the true infectious agent, *Vibrio cholerae.*

parachute reflex /per'əsho͞ot/, a variation of the **Moro reflex** or **startle reflex,** whereby an infant is tested for motor nerve development by suspending him or her in the prone position and then dropping him or her a short distance onto a soft surface. If the motor nerve development is normal, the infant at 4 to 6 months will extend the arms, hands, and fingers on both sides of the body in a protective movement.

paracme /perak'mē/, **1.** the phase of a fever or disease marked by a subsidence of symptoms. **2.** the point of involution, beyond the prime of life.

paracoccidioidomycosis /per'əkoksid'ē-oi'dōmīkō'sis/ [Gk, *para* + *kokkos*, berry, *eidos*, form, *mykes*, fungus, *osis*, condition], a chronic, occasionally fatal fungal infection caused by *Paracoccidioides brasiliensis.* It is characterized by ulcers of the oral cavity, larynx, and nose. Other effects include large, draining lymph nodes; cough, dyspnea; weight loss; and skin, genital, and intestinal lesions. The disease occurs in Mexico and Central and South America and is acquired by inhalation of spores of the fungus.

paracolitis /-kōlī'tis/, an inflammation of the outer, peritoneal coat of the colon.

paracolpium /-kol'pē-əm/, the connective and other tissues around the vagina.

paracortex /-kôr'teks/, the thymus-dependent area of a lymph node between the subscapular cortex and the medullary cord.

paracrine /per'əkrēn/, an endocrine function in which effects of a hormone are localized to adjacent or nearby cells.

paracusis /per'əko͞o'sis/, a disorder involving the sense of hearing, including distortions of pitch.

paracystitis /sistī'tis/, an inflammation of the tissues around the urinary bladder.

paradenitis /-dēnī'tis/, an inflammation of tissues around a gland.

paradidymal /-did'iməl/ [Gk, *para*, beside, *didymos*, twin], **1.** pertaining to the paradidymis. **2.** beside the testis.

paradidymis /per'ədid'imis/, *pl.* **paradidymides** /per'ədidim'idēz/ [Gk, *para* + *epi*, above, *didymos*, twin], a rudimentary structure in the male, situated on the spermatic cord of the epididymis, that consists of vestigial remains of the caudal part of the embryonic mesonephric tubules. A similar vestigial structure, the paraoöphoron, is found in the female.

paradigm /per'ədīm, -dim/, a pattern that may serve as a model or example.

paradipsia /dip'sē-ə/, an abnormal desire for fluids unrelated to body needs.

paradoxic /-dok'sik/ [Gk, *paradoxos*, strange], pertaining to a person, situation, statement, or act that may appear to have inconsistent or contradictory qualities or that may be true but appears to be absurd or unbelievable.

paradoxic aciduria, a metabolic alkalosis condition that may involve an exchange of sodium and hydrogen ions for potassium. It may occur with prolonged nasogastric suctioning or repeated vomiting.

paradoxic breathing [Gk, *paradoxos* + AS, *braeth*], a condition in which a part of the lung deflates during inspiration and inflates during expiration. The condition usually is associated with a chest trauma, such as an open chest wound or rib cage damage. In such cases the paradoxic breathing that occurs spontaneously is sometimes called internal paradoxic breathing. External paradoxic breathing may be observed during deep general anesthesia.

paradoxic bronchospasm, a constriction of the airways after treatment with a sympathomimetic bronchodilator.

paradoxic intention, a logotherapeutic technique that encourages a patient to do what he or she fears and if possible to exaggerate it to the point of humor. The technique is used in the treatment of phobias.

paradoxic pupillary reflex, the response of a pupil to light that is the reverse of a normal reflex, as when the pupil contracts in a darkened room.

paradoxic thrombosis syndrome, a condition of arterial and venous thrombi that may develop after a period of heparin therapy. It is thought to be caused by the production of antiplatelet antibodies that induce clotting.

paraffin /per'əfin/ [L, *paraum,* little + *affinis,* related], any of a group of hydrocarbons or hydrocarbon mixtures of the paraffin series as indicated by the formula, $C_nH_{(2n+2)}$. Examples include methane gas, kerosene, and paraffin wax.

paraffin bath [L, *parum,* little, *affinis,* related], the application of heat to a specific area of the body through the use of paraffin. The part is quickly immersed in heated liquid wax and then withdrawn so that the wax solidifies to form an insulating layer. The procedure is repeated until the layer is 5 to 10 mm thick, and then the entire area is wrapped in an insulating material, such as a loose-fitting plastic bag or paper towels. The technique is used primarily for patients with arthritis and rheumatism or any joint condition.

paraffin method, (in surgical pathology) a method used in preparing a selected part of tissue for pathologic examination. The tissue is fixed, dehydrated, and infiltrated by and embedded in paraffin, forming a block that is cut with a microtome into slices 8 μm thick. This method, which is more commonly used than the frozen section method, is slower and therefore not used during surgery.

paraffinoma /per'əfinō'mə/, a tumor caused by the prosthetic or therapeutic injection of paraffin beneath the skin.

paraffin section [L, *parum,* little + *affinis,* related, *sectio*], a histologic section cut from tissue that has been embedded in paraffin wax.

parafollicular C cell /-folik'yələr/, a calcitonin-secreting cell located between follicles.

paraganglioma /-gang'glē·ō'mə/, a tumor derived from the chromoreceptor tissue of a paraganglion.

paraganglion /-gang'glē·on/, *pl.* **paraganglia** [Gk, *para* + *ganglion,* knot], any one of the small groups of chromaffin cells associated with the ganglia of the sympathetic nerve trunk and situated outside the adrenal medulla, most often near the sympathetic ganglia along the aorta and its branches. The paraganglia secrete the hormones epinephrine and norepinephrine.

parageusia /-jōō'sē·ə/, a disorder involving the sense of taste.

paragonimiasis /per'əgon'imī'əsis/ [Gk, *para* + *gonimos,* generative, *osis,* condition], chronic infection by the lung fluke *Paragonimus westermani,* occurring most commonly in Asia. It is characterized by hemoptysis, bronchitis, and occasionally

abdominal masses, pain and diarrhea, or cerebral involvement with paralysis, ocular pathologic conditions, or seizures. The disease is acquired by ingesting cysts in infected freshwater crabs or crayfish, the intermediate hosts.

paragraphia /-graf'ē·ə/, a communication disorder characterized by errors of omission and transposition of letters or words or substitution of a wrong letter or word in writing or speaking.

parahormone /-hôr'mōn/, a substance that may exert a hormonal influence, although it is not a true hormone.

parahypnosis /-hipnō'sis/ [Gk, *para* + *hypnos,* sleep], a form of disordered sleep that is observed in hypnosis and narcosis.

parainfluenza virus /per'ə·in'flōō·en'zə/ [Gk, *para* + It, *influenza,* influence], a myxovirus with four serotypes, causing respiratory infections in infants and young children and less commonly in adults. Type 1 and 2 parainfluenza viruses may cause laryngotracheobronchitis or croup; type 3 is a cause of croup, tracheobronchitis, bronchiolitis, and bronchopneumonia in children; types 1, 3, and 4 are associated with pharyngitis and the common cold.

parakeratosis /-ker'ətō'sis/, an abnormal formation of horn cells of the epidermis caused by the persistence of nuclei, incomplete formation of keratin, and moistness and swelling of the horn cells. It is observed as scaling in many conditions such as psoriasis.

parakinesia /-kinē'zhə/ [Gk, *para* + *kinesis,* movement], an abnormality of movement resulting from a nerve disorder in a muscle, such as an irregularity of one of the ocular muscles.

paraldehyde /peral'dəhīd/, a clear, colorless strong-smelling liquid obtained by the polymerization of acetaldehyde with a small amount of sulfuric acid. It is used as a solvent and may be administered orally, intravenously, intramuscularly, or rectally to induce hypnotic states or sedation.

parallax /per'əlaks/ [Gk, *parallelos,* side-by-side], the apparent displacement of an object at different distances from the eyes when viewed by both eyes together. It is the basis of stereoscopic vision and depth perception.

parallel grid /per'əlel/ [Gk, *parallelos,* side-by-side; ME, *gredire*], (in radiography) an x-ray grid that has lead strips oriented parallel to each other.

parallelogram condenser /per'əlel'ə-gram'/ [Gk, *parallelos* + *gramma,* record; L, *condensare,* to make thick], (in dentistry) an instrument with a face shaped like a rectangle or parallelogram, used for compacting amalgams in filling teeth.

parallel play [Gk, *parallelos* + AS, *plegan*, to play], a form of play among a group of children, primarily toddlers, in which each engages in an independent activity that is similar to but not influenced by or shared with the others.

parallel talk, a form of speech used during children's play therapy in which the clinician verbalizes activities of the child without requiring answers to questions. The clinician repeats utterances of the child correctly and may parallel the child's actions.

parallergic /per′alur′jik/, having a non-specific sensitivity to antigens as a result of a prior sensitization with a specific allergen.

Paralympics /per′əlim′piks/, [*paraplegic* + *Olympics*], an international competitive wheelchair sports event, usually held in association with the official quadrennial Olympic Games.

paralysis /pərəl′isis/, *pl.* **paralyses** [Gk, *paralyein,* to be palsied], the loss of muscle function, loss of sensation, or both. It may be caused by a variety of problems such as trauma, disease, and poisoning. Paralyses may be classified according to the cause, muscle tone, distribution, or body part affected. —**paralytic,** *adj.*

paralytic /per′əlit′ik/, [Gk, *paralyein,* to be palsied], pertaining to the characteristics of paralysis.

paralytic ileus [Gk, *paralyein,* to be paralyzed, *eilein,* to twist], a decrease in or absence of intestinal peristalsis. It may occur after abdominal surgery or peritoneal injury or be associated with severe pyelonephritis, ureteral stone, fractured ribs, myocardial infarction, extensive intestinal ulceration, heavy metal poisoning, porphyria, retroperitoneal hematoman, especially those associated with fractured vertebrae, or any severe metabolic disease. It is the most common overall cause of intestinal obstruction. Paralytic ileus is characterized by abdominal tenderness and distension, absence of bowel sounds, lack of flatus, and nausea and vomiting.

paralytic incontinence [Gk, *paralyein,* to be palsied; L, *incontinentia,* inability to retain], urinary or fecal incontinence resulting from loss of or impaired motor nerve control of the sphincter muscles.

paralytic mydriasis [Gk, *paralyein,* to be palsied, *mydriasis,* pupil enlargement], an area of depressed vision that is on the periphery of the field.

paralytic poliomyelitis [Gk, *paralyein,* to be palsied, *polios,* gray, *myelos,* marrow, *itis,* inflammation], a flaccid paralysis of

the limbs resulting from damaged lower motor neurons. Progressive bulbar paralysis with respiratory and vasomotor failure may result when the brainstem nuclei are involved.

paralytic stroke [Gk, *paralyein,* to be palsied; AS, *strac*], a sudden attack of paralysis caused by disease or injury to the brain or spinal cord.

paralyze /per′əliz/ [Gk, *paralyein,* to be palsied], **1.** to produce or enter into a state of paralysis. **2.** to cause loss of muscle power.

paramedic /-med′ik/ [Gk, *para* + L, *medicina,* art of healing], a person who acts as an assistant to a physician or in place of a physician, especially a person in the military trained in emergency medical procedures. —**paramedical,** *adj.*

paramedical personnel, health care workers other than physicians, dentists, podiatrists, and nurses who have special training in the performance of supportive health care tasks, for example, the **emergency medical technician, audiologist,** and **radiologic technologist.**

paramesonephric duct /per′əmēz′ōnef′rik/ [Gk, *para* + *mesos,* middle, *nephros,* kidney], one of a pair of embryonic ducts that develops into the uterus and the uterine tubes.

parameter /pəram′ətər/ [Gk, *para* + *metron,* measure], **1.** a value or constant used to describe or measure a set of data representing a physiologic function or system, as in the use of acid-base relationships of the blood as parameters for evaluating the function of a patient's respiratory system. **2.** a statistical value of a population group. **3.** *informal.* limit or boundary.

paramethasone acetate /-meth′əsōn/, a glucocorticoid prescribed in the treatment of inflammatory and allergic conditions.

parametric imaging /-met′rik/ [Gk, *para* + *metron,* measure; L, *imago,* image], (in nuclear medicine) a diagnostic procedure in which an image of an administered radioactive tracer is derived according to a mathematic rule, such as by the division of one image by another.

parametric statistics, statistics that assume a population has a symmetric, such as a gaussian or normal, distribution.

parametritis /per′əmetri′tis/ [Gk, *para* + *metra,* womb, *itis*], an inflammatory condition of the tissue of the structures around the uterus.

parametrium /per′əmē′trē·əm/, *pl.* **parametria** [Gk, *para* + *metra,* womb], the lateral extension of the uterine subserous connective tissue into the broad ligament.

paramnesia /per′amnē′zhə/ [Gk, *para* + *amnesia,* forgetfulness], **1.** a perversion of memory in which one believes one re-members events and circumstances that never actually occurred. **2.** a condition in which words are remembered and used without comprehension of their meaning.

paramyloidosis /peram′iloidō′sis/, **1.** an accumulation of amyloidlike protein in the tissues. **2.** any of several hereditary forms of amyloidosis characterized by sensory changes and muscle atrophy caused by amyloid deposits in somatic and visceral nerves.

paramyxovirus /-mik′sōvī′rəs/ [Gk, *para* + *myxa,* mucus; L, *virus,* poison], a member of a family of viruses that in-cludes the organisms that cause parainflu-enza, mumps, and some respiratory infec-tions.

paranasal /-nā′zəl/ [Gk, *para* + L, *nasus,* nose], pertaining to an area near or alongside the nose, such as the paranasal sinuses.

paranasal sinus, any one of the air cavi-ties in various bones around the nose, such as the frontal sinus in the frontal bone ly-ing deep to the medial part of the super-ciliary ridge and the maxillary sinus within the maxilla between the orbit, the nasal cavity, and the upper teeth.

paraneoplastic syndromes /-nē′əplas′tik/ [Gk, *para* + *neos,* new, *plassein,* to mold, *syn,* together, *dromos,* course], indirect effects of a tumor that occur distant to the tumor or metastatic site. They may result from the production of active proteins, polypeptides, or inactive hormones by the tumor.

paranesthesia /peran′esthē′zhə/, anes-thesia affecting the lower half of the body.

paranoia /per′ənoi′ə/ [Gk, *para* + *nous,* mind], (in psychiatry) a condition char-acterized by an elaborate, overly suspi-cious system of thinking. It often includes delusions of persecution and grandeur usually centered on one major theme, such as a financial matter, a job situation, an un-faithful spouse, or another problem, such as being followed or monitored by the CIA, or outer space aliens.

paranoiac /per′ənoi′ak/, **1.** a person af-flicted with or exhibiting characteristics of paranoia. **2.** pertaining to paranoia.

paranoid /per′ənoid/ [Gk, *para* + *nous,* mind, *eidos,* form], **1.** pertaining to or resembling paranoia. **2.** a person afflicted with a paranoid disorder. **3.** *informal.* a person, or pertaining to a person, who is overly suspicious or exhibits persecutory trends or attitudes.

paranoid disorder, any of a large group of mental disorders characterized by an impaired sense of reality and persistent de-lusions.

paranoid ideation, an exaggerated, sometimes grandiose, belief or suspicion, usually not of a delusional nature, that one is being harassed, persecuted, or treated unfairly.

paranoid personality, a personality char-acterized by paranoia.

paranoid personality disorder, a psy-chiatric disorder characterized by extreme suspiciousness and distrust of others to the degree that one blames them for one's mistakes and failures and goes to abnor-mal lengths to validate prejudices, atti-tudes, or biases.

paranoid reaction, a psychopathologic condition associated with aging and char-acterized by the gradual formation of delu-sions, usually of a persecutory nature and often accompanied by related hallucina-tions. Other manifestations of senile de-generation, such as memory loss and con-fusion, do not usually accompany the reaction, and the individual maintains ori-entation for time, place, and person.

paranoid schizophrenia, a form of schizophrenia characterized by persistent preoccupation with illogical, absurd, and changeable delusions, usually of a perse-cutory, grandiose, or jealous nature, ac-companied by related hallucinations. The symptoms include extreme anxiety, exag-gerated suspiciousness, aggressiveness, anger, argumentativeness, hostility, and violence. The condition occurs most fre-quently during middle age.

paranoid state, a transitory abnormal mental condition characterized by illogical thought processes and generalized suspi-cion and distrust, with a tendency toward persecutory ideas or delusions.

paranormal /-nôr′məl/ [Gk, *para* + L, *normalis,* rule], pertaining to phenom-ena that cannot be explained by normal scientific investigation.

paraparesis /-pərē′sis/ [Gk, *para* + *pare-sis,* paralysis], a partial paralysis, usually affecting only the lower extremities.

parapedesis /-pedē′sis/, any secretion or excretion through an abnormal passage-way.

paraperitoneal /-per′itənē′əl/, near or beside the peritoneum.

paraperitoneal nephrectomy /-per′itənē′-əl/ [Gk, *para* + *peri* + *tenein,* to stretch, *nephros,* kidney, *ektome,* excision], sur-gery to remove the kidney through an ex-traperitoneal incision.

parapertussis /per′əpərtus′is/ [Gk, *para* + L, *per,* very, *tussis,* cough], an acute bac-terial respiratory infection caused by *Bor-detella parapertussis,* having symptoms closely resembling those of pertussis. It is usually milder than pertussis, although it can be fatal. It is possible to be infected with both *B. parapertussis* and *B. pertussis* at the same time.

parapharyngeal abscess /per'əfərin'jē-əl/ [Gk, *para* + *pharynx*, throat; L, *abscedere*, to go away], a suppurative infection of tissues adjacent to the pharynx, usually a complication of acute pharyngitis or tonsillitis. Infection may spread to the jugular vein, where it may cause thrombophlebitis and septic emboli.

paraphasia /-fā'zhə/ [Gk, *para* + *phrasein*, to utter], **1.** a condition in which a person hears and comprehends words but is unable to speak correctly. Incoherent words are substituted for intended words. **2.** speech that is incoherent, unintelligible, and apparently incomprehensible but may be meaningful when carefully interpreted by a psychotherapist.

paraphilia /per'əfil'yə/ [Gk, *para* + *philein*, to love], sexual perversion or deviation; a condition in which the sexual instinct is expressed in ways that are socially prohibited or unacceptable or are biologically undesirable, such as sexual relations with a nonconsenting partner. Kinds of paraphilia include **exhibitionism, fetishism, pedophilia, transvestism, voyeurism,** and **zoophilia.** —**paraphiliac,** *adj., n.*

paraphimosis /per'əfīmō'sis/ [Gk, *para* + *phimoein*, to muzzle], a condition characterized by an inability to replace the foreskin in its normal position after it has been retracted behind the glans penis. Caused by a narrow or inflamed foreskin, the condition may lead to gangrene.

paraphrenia /-frē'nē-ə/, a psychiatric condition that is primary to an affective illness or to an organic mental disorder. Gross disturbances of affect, volition, and function, which are characteristic of schizophrenia, are not prominent, but paranoid delusions and hallucinations are always present.

paraplasm /per'əplaz'əm/ [Gk, *para* + *plassein*, to mold], any abnormal growth or malformation. —**paraplasmic,** *adj.*

paraplastic /plas'tik/ [Gk, *para* + *plassein*, to mold], **1.** misshapen or malformed. **2.** showing abnormal formative power; of the nature of a paraplasm.

paraplegia /per'əplē'jē-ə/ [Gk, *para* + *plege*, stroke], paralysis characterized by motor or sensory loss in the lower limbs and trunk. The signs and symptoms of paraplegia may develop immediately from trauma and may include the loss of sensation, motion, and reflexes below the level of the lesion. Depending on the level of the lesion and whether damage to the spinal cord is complete or incomplete, the patient

may lose bladder and bowel control, and sexual dysfunctions may develop. Paraplegia less commonly results from nontraumatic lesions such as scoliosis, spina bifida, or neoplasms. —**paraplegic,** *adj., n.*

paraplegic /-plē'jik/ [Gk, *para* + *plege*, stroke], pertaining to a person affected by paraplegia or a condition resembling paraplegia.

parapraxia /-prak'sē-ə/ [Gk, *para* + *praxis*, doing], **1.** the abnormal performance of purposive actions, such as performance of one movement occurring in place of another intended movement. **2.** forgetfulness with a tendency to misplace things.

paraproctitis /-proktī'tis/, an inflammation affecting the tissues around the rectum and anus.

paraprostatitis /-pros'tətī'tis/, an inflammation of the tissues around the prostate gland.

paraprotein /-prō'tēn/, any of the incomplete monoclonal immunoglobulins that occur in plasma cell disorders.

parapsoriasis /per'əsərī'əsis/ [Gk, *para* + *psorian*, to itch], a group of chronic skin diseases resembling psoriasis, characterized by maculopapular, erythematous scaly eruptions without systemic symptoms. Parapsoriasis is resistant to all treatment.

parapsychology /-sīkol'əjē/ [Gk, *para* + *psyche*, mind, *logos*, science], a branch of psychology concerned with the study of alleged psychic phenomena such as clairvoyance, extrasensory perception, and telepathy.

paraquat poisoning /per'əkwot'/ [Gk, *para* + L, *quaterni*, four each, *potio,* drink], a toxic condition caused by the ingestion of paraquat dichloride, a highly poisonous pesticide. Characteristically progressive pulmonary fibrosis and damage to the esophagus, kidneys, and liver develop several days after ingestion. After fibrosis begins, death is inevitable, usually within 3 weeks. The mechanism of action of the poison is unknown. Most often poisoning results from accidental occupational exposure.

parareflexia /riflex'sē-ə/, any abnormal condition of the reflexes.

parasacral /-sā'krəl/ [Gk, *para* + *sacrum*], pertaining to the area around the sacrum.

parasalpingitis /-sal'pinjī'tis/, an inflammation of the tissues around the fallopian tubes.

parasite /per'əsīt/ [Gk, *parasitos*, guest], an organism living in or on and obtaining nourishment from another organism. A facultative parasite may live on a host but is capable of living independently. An ob-

P

ligate parasite is one that depends entirely on its host for survival. —**parasitic,** *adj.*

parasitemia /per´əsītē´mē-ə/ [Gk, *parasitos* + *haima,* blood], the presence of parasites in the blood.

parasitic fetus /-sit´ik/ [Gk, *parasitos* + L, *icus,* like, *fetus,* pregnant], the smaller, usually malformed member of conjoined, unequal, or asymmetric twins that is attached to and dependent on the more normal fetus for growth and development.

parasitic fibroma, a pedunculated uterine fibroid deriving part of its blood supply from the omentum.

parasitic glossitis, a mycosis of the tongue, characterized by a black or brown furry patch on the posterior dorsal surface. The patch is composed of hypertrophied filiform papillae that measure about 1 cm in length and are easily broken. The condition, caused by *Cryptococcus linguae-pilosasae* in symbiosis with *Nocardia lingualis,* produces no discomfort and may be treated with a simple mouthwash.

parasitic hemoptysis [Gk, *parasitos,* guest, *haima,* blood + *ptyein,* to spit], the spitting of bright red blood caused by a parasitic infection. The condition usually involves the lung fluke *(Paragonimus)* or tapeworms *(Echinococcus).*

parasitism /per´əsitiz´əm/ [Gk, *parasitos,* guest], an infestation or presence of parasites.

parasympathetic /-sim´pəthet´ik/ [Gk, *para* + *sympathein,* to feel with], pertaining to the craniosacral division of the autonomic nervous system, consisting of the oculomotor, facial, glossopharyngeal, vagus, and pelvic nerves. The actions of the parasympathetic division are mediated by the release of acetylcholine and primarily involve the protection, conservation, and restoration of body resources. Reactions to parasympathetic stimulation are highly localized and tend to counteract the adrenergic effects of sympathetic nerves. Parasympathetic fibers slow the heart; stimulate peristalsis; promote the secretion of lacrimal, salivary, and digestive glands; induce bile and insulin release; dilate peripheral and visceral blood vessels; constrict the pupils, esophagus, and bronchioles; and relax sphincters during micturition and defecation. Postganglionic parasympathetic fibers extend to the uterus, vagina, oviducts, and ovaries in females and to the prostate, seminal vesicles, and external genitalia in males, innervating blood vessels of pelvic organs in both sexes; stimulation of these nerves causes vasodilation in the clitoris and labia minora and erection of the penis.

parasympathetic ganglion [Gk, *para* + *sympathein,* to feel with, *gagglion,* knot], a cluster of nerve cell bodies of the parasympathetic division of the autonomic nervous system. The nerves are functionally antagonistic to those of the sympathetic division.

parasympathomimetic /per´əsim´pəthō´-mimet´ik/ [Gk, *para* + *sympathein,* to feel with, *mimesis,* imitation], **1.** pertaining to a substance producing effects similar to those caused by stimulation of a parasympathetic nerve. **2.** an agent whose effects mimic those resulting from stimulation of parasympathetic nerves, especially those produced by acetylcholine.

parasynovitis /-sinəvī´tis/, an inflammation of the tissues around a joint.

parasystole [Gk, *para* + *systole,* contraction], an independent ectopic rhythm whose pacemaker cannot be discharged by impulses of the dominant, usually the sinus, rhythm because an area of depressed conduction surrounds the parasystolic focus. In the classic parasystole the interectopic intervals are exact multiples of a common denominator reflecting the protected status of the parasystolic focus.

parataxic distortion /per´ətak´sik/ [Gk, *para* + *taxis,* arrangement], **1.** a defense mechanism in which current interpersonal relationships are perceived and judged according to a mode of reference established by an earlier experience. **2.** Harry S. Sullivan's term for inaccuracies in judgment and perception.

parataxic mode, a term introduced by H. S. Sullivan to identify a childhood perception of the physical and social environment as being illogical, disjointed, and inconsistent. The parataxic mode may persist into adulthood in some individuals.

parathion poisoning /per´əthī´on/ [Gk, *para* + *thio,* phosphate, *on* + L, *potio,* drink], a toxic condition caused by the ingestion, inhalation, or absorption through the skin of the highly toxic organophosphorus insecticide parathion. Symptoms include nausea, vomiting, abdominal cramps, confusion, headache, lack of muscular control, convulsions, and dyspnea.

parathyroidectomy /-thī´roidek´təmē/ [Gk, *para* + *thyreos,* shield, *eidos,* form, *ektome,* excision], the surgical removal of the parathyroid gland.

parathyroid gland /-thī´roid/ [Gk, *para* + *thyreos,* shield, *eidos,* form; L, *glans,* acorn], any one of several small structures, usually four, attached to the dorsal surfaces of the lateral lobes of the thyroid gland. The parathyroid glands secrete parathyroid hormone, which helps maintain the blood calcium concentration and ensures normal neuromuscular irritability, blood clotting, and cell membrane permeability.

parathyroid hormone (PH), a hormone secreted by the parathyroid glands that acts to maintain a constant concentration of calcium in the extracellular fluid. The hormone regulates absorption of calcium from the gastrointestinal tract; mobilization of calcium from the bones; deposition of calcium in the bones; and excretion of calcium in the breast milk, feces, sweat, and urine.

parathyroid injection, bovine parathyroid hormone prescribed to regulate blood levels of calcium, especially in the treatment of hypoparathyroidism with tetany.

parathyroid tetany [Gk, *para* + *thyreos,* shield, *tetanos,* convulsive tension], a form of tetany that is caused by a deficiency of parathyroid secretion.

parathyrotropic /-thī′rōtrop′ik/, pertaining to an agent that influences the growth or rate of activity of the parathyroid glands.

paratrichosis /-trikō′sis/, an abnormality in the distribution, growth, and quantity of scalp hair.

paratriptic /-trip′tik/, pertaining to an agent that causes chafing.

paratrooper fracture /-trōō′pər/ [Fr, *parasol* + *troupe,* company; L, *fractura,* break], a fracture of the distal tibia and its malleolus, commonly occurring when an individual jumps from an elevated platform such as the back of a truck or parachutes from an airplane and lands feet first on the ground, subjecting the ankles to extreme force.

paratyphlitis /tif′ilī′tis/ [Gk, *para* + *typhlos.* blind, *itis,* inflammation], an inflammation of the tissues around the cecum and vermiform appendix.

paratyphoid fever /-tī′foid/ [Gk, *para* + *typhos,* stupor, *eidos,* form; L, *febris,* fever], a bacterial infection, caused by any *Salmonella* species other than *S. typhi,* characterized by symptoms resembling typhoid fever, although somewhat milder.

paraurethral duct /-per′əyō͝orē′thrəl/ [Gk, *para* + *ourethra,* urethra; L, *ducere,* to lead], one of a pair of ducts that drain the bulbourethral glands into the vestibule of the vagina.

paravaccinia virus /-vaksin′ē-ə/, a member of a subgroup of pox viruses that can infect humans through direct contact with infected livestock. It is related to the smallpox virus and is the cause of pseudocowpox, which produces milker's nodules.

paravaginitis /vaj′inī′tis/, an inflammation of the tissues around the vagina.

paravertebral /-vur′təbrəl/ [Gk, *para* + L, *vertebra,* joint], pertaining to the area alongside the spinal column or near a vertebra.

paravertebral block [Gk, *para* + L, *vertebra* + OFr, *bloc*], **1.** the blocking of transmission of somatic impulses by the spinal nerves by injection of a local analgesic solution near the point of their emergence. **2.** the blocking of the paravertebral sympathetic chain of nerves anterolateral to the vertebral bodies.

paraxial /perak′sē·əl/, pertaining to an organ or other structure located near the axis of the body.

parchment skin /pärch′mənt/ [Fr, *parchemin* + AS, *scinn*], thin, wrinkled, or stretched atrophic skin.

paregoric /per′əgôr′ik/, a camphorated tincture of opium prescribed in the treatment of diarrhea and as an analgesic.

parencephalitis /per′ensef′əlī′tis/, an inflammation of the cerebelllum.

parencephalocele /per′ensef′əlōsēl/, a protrusion of the cerebellum through a hole in the cranium.

parenchyma /pəreng′kimə/ [Gk, *para* + *enchyma,* infusion], the functional tissue of an organ as distinguished from supporting or connective tissue.

parenchymal cell /pəreng′kiməl/, any cell that is a functional element of an organ, such as a hepatocyte.

parenchymatous /per′əngkim′ətəs/ [Gk, *para* + *enchyma,* infusion], pertaining to or resembling the functional tissues of an organ or gland.

parenchymatous neuritis [Gk, *para* + *enchyma,* infusion; L, *osus,* like], any inflammation affecting the substance, axons, or myelin of the nerve.

parenchymatous salpingitis, an inflammation and thickening of the fallopian tubes.

parent [L, *parens*], a mother or father; one who bears offspring. —**parental,** *adj.*

parental generation (P₁) /pəren′təl/, the initial cross between two varieties in a genetic sequence; the parents of any individual, organism, or plant belonging to an F_1 generation.

parental grief, the behavioral reactions that characterize the grieving process and result in the resolution of the loss of a child from expected or unexpected death. When the death of a child of terminal illness is expected, there is time for anticipatory grieving so that parents can evaluate their relationship with the child, set priorities for the duration of time involved, and prepare for the actual death of the child. In such cases parental grieving begins with the discovery of the diagnosis of a life-

P

threatening condition. The immediate reactions are shock and disbelief, followed by acute grief at the anticipation of losing the child. Periods of depression, anger, hope, fear, and anxiety alternate during induction therapy, remission, and maintenance of the disease as parents learn to accept and cope with the situation. Although families can prepare themselves for the expected loss, at the time of death there is a period of acute grief, during which parents need to express their deep sorrow and anger. An extended phase of mourning follows, with the eventual resolution of grief and integration into society. In sudden, unexpected death parents are denied the advantages of anticipatory grief and, because of the lack of time to prepare, usually have extreme feelings of guilt and remorse. The function of the nurse during all phases of parental grief is primarily supportive, and the degree of intervention depends on the family's strengths and weaknesses in coping with the crisis.

parental role conflict, a NANDA-accepted nursing diagnosis of a state in which a parent experiences role confusion and conflict in response to a crisis. Defining characteristics include an expression by the parent or parents of concerns or feelings of inadequacy to provide for the child's physical and emotional needs during hospitalization or in the home, expressions of concern about perceived loss of control over decisions relating to the child and reluctance to participate in normal caretaking activities, even with encouragement and support. Parents also verbalize or demonstrate feelings of guilt, anger, fear, anxiety, and frustration about the effect of the child's illness on the family process.

parent education, any experience geared to the thoughtful conveyance of information enabling the parent to provide high-quality childrearing.

Parent Education: Adolescent, a Nursing Interventions Classification defined as assisting parents to understand and help their adolescent children.

Parent Education: Childbearing Family, a Nursing Interventions Classification defined as preparing another to perform the role of parent.

Parent Education: Childrearing Family, a Nursing Interventions Classification defined as assisting parents to understand and promote the physical, psychologic, and social growth and development of their toddler, preschool, or school-aged child/children.

parent ego state, (in transactional analysis) an ego state that incorporates the feelings and behavior learned from the parents or other authority figures. A part of the self that offers advice like that of one's own parents, containing messages that emphasize what one "ought to" or "should not" do.

parenteral /pəren'tərəl/ [Gk, *para* + *enteron,* bowel], pertaining to treatment other than through the digestive system. **—parenterally,** *adv.*

parenteral absorption, the taking up of substances within the body by structures other than the digestive tract.

parenteral dosage, pertaining to a medication administered by a route that bypasses the gastrointestinal tract, such as a drug given by injection.

parenteral nutrition, the administration of nutrients by a route other than the alimentary canal, such as subcutaneously, intravenously, intramuscularly, or intradermally. The parenteral fluids usually consist of physiologic saline solution with glucose, amino acids, electrolytes, vitamins, and medications. They are not nutritionally complete but maintain fluid and electrolyte balance during the immediate postoperative period and in other conditions, such as shock, coma, malnutrition, and chronic renal and hepatic failures.

parent figure [L, *parens* + *figura,* form], **1.** a parent or a substitute parent or guardian who cares for a child, providing the physical, social, and emotional requirements necessary for normal growth and development. **2.** a person who symbolically represents an ideal parent, having those attributes that one conceptualizes as necessary for forming the perfect parent-child relationship.

parent image, a conscious and unconscious concept that a child forms concerning the roles and characteristics of the personality of the mother and father.

parent/infant/child attachment, altered: risk for, a NANDA-accepted nursing diagnosis of disruption of the interactive process between parent or significant other and infant that fosters the development of a protective and nurturing reciprocal relationship. The risk factors are inability of parents to meet the personal needs; anxiety associated with the parental role; substance abuse; prematurity of an infant; inability of an ill infant or child to initiate parental contact effectively because of altered behavioral organization; separation; physical barriers; and lack of privacy.

parenting, altered, a NANDA-accepted nursing diagnosis of the changes in ability of nurturing figures to create an environment that promotes the optimum growth and development of another human being.

The defining characteristics are multiple and may include constant complaints about the sex or appearance of the new child, verbal self-assessment of inadequacy in the parental role, expressed disgust about the child's body functions, failure to keep health care appointments for the child, inconsistent disciplinary practices, slow growth and development in the child, and an observed need of the parent to receive approval from others. The critical defining characteristics, at least one of which must be present to make the diagnosis, include an observed lack of actions that demonstrate attachment to the child; inattentiveness to the child's needs; inappropriate caretaking behavior, especially in toilet training and in sleep and feeding patterns; and a history of abuse or abandonment of the child.

parenting, altered, risk for, a NANDA-accepted nursing diagnosis of the possibility of changes in ability of nurturing figures to create an environment that promotes the optimum growth and development of another human being. The cause of the problem may be complex and may involve several factors. Risk factors include lack of parental attachment behaviors; inappropriate visual, tactile, or auditory stimulation; negative identification or attachment of meanings to infant or child characteristics; verbalization of disappointment in or resentment toward the infant or child; noncompliance with health appointments; inappropriate caretaking behaviors; inappropriate or inconsistent discipline practices; history of child abuse or abandonment by primary caretaker; and employment of multiple caretakers without consideration for the child's needs.

Parents Anonymous, a self-help group for parents who have abused their children or who feel that they are prone to maltreat them. The organization offers support and guidance, provides a forum for discussing mutual problems, and furnishes distressed parents with a positive mechanism for coping with anger by talking to another member rather than by releasing their emotions on the child.

Parents Without Partners, a self-help group for single parents, including those who are separated, divorced, or widowed.

paresis /pərē′sis, per′isis/ [Gk, paralyein, to be palsied], 1. motor weakness or partial paralysis related in some cases to local neuritis. 2. a late manifestation of neurosyphilis, characterized by generalized paralysis, tremulous incoordination, transient seizures, Argyll Robertson pupils, and progressive dementia caused by degeneration of cortical neurons. Paresis

resulting from untreated syphilis usually develops in the third to fifth decade but may occur at an early age in patients with congenital syphilis. —**paretic**, adj.

paresthesia /per′esthē′zhə/ [Gk, para + erethizein, to excite], any subjective sensation, experienced as numbness, tingling, or a "pins and needles" feeling. Paresthesias often fluctuate according to such influences as posture, activity, rest, edema, congestion, or underlying disease. When experienced in the extremities, it is sometimes identified as acroparesthesia.

paretic /peret′ik/ [Gk, paresis, paralysis], pertaining to or resembling partial paralysis.

pargyline hydrochloride /per′jəlēn/, a monoamine oxidase inhibitor used as an antihypertensive. It is prescribed in the treatment of moderate to severe hypertension.

paries /per′i-ēz/, pl. **parietes** /pərī′itēz/, the wall of an organ or cavity in the body.

parietal /pərī′ətəl/ [L, paries, wall], 1. pertaining to the outer wall of a cavity or organ. 2. pertaining to the parietal bone of the skull or the parietal lobe of the cerebrum.

parietal bone, one of a pair of bones forming the sides of the cranium. Each parietal bone has two surfaces, four borders, and four angles and articulates with five bones: the opposite parietal, occipital, frontal, temporal, and sphenoid.

parietal cells [L, paries, wall, cella, storeroom], the cells on the periphery of the gastric glands of the stomach. They are located on the basement membrane beneath the chief cells and secrete hydrochloric acid.

parietal lobe, a part of each cerebral hemisphere that occupies the parts of the lateral and medial surfaces that are covered by the parietal bone. On the lateral surface of the hemisphere, the parietal lobe is separated from the frontal lobe by the central sulcus and from the temporal lobe by an imaginary line that extends from the posterior ramus of the lateral sulcus toward the occipital pole. It is concerned with language mechanisms and general sensory functions.

parietal lymph node, any one of the small oval glands that filter the lymph coursing through the lymphatic vessels in the walls of the thorax or through the lymphatic vessels associated with the larger blood vessels of the abdomen and the pelvis.

parietal pain, a sharp sensation of distress in the parietal pleura, aggravated by respiration and thoracic movements and caused by pneumonia, empyema, pneumothorax, asbestosis, tuberculosis, neoplasm, or the accumulation of fluid resulting from heart, liver, or kidney disease. Pain arising from the parietal pleura lining the chest wall is perceived over the involved area, but that arising from the central part of the diaphragm is referred to the posterior shoulder area; pain from the costal parts of the diaphragm is referred to the adjacent thoracic wall.

parietal pericardium [L, *paries,* wall; Gk, *peri* + *kardia,* heart], an outer layer of the serous pericardium that is not in direct contact with the heart muscle.

parietal peritoneum, the part of the largest serous membrane in the body that lines the abdominal wall.

parietooccipital /pərī′ətō·oksip′itəl/ [L, *paries* + *occiput,* back of the head], pertaining to the parietal and occipital bones or cerebral lobes.

parietooccipital sulcus, a groove on each cerebral hemisphere marking the division of the parietal and occipital lobes of the cerebrum.

parietotemporal /-tem′pərəl/ [L, *paries,* wall, *tempus,* temple], pertaining to the temporal and parietal bones of the cranium.

parietovisceral /-vis′ərəl/, pertaining to the abdominal wall and abdominal organs.

Parinaud's syndrome /per′ənōz/ [Henri Parinaud, French ophthalmologist, 1844–1905], a term often used to refer to conjunctivitis that is usually unilateral, follicular, and followed by enlargement of the preauricular lymph nodes and tenderness. The syndrome is frequently caused by infection with a species of the microorganism *Leptothrix.* It also may be associated with other infections, such as tularemia and cat-scratch fever.

pari passu /per′ē pas′ oo/ [L, *par,* equal, *passus,* step], at the same time or in equal proportions.

parity /per′itē/ [L, *parere,* to give birth], **1.** (in obstetrics) the classification of a woman by the number of live-born children and stillbirths she has delivered at more than 20 weeks of gestation. Commonly parity is noted with the total number of pregnancies and represented by the letter *P* or the word *para.* **2.** (in epidemiology) the classification of a woman by the number of live-born children she has delivered.

parkinsonian /pär′kinsō′nē·ən/ [James Parkinson, English physician, 1755–1824], pertaining to or resembling Parkinson's disease.

parkinsonian facies [James Parkinson; L, *facies,* face], a masklike and immobile facial expression, usually occurring with

Parkinson's disease. Infrequent blinking also occurs.

parkinsonian tremor [James Parkinson; L, *tremor,* shaking], a mild resting tremor with slow, regular oscillations of three to six per second, exacerbated by fatigue, cold, or emotion. The tremors usually, but not always, cease during voluntary movement of the affected part and during sleep.

parkinsonism /pär′kənsəniz′əm/ [James Parkinson], a neurologic disorder characterized by tremor, muscle rigidity, hypokinesia, a slow shuffling gait, and difficulty in chewing, swallowing, and speaking, caused by various lesions in the extrapyramidal motor system. Signs and symptoms of parkinsonism resemble those of idiopathic Parkinson's disease and may develop during or after acute encephalitis and in syphilis, malaria, poliomyelitis, and carbon monoxide poisoning.

Parkinson's disease [James Parkinson], a slowly progressive degenerative neurologic disorder characterized by resting tremor, pill rolling of the fingers, a masklike facies, shuffling gait, forward flexion of the trunk, loss of postural reflexes, and muscle rigidity and weakness. It is usually an idiopathic disease of people over 60 years of age. Typical pathologic changes are destruction of neurons in basal ganglia, loss of pigmented cells in the substantia nigra, and depletion of dopamine in the caudate nucleus, putamen, and pallidum, structures in the neostriatum that normally contain high levels of the neurotransmitter dopamine. Signs and symptoms of Parkinson's disease, which include resting tremor, bradykinesias, drooling, increased appetite, intolerance to heat, oily skin, emotional instability, and defective judgment, are increased by fatigue, excitement, and frustration. Levodopa, a dopamine precursor that crosses the blood-brain barrier, may be used, but many patients experience side effects such as nausea, vomiting, insomnia, orthostatic hypotension, and mental confusion. Carbidopa-levodopa, which contains an inhibitor of the enzyme dopa decarboxylase, limits peripheral metabolism of levodopa and thus causes fewer side effects.

Parkinson's mask [James Parkinson; Fr, *masque*], an expressionless face with eyebrows raised, smoothing of facial muscles, but immobility of the facial muscles.

parole /pərōl′/, (in psychiatry) a system of supervision of a patient who has been physically released from a hospital setting but is still listed as an inpatient and may be returned to the hospital without further court action.

paromomycin sulfate /per′əmōmī′sin/, an oral antiamebic aminoglycoside antibiotic prescribed in the treatment of intestinal amebiasis.

paromphalocele /perom′fəlōsēl/, a hernia or tumor near the umbilicus.

paronychia /per′ənik′ē·ə/ [Gk, *para* + *onyx*, nail], an infection of the fold of skin at the margin of a nail.

paroöphoritis /per′ō·of′ərī′tis/ [Gk, *para* + *oon*, egg, *pherein*, to bear, *itis*], 1. inflammation of the paroöphoron. 2. inflammation of the tissues surrounding the ovary.

paroophoron /per′ō·of′əron/ [Gk, *para* + *oon*, egg, *pherein*, to bear], a small vestigial remnant of the mesonephros, consisting of a few rudimentary tubules lying in the broad ligament between the epoophoron and the uterus. A similar vestigial structure, the aberrant ductule, is found in the male.

parosmia /pəroz′mē·ə/ [Gk, *para* + *osme*, smell], any dysfunction or perversion concerning the sense of smell.

parosteitis /per′ostē·ī′tis/, an inflammation of the tissues adjacent to or associated with a bone.

parosteosis /per′ostē·ō′sis/, the development of bone in an abnormal location, such as in the area of the periosteum or in the skin.

parotid /pərot′id/ [Gk, *para* + *ous*, ear], near the ear.

parotid abscess, a collection of pus in a parotid salivary gland.

parotid duct /pərot′id/ [Gk, *para* + *ous*, ear; L, *ducere*, to lead], a tubular canal, about 7 cm long, that extends from the anterior part of the parotid gland to the mouth.

parotidectomy /pərot′idek′təmē/ [Gk, *para* + *ous* + *ektome*, excision], the surgical removal of the parotid gland.

parotid gland [Gk, *para* + *ous*, ear; L, *glans*, acorn], one of the largest pairs of salivary glands that lie at the side of the face just below and in front of the external ear. The main part of the gland is superficial, somewhat flattened, and quadrilateral. It is enclosed in a capsule continuous with the deep cervical fascia.

parotitis /per′ətī′tis/ [Gk, *para* + *ous*, ear, *itis*, inflammation], inflammation or infection of one or both parotid salivary glands.

parous /per′əs/, having borne one or more viable offspring.

parovarian /per′ōver′ē·ən/ [Gk, *para* + L, *ovum*, egg], pertaining to residual tissues in the area near the fallopian tubes and the ovary.

paroxetine, a mood-elevating drug that blocks the uptake of serotonin prescribed in the treatment of mental depression and panic disorder.

paroxysm /per′əksiz′əm/ [Gk, *paroxynein*, to stimulate], 1. a marked, usually episodic increase in symptoms. 2. a convulsion, fit, seizure, or spasm. —**paroxysmal**, *adj.*

paroxysmal atrial tachycardia [Gk, *paroxynein*, to stimulate], a rapid atrial rate that begins and ends abruptly but is usually present more than half the day. It can result in dilated cardiomyopathy (tachycardiomyopathy) if untreated.

paroxysmal AV nodal reentry tachycardia [Gk, *paroxysmos*, irritation; L, *nodus*, knot; Gk, *tachys*, fast, *kardia*, heart], a type of paroxysmal supraventricular tachycardia usually initiated by a premature atrial complex and sustained by an atrioventricular nodal reentry mechanism. A vagal maneuver is usually successful in restoring sinus rhythm.

paroxysmal cold hemoglobinuria (PCH), a rare autoimmune disorder characterized by hemolysis and hematuria, associated with exposure to cold.

paroxysmal cough [Gk, *paroxysmos*, irritation; AS, *cohhetan*, cough], a severe attack of coughing, as may accompany whooping cough, bronchiectasis, or a lung injury.

paroxysmal hemoglobinuria, the sudden passage of hemoglobin in urine, occurring after local or general exposure to low temperatures, as in paroxysmal cold hemoglobinuria.

paroxysmal nocturnal dyspnea (PND), a disorder characterized by sudden attacks of respiratory distress that awaken the person, usually after several hours of sleep in a reclining position. It is most commonly caused by pulmonary edema resulting from congestive heart failure. The attacks are often accompanied by coughing, a feeling of suffocation, cold sweat, and tachycardia with a gallop rhythm.

paroxysmal nocturnal hemoglobinuria (PNH), a disorder characterized by intravascular hemolysis and hemoglobinuria. It occurs in irregular episodes of several days' duration, especially at night. The basic defect in the red blood cell is an unusual sensitivity to lysis by complement or a deficiency or absence of acetylcholinesterase. It is characterized by abdominal pain, back pain, and headache. Its course may be complicated by thrombotic episodes and by iron deficiency caused by excessive loss of hemoglobin.

paroxysmal supraventricular tachycardia, an ectopic rhythm with a rate of 170 to 250 beats/min. It begins abruptly with a premature atrial or ventricular beat and is supported by an atrioventricular (AV) nodal reentry mechanism or by an AV reentry mechanism involving an accessory pathway.

paroxysmal ventricular tachycardia [Gk, *paroxysmos,* irritation; L, *ventriculus,* little belly; Gk, *tachys* + *kardia*], a sudden onset and termination of rapid heartbeat caused by a quick succession of discharges from an ectopic site in the ventricle.

pars /pärs/ [L, part], a part, such as the pars abdominalis esophagi.

Parse, Rosemarie Rizzo, a nursing theorist who, in her *Man-Living-Health: A Theory of Nursing* (1981), synthesized Martha E. Rogers' principles and concepts (Science of Unitary Human Beings) and the work of existential phenomenologists. Parse's view of nursing is based on humanism as opposed to positivism. Her theory addresses the unity of humans' lived experience, the lived experience of health. She used the term *man* to express male and female. Man chooses from options and bears responsibility for choices. Parse proposes that nursing is a human science and rejects the traditional view of nursing as an emerging natural science.

part [L, *pars*], a part of a larger area, such as the condylar part of the occipital bone.

part. aeq. abbreviation for the Latin phrase *partes aequales,* meaning 'in equal parts.'

parthenogenesis /pär´thənōjen´əsis/ [Gk, *parthenos,* virgin, *genesis,* origin], a type of nonsexual reproduction in which an organism develops from an unfertilized ovum, as in many simpler animals. The development of the unfertilized ovum may be artificially induced through mechanical or chefnical stimulation. —**parthenogenetic, parthenogenic,** *adj.*

partial cleavage /pär´shäl/, mitotic division of only part of a fertilized ovum into blastomeres, usually the activated cytoplasmic part surrounding the nucleus; restricted division.

partial crown, a restoration that replaces surfaces of a tooth.

partial denture [L, *pars,* part, *dens,* tooth], a dental prosthesis, either fixed or removable, used to replace one or more missing teeth.

partial dislocation [L, *pars* + *dis* + *locare,* to place], the partial abnormal separation of the articular surface of a joint.

partial hospitalization program, an organizational entity that provides therapeutic services to patients who use only day or night hospital services or adult day health services, rather than regular inpatient hospitalization services.

partially acid-fast /pär´shəlē/, capable of retaining the stain carbolfuchsin during mild acid decolorization. This ability is restricted to bacteria of the genus *Nocardia,* because of the presence of unusual long-chain fatty acids in their cell walls.

partially edentulous arch, a dental arch in which one or more but not all natural teeth are missing.

partial placenta previa, placenta previa in which the placenta is implanted in the lower uterine segment and partially covers the internal os of the uterine cervix. As the cervix dilates in labor, the part of the placenta that lies over the cervix is separated, causing bleeding from the villous spaces of the uterine wall. Depending on the degree of separation, the bleeding may be scant or severe, resulting in hemorrhage that is life-threatening to the mother and baby.

partial pressure, the pressure exerted by any one gas in a mixture of gases or in a liquid, with the pressure directly related to the concentration of that gas to the total pressure of the mixture. The concentration of oxygen in the atmosphere represents approximately 21% of the total atmospheric pressure, calculated at 760 mm Hg under standard conditions. Therefore, the partial pressure of atmospheric oxygen is about 160 mm Hg (760 × 0.21).

partial pressure of carbon dioxide in arterial blood (PaCO$_2$), the part of total blood gas pressure exerted by carbon dioxide. It decreases, for example, during heavy exercise, or in association with uncontrolled diabetes. It increases with chest injuries or respiratory disorders. The normal pressures of carbon dioxide in arterial blood are 35 to 45 mm Hg, and in venous blood, 40 to 45 mm Hg.

partial pressure of oxygen in arterial blood (PaO$_2$), the part of total blood gas pressure exerted by oxygen gas. It is lower than normal in patients with asthma, obstructive lung disease, or certain blood diseases. The normal partial pressure of oxygen in arterial blood is 95 to 100 mm Hg.

partial response, the condition in which the maximum decrease in treated tumor volume is at least 50% but less than 100%.

partial shadowing, (in ultrasonics) a manifestation of decreased echo signal amplitudes returning from regions lying beyond an object in which the attenuation is higher than the average attenuation in adjacent overlying regions.

partial thromboplastin time (PTT), a test for detecting coagulation defects of the intrinsic system by adding activated partial thromboplastin to a sample of test plasma and to a control sample of normal plasma. The time required for the formation of a clot in test plasma is compared with that in the normal plasma. Partial thromboplastin time is one of the basic tests used to measure specific factor activity and to detect hemophilias. The normal PTT in plasma is 60 to 85 seconds after the addition to the plasma sample of partial thromboplastin reagent and ionized calcium.

particle /pär'tikəl/ [L, *particula.* small part], **1.** any fundamental unit of matter. **2.** a minute fragment or speck.

particulate /pärtik'yəlit/, pertaining to a minute discrete particle or fragment of a substance or material.

parts per million (PPM, ppm), the ratio of the concentration of one substance to the concentration of another, as a unit of solute dissolved in one million units of solution. It may be further expressed in terms of mass-to-mass, volume-to-volume, or another relationship of units of measure.

parturient /pärt(y)ōō'rē·ənt/ [L, *parturire,* to desire to bring forth], pertaining to the act of childbirth.

parturition /pär't(y)ōōrish'ən/ [L, *parturire,* to desire to bring forth], the process of giving birth.

part. vic., abbreviation for the Latin term *partes vicibus,* meaning 'divided doses.'

paruresis, the inhibition of urination for psychologic or other reasons.

paruria /pərōōr'ē·ə/, any defect of the urination process.

parvovirus B19 /pär'vōvī'rəs/, a small single-stranded deoxyribonucleic acid virus of the Parvoviridae family that infects humans, causing erythema infectiosum and aplastic crisis in hemolytic anemia.

parvule /pär'vyōōl/, a very small pill.

PAS, PASA, abbreviation for **paraaminosalicylic acid.**

Pascal's principle /poskuls', paskals'/ [Blaise Pascal, French scientist, 1623–1662], (in physics) a law stating that a confined liquid transmits pressure applied to it from an external source equally in all directions. Pascal's principle provides the basis for all hydraulic devices.

passage /pas'ij/, **1.** an opening, channel, route, or gap. **2.** the movement of something from one place to another, as in evacuation of the bowels.

Pass Facilitation, a Nursing Interventions Classification defined as arranging a leave from a health care facility for a patient.

passiflora /pas'iflôr'ə/, the passion flower, *Passiflora incarnata.* The climbing herb has flowers and fruiting tops that are the source of medications used as antispasmodics and sedatives and for the treatment of burns, dysmenorrhea, hemorrhoids, and insomnia.

passive [L *passivus*], pertaining to behavior that subordinates the individual's own interests to the demands of others.

passive-aggressive personality [L, *passivus + aggressus,* combative, *persona,* character], a personality characterized by a chronically negativistic disposition with passive resistance and aggression with forceful actions or attitudes expressed in an indirect, nonviolent manner, such as pouting, obstructionism, procrastination, inefficiency, stubbornness, and forgetfulness.

passive-aggressive personality disorder, a *DSM-IV* psychiatric disorder characterized by the indirect expression of resistance to occupational or social demands. It results in persistent pervasive ineffectiveness, lack of self-confidence, poor interpersonal relationships, and pessimism that can lead in severe cases to major depression, alcoholism, or drug dependence.

passive carrier [L, *passivus + OFr, carier*], **1.** a healthy person whose body carries the causal organisms of an infectious disease, although the person has not contracted the disease and remains symptomless. **2.** a person who carries a gene associated with a hereditary trait, although the trait is not expressed in the person.

passive clot, a clot that forms in an aneurysm when circulation is interrupted.

passive congestion [L, *passivus + congerere,* to heap together], an excessive amount of blood accumulation in an organ resulting from increased venous pressure.

passive-dependent personality [L, *passivus + Fr, dependre,* to depend; L, *persona,* character], a personality characterized by helplessness, indecisiveness, and a tendency to cling to and seek support from others.

passive exercise, repetitive movement of a part of the body as a result of an externally applied force or the voluntary effort of the muscles controlling another part of the body.

passive expiration [L, *passivus + expirare,* to breathe out], normal expiration that occurs without direct muscular effort, as is the case in normal tidal breathing. The air is compressed from the lungs through recoil effect of elastic tissues of the chest and lungs.

passive immunity, a form of acquired immunity resulting from antibodies that are transmitted naturally through the placenta to a fetus, through the colostrum to an infant, or artificially by injection of antiserum for treatment or prophylaxis.

passive incontinence [L, *passivus* + *incontinentia*], urine overflow that may occur when the bladder (musculus detrusor vesicae) is paralyzed and greatly distended.

passive lingual arch, an orthodontic appliance that may help maintain tooth space and dental arch length when bilateral primary molars are prematurely lost.

passive lung collapse [L, *passivus* + AS, *lungen* + L, *collabi*], a condition of dyspnea, cough, and hemoptysis with pigmented cells, caused by an obstructed blood flow from the lungs to the heart.

passive motion [L, *passivus* + *motio*], involuntary motion caused by an external force, differentiated from active, voluntary muscular effort.

passive movement, the moving of parts of the body by an outside force without voluntary action or resistance by the individual.

passive play, play in which a person does not participate actively. For younger children such activity may include watching and listening to others, observing other children or animals, listening to stories, or looking at pictures. Older children are passively entertained by games and toys that require concentration and intellectual skill.

passive recoil, the normal, quiet act of exhalation caused by the rebound effect of elastic tissue of the lungs, aided by the force of surface tension.

passive sensitization [L, *passivus* + *sentire,* to feel], a temporary form of sensitization induced by injecting serum from a sensitized human or animal.

passive smoking, the inhalation by nonsmokers of the smoke from other people's cigarettes, pipes, and cigars.

passive stretching, stretching that involves only noncontractile elements such as ligaments. Examples include manipulation of a muscle, such as during therapeutic massage or during isometric exercises.

passive symptom [L, *passivus* + Gk, *symptoma,* that which happens], a symptom that attracts little or no attention.

passive transport, the movement of small molecules across the membrane of a cell by diffusion. Passive transport is essential to various processes of metabolism, such as the intake of digestive products by the cells lining the intestines.

passivity /pəsif′itē/ [L, *passivus*], a mental state of being submissive, dependent, or inactive, as a form of maladaptation.

paste /pāst/, a topical semisolid formulation containing a pharmacologically active ingredient in a fatty base, a viscous or mucilaginous base, or a mixture of starch and petrolatum.

Pasteur effect /pastŏŏr′, pästœr′/ [Louis Pasteur, French chemist, 1822–1895], the inhibiting effect of oxygen on carbohydrate fermentation by living cells.

Pasteurella /pas′tərel′ə/ [Louis Pasteur], a genus of gram-negative bacilli or coccobacilli, including species pathogenic to humans and domestic animals. *Pasteurella* infections may be transmitted to humans by animal bites.

pasteurellosis /pas′tərelō′sis/ [Louis Pasteur], a local wound infection caused by the gram-negative bacillus *Pasteurella multicide,* which may be acquired through the bite or scratch of an infected animal, usually a cat.

pasteurization /pas′tərīzā′shən/ [Louis Pasteur; Gk, *izein,* to cause], the process of applying heat, usually to milk or cheese, for a specified period for the purpose of killing or retarding the development of pathogenic bacteria. —**pasteurize,** *v.*

pasteurized milk /pas′tərīzd/ [Louis Pasteur; Gk, *izein,* to cause; AS, *moluc,* milk], milk that has been treated by heat to destroy pathogenic bacteria. By law, pasteurization requires a temperature of 145° to 150° F for not less than 30 minutes, followed by a temperature of 161° F for 15 seconds, followed by immediate cooling.

Pasteur, Louis [French chemist, 1822–1895], promoter of the "germ theory" of infection and developer the "pasteurization" process to kill pathogenic organisms in milk. Pasteur also developed several vaccines and pioneered in the development of stereochemistry by separating mirror image isomers.

Pasteur treatment [Louis Pasteur], a method of preventing rabies by daily injections of attenuated cultures of rabies virus cultured in the central nervous system tissues of rabbits. The treatment, developed by Pasteur, is no longer used.

past health [ME, *passen,* to pass; AS, *hoelth,* sound body], (in a health history) an overall summary of the person's general health to date, including past injuries, allergies, surgical procedures, immunizations, hospitalizations, and obstetric and psychiatric history.

pastille /pastēl′, pas′til/, **1.** a gelatin-based sweetened and molded medication impregnated with a therapeutic substance intended to be sucked. **2.** a chemically treated paper disk that undergoes color changes when exposed to radiation.

pastoral counseling department /pas'-tərəl/ [L, *pastor*, shepherd], the hospital chaplaincy service.

past pointing [OFr, *passer* + L, *punctus*, pricked], the inability to place a finger on another part of the body accurately, indicating a lack of coordination in voluntary movements.

patch [ME, *pacche*], a small spot of surface tissue that differs from the surrounding area in color or texture or both and is not elevated above it.

patch test, a skin test for identifying allergens, especially those causing contact dermatitis. The suspected substance (food, pollen, animal fur) is applied to an adhesive patch that is placed on the patient's skin. Another patch, with nothing on it, serves as a control.

patella /pətel'ə/ [L, small dish], a flat triangular bone at the front of the knee joint, having a pointed apex that attaches to the ligamentum patellae.

patellar /pətel'ər/ [L, *patella*, small dish], pertaining to the patella.

patellar-bearing supracondylar/suprapatellar socket (PTBSC/SP), a type of patellar-tendon below-the-knee bearing prosthesis with a socket that extends in front, medially, and laterally to accommodate both the patella and the femoral condyles. The higher socket increases knee stability, and a suspension strap is not required.

patellar bursa [L, *patella*, small dish; Gk, *byrsa*, wineskin], any of the fluid-filled connective tissue sacs around the knee cap.

patellar ligament [L, *patella* + *ligare*, to bind], the central part of the common tendon of the quadriceps femoris. The ligament is a strong, flat ligamentous band attached proximally to the apex and the adjoining margins of the patella and distally to the tuberosity of the tibia.

patellar reflex, a deep tendon reflex, elicited by a sharp tap on the tendon just distal to the patella, normally characterized by contraction of the quadriceps muscle and extension of the leg at the knee.

patellar-tendon bearing prosthesis (PTB), an ankle-foot orthosis that provides prolonged stretch to the posterior leg musculature and may create extension force at the knee joint.

patellar-tendon bearing supracondylar socket (PTB/SC), a patellar-tendon bearing prosthesis with supracondylar (above a condyle) and suprapatellar (above the patella) suspension.

patellectomy /pat'əlek'təmē/ [L, *patella*, small dish; Gk, *ektome*, excision], the surgical removal of the patella.

patency /pā'tənsē/ [L, *patens*, open], a state of being open or exposed.

patent /pā'tənt/ [L, *patens*, open], open and unblocked, such as a patent airway or a patent anus.

patent ductus arteriosus (PDA), an abnormal opening between the pulmonary artery and the aorta caused by failure of the fetal ductus arteriosus to close after birth. It is seen primarily in premature infants. The defect allows blood from the aorta to flow into the pulmonary artery and to recirculate through the lungs, where it is reoxygenated and returned to the left atrium and left ventricle, causing an increased work load on the left side of the heart and increased pulmonary vascular congestion and resistance.

patent medicine [L, *patens*, open, *medicina*], a nonprescription drug available to the general public without a prescription. The ingredients and contraindications are usually listed on the label or wrapper.

paternal /pətur'nəl/ [L, *pater*, father], pertaining to fatherhood, characteristic of a father, or related through a father.

paternity test /pətur'nitē/ [L, *pater* + *testum*, crucible], a test based on genetic blood groups and used mainly to exclude the possibility that a particular man could be the father of a specific child. For example, a man with group AB blood could not be the father of a child with group O blood, or vice versa.

Paterson-Parker dosage system [James R. K. Paterson, English radiologist; H. M. Parker, twentieth-century American-English physicist], a radiotherapy system that uses sources of specific relative loadings arranged according to defined rules, which lead to a homogenous dose in the implanted region.

path [AS, *paeth*], a route or course along which something moves, such as a circuit of the nervous system that is followed by sensory or motor nerve impulses.

path., 1. abbreviation for **pathologic**. 2. abbreviation for **pathology**.

pathetic /pəthet'ik/, pertaining to something that affects emotions of sympathy, pity, and sadness.

pathfinder, a thin, flexible cylindric instrument containing a series of filiform guides, used to locate strictures.

pathogen /path'əjən/ [Gk, *pathos*, disease, *genein*, to produce], any microorganism capable of producing disease. **—pathogenic,** *adj.*

pathogenesis /-jen'əsis/ [Gk, *pathos* + *genesis*, origin], the source or cause of an illness or abnormal condition.

pathogenic /-jen′ik/ [Gk, *pathos,* disease, *genein,* to produce], capable of causing or producing a disease.

pathogenicity /-jənis′itē/, the ability of a pathogenic agent to produce a disease.

pathogenic occlusion, an abnormal closure of the teeth, capable of producing pathologic changes in the teeth, supporting tissues, and other components of the stomatognathic system.

pathognomonic /pəthog′nəmon′ik/ [Gk, *pathos* + *gnomon,* index], (of a sign or symptom) specific to a disease or condition, such as Koplik's spots on the buccal and lingual mucosa, which are indicative of measles.

pathologic (path.) /-loj′ik/ [Gk, *pathos* + *logos,* science], pertaining to a condition that is caused by or involves a disease process.

pathologic absorption, the taking up by the blood of an excretory or morbid substance.

pathologic amenorrhea [Gk, *pathos,* disease, *logos,* science, *a* + *men,* month, *rhoia,* to flow], a stoppage or absence of menstrual discharge from the uterus resulting from a disease.

pathologic anatomy, (in applied anatomy) the study of the structure and morphologic characteristics of the tissues and cells of the body as related to disease.

pathologic diagnosis, a diagnosis arrived at by an examination of the substance and function of the tissues of the body, especially of the abnormal developmental changes in the tissues by histologic techniques of tissue examination.

pathologic histology [Gk, *pathos,* disease, *logos,* science, *histos,* tissue, *logos,* science], the specialized study of the effects of disease on minute structures, composition, and function of tissues.

pathologic microorganisms [Gk, *pathos,* disease, *logos,* science, *mikros,* small, *organon,* instrument, *ismos,* condition], any microscopic life form, from a virus to a nematode, that has the potential to cause disease.

pathologic mitosis, any cell division that is atypical, asymmetric, or multipolar and results in an unequal number of chromosomes in the nuclei of the daughter cells. It is indicative of malignancy, as occurs in cancer and the genetic anomalies.

pathologic myopia, a type of progressive nearsightedness characterized by changes in the fundus of the eye, posterior staphyloma, and deficient corrected acuity.

pathologic physiology, 1. the study of the physical and chemical processes involved in the functioning of diseased tissues. **2.** the study of the modification of the normal functioning processes of an organism caused by disease.

pathologic reflex [Gk, *pathos,* disease, *logos,* science; L, *reflectere,* to bend back], any abnormal reflex that is caused by a lesion in or an organic disease of the nervous system.

pathologic retraction ring, a ridge that may form around the uterus at the junction of the upper and lower uterine segments during the prolonged second stage of an obstructed labor.

pathologic sleep [Gk, *pathos,* disease, *logos,* science; AS, *slaep*], excessive sleep associated with a neurologic disorder such as encephalitis lethargica, or sleeping sickness.

pathologic triad, the combination of three respiratory disease conditions: bronchospasm, retained secretions, and mucosal edema.

pathologist /pəthol′əjist/, a physician specializing in the study of disease. A pathologist usually specializes in autopsy or in clinical or surgical pathology.

pathology (path.) /pəthol′əjē/ [Gk, *pathos,* disease, *logos,* science], the study of the characteristics, causes, and effects of disease, as observed in the structure and function of the body. Cellular pathology is the study of cellular changes in disease. **Clinical pathology** is the study of disease by the use of laboratory tests and methods. —**pathologic,** *adj.*

pathophysiology /-fiz′ē·ol′əjē/ [Gk, *pathos,* disease, *physis,* nature, *logos,* science], the study of the biologic and physical manifestations of disease as they correlate with the underlying abnormalities and physiologic disturbances. —**pathophysiologic,** *adj.*

pathosis, a disease condition.

pathway [AS, *paeth* + *weg*], **1.** a network of neurons that provides a transmission route for nerve impulses from any part of the body to the spinal cord and the cerebral cortex or from the central nervous system to the muscles and organs. **2.** a chain of chemical reactions that produces various compounds in critical sequence, such as the Embden-Meyerhof pathway.

patient (pt.) /pā′shənt/ [L, *pati,* to suffer], **1.** a recipient of a health care service. **2.** a health care recipient who is ill or hospitalized. **3.** a client in a health care service.

patient assignment, a specialty capitation method in which patients choose a provider in each specialty represented. Capitation payments are then distributed accordingly to the providers selected.

patient care committee, a hospital staff organization, composed of medical, nursing, and other health professionals, with responsibility for monitoring all patient care practices to ensure that predetermined standards are met.

patient care technician, a health technician working under the supervision of a registered nurse, physician, or other health professional to provide basic patient care. Duties may include taking vital signs, obtaining blood and urine samples, performing basic diagnostic tests, and assisting the physician as needed.

patient compensation fund, a fund usually established by state law and commonly financed by a surcharge on malpractice premiums and used to pay malpractice claims.

Patient Contracting, a Nursing Interventions Classification defined as negotiating with a patient an agreement that reinforces a specific behavior change.

patient-controlled analgesia (PCA), a drug-delivery system that dispenses a preset intravascular dose of a narcotic analgesic into a patient when the patient pushes a switch on an electric cord.

Patient-Controlled Analgesia (PCA) Assistance, a Nursing Interventions Classification defined as facilitating patient control of analgesic administration and regulation.

patient day (P.D.), a unit in a system of accounting used by health care facilities and health care planners. Each day represents a unit of time during which the services of the institution or facility were used by a patient; thus 50 patients in a hospital for 1 day would represent 50 patient days.

patient dumping, the premature discharge of Medicare or indigent patients from hospitals for economic reasons. A 1986 U.S. federal rule requires hospitals to advise Medicare patients on admission for treatment of their right to challenge what they consider to be premature discharge after treatment.

patient interview, a systematic interview of a patient, the purpose of which is to obtain information that can be used to develop an individualized plan for care.

patient mix, 1. the distribution of demographic variables in a patient population, often represented by the percentage of a given race, age, sex, or ethnic derivation. **2.** the distribution of indications for admission in a patient population, such as surgical, maternity, or trauma.

patient plan of care, a method, formulated beforehand, to provide for a patient's needs. It is a plan of care coordinated to include appropriate participation by each member of the health care team.

patient record, a collection of documents that provides an account of each episode in which a patient visited or sought treatment and received care or a referral for care from a health care facility. The record is confidential and is usually held by the facility, and the information in it is released only to the patient or with the patient's written permission. It may be computerized, making the documents available on video display terminals or printouts.

patient representative services, hospital services provided by designated staff members relating to the investigation and mediation of patients' complaints and the promotion and protection of patients' rights.

Patient Rights Protection, a Nursing Interventions Classification defined as protection of health care rights of a patient, especially a minor, incapacitated, or incompetent patient unable to make decisions.

Patient's Bill of Rights, a list of the patient's rights promulgated by the American Hospital Association. It offers some guidance and protection to patients by stating the responsibilities that a hospital and its staff have toward them and their families during hospitalization, but it is not a legally binding document.

Patient Self-Determination Act, an act mandating that individuals enrolled in health care facilities are informed of their rights to formulate advance directives and to consent to or refuse treatment.

Patient Zero, an individual identified by the Centers for Disease Control and Prevention (CDC) as the person who introduced the human immunodeficiency virus in the United States. According to CDC records, Patient Zero, an airline steward, infected nearly 50 other persons before he died of acquired immunodeficiency syndrome in 1984.

patrilineal /pat′rilin′ē·əl/, [L, *pater,* father, *linea,* line] pertaining to a line of descent through the male members of the family.

patten /pat′ən/, a metal support worn on a shoe to prevent weight bearing on the opposite leg.

patterning /pat′ərning/ [ME, *patron*], the method of treatment or act of establishing a system or pattern of stimuli that will evoke a new set of responses. The process is commonly used to retrain people who have suffered a brain injury that disrupts normal sensory-motor activities.

patulous /pat′yələs/ [L, *patulus,* open], pertaining to something that is open or spread apart.

Paul-Bunnell test [John R. Paul, American physician, 1893–1971; Walls W. Bunnell,

American physician, 1902–1966], a blood test for heterophil antibodies, used for confirming a diagnosis of infectious mononucleosis.

Pautrier's microabscess /pôtrēyä′/ [Lucien M. A. Pautrier, French dermatologist, 1876–1959; Gk, *mikros*, small; L, *abscedere*, to go away], an accumulation of intensely staining mononuclear cells in the epidermis, characterizing malignant lymphoma of the skin, especially mycosis fungoides.

Pauwels' fracture /pou′əlz/ [Friedrich Pauwels, twentieth-century German surgeon; L, *fractura*, break], a fracture of the proximal femoral neck with varying degrees of angulation.

Pavlov, Ivan Petrovich /pav′lôv, pä′vlôf/ (1849–1936), a Russian physiologist who discovered a pattern of conditioned stimulus-reflex learning, the manner in which the physiologic mechanism of digestion is controlled by the nervous system, and a theory of the causes and treatment of human neuroses.

pavor /pā′vôr/ [L, quaking], a reaction to a frightening stimulus characterized by excessive terror.

pavor diurnus /dī·ur′nəs/, a sleep disorder occurring in children during daytime sleep in which they cry out in alarm and awaken in fear and panic.

pavor nocturnus /noktur′nəs/, a sleep disorder occurring in children during nighttime sleep in which they cry out in alarm and awaken in fear and panic.

Payr's clamp /pī′ərz/ [Erwin Payr, German surgeon, 1871–1946; AS, *clam*, fastener], a heavy clamp used in gastrointestinal surgery.

Pb, symbol for the element **lead.**

PBI, abbreviation for **protein-bound iodine.**

PBL, abbreviation for *peripheral blood lymphocytes.*

p.c., abbreviation for the Latin *post cibum,* 'after meals.'

PC, 1. abbreviation for *professional corporation.* **2.** abbreviation for *personal computer.* **3.** abbreviation for *after meals.*

PCB, abbreviation for **polychlorinated biphenyls.**

pcc, abbreviation for *precipitated calcium carbonate.*

PCCM, abbreviation for **primary care case management.**

PCH, abbreviation for **paroxysmal cold hemoglobinuria.**

PCIS, abbreviation for *Patient Care Information System,* an online computer system that contains full medical care data on all the residents or the patients in a facility.

PCLN, abbreviation for **psychiatric consultation liaison nurse.**

PCP, 1. abbreviation for **phencyclidine hydrochloride. 2.** abbreviation for *Pneumocystis carinii pneumonia.*

PCR, abbreviation for **polymerase chain reaction.**

p.d., abbreviation for the Latin, *per diem,* 'by the day.'

Pd, symbol for the element **palladium.**

P.D., PD, 1. abbreviation for **patient day. 2.** abbreviation for *Doctor of Pharmacy.* **3.** abbreviation for *prism diopter.* **4.** abbreviation for *pupil diameter.* **5.** abbreviation for *pupillary distance.* **6.** abbreviation for *pulse duration.*

PDA, abbreviation for **patent ductus arteriosus.**

PDL, abbreviation for **periodontal ligament.**

PDR, abbreviation for *Physicians' Desk Reference.*

PE, abbreviation for **pulmonary embolism.**

peak [ME, *pec*], the amount of medication in the blood that represents the highest level during a drug administration cycle.

peak and trough specimens, serum samples collected to determine the level of an antibiotic or other pharmaceutic agent in the blood. Peak specimens, which represent the highest level, are generally collected one half-hour after the dose is given intravenously or intramuscularly. Trough specimens, representing the lowest level, are generally collected approximately one half-hour before the next dose.

peak compressional pressure, (in ultrasonics) the temporal maximum positive-pressure in a medium during the passage of a pulsed sound wave. It is expressed in pascals or megapascals.

peak concentration, the maximum amount of a substance or force, such as the highest concentration of a drug measured after it is administered.

peak height velocity, a point in pubescence in which the tempo of growth is the greatest.

peak level, the highest concentration, usually in the blood, that a substance reaches during the period under consideration, such as the highest blood glucose level attained during a glucose tolerance test.

peak method of dosing, the administration of a drug dosage so that a specified maximum level is reached to produce a desired effect, such as lowering the blood pressure.

peak mucus sign a lubricative, cloudy-to-clear white cervical mucus that occurs during periods of high estrogen levels, particularly at the time of ovulation.

peak refractional pressure, (in ultrasonics) the temporal maximum negative pressure in a medium occurring during the passage of a pulsed ultrasound wave. It is expressed in pascals or megapascals.

Pearson's product movement correlation [Karl Pearson, English mathematician, 1857–1936], (in statistics) a statistical test of the relationship between two variables measured in interval or ratio scales. Correlations computed fall between + 1.00 and − 1.00.

peau d'orange /pō'dôräNzh'/ [Fr, skin of orange], a dimpling of the skin that gives it the appearance of the skin of an orange. It is common in advanced breast cancer.

pecten, 1. a ridge extending laterally from the pubic tubercle, to which the pectineal part of the inguinal ligament is attached. **2.** a vascular pleated membrane that extends from the optic disc to the vitreous humor in some animals.

pectenitis /pek'tənī'tis/, an inflammation of the anal canal, causing interference with the anal sphincter muscle.

pectin /pek'tən/ /pek'tin/ [Gk, pektos, congealed], a gelatinous carbohydrate substance found in fruits and succulent vegetables and used as the setting agent for jams and jellies and as an emulsifier and stabilizer in many foods. It also adds to the diet bulk necessary for proper gastrointestinal functioning.

pectineus /pektin'ē·əs/ [L, pecten, comb], the most anterior of the five medial femoral muscles. It functions to flex and adduct the thigh and to rotate it medially.

pectoral /pek'tərəl/ [L, pectus, breast], pertaining to the thorax or chest.

pectoralgia /pek'tôral'jə/, a pain in the thorax.

pectoralis major /pek'torā'lis, pek'tərəlis/ [L, pectus, breast], a large muscle of the upper chest wall that acts on the joint of the shoulder. It serves to flex, adduct, and medially rotate the arm in the shoulder joint.

pectoralis minor, a thin triangular muscle of the upper chest wall beneath the pectoralis major. It functions to rotate the scapula, to draw it down and forward, and to raise the third, fourth, and fifth ribs in forced inspiration.

pectoriloquy /pek'toril'əkwē/, a phenomenon in which voice sounds, including whispers, are transmitted clearly through the pulmonary structures and are clearly audible through a stethoscope. It is often a sign of lung consolidation.

pedagogy /ped'əgōj'ē/ [Gk, pais, child, agogos, leader], the art and science of teaching children, based on a belief that the purpose of education is the transmittal of knowledge.

pedal /ped'əl/ [L, pes, foot], pertaining to the foot.

pediatric /pē'dē·at'rik/ [Gk, pais, child, iatreia, treatment], pertaining to preventive and primary health care and treatment of children and the study of childhood diseases.

Pediatric AIDS Program, an endeavor administered by the Federal Maternal and Child Health Bureau for children infected with human immunodeficiency virus (HIV), which produces acquired immunodeficiency syndrome (AIDS). Projects funded under the program provide comprehensive health services to the children and social support for affected families. Prevention of HIV infection among children is also a part of the Pediatric AIDS Program. Projects also stress the identification of HIV-positive pregnant women along with counseling and follow-up care.

pediatric advanced life support (PALS), a system of critical care procedures and facilities, such as the intensive care nursery for the basic and advanced treatment of seriously ill or injured infants and children. It includes the neonatal resuscitation program as recommended by the American Academy of Pediatrics and the American Heart Association.

pediatric anesthesia [Gk, pais, child, iatreia, treatment], a subspecialty of anesthesiology dealing with the anesthesia of neonates, infants, and children up to 12 years of age.

pediatric dosage, the determination of the correct amount, frequency, and total number of doses of a medication to be administered to a child or infant. Various formulas have been devised to calculate pediatric dosage from a standard adult dose, although the most reliable method is to use the proportional amount of body surface area to body weight, based on one of the formulas.

pediatric hospitalization, the confinement of a child or infant in a hospital for diagnostic testing or therapeutic treatment.

pediatrician /pē'dē·ətrish'ən/ [Gk, pais, child, iatreia, treatment], a physician who specializes in the development and care of infants and children and in the treatment of their diseases.

pediatric nurse practitioner (PNP), a nurse practitioner who, by advanced study and clinical practice, such as in a master's degree program or certificate program in pediatric nursing, has gained advanced knowledge in the nursing care of infants and children.

pediatric nursing, the branch of nursing concerned with the care of infants and children. Preventive care and anticipatory guidance are integral to the practice of pediatric nursing.

pediatric nutrition, the maintenance of a proper, well-balanced diet, consisting of the essential nutrients and the adequate caloric intake necessary to promote growth and sustain the physiologic requirements at the various stages of a child's development. Nutritional needs vary considerably with age, level of activity, and environmental conditions, and they are directly related to the rate of growth.

pediatrics (peds) /pē'dē·at'triks/, a branch of medicine concerned with the development and care of infants and children. Its specialties are the particular diseases of children and their treatment and prevention. —**pediatric,** *adj.*

pediatric surgery, the special preparation and care of the child undergoing surgical procedures for injuries, deformities, or disease. In addition to the usual fears and emotional trauma of illness and hospitalization, the child is especially concerned about being anesthetized.

pedicle [L, *pediculus,* little foot], a narrow stalk, stem, or tube of tissue attached to a tumor, skin flap, bone, or organ.

pedicle clamp /ped'ikəl/ [L, *pediculus,* little foot; ME, *clam,* fastener], a locking surgical forceps used for compressing blood vessels or pedicles of tumors during surgery.

pedicle flap operation, a mucogingival surgical procedure for relocating or sliding gingival tissue from a donor site to an isolated defect, usually a tooth surface denuded of attached gingiva.

pediculicide /pədik'yōōlisīd'/ [L, *pediculus,* little foot, *caedere,* to kill], any of a group of drugs that kill lice.

pediculosis /pədik'yōōlō'sis/ [L, *pediculus* + *osis,* condition], an infestation with blood-sucking lice. Pediculosis capitis is infestation of the scalp with lice. Pediculosis corporis is infestation of the skin of the body with lice. Pediculosis palpebrarum is infestation of the eyelids and eyelashes with lice. Pthirus pubis is infestation of the pubic hair region with lice. Infestation with lice causes intense itching, often resulting in excoriation of the skin and secondary bacterial infection.

pediculous /pədik'yələs/ [L, *pediculus*], infested with sucking lice.

Pediculus humanus capitis, a species of head lice.

Pediculus humanus corporis, a species of body lice.

pedicure /ped'ikyōor/, care of the feet, especially trimming of the toenails.

pedigree /ped'əgrē/ [Fr, *pied de grue,* crane's foot pattern], **1.** line of descent; lineage; ancestry. **2.** (in genetics) a chart that shows the genetic makeup of a person's ancestors, used in the mendelian analysis of an inherited characteristic or disease in a particular family.

pedodontics /ped'ədon'tiks/ [Gk, *pais,* child, *odius,* tooth], a field of dentistry devoted to the diagnosis and treatment of dental problems affecting children.

pedogenesis /pē'dōjen'əsis/ [Gk, *pais,* child, *genesis,* origin], the production of offspring by young or larval forms of animals, often by parthenogenesis, as in certain amphibians. —**pedogenetic,** *adj.*

pedophilia /ped'əfil'ē·ə/ [Gk, *pais,* child, *philein,* to love], **1.** an abnormal interest in children. **2.** (in psychiatry) a psychosexual disorder in which the fantasy or act of engaging in sexual activity with prepubertal children is the preferred or exclusive means of achieving sexual excitement and gratification. —**pedophilic,** *adj.*

peds, *(informal)* abbreviation for **pediatrics.**

peduncle /pədung'kəl/ [L, *pes,* foot], a stemlike connecting part, such as the pineal peduncle or a peduncle graft. —**peduncular, pedunculate,** *adj.*

peduncular /pədung'kyələr/, pertaining to a pedicle or peduncle.

pedunculated /pədung'kyəlā'tid/ [L, *pes,* foot], pertaining to a structure with a stalk or peduncle.

pedunculotomy /pədung'kyəlot'əmē/, a surgical incision in a cerebral peduncle.

pedunculus /pədung'kyələs/ [L, *pes,* foot], a stalk, stem, or stalklike anatomic structure.

peeling, the loss of epidermis, as may occur after a sunburn or exposure to a chemical.

PEEP, abbreviation for **positive end expiratory pressure.**

peer [L, *par,* equal], a person deemed an equal for the purpose at hand. It is usually an "age mate" or a companion or associate on roughly the same level of age or mental endowment.

peer review, an appraisal by professional co-workers of equal status of the way an individual nurse or other health professional conducts practice, education, or research.

Peer Review, a Nursing Interventions Classification defined as systematic evaluation of a peer's performance compared with professional standards of practice.

pegaspargase, an oncolytic agent and modified version of the enzyme l-asparaginase. It is prescribed in the treatment of patients with acute lymphoblastic leukemia who are hypersensitive to other forms of the enzyme.

PEL, abbreviation for *permissible exposure limit.*

Pel-Ebstein fever /pel′eb′stēn/ [Pieter K. Pel, Dutch physician, 1852–1919; Wilhelm Ebstein, German physician, 1836–1912], a recurrent fever, occurring in cycles of several days or weeks, characteristic of Hodgkin's disease or malignant lymphoma.

Pelger-Huët anomaly /pel′gərhyōō′ət/ [Karel Pelger, Dutch physician, 1885–1931; G. J. Huët, Dutch physician, 1879–1970; Gk, *anomalia,* irregular], an inherited disorder characterized by granulocytes with unusually coarse nuclear material and dumbbell-shaped or peanut-shaped nuclei.

pelidnoma /pel′idnō′mə/, a circumscribed elevated dark patch on the skin.

peliosis hepatitis /pel′ē·ō′sis/, the presence of blood-filled cavities in the liver. The cavities may become lined by endothelium and may be found in patients who are infected with human immunodeficiency virus or who use oral contraceptives or anabolic steroids.

pellagra /pəlā′grə, pəlag′rə/ [It, *pelle,* skin, *agra,* rough], a disease resulting from a deficiency of niacin or tryptophan or a metabolic defect that interferes with the conversion of the precursor tryptophan to niacin. It is characterized by scaly dermatitis, especially of the skin exposed to the sun; glossitis; inflammation of the mucous membranes; diarrhea; and mental disturbances, including depression, confusion, disorientation, hallucination, and delirium. —**pellagrous,** *adj.*

pellagra sine pellagra /sī′nē, sē′nə/, a form of pellagra in which the characteristic dermatitis is not present.

Pellegrini's disease /pel′əgrē′nēz/ [Augusto Pellegrini, Italian surgeon, b. 1877], ossification of the upper part of the medial collateral ligament, sometimes accompanied by bony growth at the internal condyle of the femur. The condition usually follows a leg injury.

pellet /pel′it/, a pilule or very small pill.

pellicle /pel′ikəl/, **1.** a thin film or skin. **2.** a scum or crust on a solution.

pelotherapy /pē′lōther′əpē/, the treatment of certain conditions with baths or packs of mud, peat, or earth on part or all of the body surface.

pelvic /pel′vik/ [L, *pelvis,* basin], pertaining to the pelvis.

pelvic abscess [L, *pelvis,* basin, *abscedere,* to go away], a pus-producing lesion in the pelvic peritoneum, usually originating in the rectouterine pouch.

pelvic axis, an imaginary curved line that passes through the centers of the various anteroposterior diameters of the pelvis.

pelvic bones [L, *pelvis,* basin; AS, *ban*], a combination of the ilium, ischium, and pubis.

pelvic brim, the curved top of the bones of the hip extending from the anterosuperior iliac crest in front on one side around and past the sacrum to the crest on the other side. Below the brim is the pelvis.

pelvic cellulitis, bacterial infection of the parametrium, occurring after childbirth or spontaneous therapeutic abortion. It represents an extension of infection via the blood vessels and lymphatics from a primary wound infection in the external genitalia, perineum, vagina, cervix, or uterus. It is characterized by fever, uterine subinvolution, chills and sweats, abdominal pain that spreads laterally, and, if untreated, the formation of a large abscess and signs of peritonitis.

pelvic classification, 1. a process in which the anatomic and spatial relationships of the bones of the pelvis are evaluated, usually to assess the adequacy of the pelvic structures for vaginal delivery. **2.** one of the types in a classification system of the pelvis.

pelvic congestion syndrome, an abnormal gynecologic condition characterized by chronic low back pain, dysuria, dysmenorrhea, vague lower abdominal pain, vaginal discharge, and dyspareunia.

pelvic diameter [L, *pelvis,* basin; Gk, *diametros,* measuring across], **1.** at the rim of the pelvis, a line from the lumbosacral angle to the symphysis pubis. **2.** at the pelvic outlet, a line from the tip of the coccyx to the lower border of the symphysis pubis.

pelvic diaphragm, the inferior aspect of the body wall, stretched like a hammock across the pelvic cavity and comprising the levator ani and the coccygeus muscles. It holds the abdominal contents; supports the pelvic viscera; and is pierced by the anal canal, the urethra, and the vagina.

pelvic examination, a diagnostic procedure in which the external and internal genitalia are physically examined by inspection, palpation, percussion, and auscultation. It should be performed regularly throughout a woman's life. Pelvic examination may demonstrate many pelvic abnormalities and diseases. Cytologic and bacteriologic specimens are conveniently obtained. A pelvic examination cannot be satisfactorily performed without the cooperation of the woman being examined; inadequate relaxation, obesity, extensive scarring, pelvic tenderness, and heavy vaginal discharge also may preclude an adequate examination.

pelvic exenteration /eksen'tərā'shən/, the surgical removal of all reproductive organs and adjacent tissues.

pelvic floor, the soft tissues enclosing the pelvic outlet.

Pelvic Floor Exercise, a Nursing Interventions Classification defined as strengthening the pubococcygeal muscles through voluntary repetitive contraction to decrease stress or urge incontinence.

pelvic girdle [L, *pelvis,* basin; AS, *gyrdel*], a bony ring formed by the hip bones, the sacrum, and the coccyx.

pelvic hematoma, an accumulation of blood in the soft tissues of the pelvis, as may occur during childbirth.

pelvic inflammatory disease (PID), any inflammatory condition of the female pelvic organs, especially one caused by bacterial infection. Characteristics of the condition include fever; foul-smelling vaginal discharge pain in the lower abdomen; abnormal uterine bleeding; pain with coitus; and tenderness or pain in the uterus, affected ovary, or fallopian tube on bimanual pelvic examination. If an abscess has already developed, a soft, tender fluid-filled mass may be palpated.

pelvic inlet, (in obstetrics) the inlet to the true pelvis, bounded by the sacral promontory, the horizontal rami of the pubic bones, and the top of the symphysis pubis. Because the infant must pass through the inlet to enter the true pelvis and be born vaginally, the anteroposterior, transverse, and oblique dimensions of the inlet are important measurements to be made in assessing the pelvis in pregnancy.

pelvic minilaparotomy /min'ēlap'ərot'-əmē/, a surgical operation in which the lower abdomen is entered through a small suprapubic incision. It is performed most often for tubal sterilization but also for diagnosis and treatment of ectopic pregnancy, ovarian cyst, endometriosis, and infertility. It may be performed as an alternative to laparoscopy, often on an outpatient basis.

pelvic outlet, the space surrounded by the bones of the lower part of the true pelvis. In women the shape and size of the pelvis vary and are of importance in childbirth. The shapes are classified by the length of the diameters as compared with each other and by the thickness of the bones.

pelvic pain, pain in the pelvis, as occurs in appendicitis, oophoritis, and endometri-

tis. The character and onset of pelvic pain and any factors that alleviate or aggravate it are significant in making a diagnosis.

pelvic pole, the end of the axis at which the breech of the fetus is located.

pelvic presentation [L, *pelvis,* basin, *praesentare,* to show], a breech presentation.

pelvic rotation, one of the five major kinematic determinants of gait, involving the alternate rotation of the pelvis to the right and left of the body's central axis. The usual pelvic rotation occurring at each hip joint in most healthy individuals is approximately 4 degrees to each side of the central axis. Pelvic rotation occurs during the stance phase of gait and involves a medial to lateral circular motion.

pelvic rotunda [L, *pelvis,* basin, *rotundus,* wheel], a part of the ear appearing as a funnel-shaped depression of the tympanum above the fenestra cochlea.

pelvic tilt, one of the five major kinematic determinants of gait that lowers the pelvis on the side of the swinging lower limb during the walking cycle. Through the action of the hip joint, the pelvis tilts laterally downward, adducting the lower limb in the stance phase of gait and abducting the opposite extremity in the swing phase of gait. The knee joint of the nonweight-bearing limb flexes during its swing phase to allow the pelvic tilt. Pelvic tilt helps minimize the vertical displacement of the body's center of gravity, thus conserving energy during walking.

pelvifemoral /pel'vēfem'ərəl/ [L, *pelvis,* basin, *femur,* thigh], pertaining to the structures of the hip joint, especially the muscles and the area around the bony pelvis and the head of the femur that make up the pelvic girdle.

pelvimeter /pelvim'ətər/ [L, *pelvis,* basin; Gk, *metron,* measure], a device for measuring the diameter and capacity of the pelvis.

pelvimetry /pelvim'ətrē/, the act or process of determining the dimensions of the bony birth canal. Kinds of pelvimetry are **clinical pelvimetry** and **x-ray pelvimetry.**

pelvis /pel'viz/, *pl.* **pelves** [L, basin], the lower part of the trunk of the body, composed of four bones, the two innominate bones laterally and ventrally and the sacrum and coccyx posteriorly. It is divided into the greater or false pelvis and the lesser or true pelvis by an oblique plane passing through the sacrum and the pubic symphysis. The greater pelvis is the expanded part of the cavity situated cranially and ventral to the pelvic brim. The lesser pelvis is situated distal to the pelvic brim, and its bony walls are more complete than those of the greater pelvis. The inlet and outlet of the pelvis have three important diameters: anteroposterior, oblique, and transverse. The pelvis of a woman is usually less massive but wider and more circular than that of a man. —**pelvic,** *adj.*

pelvisacral /pel'visā'krəl/, pertaining to the pelvis and sacrum.

pelvospondylitis ossificans /pel'vōspon'dili'tis/, inflammation of the pelvic part of the spine with deposits of bony material between the sacral vertebrae.

PEM, abbreviation for **protein-energy malnutrition.**

pemoline /pem'əlēn/, a central nervous system stimulant prescribed in the treatment of minimal brain dysfunction and attention-deficit disorder in children.

pemphigoid /pem'figoid/ [Gk, *pemphix,* bubble, *eidos,* form], a bullous disease resembling pemphigus, distinguished by thicker walled bullae arising from erythematous macules or urticarial bases. Oral lesions are uncommon.

pemphigus /pem'figəs, pemfī'gəs/ [Gk, *pemphix,* bubble], an uncommon, severe disease of the skin and mucous membranes, characterized by thin-walled bullae arising from apparently normal skin or mucous membrane. The bullae rupture readily, leaving raw patches. The person loses weight, becomes weak, and is subject to major infections.

pemphigus vulgaris [Gk, *pemphix,* bubble; L, *vulgus,* common], a chronic progressive, often fatal disease, characterized by the formation of bullae on otherwise normal skin.

Pender, Nola J., a nursing theorist who first presented her Health Promotion Model for nursing in her book *Health Promotion in Nursing Practice* (1982). She developed the idea that promoting optimal health supersedes preventing disease. Pender's theory identifies cognitive-perceptual factors in the individual, such as importance of health, perceived benefits of health-promoting behaviors, and perceived barriers to health-promoting behaviors. A major assumption in Pender's theory is that health, as a positive high-level state, is assumed to be a goal toward which individual strives.

pendular nystagmus [L, *pendulus,* hanging down; Gk, *nystagmos,* nodding], an undulating involuntary movement of the eyeball.

pendulous /pen'dələs/, hanging loose or lacking proper support.

pendulous abdomen [L, *pendulus,* hanging down, *abdomen*] an abnormal condition in which the anterior abdominal wall becomes relaxed and hangs down over the pubic region.

penetrance /pen'ətrəns/ [L, *penetrare,* to penetrate], (in genetics) a variable factor that modifies basic patterns of inheritance. It is the regularity with which an inherited trait is manifest in the person who carries the gene. —**penetrant,** *adj.*

penetrate /pen'ətrāt/ [L, *penetrare*], **1.** to enter or pierce a barrier. **2.** pertaining to the degree to which x-rays pass through matter.

penetrating wound /pen'ətrā'ting/ [L, *penetrare* + AS, *wund*], a wound that breaks the skin and enters into a body area, organ, or cavity.

penetration /pen'ətrā'shən/, **1.** a piercing or entering. **2.** intellectual discernment. **3.** a stage in establishment of a viral infection in which the viral genetic material enters the host cell through fusion, phagocytosis, or injection.

penfluridol /penflŏŏ'ridol/, an antipsychotic drug, chemically similar to pimozide.

penicillamine (D-penicillamine) /pen'isil'-əmēn/, a chelating agent prescribed to bind with and remove metals from the blood in the treatment of heavy metal (especially lead) poisoning, in cystinuria, and in Wilson's disease. It is also prescribed as a palliative in the treatment of sclerosis and rheumatoid arthritis when other medications have failed.

penicillic acid /pen'isil'ik/, an antibiotic compound isolated from various species of the fungus *Penicillium.*

penicillin /pen'isil'in/ [L, *penicillus,* paintbrush], any one of a group of antibiotics derived from cultures of species of the fungus *Penicillium* or produced semisynthetically. Various penicillins administered orally or parenterally for the treatment of bacterial infections exert their antimicrobial action by inhibiting the biosynthesis of cell wall mucopeptides during active multiplication of the organisms.

penicillinase /pen'əsil'ənās/, an enzyme elaborated by certain bacteria, including many strains of staphylococci, that inactivates penicillin and thereby promotes resistance to the antibiotic. A purified preparation of penicillinase is used in the treatment of adverse reactions to penicillin.

penicillinase-producing *Neisseria gonorrhoeae* **(PPNG),** those strains of *Neisseria gonorrhoeae* that are resistant to the effects of penicillin through the production of penicillinase or beta-lactamase.

penicillinase-producing staphylococci, strains of staphylococcal organisms that elaborate the penicillin-inactivating enzyme penicillinase (beta-lactamase) and thereby resist the bactericidal action of the antibiotic.

penicillinase-resistant antibiotic, an antimicrobial agent that is not rendered inactive by penicillinase, an enzyme produced by certain bacteria, especially by strains of staphylococci. The semisynthetic penicillins resist the action of penicillinase and are used in treating infections caused by staphylococci that elaborate the enzyme.

penicillinase-resistant penicillin, one of the semisynthetic penicillins derived from *Penicillium,* a genus of mold. Among these drugs are cloxacillin sodium, dicloxacillin sodium, methicillin sodium, nafcillin sodium, and oxacillin sodium.

penicillin G benzathine, a long-acting depot form of penicillin. It is used in the treatment of group A beta-hemolytic streptococcal pharyngitis, group A beta-hemolytic streptococcal pyoderma, and syphilitic infection outside the central nervous system. It is given by deep intramuscular injection to achieve steady concentrations in the plasma and to slow systemic absorption from the repository in the muscle over a period of 12 hours to several days.

penicillin G potassium, an antibacterial prescribed in the treatment of many infections, including syphilis, rheumatic fever, and glomerulonephritis.

penicillin V, an antibacterial prescribed in the treatment of susceptible infections.

penicilliosis /pen'isil'ē-ō'sis/ [L, *penicillus,* paintbrush; Gk, *osis,* condition], pulmonary infection caused by fungi of the genus *Penicillium.*

Penicillium /pen'isil'ē-əm/ [L, *penicillus,* paintbrush], a genus of fungi, some species of which have been tentatively linked to disease in humans. Penicillin G is obtained from *Penicillium chrysogenum* and *P. notatum.*

penile /pē'nīl/ [L, penis], pertaining to the penis.

penile cancer /pē'nīl/ [L, *penis,* penis, *cancer,* crab], a rare malignancy of the penis generally occurring in uncircumcised men and associated with genital herpesvirus infection and poor hygiene. Leukoplakia or the flat-topped papules of balanitis xerotica obliterans may be premalignant lesions, and the velvety red painful papules of Queyrat's erythroplasia are penile squamous cell carcinoma in situ. Cancer of the penis usually presents as a local mass or a bleeding ulcer and metastasizes early in its course.

penile prosthesis [L, *penis* + Gk, *prosthesis,* addition], a device that can be surgically implanted in the penis to treat impotence. Penile implants may consist of inflatable plastic cavernosal cylinders attached to a fluid reservoir and a pump mechanism. The pump forces fluid into the cylinders to produce an erection.

penis /pē'nis/ [L, male sex organ], the external reproductive organ of a man, homologous with the clitoris of a woman. It is attached with ligaments to the front and sides of the pubic arch and is composed of three cylindric masses of cavernous tissue covered with skin. The corpora cavernosa penis surrounds a median mass called the corpus spongiosum penis, which contains the greater part of the urethra.

penischisis /pēnis'kisis/ [L, *penis* + Gk, *schisis,* splitting], a penis with a fissure resulting in an abnormal opening, such as into the urethra in epispadias.

penis envy, literally, female envy of the male penis, but generally a female wish for male attributes, position, and advantages. It is believed by some psychologists to be a significant factor in female personality development.

penniform /pen'ifôrm/ [L, *penna,* feather, *forma,* form], pertaining to the shape of a feather, especially the patterns of muscular fasciculi that correlate with the range of motion and the power of muscles.

Penrose drain [Charles B. Penrose, American surgeon, 1862–1925; AS, *draehen,* teardrop], a thin rubber tube used as a surgical drain device. It is surrounded by rubber or other waterproof materials.

pentachlorophenol poisoning /pen'tə-klôr'ōfē'nol/, a toxic effect of skin absorption of sodium pentachlorophenate, an antimildew agent sometimes used in laundering. The condition has affected newborns with occasionally fatal symptoms of fever and profuse sweating, caused by skin contact with pentachlorophenate residue on diapers and nursery linens.

pentad /pen'tad/, **1.** a pentavalent chemical element. **2.** a relationship among five things.

pentadactyl /pen'tədak'til/ [Gk, *pente,* five, *daktylos,* fingers or toes], having five fingers per hand and five toes per foot.

pentaerythritol tetranitrate /pen'tə·erith'-rətol/, a coronary vasodilator prescribed for the relief of angina pectoris.

pentamidine, /pentam'idēn/, an antiprotozoal. It is sometimes prescribed in the treatment of trypanosomiasis and leishmaniasis, and of *Pneumocystis carinii* pneumonia in immune-compromised patients.

pentamidine isethionate a parenteral antiprotozoal drug prescribed in the treatment of pneumonia caused by *Pneumocys-*

tis carinii, particularly in patients who have human immunodeficiency syndrome.

Pentatrichomonas hominis /pen'tətrik'-əmō'nəs/, a species of parasitic protozoan flagellate, formerly part of the genus *Trichomonas* that lives symbiotically in the colon of humans.

pentavalent /pəntav'ələnt/ [GK, *pente,* five; L, *valere,* to have worth], **1.** a chemical radical or element that has a valency of 5. **2.** pertaining to a body formed by the association of five chromosomes held together by chiasmata at the first division of meiosis.

pentazocine hydrochloride /pentā'zəsēn/, an agonist/antagonist narcotic analgesic prescribed for the relief of moderate to severe pain.

pentobarbital /pen'təbär'bitol/, a sedative and hypnotic prescribed as a preoperative sedative, in the treatment of insomnia, and in the control of acute convulsive disorders.

pentose /pen'tōs/ [GK, *pente,* five; L, *osus,* having], a monosaccharide made of carbohydrate molecules, each containing five carbon atoms. It is produced by the body and is elevated after the ingestion of certain fruits such as plums and cherries and in certain rare diseases.

pentosuria /pen'təsŏŏr'ē·ə/ [GK, *pente* + L, *osus,* having; Gk, *ouron,* urine], a rare condition in which the monosaccharide pentose is found in the urine. Essential or idiopathic pentosuria is caused by a genetically transmitted error of metabolism.

pentoxifylline /pentok'səfil'ēn/, an oral hemorheologic drug prescribed for the treatment of intermittent claudication associated with chronic occlusive arterial limb disease.

pentylenetetrazol /pen'tilē'nətet'rəzol/, a central nervous system stimulant prescribed as an analeptic to stimulate the respiratory, vagal, and vasomotor centers of the brain; to counter the effects of depressants; and to increase cerebral blood flow, especially in geriatric patients.

Peplau, Hildegard E., a pioneer in nursing theory development and a proponent in the 1950s of the concept that nursing is an interpersonal process. In a 1952 work Peplau wrote that the nurse-patient relationship occurs in phases during which the nurse functions as a resource person, a counselor, and a surrogate. The four phases of the process are orientation, identification, exploitation, and resolution. Thus the nurse assists in orientation when a patient with a need seeks help. Identification assures the patient that the nurse can understand his or her situation. Exploitation begins when the patient uses the

services available. Resolution is marked as old needs are met and newer ones emerge.

peplos /pep'los/, a lipoprotein coat that may surround a virion.

peppermint, the dried leaves and flowering tops of an herb, *Mentha piperita.* It is a source of a volatile oil, used as a carminative and antiemetic.

Pepper syndrome [William Pepper, American physician, 1874–1947], a neuroblastoma of the adrenal glands that usually metastasizes to the liver.

pep pills, *slang.* amphetamines.

pepsin /pep'sin/ [Gk, *pepsis,* digestion], an enzyme secreted in the stomach that catalyzes the hydrolysis of protein. Preparations of pepsin obtained from pork and beef stomachs are sometimes used as digestive aids.

pepsinogen /pəpsin'əjən/ [Gk, *pepsis* + *genein,* to produce], a zymogenic substance secreted by pyloric and gastric chief cells. It is converted to the enzyme pepsin in an acidic environment, as in the presence of hydrochloric acid produced in the stomach.

pepsinuria /pep'sinŏŏr'ē·ə/ [Gk, *pepsis,* digestion + *ouron,* urine], the presence of pepsin in urine.

peptic [Gk, *peptein,* to digest], pertaining to digestion or to the enzymes and secretions essential to digestion.

peptic ulcer /pep'tik/, a sharply circumscribed loss of the mucous membrane of the stomach, duodenum, or any other part of the gastrointestinal system exposed to gastric juices containing acid and pepsin. Acute lesions are almost always multiple and superficial. They may be totally asymptomatic and usually heal without scarring or other sequelae. Chronic ulcers are true ulcers. They are deep, single, persistent, and symptomatic; the muscular coat of the wall of the organ does not regenerate; a scar forms, marking the site, and the mucosa may heal completely. Peptic ulcers are caused by a combination of factors, including an excessive secretion of gastric acid; inadequate protection of the mucous membrane; stress; heredity; and the use of certain drugs, including the corticosteroids, certain antihypertensives, and antiinflammatory medications. There is growing evidence from research that a bacterium *(Helicobacter pylori)* present in the gut may be responsible for peptic ulcer disease. Characteristically ulcers cause a gnawing pain in the epigastrium that does not radiate to the back, is not aggravated by a change in position, and has a temporal pattern that mimics the diurnal rhythm of gastric acidity.

P

peptidase /pep'tidās/ [Gk, *peptein,* to digest, *ase,* enzyme suffix], a protein-splitting enzyme that breaks peptides into amino acids. It occurs naturally in plants, yeasts, certain microorganisms, and digestive juices.

peptide /pep'tīd/ [Gk, *peptein,* to digest], a molecular chain compound composed of two or more amino acids joined by peptide bonds.

peptidergic /pep'tidur'jik/, using small peptides as neurotransmitters.

peptogenic /pep'təjen'ik/, pertaining to an agent that produces peptones or pepsin.

peptone /pep'tōn/, a derived protein, which may be produced by hydrolysis of a native protein with an acid or enzyme.

Peptostreptococcus /pep'tastrep'tɔkok'əs/, a genus of gram-positive anaerobic chemoorganotrophic bacteria that occur in pairs or chains. The potentially pathogenic organisms are found in normal and pathologic female genital tracts and in the intestinal and respiratory tracts of normal humans. They have been associated with a variety of disorders ranging from appendicitis to putrefactive wounds.

Peptostreptococcus anaerobius, a potentially pathogenic species of anaerobic bacterium found throughout the body, including the mouth, the intestinal and respiratory tracts, and body cavities, particularly the vagina.

per, [Gk, *peri*], around, near, enclosing.

peracephalus /pur'əsef'ələs/, *pl.* **peracephali** [L, *per,* completely; Gk, *a + kephale,* not head], a fetus or individual with a malformed head.

per an., abbreviation for the Latin phrase *per annum,* 'yearly.'

perceived severity /pərsēvd'/ [L, *percipere,* to perceive, *severus,* serious], (in health belief model) a person's perception of the seriousness of the consequences of contracting a disease.

perceived susceptibility, (in health belief model) a person's perception of the likelihood of contracting a disease.

percentage depth dose /pərsen'tij/ [L, *per,* completely, *centum,* hundred; ME, *dep,* deep; L, *dosis,* something given], (in radiotherapy) the amount of radiation delivered at a specified dose, expressed as a percentage of the skin dose.

percentile, the 100th part of a statistical distribution. A percentile rank of 80 indicates that 20% of the total number of cases scored above and 80% scored below in whatever characteristics were being studied.

percent solution, a relationship of a solute to a solution, expressed in terms of mass of solute per mass of solution. An example of a 5% by mass solution is 5 g of glucose dissolved in 95 g of water, forming 100 g of solution.

percent systole [L, *per + centum +* Gk, *systole,* contraction], an amount of time of each heartbeat that is devoted to the ejection of blood from the ventricle.

percept /pur'sept/ [L, *percipere,* to perceive], the mental impression of an object that is gained through the use of the senses.

perception /pərsep'shən/ [L, *percipere,* to perceive], **1.** the conscious recognition and interpretation of sensory stimuli that serve as a basis for understanding, learning, and knowing or for motivating a particular action or reaction. **2.** the result or product of the act of perceiving. —**perceptive, perceptual,** *adj.*

perceptivity /pur'səptiv'itē/, the ability to receive sense impressions.

perceptual constancy /pərsep'chŏŏ·əl/ [L, *percipere,* to perceive, *cum,* together with, *stare,* to stand], (in Gestalt psychology) the phenomenon in which an object is seen in the same way under varying circumstances.

perceptual defect, any of a broad group of disorders or dysfunctions of the central nervous system that interfere with the conscious mental recognition of sensory stimuli. Such conditions are caused by lesions at specific sites in the cerebral cortex that may result from any illness or trauma affecting the brain at any age or stage of development.

perceptual deprivation, the absence of or decrease in meaningful groupings of stimuli, which may result from a constant background noise or constant inadequate illumination.

perceptual monotony, a mental state characterized by a lack of variety in the normal pattern of everyday stimuli.

percolation /pur'kəlā'shən/ [L, *percolare,* to strain], **1.** the act of filtering any liquid through a porous medium. **2.** (in pharmacology) the removal of the soluble parts of a crude drug by passing a liquid solvent through it.

per con., abbreviation for the Latin phrase *per contra,* 'the other side.'

per contiguum, spreading from one body structure to a contiguous area.

per continuum, describing the spread of an inflammation or other disease process from one body part to another through continuous tissue.

percuss /pərkus'/ [L, *percutere,* to strike hard], to perform percussion by striking, for example, the thoracic or abdominal wall, thereby producing sound vibrations that aid in diagnosis.

percussion /pərkush'ən/ [L, *percutere,* to strike hard], a technique in physical examination of tapping the body with the fingertips or fist to evaluate the size, borders, and consistency of some of the internal organs and to discover the presence and evaluate the amount of fluid in a body cavity. Immediate or direct percussion is percussion performed by striking the fingers directly on the body surface; indirect, mediate, or finger percussion involves striking a finger of one hand on a finger of the other hand as it is placed over the organ. —**percuss,** *v.,* **percussible,** *adj.*

percussor /pərkus'ər/ [L, a striker], a small hammerlike diagnostic tool having a rubber head that is used to tap the body lightly in percussion.

percutaneous /pur'kyo͞otā'nē·əs/ [L, *per* + *cutis,* skin], performed through the skin, such as a biopsy; aspiration of fluid from a space below the skin using a needle, catheter, and syringe; or instillation of a fluid in a cavity or space by similar means.

percutaneous absorption, the process of absorption through the skin from topical application.

percutaneous catheter placement, (in arteriography) the technique in which an intracatheter is introduced through the skin into an artery and placed at the site or structure to be studied.

percutaneous endoscopic gastrostomy, the creation of a new opening in the stomach, accomplished by puncturing the abdominal wall after the stomach has been distended by endoscopy.

percutaneous nephrolithotomy, a uroradiologic procedure performed to extract stones from within the kidney or proximal ureter by percutaneous surgery after the stones have been visualized radiologically.

percutaneous nephroscope, a thin fiberoptic probe that can be inserted into the kidney through an incision in the skin. Light transmitted along the fibers allows visualization of the inside of the kidney. The device is equipped with a tool that can be used to grasp and remove small kidney stones.

percutaneous transhepatic cholangiography (PTC), a radiographic examination of the structure of the bile ducts. A needle is passed directly into a hepatic duct, after which a contrast medium is injected.

percutaneous transluminal angioplasty (PTA), a procedure for dilating blood vessels in the treatment of peripheral artery disease. Under fluoroscopic guidance a balloon-tipped catheter is inserted into a stenotic artery, and the balloon is inflated. The inflated balloon may dilate the artery by stretching its elastic fibers or by flattening accumulation of plaque.

percutaneous transluminal coronary angioplasty (PTCA), a technique in the treatment of atherosclerotic coronary heart disease and angina pectoris in which some plaques in the arteries of the heart are flattened against the arterial walls, resulting in improved circulation. The procedure involves threading a catheter through the vessel to the atherosclerotic plaque and inflating and deflating a small balloon at the tip of the catheter several times, then removing the catheter. The procedure is performed under radiographic or ultrasonic visualization.

per diem rate /pər dē'əm, dī'əm/ [L, *per diem,* daily, *ratus,* reckoned], an established rate of payment for hospital services determined by dividing the total cost of providing routine inpatient services for a given period by the total number of inpatient days of care during the period.

per discharge payment, a payment method in which costs of resources used for the entire hospital stay are the responsibility of the hospital. The hospital is then compensated according to a contractually determined amount per discharge.

perencephaly /per'ensef'əlē/, a condition characterized by one or more cerebral cysts.

Perez reflex /pərez', per'ez/ [Bernard Perez, French physician, 1836–1903; L, *reflectere,* to bend back], the normal response of an infant to cry, flex the limbs, and elevate the head and pelvis when supported in a prone position with a finger pressed along the spine from the sacrum to the neck.

perfectionism /pərfek'shəniz'əm/ [L, *perficere,* to complete], a subjective state in which a person pursues an extremely high standard of performance and in many cases demands the same standards of others. Failure to attain the goals may lead to feelings of defeat and other adverse psychologic consequences.

perflation /pərflā'shən/, a method of opening a passage or cavity entrance with air pressure.

perfloxacin /pərflok'səsin/, an antibiotic of the carboxyfluoroquinolone type.

perfluorocarbons /pərflo͞or'ōkär'bəns/, a group of chemicals with limited capacity for performing the function of hemoglobin in red blood cells by transporting oxygen through the circulatory system. They can be used for certain blood substitute purposes.

perforans /pur'fôrənz/ [L, *perforare,* to pierce], penetrating. The term applies mainly to nerves, muscles, or other anatomic features that penetrate other structures, such as perforans gasseri, or nerves of the musculocutaneous tissues.

perforate [L, *perforare,* to pierce], **1.** /pur′fôrāt/ to pierce, punch, puncture, or otherwise make a hole. **2.** /pur′fôrit/ riddled with small holes. **3.** /pur′fôrit/ (of the anus) having a normal opening; not imperforate. —**perforation,** *n.*

perforating fracture, an open fracture caused by a projectile, making a small surface wound.

perforating ulcer /pur′fôrā′ting/ [L, *perforare,* to pierce, *ilcus*], **1.** an ulcer that penetrates the thickness of a wall or membrane, such as a peptic ulcer of the digestive tract. **2.** a deep painless ulcer, often on the sole of the foot, of a person whose skin is insensitive because of a disease such as diabetes.

perforation /pur′fôrā′shən/ [L, *perforare,* to pierce], a hole or opening made through the entire thickness of a membrane or other tissue or material.

perforation of stomach or intestines, a condition in which disease or injury has resulted in a leakage of digestive tract contents into the peritoneal cavity. A common cause is a ruptured appendix or perforating peptic ulcer. Immediate surgical intervention is needed to prevent peritonitis.

perforation of the uterus, an accidental puncture of the uterus, as may be caused by a curet or by an intrauterine contraceptive device.

perfusion /pərfyoo̅′zhən/ [L, *perfundere,* to pour over], **1.** the passage of a fluid through a specific organ or an area of the body. **2.** a therapeutic measure whereby a drug intended for an isolated part of the body is introduced via the bloodstream.

perfusionist /pərfyoo̅′zhənist/ [L, *perfundere,* to pour over], an allied health professional who assists in performing procedures that involve extracorporeal circulation, such as during open-heart surgery, or hypothermia.

perfusion lung scan, a radiographic examination of the lungs and their function, performed after an intravenous injection of a contrast medium, such as radioactive albumin, and used to aid in the diagnosis of pulmonary embolism.

perfusion rate, the rate of blood flow through the capillaries per unit mass of tissue, expressed in milliliters/minute per 100 g.

perfusion technologist, a person who, under the supervision of a physician, operates a heart-lung machine used for cardiopulmonary bypass during surgery.

per gene, a segment of nucleic acid that is associated with circadian rhythms of some animal species. Mutations of the per gene locus result in alterations of their biorhythms. A similar deoxyribonucleic acid sequence occurs in human genes, but it is not known whether it affects human circadian rhythms.

periadenitis /per′i·ad′ənī′tis/, an inflammation of tissues around a gland.

perianal /per′i·ā′nəl/ [Gk, *peri,* around; L, *anus*], pertaining to the area around the anus.

perianal abscess [Gk, *peri,* around; L, *anus* + *abscedere,* to go away], a focal purulent subcutaneous infection in the region of the anus.

periaortic /per′i·ā·ôr′tik/ [Gk, *peri,* around, *aerein,* to raise], pertaining to the area around the aorta.

periaortitis /per′i·ā′ôrtī′tis/, an inflammation of the adventitia or surrounding tissues of the aorta.

periapical /per′i·ap′ikəl/ [Gk, *peri* + L, *apex,* top], pertaining to the tissues around the apex of the anatomic root of a tooth, including the periodontal membrane and the alveolar bone.

periapical abscess, an infection around the root of a tooth, usually a result of spreading of dental caries. The abscess may extend into nearby bone, causing osteomyelitis, or, more often, it may spread to soft tissues, causing cellulitis and a swollen face.

periapical fibroma, a mass of benign connective tissue that may form at the apex of a tooth with normal pulp.

periapical infection, infection surrounding the root of a tooth, often accompanied by toothache.

periapical radiograph, a dental X-ray film used to detect changes in the bone support surrounding the roots of the teeth.

periappendicitis decidualis /per′i·apen′-disī′tis/, an inflammation of the vermiform appendix with the presence of decidual cells in the peritoneum of the appendix. It occurs in cases of right tubal pregnancy with adhesions between the appendix and the fallopian tubes.

periappendicular /per′i·ap′əndik′yələr/ [Gk, *peri,* around; L, *appendere,* to hang upon], pertaining to the area around the appendix.

periarterial /per′i·ärtir′ē·əl/ [Gk, *peri,* around, *arteria,* airpipe], pertaining to the area around an artery.

periarteritis /per′i·är′təri′tis/ [Gk, *peri* + *arteria,* airpipe, *itis*], an inflammatory condition of the outer coat of one or more arteries and the tissue surrounding the vessel.

periarteritis nodosa, a progressive polymorphic disease of the connective tissue that is characterized by numerous large and palpable nodules or clusters of visible nodules along segments of middle-sized arteries, particularly near points of bifurcation. This process causes occlusion of vessels, resulting in regional ischemia, hemorrhage, necrosis, and pain. Early signs of the disease include tachycardia, fever, weight loss, and pain in the viscera.

periarthritis /per′i·ärthrī′tis/, inflammation of tissues around a joint.

periarticular /per′i·ärtik′yələr/ [Gk, peri, around; L, articulus, joint], pertaining to the area around a joint.

peribronchial /-brong′kē·əl/, surrounding a bronchus.

peribronchiolar /-brong′kē·ō′lər/ [Gk, peri, around, bronchiolus], pertaining to the area around the bronchioles.

pericardiac /-kär′dē·ak/ [Gk, peri, around, kardia, heart], **1.** pertaining to the pericardium. **2.** pertaining to the area around the heart.

pericardial adhesion /-kär′dē·əl/ [Gk, peri, around, kardia, heart; L, adhesio, sticking to], an attachment of the pericardium to the heart muscle, sometimes restricting action of the heart muscle. The condition may be general or localized and may involve adhesion between the two layers of pericardium (internal adhesive pericarditis) or between one layer and surrounding tissues (external adhesive pericarditis).

pericardial artery [Gk, peri + kardia, heart, arteria, airpipe], one of several small vessels branching from the thoracic aorta, supplying the dorsal surface of the pericardium.

pericardial effusion [Gk, peri, around, kardia, heart; L, effundere, to pour out], a collection of blood or other fluid into the pericardium.

pericardial friction rub [Gk, peri, around, kardia, heart, L, fricare, to rub; ME, rubben], the rubbing together of inflamed membranes of the pericardium, as may occur in pericarditis or after a myocardial infarction. It produces a sound audible on auscultation.

pericardiocentesis /per′ikär′dē·ō′sintē′sis/ [Gk, peri + kardia, heart, kentesis, pricking], a procedure for drawing fluid into the pericardial space between the serous membranes by surgical puncture and aspiration of the pericardial sac.

pericardiotomy /-kär′di·ot′əmē/, a surgical incision in the pericardium.

pericarditis /per′ikärdī′tis/ [Gk, peri + kardia, heart, itis], an inflammation of the pericardium associated with trauma, malignant neoplastic disease, infection, uremia, myocardial infarction, collagen disease, or idiopathic causes. Two stages

are observed if treatment in the first stage does not halt progress of the condition. The first stage is characterized by fever, substernal chest pain that radiates to the shoulder or neck, dyspnea, and a dry nonproductive cough. On examination a rapid and forcible pulse, a pericardial friction rub, and a muffled heartbeat over the apex are noted. During the second stage a serofibrinous effusion develops within the pericardium, restricting cardiac activity; the heart sounds become muffled, weak, and distant on auscultation. A bulge is visible on the chest over the precordial area. If the effusion is purulent, caused by bacterial infection, a high fever, sweat, chills, and prostration also occur.

pericardium /per′ikär′dē·əm/, pl. **pericardia** [Gk, peri + kardia, heart], a fibroserous sac that surrounds the heart and the roots of the great vessels. It consists of the serous pericardium and the fibrous pericardium. The serous pericardium consists of the parietal layer and the visceral layer. Between the two layers is the pericardial space containing a few drops of pericardial fluid, which lubricates opposing surfaces of the space and allows the heart to move easily during contraction. The fibrous pericardium, which constitutes the outermost sac and is composed of tough, white fibrous tissue lined by the parietal layer of the serous pericardium, fits loosely around the heart and attaches to large blood vessels emerging from the top of the heart but not to the heart itself. —**pericardial,** adj.

pericholangitis /per′əkō′lanjī′tis/ [Gk, peri + chole, bile, angeion, vessel, itis, inflammation], an inflammatory condition of the tissues surrounding the bile ducts in the liver. Pericholangitis is a complication of ulcerative colitis and portal hypertension.

perichondrial bone /-kon′drē·əl/ [Gk, peri, around, chondros, cartilage; AS, ban], bone that forms in the perichondrium of the cartilaginous template.

perichondrium /-kon′drē·əm//, a fibrous connective tissue sheath and membrane surrounding both hyaline and elastic cartilages.

perichrome /per′ikrōm/, a nerve cell in which the stainable chromophil substance is scattered throughout the cytoplasm.

pericolitis /-kōli′tis/, an inflammation of the connective tissue around the colon.

pericoronitis /-kôr′ənī′tis/, an inflammation of the gingival flap (gum tissue) around the crown of a tooth, usually associated with the eruption of a third molar.

pericranium /-krā′nē·əm/, the connective tissue membrane that surrounds the skull.

pericystium /-sis'tē-əm/, the tissues around a gallbladder or urinary bladder.

periderm /per'idurm/, the outermost layer of flattened epidermis on an embryo or fetus during the first 6 months of gestation.

perididymis /-did'imis/, the three coats of fibrous tissue surrounding the testis.

perididymitis /-did'imi'tis/, an inflammation of the perididymis.

periencephalitis /per'i·ensef'əlī'tis/, an inflammation of the membranes and surface of the brain, including the cortex.

perifocal /-fō'kəl/, pertaining to tissues situated around a focus of infection.

perifollicular /-folik'yələr/ [Gk, *peri,* around; L, *folliculus,* small bag], pertaining to the area around a follicle.

perifolliculitis /-folik'yəlī'tis/ [Gk, *peri* + L, *folliculus,* small bag; Gk, *itis*], inflammation of the tissue surrounding a hair follicle.

periglottic /-glot'ik/, around the tongue, particularly the base of the tongue.

peri-implantoclasia /per'i·implan'tōklā'-zhə/, (in dentistry) a pathologic tissue reaction surrounding implanted foreign material, characterized by local inflammation.

perikaryon /per'iker'ē·on/ [Gk, *peri* + *karyon,* nut], the cytoplasm of a cell body exclusive of the nucleus and any processes, specifically the cell body of a neuron. —**perikaryontic,** *adj.*

perilymph /per'ilimf/ [Gk, *peri* + L, *lympha,* water], the clear fluid separating the osseous labyrinth from the membranous labyrinth in the internal ear.

perimenopause /-men'əpôs/, a span of 4 to 6 years preceding menopause when menstrual cycles and blood flow may be irregular. As estrogen levels decline, osteoporosis begins to develop, and depressive symptoms may occur.

perimeter /pərim'ətər/ [Gk, *peri,* around, *metron,* measure], **1.** the circumference, outer edge, or periphery of an object. **2.** an instrument for measuring visual fields. **3.** an instrument for measuring the circumference of teeth.

perimetrium /per'imē'trē·əm/ [Gk, *peri* + *metra,* womb], the serous membrane enveloping the uterus.

perimetry /pərim'ətrē/, the determination and mapping of the limits of the visual field.

perimolysis /-mol'isis/, decalcification of the teeth caused by exposure to gastric acid in patients with chronic vomiting, as may occur in anorexia or bulimia.

perinatal /per'inā'təl/ [Gk, *peri* + L, *natus,* birth], pertaining to the time and process of giving birth or being born.

perinatal AIDS, acquired immunodeficiency syndrome acquired by infants and children from their mothers during pregnancy, during delivery, or from ingesting infected breast milk.

perinatal death, 1. the death of a fetus weighing more than 1000 g at 28 or more weeks of gestation. **2.** the death of an infant between birth and the end of the neonatal period.

perinatal mortality, the statistical rate of fetal and infant death, including stillbirth, from 28 weeks of gestation to the end of the neonatal period of 4 weeks after birth. Perinatal mortality is usually expressed as the number of deaths per 1000 live births in a specific geographic area or program in a given period.

perinatal period, an interval extending approximately from the twenty-eighth week of gestation to the twenty-eighth day after birth.

perinatal physiology, the physiology of the process of giving birth or being born.

perinatologist /-nātol'əjəst/, a physician who specializes in the diagnosis and treatment of disorders of pregnancy, childbirth, and the puerperium in the mother and child.

perinatology /-nātol'əgē/ [Gk, *peri* + L, *natus,* birth; Gk, *logos,* science], a branch of medicine concerned with the study of the anatomic and physiologic characteristics of the mother and her unborn and newborn and with the diagnosis and treatment of disorders occurring in them during pregnancy, childbirth, and the puerperium. —**perinatologic, perinatological,** *adj.*

perineal /per'inē'əl/ [Gk, *perineos,* perineum], pertaining to the perineum.

perineal body [Gk, *perineos,* perineum; AS, *bodig*], a mass of tissue composed of muscle and fascia between the vagina and rectum in females and between the scrotum and rectum in males.

perineal care [Gk, *perineos,* perineum], a cleansing procedure prescribed for cleansing the perineum after various obstetric and gynecologic procedures. Sterile or clean perineal care may be prescribed. Sterile and clean perineal care is practiced to remove secretions or dried blood from a wound and to prevent contamination of the urethral and vaginal areas or perineal wounds with fecal matter or urine.

Perineal Care, a Nursing Interventions Classification defined as maintenance of perineal skin integrity and relief of perineal discomfort.

perineal pad [Gk, *perineos,* perineum], a cushion of soft material used to cover the perineum to absorb the menstrual flow or to protect a wound or incision.

perineorrhaphy /per'ine·ôr'əfē/ [Gk, *perineos* + *rhaphe,* suture], a surgical procedure in which an incision, tear, or defect in the perineum is repaired by suturing.

perineostomy /per'ine·os'təmē/, the surgical creation of an opening between the urethra and the skin of the perineal region.

perineotomy /per'ine·ot'əmē/ [Gk, *perineos* + *temnein,* to cut], a surgical incision into the perineum.

perinephric abscess /-nef'rik/ [Gk, *peri,* around, *nephros,* kidney; L, *abscedere,* to go away], an abscess that develops in the fatty tissue around a kidney. It is usually secondary to an abscess originating earlier in the cortex of the organ.

perinephrium /-nef're·əm/, the connective tissue around the kidneys.

perineum /per'ine'əm/ [Gk, *perineos*], the part of the body situated dorsal to the pubic arch and the arcuate ligaments, ventral to the tip of the coccyx, and lateral to the inferior rami of the pubis and the ischium and sacrotuberous ligaments. The perineum supports and surrounds the distal parts of the urogenital and gastrointestinal tracts of the body. —**perineal,** *adj.*

perinocele, a hernia in the perineum.

perinodal fibers /-nō'dəl/ [Gk, *peri* + L, *nodus,* knot], the atrial fibers surrounding the atrioventricular or sinoatrial node.

period /pir'ē·od/, **1.** an interval of time. **2.** one of the stages of a disease. **3.** (in physics) the duration of a single cycle of a periodic wave or event. **4.** *(informal).* menses.

periodic /pir'ē·od'ik/ [Gk, *peri* + *hodos,* way], (of an event or phenomenon) recurring at regular or irregular intervals. —**periodicity,** *n.*

periodic apnea of the newborn, a normal condition in the full term newborn, characterized by an irregular pattern of rapid breathing followed by a brief period of apnea, usually associated with rapid eye movement sleep.

periodic deep inspiration, (in respiratory therapy) periodic deep forced inspiration of compressed gas or air in controlled ventilation.

periodic fever [Gk, *peri,* around, *hodos,* way; L, *febris*], a hereditary illness with intermittent episodes of fever accompanied by abdominal or pleuritic pain. Onset occurs between 10 and 20 years of age. Some cases are complicated by symptoms of arthritis, splenomegaly, and renal amyloidosis that may progress to a fatal kidney disorder.

periodic hyperinflation, a normal phenomenon of an unconscious sighing or deep breathing. Because of the natural need for periodic hyperinflation of the lungs, an artificial sigh is often programmed into the mechanism of mechanical ventilators.

periodicity /pir'ē·ədis'itē/ [Gk, *periodikos,* periodical], events or episodes that tend to repeat at predictable intervals; for example, filarial worms may appear in cutaneous blood vessels at night but not in daylight hours, and malaria may cause paroxysms at 24-, 48-, or 72-hour intervals, depending on the species of pathogen.

periodic table, a systematic arrangement of the chemical elements. An earlier version was devised in 1869 by Dmitry Ivanovich Mendeleyev (Russian chemist, 1834–1907). By arranging the elements in order of their atomic weights, he was able to show relationships, such as valency, that occurred at regular intervals and was able to predict the properties of elements still undiscovered in the nineteenth century.

periodontal /per'ē·ōdon'təl/ [Gk, *peri* + *odous,* tooth], pertaining to the area around a tooth, such as the periodontium.

periodontal abscess [Gk, *peri,* around, *odous,* tooth; L, *abscedere,* to go away], a localized collection or pocket of inflammatory material, including pus, in the periodontal tissue. It is usually classified according to its location in the periodontal tissues, such as lateral alveolar, parietal, peridental, or lateral.

periodontal cyst, an epithelium-lined sac that contains fluid, most often occurring at the apex of a tooth that has an infected pulp. Periodontal cysts that occur lateral to a tooth root are less common.

periodontal disease, a pathologic condition of the tissues around a tooth or teeth, such as an inflammation of the periodontal membrane or periodontal ligament.

periodontal index, a measure of an individual's periodontal condition. It is determined by adding scores based on the condition of the gingiva and dividing by the number of teeth present. Individuals with clinically normal gingiva have an index of 0 to 0.2. The index reaches a maximum of 8.0 in persons with severe terminal destructive periodontitis.

periodontal ligament (PDL), the fibrous tissue that attaches the tooth to the alveolus. It is composed of many bundles of collagenous tissue arranged in groups between which lies loose connective tissue interwoven with blood vessels, lymph vessels, and nerves. The periodontal ligament invests and supports the teeth.

P

periodontal pocket [Gk, *peri,* around, *odous,* tooth; Fr, *pochette*], a pathologic increase in the depth of the gingival crevice or sulcus surrounding the tooth at the gingival margin.

periodontal probe [Gk, *peri,* around, *odous,* tooth; L, *probare,* to test], **1.** a slender, tapered flat or cylindric instrument with indentations spaced in millimeters designed for introduction into the gingival sulcus for the purpose of measuring its depth around the tooth. **2.** a slender tapered instrument with or without millimeter indentations for measuring furcations of the roots or premolars (bicuspids) and molars.

periodontics /-don'tiks/ [Gk, *peri,* around, *odous,* tooth], a branch of dentistry concerned with the diagnosis, treatment, and prevention of diseases of the periodontium.

periodontist /-don'tist/, a dentist who specializes in treatment of the supporting structures of the teeth.

periodontitis /per'ē·ō·dontī'tis/, inflammation of the periodontium, which includes the periodontal ligament, the gingiva, and the alveolar bone.

periodontoclasia [Gk, *peri* + *odous,* tooth, *klasis,* breaking], the loosening of permanent teeth caused by breakdown and absorption of the supporting bone.

periodontosis /-dontō'sis/ [Gk, *peri* + *odous,* tooth, *osis,* condition], a rare disease that affects young people, especially women, and is characterized by idiopathic destruction of the periodontium without inflammation.

perioperative /per'i·op'ərətiv/ [Gk, *peri,* around; L, *operari,* to work], pertaining to the time of the surgery.

perioperative nursing [Gk, *peri* + L, *operari,* to work, *nutrix,* nurse], nursing care provided to surgery patients during the entire inpatient period, from admission to date of discharge.

periorbita /per'i·ôr'bitə/ [Gk, *peri* + L, *orbita,* wheel mark], the periosteum of the orbit of the eye. It is continuous with the dura mater and the sheath of the optic nerve.

periorbital /per'i·ôr'bitəl/, pertaining to the area surrounding the socket of the eye.

periosteal /per'i·os'tē·əl/ [Gk, *peri,* around, *osteon,* bone], pertaining to the periosteum, the membrane covering the bone.

periosteum /per'i·os'tē·əm/ [Gk, *peri* + *osteon,* bone], a fibrous vascular membrane covering the bones, except at their extremities. It consists of an outer layer of collagenous tissue containing a few fat cells and an inner layer of fine elastic fibers. Periosteum is permeated with the nerves and blood vessels that innervate and nourish underlying bone. The membrane is thick and markedly vascular over young bones but thinner and less vascular in later life.

periostitis /per'i·ostī'tis/ [Gk, *peri* + *osteon,* bone, *itis*], inflammation of the periosteum. The condition is caused by chronic or acute infection or trauma and is characterized by tenderness and swelling of the affected bone, pain, fever, and chills.

peripatetic /-pətet'ik/ [Gk, *peripatein,* to walk about], pertaining to an ambulatory patient.

peripheral /pərif'ərəl/ [Gk, *periphereia,* circumference], pertaining to the outside, surface, or surrounding area of an organ, other structure, or field of vision.

peripheral acrocyanosis of the newborn, a normal transient condition of the newborn, characterized by pale cyanotic discoloration of the hands and feet, especially the fingers and toes.

peripheral angiography [Gk, *peri,* around, *phereia,* boundary, *angeion,* vessel, *graphein,* to record], the study of the peripheral blood vessels by radiography after an opaque dye is injected into the circulation.

peripheral arterial disease (PAD), a systemic form of atherosclerosis producing symptoms in cardiac, cerebral, and renal vascular systems. It affects up to 2% of individuals between 37 and 69 years of age and about 10% of persons over 70 years of age. The incidence is highest among males with diabetes mellitus. Other risk factors include obesity and stress. Blood flow is restricted by an intraarterial accumulation of soft deposits of lipids and fibrin that harden over time, particularly at bends or bifurcations of the arterial walls. Patients are generally not aware of the changes until the diameter of the arterial lumen has been reduced by half. Early symptoms include two types of reproducible pain, intermittent claudication, and ischemic rest pain.

peripheral arteriovenography, a radiographic examination of the blood vessels in the peripheral parts of the body such as the arms and legs after the injection of a contrast medium into these vessels.

peripheral device, any hardware device that may be attached to the central processing unit, such as a printer, monitor, or drive.

peripheral lesion [Gk, *perphereia* + L, *laesio,* hurting], an injury to any tissues distal to the main organ systems.

Peripherally Inserted Central (PIC) Catheter Care, a Nursing Interventions

Classification defined as insertion and maintenance of a peripherally inserted central catheter.

peripheral motor neuron [Gk, *periphereia* + L, *motor,* mover; Gk, *neuron,* nerve], an effector neuron located outside the central nervous system, usually in a ganglion of a sympathetic or parasympathetic nervous system.

peripheral neurovascular dysfunction, risk for, a NANDA-accepted nursing diagnosis of a state in which an individual is in danger of experiencing a disruption in circulation, sensation, or motion of an extremity. Risk factors include fractures, mechanical compression (e.g., tourniquet, cast, brace, dressing, or restraint), orthopedic surgery, trauma, immobilization, burns, and vascular obstruction.

peripheral nervous system, the motor and sensory nerves and ganglia outside the brain and spinal cord. The system consists of 12 pairs of cranial nerves, 31 pairs of spinal nerves, and their various branches in body organs. Sensory, or afferent, peripheral nerves transmitting information to the central nervous system and motor, or efferent, peripheral nerves carrying impulses from the brain usually travel together but separate at the cord level into a posterior sensory root and an anterior motor root. Fibers innervating the body wall are designated somatic; those supplying internal organs are termed visceral. The autonomic system includes the peripheral nerves involved in regulating cardiovascular, respiratory, endocrine, and other automatic body functions. Nerves in the sympathetic or thoracolumbar division of the autonomic system secrete norepinephrine and cause peripheral vasoconstriction, cardiac acceleration, coronary artery dilation, bronchodilation, and inhibition of peristalsis. Parasympathetic nerves, which constitute the craniosacral division of the autonomic system, secrete acetylcholine; cause peripheral vasodilation, cardiac inhibition, and bronchoconstriction; and stimulate peristalsis.

peripheral neuropathy, any functional or organic disorder of the peripheral nervous system. A kind of peripheral neuropathy is **paresthesia.**

peripheral odontogenic fibroma, a fibrous connective tissue tumor associated with the gingival margin. It is a localized form of fibromatosis gingivae and commonly contains areas of calcification.

peripheral pulse [Gk, *periphereia* + L, *pulsare,* to beat], the series of waves of arterial pressure caused by left ventricle systoles as measured in the limbs.

peripheral resistance, a resistance to the flow of blood determined by the tone of the vascular musculature and the diameter of the blood vessels.

peripheral scotoma [Gk, *periphereia* + *skotos,* darkness, *oma* tumor], a lost area of the visual field that is located peripherally and does not involve the central region.

peripheral vascular disease (PVD), any abnormal condition that affects the blood vessels outside the heart and the lymphatic vessels. Different kinds and degrees of peripheral vascular disease are characterized by a variety of signs and symptoms such as numbness, pain, pallor, elevated blood pressure, and impaired arterial pulsations. Various causative factors include obesity, cigarette smoking, stress, sedentary occupations, and numerous metabolic disorders. Peripheral vascular disease in association with bacterial endocarditis may involve emboli in terminal arterioles and produce gangrenous infarctions of various distal parts of the body, such as the tips of the nose, the pinna of the ear, the fingers, and the toes. Large emboli may occlude peripheral vessels and cause atherosclerotic occlusive disease.

peripheral vision, a capacity to see objects in the outer aspects of the field of use caused by reflected light waves that fall on areas of the retina distant from the macula.

periphery /pərif'ərē/ [Gk, *peri,* around, *phereia,* boundary], **1.** parts or areas near or outside a perimeter or boundary **2.** the outer body parts, such as the skin or limbs.

perirectal /-rek'təl/ [Gk, *peri,* around; L, *rectus,* straight], pertaining to the area around the rectum.

perisinusitis /-sī'nəsī·tis/ [Gk, *peri,* around; L, *sinus,* hollow], an inflammation of the structures around a sinus.

peristalsis /-stal'ʊ̄is, ·stôl'sis/ [Gk, *peri* + *stalsis,* contraction], the coordinated, rhythmic serial contraction of smooth muscle that forces food through the digestive tract, bile through the bile duct, and urine through the ureters.

peristaltic /-stal'tik, -stôl'tik/ [Gk, *peri* + *stalsis,* contraction], pertaining to peristalsis.

peristomal /per'istō'məl/, pertaining to the area of skin surrounding a stoma, or surgically created opening in the abdominal wall.

peritoneal /-tənē'əl/ [Gk, *peri* + *tenein,* to stretch], pertaining to the peritoneum.

peritoneal abscess [Gk, *peri* + *tenein* + L, *abscedere,* to go away], an abscess in the peritoneal cavity, the result of peritonitis and usually complicated by adhesions.

peritoneal cavity /per'itōnē'əl/ [Gk, *peri* +

teinein, to stretch], the potential space between the parietal and visceral layers of the peritoneum. Normally the two layers are in contact.

peritoneal dialysis, a dialysis procedure performed to correct an imbalance of fluid or of electrolytes in the blood or to remove toxins, drugs, or other wastes normally excreted by the kidney. The peritoneum is used as a diffusible membrane. Under local anesthesia a many-eyed catheter is sutured in place in the peritoneum, and a sterile dressing is applied. The catheter is connected to the inflow and outflow tubing with a Y connector. During inflow the dialysate is introduced into the peritoneal cavity. By means of osmosis, diffusion, and filtration, the needed electrolytes pass to the bloodstream via the vascular peritoneum to the blood vessels of the abdominal cavity, and the waste products pass from the blood vessels through the vascular peritoneum into the dialysate. During outflow the dialysate is allowed to drain from the peritoneal cavity by gravity.

peritoneal dialysis solution, a solution of electrolytes and other substances that is introduced into the peritoneum to remove toxic substances from the body.

Peritoneal Dialysis Therapy, a Nursing Interventions Classification defined as administration and monitoring of dialysis solution into and out of the peritoneal cavity.

peritoneal endometriosis [Gk, *peri* + *teinein,* to stretch, *endon,* within, *metra,* womb], ectopic endometrial tissue found in the pelvic cavity.

peritoneal fluid, a naturally produced fluid in the abdominal cavity that lubricates surfaces, thereby preventing friction between the peritoneal membrane and internal organs.

peritoneoscopy /-tō′nē·os′kəpē/ [Gk, *peri* + *teinein* + *skopein,* to view], the use of an endoscope to inspect the peritoneum through a stab incision in the abdominal wall.

peritoneum /per′itōnē′əm/ [Gk, *peri* + *teinein,* to stretch], an extensive serous membrane that lines the entire abdominal wall of the body and is reflected over the contained viscera. It is divided into the parietal peritoneum and the visceral peritoneum. In men the peritoneum is a closed membranous sac. In women it is perforated by the free ends of the uterine tubes. The free surface of the peritoneum is smooth mesothelium, lubricated by serous fluid that permits the viscera to glide easily against the abdominal wall and against one another. The mesentery of the peritoneum fans out from the main membrane to suspend the small intestine. Other parts of the peritoneum are the transverse mesocolon, the greater omentum, and the lesser omentum. —**peritoneal,** *adj.*

peritonitis /per′itəni′tis/ [Gk, *peri* + *teinein,* to stretch, *itis*], an inflammation of the peritoneum. It is produced by bacteria or irritating substances introduced into the abdominal cavity by a penetrating wound or perforation of an organ in the gastrointestinal or reproductive tract. Peritonitis is caused most commonly by rupture of the vermiform appendix but also occurs after perforations of intestinal diverticula, peptic ulcers, gangrenous gallbladders, gangrenous obstructions of the small bowel, or incarcerated hernias, as well as ruptures of the spleen, liver, ovarian cyst, or fallopian tube, especially in ectopic pregnancy. Characteristic signs and symptoms include abdominal distension, rigidity and pain, rebound tenderness, decreased or absent bowel sounds, nausea, vomiting, and tachycardia. The patient has chills and fever; breathes rapidly and shallowly; is anxious, dehydrated, and unable to defecate; and may vomit fecal material. Leukocytosis, an electrolyte imbalance, and hypovolemia are usually present; and shock and heart failure may ensue.

peritonitis meconium [Gk, *peri* + *teinein, itis,* inflammation, *mekon,* poppy], a condition of peritonitis in a newborn resulting from rupture of the digestive tract. The inflammation is caused by leakage of meconium, or fetal contents, into the peritoneal cavity.

peritonsillar /-ton′silər/ [Gk, *peri* + L, *tonsilla*], pertaining to the area around a tonsil.

peritonsillar abscess [Gk, *peri* + L, *tonsilla,* tonsil, *abscedere,* to go away], an infection of tissue between the tonsil and pharynx, usually after acute follicular tonsillitis. The symptoms include dysphagia, pain radiating to the ear, and fever. Redness and swelling of the tonsil and adjacent soft palate are present.

periumbilical /per′i·umbil′ikəl/ [Gk, *peri,* around, *umbilicus,* navel], pertaining to the area around the umbilicus.

periungual /per′i·ung′gwəl/ [Gk, *peri* + L, *unguis,* nail], pertaining to the area around the fingernails or the toenails.

perivascular goiter /per′ivas′kyŏŏlər/ [Gk, *peri* + L, *vasculum,* little vessel, *guttur,* throat], an enlargement of the thyroid gland surrounding a large blood vessel.

perivascular spaces [Gk, *peri,* around; L, *vasculum,* little vessel, *spatium,* space], spaces that surround blood vessels as they enter the brain. They communicate with the subarachnoid space.

perivertebral /-var′təbrəl/ [Gk, *peri,*

around, *vertebra*, joint], pertaining to the area around a vertebra.

perivitelline /-vitel′ēn/ [Gk, *peri* + L, *vitellus*, yolk], surrounding the vitellus or yolk mass.

perivitelline space, the space between the ovum and the zona pellucida of mammals into which the polar bodies are released at the time of maturation.

perle /purl, perl/ [Fr, pearl], a soft capsule filled with medicine.

perlingual /pərling′gwəl/ [L, *per* + *lingua*, tongue], pertaining to the administration of drugs through the tongue, which absorbs substances through its surface.

permanent dentition /pur′mənənt/ [L, *permanere*, to remain], the eruption of the 32 permanent teeth, beginning with the appearance of the first permanent molars at about 6 years of age. The process is completed by 12 or 13 years of age, except that the four wisdom teeth usually do not erupt until 18 to 25 years of age or later.

permanent pacemaker [L, *permanere,* to remain, *passus*, step; ME, *maken*], any pacemaker implanted inside a patient's body for permanent long-term use.

permanent tooth, one of the set of 32 teeth that appear during and after childhood and usually last until old age. In each jaw they include four incisors, two canines, four premolars, and six molars. They are divided into the permanent teeth, which replace the 20 deciduous teeth of infancy, and the superadded teeth, which include 12 molars, 3 on each side of the upper and lower jaws. The permanent teeth start to develop in the ninth week of fetal life with the thickening of the epithelium along the line of the future jaw and start to calcify soon after birth. They erupt first in the lower jaw; the first molars in about the sixth year; the two central incisors about the seventh year, the two lateral incisors about the eighth year; the first premolars about the ninth year; the second premolars about the tenth year; the canines between the eleventh and the twelfth years; the second molars between the twelfth and the thirteenth years; and the third molars between the seventeenth and twenty-fifth years.

permeability /pur′mē-əbil′itē/ [L, *permeare*, to pass through], the degree to which one substance allows another substance to pass through it.

permeable /pur′mē-əbəl/ [L, *permeare*, to pass through], a condition of allowing fluids and certain other substances to pass through, such as a permeable membrane.

per member per month (PMPM), usual unit of measure for capitation payments that payers provide to providers, both hospitals and physicians. These payments also include ancillary services.

permethrin /pərməth′rin/, a topical pediculicide used for the treatment of head lice and nits.

permissible dose /pərmis′ibəl/ [L, *permittere,* to permit, *dosis,* something given], (in radiotherapy) the amount of radiation that may be received by an individual in a specified period with the expectation of no significantly harmful results.

permissible exposure limit (PEL), an occupational health standard instituted to safeguard workers against exposure to toxic material in the workplace. PELs are the result of the 1970 U.S. Occupational Safety and Health Act, which established the Occupational Safety and Health Administration (OSHA), the policing and enforcing arm of the act, and the National Institute for Occupational Safety and Health (NIOSH), which represents the research arm. OSHA publishes PELs and short-term exposure limits based on recommendations of NIOSH.

pernicious /pərnish′əs/ [L, *perniciosus*, destructive], potentially injurious, destructive, or fatal unless treated, such as pernicious anemia.

pernicious anemia [L, *perniciosus,* destructive; Gk, *a* + *haima,* not blood], a progressive megaloblastic macrocytic anemia that results from a lack of intrinsic factor essential for the absorption of cyanocobalamin (vitamin B_{12}). The maturation of red blood cells in bone marrow becomes disordered, the posterior and lateral columns of the spinal cord deteriorate, the white blood cell count is reduced, and the polymorphonuclear leukocytes become multilobed. Extreme weakness, numbness and tingling in the extremities, fever, pallor, anorexia, and loss of weight may occur.

pernicious vomiting [L, *perniciosus,* destructive, *vomere,* to vomit], a severe life-threatening episode of vomiting that may occur during pregnancy.

perobrachius /pe′rōbrā′kē-əs/ [Gk, *peros,* damaged, *brachion,* arm], a fetus or individual with malformed arms.

perochirus /pe′rōkī′rəs/ [Gk, *peros* + *cheir,* hand], a fetus or individual with malformed hands.

perodactylus /pe′rōdak′tiləs/, a fetus or an individual with a deformity of the fingers or the toes, especially the absence of one or more digits.

perodactyly /pe′rōdak′tilē/ [Gk, *peros* + *daktylos,* finger], a congenital anomaly characterized by a deformity of the digits, primarily the complete or partial absence of one or more of the fingers or toes.

peromelia /pē'rōmē'lyə/ [Gk, *peros* + *melos,* limb], a congenital anomaly characterized by the malformation of one or more of the limbs. **—peromelus,** *n.*

peroneal /per'ənē'əl/ [Gk, *perone,* brooch], pertaining to the outer part of the leg, over the fibula and the peroneal nerve.

peroneal muscular atrophy, symmetric weakening or atrophy of the foot and ankle muscles and hammertoes. Affected individuals usually have high plantar arches and an awkward gait, caused by weak ankle muscles.

peroneus brevis /per'ənē'əs/ [Gk, *perone* + L, *brevis,* short], the smaller of the two lateral muscles of the leg, lying under the peroneus longus. It pronates and plantar flexes the foot.

peroneus longus, the more superficial of the two lateral muscles of the leg. The muscle pronates and plantar flexes the foot.

peronia /pərō'nē·ə/ [Gk, *peros,* damaged], a congenital malformation or developmental anomaly.

peropus /pərō'pəs/ [Gk, *peros* + *pous,* foot], a fetus or individual with malformed feet, often in association with some defect of the legs.

per os /pər os'/ [L], by mouth.

perosomus /pē'rōsō'məs/ [Gk, *peros* + *soma,* body], a fetus or individual whose body, especially the trunk, is severely malformed.

perosplanchnia /pē'rōsplangk'nē·ə/ [Gk, *peros* + *splanchnon,* viscera], a congenital anomaly characterized by the malformation of the viscera.

perphenazine /pərfen'əzēn/, an antipsychotic prescribed in the treatment of psychotic disorders and in the control of severe nausea and vomiting in adults.

per primam intentionem [L], by primary (first) intention.

per pro., abbreviation for the Latin term *per procurationem,* 'on behalf of.'

per rectum [L], by rectum.

PERRLA /pur'lə/, abbreviation for *pupils equal, round, react to light, accommodation.* In the process of performing an assessment of the eyes, one evaluates the size and shape of the pupils, their reaction to light, and their ability to accommodate. If all findings are normal, the acronym is noted in the account of the physical examination.

per se [L], by itself, or of itself.

per secundum intentionem [L], by second intention.

perseveration /pur'səvərā'shən/ [L, *persevero,* to persist], the involuntary and pathologic persistence of the same verbal response or motor activity, regardless of the stimulus or its duration.

Persian Gulf syndrome, a diffuse collection of symptoms reported by many veterans of the 1991 Persian Gulf war. Symptoms vary widely but include fatigue, joint pain, headache, and sleep disturbances. Musculoskeletal and connective tissue diseases are also common. The specific cause is unknown, but explanations include exposure to chemicals from burning oil wells, insecticides, and poisons linked to inoculations against biologic warfare or to chemical weapons used by the Iraqi army.

persistent cloaca /pərsis'tənt/ [L, *persistere,* to persist, *cloaca,* sewer], a congenital anomaly in which the intestinal, urinary, and reproductive ducts open into a common cavity resulting from the failure of the urorectal septum to form during prenatal development.

persistent vegetative state, a state of wakefulness accompanied by an apparent complete lack of cognitive function, experienced by some patients in an irreversible coma. Vegetative functions and brainstem reflexes are intact, but the cortex is permanently damaged.

persona /pərsō'nə/, *pl.* **personae** /-nē/ [L, mask], (in analytic psychology) the personality façade or role that a person assumes and presents to the outer world to satisfy the demands of the environment or society or to express some intrapsychic conflict.

personal and social history /pur'sənəl/, (in a health history) an account of the personal and social details of a person's life that serves to identify the person. Place of birth, religion, race, marital status, number of children, military status, occupational history, and place of residence are the usual components of this part of the history.

personal care services, the services performed by health care workers to assist patients in meeting the requirements of daily living.

personal identity disturbance, a NANDA-accepted nursing diagnosis of the inability to distinguish between self and nonself. The defining characteristics and related factors are to be developed at a later conference.

personality /pur'sənal'itē/ [L, *personalis,* role], **1.** the composite of the behavioral traits and attitudinal characteristics by which one is recognized as an individual. **2.** the behavior pattern each person develops, both consciously and unconsciously, as a means of adapting to a particular environment and its cultural, ethnic, national, and provincial standards.

personality disorder, a *DSM-IV* psychiatry disorder characterized by disruption in relatedness. It is manifested in any of a large group of mental disorders characterized by rigid, inflexible, and maladaptive behavior patterns and traits that impair a person's ability to function in society by severely limiting adaptive potential.

personality test, any of a variety of standardized tests used in the evaluation or assessment of various facets of personality structure, emotional status, and behavioral traits.

personal orientation, 1. a continually evolving process in which a person determines and evaluates the relationships that appear to exist between him or her and other people. **2.** the assessment of those relationships derived by a person.

personal protective equipment, a part of standard precautions for all health care workers to prevent skin and mucous membrane exposure when in contact with blood and body fluid of any patient. Personal equipment includes protective laboratory clothing, disposable gloves, eye protection, and face masks.

personal space, the area surrounding an individual that is perceived as private by the individual, who may regard a movement into the space by another person as intrusive. Personal space boundaries vary somewhat in different cultures, but in general they are regarded as a distance of about 1 meter (3 feet) around the individual.

personal unconscious, (in analytic psychology) the thoughts, ideas, emotions, and other mental phenomena acquired and repressed during one's lifetime.

personal zone, an individual protective zone in which the boundaries may contract or expand according to contextual characteristics, usually between 18 inches and 4 feet.

person year, a statistical measure representing one person at risk of development of a disease during a period of 1 year.

perspiration /pur'spirǎ'shǝn/ [L, *per* + *spirare,* to breath], **1.** the act or process of perspiring; the excretion of fluid by the sweat glands through pores in the skin. **2.** the fluid excreted by the sweat glands. It consists of water containing sodium chloride, phosphate, urea, ammonia, and other waste products. Perspiration serves as a mechanism for excretion and for regulation of body temperature.

perspire /pǝrspī'ǝr/ [L, *per* + *spirare,* to breathe], to sweat or excrete sweat.

per tertiam intentionem [L], by tertiary (third) intention.

perturbation /pur'tǝrbā'shǝn/ [L, *per* + *tubare,* to disturb], a cause or a condition of disturbance, disorder, or confusion.

pertussis /pǝrtus'is/ [L, *per* + *tussis,* cough], an acute, highly contagious respiratory disease characterized by paroxysmal coughing that ends in a loud whooping inspiration. It occurs primarily in infants and in children less than 4 years of age who have not been immunized. The causative organism, *Bordetella pertussis,* is a small, nonmotile gram-negative coccobacillus. A similar organism, *B. parapertussis,* causes a less severe form of the disease called parapertussis.

pertussis immune globulin, a passive immunizing agent prescribed for immunization against whooping cough.

pertussis vaccine, an active immunizing agent prescribed for immunization against pertussis when the administration of diphtheria, pertussis, and tetanus vaccine is contraindicated.

per vaginam [L], via the vagina.

pervasive developmental disorder /pǝrvā'siv/ [L, *pervadere,* to go through], any of certain disorders of infancy and childhood that are characterized by severe impairment of relatedness and behavioral aberrations previously identified as childhood psychoses. The group of disorders includes infantile autism, childhood schizophrenia, and symbiotic psychosis.

perversion /pǝrvur'shǝn/ [L, *pervertere,* to turn about], **1.** any deviation from what is considered normal or natural. **2.** the act of causing a change from what is normal or natural. **3.** *informal.* (in psychiatry) any of a number of sexual practices that deviate from what is considered normal adult behavior.

pervert /pur'vǝrt/ [L, *pervertere*], **1.** *informal.* a person whose sexual pleasure is derived from stimuli almost universally regarded as unnatural, such as a fetishist or sadomasochist; a paraphiliac. **2.** one whose sexual behavior deviates from a social or statistical norm but is not necessarily pathologic.

pes /pēz, pās/, *pl.* **pedes** /pē'dēz/ [L, foot], the foot or a footlike structure.

pes cavus, a deformity of the foot characterized by an excessively high arch with hyperextension of the toes at the metatarsophalangeal joints, flexion at the interphalangeal joints, and shortening of the Achilles tendon. The condition may be present at birth or appear later as a result of contractures or an imbalance of the muscles of the foot, as in neuromuscular

P

diseases such as Friedreich's ataxia or peroneal muscular atrophy.

pes equinus [L, *pes* foot, *equinus*, pertaining to a horse], a foot deformity in which the toes are extremely flexed, walking is done on the dorsal surface, and the heel does not touch the ground.

pes planus, an abnormal but relatively common condition characterized by the flattening out of the arch of the foot.

pessary /pes'ərē/ [Gk, *pessos*, oval stone], a device inserted in the vagina to treat uterine prolapse, uterine retroversion, or cervical incompetence. It is used in the treatment of women whose advanced age or poor general condition precludes surgical repair. Pessaries are also used in younger women in evaluating symptomatic uterine retroversion and in managing cervical incompetence in pregnancy. A pessary must be removed, usually daily, for cleaning. A Smith-Hodge pessary is a rubber- or vinyl-covered wire rectangle that fits between the pubic bone and the posterior vaginal fornix, supporting the uterus and holding the cervix in a posterior position. A Gellhorn pessary is an inflexible device made of acrylic resin or plastic (Lucite) in the form of a large collar button. It has a canal through the stem that allows drainage of vaginal secretions. A doughnut pessary is a permanently inflated flexible rubber doughnut that is inserted to support the uterus by blocking the canal of the vagina. An inflatable pessary is a collapsible rubber doughnut to which a flexible stem containing a rubber valve is attached. The collapsed pessary is inserted, inflated with a bulb similar to that of a sphygmomanometer, and deflated for removal. A bee cell pessary is a soft rubber cube; in each face of the cube is a conical depression that acts as a suction cup when the pessary is in the vagina. A diaphragm pessary is a contraceptive diaphragm used for uterovaginal support. A stem pessary, a slim curved rod, is rarely used today.

pessimism /pes'imiz'əm/ [L, *pessimus*, worst], the inclination to anticipate the worst possible results from any action or situation or to emphasize unfavorable conditions, even when progress or gain might reasonably be expected. —**pessimist**, *n.*

pesticide poisoning /pes'tisīd/ [L, *pestis*, plague, *caedere*, to kill, *potio*, drink], a toxic condition caused by the ingestion or inhalation of a substance used for the eradication of pests. Kinds of pesticide poisoning include **malathion poisoning** and **parathion poisoning.**

pestilence /pes'tiləns/ [L, *pestilentia*, infectious disease], any epidemic of a virulent infectious or contagious disease.

pes valgus [L, *pes*, foot, *valgus*, bent outward], deviation of the foot outward at the talocalcanean joint.

PET /pet/, abbreviation for **positron emission tomography.**

petaling /pet'əling/, a process of smoothing the raw or ragged edges of a plaster cast to prevent skin irritation.

petechiae /pētē'kē·ē/, *sing.* **petechia** /-kē·ə/ [It, *petecchie*, flea-bite], tiny purple or red spots appearing on the skin as a result of tiny hemorrhages within the dermal or submucosal layers. —**petechial**, *adj.*

petechial [It, *petecchie*], pertaining to tiny red or purple spots caused by an extravasation of blood into the skin.

petechial fever /pitē'kē·əl/ [It, *petecchie* + L, *febris*, fever], any febrile illness accompanied by small petechiae on the skin, such as seen with meningococcemia or in the late stage of typhoid fever.

petechial hemorrhage [It, *petecchie* + Gk, *haima*, blood, *rhegnynei*, to gush], a small discrete hemorrhage under the skin.

petit pas gait /pet'ē pä, ptē'pä/, a manner of walking with short, mincing steps and shuffling with loss of associated movements. It is seen in cases of parkinsonism as well as in diffuse cerebral disease resulting from multiple small infarcts.

Petren's gait /pet'rənz/, a hesitant form of walking in which a patient takes a few steps, halts, and then takes a few more steps. In some cases the patient must be encouraged to begin the next brief walking period.

Petri dish /pē'trē, pä'trē/ [Julius R. Petri, German bacteriologist, 1852–1921], a shallow circular glass dish used to hold solid culture media.

petrification /pet'rifikā'shən/, the process of becoming calcified or stonelike.

pétrissage /pā'trisäzh'/ [Fr, *petrir*, to knead], a technique in massage in which the skin is gently lifted and squeezed. Pétrissage promotes circulation and relaxes muscles.

petrolatum /pet'rəlā'təm/ [L, *petra*, rock, *oleum*, oil], a purified mixture of semisolid hydrocarbons obtained from petroleum and commonly used as an ointment base or skin emollient.

petrolatum gauze /pet'rəlā'təm/, absorbent gauze permeated with white petrolatum.

petroleum distillate poisoning /pətrō'lē·əm/ [L, *petra* + *oleum* + *distillare*, to drop down, *potio*, drink], a toxic condition caused by the ingestion or inhalation of a petroleum distillate such as fuel oil, lubricating oil, glue used in making model airplanes or the like, and various solvents. Nausea, vomiting, chest pain, dizziness, and severe depression of the central nervous system characterize the condition. Severe or fatal pneumonitis may occur if the substance is aspirated.

petroleum jelly, a nonliquid colloidal solution or gel of soft paraffin. It is an intermediate product of the distillation of petroleum and is used as a topical soothing medication for burns and abrasions.

petrosphenoidal fissure /pet′rōsfēnoi′dəl/ [L, *petra*, rock; Gk, *sphen*, wedge, *eidos*, form], a fissure on the floor of the cranial fossa between the posterior edge of the great wing of the sphenoid bone and the petrous part of the temporal bone.

petrous /pet′rəs/ [L, *petra*, rock], resembling a rock or stone.

Peutz-Jeghers' syndrome /poits′jeg′ərz/ [J. L. A. Peutz, Dutch physician, 1886–1957; Harold J. Jeghers, American physician, b. 1904], an inherited disorder transmitted as an autosomal-dominant trait, characterized by multiple intestinal polyps and abnormal mucocutaneous pigmentation, usually over the lips and buccal mucosa.

Peyer's patches, one of a group of lymphatic nodules forming a single layer in the mucous membrane of the ileum opposite the mesenteric attachment. In most individuals they appear in the distal ileum, but they also appear in the jejunum of a few individuals.

peyote /pā-ō′tē/ [Aztec, *peyotl*], **1.** a cactus from which a hallucinogenic drug, mescaline, is derived. **2.** mescaline.

Peyronie's disease /pārōnēz′/ [François de la Peyronie, French physician, 1678–1747], a disease of unknown cause resulting in fibrous induration of the corpora cavernosa of the penis. The chief symptom of Peyronie's disease is painful erection.

pF, abbreviation for *picofarad.*

PFT, abbreviation for **pulmonary function test**

PG, abbreviation for **prostaglandin.**

PGI$_2$, abbreviation for **prostacyclin.**

PGY, abbreviation for *postgraduate year,* describing medical school graduates during their postgraduate training as interns (PGY-1, first year), residents (PGY-2, 3, 4), or fellows (PGY-4, 5).

pH, abbreviation for *potential hydrogen,* a scale representing the relative acidity (or alkalinity) of a solution, in which a value of 7.0 is neutral, below 7.0 is acid, and above 7.0 is alkaline. The numeric pH value is equal to the negative log of the hydrogen ion concentration expressed in moles per liter.

Ph, symbol for **phenyl.**

Ph^1, symbol for **Philadelphia chromosome.**

PH, abbreviation for **parathyroid hormone.**

PHA, 1. abbreviation for **paraaminohippuric acid. 2.** abbreviation for **phytohemagglutinin.**

phacomalacia /fak′ōməlā′shə/ [Gk, *phalos*, lens, *malkia*, softness], an abnormal condition of the eye in which the lens becomes soft as a result of the presence of a soft cataract.

phaeohyphomycosis /fē′ōhī′fōmīkō′sis/, an opportunistic fungal infection other than mycetoma and chromoblastomycosis caused by the dematiaceous or darkly pigmented molds.

phage typing /fāj/ [Gk, *phagein*, to eat, *typos*, mark], the identification of bacteria by testing their vulnerability to bacterial viruses.

phagocyte /fag′əsīt/ [Gk, *phagein* + *kytos*, cell], a cell that is able to surround, engulf, and digest microorganisms and cellular debris. Fixed noncirculating phagocytes include the fixed macrophages and the cells of the reticuloendothelial system. Free circulating phagocytes include the leukocytes. —**phagocytic,** *adj.*

phagocytic /-sit′ik/ [Gk, *phagein*, to eat, *kytos*, cell], pertaining to phagocytes or phagocytosis.

phagocytize /fag′əsitīz/ [Gk, *phagein*, to eat, *kytos*, cell], to engulf and destroy bacteria or other foreign materials.

phagocytosis /fag′əsītō′sis/ [Gk, *phagein* + *kytos* + *osis*, condition], the process by which certain cells engulf and destroy microorganisms and cellular debris.

phagolysosome, a cytoplasmic body formed by the fusion of a phagosome or ingested particle with a lysosome containing hydrolytic enzymes. The enzymes digest most of the material within the phagosome.

phagosome /fag′əsōm/, a membrane-bound cytoplasmic vesicle within the phagocyte that engulfs it. The vesicle contains phagocytized materials and may fuse with a lysosome, forming a phagolysosome within which the lysosome digests the phagocytized material.

phakomatosis /fak′ōmatō′sis/, *pl.* **phakomatoses** [Gk, *phako*, lens, *oma*, tumor, *osis*, condition], (in ophthalmology) any of several hereditary syndromes characterized by benign tumorlike nodules of the eye, skin, and brain. The four disorders designated phakomatoses are neurofibromatosis (Recklinghausen's disease), tuberous sclerosis (Bourneville's disease), encephalotrigeminal angiomatosis (Sturge-Weber's syndrome), and cerebroretinal angiomatosis (von Hippel-Lindau's disease).

P

phal, 1. abbreviation for **phalanges.** 2. abbreviation for **phalanx.**

phalangeal /fəlan′jē·al/ [Gk, *phalanx,* line of soldiers], pertaining to a phalanx.

phalanx (phal) /fā′langks/, *pl.* **phalanges (phal)** /fəlan′jēz/ [Gk, line of soldiers], any of the 14 tapering bones composing the fingers of each hand and the toes of each foot. They are arranged in three rows at the distal end of the metacarpus and the metatarsus. The fingers each have three phalanges; the thumb has two. The toes each have three phalanges; the great toe has two.

phallic /fal′ik/ [Gk, *phallos,* penis], pertaining to the penis or penis-shaped.

phallic stage [L, *phallos,* penis, *stare,* to stand], (in psychoanalysis) the period in psychosexual development occurring between 3 and 6 years of age when emerging awareness and self-manipulation of the genitals are the predominant source of pleasurable experience.

phallic symbol [Gk, *phallos,* penis, *symbolon,* sign], (in psychoanalysis) any object that may be thought to resemble a penis.

phalloidine /faloi′din/, a poison present in the mushroom *Amanita phalloides.* Ingestion of phalloidin results in bloody diarrhea, vomiting, severe abdominal pain, kidney failure, and liver damage.

phalloplasty /fal′ōplas′tē/, a plastic surgery procedure to lengthen, thicken, reconstruct, or otherwise reshape the penis. It may be performed to correct congenital defects such as epispadias.

phantasm /fan′taz′əm/ [Gk, *phantasma,* vision], an illusory image, such as an optical illusion of something that does not exist.

phantom /fan′təm/ [Gk, *phantasma,* vision], a mass of material similar to human tissue used to investigate the interaction of radiation beams with human beings. Phantom materials can range from water to complex chemical mixtures that faithfully mimic the human body as it would interact with radiation.

phantom images, (in computed tomography) false images that appear but are not actually in the focal plane. They are created by the incomplete blurring or fusion of the blurred margins of some structures characteristic of the type of tomographic motion used.

phantom limb syndrome, a phenomenon common after amputation of a limb in which sensation or discomfort is experienced in the missing limb.

phantom tumor, a swelling resembling a tumor, usually caused by muscle contraction or gaseous distension of the intestines.

phantom vision, a sense perception occurring in the form of a visual illusion or hallucination. It is usually regarded as a pseudohallucination in that the person sensing the perception is aware that the phenomenon is illusory.

phar, 1. abbreviation for **pharmacy.** 2. abbreviation for **pharmacology.** 3. abbreviation for **pharmaceutic.**

Phar.B., abbreviation for *Bachelor of Pharmacy.*

Phar.D., abbreviation for *Doctor of Pharmacy.*

pharmaceutic (phar) /fär′məsoo͞′tik/ [Gk, *pharmakeuein,* to give drugs], 1. pertaining to pharmacy or drugs. 2. a drug.

pharmaceutical chemistry, the science dealing with the composition and preparation of chemical compounds used in medical diagnoses and therapies.

pharmacist /fär′məsist/ [Gk, *pharmakon,* drug], a person prepared to formulate, dispense, and provide clinical information on drugs or medications to health professionals and patients, through completion of a university program in pharmacy of at least 4 years' duration.

pharmacodynamics /-dīnam′iks/ [Gk, *pharmakon,* drug, *dynamis,* power], the study of how a drug acts on a living organism, including the pharmacologic response observed relative to the concentration of the drug at an active site in the organism.

pharmacogenetics /-jənet′iks/ [Gk, *pharmakon,* drug, *genesis,* origin], the study of the effect of the genetic factors belonging to a group or an individual on the response of the group or the individual to certain drugs.

pharmacokinetics /fär′məkōkinet′iks/ [Gk, *pharmakon* + *kinesis,* motion], (in pharmacology) the study of the action of drugs within the body, including the routes and mechanisms of absorption, distribution, excretion, and metabolism; onset of action; duration of effect; biotransformation; and effects and routes of excretion of the metabolites of the drug.

pharmacologic agent /-loj′ik/, any oral, parenteral, or topical substance used to alleviate symptoms and treat or control a disease process or aid recovery from an injury.

pharmacologic vagotomy, the use of medications to curtail functions of the vagus nerve.

pharmacologist /fär′məkol′əjist/, a specialist in the preparation, properties, uses, and actions of drugs.

pharmacology (phar) /-kol′əjē/ [Gk, *pharmakon* + *logos,* science], the study of the preparation, properties, uses, and actions of drugs.

pharmacopoeia /fär'məkəpē'ə/ [Gk, *pharmakon* + *poiein,* to make], **1.** a compendium containing descriptions, recipes, strengths, standards of purity, and dosage forms for selected drugs. **2.** the available stock of drugs in a pharmacy. **3.** the total of all authorized drugs available within the jurisdiction of a given geographic or political area.

pharmacotherapy /-ther'əpē/ [Gk, *pharmakon,* drug, *therapeia*], the use of drugs to treat diseases.

pharmacy (phar) /fär'məsē/ [Gk, *pharmakon*], **1.** the study of preparing and dispensing drugs. **2.** a place for preparing and dispensing drugs.

pharyngeal /ferin'jē·əl/ [Gk, *pharynx,* throat], pertaining to the pharynx.

pharyngeal aponeurosis [Gk, *pharynx,* throat, *apo,* from, *neuron,* sinew], a sheet of connective tissue immediately beneath the mucosa of the pharynx.

pharyngeal bursa, a blind sac at the base of the pharyngeal tonsil.

pharyngeal membrane, a thin fold of ectoderm and endoderm that separates the pharyngeal pouches from the branchial clefts in a developing embryo.

pharyngeal suction catheter, a device that allows direct visualization of a pharyngeal suctioning procedure.

pharyngeal tonsil, one of two masses of lymphatic tissue situated on the posterior wall of the nasopharynx behind the posterior nares.

pharyngitis /fer'inji'tis/ [Gk, *pharynx* + *itis*], inflammation or infection of the pharynx, usually causing symptoms of a sore throat. Some causes of pharyngitis are diphtheria, herpes simplex virus, infectious mononucleosis, and streptococcal infection.

pharyngoconjunctival fever /fəring'gō-kon'jungktī'vəl/ [Gk, *pharnyx* + L, *conjunctivus,* connecting, *febris,* fever], an adenovirus infection characterized by fever, sore throat, and conjunctivitis. Contaminated water in lakes and swimming pools is a common source of infection.

pharyngoscope /fəring'gəskōp/ [Gk, *pharynx* + *skopein,* to view], an endoscopic device for examining the lining of the pharynx.

pharyngoscopy /fer'ing·gos'kəpē/ [Gk, *pharynx,* throat, *skopein,* to view], the examination of the throat with a pharyngoscope.

pharyngotonsillitis /-ton'silī'tis/ [Gk, *pharynx* + L, *tonsilla* + Gk, *itis,* inflammation], an inflammation involving the pharynx and the tonsils.

pharynx /fer'inks/ *pl.* **pharynxes, pharynges** [Gk], the throat, a tubular structure that extends from the base of the skull to the esophagus and is situated immediately in front of the cervical vertebrae. The pharynx serves as a passageway for the respiratory and digestive tracts and changes shape to allow the formation of various vowel sounds. The pharynx is composed of muscle; lined with mucous membrane; and divided into the nasopharynx, the oropharynx, and the laryngopharynx. It contains the openings of the right and left auditory tubes, the openings of the two posterior nares, the fauces, the opening into the larynx, and the opening into the esophagus. It also contains the pharyngeal tonsils, the palatine tonsils, and the lingual tonsils.

phase /fāz/ [Gk, *phasis,* appearance], in a periodic function such as rotational or sinusoidal motion, the position relative to a particular part of the cycle.

phase 0, (in cardiology) the upstroke of the action potential.

phase 1, (in cardiology) the initial rapid repolarization phase of the action potential; seen in ventricular and His-Purkinje action potentials.

phase 2, (in cardiology) the plateau of the action potential; occurs during repolarization.

phase 3, (in cardiology) the terminal rapid repolarization phase of the action potential.

phase 4, (in cardiology) the period of electrical diastole. A graph of phase 4 shows a gradual upward slope in a pacemaker cell, whereas phase 4 in a nonpacemaker cell is flat.

phase-contrast microscopy, a type of light microscopy in which a special condenser and objective with a phase-shifting ring are used to visualize small differences in refractive index as differences in intensity or contrast. It is useful in viewing unstained specimens that appear transparent.

phased array /fāzd/, an array transducer assembly that has very thin rectangular elements arranged side by side. It relies on electronic beam steering to sweep sound beams over a sector-shaped scanned region. Beam steering is done using electronic time delays in the transmitting and receiving circuits.

phase microscope, a microscope with a special condenser and objective containing a phase-shifting ring that allows the viewer to see small differences in refraction indexes as differences in image intensity or contrast.

phase of maximum slope, the time of

rapid cervical dilation and rapid fetal descent in the active phase of labor.

phase one study, a clinical trial to assess the risk that may arise from administering a new treatment modality. A phase two study evaluates the clinical effectiveness of the new modality, and a phase three study compares its effectiveness with that of the best existing treatment.

phasic /fā′zik/ [Gk, *phasis*], **1.** pertaining to a process proceeding in stages or phases. **2.** pertaining to a type of afferent or sensory nerve receptor of the proprioceptive system that responds to rate versus length changes in a muscle spindle.

Ph.D., abbreviation for *Doctor of Philosophy.*

phenacemide /fənas′əmīd/, an anticonvulsant prescribed in the treatment of mixed seizures, particularly mixed forms of psychomotor seizures refractory to other drugs.

phenacetin /fənas′itin/, an analgesic now little used because of its toxicity.

phenazopyridine hydrochloride /fen′əzō-pī′ridēn/, a urinary tract analgesic prescribed to reduce the pain of cystitis or other urinary tract infections.

phencyclidine hydrochloride (PCP) /fen-sī′klidēn/, a piperidine derivative administered parenterally to achieve neuroleptic anesthesia. Because of its marked hallucinogenic properties, it is not used therapeutically in the United States.

phendimetrazine tartrate /fen′dīmet′rə-sēn/, a sympathomimetic amine used as an anorectic agent. It is prescribed to decrease the appetite in the treatment of exogenous types of obesity.

phenelzine sulfate /fē′nəlzēn/, a monoamine oxidase inhibitor prescribed in the treatment of endogenous and other types of depression.

pheniramine maleate /fənir′əmēn, -min/, an antihistamine prescribed in the treatment of hypersensitivity reactions, including rhinitis, skin rash, and pruritus.

phenmetrazine hydrochloride /fənmet′rə-zēn/, a sympathomimetic amine used as an anorectic agent. It is prescribed for reduction of appetite and in the short-term treatment of exogenous obesity.

phenobarbital /fē′nəbär′bital/, a barbiturate anticonvulsant and sedative-hypnotic prescribed in the treatment of seizure disorders and as a long-acting sedative.

phenobarbital-phenytoin serum levels /-fen′itō′in/, the concentration of phenobarbital and phenytoin in the serum, monitored to maintain concentrations sufficient to control seizures but not high enough to cause toxic reactions.

phenocopy /fē′nōkop′ē/ [Gk, *phainein,* to appear; L, *copia,* plenty], a phenotypic trait or condition that is induced by environmental factors but closely resembles a phenotype usually produced by a specific genotype. The trait is neither inherited nor transmitted to offspring. Because phenocopies may present problems in genetic screening and genetic counseling, all exogenous factors must be ruled out before any congenital trait or defect is labeled hereditary.

phenol /fē′nol/ [Gk, *phainein,* to appear; L, *oleum,* oil], **1.** a highly poisonous caustic crystalline chemical derived from coal tar or plant tar or manufactured synthetically. It has a distinctive pungent odor and in solution is a powerful disinfectant, commonly called carbolic acid. **2.** any of a large number and variety of chemical products closely related in structure to the alcohols and containing a hydroxyl group attached to a benzene ring.

phenol block, a type of nerve block using hydroxybenzene (phenol) intended to anesthetize a particular nerve permanently. The technique is sometimes used to control spasticity in specific muscle groups or to block transmission of nerve impulses in chronic pain conditions such as cancers.

phenol camphor, an oily mixture of camphor and phenol, used as an antiseptic and toothache remedy.

phenol coefficient, a measure of the disinfectant activity of a given chemical in relation to carbolic acid.

phenolphthalein /fē′nolthal′ē·in, -thā′lēn/, **1.** a laxative that acts by stimulating the motor activity of the lower intestinal tract. **2.** an indicator of hydrogen ion in urine and gastric juice.

phenolphthalein laxative, a purgative that acts on the wall of the bowel. It is prescribed to treat chronic constipation and to prevent straining at the stool for postoperative patients and those with heart disease or hypertension.

phenol poisoning, corrosive poisoning caused by the ingestion of compounds containing phenol, such as carbolic acid, creosote, cresol, guaiacol, and naphthol. Characteristic of phenol poisoning are burns of the mucous membranes; weakness; pallor; pulmonary edema; seizures; and respiratory, circulatory, cardiac, and renal failure.

phenolsulfonphthalein/fē′nəlsul′fōnfthal′-ē·in/, a bright red dye used as a test for renal function.

phenomenon /finom′ənən/, *pl.* **phenomena** /finom′ənnl/ [Gk, *phainomenon,* something seen], a sign that is often associated with a specific illness or condition and is therefore diagnostically important.

phenothiazine /fē′nōthī′əzēn/, a yellow to green crystalline compound that is a source of dyes and is used in veterinary medicine. It is too toxic for human use, but derivatives of phenothiazine are used in tranquilizers and antihistamine medications.

phenothiazine derivatives, any of a group of drugs that have a three-ring structure in which two benzene rings are linked by a nitrogen and a sulfur. They represent the largest group of antipsychotic compounds in clinical medicine. Of the many phenothiazines and their congeners that are used as adjuncts to general anesthesia, antiemetics, major tranquilizers (antipsychotic agents), and antihistamines, the most widely used are the two prototypes, chlorpromazine and prochlorperazine.

phenotype /fē′nətīp/ [Gk, phainein, to appear, typos, mark], 1. the complete observable characteristics of an organism or group, including anatomic, physiologic, biochemical, and behavioral traits, as determined by the interaction of both genetic makeup and environmental factors. 2. a group of organisms that resemble each other in appearance. —phenotypic, adj.

phenoxybenzamine hydrochloride /fē-nok′sēben′zə-mēn/, an antihypertensive prescribed in the control of hypertension and sweating in pheochromocytoma. If tachycardia is excessive, concomitant administration of propranolol may be necessary.

phensuximide /fensuk′simīd/, an anticonvulsant prescribed to prevent and treat seizures in petit mal epilepsy.

phentermine hydrochloride /fen′tərmēn/, a sympathomimetic amine used as an anorectic agent. It is prescribed to decrease the appetite in the short-term treatment of exogenous obesity.

phentolamine /fentol′əmēn/, an antiadrenergic. It is administered as the hydrochloride form in tablets and as the mesylate form for injections. It is prescribed in the control of symptoms of pheochromocytoma before and during surgery and for dermal necrosis and sloughing after extravasation of parenteral norepinephrine.

phenyl (Ph) /fē′nil, fen′il/, a monovalent organic radical, C_6H_5, derived from benzene.

phenylacetic acid /fen′iləsē′tik/, a metabolite of phenylalanine excreted in urine together with glutamine.

phenylalanine (Phe) /fen′ilal′ənēn/, an essential amino acid necessary for the normal growth and development of infants and children and for normal protein metabolism throughout life.

phenylalaninemia /fen′ilaləninē′mē-ə/,

the presence of phenylalanine in the blood.

phenylbutazone /-bōō′təzōn/, a nonsteroidal antiinflammatory agent prescribed in the treatment of severe symptoms of arthritis, bursitis, and other inflammatory conditions.

phenylephrine hydrochloride /-ef′rēn/, an alpha-adrenergic agent prescribed for maintenance of blood pressure that is used locally as a nasal or ophthalmic vasoconstrictor.

phenylethyl alcohol /-eth′il/, a colorless fragrant liquid with a burning taste, used as a bacteriostatic agent and preservative in medicinal solutions.

phenylketonuria (PKU) /fen′əlkē′tōn-yōōr′ē-ə, fē′nəl-/, abnormal presence of phenylketone and other metabolites of phenylalanine in the urine, characteristic of an inborn metabolic disorder caused by the absence or a deficiency of phenylalanine hydroxylase, the enzyme responsible for the conversion of the amino acid phenylalanine into tyrosine. Accumulation of phenylalanine is toxic to brain tissue. Untreated individuals have very fair hair, eczema, a mousy odor of the urine and skin, and progressive mental retardation. —phenylketonuric, adj.

phenyl-methoxypropyl adenine (PMPA), a drug used in acquired immunodeficiency syndrome treatment. It blocks an enzyme that helps human immunodeficiency virus spread through the body. Unlike some other remedies that must be absorbed into the body's cells to be effective, PMPA can begin blocking the virus as soon as it enters the body.

phenylpropanolamine hydrochloride /fen′əlprō′pənol′-əmēn/, a sympathomimetic amine with vasoconstrictor action. It is prescribed to relieve nasal congestion and related cold symptoms.

phenylpyruvic acid /fen′ilpīrōō′vik/, a product of the metabolism of phenylalanine. The presence of phenylpyruvic acid in the urine is indicative of phenylketonuria.

phenyl salicylate, the salicylic ester of phenol.

phenyltoloxamine citrate /fen′iltəlok′sə-mēn/, an antihistamine usually used in a fixed-combination drug with an analgesic.

phenytoin /fen′ətō′in/, an anticonvulsant prescribed as an anticonvulsant in grand mal and psychomotor seizure disorders and as an antiarrhythmic agent, particularly in digitalis-induced arrhythmias.

pheochromocytoma /fē′ōkrō′mōsītō′mə/ [Gk, phaios, dark, chroma, color, kytos, cell, oma, tumor], a vascular tumor of chromaffin tissue of the adrenal medulla or sympathetic paraganglia, characterized by hypersecretion of epinephrine and norepinephrine, causing persistent or intermittent hypertension. Typical signs include headache, palpitation, sweating, nervousness, hyperglycemia, nausea, vomiting, and syncope. Weight loss, myocarditis, cardiac arrhythmia, and heart failure may occur. The tumor occurs most commonly at 40 to 60 years of age, and only a small percentage of the lesions are malignant.

pheromone /fer'əmōn'/ [Gk, *pherein,* to carry, *hormaein,* to stimulate], a hormonal substance secreted by an organism that elicits a particular response from another individual of the same species, but usually of the opposite sex.

phi /fī/, Φ, φ, the twenty-first letter of the Greek alphabet.

Philadelphia chromosome (Ph^1) [Philadelphia, Pennsylvania], a translocation of the long arm of chromosome 22, often seen in the abnormal myeloblasts, erythroblasts, and megakaryoblasts of patients who have chronic myelocytic leukemia.

philtrum /fil'trəm/, the vertical groove in the center of the upper lip.

phimosis /fīmō'sis/ [Gk, muzzle], tightness of the prepuce of the penis that prevents the retraction of the foreskin over the glans. The condition is usually congenital but may be the result of infection.

phimosis vaginalis /vaj'inā'lis/, congenital narrowness or closure of the vaginal opening.

phlebectomy /fləbek'əmē/ [Gk, *phleps,* vein, *ektome,* cutting out], the surgical removal of a vein or part of a vein.

phlebogram /fleb'əgram/ [Gk, *phleps,* vein, *gramma,* record], 1. a radiograph obtained by phlebography. 2. a graphic representation of the venous pulse, obtained by phlebograph.

phlebograph /fleb'əgraf'/, a device for producing a graphic record of the venous pulse.

phlebography /fləbog'rəfē/ [Gk, *phleps + graphein,* to record], 1. the technique of preparing a radiographic image of veins injected with a radiopaque contrast medium. 2. the technique of preparing a graphic record of the venous pulse by means of a phlebograph.

phlebostasis /-stāsis/, an abnormally slow flow of blood in the veins, which are usually distended.

phlebostatic axis /-stat'ik/ [Gk, *phleps + stasis,* standing still], the approximate location of the right atrium, found by drawing an imaginary line from the fourth intercostal space at the right side of the

sternum to an intersection with the midaxillary line.

phlebothrombosis /fleb'ōthrombō'sis/ [Gk, *phleps + thrombos,* lump, *osis,* condition], an abnormal venous condition in which a clot forms within a vein. It is usually caused by hemostasis, hypercoagulability, or occlusion. In contrast to that in thrombophlebitis, the wall of the vein is not inflamed.

phlebotomist /fləbot'əmist/ [Gk, *phleps,* vein + *ektome*], a person with special training in the practice of drawing blood.

phlebotomize /fləbot'əmīz/ [Gk, *phleps,* vein, *ektome,* excision], to open a vein to remove blood.

phlebotomus fever /fləbot'əməs/ [Gk, *phleps + tomos,* cutting; L, *febris,* fever], an acute mild infection, caused by one of five distinct arboviruses transmitted to humans by the bite of an infected sandfly, characterized by rapidly developing fever, headache, eye pain, conjunctivitis, myalgia, and occasionally a macular or urticarial rash.

phlebotomy /fləbot'əmē/ [Gk, *phleps + temnein,* to cut], the incision of a vein for the letting of blood, as in collecting blood from a donor. Phlebotomy is the chief treatment for polycythemia vera and may be performed every 6 months or more frequently if required.

Phlebotomy: Arterial Blood Sample, a Nursing Interventions Classification defined as obtaining a blood sample from an uncannulated artery to assess oxygen and carbon dioxide levels and acid-base balance.

Phlebotomy: Blood Unit Acquisition, a Nursing Interventions Classification defined as procuring blood and blood products from donors.

Phlebotomy: Venous Blood Sample, a Nursing Interventions Classification defined as removal of a sample of venous blood from an uncannulated vein.

phlegm /flem/ [Gk, *phlegma,* mucus, sluggishness], thick mucus secreted by the tissues lining the airways of the lungs.

phlegmasia alba dolens [Gk, *phlegmone,* inflammation; L, *albus,* white, *dolens,* painful], thrombophlebitis of the femoral vein, resulting in edema of the leg and pain. It may occur after childbirth or after a severe febrile illness.

phlegmasia cerulea dolens, a severe form of thrombosis of a deep vein, usually the femoral vein. The condition is acute and fulminating and is usually accompanied by cyanosis of the limb distal to the occluding thrombosis.

phlegmatic /flegmat'ik/ [Gk, *phlegma,* mucus, sluggishness], pertaining to a person who may be dull or apathetic, or calm and composed to an extent that excitation is difficult.

phlegmon /fleg'mon/ [Gk, *phlegmone,* inflammation], an inflammation of connective tissue.

phlegmonous gastritis /fleg'mənsəs/ [Gk, *phlegmone + osis,* condition], a rare but severe form of gastritis, involving the connective tissue layer of the stomach wall.

phlyctenular keratoconjunctivitis /flikten'yələr/ [Gk, *phlyktaina,* blister], an inflammatory condition of the cornea, characterized by tiny ulcerating nodules. It is seen most often in children as a response to allergens found in tuberculin, gonococci, *Candida albicans,* or various parasites.

PHO, abbreviation for **physician-hospital organization.**

phobia /fō'bē·ə/ [Gk, *phobos,* fear], an obsessive, irrational, and intense fear of a specific object, such as an animal or dirt; of an activity, such as leaving the familiar setting of the home; or of a physical situation, such as heights. Typical manifestations of phobia include faintness, fatigue, palpitations, perspiration, nausea, tremor, and panic. **—phobic,** *adj.*

phobiac /fō'bē·ak/, a person who exhibits or is afflicted with a phobia.

phobic /fō'bik/ [Gk, *phobos,* fear], pertaining to or resembling phobia.

phobic desensitization [Gk, *phobos,* fear; L, *de + sentire,* to feel], a method of resolving an ego dystonic or uncomfortable behavior pattern by reentry into the emotionally upsetting life situation in stages, first in fantasy and again in real life. It is similar to the psychotherapeutic techniques of **flooding** and implosive therapy.

phobic state, a condition characterized by extreme anxiety resulting from the excessive, irrational fear of a particular object, situation, or activity.

phocomelia /fō'kəmē'lyə/ [Gk, *phoke,* seal, *melos,* limb], a developmental anomaly characterized by absence of the upper part of one or more of the limbs so that the feet or hands or both are attached to the trunk of the body by short, irregularly shaped stumps, resembling the fins of a seal. **—phocomelic,** *adj.*

phocomelic dwarf /fō'kəmē'lik/, a dwarf in whom the long bones of any or all of the extremities are abnormally short.

phocomelus /fōkom'ələs/, an individual who has phocomelia.

phonation /fōnā'shən/ [Gk, *phone,* sound; L, *atio,* process], the production of speech sounds through the vibration of the vocal folds of the larynx.

phonetics /fōnet'iks/ [Gk, *phone,* voice], the science of speech sounds used in language.

phonic, pertaining to voice, sounds, or speech.

phonocardiogram /-kär'dē·əgram'/, a graphic recording obtained from a phonocardiograph.

phonocardiograph /-kär'dē·əgraf'/ [Gk, *phone,* sound, *kardia,* heart, *graphein,* to record], an electroacoustic device that produces graphic heart sound recordings, used in the diagnosis and monitoring of heart disorders. This instrument produces phonocardiograms by using a system of microphones and associated recording equipment. **—phonocardiographic,** *adj.*

phonocardiography /-kär'dē·og'rəfē/ [Gk, *phone + kardia + graphein,* to record], the recording of heart sounds and murmurs by an electromechanical apparatus.

phonology /fōnol'əjē/, the study of speech sounds, particularly the principles governing the way speech sounds are used in a given language.

phonophoresis /fō'nōfərē'sis/, an ultrasound therapeutic technique in which the high-frequency sound waves are used to force topical medicines into subcutaneous tissues. The technique is used with caution.

phonoreceptor /-risep'tər/ [Gk, *phone,* sound; L, *recipere,* to receive], a device for receiving sound impulses.

phosphatase /fos'fətāz/, an enzyme that acts as a catalyst in chemical reactions involving phosphorus. It is essential in the calcification of bone.

phosphate /fos'fāt/, a salt of phosphoric acid. Phosphates are extremely important in living cells, particularly in the storage and use of energy and the transmission of genetic information.

phosphate-bond energy, the Gibbs energy for hydrolysis of a phosphate compound; a measure of relative phosphorylation power.

phosphatemia /fos'fātē'mē·ə/ [Gk, *phosphoros,* bringer of light; Gk, *haima,* blood], a condition of excessive levels of phosphates in the blood.

phosphatide /fos'fətīd/, a phosphatidic acid from which the choline or colamine part has been removed. It may occur as an intermediate in the biosynthesis of triglycerides and phospholipids.

phosphaturia /fos'fətōōr'ē·ə/ [Gk, *phosphoros,* bringer of light, *ouron,* urine], an excessive level of phosphates in the urine.

phosphoglycerate kinase /fos'fōglis'ərāt/, an enzyme that catalyzes the reversible transfer of a phosphate group from adenosine triphosphate to D-3-phosphoglycerate, forming D-1,3-diphosphoglycerate. The reaction is one of the steps in glycolysis.

phospholipase /fos'fōlī'pās/, any of a group of enzymes that catalyze the hydrolysis of phospholipids. Various phospholipases digest cell membranes, aid in the synthesis of prostaglandins, and help produce arachidonic acid, one of the essential fatty acids.

phospholipid /fos'fōlip'id/ [Gk, *phos*, light, *pherein*, to bear, *lipos* fat], one of a class of compounds, widely distributed in living cells, containing phosphoric acid, fatty acids, and a nitrogenous base. Two kinds of phospholipids are **lecithin** and **sphingomyelin.**

phosphomevalonate kinase /fos'fōməval'-ənāt/, an enzyme that catalyzes the transfer of a phosphate group from adenosine triphosphate to produce adenosine diphosphate and 5-pyrophosphomevalonate.

phosphorescence /fos'fôres'əns/ [Gk, *phos*, light, *pherein*, to bear], **1.** a glow of yellow phosphorus caused by slow oxidation. **2.** the emission of visible light without accompanying heat as observed in phosphorus that has been exposed to radiation, which continues after radiation has ceased.

phosphoric acid /fosfôr'ik/, a clear, colorless, odorless liquid that is irritating to the skin and eyes and moderately toxic if ingested.

phosphorus (P) /fos'fərəs/ [Gk, *phos*, light, *pherein*, to bear], a nonmetallic chemical element occurring extensively in nature as a component of phosphate rock. Its atomic number is 15; its atomic mass (weight) is 30.975. Phosphorus is essential for the metabolism of protein, calcium, and glucose; and to the body for the production of adenosine triphosphate and for the process of glycolysis. A nutritional deficiency of phosphorus can cause weight loss, anemia, and abnormal growth.

phosphorus poisoning, a toxic condition caused by the ingestion of white or yellow phosphorus, sometimes found in rat poisons, certain fertilizers, and fireworks. Intoxication is characterized initially by nausea, throat and stomach pain, vomiting, diarrhea, and an odor of garlic on the breath.

phosphorylase /fosfôr'ilās/ [Gk, *phosphoros*, bringer of light + *ase*, enzyme suffix], any of a group of physiologically important enzymes that catalyze reactions between phosphates and glycogen or other starch components, yielding glucose-1-phosphate.

phosphorylation /fosfôr'ilā'shən/, the process of attaching a phosphate group to a protein, sugar, or other compound.

photic /fō'tik/ [Gk, *phos*, light], pertaining to light.

photic epilepsy [Gk, *phos*, light, *epilepsia*, seizure], a condition in which epileptic attacks may be triggered by flickering light.

photoallergic /-əlur'gik/ [Gk, *phos*, light, *allos*, other, *ergein*, to work], exhibiting a delayed hypersensitivity reaction after exposure to light.

photoallergic contact dermatitis, a papulovesicular, eczematous, or exudative skin reaction that occurs 24 to 48 hours after exposure to light in a previously sensitized person. The sensitizing substance concentrates in the skin and requires chemical alteration by light to become an active antigen. Among common photosensitizers are phenothiazines, hexachlorophene, oral hypoglycemic agents, and sulfanilamide.

photoallergy /-al'ərjē/ [Gk, *phos*, light, *allos*, other + *ergein*, to work], a sensitivity to light that causes allergic reactions.

photobiology /-bī·ol'əjē/, the study of the effects of light on living organisms.

photochemotherapy /-kē'mōther'əpē/ [Gk, *phos* + *chemeia*, alchemy, *therapeia*, treatment], a kind of chemotherapy in which the effect of the administered drug is enhanced by exposing the patient to light.

photochromogen /-krō'məjen/, **1.** a pigment that develops as a result of exposure to light. **2.** a type of mycobacterium that is nonpigmented in the dark but produces a yellow pigment on constant exposure to light.

photodisintegration /-disin'təgrā'shən/, (in radiology) the interaction of a high-energy x-ray photon with the nucleus of a target atom, resulting in the emission of a nucleon or other nuclear fragment.

photoelectron /-ilek'tron/ [Gk, *phos*, light + *elektron*, amber], any electron that is discharged when light strikes a metal surface.

photokinetic /-kinet'ik/ [Gk, *phos*, light, *kinesis*, movement], pertaining to any movement that is stimulated by light rays.

photometer /fōtom'ətər/ [Gk, *phos* + *metron*, measure], an instrument that measures light intensity.

photomultiplier /-mul'tiplī'ər/ [Gk, *phos*, light; L, *multiplex*, many folds], a device used in many radiation detection applications that converts low levels of light into electrical pulses.

photon /fō'ton/ [Gk, *phos*, light], the smallest quantity of electromagnetic energy. It has no mass and no charge but travels at the speed of light. Photons may occur in the form of x-rays, gamma rays, or quanta of light.

photophobia /-fō'bē-ə/ [Gk, *phos* + *phobos*, fear], **1.** abnormal sensitivity to light, especially by the eyes. The condition is prevalent in albinism and various diseases of the conjunctiva and cornea and may be a symptom of such disorders as measles, psittacosis, encephalitis, Rocky Mountain spotted fever, and Reiter's syndrome. **2.** (in psychiatry) a morbid fear of light with an irrational need to avoid light places. —**photophobic,** *adj.*

photopic vision /fōtop'ik/, daylight vision, which depends primarily on the function of the retinal cone cells.

photoprotective /-prətek'tiv/, protective against the potential adverse effects of ultraviolet light.

photoreaction /-rē·ak'shən/ [Gk, *phos* + L, *re,* again, *agere,* to act], any chemical reaction that is stimulated by the influence of light.

photoreceptor /-risep'tər/ [Gk, *phos,* light; L, *recipere,* to receive], a nerve cell that is receptive to light stimuli.

photorefractive keratectomy (PRK) /-re-frak'tiv/, a surgical procedure in which an excimer laser is used to reshape the human cornea to improve the refractive properties of the eye and reduce or eliminate the need for eye glasses. Rather than cutting, the laser shaves off preprogrammed outer layers of corneal tissue.

photoscan /fo'tōskan'/, a radiograph that shows the distribution of a radiopharmaceutical in the body.

photosensitive /-sen'sitiv/ [Gk, *phos* + L, *sentire,* to feel], pertaining to increased reactivity of skin to sunlight caused by a disorder such as albinism or porphyria, or more frequently resulting from the use of certain drugs. Relatively brief exposure to sunlight or to an ultraviolet lamp may cause edema, papules, urticaria, or acute burns in individuals with endogenous or acquired photosensitivity.

photosensitivity /-sen'sitiv'itē/, any abnormal response to exposure to light, specifically, a skin reaction requiring the presence of a sensitizing agent and exposure to sunlight or its equivalent.

photosensitization /-sen'sitīzā'shən/ [Gk, *phos,* light; L, *sentire,* to feel], the process of rendering an organism sensitive to the effects of light rays.

photosynthesis /fōtōsin'thəsis/ [Gk, *phos* + *synthesis,* putting together], a process by which green plants containing chlorophyll synthesize chemical substances, chiefly carbohydrates, from atmospheric carbon dioxide and water, using light for

energy and liberating oxygen in the process.

phototherapy /-ther'əpē/ [Gk, *phos* + *therapeia* treatment], the treatment of disorders by the use of light, especially ultraviolet light. Ultraviolet light may be used in the therapy of acne, pressure ulcers and other indolent ulcers, psoriasis, and hyperbilirubinemia. —**phototherapeutic,** *adj.*

phototherapy in the newborn, a treatment for hyperbilirubinemia and jaundice in the newborn that involves the exposure of an infant's bare skin to intense fluorescent light. The blue range of light accelerates the excretion of bilirubin in the skin, decomposing it by photooxidation.

Phototherapy: Neonate, a Nursing Interventions Classification defined as use of light therapy to reduce bilirubin levels in newborn infants.

phototoxic /-tok'sik/ [Gk, *phos* + *toxikon,* poison], characterized by a rapidly developing nonimmunologic reaction of the skin when it is exposed to a photosensitizing substance and light.

phototoxic contact dermatitis, a rapidly appearing, sunburnlike response of areas of skin that have been exposed to the sun after contact with a photosensitizing substance. Hyperpigmentation may follow the acute reaction. Coal tar derivatives, oil of bergamot (often used in cosmetics and beverages), and many plants containing furocoumarin (cowslip, buttercup, carrot, parsnip, mustard, and yarrow) are known photosensitizing materials.

phren /fren/ [Gk, mind], **1.** the diaphragm. **2.** the mind.

phrenetic /frənet'ik/ [Gk, *phren*], frenzied, delirious, maniacal.

phrenic /fren'ik/ [Gk, *phren,* mind], **1.** pertaining to the diaphragm. **2.** pertaining to the mind.

phrenic nerve, one of a pair of branches of the cervical plexus, arising from the first four cervical nerves. It contains about half as many sensory as motor fibers and is generally known as the motor nerve to the diaphragm, although the lower thoracic nerves also help to innervate the diaphragm.

phrenology [Gk, *phren,* mind], the study of the conformation of the skull based on the assumption that mental faculties are localized in particular sites on the surface of the brain. According to phrenologists, intelligence or other faculties of a person may be mirrored through elevations in the skull overlying the particular area of the brain.

PHSP, abbreviation for **physician health service plan.**

Phthirus /thī′rəs/ [Gk, *phtheir,* louse], a genus of blood-sucking lice that includes the species *Phthirus pubis,* the pubic louse, or crab.

phthisis /tis′is, thī′sis/ [Gk, *phthisis,* wasting away], any wasting disease involving all or part of the body, such as pulmonary tuberculosis.

phycologist /fēkol′əjist/, a person who specializes in the study of algae.

phycology /fēkol′əjē/ [Gk, *phykos,* seaweed, *logos,* science], the branch of science that is concerned with algae.

phycomycosis /fī′kōmīkō′sis/ [Gk, *phykos* + *mykes,* fungus, *osis* condition], a fungal infection caused by a species of the order Phycomycetes. These organisms are common in the soil and are not usually pathogenic.

phylactic /filak′tik/ [Gk, *phylax,* guard], 1. serving to protect. 2. something that produces phylaxis.

phylogenetic /fī′lōgənet′ik/ [Gk, *phylon,* tribe, *genesis,* origin], 1. relating to or acquired during phylogeny. 2. based on a natural evolutionary relationship, such as a system of classification.

phylogeny /filoj′ənē/ [Gk, *phylon* + *genesis*], the development of the structure of a particular race or species as it evolved from simpler forms of life.

phylum /fī′ləm/ [Gk, *phylon,* tribe], a major classification category of the plant and animal kingdoms, representing one or more classes.

physiatrics /fiz′ē·at′riks/ [Gr, *physis,* nature, *iatrikos,* treatment], a specialized field of physical medicine and rehabilitation. It includes the diagnosis and treatment of disease by the use of physical agents such as heat, cold, light, water, electricity, and mechanical devices.

physiatrist /fiz′ē·at′rist/, a physician specializing in physical medicine and rehabilitation who has been certified by the American Board of Physical Medicine and Rehabilitation after completing residency and other requirements.

physical abuse /fiz′ikəl/ [Gk, *physikos,* natural; L, *abuti,* to abuse], one or more episodes of aggressive behavior, usually resulting in physical injury with possible damage to internal organs, sense organs, the central nervous system, or the musculoskeletal system of another person.

physical allergy, an allergic response to physical factors, such as cold, heat, light, or trauma. Usually specific antibodies are found in people having physical allergies. Common characteristics include pruritus, urticaria, and angioedema.

physical assessment, the part of the health assessment representing a synthesis of the information obtained in a physical examination.

physical chemistry, the natural science dealing with the relationship between chemical and physical properties of matter.

physical diagnosis, the diagnostic process accomplished by the study of the physical manifestations of health, disease, and illness revealed in the physical examination, as guided by the patient's complete history and supported by various laboratory tests.

physical examination, an investigation of the body to determine its state of health, using any or all of the techniques of inspection, palpation, percussion, auscultation, and smell. The physical examination, history, and initial laboratory tests constitute the data base on which a diagnosis is made and on which a plan of treatment is developed.

physical fitness, the ability to carry out daily tasks with alertness and vigor, without undue fatigue, and with enough energy reserve to meet emergencies or to enjoy leisure time pursuits.

physical medicine, the use of rehabilitation specialties, including physical therapy, occupational therapy, speech therapy, and recreational therapy to return physically diseased or injured patients to their maximum potential.

Physical Restraint, a Nursing Interventions Classification defined as application, monitoring, and removal of mechanical restraining devices or manual restraints that are used to limit physical mobility of a patient.

physical science, the study of the properties and behavior of nonliving matter. Some kinds of physical science are **chemistry,** geology, and **physics.**

physical sign [Gk, *physikos,* natural; L, *signum*], an objective indicator found during physical diagnosis or detected by palpation, percussion, or auscultation.

physical therapist, a person who is licensed in the examination, testing, and treatment of physical impairments through the use of special exercise, application of heat or cold, and other physical modalities. A physical therapist becomes qualified by studying a 4- to 7-year college curriculum leading to a bachelor's or master's degree in physical therapy (usually B.S, M.S. or M.P.T.).

physical therapist assistant, a person who, under the supervision of a licensed physical therapist, assists in carrying out patient treatment programs and performing related clerical tasks.

physical therapy, the treatment of disorders with physical agents and methods, such as massage, manipulation, therapeutic exercises, cold, heat (including shortwave and microwave diathermy and ultrasonic heat), hydrotherapy, electrical stimulation, and light to assist in habilitating or rehabilitating patients and in restoring function after an illness or injury.

physician /fizish'ən/ [Gk, *physikos,* natural], a health professional who has earned a degree of Doctor of Medicine (M.D.) after completing an approved course of study at an approved medical school. Satisfactory completion of National Board Examinations, usually given during both the second and the final years of medical school and after graduation, is also required. An M.D. usually enters a hospital internship or residency program for 1 year of postgraduate training before beginning practice or further training in a specialty. To practice medicine, an M.D. is required to obtain a license from the state in which professional services will be performed.

physician extender, a health care provider who is not a physician but who performs medical activities typically performed by a physician.

physician health service plan, (in the United States) a general term relating to an arrangement for provision of professional (physician) services only.

physician-hospital organization (PHO), (in the United States) a management service organization in which the partners are physicians and a hospital. The PHO organization contracts for physician and hospital services.

physician's assistant (PA), a person trained in certain aspects of the practice of medicine to provide assistance to a physician. A physician's assistant is trained by physicians and practices under the direction and supervision and within the legal license of a physician. Training programs vary in length from a few months to 2 years. National certification is available to qualified graduates of approved training programs. The national organization is the American Association of Physician's Assistants.

Physician's Desk Reference (PDR), a compendium compiled annually, containing information about drugs, primarily prescription drugs and products used in diagnostic procedures in the United States, supplied by their manufacturers.

Physician Support, a Nursing Interventions Classification defined as collaborating with physicians to provide high-quality patient care.

physicist /fis'isist/, a scientist who specializes in physics.

physics /fiz'iks/ [Gk, *physikos,* natural], the study of matter and energy, particularly as related to motion and force.

physiognomy /fiz'ē·og'nəmē/ [Gk, *physis,* nature, *gnosis,* knowledge], a method of judging the personality and other characteristics of a client by studying the face and general carriage of the body.

physiologic /fiz'ē·əloj'ik/ [Gk, *physis,* nature, *logos,* science], pertaining to physiology, particularly normal functions as opposed to the pathologic.

physiologic age [Gk, *physis,* nature, *logos,* science; L, *aetas,* age], the age of the body as determined by its stage of development in terms of functional norms for various systems.

physiologic albuminuria [Gk, *physis,* nature, *logos,* science; L, *albus,* white; Gk, *ouron,* urine], the presence of albumin in the urine in the absence of any disease.

physiologic amenorrhea [Gk, *physis,* nature, *logos,* science, *a* + *men,* month, *rhoia,* to flow], an absence of menstruation having a nonpathologic cause such as pregnancy, lactation, menopause, or a prepubertal state of maturity.

physiologic antidote [Gk, *physis* + *logos* + *anti,* against, *dotos,* that which is given], a drug that has the opposite effect on the body from that caused by a poisonous or toxic substance.

physiologic contracture [Gk, *physis* + *logos,* science; L, *contractio,* drawing together], a temporary condition in which muscles may contract and shorten for a considerable period. Drugs, temperature extremes, and local accumulation of lactic acid are possible causes.

physiologic flexion, an excessive amount of flexor tone that is normally present at birth because of the existing level of central nervous system maturation and fetal positioning in the uterus.

physiologic hypertrophy, a temporary increase in the size of an organ or part caused by normal physiologic functions, such as occurs in the walls of the uterus and in the breasts during pregnancy.

physiologic incompatibility, a condition in which substances such as drugs may have mutually antagonistic effects on the body.

physiologic jaundice [Gk, *physis,* nature, *logos,* science; Fr, *jaune,* yellow], a simple jaundice of newborns that involves the breaking down of the excessive number of red blood cells that may be present at birth.

physiologic motivation, a body need, such as for food or water, that initiates behavior directed toward satisfying the particular need.

physiologic murmur [Gk, *physis* + *logos* + L, *murmur*, humming], a functional murmur produced by an alteration of function without evidence of heart damage or disease.

physiologic occlusion, 1. a closure of the teeth that complements and enhances the functions of the masticatory system. 2. a closure of the teeth that produces no pathologic effects on the stomatognathic system, normally dissipating the stresses placed on the teeth and creating a balance between the stresses and the adaptive capacity of the supporting tissues. 3. an acceptable occlusion in a healthy gnathic system.

physiologic psychology, the study of the interrelationship of physiologic and psychologic processes, especially the effects of a change from normal to abnormal.

physiologic retraction ring, a ridge around the inside of the uterus that forms during the second stage of normal labor at the junction of the thinned lower uterine segment and thickened upper segment. It forms as a result of progressive lengthening of the muscle fibers of the lower segment and concomitant shortening of the muscle fibers of the upper segment.

physiologic salt solution, a normal saline solution, usually consisting of a sterile 0.9% w/v solution of sodium chloride in distilled water. It is isotonic with normal body fluids.

physiologic third heart sound, a low-pitched extra heart sound heard early in diastole in a healthy child or young adult. The same sound, heard in an older person who has heart disease, is an abnormal finding called a ventricular gallop.

physiologic tremor [Gk, *physis* + *logos*; L, *tremor*, shaking], any shaking or trembling caused by physiologic factors such as fatigue, fear, or cold.

physiologist /fiz′ē·ol′əjist/ [Gk, *physis*, nature, *logos*, science], a person who specializes in the science of living organisms.

physiology /fix′ē·ol′əjē/ [Gk, *physis* + *logos*, science], 1. the study of the processes and function of the human body. 2. the study of the physical and chemical processes involved in the functioning of living organisms and their component parts.

physiopathologic /fiz′ē·əpath′əloj′ik/ [Gk, *physis*, nature, *pathos*, disease, *logos*, science], pertaining to the physiologic approach to disease.

physique /fizēk′/, the body structure and development of a person.

physostigmine /fī′sōstig′min/, an acetyl-cholinesterase inhibitor prescribed to treat some forms of glaucoma and to reverse effects of neuromuscular blocking agents.

physostigmine salicylate, an anticholinergic drug antidote prescribed in the treatment of central nervous system effects caused by drugs in clinical or toxic dosages capable of producing anticholinergic poisoning.

phytanic acid storage disease /fītan′ik/, a rare genetic disorder of lipid metabolism in which phytanic acid accumulates in the plasma and tissues. The condition is characterized by ataxia, peripheral neuropathy, retinitis pigmentosa, and abnormalities of the bone and skin.

phytogenesis /fī′tōjen′əsis/ [Gk, *phyton*, plant, *genein*, to produce], the origin and evolution of plant organisms.

phytogenous /fītoj′ənəs/ [Gk, *phyton*, plant, *genein*, to produce], pertaining to production by plant growth, origin in a plant, or origin or formation of plant organisms.

phytohemagglutinin (PHA) /fī′tōhem′-əgloo′tinin/ [Gk, *phyton*, plant, *haima*, blood; L, *agglutinare*, to glue], a hemagglutinin that is derived from a plant, specifically the lectin obtained from the red kidney bean.

phytohemagglutinin test, a test to identify genetic carriers of cystic fibrosis, performed by exposing white blood cells to phytohemagglutinin. A normal reaction involves a noticeable increase of cell protein.

pi /pī/, Π, π, the sixteenth letter of the Greek alphabet.

P.I., 1. (in patient records) abbreviation for *present illness*. 2. abbreviation for *International Pharmacopeia*.

pia, abbreviation for **pia mater.**

piaarachnoid /pī′ə·arak′noid/ [L, *pia*, tender; Gk, *arachne*, spider, *eidos*, form], pertaining to both the pia mater and arachnoid layers of the meninges covering the brain and spinal cord.

Piaget, Jean, (1896–1980) a Swiss psychologist and genetic epistemologist who established the Genevan school of developmental psychology. From his original training in zoology and his early work in testing laboratory schoolchildren, Piaget developed a premise that human intelligence is an extension of biologic adaptation. He assumed that human intelligence evolves in a series of stages that are related to age. At each successive stage intellectual adaptation is more general and shows a higher level of logical organization.

piagetian, pertaining to the theories and viewpoints of **Jean Piaget.**

pia mater (pia) /pē'ə mā'tər/ [L, *pia,* tender, *mater,* mother], the innermost of the three meninges covering the brain and spinal cord. It is closely applied to both structures and carries a rich supply of blood vessels, which nourish the nervous tissue. The cranial pia mater covers the surface of the brain and dips into the fissures and sulci of the cerebral hemispheres. The spinal pia mater is thicker, firmer, and less vascular than the cranial pia mater.

pica /pī'kə/ [L, magpie], a craving to eat nonfood substances such as dirt, clay, chalk, glue, ice, starch, or hair. The appetite disorder may occur with some nutritional deficiency states (particularly iron deficiency), with pregnancy, and in some forms of mental illness.

Pick's disease [Arnold Pick, Czech neurologist, 1851–1924], a form of dementia occurring in middle age. This disorder mainly affects the frontal and temporal lobes of the brain and characteristically produces neurotic behavior; slow disintegration of intellect, personality, and emotions; and degeneration of cognitive abilities.

Pick's disease [Friedel Pick, Czech physician, 1867–1926], a condition of constrictive inflammation of the mediastinum and pericardium, leading to chronic venous congestion and cirrhosis.

pickwickian syndrome /pikwik'ē-ən/ [*Pickwick Papers* by Charles Dickens], an abnormal condition characterized by obesity, decreased pulmonary function, somnolence, and polycythemia.

picogram (pg) /pī'kəgram/, a unit of measure equal to one trillionth of a gram, or 10^{-12} gram.

picornavirus /pīkôr'nəvī'rəs/ [It, *pico,* small; *RNA,* ribonucleic acid; L, *virus,* poison], a member of a group of small ribonucleic acid viruses that are ether-resistant. The two main genera are *Enterovirus* and *Rhinovirus.* These viruses cause poliomyelitis, herpangina, aseptic meningitis, encephalomyocarditis, and foot-and-mouth disease.

picosecond (ps), a unit of measure equal to one trillionth of a second.

picrotoxin /pik'rōtok'sin/ [Gk, *pikros,* bitter, *toxikon,* poison], a central nervous system stimulant obtained from the seeds of *Anamirta cocculus,* formerly used as an antidote for acute barbiturate poisoning.

PID, abbreviation for **pelvic inflammatory disease.**

PIE, abbreviation for *pulmonary infiltrate with eosinophilia,* a hypersensitivity reaction characterized by infiltration of alveoli with eosinophils and large mononuclear cells, edema, and inflammation of the lungs. Simple pulmonary eosinophilia, in which patchy, migratory infiltrates cause minimal symptoms, is a self-limited reaction that is elicited by helminthic infections and certain drugs. A more prolonged illness, characterized by fever, night sweats, cough, dyspnea, weight loss, and more severe tissue reaction, occurs in certain drug allergies and bacterial, fungal, and parasitic infections.

piebald /pī'bôld/ [L, *pica,* magpie; ME, *balled,* smooth], having patches of white hair or skin caused by an absence of melanocytes in those nonpigmented areas. It is a hereditary condition. —**piebaldism,** *n.*

Piedmont fracture /pēd'mənt/, an oblique fracture of the distal radius, with fragments of bone pulled into the ulna.

piedra /pē·ā'drə/, fungal disease of the hair characterized by the presence of small black or white nodules. Black piedra is caused by *Piedria bortae.* White piedra (called trichosporosis) is caused by *Trichosporon biegetii.*

Pierre Robin's syndrome /pyerob'inz, pyerōbaNs'/ [Pierre Robin, French histologist, 1867–1950], a complex of congenital anomalies, including a small mandible, cleft lip, cleft palate, other craniofacial abnormalities, and defects of the eyes and ears, including glaucoma. Intelligence is usually normal.

piezochemistry /pī·ē'zōkem'istrē/ [Gk, *piezein,* to press, *chemeia* alchemy], a branch of chemistry concerned with reactions that occur under pressure.

piezoelectric effect /pī·ē'zō·ilek'trik/ [Gk, *piezein,* to press, *elektron* amber; L *effectus*], **1.** the generation of a voltage across a solid when a mechanical stress is applied. **2.** the dimensional change resulting from the application of a voltage. **3.** (in ultrasound) the conversion of one form of energy into another, such as the conversion of electrical energy into mechanical energy.

pigeon breast /pij'ən/ [L, *pipio,* young bird; AS, *broest,* breast], a congenital structural defect characterized by a prominent anterior projection of the xiphoid and the lower part of the sternum and by a lengthening of the costal cartilages. It may cause cardiorespiratory complications. —**pigeon-breasted,** *adj.*

pigeon breeder's lung, a respiratory disorder caused by acquired hypersensitivity to antigens in bird droppings.

piggyback port [AS, *piken,* pick; ME, *pakke,* pack; L, *portus,* haven], a special coupling for the primary intravenous (IV) tubing that allows a supplementary, or piggyback, solution to run into the IV system.

pigment /pig'mənt/ [L, *pigmentum,* paint],

P

1. any organic coloring material produced in the body, such as melanin. **2.** any colored, paintlike medicinal preparation applied to the skin surface. —**pigmentary, pigmented,** *adj.,* **pigmentation,** *n.*

pigmentary retinopathy /pig'mənter'ē/, a disorder of the retina characterized by deposits of pigment and increasing loss of vision.

pigmented villonodular synovitis /pig'-məntid/, a disease of the joints characterized by fingerlike proliferative growths of synovial tissue, with hemosiderin deposition within the synovial tissue.

pigment layers, the parts of the eye comprising the pigmented strata of the ciliary body, iris, and retina.

pil, abbreviation for the Latin words *pilula,* 'pill,' and *pilulae,* 'pills.'

pilar cyst /pī'lər/ [L, *pilus,* hair; Gk, *kystis,* bag], an epidermoid cyst of the scalp. The cyst originates from the middle part of the epithelium of a hair follicle.

piliform /pī'lifôrm/ [L, *pilus,* hair], having the appearance of hair.

pi lines /pī/, radiograph artifacts that result from dirt or chemical stains on a processing roller.

pillion fracture /pil'yən/ [Gael, *pillean,* couch; L, *fractura,* break], a T-shaped fracture of the distal femur with displacement of the condyles posterior to the femoral shaft, caused by a severe blow to the knee.

pilocarpine and epinephrine /-kär'pēn/, a fixed-combination drug used in the treatment of glaucoma, containing a cholinergic (pilocarpine hydrochloride) and an adrenergic (epinephrine bitartrate) vasoconstrictor.

pilocarpine and physostigmine, a fixed-combination drug used in the treatment of glaucoma, containing a cholinergic (pilocarpine hydrochloride) and a short-acting (physostigmine salicylate) cholinesterase inhibitor. Both ingredients reduce intraocular pressure.

pilocarpine hydrochloride, a cholinergic derived from the leaves of the jaborandi tree and other species of *Pilocarpus.* It is used mainly as a miotic to contract the pupil in cases of glaucoma. The drug also increases the secretion of salivary, intestinal, and gastric glands when injected; reduces the heartbeat; and constricts the bronchioles.

pilomotor reflex /pī'lōmō'tər/ [L, *pilus,* hair, *motor,* mover, *reflectere,* to bend back], erection of the hairs of the skin caused by contraction of small involuntary arrector muscles (arrectores pilorum) in response to a chilly environment, emotional stimulus, or skin irritation.

pilonidal /pī'lənī'dəl/ [L, *pilus,* hair, *nidus,* nest], a growth of hair in a cyst or other internal structure.

pilonidal cyst [L, *pilus* + *nidus,* nest], a cyst that often develops in the sacral region of the skin. Pilonidal cysts may sometimes be recognized at birth by a depression; sometimes by a hairy dimple in the midline of the back in the sacrococcygeal area.

pilonidal fistula, an abnormal channel containing a tuft of hair, situated most frequently over or close to the tip of the coccyx but also occurring in other regions of the body.

pilonidal sinus [L, *pilus* + *nidus* + *sinus,* curve], a cavity or sinus containing hair, such as the axilla or navel. In most instances the hair originates in another area and becomes lodged in the sinus.

pilosebaceous /pī'lōsibā'shəs/ [L, *pilus* + *sebum,* fat], pertaining to a hair follicle and its oil gland.

pilus /pē'ləs/, *pl.* **pili** [L, hair], **1.** a hair or hairlike structure. **2.** (in microbiology) a fine filamentous appendage found on certain bacteria and similar to flagellum, except that it is shorter, straighter, and found in greater quantities in the organism.

pimozide /pim'əzīd/, an oral neuroleptic agent prescribed for the suppression of motor and phonic tics associated with Gilles de la Tourette's syndrome.

pimple [ME, *pinple*], a small papule, pustule, or furuncle.

pin [AS, *pinn*], **1.** (in orthopedics) to secure and immobilize fragments of bone with a nail. **2.** (in dentistry) a small metal rod or peg, used as a support in rebuilding a tooth.

pin and tube fixed orthodontic appliance, an orthodontic appliance for correcting and improving malocclusion. It uses a labial arch with vertical posts that insert into tubes attached to bands on the teeth.

pinch, a compression or squeezing of the end of the thumb in opposition to the end of one or more of the fingers.

pinch graft [Fr, *pince* + Gk, *graphion,* stylus], a small, circular deep graft of skin only a few millimeters in diameter. It is cut so that the center is of whole skin but the edges consist of only epidermis.

pinch meter, a type of dynamometer that measures the strength of a finger pinch.

pindolol /pin'dəlol/, a beta-adrenergic blocker with sympathomimetic activity. It is prescribed in the treatment of hypertension, alone or concomitantly with a diuretic.

pineal /pin'ē·əl/ [L, *pineus,* pine cone],

1. pertaining to the pineal body. **2.** resembling a pine cone.

pineal body [L, *pineas,* pine cone; AS, *bodig,* body], a cone-shaped structure in the brain, situated between the superior colliculi, the pulvinar, and the splenicum of the corpus callosum. Its precise function has not been established.

pinealectomy /pin'ē-əlek'təme/ [L, *pineus* + Gk, *ektome,* excision], the surgical removal of the pineal body.

pineal hyperplasia syndrome, an abnormal condition caused by overgrowth of the pineal gland. It is characterized by severe insulin resistance, dry skin, thick nails, hirsutism, early dentition, and sexual precocity.

pinealoma /pin'ē-əlō'mə/ [L, *pineas* + Gk, *oma,* tumor], a rare neoplasm of the pineal body in the brain, characterized by hydrocephalus, pupillary changes, gait disturbances, headache, nausea, and vomiting.

pineal peduncle [L, *pineus,* pine cone, *peduncle,* small foot], the stalk of the pineal body.

pineal tumor, a neoplasm of the pineal body.

pine tar [L, *pinus,* pine; AS, *teoru,* tar], a topical antieczematic and a rubefacient. It is a common ingredient in creams, soaps, and lotions used in the treatment of chronic skin conditions such as eczema or psoriasis.

pinhole pupil [ME, *pyn* + *hol* + L, *pupilla,* little girl], a very small pupil, which may be a congenital condition, an effect of the use of miotics, or the result of an inflamed iris.

pinhole retention [ME, *pyn* + *hol* + L, *retinere,* to hold], retention developed by drilling one or more holes, 2 to 3 mm in depth, in suitable areas of a cavity preparation to supplement resistance and retention form.

pinhole test, 1. a test performed in examining a person who has diminished visual acuity to distinguish a refractive error from organic disease. Several pinholes, 0.5 to 2 mm in diameter, are punched in a card; the patient selects one and looks through it with one eye at a time, without wearing glasses. If visual acuity is improved, the defect is refractive; if not, it is organic. The pinhole effect results from blocking peripheral light waves, those most distorted by refractive error. **2.** (in radiology) a test to identify the size of the focal spot of the x-ray tube. Also, a tomography test used to trace the path of the tube movement.

Pin-Index Safety System (PISS), a system for identifying connectors for certain small cylinders of medical gases that have flush valve outlets rather than threaded outlets.

pinocytic /pī'nəsit'ik/ [Gk, *pinein,* to drink, *kytos,* cell], pertaining to a pinocyte, particularly its ability to absorb liquids by phagocytosis in cellular metabolic processes.

pinocytosis /pī'nōsītō'sis/ [Gk, *pinein* + *kytos* + *osis,* condition], the process by which extracellular fluid is taken into a cell. The plasma membrane develops a saccular indentation filled with extracellular fluid, then closes around it, forming a vesicle or a vacuole of fluid within the cell.

pinprick test, a test of a person's ability to detect a cutaneous pain sensation and to differentiate such sensations from pressure stimuli. The test is performed with a pin or needle gently applied to a skin area where it cannot be observed by the subject. The application of the pin or needle is alternated with the pressing of a dull object against the skin.

pinta /pēn'tə/ [Sp, spot], an infection of the skin caused by *Treponema carateum,* a common organism in South and Central America. The bacterium gains entry into the body through a break in the skin. The primary lesion is a slowly enlarging papule with regional lymph node enlargement, followed in 1 to 12 months by a generalized red to slate-blue macular rash.

pin track infection [ME, *pyn* + *trak,* trace; L, *inficere,* to taint], an abnormal condition associated with skeletal traction and characterized by infection of superficial, deeper, or soft tissues or by osteomyelitis. These infections may develop at skeletal traction pin sites.

PIO$_2$, symbol for *partial pressure of inspired oxygen.*

pions /pī'onz/ [Gk, *pi,* 16th letter of Greek alphabet, *meson,* nuclear particle], a family of particles that can be created in nuclear reactions. Pions are unstable but can survive long enough to be formed into beams and used in certain types of medical therapy, such as the treatment of brain tumors.

pipette /pīpet', pipet'/ [Fr, little pipe], **1.** a calibrated transparent open-ended tube of glass or plastic used for measuring or transferring small quantities of a liquid or gas. **2.** use of a pipette to dispense liquid.

piriform /pir'ifôrm/ [L, *pirum,* pear, *forma*], pear-shaped.

piriform aperture [L, *pirum,* pear, *forma,* form, *apertura,* opening], the anterior nasal opening in the skull.

piriformis /pir'ifôr'mis/ [L, *pirum* + *forma*], a flat pyramidal muscle lying almost parallel with the posterior margin of the gluteus medius. It functions to rotate the thigh laterally and to abduct and help extend it.

Pirogoff's amputation [Nikolai I. Pirogoff, Russian surgeon, 1810–1881], an ankle joint amputation in which the posterior process of the calcaneum is retained at the skin flap and opposed to the cut end of the tibia.

Pirquet's test /pirkāz'/ [Clemens P. von Pirquet, Austrian physician, 1874–1929], a tuberculin skin test that consists of scratching the tuberculin material onto the skin.

pisiform /pī'sifôrm, pē'-/ [L, *pisum,* pea, *forma*], pea-shaped.

pisiform bone [L, *pisa,* pea, *forma,* form; AS, *ban,* bone], a small spheroidal carpal bone in the proximal row of carpal bones.

PISS, abbreviation for **Pin-Index Safety System.**

pistol-shot sound, a sharp slapping sound heard by auscultation over the femoral pulse of a patient with aortic incompetence. It is caused by a large-volume pulse with a sharp rise in pressure.

pit and fissure cavity [AS, *pytt* + L, *fissura,* cleft, *cavum,* cavity], a cavity that starts in tiny faults in tooth enamel, usually on occlusal surfaces of molars and premolars.

pitch [ME, *picchen*], **1.** the frequency of vibrations per unit of time. **2.** the quality of a tone or sound dependent on the relative rapidity of the vibrations by which it is produced.

pithing /pith'ing/ [AS, *pitha*], the destruction of the central nervous system of an experimental animal in preparation for physiologic research. It is usually done by inserting a blunt probe through a foramen.

pitting [AS, *pytt*], **1.** small, punctate indentations in fingernails or toenails, often a result of psoriasis. **2.** an indentation that remains for a short time after pressing edematous skin with a finger. **3.** small depressed scars in the skin or other organ of the body. **4.** the removal by the spleen of material from within erythrocytes without damage to the cells.

pitting edema [AS, *pytt* + Gk, *oidema,* swelling], an edema characterized by a condition in which a finger pressed into the skin over an accumulation of fluid will result in a temporary depression in the skin; normal skin and subcutaneous tissues quickly rebound when the pressure is released.

pituicyte /pit(y)o͞o'isīt/ [L, *pituita,* phlegm; Gk, *kytos,* cell], a cell of the neurohypophysis.

pituitarism /pit(y)o͞o'itəriz'əm/ [L, *pituita,* phlegm], any condition caused by a defect or failure of the pituitary gland.

pituitary, pertaining to the pituitary gland.

pituitary dwarf /pit(y)o͞o'iter'ē/ [L, *pituita,* phlegm; AS, *dweorge*], a dwarf whose retarded development is caused by a deficiency of growth hormone resulting from hypofunction of the anterior lobe of the pituitary. The body is properly proportioned, with no facial or skeletal deformities, and mental and sexual development is normal.

pituitary eunuchism, a form of impotence resulting from disease or dysfunction of the pituitary gland.

pituitary gland [L, *pituita,* phlegm], an endocrine gland suspended beneath the brain in the pituitary fossa of the sphenoid bone, supplying numerous hormones that govern many vital processes. It is divided into an anterior adenohypophysis and a smaller posterior neurohypophysis.

pituitary myxedema [L, *pituita* + Gk, *myxa,* mucus, *oidema,* swelling], a type of hypothyroid condition secondary to an anterior pituitary disease.

pituitary nanism, a type of dwarfism associated with hypophyseal infantilism.

pituitary snuff lung, a type of hypersensitivity pneumonitis that sometimes occurs among users of pituitary snuff. Symptoms of the acute form of the disease include chills, cough, fever, dyspnea, anorexia, nausea, and vomiting. The chronic form of the disease is characterized by fatigue, chronic cough, weight loss, and dyspnea on exercise.

pituitary stalk, a structure that connects the pituitary gland with the hypothalamus.

pit viper [AS, *pytt* + L, *vipera,* snake], any one of a family of venomous snakes found in the Western Hemisphere and Asia, characterized by a heat-sensitive pit between the eye and nostril on each side of the head and hollow perforated fangs that are usually folded back in the roof of the mouth. With the exception of coral snakes, all indigenous poisonous snakes in the United States are pit vipers.

pityriasis /pitərī'əsis/ [Gk, *pityron,* bran], any of a number of skin diseases that have in common lesions that resemble dandifflike scales without obvious signs of inflammation.

pityriasis alba [Gk, *pityron,* bran; L, *albus,* white], a common idiopathic dermatosis characterized by round or oval finely scaling patches of hypopigmentation, usually on the cheeks.

pityriasis rosea, a self-limited skin disease in which a slightly scaling pink macular rash spreads over the trunk and other unexposed areas of the body. A characteristic feature is the **herald patch,** a larger, more scaly lesion that precedes the diffuse rash by several days. The smaller lesions tend to line up with the long axis parallel to normal lines of cleavage of the skin. Mild itching is the only symptom.

pivot joint /piv′ət/ [Fr, hinge; L, *jungere,* to join], a synovial joint in which movement is limited to rotation. The joint is formed by a pivotlike process that may turn within a ring composed partly of bone and partly of ligament. The proximal radioulnar articulation is a pivot joint.

pivot transfer, the movement of a person from one site to another, such as from a bed to a wheelchair, when there is a loss of control of one side of the body or one side of the body is immobile. The person is helped to a position on the strong side of the body with both feet on the floor, heels behind the knees, and knees lower than the hips. The person stands with the weight on the strong leg, pivots on it, and carefully lowers the body into the wheelchair.

PJC, abbreviation for *premature junctional complex.*

PK, abbreviation for **psychokinesis.**

pK$_a$, the negative logarithm of the ionization constant of an acid. A measure of the strength of an acid.

PKA, abbreviation for **protein kinase.**

PKD, abbreviation for **polycystic kidney disease.**

PK test, abbreviation for **Prausnitz-Küstner test.**

PKU, abbreviation for **phenylketonuria.**

placebo /pləsē′bō/ [L, shall please], an inactive substance such as saline solution, distilled water, or sugar or a less than effective dose of a harmless substance, such as a water-soluble vitamin, prescribed as if it were an effective dose of a needed medication. Placebos are prescribed for patients who cannot be given the medication they request or who, in the judgment of the health care provider, do not need that medication.

placebo effect, a physical or emotional change occurring after a substance is taken or administered that is not the result of any special property of the substance. The change may be beneficial, reflecting the expectations of the person.

placement /plās′mənt/ [Fr, *placer,* to place], the positioning of a dental prosthesis, such as a removable denture in its planned site on the dental arch.

placement path, the direction of insertion and removal of a removable partial denture on its supporting oral structures.

placenta /pləsen′tə/ [L, flat cake], a highly vascular fetal organ that exchanges with the maternal circulation, mainly by diffusion of oxygen, carbon dioxide, and other substances. It begins to form on approximately the eighth day of gestation when the blastocyst touches the wall of the uterus and adheres to it. At term the normal placenta is one seventh to one fifth of the weight of the infant. The maternal surface is lobulated and has a dark red rough, liverlike appearance. The fetal surface is smooth and shiny, covered with the fetal membranes, and marked by the large white blood vessels beneath the membranes that fan out from the centrally inserted umbilical cord. The time between the infant's birth and the expulsion of the placenta is the third and last stage of labor.

placenta accreta, a placenta that invades the uterine muscle, making separation from the muscle difficult.

placental /pləsen′təl/ [L, *placenta,* flat cake], pertaining to the placenta.

placental bruit [L, *placenta,* flat cake; Fr, *bruit,* noise], a humming noise caused by fetal circulation, heard in the pregnant uterus. It is synchronized with the mother's pulse.

placental dystocia, a prolonged or otherwise difficult delivery of the placenta.

placental hormone, one of the several hormones produced by the placenta, including human placental lactogen, chorionic gonadotropin, estrogen, progesterone, and a thyrotropin-like hormone.

placental infarct, a localized ischemic hard area on the fetal or maternal side of the placenta.

placental insufficiency, an abnormal condition of pregnancy, manifested clinically by a retarded rate of fetal and uterine growth. Some of the abnormalities that can result in placental insufficiency are abnormal implantation of the placenta, multiple pregnancy, abnormal attachments of the umbilical cord or anomalies of the cord itself, and abnormalities of the placental membranes.

placental membrane, a layer of tissue in the placenta between the fetal and maternal blood systems. The membrane regulates the diffusion of materials between the two systems.

placental presentation [L, *placenta,* flat cake, *praesentare,* to show], a complication of childbirth in which the placenta is located in or near the lower uterine segment.

placental scan, a scan of the uterus of a pregnant woman, performed after an intravenous injection of a contrast medium, used for locating the fetus and placenta and for detecting intrauterine bleeding.

P

placental stage of labor, the third stage of labor when the placenta and membranes are expelled from the uterus after birth of the child.

placental thrombosis [L, *placenta,* flat cake; Gk, *thrombos,* lump, *osis,* condition], intravascular coagulation that occurs in the placenta and veins of the uterus.

placental transmission [L, *placenta,* flat cake; L, *transmittere,* to transmit], the transference of a drug or other substance across the placenta.

placenta previa /prē′vē·ə/, a condition of pregnancy in which the placenta is implanted abnormally in the uterus so that it impinges on or covers the internal os of the uterine cervix. It is the most common cause of painless bleeding in the third trimester of pregnancy. Its cause is unknown. Even slight dilation of the internal os can cause enough local separation of an abnormally implanted placenta to result in bleeding. Complete previa refers to a placenta that has grown to cover the internal cervical os completely; low-lying placenta identifies a placenta that is just within the lower uterine segment; and **partial** or **marginal previa** is a condition in which the placenta partially covers the internal cervical os.

placenta previa partialis, a placenta that partially obstructs the internal cervical os.

placenta souffle [L, *placenta,* flat cake; Fr, *souffle,* puff], a soft blowing or humming sound produced by fetal circulation at the placenta.

placenta succenturiate, an accessory placenta.

Plafon fracture, a fracture that involves the buttress part of the malleolus of a bone.

plagiocephaly /plā′jē·ōsef′əlē/ [Gk, *plagios,* askew, *kephale,* head], a congenital malformation of the skull in which premature or irregular closure of the coronal or lambdoidal sutures results in asymmetric growth of the head, giving it a twisted, lopsided appearance. —**plagiocephalic, plagiocephalous,** *adj.*

plague /plāg/ [L, *plaga,* blow], an infectious disease transmitted by the bite of a flea from a rodent infected with the bacillus *Yersinia pestis.* Plague is primarily an infectious disease of rats. The rat fleas feed on humans only when their preferred rodent hosts, usually rats, have been killed by the plague in a rat epizootic; therefore epidemics occur after rat epizootics. Kinds of plague include **bubonic plague, pneumonic plague,** and **septicemic plague.**

plague vaccine, an active immunizing agent prepared with killed plague bacilli.

It is prescribed for immunization against plague after probable exposure or as protection for travelers in endemic areas such as Southeast Asia.

plaintiff /plān′tif/ [ME, *plaintif,* one who complains], (in law) a person who files a lawsuit initiating a legal action.

planar xanthoma /plā′nər/ [L, *planum,* level; Gk, *xanthos,* yellow, *oma,* tumor], a yellow or orange flat macule or slightly raised papule containing foam cells and occurring in clusters in localized areas such as the eyelids. These lesions may be widely distributed over the body.

Planck's constant (h), /plangks′/ [Max Planck, German physicist, 1858–1947], a fundamental physical constant that relates the energy of radiation to its frequency. It is expressed as 6.63×10^{-27} erg-seconds or 6.63×10^{-34} joule-seconds.

plane [L, *planum,* level], **1.** a flat surface determined by three points in space. **2.** an extension of a longitudinal section through an axis, such as the coronal, horizontal, transverse, frontal, and sagittal planes, used to identify the position of various parts of the body in the study of anatomy. **3.** the act of paring or rubbing away. **4.** a superficial incision in the wall of a cavity or between tissue layers, especially in plastic surgery. —**planar,** *adj.*

planigraphic principle /plan′igraf′ik/, a rule of tomography in which the fulcrum or axis of rotation is raised or lowered to alter the level of the focal plane, but the tabletop height remains constant.

plankton /plangk′tən/ [Gk, *planktos,* wandering], nearly microscopic floating or weakly swimming organisms (both plant and animal) found in lakes and oceans that provide the initial rung in the food chain for aquatic animals.

planned change, an alteration of the status quo by means of a carefully formulated program that follows four steps: unfreezing the present level, establishing a change relationship, moving to a new level, and freezing at the new level.

planned parenthood, a philosophic framework central to the development of contraceptive methods, contraceptive counseling, and family planning programs and clinics. Advocates hold that it is the right of each woman to decide when to conceive and bear children and that contraceptive and gynecologic care and information should be available to her to help her become or prevent becoming pregnant.

planning [L, *planum*], (in five-step nursing process) a category of nursing behavior in which a strategy is designed to achieve the goals of care for an individual patient, as established in assessing and analyzing. Planning includes developing and modifying a care plan for the patient, cooperating with other personnel, and recording relevant information.

plantago seed /plantā′gō/, a bulk-forming laxative derived from *Plantago psyllium* seeds. It is prescribed in the treatment of constipation and nonspecific diarrhea.

plantar /plan′tər/ [L, *planta*, sole], pertaining to the sole of the foot.

plantar aponeurosis, the tough fascia surrounding the muscles of the soles of the feet.

plantar arch [L, *planta*, sole, *arcus*, bow], the arterial arch in the sole of the foot, over the metatarsal bone.

plantar flexion [L, *planta*, sole, *flectere*, to bend], a toe-down motion of the foot at the ankle. It is measured in degrees from the 0-degree position of the foot at rest on the ground in a standing position.

plantar grasp reflex, a reflex characterized by the flexion of the toes when the sole of the foot is stroked gently. It is present in babies at birth but should disappear after 6 weeks.

plantaris /planter′is/ /plantä′ris/ [L, *planta*], one of three superficial muscles at the back of the leg, between the soleus and the gastrocnemius. It flexes the foot and the leg.

plantar neuroma, a neuroma of the sole of the foot.

plantar reflex, the normal response, elicited by firmly stroking the outer surface of the sole of the foot from heel to toes, characterized by flexion of the toes.

plantar wart, a painful verrucous lesion on the sole of the foot, primarily at points of pressure, such as over the metatarsal heads and the heel. Caused by the common wart virus, it appears as a soft central core and is surrounded by a firm hyperkeratotic ring resembling a callus.

plantigrade /plan′tigrād′/ [L, *planta*, sole, *gradi*, to walk], 1. pertaining to or characterizing the human gait; walking on the sole of the foot with the heel touching the ground. 2. a position in which an individual is standing flexed at the hips and bearing some weight through the upper extremities.

plant toxin [ME, *plante* + Gk, *toxikon*, poison], any poisonous substance derived from a plant, such as the ricin of castor-oil seeds.

plaque /plak/ [Fr, plate], 1. a flat, often raised patch on the skin or any other organ of the body. 2. a patch of atherosclerosis. 3. a usually thin film on the teeth. It is

made up of mucin and colloidal material found in saliva and often secondarily invaded by bacteria.

plasma /plaz′mə/ [Gk, something formed], the watery straw-colored fluid part of the lymph and the blood in which the leukocytes, erythrocytes, and platelets are suspended. Plasma is made up of water, electrolytes, proteins, glucose, fats, bilirubin, and gases and is essential for carrying the cellular elements of the blood through the circulation, transporting nutrients, maintaining the acid-base balance of the body, and transporting wastes from the tissues.

plasma cell, a lymphoid or lymphocyte-like cell found in the bone marrow, connective tissue, and sometimes the blood. Plasma cells are involved in the immunologic mechanism.

plasma cell leukemia, an unusual neoplasm of blood-forming tissues in which the predominant cells are plasmacytes. The disease may develop with multiple myeloma or arise independently.

plasmacytoma /plaz′məsītō′mə/, a focal neoplasm containing plasma cells that may develop in the bone marrow, as in multiple myeloma, or outside the bone marrow, as in tumors of the viscera and the mucosa of the nasal, oral, and pharyngeal areas.

plasma exchange therapy [Gk, *plassein*, to mold; L, *ex* + *cambire*, to change; Gk, *therapeia*, treatment], a method of treating certain diseases by removing a part of plasma from the blood supply of a patient and replacing it with plasma from a disease-free person.

plasma expander, a substance, usually a high-molecular-weight dextran, that is administered intravenously to increase the oncotic pressure of a patient.

plasma membrane, the outer covering of a cell, often having projecting microvilli and containing the cellular cytoplasm. The plasma membrane is so thin and delicate that it is barely visible with a light microscope and can be studied in detail only with an electron microscope. The membrane controls the exchange of materials between the cell and its environment by various processes such as osmosis, phagocytosis, pinocytosis, and secretion.

plasmapheresis /plaz′məfərē′sis/, the removal of plasma from previously withdrawn blood by centrifugation, reconstitution of the cellular elements in an isotonic solution, and reinfusion of this solution into the donor or another client who needs red cells rather than whole blood.

plasma protein, any of the proteins, including albumin, fibrinogen, prothrombin, and the gamma globulins. These sub-

P

stances help maintain water balance that affects osmotic pressure, increase blood viscosity, and help maintain blood pressure.

plasma renin activity, the action of the enzyme renin (produced by the kidney), measured in plasma to aid in the diagnosis of adrenal disease associated with hypertension.

plasma volume, the total volume of plasma in the body, elevated in diseases of the liver and spleen and in vitamin C deficiency and lowered in Addison's disease, dehydration, and shock.

plasma volume extender [Gk, *plassein* + L, *volumen,* paper roll, *extendere,* to stretch], an intravenous solution of dextran, proteins, or other substances used to treat shock caused by blood volume loss.

plasmid /plaz′mid/ [Gk, *plasma,* something formed], (in bacteriology) any type of intracellular inclusion considered to have a genetic function, especially a molecule of deoxyribonucleic acid that is separate from the bacterial chromosome that determines traits not essential for the viability of the organism but that in some way changes the organism's ability to adapt.

Plasmodium /plazmō′dē·əm/ [Gk, *plasma* + *eidos,* form], a genus of protozoa, several species of which cause malaria, transmitted to humans by the bite of an infected *Anopheles* mosquito. *Plasmodium falciparum* causes falciparum malaria, the most severe form of the disease; *P. malariae* causes quartan malaria; *P. ovale* causes mild tertian malaria with oval red blood cells; and *P. vivax* causes common tertian malaria.

plasmosome /plaz′məsōm/ [Gk, *plasma* + *soma,* body], the true nucleolus of a cell as distinguished from the karyosomes in the nucleus.

plaster [Gk, *emplastron*], **1.** any composition of a liquid and a powder that hardens when it dries, used in shaping a cast to support a fractured bone as it heals, such as plaster of paris. **2.** a home remedy consisting of a semisolid mixture applied to a part of the body as a counterirritant or for other therapeutic reasons, such as a mustard plaster.

plaster cast [Gk, *emplastron,* plaster; ONorse, *kasta*], a traditional cast designed to encase and immobilize a part of the body in a gauze roll impregnated with plaster of paris. The gauze is dipped in warm water and circumferentially wrapped.

plaster of paris [Gk, *emplastron,* plaster; Paris, France], a white powder, calcium sulfate hemihydrate, which is mixed with water to make a paste that can be molded to encase a body part.

plasticity /plastis′itē/ [Gk, *plassein,* to mold], the quality of being plastic or formative.

plastic surgery [Gk, *plassein,* to mold, *cheirourgia,* surgery], the alteration, replacement, or restoration of visible parts of the body, performed to correct a structural or cosmetic defect. In performing corrective plastic surgery, the surgeon may use tissue from the patient or from another person or an inert material that is nonirritating, has a consistency appropriate to the use, and is able to hold its shape and form indefinitely.

plate [Fr, *plat,* flat dish], **1.** a flat structure or layer, such as a thin layer of bone or the frontal plate between the sides of the ethmoid cartilage and the sphenoid bone in the fetus. **2.** a single partitioning unit of a chromatographic system.

platelet /plāt′lit/ [Fr, small plate], the smallest cells in the blood. They are formed in the red bone marrow, and some are stored in the spleen. Platelets are disk-shaped, contain no hemoglobin, and are essential for the coagulation of blood and in maintenance of hemostasis.

plateletpheresis /plāt′litfer′əsis/ [Fr, *platelet* + Gk, *aphairesis,* to carry away], the removal of platelets from withdrawn blood. The remainder of the blood is reinfused into the donor.

platinized gold foil /plat′inīzd/ [Sp, *plata,* silver; AS, *geolu,* gold; L, *folium,* leaf], a thin sheet rolled or hammered from platinum sandwiched between two sheets of gold, used for making parts of dental restorations requiring greater hardness than that obtained by using other materials such as copper amalgam.

platinum (Pt) /plat′ənəm/ [Sp, *plata,* silver], a silver-white soft metallic element. Its atomic number is 78; its atomic mass (weight) is 195.09. Platinum is used in dentistry and is a good catalyst for a variety of chemical reactions.

platinum foil, a very thin sheet of rolled pure platinum that has a high fusing point, making it an ideal matrix in various soldering procedures for fabricating orthodontic appliances and dentures.

Platyhelminthes /plat′ihelmin′thēz/ [Gk, *platys,* broad, *helmins,* worm], a phylum of parasitic flatworms that includes the Monogenea and Cestoidea classes of tapeworms and Trematoda class of flukes.

platypelloid pelvis /plat′əpel′oid/ [Gk, *platys,* broad, *pella,* bowl, *eidos,* form; L, *pelvis,* basin], a rare type of pelvis in which the inlet is round like the gynecoid type in the anterior section, but the posterior section is foreshortened by its flat and heavy border. The sacrum is hollow and inclines posteriorly, and the sidewalls are convergent.

platysma /plətiz'mə/ [Gk, *platys,* broad], one of a pair of wide muscles at the side of the neck. It serves to draw down the lower lip and the corner of the mouth. When the platysma fully contracts, the skin over the clavicle is drawn toward the mandible, increasing the diameter of the neck.

play [AS, *plegan,* sport], any spontaneous or organized activity that provides enjoyment, entertainment, amusement, or diversion. It is essential in childhood for the development of a normal personality and as a means for physical, intellectual, and social development. Play provides an outlet for releasing tension and stress, as well as a means for testing and experimenting with new or fearful roles or situations.

Play Support, a Nursing Interventions Classification defined as purposeful use of toys or other equipment to assist a patient in communicating his or her perception of the world and mastering the environment.

play therapy, a form of psychotherapy in which a child plays in a protected and structured environment with games and toys provided by a therapist, who observes the behavior, affect, and conversation of the child to gain insight into thoughts, feelings, and fantasies.

pleasure principle /plezh'ər/ [Fr, *plaisir,* pleasure; L, *principium*], (in psychoanalysis) the need for immediate gratification of instinctual drives.

pledget /plej'ət/, a small flat compress made of cotton gauze, a tuft of cotton wool, lint, or a similar synthetic material used to wipe the skin, absorb drainage, or clean a small surface.

pleiotropic gene /plī'ətrop'ik/, a gene that produces a complex of unrelated phenotypic effects.

pleiotropy /plī-ot'rəpē/ [Gk, *pleion,* more, *trepein* to turn], (in genetics) the production by a single gene of a multiple, different, and apparently unrelated manifestation of a particular disorder, such as the cluster of symptoms in Marfan's syndrome, aortic aneurysm, dislocation of the optic lens, skeletal deformities, and arachnodactyly, any or all of which may be present.

plerocercoid /plir'ōsur'koid/, second larval stage of the cestode *Diphyllobothrium latum* that develops in the second intermediate host, the freshwater fish. It is infective to humans if ingested.

plethora /pleth'ərə/ [Gk, *plethore,* fullness], a term applied to the beefy red coloration of a newborn. The "boiled lobster" hue of the infant's skin is caused by an unusually high proportion of erythrocytes per volume of blood. **—plethoric,** *adj.*

plethysmogram /pləthiz'məgram'/ [Gk, *plethynein,* to increase, *gramma,* to record], a tracing produced by a plethysmograph.

plethysmograph /pləthiz'məgraf'/, an instrument for measuring and recording changes in the size and volume of extremities and organs by measuring changes in their blood volume. **—plethysmographic,** *adj.,* **plethysmography,** *n.*

plethysmography /pleth'izmog'rəfē/ [Gk, *plethynein,* to increase, *graphein,* to record], the measurement of changes in the volume of organs or other body parts, particularly those changes resulting from blood flow.

pleura /plŏŏr'ə/, *pl.* **pleurae** [Gk, rib], a delicate serous membrane enclosing the lung, composed of a single layer of flattened mesothelial cells resting on a delicate membrane of connective tissue. The pleura divides into the visceral pleura, which covers the lung, dipping into the fissures between the lobes, and the parietal pleura, which lines the chest wall, covers the diaphragm, and reflects over the structures in the mediastinum. **—pleural,** *adj.*

pleural [Gk, *pleura,* rib], pertaining to the pleurae.

pleural cavity /plŏŏr'əl/ [Gk, *pleura,* rib; L, *cavum,* cavity], the space within the thorax that contains the lungs. Between the ribs and the lungs are the visceral and parietal pleurae.

pleural effusion, an abnormal accumulation of fluid in the intrapleural spaces of the lungs. It is characterized by fever, chest pain, dyspnea, and nonproductive cough. The fluid involved is an exudate or a transudate from inflamed pleural surfaces.

pleural friction rub [Gk, *pleura,* rib; L, *fricare,* to rub; ME, *rubben*], a rubbing, grating sound that occurs with pleurisy as one layer of the pleural membrane slides over the other during breathing.

pleural space, the potential space between the visceral and parietal layers of the pleurae. The space contains a small amount of fluid that acts as a lubricant, allowing the pleurae to slide smoothly over each other as the lungs expand and contract with respiration.

pleura pulmonalis [Gk, *pleura,* rib; L, *pulmo,* lung], the part of the pleural membrane that covers the lungs, as distinguished from the parietal layer of pleura that lines the inner aspect of the thoracic cavity.

P

pleurisy /plŏŏr'əsē/ [Gk, *pleura* + *itis*, inflammation], inflammation of the parietal pleura of the lungs. It is characterized by dyspnea and stabbing pain, leading to restriction of ordinary breathing with spasm of the chest on the affected side. A pleural friction rub may be heard on auscultation. Common causes of pleurisy include bronchial carcinoma, lung or chest wall abscess, pneumonia, pulmonary infarction, and tuberculosis.

pleurisy with effusion [Gk, *pleura* + *itis,* inflammation; L, *effundere,* to pour out], pleurisy in which inflammation has progressed to an effusion into the intrapleural space, characterized by fluid with a high specific gravity caused by a high concentration of fibrin and clots.

pleuritic /plŏŏri'tik/ [Gk, *pleura,* rib], pertaining to a condition of pleurisy.

pleurodynia /plŏŏr'ōdin'ē·ə/ [Gk, *pleura* + *odyne,* pain], acute inflammation of the intercostal muscles and the muscular attachment of the diaphragm to the chest wall. It is characterized by sudden severe pain and tenderness, fever, headache, and anorexia. These symptoms are aggravated by movement and breathing.

pleuropericardial rub /-per'ikär'dē·əl/ [Gk, *pleura* + *peri,* around, *kardia,* heart; ME, *rubben,* to scrape], an abnormal coarse friction sound heard on auscultation of the lungs during late inspiration and early expiration. It occurs when the visceral and parietal pleural surfaces rub against each other.

pleuropneumonia /plŏŏr'ōnŏŏmō'nē·ə/ [Gk, *pleura* + *pneumon,* lung], **1.** a combination of pleurisy and pneumonia. **2.** an infection of cattle resulting in inflammation of both the pleura and lungs, caused by microorganisms of the *Mycoplasma* group.

pleuropneumonia-like organism (PPLO), a group of filterable organisms of the genus *Mycoplasma* similar to *M. mycoides,* the cause of pleuropneumonia in cattle.

pleurothotonos /plŏŏr'əthot'ənəs/ [Gk, *pleurothen,* side of the body, *tonos,* tension], an involuntary severe prolonged contraction of the muscles of one side of the body, resulting in an acute arch to that side. **—pleurothotonic,** *adj.*

plexiform neuroma /plek'sifôrm/ [L, *plexus,* braided, *forma,* form; Gk, *neuron,* nerve, *oma,* tumor], a neoplasm composed of twisted bundles of nerves.

pleximeter /pleksim'ətər/ [Gk, *plessein,* to strike, *metron,* measure], a mediating device such as a percussor or finger used to receive light taps in percussion.

plexus /plek'səs/, *pl.* **plexuses** [L, braided], a network of intersecting nerves and blood vessels or of lymphatic vessels.

plica /plī'kə/, *pl.* **plicae** /plī'sē/[L, plicare, to fold], a fold of tissue within the body, such as the plicae transversales of the rectum and the plicae circulares of the small intestine. **—plical,** *adj.*

plicae transversales recti /plī'sē/, semilunar transverse folds in the rectum that support the weight of feces.

plicamycin /plī'kəmī'sin/, an antineoplastic agent prescribed primarily in the treatment of malignant tumors of the testis. It is also prescribed in the treatment of hypercalcemia and hypercalciuria associated with cancer.

plication /plīkā'shən/, any operation that involves folding, shortening, or decreasing the size of a muscle or hollow organ, such as the stomach, by taking in tucks.

plication of stomach [L, *plicare,* to fold; Gk, *stomakhos,* gullet], a surgical treatment for obesity in which tucks are created in the wall of the stomach.

Plimmer's bodies [Henry G. Plimmer, English biologist, 1857–1918], small round encapsulated bodies found in cancers and once thought to be the causative parasites.

ploidy /ploi'dē/, [Gk, *eidos,* form], the status of a cell nucleus in regard to the number of complete chromosome sets it contains.

plug [D, *plugge,* stopper], a mass of tissue cells, mucus, or other matter that blocks a normal opening or passage of the body, such as a cervical plug.

plugger, an instrument for condensing or consolidating a filling material, such as a dental amalgam into a tooth restoration.

plumbism /plum'izəm/ [L, *plumbum,* lead], a chronic form of lead poisoning caused by absorption of lead or lead salts.

Plummer's disease [Henry S. Plummer, American physician, 1874–1937], goiter characterized by a hyperfunctioning nodule or adenoma and thyrotoxicosis.

Plummer-Vinson's syndrome /plum'ərvin'sən/ [Henry S. Plummer; Porter P. Vinson, American physician, 1890–1959], a rare disorder associated with severe and chronic iron deficiency anemia, characterized by glossitis, koilonychia, and dysphagia caused by esophageal webs at the level of the cricoid cartilage.

pluripara /plŏŏrip'ərə/ [L, *plus,* more, *parere,* to bear], a woman who has borne several children.

plutonium (Pu) /plŏŏtō'nē·əm/ [planet, *Pluto*], a synthetic transuranic metallic element. Its atomic number is 94; its atomic mass (weight) is 242. A highly toxic waste product of nuclear power plants, plutonium was used in the assembly of early nuclear weapons.

plyometrics, bounding or high-velocity exercise that entails eccentric and rapid concentric contractions, such as jumping or weighted ball throwing and catching.

pm, abbreviation for *picometer.*

Pm, symbol for the element **promethium.**

P.M.D., abbreviation for *private medical doctor.*

PMDD, abbreviation for **premenstrual dysphoric disorder.**

pmh, abbreviation for *past medical history.*

PMI, abbreviation for **point of maximum impulse.**

PMN, abbreviation for **polymorphonuclear cell.**

PMPA, abbreviation for **phenyl-methoxypropyl adenine.**

PMS, pms, abbreviation for **premenstrual syndrome.**

PMT, abbreviation for *premenstrual tension.*

PND, 1. abbreviation for **paroxysmal nocturnal dyspnea. 2.** abbreviation for **postnasal drip.**

pneopneic reflex /nē'ōnē'ik/ [Gk, *pnoe,* breath; L, *reflectere,* to bend back], a change in the normal breathing rhythm when an irritating gas is introduced into the lungs.

pneumatic /nōomat'ik/ [Gk, *pneuma,* air], pertaining to air or gas.

pneumatic condenser [Gk, *pneuma,* air; L, *condensare,* to thicken], (in dentistry) a pneumatic device developed by George M. Hollenback to deliver a compacting force to restorative material used in filling tooth cavities.

pneumatic heart driver, a mechanical device that regulates compressed air delivery to an artificial heart, controlling heart rate, percentage systole, and delay in systole.

Pneumatic Tourniquet Precautions, a Nursing Interventions Classification defined as applying a pneumatic tourniquet while minimizing the potential for patient injury from use of the device.

pneumatocele /nōomat'əsēl'/, **1.** a thin-walled cavity in the lung parenchyma caused by partial airway obstruction. **2.** hernial protrusion of lung tissue. **3.** a tumor or sac containing gas, especially of the scrotum.

pneumatogram /nōomat'əgram'/ [Gk, *pneuma,* air, *gramma,* to record], a tracing made by a pneumograph of chest movements during breathing.

pneumobelt /nōo'mōbelt/, a corset with an inflatable bladder that fits over the abdominal area. The bladder is connected by a hose to a ventilator that delivers positive pressure at an adjustable rate and pressure. It is used to assist in the respiratory rehabilitation of patients with high cervical injuries.

pneumocentesis /-sentē'sis/ [Gk, *pneumon,* lung, *kentesis,* pricking], a procedure in which a lung is punctured to drain fluid contents.

pneumococcal /nōo'mōkok'əl/ [Gk, *pneumon,* lung, *kokkos,* berry], pertaining to bacteria of the genus *Pneumococcus.*

pneumococcal meningitis [Gk, *pneumon,* lung, *kokkos,* berry, *meningx,* membrane, *itis,* inflammation], meningitis caused by pneumococcal infection.

pneumococcal pneumonitis, an inflammation of the lung caused by an infection of pneumococcal bacteria.

pneumococcal vaccine, an active immunizing agent containing antigens of the 14 types of *Pneumococcus* associated with 80% of the cases of pneumococcal pneumonia. It is prescribed for persons over 2 years of age who are at high risk of development of severe pneumococcal pneumonia, all adults over 65 years of age, and immunocompromised adults.

pneumococcus /nōo'mōkok'əs/, *pl.* **pneumococci** /'kok'sī/ [Gk, *pneumon* + *kokkos,* berry], a gram-positive diplococcal bacterium of the species *Streptococcus pneumoniae,* the most common cause of bacterial pneumonia.

pneumoconiosis /nōo·mōkō'nē·ō'sis/ [Gk, *pneumon* + *konis,* dust, *osis,* condition], any disease of the lung caused by chronic inhalation of dust, usually mineral dust of occupational or environmental origin. Some kinds of pneumoconioses are anthracosis, asbestosis, silicosis.

pneumoconstriction /nōo'mōkənstrik'-shən/, an area of collapsed lung tissue that results from mechanical stimulation of an exposed part of the lung. It is produced by local reflex muscular closure of alveolar ducts and alveoli.

Pneumocystis carinii /nōo'mōsis'tis kərin'ē·ī/, a microorganism that causes pneumocystosis, a type of interstitial cell pneumonitis.

pneumocystis pneumonia [Gk, *pneuma,* air, *kystis,* bag, *pneumon,* lung], a type of interstitial plasma cell pneumonia in which the alveoli become honeycombed with an acidophilic material. The patient may or may not be febrile but usually is weak, dyspneic, and cyanotic.

pneumocystosis /nōo'mōsistō'sis/ [Gk, *pneuma,* air, *kystis,* bag, *osis,* condition], infection with the parasite *Pneumocystis carinii,* usually seen in patients with hu-

P

man immunodeficiency virus infection, infants, or debilitated or immunosuppressed people, particularly those with lymphomas. It is characterized by fever, cough, tachypnea, and frequently cyanosis.

pneumoencephalography /nōō'mō·ensef'-əlog'rəfē/ [Gk, *pneuma,* air, *enkephalos,* brain, *graphein,* to record], a procedure for the radiographic visualization of the ventricular space, basal cisterns, and subarachnoid space overlying the cerebral hemispheres of the brain. Air, helium, or oxygen is injected into the lumbar subarachnoid space after the intermittent removal of the cerebrospinal fluid by lumbar puncture. —**pneumoencephalographic,** *adj.*

pneumograph /nōō'məgraf/, a device that records breathing movements by means of an inflated coil around the chest.

pneumohemothorax /-hem'ōthôr'aks/ [Gk, *pneuma,* air, *haima,* blood, *thorax,* chest], an accumulation of air and blood in the pleural cavity.

pneumolysin /mōōmol'isin/, virulence factor produced by *Streptococcus pneumoniae* associated with cytolysis.

pneumomediastinum /nōō'mōmē'dē·əstī'-nəm/ [Gk, *pneuma,* air, *mediastinus,* midway], the presence of air or gas in the mediastinal tissues. The condition may result from bronchitis, acute asthma, pertussis, cystic fibrosis, or bronchial rupture from cough or trauma.

pneumonectomy /nōō'mənek'təmē/ [Gk, *pneumon,* lung, *ektome,* excision], the surgical removal of all or part of a lung.

pneumonia /nōōmō'nē·ə/ [Gk, *pneumon,* lung], an acute inflammation of the lungs, often caused by inhaled pneumococci of the species *Streptococcus pneumoniae.* The alveoli and bronchioles of the lungs become plugged with a fibrous exudate. Pneumonia may be caused by other bacteria, as well as by viruses, rickettsiae, and fungi. Kinds of pneumonia are **aspiration pneumonia, bronchopneumonia, eosinophilic pneumonia, interstitial pneumonia, lobar pneumonia, mycoplasma pneumonia,** and **viral pneumonia.**

pneumonic plague /nōōmon'ik/ [Gk, *pneumon,* lung; L, *plaga,* stroke], a highly virulent and rapidly fatal form of plague characterized by bronchopneumonia. There are two forms: primary pneumonic plague results from involvement of the lungs in the course of bubonic plague; secondary pneumonic plague results from the inhalation of infected particles of sputum from a person having pneumonic plague.

pneumonitis /nōō'mənī'tis/, *pl.* **pneumonitides** [Gk, *pneumon* + *itis*], inflammation of the lung. Pneumonitis may be caused by a virus or may be a hypersensitivity reaction to chemicals or organic dusts, such as bacteria, bird droppings, or molds. It is usually an interstitial, granulomatous, fibrosing inflammation of the lung, especially of the bronchioles and alveoli. Dry cough is a common symptom.

pneumonopathy /nōō'mənop'əthē/, any disease or disorder involving the lung.

pneumonopleuritis /-plōōrī'tis/, a combined disorder of pneumonia and pleurisy.

pneumonotherapy /-ther'əpē/, the treatment of disease of the lung.

pneumopericardium /-per'ikär'dē·əm/, the presence of air or gas in the pericardial sac.

pneumoperitoneum /nōō'mōper'itənē'əm/ /-per'itənē'əm/ [Gk, *pneuma,* air, *peri,* around, *teinein,* to stretch], the presence of air or gas within the peritoneal cavity of the abdomen. It may be spontaneous, such as from rupture of a hollow gas-containing organ, or induced for diagnostic or therapeutic purposes.

pneumoperitonitis /nōō'mōper'itənī'tis/, an acute inflammation of the peritoneal cavity accompanied by the presence of air or gas.

pneumotachometer /-takom'ətər/, a device that measures the flow of respiratory gases. The pressure gradient is directly related to flow, thus allowing a computer to derive a flow curve measured in liters per minute.

pneumothorax /nōō'mōthôr'aks/ [Gk, *pneuma,* air, *thorax,* chest], a collection of air or gas in the pleural space, causing the lung to collapse. Pneumothorax may be the result of an open chest wound that permits the entrance of air, the rupture of an emphysematous vesicle on the surface of the lung, or a severe bout of coughing, or it may occur spontaneously without apparent cause. The onset of pneumothorax is accompanied by a sudden sharp chest pain, followed by difficult, rapid breathing; cessation of normal chest movements on the affected side; tachycardia; a weak pulse; hypotension; diaphoresis; an elevated temperature; pallor; dizziness; and anxiety.

PNF, abbreviation for **proprioceptive neuromuscular facilitation.**

PNH, abbreviation for **paroxysmal nocturnal hemoglobinuria.**

PNP, abbreviation for **pediatric nurse practitioner.**

p.o., an abbreviation for the Latin phrase *per os,* 'by mouth'; a route for administration of medications.

Po, symbol for the element **polonium.**

PO₂, symbol for *partial pressure of oxygen*.

pockmark [AS, *pocc + meark*], a pitted scar on the skin, usually the result of a smallpox pustule at the site.

podalic /pōdal′ik/ [Gk, *pous*, foot], pertaining to the feet.

podalic version, the shifting of the position of a fetus to position the feet at the outlet during labor.

podiatrist, a health professional who diagnoses and treats disorders of the feet. Podiatrists complete a 4-year postgraduate educational program leading to a degree of Doctor of Podiatric Medicine (D.P.M.). Also called *chiropodist* in Canada.

podiatry /pədī′ətrē/ [Gk, *pous + iatros*, healer], the diagnosis and treatment of diseases and other disorders of the feet. Also called *chiropody* in Canada.

podophyllotoxin /pō′dōfil′ətok′sin/ [Gk, *pous + phyllon*, leaf, *toxikon*, poison], any one of a group of substances derived from the roots of *Podophyllum peltatum*, a common plant species known as mayapple or American mandrake. Podophyllin, a resinous preparation of podophyllotoxin, is prescribed in the topical treatment of condyloma acuminatum and other types of warts. Several podophyllotoxin derivatives have been used as purgatives.

podophyllum /pod′əfil′əm/ [Gk, *pous + phyllon*, leaf], the dried rhizome and roots of *Podophyllum peltatum*, from which a caustic resin is derived for use in removing certain warts.

poikilocytosis /poi′kilō′sītō′sis/ [Gk, *poikilos*, variation, *kytos*, cell, *osis*, condition], an abnormal degree of variation in the shape of the erythrocytes in the blood.

poikiloderma atrophicans vasculare /-dur′mə/ [Gk, *poikilos*, variation, *derma*, skin, *a + trophe*, not nourishment; L, *vasculum*, little vessel], an abnormal skin condition characterized by hyperpigmentation or hypopigmentation, telangiectasia, and atrophy of the epidermis.

poikiloderma of Civatte, a common benign progressive dermatitis characterized by erythematous patches on the face and neck that become dry and scaly. As the condition progresses, pigment is deposited around the hair follicles, extending down the lateral aspects of the neck.

point [L, *punctus*, pricked], a small spot or designated area.

point behavior [L, *punctus*, pricked; AS, *bihabban*, to behave], the orientation of body parts in a certain direction within a quantum of space.

point forceps, a dental instrument used in filling root canals. It holds the filling cones during their placement.

point lesion, a disruption of single chemical bonds caused by effects of ionizing radiation on a macromolecule.

point mutation [L, *punctus*, pricked, *mutare*, to change], a mutation in which only a single base-pair of deoxyribonucleic acid is changed.

point of maximum impulse (PMI), the place where the apical pulse is palpated as strongest, often in the fifth intercostal space of the thorax, just medial to the left midclavicular line.

point-of-service plan, (in the United States) a plan in which the member may seek care outside the network or directly from preferred providers with initial evaluation by a primary care provider, but must pay a deductible and/or co-payment.

point system, (in the United States) a specialty capitation method in which points are assigned for each patient seen in specific diagnostic or service categories. Periodically points are totaled, and income distributed proportionally.

poise /poiz/ [Jean L. M. Poiseuille, French physiologist, 1799–1869], a unit of liquid or gas (fluid) viscosity expressed in terms of grams per centimeter per second (g × cm⁻¹ × sec⁻¹). The centipoise, or 1/100 of a poise, is more commonly used.

poison /poi′zən/ [L, *potio*, drink], any substance that impairs health or destroys life when ingested, inhaled, or absorbed by the body in relatively small amounts. **—poisonous,** *adj.*

poison control center, one of a nearly worldwide network of facilities that provide information regarding all aspects of poisoning or intoxication, maintain records of their occurrence, and refer patients to treatment centers.

poisoning, **1.** the act of administering a toxic substance. **2.** the condition or physical state produced by the ingestion of, injection of, inhalation of, or exposure to a poisonous substance. Identification of the poison and presentation of a container label are critical to expeditious diagnosis and treatment.

poisoning, risk for, a NANDA-accepted nursing diagnosis of the accentuated risk of accidental exposure to or ingestion of drugs or dangerous products in doses sufficient to cause poisoning. The risk factors may be internal (individual) or external (environmental). Internal risk factors include reduced vision without adequate safeguards, lack of safety or drug education, lack of proper precautions, cognitive or emotional difficulties, and insufficient finances. External risk factors include large supplies of drugs in the house; medicines or dangerous products stored in unlocked cabinets accessible to children or confused people; availability of illicit drugs potentially contaminated by poisonous additives; flaking, peeling paint or plaster in the environment of young children; chemical contamination of food and water; unprotected contact with heavy metals or chemicals; paint or lacquer in poorly ventilated areas or without effective protection; presence of poisonous vegetation; and presence of atmospheric pollutants.

poisoning treatment, the symptomatic and supportive care given a patient who has been exposed to or who has ingested a toxic drug, commercial chemical, or other dangerous substance. In the case of oral poisoning, a primary effort should be directed toward recovery of the toxic substance before it can be absorbed into the body tissues. If vomiting does not occur spontaneously, it should be induced after first identifying the poison, if possible, and calling a poison control center. If the poison is a petroleum distillate, such as kerosene, or a caustic or corrosive substance, vomiting should *not* be induced.

poison ivy, any of several species of climbing vine of the genus *Rhus,* characterized by shiny three-pointed leaves. It is common in North America and causes severe allergic contact dermatitis in many people. Localized vesicular eruption with itching and burning results.

poison ivy dermatitis [L, *potio,* drink; ME, *ivi* + Gk, *derma,* skin, *itis,* inflammation], a type of skin eruption caused by exposure to a nonvolatile oil, toxicodendrol, present in the leaves and other plant parts of poison ivy, a member of the *Rhus toxicodendron* species. Other *Rhus* species producing the same kind of contact dermatitis are poison oak and poison sumac.

poison oak, any of several species of shrub of the genus *Rhus,* common in North America. Skin contact results in allergic dermatitis in many people. The characteristics and treatment of the condition are similar to those of poison ivy.

poison sumac /sōō'mak/, a shrub of the genus *Rhus,* common in North America. Skin contact results in allergic dermatitis in many people. The characteristics and treatment of the condition are similar to those of poison ivy.

polar [L, *polus,* pole], pertaining to molecules that are hydrophilic, or "water-loving." Polar substances tend to dissolve in polar solvents.

polar body, one of the small cells produced during the two meiotic divisions in the maturation process of female gametes, or ova. It is nonfunctional and incapable of being fertilized.

polarity /pōler'itē/ [L, *polus*], **1.** the existence or manifestation of opposing qualities, tendencies, or emotions, such as pleasure and pain, love and hate, strength and weakness, dependence and independence, masculinity and femininity. **2.** (in physics) the distinction between a negative and a positive electric charge.

polarity therapy, a technique of massage based on the theory that the body has positive and negative energy patterns that must be balanced to establish physical harmony.

polarization /pōlərīzā'shən/ [L, *polus* + Gk, *izein,* to cause], the concentration, within a population or group, of members' interests, beliefs, and allegiances around two conflicting positions.

polarization microscope [L, *polus,* pole; Gk, *mikros,* small, *skopein* to view], a microscope that uses polarized light for special diagnostic purposes, such as examining crystals of chemicals found in patients with gout and related disorders.

polarized light /po'lərīzd/ [L, *polus* + AS, *leoht*], light that is propagated in such a way that the radiation waves occur in only one direction in the vibration plane and not at random.

polarographic oxygen analyzer /pō'-lərōgraf'ik/, an electrochemical device used to analyze the proportion of oxygen molecules in respiratory care systems. The oxygen is measured in terms of an electron current produced after it acquires electrons from a negative electrode in a hydroxide bath.

pole [L, *polus*], **1.** (in biology) an end of an imaginary axis drawn through the symmetrically arranged parts of a cell, organ, ovum, or nucleus. **2.** one of a pair of opposite forces or attractants as in magnetism or electricity. **3.** (in anatomy) the point on a nerve cell at which a dendrite originates. **—polar,** *adj.*

poles of kidney, either end of an axis through the length of a kidney. They are designated as the upper pole of the kidney (extremitas superior renis) and the inferior pole of the kidney (extremitas inferior renis).

pol gene, a segment of a retrovirus, such as the human T cell leukemia virus, that encodes its reverse transcriptase enzyme.

policy /pol'isē/ [L, *politia,* the state], a principle or guideline that governs an activity and that employees or members of an institution or organization are expected to follow.

polioencephalitis /pō'lē-ō'ensef'əlī'tis/ [Gk, *polios,* gray, *enkephalos,* brain, *itis*], an inflammation of the gray matter of the brain caused by infection of the brain by a poliovirus.

polioencephalomeningomyelitis /pō'lē-ō'-ensef'əlō'məning'gōm'īəlī'tis/ [Gk, *polios*, gray, *enkephalos*, brain, *menigx*, membrane, *myelos*, marrow, *itis*, inflammation], an inflammation that involves the gray matter of the brain and spinal cord and also the meninges.

polioencephalomyelitis /pō'lē-ō'ensef'-əlōmī'əlī'tis/ [Gk, *polios* + *enkephalos* + *myelos*, marrow, *itis*], inflammation of the gray matter of the brain and the spinal cord, caused by a poliovirus.

polioencephalopathy /pō'lē-ō'ensef'əlop'-əthē/ [Gk, *polios*, gray, *enkephalos*, brain, *pathos*, disease], a pathologic condition affecting the gray matter of the brain.

poliomyelitis /pō'lē-ōmī'əlī'tis/ [Gk, *polios* + *myelos*, marrow, *itis*], an infectious disease caused by one of the three polioviruses. Asymptomatic, mild, and paralytic forms of the disease occur. It is transmitted from person to person through fecal contamination or oropharyngeal secretions. Abortive poliomyelitis lasts only a few hours and is characterized by minor illness with fever, malaise, headache, nausea, vomiting, and slight abdominal discomfort. Nonparalytic poliomyelitis is longer lasting and is marked by meningeal irritation with pain and stiffness in the back and by all the signs of abortive poliomyelitis. Paralytic poliomyelitis begins as abortive poliomyelitis. The symptoms abate, and for several days the person seems well. Malaise, headache, and fever recur; pain, weakness, and paralysis develop. The peak of paralysis is reached within the first week. In spinal poliomyelitis viral replication occurs in the anterior horn cells of the spine, causing inflammation, swelling, and, if severe, destruction of the neurons. The large proximal muscles of the limbs are most often affected. Bulbar poliomyelitis results from viral multiplication in the brainstem. Bulbar and spinal poliomyelitis often occur together.

poliosis /pō'lē-ō'sis/ [Gk, *polios* + *osis*, condition], depigmentation of the hair on the scalp, eyebrows, eyelashes, mustache, beard, or body. The condition may be inherited and generalized or acquired and localized in patches. Acquired localized poliosis occurs in alopecia areata.

poliovirus /-vī'rəs/ [Gk, *polios* + L, *virus*, poison], the causative organism of poliomyelitis. This very small ribonucleic acid virus has three serologically distinct types. Infection or immunization with one type does not protect against the others.

poliovirus vaccine, a vaccine prepared from poliovirus to confer immunity to it. The trivalent live oral form of vaccine, TOPV, is recommended for all children less than 18 years of age who have no specific contraindications. The inactivated poliovirus vaccine (IPV) is recommended for infants and children who are immunodeficient, including human immunodeficiency virus–infected infants, and for unvaccinated adults. TOPV is called Sabin vaccine; IPV is called Salk vaccine. IPV is given subcutaneously.

polishing [L, *polire*, to make smooth], a tendency of patients with right temporal lobe lesions to deny dysphoric affect and minimize socially disapproved behavior while exaggerating other qualities.

political nursing /pəlit'ikəl/ [L, *politia*, the state, *nutrix*, nurse], the use of knowledge about power processes and strategies to influence the nature and direction of health care and professional nursing.

pollakiuria /pol'əkēyŏŏr'ē-ə/ [Gk, *pollache*, frequent, *ouron*, urine], an abnormal condition characterized by unduly frequent passage of urine.

pollen coryza /pol'ən/ [L, dust; Gk, *koryza*, runny nose], acute seasonal rhinitis caused by exposure to an allergenic.

pollenogenic, pertaining to an agent that produces pollen or is produced by pollen.

pollex /pol'eks/, *pl.* **pollices** ', the thumb; also, the big toe.

pollutant /pəlŏŏ'tənt/ [L, *polluere*, to defoul], an unwanted substance that occurs in the environment, usually with health-threatening effects. Pollutants may exist in the atmosphere as gases or fine particles that may be irritating to the lungs, eyes, and skin; as dissolved or suspended substances in drinking water; and as carcinogens or mutagens in foods or beverages.

polonium (Po) /pəlō'nē-əm/ [Polonia, Poland], a radioactive element that is one of the disintegration products of uranium. Its atomic number is 84; its atomic mass (weight) is approximately 210.

polus /pō'ləs/, *pl.* **poli** [L, pole], either of the opposite ends of any axis; the official anatomic designation for the extremity of an organ. **—polar,** *adj.*

polyacrylamide /-akril'əmīd/, a polymer of acrylamide and usually some cross-linking derivative.

polyamine /pol'ē·am'ēn/, any compound that contains two or more amine groups, such as spermidine and spermine, which are normally occurring tissue constituents in humans.

polyanionic /pol'ē·an'ī·on'ik/ [Gk, *polys*, many, *ana*, again, *ion*, going], pertaining to multiple negative electric charges.

polyarteritis /pol′ē·är′tərī′tis/ [Gk, *polys* + *arteria*, airpipe, *itis* inflammation, an abnormal inflammatory condition of several arteries.

polyarteritis nodosa, a severe and poorly understood collagen vascular disease in which widespread inflammation and necrosis of small and medium-sized arteries and ischemia of the tissues they serve occur. It is characterized by fever, abdominal pain, weight loss, neuropathy, and, if the kidneys are affected, hypertension, edema, and uremia. Some symptoms may mimic those of gastrointestinal or cardiac disorders.

polyarthritis /-ärthrī′tis/, an inflammation that involves more than one joint. The inflammation may migrate from one joint to another, or there may be simultaneous involvement of two or more joints.

polyarticular /-ärtik′yələr/ [Gk, *polys, many, articulus,* joint], pertaining to many joints.

polychlorinated biphenyls (PCBs) /-klôr′-inā′tid/, a group of more than 30 isomers and compounds used in plastics, insulation, and flame retardants and varying in physical form from oily liquids to crystals and resins. All are potentially toxic and carcinogenic.

polychromatic /-krōmatik/ [Gk, *polys* + *chroma,* color], a light of many colors or wavelengths. The term is usually applied to white light, although it may also refer to a defined part of the spectrum.

polychromatophil /pol′ēkrōmat′əfil/, any cell that may be stained by several different dyes.

polychromatophilia /pol′ēkrō′matəfil′yə/ [Gk, *polys* + *chroma* + *philein,* to love], an abnormal tendency of a cell, particularly an erythrocyte, to be dyed by a variety of laboratory stains.

polyclonal /pol′ēklō′nəl/ [Gk, *polys* + *klon,* cutting], **1.** pertaining to or designating a group of identical cells or organisms derived from several identical cells. **2.** pertaining to or designating several groups of identical cells or organisms (clones) derived from a single cell.

polycystic /-sis′tik/ [Gk, *polys* + *kystis,* bag], characterized by the presence of many cysts.

polycystic kidney disease (PKD), an abnormal condition in which the kidneys are enlarged and contain many cysts. There are three forms of the disease: Childhood polycystic disease is uncommon and may be differentiated from adult or congenital polycystic disease by genetic, morphologic, and clinical facets. Death usually occurs within a few years as the result of portal hypertension and liver and kidney failure. Adult polycystic disease may be unilateral, bilateral, acquired, or congenital. The condition is characterized by flank pain and high blood pressure. Kidney failure eventually develops and progresses to uremia and death. Congenital polycystic disease is a rare congenital aplasia of the kidney involving all or only a small segment of one or both kidneys.

polycystic ovary syndrome, an endocrine disturbance characterized by anovulation, amenorrhea, hirsutism, and infertility. It is caused by increased levels of testosterone, estrogen, and luteinizing hormone and decreased secretion of follicle-stimulating hormone (FSH). The depressed but continuous production of FSH associated with this disorder causes continuous partial development of ovarian follicles.

polycythemia /pol′ēsīthē′mē·ə/ [Gk, *polys* + *kytos,* cell, *haima,* blood], an increase in the number of erythrocytes in the blood that may be primary or secondary to pulmonary disease, heart disease, or prolonged exposure to high altitudes.

polycythemia rubra vera (PV) [Gk, *polys, many, kytos,* cell, *haima,* blood], a condition of unknown cause characterized by a marked increase in the red blood cell count, packed cell volume, cellular hemoglobin, leukocytes, platelets, and total blood volume. The skin and mucous membranes acquire a maroon or plum color; and hepatomegaly, splenomegaly, hypertension, and neurologic symptoms develop. The condition is associated with an F chromosome defect.

polydactyly /-dak′tilē/ [Gk, *polys* + *daktylos,* finger], a congenital anomaly characterized by the presence of more than the normal number of fingers or toes. The condition is usually inherited and can usually be corrected by surgery shortly after birth.

polydipsia /pol′ēdip′sē·ə/ [Gk, *polys* + *dipsa,* thirst], **1.** excessive thirst. It is characteristic of several different conditions, including diabetes mellitus, in which an excessive concentration of glucose in the blood osmotically increases the excretion of fluid via increased urination, which leads to hypovolemia and thirst. **2.** *(informal)* alcoholism.

polyelectrolyte /pol′ē·ilek′trəlīt/ [Gk, *polys* + *elektron,* amber, *lytos,* soluble], a substance with many charged or potentially charged groups.

polyesthesia /pol′ē·esthē′zhə/ [Gk, *polys* + *aisthesis,* feeling], a sensory disorder involving the sense of touch in which a stimulus to one area of the skin is also felt at nonstimulated sites.

polyestradiol phosphate /-es′trədī′ôl/, an antineoplastic estrogen compound prescribed for cancer of the prostate and postmenopausal breast cancer.

polyethylene /pol′ē·eth′ilēn/, a strong but flexible synthetic resin produced by the polymerization of ethylene. Polyethylene materials have been used in surgery.

polygene /pol′ējēn′/ [Gk, *polys* + *genein*, to produce], any of a group of nonallelic genes that individually exert a small effect but together interact in a cumulative manner to produce a particular characteristic within an individual, usually of a quantitative nature, such as size, weight, skin pigmentation, or degree of intelligence. — **polygenic,** *adj.*

polyglandular autoimmune syndromes, disorders manifested by subnormal functioning of more than one endocrine gland. Type I is characterized by the appearance of mucocutaneous candidiasis, often occurring in childhood, and is associated with hypoparathyroidism and adrenal insufficiency. The type I condition occurs in siblings, without involvement of other generations in the family. Type II involves primary adrenal insufficiency and primary thyroid failure occurring in the same patient for unclear reasons. It has been demonstrated that many of these patients have an autoimmune disorder, with formation of antibodies against cellular fractions of many endocrine glands.

polyglucosan /-gloo′kəsan/ [Gk, *polys* + *glykys*, sweet], a large molecule consisting of many anhydrous polysaccharides.

polyhybrid /-hī′brid/ [Gk, *polys* + L, *hybrida*, offspring of mixed parents], (in genetics) pertaining to or describing an individual, organism, or strain that is heterozygous for more than three specific traits.

polyhybrid cross, (in genetics) the mating of two individuals, organisms, or strains that have different gene pairs that determine more than three specific traits.

polyleptic /pol′ēlep′tik/ [Gk, *polys* + *lambanein*, to seize], describing any disease or condition marked by numerous remissions and exacerbations.

polyleptic fever, a fever occurring paroxysmally, such as smallpox and relapsing fever.

polymenorrhea, an abnormally frequent recurrence of the menstrual cycle.

polymer /pol′imər/ [Gk, *polys* + *meros*, part], a compound formed by combining or linking a number of monomers, or small molecules. A polymer may be composed of various monomers or of many units of the same monomer.

polymerase chain reaction (PCR) /pol′ē-

mer′ās, polim′ərās/, a process whereby a strand of deoxyribonucleic acid can be cloned millions of times within a few hours. The process can be used to make prenatal diagnoses of genetic diseases and to identify an individual by analysis of a single tissue cell.

polymerize /pol′əmərīz/ [Gk, *polys*, many, *meros*, parts], to convert two or more molecules into a polymer.

polymicrobial /-mīkrō′bē·əl/ [Gk, *polys*, many, *mikros*, small, *bios*, life], pertaining to a number of species of microbes.

polymicrobic infection /-mīkrō′bik/ [Gk, *polys*, many, *mikros*, small, *bios*, life; L, *inficere*, to stain], an infection involving more than one species of pathogens.

polymorphic /-môr′fik/ [Gk, *polys*, many, *morphe*, form], pertaining to the ability to assume two or more distinct forms, such as the existence of two or more forms of chromosomes or hemoglobins in a population.

polymorphism /pol′ēmôr′fizəm/ [Gk, *polys* + *morphe*, form], **1.** the state or quality of existing or occurring in several different forms. **2.** the state or quality of appearing in different forms at different stages of development. —**polymorphic,** *adj.*

polymorphocytic leukemia /pol′ēmôr′fəsit′ik/ [Gk, *polys* + *morphe* + *kytos*, cell, *leukos*, white, *haima*, blood], a neoplasm of blood-forming tissues in which mature segmented granulocytes are predominant.

polymorphonuclear /pol′ēmôr′fōnoo′klē·ər/ [Gk, *polys* + *morphe* + L, *nucleus*, nut kernel], having a nucleus with a number of lobules or segments connected by a fine thread.

polymorphonuclear cell (PMN), a leukocyte with a multilobed nucleus such as a neutrophil.

polymorphonuclear leukocyte, a white blood cell containing a segmented lobular nucleus; an eosinophil, basophil, or neutrophil.

polymorphous /pol′ēmôr′fəs/ [Gk, *polys* + *morphe*, form], occurring in many varying forms, possibly changing in structure or appearance at different stages.

polymorphous light eruption, a common recurrent superficial vascular reaction to sunlight or ultraviolet light in susceptible individuals. Within 1 to 4 days after exposure to the light, small erythematous papules and vesicles appear on otherwise normal skin, then disappear within 2 weeks.

polymyalgia rheumatica /-mī·al′jə/ [Gk, *polys* + *mys*, muscle, *algos*, pain, *rheuma*,

P

flux], a chronic episodic inflammatory disease of the large arteries that usually develops in people over 60 years of age. Polymyalgia rheumatica primarily affects the muscles. It is characterized by pain and stiffness of the back, shoulder, or neck; it is usually more severe on rising in the morning. There may also be a cranial headache, which affects the temporal and occipital arteries, causing a severe throbbing headache.

polymyositis /pol'ēmī'ōsī'tis/ [Gk, *polys* + *mys*, muscle, *itis*], inflammation of many muscles, usually accompanied by deformity, edema, insomnia, pain, sweating, and tension. Some forms of polymyositis are associated with malignancy.

polymyxin /-mik'sin/, an antibiotic used topically and systemically in the treatment of gram-negative bacterial infections, including meningitis, corneal ulcerations, and otitis media.

polymyxin B sulfate, an antibiotic prescribed for infections caused by microorganisms sensitive to this drug, including urinary tract infections, septicemia, and conjunctivitis.

polyneuralgia /-nŏŏral'jə/ [Gk, *polys*, many, *neuron*, nerve, *algos*, pain], a type of neuralgia that affects several nerves at the same time.

polyneuritis /-nŏŏrī'tis/ [Gk, *polys*, many, *neuron*, nerve, *itis*, inflammation], an inflammation involving many nerves.

polyneuropathy /-nŏŏrop'əthē/ [Gk, *polys*, many, *neuron*, nerve, *pathos*, disease], a condition in which many peripheral nerves are afflicted with a disorder.

polynuclear, having many nuclei.

polyopia /pol'ē·ō'pē·ə/ [Gk, *polys* + *ops*, eye], a defect of sight in which one object is perceived as many images; multiple vision. The condition can occur in one or both eyes.

polyp /pol'ip/ [Gk, *polys* + *pous*, foot], a small tumorlike growth that projects from a mucous membrane surface.

polypapilloma /-pap'ilō'mə/ [Gk, *polys*, many; L, *papilla*, nipple; Gk, *oma*], multiple papillomas or stalked tumors.

polypeptide /pol'ēpep'tīd/, a chain of amino acids joined by peptide bonds. A polypeptide has a greater molecular weight than a peptide but a lesser molecular weight than a protein.

polyphagia /pol'ēfā'jē·ə/ [Gk, *polys* + *phagein*, to eat], excessive uncontrolled eating.

polypharmacy /-fär'məsē/, the use of a number of different drugs by a patient who may have one or several health problems.

polyploid /pol'əploid/ [Gk, *polys* + *plous*, times], **1.** pertaining to an individual, organism, strain, or cell that has more than the two complete sets of chromosomes normal for the somatic cell. The multiple of the haploid number characteristic of the species is denoted by the appropriate prefix, as in triploid, tetraploid, pentaploid, hexaploid, heptaploid, octaploid, and so on. **2.** such an individual, organism, strain, or cell.

polyploidy /pol'iploi'dē/ /pol'əploi'dē/, the state or condition of having more than two complete sets of chromosomes.

polypoid [Gk, *polys,* many, *pous,* foot, *eidos,* form], like a polyp or tumor on a stalk.

polyposis /-pōsis/ [Gk, *polys* + *pous,* foot, *osis,* condition], an abnormal condition characterized by the presence of numerous polyps on a part.

polyposis coli [Gk, *polys,* many, *pous,* foot, *osis,* condition, *kolikos* colon], a condition of multiple polyps in the large intestine.

polyradiculitis /pol'ērədik'yŏŏlī'tis/ [Gk, *polys* + L, *radicula,* rootlet; Gk, *itis*], inflammation of many nerve roots, such as found in Guillain-Barré's syndrome.

polysaccharide /-sak'ərīd/ [Gk, *polys* + *sakcharon,* sugar], a carbohydrate that contains three or more molecules of simple carbohydrates. Examples of polysaccharides are dextrins, starches, and glycogens.

polysome /pol'isōm/ [Gk, *polys* + *soma,* body], (in genetics) a group of ribosomes joined together by a molecule of messenger ribonucleic acid containing the genetic code.

polysomy /pol'isō'mē/, the presence of a chromosome in at least triplicate in an otherwise diploid somatic cell as the result of chromosomal nondisjunction during meiotic division in the maturation of gametes. The chromosome may be duplicated three times (trisomy), four times (tetrasomy), or more times.

polysynaptic /-sinap'tik/ [Gk, *polys,* many, *synaptein,* to join], pertaining to nerve cells that end in synapses.

polysyndactyly /-sindak'tilē/ [Gk, *polys,* many, *syn,* together, *daktylos,* finger or toe], multiple webbing or fusion between fingers or toes.

polytene chromosome /pol'itēn/ [Gk, *polys* + *tainia,* band], an excessively large type of chromosome consisting of bundles of unseparated chromonemata filaments. It is found primarily in the saliva of certain insects.

polythiazide /-thī·az'īd/, a diuretic and antihypertensive prescribed in the treatment of hypertension and edema.

polyunsaturated /-unsach'ərā'tid/ [Gk,

polys, many; AS, *un,* not; L, *saturare,* to fill], pertaining to a chemical compound containing double or triple valency bonds that can be opened to accept more atoms in the molecule, thereby becoming saturated. A polyunsaturated fatty acid is one in which there are two or more links in the chain of carbon atoms that can be opened to accept hydrogen atoms.

polyuria /pol′ēyŏŏr′ē·ə/ [Gk, *polys* + *ouron,* urine], the excretion of an abnormally large quantity of urine. Some causes of polyuria are diabetes insipidus, diabetes mellitus, use of diuretics, excessive fluid intake, and hypercalcemia.

polyvalent vaccine /-vā′lənt/ [Gk, *polys,* many; L, *valere,* worth, *vaccinus,* cow], a vaccine prepared from several different antigenic types of a species.

polyvinyl chloride (PVC) /-vī′nil/, a common synthetic thermoplastic material that releases hydrochloric acid when burned and that may contain carcinogenic vinyl chloride molecules as a contaminant.

polyvinylidene (PVF$_2$) /-vīnil′idēn/, a commonly used piezoelectric material in a hydrophone. It is also used in imaging transducers.

POMP /pomp/, an abbreviation for a combination drug regimen used in the treatment of cancer, containing three antineoplastics—Purinethol (mercaptopurine), Oncovin (vincristine sulfate), and methotrexate—and prednisone (a glucocorticoid).

Pompe's disease [J. C. Pompe, twentieth-century Dutch physician; L, *dis,* opposite of; Fr, *aise,* ease], a form of muscle glycogen storage disease. There is a generalized accumulation of glycogen, resulting from a deficiency of acid maltase (alpha-1, 4-glucosidase). Children with Pompe's disease appear mentally retarded and hypotonic, seldom living beyond 20 years of age. In adults muscle weakness is progressive, but the disease is not fatal.

POMR, abbreviation for **problem-oriented medical record.**

pons /ponz/, *pl,* pontes /pon′tēz/ [L, bridge], **1.** a prominence on the ventral surface of the brainstem, between the medulla oblongata and the cerebral peduncles of the midbrain. The pons consists of white matter and a few nuclei and is divided into a ventral part and a dorsal part. The ventral part consists of transverse fibers separated by longitudinal bundles and small nuclei. The dorsal part comprises the tegmentum, which is a continuation of the reticular formation of the medulla. **2.** any slip of tissue connecting two parts of a structure or an organ of the body.

pontic /pon′tik/ [L, *pons,* bridge], the suspended member of a removable partial denture or fixed bridge, such as an artificial tooth, usually occupying the space previously occupied by the natural tooth crown.

pontine /pon′tīn/ [L, *pons,* bridge], pertaining to the pons.

pontine nucleus [L, *pons,* bridge, *nucleus,* nut kernel], nerve cells in the basilar part of the pons where impulses are relayed between the cerebrum and cerebellum.

pooled plasma [AS, *pol* + Gk, *plasma,* something formed], a liquid component of whole blood, collected and pooled to prepare various plasma products or to use directly as a plasma expander when whole blood is unavailable or is contraindicated.

poorly differentiated lymphocytic malignant lymphoma, a lymphoid neoplasm containing cells resembling lymphoblasts that have a fine nuclear structure and one or more nucleoli.

popliteal /poplit′ē-əl, pop′litē′əl/ [L, *poples,* ham of the knee], pertaining to the area behind the knee.

popliteal artery /pop′litē′əl/ [L, *poples,* ham of the knee; Gk, *arteria,* airpipe], a continuation of the femoral artery, extending from the opening in the abductor magnus; passing through the popliteal fossa at the knee; dividing into eight branches; and supplying various muscles of the thigh, leg, and foot.

popliteal node, a node in one of the groups of lymph glands in the leg.

popliteal pulse, the pulsation of the popliteal artery, behind the knee, best palpated with the patient lying prone with the knee flexed.

population /pop′yəlā′shən/ [L, *populus,* the people], **1.** (in genetics) an interbreeding group of individuals, organisms, or plants characterized by genetic continuity through several generations. **2.** a group of individuals collectively occupying a particular geographic locale. **3.** any group that is distinguished by a particular trait or situation. **4.** any group measured for some variable characteristic from which samples may be taken for statistical purposes.

population at risk, a group of people who share a characteristic that causes each member to be susceptible to a particular event, such as nonimmunized children who are exposed to poliovirus.

population genetics, a branch of genetics that applies mendelian inheritance to groups and studies the frequency of alleles and genotypes in breeding populations.

porcine /pôr′sīn/ [L, *porcinus,* pig-like], obtained from or related to hogs, such as porcine insulin.

P

porcine graft [L, *porcinus,* pig-like; Gk, *graphion,* plant stylus], a temporary biologic heterograft made from the skin of a pig.

poriomania /pôr'ē·ōmā'nē·ə/, a tendency to leave home impulsively or to be a vagabond.

pork tapeworm infection [L, *porcus,* pig, hog (male); AS, *taeppe,* tape, *wyrm,* worm; L, *inficere,* to stain], an infection of the intestine or other tissues caused by adult and larval forms of the tapeworm *Taenia solium.* The pork tapeworm is unique in that it can use humans as both intermediate hosts for larvae and definitive hosts for the adult worm. Humans are usually infected with the adult worm after eating contaminated undercooked pork.

porosis /pərō'sis/ [Gk, *poros,* passage], a condition of thinning bone tissue, particularly its supporting connective tissue, as in osteoporosis.

porous /pôr'əs/ [Gk, *poros,* passage], pertaining to something with pores or openings.

porphobilinogen /pôr'fōbilin'əjən/, a chromogen substance that is an intermediate in the biosynthesis of heme and porphyrins. It appears in the urine of people with porphyria.

porphyria /pôrfir'ē·ə/ [Gk, *porphyros,* purple], a group of inherited disorders in which there is abnormally increased production of substances called porphyrins. Two major classifications of porphyria are erythropoietic porphyria, characterized by the production of large quantities of porphyrins in the blood-forming tissue of the bone marrow, and hepatic porphyria, in which large amounts of porphyrins are produced in the liver. Clinical signs common to both classifications of porphyria are photosensitivity, abdominal pain, and neuropathy.

porphyrin /pôr'fərin/ [Gk, *porphyros,* purple], any iron- or magnesium-free pyrrole derivative occurring in many plant and animal tissues.

portacaval shunt /pôr'təkā'vəl/ [L, *porta,* gateway, *cavus,* cavity; ME, *shunten*], a shunt created surgically to increase blood flow from the portal circulation by carrying it into the vena cava.

portal /pôr'təl/ [L, *porta,* gateway], **1.** an entrance. **2.** pertaining to the porta hepatis, or portal vein.

portal circulation [L, *porta,* gateway, *circulare,* to go around], the pathway of blood flow from the gastrointestinal tract and spleen to the liver via the portal vein and its tributaries.

portal fissure [L, *porta* + *fissura,* cleft], a fissure on the visceral surface of the liver along which the portal vein, the hepatic artery, and the hepatic ducts pass.

portal hypertension, an increased venous pressure in the portal circulation caused by compression or occlusion in the portal or hepatic vascular system. It results in splenomegaly, large collateral veins, ascites, and in severe cases systemic hypertension and esophageal varices.

portal of entry, the route by which an infectious agent enters the body, such as through nonintact skin.

portal system, arrangement of blood vessels in which blood exiting one tissue is immediately carried to a second tissue before being returned to the heart and lungs for oxygenation and redistribution.

portal vein, a vein from the small intestine that ramifies in the liver and ends in capillary-like sinusoids that convey the blood to the inferior vena cava through the hepatic veins. The right branch of the portal vein enters the right lobe of the liver, and the left branch enters the left lobe.

Porter-Silber reaction [Curt C. Porter, American biochemist, b. 1914; Robert H. Silber, American biochemist, b. 1915], a reaction, visible as a change in color to yellow, that indicates the amount of adrenal steroids (the 17-hydroxycorticosteroids) excreted per day in the urine. The test is used to evaluate adrenocortical function but is now largely supplanted by immunoassay techniques.

portoenterostomy /pôr'tō·en'təros'təmē/ [L, *porta* + Gk, *enteron,* bowel, *stoma,* mouth, *temnein,* to cut], a procedure to correct biliary atresia in which the jejunum is anastomosed by a Roux-en-Y loop to the portal fissure region to establish bile flow from the bile ducts to the intestine.

position /pəzish'ən/ [L, *positio*], **1.** any one of many postures of the body, such as the anatomic position, lateral recumbent position, or semi-Fowler's position. **2.** (in obstetrics) the relationship of an arbitrarily chosen fetal reference point, such as the occiput, sacrum, chin, or scapula, on the presenting part of the fetus to its location in the maternal pelvis.

positional behavior /pəzish'ənəl/, the orientation of the body regions to claim a quantum of space. Positional behavior involves four body regions: head and neck, upper torso, pelvis and thighs, and lower legs and feet.

Positioning, a Nursing Interventions Classification defined as moving the patient or a body part to provide comfort, reduce the risk of skin breakdown, promote skin integrity, and/or promote healing.

Positioning: Intraoperative, a Nursing Interventions Classification defined as moving the patient or body part to promote surgical exposure while reducing the risk of discomfort and complications.

Positioning: Neurologic, a Nursing Interventions Classification defined as achievement of optimal appropriate body alignment for the patient experiencing or at risk for spinal cord injury or vertebral irritability.

Positioning: Wheelchair, a Nursing Interventions Classification defined as placement of a patient in a properly selected wheelchair to enhance comfort, promote skin integrity, and foster independence.

positive /poz'itiv/ [L, *positivus,*], **1.** (of a laboratory test result) indicating that a substance or a reaction is present. **2.** (of a sign) indicating on physical examination that a finding is present, often meaning that there is pathologic change. **3.** (of a substance) tending to carry or carrying a positive chemical charge.

positive end expiratory pressure (PEEP), (in respiratory therapy) the addition of positive airway pressure at the end of the exhalation phase. Each successive breath begins from a new baseline. Ventilation is controlled by a flow of air delivered in cycles of constant pressure through the respiratory cycle. PEEP is used for the relief of respiratory distress secondary to prematurity, pancreatitis, shock, pulmonary edema, trauma, surgery, or other conditions in which spontaneous respiratory efforts are inadequate and arterial levels of oxygen are deficient.

positive feedback, 1. (in physiology) an increase in function in response to a stimulus; for example, micturition increases after the flow of urine has started. **2.** *informal.* an encouraging, favorable, or otherwise positive response from one person to what another person has communicated.

positive identification, the unconscious modeling of one's personality on that of another who is admired and esteemed.

positive pressure, 1. a greater than ambient atmospheric pressure. **2.** (in respiratory therapy) any technique in which compressed gas or air is delivered to the airways at greater than ambient pressure.

positive relationship, (in research) a direct relationship between two variables; as one increases, the other can be expected to increase.

positive signs of pregnancy, three unmistakable signs of pregnancy: fetal heart tones, heard on auscultation; fetal skeleton, seen on X-ray film or ultrasonogram; and fetal parts, felt on palpation.

positron /pos'itron/, a positive electron,

or positively charged particle emitted from neutron-deficient radioactive nuclei.

positron emission tomography (PET) [L, *positivus* + Gk, *elektron,* amber; L, *emittere,* to send out; Gk, *tome,* section, *graphein* to record], a computerized radiographic technique that uses radioactive substances to examine the metabolic activity of various body structures. In PET studies the patient either inhales or is injected with a biochemical such as glucose that carries a radioactive substance that emits positively charged particles, or positrons. When these positrons combine with negatively charged electrons normally found in the cells of the body, gamma rays are emitted. The electronic circuitry and computers of the PET device detect the gamma rays and convert them into color-coded images that indicate the intensity of the metabolic activity of the organ involved.

Postanesthesia Care, a Nursing Interventions Classification defined as monitoring and management of the patient who has recently undergone general or regional anesthesia.

postcaval shunt /-kā'vəl/ [L, *post,* after, *vena cava* + ME, *shunten*], any of several surgical anastomoses of the portal and systemic circulations to relieve symptoms of portal hypertension.

postcentral gyrus /-sen'trəl/ [L, *post,* after; Gk, *kentron,* center, *gyros,* turn], a convolution of the brain immediately posterior to the central sulcus of the cerebrum.

postcoital /-kō'itəl/ [L, *post,* after, *coire,* to come together], after sexual intercourse.

postcommissurotomy syndrome /-kəmis'-yərot'əmē/ [L, *post,* after, *commissura,* a union; Gk, *temnein,* to cut], a condition of unknown cause occurring within the first few weeks after cardiac valvular surgery, characterized by intermittent episodes of pain and fever, which may last weeks or months and then resolve spontaneously.

postconcussional syndrome /-kənkush'-ənəl/ [L, *post* + *concussio,* shake violently], a condition that follows head trauma, characterized by dizziness, poor concentration, headache, hypersensitivity, and anxiety.

postdate pregnancy /-dāt'/ [L, *post,* after, *data* + *praegnans,* bearing child], a pregnancy that lasts more than 42 weeks.

posterior /postir'ē·ər/ [L, behind], **1.** in the back part of a structure, such as of the dorsal surface of the human body. **2.** the back part of something. **3.** toward the back.

posterior Achilles bursitis, a painful heel condition caused by inflammation of the bursa between the Achilles tendon and the calcaneus. It is commonly associated with Haglund's deformity.

posterior atlantoaxial ligament, one of five ligaments connecting the atlas to the axis.

posterior atlantooccipital membrane, one of a pair of thin, broad fibrous sheets that form part of the atlantooccipital joint between the atlas and the occipital bone.

posterior auricular artery, one of a pair of small branches from the external carotid arteries, dividing into auricular and occipital branches and supplying parts of the ear, scalp, and other structures in the head.

posterior column [L, behind, *columna*], the posterior horns of the gray substance in the spinal cord.

posterior costotransverse ligament, one of the five ligaments of each costotransverse joint, comprising a fibrous band passing from the neck of each rib to the base of the vertebra above.

posterior drawer sign, an orthopedic test in which the patient is positioned with hips at 45 degrees and knees flexed at 90 degrees while the examiner stabilizes the foot and pushes the tibia backward. Also, with both the hips and knees flexed at 90 degrees, the heels are held together, and the knees are observed for comparison of relative posterior sag of the tibia.

posterior fontanel, a small triangular area between the occipital and parietal bones at the junction of the sagittal and lambdoidal sutures.

posterior fossa, a depression on the posterior surface of the humerus, above the trochlea, that lodges the olecranon of the ulna when the elbow is extended.

posterior horn [L, behind, *cornu*, horn], the horn-shaped projections of gray matter in the posterior region of the spinal cord.

posterior longitudinal ligament, a thick strong ligament attached to the dorsal surfaces of the vertebral bodies, extending from the occipital bone to the coccyx.

posterior mediastinal node, a node in one of three groups of thoracic visceral nodes, connected to the part of the lymphatic system that serves the esophagus, pericardium, diaphragm, and convex surface of the liver.

posterior mediastinum, the irregularly shaped lower part of the mediastinum, parallel with the vertebral column.

posterior nares, a pair of posterior openings in the nasal cavity connecting it with the nasopharynx and allowing the inhalation and exhalation of air.

posterior neuropore, the opening at the inferior end of the embryonic neural tube.

posterior palatal seal area, the area of soft tissues along the junction of the hard and soft palates on which displacement, within the physiologic tolerance of the tissues, can be applied by a denture to aid its retention.

posterior rhizotomy [L, behind; Gk, *rhiza*, root, *temnein*, to cut], a surgical procedure for cutting the posterior, or sensory, nerve root for the relief of intractable pain.

posterior tibial artery, one of the divisions of the popliteal artery, supplying various muscles of the lower leg, foot, and toes.

posterior tibialis pulse, the pulse of the posterior tibialis artery palpated on the medial aspect of the ankle, just posterior to the prominence of the ankle bone.

posterior tooth, any of the maxillary and mandibular premolars and molars of the deciduous or permanent dentition, or of prostheses.

posterior vein of left ventricle, one of the five tributaries of the coronary sinus that drain blood from the capillary bed of the myocardium.

posteroanterior /-antir′ē·ər/ [L, *posterus*, coming after, *anterior*, before], the direction from back to front.

posteroinferior /-infir′ē·ər/ [L, *posterus*, coming after, *inferior*, lower], pertaining to a position that is both lower and behind.

posterolateral /-lat′ərəl/ [L, *posterus*, coming after, *latus*, side], pertaining to a position behind and to the side.

posterolateral thoracotomy /pos′tərōlat′-ərəl/, a chest surgery technique in which an incision is made in the submammary fold, below the tip of the scapula.

postganglionic /-gang′glē·on′ik/ [L, *post*, after; Gk, *ganglion*, knot], distal to a ganglion.

postganglionic fiber, the axon of a nerve cell whose cell body is situated in a ganglion.

postganglionic neuron [L, *post*, after; Gk, *ganglion*, knot, *neuron*, nerve], a neuron that is distal to or beyond a ganglion.

posthepatic jaundice /pōst′hepat′ik/ [L, *post*, after; Gk, *hepar*, liver; Fr, *jaune*, yellow], jaundice caused by obstruction of the bile ducts.

posthumous /pos′chəməs/ [L, *post*, after, *humare*, to bury], after a person's death.

posthypnotic suggestion /-hipnot′ik/ [L, *post*, after; Gk, *hypnos*, sleep; L, *suggerere*, to suggest], an action suggested to a hypnotized subject during a trance that the subject carries out on awakening from the trance. The action is in response to a cue, and the subject usually does not know why he or she is performing it.

postictal /pōst'iktəl/ [L, *post* + Gk, *ikteros,* jaundice], after a seizure. **—postictus,** *n.*

postinfectious /-infek'shəs/ [L, *post* + *inficere,* to stain], after an infection.

postinfectious glomerulonephritis, the acute form of glomerulonephritis, which may follow 1 to 6 weeks after a streptococcal infection, most often in childhood. Characteristics of the disease are hematuria, oliguria, edema, and proteinuria, especially in the form of granular casts.

postinfectious psychosis [L, *post,* after, *inficere,* to stain; Gk, *psyche,* mind, *osis,* condition], psychotic behavior that follows a severe infection such as pneumonia, scarlet fever, malaria, uremia, or typhoid fever.

postlumbar puncture headache /-lum'bar/ [L, *post,* after, *lumbus,* loin, *punctura;* AS, *heafod + acan*], a headache that occurs within a few hours of a lumbar puncture and usually lasts 1 or 2 days to several weeks. It may be accompanied by nausea and vomiting and improves when the patient lies down.

postmastectomy exercises /-məstek'təmē/ [L, *post* + Gk, *mastos,* breast, *ektome,* excision], exercises essential to the prevention of shortening of the muscles, contracture of the joints, and improvement in lymph and blood circulation after mastectomy. The woman is asked to flex and extend the fingers of the affected arm and to pronate and supinate the forearm immediately on return to her room after recovery from anesthesia and surgery. Brushing her teeth and hair is encouraged as effective exercise. Other exercises are usually taught, including four specific exercises: climbing the wall, arm swinging, rope pulling, and elbow spreading.

postmature /-məchoor'/ [L, *post + matu rare,* to become ripe], **1.** overly developed or matured. **2.** pertaining to a postmature infant. **—postmaturity,** *n.*

postmature infant, an infant born after the end of the forty-second week of gestation, bearing the physical signs of placental insufficiency. Characteristically the baby has dry, peeling skin; long fingernails and toenails; and folds of skin on the thighs and sometimes on the arms and buttocks. Hypoglycemia and hypokalemia are common. Postmature infants often look as if they have lost weight in utero.

postmaturity /-məchoo'ritē/ [L, *post,* after, *maturare,* to make ripe], beyond the normal date for maturity.

postmenopausal /-men'əpô'səl/ [L, *post* + *men,* month; Gk, *pauein,* to cease], pertaining to the period of life after the menopause.

postmenopausal hemorrhage, bleeding from the uterus after menopause.

postmenopausal vaginitis [L, *post,* after, *men,* month; Gk, *pauein,* to cease; L, *vagina,* sheath; Gk, *itis,* inflammation], an inflammation caused by degenerative changes in the vaginal mucosa after menopause.

postmortem /môr'təm/ [L, *post* + *mors,* death], **1.** after death. **2.** *(informal)* **postmortem examination.**

Postmortem Care, a Nursing Interventions Classification defined as providing physical care of the body of an expired patient and support for the family viewing the body.

postmortem cesarean section [L, *post,* after, *mors,* death, *secare,* to cut, *sectio*], delivery of a fetus by incision into the uterus after death of a woman.

postmortem examination [L, *post,* after, *mors,* death, *examinatio*], an examination of a body after death by a person trained in pathology.

postmortem graft [L, *post,* after, *mors,* death; Gk, *graphion,* stylus], the transplanting of a cornea, artery, or other body part from a dead person to repair a defect in a living body.

postmortem lividity, the black and blue discoloration of the skin of a cadaver resulting from an accumulation of deoxygenated blood in subcutaneous vessels.

postmyocardial infarction syndrome /-mī'əkär'dē-əl/ [L, *post* + Gk, *mys,* muscle, *kardia,* heart; L, *infarcire,* to stuff], a condition that may occur days or weeks after an acute myocardial infarction. It is characterized by chest pain, fever, pericarditis with a friction rub, pleurisy, pleural effusion, joint pain, elevated white blood cell count, and sedimentation rate. It tends to recur and often provokes severe anxiety, depression, and fear that another heart attack is occurring.

postnasal /-nā'zəl/ [L, *post,* after, *nasus,* nose], pertaining to the region behind the nose, or the posterior part of the nasal fossae.

postnasal drip (PND) [L, *post + nasus,* nose; AS, *dryppan*], a drop-by-drop discharge of nasal mucus into the posterior pharynx. It is often accompanied by a feeling of obstruction, an unpleasant taste, and fetid breath, caused by rhinitis, chronic sinusitis, or hypersecretion by the nasopharyngeal mucosa.

postnecrotic cirrhosis /-nekrot'ik/ [L, *post* + Gk, *nekros,* dead; *kirrhos,* yellowish, *osis,* condition], a nodular form of cirrhosis that may follow hepatitis or other inflammation of the liver.

postoperative /-op'ərətiv'/ [L, *post + op-*

P

erari, to work], pertaining to the period of time after surgery. It begins with the patient's emergence from anesthesia and continues through the time required for the acute effects of the anesthetic or surgical procedures to abate.

postoperative atelectasis, a form of atelectasis in which collapse of lung tissue is caused by the depressant effects of anesthetic drugs. Deep breathing and coughing are encouraged at frequent postoperative intervals to prevent this condition.

postoperative bed, a surface prepared for a patient who is weak or unconscious, as when recovering from anesthesia. The bed is in the flat position. The bottom sheet may be covered with a cotton bath blanket that is tucked tightly beneath the mattress. The top linen is fan-folded to the far side of the bed and not tucked in. The bed is made in this way to simplify transferring a patient from a stretcher into the bed.

postoperative care, the management of a patient after surgery. Before the patient's discharge from the operating room, the surgical drapes, ground plate, and restraints are removed; and a sterile dressing may be applied to the incision. The patency and connections of all drainage tubes and the flow rate of parenteral infusions are checked. The patient's cleanliness and dryness are given attention, and the gown is changed, avoiding exposing the individual. The patient is transferred slowly and cautiously to a recovery room bed, maintaining body alignment and protecting the limbs. When indicated, an oral or nasal airway is inserted, or a previously inserted endotracheal tube is suctioned; respiration may be supported with a pulmonator or pulse oximeter; if respiration remains impaired, the anesthetist is notified. The blood pressure, pulse, and respirations are initially reported to the anesthetist and are then checked every 15 minutes or as ordered. At similar intervals the level of consciousness, reflexes, and movements of extremities are observed; and the incision, drainage tubes, and intravenous infusion site are inspected. Nothing is given orally; medication, blood or blood components, and oxygen are administered as ordered; and fluid intake and output are measured. Pain is controlled by administration of analgesics.

postoperative cholangiography, (in diagnostic radiology) a procedure for outlining the major bile ducts. A radiopaque contrast material is injected into the common bile duct via a T-tube inserted during surgery. It is usually performed after a cholecystectomy to discover any residual calculi.

postoperative ileus [L, *post* + *operari,* to work; Gk, *eilein,* to twist], an obstruction to normal intestinal function caused by a loss of peristaltic muscular action of the ileus after surgery.

postparalytic /-perʹəlitʹik/ [L, *post* + Gk, *paralyein,* to be palsied], pertaining to something that occurred after paralysis.

postpartal care /-pärʹtəl/ [L, *post* + *partus,* bringing forth], care of the mother and her newborn during the first few days of the puerperium. The physical and physiologic changes of involution in the mother are observed for deviation from the normal. The uterus contracts after delivery, causing bleeding from the site of placental implantation to diminish. It is the size of a softball; the fundus is below the umbilicus. The lochia changes color and consistency during the first few days. Lochia rubra flows for 2 to 4 days, followed by pinkish brown lochia serosa and finally by clear, sticky lochia alba. The abdominal wall is soft, but muscle tone returns with time and exercise. On the third day the milk usually begins to fill the breasts.

Postpartal Care, a Nursing Interventions Classification defined as monitoring and management of the patient who has recently given birth.

postpartum /pōstpärʹtəm/, after childbirth.

postpartum blues [L, *post,* after, *parturire,* labor pains; ME, *bleu*], an emotional effect of childbirth experienced by mothers, consisting mainly of transient feelings of sadness for a period of about 72 hours. If the symptom persists for a longer period, the diagnosis of depression may apply. The condition may require psychotherapy, use of antidepressant medications, or both.

postpartum depression [L, *post* + *partus* + *deprimere,* to press down], an abnormal psychiatric condition that occurs after childbirth, typically from 3 days to 6 weeks after delivery. It is characterized by symptoms that range from mild "postpartum blues" to an intense suicidal depressive psychosis. Some women at risk for postpartum depression may be identified during the prenatal period: those who have made no preparations for the expected baby, expressed unrealistic plans for postpartum work or travel, or denied the reality of the responsibilities of parenthood.

postpartum hemorrhage [L, *post,* after, *parturire,* labor pains; Gk, *haima,* blood, *rhegnynai,* to burst forth], excessive bleeding (a loss of more than 500 ml of blood) after childbirth.

postpartum iliofemoral thrombophlebitis [L, *post,* after, *parturire,* labor pains, *ilia,* flank, *femur,* thigh; Gk, *thrombos,* lump, *phleps,* vein, *itis,* inflammation], a condition of thrombophlebitis involving the iliofemoral artery after childbirth.

postpartum pituitary necrosis [L, *post + parturire + pituita,* phlegm; GK, *nekros,* dead, *osis,* condition], a condition of hypopituitarism resulting from hypovolemia and shock in the immediate postpartum period. Lactation may not develop, pubic and axillary hair may be lost, and symptoms of hypoglycemia and amenorrhea are experienced.

postpartum psychosis [L, *post,* after, *parturire,* labor pains; Gk, *psyche,* mind], an episode of psychosis, either depressive or schizophrenic, after childbirth. Because the condition usually develops in the month after childbirth, endocrinologic factors are believed to be a cause.

postperfusion syndrome /-pərfyōo′zhən/ [L, *post + perfundere,* to pour over], a cytomegalovirus (CMV) infection occurring between 2 and 4 weeks after the transfusion of fresh blood containing CMV. It is characterized by prolonged fever, hepatitis, rash, atypical lymphocytosis, and occasionally jaundice.

postpericardiotomy syndrome /pōst′-perikär′dē·ot′əmē/ [L, *post +* Gk, *peri,* around, *kardia,* heart, *temnein,* to cut], a condition that sometimes occurs days or weeks after pericardiotomy, characterized by symptoms of pericarditis, often without any fever. It appears to be an autoimmune response to damaged muscle cells of the myocardium and pericardium.

postpill amenorrhea /-pill′/ [L, *post + pilla,* ball; Gk, *a,* not, *men,* month, *rhoia,* flow], failure of normal menstrual cycles to resume within 3 months after discontinuation of oral contraception.

postpoliomyelitis muscular atrophy (PPMA) /-pō′lēomī′əlī′tis/ [L, *post,* after; Gk, *polios,* gray, *myelos,* marrow, *itis,* inflammation; L, *musculus +* Gk, *a,* not, *trophe,* nourishment], a recurrence of neuromuscular symptoms in people who had recovered from acute paralytic polio many years earlier. The chief symptom is muscular weakness, and the condition may affect the same muscles or muscles that were not damaged in the earlier polio attack.

postpolycythemic myeloid metaplasia /-pol′isithē′mik/ [L, *post +* Gk, *polys,* many, *kytos,* cell, *haima,* blood, *myelos,* marrow, *eidos,* form, *meta,* with, *plassein,* to mold], a late development in polycythemia vera, characterized by anemia caused by sclerosis of the bone marrow. The production of red blood cells occurs only in the liver and spleen.

postprandial, after a meal.

postprandial pain [L, *post,* after, *prandium,* meal, *poena,* penalty], pain that occurs after a meal.

postprocessing /-pros′əsing/, (in ultrasonics) manipulation and conditioning of signals and image data after they emerge from the scan converter and before they are displayed. Postprocessing is used to change the assignment of image brightness versus echo signal amplitude in memory.

postpubertal panhypopituitarism /-pyōo′-bərtəl/ [L, *post + pubertas,* maturation; Gk, *pan,* all, *hypo,* below, *pituita,* phlegm], insufficiency of pituitary hormones, caused by postpartum pituitary necrosis resulting from thrombosis of the circulation of the gland during or after birth. The disorder, characterized initially by weakness, lethargy, failure to lactate, amenorrhea, loss of libido, and intolerance to cold, leads to loss of axillary and pubic hair, bradycardia, hypotension, premature wrinkling of the skin, and atrophy of the thyroid and adrenal glands.

postpuberty /-pyōo′bərtē/ [L, *post + pubertas*], a period of approximately 1 to 2 years after puberty during which skeletal growth slows and the physiologic functions of the reproductive years are established. **—postpuberal, postpubertal, postpubescent,** *adj.*

postrenal anuria /-rē′nəl/ [L, *post + renes,* kidney; Gk, *a + ouron,* not urine], cessation of urine production caused by obstruction in the ureters.

poststeroid lobular panniculitis [L, *panniculus,* piece of cloth], subcutaneous nodules that may develop in a layer of fatty connective tissue in children 1 to 13 days after discontinuation of steroid therapy. The condition resolves spontaneously with or without readministration of the medication.

postsynaptic /-sinap′tik/ [L, *post +* Gk, *synaptein,* to join], **1.** situated after a synapse. **2.** occurring after a synapse has been crossed.

posttransfusion syndrome /-transfyōo′-zhən/ [L, *post,* after, *transfundere,* to pour through; Gk, *syn,* together, *dromos,* course], a complex of adverse reactions that may accompany or follow intravenous administration of blood or blood components. Reactions may include hemolytic effects, headache and back pain, allergies to an unknown component in donor blood, circulatory overloading, effects of cold blood that chill the patient's cardiovascular system, and effects of microaggregates in stored blood.

posttrauma response /-trô′mə/, a

NANDA-accepted nursing diagnosis of the state of an individual experiencing a sustained painful response to overwhelming traumatic events. Critical defining characteristics include reexperience of the traumatic event, which may be identified in cognitive, affective, or sensory motor activities (flashbacks, intrusive thoughts, repetitive dreams or nightmares, excessive verbalization of the traumatic event, or verbalization of survival guilt or guilt about behavior required by survival).

posttraumatic /pōst'trômat'ik/ [L, *post,* after, Gk, *trauma,* wounded], pertaining to any emotional, mental, or physiologic consequences after a major illness or injury.

posttraumatic amnesia [L, *post* + Gk, *trauma,* wound], a period of amnesia between a brain injury resulting in memory loss and the point at which the functions concerned with memory are restored.

posttraumatic osteoporosis /-trômat'ik/ [L, *post,* after; Gk, *trauma,* wound, *osteon,* bone, *poros,* passage, *osis,* condition], osteoporosis that develops after an injury or other severe health episode.

posttraumatic stress disorder (PTSD), a DSM-IV psychiatric disorder characterized by an acute emotional response to a traumatic event or situation involving severe environmental stress, such as a natural disaster, airplane crash, serious automobile accident, military combat, or physical torture.

postulate /pos'chəlāt/ [L, *postulare,* to demand], a hypothesis that is offered as true without proof or as a basis for argument or debate.

postural background movements /pos'-chərəl/ [L, *ponere,* to place], the spontaneous body adjustments, requiring vestibular and proprioceptive integration, that maintain the center of gravity, keep the head and body in alignment, and stabilize body parts.

postural drainage, the use of positioning to drain secretions from specific segments of the bronchi and the lungs into the trachea. Coughing usually expels secretions from the trachea. Positions that promote drainage from the affected parts of the lungs are selected. Pillows and raised sections of the hospital bed are used to support or elevate parts of the body. The procedure is begun with the patient level, and the head is gradually lowered to a full Trendelenburg position. Inhalation through the nose and exhalation through the mouth are encouraged. Simultaneously the nurse or other health care provider may use cupping and vibration over the affected area of the lungs to dislodge and mobilize secretions. The person is then helped to a position conducive to coughing and is asked to breathe deeply at least three times and to cough at least twice.

postural reflex [L, *ponere,* to place, *reflectere,* to turn back], any of several reflexes associated with maintaining normal body posture.

postural vertigo, a severe but brief episode of vertigo associated with a change of body position, as when a patient lies down. It may be caused by an injury or disease of the utricle.

posture /pos'chər/ [L, *ponere,* to place], the position of the body with respect to the surrounding space. A posture is determined and maintained by coordination of the various muscles that move the limbs, by proprioception, and by the sense of balance.

postvaccinal encephalitis /-vak'sinəl/ [L, *post,* after, *vaccinus,* of a cow; Gk, *enkephalos,* brain, *itis,* inflammation], acute encephalitis after vaccination.

postvaccinal encephalomyelitis [L, *post,* after, *vaccinus,* of a cow; Gk, *enkephalos,* brain, *myelos,* marrow, *itis,* inflammation], acute encephalomyelitis after vaccination.

postviral fatigue syndrome /-vīrəl/ [L, *post,* after, *virus,* poison, *fatigare,* to tire; Gk, *syn,* together, *dromos,* course], a condition of chronic muscle fatigue unrelieved by rest after a viral infection. Other symptoms may include visual and hearing difficulties, low-grade fever, stiff neck, urinary frequency, and insomnia.

potable water /pō'təbəl/ [L, *potare,* to drink], water that can be consumed without concern for adverse health effects. Potable water does not have to taste good; palatable water may taste good but is not necessarily safe to drink.

potassemia /pōt'əsē'meiə/ [D, *potasschen,* potash; Gk, *haima,* blood], an excess of potassium in the blood.

potassium (K) /pətas'ē·əm/ [D, *potasschen,* potash], an alkali metal element, the seventh most abundant element in the earth's crust. Its atomic number is 19; its atomic mass (weight) is 39.1. Potassium salts are necessary to the life of all plants and animals. Potassium in the body constitutes the predominant intracellular cation, helping to regulate neuromuscular excitability and muscle contraction.

potassium chloride (KCl), a white crystalline salt used as a substitute for table salt in the diet of people with cardiovascular disorders, in administration of the potassium ion, and as a constituent of Ringer's solution. It is prescribed in the treatment of hypokalemia resulting from a variety of causes and of digitalis intoxication.

potassium hydroxide (KOH), a white, soluble, highly caustic compound. Occasionally used in solution as an escharotic for bites of rabid animals, KOH has many laboratory uses as an alkalinizing agent, including the preparation of clinical specimens for examination for fungi under the microscope.

potassium iodide, a bronchodilator prescribed in the treatment of bronchitis, bronchiectasis, and asthma and in various thyroid disorders.

potassium pump, a mechanism that involves energy-dependent pumping of potassium or the active transport of the potassium ion (K^+) across a biologic membrane using the energy of K^+-activated adenosine triphosphatase.

potency /pō'tənsē/ [L, *potentia,* power], (in embryology) the range of developmental possibilities of which an embryonic cell or part is capable, regardless of whether the stimulus for growth or differentiation is natural, artificial, or experimental.

potent /pō'tənt/ [L, *potentia,* power], powerful or strong.

potential /pəten'shəl/ [L, *potentia*], an expression of the energy involved in transferring a unit of electrical charge. The gradient or slope of a potential causes the charge to move.

potential abnormality of glucose tolerance, a classification that includes people who have never had abnormal glucose tolerance but who have an increased risk of diabetes or impaired glucose tolerance. Factors associated with an increased risk of insulin-dependent diabetes mellitus (IDDM) include having circulating islet cell antibodies, being a monozygotic twin or sibling of an IDDM patient and being the offspring of an IDDM patient. Factors associated with an increased risk of noninsulin-dependent diabetes mellitus (NIDDM) include being a first-degree relative of an NIDDM patient (particularly in a family in which there are several generations with NIDDM), giving birth to a neonate weighing more than 9 pounds, being a member of a racial or ethnic group with a high prevalence of diabetes such as some Native American groups, and being an obese adult.

potential difference, the difference in electrical potential between two points.

potential energy [L, *potentia,* power; Gk, *energeia*], the energy contained in a body as a result of its position in space, its internal structure, and the stresses imposed on it.

potential life, a criterion used by the federal Centers for Disease Control and Prevention to gauge premature death rates. Among younger individuals, it is based on an assumption that the person would have lived to 65 years of age if life had not been interrupted by a particular disease or injury. For older people the system is based on years of potential life lost before 85 years of age, in which case cancer and heart disease rank first and second.

potential trauma, (in dentistry) a change in tissue that may occur because of existing malocclusion or dental disharmony.

potentiate /pōten'shē-āt/, to increase the strength or degree of activity of something.

potentiation /pōten'shē-ā'shən/ [L, *potentia*], a synergistic action in which the effect of two drugs given simultaneously is greater than the effect of the drugs given separately.

potentiometer /pōten'shē-om'ətər/ [L, *potentia* + Gk, *metron,* measure], a voltage-measuring device.

Potter-Bucky grid [Hollis E. Potter; Gustav Bucky; twentieth-century American radiologists; ME, *gredire,* grate], (in radiography) an x-ray grid designed on the principle of a moving grid, which oscillates during the exposure of a radiographic film.

Pott's fracture [Percival Pott, English physician, 1713–1788], a fracture of the fibula near the ankle, often accompanied by a break of the malleolus of the tibia or rupture of the internal lateral ligament.

potty chair [AS, *pott* + ME, *chaire*], a small chair that has an open seat over a removable pot, used for the toilet training of young children.

pouch [OFr, *pouche*], any small saclike appendage or pocket, such as Rathke's pouch in the roof of the embryonic roof cavity.

poultice /pōl'tis/ [L, *puls,* porridge], a soft moist pulp spread between layers of gauze or cloth and applied hot to a surface to provide heat or to counter irritation. A kind of poultice is a **mustard plaster.**

pound [L, *pondus,* weight], a unit of measure equal to 16 ounces, avoirdupois; 0.45359 kg; 7000 grains.

poverty /pov'ərtē/ [L, *paupertas*], **1.** a lack of material wealth needed to maintain existence. **2.** a loss of emotional capacity to feel love or sympathy.

povidone /pō'vidōn/, a polymerized form of vinylpyrrolidone, a white hygroscopic powder readily soluble in water, used as a dispersing and suspending agent in drugs. It also has been used as a blood volume

P

extender and, in a complex with iodine, as a topical antiseptic.

povidone-iodine /pō′vidōnī′ədīn/, an antiseptic microbicide prescribed as a topical microbicide for disinfection of wounds, as a preoperative surgical scrub, for vaginal infections, and for antiseptic treatment of burns.

Powassan virus infection [Powassan, Ontario], an uncommon form of encephalitis caused by a tickborne arbovirus found in eastern Canada and the northern United States.

powder bed [L, *pulvis*, dust; AS, *bedd*], a treatment in which large areas of a patient's body are kept in contact with a powdered medication for a certain time. The patient lies supine on the powdered sheet. Areas of skin that are apposed are separated with gauze, and powder is shaken over the patient's body. The powdered sheet is then wrapped around the limbs and the trunk from the side to keep the powder in contact with the body.

powerlessness /pow′ərləsnes′/ [Fr, *pouvoir,* to have power; AS, *loes,* limited, *nes,* condition], a NANDA-accepted nursing diagnosis of a perceived lack of control over a current situation or problem and the client's perception that any action he or she takes will not affect the outcome of the particular situation. The defining characteristics may be of a severe, moderate, or passive nature. Severe characteristics include the client's verbal expression of having no control or influence over self-care, the particular situation, or its outcome; apathy; or depression about physical deterioration that occurs despite compliance with regimens. Moderate characteristics include the client's nonparticipation in or lack of interest in the mode of care, in decision making regarding regimens, or in monitoring progress; the client's verbal expression of dissatisfaction and frustration regarding the inability to perform previous activities; the reluctance to express true feelings, fearing alienation of others; general irritability or passivity; and expressions of resentment, anger, guilt, or doubt regarding role performance. Passive characteristics involve expressions of uncertainty about fluctuating energy levels.

power mode, a method of color flow processing and display in which the Doppler signal amplitude or the signal intensity, averaged over a small interval, is displayed rather than the average Doppler frequency. Velocity and flow direction are not displayed, and artefacts do not affect the image.

power of attorney [Fr, *pouvoir* + OFr,

atorne, legal agent], a document authorizing one person to take legal actions on behalf of another, to act as an agent for the grantor.

power stroke, a working stroke with a dental scaling instrument, used for splitting or dislodging calculus from the surface of a tooth or tooth root.

pox [ME, *pokkes,* pustules], **1.** any of several vesicular or pustular exanthematous diseases. **2.** the pitlike scars of smallpox.

poxvirus /poksvī′rəs/ [ME, *pokkes* + L, *virus,* poison], a member of a family of viruses that includes the organisms that cause molluscum contagiosum, smallpox, and vaccinia.

PPD, abbreviation for **purified protein derivative.**

PPLO, abbreviation for **pleuropneumonia-like organism.**

PPM, ppm, abbreviation for **parts per million.**

PPMA, abbreviation for **postpoliomyelitis muscular atrophy.**

PPO, abbreviation for **preferred provider organization.**

PPNG, abbreviation for **penicillinase-producing** *Neisseria gonorrhoeae.*

PPS, abbreviation for **prospective payment system.**

PPV, abbreviation for *positive pressure ventilation.*

Pr, symbol for the element **praseodymium.**

practice guideline, a detailed description of a process of patient care management that will facilitate improvement or maintenance of health status or slow the decline in health status in certain chronic clinical conditions. The purpose of a practice guideline is to assist health care providers to identify preferred treatment by providing linkages among diagnoses, treatments, and outcomes and by describing alternatives available for each patient.

practice models /prak′tis/ [Gk, *praktikos,* practical], the different patterns in delivery of health care services by means of which health care is made available to diverse groups of people in different settings.

practice setting, the context or environment within which nursing care is given.

practice theory, (in nursing research) a theory that describes, explains, and prescribes nursing practice in general. It serves as the basis for specific items in the curriculum of nursing education and for the development of theories in the administration of nursing and nursing education.

practicing /prak′tising/, the second subphase of the separation-individuation phase in Mahler's system of preoedipal development, when the child is able to move away from the mother and return to her for emotional nurturing.

practicing medicine without a license, (in law) practicing activities defined under state law in the medical practice act without physician supervision, direction, or control.

practitioner /praktish'ənər/ [Gk, *praktikos*], a person qualified to practice in a special professional field, such as a nurse practitioner.

Prader-Willi's syndrome /prä'dər wil'ē/ [A. Prader, twentieth-century Swiss physician; H. Willi; Gk, *syn*, together, *dromos*, course], a metabolic condition characterized by congenital hypotonia, hyperphagia, obesity, and mental retardation. The syndrome is associated with a below-normal secretion of gonadotropic hormones by the pituitary gland.

praecox [L, premature], pertaining to something that occurred at an earlier stage of life or development.

praevia /prē'vē-ə/, [L], having occurred at an earlier time or in front of a place.

pragmatic /pragmat'ik/, pertaining to a belief that ideas are valuable only in terms of their consequences.

pragmatism /prag'mətizəm/ [Gk, *pragma*, deed], a philosophy concerned with actual practice and practical results as opposed to theory and speculation.

pralidoxime chloride /pral'ədok'sēm/, a cholinesterase reactivator prescribed as an antidote for organophosphate poisoning and drug overdosage in the treatment of myasthenia gravis.

pramoxine hydrochloride /prəmok'sēn/, a local anesthetic for the relief of pain and itching associated with dermatoses, anogenital pruritus, hemorrhoids, anal fissure, and minor burns.

prandial /pran'dē-əl/ [L, *prandium,* meal], pertaining to a meal. The term is used in relation to timing, such as postprandial or preprandial. —**prandiality,** *n.*

praseodymium (Pr) /prä'sē-ōdīm'ē-əm/ [Gk, *prasaios*, light-green, *didymos*, twin], a rare earth metallic element. Its atomic number is 59; its atomic mass (weight) is 140.91.

Prausnitz-Küstner (PK) test /prous'-nitskist'nər/ [Otto C. Prausnitz, German hygienist, 1876–1963; Heinz Küstner, German gynecologist, 1897–1963], a skin test formerly used to measure the presence of immunoglobulin E. It is no longer used because of the high risk of transfer of hepatitis or blood-borne diseases such as acquired immunodeficiency syndrome.

praxis [Gk, action], a concept that deals with actions and overt behavior, or the performance of an action, to the exclusion of metaphysical thought.

prazepam /praz'əpam/, an antianxiety agent derived from benzodiazepine. It is prescribed for the treatment of anxiety disorders or the short-term relief of symptoms of anxiety.

prazosin hydrochloride /prä'zəsin/, an antihypertensive alpha-adrenergic blocker prescribed to treat hypertension and to decrease afterload in congestive heart disease.

preadmission certification /prē'ədmish'-ən/, a system whereby physicians are required to obtain advance approval for nonemergency admission of Medicare and managed care patients to hospitals. The system is intended to determine whether the patient can be treated as an outpatient or in another, less expensive manner than hospitalization. Emergency admissions require post hoc approval.

preagonal ascites /prē-ag'ənəl/ [L, *prae,* before; Gk, *agon,* struggle, *askos,* bag], a rapid accumulation of fluid within the peritoneal cavity, representing the transudation of serum from the circulatory system.

preanal /prē-ā'nəl/, located anterior to the anus.

preaortic node /prē'ā-ôr'tik/ [L, *prae* + Gk, *aerein,* to raise; L, *nodus,* knot], a node in one of the three sets of lumbar lymph nodes that serve various abdominal viscera supplied by the celiac, superior mesenteric, and inferior mesenteric arteries.

preauricular /prē'ôrik'yələr/, located anterior to the auricle of the ear.

precancerous /-kan'sərəs/ [L, *prae* + *cancer,* crab], pertaining to a stage of abnormal tissue growth that is likely to develop into a malignant tumor.

precautionary labels /prikô'shənər'ē/, information and identification that must be applied to the containers of all hazardous chemicals, including flammables, combustibles, corrosives, carcinogens, and potential carcinogens.

precedent /pres'ədənt/ [L, *praecedere,* to go before], a previously adjudged decision that serves as an authority in a similar case.

precentral gyrus /-sen'trəl/ [L, *prae* + Gk, *kentron,* center, *gyros,* turn], a convolution of the cerebral hemisphere immediately anterior to the central sulcus of the cerebrum in each hemisphere. It is the location of the motor strip that controls voluntary movements of the contralateral side of the body.

P

Preceptor: Employee, a Nursing Interventions Classification defined as assisting and supporting a new or transferred employee through a planned orientation to a specific clinical area.

Preceptor: Student, a Nursing Interventions Classification defined as assisting and supporting learning experiences for a student.

preceptorship /-sep'tərship'/ [L, *prae* + *capere,* to take up], the position of teacher or instructor; also a nurse who serves as a preceptor for a new graduate.

precertification, authorization for a specific medical procedure before it is done or for admission to an institution for care. It is required for payment by most U.S. managed care organizations.

precession /-sesh'ən/ [L, *praecedere,* to go before], a comparatively slow gyration of the axis of a spinning body, so as to trace out a cone, caused by the application of a torque.

precipitant /-sip'ətənt/ [L, *praecipitare,* to cast down], a substance that causes another substance to settle, separate, or deposit from a solution, such as a reagent that causes certain metals to precipitate.

precipitate /prəsip'itāt, -it/ [L, *praecipitare,* to cast down], 1. to cause a substance to separate or to settle out of solution. 2. a substance that has separated from or settled out of a solution. 3. occurring hastily or unexpectedly.

precipitate delivery /-sip'itit/, childbirth that occurs with such speed or in such a situation that the usual preparations cannot be made.

precipitating factor /-sip'itā'ting/, an element that causes or contributes to the occurrence of a disorder.

precipitation /-sip'itā'shən/ [L, *praecipitare,* to cast down], a process whereby solid particles are made to settle out of a solution so they can be separated from other dissolved substances.

precipitin /prəsip'itin/ [L, *praecipitare* + Gk, *anti,* against; AS, *bodig,* body; Gk, *genein,* to produce], an antibody that causes formation of an insoluble complex when combined with a specific soluble antigen.

precision rest /prisish'ən/ [L, *praecidere,* to cut short; AS, *rest*], a rigid denture support consisting of two tightly fitting parts, the insert of which rests firmly against the gingival part of the device.

preclinical /-klin'ikəl/ [L, *prae* + Gk, *kline,* bed], a stage in a disease when a specific diagnosis cannot be made because adequate signs and symptoms have not yet developed.

precocious /-kō'shəs/ [L, *praecoquere,* to

mature early], pertaining to the early, often premature, development of physical or mental qualities.

precocious dentition, the abnormal acceleration of the eruption of the deciduous or permanent teeth, usually associated with an endocrine imbalance, such as excess pituitary growth hormone or hyperthyroidism.

precocious puberty [L, *praecoquere,* to mature early, *pubertas*], abnormally early development of sexual maturity. It is usually marked by early breast development and ovulation in girls before 8 years of age and the production of mature sperm in boys before 10 years of age.

precognition /-kognish'ən/, the alleged intuitive foreknowledge of events.

Preconception Counseling, a Nursing Interventions Classification defined as screening and counseling done before pregnancy to prevent or decrease the risk for birth defects.

preconscious /-kon'shəs/ [L, *prae,* before, *conscire,* to be aware], 1. before the development of self-consciousness and self-awareness. 2. (in psychiatry) the mental function in which thoughts, ideas, emotions, or memories not in immediate awareness can be brought into the consciousness without encountering any intrapsychic resistance or repression. 3. the mental phenomena capable of being recalled, although not present in the conscious mind.

precordia /prekôr'dē·ə/ [L, *prae* + *cor,* heart], pertaining to the front area of the thorax that lies over the heart.

precordial /prēkôr'dē·əl/ [L, *prae* + *cor,* heart], pertaining to the precordium, which forms the region over the heart and the lower part of the thorax.

precordial lead /lēd/ [L, *prae,* before, *cor,* heart; AS *laedan*], an electrocardiographic lead from the chest wall over the heart.

precordial movement, any motion of the anterior wall of the thorax localized in the area over the heart. Variations of precordial movements include apical impulse, left ventricular thrust, and right ventricular thrust.

precordial pain [L, *prae,* before, *cor,* heart; *poena,* penalty], a pain in the chest wall area over the heart.

precordium /-kôr'dē·əm/ [L, *prae,* before, *cor,* heart], the part of the front of the chest wall that overlays the heart and the epigastrium.

precursor /-kur'sər/ [L, *prae* + *currere,* to run], a prognostic characteristic or feature of a patient's health data, such as a radiographic or laboratory finding, that is associated with a higher or lower risk of death than the average.

precursor therapy, a type of treatment involving the use of nutrients that may influence neurologic clinical conditions.

predeciduous dentition /-disid'yŏŏ·əs/ [L, *prae* + *decidere,* to fall off], the epithelial structures in the mouth of the infant before the eruption of the deciduous teeth.

prediastole /-dī·as'təlē/ [L, *prae,* before; Gk, *dia* + *stellein,* to set], the part of the cardiac cycle between the late systolic phase and the early diastolic phase.

prediastolic murmur /-dī·əstol'ik/ [L, *prae* + Gk, *dia* + *stellein,* to set; L, *murmur,* humming], a murmur heard during cardiac systole.

predictive hypothesis /-dik'tiv/ [L, *prae* + *dicere,* to say; Gk, foundation], (in research) a hypothesis that predicts the nature of a relationship among the variables to be studied.

predictive validity, validity of a test or a measurement tool that is established by demonstrating its ability to predict the results of an analysis of the same data using another test instrument or measurement tool.

predisposing cause /-dispō'sing/ [L, *prae* + *disponere,* to arrange, *causa*], any condition that enhances the specific cause of a disease, such as susceptibility caused by hereditary or life-style factors.

predisposing factor [L, *prae* + *disponere,* to dispose], any conditioning factor that influences both the type and the amount of resources that the individual can elicit to cope with stress. It may be biologic, psychologic, or sociocultural.

predisposition /-dis'pəzish'ən/ [L, *prae* + *disponere,* to dispose], a state of being particularly susceptible.

prednisolone /prednis'əlōn/, a glucocorticoid prescribed as treatment for inflammation of the skin, conjunctiva, and cornea and for immunosuppression.

prednisone /pred'nisōn/, a glucocorticoid prescribed in severe inflammation and immunosuppression.

preeclampsia /prē'iklamp'sē·ə/ [L, *prae* + Gk, *ek,* out, *lampein,* to flash], an abnormal condition of pregnancy characterized by the onset of acute hypertension after the twenty-fourth week of gestation. The classic triad of preeclampsia is hypertension, proteinuria, and edema. Preeclampsia is classified as mild or severe. It commonly causes abnormal metabolic function, including negative nitrogen balance, increased central nervous system irritability, hyperactive reflexes, compromised renal function, hemoconcentration, and alterations of fluid and electrolyte bal-

ance. Complications include premature separation of the placenta, hypofibrinogenemia, hemolysis, cerebral hemorrhage, ophthalmologic damage, pulmonary edema, hepatocellular changes, fetal malnutrition, and lowered birth weight. The most serious complication is eclampsia, which can result in maternal and fetal death.

preexcitation /prē'eksitā'shən/ [L, *prae* + *excitare,* to arouse], activation of part of the ventricular myocardium earlier than would be expected if the activating impulses traveled only down the normal routes and had experienced a normal delay within the atrioventricular (AV) node. The degree of preexcitation is determined by the speed at which the impulse traverses the atrial tissue and the accessory pathway or the AV node.

preexisting condition /prē'iksis'ting/ [L, *prae* + *existere,* to have reality, *conditio*], any injury, disease, or disability that may have occurred at some time in the past and may predispose an individual to limited health in the future.

preferential anosmia /pref'əren'shəl/ [L, *praeferens,* being preferred; Gk, *a* + *osme,* not smell], the inability to smell certain odors. The condition is often caused by psychologic factors concerning either a particular smell or the situation in which the smell occurs.

preferred provider organization (PPO) /-furd'/ [L, *praeferre,* to put before], an organization of physicians, hospitals, and pharmacists whose members discount their health care services to subscriber patients.

preformation /-fôrmā'shən/ [L, *prae* + *formatio,* formation], an early theory in embryology in which the organism is contained in minute and complete form within the germ cell and after fertilization grows from microscopic to normal size.

preformed water /-fôrmd'/ [L, *prae* + *forma,* form; AS, *waeter*], the water that is contained in foods.

prefrontal lobotomy /-frôn'təl/ [L, *prae* + *frons,* forehead; Gk, *lobos, lobe, temnein,* to cut], a surgical procedure in which connecting fibers between the prefrontal lobes of the brain and the thalamus are severed. It is rarely used today but formerly was an accepted procedure for treating schizophrenic patients with uncontrollable, destructive behavior.

preg. abbreviation for **pregnancy.**

preganglionic neuron /-gang'glē·on'·ik/ [L, *prae* + Gk, *gagglion,* knot, *neurom,* nerve], a neuron whose axon terminates in contact with another nerve cell located in a peripheral ganglion.

pregnancy (preg) /preg'nənse/ [L, *praegnans,* pregnant], the gestational process, comprising the growth and development within a woman of a new individual from conception through the embryonic and fetal periods to birth. Pregnancy lasts approximately 266 days (38 weeks) from the day of fertilization, but it is clinically considered to last 280 days (40 weeks; 10 lunar months; 9⅓ calendar months) from the first day of the last menstrual period. The expected date of delivery (EDD) is calculated on the latter basis even if a woman's periods are irregular. The emotional experiences of pregnancy, as reported by pregnant women, are normal and healthy, but extraordinary. Cardiac output increases 30% to 50% in pregnancy. The increase begins at about the sixth week, reaches a maximum about the sixteenth week, declines slightly after the thirtieth week, and rapidly falls off after delivery. Although vital capacity and PO_2 remain the same in pregnancy, respiratory rate, tidal and minute volumes, and plasma pH increase. Inspiratory and expiratory reserves, residual volume and residual capacity, and plasma PCO_2 diminish. The glomerular filtration rate and the renal plasma flow increase approximately 30% to 50% in pregnancy; the pattern of change closely parallels that of cardiac function. A marked dilation of the excretory tract, called *hydronephrosis of pregnancy,* often occurs. Progesterone, the level of which increases in pregnancy, causes some relaxation of gastrointestinal smooth muscle. Heartburn may result from delayed gastric emptying and relaxation of the sphincter at the gastroesophageal junction. Protein binding is increased in pregnancy. Because most hormones are circulated in protein-bound forms, the function of most endocrine glands is altered. The breasts become firm and tender early in pregnancy. This tenderness constitutes a subjective symptom of pregnancy. As the breasts enlarge and soften, the tenderness disappears. Perspiration increases. Erythema of the thenar and hypothenar eminences of the palms becomes apparent. Hair growth may be stimulated. Normal weight gain may vary within wide limits in pregnancy. Average weight gain is 25 to 30 pounds, but greater increases are common without ill effects. Requirements for dietary iron, protein, and calcium increase out of proportion to the need for an overall increase in intake of calories and other nutrients.

pregnancy gingivitis, an enlargement or hyperplasia of the gingivae caused by hormonal imbalance during pregnancy.

pregnancy rate, (in statistics) the ratio of pregnancies per 100 woman-years, calculated as the product of the number of pregnancies in the women observed multiplied by 12 (months), divided by the product of the number of women observed multiplied by the number of months observed.

Pregnancy Termination Care, a Nursing Interventions Classification defined as management of the physical and psychologic needs of a woman undergoing a spontaneous or elective abortion.

pregnanediol /pregnān'dē·ol/, a crystalline biologically inactive compound in the urine of women during pregnancy or during the secretory phase of the menstrual cycle.

pregnant /preg'nənt/ [L, *praegnans*], gravid, with child.

prehensile /-hen'sil/ [L, *prehendre,* to seize], able to grasp.

prehension /-hen'shən/, the use of the hands and fingers to grasp or pick up objects.

prehospital care, any initial medical care given an ill or injured patient by a paramedic or other person before the patient reaches the hospital emergency department.

preload /prē'lōd/ [L, *prae* + AS, *lad*], the stretch of myocardial fiber at end diastole. The ventricular end diastolic pressure and volume reflect this parameter.

preload filling pressure, the load on the ventricular muscle fibers at the end of diastole or just before contraction. The preload on the heart is estimated by the left ventricular filling pressure.

premalignant fibroepithelioma /-məlig'-nənt/ [L, *prae* + *malignus,* bad disposition, *fibra,* fiber; Gk, *epi,* above, *thele,* nipple, *oma,* tumor], an elevated white flesh-colored sessile neoplasm formed of interlacing ribbons of epithelial cells on a hyperplastic mesodermal stroma. The tumor occurs most often on the lower trunk of older people.

premarket approval (P.M.A.) /-mâr'kit/, permission given by the federal government to equipment manufacturers to sell their devices to the medical profession.

premature /-məchŏŏr'/ [L, *prae* + *maturare,* to ripen], **1.** not fully developed or mature. **2.** occurring before the appropriate or usual time. —**prematurity,** *n.*

premature alopecia [L, *praematurus,* too soon; Gk, *alopex,* fox mange], acquired baldness in a person who is not old.

premature atrial complex (PAC), an atrial depolarization occurring earlier than expected. It is indicated electrocardiographically by an early P' wave followed by a normal QRS. They may be the result of atrial enlargement or ischemia or may be caused by stress, caffeine, or nicotine.

premature beat [L, *praematurus,* too soon; AS, *beatan*], an ectopic electrocardiogram complex that occurs earlier than expected in the ongoing rhythm pattern.

premature complex, any electrocardiogram deflection representing either the ventricles or atria that occurs early with respect to the dominant rhythm.

premature ejaculation, uncontrollable untimely ejaculation of semen often caused by anxiety during sexual intercourse.

premature impulse, any impulse that occurs early with respect to a dominant rhythm.

premature infant, any neonate, regardless of birth weight, born before 37 weeks of gestation. Predisposing factors associated with prematurity include multiple pregnancy, toxemia, chronic or acute infection, sensitization to blood incompatibility, any severe trauma that may interfere with normal fetal development, substance abuse, and teenage pregnancy. The premature infant usually appears small and scrawny, with a large head in relation to body size, and weighs less than 2500 g. The skin is shiny and translucent with the underlying vessels clearly visible. The arms and legs are extended, not flexed, as in the full-term infant. There is little subcutaneous fat, sparse hair, few creases on the soles and palms, and poorly developed ear cartilage. Among the common problems of the premature infant are variations in thermoregulation, chilling, apnea, respiratory distress, sepsis, poor sucking and swallowing reflexes, small stomach capacity, lowered tolerance of the alimentary tract that may lead to necrotizing enterocolitis, immature renal function, hepatic dysfunction often associated with hyperbilirubinemia, incomplete enzyme systems, and susceptibility to various metabolic upsets, such as hypoglycemia, hyperglycemia, and hypocalcemia.

premature rupture of membranes, the spontaneous rupture of the amniotic sac before the onset of labor.

premature systole [L, *praematurus* + Gk, *systole,* contraction], a contraction that occurs too early as a result of a discharge of an ectopic focus in the atria, atrioventricular junction, or ventricle.

premature ventricular complex (PVC), a cardiac sinus-conducted arrhythmia characterized by ventricular depolarization occurring earlier than expected. It appears on the electrocardiogram as an early wide QRS complex without a preceding related P wave. It may be caused by stress,

electrolyte imbalance, ischemia, hypoxemia, hypercapnia, ventricular enlargement, or a toxic reaction to drugs.

prematurity /-məchoo′ritē/ [L, *praematurus,* too soon], pertaining to an event that occurs before the usual or expected time, such as a premature birth.

premed /-med′/, abbreviation for *premedical student.*

premedication /-med′ikā′shən/ [L, *prae* + *medicare,* to heal], **1.** any sedative, tranquilizer, hypnotic, or anticholinergic medication administered before anesthesia. The choice of drug depends on such variables as the patient's age and physical condition and the specific operative procedure. **2.** the administration of such medications. —**premedicate,** *v.*

premenarchal /-mənär′kəl/ [L, *prae,* before, *men,* month; Gk, *archaios,* from the beginning], before the start of the first menstrual period.

premenopausal /-men′əpô′səl/ [L, *prae* + *men,* month; Gk, *pauein,* to cease], before the start of menopause.

premenstrual /-men′stroo·əl/ [L, *prae,* before, *menstrualis,* monthly], before the start of menstruation each month.

premenstrual dysphoric disorder (PMMD), a mental health condition in women that begins 1 or 2 weeks before menstrual flow. Symptoms include depression, tension, mood swings, irritability, decreased interest, difficulty in concentrating, fatigue, changes in appetite or sleep, physical symptoms, and a sense of being overwhelmed. The condition affects 3% of menstruating women, usually between 25 and 30 years of age.

premenstrual syndrome (PMS) [L, *prae* + *menstrualis,* monthly, *tendere,* to stretch], a syndrome of nervous tension, irritability, weight gain, edema, headache, mastalgia, dysphoria, and lack of coordination occurring during the last few days of the menstrual cycle before the onset of menstruation.

premise /prem′is/ [L, *prae* + *mittere,* to send], a proposition that is presented as the base of an argument and usually established beforehand.

premolar /prēmō′lər/ [L, *prae* + *mola,* mill], one of eight teeth, four in each dental arch, located lateral and posterior to the canine teeth. The term refers to a position in front of the molars. They are smaller and shorter than the canine teeth.

premonition /-mənish′ən/, a sense of an impending event without prior knowledge of it.

premonitory /-mon′iter′ē/ [L, *prae* + *monere,* to warn], an early symptom or sign of a disease. The term is commonly used

P

to describe minor symptoms that precede a major health problem.

premorbid personality /-môr'bid/, a personality characterized by early signs or symptoms of a mental disorder. The specific defects may indicate whether the condition will progress to schizophrenia, a bipolar disorder, or another type of condition.

prenatal /-nā'təl/ [L, *prae* + *natus,* birth], before birth; occurring or existing before birth, referring to both the care of the woman during pregnancy and the growth and development of the fetus.

Prenatal Care, a Nursing Interventions Classification defined as monitoring and management of a patient during pregnancy to prevent complications of pregnancy and promote a healthy outcome for both mother and infant.

prenatal development, the entire process of growth, maturation, differentiation, and development that occurs between conception and birth. On approximately the fourteenth day before the next expected menstrual period, ovulation usually occurs. If the egg is fertilized, it immediately begins the course to fetal maturity and birth. During the first 14 days the fertilized ovum undergoes cell division several times, becoming a morula and then a blastocyst that is able to implant in the uterine wall. From the beginning of the third to the end of the seventh week of embryonic development, implantation deepens and completes. By the end of the seventh week all essential systems are present. The period from the eighth week to birth is called the *fetal stage.* From the thirteenth to the sixteenth week the arms, legs, and trunk grow rapidly; and the fetus is active. The skeleton of the fetus is calcified and may be seen on a x-ray film. Between the seventeenth and the twentieth week of pregnancy the mother usually first feels the baby move. The fetus looks like a very small baby at this time. At 28 weeks subcutaneous fat begins to develop, fingernails and toenails are present, the eyelids are separate, the eyes may open, scalp hair is well developed, and in males the testes are at the internal inguinal ring or below. By the thirty-second week, the hair is fine and woolly, the fingernails and toenails have grown to the tips of the fingers and toes, and there are one or two creases on the anterior part of the soles of the feet. At 36 weeks the body and the limbs are fuller and more rounded, and the skin is thicker and less translucent. As the fetus reaches term, between 38 and 42 weeks, the vernix decreases, and the ear cartilage is developed. In males the testes are in the scro-

tum; in females the labia majora meet in the midline and cover the labia minora and the clitoris. At 40 weeks the average fetus weighs 7¼ pounds and is between 19 and 22 inches long. Prenatal development may be adversely affected by several factors. Between 2 and 14 weeks of gestation ionizing radiation and some drugs may have profound effects on morphologic and functional development. After 14 weeks, when all of the organs, systems, and body parts have formed, any adverse effects are largely functional; major morphologic damage does not occur.

prenatal diagnosis, any of various diagnostic techniques to determine whether a developing fetus in the uterus is affected with a genetic disorder or other abnormality. Such procedures as radiographic examination and ultrasound scanning can be used to follow fetal growth and detect structural abnormalities; amniocentesis enables fetal cells to be obtained from the amniotic fluid for culture and biochemical assay for detection of metabolic disorders and chromosomal analysis; fetoscopy enables fetal blood to be withdrawn from a blood vessel of the placenta and examined for disorders such as thalassemia, sickle cell anemia, and Duchenne's muscular dystrophy.

prenatal surgery, any surgical procedure that is performed on a fetus. The technique has been used to correct hydrocephalus and urinary tract obstructions.

preoccupation /prē·ok'yəpā'shən/, a state of being self-absorbed or engrossed in one's own thoughts to a degree that hinders effective contact with or relationship to external reality.

pre-op /prē·op'/, abbreviation for *preparation for operation.*

preoperational thought phase /prē·op'-ərā'shənəl/ [L, *prae* + *operari,* to work; AS, *thot* + Gk, *phainein,* to show], a piagetian phase of child development, during the period of 2 to 7 years of age, when the child focuses on the use of language as a tool to meet his or her needs.

preoperative /prē·op'ərətiv'/ [L, *prae* + *operari,* to work], pertaining to the period before a surgical procedure. Commonly the preoperative period begins with the first preparation of the patient for surgery, such as when, several hours before the scheduled procedure, ingestion of fluids or food by mouth is forbidden. It ends with the induction of anesthesia in the operating suite.

preoperative care, the preparation and management of a patient before surgery. The patient's nutritional and hygienic state, medical and surgical history, allergies, current medication, physical handicaps, signs of infection, and elimination habits are noted and recorded. The patient's understanding of the operative, preoperative, and postoperative procedures; the patient's ability to verbalize anxieties; and the family's knowledge of the planned surgery are ascertained. The signed informed consent statement, the physician's preoperative orders, and the patient's identification bands and willingness to receive blood if necessary are checked. Vital signs are recorded, and any abnormalities are reported to the physician. The physician is also informed if the electrocardiogram, chest radiographic study, or laboratory tests show any abnormalities. On completion of the patient's blood typing, the number of matched blood units required to be held for a possible blood transfusion is determined. When ordered, an enema is given, a bowel preparation is completed, a nasogastric tube or indwelling catheter is inserted, and parenteral fluids are administered. Nothing is given orally for several hours before surgery unless ordered. After preoperative medication is administered, the side rails of the bed are raised. Before transfer to the operating room with the completed chart the patient voids, and any dentures, contact lenses, and valuables are removed for safekeeping.

Preoperative Coordination, a Nursing Interventions Classification defined as facilitating preadmission diagnostic testing and preparation of the surgical patient.

prep, 1. abbreviation for *prepare*. 2. abbreviation for preparation, particularly when referring to preparation for surgery.

preparatory prosthesis /prep′ərətôr′ē/, a temporary artificial limb that is fitted to the stump soon after amputation. It permits ambulation and biomechanical adaptation during the first several weeks after surgery.

Preparatory Sensory Information, a Nursing Interventions Classification defined as describing both the subjective and objective physical sensations associated with an upcoming stressful health care procedure/treatment.

prepared cavity /priperd′/ [L, *praeparare,* to make ready, *cavum,* cavity], a tooth cavity that has been carved with an electric handpiece and hand instruments to receive and retain a restoration.

prepartum /-pär′təm/, before childbirth.

prepatellar /-pətel′ər/ [L, *prae,* before, *patella,* small dish], pertaining to the area in front of the patella.

prepatellar bursa [L, *prae* + *patella,* small dish; Gk, *byrsa,* wineskin], a bursa between the tendon of the quadriceps muscle group and the lower part of the femur continuous with the cavity of the knee joint.

prepatellar bursitis [L, *prae,* before, *patella* + Gk, *byrsa,* wineskin, *itis* inflammation], an inflammation of the bursa in front of the patella and beneath the skin over the site.

prepayment /-pā′mənt/ [L, *prae* + *pacere,* to pacify], the payment in advance for health care services by subscribers to a third-party insurance program such as Blue Cross.

preprandial /-pran′dē-əl/ [L, *prae* + *prandium,* meal], before a meal.

preprocessing /prēpros′əsing/, (in ultrasonics) conditioning and manipulation of echo signals before their storage in the scan memory.

prepubertal panhypopituitarism /-pyoo′-bərtəl/ [L, *prae,* + *pubertas,* maturity; Gk, *pan,* all, *hypo,* under, *pituita,* phlegm], insufficiency of pituitary hormones, caused by damage to the gland usually associated with a suprasellar cyst or craniopharyngioma, occurring in childhood. The disorder is characterized by dwarfism with normal body proportions, subnormal sexual development, impaired thyroid and adrenal function, and yellow, wrinkled skin.

prepuberty /-pyoo′bərtē/ [L, *prae* + *pubertas,* maturity], the period immediately before puberty, lasting approximately 2 years. It is characterized by preliminary physical changes, such as accelerated growth and appearance of secondary sex characteristics that lead to sexual maturity. —**prepuberal, prepubertal,** *adj.*

prepubescence /prē′pyoobes′əns/, the state of being prepubertal. —**prepubescent,** *adj.*

prepuce /prē′pyoos/ [L, *praeputium,* foreskin], a fold of skin that forms a retractable cover, such as the foreskin of the penis or the fold around the clitoris. —**prepucial, preputial,** *adj.*

prerenal /-rē′nəl/ [L, *prae,* before, *ren,* kidney], 1. pertaining to the area in front of the kidney. 2. pertaining to events occurring before reaching the kidney.

prerenal anuria [L, *prae* + *renes,* kidneys; Gk, *a* + *ouron,* not urine], cessation of urine production that results when the blood pressure in the kidney is too low to maintain glomerular filtration pressure.

prerenal uremia [L, *prae,* before, *ren,* kidney; Gk, *ouron,* urine, *haima,* blood], a condition of kidney failure in which the primary cause may be outside the kidney, as in some severe cases of alkalosis.

P

presbycardia /prez'bēkär'dē·ə/ [Gk, *presbys*, old man, *kardia*, heart], an abnormal cardiac condition, especially affecting elderly individuals and associated with heart failure in the presence of other complications, such as heart disease, fever, anemia, mild hyperthyroidism, and excess fluid administration. Presbycardia may be associated with decreased elasticity of the musculature of the heart and with mild fibrotic changes of the heart valves, but the basis for these changes is not known.

presbycusis /-kōō'sis/ [Gk, *presbys* + *akousis*, hearing], hearing loss associated with aging.

presbyopia /prez'bē·ō'pē·ə/ [Gk, *presbys* + *ops*, eye], a hyperopic shift to farsightedness resulting from a loss of elasticity of the lens of the eye. The condition commonly develops with advancing age. —**presbyopic,** *adj.*

presbyopic /prez'bē·op'ik/ [Gk, *presbys*, old man, *ops*, eye], pertaining to a decrease in accommodation of the lens as one grows older and usually resulting in hyperopia or farsightedness.

preschizophrenic state /prēskit'səfren'ik, prē'-/ [L, *prae* + Gk, *schizein*, to split, *phren*, mind], a period before psychosis is evident when the patient deviates from normal behavior but does not demonstrate psychotic symptoms of delusions, hallucinations, or stupor.

prescreen /-skrēn/ [L, *prae* + ME, *scren*], **1.** to evaluate a patient or a group of patients to identify those who are at greater risk of development of a specific condition in order to select those who are in particular need of special diagnostic procedures or health care. **2.** *informal.* a rapid, superficial examination of a person who does not appear to be acutely ill. It may include taking a medical history.

prescribe /priskrīb'/ [L, *prae* + *scribere*, to write], **1.** to write an order for a drug, treatment, or procedure. **2.** to recommend or encourage a course of action.

prescription /priskrip'shən/, an order for medication, therapy, or therapeutic device given by a properly authorized person to a person properly authorized to dispense or perform the order. A prescription is usually in written form and includes the patient's name and address, the date, the ℞ symbol (superscription), the medication prescribed (inscription), directions to the pharmacist or other dispenser (subscription), directions to the patient that must appear on the label, prescriber's signature and, in some instances an identifying number.

prescription drug [L, *prae* + *scribere* + Fr, *drogue*], a drug that can be dispensed to the public only with an order given by a properly authorized person. The designation of a medication as a prescription drug is made by the U.S. Food and Drug Administration.

prescriptive intervention mode /priskrip'-tiv/ [L, *praescriptus*, prescribed, *intervenire*, to come between, *modus*, measure], a therapeutic situation in which the health professional tells the patient explicitly how to solve a problem, so that less collaboration between the consultant and patient is needed.

prescriptive theory, a theory that comprises a description of a specific activity, a statement of the goal of the activity, and an analysis of the elements of the activity, which together constitute a prescription for reaching the goal.

presence /prez'əns/ a mode of being available in a situation with the wholeness of one's individual being; a gift of self that can be given freely, invoked, or evoked.

Presence, a Nursing Interventions Classification defined as being with another during times of need.

presenile /-sē'nīl/ [L, *prae*, before, *senex*, aged], pertaining to a condition in which a person manifests signs of aging in early or middle life.

present health [L, *praesentare*, to show; AS, *haelth*], (in a health history) a succinct chronologic account of any recent changes in the health of the patient and of the circumstances or symptoms that prompted the person to seek health care.

presenting part /prəsen'ting/ [L, *praesentare* + *pars*, part], the part of the fetus that lies closest to the internal os of the cervix.

preservative /prisur'vətiv/ [L, *praeservare*, to keep], a chemical or other agent that reduces the rate of decomposition of a substance.

presomite embryo /prēsō'mīt/ [L, *prae* + Gk, *soma*, body, *en*, in, *bryein*, to grow], an embryo in any stage of development before the appearance of the first pair of somites (segments), which in humans usually occurs around 19 to 21 days after fertilization of the ovum.

pressor /pres'ər/ [L, *premere*, to press], describing a substance that tends to cause a rise in blood pressure.

pressure /presh'ər/ [L, *premere*, to press], a force, or stress, applied to a surface by a fluid or an object, usually measured in units of mass per unit of area, such as pounds per square inch.

pressure acupuncture, a system of acupuncture involving the application of pressure, such as by the tip of a finger, to certain specified points of the body.

pressure area, an oral area that is subject to excessive displacement of soft tissue by a prosthesis.

pressure dressing, a bandage or cloth material firmly applied to exert pressure to stop bleeding, prevent edema, and provide support for varicose veins. It also is commonly used after skin grafting, in the treatment of burns, and on wounds for hemostasis.

pressure edema, 1. edema of the lower extremities caused by pressure of a pregnant uterus against the large veins of the area. 2. edema of the fetal scalp after cephalic presentation.

Pressure Management, a Nursing Interventions Classification defined as minimizing pressure to body parts.

pressure point, 1. a point over an artery where the pulse may be felt. Pressure on the point may be helpful in stopping the flow of blood from a wound distal to it. 2. a site that is extremely sensitive to pressure, such as the phrenic pressure point along the phrenic nerve between the sternocleidomastoid and the scalenus anticus on the right side.

pressure-sensitive adhesive, a drug-delivery device that uses polymers that are permanently tacky at room temperature and adhere to the skin when slight pressure is applied.

pressure support ventilation (PSV), the augmentation of spontaneous breathing effort with a specific amount of positive airway pressure. The patient initiates the inspiratory flow, generating his or her own V_t and frequencies.

pressure ulcer, an inflammation, sore, or ulcer in the skin over a bony prominence. It results from ischemic hypoxia of the tissues caused by prolonged pressure on them. Pressure ulcers are most often seen in aged, debilitated, immobilized, or cachectic patients. The sores are graded by stages of severity. Prevention of pressure ulcers is a cardinal aspect of nursing care; treatment specific to the location and extent of the condition is planned.

pressure ulcer care, the management and prevention of pressure ulcers that occur most frequently on the sacrum, elbows, heels, outer ankles, inner knees, hips, shoulder blades, and ear rims of immobilized patients, especially those who are obese, elderly, or suffering from infections, injuries, or a poor nutritional state. Pressure ulcers may be prevented by repositioning the immobile patient every 2 hours or less, keeping the skin dry, and inspecting pressure areas every 4 to 6 hours for signs of redness. Bed linen is kept dry and wrinkle-free; a sheet or mechanical lift is used to raise the patient, who is moved frequently from the bed but is not allowed to sit in one place for more than 30 minutes. A prophylactic measure is daily skin care, in which all areas are washed, rinsed, and dried thoroughly and lotion is gently rubbed on bony prominences. The importance of frequent change of position, dryness, cleanliness, and good nutrition is emphasized.

Pressure Ulcer Care, a Nursing Interventions Classification defined as facilitation of healing in pressure ulcers.

Pressure Ulcer Prevention, a Nursing Interventions Classification defined as prevention of pressure ulcers for a patient at high risk for their development.

pressure ventilator, a ventilator in which gas delivery is limited by a predetermined pressure.

presumptive signs /-sump′tiv/ [L, *praesumere,* to take beforehand, *signum,* mark], manifestations that indicate a pregnancy, although they are not necessarily positive. Presumptive signs may include cessation of menses and morning sickness.

preswing stance stage /prē′swing/ [L, *prae* + AS, *swingan,* to fling; L, *stare,* to stand; OFr, *estage,* stage], one of the five stages in the stance phase of walking or gait, involving a brief transitional period of double limb support during which one leg of the body is rapidly relieved of body-bearing weight and prepared for the swing forward.

presymptomatic disease /-simp′təmat′ik/ [L, *prae* + Gk, *symptoma,* a happening], an early stage of disease when physiologic changes have begun, although no signs or symptoms are observed.

presynaptic /-sinap′tik/ [L, *prae* + *synaptein,* to join], 1. situated near or before a synapse. 2. before a synapse is crossed.

presystole /-sis′təlē/ [L, *prae,* before; Gk, *systole,* contraction], an interval in the cardiac cycle immediately before systole.

presystolic /-sistol′ik/ [L, *prae* + Gk, *systole,* contraction], pertaining to the period preceding systole.

presystolic murmur [L, *prae,* before; Gk, *systole,* contraction; L, *murmur,* humming], a heart murmur in cases of mitral stenosis, before diastole.

preterm /prēturm′/ [L, *prae,* before; Gk, *terma,* limit], 1. events before a specific date. 2. pertaining to a shorter than normal period of gestation.

preterm birth, any birth that occurs before the thirty-seventh week of gestation.

preterm contractions, irregular tightening of the pregnant uterus that begins in the first trimester and increases in frequency, duration, and intensity as pregnancy progresses. Contractility of uterine muscle increases in pregnancy. Strong preterm contractions near-term are often difficult to distinguish from the contractions of true labor.

preterm labor, labor that occurs earlier in pregnancy than normal, either before the fetus has reached a weight of 2000 to 2500 g or before the thirty-seventh or thirty-eighth week of gestation. No single measure of fetal weight or gestational age is used universally to designate preterm birth; local or institutional policy dictates which of several standards is applied. The incidence of preterm labor increases in inverse proportion to maternal age, weight, and socioeconomic status. Predisposing conditions include maternal infection, low weight gain, uterine bleeding, multiple gestation, polyhydramnios, uterine abnormalities, incompetent cervix, premature rupture of membranes, and intrauterine fetal growth retardation. The cause of preterm labor is poorly understood; in some cases there may be several contributing causes. In some pregnancies preterm labor may be homeostatic, resulting in the best possible outcome under the particular abnormal conditions. If preterm labor itself constitutes a threat to the fetus, the outcome of pregnancy may be improved if labor can be inhibited.

pretibial /prētib′ē·əl/ [L, *prae* + *tibia,* shinbone], pertaining to the area of the leg in front of the tibia.

pretibial fever, an acute infection caused by *Leptospira autumnalis.* It is characterized by headache, chills, fever, enlarged spleen, myalgia, low white blood cell count, and rash on the anterior surface of the legs.

prevalence /prev′ələns/ [L, *praevalentia,* a powerful force], (in epidemiology) the number of all new and old cases of a disease or occurrences of an event during a particular period.

prevention /-ven′shən/ [L, *praevenire,* to anticipate], (in nursing care) any action directed to preventing illness and promoting health to eliminate the need for secondary or tertiary health care.

preventive /-ven′tiv/ [L, *praevenire,* to anticipate], tending to slow, stop, or interrupt the course of an illness or to decrease the incidence of a disease.

preventive care, a pattern of nursing and medical care that focuses on disease prevention and health maintenance. It includes early diagnosis of disease, discovery and identification of people at risk of development of specific problems, coun-

seling, and other necessary intervention to avert a health problem.

preventive dentistry [L, *praevenire,* to anticipate, *dens,* tooth], the science of the care required to prevent disease affecting the teeth and supporting structures.

preventive medicine [L, *praevenire,* to anticipate, *medicina*], the branch of medicine that is concerned with the prevention of disease and methods for increasing the power of the patient and community to resist disease and prolong life.

preventive nursing [L, *praevenire,* to anticipate, *nutrix,* nurse], the branch of nursing concerned with general health promotion, teaching of early recognition and treatment of disease, encouragement of life-style modification, and prevention of further deterioration of the disabled.

preventive psychiatry, the use of theoretic knowledge and skills to plan and implement programs designed to achieve primary, secondary, and tertiary prevention of the onset of psychiatric disorders.

preventive treatment, a procedure, measure, substance, or program designed to prevent a disease from occurring or a mild disorder from becoming more severe. Various diseases are prevented by immunizations with vaccines, antiseptic measures, the avoidance of smoking, regular exercise, prudent diet, adequate rest, correction of congenital anomalies, and screening programs for the detection of preclinical signs of disorders.

previllous embryo /prēvil′əs/ [L, *prae* + *villus,* hairy; Gk, *en* in, *bryein,* to grow], an embryo of a placental mammal at any stage before the development of the chorionic villi, which in humans begin to form between the first and second months after fertilization of the ovum.

previous abnormality of glucose tolerance /prē′vē·əs/, a classification that includes people who previously had diabetic hyperglycemia or impaired glucose tolerance but whose fasting plasma glucose level has returned to normal. Included in this category are people who had gestational diabetes but whose plasma level returned to normal.

prevocational evaluation /-vōkā′shənəl/, an evaluation of the abilities and limitations of a patient undergoing rehabilitation from a disabling disorder. The goal is to find eventual employment in a sheltered workshop or in the general community.

prevocational training, a rehabilitation program designed to prepare a patient for the performance of useful paid work in a sheltered setting or community. It may involve training in basic work skills and counseling as required for a typical employment setting.

PRF, abbreviation for **pulse repetition frequency.**

priapism /prī′əpiz′əm/ [Gk, *priapos,* phallus], an abnormal condition of prolonged or constant penile erection, often painful and seldom associated with sexual arousal. It may result from urinary calculi or a lesion within the penis or the central nervous system.

priapitis /prī′əpī′tis/, inflammation of the penis.

prilocaine hydrochloride /pril′ōkān/, a local anesthetic agent of the amide family, used for nerve block, epidural, and regional anesthesia. It is not used for spinal or topical anesthesia.

prima facie rights /prī′mə fā′shē·ə/, rights on the surface, or face, that may be overridden by stronger conflicting rights or by other values.

primal scream therapy /prī′məl/, a nonmainstream form of psychotherapy developed by Arthur Janov that focuses on repressed pain of infancy or childhood. The goal of the therapy is that the patient will surrender his or her anxiety defenses and "become real."

primaquine phosphate /prī′məkwin/, an antimalarial prescribed in the treatment of malaria and prevention of relapse during recovery from the disease.

primary /prī′mərē/ [L, *primus,* first], **1.** first in order of time, place, development, or importance. **2.** not derived from any other source or cause, specifically the original condition or set of symptoms in disease processes, such as a primary infection or a primary tumor. **3.** (in chemistry) noting the first and most simple compound in a related series, formed by the substitution of one of two or more atoms or of a group in a molecule.

primary abscess [L, *primus + abscedere,* to go away], an abscess that develops at the original point of infection by a pus-producing microorganism.

primary amputation, amputation performed after severe trauma, after the patient has recovered from shock, and before infection occurs.

primary anesthesia [L, *primus,* first; Gk, *anaisthesia,* lack of feeling], any anesthetic or analgesic given a surgical patient before the administration of chemical agents that produce reversible unconsciousness.

primary apnea, a self-limited condition characterized by an absence of respiration. It may follow a blow to the head and is common immediately after birth in the newborn who breathes spontaneously when the carbon dioxide in the circulation reaches a certain level. Reflexes are present, and the heart is beating, but the skin color may be pale or blue and muscle tone is diminished.

primary atelectasis, failure of the lungs to expand fully at birth, most commonly seen in premature infants or those narcotized by maternal anesthesia. The infant is usually cared for in an incubator in which the temperature and humidity may be closely monitored.

primary biliary cirrhosis, a chronic inflammatory condition of the liver. It is characterized by generalized pruritus, enlargement and hardening of the liver, weight loss, and diarrhea with pale, bulky stools. Petechiae, epistaxis, or hemorrhage resulting from hypoprothrombinemia may also be evident. Jaundice, dark urine, pale stools, and cutaneous xanthosis may occur in the later stages of this disease.

primary bronchus, one of the two main air passages that branch from the trachea and convey air to the lungs as part of the respiratory system. The right primary bronchus enters the right lung nearly opposite the fifth thoracic vertebra. The left primary bronchus divides into bronchi for the superior and anterior lobes of the lung.

primary carcinoma, a neoplasm at the site of origin.

primary care, the first contact in a given episode of illness that leads to a decision regarding a course of action to resolve the health problem.

primary care physician [L, *primus +* ME, *caru,* sorrow; Gk, *physikos,* natural], a physician who usually is the first health professional to examine a patient and who recommends secondary care physicians, medical or surgical specialists with expertise in the patient's specific health problem, if further treatment is needed.

primary care case management (PCCM) (in the United States) a situation in which primary care receives concurrent utilization management review and discharge planning is used to minimize resource consumption while maintaining quality of care.

primary cell culture, a cell line derived directly from the parent tissue. Cells in primary culture have the same karyotype and chromosome number as those in the original tissue.

primary colors, (in physiology and physics) a small number of fundamental colors: red, green, and blue-violet. In humans the retinal receptor cones contain pigments most sensitive to red, green, or blue light.

primary cutaneous melanoma, the site

of origin of a malignant neoplasm on the skin.

primary dental caries, dental caries developing in the enamel of a tooth that was previously unaffected.

primary dermatitis [L, *primus* + Gk, *derma,* skin, *itis,* inflammation], skin eruption caused by a substance that can produce cell damage on initial contact, as opposed to that which develops as a sensitivity reaction to an allergen.

primary endometriosis [L, *primus* + Gk, *endon,* within, *metra,* womb, *osis,* condition], an ingrowth of the muscle walls of the uterus by the mucous membrane lining of the organ.

primary fissure, a fissure that marks the division of the anterior and posterior lobes of the cerebellum.

primary gain, a benefit, primarily relief from emotional conflict and freedom from anxiety, attained through the use of a defense mechanism or other psychologic process.

primary gangrene [L, *primus* + Gk, *gaggraina*], a form of gangrene that occurs without preceding inflammation.

primary health care, a basic level of health care that includes programs directed at the promotion of health, early diagnosis of disease or disability, and prevention of disease. Primary health care is provided in an ambulatory facility to limited numbers of people, often those living in a particular geographic area. It includes continuing health care, as provided by a family nurse practitioner.

primary hemorrhage [L, *primus* + Gk, *haima,* blood, *rhegnynei,* to burst forth], a hemorrhage immediately after an injury.

primary iritis [L, *primus* + Gk, *iris,* rainbow, *itis,* inflammation], an inflammation of the iris that results from a source within the body, such as a systemic disease.

primary lateral sclerosis, a slowly progressing degenerative brain disease characterized by weakness, spasticity, hyperreflexia, and a positive Babinski's sign. It involves neurons of the motor cortex but not the brainstem or spinal cord neurons.

primary lesion [L, *primus* + *laesio,* hurting], a sore or wound that develops at the point of inoculation of the disease, usually applied to a syphilis chancre.

primary nurse, a nurse who is responsible for the planning, implementation, and evaluation of the nursing care of one or more clients 24 hours a day for the duration of the hospital stay.

primary nursing, a system for the distribution of nursing care in which care of one patient is managed for the entire 24-hour day by one nurse who directs and coordinates nurses and other personnel; schedules all tests, procedures, and daily activities for that patient; and cares for that patient personally when on duty. In acute care the primary care nurse may be responsible for only one patient; in intermediate care the primary care nurse may be responsible for three or more patients.

primary organizer, the part of the dorsal lip of the blastopore that is self-differentiating and induces the formation of the neural plate that gives rise to the main axis of the embryo.

primary palate, a shelf formed from the medial nasal process of an embryo that separates the primitive nasal cavity from the oral cavity.

primary physician, 1. the physician who usually takes care of a patient; the physician who first sees a patient for the care of a given health problem. **2.** a family practice physician or general practitioner.

primary prevention, a program of activities directed to improving general well-being while also involving specific protection for selected diseases, such as immunization against measles.

primary processes, (in psychoanalytic theory) unconscious processes, originating in the id, that obey laws different from those of the ego. These processes occur in the least disguised form in infancy and in the dreams of the adult.

primary relationships, relationships with intimates, close friends, and family.

primary sensation, a feeling or impression resulting directly from a particular stimulus.

primary sequestrum, a piece of dead bone that completely separates from sound bone during the process of necrosis.

primary sex character, an inherited trait directly concerned with the reproductive function of the primary sex organs of the individual.

primary shock, a state of physical collapse comparable to fainting. It may be the result of slight pain, such as that produced by venipuncture, or may be caused by fright. Primary shock is usually mild, self-limited, and of short duration.

primary sterility [L, *primus* + *sterilis,* barren], the inability to produce offspring caused by a functional failure of the ovaries or testes.

primary triad, in A. T. Beck's theory of depression the three major cognitive patterns that force the individual to view self, environment, and future in a negativistic manner.

primary tuberculosis, the childhood

form of tuberculosis, most commonly occurring in the lungs, the posterior pharynx, or rarely the skin. Infants lack resistance to the disease and are readily infected and especially vulnerable to rapid and extensive spread of infection through the body. In childhood the disease is usually brief and benign, characterized by regional lymphadenopathy, calcification of the tubercles, and residual immunity.

primate /prī′māt, prī′mit/ [L, *primus,* first], a member of the biologic order of animals of the chordate class Mammalia. The primate order includes lemurs, monkeys, apes, and humans. Most primates a have large brain, stereoscopic vision, and hands and feet developed for grasping.

prime mover /prīm′/ [L, *primus + movere,* to move], a muscle that acts directly to produce a desired movement amid other muscles acting simultaneously to produce the same movement indirectly. Most movements of the body require the combined action of numerous muscles.

primer /prī′mər/, **1.** a short piece of deoxyribonucleic acid (DNA) or ribonucleic acid complementary to a given DNA sequence. It acts as a point at which replication can proceed, as in a polymerase chain reaction. **2.** a molecule such as a small polymer that induces the synthesis of a larger structure.

primidone /prī′mədōn/, an anticonvulsant prescribed in the treatment of seizure disorders, including grand mal, psychomotor, and focal epilepsy-like seizures.

primigravida /prim′igrav′idə/ [L, *primus + gravidus,* pregnant], a woman pregnant for the first time. —**primigravid,** *adj.*

primipara /primip′ərə/, *pl.* **primiparae** [L, *primus + parere,* to bear], a woman who has given birth to one viable infant, indicated by the notation *para 1* on the patient's chart.

primiparity /prim′iper′itē/ [L, *primus + parere,* to bear], the condition of having borne one child.

primiparous /primip′ərəs/ [L, *primus + parere,* to bear], pertaining to a woman who has borne one child.

primitive /prim′itiv/ [L, *primivus*], **1.** undeveloped; undifferentiated; rudimentary; showing little or no evolution. **2.** embryonic; formed early in the course of development; existing in an early or simple form.

primitive groove, a furrow in the posterior region of the embryonic disk. It indicates the cephalocaudal axis that results from the active involution of cells forming the primitive streak.

primitive node, a knoblike accumulation of cells at the cephalic end of the primitive streak in the early stages of embryonic development in humans and higher animals.

primitive pit, a minute indentation at the anterior end of the primitive groove in the early developing embryo.

primitive reflex, any reflex normal in an infant or fetus. Its presence in an adult usually indicates serious neurologic disease. Some kinds of primitive reflexes are **grasp reflex, Moro reflex,** and **sucking reflex.**

primitive ridge, a ridge that bounds the primitive groove in the early stages of embryonic development.

primitive streak, a dense area on the central posterior region of the embryonic disk. It is formed by the morphogenetic movement of a rapidly proliferating mass of cells that spreads between the ectoderm and endoderm, giving rise to the mesoderm layer.

primordial /prīmôr′dē·əl/ [L, *primordium,* origin], **1.** characteristic of the most undeveloped or primitive state, specifically those cells or tissues that are formed in the early stages of embryonic development. **2.** first or original; primitive.

primordial cyst, a follicular cyst, consisting of an epithelium-lined sac that contains fluid and appears radiographically as a light area in the affected jaw. It develops from a dental enamel organ before the formation of hard tissue.

primordial dwarf, a person of extremely short stature who is otherwise perfectly formed, with the usual proportions of body parts and normal mental and sexual development.

primordial germ cell, any of the large spheric diploid cells that are formed in the early stages of embryonic development and are precursors of the oogonia and spermatogonia.

primordial image, (in analytic psychology) the archetype or original parent, representing the source of all life.

primordium /prīmôr′dē·əm/, *pl.* **primordia** [L, origin], the first recognizable stage in the embryonic development and differentiation of a particular organ, tissue, or structure.

principal /prin′sipəl/ [L, *principalis,* first in rank], first in authority or importance.

principle /prin′sipəl/ [L, *principium,* foundation], **1.** a general truth or established rule of action. **2.** a prime source or element from which anything proceeds. **3.** a law on which others are founded or from which others are derived.

principles of instrumentation, (in dentistry and dental hygiene) the six principles for the use of mirrors and other hand and motor-driven devices: (1) grasp,

P

(2) fulcrum, (3) insertion, (4) adaptation and angulation, (5) activation (lateral pressure and working stroke), (6) rest.

P-R interval, (in electrocardiography) the interval measured from the beginning of the P wave to the beginning of the QRS complex, representing atrioventricular conduction time. It is between 0.12 to 0.20 seconds.

Prinzmetal's angina [Myron Prinzmetal, American cardiologist, b. 1908], chest pain that is caused by reversible severe coronary artery spasm. It is associated with ST segment elevation that reverts to normal within minutes. The ST elevation indicates total occlusion through the epicardial coronary artery.

prion /prī′on/, one of several kinds of proteinaceous particles believed to be responsible for transmissible neurodegenerative diseases, including scrapie in sheep and kuru and Creutzfeldt-Jakob's disease in humans. Because prions lack detectable nucleic acid, they are not inactivated by the usual procedures for destroying viruses. They also do not trigger an immune response.

priority /prī·ôr′itē/ [L, *prius,* previously], actions established in order of importance or urgency to the welfare or purposes of the organization, patient, or other person at a given time.

prism /priz′əm/ [Gk, *prisma* that which is sawn through], **1.** a solid figure, with a triangular or polygonal cross section, bounded by parallelograms. **2.** enamel prism, or calcified rods, surrounded by organic prism cuticle joined together to form tooth enamel. **3.** an adverse prism or verger prism used to test and train ocular muscles.

prismatic colors /prizmat′ik/, the seven rainbow hues (red, orange, yellow, green, blue, indigo, and violet) produced from white light when it is reduced to its component wavelengths by the dispersion effect of a prism.

privacy /prī′vəsē/, a culturally specific concept defining the degree of one's personal responsibility to others in regulating behavior that is regarded as intrusive. Some privacy-regulating mechanisms are physical barriers (closed doors or drawn curtains, such as around a hospital bed) and interpersonal types (lowered voices or cessation of smoking).

private duty nurse /prī′vit/, a nurse who may work in an institution caring for a patient on a fee-for-service basis. The private duty nurse is not a member of the institution staff. Private duty care also occurs in the home.

private practice, the work of a profes-sional health care provider who is independent of economic or policy control by professional peers, except for licensing and other legal restrictions.

privileged communication /priv′ilijd/, a legal term used in court-related proceedings concerning the right to reveal information that belongs to the person who spoke. Privileged communication may exist between a patient and a health professional only if the law specifically establishes it.

privileges /priv′ilij′əs/ [L, *privilegium,* private law], authority granted to a physician or dentist by a hospital governing board to provide patient care in the hospital. Clinical privileges are limited to the individual's professional license, experience, and competence. Emergency privileges may be granted by a hospital governing board or chief executive officer in an emergency and without regard to the physician's or dentist's regular service assignment or status. Temporary privileges may be granted a physician or dentist to provide health care to patients for a limited period or to a specific patient.

PRK, abbreviation for **photorefractive keratectomy.**

PRL, abbreviation for **prolactin.**

prn, (in prescriptions) abbreviation for *pro re nata,* a Latin phrase meaning 'as needed.' The administration times are determined by the patient's needs.

Pro, abbreviation for the amino acid **pro-line.**

probability /prob′əbil′itē/ [L, *probabilitas*], **1.** a measure of the increased likelihood that something will occur. **2.** a mathematic ratio of the number of times something will occur to the total number of possible occurrences.

probable signs /prob′əbəl/ [L, *probabalis,* credible, *signum,* mark], clinical signs that there is a definite likelihood of pregnancy. Examples include enlargement of the abdomen, Goodell's sign, Hegar's sign, Braxton Hicks' sign, and positive hormonal test results.

probe, 1. any device used to explore an opening such as a sinus or wound. Common types of probes include a probe with a blunt leading end, a drum probe with a sounding device for the detection of metallic foreign particles, and an eyed probe with a small opening at one end for introducing a guiding thread along a fistula. **2.** any device or agent, such as a radioactively tagged isotope or a molecular deoxyribonucleic acid fragment probe, inserted into a medium to obtain information about a structure or substance. **3.** a Doppler probe used to detect blood flow in a vessel. **4.** the act of exploring or investigating an action or unfamiliar matter.

probenecid /prōben'əsid/, a uricosuric and adjunct to antibiotics prescribed in the treatment of gout and as an adjunct to prolong the activity of penicillin or cephalosporins in some infections such as gonorrhea.

problem /prob'ləm/ [Gk, *proballein*, to throw forward], any health care condition that requires diagnostic, therapeutic, or educational action. An active problem requires immediate action, whereas an inactive problem is one that occurred in the past. A subjective problem is one reported by the patient, whereas one noted by an observer is regarded as an objective problem.

problem-oriented medical record (POMR), a method of recording data about the health status of a patient in a problem-solving system. The POMR preserves the data in an easily accessible way that encourages ongoing assessment and revision of the health care plan by all members of the health care team. The particular format of the system used varies from setting to setting, but the components of the method are similar. A data base is collected before beginning the process of identifying the patient's problems. The data base consists of all information available that contributes to this end, such as that collected in an interview with the patient and family or others, that from a health assessment or physical examination of the patient, and that from various laboratory tests. The next section of the POMR is the master problem list. The formulation of the problems on the list is similar to the assessment phase of the nursing process. Each problem as identified represents a conclusion or a decision resulting from examination, investigation, and analysis of the data base. The third major section of the POMR is the initial plan, in which each separate problem is named and described, usually on the progress note in a SOAP format. A discharge summary is formulated and written, relating the overall assessment of progress during treatment and the plans for follow-up or referral. The summary allows a review of all the problems initially identified and encourages continuity of care for the patient.

problem-solving approach to patient-centered care, (in nursing) a conceptual framework that incorporates the overt physical needs of a patient with covert psychologic, emotional, and social needs. It provides a model for caring for the whole person as an individual, not as an example of a disease or medical diagnosis.

Nursing is defined within this model as a problem-solving process. The patient is viewed as a person who is in an impaired state, less than able to perform self-care activities.

probucol /prōbyoo'kəl/, a cholesterol-lowering agent prescribed in the treatment of primary hypercholesterolemia in patients who have not responded to diet, weight control, or other therapies.

procainamide hydrochloride /prōkān'-əmīd/, an antiarrhythmic agent prescribed in the treatment of a variety of cardiac arrhythmias, including premature ventricular contractions, ventricular tachycardia, and atrial fibrillation.

procaine hydrochloride /prō'kān/, a local anesthetic of the ester family administered for local anesthesia by infiltration and injection and for caudal, epidural, and other regional anesthetic procedures. It is not used for topical anesthesia.

procarbazine hydrochloride /prōkär'-bəzēn/, an antineoplastic prescribed in the treatment of a variety of neoplasms, including Hodgkin's disease and lymphomas.

Procaryotae /prōker'ē-ō'tē/, (in bacteriology) a kingdom of bacteria, viruses, and blue-green algae that includes all microorganisms in which the nucleoplasm has no basic protein and is not surrounded by a nuclear membrane. The kingdom has two divisions: cyanobacteria, which includes the blue-green bacteria, and bacteria.

procedure /prəsē'jər/ [L, *procedere*, to proceed], the sequence of steps to be followed in establishing some course of action.

procerus /prəsir'əs/ [L, stretched], one of three muscles of the nose. The procerus functions to draw down the eyebrows and wrinkle the nose.

process /pros'əs/ [L, *processus*], **1.** a series of related events that follow in sequence from a particular state or condition to a conclusion or resolution. **2.** a natural growth that projects from a bone or other part. **3.** to put through a particular series of interdependent steps, as in preparing a chemical compound.

process criteria, standards identified by the American Nurses Association Division on Psychiatric and Mental Health Nursing Practice that focus on nursing activities.

process recording, (in nursing education) a system used for teaching nursing students to understand and analyze verbal and nonverbal interaction. The conversation between nurse and patient is written on special forms or in a special format.

processus vaginalis peritonei /prəses'əs/

[L, *processus,* process, *vagina,* sheath; Gk, *peri,* around, *tenein,* to stretch], a diverticulum of the peritoneal membrane that during embryonic development extends through the inguinal canal. In males it descends into the scrotum to form the processus vaginalis testis; in females it is usually completely obliterated.

prochlorperazine /-klôrper′əzēn/, a phenothiazine antipsychotic and antiemetic prescribed in the treatment of psychotic disorders and the control of nausea and vomiting.

procidentia /-siden′shə/ [L, *procidere,* to fall forward], the prolapse of an organ. The term is usually applied to a prolapsed uterus.

procoagulant /-ko·ag′yələnt/, a precursor or other agent that mediates the coagulation of blood. Examples include fibrinogen and prothrombin.

procreate /prō′krē·āt/ [L, *procreare,* to create], to produce offspring.

procreation /-krē·ā′shən/ [L, *procreare,* to create], the entire reproductive process of producing offspring. **—procreate,** *v.*

proctalgia /proktal′jə/ [Gk, *proktos, algos,* pain], a neurologic pain in the anus or lower rectum.

proctalgia fugax [Gk, *proktos + algos,* pain; L, *fugax,* fleeting], periodic pain in the anus, possibly muscular in origin, that follows a pattern and is sometimes relieved by food and drink.

proctitis /proktī′tis/ [Gk, *proktos,* anus, *itis*], inflammation of the rectum and anus caused by infection, trauma, drugs, allergy, or radiation injury. Acute or chronic, it is accompanied by rectal discomfort and the repeated urge to pass feces and inability to do so. Pus, blood, or mucus may be present in the stools; and tenesmus may occur.

proctocolectomy /prok′tōkəlek′təmē/, a surgical procedure in which the anus, rectum, and colon are removed. An ileostomy is created for the removal of digestive tract wastes. The procedure is a common treatment for severe, intractable ulcerative colitis.

proctodeum /proktō′dē·əm/, *pl.* **proctodea** [Gk, *proktos + hodiaos,* a route], an invagination of the ectoderm, behind the urorectal septum of the developing embryo, that forms the anus and anal canal when the cloacal membrane ruptures. **—proctodeal, proctodaeal,** *adj.*

proctodynia /-din′ē·ə/ [Gk, *proktos + odyne,* pain], pain in or around the anus.

proctologist /proktol′əjist/, a physician who specializes in proctology.

proctology /proktol′əjē/ [Gk, *proktos + logos,* science], the branch of medicine concerned with treating disorders of the colon, rectum, and anus.

proctoplasty /prok′təplas′tē/ [Gk, *proktos,* anus, *plassein,* to mold], a plastic surgery procedure performed on the anus and rectum.

proctoscope /prok′təskōp′/ [Gk, *proktos + skopein,* to look], an instrument used to examine the rectum and the distal part of the colon. It consists of a light mounted on a tube or speculum.

proctoscopy /proktos′kəpē/, the examination of the rectum with an endoscope inserted through the anus.

proctosigmoidoscopy /prok′tōsig′moidos′-kəpē/ [Gk, *proktos + sigmoid + skopein,* to view], the use of a sigmoidoscope to examine the rectum and pelvic colon.

procyclidine hydrochloride /prōsī′-klədēn/, an anticholinergic prescribed in the treatment of parkinsonism and the extrapyramidal dysfunction and sialorrhea that are side effects of other medications.

prodromal /-drō′məl/ [Gk, *pro,* before, *dromos,* course], pertaining to early symptoms that may mark the onset of a disease.

prodromal labor [Gk, *prodromos,* running before; L, *labor,* work], the early period in parturition before uterine contractions become forceful and frequent enough to result in progressive dilation of the uterine cervix.

prodromal myopia /prōdrō′məl/, an optical condition in which the ability to do close work without eyeglasses returns, but usually as a symptom of developing cataracts.

prodromal phase, a clear deterioration in function before the active phase of a mental disturbance that is not caused by a disorder in mood or a psychoactive substance. It includes some residual phase symptoms.

prodromal rash, a rash that precedes a potentially more serious skin eruption caused by an infectious disease.

prodromal symptom [Gk, *pro + dromos,* course, *symptoma,* that which happens], a symptom that may be the first indication of the onset of a disease.

prodrome /prō′drōm/ [Gk, *prodromos,* running before], **1.** an early sign of a developing condition or disease. **2.** the earliest phase of a developing condition or disease. **—prodromal,** *adj.*

prodrug /prō′drug/, an inactive or partially active drug that is metabolically changed in the body to an active drug.

Product Evaluation, a Nursing Interventions Classification defined as determining the effectiveness of new products or equipment.

product evaluation committee /prod'əkt/, a hospital committee composed of medical, nursing, purchasing, and administrative staff members whose purpose is to evaluate health care–related products and advise on their procurement.

productive cough /prəduk'tiv/ [L, *producere* + AS, *cohhetan,* to cough], a sudden noisy expulsion of air from the lungs that effectively removes sputum from the respiratory tract and helps clear the airways, permitting oxygen to reach the alveoli. Coughing is stimulated by irritation or inflammation of the respiratory tract, which is caused most frequently by infection. Deep breathing, with contraction of the diaphragm and intercostal muscles and forceful exhalation, promotes productive coughing in patients with respiratory infections.

professional corporation (PC) /prəfesh'-ənəl/ [L, *professio,* profession], a corporation formed according to the law of a particular state for the purpose of delivering a professional service. In some states corporations may not practice law, medicine, surgery, or dentistry; in some states nurses may form or be partners in a professional corporation.

professional liability, the legal obligation of health care professionals, or their insurers, to compensate patients for injury or suffering caused by acts of omission or commission by the professionals. Professional liability is a better characterization of the responsibility of all professionals to their clients than is the concept of malpractice, but the idea of professional liability is central to malpractice.

professional network, (in psychiatric nursing) the network of professional resources available to support the psychiatric outpatient in the community. The network may include a therapist, hospital day treatment program, social work agency, and other agencies.

professional organization, an organization whose members share a professional status, created to deal with issues of concern to the professional group or groups involved.

Professional Standards Review Organization (PSRO), an organization formed under the U.S. Social Security Act Amendments of 1972 to review the services provided under Medicare, Medicaid, and Maternal Child Health programs. Review is conducted by physicians to ascertain the need for the program and to ensure that it is carried out in accord with certain criteria, norms, and standards, and, in institutional situations in a proper setting.

profile /prō'fīl/ [L, *profilare,* to outline], a short sketch, diagram, or summary relating to a person or thing.

profunda /prōfun'də/ [L, *profundus,* deep], pertaining to structures, mainly blood vessels, that are deeply embedded in tissues.

profuse sweat /prəfyo͞os'/ [L, *profundere,* to pour out; AS, *swaetan*], excessive perspiration.

progenitive /-jen'itiv/ [Gk, *pro,* before, *genein,* to produce], capable of producing offspring; reproductive.

progenitor /-jen'itər/ [Gk, *pro* + *genein*], **1.** a parent or ancestor. **2.** someone or something that begets or creates.

progeny /proj'ənē/ [L, *progenies*], **1.** offspring; an individual or organism resulting from a particular mating. **2.** the descendants of a known or common ancestor.

progeria /prōjir'ē·ə/ [Gk, *pro* + *geras,* old age], an abnormal congenital condition characterized by premature aging, appearance in childhood of gray hair and wrinkled skin, small stature, absence of pubic and facial hair, and posture and habitus of an aged person. Death usually occurs before 20 years of age.

progestational /prō'jestā'shənəl/ [Gk, *pro* + L, *gestare,* to bear], pertaining to a drug with effects similar to those of progesterone, the hormone produced by the corpus luteum and adrenal cortex during the luteal phase of the menstrual cycle that prepares the uterus for reception of the fertilized ovum.

progestational agent [L, *pro* + *gestare,* to bear, *agere,* to do], any chemical having the same action as progesterone produced by the corpus luteum and the placenta.

progesterone /prəjes'tərōn/, a natural progestational hormone prescribed in the treatment of various menstrual disorders, infertility associated with luteal phase dysfunction, and repeated spontaneous abortion.

progestin /-jes'tin/, **1.** progesterone. **2.** any of a group of hormones, natural or synthetic, secreted by the corpus luteum, placenta, or adrenal cortex that have a progesterone-like effect on the uterine endometrial lining to prepare it for implantation of the blastocyst.

progestogen /-jes'təjən/, any natural or synthetic progestational hormone.

proglottid /prōglot'id/ [Gk, *pro* + *glossa,* tongue], a sexual segment of an adult tapeworm, containing both male and female reproductive organs.

prognathism /prog'nəthiz'əm/ [Gk, *pro* + *gnathos,* jaw], an abnormal facial configuration in which one or both jaws project forward. It is considered real or imaginary, depending on anatomic and de-

P

velopmental factors involved. —**prognathic,** *adj.*

prognosis /progno̅'sis/ [Gk, *pro* + *gnosis,* knowledge], a prediction of the probable outcome of a disease based on the condition of the person and the usual course of the disease as observed in similar situations.

prognostic /prognos'tik/ [Gk, *pro* + *gnosis,* knowledge], pertaining to signs and symptoms that may indicate the outcome of an illness or injury.

prognosticate /prognos'tikāt/ [Gk, *pro,* before, *gnosis,* knowledge], to forecast or predict from facts, present indications, or signs, such as the course a disease may take and the final outcome.

programmable pacemaker /-gram'əbəl/ [Gk, *pro* + *graphein,* to record; L, *passus,* step; ME, *maken*], an electronic pacemaker with multiple settings that can be changed after implantation.

programmed pacing, control of the heart rate by an electronic pacemaker whose output characteristics can be changed.

Program of All-inclusive Care of the Elderly (PACE), a U.S. federally supported program of comprehensive care with a primary objective of keeping clients in the community as long as medically, socially, and financially possible. It is a team approach in which professionals assess client needs, develop a care plan, integrate primary care and other services, and arrange for implementation of services. PACE is sponsored by one or more facilities and community groups and receives funds from Medicare, Medicaid, and private donations. A forerunner of PACE is the San Francisco On Lok program, which provides comprehensive adult day care, custodial or personal care, drug treatment, dentistry, and housekeeping for older persons who have a level of impairment that usually requires admission to a nursing facility.

progravid /-gravid/ [L, *pro* + *gravid,* pregnant], before pregnancy.

progression /-gresh'ən/, a carcinogenic process whereby cells genetically altered by initiators undergo a second (nongenetic) cell expansion that allows uncontrollable growth.

progressive /-gres'iv/ [L, *progredi,* to advance], describing the course of a disease or condition in which the characteristic signs and symptoms become more prominent and severe, such as progressive muscular atrophy.

progressive assistive exercise, an exercise designed to improve the strength of a muscle group progressively by gradually decreasing assistance required of a thera-

pist for an active motion, thereby increasing the patient's active effort.

progressive bulbar paralysis [L, *progredi,* to advance, *bulbus,* swollen root; Gk, *paralyein* to be palsied], a motor neuron disease characterized by weakness of the laryngeal, pharyngeal, tongue, and facial muscles. The patient experiences progressive dysarthria and dysphagia.

Progressive Muscle Relaxation, a Nursing Interventions Classification defined as facilitating the tensing and releasing of successive muscle groups while attending to the resulting differences in sensation.

progressive myopia [L, *progredi* + Gk, *myops,* nearsighted], a condition in which myopia increases at a more rapid rate than normal, often continuing into adulthood.

progressive ophthalmoplegia [L, *progredi*], a form of ocular muscle paralysis that usually begins with ptosis and gradually involves all of the extraocular muscles.

progressive patient care, a system of care in which patients are placed in units on the basis of their needs for care as determined by the degree of illness rather than in units based on a medical specialty.

progressive relaxation, a technique for combating tension and anxiety by systematically tensing and relaxing muscle groups.

progressive resistance exercise (PRE), a method of increasing the strength of a weak or injured muscle by gradually increasing the resistance against which the muscle works, such as by using graduated weights over a period.

progressive supranuclear palsy [L, *supra,* above, *nucleus,* nut kernel; Gk, *paralyein*], a mild form of paralysis involving muscles innervated by the cranial nerves and primarily affecting the face, throat, and tongue.

progressive systemic sclerosis (PSS), the most common form of scleroderma.

progress notes [L, *progredi* + *nota,* mark], (in the patient record) notes made by a nurse, physician, social worker, physical therapist, and others that describe the patient's condition and the treatment given or planned. Progress notes may follow the problem-oriented medical record format. The physician's progress notes usually focus on the medical or therapeutic aspects of the patient's condition and care; the nurse's progress notes, although recording the medical conditions of the patient, usually focus on the objectives stated in the nursing care plan.

proinsulin /prō·in's(y)əlin/ [L, *pro* + *in-*

sula, island], a single-chain protein molecule that is a precursor of insulin.

projectile vomiting /-jek′til/, expulsive vomiting that is extremely forceful.

projection /-jek′shən/ [L, *projectio,* thrown forward], **1.** a protuberance; anything that thrusts or juts outward. **2.** the act of perceiving an idea or thought as an objective reality. **3.** (in psychology) an unconscious defense mechanism by which an individual attributes his or her own unacceptable traits, ideas, or impulses to another.

projection reconstruction imaging, the techniques used in magnetic resonance (MR) imaging to obtain a cross-sectional image of an object. Such an image is computer reconstructed from a series of projections, MR profiles, recorded all around the object by rotating the direction of the gradient field superimposed on the static magnetic field.

projective test /-jek′tiv/ [L, *projectio,* thrown forward], a kind of diagnostic, psychologic, or personality test that uses unstructured or ambiguous stimuli such as inkblots, a series of pictures, abstract patterns, or incomplete sentences to elicit responses that reflect a projection of various aspects of the individual's personality.

prokaryocyte /prōker′ē-əsīt′/ [Gk, *protos,* first, *karyon,* nut, *kytos,* cell], a cell without a true nucleus and with nuclear material scattered throughout the cytoplasm.

prokaryon /prōker′ē-on/ [Gk, *protos* + *karyon,* nut], **1.** nuclear elements that are not bound by a membrane but are spread throughout the cytoplasm. **2.** an organism containing such unbound nuclear elements.

prokaryosis /′kεr′ə ō′sis/ [Gk, *protos* + *karyon* + *osis,* condition], the condition of not containing a true nucleus surrounded by a nuclear membrane.

prokaryote /prōker′ē-ōt/ [Gk, *protos* + *karyon*], an organism that does not contain a true nucleus surrounded by a nuclear membrane, characteristic of lower forms, such as bacteria, viruses, and blue-green algae. Division occurs through simple fission. —**prokaryotic,** *adj.*

prolactin (PRL) /prōlak′tin/ [Gk, *pro,* before, *lac,* milk], a hormone produced and secreted into the bloodstream by the anterior pituitary gland. Prolactin, acting with estrogen, progesterone, thyroxine, insulin, growth hormone, glucocorticoids, and human placental lactogen, stimulates the development and growth of the mammary glands. After parturition prolactin, together with glucocorticoids, is essential for the initiation and maintenance of milk production.

prolapse /prō′laps, prōlaps′/ [L, *prolapsus,* falling], the falling, sinking, or sliding of an organ from its normal position or location in the body, such as a prolapsed uterus.

prolapsed cord /prōlapst/, an umbilical cord that protrudes beside or ahead of the presenting part of the fetus.

prolapsed hemorrhoid [L, *prolapsus,* falling; Gk, *haim orrhois,* a vein that loses blood], an internal hemorrhoid that protrudes through the anal orifice.

prolapse of anus [L, *prolapsus,* falling, *anus*] the protrusion of the mucous membrane of the anus through the external sphincter.

prolapse of rectum [L, *prolapsus,* falling, *rectus,* straight], a protrusion of the mucous membrane of the lower part of the rectum through the anal orifice.

prolapse of uterus [L, *prolapsus,* falling, *uterus,* womb], the descent of the uterine cervix into the vagina, partly into the vagina, or outside the vagina.

proliferate /-lif′ərāt/ [L, *proles,* offspring, *ferre,* to bear], to grow by multiplication of cells, parts, or organisms.

proliferation /-lif′ərā′shən/ [L, *proles,* offspring, *ferre,* to bear], the reproduction or multiplication of similar forms. The term is usually applied to increases of cells or cysts.

proliferation inhibiting factor, a lymphokine that restricts cell division in tissue cultures.

proliferative phase /-lif′ərətiv/, the phase of the menstrual cycle after menstruation. Under the influence of follicle-stimulating hormone from the pituitary, the ovary produces increasing amounts of estrogen, causing the lining of the uterus to become dense and richly vascular.

prolific /lif′ik/ [L, *proles,* offspring, *ferre,* to bear], highly productive.

proline (Pro) /prō′lēn/, a nonessential amino acid found in many proteins of the body, particularly collagen.

prolonged gestation /-longd′/ [L, *prolongare,* to lengthen, *gestare,* to bear], a pregnancy that lasts longer than the usual period of 41 weeks.

prolonged release [Gk, *pro,* before, *longus,* long], a term applied to a drug that is designed to deliver a dose of a medication over an extended period. The most common device for this purpose is a soft, soluble capsule containing minute pellets of the drug for release at different rates in the gastrointestinal tract, depending on the thickness and nature of the oil, fat, wax, or resin coating on the pellets.

P

promastigote /prōmas'tigōt/, the flagellate stage of a trypanosomatid protozoan. It is found in the insect intermediate host (or in culture) of *Leishmania* parasites.

promethazine hydrochloride /-meth'-əzēn/, a phenothiazine antiemetic, antihistamine, and sedative. It is prescribed in the treatment of motion sickness, nausea, rhinitis, itching, and skin rash and as an adjunct to anesthesia.

promethium (Pm) /-mē'thē·əm/ [L, *Prometheus,* mythic character who gave fire to humans], a radioactive rare earth metallic element. Its atomic number is 61; its atomic mass (weight) is 145.

prominence /prom'inəns [L, *prominentia,* sticking out], any elevation or projection of a structural feature.

promontory of the sacrum /prom'əntôr'ē/ [L, *promontorium,* headland], the superior projecting part of the sacrum at its junction with the L5 vertebra.

promoter /-mō'tər/ [L, *promovere,* to move forward], **1.** (in molecular genetics) a deoxyribonucleic acid sequence that initiates ribonucleic acid transcription of the genetic code. **2.** a cocarcinogenic factor that encourages cells altered by initiators to reproduce at a faster than normal rate, increasing the probability of malignant transformation.

prompt insulin zinc suspension [L, *promptus,* ready], a fast-acting noncrystalline semilente insulin prescribed in the treatment of diabetes mellitus when a prompt, intense, and short-acting response is desired.

promyelocyte /prōmī'ələsīt'/, a large mononuclear blood cell that contains a single regular, symmetric nucleus and a few undifferentiated cytoplasmic granules.

pronate /prō'nāt/ [L, *pronare,* to bend forward], to place in a prone position of lying flat with the face forward.

pronation /prōnā'shən/ [L, *pronare,* to bend forward], **1.** assumption of a prone position, one in which the ventral surface of the body faces downward. **2.** (of the arm) the rotation of the forearm so that the palm of the hand faces downward and backward. **3.** (of the foot) the lowering of the medial edge of the foot by turning it outward and through abduction movements in the tarsal and metatarsal joints. **—pronate,** *v.*

pronator quadratus, a muscle of the forearm. It functions to pronate the forearm and hand.

pronator reflex /prōnā'tər/ [L, *pronare + reflectere,* to bend back], a reflex elicited by holding the patient's hand vertically and tapping the distal end of the radius or ulna, resulting in pronation of the forearm.

pronator syndrome [L, *pronare,* to bend forward; Gk, *syn,* together, *dromos,* course], the compression of the median nerve between the two heads of the pronator teres muscle.

pronator teres, /ter'əs/, a superficial muscle of the forearm. It functions to pronate the hand.

prone /prōn/ [L, *pronare,* to bend forward], **1.** having a tendency or inclination. **2.** (of the body) being in horizontal position when lying face downward.

proneness profile /prōn'nəs/ [L, *pronare,* to bend forward, *profilare,* to outline], a screening process that evaluates the probability of developmental problems in the early years of a child's life. Several of the variables in the proneness profile that appear to be significant in selecting the infants who are at risk are the perinatal health status of the mother and infant, especially complications of pregnancy, delivery, the neonatal period, and the puerperium; characteristics of the mother, especially her temperament, educational level, perception of the life situation, and perception of the infant; characteristics of the infant, including alertness, activity pattern, and responsiveness; and behaviors of the infant and caregiver as they interact.

prone-on-elbows, a body position in which the person rests the upper part of the body on the elbows while lying face down. The position is used as an initial rehabilitation exercise in training a person with a cerebellar dysfunction to achieve ambulation.

pronephric duct /-nef'rik/ [Gk, *pro,* before, *nephros,* kidney; L, *ducere,* to lead], one of the paired ducts that connect the tubules of each of the pronephros with the cloaca in the early developing vertebrate embryo.

pronephric tubule, any of the segmentally arranged excretory units of the pronephros in the early developing vertebrate embryo.

pronephros /-nef'rəs/, *pl.* **pronephroi** [Gk, *pro + nephros,* kidney], the primordial excretory organ in the developing vertebrate embryo. **—pronephric,** *adj.*

prone position [L, *pronare,* to bend forward, *positio*], a postural position of facing downward while lying flat.

prone posture [L, *pronare,* to bend forward, *ponere,* to place], a posture assumed by lying flat with the face forward during certain disorders of the spine or viscera.

pronucleus /-nōō'klē·əs/, *pl.* **pronuclei** [Gk, *pro + L, nucleus,* nut kernel], the nucleus of the ovum or the spermatozoon after fertilization but before fusion of the chromosomes to form the nucleus of the zygote.

propagation /prop'əgā'shən/ [L, *propagare,* to generate], the process of increasing or causing to increase.

propantheline bromide /-pan'thəlēn/, an anticholinergic prescribed as an adjunct in peptic ulcer therapy.

proparacaine hydrochloride /prōper'-əkān/, a rapid-acting topical anesthetic of the amide family. It is used for tonometry, gonioscopy, removal of foreign objects from the eye, and other minor ophthalmologic procedures and preoperatively for major eye surgery.

prophase /prō'fāz/ [Gk, *pro* + *phasis,* appearance], the first of four stages of nuclear division in mitosis and in each of the two divisions of meiosis.

prophylactic /prō'filak'tik/ [Gk, *prophylax,* advance guard], 1. preventing the spread of disease. 2. an agent that prevents the spread of disease. —**prophylactically,** *adv.*

prophylactic odontomy, (in dentistry) the surgical removal of harmful pits and fissures in the posterior primary and permanent molars.

prophylaxis /prō'filak'sis/ [Gk, *prophylax,* advance guard], prevention of or protection against disease, often involving the use of a biologic, chemical, or mechanical agent to destroy or prevent the entry of infectious organisms.

Propionibacterium /prō'pē·on'ēbaktir'ē--əm/ [Gk, *pro* + *pion,* fat, *bakterion* small rod], a genus of nonmotile anaerobic gram-positive bacteria found on the skin of humans, in the intestinal tract of humans and animals, and in dairy products. *Propionibacterium acnes* is common in acne pustules

propionic acid /prō'pē·on'ik/, a saturated fatty acid, methylacetic acid, a chemical component of sweat. It can be fermented by several species of bacteria.

propionicacidemia /prō'pē·on'ikas'idē'-mē·ə/ [Gk, *pro* + *pion,* fat; L, *acidus,* sour; Gk, *haima,* blood], a rare inherited metabolic defect caused by the failure of the body to metabolize the amino acids threonine, isoleucine, and methionine, characterized by lethargy and mental and physical retardation. Acidosis results from the accumulation of propionic acid in the body. —**propionicacidemic,** *adj.*

propionic fermentation /prō'pē·on'ik/ [Gk, *pro* + *pion* + L, *fermentare,* to cause to ferment], the production of propionic acid by the action of certain bacteria on sugars or lactic acid.

proportional /prəpôr'shənəl/, pertaining to the relationship between two quantities when a fractional variation of one is always accompanied by the same factional change in the other.

proportional gas detector /-pôr'shənəl/, a device for measuring alpha and beta forms of radioactivity.

proportional mortality [L, *pro* + *portio,* part, *mortalis,* subject to death], a statistical method of relating the number of deaths from a particular condition to all deaths within the same population group for the same period.

proposition /prop'əzish'ən/ [L, *proponere,* to place forward], 1. a statement of a truth to be demonstrated or an operation to be performed. 2. to bring forward or offer for consideration, acceptance, or adoption.

propositus /prōpoz'itəs/ [L, *proponere,* to place forward], a person from whom a genealogic lineage is traced, as is done to discover the pattern of inheritance of a familial disease or a physical trait.

propoxyphene /prōpok'səfēn/, a mild, centrally acting narcotic analgesic prescribed to relieve mild to moderate pain.

propoxyphene hydrochloride, an analgesic prescribed for the relief of mild to moderate pain.

propranolol hydrochloride /-pran'əlol/, a beta-adrenergic blocking agent prescribed in the treatment of angina pectoris, cardiac arrhythmias, and hypertension.

proprietary /-prī'əterē/ [L, *proprietas,* property], 1. pertaining to an institution or other organization that is operated for profit. 2. pertaining to a product, such as a drug or device, that is made for profit.

proprietary hospital, a hospital operated as a profit-making organization. Many proprietary hospitals are owned by physicians who operate them primarily for their own patients but also accept patients from other physicians. Some proprietary hospitals are owned by investor groups or large corporations.

proprietary medicine, any pharmaceutic preparation or medicinal substance that is protected from commercial competition because its ingredients or method of manufacture is kept secret or protected by trademark or copyright.

proprioception /prō'prē·əsep'shən/ [L, *proprius,* one's own, *capere,* to take], sensation pertaining to stimuli originating from within the body related to spatial position and muscular activity or to the sensory receptors that they activate.

proprioceptive /-prē·ə·sep'tiv/ [L, *proprius,* one's own, *capere,* to take], pertaining to the sensations of body movements and awareness of posture, enabling the body to orient itself in space without visual clues.

proprioceptive impulse /prō′prē·əsep′tiv/, a nerve impulse that originates with a sensory ending in muscle, joint, or tendon. Such impulses provide information to the central nervous system about the relative position of body parts.

proprioceptive neuromuscular facilitation (PNF), an activity, such as a therapeutic technique, that helps initiate a proprioceptive response in a person.

proprioceptive reflex [L, *proprius* + *capere,* to take, *reflectere,* to bend back], any reflex initiated by stimulation of proprioceptors, such as the increase in respiratory rate and volume induced by impulses arising from muscles and joints during exercise.

proprioceptive sensation [L, *propius* + *capere* + *sentire,* to feel], the feeling of body movement and position, including motion of the arms and legs, resulting from stimuli received by special sense organs in the muscles, tendons, joints, and inner ear.

proprioceptor /prō′prē·əsep′tər/ [L, *proprius* + *capere*], any sensory nerve ending, such as those located in muscles, tendons, joints, and the vestibular apparatus, that responds to stimuli originating from within the body related to movement and spatial position.

proptosis /proptō′sis/ [L, *pro* + *ptosis,* falling], bulging, protrusion, or forward displacement of a body organ or area.

propulsion /-pul′shən/ [L, *propellere,* to drive forward], **1.** the process of pushing forward. **2.** the tendency of some patients, particularly those afflicted with nervous disorders, to push or fall forward while walking as their center of gravity is displaced.

propylene glycol /prop′ilēn/, a colorless viscous liquid used as a solvent in the preparation of certain medications. It also inhibits the growth of fungi and microorganisms and is used commercially as an antifreeze.

propylthiouracil /prō′pilthī′əyŏŏr′əsil/, an inhibitor of thyroid hormone biosynthesis prescribed in treatment of hyperthyroidism and thyrotoxic crisis and in preparation for thyroidectomy.

proscribe /prōskrīb′/, to forbid. **—proscriptive,** *adj.*

prosector /-sek′tər/ [L, *prosecare,* to cut off], a person who, under the supervision of a pathologist, performs gross dissections and prepares autopsy specimens for pathologic examination.

prosencephalon /pros′ensef′əlon/ [Gk, *pro* + *enkephalon,* brain], the part of the brain that includes the diencephalon and the telencephalon. It contains various

structures, such as the thalamus and hypothalamus, that control important body functions and affect the consciousness, the appetite, and the emotions. **—prosencephalic,** *adj.*

prosopopilary virilism /pros′əpōpī′lərē/, a heavy growth of facial hair.

prosopospasm /pros′əpōspaz′əm/ [Gk, *prosopon,* face, *spasmos*], a spasm of the facial muscles, such as may occur in tetanus.

prosoposternodidymus /pros′əpōstur′nədid′əməs/ [Gk, *prosopon,* face, *sternon,* chest, *didymos,* twin], a fetus consisting of conjoined twins united laterally from the head through the sternum.

prosopothoracopagus /pros′əpōthôr′əkop′əgəs/ [Gk, *prosopon* + *thorax,* chest, *pagos,* fixed], conjoined symmetric twins who are united laterally in the frontal plane from the thorax through most of the head region.

prospective medicine /-spek′tiv/ [L, *proscipere,* to look forward, *medicina,* art of healing], the early identification of pathologic or potentially pathologic processes and the prescription of intervention to stop them.

prospective payment system (PPS), a payment mechanism for reimbursing hospitals for inpatient health care services in which a predetermined rate is set for treatment of specific illnesses. The system was originally developed by the U.S. federal government for use in treatment of Medicare recipients.

prospective reimbursement, a method of payment to an agency for health care services to be delivered that is based on predictions of what the agency's costs will be for the coming year.

prospective study, an analytic study designed to determine the relationship between a condition and a characteristic shared by some members of a group. The population selected is healthy at the beginning of the study. Some of the members of the group share a particular characteristic, such as cigarette smoking. The researcher follows the population group over a period, noting the rate at which a condition, such as lung cancer, occurs in the smokers and in the nonsmokers. Prospective studies produce a direct measure of risk called *relative risk.*

prostacyclin (PGI$_2$) /pros′təsī′klin/, a prostaglandin. It is a biologically active product of arachidonic acid metabolism in human vascular walls and a potent inhibitor of platelet aggregation.

prostaglandin (PG) /pros′təglan′din/ [Gk, *prostates,* standing before; L, *glans,* acorn], one of several potent unsaturated fatty acids that act in exceedingly low concentrations on local target organs. Prostaglandins are produced in small amounts and have a large array of significant effects. Some of the pharmacologic uses of the prostaglandins are termination of pregnancy and treatment of asthma and gastric hyperacidity.

prostaglandin inhibitor, an agent that prevents the production of prostaglandins. An example is a nonsteroidal antiinflammatory drug.

prostanoic acid /pros'tənō'ik/, a 20-carbon aliphatic acid that is the basic framework for prostaglandin molecules, which differ according to the location of hydroxyl and keto substitutions at various positions along the molecule.

prostate /pros'tāt/ [Gk, *prostates,* standing before], a gland in men that surrounds the neck of the bladder and the deepest part of the urethra and produces a secretion that liquefies coagulated semen. It is a firm structure about the size of a chestnut, composed of muscular and glandular tissue. It is located in the pelvic cavity, below the inferior part of the symphysis pubis and ventral to the rectum, through which it can be felt, especially when enlarged. In most men the urethra lies along the junction of the anterior part and the middle third of the prostate. The prostatic secretion consists of alkaline phosphatase, citric acid, and various proteolytic enzymes. It contracts during ejaculation of seminal fluid.

prostate cancer, a slowly progressive adenocarcinoma of the prostate that affects an increasing proportion of American males after 50 years of age. It is the third leading cause of cancer deaths; more than 120,000 new cases are reported in the United States each year. The cause is unknown, but it is believed to be hormone-related. The disease may cause no direct symptoms but can be detected in the course of diagnosing bladder or ureteral obstruction, hematuria, or pyuria. The cancer can spread to cause bone pain in the pelvis, ribs, or vertebrae.

prostatectomy /pros'tətek'təmē/ [Gk, *prostates + ektome,* excision], surgical removal of a part of the prostate gland, such as performed for benign prostatic hypertrophy, or the total excision of the gland, as performed for malignancy. Kinds of approaches include transurethral, the most common, in which a resectoscope is inserted and through it shavings of prostatic tissue are cut off at the bladder opening. The perineal approach is used for biopsy when early cancer is suspected or for the removal of calculi.

prostate-specific antigen (PSA), a protein produced by the prostate that may be present at elevated levels in patients with cancer or other disease of the prostate.

prostatic /prostat'ik/, pertaining to the prostate.

prostatic calculus [Gk, *prostates,* standing before; L, *calculus,* pebble], a solid pathologic calcification formed in the prostate, usually of calcium carbonate and/or calcium phosphate.

prostatic catheter, a catheter that is approximately 16 inches long and has an angled tip. It is used in male urinary bladder catheterization to pass an enlarged prostate gland obstructing the urethra.

prostatic ductule /duk'tyōōl/ [Gk, *prostates* + L, *ductulus,* little duct], any of 12 to 20 tiny excretory tubes that convey the alkaline secretion of the prostate and open into the floor of the prostatic part of the urethra.

prostatic syncope [Gk, *prostates,* standing before, *syn,* together, *koptein,* to cut], a temporary loss of consciousness caused by restricted cerebral blood flow that may occur during a prostate examination.

prostatic utricle, the part of the urethra in men that forms a cul-de-sac about 6 mm long behind the middle lobe of the prostate. It is homologous with the uterus in women.

prostatism /pros'tətiz'əm/ [Gk, *prostates,* standing before], an abnormal condition of the prostate, particularly an enlargement of the gland, resulting in an obstruction to the urinary flow.

prostatitis /pros'tətī'tis/ [Gk, *prostates + itis,* inflammation], acute or chronic inflammation of the prostate gland, usually the result of infection. The patient complains of burning, frequency, and urgency.

prostatomegaly /pros'tətōmeg'əlē/ [Gk, *prostates + megas,* large], the hypertrophy or enlargement of the prostate.

prosthesis /prosthē'sis/, *pl.* **prostheses** [Gk, addition], **1.** an artificial replacement for a missing body part, such as an artificial limb or total joint replacement. **2.** a device designed and applied to improve function, such as a hearing aid.

Prosthesis Care, a Nursing Interventions Classification defined as care of a removable appliance worn by a patient and prevention of complications associated with its use.

prosthetic heart valve /prosthet'ik/ [Gk, *prosthesis,* addition; AS, *hoerte* + L, *valva,* door, leaf], an artificial heart valve.

prosthetics /prosthet'iks/ [Gk, *prosthesis,* addition], the branch of surgery concerned with the design, construction, and attachment of artificial limbs or other systems to assume the function of a missing body part.

prosthetist /pros′thətist/, a person who fabricates and fits artificial limbs and similar devices prescribed by a physician. A certified prosthetist is one who has successfully completed the examination of the American Orthotic and Prosthetic Association.

prosthodontics /pros′thədon′tiks/ [Gk, *prosthesis* + *odous,* tooth], a branch of dentistry devoted to the construction of artificial appliances that replace missing teeth or restore parts of the face.

prostration /prostrā′shən/ [L, *prosternere,* to throw down], a condition of extreme exhaustion and inability to exert oneself further, as in heat or nervous prostration. —**prostrate,** adj.

protactinium (Pa) /-taktin′ē·əm/ [Gk, *protos,* first, *aktis,* ray], a radioactive element. Its atomic number is 91; its atomic mass (weight) is 231.04. Its decay products are actinium and an alpha particle.

protamine sulfate /prō′təmēn/, a heparin antagonist derived from fish sperm. It is prescribed to diminish or reverse the anticoagulant effect of heparin, particularly in cases of heparin overdosage.

protamine zinc insulin (PZI) suspension, a long-acting insulin that is absorbed slowly at a steady rate. Some patients can be treated with only one injection daily, but combination therapy with regular insulin may be necessary for adequate control.

protanopia /-tənō′pē·ə/, a form of color blindness in which the person is unable to distinguish shades of red.

protaxic mode of experience /-tak′sik/ (in psychology) a type of primitive experience characterized by sensations, feelings, and fragmented images of short duration that are not logically connected.

protease /prō′tē·ās/, an enzyme that is a catalyst in the breakdown of peptide bonds that join the amino acids in a protein.

protease inhibitors, a class of antiretroviral drugs that block the process by which human immunodeficiency virus reassembles itself inside a cell. Specifically protease inhibitors disable protease, an enzyme necessary for cutting large viral peptides into smaller functional units to create active new viral particles. The resulting virus is defective and not infectious. Examples of protease inhibitors include saquinavir, ritonavir, and indinavir.

protection, altered, a NANDA-accepted nursing diagnosis of a state in which an individual experiences a decrease in the ability to guard the self from internal or external threats such as illness or injury. Defining characteristics include deficient immunity, impaired healing, altered clotting, maladaptive stress response, neurosensory alterations, chilling, perspiration, dyspnea, cough, itching, restlessness, insomnia, fatigue, anorexia, weakness, immobility, disorientation, and pressure sores.

protective /-tek′tiv/ [L, *protegere,* to cover], guarding another person from danger or injury and providing a safe environment.

protective isolation [L, *protegere,* to cover in front; It, *isolare,* detached], **1.** the practice of confining a patient with a virulent infectious disease in a separate area so that contact with other people can be minimized. **2.** the practice of placing a highly susceptible person, such as an immunodeficient patient, in a separate area where the risk of contact with pathogenic microorganisms can be controlled.

protein /prō′tē·in, prō′tēn/ [Gk, *proteios,* first rank], any of a large group of naturally occurring complex organic nitrogenous compounds. Each is composed of large combinations of amino acids containing the elements carbon, hydrogen, nitrogen, oxygen, and occasionally sulfur, phosphorus, iron, iodine, or other essential constituents of living cells. Twenty-two amino acids have been identified as vital for proper growth, development, and maintenance of health. The body can synthesize 13 of these, the nonessential amino acids, whereas the remaining 9 must be obtained from dietary sources and are termed *essential.* Protein is the major source of building material for muscles, blood, skin, hair, nails, and the internal organs. It is necessary for the formation of hormones, enzymes, and antibodies; may act as a source of heat and energy; and functions as an essential element in proper elimination of waste materials. Excessive intake of protein may in some conditions result in fluid imbalance. Normal adult findings of total blood protein are 6 to 8 g/dl.

proteinase /prō′tē·inās/ [Gk, *proteios,* first rank, *ase,* enzyme suffix], a proteolytic enzyme that splits protein molecules at central linkages.

protein-bound iodine (PBI), iodine that is firmly bound to protein in serum, the measurement of which indirectly indicates the concentration of circulating thyroxine (T_4).

proteinemia /prōtē·inē′mē·ə/ [Gk, *proteios,* first rank, *haima,* blood], an excessive level of protein in the blood.

protein-energy malnutrition (PEM), a wasting condition resulting from a diet deficient in either protein or energy (calories) or both. These deficits are major problems for children in Third World countries.

protein hydrolysate injection, a fluid and nutrient replenisher prescribed to correct a negative nitrogen balance and to provide parenteral nutrition in other clinical situations.

protein kinase, a protein that catalyzes the transfer of a phosphate group from adenosine triphosphate to produce a phosphoprotein.

protein metabolism, the processes whereby protein foods are used by the body to make tissue proteins, together with the processes of breakdown of tissue proteins in the production of energy. Food proteins are first broken down into amino acids, then absorbed into the bloodstream, and finally used in body cells to form new proteins. Amino acids in excess of the body's needs may be converted by liver enzymes into keto acids and urea.

protein sensitization [Gk, *proteios,* first rank; L, *sentire,* to feel], a reaction that follows parenteral introduction of a foreign protein into the body. Symptoms of varying severity, including serum sickness, occur when the same foreign protein is reintroduced into the body at a later date.

proteinuria /prō'tēnyŏŏr'ē·ə/ [Gk, *proteios* + *ouron,* urine], the presence in the urine of abnormally large quantities of protein, usually albumin. Healthy adults excrete less than 250 mg of protein per day. Persistent proteinuria is usually a sign of renal disease or renal complications of another disease.

proteolipid /prō'tē·ōlip'id/ [Gk, *proteios* + *lipos,* fat], a type of lipoprotein in which lipid material forms more than half of the molecule. It is insoluble in water and occurs primarily in the brain.

proteolysis /prō'tē·ol'isis/ [Gk, *proteios* + *lysis,* loosening], a process in which water added to the peptide bonds of proteins breaks down the protein molecule into simpler substances. Numerous enzymes may catalyze this process.

proteolytic /prō'tē·əlit'ik/, pertaining to any substance that promotes the breakdown of protein.

Proteus /prō'tē·əs/ [Gk, *Proteus,* mythic god who changed shapes], a genus of motile, gram-negative bacilli often associated with nosocomial infections, normally found in feces, water, and soil. *Proteus* may cause urinary tract infections, pyelonephritis, wound infections, diarrhea, bacteremia, and endotoxic shock.

Proteus mirabilis a species of anaerobic

motile rod-shaped bacteria found in putrid meat, abscesses, and fecal material. It is a leading cause of urinary tract infections.

Proteus morgani, a species of bacteria associated with infectious diarrhea in infants.

Proteus vulgaris, a species of bacteria that is a frequent cause of urinary tract infections. The bacteria are found in feces, water, and soil.

prothrombin /prōthrom'bin/ [L, *pro,* before; Gk, *thrombos,* lump], a plasma protein that is the precursor to thrombin. It is synthesized in the liver if adequate vitamin K is present.

prothrombinemia /-ē'mē·ə/ [L, *pro,* before; Gk, *thrombos,* lump, *haima* blood], the presence of prothrombin in the blood.

prothrombin time (PT), a one-stage test for detecting certain plasma coagulation defects caused by a deficiency of factors V, VII, or X. Thromboplastin and calcium are added to a sample of the patient's plasma and simultaneously to a sample from a normal control. The amount of time required for clot formation in both samples is observed.

protocol /prō'təkôl/ [Gk, *protos,* first, *kolla,* glued page], a written plan specifying the procedures to be followed in giving a particular examination, in conducting research, or in providing care for a particular condition.

proton /prō'ton/ [Gk, *protos,* first], a positively charged particle that is a fundamental component of the nucleus of all atoms. The number of protons in the nucleus of an atom equals the atomic number of the element.

proton density, a measure of proton concentration, or the number of atomic nuclei per given volume. It is one of the major determinants of magnetic resonance signal strength in hydrogen imaging.

protopathic sensibility /prō'təpath'ik/, pertaining to the somatic sensations of fast localized pain; slow, poorly localized pain; and temperature.

protoplasm /prō'təplaz'əm/ [Gk, *protos* + *plasma,* something formed], the living substance of a cell, usually composed of myriad molecules of water, minerals, and organic compounds.

protoplasmic /-plaz'mik/ [Gk, *protos,* first, *plasma,* something formed], pertaining to or composed of protoplasm.

protoplast /prō'təplast/ [Gk, *protos* + *plassein,* to mold], **1.** (in biology) the protoplasm of a cell without its containing membrane. **2.** a first entity or an original. —**protoplastic,** *adj.*

protoporphyria /prō'tōpôrfir'ē·ə/ [Gk, *protos* + *porphyros,* purple, *haima,* blood],

P

increased levels of protoporphyrin in the blood and feces.

protoporphyrin /prō'tōpôr'firin/ [Gk, *protos* + *porphyros*], a kind of porphyrin that combines with iron and protein to form various important organic molecules, including catalase, hemoglobin, and myoglobin.

prototaxic mode /prōtətak'sik/ [Gk, *protos* + *taxis*, arrangement, *modus,* measure], a stage in infancy characterized by a lack of differentiation between the self and the environment.

prototype /prō'tətīp/ [Gk, *protos,* first, *typos,* mark], the primary or original form of an object or organism.

protozoa /prō'təzō'ə/, *sing.* **protozoon** [Gk, *protos* + *zoon,* animal], single-celled microorganisms of the subkingdom Protozoa (within the kingdom Protista). Protozoa, the lowest form of animal life, are more complex than bacteria, forming a self-contained unit with organelles that carry on such functions as locomotion, nutrition, excretion, respiration, and attachment to other objects or organisms. Approximately 30 protozoa are pathogenic to humans. —**protozoal, protozoan,** *adj.*

protozoal infection /-zō'əl/, any disease caused by single-celled organisms of the subkingdom Protozoa. Some kinds of protozoal infections are **amebic dysentery, kala-azar, malaria,** and Trichomoniasis.

protozoan /-zō'ən/ [Gk, *protos,* first, *zoon,* animal], pertaining to or caused by protozoa.

protracted dose /prōtrak'tid/ [L, *pro,* before, *trahere,* to draw, *dosis,* something given], (in radiotherapy) a low amount of radiation delivered continuously over a relatively long period.

protriptyline hydrochloride /-trip'tilēn/, a tricyclic antidepressant prescribed in the treatment of endogenous depression marked by withdrawal and anergy.

protrusion /-trōō'zhən/ [L, *protrudere,* to push forward], a state or condition of being forward or projecting.

protrusive incisal guide angle /-trōō'siv/, (in dentistry) the inclination of the incisal guide in the sagittal plane.

protuberance /-t(y)ōō'bərəns/ [L, *pro* + *tuberare,* to swell], an anatomic landmark that appears as a blunt projection or swelling, such as the chin, buttock, or bulge of the frontal bone above the eyebrow.

proud flesh [AS, *prud* + *flaesc*], excessive granulation tissue.

provider, a hospital, clinic, health care professional, or group of health care professionals who provide a service to patients.

Provincial/Territorial Nurses Association (PTNA), an association of Canadian nurses organized at the provincial or territorial level. The Canadian Nurses' Association is a federation of the 11 PTNAs.

provirus /-vī'rəs/, a stage of viral replication in which the viral genetic information has been integrated into the genome of the host cell.

provitamin /prōvī'təmin/, a precursor of a vitamin; a substance found in certain foods that in the body may be converted into a vitamin.

provocative diagnosis /-vok'ətiv/ [L, *provocare,* to call forth; Gk, *dia,* through, *gnosis,* knowledge], a diagnosis in which the identity and cause of an illness are discovered by inducing an episode of the condition.

prox, abbreviation for **proximal.**

proxemics /proksē'miks/ [L, *proximus,* nearest], the study of spatial distances between people and their effect on interpersonal behavior, especially in relation to population density, placement of people within an area, territoriality, personal space, and the opportunity for privacy.

proximal /prok'siməl/ [L, *proximus*], nearer to a point of reference or attachment, usually the trunk of the body, than other parts of the body. Proximal interphalangeal joints are those closest to the hand.

proximal cavity, a cavity that occurs on the mesial or distal surface of a tooth.

proximal contact [L, *proximus,* nearest, *contingere,* to touch], the contact between the distal surface of one tooth and the mesial surface of an adjacent tooth.

proximal contour, the shape or form of the mesial or the distal surface of a tooth.

proximal dental caries, decay that may occur in the mesial or distal surface of a tooth.

proximal radioulnar articulation, the pivot joint between the circumference of the head of the radius and the ring formed by the radial notch of the ulna and the annular ligament. The joint allows the rotary movements of the head of the radius in pronation and supination.

proximal renal tubular acidosis (proximal RTA), an abnormal condition characterized by excessive acid accumulation and bicarbonate excretion. It is caused by the defective resorption of bicarbonate in the proximal tubules of the kidney and the resulting flow of excessive bicarbonate into the distal tubules, which normally secrete hydrogen ions. In **primary proximal RTA** the defective resorption of bicarbonate is the sole causative factor. In **second-**

ary proximal RTA the resorptive defect is one of several causative factors and may result from tubular cell damage produced by various disorders, such as Fanconi's syndrome.

proximate /prok'simit/ [L, *proximus*, nearest], the nearest to a point of origin or attachment.

proximate cause [L, *proximus*, nearest], a legal concept of cause-and-effect relationships in determining, for example, whether an injury would have resulted from a particular cause.

proximity principle /proksim'itē/ [L, *proximus* + *principium*, origin], a rule that when two or more objects are close to each other, they may be seen as a perceptual unit.

PrP, abbreviation for *prion protein*, a viruslike infectious agent associated with Creutzfeldt-Jakob's disease.

prurigo /prŏŏrī'gō/ [L, an itch], any of a group of chronic inflammatory conditions of the skin characterized by severe itching and multiple dome-shaped small papules capped by tiny vesicles. Later (as a result of repeated scratching), crusting and lichenification may occur. Some causes of prurigo are allergies, drugs, endocrine abnormalities, malignancies, and parasites. A mild form of the disease is called prurigo mitis, a more severe form, prurigo agria or prurigo ferox. —**pruriginous,** *adj.*

pruritic urticarial papules and plaques of pregnancy (PUPPP) /prŏŏrit'ik/, small, semisolid, intensely itching blisters that may appear on the abdomen of a pregnant woman and spread peripherally. They begin in the third trimester and resolve spontaneously after delivery.

pruritus /prŏŏrī'təs/ [L, *prurire*, to itch], the symptom of itching, an uncomfortable sensation leading to the urge to scratch. Scratching may result in secondary infection. Some causes of pruritus are allergy, infection, jaundice, chronic renal disease, lymphoma, and skin irritation. —**pruritic,** *adj.*

pruritus ani, a common chronic condition of itching of the skin around the anus. Some causes are candidal infection, contact dermatitis, external hemorrhoids, pinworms, psoriasis, and psychogenic illness.

pruritus vulvae, itching of the external genitalia of a female. The condition may become chronic and result in lichenification, atrophy, and occasionally malignancy. Some causes of pruritus vulvae are contact dermatitis, lichen sclerosus et atrophicus, psychogenic pruritus, trichomoniasis, and vaginal candidiasis.

Prussian blue /prush'ən/ [Prussia, Germany; ME, *blew*], a chemical stain used on microscopic preparations. It demonstrates the presence of copper by developing a bright blue color.

ps, abbreviation for **picosecond.**

PSA, 1. abbreviation for **pressure-sensitive adhesive. 2.** abbreviation for **prostate-specific antigen.**

P sac, abbreviation for *pericardial cavity.*

psammoma /samō'mə/ [Gk, *psammos*, sand, *oma*, tumor], a neoplasm containing small calcified granules (psammoma bodies) that occurs in the meninges, choroid plexus, pineal body, and ovaries.

psammoma body, a round layered mass of calcareous material occurring in benign and malignant epithelial and connective tissue neoplasms and in some chronically inflamed tissue.

pseudarthritis /sŏŏ'därthrī'tis/ [Gk, *pseudes*, false, *arthron*, joint, *itis*, inflammation], musculoskeletal pain that does not involve the joints.

pseudesthesia /sŏŏ'desthē'zhə/ [Gk, *pseudes*, false, *aisthesis*, feeling], a sensation experienced without an external stimulus or a sensation that does not correspond to the causative stimulus, such as phantom limb pain occurring after an amputation.

pseudoacanthosis nigricans /sŏŏ'dō·ak'-ənthō'sis/, a condition of pigmented velvety thickening of the flexural skin, often with skin tags. It occurs most commonly in obese persons with dark complexions or in persons with endocrine disorders, and secondary to maceration of the skin from sweating.

pseudoallele /-əlēl'/ [Gk, *pseudes* + *allelon*, of one another], (in genetics) one of two or more closely linked genes on a chromosome that appear to function as a single member of an allelic pair but occupy distinct, nearly corresponding loci on homologous chromosomes. —**pseudoallelic,** *adj.,* **pseudoallelism,** *n.*

pseudoaneurysm /sŏŏ'dō·an'yəriz'əm/, **1.** a dilation of an artery caused by damage to one or more layers of the artery as a result of arterial trauma or rupture of a true aneurysm. **2.** a tortuosity of a blood vessel or cavity resulting from a herniated infarction.

pseudoankylosis /-ang'kilō'sis/ [Gk, *pseudes*, false, *ankylosis*, joint stiffness], fibrous ankylosis, or false ankylosis caused by inflexibility of body structures outside the joint.

pseudoanodontia /sŏŏ'dō·an'odon'shə/, an absence of teeth caused by an eruption failure.

pseudoanorexia /-an'ərek'sē·ə/ [Gk, *pseudes* + *a* + *orexis*, without appetite], a condition in which an individual eats se-

P

cretly while claiming a lack of appetite and inability to eat.

pseudoataxia /-ətak'sē·ə/ [Gk, *pseudes,* false, *ataxia,* without order], a loss of control over voluntary movements that does not involve an organic lesion.

pseudobulbar paralysis /-bul'bər/ [Gk, *pseudes,* false; L, *bulbus,* swollen root, *paralyein,* to be palsied], a condition resembling progressive bulbar paralysis, with dysarthria and dysphagia, but in which weakness of the bulbar muscles is of the upper motor neuron type. It may result from multiple bilateral infarcts of the cerebral cortex in some cases.

pseudocephalocele /-sef'əlōsēl'/, a noncongenital cerebral hernia resulting from a skull injury or disease.

pseudochancre /-shang'kər/, an indurated genital sore resembling a chancre.

pseudochondroplasia /sōō'dō·akon'drō-plā'zhə/, a hereditary condition resembling achondroplasia but developing after birth.

pseudochylous ascites /sōō'dōkī'ləs/ [Gk, *pseudes + chylos,* juice, *askos,* bag], the abnormal accumulation in the peritoneal cavity of a milky fluid that resembles chyle.

pseudoclaudication /-klô'dika'shən/, painful cramps that are not caused by peripheral artery disease but rather by spinal, neurologic, or orthopedic disorders, such as spinal stenosis, diabetic neuropathy, or arthritis.

pseudocyesis /sōō'dōsī·ē'sis/ [Gk, *pseudes + kyesis,* pregnancy], a condition in which a woman believes she is pregnant when she is not. The condition may be psychogenic in origin or caused by a tumor or endocrine dysfunction.

pseudocyst /sōō'dəsist/ [Gk, *pseudes + kystis,* bag], a space or cavity containing gas or liquid but without a lining membrane. Pseudocysts commonly occur after pancreatitis when digestive juices break through the normal ducts of the pancreas and collect in spaces lined by fibroblasts and surfaces of adjacent organs.

pseudodementia /-dimen'shə/, a syndrome that mimics dementia. It needs to be differentiated from depression.

pseudoephedrine hydrochloride /-ef'ədrēn/, an adrenergic that acts as a vasoconstrictor and bronchodilator. It is prescribed for the relief of nasal congestion and eustachian tube congestion.

pseudofracture /-frak'shər/ [Gk, *pseudes,* false; L, *fractura*], radiologic evidence of a thickened periosteum and new bone formation over what looks like an incomplete fracture.

pseudogene /sōō'dōjēn'/ [Gk, *pseudes + genein,* to produce], (in molecular genetics) a sequence of nucleotides that resembles a gene and may be derived from one but lacks a genetic function.

pseudogynecomastia /-gī'nəmas'tē·ə/, enlarged breasts in a male caused by fat accumulation.

pseudohermaphrodite /-hərmaf'redīt/ [Gk, *pseudes,* false, *Hermaphroditos,* son of Hermes and Aphrodite], a congenital condition in which a person has either male or female gonads but external genitalia of the opposite sex, or both.

pseudohermaphroditism /-hərmaf'rəditiz'əm/ [Gk, *pseudes + Hermaphroditos,* son of Hermes and Aphrodite], a condition in which a person exhibits the somatic characteristics of both sexes though possessing the physical characteristics of either males (testes) or females (ovaries).

pseudohyperkalemia /-hī'pərkəlē'mē·ə/, a laboratory artifact indicating an elevated blood potassium level caused by potassium released in vitro from cells in the blood sample.

pseudohyperparathyroidism /hī'pərper'-əthī'roidiz'əm/, signs of hypercalcemia in a cancer patient in the absence of primary hyperparathyroidism or skeletal metastases.

pseudohypertension /-hī'pərten'shən/, a blood pressure reading that erroneously appears elevated as a result of arterial compliance. The condition occurs most often in elderly patients.

pseudohypertrophy /-hīpur'trəfē/, abnormal enlargement of an organ or body structure caused by an overgrowth of fatty and fibrous tissues.

pseudohyponatremia /-hī'pōnātrē'mē·ə/, a decreased sodium concentration that does not correspond to a true hypotonic disorder. It may result instead from volume displacement by massive hyperlipidemia or hyperproteinemia.

pseudohypoparathyroidism /-hī'pōper'ə-thī'roidiz'əm/, a condition of end-organ resistance characterized by hypocalcemia, growth failure, and skeletal abnormalities such as short fingers.

pseudoileus /sōō'dō·il'ē·əs/ **1.** a condition resembling an intestinal obstruction caused by paralysis of a part of the bowel wall. **2.** an adynamic bowel obstruction.

pseudoisochromatic /sōō'dō·ī'sōkrōmat'-ik/, pertaining to visual test materials in which dots that differ in color appear similar to a person with color blindness.

pseudojaundice /-jôn'dis/ [Gk, *pseudes + Fr, jaune,* yellow], a yellow discoloration of the skin that is not caused by hyperbilirubinemia. The excessive ingestion of carotene results in a form of pseudojaundice.

pseudolymphoma /-limfō'mə/, a benign disorder of lymphoid cells or histiocytes that produces clinical features of a malignant lymphoma.

pseudolysogeny /-līsoj'ənē/, a condition in which a bacteriophage is carried in a culture of a bacterial strain by infecting susceptible variants of the strain.

pseudomamma /-mam'ə/, a glandular structure resembling a nipple or mammary gland, sometimes found in a dermoid ovarian cyst.

pseudomania /-mā'nē·ə/, **1.** a condition in which a person may claim to have committed crimes of which he or she is really innocent. **2.** a deliberately pretended condition of mental illness.

pseudomegacolon /-meg'əkō'lon/, a dilation of the colon in an adult patient.

pseudomembrane /-mem'brān/ [Gk, pseudes, false; L, membrana], a membrane consisting of coagulated fibrin, bacteria, and leukocytes that forms in the throats of diphtheria patients.

pseudomembranous colitis /-mem'brənəs/ [Gk, pseudes + L, membrana, thin skin], a diarrheal disease frequently found in hospitalized patients who have received antibiotics that caused overgrowth of the anaerobic spore-forming toxin producing *Clostridium difficile*. Patients have profuse watery diarrhea, fever, and cramping and are found to have exudates of the colon on endoscopy.

pseudomembranous stomatitis, a severe inflammation of the mouth that produces a membranelike exudate. The inflammation may be caused by various bacteria or by chemical irritants. It may produce dysphagia, pain, fever, and swelling of the lymph glands.

pseudomenstruation /-men'strōo·ā'shən/, bleeding from the uterus that resembles menstruation but is not associated with the usual changes in endometrial tissues.

pseudomnesia /sōo'domnē'zhə/, a memory aberration in which a client claims to remember events that actually have not taken place.

pseudomonad /sōo'dōmō'nad, sōodom'-ənad/, a bacterium of the genus *Pseudomonas*.

Pseudomonas /sōodom'ənas/ [Gk, pseudes + monas, unit], a genus of gram-negative bacteria that includes several free-living species in soil and water and some opportunistic pathogens. Pseudomonads are notable for their fluorescent pigments and their resistance to disinfectants and antibiotics.

Pseudomonas aeruginosa [Gk, pseudes, false, monas, unity], a species of gram-negative nonspore-forming motile bacteria that may cause various human diseases ranging from purulent meningitis to nosocomial infected wounds.

pseudomutuality /-mōo'tyōo·al'itē/ [Gk, pseudes + L, mutuus, reciprocal], (in psychotherapy) an atmosphere maintained by family members in which there is surface harmony and a high degree of agreement with one another, but deep and destructive intrapsychic and interpersonal conflicts are hidden.

pseudomyopia /-mī·ō'pē·ə/, a condition in which a person holds objects close to the eyes to see them, although he or she does not have myopia.

pseudomyxoma /-miksō'mə/, a mucus-rich tumor.

pseudopapilledema /-pap'ilēdē'mə/, a congenitally swollen optic disc that resembles papilledema.

pseudoparalysis /-pəral'isis/, a condition in which a person appears to be unable to move the arms or legs but there is no "true" paralysis. In infants the condition may be caused by pain in joints resulting from a disease such as rickets or scurvy.

pseudopelade /-pelād', -pē'lad/, a scarring type of alopecia, preceded by folliculitis, in which one or more areas of baldness may appear and spread to become joined, forming an area of smooth fingerlike projections that are slightly depressed in the skin.

pseudophakia /-fā'kē·ə/, a failure of development of an eye in which the natural crystalline lens has been replaced by mesodermal tissue.

pseudophakodonesis /-fā'kōdənē'sis/, excessive movement by an intraocular lens implant.

Pseudophyllidea /-filid'ē·ə/, an order of tapeworms with an aquatic life cycle. The scolex usually has two opposing sucking organs.

pseudopod /sōo'dəpod/ [Gk, pseudes, false, pous, foot], a temporary protoplasmic limblike process of an amoeba that can be extended to propel itself or to engulf food.

pseudopolyp /-pol'ip/, a projecting mass of granulation tissue that may develop in ulcerative colitis and become covered by regenerating epithelium.

pseudoprognathism /-prog'nəthiz'əm/, a condition in which the mandible is forced forward of its normal position by an occlusal disorder.

P

pseudopsychosis /-sīkō'sis/, a condition such as malingering that may resemble a true mental and behavioral disorder.

pseudoptosis /soo'doptō'sis/, an abnormally small palpebral fissure.

pseudopterygium /soo'dopterij'ē·əm/, a fold of conjunctiva that has become attached to the cornea after an injury or disease.

pseudopuberty /-p(y)oo'pərtē/, the appearance of somatic and functional changes in an individual before the chronologic age of puberty.

pseudoretinitis pigmentosa /-ret'inī'tis/, a pigmentary mottling of the retina that may follow an eye injury.

pseudosarcoma /-särkō'mə/, a spindle cell epithelioma on skin that has been exposed to irradiation.

pseudostrabismus /-strəbiz'məs/, an appearance of strabismus caused by a fold of skin of the lower eyelid, which narrows the visible width of the sclera medial to the iris.

pseudostratified /-stra'tifīd/ [Gk, *pseudes,* false, *stratum,* cover], pertaining to a type of columnar epithelium in which the nuclei of adjacent cells are at different levels.

pseudotabes /-tā'bēz/, any neuropathy with symptoms like those of tabes dorsalis.

pseudotruncus arteriosus /-trung'kəs/, a condition in which blood is carried to the pulmonary arteries by collateral vessels.

pseudotubercle /-t(y)oo'bərkəl/, a nodule that resembles a tuberculosis granule but is caused by a microorganism other than *Mycobacterium tuberculosis.*

pseudotuberculosis /-t(y)oobur'kyəlō'sis/, a pulmonary condition with symptoms resembling those of tuberculosis but not caused by *Mycobacterium tuberculosis.*

pseudotumor /-t(y)oo'mər/ [Gk, *pseudes* + L, *tumor,* swelling], a false tumor.

pseudotumor cerebri, a condition characterized by increased intracranial pressure, headache, blurring of the optic disc margins, vomiting, and papilledema without neurologic signs, except palsy of the sixth cranial nerve.

pseudovitamin /-vī'təmin/, a substance that has a chemical structure similar to that of a vitamin but lacks the physiologic effects.

psi /sī/, Ψ, ψ, the twenty-third letter of the Greek alphabet.

p.s.i., abbreviation for *pounds per square inch.*

psia, abbreviation for *pounds per square inch, absolute.*

psig, abbreviation for *pounds per square inch, gauge.*

psilocin /sī'ləsin/, one of several indole-derived psychomimetic drugs. It is related chemically to psilocybin.

psilocybin /sī'lōsī'bin,-sib'in/, a psychedelic drug and an active ingredient of various Mexican hallucinogenic mushrooms of the genus *Psilocybe mexicana.* It can produce altered states of mood and consciousness and has no acceptable medical use in the United States. Psilocybin is controlled under Schedule I of the Controlled Substances Act of 1970, which bans the prescription of psilocybin.

psittacosis /sit'əkō'sis/ [Gk, *psittakos,* parrot], an infectious illness caused by the bacterium *Chlamydia psittaci.* It is characterized by respiratory pneumonia-like symptoms and transmitted to humans by infected birds, especially parrots. The clinical manifestations of the disease are extremely variable and resemble those of a great number of infectious diseases, but fever, cough, anorexia, and severe headache are almost always present.

psm, abbreviation for **presystolic murmur.**

psoas major /sō'əs/ [Gk, *psoa,* loin], a long muscle originating from the transverse processes of the lumbar vertebrae and the fibrocartilages and sides of the vertebral bodies of the lower thoracic vertebrae and the lumbar vertebrae. It acts to flex and rotate the thigh and to flex and laterally bend the spine laterally.

psoas minor, a long, slender muscle of the pelvis, ventral to the psoas major. The psoas minor functions to flex the spine.

psomophagia /sō'mōfā'jē·ə/, the swallowing of food that has not been chewed properly.

psoralen-type photosensitizer /sôr'ələn/, any one chemical compound that contains photosensitizing psoralen and that reacts on exposure to ultraviolet light to increase the melanin in the skin. Some psoralen-type photosensitizers produced as pharmaceutics are methoxsalen and trioxsalen; both are used to enhance skin pigmentation or tanning in the treatment of skin diseases such as psoriasis and vitiligo.

psorelcosis /sôr'əlkō'sis/, an ulceration of the skin caused by scabies.

psorenteritis /sôr'enterī'tis/, an inflammation of the intestines.

psoriasis /sərī'əsis/ [Gk, itch], a common chronic skin disorder characterized by circumscribed red patches covered by thick, dry silvery adherent scales that are the result of excessive development of epithelial cells. Exacerbations and remissions are typical. Lesions may be anywhere on the body but are more common on extensor surfaces, bony prominences, scalp, ears, genitalia, and the perianal area. An arthritis, particularly of distal small joints, may accompany the skin disease. —**psoriatic** /sôr'ē·at'ik/, *adj.*

psoriasis universalis [Gk, *psoriasis,* itch; L, *universus,* on the whole], a severe attack of psoriasis in which most or all of the skin is involved.

psoriatic arthritis /sôr'ī·at'ik/, a form of arthritis associated with psoriatic lesions of the skin and nails, particularly at the distal interphalangeal joints of the fingers and toes.

PSRO, abbreviation for **Professional Standards Review Organization.**

PSS, abbreviation for **progressive systemic sclerosis.**

PSSO, abbreviation for *peer specialist second opinion.*

PSV, abbreviation for **pressure support ventilation.**

PSW, abbreviation for **psychiatric social worker.**

psych, abbreviation for **psychology.**

psyche /sī'kē/ [Gk, mind], **1.** the aspect of one's mental faculty that encompasses the conscious and unconscious processes. **2.** the vital mental or spiritual entity of the individual as opposed to the body or soma. **3.** (in psychoanalysis) the total components of the id, ego, and superego, including all conscious and unconscious aspects.

psychedelic /sī'kədel'ik/ [coined in 1956 by Humphry Osmond from Gk, *psyche* + *deloun,* to reveal], **1.** describing a mental state characterized by altered sensory perception and hallucination, accompanied by euphoria or fear, usually caused by the deliberate ingestion of drugs or other substances known to produce this effect. **2.** describing any drug or substance that causes this state, such as mescaline or psilocybin.

psychiatric /sī'kē·at'rik/ [Gk, *psyche,* mind, *iatreia,* treatment], pertaining to psychiatry.

psychiatric consultation liaison nurse (PCLN), an advanced practice nurse with a master's degree in psychiatric/ mental health nursing. The practice focuses on emotional, spiritual, developmental, cognitive, and behavioral responses of patients with actual or potential physical dysfunction.

psychiatric emergency service [Gk, *psyche* + *iatreia,* treatment], a hospital service that provides immediate initial evaluation and treatment to acutely disturbed mental patients on a 24-hour-a-day basis.

psychiatric foster care, a service for discharged psychiatric patients who receive observation and care in an approved foster home.

psychiatric home care, a service whereby a discharged psychiatric patient is provided observation and care in his or her place of residence.

psychiatric hospital, a health care facility providing inpatient and outpatient therapeutic services to clients with behavioral or emotional illnesses.

psychiatric inpatient unit, a hospital ward or similar area used for the treatment of inpatients who require psychiatric care.

psychiatric nurse practitioner, a nurse practitioner who, by advanced study and clinical practice, such as in a master's program in psychiatric nursing, has gained expert knowledge in the care and prevention of mental disorders.

psychiatric nursing, the branch of nursing concerned with the prevention and cure of mental disorders and their sequelae. Psychiatric nurses work in many settings; their responsibilities vary with the setting and with the level of expertise, experience, and training of the individual nurse.

psychiatric social worker (PSW), a social worker who specializes in or works exclusively with the mentally ill.

psychiatrist /sīkī'ətrist/ [Gk, *psyche,* mind, *iatreia,* treatment], a physician with additional medically qualified training and experience in the diagnosis, prevention, and treatment of mental disorders.

psychiatry /sīkī'ətrē/ [Gk, *psyche* + *iatreia,* treatment], the branch of medical science that deals with the causes, treatment, and prevention of mental, emotional, and behavioral disorders. —**psychiatric,** *adj.*

psychic /sī'kik/ [Gk, *psyche,* mind], a practitioner of the systematic study of parapsychology, a category of usually alleged psychologic phenomena that cannot be explained by scientific thinking.

psychic blindness [Gk, *psyche,* mind; AS, *blind*], a somatoform disorder that is manifested by the total or partial loss of vision in eyes that are organically normal. Despite the symptoms claimed, the patient usually reacts to light and avoids objects that might cause injury.

psychic energy, body energy such as thinking, perceiving, and remembering.

psychic impotence [Gk, *psyche,* mind; L, *in* + *potentia,* power], a functional disorder of the male who is unable to perform sexual intercourse despite normal genitalia and sexual desire. The term generally applies to an inability to achieve and maintain an erection, but the disorder may be manifested in other forms such as prema-

P

ture ejaculation or the need for certain conditions.

psychic infection, [Gk, *psyche* + L, *inficere,* to stain], the spread of psychic effects or influences on others on a small scale, as in folie á deux, or on a large scale, as in the spread of hysteric or panic reactions in a crowd.

psychic pain [Gk, *psyche,* mind; L, *poena,* penalty], a functional pain that, in the absence of any organic cause, is usually associated with feelings of acute anxiety. In some cases, the person may experience hallucinations or obsessions.

psychic suicide, the termination of one's own life without the use of physical means or agents, such as by an older person who becomes sufficiently depressed to lose "the will to live."

psychic trauma, an emotional shock or injury or a distressful situation that produces a lasting impression, especially on the subconscious mind. Some causes of psychic trauma may include abuse or neglect in childhood, rape, and loss of a loved one.

psychoacoustics /sīkō·ək ōōs'tiks/, the branch of science concerned with the physical features of sound as it relates to the psychologic and physiologic aspects of the sense of hearing.

psychoactive /sīkō·ak'tiv/ [Gk, *psyche,* mind; L, *activus*], pertaining to a drug or other agent that affects such normal mental functioning as mood, behavior, or thinking processes. Examples include stimulants, sedatives, or hallucinogens.

psychoanalysis /sīkō·ənal'isis/ [Gk, *psyche* + *analyein,* to separate parts], a branch of psychiatry founded by Sigmund Freud, devoted to the study of the psychology of human development and behavior. From its systematized method for investigating the processes of the mind evolved a system of psychotherapy based on the concepts of a dynamic unconscious. Using such techniques as free association, dream interpretation, and analysis of defense mechanisms, emotions and behavior are traced to the influence of repressed instinctual drives in the unconscious.

psychoanalyst /sīkō·an'əlist/, a psychotherapist, usually a psychiatrist, who has had special training in psychoanalysis and who applies the techniques of psychoanalytic theory.

psychoanalytic /sīkō·an'əlit'ik/, **1.** pertaining to psychoanalysis. **2.** using the techniques or principles of psychoanalysis.

psychobiologic resilience /-bī·əloj'ik/, a concept that proposes a recurrent human need to weather periods of stress and change successfully throughout life. The ability to weather each period of disruption and reintegration leaves the person better able to deal with the next change.

psychobiology /-bī'ol'əjē/ [Gk, *psyche* + *bios,* life, *logos,* science], **1.** the study of biochemical foundations of thought, mood, emotion, affect, and behavior. **2.** personality development and functioning in terms of the interaction of the body and the mind. **3.** a school of psychiatric thought that stresses total life experience, including biologic, emotional, and sociocultural factors, in assessing the psychologic makeup or mental status of an individual.

psychodiagnosis /-dī'agnō'sis/ [Gk, *psyche,* mind, *dia* + *gnosis,* knowledge], the study of a personality through observations of behavior and mannerisms, combined with various tests.

psychodrama /-dram'ə/, a form of group psychotherapy, originated by J. L. Moreno, in which people act out their emotional problems through improvisational dramatizations.

psychodynamics /-dīnam'iks/ [Gk, *psyche* + *dynamis,* power], the study of the forces that motivate behavior.

psychoendocrinology /sī'kō·en'dōkrinol'-əjē/, the study of the relationship between endocrinology and psychology.

psychoesthesia, a sensation of cold perceived although the body is warm.

psychogalvanic /-galvan'ik/, pertaining to the effects of psychologic influences on the electrical properties of skin.

psychogender /-jen'dər/, the psychologic sex as expressed in gender attitudes of a person as distinguished from biologic or somatic sex.

psychogenesis /sī'kōjen'əsis/ [Gk, *psyche* + *genesis,* origin], **1.** the development of the mind or of a mental function or process. **2.** the development or production of a physical symptom or disease having a mental or psychic origin rather than an organic cause. **3.** the development of emotional states, either normal or abnormal, from the interaction of conscious and unconscious psychologic forces.

psychogenic /sī'kōjen'ik/ [Gk, *psyche* + *genein,* to produce], **1.** originating within the mind. **2.** referring to any physical symptom, disease process, or emotional state that is of psychologic rather than physical origin.

psychogenic pain [Gk, *psyche,* mind; L, *poena,* penalty], a functional pain that does not have any known organic cause.

psychogenic pain disorder, a *DSM-IV* psychiatric disorder characterized by persistent pain for which there is no apparent organic cause. The condition is often accompanied by other sensory or motor dysfunction, such as paresthesia or muscle spasm.

psychogenic vomiting, vomiting that is stimulated by anxiety and emotional distress.

psychogeusic /-jōō'sik/, pertaining to the psychologic influences in taste.

psychokinesia /sī'kōkinē'zhə, -kīnē'zhə/ [Gk, *psyche* + *kinesis,* motion], **1.** impulsive behavior resulting from deficient or defective inhibitions without benefit of processing between the stimulus and the response. **2.** (in parapsychology) psychokinesis.

psychokinesis (PK) /sī'kōkinē'sis, -kīnē'-sis/ [Gk, *psyche* + *kinesis,* motion], the alleged direct influence of the mind or will on matter to produce motion in objects without the intervention of the physical senses or a physical force.

psychokinetics /sī'kōkinet'iks, -kīnet'iks/, the study of psychokinesis.

psycholinguistics /-ling·gwis'tiks/, the study of language as a form of behavior, including language development, speech, and personality.

psychologic /sī'kōloj'ik/ [Gk, *psyche,* mind, *logos,* science], pertaining to or involving psychology.

psychologic miscarriage, an absence or deficiency of a mother's love for her infant or absence of mother-child bonding.

psychologic test [Gk, *psyche* + *logos,* science; L, *testum,* crucible], any of a group of standardized tests designed to measure or ascertain such characteristics of an individual as intellectual capacity, motivation, perception, role behavior, values, level of anxiety or depression, coping mechanisms, and general personality integration.

psychologist /sīkol'əjist/, a person who specializes in the study of the structure and function of the brain and related mental processes of animals and humans. A clinical psychologist is one who is qualified by graduate study in psychology and training in clinical psychology and who provides testing and counseling services to patients with mental and emotional disorders.

psychology (psych) /sīkol'əjē/ [Gk, *psyche* + *logos,* science], **1.** the study of behavior and of the functions and processes of the mind, especially as related to the social and physical environment. **2.** a profession that involves the practical applications of knowledge, skills, and techniques in the understanding of, prevention of, or solution to individual or social problems, especially in regard to the interaction between the individual and the physical and social environment. **3.** the mental, motivational, and behavioral characteristics and attitudes of an individual or group of individuals. —**psychologic, psychological,** *adj.,* **psychologically,** *adv.*

psychometrician /-mətrish'ən/ [Gk, *psyche,* mind, *metron,* measure], a specialist who performs quantitative estimation or measurement of personality and intelligence.

psychometrics /sī'kōmet'riks/ [Gk, *psyche* + *metron,* measure], the development, administration, or interpretation of psychologic and intelligence tests.

psychomotor /-mō'tər/ [Gk, *psyche* + L, *motare,* to move about], pertaining to or causing voluntary movements usually associated with neural activity.

psychomotor and physical development of infants, a branch of pediatric psychiatry that is concerned with the development of skills requiring coordination of sensory processes and motor activities, including infant reflexes, developmental timetables, and emotional and behavioral disorders.

psychomotor development, the progressive attainment by the child of skills that involve both mental and muscular activity, such as the ability of the infant to turn over, sit, or crawl at will and of the toddler to walk, talk, control bladder and bowel functions, and begin solving cognitive problems. The mean chronologic ages at which certain psychomotor skills are attained by most children follow.

12 weeks	Looks at own hand.
20 weeks	Able to grasp objects voluntarily.
24 weeks	Able to roll from back to front at will.
11 months	Creeps with abdomen off the floor and imitates speech sounds.
15 months	Able to walk without help.
24 months	Has a vocabulary of 300 or more words and uses pronouns.
30 months	Able to jump with both feet.
3 years	Able to ride a tricycle and to feed self well.
4 years	Able to hop and skip on one foot, catch and throw a ball; is independent, boasts, tattles, and shows off.
5 years	Able to tie shoelaces and cut with scissors, tries to please, interested in facts about world, gets along more easily with parents.

psychomotor domain, the area of observable performance of skills that require some degree of neuromuscular coordination.

psychomotor learning, the acquisition of ability to perform motor skills.

psychomotor retardation, a generalized slowing of motor activity related to a state of severe depression.

psychomotor seizure, a temporary impairment of consciousness, characterized by psychic symptoms, loss of judgment, automatic behavior, and abnormal acts. It is often associated with temporal lobe disease. No apparent convulsions occur, but there may be loss of consciousness or amnesia for the episode. During the seizure the individual may appear drowsy, intoxicated, or violent; asocial acts or crimes may be committed, but normal activities such as driving a car, typing, or eating may continue at an automatic level.

psychoneuroimmunology /-nŏŏr′ŏ-imyōōnol′əjē/, a discipline that studies the relationships between psychologic states and the immune response.

psychooncology /sīkō-ongkol′əjē/, the psychologic effects of cancer, particularly the psychosocial needs of the patient and the patient's family.

psychopath /sī′kōpath/ [Gk, *psyche* + *pathos,* disease], a person who has an antisocial personality disorder. —**psychopathic** /sī′kōpath′ik/, adj.

psychopathia sexualis /sī′kōpā′thē-ə sek′-shōō-al′is/ [Gk, *psyche* + *pathos,* disease; L, *sexus,* male or female], a mental disease characterized by sexual perversion.

psychopathologist /-pathol′əjist/, one who specializes in the study and treatment of mental disorders.

psychopathology /-pathol′əjē/, **1.** the study of the causes, processes, and manifestations of mental disorders. **2.** the behavioral manifestation of any mental disorder.

psychopathy /sīkop′əthē/, any disease of the mind, congenital or acquired, not necessarily associated with subnormal intelligence.

psychopharmaceutical /-fär′məsōō′tikəls/ a drug used in the treatment of mental health disorders.

psychopharmacology /-fär′məkol′əjē/ [Gk, *psyche* + *pharmakon,* drug, *logos,* science], the scientific study of the effects of psychoactive drugs on behavior and normal and abnormal mental functions.

psychophysical /-fiz′ikəl/, pertaining to the psychosocial and physical aspects of a client's health and illness.

psychophysical preparation for childbirth, a program that prepares women for giving birth by teaching them the physiologic characteristics of the process, exercises to improve muscle tone and physical stamina, and various techniques of breathing and relaxation to promote control and comfort during labor and delivery. Methods of psychophysical preparation for childbirth include the **Bradley method, Lamaze method, Leboyer method,** and **Read method.**

psychophysics /-fiz′iks/ [Gk, *psyche* + *physikos,* natural], the branch of psychology concerned with the relationships between physical stimuli and sensory responses.

psychophysiologic /-fiz′ē-əloj′ik/ [Gk, *psyche* + *physikos,* natural], having physical symptoms, usually under the control of the autonomic nervous system, having emotional origins, and involving a single organ system; psychosomatic.

psychophysiologic disorder, any of a large group of mental disorders that is characterized by the dysfunction of an organ or organ system controlled by the autonomic nervous system and that may be caused or aggravated by emotional factors.

psychophysiology /-fiz′ē-ol′əjē/, **1.** the study of physiology as it relates to various aspects of psychologic or behavioral function. **2.** the study of mental activity by physical examination and observation.

psychoprophylactic preparation for childbirth /-prō′-filak′tik/, a system of prenatal education for giving birth using the Lamaze method of natural childbirth.

psychoprophylaxis /-prō′filak′sis/, a type of psychotherapy that is directed to prevention of emotional disorders. For example, it is used in the preparation for childbirth to reduce a woman's anxiety about pain and birth of a normal child.

psychorelaxation /-ri′laksā′shən/, the systematic desensitization of stress and anxiety by the practice of general body relaxation.

psychosensory /-sen′sərē/, pertaining to the perception and interpretation of sensory stimuli.

psychosexual /-sek′shōō-əl/ [Gk, *psyche* + L, *sexus,* male or female], pertaining to the psychologic and emotional aspects of sex. —**psychosexuality,** *n.*

psychosexual development, (in psychoanalysis) the emergence of the personality through a series of stages from infancy to adulthood. Each stage is relatively fixed in time and characterized by a dominant mode of achieving libidinal pleasure through the interaction of the person's biologic drives and the environmental restraints.

psychosexual disorder, any condition characterized by abnormal sexual attitudes, desires, or activities resulting from psychologic rather than organic causes.

psychosexual dysfunction, any of a large group of sexual maladjustments or disorders caused by an emotional or psychologic problem.

psychosis /sīkō′sis/, *pl.* **psychoses** [Gk, *psyche + osis,* condition], any major mental disorder of organic or emotional origin characterized by a gross impairment in reality testing; the individual incorrectly evaluates the accuracy of his or her perceptions and thoughts and makes incorrect references about external reality, even in the face of contrary evidence. It is often characterized by regressive behavior, inappropriate mood and affect, and diminished impulse control.

psychosocial /-sō′shəl/, [Gr, *psyche + L, socialis,* partners], pertaining to a combination of psychologic and social factors.

psychosocial assessment, an evaluation of a person's mental health, social status, and functional capacity within the community.

psychosocial development, (in child development) a description devised by Erik Erikson of the normal serial development of trust, autonomy, initiative, industry, identity, intimacy, generativity, and integrity; the development begins in infancy and progresses as the infantile ego interacts with the environment. For the child to reach a new stage successfully, the tasks of the preceding one should be fully mastered.

psychosomatic /sī′kōsəmat′ik/ [Gk, *psyche + soma,* body], **1.** pertaining to psychosomatic medicine. **2.** relating to, characterized by, or resulting from the interaction of the mind or psyche and the body. **3.** the expression of an emotional conflict through physical symptoms.

psychosomatic approach, the interdisciplinary or holistic study of physical and mental disease from a biologic, psychosocial, and sociocultural point of view.

psychosomatic medicine, the branch of medicine concerned with the interrelationships between mental and emotional reactions and somatic processes, in particular the manner in which intrapsychic conflicts influence physical symptoms.

psychosomatic pain [Gk, *psyche,* mind, *soma,* body; L, *poena,* penalty], pain that is caused in part by psychologic factors.

psychosomatogenic /-sōmat′əjen′ik/, pertaining to factors that cause or lead to the development of psychophysiologic coping measures as learned responses to stressors.

psychostimulant /-stim′yələnt/, an agent with mood-elevating or antidepressant effects.

psychosurgery /-sur′jərē/ [Gk, *psyche + cheirourgia*], surgical interruption of certain nerve pathways in the brain, performed to treat selected cases of chronic unremitting anxiety, agitation, or obsessional neuroses. Psychosurgery is performed when the condition is severe and when alternative treatments such as psychotherapy, drugs, and electroshock have proved ineffective.

psychosynthesis /-sin′thəsis/, a form of psychotherapy that focuses on three levels of the unconscious—lower, middle, and higher unconscious, or superconscious. The goal of the treatment is the re-creation or integration of the personality.

psychotaxia, a condition of mental confusion and inability to concentrate or fix attention.

psychotherapeutic drugs /-ther′əp(y)ōō′-tik/ [Gk, *psyche,* mind, *therapeutike,* medical practice; Fr, *drogue*], drugs that are prescribed for their effects in relieving symptoms of anxiety, depression, or other mental disorders.

psychotherapeutics /-tiks/ [Gk, *psyche + therapeia,* treatment], the treatment of personality disorders by means of psychotherapy.

psychotherapist /-ther′əpist/, one who practices psychotherapy, including psychiatrists, licensed psychologists, psychiatric nurses, psychiatric social workers, and individuals trained in counseling.

psychotherapy /-ther′əpē/ [Gk, *psyche + therapeia,* treatment], any of a large number of related methods of treating mental and emotional disorders by psychologic techniques rather than by physical means.

psychotic /sīkot′ik/ [Gk, *psyche + osis,* condition], **1.** pertaining to psychosis. **2.** a person exhibiting the characteristics of a psychosis.

psychotic insight, a stage in the development of a psychosis that follows an initial experience of confusion, bizarreness, and apprehension. At this point, an insight is reached that enables the patient to interpret the external world in terms of a delusional system of thinking. The factors that had previously been confusing become a part of the systematized pattern of the delusion, which, although irrational to an observer, is perceived by the patient as the attainment of exceptionally lucid thinking.

psychotogenic /sīkot′əjen′ik/, pertaining to an agent that is capable of inducing symptoms of psychosis.

psychotomimetic /sīkot′ōmimet′ik/, a drug or other substance whose effects mimic the symptoms of psychosis, such as hallucinations.

psychotropic /-trop′ik/ [Gk, *psyche* + *trepein,* to turn], exerting an effect on the mind or modifying mental activity, as in psychotropic medications.

psychotropic drugs, drugs that affect the psychic functions, behavior, or experience of a person using them.

psychrometer /sīkrom′ətər/, an instrument for calculating the degree of humidity in the atmosphere by comparing the temperatures of two thermometers. The bulb of one thermometer is wet; that of the other is dry. The difference in temperatures between the two thermometers indicates the dryness of the atmosphere. No difference indicates 100% humidity.

psychrometry /sīkrom′ətrē/, the calculation of relative humidity and water vapor pressure from psychrometer data and barometric pressure.

psychrophore /sī′krəfôr′/, a double-lumen catheter through which cold water is circulated.

pt., 1. abbreviation for *pint.* **2.** abbreviation for **patient.**

Pt, symbol for the element **platinum.**

PT, 1. abbreviation for **physical therapist 2.** abbreviation for **physical therapy. 3.** abbreviation for **prothrombin time.**

PTA, 1. abbreviation for **percutaneous transluminal angioplasty. 2.** abbreviation for *plasma thromboplastin antecedent.*

PTB, abbreviation for **patellar-tendon bearing prosthesis.**

PTB/SC, abbreviation for **patellar-tendon bearing supracondylar socket.**

PTCA, abbreviation for **percutaneous transluminal coronary angioplasty.**

pterion /tir′ē-on/, a point near the sphenoid fontanel of the skull, at the junction of the greater wing of the sphenoid, squamous, temporal, frontal, and parietal bones. It also intersects the course of the anterior division of the middle meningeal artery.

pterygium /tərij′ē-əm/ [Gk, *pterygion,* wing], a thick triangular piece of pale tissue that extends medially from the nasal border of the cornea to the inner canthus of the eye.

pterygoid /ter′igoid/ [Gk, *pteryx,* wing, *eidos,* form], pertaining to a winglike structure.

pterygoid plexus, one of a pair of extensive networks of veins between the temporalis and the pterygoideus lateralis muscles, extending between surrounding structures in the infratemporal fossa.

pterygoid process [Gk, *pteryx,* wing, *eidos,* form; L, *processus*], any one of the paired processes of the sphenoid bone.

pterygomandibular /ter′igōmandib′yələr/ [Gk, *pteryx,* wing, *eidos,* form; L, *mandere,* to chew], pertaining to the pterygoid process and the mandible.

pterygomaxillary /-mak′silerē/ [Gk, *pteryx,* wing, *eidos,* form; L, *maxilla,* jaw], pertaining to the sphenoid bone and the maxilla.

pterygomaxillary notch, a fissure at the junction of the maxilla and the pterygoid process of the sphenoid bone.

PTH, abbreviation for **parathyroid hormone.**

PTNA, abbreviation for **Provincial/ Territorial Nurses Association.**

ptomaine /tō′mān/ [Gk, *ptoma,* corpse], an imprecise term introduced in the nineteenth century to identify a group of nitrogenous substances found in putrefied proteins.

ptomainemia /tō′mānē′mē-ə/, a condition caused by the presence of a ptomaine, a potentially toxic amine, in the blood.

ptosis /tō′sis/ [Gk, falling], an abnormal condition of one or both upper eyelids in which the eyelid droops because of a congenital or acquired weakness of the levator muscle or paralysis of the third cranial nerve.

ptotic kidney /tot′ik/, a kidney that is abnormally situated in the pelvis, usually over the sacral promontory behind the peritoneum.

ptyalin /tī′əlin/ [Gk, *ptyalon,* spittle], a starch-digesting enzyme present in saliva. It hydrolyzes starch and glycogen.

ptyalism /tī′əliz′əm/ [Gk, *ptyalon,* spittle], excessive salivation, such as sometimes occurs in the early months of pregnancy. It is also a clinical sign of mercury poisoning.

ptyocrinous /tī-ok′rinəs/, the secretion of the contents of a unicellular gland in the form of extruded granules.

Pu, symbol for the element **plutonium.**

pubarche /pyoobär′kē, pyoo′bärkē/ [L, *puber,* maturity, *arch,* beginning], onset of puberty. It is marked by the beginning of the development of secondary sexual characteristics.

pubertal /p(y)oo′bərtəl/ [L, *pubertas,* age of maturity], pertaining to puberty.

puberty /p(y)oo′bərtē/ [L, *pubertas,* age of maturity], the period of life at which the ability to reproduce begins. It is a stage of development when genitalia reach maturity and secondary sex characteristics appear. The onset normally occurs in females between 9 and 13 years of age with the development of breasts and during the phase of menarche. In males puberty usually occurs between 12 and 14 years of age and is characterized by the ejaculation of sperm.

puberulic acid /pyo͞ober′yo͞olik/, an antibiotic isolated from the mold *Penicillium puberulum* that prevents the replication of gram-positive bacteria.

pubescent /p(y)o͞obes′ənt/ [L, *pubescere,* to reach puberty], pertaining to the beginning of puberty.

pubescent uterus [L, *pubescere,* to reach puberty, *uterus,* womb], a uterus in which the cervix and body remain of equal length, the premenstruation state, in adult life.

pubic /p(y)o͞o′bik/ [L, *pubis*], pertaining to or involving the region of the pubic symphysis.

pubic hair /p(y)o͞o′bik/ [L, *pubis* + AS, *haer*], hair of the pubic region.

pubic region [L, *pubes,* signs of maturity, *regio,* territory], the most inferior part of the abdomen in the lower zone between the right and left inguinal regions and below the umbilical region.

pubic symphysis, the slightly movable interpubic joint of the pelvis, consisting of two pubic bones separated by a disk of fibrocartilage and connected by two ligaments.

pubiotomy /p(y)o͞o′bi·ot′əmē/, the separation of the pubic bone, performed to increase the capacity of the pelvis to permit passage of a fetus.

pubis /pyo͞o′bis/, *pl.* **pubes** [L, *pubes*], one of a pair of pubic bones that, with the ischium and the ilium, form the hip bone and join the pubic bone from the opposite side at the pubic symphysis. The pubis forms one fifth of the acetabulum and is divisible into the body, the superior ramus, and the inferior ramus.

public health [L, *publicus,* of the people; AS, *haelth*], a field of medicine that deals with the physical and mental health of the community, particularly in such areas as water supply, waste disposal, air pollution, and food safety.

public health nursing, a field of nursing that is concerned with the health needs of the community as a whole. Public health nurses may work with families in the home, in schools, at the workplace, in government agencies, and at major health facilities. A home care nursing service is provided by nurses who have special training in public health and are employed by such voluntary agencies as the Visiting

Nurses Association, the Visiting Nurse Service, or the Victorian Order of Nurses for Canada.

public sector, (in health care) typically, government at the federal, state, provincial, and local levels; may refer to other community organizations and lobbying groups.

publish or perish [L, *publicare,* to make public, *perire,* to come to naught], *informal.* a practice followed in many academic institutions in which a contract for employment is renewed at the same rank only if a candidate has demonstrated scholarship and professional status by having had work published in a book or in a reputable refereed professional or scientific journal.

pubocapsular /p(y)o͞o′bōkap′sələr/, pertaining to the pubis and articular capsule of the hip joint.

pubococcygeal /p(y)o͞o′bōkoksïjē·əl/ [L, *pubis* + Gk, *kokkyx,* cuckoo's beak], pertaining to the pubis and the coccyx.

pubococcygeus exercises /pyo͞o′bōkoksij′-ē·əs/ [L, *pubes* + Gk, *kokkyx,* cuckoo's beak; L, *exercere,* to make strong], a regimen of isometric exercises in which a woman executes a series of voluntary contractions of the muscles of her pelvic diaphragm and perineum in an effort to increase the contractility of her vaginal introitus or to improve retention of urine. The exercise involves the familiar muscular squeezing action that is required to stop the urinary stream while voiding; that action is performed in an intensive, repetitive, and systematic way throughout each day.

puboprostatic /p(y)o͞o′bōprostat′ik/, pertaining to the pubis and prostate gland.

pudendal block /p(y)o͞oden′təl/ [L, *pudendus,* shameful; Fr, *bloc,* lump], a form of regional anesthetic block administered to provide anesthesia of the perineum, which is particularly useful during the expulsive second stage of labor. Pudendal block anesthetizes the perineum, vulva, clitoris, labia majora, and perirectal area without affecting the muscular contractions of the uterus. When the block is properly administered, the risk is minimal.

pudendal nerve, one of the branches of the pudendal plexus that arises from the second, third, and fourth sacral nerves; passes between the piriformis and coccygeus; and leaves the pelvis through the greater sciatic foramen.

pudendal plexus, a network of motor and sensory nerves formed by the anterior branches of the second, the third, and all of the fourth sacral nerves. It is often considered part of the sacral plexus. The pu-

P

dendal plexus lies in the posterior hollow of the pelvis.

pudendum /p(y)ōōden'dəm/, *pl.* **pudenda** [L, *pudendus,* shameful], the external genitalia, especially of women. In a woman it comprises the mons veneris, the labia majora, the labia minora, the vestibule of the vagina, and the vestibular glands. In a man it comprises the penis, scrotum, and testes. —**pudendal,** *adj.*

puericulture /pyōō'ərikul'chər/ [L, *pueri,* children, *colere,* to cultivate], the rearing and training of children. —**puericulturist,** *n.*

puerile /pyōō'əril, -īl/ [L, *puerilis,* childish], pertaining to children or childhood; juvenile. —**puerility,** *n.*

puerilism /pyōō'əriliz'əm/ [L, *puerilis,* childish], childishness, particularly when manifested in an older adult.

puerpera /pyōō·er'pərə/ [L, *puerpus,* childbirth], a woman who has just given birth.

puerperal /pyōō·er'pərəl/ [L, *puerpus,* childbirth], **1.** pertaining to the period immediately after childbirth. **2.** pertaining to a woman (a puerpera) who has just given birth to an infant.

puerperal eclampsia [L, *puerpus,* childbirth; Gk, *ek,* out, *lampein* to flash], a condition of coma and convulsive seizures occurring after childbirth. It is associated with hypertension, edema, and proteinuria.

puerperal fever, a syndrome associated with systemic bacterial infection and septicemia that occurs after childbirth, usually as a result of unsterile obstetric technique. It is characterized by endometritis, fever, tachycardia, uterine tenderness, and foul lochia; if it is untreated, prostration, renal failure, bacteremic shock, and death may occur. The causative organism is most often one of the hemolytic streptococci.

puerperal mania, a rare acute mood disorder that sometimes occurs in women after childbirth, characterized by a severe manic reaction.

puerperal mastitis [L, *puerpus,* childbirth; Gk, *mastos,* breast, *itis,* inflammation], a form of acute mastitis in a nursing mother.

puerperal phlebitis [L, *puerpus,* childbirth; Gk, *phleps,* vein, *itis,* inflammation], an inflammation that begins in a uterine vein after childbirth and spreads to other veins, particularly the iliac and femoral veins.

puerperal sepsis, an infection acquired during the puerperium.

puerperium /pyōō'ərpir'ē·əm/ [L, *puerperus*], the time after childbirth, lasting approximately 6 weeks, during which the anatomic and physiologic changes brought about by pregnancy resolve and a woman adjusts to the new or expanded responsibilities of motherhood and nonpregnant life.

PUFA, abbreviation for *polyunsaturated fatty acid.*

puff [ME *puf*] a short, soft, blowing sound heard on auscultation.

Pulex /pyōō'leks/ [L, flea], a genus of fleas, some species of which transmit arthropod-borne infections such as plague and epidemic typhus.

pulmoaortic /pŏŏl'mō·ā·ôr'tik/, pertaining to the lungs and aorta.

pulmonary /pŏŏl'məner'ē/ [L, *pulmoneus,* lungs], pertaining to the lungs or the respiratory system.

pulmonary alveolar proteinosis [L, *pulmoneus,* lungs, *alveolus,* little hollow; Gk, *proteios,* first rank, *osis,* condition], a condition in which the air sacs of the lungs become filled with protein and lipids, progressing to respiratory failure.

pulmonary alveolus, one of the numerous terminal air sacs in the lungs where oxygen and carbon dioxide are exchanged.

pulmonary angiography [L, *pulmoneus,* lungs; Gk, *angeion,* vessel, *graphein,* to record], the radiographic study of the blood vessels of the lungs after the injection of an opaque contrast medium into the pulmonary circulation.

pulmonary arteriolar resistance (PAR), pressure loss per unit of blood flow from the pulmonary artery to a pulmonary vein.

pulmonary artery [L, *pulmoneus,* lungs; Gk, *arteria,* airpipe], either the left pulmonary artery supplying the left lung or the right pulmonary artery supplying the right lung. The lobar branches are named according to the lobe they supply, such as apical (*ramus apicalis*).

pulmonary artery catheter [L, *pulmoneus,* lungs; Gk, *arteria* + *katheter,* a thing lowered], a catheter inserted into a pulmonary artery to measure cardiac output, pulmonary arterial pressure, and capillary wedge pressure.

pulmonary artery wedge pressure [L, *pulmoneus* + Gk, *arteria* + ME, *wegge* + L, *premere,* to press], the blood pressure as measured by a transducer when a catheter is wedged into a distal branch of the pulmonary artery. The pressure measured is that of the pulmonary vein and, indirectly, that of the left atrium and left ventricle during diastole.

pulmonary atresia [L, *pulmoneus,* lungs; Gk, *a* + *tresis,* without perforation], a congenital heart defect of the right ventricular outflow tract. In one form there is an intact ventricular septum with an interatrial communication and a persistent patent ductus arteriosus. A more extreme form is the four-defect **tetralogy of Fallot.**

pulmonary atrium, any of the spaces at the end of an alveolar duct into which alveoli open.

pulmonary circulation [L, *pulmoneus,* lungs, *circulare*], the blood flow through a network of vessels between the heart and lungs for the oxygenation of blood and removal of carbon dioxide.

pulmonary compliance, a measure of the elasticity or expansibility of the lungs.

pulmonary congestion [L, *pulmoneus,* lungs, *congerere,* to heap together], an excessive accumulation of fluid in the lungs, usually associated with either an inflammation or congestive heart failure.

pulmonary disease, an abnormal condition of the respiratory system, characterized by cough, chest pain, dyspnea, hemoptysis, sputum production, stridor, and wheezing. Less common symptoms may be anxiety, arm and shoulder pain, tenderness in the calf of the leg, erythema nodosum, swelling of the face, headache, hoarseness, joint pain, and somnolence. Obstructive respiratory disease is the result of a reduction of airway size that impedes the air flow. Obstructive disease is characterized by reduced expiratory flow rates and increased total lung capacity. Restrictive respiratory disease is caused by conditions that limit lung expansion such as fibrothorax, obesity, a neuromuscular disorder, kyphosis, scoliosis, spondylitis, or surgical removal of lung tissue. Characteristic features of restrictive respiratory disease are decreased forced vital capacity and total lung capacity, with increased work of breathing and inefficient exchange of gases.

pulmonary dysmaturity syndrome, a respiratory disorder of premature infants in which the lungs contain focal emphysematous blebs and thickened alveolar walls. The infants commonly die of hypoxia.

pulmonary edema, the accumulation of extravascular fluid in lung tissues and alveoli, caused most commonly by congestive heart failure. The condition also may occur in barbiturate and opiate poisoning, diffuse infections, hemorrhagic pancreatitis, and renal failure and after a stroke, skull fracture, near-drowning, inhalation of irritating gases, and rapid administration of whole blood, plasma, serum albumin, or intravenous fluids. Signs and symptoms of pulmonary edema include tachypnea, labored shallow respirations, restlessness, apprehensiveness, air hunger, or cyanosis and blood-tinged or frothy pink sputum. The peripheral and neck veins are usually engorged; the blood pressure and heart rate are increased; and the pulse may be full and pounding or weak and thready. There may be edema of the extremities, crackles in the lungs, respiratory acidosis, and profuse diaphoresis.

pulmonary embolism (PE), the blockage of a pulmonary artery by foreign matter. The obstruction may be fat, air, tumor tissue, or a thrombus that usually arises from a peripheral vein. Predisposing factors include an alteration of blood constituents with increased coagulation, damage to blood vessel walls, and stagnation or immobilization, especially when associated with childbirth, congestive heart failure, polycythemia vera, or surgery. Pulmonary embolism is difficult to distinguish from myocardial infarction and pneumonia. It is characterized by dyspnea, sudden chest pain, shock, and cyanosis.

pulmonary emphysema, a chronic obstructive disease of the lungs, marked by an overdistension of the alveoli and destruction of the supporting alveolar structure.

pulmonary function laboratory, an area of a hospital or other health facility used for examination and evaluation of patients' respiratory function.

pulmonary function test (PFT), a procedure for determining the capacity of the lungs to exchange oxygen and carbon dioxide efficiently. There are two general kinds of respiratory function tests. One measures ventilation, or the ability of the bellows action of the chest and lungs to move gas in and out of alveoli; the other kind measures the diffusion of gas across the alveolar capillary membrane and the perfusion of the lungs by blood. Efficient gas exchange in the lungs requires a balanced ventilation-perfusion ratio, with areas receiving ventilation well perfused and areas receiving blood flow capable of ventilation.

pulmonary hypertension, a condition of abnormally high pressure within the pulmonary circulation.

pulmonary infarction (PI) [L, *pulmoneus,* lungs, *infarcire,* to stuff], an obstruction in a branch of a pulmonary artery resulting from a thrombus that may have originated in a leg or pelvic vein. After it is released into the venous circulation, the thromboembolus is carried in the bloodstream to one of the lungs, where it is filtered by the pulmonary vascular system.

pulmonary insufficiency [L, *pulmoneus,* lungs, *in* + *sufficere,* to suffice], a failure of the pulmonary valve to close properly.

P

pulmonary oxygen toxicity [L, *pulmoneus*, lungs; Gk, *toxikon*, poison], a form of oxygen poisoning caused by breathing high partial pressures of oxygen. Pathophysiologic effects include pulmonary capillary endothelial damage and alveolar epithelial cell destruction. Clinical manifestations include cough, substernal pain, nausea, vomiting, and atelectasis.

pulmonary stenosis, an abnormal cardiac condition, generally characterized by concentric hypertrophy of the right ventricle with relatively little increase in diastolic volume. When the ventricular septum is intact, this condition may be caused by valvular stenosis, by infundibular stenosis, or by both; it produces a pressure difference during systole between the right ventricular cavity and the pulmonary artery.

pulmonary sulcus tumor, a destructive invasive neoplasm that develops at the apex of the lung and infiltrates the ribs, vertebrae, and brachial plexus.

pulmonary surfactant, a chemical found in the lungs that reduces the surface tension of the fluid on the surface of the cells of the lower respiratory system, enhancing the elasticity of the alveoli and bronchioles and thus the exchange of gases in the lungs.

pulmonary trunk, the short, wide vessel that conveys venous blood from the right ventricle of the heart to the lungs.

pulmonary valve, a cardiac structure composed of three semilunar cusps that close during each heartbeat to prevent blood from flowing back into the right ventricle from the pulmonary trunk. The cusps are separated by sinuses that resemble tiny buckets when they are closed and filled with blood. These flaps grow from the lining of the pulmonary trunk.

pulmonary vascular resistance (PVR), the resistance in the pulmonary vascular bed against which the right ventricle must eject blood.

pulmonary vein, one of two pairs of large vessels that return oxygenated blood from each lung to the left atrium of the heart. The right pulmonary veins pass dorsal to the right atrium and the superior vena cava. The left pulmonary veins pass ventral to the descending thoracic aorta.

pulmonary ventilation [L, *pulmoneus*, lungs; *ventilare*, to fan], the process of inhaling and exhaling air through the lungs.

pulmonary wedge pressure (PWP), the pressure produced by an inflated latex balloon against a pulmonary artery, as part of a procedure used in the diagnosis of congestive heart failure, myocardial infarction, and other conditions. A balloon-tipped catheter is inserted through a subclavian, jugular, or femoral vein to the vena cava and on through the right atrium and ventricle to the pulmonary artery. When the balloon is inflated, it can continuously measure pulmonary pressure.

pulmonary Wegener's granulomatosis, a rare fatal disease of young or middle-aged men, characterized by granulomatous lesions of the respiratory tract, focal necrotizing arteritis, and finally widespread inflammation of body organs.

pulp [L, *pulpa*, flesh], any soft spongy tissue, such as that contained within the spleen, the pulp chamber of the tooth, or the distal subcutaneous pads of the fingers and toes. —**pulpy,** *adj.*

pulp abscess [L, *pulpa*, flesh + *abscedere*, to go away], a pus-producing abscess that develops in the center of a tooth.

pulpal /pul′pəl/, pertaining to pulp.

pulp canal, the space occupied by the nerves, blood vessels, and lymph in the radicular part of the tooth.

pulp cavity, the space in a tooth bounded by the dentin and containing the dental pulp. It is divided into the pulp chamber and the pulp or root canal.

pulpectomy /pulpek′təmē/ [L, *pulpa*, flesh; Gk, *ektome*, excision], the surgical removal, either complete or partial, of the pulp from a tooth.

pulpifaction /pul′pifak′shən/, the act of reducing something to a pulp.

pulpitis /pulpī′tis/, infection or inflammation of the dental pulp.

pulpless tooth /pulp′ləs/, a tooth in which the dental pulp is necrotic or has been removed.

pulpodontia /pul′pədon′shə/, the branch of dentistry that specializes in root canal therapy.

pulsate /pul′sāt/ [L, *pulsare*, to beat], to throb or vibrate rhythmically, such as the expansion and contraction rhythm of the heart.

pulsatile /pul′sətil/ [L, *pulsare*, to beat], pertaining to an activity characterized by a rhythmic pulsation.

pulsatile assist device (PAD), a flexible valveless balloon conduit contained within a rigid plastic cylinder that is inserted into the arterial circulation to provide pulsatile cardiopulmonary bypass support.

pulsatility index /pul′sətil′itē/, a parameter of blood flow in a vessel. It is equal to the difference between the peak and minimum diastolic velocities, divided by the mean flow during the cardiac cycle.

pulsating exophthalmos /pul′sāting/ [L, *pulsare*, to beat; Gk, *ex* + *ophthalmos*, eye], an eye disorder characterized by a bulging, pulsating eyeball. The cause is an arteriovenous aneurysm involving the internal carotid artery and the cavernous sinus of the orbit.

pulse [L, *pulsare,* to beat], **1.** a rhythmic beating or vibrating movement. **2.** a brief electromagnetic wave. **3.** the regular, recurrent expansion and contraction of an artery produced by waves of pressure caused by the ejection of blood from the left ventricle of the heart as it contracts. The phenomenon is easily detected on superficial arteries, such as the radial and carotid arteries, and corresponds to each beat of the heart. The normal number of pulse beats per minute in the average adult varies from 60 to 80, with fluctuations occurring with exercise, injury, illness, and emotional reactions.

pulsed Doppler, a type of Doppler device involving the transmission of a short-duration burst of sound into the region to be examined. The Doppler-shifted signals are processed from a limited depth range. The depth range is determined by a sample gate whose position and size usually can be selected by the instrument operator.

pulse deficit, a condition that exists when a peripheral pulse is less than the ventricular rate as auscultated at the apex of the heart or seen on the electrocardiogram. The condition indicates a lack of peripheral perfusion.

pulse duration, (in ultrasonics) a measure of the time a transducer oscillates for each pulse. The shorter the pulse duration, the better the axial resolution.

pulse-echo response profile, a graph of the amplitude of an ultrasound echo from a small reflector versus the distance from the reflector beam axis. The reflector is scanned perpendicular to the axis of the ultrasound transducer beam.

pulse-echo ultrasound, a diagnostic technique in which short-duration ultrasound pulses are transmitted into the region to be studied and echo signals resulting from scattering and reflection are detected and displayed. The depth of a reflective structure is inferred from the delay between pulse transmission and echo reception.

pulse height analyzer, (in radiology) a device that accepts or rejects electronic pulses according to their amplitude or energy.

pulse MR, magnetic resonance (MR) technique that uses radiofrequency pulses and Fourier transformation of the MR signal. Pulse MR has largely replaced the older continuous wave techniques.

pulse point, any one of the sites on the surface of the body where arterial pulsations can be easily palpated. The most commonly used pulse point is over the radial artery at the wrist. Other pulse points include the temporal artery in front of the ear, the common carotid artery at the lower level of the thyroid cartilage, the facial artery at the lower margin of the jaw, and the femoral, popliteal, posterior tibialis, and dorsalis pedis points.

pulse pressure, the difference between the systolic and diastolic pressures, normally 30 to 40 mm Hg.

pulser /pul′sər/, a component of an ultrasound instrument that provides signals for exciting the piezoelectric transducer in order to transmit an ultrasound beam.

pulse rate [L, *pulsare* + *reri,* to calculate], the number of beats per minute as measured on the radial, carotid, femoral, and pedal arteries. Normally it is the same rate as the heartbeat, but pulses in various body areas may differ slightly.

pulse repetition frequency (PRF), (in ultrasonics) the number of acoustic pulses transmitted per second.

pulse wave [L, *pulsare,* to beat; AS, *wafian*], a local blood pressure change caused by the passage of blood from the left ventricle into the aorta. It is accompanied by a wave action through the artery.

pulsus alternans /pul′səs ôl′tərnanz/ [L, *pulsare* + *alternare,* to alternate], a pulse characterized by a regular alternation of weak and strong beats without changes in the cycle length.

pulsus paradoxus, an abnormal decrease in systolic pressure and pulse wave amplitude during inspiration.

pulsus parvus et tardus [L, *pulsus,* beat, *parvus,* small, *tardus,* slow], a small pulse with low pressure that rises and falls slowly. The condition occurs in aortic stenosis.

pulsus tardus [L, *pulsus,* beat, *tardus,* slow], a pulse with a gradual rise and fall in amplitude.

pultaceous, pertaining to a substance that is pulpy or macerated.

pulverize /pul′vəriz/ [L, *pulvis,* dust], to reduce to a fine powder.

pulverulent /pulver′ələnt/, having the form of a fine powder.

pulvule /pul′vyool/ [L, *pulvis,* dust], a proprietary capsule containing a dose of a drug in powder form.

pumice /pum′is/ [L, *pumex*], a very finely divided volcanic rock, used in powdered or solid form for smoothing or polishing surfaces.

pump [ME, *pumpe*], **1.** an apparatus used to move fluids or gases by suction or by positive pressure, such as an infusion pump or stomach pump. **2.** a physiologic mechanism by which a substance is moved, usually by active transport across a cell membrane, such as a sodium pump. **3.** to move a liquid or gas by suction or positive pressure.

pump oxygenator [ME, *pumpe* + Gk, *oxys*, sharp, *genein*, to produce], a device that pumps oxygenated blood through the body during cardiopulmonary surgery.

punch biopsy [L, *pungere*, to prick; Gk, *bios*, life, *opsis*, view], the removal of living tissue for microscopic examination, usually bone marrow aspirates from the sternum, by means of a punch.

punchdrunk syndrome, a condition in which repeated cerebral concussions result in an abnormal gait, slow movement, tremor, and slurred or halting speech.

punch forceps, a surgical instrument used to cut out a disk of dense or resistant tissue, such as bone and cartilage. The ends of the blades of the punch forceps are perforated to grip the involved tissue.

punctate /pungk′tāt/ [L, *punctum*, point], marked with elevated or colored dots or punctures.

punctiform /pungk′tifôrm/, of very small size, as is a bacterial colony in a solid medium.

punctum /pungk′təm/, a physiologic area or point.

punctum caecum, blind spot.

punctum lacrimale /pungk′təm/, *pl.* **puncta lacrimalia** [L, *punctum*, prick, *lacrima*, tear], a tiny aperture in the medial margin of each eyelid that opens into the nasolacrimal sac. The puncta drain the tears that travel from the lacrimal glands through the lacrimal ducts to the conjunctiva.

puncture /pungk′chər/ [L, *punctura*], **1.** to prick or pierce a surface, as with a needle or knife. **2.** a wound or opening made by piercing.

puncture of the antrum [L, *punctura* + Gk, *antron*, cave], a cavity or hollow, as is made in piercing the wall of the maxillary sinus to drain pus.

puncture wound [L, *punctura* + AS, *wund*], a traumatic injury caused by the penetration of the skin by a narrow object such as a knife, nail, or slender fragment of metal, wood, glass, or other material.

Punnett square [Reginald C. Punnett, English geneticist, 1875–1967; OFr, *esquarre*], a checkerboard, graphlike diagram, used in charting genetic ratios, that shows all of the possible combinations of male and female gametes when one or more pairs of independent alleles are crossed.

P.U.O., abbreviation for *pyrexia of unknown origin.*

pupa /pyoo′pə/ [L, doll], a second stage

in the life cycle of certain (endopterytgote) insects between a larva and adult.

pupil /pyoo′pəl/ [L, *pupa*, doll], a circular opening in the iris of the eye, located slightly to the nasal side of the center of the iris. The pupil lies posterior to the cornea and the anterior chamber of the eye and is anterior to the lens. Its diameter changes with contraction and relaxation of the muscular fibers of the iris as the eye responds to changes in light, emotional states, and autonomic stimulation. —**pupillary,** *adj.*

pupilla /pyoopil′ə/ ′, the pupil of the eye.

pupillary /pyoo′pilerē/ [L, *pupilla*] pertaining to the pupil.

pupillary ruff, a brown wrinkled rim on the edge of the pupil, derived from posterior pigment epithelium of the iris.

pupillometry /pyoo′pilom′ətrē/, the measurement of the pupil.

pupillomotor /pyoo′pilōmō′tər/, pertaining to the autonomic nerve fibers of the smooth muscles of the iris.

PUPPP /pup/, abbreviation for **pruritic urticarial papules and plaques of pregnancy.**

PUPs, abbreviation for *previously untreated patients,* usually infants participating in clinical trials.

pure /pyoor/, **1.** free of contamination by extraneous matter. **2.** a state in which a substance contains nothing other than itself.

purgative /pur′gətiv/ [L, *purgare*, to purge], a strong medication usually administered by mouth to promote evacuation of the bowel or several bowel movements.

purge /purj/ [L, *purgare*], **1.** to evacuate the bowels, as with a cathartic. **2.** a cathartic. **3.** to make free of an unwanted substance. —**purgative,** *n., adj.*

purified protein derivative (PPD) /pyoo′-rifīd/, a dried form of tuberculin used in testing for past or present infection with tubercle bacilli. This product is usually introduced into the skin during such tests.

purine /pyoo′rēn/ [L, *purus*, pure, *urina*, urine], any one of a large group of nitrogenous compounds. Purines are produced as end products in the digestion of certain proteins in the diet, but some are synthesized in the body. Purines are also present in many medications and other substances, including caffeine, theophylline, and various diuretics, muscle relaxants, and myocardial stimulants.

purine base [L, *purus*, pure], any of the purine derivatives found in animal waste products. They include hypoxanthine, xanthine, and uric acid.

purine-free diet, a diet that excludes

foods that are rich sources of purines, end products of digestion of certain proteins. Foods high in purines particularly include organ meats such as liver, kidney, and sweetbreads, as well as red meats, poultry, and fish. These items can be replaced by milk, eggs, cheese, and some vegetable sources of protein.

purine-low diet, a diet that excludes some foods rich in purines, such as certain meat products, fish, and poultry, and particularly anchovies, meat extracts, sardines, and organ meats.

Purkinje's cells /pərkin'jəz/ [Johannes E. Purkinje, Czech physiologist, 1787–1869], large neurons that provide the only output from the cerebellar cortex after the cortex processes sensory and motor impulses from the rest of the nervous system.

Purkinje's fibers [Johannes E. Purkinje], myocardial fibers that are the termination of the bundle branches.

Purkinje's network /pərkin'jēz, pur'kinjēz, -jāz/ [Johannes E. Purkinje], a complex network of specialized cardiac muscle fibers that spread through the right and left ventricles of the heart and carry the impulses that contract those chambers almost simultaneously.

purposeful activity /pur'pəsfool/, activity that depends on consciously planned and directed involvement of the person.

purpura /pur'pyərə/ /pur'pyŏŏrə/ [L, purple], any of several bleeding disorders characterized by hemorrhage into the tissues, particularly beneath the skin or mucous membranes, producing ecchymoses or petechiae. —**purpuric,** *adj.*

purpura rheumatica [L, *purpura,* purple; Gk, *rheum,* flow], a distinctive clinical sign associated with hemorrhages of the skin and other tissues. The lesions are red or purple and do not blanche on pressure. Purpura is related to either a disorder of the blood or an abnormality affecting the blood vessels.

purpura senile /senē'lā/ [L, *purpura,* purple, *senilis,* aged], a skin condition affecting older people and characterized by fragile blood vessel walls that rupture on minimal trauma.

pursed-lip breathing /purst-/, respiration characterized by deep inspirations followed by prolonged expirations through pursed lips. It is done to increase expiratory airway pressure, improve oxygenation, and help prevent early airway closure.

purse-string suture [L, *sutura*], a continuous suture inserted in a circle about a round wound. The opening is closed by tightly drawing the ends of the suture together.

purulence /pyoor'(y)ələns/ [L, *purulentus,* pus formation], the condition of producing or discharging pus.

purulent /pyoor'(y)ələnt/[L, containing pus], producing or containing pus.

purulent conjunctivitis [L, *purulentus,* pus formation, *conjunctivus,* connecting; Gk, *itis,* inflammation], an inflammation of the conjunctiva caused by suppurative microorganisms, including species of streptococci, gonococci, and pneumococci.

purulent diarrhea [L, *purulentus,* pus formation; Gk, *dia* + *rhein,* to flow], diarrhea in which stools contain pus, a sign of a purulent gastrointestinal tract infection.

purulent inflammation [L, *purulentus,* pus formation, *inflammare,* to set afire], an inflammation that is accompanied by the formation of pus.

purulent iritis [L, *purulentus,* pus formation; Gk, *iris,* rainbow, *itis,* inflammation], an inflammation of the iris accompanied by the formation of pus.

purulent keratitis [L, *purulentus,* pus formation; Gk, *keras,* horn, *itis,* inflammation], a severe form of keratitis leading to disintegration of the cornea if untreated. The condition commonly begins with a bacterial infection of the lacrimal sac, occurs frequently in elderly patients who have poor nutrition, and spreads into a pus-producing ulcer.

purulent pancreatitis [L, *purulentus,* pus formation; Gk, *pan,* all, *kreas,* flesh, *itis,* inflammation], inflammation of the pancreas accompanied by pus formation.

purulent rhinitis [L, *purulentus,* pus formation; Gk, *rhis,* nose, *itis,* inflammation], an infection of the nasal mucosa that is accompanied by pus formation. The condition is often secondary to a systemic infection, such as measles.

purulent synovitis [L, *purulentus,* pus formation; Gk, *syn,* together; L, *ovum,* egg], an inflammation of the synovial membrane of a joint with pus formation in the cavity.

pus [L, corrupt matter], a creamy, viscous fluid exudate that is the result of fluid remains of liquefactive necrosis of tissues. It is usually pale yellow to yellow green, sometimes whitish, and sometimes bloody. Its main constituent is an abundance of polymorphonuclear leukocytes. Bacterial infection is its most common cause.

pus cell, a necrotic polymorphonuclear leukocyte, a major component of pus.

pus in urine [L, *pus* + Gk, *ouron,* urine], the presence of pus in a urine sample, indicating a urinary tract infection anywhere from the kidneys to the urethra.

P

pustular /pus'chələr/ [L, *pustula*, blister], pertaining to or resembling pustules.

pustular psoriasis [L, *pustula*, blister; Gk, *psoriasis*, itch], a severe form of psoriasis consisting of bright red patches and sterile pustules all over the body. Crops of lesions lasting 4 to 7 days occur every few days in cycles over weeks or months. Fever, leukocytosis, and hypoalbuminemia are associated.

pustule /pus'chool/ /pus'chŏŏl/ [L, *pustula*], a small circumscribed elevation of the skin containing fluid that is usually purulent. —**pustular,** *adj.*

putamen /pyŏŏtā'mən/ [L, *putamen*, husk], a part of the lentiform nucleus that is lateral to the globus pallidus. It is associated with the corpus striatum and receives connections from the suppressor centers of the cortex.

putrefaction /pyŏŏ'trəfak'shən/ [L, *puter,* rotten, *facere,* to make], the decay of enzymes, especially proteins, that produces foul-smelling compounds such as ammonia, hydrogen sulfide, and mercaptans. —**putrefactive,** *adj.*

putrefactive /-fak'tiv/ [L, *puter,* rotten, *facere,* to make], causing, promoting, or relating to putrefaction.

putrefy /pyŏŏ'trəfī/ [L, *puter,* rotten, *facere,* to make], to decay, with the production of foul-smelling substances, especially putrescine and mercaptans associated with the decomposition of animal tissues and proteins.

putrescine /pyŏŏ'tresēn/, a foul-smelling toxic ptomaine produced by the decomposition of the amino acid ornithine during the decay of animal tissues, bacillus cultures, and fecal bacteria.

putrid /pyŏŏ'trid/ [L, *putridus,* rotten], decomposed.

putromaine /pyŏŏtrō'mān/, any toxin produced by the decay of food within a living body.

PUVA, an abbreviation for a psoriasis treatment consisting of a medication called *p*soralen plus *u*ltraviolet light of *A* (long) wavelength.

P value, (in research) the statistical probability of the occurrence of a given finding by chance alone in comparison with the known distribution of possible findings, considering the kinds of data, the technique of analysis, and the number of observations.

PVC, 1. abbreviation for **polyvinyl chloride.** 2. abbreviation for **premature ventricular complex.**

PVR, abbreviation for **pulmonary vascular resistance.**

pW, abbreviation for *picowatt.*

PWA, abbreviation for *person with AIDS.*

P wave, the component of the cardiac cycle shown on an electrocardiogram as an inverted U-shaped curve that follows the T wave and precedes the QRS complex. It represents atrial depolarization.

P′ wave (P prime wave), a P wave that is generated from other than the sinus node; an ectopic P wave.

PWP, abbreviation for **pulmonary wedge pressure.**

pyelogram /pī'əlōgram'/ [Gk, *pyelos,* pelvis, *gramma,* record], a radiographic picture of the kidneys and ureters. An intravenous pyelogram, taken after the injection of a radiopaque dye, shows the size and location of the kidneys, the outline of the ureters and bladder, the filling of the renal pelves, the patency of the urinary tract, and any cysts or tumors within the kidneys.

pyelolithotomy /pī'əlō'lithot'əmē/, a surgical procedure in which renal calculi are removed from the pelvis of the ureter.

pyelonephritis /pī'əlōnəfrī'tis/ [Gk, *pyelos* + *nephros,* kidney, *itis,* inflammation], a diffuse pyogenic infection of the pelvis and parenchyma of the kidney. Acute pyelonephritis is usually the result of an infection that ascends from the lower urinary tract to the kidney. The onset of acute pyelonephritis is rapid, characterized by fever, chills, pain in the flank, nausea, and urinary frequency. Chronic pyelonephritis develops slowly after bacterial infection of the kidney and may progress to renal failure. Most cases are associated with some form of obstruction, such as a stone or a stricture of the ureter.

pyeloplasty /pī'əlōplas'tē/, the surgical reconstruction of the kidney pelvis.

pyelorostomy, the surgical establishment of a fistula from the abdominal surface to the stomach at a point near the pylorus.

pyemesis /pī·em'əsis/, the action of vomiting purulent material.

pyemic embolism /pī·ē'mik/ [Gk, *pyon,* pus, *haima,* blood, *embolos,* plug], an infective embolus producing an abscess.

pygmalianism /pigmā'lē·əniz'əm/ [Gk, *Pygmalion,* mythic sculptor who fell in love with his statue], a psychosexual abnormality in which the individual directs erotic fantasies to an object that he or she has created.

pygmy /pig'mē/ [L, *pygmaeus,* dwarf], an extremely small person whose body parts are proportioned accordingly; a primordial dwarf.

pygoamorphus /pī'gō·əmôr'fəs/ [Gk, *pyge,* buttocks, *a* + *morphe,* not form], asymmetric, conjoined twins in which the parasitic member is represented by an undifferentiated amorphous mass attached to the autosite in the sacral region.

pygodidymus /pī'gōdid'əməs/ [Gk, *pyge*, buttocks, *didymos*, twin], **1.** a malformed fetus that has a double pelvis and hips. **2.** conjoined twins who are fused in the cephalothoracic region but separated at the pelvis.

pygomelus /pīgom'ələs/ [Gk, *pyge* + *melos*, limb], a malformed fetus that has an extra limb or limbs attached to the buttock.

pygopagus /pīgop'əgəs/ [Gk, *pyge* + *pegos*, fixed], conjoined twins consisting of two fully formed or nearly formed fetuses united in the sacral region so that they are positioned back to back.

pyknic /pik'nik/ [Gk, *pyknos*, thick], describing a body structure characterized by short, round limbs; a full face; a short neck; stockiness; and a tendency to obesity.

pyknosis /piknō'sis/, the condensation of nuclear material into a solid, darkly staining mass in a dying cell.

pyla /pī'lə/, the opening between the third ventricle and the cerebral aqueduct.

pylethrombophlebitis /pī'ləthrom'bōflə-bī'tis/, an inflammation of the portal vein with formation of a thrombus.

pylon /pī'lon/ [Gk, gate], an artificial lower limb, often a narrow vertical support consisting of a socket with wooden side supports and a rubber-clad peg end. It may be used as a temporary prosthesis.

pyloric /pīlôr'ik/ [Gk, *pyle*, gate, *ouros*, guard], pertaining to the pylorus.

pyloric canal, the lumen of the pyloric part of the stomach.

pyloric obstruction and dilation /pīlôr'ik/ [Gk, *pyle*, gate, *ouros*, guard; L, *obstruere*, to build against, *dilatare*, to widen], a reaction of the stomach to pyloric obstruction, which increases the resistance to the expulsion of partly digested food from the stomach. As a result, the stomach may become hypertrophied, then dilated. Excessive consumption of food and beverages contributes to the condition.

pyloric orifice [Gk, *pyle*, gate, *ouros*, guard; L, *orificium*, opening], the opening of the stomach into the duodenum lying to the right of the midline at the level of the upper border of the first lumbar vertebra.

pyloric sphincter, a thickened muscular ring in the stomach, separating the pylorus from the duodenum.

pyloric stenosis, a narrowing of the pyloric sphincter at the outlet of the stomach, causing an obstruction that blocks the flow of food into the small intestine.

pyloroduodenitis /pilôr'ōdoo'ōdənī'tis/,

an inflammation of the pylorus and the duodenum.

pyloromyotomy /pīlôr'ōmī-ot'əmē/ [Gk, *pyle* + *ouros* + *mys*, muscle, *temnein*, to cut], the incision of the longitudinal and circular muscle of the pylorus, which leaves the mucosa intact but separates the incised muscle fibers.

pyloroplasty /pīlôr'əplas'tē/ [Gk, *pyle* + *ouros* + *plassein*, to mold], a surgical procedure performed to relieve pyloric stenosis.

pylorospasm /pīlôr'əspaz'əm/ [Gk, *pyle*, *ouros* + *spasmos*], a spasm of the pyloric sphincter of the stomach, as occurs in pyloric stenosis.

pylorotomy /pī'lôrot'əmē/ [Gk, *pyle*, gate, *ouros*, guard, *temnein*, to cut], a surgical incision of the pylorus, usually performed to remove an obstruction.

pylorus /pīlôr'əs/, *pl.* **pylori, pyloruses** [Gk, *pyle*, gate, *ouros*, guard], a narrow, nearly tubular part of the stomach that angles to the right from the body of the stomach toward the duodenum. —**pyloric,** *adj.*

pyocele, an accumulation of pus in the scrotum.

pyocolpos, an accumulation of pus in the vagina.

pyocyanic /pī'ōsī-an'ik/, pertaining to pus that is blue or to an organism that produces blue pus, such as *Pseudomonas pyocyanea.*

pyocyanin /pī'ōsī'ənin/, a blue or blue-green pigment that may be extracted from *Pseudomonas aeruginosa* with chloroform.

pyocyst /pī'əsist/ [Gk, *pyon*, pus, *kytos*, cell], a pus-filled cyst.

pyocystitis /-sistī'tis/, an inflammation involving a pus-filled cyst within the urinary bladder.

pyoderma /pī'ōdur'mə/ [Gk, *pyon*, pus, *derma*, skin], any purulent skin disease such as impetigo.

pyogenic /pī'əjen'ik/ [Gk, *pyon* + *genein*, to produce], pus-producing.

pyogenic exotoxin, extracellular toxin secreted by *Streptococcus pyogenes* that may be associated with fever and the development of renal failure, respiratory distress, and necrosis.

pyogenic granuloma, a small nonmalignant mass of excessive granulation tissue, usually found at the site of an injury. Most often a dull red color, it contains numerous capillaries, bleeds readily, and is very tender; it may be attached by a narrow stalk.

pyogenic infection [Gk, *pyon*, pus, *genein*, to produce; L, *inficere*, to stain], any infection that results in pus production.

pyogenic microorganisms [Gk, *pyon*, pus,

P

genein, to produce, *mikros,* small, *organon,* instrument], microorganisms that produce pus. They include species of bacilli, clostridia, gonococci, meningococci, pseudomonas, staphylococci, and streptococci.

pyohemothorax /-hem'ōthôr'aks/ [Gk, *pyon,* pus, *haima,* blood, *thorax,* chest], an accumulation of blood and pus in the pleural cavity.

pyonephrolithiasis /-nef'rōlithī'əsis/, an accumulation of pus and calculi in the kidney.

pyophylactic /-filak'tik/ [Gk, *pyon,* pus, *phylax,* protector], providing protection against purulent infections, such as administering an antibiotic before the onset of an infection.

pyophysometra /-fī'sōmē'trə/, an accumulation of pus and gas in the uterus.

pyopneumopericardium /pī'ōn oo'mōper'-ikär'dē-əm/, the presence of pus and air or gas in the pericardial sac.

pyopneumoperitonitis /pī'ōnoo'mōper'-itonī'tis/, inflammation of the peritoneal cavity caused by an accumulation of air and pus in the cavity.

pyopyelectasis /-pī'əlek'təsis/, a dilation of the renal pelvis of the kidney due to an accumulation of pus.

pyorrhea /pī'ərē'ə/ [Gk, *pyon* + *rhoia,* flow], **1.** a discharge of pus. **2.** a purulent inflammation of the tissues surrounding the teeth. **—pyorrheal,** *adj.*

pyosalpinx /pī'ōsal'pingks/ [Gk, *pyon* + *salpinx,* tube], an accumulation of pus in a fallopian tube.

pyospermia, a complication of chronic prostatitis marked by pus in the seminal fluid.

pyostatic /-stat'ik/, the formation of pus.

pyostomatitis /-stō'mətī'tis/, an inflammation of the mouth.

pyothorax, 1. a collection of pus in the pleural cavity. **2.** purulent pleurisy.

pyoureter /pī'ōyōō'ətər, -yōorē'tər/, the presence of pus in the ureter.

pyoverdin /-vur'din/, a yellow pigment produced by some strains of *Pseudomonas aeruginosa.*

pyramid /pir'əmid/ [Gr, *pyramis*], a mass of tissue rising to an apex, such as the pyramids of the cerebellum and kidneys.

pyramidal /piram'idəl/ [Gk, *pyramis*], pertaining to the shape of a pyramid.

pyramidal cell [Gk, *pyramis* + L, *cella,* storeroom], a neuron with a pyramid-shaped cell body in the gray matter of the cerebral cortex.

pyramidalis /piram'idā'lis/, one of a pair of anterolateral muscles of the abdomen, contained in the lower end of the sheath of the rectus abdominis.

pyramidal nucleus [Gk, *pyramis* + L, *nucleus,* nut kernel], a band of gray matter lying between the olivary nucleus and the midline that projects fibers contralaterally to the vermis or part of the cerebellum.

pyramidal tract, a pathway composed of groups of nerve fibers in the white matter of the spinal cord through which motor impulses are conducted to the anterior horn cells from the opposite side of the brain. These descending fibers regulate the voluntary and reflex activity of the muscles through the anterior horn cells.

pyramidotomy /piram'idot'əmē/, the surgical severance of pyramidal tracts in the treatment of disorders associated with involuntary muscle contractions.

pyrantel pamoate /pīran'təl/, an anthelmintic prescribed in the treatment of infestation by roundworms or pinworms.

pyrazinamide /pī'rəzin'əmīd/, an antimycobacterial prescribed in combination chemotherapy in the treatment of tuberculosis of hospitalized patients who fail to respond to other medications.

pyrectic /pīrek'tik/ [Gk, *pyretos* fever], pertaining to or characterized by fever.

pyrenemia /pī'rənē'mē-ə/, a condition in which nucleated erythrocytes are present in the blood.

pyrethrin and piperonyl butoxide /pī'-rəthrin, piper'ənil/, a fixed-combination scabicide and pediculicide prescribed in the treatment of infestations of head, body, and pubic lice.

pyretogenic /pī'rətojen'ik/ [Gk, *pyretos,* fever, *genein,* to produce], inducing, causing, or resulting from a fever.

pyridostigmine bromide /pir'idōstig'mēn/, a cholinergic prescribed in the treatment of myasthenia gravis and used as an antagonist to nondepolarizing muscle relaxants such as curare.

pyridoxal phosphate /pir'ədok'səl/, an enzyme that acts with pyridoxamine phosphate and transaminase to catalyze the reversible transfer of an amino group from an alpha-amino acid to an alpha-keto acid, especially alpha-ketoglutaric acid. Such processes are essential to metabolism.

pyridoxamine phosphate /pir'ədok'sə-mēn/, an enzyme that participates with pyridoxal phosphate and transaminase in the reversible transfer of an amino group from an alpha-amino acid to an alpha-keto acid.

pyridoxine /pir'ədok'sēn/, a water-soluble white crystalline vitamin that is part of the B complex (vitamin B_6). It is derived from pyridine and converted in the body to pyridoxal and pyridoxamine for synthesis. It functions as a coenzyme essential for the synthesis and breakdown of amino acids, the conversion of tryptophan to niacin, the breakdown of glycogen to glucose 1-phosphate, the production of antibodies, the formation of heme in hemoglobin, the formation of hormones important in brain function, the proper absorption of vitamin B_{12}, the production of hydrochloric acid and magnesium, and the maintenance of the balance of sodium and potassium, which regulates body fluids and the functioning of the nervous and musculoskeletal systems.

pyrilamine maleate /piril'əmēn/, an antihistamine prescribed in the treatment of hypersensitivity reactions, including rhinitis, skin rash, and pruritus.

pyrimethamine /pir'imeth'əmēn/ an antimalarial prescribed in the treatment of malaria and toxoplasmosis.

pyrimethamine and sulfadoxine, /sulfə-dok'sēn, a fixed-combination antimalarial drug prescribed for prophylaxis and treatment of malaria and other opportunistic infections.

pyrimidine /pərim'ədēn/, an organic compound of heterocyclic nitrogen found in nucleic acids and in many drugs, including the antiviral drugs acyclovir, ribavirin, and trifluridine.

pyrogen /pī'rəjən/ [Gk, *pyr,* fire, *genein,* to produce], any substance or agent that tends to cause a rise in body temperature, such as some bacterial toxins. —**pyrogenic,** *adj.*

pyroglobulin /pī'rōglob'yəlin/, an immunoglobulin that precipitates irreversibly when heated.

pyrolagnia /pī'rōlag'nē·ə/ [Gk, *pyr* + *lagneia,* lust], sexual stimulation or gratification from watching or setting fires.

pyrolysis /pīrol'isis/, the decomposition of a chemical compound by the application of heat.

pyromania /pī'rōmā'nē·ə/ [Gk, *pyr* + *mania,* madness], an impulse-control disorder characterized by an uncontrollable urge to set fires.

pyromaniac /pī'rōmā'nē·ak/, **1.** a person having or displaying characteristics of pyromania. **2.** pertaining to or exhibiting pyromania. —**pyromaniacal,** *adj.*

pyropoikilocytosis /pī'rōpoi'kilō'sītō'sis/, a recessive inherited disorder characterized by severe hemolysis, irregular shapes of red blood cells, and sensitivity of blood cells to fragmentation in vitro after minor temperature variations.

pyrotherapy /pī'rōther'əpē/, a method of treatment in which the temperature of a patient is raised to a fever level.

pyrrole /pirōl', pir'ōl/ [Gk, *pyrrhos,* red], a heterocyclic substance occurring naturally in many compounds in the body. Heme and porphyrin are pyrrole derivatives.

pyruvate kinase /pī'rəvāt/, an enzyme essential for anaerobic glycolysis in red blood cells. It catalyzes the transfer of a phosphate group from adenosine triphosphate to produce adenosine diphosphate.

pyruvate kinase deficiency, a congenital hemolytic disorder transmitted as an autosomal-recessive trait. The homozygous condition is characterized by severe chronic hemolysis.

pyruvic acid /pīroo'vik/, a compound formed as an end product of glycolysis, the anaerobic stage of glucose metabolism.

pyuria /pīyoor'ē·ə/, the presence of white blood cells in the urine, usually a sign of an infection in the urinary tract.

PZI, abbreviation for **protamine zinc insulin.**

Q

Q, 1. symbol for *blood volume.* 2. symbol for *quantity.* 3. symbol for *coulomb.*

Q̇, symbol for *rate of blood flow.*

Q angle, the angle of incidence of the quadriceps muscle relative to the patella. The Q angle determines the tracking of the patella through the trochlea of the femur. As the angle increases, the chance of patellar compression problems increases.

QCT, abbreviation for **quantitative computed tomography.**

q.d., 1. (in prescriptions) abbreviation for *quaque die* /dē'ā/, a Latin phrase meaning 'every day.' 2. abbreviation for *quartile deviation.*

qdrnt, abbreviation for **quadrant.**

Q fever [L, *febris*], an acute febrile illness, usually respiratory, caused by the rickettsia *Coxiella burnetii (Rickettsia burnetii).* The disease is spread through contact with infected domestic animals, by inhaling the rickettsiae from their hides, by drinking their contaminated milk, or by being bitten by a tick harboring the organism.

q.h., (in prescriptions) abbreviation for *quaque hora,* a Latin phrase meaning 'every hour.'

q.2h, (in prescriptions) abbreviation for *quaque secunda hora,* a Latin phrase meaning 'every 2 hours.'

q.3h, (in prescriptions) abbreviation for *quaque tertia hora,* a Latin phrase meaning 'every 3 hours.'

q.4h, (in prescriptions) abbreviation for *quaque quarta hora,* a Latin phrase meaning 'every 4 hours.'

q.6h, (in prescriptions) abbreviation for *quaque sex hora,* a Latin phrase meaning 'every 6 hours.'

q.8h, (in prescriptions) abbreviation for *quaque octa hora,* a Latin phrase meaning 'every 8 hours.'

q.i.d., (in prescriptions) abbreviation for *quater in die* /dē'ā/, a Latin phrase meaning 'four times a day.'

q.l., abbreviation for the Latin phrase *quantum libet,* 'as much as one pleases.'

qli, abbreviation for *quality of life index.*

Q-R interval, in an electrocardiogram, the period from the start of the QRS complex to the peak of the R wave.

QRS complex, a series of wave forms on an electrocardiogram that represent depolarization of ventricular muscle cells. The term, 'QRS complex,' is assigned by convention to describe both normal and abnormal ventricular depolarization. The variable morphologies of the QRS complex are described in detail by labeling each deflection above and below the baseline as Q, R, or S wave; upper and lower case letters are used to describe the amplitude of each waveform. In the QRS complex, a Q wave is the negative deflection preceding the first R wave; an R wave is any positive deflection, and an S wave is the negative deflection following an R wave.

QRST complex [L, *complexus*], components of an electrocardiogram, consisting of the QRS complex, the S-T segment and the T wave. It represents depolarization and repolarization of the ventricles.

q.s., (in prescriptions) abbreviation for *quantum sufficit,* a Latin phrase meaning 'quantity required.'

Q-switching, a laser technique used in corneal surgery to achieve high-peak power in nanosecond pulses of energy.

qt, abbreviation for **quart.**

Q-T interval, the part on an electrocardiogram from the beginning of the QRS complex to the end of the T wave, reflecting the length of the refractory period of the heart. A long Q-T interval is associated with the life-threatening ventricular tachycardia known as torsades de pointes.

quad, 1. abbreviation for *quadriceps.* 2. abbreviation for *quadrilateral.* 3. abbreviation for *quadrant.* 4. abbreviation for **quadriplegia.**

quad coughing /kwod/, a form of assisted coughing for patients with central nervous system disorders who are unable to generate sufficient force to clear respiratory secretions. After a maximal inspiration, the patient coughs while an assistant exerts gentle upward and inward pressure with both hands on the abdomen. The increased intraabdominal pressure produces a more forceful cough.

quadrangular bandage /kwodrang'gələr/, a towel or other large rectangular sheet of cloth folded over for use as a wrapping for a wound of the abdomen, chest, or head.

quadrant (gdrnt, quad.) /kwod'rənt/ [L, *quadrans,* a fourth part], **1.** one quarter of a circle. **2.** one quarter of an anatomic area formed by the division of the area by imaginary vertical and horizontal lines bisecting each other.

quadrantanopsia /kwodran'tənop'sē·ə/, a loss of vision in a quarter section of the visual field of one or both eyes. The cause may vary with the quadrant affected.

quadrantectomy /kwod'rantek'təmē/, a partial mastectomy in which a tumor is excised in one quadrant of a breast along with the pectoralis muscle fascia.

quadrant streak, a technique for microbial inoculation in which a single colony is isolated on a culture plate divided into four sections.

quadriceps femoris /kwod'riseps/ [L, *quattuor,* four, *caput,* head, *femur,* thigh], the great extensor muscle of the anterior thigh, composed of the rectus femoris, the vastus lateralis, the vastus medialis, and the vastus intermedius. The muscle functions to extend the leg.

quadrigeminal /kwod'rijem'inəl/ [L, *quadrigeminum,* fourfold], **1.** in four parts. **2.** a fourfold increase in size or frequency. **3.** having four symmetric parts.

quadrigeminal pulse, a pulse in which a pause occurs after every fourth beat.

quadrilateral socket /kwod'rilat'ərəl/, a four-sided prosthetic socket design for people with above-the-knee amputations. The posterior brim is designed to fit directly beneath the ischial tuberosity so that the person literally sits on it.

quadriplegia (quad) /kwod'rəplē'jē·ə/ [L, *quattuor,* four; Gk, *plege,* stroke], paralysis of the arms, legs, and trunk of the body below the level of an associated injury to the spinal cord. This disorder is usually caused by spinal cord injury, especially in the area of the fifth to the seventh vertebrae. Automobile accidents and sporting mishaps are common causes. Signs and symptoms commonly include flaccidity of the arms and legs and the loss of power and sensation below the level of the injury. Cardiovascular complications also may develop from any injury that damages the spinal cord above the fifth cervical vertebra because of an associated block of the sympathetic nervous system. Other symptoms may include low body temperature, bradycardia, impaired peristalsis, and autonomic dysreflexia.

quadrivalent /kwod'rivā'lənt/ **1.** a chemical element or radical with a valence of four. **2.** a body formed in the first meiotic division by the association of four chromosomes.

quadruped /kwod'rŏŏped'/ [L, *quattuor,*

four, *pes,* foot], **1.** any four-footed animal. **2.** a human whose body weight is supported by both arms as well as both legs.

quadruplet /kwod'rŏŏplit, kwodrŏŏ'plit/ [L, *quadruplex,* fourfold], any one of four offspring born of the same gestation period during a single pregnancy.

quadrupole mass filter, a four-pole magnet system used to separate charged mass fragments in a mass spectrometer.

qual anal, abbreviation for **qualitative analysis.**

quale /kwä'lē/, *pl.* **qualia** /kwä'lē·ə/ [L, *qualis,* what kind], **1.** the quality of a particular thing. **2.** a quality considered as an independent entity. **3.** (in psychology) a feeling, sensation, or other conscious process that has its unique particular quality, regardless of its external meaning or frame of reference.

qualified /kwol'ifīd/ [L, *qualis*], pertaining to a health professional or health facility that is formally recognized by an appropriate agency or organization as meeting certain standards of performance related to the professional competence of an individual or the eligibility of an institution to participate in an approved health care program.

qualitative /kwol'itā'tiv/ [L, *qualis*], pertaining to the quality, value, or nature of something.

qualitative analysis (qual anal) [L, *qualis,* what kind; Gk, *analysis* a loosening] **1.** (in chemistry) the study of a sample of material to determine what chemical substances are present. **2.** (in research) the analysis and interpretation of data that cannot be analyzed by statistical methods.

qualitative melanin test, a test for detecting melanin in the urine of patients with malignant melanomas.

qualitative test, a test that determines the presence or absence of a substance.

quality /kwol'itē/ [L, *qualis*], (in radiotherapy and radiography) a descriptive specification of the penetrating nature of the x-ray beam as influenced by kilovoltage and filtration. Kilovoltage produces more penetration. Filtration removes the 'softer' wavelengths and 'hardens' the beam.

quality assessment measures, formal systematic organizational evaluation of overall patterns or programs of care, including clinical, consumer, and systems evaluation.

quality control, a method of repeated assay of known standard materials and monitoring reaction parameters to ensure precision and accuracy.

quality factor, (in radiotherapy) evalua-

Q

tion of the biologic damage that radiation can produce. In the field of radiation protection, biologically equivalent doses are set equal to one another by multiplying the actual absorbed dose by a number called the quality factor. The resulting quantity is called dose equivalent, measured in sieverts or rem.

quality management, 1. (in health care) any evaluation of services provided and the results achieved as compared with accepted standards. In one form of quality assurance, various attributes of health care such as cost, place, accessibility, treatment, and benefits are scored in a two-part process. **2.** a system of review of selected hospital medical/nursing records by medical/nursing staff members, performed for the purposes of evaluating the quality and effectiveness of medical/nursing care in relation to accepted standards.

Quality Monitoring, a Nursing Interventions Classification defined as systematic collection and analysis of an organization's quality indicators for the purpose of improving patient care.

quality of life [L, *qualis,* what kind; AS, *lif*], a measure of the optimum energy or force that endows a person with the power to cope successfully with the full range of challenges encountered in the real world. The term applies to all individuals, regardless of illness or handicap, on the job, at home, or in leisure activities. Quality enrichment methods can include activities that reduce boredom and allow a maximum amount of freedom in choosing and performing various tasks.

quantitative /kwon'titā'tiv/ [L, *quantus,* how much], capable of being measured.

quantitative analysis [L, *quantum,* how much; Gk, *analysis,* a loosening], **1.** (in chemistry) the determination of the amounts of constituents in a sample of material. Kinds of quantitative analysis include gravimetric analysis, volumetric analysis, and spectrophotometric analysis. **2.** (in research) the use of statistical methods to analyze data.

quantitative computed tomography (QCT), a type of computed tomography of bone mineral densities that allows for a three-dimensional density measurement. It calculates true densities in grams per cubic centimeter. QCT is used mainly for lumbar spine studies but can also be applied in hip and peripheral bone mineral evaluations.

quantitative test [L, *quantum,* how much, *testum,* crucible], a test that determines the amount of a substance per unit volume or unit weight.

quantitative ultrasound, an ultrasound technique for assessing bone mineral density. The main advantage of ultrasound is the complete absence of radiation; a disadvantage is the confounding influence of soft tissue.

quantum theory /kwon'təm/ [L, *quantum,* how much; Gk, *theoria,* speculation], (in physics) the theory dealing with the interaction of matter and electromagnetic radiation, particularly at the atomic and subatomic levels, according to which radiation consists of small units of energy called quanta.

quarantine /kwor'əntēn/ [It, *quarantina,* forty], **1.** isolation of people with communicable disease or those exposed to communicable disease during the contagious period in an attempt to prevent spread of the illness. **2.** the practice of detaining travelers or vessels coming from places of epidemic disease, originally for 40 days, for the purpose of inspection or disinfection.

quart (qt) /kwôrt/ [L, *quartus,* one-fourth], a unit of volume fluid measure equivalent to ¼ gallon, 2 pints, 32 ounces, or 946.24 milliliters. The British Imperial quart is equal to 1.136 liters, and the American quart for dry measure is 1.101 liters.

quartan /kwôr'tən/ [L, *quartanus,* relating to the fourth], recurring on the fourth day, or at about 72-hour intervals.

quartan malaria, a form of malaria, caused by the protozoan *Plasmodium malariae,* characterized by febrile paroxysms that occur every 72 hours.

quartile /kwôr'təl, kwôr'tīl/ [L, *quartus,* one-fourth], one-fourth of the distribution of scores. The first quartile would be the lowest 25% of scores, the second quartile would represent the 26% to 50% range of scores, and so on.

quaternary /kwot'əner'ē, kwətur'nərē/ [L, *quattuor,* four], **1.** pertaining to a chemical compound in which four atoms or groups of elements are bonded to one atom, such as a quaternary ammonium compound in which four organic radicals are substituted for the four hydrogen molecules on an ammonium ion. **2.** fourth-level structure in proteins as in the structure of hemoglobin made up of two alpha and two beta globulins.

quaternary ammonium derivative, a substance whose chemical structure has four carbon groups attached to a nitrogen atom. It is usually a strong emulsifying agent, highly water soluble but relatively insoluble in lipids.

Queckenstedt's test /kwek'ənstets/ [Hans H. G. Queckenstedt, German physician, 1876–1918], a test for an obstruction in the spinal canal in which the jugular veins on each side of the neck are compressed alternately. Normally occlusion of the veins of the neck causes an immediate rise in spinal fluid pressure; if the vertebral canal is blocked, no rise occurs.

Queensland tick typhus, an infection caused by *Rickettsia australis,* occurring in Australia, transmitted by ticks, and resembling mild Rocky Mountain spotted fever.

quellung reaction /kwel'ung/ [Ger, *Quellung,* swelling; L, *re,* again, *agere,* to act], the swelling of the capsule of a bacterium, seen in the laboratory when the organism is exposed to specific antisera. This phenomenon is used to identify the genera, species, or subspecies of the bacteria causing a disease.

quenching /kwen'ching/, **1.** a process of removing or reducing an energy source such as heat or light. **2.** stopping or diminishing a chemical or enzymatic reaction. **3.** decreasing counting efficiency in beta liquid scintillation caused by interfering materials.

Quengle cast /kwen'gəl/, a two-section, hinged orthopedic cast for immobilizing the lower extremities from the foot or ankle to below the knee and the upper thigh to a level just above the knee. The two parts of the cast are connected by special hinges at knee level.

quercetin /kwur'sitin/, a yellow, crystalline, flavonoid pigment found in oak bark, the juice of lemons, asparagus, and other plants. It is used to reduce abnormal capillary fragility.

querulous paranoia /kwer'(y)ələs/ [L, *queri,* to complain; Gk, *para,* beside, *nous,* mind], a form of paranoia characterized by extreme discontent and habitual complaining, usually about imagined slights by others.

Quervain's disease /kervānz', kervɛNz'/ [Fritz de Quervain, Swiss surgeon, 1868–1940; L, *dis;* Fr, *aise,* ease], chronic tenosynovitis of the abductor pollicis longus and extensor pollicis brevis muscles of the thumb.

quick connect [ME, *quic,* living; L, *connectere,* to bind], a plastic or similar connecting device that is attached to or implanted in a patient who will be joined to an electromechanical or other apparatus.

quickening /kwik'(ə)ning/ [ME, *quic,* living], the first feeling by a pregnant woman of movement of her baby in utero, usually occurring between 16 and 20 weeks of gestation.

Quick's test [Armand J. Quick, American physician, 1894–1978], **1.** a test for jaundice. The patient is given an oral dose of sodium benzoate, which is conjugated in the liver with glycine to form hippuric acid. The amount of hippuric acid excreted in the urine is inversely proportional to the degree of liver damage. **2.** a test for hemophilia. A solution of thromboplastin is added to oxalated blood plasma and calcium chloride. The amount of time required for formation of a firm clot is inversely proportional to the amount of prothrombin in the plasma.

quiescent /kwī-es'ənt/, **1.** inactive, quiet, or at rest. **2.** latent. **3.** dormant.

quiet alert /kwī'ət/, a period when a neonate is calm and attentive, with eyes open, ready to become acquainted with an adult person. Newborns spend about 10% of their time in this state.

Quigley traction /kwig'lē/, a type of traction for lateral malleolar and trimalleolar fractures in which a stockinette is placed around the leg and ankle and attached to an overhead frame, thus suspending the leg by the ankle.

quinacrine hydrochloride /kī'nəkren/, an anthelmintic and antimalarial prescribed in the treatment of giardiasis and cestodiasis and the treatment and suppression of malaria.

Quincke's disease [Heinrich I. Quincke, German physician, 1842–1922; L, *dis* + Fr, *aise,* ease], angioneurotic edema, a potentially fatal chronic condition of subcutaneous edema, abdominal pain, urticaria, and laryngeal edema.

Quincke's pulse /kwing'kēz/ [Heinrich I. Quincke], an abnormal alternate blanching and reddening of the skin or nails that may be observed in several ways, such as by pressing the front edge of the fingernail and watching the blood in the nail bed recede and return. This pulsation is characteristic of aortic insufficiency.

quinidine /kwin'ədēn, -din/, an antiarrhythmic agent used as a bisulfate, gluconate, polygalacturonate, or sulfate. It is prescribed in the treatment of atrial flutter, atrial fibrillation, premature ventricular contractions, and tachycardias.

quinine /kwī'nīn/ [Sp, *quina,* bark], a white bitter crystalline alkaloid made from cinchona bark.

quinolone /kwin'əlōn/, any of a class of antibiotics that act by interrupting the replication of deoxyribonucleic acid molecules in bacteria.

quintan /kwin'tən/ [L, *quintanus,* relating to the fifth], recurring on the fifth day, or at about 96-hour intervals.

quintessence /kwintes'əns/ [L, *quinta* + *essentia,* the fifth essence], **1.** a highly concentrated extract of any substance. **2.** a tincture or extract containing the most essential components of plant materials.

Q

quintuplet /kwin'tŏŏplit, kwintŏŏ'plit/ [L, *quintuplex*, fivefold], any one of five offspring born of the same gestation period during a single pregnancy.

quotidian /kwōtid'ē·ən/ [L, *quotidianus*, daily], occurring every day; for example, a malarial fever with daily attacks.

quotient /kwō'shənt/, the number obtained by dividing one number by another.

quot. op sit, abbreviation for the Latin phrase *quoties opus sit,* 'as often as necessary.'

q.v.,   **1.** abbreviation for the Latin phrase *quantum vis,* 'as much as you please.' **2.** abbreviation for the Latin phrase *quod vide,* 'which see.'

Q wave, the first negative component of the QRS complex preceding an R wave. Lengthening of the wave indicates myocardial infarction.

R

r, 1. abbreviation for *right.* 2. symbol for *resistance ohm.*

R, 1. abbreviation for **resolution.** 2. abbreviation for **respiratory exchange ratio.** 3. abbreviation for **roentgen.** 4. symbol for *gas constant.*

R$_f$, symbol for a ratio used in paper and thin-layer chromatography, representing the distance from the origin to the center of the separated zone divided by the distance from the origin to the solvent front. 2. abbreviation for **radiofrequency.**

R$_i$, symbol for *inhibitory receptor* molecule.

R$_s$, symbol for *stimulatory receptor* molecule.

R$_x$, symbol for the Latin *recipe,* 'take.'

Ra, symbol for the element **radium.**

RA, 1. abbreviation for **rheumatoid arthritis;** 2. abbreviation for *right atrium.*

rabid /rab′id/ [L, *rabidus,* raving], pertaining to or suffering from rabies, displaying signs of madness, agitation, delirium, hallucinations, and bizarre behavior.

rabies /rā′bēz/ [L, *rabere,* to rave], an acute, usually fatal viral disease of the central nervous system of animals. It is transmitted from animals to people by infected blood, tissue, or, most commonly, saliva. The reservoir of the virus is chiefly wild animals, including skunks, bats, foxes, dogs, raccoons, and cats. After introduction into the human body, often by a bite of an infected animal, the virus travels along nerve pathways to the brain and later to other organs. An incubation period ranges from 10 days to 1 year and is followed by a prodromal period characterized by fever, malaise, headache, paresthesia, and myalgia. After several days severe encephalitis, delirium, agonizingly painful muscular spasms, seizures, paralysis, coma, and death ensue. —**rabid**/rab′id/, *adj.*

rabies immune globulin (RIG), a solution of antirabies immune globulin used in conjunction with rabies duck embryo vaccine for possible protection against rabies in persons suspected of exposure to rabies.

rabies vaccine (DEV), a sterile suspension of killed rabies virus prepared from duck embryo. It is prescribed for immunization and postexposure prophylaxis against rabies.

rabies virus group [L, *rabere,* to rave, *virus,* poison; It, *gruppo,* knot], the genus of viruses that includes the organism that causes rabies in humans, the *lyssa* virus.

race [It, *razza*], 1. a vague unscientific term for a group of genetically related people who share certain physical characteristics. 2. a distinct ethnic group characterized by traits that are transmitted through their offspring.

racemic /rāsē′mik/ [L, *racemus,* bunch of grapes], pertaining to a compound made up of dextrorotatory and levorotatory isomers, rendering it optically inactive under polarized light.

racemose /ras′əmōs′/ [L, *racemus*], like a bunch of grapes. The term is used in describing a structure in which many branches terminate in nodular cystlike forms such as pulmonary alveoli.

racemose aneurysm, a pronounced dilation of lengthened and tortuous blood vessels, which may form a tumor.

rachial /rā′kē·əl/ [Gk, *rhachis,* backbone], pertaining to the spinal column.

rachiopagus /rā′kē·op′əgəs/ [Gk, *rachis,* backbone, *pagos,* fixed], conjoined symmetric twins united back to back along the spinal column.

rachiresistance /rākēresis′təns/ [Gk, *rachis,* backbone], a failure to respond adequately to spinal anesthesia.

rachischisis /rəkis′kəsis/ [Gk, *rachis* + *schizein,* to split], a congenital fissure of one or more vertebrae.

rachitic /rəkit′ik/, 1. pertaining to rickets. 2. resembling or suggesting the condition of one afflicted with rickets.

rachitic dwarf, a person whose retarded growth is caused by rickets.

rachitis /rəkī′tis/ [Gk, *rachis* + *itis,* inflammation], 1. rickets. 2. an inflammatory disease of the vertebral column.

rachitis fetalis annularis, congenital enlargement of the epiphyses of the long bones.

rachitis fetalis micromelia, congenital shortening of the long bones.

racial immunity /rā′shəl/ [It, *razza* + L, *immunis,* free], a form of natural immunity shared by most of the members of a genetically related population.

rad /rad/, abbreviation for *radiation absorbed dose*; the basic unit of absorbed dose of ionizing radiation. One rad is equal to the absorption of 100 ergs of radiation energy per gram of matter and therefore differs from the roentgen.

radappertization /rad'apur'tizā'shən/, the irradiation of food for the destruction of *Clostridium botulinum*.

radarkymography /rā'därkīmog'rəfē/ [radar + Gk, *kyma*, wave, *graphein*, to record], a radar (radio detection and ranging) technique for showing the size and outline of the heart, using a radar tracking device and a fluoroscopic screen to display images produced by electrical impulses passed over the chest surface.

Radford nomogram [Edward P. Radford, Jr., American physiologist, b. 1922], a mathematic chart device used in respiratory therapy to estimate combined tidal volumes and rates for mechanical ventilation. It is based on three parameters of body weight, sex, and respiratory rate.

radial /rā'dē-əl/ [L, *radius*, ray], pertaining to the radius.

radial artery [L, *radius*, ray], an artery in the forearm, starting at the bifurcation of the brachial artery and passing in 12 branches to the forearm, wrist, and hand.

radial keratotomy (RK), a surgical procedure in which a series of tiny shallow incisions are made on the cornea, causing it to bulge slightly to correct for nearsightedness.

radial nerve, the largest branch of the brachial plexus, arising on each side as a continuation of the posterior cord. It supplies the skin of the arm and forearm and their extensor muscles.

radial nerve palsy, a type of mononeuropathy characterized by radial nerve damage with symptoms of forearm muscle weakness and sensory loss. It may be caused by excessive compression of the radial nerve against a hard surface in individuals insensitized by the intake of alcohol or sedatives. It may also be caused by the repeated compression of the nerve by various weights.

radial notch of ulna, the narrow lateral depression in the coronoid process of the ulna that receives the head of the radius.

radial paralysis [L, *radius* + Gk, *paralyein*], musculospiral paralysis involving muscles supplied by the radial nerve, mainly the wrist and finger extensors.

radial pulse, the pulse of the radial artery palpated at the wrist over the radius. The radial pulse is the one most often taken, because of the ease with which it is palpated.

radial recurrent artery, a branch of the radial artery arising just distal to the elbow, ascending between the branches of the radial nerve, and supplying several muscles of the arm and the elbow.

radial reflex, a normal reflex elicited by tapping over the distal radius, with the response being flexion of the forearm.

radial symmetry, a form of symmetry in which body parts are arranged around a central axis, as found in animals such as jellyfish and sea urchins.

radiant /rā'dē-ənt/ [L, *radiare*, to emit rays], pertaining to any object that emits rays or is the center of rays that spread outward.

radiant energy [L, *radiare*, to emit rays; Gk *energeia*], energy emitted as electromagnetic radiation such as radio waves, infrared radiation, visible light, ultraviolet light, x-rays, and gamma rays.

radiant heat, a form of infrared energy that is emitted in electromagnetic waves from a central source. It proceeds outward in wavelengths greater than those of visible light. Objects absorbing the energy experience a rise in temperature.

radiate /rā'dē-āt/ [L, *radiare*, to emit rays], to diverge or spread from a common point.

radiate ligament, a ligament that connects the head of a rib with a vertebra and an associated intervertebral disk.

radiation /rā'dē-ā'shən/ [L, *radiatio*], **1.** the emission of energy, rays, or waves. **2.** (in medicine) the use of a radioactive substance in the diagnosis or treatment of disease.

radiation absorbed dose (rad), a unit of absorbed dose of ionizing radiation. One rad is equal to 0.01 joules per kilogram, or 100 ergs of ionizing radiation per gram of tissue or other substance.

radiation burn, a burn resulting from exposure to radiant energy in the form of sunlight, x-rays, or nuclear emissions or explosion. Ionizing radiation can produce tissue damage directly by striking a vital molecule such as deoxyribonucleic acid.

radiation caries, a morbid increase in tooth decay, especially affecting the coronal root area caused by ionizing radiation of the oral and maxillary structure. Radiation caries is often a side effect of treatment for oral malignancies.

radiation cataract [L, *radiare*, to emit rays; Gk, *katarrhaktes*, portcullis], a cataract that is caused by excessive exposure of the eye to x-rays or other types of radiation that cause a change in the protein molecules of the lens.

radiation dermatitis [L, *radiare,* to emit rays; Gk, *derma,* skin, *itis,* inflammation], an acute or chronic inflammation of the skin caused by exposure to ionizing radiation, as in cancer radiation therapy. Symptoms, which may not appear until 3 weeks after exposure, include redness, blistering, and sloughing of the skin. In severe cases the condition can progress to scarring, fibrosis, and atrophy.

radiation detector, a device for converting radiant energy to an observable form, used for detecting the presence and sometimes the amount of radiation.

Radiation Effects Research Foundation (RERF), an organization that studies the long-term effects of atomic bombings of Hiroshima and Nagasaki during World War II on survivors.

radiation exposure, a measure of the ionization produced in air by x-rays or gamma rays. It is the sum of the electric charges on all ions of one sign that are produced when all electrons liberated by photons in a volume of air are completely stopped, divided by the mass of air in the volume element. The unit of exposure is the roentgen. Acute radiation exposure is exposure of short duration to intense ionizing radiation, usually occurring as the result of an accidental spill of radioactive material.

radiation exposure, emergency procedures, first aid treatment of a person who has received external body radiation through exposure to radioactive material or internal radiation contamination by inhaling or ingesting radioactive material. External radiation exposure is treated initially by cleansing and surgical isolation to protect others. One who has inhaled or ingested radioactive material should be given emergency treatment similar to a person who has been exposed to chemical poisons. But body wastes should be collected and checked for radiation levels. If the victim has also suffered a wound, care must be taken to avoid cross-contamination of exposed surfaces. In general, except for taking special precautions to control the spread of radiation effects, the patient should be given any lifesaving emergency treatment needed, and personnel handling the patient should wear surgical gowns, caps, and gloves.

radiation force, a small steady force that is produced when a sound beam strikes a reflecting or absorbing surface. It is proportional to the acoustic power.

radiation hygiene, the art and science of protecting human beings from injury by radiation. It reduces clinical exposure from external radiation through protective barriers of radiation-absorbing material, ensures safe distances between people and radiation sources, reduces radiation exposure times, or uses combinations of all these measures.

radiation oncologist, a physician with special training in the use of ionizing radiation in the treatment of cancers.

radiation oncology, the study of the treatment of cancer using ionizing radiation.

radiation protection, use of devices, equipment, distance, and barriers to reduce the risk of exposure to ionizing radiation in a health care facility, research center, or industrial site where radiation-emitting devices are used. The risk also varies with the type and intensity of radiation.

radiation risk, a hazard to health resulting from exposure to natural and synthetic radioactive materials. Radiation sources include cosmic rays, radon, radium, and other radionuclides in the soil, nuclear reactors, accelerators, and weapons; uranium mining and milling; and diagnostic and therapeutic x-ray devices.

radiation safety committee, an organization responsible for monitoring and maintaining a safe radiation environment. It is used in institutions where radiation is produced and/or used.

radiation sensitivity, a measure of the response of tissue to ionizing radiation.

radiation sickness, an abnormal condition resulting from exposure to ionizing radiation. Moderate exposure may cause headache, nausea, vomiting, anorexia, and diarrhea; long-term exposure may result in sterility, damage to the fetus in pregnant women, leukemia or other forms of cancer, alopecia, and cataracts.

radiation symbol, a universal symbol consisting of a 'purple propeller' pattern of three fan-shaped images arranged at positions 120° apart as if radiating from a solid dark circle on a yellow background. The symbol is intended to identify sources or containers of radioactive materials and areas of potential radiation exposure.

radiation therapist, an allied health professional who administers radiation therapy services to patients, observing patients during treatment and maintaining records. Duties may include tumor localization, dosimetry, patient follow-up, and patient education.

Radiation Therapy Management, a Nursing Interventions Classification defined as assisting the patient to understand

R

and minimize the side effects of radiation treatments.

radical /rad'ikəl/ [L, *radix,* root], **1.** an atom or group of atoms that contains an unpaired electron. A radical does not exist freely in nature. **2.** pertaining to drastic therapy, such as the surgical removal of an organ, limb, or other part of the body.

radical dissection, the surgical removal of tissue in an extensive area surrounding the operative site. Most often it is performed to identify and excise all tissue that may possibly be malignant to decrease the chance of recurrence.

radical mastectomy, surgical removal of an entire breast; pectoral muscles; axillary lymph nodes; and all fat, fascia, and adjacent tissues. It is one kind of surgical treatment for breast cancer.

radical neck dissection, dissection and removal of all lymph nodes and removable tissues under the skin of the neck, performed to prevent the spread of malignant tumors of the head and neck that have a reasonable chance of being controlled.

radical nephrectomy, the surgical removal of a kidney, usually performed in the treatment of cancer of the kidney.

radical surgery [L, *radix,* root; Gk, *cheirourgia,* surgery], surgery that is usually extensive and complex and intended to correct a severe health threat such as a rapidly growing cancer.

radical therapy, 1. a treatment intended to cure, not palliate. **2.** a definitive extreme treatment; not conservative, such as radical mastectomy rather than simple or partial mastectomy.

radicidation /rādisidā'shən /, the irradiation of food to inactivate nonsporing pathogens of *Salmonella* and other microorganisms.

radicular /rədik'yələr/ [L, *radix,* root], pertaining to a root, such as a spinal nerve root.

radicular cyst [L, *radix,* root; Gk, *kystis.* bag], (in dentistry) a cyst with a wall of fibrous connective tissue and a lining of stratified squamous epithelium that is attached to the apex of the root of a tooth with dead pulp or a defective root canal filling.

radicular retainer, a type of retainer that lies within the body of a tooth, usually in the root part, such as a dowel crown.

radicular retention, a resistance to displacement developed by placing metal projections into the root canals of pulpless teeth.

radiculitis /rədik'yəlī'tis/ [L, *radix,* root; Gk, *itis,* inflammation], an inflammation involving a spinal nerve root, resulting in pain and hyperesthesia.

radiculopathy /rədik'yəlop'əthē/ [L, *radix,* root; Gk, *pathos,* disease], a disease involving a spinal nerve root.

radioactive /-ak'tiv/ [L, *radius,* ray, *activus,* active], giving off radiation as the result of the disintegration of the nucleus of an atom.

radioactive contamination, the undesirable addition of radioactive material to the body or part of the environment, such as clothing or equipment. Beta radiation contamination of the body of health care personnel is only possible through the ingestion, inhalation, or absorption of the source, as when the skin is contaminated with a beta emitter contained in an absorbable chemical form. Instruments, drapes, surgical gloves, and clothing that come in contact with serous fluids, blood, and urine of patients containing beta or gamma radiation emitters may be contaminated.

radioactive contrast media, a solution or colloid containing material of high atomic number, used for visualizing soft tissue structures.

radioactive decay, the disintegration of the nucleus of an unstable nuclide by the spontaneous emission of charged particles, photons, or both.

radioactive element, an element subject to spontaneous degeneration of its nucleus accompanied by the emission of alpha particles, beta particles, or gamma rays. All elements with atomic numbers greater than 83 are radioactive.

radioactive implant, a small container holding a radioactive isotope to be embedded in tissues for purposes of interstitial radiotherapy.

radioactive iodine (RAI), a radioactive isotope of iodine, used as a tracer in biology and medicine.

radioactive iodine excretion, the elimination by the body of radioactive iodine (RAI) administered in a test of thyroid function and in the treatment of hyperthyroidism. Most RAI is excreted in urine, but small amounts may be found in sputum, perspiration, feces, and vomitus.

radioactive iodine excretion test, a method of evaluating thyroid function by measuring the amount of radioactive iodine (RAI) in urine after the patient is given an oral tracer dose of the radioisotope ^{131}I. After administration of the tracer, a scintillation detector is placed over the patient's neck at 2, 6, and 24 hours to measure the RAI accumulated by the thyroid.

radioactive iodine uptake (RAIU), the absorption and incorporation by the thyroid of radioactive iodine (RAI), administered orally as a tracer dose in a test of thyroid function and as larger doses for the treatment of hyperthyroidism.

radioactive tracer, a molecule to which a radioactive atom, or tag, has been attached so it can be followed through a physiologic system with radiation detectors.

radioactivity /-activ′itē/, the emission of corpuscular α or β or electromagnetic γ radiations as a consequence of nuclear disintegration.

radioallergosorbent test (RAST) /rā′-dē·ō′alur′gōsôr′-bənt/ [L, *radius* + Gk, *allos,* other, *ergein,* to work; L, *absorbere,* to swallow], a test in which a technique of radioimmunoassay is used to identify and quantify IgE in serum that has been mixed with any of 45 known allergens. If an atopic allergy to a substance exists, an antigen-antibody reaction occurs with characteristic conjugation and clumping.

radiobiology /-bī·ol′əjē/ [L, *radius* + *bios,* life, *logos,* science], the branch of the natural sciences dealing with the effects of radiation on biologic systems. —**radiobiologic, radiobiological,** *adj.*

radiocarcinogenesis /-kär′sinəjen′əsis/, the production of cancer by exposure to ionizing radiation.

radiocarpal articulation /-kär′pəl/ [L, *radius* + Gk, *karpos,* wrist], the condyloid joint at the wrist that connects the radius and distal surface of an articular disk with the scaphoid, lunate, and triangular bones. The joint involves four ligaments and allows all movements but rotation.

radiochemistry /-kem′istrē/ [L, *radius* + Gk, *chemiea,* alchemy], the branch of chemistry that deals with the properties and behavior of radioactive materials and the use of radionuclides in the study of chemical and biologic problems.

radiocurable /·kyoō′rəbəl/, pertaining to the susceptibility of tumor cells to destruction by ionizing radiation.

radiodermatitis /-dur′mətī′tis/, a skin inflammation caused by exposure to ionizing radiation. The skin changes resemble those of thermal damage.

radiofrequency (rf) /-frē′kwənsē/ [L, *radius* + *frequens*], the part of the electromagnetic spectrum with frequencies lower than about 10^{10} Hz, used to produce magnetic resonance images.

radiofrequency ablation, unmodulated high-frequency alternating current flow that is applied to tissue to cause heat and cell injury for the purpose of destroying areas of extra stimuli and pathways to the heart. The technique has replaced surgical ablation.

radiofrequency (rf) signal, 1. an electri-

cal signal whose frequency is in the rf range. 2. a signal within an ultrasound instrument between the transducer terminals and components where rectification and filtering occur.

radiograph /rā′dē·əgraf′/, an x-ray image.

radiographer /rā′dē·og′rəfər/, an allied health professional who performs diagnostic examinations on patients using a variety of modalities, including radiography, computed tomography, magnetic resonance imaging, mammography, and cardiovascular interventional technology. In addition to the technical duties of evaluating radiographs, evaluating equipment performance, and managing a quality assurance program, radiographers also play significant roles in patient assessment and education.

radiographic grid /-graf′ik/, a device used to reduce the amount of scatter radiation reaching the x-ray film. Grids are fabricated using parallel strips of radiopaque materials with alternating strips of radiolucent materials.

radiographic magnification, a radiographic procedure used to improve visualization of fine blood vessels and small bony structures. Magnification is achieved by increasing the distance of the object from the radiographic image receptor.

radiographic position, the specific position of the body or body part in relation to the table or the image receptor.

radiographic projection, the path taken by an x-ray beam as it passes through the body. It is described as if the body were in the anatomic position.

radiographic view, the body image as seen by the image receptor. It is the opposite of the radiographic projection.

radiography /rā′dē·og′rəfē/ [L, *radius* + Gk, *graphein,* to record], the production of shadow images on photographic emulsion through the action of ionizing radiation. —**radiographic,** *adj.*

radioimmunoassay (RIA) /rā′dē·ō·im′-yənō·os′ā/imyoo͞o′nō·as′ā/ [L, *radius* + *immunis,* free; Fr, *essayer,* to try], a technique in radiology used to determine the concentration of an antigen, antibody, or other protein in the serum.

radioimmunofluorescence assay (RIPA) /rā′dē·ō·im′yənō′flŏŏres′əns/, a test for the presence of antibodies sometimes used to confirm the results of ELISA or other methods.

radioimmunosorbent test (RIST) /rā′-dē·ō·im′yənōsôr′bənt/ [L, *radius* + *immunis* + *absorbere,* to swallow], a test that uses serum immunoglobulin E to detect allergies to various substances such as

R

certain cosmetics, animal fur, dust, and grasses.

radioiodine /rā'dē·ō·ī'ədīn/ [L, *radius* + Gk, *ioeides,* violet], a radioactive isotope of iodine used in nuclear medicine and radiotherapy. A common form of radioiodine is ^{131}I.

radioisotope /rā'dē·ō·ī'sətōp/ [L, *radius* + Gk, *isos,* equal, *topos* place], a radioactive isotope of an element, used for therapeutic and diagnostic purposes.

radioisotope scan, a two-dimensional representation of the gamma rays emitted by a radioisotope, showing its concentration in a body site such as the thyroid gland, brain, or kidney.

Radiological Society of North America (RSNA), a professional organization of radiologists. The group originated the certification of operators of x-ray equipment in 1920 but is no longer involved in such certification.

radiologic anatomy /-loj'ik/ [L, *radius* + Gk, *logos,* science], (in applied anatomy) the study of the structure and morphology of the tissues and organs of the body based on their x-ray visualization.

radiologic technologist, a person who, under the supervision of a physician radiologist, operates radiologic equipment and assists radiologists and other health professionals, and whose competence has been tested and approved by the American Registry of Radiologic Technologists.

radiologist /rā'dē·ol'əjist/, a physician who specializes in radiology. A certified radiologist is one whose competence has been tested and approved by the American Board of Radiology.

radiology /-ol'əjē/ [L, *radius* + *logos,* science], the branch of medicine concerned with radioactive substances and, using various techniques of visualization, with the diagnosis and treatment of disease using any of the various sources of radiant energy. Three subbranches of radiology are **diagnostic radiology,** which concerns itself with imaging using external sources of radiation; **nuclear medicine,** which is involved with imaging radioactive materials that are placed into body organs; and therapeutic radiology, which is concerned with the treatment of cancer using radiation. —**radiologic, radiological,** *adj.*

radiolucency /-lōō'sənsē/ [L, *radiare* + *lucere,* to shine], a characteristic of materials of relatively low atomic number that have low attenuation characteristics, allowing most x-rays to pass through them, producing relatively dark images. —**radiolucent,** *adj.*

radiolucent /-lōō'sənt/ [L, *radiare,* to emit rays, *lucere,* to shine], pertaining to materials that allow x-rays to penetrate with a minimum of absorption.

radionecrosis /-nəkrō'sis/, tissue death caused by radiation.

radionuclide /-nōō'klīd/ [L, *radiare* + *nucleus,* nut kernel], **1.** an isotope (or nuclide) that undergoes radioactive decay. **2.** any of the radioactive isotopes of cobalt, iodine, phosphorus, strontium, and other elements used in nuclear medicine for treatment of tumors and cancers and for nuclear imaging of internal parts of the body.

radionuclide angiocardiography, the radiographic examination of cardiac blood vessels after an intravenous injection of a radiopharmaceutical.

radionuclide imaging, the noninvasive examination of various parts of the body, especially the heart, using a radiopharmaceutical such as thallium 201 and a detection device such as a gamma camera, rectilinear scanner, or positron camera.

radiopacity /-pas'itē/ [L, *radiare,* to emit rays, *opacus,* obscure], the quality of being radiopaque, or having the ability to stop or reduce the passage of x-radiation.

radiopaque /-pāk'/ [L, *radiare* + *opacus,* obscure], not permitting the passage of x-rays or other radiant energy. Bones are relatively radiopaque and therefore show as white areas on an exposed x-ray film. —**radiopacity,** *n.*

radiopaque contrast medium, a chemical substance that does not permit the passage of x-rays. Various radiopaque compounds are used to outline the interior of hollow organs such as heart chambers, blood vessels, respiratory passages, and the biliary tract in x-ray or fluoroscopic pictures.

radiopathology /-pəthol'əjē/, a branch of medicine involving both pathology and radiology and concerned with the effects of ionizing radiation on body tissues.

radiopharmaceutical /-fär'məsōō'tikəl/ [L, *radiare* + Gk, *pharmakeuein,* to give a drug], a drug that contains radioactive atoms. Kinds of radiopharmaceuticals are **diagnostic radiopharmaceutical, research radiopharmaceutical,** and **therapeutic radiopharmaceutical.**

radiopharmacist /-fär'məsist/, a trained professional responsible for formulating and dispensing prescribed radioactive tracers and for the clinical aspects of radiopharmacy. Radiopharmacists are required to receive training in radioactive tracer techniques, in the safe handling of radioactive materials, in the preparation and quality control of drugs for administration to humans, and in the basic principles of nuclear medicine.

radiopharmacy /-fär'məsē/ [L, *radiare* + Gk, *pharmakeuein,* to give a drug], a facility for the preparation and dispensing of radioactive drugs and for the storage of radioactive materials, inventory records, and prescriptions of radioactive substances. The radiopharmacy is usually the correlation point for radioactive wastes.

radioprotective drugs /-prətek'tiv/ [L, *radiare,* to emit rays, *protegere,* to cover; Fr, *drogue*], pharmaceuticals that protect the body against ionizing radiation. An example is Lugol's solution, an aqueous solution of iodine used to supply iodine internally, thereby blocking the uptake of radioactive iodine.

radioresistance /-risis'təns/ [L, *radiare* + *resistare,* to withstand], the relative resistance of cells, tissues, organs, organisms, chemical compounds, or any other substances to the effects of radiation.

radioresistant /-risis'tənt/, unchanged by or protected against damage by radioactive emissions such as x-rays, alpha particles, or gamma rays.

radioresponsive /-rispon'siv/, pertaining to the sensitivity of a chemical or tissue to radiation, whether harmful or beneficial.

radiosensitive /-sen'sitiv/ [L, *radiare* + *sentire,* to feel], capable of being changed by or reacting to radioactive emissions such as x-rays, alpha particles, or gamma rays.

radiosensitivity /-sen'sitiv'itē/, the relative susceptibility of cells, tissues, organs, organisms, or any other living substances to the effects of radiation. Cells of self-renewing systems, as those in the crypts of the intestine, are the most radiosensitive. Cells that divide regularly but mature between divisions, such as spermatogonia and spermatocytes, are next in radiosusceptibility. Long-lived cells that usually do not undergo mitosis unless there is a suitable stimulus include the less radiosensitive liver, kidney, and thyroid cells. Least sensitive are fixed postmitotic cells that have lost the ability to divide, such as neurons.

radiosensitizers /-sen'sitī'zərs/ [L, *radiare* + *sentire* + Gk, *izein,* to cause], drugs that enhance the killing effect of radiation on cells.

radiotherapist /-ther'əpist/, a health professional who specializes in the use of electromagnetic or particulate radiation, including the application of radiopharmaceuticals, in the treatment of disease..

radiotherapy /-ther'əpē/ [Gk, *radiare,* to emit rays; Gk, *therapeia,* treatment], the treatment of neoplastic disease by using x-rays or gamma rays, usually from a cobalt source, to deter the proliferation of malignant cells by decreasing the rate of mitosis or impairing deoxyribonucleic acid synthesis.

radioulnar articulation /-ul'nər/ [L, *radius,* ray, *ulna,* elbow], the articulation of the radius and ulna, consisting of a proximal articulation, a distal articulation, and three sets of ligaments.

radium (Ra) /rā'dē·əm/ [L, *radius,* ray], a radioactive metallic element of the alkaline earth group. Its atomic number is 88. Four radium isotopes occur naturally and have different atomic masses (weights): 223, 224, 226, and 228.

radium insertion, the introduction of metallic radium (Ra) into a body cavity, such as the uterus or cervix, to treat cancer.

radium therapy [L, *radius,* ray; Gk, *therapeia,* treatment], the use of radium and its radioactive emissions to treat disease.

radium 226, a radioactive substance used for most of this century to fill the needles and tubes required for brachytherapy. Radium use is now being replaced by cesium 137 and cobalt 60, which have similar energy characteristics and are not subject to hazardous leakage as radium sources sometimes are.

radius /rā'dē·əs/, *pl.* **radii** /rā'dē·ī/ [L, ray], one of the bones of the forearm lying parallel to the ulna. Its proximal end is small and forms a part of the elbow joint. The distal end is large and forms a part of the wrist joint.

radon (Rn) /rā'don/ [L, *radiare,* to emit rays], a radioactive, inert, gaseous, nonmetallic element. Its atomic number is 86; its atomic mass (weight) is 222. Radon, a decay product of radium, is used in radiation cancer therapy.

radon daughters, electrically charged ions that are decay products of radon gas. Radon daughters are regarded as a potential health hazard by the U.S. Environmental Protection Agency because they tend to adhere to surfaces such as alveoli of the lungs, where they can cause ionizing radiation damage. Radon is released by rocks, soil, and groundwater.

radon seed, a small sealed tube of glass or gold containing radon and visible radiographically, for insertion into body tissues in the treatment of malignancies.

radon 222, the radioactive daughter of radium 226 that has been used to fill seeds for permanent implantation into tumors. This material is being replaced by the more manageable radionuclide iodine 125.

RAI, abbreviation for **radioactive iodine.**

RAIU, abbreviation for **radioactive iodine uptake.**

RA latex test, abbreviation for *rheumatoid arthritis latex test.*

rale /rāl, ral, räl/ [Fr, *râle* rattle], a common abnormal respiratory sound heard on auscultation of the chest during inspiration, characterized by discontinuous bubbling noises. Although the term rale is commonly used, the American Thoracic Society now prefers **crackle,** as this term is more descriptive of the actual sound heard.

ramification /ram'ifikā'shən/ [L, *ramus,* branch, *facere,* to make], a branching, distribution.

Ramsay Hunt's syndrome [James Ramsay Hunt, American neurologist, 1872–1937], a neurologic condition resulting from invasion of the seventh nerve ganglia and the geniculate ganglion by varicella zoster virus, characterized by severe ear pain, facial nerve paralysis, vertigo, hearing loss, and often mild generalized encephalitis.

ramus /rā'məs/, *pl.* **rami** [L, branch], a small branchlike structure extending from a larger one or dividing into two or more parts, such as a branch of a nerve or artery or one of the rami of the pubis. — **ramification,** *n.* **ramify,** *v.*

Ranchos Los Amigos Scale, a scale of cognitive functioning, developed as a behavioral rating scale to aid in assessment and treatment of head-injured persons. Eight levels of cognitive functioning are identified, from I (no response) to VIII (purposeful and appropriate behavioral response).

rancidity /ransid'itē/, the unpleasant taste and smell of fatty foods that have undergone decomposition, liberating butyric acid and other volatile lipids.

random controlled trial [ME, *randoun,* run violently; Fr, *controle,* check, *trier,* to grind], a study plan for a proposed new treatment in which subjects are assigned on a random basis to participate either in an experimental group receiving the new treatment or in a control group that does not.

randomization [ME, *randoun,* run violently], the process of assigning subjects or objects to a control or experimental group on a random basis.

random mating [ME, *randoun,* run violently, *gemate*], a pairing of subjects when each individual has an equal chance of mating with those of other genetic backgrounds.

random sampling [ME, *randoun,* run violently; L, *exemplum*], a method of sampling for a study in which each individual has the same chance of being selected and the choice of a particular individual does not affect the chances of the others.

random selection, a method of choosing subjects for a research study in which all members of a particular group have an equal chance of being selected.

random voided specimen, a voided urine specimen obtained at any point of a 24-hour period.

range /rānj/ [OFr, *ranger,* to arrange in a row], the interval between the lowest and highest values in a series of data.

range abnormalities, uncertainties in the actual range from which Doppler signals or echo signals originate. In pulsed Doppler instruments a high pulse repetition frequency can result in range ambiguities.

range equation, a relationship between the distance to a reflector and the time it takes for a pulse of ultrasound to propagate to the reflector and return to the transducer.

range of accommodation [OFr, *ranger* + L, *accommodatio*], the distance between the farthest point that an object can be seen clearly with accommodation fully relaxed and the nearest distance that an object can be observed with full accommodation, measured in inches or centimeters.

range of motion (ROM) [OFr, *ranger* + L, *motio*], the extent of movement of a joint, from maximum extension to maximum flexion, as measured in degrees of a circle.

range-of-motion exercise [OFr, *ranger,* to arrange in a row; L, *motio,* movement], any body action involving the muscles, joints, and natural directional movements such as abduction, extension, flexion, pronation, and rotation. Such exercises are usually applied actively or passively in the prevention and treatment of orthopedic deformities, in the assessment of injuries and deformities, and in athletic conditioning.

ranitidine /ranit'idēn/, a histamine H_2 receptor antagonist prescribed in the treatment of duodenal and gastric ulcers and gastric hypersecretory conditions.

Rankine scale [William J. M. Rankine, Scottish physicist, 1820–1870], an absolute temperature scale calculated in degrees Fahrenheit. Absolute zero on the Rankine scale is −460° F, equivalent to −273° C.

ranula /ran'yōōlə/, *pl.* **ranulae** [L, *rana,* frog], a large mucocele in the floor of the mouth, usually caused by obstruction of the ducts of the sublingual salivary glands and less commonly caused by obstruction of the ducts of the submandibular salivary glands.

Ranvier's nodes /ränvē·āz'/, räN-/ [Louis A. Ranvier, French pathologist, 1835–1922], constrictions in the medullary substance of a nerve fiber at more or less regular intervals.

rape [L, *rapere*, to seize], a sexual assault, homosexual or heterosexual, the legal definitions for which vary from state to state. Rape is a crime of violence or one committed under the threat of violence, and its victims are treated for medical and psychologic trauma.

rape counseling, counseling by a trained person provided to a victim of rape. Rape counseling ideally begins at the time the crime is first reported, as in an emergency room. Initially the counselor offers sensitive support for the victim by accepting the victim in a nonprejudicial, noncritical way. Counseling personnel may provide supportive services and advocacy and liaison between the victim and medical, legal, and law enforcement authorities. This involves staying with the victim during medical examination, during questioning by police or the district attorney, and throughout the criminal justice process.

rape-trauma syndrome, a NANDA-accepted nursing diagnosis of the experience of being raped, which is defined as forced, violent sexual penetration against the victim's will and consent. The trauma syndrome that develops from this attack includes an acute phase of disorganization and a longer phase of reorganization in the victim's life. The defining characteristics are divided into three subcomponents: rape trauma, compound reaction, and silent reaction. Rape trauma in the acute phase consists of emotional reactions of anger, guilt, and embarrassment; fear of physical violence and death; humiliation; wish for revenge; and multiple physical complaints. The compound reaction is characterized by all of the defining characteristics of rape trauma, reliance on alcohol or drugs, or recurrence of the symptoms of previous conditions, including psychiatric illness. The silent reaction sometimes occurs in place of the rape trauma or compound reaction. The defining characteristics of the silent reaction are an abrupt change in the victim's usual sexual relationships, an increase in nightmares, an increasing anxiety during the interview about the rape incident, a marked change in sexual behavior, denial of the rape or refusal to discuss it, and the sudden development of phobic reactions.

Rape-Trauma Treatment, a Nursing Interventions Classification defined as provision of emotional and physical support immediately following an alleged rape.

raphe /rā′fē/ [Gk, *rhaphe*, seam], a line of union of the halves of various symmetric parts, such as the abdominal raphe of

the linea alba or the raphe penis, which appears as a narrow dark streak on the inferior surface of the penis.

raphe of tongue [Gk, *rhaphe*, seam; AS, *tunge*], a fibrous wall that forms a line of union between the right and left sides of the tongue.

rapid grower /rap′id/, a saprophytic mycobacterium in group IV of the Runyon classification system that grows within 3 to 5 days.

rapid plasma reagin (RPR) test, an agglutination examination used in screening for syphilis. The test detects two groups of antibodies. The first is a nontreponemal antibody (reagin) directed against a lipoidal agent resulting from the *Treponema pallidum* infection. The second is an antibody directed against the *Treponema pallidum* organism itself.

rapid pulse [L, *rapidus*, rush, *pulsare,* to beat], a pulse faster than normal.

rapport /rapôr′/ [Fr, agreement], a sense of mutuality and understanding; harmony, accord, confidence, and respect underlying a relationship between two persons, which is an essential bond between a therapist and patient.

rapprochement /räprôshmäN′/ [Fr, *rapprocher*, to bring together], (in psychology) the third subphase of the separation-individuation phase of Mahler's system of preoedipal development. This stage is characterized by a rediscovery of and reestablishment with mother or a significant nurturer.

raptus /rap′təs/ [L, *rapere,* to seize], **1.** a state of intense emotional or mental excitement, often characterized by uncontrollable activity or behavior resulting from an irresistible impulse; ecstasy; rapture. **2.** any sudden or violent seizure or attack.

rare-earth element [L, *rarus,* thin; AS, *earthe* + L, *elementum*], a metallic element having an atomic number between 57 to 71 inclusively.

rare earth screen, a fluorescent material used as the basis of x-ray intensifying screens. In recent years new materials, including the rare earths yttrium and gadolinium, also have found application in such devices. These rare earths enable lower radiation doses to be used while producing acceptable film densities.

rarefaction /rer′əfak′shən/, reductions of density of a medium at a location in the medium accompanying the cyclic pressure reductions during the passage of a sound wave.

RAS, abbreviation for **reticular activating system.**

rash [OFr, *rasche,* scurf], a skin eruption.

R

Kinds of rashes are **butterfly rash, diaper rash, drug rash,** and **heat rash.**

Rashkind procedure /rash'kind/ [William J. Rashkind, American physician, b. 1922; L, *procedere,* to go forth], the enlargement of an opening in the cardiac septum between the right and left atria. It is performed to relieve congestive heart failure in newborns with certain congenital heart defects by improving the oxygenation of the blood.

raspberry tongue /raz'berē/, a dark red tongue with a smooth surface and prominent papillae, seen after shedding of the white coating characteristic of the early stage of scarlet fever.

rat-bite fever [AS, *raet* + *bitan,* to bite], either of two distinct infections transmitted to humans by the bite of a rat or mouse, characterized by fever, headache, malaise, nausea, vomiting, and rash. In the United States the disease is more commonly caused by *Streptobacillus moniliformis;* its unique features are a rash on palms and soles, painful joints, prompt healing of the wound, and a duration of 2 weeks. Rat-bite fever resulting from infection caused by *Streptobacillus moniliformis* is also called **Haverhill fever;** infection caused by *Spirillum minus* is also called sodoku.

rate [L, *ratus,* reckoned], a numeric ratio, often used in the compilation of data concerning the prevalence and incidence of events, in which the number of actual occurrences appears as the numerator and the number of possible occurrences appears as the denominator. Standard rates are stated in conventional units of population such as neonatal mortality per 1000 or maternal mortality per 100,000.

rate-pressure product, the heart rate multiplied by the systolic blood pressure. It is a clinical indicator of myocardial oxygen demand.

rate-responsive pacer, an artificial pacemaker whose rate can be adjusted as required to meet physiologic demands.

Rathke's pouch /rät'kēz/ [Martin H. Rathke, German anatomist, 1793–1860; OFr, *pouche*], a depression that forms in the roof of the mouth of an embryo, anterior to the buccopharyngeal membrane, around the fourth week of gestation. The walls of the diverticulum develop into the anterior lobe of the pituitary gland.

rating of perceived exertion (RPE), a scale on which perceived exertion is quantified, with 6 being extremely light exertion and 20 being extremely hard. The American College of Sports Medicine (ACSM) has modified the scale, using a system of 1 to 10. The ACSM has also es-

tablished minimal guidelines of frequency, intensity, and duration of exercise needed to obtain a training effect.

ratio /rā'shō/ [L, a reckoning], the relationship of one quantity to one or more other quantities expressed as a proportion of one to the others and written either as a fraction (⅜) or linearly (8:3).

rational /rash'ənəl/ [L, *rationalis,* reasonable], **1.** pertaining to a measure, method, or procedure based on reason. **2.** pertaining to a therapeutic method based on an understanding of the cause and mechanisms of a specific disease and the potential effects of the drugs or procedures used in treating the disorder. **3.** sane; capable of normal reasoning or behavior.

rationale /rash'ənal'/ [L, *rationalis,* reasonable], a system of reasoning or a statement of the reasons used in explaining data or phenomena.

rational emotive therapy (RET), a form of cognitive therapy, originated by Albert Ellis, that emphasizes a reorganization and challenge of one's cognitive and emotional functions, a redefinition of one's problems, and a change in one's attitudes to develop more effective and suitable patterns of behavior.

rationalization /rash'ənal'izā'shən/, the most commonly used defense mechanism in which an individual justifies ideas, actions, or feelings with seemingly acceptable reasons or explanations. It is often used to preserve self-respect, reduce guilt feelings, or obtain social approval or acceptance.

ratio solution, the relationship of a solute to a solution expressed as a proportion, such as 1:1000, or parts per thousand.

rattle [ME, *ratelen*], an abnormal sound heard by auscultation of the lungs in some forms of pulmonary disease. It consists of a coarse vibration, more intense than a crackle, very much like a rhonchus, caused by the movement of moisture and the separation of the walls of small air passages during respiration.

rattlesnake [ME, *ratelen* + AS, *snacan,* to creep], a poisonous pit viper with a series of loosely connected, horny segments at the end of the tail that make a noise like a rattle when shaken. More than 25 species of rattlesnakes are found in the Americas, including most parts of the United States. They have a hematoxin in their venom, and they are responsible for most of the poisonous snake bites in the United States.

rauwolfia /rôwol'fē·ə, rou-, rä-/ [Leonhard Rauwolf, sixteenth-century German botanist], the dried roots of *Rauwolfia serpentina* that provide the extracts for hypo-

rauwolfia alkaloid, any one of more than 20 alkaloids derived from the root of a climbing shrub, *Rauwolfia serpentina*, indigenous to India and the surrounding area. Formerly used as an antipsychotic agent, it is today confined to the treatment of hypertension.

rauwolfia serpentina, the dried root from *Rauwolfia serpentina*, used as an antihypertensive. It is prescribed in the treatment of mild hypertension and hypertensive emergencies.

raw data, (in magnetic resonance [MR] imaging) the information obtained by radio reception of the MR signal as stored by a computer. Specific computer manipulation of these data is required to construct an image from it.

ray [L, *radius*], a beam of radiation, such as heat or light, moving away from a source.

rayl /rāl/ [John W. S. Rayleigh, English physicist, 1842–1919], the unit for characteristic acoustic impedance. Its fundamental units are $kg/m^2/s$.

Rayleigh scatterer /rā′lē/ [John Rayleigh, English physicist], reflecting objects whose dimensions are much smaller than the ultrasonic wavelength. The scattered intensity from a volume of Rayleigh scatterers increases rapidly with increasing frequency, being related to frequency raised to the fourth power.

Raynaud's phenomenon /rānōz′/ [Maurice Raynaud, French physician, 1834–1881], intermittent attacks of ischemia of the extremities of the body, especially the fingers, toes, ears, and nose, caused by exposure to cold or by emotional stimuli. The attacks are characterized by severe blanching of the extremities, followed by cyanosis, then redness, they are usually accompanied by numbness, tingling, burning, and often pain. The condition is called Raynaud's disease when there is a history of symptoms for at least 2 years with no progression of symptoms and no evidence of an underlying cause.

Rb, symbol for the element **rubidium.**

RBBB, abbreviation for **right bundle branch block.**

RBC, abbreviation for *red blood cell.*

RBE, abbreviation for **relative biologic effectiveness.**

RBRVS, abbreviation for **resource-based relative value scale.**

RCEEM, abbreviation for **Recognized Continuing Education Evaluation Mechanism.**

R.C.P., abbreviation for **Royal College of Physicians.**

RCPSC, abbreviation for **Royal College of Physicians and Surgeons of Canada.**

R.C.S., abbreviation for **Royal College of Surgeons.**

RD, abbreviation for **registered dietitian.**

RDAs, abbreviation for **recommended dietary allowances.**

rdi, abbreviation for *recommended daily intake.*

RDS, abbreviation for *respiratory distress syndrome.*

Re, symbol for the element **rhenium.**

reabsorption /rē′əbsôrp′shən/, the process of something being absorbed again, such as the removal of calcium from the bone back into the blood.

reacher /rē′chər/, a pair of extended tongs that can be used by persons with upper extremity disabilities or those who lose the ability to bend and stoop to grasp objects on shelves, the floor, and similar areas beyond their usual reach.

Reach to Recovery [AS, *reacan*, to reach; ME, *recoveren*, to get back], a national volunteer organization that offers counseling and support to women with breast cancer and their families. Many of the members have had mastectomies themselves.

reaction /rē·ak′shən/ [L, *re*, again, *agere*, to act], a response in opposition to a substance, treatment, or other stimulus, such as an antigen-antibody reaction in immunology, a hypersensitivity reaction in allergy, or an adverse reaction in pharmacology. —**react,** *v.,* **reactive,** *adj.*

reaction formation, an unconscious defense mechanism in which a person expresses toward another person or situation feelings, attitudes, or behaviors that are the opposite of what would normally be expected.

reaction time [L, *re*, again, *agere*, to act; AS *tima*], the interval between the application of a stimulus and the beginning of a response.

reactivate /rē·ak′tivāt/ [L, *re* + *activus*], to make active again, as in adding fresh serum to restore the potency of an original supply of the serum.

reactivation /rē·ak′tivā′shən/, the restoration of impaired biologic activity caused by chemical reaction, thermal application, genetic recombination, or helper elements.

reactivation tuberculosis, a form of secondary tuberculosis that recurs as a result of the activation of a dormant endogenous infection. Causes of the reactivation may include loss of immunity, hormonal changes, or poor nutrition.

reactive decision /rē·ak′tiv/ [L, *re* + *activus*], (in psychology) a decision made

R

by an individual in response to the influence or goals of others.

reactive depression, an emotional condition characterized by an acute feeling of despondency, sadness, and depressive dysphoria, which varies in intensity and duration. The condition is caused by some identifiable external situation or environmental stress and is generally relieved when the circumstance is altered or the conflict understood and resolved.

reactive hypoglycemia low levels of glucose in the circulating blood (<45 to 50 mg/dl) in an arterialized specimen after ingestion of carbohydrates. It may be related to increased insulin sensitivity or excess counterregulatory hormone secretion.

reactive inflammation [L, *re* + *activus* + *inflammare,* to set afire], an inflammation that develops as a reaction to an antigen.

reactive schizophrenia, a form of schizophrenia caused by environmental factors rather than organic changes in the brain. Disease onset is usually rapid; symptoms are of brief duration, and the affected individual appears well immediately before and after the schizophrenic episode.

reactor /rē·ak'tər/, **1.** (in psychology) a family therapist who lets a family in therapy take the lead and then follows in that direction. **2.** (in radiology) a cubicle in which radioisotopes are artificially produced.

reading [AS, *raedan*], (in molecular genetics) the linear process in which the genetic information contained in a nucleotide sequence is decoded, as in the translation of the messenger ribonucleic acid directives for the sequence of the amino acids in a polypeptide.

reading disorder, a language disorder in which one's reading ability is significantly below intellectual capacity. Tests show the problem does not involve mental retardation, chronologic age, or inadequate schooling but is marked by faulty oral reading, slow reading, and reduced comprehension.

Read method [Grantley Dick-Read, twentieth century English obstetrician], a method of psychophysical preparation for childbirth. It was the first 'natural childbirth' program, a term coined by Dr. Read in the 1930s. Basically Read held that childbirth is a normal, physiologic procedure and that the pain of labor and delivery is of psychologic origin—the fear-tension-pain syndrome. He countered women's fears with education about the physiologic process, encouraged a positive welcoming attitude, corrected false information, and led tours of the hospital. To decrease tension he developed a series of breathing exercises for use during the various stages of labor. To foster relaxation and optimal physical function in labor and recovery after delivery, he incorporated a series of physical exercises to be performed regularly in classes and in practice at home during pregnancy.

readthrough [AS, *raedan* + *thurh,* through], (in molecular genetics) transcription of ribonucleic acid (RNA) beyond the normal termination sequence in the deoxyribonucleic acid template, caused by the occasional failure of RNA polymerase to respond to the end-point signal.

reagent /rē·ā'jənt/ [L, *re,* again, *agere,* to act], a chemical substance known to react in a specific way. A reagent is used to detect or synthesize another substance in a chemical reaction.

reagin /rē'ājin/ [L, *re* + *agere*], **1.** an antibody associated with human atopy such as asthma and hay fever. It attaches to mast cells and basophils and sensitizes the skin and other tissues. **2.** a nonspecific, nontreponemal antibody-like substance found in the serum of individuals with syphilis. —**reaginic,** *adj.*

reaginic antibody /rē'əgin'ik/, an IgE immunoglobulin that is elevated in hypersensitive individuals.

reagin-mediated disorder, a hypersensitivity reaction such as hay fever or an allergic response to an insect sting produced by reaginic antibodies (IgE immunoglobulins), causing degranulation and the release of histamine, bradykinin, serotonin, and other vasoactive amines. An initial sensitizing dose of the antigen induces the formation of specific IgE antibodies, and their attachment to mast cells and basophils results in hypersensitivity to a subsequent challenging dose of the antigen. Reactions range from a simple wheal and flare on the skin to life-threatening anaphylactic shock, depending on the amount and route of entrance of the sensitizing dose and challenging dose, the amount and distribution of IgE antibodies, the responsiveness of the host, the timing of exposure to the allergen, and the tissues in which the antigen-antibody reaction occurs.

reality /rē·al'itē/ [L, *res,* factual], the culturally constructed world of perception, meaning, and behavior that members of a culture regard as an absolute.

reality orientation, a formal activity that uses specific approaches to assist confused or disoriented persons toward an awareness of reality, or the 'here and now' as by emphasizing, for example, the time, day, month, year, situation, and weather.

Reality Orientation, a Nursing Interventions Classification defined as promotion of patient's awareness of personal identity, time, and environment.

reality principle, an awareness of the demands of the environment and the need for an adjustment of behavior to meet those demands, expressed primarily by the renunciation of immediate gratification of instinctual pleasures to obtain long-term and future goals.

reality testing, an ego function that enables one to differentiate between external reality and any inner imaginative world and to behave in a manner that exhibits an awareness of accepted norms and customs. Impairment of reality testing is indicative of a disturbance in ego functioning that may lead to psychosis.

reality therapy, a form of psychotherapy developed by William Glassner. The aims are to help define and assess basic values within the framework of a current situation and to evaluate the person's present behavior and future plans in relation to those values.

real time [L, *res,* factual; AS, *tid,* tide], an application of computerized equipment that allows data to be processed with relation to ongoing external events, so that the operators can make immediate diagnostic or other decisions based on the current data output. Ultrasound scanning uses real-time control systems.

real-time scanning, the scanning or imaging of an entire object, or a cross-sectional slice of the object, at a single moment. To produce such a 'snapshot' image, scanning data must be recorded quickly over a very short time rather than by accumulation over a longer period.

reamer [AS, *ryman,* to make room], **1.** a tool with a straight or spiral cutting edge, used in a rotating motion to enlarge a hole or clear an opening. **2.** (in dentistry) an instrument with a tapered and loosely spiraled metal shaft used for enlarging and cleaning root canals.

reapproximate /rē'əprok'simāt/ [L, *re,* again; *approximare,* to come near], to rejoin tissues separated by surgery or trauma so that their anatomic relationship is restored. **—reapproximation,** *n.*

reasonable accommodation, an interpretation of the U.S. Americans With Disabilities Act regarding responsibility of an employer to provide an adequate work environment for a disabled but otherwise competent employee. The rule may apply in making facilities accessible, restructuring jobs, reassigning disabled employees to vacant positions, modifying work schedules, acquiring or modifying equipment, and adjusting training materials and examinations. The employer may not be required to provide reasonable accommodation if it can be shown to impose an "undue hardship" on the business operation.

reasonable care /rē'zənəbəl/ [L, *rationalis*], the degree of skill and knowledge used by a competent health practitioner in treating and caring for the sick and injured.

reasonable charge, 1. (in Medicare) the lowest customary charge by a physician for a service. **2.** the prevailing charge by a group of physicians in the area for a particular service.

reasonable cost, the amount a medical insurer will reimburse for a particular health service based on the cost to the provider for delivering that service.

reasonable person, (in law) a hypothetical person who possesses the qualities that are used as an objective standard on which to judge a defendant's action in a negligence suit.

reasonably prudent person doctrine /rē'zənəblē'/, a concept that a person of ordinary sense will use ordinary care and skill in meeting the health care needs of a patient.

reattachment /rē'ətach'mənt/ [L, *re,* again; OFr, *attachier*], **1.** the rejoining of accidentally severed body parts. **2.** the rejoining of periodontal membrane fibers to the cementum of a tooth and the alveolar bone to restore a loosened tooth.

rebase /rēbās'/ [L, *re,* again, *basis,* base], a process of refitting a denture by replacing or adding to its base material without changing the occlusal relationships of the teeth.

rebirthing /rēbur'thing/, a form of psychotherapy developed by Leonard Orr that focuses on the breath and breathing apparatus. The goal of treatment is to overcome the trauma of the birth-damaged breathing apparatus so the person is able to use the breath as a supportive and creative part of life.

rebound /rē'bound/ [Fr, *rebondir,* to bounce], **1.** recovery from illness. **2.** a sudden contraction of muscle after a period of relaxation, often seen in conditions in which inhibitory reflexes are lost.

rebound congestion, swelling and congestion of the nasal mucosa that follows the vasodilator effects of decongestant medications.

rebound phenomenon [OFr, *rebondir* + Gk, *phainomenon,* anything seen], a renewal of reflex activity after the stimulus

R

that triggered the original action has been removed. It may be indicative of a lesion of the cerebellum.

rebound tenderness, a sign of inflammation of the peritoneum in which pain is elicited by the sudden release of a hand pressing on the abdomen.

rebreathing /rēbrē'thing/ [L, *re* + AS, *braeth*, breath], breathing into a closed system. Exhaled gas mixes with the gas in the closed system, and some of this mixture is then reinhaled. Rebreathing may result in progressively decreasing concentrations of oxygen and progressively increasing concentrations of carbon dioxide.

rebreathing bag, (in anesthesia) a flexible bag attached to a mask. It may function as a reservoir for anesthetic gases during surgery or for oxygen during resuscitation.

recalcification /rēkal'sifikā'shən/ [L, *re* + *calx*, lime, *facere*, to make], the restoration of lost calcium salts in the body needed for normal neuromuscular excitability, excitation-coupling contraction in cardiac and smooth muscle stimulus-secretion coupling, maintenance of tight junctions between cells, blood clotting, and compressional strength of bone.

recannulate /rēkan'yəlāt/ [L, *re* + *cannula*, small reed], to make a new opening through an organ or tissue, such as opening a passage through an occluded blood vessel.

recapitulation theory /rē'kəpit'yəlā'shən/ [L, *re* + *capitulum*, small head], the theory, formulated by German naturalist Ernst Heinrich Haeckel (1834–1919), that an organism during the course of embryonic development passes through stages that resemble the structural form of several ancestral types of the species as it evolved from a lower to a higher form of life. It is summarized by the statement 'Ontogeny recapitulates phylogeny.'

receiver /risē'vər/ [L, *recipere*, to receive], **1.** (in communication theory) the person or persons to whom a message is sent. **2.** the part of a hearing aid that converts electric signals to acoustic signals.

receiving sensitivity pattern /risē'ving/, the spatial response of a transducer as an echo detector. For a single-element transducer it is essentially the same as the transmitted beam. For transducer arrays it can be quite different from the transmitted beam.

receptive aphasia /risep'tiv/, a form of sensory aphasia marked by impaired comprehension of language.

receptor /risep'tər/ [L, *recipere*, to receive], **1.** a chemical structure usually

of protein/carbohydrate on the surface of a cell that combines with an antigen to produce a discrete immunologic component. **2.** a sensory nerve ending that responds to various kinds of stimulation. **3.** a specific cellular protein that must first bind a hormone before cellular response can be elicited.

receptor site [L, *recipere*, to receive, *situs*], a location on a cell surface where certain molecules such as enzymes, neurotransmitters, or viruses attach to interact with cellular components.

receptor theory of drug action, the concept that certain drugs produce their effects by acting specifically at a receptor site on a cell or within the cell or its membrane.

recess /rē'ses, rises'/ [L, *recedere*, to retreat], a small hollow cavity, such as the epitympanic recess in the tympanic cavity of the inner ear or the retrocecal recess extending as a small pocket behind the cecum.

recessive /rises'iv/ [L, *recedere*], pertaining to or describing a gene, the effect of which is masked or hidden if there is a dominant gene at the same locus.

recessive gene, the member of a pair of genes that lacks the ability to express itself in the presence of its more dominant allele; it is expressed only in the homozygous state.

recessive trait, a genetically determined characteristic that is expressed only when present in the homozygotic state.

recidivism (recid) /risid'iviz'əm/ [L, *recidivus,* falling back], a tendency by an ill person to relapse or return to a hospital.

recipient /risip'ē-ənt/ [L, *recipere*, to receive], the person who receives a blood transfusion, tissue graft, or organ.

reciprocal beat, an atrial or ventricular complex resulting from return of an impulse to its chamber of origin.

reciprocal changes, the changes seen in electrocardiograph leads facing the opposite wall to a myocardial infarction.

reciprocal inhibition, the theory in behavior therapy that, if an anxiety-producing stimulus occurs simultaneously with a response that diminishes anxiety, the stimulus may cause less anxiety.

reciprocal roentgens, (in radiology) the measure of x-ray film speed, used in the formula: speed = 1/number of roentgens needed to produce a density of 1.

reciprocal translocation, the mutual exchange of genetic material between two nonhomologous chromosomes.

reciprocity /res'ipros'itē/ [Fr, *réciprocité*], a mutual agreement to exchange privileges, dependence, or relationships. An example is an agreement between two governing bodies to accept the medical credentials of physicians licensed in either community.

Recklinghausen's canal /rek'linghou'-sənz/ [Friedrich D. von Recklinghausen, German pathologist, 1833–1910], the small lymph space in the connective tissues of the body.

Recklinghausen's tumor [Friedrich D. von Recklinghausen], a benign tumor, derived from smooth muscle containing connective tissue and epithelial elements.

reclining /riklī'ning/, leaning backward. **—recline,** v.

recognition site /rek'əgnish'ən/, a location on a nucleic acid or protein to which a specific ligand binds.

Recognized Continuing Education Evaluation Mechanism (RCEEM), a control process for checking that educational activities meet certain standards and establishing programs for evaluating educational opportunities and activities.

recombinant /rēkom'binənt/ [L, re, again, combinare, to combine], **1.** the cell or organism that results from the recombination of genes within the deoxyribonucleic acid molecule, regardless of whether naturally or artificially induced. **2.** pertaining to such an organism or cell.

recombinant DNA, a deoxyribonucleic acid (DNA) molecule in which rearrangement of the genes has been experimentally induced. Enzymes are used to break isolated DNA molecules into fragments that are then rearranged in the desired sequence. Parts of DNA material from another organism of the same or a different species may also be introduced into the molecule.

recombinant Lyme test, a method of identifying a component of the *Borrelia burgdorferi* spirochete by use of deoxyribonucleic acid (DNA) from the bacterium. The DNA is divided and spliced back in another bacterium, forcing it to produce a new protein. The new protein, P-39, belongs only to the *B. burgdorferi* disease agent and causes a strong reaction in cells from Lyme-infected blood.

recombinant vaccine, a suspension of attenuated or killed microorganisms developed through recombinant deoxyribonucleic acid techniques.

recombination /rē'kombinā'shən/ [L, re + combinare], **1.** (in genetics) the formation of new combinations and arrangements of genes within the chromosome as a result of independent assortment of unlinked genes, crossing over of linked genes, or intracistronic crossing over of nucleotides. **2.** a method of measurement

of radiation by ionimetric techniques in which it is necessary to collect the liberated charges to arrive at a value of total charge per unit mass of air. Recombination of ions lowers the value collected.

recommended dietary allowances (RDAs) /rek'əmen'did/ [L, re + commendere, to commend], levels of daily intake of essential nutrients judged by the Food and Nutrition Board of the National Research Council to be adequate to meet the known nutrient needs of practically all healthy people.

recon /rē'kon/ [L, re + combinare + Gk, ion, going], (in molecular genetics) the smallest genetic unit that is capable of recombination, thought to be a triplet of nucleotides.

reconstitution /rē'konstit(y)oo'shən/ [L, re + constituere, to establish], the continuous repair of tissue damage.

reconstruction time /rē'kənstruk'shən/, (in computed tomography) the period between the end of a scan and the appearance of an image.

record /ricôrd'/, a written form of communication that permanently documents information relevant to the care of a patient.

recorded detail, the sharpness of structural lines as recorded on a radiograph.

Recovery /rikuv'əry/, a self-help group that provides support for persons discharged from inpatient psychiatric hospitals.

recovery room (RR, R.R.) [ME, recoveren + AS rum], an area adjoining the operating room to which surgical patients are taken while recovering from anesthesia, before being returned to their rooms. It is also identified as the postanesthesia recovery area, or postanesthesia care unit.

recreational drug, any substance with pharmacologic effects that is taken voluntarily for personal pleasure or satisfaction rather than for medicinal purposes. The term is generally applied to alcohol, barbiturates, amphetamines, THC, PCP, cocaine, and heroin; but it also includes caffeine in coffee and cola beverages.

recreational therapy /rē'krē·ā'shənəl/ [L, recreare, to renew], a form of adjunctive treatment in which games or other group activities are used as a means of modifying maladaptive behavior, awakening social interests, or improving the ability to interact and function in socially acceptable ways.

Recreation Therapy, a Nursing Interventions Classification defined as purposeful use of recreation to promote relaxation and enhancement of social skills.

recrudescence /rē'krooes'əns/ [L, re +

R

crudescere, to become hard], a return of symptoms of a disease during a period of recovery.

recrudescent /-ənt/ [L, *re* + *crudescere,* to become hard], the return of disease symptoms after a period of remission.

recrudescent hepatitis, a form of acute viral hepatitis marked by a relapse during the period of recovery.

recruitment /rikro͞ot'mənt/, **1.** the perception of a rapid growth of loudness, commonly seen in sensorineural hearing losses that are cochlear in nature. The impaired ear cannot hear faint sounds but hears intense sounds as loudly as a normal ear. **2.** in muscle contractions, the ability to recruit additional motor units into action as the need to overcome resistance increases.

rectal abscess /rek'təl/ [L, *rectus,* straight, *abscedere,* to go away], an abscess in the perianal area.

rectal alimentation [L, *rectus,* straight, *alimentum,* nourishment], the delivery of nourishment in concentrated form by injection or installation through the rectum.

rectal anesthesia [L, *rectus,* straight], general anesthesia achieved by the insertion, injection, or infusion of an anesthetic agent into the rectum; this procedure is sometimes used in children because it is less painful than starting an IV.

rectal instillation of medication, the instillation of a medicated suppository, cream, or gel into the rectum. Some conditions treated by this method are constipation, pruritus ani, and hemorrhoids. Occasionally a drug may be given in a medicated enema.

Rectal Prolapse Management, a Nursing Interventions Classification defined as prevention and/or manual reduction of rectal prolapse.

rectal reflex, the normal response (defecation) to the presence of an accumulation of feces in the rectum.

rectal temperature [L, *rectus,* straight, *temperatura*], body temperature as measured by a clinical thermometer placed in the rectum. Rectal temperatures average 0.5 to 0.75° F (0.3 to 0.4° C) higher than oral temperatures.

rectal thermometer [L, *rectus* + Gk, *therme,* heat, *metron,* measure], a clinical thermometer suitable for measuring body temperature in the rectum.

rectification /rek'tifikā'shən/, a step in echo signal processing in a pulse-echo ultrasound instrument in which radiofrequency signals, which oscillate both above and below zero volts, are converted.

rectifier /rek'tifī'ər/, an electrical device

that converts alternating current into pulsating direct current.

rectilinear scanner /rek'tilin'ē·ər/, (in nuclear medicine) a device that generates an image of an anatomic structure by detecting radioactivity within the structure.

rectocele /rek'təsēl'/ [L, *rectus* + Gk, *koilos,* hollow], a protrusion of the rectum and posterior wall of the vagina into the vagina. The condition, which occurs after the muscles of the vagina and pelvic floor have been weakened by childbearing, old age, or surgery, may reflect a congenital weakness in the wall.

rectosigmoid /-sig'moid/ [L, *rectus* + Gk, *sigma,* S-shaped, *eidos* form], pertaining to the part of the large intestine that includes the lower part of the sigmoid and the upper part of the rectum.

rectosigmoidoscopy /-sig'moidəs'kəpē/ [L, *rectus,* straight; Gk, *sigma,* S-shaped, *eidos,* form, *skopein,* to view], the examination of the rectum and pelvic colon with a sigmoidoscope.

rectovaginal fistula /-vaj'ənəl/ [L, *rectus,* straight, *vagina,* sheath, *fistula,* pipe], an abnormal passage or opening between the rectum and the vagina.

rectovaginal ligament, one of the four main uterine support ligaments. It helps hold the uterus in position by maintaining traction on the cervix.

rectovaginal septum, a band of loose connective tissue between the vagina and the ampulla of the rectum.

rectovesical /-ves'ikəl/ [L, *rectus,* straight, *vesica,* bladder], pertaining to the rectum and bladder.

rectum /rek'təm/, *pl.* **rectums, recta** [L, *rectus*], the part of the large intestine, about 12 cm long, continuous with the descending sigmoid colon, proximal to the anal canal. It follows the sacrococcygeal curve and ends in the anal canal. —**rectal,** *adj.*

rectus abdominis /rek'təs/, one of a pair of anterolateral muscles of the abdomen, extending the whole length of the ventral aspect of the abdomen. It functions to flex the vertebral column, tense the anterior abdominal wall, and assist in compressing the abdominal contents.

rectus femoris, a fusiform muscle of the anterior thigh, one of the four parts of the quadriceps femoris. With the quadriceps group it functions to extend the lower leg.

rectus muscle [L, straight, *musculus*], a muscle of the body that has a relatively straight form.

recumbency /rikum'bənsē/ [L, *recumbere,* to lie down], the state of lying down or leaning against something.

recumbent /rikum'bənt/ [L, *recumbere,* to

lie down], lying down or leaning back-ward. —**recumbency,** *n.*

recuperate /rikōō′pərāt/ [L, *recupare,* to regain], to recover one's health and strength.

recuperation /rikōō′pərā′shən/ {L, *recupare,* to regain], the process of recover-ing health and strength.

recurrence /rikur′əns/ [L, *recurrere,* to run back], the reappearance of a sign or symptom of a disease after a period of re-mission.

recurrence risk, the chance that a disease found in one member of a proband will appear in other members of the same pedi-gree.

recurrent /rikur′ənt/ [L, *recurrere,* to run back], a disease sign or symptom that re-turns periodically.

recurrent bandage [L, *recurrere,* to run back], a strip of cloth that is wrapped several times around itself, usually applied to the head or amputated limb.

recurvatum /rē′kərvā′təm/ [L, *recurvare,* to bend back], backward thrust, or bend-ing, for example, of the knee caused by weakness of the quadriceps or a joint dis-order.

red blood cell count [AS, *read* + *blod* + L, *cella,* storeroom; Fr, *conter,* to count], a count of the erythrocytes in a specimen of whole blood, commonly made with an electronic counting device. The normal concentrations of red blood cells in the whole blood of males are 4.6 to 6.2 million/mm^3; in females the concentra-tions are 4.2 to 5.4 million/mm^3.

Red Book of the American Academy of Pe-diatrics, a book published by the Ameri-can Academy of Pediatrics, Inc., that serves as the standard reference source of immunization procedures for children and adults.

red cell indexes, a series of relationships that characterize the red cell population in terms of size, hemoglobin content, and he-moglobin concentration. The indexes are useful in making differential diagnoses of several kinds of anemia.

redia /rē′dē·ə/, an elongated second or third larval stage of a trematode that de-velops in a sporocyst and matures into nu-merous cercariae.

red infarct [AS, *read* + L, *infarcire,* to stuff], a pathologic change that occurs in brain tissue that has been rendered isch-emic by lack of blood. With restricted blood flow, diapedesis of red blood cells occurs into the parenchyma of the brain without actually producing a well-formed hematoma but only infiltration of erythro-cytes.

red marrow [AS, *read* + AS, *mearh,* mar-row], the red vascular substance consist-ing of connective tissue and blood vessels containing primitive blood cells, macro-phages, megakaryocytes, and fat cells. It is found in the cavities of many bones, in-cluding flat and short bones, bodies of the vertebrae, sternum, ribs, and articulating ends of long bones. Red marrow manufac-tures and releases leukocytes, erythro-cytes, and thrombocytes into the blood-stream.

red neck syndrome, an allergic reaction to a rapid infusion of the antimicrobial agent vancomycin. It is characterized by flushing, pruritus, and erythema of the head and upper body due to histamine re-lease.

redon /rē′don/, the smallest unit of the deoxyribonucleic acid molecule capable of recombination; it may be as small as one deoxyribonucleotide pair.

redox, an abbreviation for *reduction-oxidation* (reaction).

reduce /rid(y)ōōs′/ [L, *reducere,* to lead back], **1.** (in surgery) the restoration of a part to its original position after dis-placement, as in the reduction of a frac-tured bone by bringing ends or fragments back into alignment. **2.** to decrease the amount, size, extent, or number of some-thing, as of body weight.

reducible hernia /rid(y)ōō′səbəl/ [L, *re-ducere,* to lead back, *hernia,* rupture], a hernia in which the protruding tissues can be manipulated into a normal position.

reducing agent /rid(y)ōō′sing/ [L, *re-ducere,* to lead back, *agere,* to do], a substance that donates electrons to another substance in a chemical reaction.

reduction /riduk′shən/ [L, *reducere*], **1.** the addition of hydrogen to a substance. **2.** the removal of oxygen from a substance. **3.** the decrease in the valence of the elec-tronegative part of a compound. **4.** the ad-dition of one or more electrons to a mol-ecule or atom of a substance. **5.** the correction of a fracture, hernia, or luxa-tion. **6.** the reduction of data, as in con-verting interval data to an ordinal or nomi-nal scale of measurement.

reduction diet, a diet that is low in calo-ries, used to decrease body weight. The diet must supply fewer calories than the individual expends each day while supply-ing all the essential nutrients for maintain-ing health. A diet of this type may provide 1200 calories per day from the food guide pyramid.

reductionism /riduk′shəniz′əm/, an ap-proach that tries to explain a form of be-havior or an event in terms of a specific category of phenomena, such as biologic, psychologic, or cultural, negating the pos-

R

sibility of an interrelation of causal phenomena.

Reed-Sternberg cell [Dorothy M. Reed, American pathologist, 1874–1964; Karl Sternberg, Austrian pathologist, 1872–1935], one of a number of large, abnormal, multinucleated reticuloendothelial cells in the lymphatic system found in Hodgkin's disease. The number and proportion of Reed-Sternberg cells identified are the basis for the histopathologic classification of Hodgkin's disease.

reentry /rē·en'trē/ [L, *re*, again; Fr, *entree*], (in cardiology) the reactivation of myocardial tissue for the second or subsequent time by the same impulse. Reentry is one of the most common arrhythmogenic mechanisms.

refereed journal /ref'ərēd'/ [L, *referre*, to bring back, *diunalis*, daily record], a professional or literary journal in which articles or papers are selected for publication by a panel of referees who are experts in the field.

reference electrode /ref'ərəns/ [L, *referre*, to bring back; Gk, *elektron*, amber, *hodos*, way], an electrode that has an established potential and is used as a reference against which other potentials may be measured.

reference group, a group with which a person identifies or wishes to belong.

reference value, one of a battery of test results that are assumed to be typical for a population of asymptomatic persons. Each value is usually given as a range and should be interpreted according to age, sex, and race.

referential index deletions /ref'ərən'shəl/, a neurolinguistic programing term that pertains to the omission of the specific person being discussed.

referral /rifur'əl/ [L, *referre*, to bring back], a process whereby a patient or the patient's family is introduced to additional health resources in the community, as in helping a patient find an appropriate community health nurse after discharge from a hospital.

Referral, a Nursing Interventions Classification defined as arrangement for services by another care provider or agency.

referred pain /rifurd'/ [L, *referre* + *poena*, pain], pain felt at a site different from that of an injured or diseased organ or body part. Angina, the pain of coronary artery insufficiency, may be felt in the left shoulder, arm, or jaw. In gallbladder disease, pain may be felt in the right shoulder or scapular region.

referred sensation, a feeling or impression that occurs at a site other than where the stimulus is initiated.

refined birth rate /rifīnd/ [L, *re* + *finire*, to finish], the ratio of total births to the total female population, considered during a period of 1 year.

refl, abbreviation for *reflexive.*

reflecting /riflek'ting/, a communication technique in which the listener picks up the feeling tone of the patient's message and repeats it back to the patient. It encourages the patient to continue with clarifying comments.

reflection /riflek'shən/ [L, *reflectere*, to bend back], **1.** (in cardiology) a form of reentry in which, after encountering delay in one fiber, an impulse enters a parallel fiber and returns retrogradely to its source. **2.** (in ultrasonography) the return or reentry of acoustic energy where there is a discontinuity in the characteristic acoustic impedance along the propagation path.

reflective layer /riflek'tiv/, (in radiology) a thin layer of magnesium oxide or titanium oxide between the phosphor and the base of an intensifying screen. Its function is to intercept and redirect isotropically emitted light from the phosphor to the x-ray film.

reflex /rē'fleks/ [L, *reflectere*, to bend back], **1.** a backward or return flow of energy or of an image, as a reflection. **2.** a reflected action, particularly an involuntary action or movement.

reflex action, the involuntary functioning or movement of any organ or body part in response to a particular stimulus.

reflex apnea, involuntary cessation of respiration caused by irritating, noxious vapors or gases.

reflex arc [L, *reflectere*, to bend back, *arcus*, bow], a simple neurologic unit of a sensory neuron that carries a stimulus impulse to the spinal cord, where it connects with a motor neuron that carries the reflex impulse back to an appropriate muscle or gland.

reflex center [L, *reflectere*, to bend back; Gk, *kentron*], any part of the nervous system in which reception of afferent impulses results in a discharge of efferent impulses leading to some change in a muscle or gland.

reflex dyspepsia, an abnormal condition characterized by impaired digestion associated with the disease of an organ not directly involved with digestion.

reflex emesis [L, *reflectere*, to bend back; Gk, *emesis*, vomiting], vomiting or gagging that is induced by touching the mucous membrane of the throat or as a result of other noxious stimuli.

reflex hammer [L, *reflectere*, to bend back; AS, *hamer*], a percussion mallet with a rubber head used to tap tendons, nerves, or muscles to elicit reflex reactions.

reflex inhibiting pattern (RIP), a conscious set of neuromuscular actions directed toward inhibition of a natural reflex. Examples include actions taken to suppress a sneeze and the learned inhibitions of toilet training.

reflexology /rē'fleksol'əjē/, a system of treating certain disorders by massaging the soles of the feet, using principles similar to those of acupuncture.

reflex sympathetic dystrophy (RSD), a diffuse, persistent pain involving central reorganization of sensory processing. It is characterized by vasomotor disorders, limited joint mobility, and trophic changes. The condition usually follows an injury to an afferent pathway and affects an extremity.

reflex tachycardia [L, *reflectere,* to bend back; Gk, *tachys,* fast, *kardia,* heart], a rapid heart sinus rhythm caused by a variety of autonomic nervous system effects such as blood pressure changes, fever, or emotional stress.

reflex vasodilation [L, *reflectere,* to bend back, *vas,* vessel, *dilatare,* to spread out], any blood vessel dilation that results from stimulation of vasodilator nerves or inhibition of vasoconstrictors of the sympathetic nervous system, including epinephrine-type drugs.

reflux /rē'fluks/ [L, *refluere,* to flow back], an abnormal backward or return flow of a fluid.

reflux esophagitis, esophageal irritation and inflammation that result from reflux of the stomach contents into the esophagus.

reflux laryngitis, a burning sensation in the hypopharynx and larynx caused by nocturnal gastric reflux. It occurs most commonly in older patients who sleep in the recumbent position.

refraction /rifrak'shən/ [L, *refringere,* to break apart], **1.** the change of direction of energy as it passes from one medium to another of different density. **2.** an examination to determine and correct refractive errors of the eye. **3.** (in ultrasonography) the phenomenon of bending wave fronts as the acoustic energy propagates from the medium of one acoustic velocity to a second medium of differing acoustic velocity.

refraction of eye [L, *refringere,* to break apart; AS, *eage*], the deflection of light from a straight path through the eye by various ocular tissues, including the cornea, lens, aqueous humor, and vitreous body.

refractive error /rifrak'tiv/, a defect in the ability of the lens of the eye to focus an image accurately, as occurs in nearsightedness and farsightedness.

refractive index, a numeric expression of the refractive power of a medium, as compared with that of air, which has a refractive index value of 1. The refractive index is related to the number, charge, and mass of vibrating particles in the material through which light is passing.

refractive keratotomy (RK), a surgical procedure in which incisions are made to flatten the cornea, resulting in the elimination or reduction of myopia or astigmatism. Eight or 16 incisions, each about 4 mm long, are made partially through the cornea around the periphery, sparing the central cornea. Uncorrected visual acuity in myopic patients with minor degrees of ametropia is improved, and myopia is reduced by about 2.5 diopters.

refractometer /rē'frəktom'ətər/ [L, *refringere,* to break apart; Gk, *metron,* measure], an instrument for measuring the refractive index of a substance and used primarily for measuring the refractivity of solutions.

refractoriness /rifrak'tōrines'/, the property of excitable tissue that determines how closely together two action potentials can occur.

refractory /rifrak'tərē/ [L, *refringere*], pertaining to a disorder that is resistant to treatment.

refractory period, the time from phase 0 to the end of phase 3 of the action potential, divided into effective and relative. In pacing terminology, the period during which a pulse generator is unresponsive to an input signal of specified amplitude.

reframing /rēfrā'ming/, changing the viewpoint in relation to which a situation is experienced and placing it in a different frame that fits the "facts" of a concrete situation equally well, thereby changing its entire meaning.

Refsum's syndrome /ref'sŏŏmz/ [Sigvald Refsum, Norwegian physician, b. 1907], a rare hereditary disorder of lipid metabolism in which phytanic acid cannot be broken down. It is characterized by ataxia, abnormalities of the bones and skin, peripheral neuropathy, and retinitis pigmentosa.

refusal of treatment, the right of a patient to refuse treatment after the physician has informed the patient of the diagnosis, prognosis, available alternative interventions, risks and benefits of those options, and risk and probable outcome of no intervention.

regeneration / /rijen'ərā'shən/, the process of repair, reproduction, or replacement of lost or injured cells, tissues, or organs.

regimen /rej′imən/ [L, guidance], a strictly regulated therapeutic program such as a diet or exercise schedule.

regional /rē′jənəl/ [L, *regio,* territory], pertaining to a geographic area such as a regional medical facility or to a part of the body such as regional anesthesia.

regional anatomy, the study of the structural relationships among the organs and the parts of the body.

regional anesthesia, anesthesia of an area of the body by injecting a local anesthetic to block a group of sensory nerve fibers.

regional control, the control of cancer in sites that represent the first stages of spread from the local origin.

regional hyperthermia, the elevation of temperature over an extended volume of tissue.

regionalization /rē′jənal′īzā′shən/, (in health care planning) the organization of a system for the delivery of health care within a region to avoid costly duplication of services and to ensure availability of essential services.

regional medical program (RMP), a program of community health planning that includes all the medical resources available in a region that may be mobilized to meet a specific medical objective. The RMP was authorized by the Health, Disease, Cancer and Stroke Amendments passed by the U.S. Congress in 1965.

region of interest (ROI), (in positron emission tomography) an area that circumscribes a desired anatomic location. Image processing systems permit drawing of ROIs on images.

region of recombination, the first stage of amplitude of an electric signal in a gas-filled radiation detector, when the voltage is very low. No electrons are attracted to the central electrode, and ion pairs produced in the chamber will recombine.

register /rej′istər/ [L, *regerere,* to bring back], (in computed tomography) a device in the central processing unit that stores information for future use.

registered dietitian (RD), a professional trained in foods and the management of diets (dietetics) who is credentialed by the Commission on Dietetic Registration of the American Dietetic Association. Credentialing is based on completion of a BS degree from an approved program, clinical and administrative training, and passing a registration examination.

registered nurse (RN) /rej′istərd/, **1.** (*U.S.*) a nurse who has completed a course of study at a state approved school of

nursing and passed the National Council Licensure Examination (NCLEX-RN). A registered nurse may use the initials RN after the signature. RNs are licensed to practice by individual states. **2.** (*Canada.*) a nurse who has completed a course of study at an approved school of nursing and who has taken and passed an examination administered by the Canadian Nurses Association Testing Service, called the Comprehensive Examination for Nurse Registration Licensure.

registered record administrator (RRA), a medical record administrator who has successfully completed the credentialing examination conducted by the American Medical Record Association.

registered respiratory therapist (RRT), an allied health professional who has successfully completed the registry examination of the National Board for Respiratory Care and who specializes in scientific knowledge and theory of clinical problems of respiratory care. Usually a 2-or 4-year college affiliation leading to an associate or bachelor's degree is required.

registered technologist (RT), a medical professional who is certified by the American Registry of Radiologic Technologists or equivalent certifying agency in one or more of the following disciplines: radiography, nuclear medicine, radiation therapy, mammography, computed tomography, magnetic resonance imaging, or cardiovascular interventional technology.

registrar /rej′isträr/, an administrative officer whose responsibility is to maintain the records of an institution.

registration /rej′istrā′shən/ [L, *registratio*], **1.** a learning or memory recording made in the central nervous system of an impression resulting from a stimulus. **2.** the recording of vital personal information such as health data. **3.** the recording of professional qualification information relevant to government licensing regulations.

registry /rej′istrē/ [L, *regerere,* to bring back], **1.** an office or agency in which lists of nurses and records pertaining to nurses seeking employment are maintained. **2.** (in epidemiology) a listing service for incidence data pertaining to the occurrence of specific diseases or disorders, such as a tumor registry.

regression /rigresh′ən/ [L, *regredi,* to go back], **1.** a retreat or backward movement in conditions, signs, or symptoms. **2.** a return to an earlier, more primitive form of behavior. **3.** a tendency in physical development to become more typical of the population than of the parents. **—regress,** *v.*

regular diet /reg′yələr/ [L, *regula,* rule],

a full, well-balanced diet containing all of the essential nutrients needed for optimal growth, repair of the tissues, and normal functioning of the organs.

regular insulin, a fast-acting insulin prescribed in the treatment of diabetes mellitus when the desired action is prompt, intense, and short-acting.

regulative development /reg′yəlā′tiv/ [L, *regula,* rule], a type of embryonic development in which the fertilized ovum undergoes indeterminate cleavage, producing blastomeres that have similar developmental potencies and are each capable of giving rise to a single embryo. Determination of the particular organs and parts of the embryo occurs during later stages of development and is influenced by inductors and intercellular interaction.

regulator gene /reg′yəlā′tər/, (in molecular genetics) a genetic unit that regulates or suppresses the activity of one or more structural genes.

regulatory HIV gene, one of a set of genes in the genome of the human immunodeficiency virus (HIV) that influence the expression of other HIV genes. One (tat) regulatory gene stimulates expression, a second (nef) may inhibit expression, and a third (rev) provides feedback to the others.

regulatory sequence /reg′yələtôr′ē/ [L, *regula + sequi,* to follow], (in molecular genetics) a series of deoxyribonucleic acid nucleotides that regulate the expression of a gene.

regurgitant murmur /rigur′jitənt/ [L, *re + gurgitare,* to flow back; *murmur,* humming], a heart murmur caused by a defective valve as blood flows backward through the partly closed valve cusps. Kinds of regurgitant murmurs include **diastolic, pansystolic,** and **systolic.**

regurgitation [L, *re,* again, *gurgitare,* to flow back], **1.** the backward flow from the normal direction, as the return of swallowed food into the mouth. **2.** the backward flow of blood through a defective heart valve, named for the affected valve, as in **aortic regurgitation.**

regurgitation jaundice /rēgur′jitā′shən/ [L, *re + gurgitare,* again to flow back; Fr, *jaune,* yellow], jaundice caused by bile pigment entering the blood and lymphatic systems as a result of biliary obstruction.

rehabilitation (rehab) /rē′habilitā′shən/ [L, *re + habitalas,* aptitude], the restoration of an individual or a part to normal or near normal function after a disabling disease, injury, addiction, or incarceration. **—rehabilitate,** *v.*

rehabilitation center, a facility providing therapy and training for rehabilitation.

The center may offer occupational therapy, physical therapy, vocational training, and special training such as speech therapy.

Rehfuss stomach tube /rā′fəs/ [Martin E. Rehfuss, American physician, 1887–1964], a specially designed gastric tube with a graduated syringe, used for withdrawing specimens of the contents of the stomach for study after a test meal.

rehydration /rē′hīdrā′shən/ [L, *re* + Gk, *hydor,* water], restoration of normal water balance in a patient by giving fluids orally or intravenously.

Reid's base line [Robert W. Reid, Scottish anatomist, 1851–1939], the base line of the skull, a hypothetic line extending from the infraorbital point to the superior border of the external auditory meatus.

Reifenstein's syndrome /rī′fənstīnz/ [Edward C. Reifenstein, Jr., American physician, 1908–1975], male hypogonadism of unknown origin, marked by azoospermia, undescended testes, gynecomastia, testosterone deficiency, and elevated gonadotropin titers.

Reiki therapy /rī′kē/, a complementary therapy in which a trained practitioner places his or her hands on or above a specific body area and transfers what is called "universal life energy" to the patient. That energy, it is claimed, provides "strength, harmony, and balance" necessary to treat health disturbances. The therapy, derived from an ancient Buddhist practice, involves a total of 15 hand positions covering all the body systems.

reimbursement /rē′imburs′mənt/ [L, *re* + *im,* in; Fr, *bourse,* purse], a method of payment, usually by a third-party payer, for medical treatment or hospital costs. Cost-based reimbursement covers payment for all allowable costs incurred in the provision of services to patients included in a contract. Prospective reimbursement provides for additional payment by which costs incurred in providing services to patients are based on actual costs determined at the end of a fiscal period.

reinfection /rē′infek′shən/, a second infection by the same microorganism, either after recovery or during the original infection.

reinforcement /rē′infôrs′mənt/ [L, *re* + Fr, *enforcir,* to strengthen], (in psychology) a process in which a response is strengthened by the fear of punishment or the anticipation of reward.

reinforcement-extinction, a process of socialization in which one learns to engage in certain behaviors (reinforcement) or to avoid certain behaviors (extinction).

reinforcer /rē′infôr′sər/, (in psychology)

R

a consequence that increases the probability that an operant will recur.

Reiter's syndrome /rī'tərz/ [Hans Reiter, German physician, 1881–1969], an arthritic disorder of adult males, believed to result from *Chlamidia*, myxovirus, or *Mycoplasma* infection. It most often affects the ankles, feet, and sacroiliac joints and is usually associated with conjunctivitis and urethritis. Superficial ulcers may form lesions on the palms and the soles. Arthritis usually persists after the conjunctivitis and urethritis subside, but it may become episodic.

reject analysis /rē'jekt/, (in radiology) the study of repeated radiographs to determine the cause for their being discarded.

rejection /rijek'shən/ [L, *re* + *jacere*, to throw], **1.** (in medicine) an immunologic response to organisms or substances that the system recognizes as foreign, including grafts or transplants. **2.** (in psychiatry) the act of excluding or denying affection to another person.

rejunctive /rijungk'tiv/, (in contextual psychotherapy) pertaining to a relationship that is characterized by moves toward trustworthy relatedness.

rejuvenation /rējōō'vənā'shən/ [L, *re* + *juvenis*, youth], the restoration of youthful health and vitality.

relapse /rilaps'/ [L, *relabi*, to slide back], **1.** to exhibit again the symptoms of a disease from which a patient appears to have recovered. **2.** the recurrence of a disease after apparent recovery.

relapsing [L, *relabi*, to slide back], pertaining to the return of disease after a period of apparent recovery.

relapsing fever, any one of several acute infectious diseases, marked by recurrent febrile episodes, caused by various strains of the spirochete *Borrelia*. The disease is transmitted by both lice and ticks and is often seen during wars and famines. The first episode usually starts with a sudden high fever (104° to 105° F, or 40° to 40.56° C), accompanied by chills, headache, neuromuscular pains, and nausea. A rash may appear over the trunk and extremities, and jaundice is common during the later stages. Each attack lasts 2 or 3 days and culminates in a crisis of high fever, profuse sweating, and a rise in heart and respiratory rate. This is followed by an abrupt drop in temperature and a return to normal blood pressure. People typically relapse after 7 to 10 days of normal temperature and eventually recover completely.

relapsing polychondritis, a rare disease of unknown cause resulting in inflammation and destruction of cartilage with re-

placement by fibrous tissue. Autoimmunity may be involved in this condition. Most commonly the ears and noses of middle-aged people are affected with episodes of tender swelling, often accompanied by fever, arthralgias, and episcleritis.

relation searching /rilā'shən/ [L, *relatio*], (in nursing research) a study design used to discover and describe relationships between and among variables.

relationship therapy /rilā'shənship'/ [L, *relatio* + AS, *scieppan*, to shape], a therapy that is based on a totality of client-therapist relationship and encourages the growth of self in the client.

relative biologic effectiveness (RBE) /rel'ətiv/ [L, *relatio*], (in radiotherapy) a measure of the cell-killing ability of a particular radiation compared with a reference radiation. The reference is 250 keV x-rays. The ratio of cells killed with the test radiation over that of the 250 keV radiation is the RBE.

relative centrifugal force (RCF), a method of comparing the force generated by various centrifuges based on the speeds of rotation and distances from the center of rotation.

relative growth, the comparison of the various increases in size of similar organisms, tissues, or structures at different time intervals.

relative humidity, the amount of moisture in the air compared with the maximum the air could contain at the same temperature.

relative risk, the ratio of the chance of a disease developing among members of a population exposed to a factor compared to a similar population not exposed to the factor.

relative sterility [L, *relatio* + *sterilis*, barren], a condition of infertility in which one or more factors tend to reduce the chances of becoming pregnant.

relative value unit, a comparable service measure used by hospitals to permit comparison of the amounts of resources required to perform various services within a single department or between departments.

relax /rilaks'/ [L, *relaxare*, to ease], to reduce tension.

relaxant /rilak'sənt/ [L, *relaxare*, to ease], a drug or other agent that tends to reduce tension, as a muscle or bowel relaxant.

relaxation /rē'laksā'shən/ [L, *relaxare,* to ease], **1.** a reducing of tension, as when a muscle relaxes between contractions. **2.** (in magnetic resonance imaging) the return of excited nuclei to their normal unexcited state by the release of energy.

relaxation oven, (in mammography) a

part of the xerographic plate conditioner system used to eliminate ghost images. The plate is heated in the oven so that any residual electrostatic charge on the surface will be removed.

relaxation response, a protective mechanism against stress that brings about decreased heart rate, lower metabolism, and decreased respiratory rate. It is the physiologic opposite of the 'fight or flight,' or stress, response.

relaxation therapy, treatment in which patients are taught to perform breathing and relaxation exercises and to concentrate on a pleasant situation. Some patients learn through relaxation therapy to relax taut muscles at will, to abort migraine attacks, or to reduce their blood pressure.

relaxation time, (in magnetic resonance imaging) the characteristic time it takes for a sample of atoms whose nuclei have first been aligned along a static magnetic field and then excited to a higher energy (MR) state by a radiofrequency (rf) signal to return to a lower energy equilibrium state.

relaxin /rilak′sin/, a hormone obtained from the corpora lutea of swine and used to relax the pelvic ligaments and dilate the cervix during labor. The medication has also been used to treat dysmenorrhea.

release therapy /rilēs′/ [ME, *relesen,* to release], a type of pediatric psychotherapy used to treat children with stress and anxiety related to a specific recent event.

releasing hormone (RH), one of several peptides produced by the hypothalamus and secreted directly into the anterior pituitary gland via a connecting vein. Each of the releasing hormones stimulates the pituitary to secrete a specific tropic hormone; thus corticotropic-releasing hormone stimulates the pituitary to secrete adrenocorticotropic hormone.

releasing stimulus, (in psychology) an action or behavior by one individual that serves as a cue to trigger a response in others. An example is yawning by one person, which results in yawning by others in the group.

reliability /rilī′əbil′itē/ [L, *religare,* to fasten behind], (in research) the extent to which a test measurement or device produces the same results with different investigators, observers, or administration of the test over time.

relief area [L, *relevare,* to lighten], the part of the tissue surface under prosthesis on which pressures are reduced or eliminated.

relieving factor /rilē′ving/, an agent that alleviates a symptom.

religiosity /rilij′ē·os′itē/ [L, *religiosus*], a psychiatric symptom characterized by the demonstration of excessive or affected piety.

reline /rēlīn′/ [L, *re* + *linea*], the resurfacing of the tissue side of a denture with new base material.

relocation stress syndrome /rē′lōkā′shən/, a NANDA-accepted nursing diagnosis of physiologic and/or psychosocial disturbances as a result of a transfer from one environment to another. Defining characteristics include a change in environment or location, anxiety, apprehension, increased confusion (elderly population), depression, loneliness, a verbalization of unwillingness to relocate, sleep disturbance, change in eating habits, dependency, gastrointestinal disturbances, increased verbalization of needs, insecurity, lack of trust, restlessness, sad affect, unfavorable comparison of post/pretransfer staff, verbalization of being concerned or upset about the transfer, vigilance, weight change, and withdrawal.

rem /rem, är′ē′em′/, abbreviation for *roentgen equivalent man.* A dose of ionizing radiation that produces in humans the same effect as one roentgen of x-radiation or gamma radiation.

REM /rem, är′ē′em′/, abbreviation for *rapid eye movement.*

remasking /rēmas′king/, (in digital fluoroscopy) the production of one or more additional mask images if the first is inadequate because of patient motion, noise, or other factors.

remedial /rimē′dē·əl/ [L, *remediare,* to cure], designed to improve or cure.

reminiscence /rem′inis′əns/ [L, *reminisci,* to remember], the recollection of past personal experiences and significant events.

reminiscence therapy, a psychotherapeutic technique in which self-esteem and personal satisfaction are restored, particularly in older persons, by encouraging patients to review past experiences of a pleasant nature.

Reminiscence Therapy, a Nursing Interventions Classification defined as using the recall of past events, feelings, and thoughts to facilitate adaptation to present circumstances.

remission /rimish′ən/ [L, *remittere,* to abate], the partial or complete disappearance of the clinical and subjective characteristics of a chronic or malignant disease. Remission may be spontaneous or the result of therapy.

remittent fever /rimit′ənt/ [L, *remittere* + *febris,* fever], diurnal variations of an elevated temperature with exacerbations and remissions but never a return to normal.

R

remnant radiation /rem'nənt/ [L, *remanere,* to remain], the measurable radiation that passes through an object and can produce an image on an x-ray film.

remodeling /rēmod'əling/ [L, *re + modus,* to copy again], the process of changing a body part or area, as in reconstructive surgery.

remote afterloading /rimōt'/ [L, *removere,* to remove], (in radiotherapy) a technique in which an applicator such as an acrylic mold of an area to be irradiated is placed in or on the patient and then loaded from a safe source with a high-activity radioisotope. Remote afterloading is used in the treatment of head, neck, vaginal, and cervical tumors.

remotivation /rē'mōtivā'shən/ [L, *re + motus,* movement], the use of special techniques that stimulate patients to become motivated to learn and interact.

remotivation group, a treatment group that is organized with the purpose of stimulating the interest, awareness, and communication of withdrawn and institutionalized mental patients who experience amotivation.

removable lingual arch /rimoo'vəbəl/ [L, *removere,* to remove], an orthodontic arch wire designed to fit the lingual surface of the teeth and aid orthodontic movement of the dentition involved.

removable orthodontic appliance, a device placed inside the mouth to correct or alleviate malocclusion and designed to be removed or replaced by the patient.

removable rigid dressing, a dressing similar to a cast used to encase the stump of an amputated limb. It is usually applied to permit the fitting of a temporary prosthesis so that ambulation can begin soon after surgery.

renal /rē'nəl/ [L, *ren,* kidney], pertaining to the kidney.

renal acidosis [L, *ren,* kidney, *acidus,* sour; Gk, *osis,* condition], an excessive increase in the H^+ ions in body fluids because of impaired kidney function. The acidosis can result from excessive loss of bicarbonate or from the inability to excrete phosphoric and sulfuric acid.

renal angiography, a radiographic examination of the renal artery and associated blood vessels after the injection of a contrast medium.

renal anuria, cessation of urine production caused by intrinsic renal disease.

renal artery, one of a pair of large, visceral branches of the abdominal aorta. The renal arteries supply the kidneys, suprarenal glands, and the ureters.

renal biopsy, the removal of kidney tissue for microscopic examination. It is conducted to establish the diagnosis of a renal disorder and to aid in determining the stage of the disease, the appropriate therapy, and the prognosis. An open biopsy involves an incision, permits better visualization of the kidney, and carries a lower risk of hemorrhage; a closed or percutaneous biopsy performed by aspirating a specimen of tissue with a needle requires a shorter period of recovery and is less likely to cause infection.

renal calculus, a concretion occurring in the kidney.

renal calyx, the first unit in the system of ducts in the kidney carrying urine from the renal pyramid of the medulla to the renal pelvis for excretion through the ureters. There are two divisions: the minor renal calyx, with several others, drains into a larger major renal calyx, which in turn joins other major calyces to form the renal pelvis.

renal capsule [L, *ren,* kidney, *capsula,* little box], a protective connective tissue capsule surrounding the kidney.

renal cell carcinoma, a malignant neoplasm of the kidney.

renal colic, sharp, severe pain in the lower back over the kidney, radiating forward into the groin. Renal colic usually accompanies forcible dilation of a ureter, followed by spasm as a stone is lodged or passed through it.

renal cortex, the highly vascularized granular outer layer of the kidney, containing approximately 1.25 million glomeruli and convoluted tubules that filter body wastes from the blood, reclaim useful materials, and dispose of the remainder as urine.

renal dialysis [L, *ren,* kidney; Gk, *dia,* + *lysis,* loosening], a process of diffusing blood across a semipermeable membrane to remove substances that a normal kidney would eliminate, including poisons, drugs, urea, uric acid, and creatinine. Renal dialysis may restore electrolytes and acid-base imbalances.

renal diet, a diet prescribed in chronic renal failure and designed to control intake of protein, potassium, sodium, phosphorus, and fluids, depending on individual conditions. Carbohydrates and fats are the principal sources of energy. Protein is limited; the amount is determined by the patient's condition.

renal dwarf, a dwarf whose retarded growth is caused by renal failure.

renal failure, inability of the kidneys to excrete wastes, concentrate urine, and conserve electrolytes. The condition may be acute or chronic. Acute renal failure is characterized by oliguria and by the rapid accumulation of nitrogenous wastes in the blood (azotemia). It results from hemorrhage, trauma, burn, toxic injury to the kidney, acute pyelonephritis or glomerulonephritis, or lower urinary tract obstruction. Chronic renal failure may result from many other diseases. The early signs include sluggishness, fatigue, and mental dullness. Later, anuria, convulsions, gastrointestinal bleeding, malnutrition, and various neuropathies may occur. The skin may turn yellow-brown. Congestive heart failure and hypertension are frequent complications, the results of hypervolemia.

renal glycosuria [L, *ren,* kidney; Gk, *glykys,* sweet, *ouron,* urine], a familial condition characterized by lowered renal threshold to sugar. Blood sugar levels may be normal, although sugar is excreted in the urine.

renal hematuria [L, *ren,* kidney; Gk, *haima,* blood, *ouron,* urine], presence of blood in the urine because of a kidney disorder.

renal hypertension, hypertension resulting from kidney disease, including chronic glomerulonephritis, chronic pyelonephritis, renal carcinoma, and renal calculi. Analgesic abuse and certain drug reactions may also result in renal hypertension.

renal insufficiency [L, *ren,* kidney; *in + sufficere,* to suffice], partial kidney function failure characterized by less than normal urine excretion.

renal nanism, dwarfism associated with infantile renal osteodystrophy.

renal osteodystrophy, a condition resulting from chronic renal failure and characterized by uneven bone growth and demineralization.

renal pelvis [L, *ren + pelvis,* basin], a funnel-shaped dilation that drains urine from the kidney into the ureter.

renal plasma flow (RPF), the rate at which plasma flows through the renal tubules. It may be measured by p-aminohippurate clearance.

renal pyramid [L, *ren,* kidney; Gk, *pyramis*], any one of several conical masses of tissue that form the kidney medulla. The base of each pyramid adjoins the kidney's cortex; the apex terminates at a renal calyx. The pyramids consist of the loops of Henle and the collecting tubules of the nephrons.

renal rickets, a condition characterized by rachitic changes in the skeleton and caused by chronic nephritis.

renal scan, a scan of the kidneys to determine their size, shape, and exact position.

It is used to aid in the diagnosis of a tumor or other abnormalities and performed after the intravenous injection of a radioactive substance.

renal sclerosis [L, *ren,* kidney; Gk, *skerosis,* hardening], arteriosclerosis or fibrosis of the arterioles of the kidney.

renal transplantation [L, *ren,* kidney, *transplantare*], the surgical transfer of a complete kidney from a donor to a recipient.

renal tubular acidosis (RTA), an abnormal condition associated with persistent dehydration, metabolic acidosis, hypokalemia, hyperchloremia, and nephrocalcinosis. It is caused by the kidney's inability to conserve bicarbonate and to adequately acidify the urine. Some common signs and symptoms of RTA, especially in children, include anorexia, vomiting, constipation, retarded growth, excessive urination, nephrocalcinosis, and rickets. In children and adults RTA can also cause urinary tract infections and pyelonephritis.

renal tubule [L, *ren,* kidney, *tubulus,* small tube], the part of the kidney's nephron that leads from the glomerulus to the collecting tubules. It consists of a looping segment and two convoluted sections. These canals resorb selected materials back into the blood and secrete, collect, and conduct urine.

renin /rē'nin/ [L, *ren,* kidney], a proteolytic enzyme, produced by and stored in the juxtaglomerular apparatus that surrounds each arteriole as it enters a glomerulus. The enzyme affects the blood pressure by catalyzing the change of angiotensinogen to angiotensin.

rennin /ren'in/ [ME, *rennen,* to run], a milk-curdling enzyme that occurs in the gastric juices of infants and is also contained in the rennet produced in the stomach of calves and other ruminants. It is an endopeptidase that converts casein to paracasein.

renogram /rē'nəgram/, a graphic image made by a radiographic scan of the kidneys after injection of a radiopharmaceutical. It represents radioactivity versus time and is used to assess renal function.

Renshaw cells /ren'shô/ [B. Renshaw, American neurologist, b. 1911; L, *cella,* storeroom], small cells that reduce motor neuron discharge through a feedback circuit involving axon collaterals that excite interneurons. The system prevents rapid repeated firing of motor neurons.

reovirus /rē'ōvī'rəs/ [respiratory enteric orphan + L, *virus*], any one of three ubiquitous, double-stranded ribonucleic acid viruses found in the respiratory and

R

alimentary tracts in healthy and sick people. Reoviruses have been implicated in some cases of upper respiratory tract disease and infantile gastroenteritis.

repercussion /rē'pərkush'ən/ [L, *repercussio,* rebounding], **1.** (in obstetrics) ballottement. **2.** being driven back by a powerful resistance. **3.** the reduction of a swelling or tumor.

reperfusion /rē'pərfyōō'zhən/, a procedure in which blocked arteries are opened to reestablish blood flow. It may be accomplished through thrombolytic therapy or percutaneous transluminal angioplasty.

repetition compulsion /rep'ətish'ən/ [L, *repetere,* to repeat], an unconscious need to revert to and repeat earlier situations, behavior patterns, and acts to experience previously felt emotions or relationships.

repetitive stress injuries /ripet'ətiv/, tissue damage to the neck and arms associated with tasks that require repeated manipulations of the hands, such as meat cutting, computer keyboarding, or playing musical instruments. Injuries include chronic nerve and joint pain, cervical spine damage, and carpal tunnel syndrome. Among recommended preventive measures are frequent rest breaks and improved ergonomic rules for the workplace.

replacement /riplās'mənt/ [Fr, *replacer,* to put in place again], the substitution of a missing part or substance with a similar structure or substance, such as the replacement of an amputated limb with a prosthesis or the replacement of lost blood with donor blood.

replacement therapy, 1. the use of a medicinal product to replace a natural hormone or enzyme that the body is no longer able to produce in sufficient amounts. **2.** a psychotherapeutic technique of replacing abnormal behavior with healthy, constructive activities.

replacement transfusion, the removal of all or most of a patient's diseased blood and its simultaneous replacement with an equal volume of normal blood.

replication /rep'likā'shən/ [L, *replicare,* to fold back], **1.** a process of duplicating, reproducing, or copying; literally, a folding back of a part to form a duplicate. **2.** (in research) the exact repetition of an experiment performed to confirm the initial findings. **3.** (in genetics) the duplication of the polynucleotide strands of deoxyribonucleic acid (DNA) or the synthesis of DNA. —**replicate,** *v.*

replicator /rep'likā'tər/ [L, *replicare*], (in genetics) the segment of the deoxyribonucleic acid molecule that initiates and controls the replication of the polynucleotide strands.

replicon /rep'ləkon/ [L, *replicare*], (in genetics) a replication unit; the segment of the deoxyribonucleic acid molecule that is undergoing replication.

repolarization /rēpō'lərizā'shən/ [L, *re* + *polus,* pole; Gk, *izein,* to cause], the process by which the cell is restored to its resting potential. In cardiology it encompasses the effective and relative refractory periods and correlates with the QT interval on the electrocardiogram.

report /ripôrt'/ [L, *re* + *portare,* to carry], (in nursing) the transfer of information from the nurses on one shift to the nurses on the following shift. Report is given systematically at the time of change of shift.

reportable diseases /ripôr'təbəl/, diseases that must be reported by the physician to public health authorities, given their contagious nature. They include but are not limited to malaria, influenza, poliomyelitis, relapsing fever, typhus, yellow fever, cholera, and bubonic plague.

repositioning /rē'pəzish'əning/ [L, *reponere,* to put back], the restoration of an organ or body part to its natural position, as reposing an inverted uterus or changing the position of the jaws.

representative group /rep'rəsen'tətiv/, a group of individuals whose members represent all the various sectors of a community.

repression /ripresh'ən/ [L, *reprimere,* to press back], **1.** the act of restraining, inhibiting, or suppressing. **2.** (in psychoanalysis) an unconscious defense mechanism that also underlies all defense mechanisms whereby unacceptable thoughts, feelings, ideas, impulses, or memories, especially those concerning some traumatic past event, are pushed from the consciousness because of their painful guilt association or disagreeable content and are submerged in the unconscious, where they remain dormant but operant. —**repress,** *v.* **repressive,** *adj.*

repressive-inspirational approach /ripres'iv/, a psychotherapeutic approach used in some groups to discourage the breaking down of defense mechanisms. Members are encouraged to focus on positive feelings and group strengths.

repressor /ripres'ər/ [L, *reprimere,* to press back], (in molecular genetics) a protein produced by the regulator gene. It binds to a sequence of nucleotides in the operator gene, which regulates the structural gene.

reproduction /rē'prəduk'shən/ [L, *re* + *producere,* to produce], **1.** the process by which animals and plants give rise to offspring; procreation; the sum total of the cellular and genetic phenomena involved in the transmission of organic life from one organism to successive generations similar to the parents so that the perpetuation and continuity of the species is maintained. **2.** the creation of a similar structure, situation, or phenomenon; duplication; replication. **3.** (in psychology) the recalling of a former idea, impression, or something previously learned. —**reproductive,** *adj.*

reproductive /rē′prəduk′tiv/ [L, *re + producere,* again to produce], pertaining to the process of reproduction.

reproductive endocrinology, the study of the maternal female hormone system, including the activities of the hypothalamus, pituitary, and ovaries from puberty through menopause.

reproductive system, the male and female gonads, associated ducts and glands, and external genitalia that function in the procreation of offspring. In women these include the ovaries, fallopian tubes, uterus, vagina, clitoris, and vulva. In men they include the testes, epididymis, vas deferens, seminal vesicles, ejaculatory duct, prostate, and penis.

Reproductive Technology Management, a Nursing Interventions Classification defined as assisting a patient through the steps of complex infertility treatment.

repulsion /ripul′shən/ [L, *repellere,* to drive away], **1.** the act of repelling, disjoining. **2.** a force that separates two bodies or things. **3.** (in genetics) the situation in linked inheritance in which the alleles of two or more mutant genes are located on homologous chromosomes so that each chromosome of the pair carries one or more mutant and wild-type genes, which are located close enough to be inherited together.

request for proposal (RFP) /rikwest′ [L, *requaerere,* to require; *propronere,* to propound], a solicitation by a funding agency for proposals to accomplish a particular goal. The RFP lists the requirements a project must meet to receive funding.

required arch length /rikwī′ərd/ [L, *requaerere,* to require], the sum of the mesiodistal widths of all the natural teeth in a dental arch.

RES, abbreviation for **reticuloendothelial system.**

research /risurch′, rē′surch/ [Fr, *rechercher,* to investigate], the diligent inquiry or examination of data, reports, and observations in a search for facts or principles.

Research Data Collection, a Nursing Interventions Classification defined as assisting a researcher to collect patient data.

research instrument, a testing device for measuring a given phenomenon, such as a

paper and pencil test, a questionnaire, an interview, or a set of guidelines for observation.

research measurement, an evaluation of the quantity or incidence of a given variable as obtained by using a research instrument.

research radiopharmaceutical, a drug that is labeled with a small quantity of a radioactive tracer to allow its biodistribution to be studied; it may later be used in a nonradioactive form.

resect /risekt′/ [L, *re + secare,* to cut], to remove tissue from the body by surgery.

resection /risek′shən/, the cutting out of a significant part of an organ or structure. Resection of an organ may be partial or complete.

reserpine /res′ərpēn/, an antihypertensive prescribed in the treatment of high blood pressure and certain neuropsychiatric disorders.

reserve /rizurv′/ [L, *reservare,* to save], a potential capacity to maintain vital body functions in homeostasis by adjusting to increased need, such as cardiac reserve, pulmonary reserve, and alkali reserve.

reserve capacity [L, *reservare,* to save; Gk, *aer*], the volume of air that can be exhaled with maximum effort after completion of a normal expiration.

reservoir /rez′əvwär/ [Fr, réservoir], a chamber or receptacle for holding or storing a fluid.

reservoir bag, a component of an anesthesia machine in which gas accumulates, forming a reserve supply of gas for use during bagging, or manual control of ventilation. It serves as a visible monitor of respiratory rate and depth.

reservoir host, a nonhuman host that serves as a means of sustaining an infectious organism as a potential source of human infection. Wild monkeys are reservoir hosts for the yellow fever virus.

reservoir of infection, a continuous source of infectious disease. People, animals, and plants may be reservoirs of infection.

resident /rez′idənt/ [L, *residere,* to remain], a physician in one of the postgraduate years of clinical training after the first, or internship, year. The length of residency varies according to the specialty.

resident bacteria, bacteria living in a specific area of the body.

residential care facility /rez′iden′shəl/, a facility that provides custodial care to persons who, because of physical, mental, or emotional disorders, are not able to live independently.

residual /rizij′ $\overline{oo}$ ·əl/ [L, *residuum,* remainder], pertaining to the part of something

R

that remains after an activity that removes the bulk of the substance.

residual cyst, an odontogenic cyst that remains in the jaw after the removal of a tooth.

residual dental caries, any decayed material left in a prepared tooth cavity.

residual function [L, *residuum,* remainder, *functio,* performance], the remaining ability to function after a serious illness or injury.

residual ridge, the part of the dental ridge that remains after the alveolar process has disappeared after extraction of the teeth.

residual urine, urine that remains in the bladder after urination.

residual volume [L, *residuum,* remainder, *volumen,* papyrus roll], the amount of air remaining in the lungs at the end of a maximum expiration.

residue-free diet /rez′id(y)o͞o/ [L, *residuum,* remainder; AS, *freo* + Gk, *diaita,* way of life], a diet free of nondigestible cellulose or fiber, such as found in semisolid bland food.

residue schizophrenia [L, *residuum*], a form of schizophrenia in which the essential features include the presence of residual symptoms without evidence of delusions, hallucinations, incoherence, or gross disorganization.

resilience /rizil′yənt/ [L, *resilere,* to spring back], the ability of a body to return to its original form after being stretched or compressed.

resins /rez′ins/, substances used in a kind of drug therapy for lowering low-density lipoprotein C (LDL-C) levels. Bile-acid binding resins such as cholestyramine and colestipol interrupt the normal enterohepatic circulation of bile acids and indirectly increase the liver's breakdown of LDL-C.

res ipsa loquitur /räs′ ip′sə lok′witȯr/ [L, the thing speaks for itself], a legal concept that is important in many malpractice suits, describing a situation in which an injury occurred when the defendant was solely and exclusively in control and in which the injury would not have occurred had due care been exercised.

resistance /rizis′təns/ [L, *resistere,* to withstand], **1.** an opposition to a force, such as the resistance offered by the constriction of peripheral vessels to the blood flow in the circulatory system. **2.** the frictional force that opposes the flow of an electric charge, as measured in ohms. **3.** (in respiratory therapy) the process or power of acting against a force placed on it, pertaining to thoracic resistance, tissue resistance, and airway resistance.

resistance form, the shape given to a prepared tooth cavity to impart strength and durability to the restoration and remaining tooth structure.

resistance-inducing factor (RIF), an agent that interferes with multiplication of a virus or other pathogen.

resistance to flow, (in respiratory therapy) the pressure differential required to produce a unit flow change.

resistance training, any method or form of strength training used to resist, overcome, or bear force.

resistance vessels, the blood vessels, including small arteries, arterioles, and metarterioles that form the major part of the total peripheral resistance to blood flow.

resistant /rizis′tənt/, pertaining to an ability of a microorganism to remain unaffected by an antimicrobial agent.

resistive magnet /resis′tiv/, a simple electromagnet in which electricity passing through coils of wire produces a magnetic field.

resocialization /rēsō′shəlīzā′shən/ [L, *re* + *socialis,* partners; Gk, *izein,* to cause], the reintegration of a client into family and community life after critical or long-term hospitalization.

resolution [L, *re* + *solvere,* to solve], **1.** the ability of an imaging process to distinguish adjacent structures in the object. **2.** the state of having made a firm determination or decision on a course of action. **3.** the ability of a chromatographic system to separate two adjacent peaks.

resolving power /rizol′ving/, **1.** the ability to separate closely migrating substances, as in electrophoresis. **2.** the ability to distinguish closely positioned objects as distinct entities.

resolving time, (in radiology) the minimum time between ionization that can be detected by a Geiger-Müller-type scintillation device.

resonance /rez′ənəns/ [L, *resonare,* to sound again], **1.** an echo or other sound produced by percussion of an organ or cavity of the body during a physical examination. **2.** the process of energy absorption by an object that is tuned to absorb energy of a specific frequency only. Other frequencies do not affect the object. —**resonant,** *adj.*

resonance frequency, 1. in an ultrasound transducer, the frequency for which the response of a transducer to an ultrasound beam is a maximum. **2.** the frequency at which the transducer most efficiently converts electrical signals to mechanical vibrations. **3.** (in magnetic resonance) the frequency at which a

resonant /rez'ənənt/ [L, *resonare*, to sound again], pertaining to a sound that vibrates on percussion or is amplified by sympathetic vibrations in another medium.

resonating /rez'ənā'ting/ [L, *resonare*, to sound again], pertaining to vibrations or pulsations that are synchronous with a source of sound waves or electromagnetic oscillations.

resorb /risôrb'/ [L, *resorbere*, to swallow again], to absorb again.

resorbent /risôr'bənt/ [L, *resorbere*], a material or agent that is used to absorb blood or other substances.

resorcinated camphor /rizôr'sinā'tid/, a mixture of camphor and resorcinol, used for the treatment of pediculosis and itching.

resorcinol /rizôr'sinol/, an antiseptic substance used as a keratolytic agent in the dermatoses.

resorption /risôrp'shən/ [L, *resorbere*, to swallow again], **1.** the loss of substance or bone by physiologic or pathologic means. **2.** the cementoclastic and dentinoclastic action that may occur on a tooth root.

resource-based relative value scale (RBRVS), a system for a Medicare fee schedule designed to address the promise of compensation to a physician for the time involved in giving physical and mental status examinations and obtaining patient history from family members.

Res. Phys., abbreviation for *resident physician.*

respiration /res'pirā'shən/ [L, *respirare*, to breathe], the process of the molecular exchange of oxygen and carbon dioxide within the body's tissues, from the lungs to cellular oxidation processes. Certain types of rhythmic and dysrhythmic breathing patterns commonly referred to as 'respiration' are **Biot's respiration, Cheyne-Stokes respiration,** and **Kussmaul breathing.**

respiration of infants [L, *respirare*, to breathe, *infans*, unable to speak], a rate of breathing that averages 40 to 50 breaths per minute at birth and declines to 15 to 20 breaths per minute at puberty.

respiration rate [L, *respirare*, to breathe, *ratum*, rate], the number of inspirations per minute, ranging from a rapid 40 to 50 breaths/min for newborns, through 20 to 25 breaths/min for older children, and 15 to 20 breaths/min for most teenagers and adults. An adult rate of 25 breaths/min may be regarded as accelerated, whereas a rate of less than 12 breaths/min is abnormally slow.

respirator /res'pirā'tər/ [L, *respirare*], an apparatus used to modify air for inspiration or to improve pulmonary ventilation.

respiratory /res'pərətôr'ē, rispī'rətôr'ē/ [L, *respirare*], pertaining to respiration.

respiratory acidosis, an abnormal condition characterized by increased arterial PCO_2, excess carbonic acid, and increased plasma hydrogen ion concentration. It is caused by reduced alveolar ventilation or the suppression of respiratory reflexes with narcotics, sedatives, hypnotics, or anesthetics. The hypoventilation inhibits the excretion of carbon dioxide, which consequently combines with water in the body to produce excessive carbonic acid and thus reduces blood pH. Some common signs and symptoms of respiratory acidosis are headache, dyspnea, fine tremors, tachycardia, hypertension, and vasodilation. Ineffective treatment of acute respiratory acidosis can lead to coma and death.

respiratory alkalosis, an abnormal condition characterized by decreased PCO_2, decreased hydrogen ion concentration, and increased blood pH. Some pulmonary causes are acute asthma, pulmonary vascular disease, and pneumonia. Some nonpulmonary causes are aspirin toxicity, anxiety, fever, metabolic acidosis, inflammation of the central nervous system, gram-negative septicemia, and hepatic failure. Deep and rapid breathing at rates as high as 40 respirations per minute is a major sign of respiratory alkalosis. Other symptoms are light-headedness, dizziness, peripheral paresthesia, tingling of the hands and the feet, muscle weakness, tetany, and cardiac arrhythmia.

respiratory arrest, the cessation of breathing.

respiratory assessment, an evaluation of the condition and function of a person's respiratory system. Signs of confusion, anxiety, restlessness, flaring nostrils, cyanotic lips, gums, earlobes, or nails, clubbing of extremities, fever, anorexia, and a tendency to sit upright are noted if present. The person's breathing is closely observed. The thorax is examined. Percussion is performed to evaluate resonance, hyperresonance, tympany, and dull or flat sounds. Crackles, rhonchi, wheezing, friction rubs, the transmission of spoken words through the chest wall, and decreased or absent breath sounds are detected by auscultation. Background information pertinent to the evaluation includes allergies, recent exposure to infection, immunizations, exposure to environmental irritants, previous respiratory disorders and operations, preexisting chronic conditions, medication currently taken, the per-

R

son's smoking habits, and the family history. An accurate and thorough assessment of respiratory function is an essential component of the physical examination and is vital to the diagnosis or ongoing care of a respiratory illness.

respiratory burn, tissue damage to the respiratory system resulting from the inhalation of a hot gas or burning particles, as may occur in a fire or explosion.

respiratory care practitioner, a health professional with special training and experience in the treatment and rehabilitation of patients with respiratory disorders. The respiratory care practitioner typically does not diagnose but must be competent with patient assessment skills in a variety of clinical settings.

respiratory center, a group of nerve cells in the pons and medulla of the brain that control the rhythm of breathing in response to changes in levels of oxygen and carbon dioxide in the blood and cerebrospinal fluid. Change in the concentration of oxygen and carbon dioxide or hydrogen ion levels in the arterial circulation and cerebrospinal fluid activate central and peripheral chemoreceptors; these send impulses to the respiratory center, increasing or decreasing the breathing rate.

respiratory component (αPco_2), the acid component of an acid-base control system that is modified by the respiratory status.

respiratory cycle, an inspiration followed by an expiration.

respiratory depressant [L, *respirare,* to breathe, *depremere,* to press down], a drug or other agent that diminishes normal breathing functions. Most respiratory depressants such as alcohol and opiates act by depressing the central nervous system.

respiratory depression [L, *respirare,* to breathe, *depremere,* to press down], respiration that is slow, below 12 inspirations per minute, or feeble, failing to provide full ventilation and perfusion of the lungs.

respiratory distress syndrome of the newborn (RDS), an acute lung disease of the newborn, characterized by airless alveoli, inelastic lungs, more than 60 respirations per minute, nasal flaring, intercostal and subcostal retractions, grunting on expiration, and peripheral edema. It is caused by a deficiency of pulmonary surfactant, resulting in overdistended alveoli and at times hyaline membrane formation, alveolar hemorrhage, severe right-to-left shunting of blood, increased pulmonary resistance, decreased cardiac output, and severe hypoxemia.

respiratory exchange ratio (R), the ratio of carbon dioxide product to that of oxygen consumption or uptake, expressed by the formula VCO_2/V_2.

respiratory failure, the inability of the cardiac and pulmonary systems to maintain an adequate exchange of oxygen and carbon dioxide in the lungs. Respiratory failure may be oxygenation or hypercapnic. Oxygenation failure is characterized by hyperventilation and occurs in diseases that affect the alveoli or interstitial tissues of the lobes of the lungs, such as alveolar edema, emphysema, fungal infections, leukemia, lobar pneumonia, or tuberculosis. Ventilatory failure, characterized by increased arterial tension of carbon dioxide, occurs in acute conditions in which retained pulmonary secretions cause increased airway resistance and decreased lung compliance, as in bronchitis and emphysema.

respiratory insufficiency [L, *respirare,* to breathe, *in* + *sufficere,* to suffice], a failure of the respiratory system to maintain adequate ventilation and perfusion of the lungs.

Respiratory Monitoring, a Nursing Interventions Classification defined as collection and analysis of patient data to ensure airway patency and adequate gas exchange.

respiratory muscles, the muscles that produce volume changes of the thorax during breathing. The inspiratory muscles include the hemidiaphragms, external intercostals, scaleni, sternomastoids, trapezius, pectoralis major, pectoralis minor, subclavius, latissimus dorsi, serratus anterior, and muscles that extend the back. The expiratory muscles are the internal intercostals, the abdominals, and the muscles that flex the back.

respiratory quotient (RQ), the body's total exchange of oxygen for carbon dioxide, expressed as the ratio of the volume of carbon dioxide produced to the volume of oxygen consumed per unit of time at steady-state conditions.

respiratory rate, the normal rate of breathing at rest, about 12 to 20 inspirations per minute. The hydrogen ion concentration in the cerebrospinal fluid controls the rate of respiration. The rate may be more rapid in fever, acute pulmonary infection, diffuse pulmonary fibrosis, gas gangrene, left ventricular failure, thyrotoxicosis, and states of tension. Slower breathing rates may result from head injury, coma, or narcotic overdose.

respiratory rhythm, a regular oscillating cycle of inspiration and expiration, controlled by neuronal impulses transmitted between the muscles of inspiration in the chest and the respiratory centers in the brain.

respiratory standstill, the cessation of respiratory movements.

respiratory syncytial virus (RSV, RS virus), a member of a subgroup of myxoviruses that in tissue culture cause formation of giant cells or syncytia. It is a common cause of epidemics of acute bronchiolitis, bronchopneumonia, and the common cold in young children and sporadic acute bronchitis and mild upper respiratory tract infections in adults. Symptoms of infection with this virus include fever, cough, and severe malaise.

respiratory therapist, a graduate of a school approved by the American Medical Association designed to qualify the person for the registry examination of the National Board of Respiratory Care (NBRC).

respiratory therapy (RT), 1. any treatment that maintains or improves the ventilatory function of the respiratory tract. 2. *informal.* the department in a health care facility that provides respiratory therapy for the patients of the facility.

respiratory therapy technician, a graduate of an AMA-approved school designed to qualify the person for the technician certification examination of the National Board for Respiratory Care. It usually requires a 1-year hospital-based program combining a special curriculum of basic sciences with supervised clinical experience.

respiratory therapy technician, certified (CRTT), an allied health professional who administers general respiratory care. Duties can include collection and review of clinical data; examination of the patient by inspection, palpation, percussion, and auscultation; and assembling and maintaining equipment used in respiratory care.

respiratory tract, the complex of organs and structures that performs the pulmonary ventilation of the body and the exchange of oxygen and carbon dioxide between ambient air and blood circulating through the lungs. It also warms the air passing into the body and assists in the speech function by providing air for the larynx and the vocal cords.

respiratory tract infection, any infectious disease of the upper or lower respiratory tract. Upper respiratory tract infections include the common cold, laryngitis, pharyngitis, rhinitis, sinusitis, and tonsillitis. Lower respiratory tract infections include bronchitis, bronchiolitis, pneumonia, and tracheitis.

respiratory zone, the terminal air units where gas exchange actually occurs, usually below the seventeenth division of bronchi.

respirometer /res′pirom′ətər/ [L, *respirare,* to breath; Gk, *metron,* measure], an instrument used to analyze the quality of a patient's respirations.

respite care /res′pit/ [L, *respicere,* to look back], 1. short-term health services provided to the dependent older adult, either at home or in an institutional setting. 2. the provision of temporary care for a patient who requires specialized or intensive care or supervision that is normally provided by his or her family at home.

Respite Care, a Nursing Interventions Classification defined as provision of short-term care to provide relief for family caregiver.

respite time /res′pit/, relief time from responsibilities for the care of a patient, an individual, or a family member.

respondeat superior /respon′dē·at/ [L, let the master answer], the concept that an employer may be held liable for torts committed by employees acting within the scope of their employment.

responder /rispon′dər/ [L, *respondere,* to promise in return], a person whose tumor shrinks in volume by at least 50% as a result of chemotherapy, radiation, or other treatment.

response /rispons′/ [L, *responsum,* reply], 1. a reaction of an organism to a stimulus. 2. (in psychology) a category of negative punishment in which the reinforcer is lost or withdrawn after an operant.

response time, the period between the application of a stimulus and the response of a cell or cells.

rest [AS, *restan,* to rest], an extension from a prosthesis that affords vertical support for a dental restoration.

rest area, a surface prepared on a tooth or fixed restoration into which the rest fits, providing vertical support for a removable partial denture.

resting cell, a cell that is not undergoing division.

resting membrane potential, the transmembrane voltage that exists when the heart muscle is at rest.

resting potential [AS, *rest* + L, *potentia,* power], the electrical potential across a nerve cell membrane before it is stimulated to release the charge. The resting potential for a neuron is between 50 and 100 mV, with the excess of negatively charged ions inside the cell membrane.

resting tremor, an involuntary tremor occurring when the person is at rest; one of the signs of Parkinson's disease.

restitution /res′tit(y)o͞o′shən/, the spontaneous turning of the fetal head to the right or left after it has extended through the vulva.

rest jaw relation, (in dentistry) the postural relation of the mandible to the maxilla when the patient is resting comfortably in the upright position.

rest joint position, the position of a joint where the joint surfaces are relatively incongruent and the support structures are relatively lax. The position is used extensively in passive mobilization procedures.

restless legs syndrome [AS, *restlaes* + ONorse, *leggr*], a benign condition of unknown origin characterized by an irritating sensation of uneasiness, tiredness, and itching deep within the muscles of the leg, especially the lower part of the limb, accompanied by twitching and sometimes pain. The only relief is walking or moving the legs.

restoration /res′tôrā′shən/ [L, *restaurare,* to restore], any tooth filling, inlay, crown, partial or complete denture, or prosthesis that restores or replaces lost tooth structure, teeth, or oral tissues.

restoration contour, the profile of the surfaces of teeth that have been restored.

restoration of cusps, a reduction and inclusion of tooth cusps within a tooth cavity preparation and their restoration to functional occlusion with an artificial dental material.

restorative /ristôr′ətiv/ [L, *restaurare*], pertaining to the power or ability to restore or renew a person to a normal state of health or consciousness.

restraint /ristrānt′/ [L, *restringere,* to confine], any one of numerous devices used in aiding immobilized patients, especially children in traction. Examples of restraints are specially designed slings, jackets, or diapers.

restraint in bed [L, *restringere,* to confine; AS, *bedd*], the confinement of a person to bed rest by the use of mechanical, physical, or chemical means, if needed.

restraint of trade, an illegal act that interferes with free competition in a commercial or business transaction so as to restrict the production of a product or the provision of a service, affect the cost of a product or a service, or control the market in any way to the detriment of the consumers or purchasers of the service or product.

restriction endonuclease /ristrik′shən en′- dōnoo̅′klē-ās/ [L, *restringere* + Gk, *endon,* within; L, *nucleus* nut kernel; Fr, *diastase,* enzyme], (in molecular genetics) an enzyme that cleaves deoxyribonucleic acid (DNA) at a specific site. Each of the many different endonucleases isolated

from various bacteria acts at a species-specific cleavage site.

restriction fragment, a fragment of viral or cellular nucleic acid produced by cleavage of the deoxyribonucleic acid molecule by specific endonucleases.

restriction fragment length polymorphism (RFLP), a marker for a deoxyribonucleic acid (DNA) segment of a chromosome that may act as a marker associated with a hereditary disease. RFLPs are used in the detection of sequence variations in human genomic DNA segments.

restrictive cardiomyopathy /ristrik′tiv/ [L, *restringere,* to confine; Gk, *kardia,* heart, *mys,* muscle, *pathos,* disease], a form of heart disease characterized by diastolic noncompliance or poor compliance of the ventricles, as in constrictive pericarditis.

restrictive disease, a respiratory disorder characterized by restriction of expansion of the lungs or chest wall, resulting in diminished lung volumes and capacities.

resuscitation /risus′itā′shən/ [L, *resuscitare,* to revive], the process of sustaining the vital functions of a person in respiratory or cardiac failure while reviving him or her, using techniques of artificial respiration and cardiac massage, correcting acid-base imbalance, and treating the cause of failure. **—resuscitate,** *v.*

Resuscitation: Fetus, a Nursing Interventions Classification defined as administering emergency measures to improve placental perfusion or correct fetal acid-base status.

Resuscitation: Neonate, a Nursing Interventions Classification defined as administering emergency measures to support newborn adaptation to extrauterine life.

resuscitator /risus′itā′tər/, an apparatus for pumping air into the lungs. It consists of a mask snugly applied over the mouth and nose, a reservoir for air, and a manually or electrically powered pump.

RET, abbreviation for **rational emotive therapy.**

retail dentistry /rē′tāl/ [ME, *retailen,* to divide into pieces], the practice of fee-for-service dentistry in an exclusively retail environment such as a shopping center, with the specific intention of attracting the customers of such retail centers and by using the marketing techniques of the retailers involved.

retained placenta /ritānd′/ [L, *retinere,* to hold, *placenta,* flat cake], the failure of the placenta to be delivered during an appropriate period, usually 30 minutes, following birth of the infant.

retainer [L, *retinere,* to hold], **1.** the part

of a dental prosthesis that connects an abutment tooth with the suspended part of a bridge. **2.** an appliance for maintaining teeth and jaw positions gained by orthodontic procedures. **3.** the part of a fixed prosthesis that attaches a pontic to the abutment teeth. **4.** any clasp, attachment, or device for fixing or stabilizing a dental prosthesis.

retaining orthodontic appliance, an orthodontic device for holding the teeth in place, following orthodontic tooth movement, until the occlusion is stabilized.

retake /rē'tāk/, the repeat of a radiograph because of inadequate technical quality, patient motion, mispositioning of the body part, or equipment malfunction.

retardation /rē'tärdā'shən/ [L, *retardare,* to check], the slowing down of any mental or physical activity or failure of intellectual abilities to develop normally, as in mental retardation. Psychomotor retardation may occur in depression, and a conditioned response to an unconditioned stimulus may be retarded in appearance.

retarded /ritär'did/, [L, *retardare,* to check], (of physical, intellectual, social, or emotional development) abnormally slow. **—retard** /ritärd'/, *v.*

retarded dentition, the abnormal delay of the eruption of the deciduous or permanent teeth resulting from malnutrition, malposition of the teeth, a hereditary factor, or a metabolic imbalance such as hypothyroidism.

retarded depression, the depressive phase of bipolar disorder.

retarded ejaculation, the inability of a male to ejaculate after having achieved an erection. This often accompanies the aging process.

retch [AS, *hraecan,* to spit], a strong, wrenching attempt to vomit that does not bring up anything.

rete /rē'tē/ [L, net], a network, especially of arteries or veins. **—retial** /rē'tē·əl/, *adj.*

rete arteriosum [L, *rete,* net: Gk, *arteria*], an anastomotic network of small arteries at a point before they branch into arterioles and capillaries.

retention /riten'shən/, **1.** a resistance to movement or displacement. **2.** the ability of the digestive system to hold food and fluid. **3.** the inability to urinate or defecate. **4.** the ability of the mind to remember information acquired from reading, observation, or other processes. **5.** the inherent property of a dental restoration to maintain its position without displacement under axial stress. **6.** a characteristic of proper tooth cavity preparation in which provision is made for preventing vertical

displacement of the cavity filling. **7.** a period of treatment during which an individual wears an appliance to maintain teeth in positions to which they have been moved by orthodontic procedures. **—retain,** *v.*

retention enema [L, *retinere,* to hold; Gk, *enema,* clyster], a medicinal or nutrient enema specially formulated so it will remain in the bowel without stimulating the nerve endings that would ordinarily result in evacuation.

retention form, the provision made in a prepared tooth cavity to hold in place a restoration and to prevent its displacement.

retention groove, a depression formed by the opposing vertical constrictions in the preparation of a tooth, which improves the holding ability of a restoration.

retention of urine, an abnormal, involuntary accumulation of urine in the bladder as a result of a loss of muscle tone in the bladder, neurologic dysfunction or damage to the bladder, obstruction of the urethra, or administration of a narcotic analgesic.

retention pin, a small metal projection that extends from a dental metal casting into the dentin of a tooth to improve the holding ability of a tooth restoration.

retention procedure, a method established by state laws or mental health codes for committing a person to a psychiatric institution.

retention time (t$_a$), **1.** (in chromatography) the amount of time elapsed from the injection of a sample into the chromatographic system to the recording of the peak (band) maximum of the component in the chromatogram. **2.** the length of time a compound is retained on a chromatography column.

retention with overflow [L, *retinere,* to hold; AS, *ofer + flowan*], a complication of urinary incontinence in which the pressure of retained urine after a voiding results in dribbling.

reticular /ritik'yələr/ [L, *reticulum,* little net], (of a tissue or surface) having a netlike pattern or structure.

reticular activating system (RAS), a functional system in the brain essential for wakefulness, attention, concentration, and introspection. A network of nerve fibers in the thalamus, hypothalamus, brainstem, and cerebral cortex contribute to the system.

reticular formation, a small, thick cluster of neurons nestled within the brainstem, including the medulla that controls the level of consciousness and other vital

R

functions of the body. The reticular formation constantly monitors the state of the body through connections with the sensory and motor tracts.

reticulation film fault /ritik′yəlā′shən/ [L, *reticulum + atio,* process], a defect in a radiograph or developed photographic film that appears as a network of corrugations. It is usually caused by film development with an excessive temperature difference between any two of the three darkroom solutions.

reticulin /ritik′yəlin/ [L, *reticulum,*], an albuminoid substance found in the connective fibers of reticular tissue.

reticulocyte /ritik′yələsīt′/ [L, *reticulum* + Gk, *kytos,* cell], an immature erythrocyte characterized by a meshlike pattern of threads and particles at the former site of the nucleus.

reticulocyte count, a count of the number of reticulocytes in a whole blood specimen, used in determining bone marrow activity. The reticulocyte count is lowered in hemolytic diseases and chronic infection; it is elevated after hemorrhage or during recovery from anemia.

reticulocytopenia /ritik′yəlōsī′təpē′nē·ə/ [L, *reticulum* + Gk, *kytos,* cell, *penia,* poverty], a decrease below the normal range of 0.5% to 1.5% in the number of reticulocytes in a blood sample.

reticulocytosis /-sītō′sis/, an increase in the number of reticulocytes in the circulating blood.

reticuloendothelial cells /ritik′yəlō·en′dō-thē′lē·əl/ [L, *reticulum* + Gk, *endon,* within, *thele,* nipple], cells lining vascular and lymph vessels capable of phagocytosing bacteria, viruses, and colloidal particles or of forming immune bodies against foreign particles.

reticuloendothelial system (RES), a functional rather than anatomic system of the body involved primarily in defense against infection and disposal of the products of the breakdown of cells. It is made up of macrophages; the Kupffer cells of the liver; and the reticulum cells of the lungs, bone marrow, spleen, and lymph nodes.

reticuloendotheliosis /ritik′yəlō·en′dōthē′-lē·ō′sis/, an abnormal condition characterized by increased growth and proliferation of the cells of the reticuloendothelial system.

reticulogranular /-gran′yələr/ [L, *reticulum* + *granulum,* little grain], pertaining to a cloudy appearance of the lungs on a chest radiograph of a patient with respiratory distress syndrome.

retina /ret′inə/ [L, *rete,* net], a 10-layered, delicate nervous tissue membrane

of the eye, continuous with the optic nerve, that receives images of external objects and transmits visual impulses through the optic nerve to the brain. The retina is soft and semitransparent and contains rhodopsin. It consists of the outer pigmented layer and the nine-layered retina proper. These nine layers, starting with the most internal, are the internal limiting membrane, the stratum opticum, the ganglion cell layer, the inner plexiform layer, the inner nuclear layer, the outer plexiform layer, the outer nuclear layer, the external limiting membrane, and the layer of rods and cones. The outer surface of the retina is in contact with the choroid; the inner surface with the vitreous body.

retinaculum /ret′inak′yələm/, *pl.* **reti-nacula** [L, halter], 1. a structure that retains an organ or tissue. 2. an instrument for retracting tissues during surgery.

retinal /ret′inəl, ret′inal′/ [L, *rete*], 1. an aldehyde precursor of vitamin A produced by the enzymatic dehydration of retinol. 2. pertaining to the retina.

retinal detachment, a separation of the retina from the choroid in the back of the eye. It usually results from a hole in the retina that allows the vitreous humor to leak between the choroid and the retina. Severe trauma to the eye such as a contusion or penetrating wound may be the proximate cause, but in the great majority of cases retinal detachment is the result of internal changes in the vitreous chamber associated with aging or less frequently with inflammation of the interior of the eye. The first symptom is often the sudden appearance of a large number of floating spots loosely suspended in front of the affected eye. The person may not seek help because the number of spots tends to decrease during the days and weeks after the detachment. The person may also notice a curious sensation of flashing lights as the eye is moved. Because the retina does not contain sensory nerves that relay sensations of pain, the condition is painless. If the process of detachment is not halted, total blindness of the eye ultimately results.

retinene /ret′inin/ [L, *rete*], either of the two carotenoid pigments found in the rods of the retina that are precursors of vitamin A and are activated by light.

retinitis /ret′inī′tis/ [L, *rete,* net; Gk, *itis,* inflammation], an inflammation of the retina.

retinitis pigmentosa [L, *rete,* net; Gk, *itis,* inflammation; L, *pigmentum,* paint], a group of diseases, often hereditary, characterized by bilateral primary degeneration of the retina, beginning in childhood and progressing to blindness by middle age. Clinical signs include night blindness, reduced visual fields, pigmentation of the retina, macular degeneration, and eventually total loss of vision.

retinoblastoma /ret'inōblastō'mə/ [L, *rete* + Gk, *blastos,* germ, *oma,* tumor], a congenital hereditary neoplasm developing from retinal germ cells. Characteristic signs are diminished vision, strabismus, retinal detachment, and an abnormal pupillary reflex. The rapidly growing tumor may invade the brain and metastasize to distant sites.

retinochoroiditis /-kôr'oidī'tis/ [L, *rete,* net; Gk, *chorion,* skin, *itis,* inflammation], an inflammation of the retina and choroid coat of the eye.

retinodialysis /ret'inō'dī·al'isis/ [L, *rete* + Gk, *dia,* through, *lysis,* loosening], a separation or tear in the retina in its anterior part, in the area of the ora serrata, just behind the ciliary body.

retinoid /ret'inoid/, [L, *rete,* net; Gk, *eidos,* form], **1.** resembling the retina. **2.** pertaining to any of a group of compounds whose molecules contain 20 carbon atoms structurally related to retinal, retinol, and other substances, some of which exhibit vitamin A activity. **3.** resinlike or having a resemblance to resin.

retinol /ret'inol/ [L, *rete*], the cis-trans form of vitamin A. It is found in the retinas of mammals.

retinol equivalent (RE), a unit used for quantifying the vitamin A value of sources of vitamin A, with RE defined as 3.3 International Units of vitamin A.

retinopathy /ret'inop'əthē/ [L, *rete* + Gk, *pathos,* disease], a noninflammatory eye disorder resulting from changes in the retinal blood vessels.

retinoscope /ret'inəskōp'/ [L, *rete,* net; Gk, *skopein,* to view], an instrument used in retinoscopy to determine errors of refraction.

retinoscopy /ret'inos'kəpē/ [L, *rete,* net; Gk, *skopein,* to view], a procedure for examining the eyes for possible errors of refraction. The examiner shines a light into the eyeball and notes the movements of reflex from the fundus. This indicates the types of lenses needed to neutralize the refractive errors.

retirement center /ritī'ərmənt/ [Fr, *retirer,* to withdraw; Gk, *kentron,* center], a facility or organized program to provide social services and activities for senior citizens who generally do not require ongoing health care.

retract /ritrakt/ [L, *retractare,* to draw back], to shrink, make shorter, or pull back.

retracted nipple [L, *retractare,* to draw back; ME, *neb*], a nipple drawn inward, resulting from cancer or adhesions below the skin surface or a natural condition present at birth.

retraction /ritrak'shən/ [L, *retractare,* to draw back], **1.** the displacement of tissues to expose a part or structure of the body. **2.** a distal movement of the teeth. **3.** a distal or retrusive position of the teeth, dental arch, or jaw.

retraction of the chest, the visible sinking in of the soft tissues of the chest between and around the firmer tissue of the cartilaginous and bony ribs, as occurs with increased inspiratory effort or obstruction at some level of the respiratory tract.

retractor /ritrak'tər/ [L, *retractare*], an instrument for holding back the edges of tissues and organs to maintain exposure of the underlying anatomic parts, particularly during surgery.

retroanterograde amnesia /retrō·anter'-ōgrād/ [L, *retro,* backward, *antero,* foremost, *gradus,* step; Gk, *amnesia,* forgetfulness], a memory disorder in which current events may be assigned to the past and past events may be regarded as current.

retroaortic node /ret'rō·ā·ôr'tik/ [L, *retro,* backward; Gk, *aerein,* to raise], a node in one of three sets of lumbar lymph nodes that serve various structures in the abdomen and pelvis.

retroauricular /ret'rō·ôrik'yələr/ [L, *retro,* backward, *auricula,* little ear], pertaining to a location behind the ear.

retrobulbar /-bul'bər/ [L, *retro,* backward, *bulbus,* swollen root], **1.** pertaining to the area behind the pons. **2.** pertaining to the area behind the eyeball.

retrobulbar neuritis [L, *retro,* backward, *bulbus,* swollen root; Gk, *neuron* + *itis,* inflammation], a form of neuritis that involves the optic nerve or the optic disc.

retrobulbar pupillary reflex, an abnormal response of a pupil to light. After initial constriction of the pupil, dilation occurs as the stimulus continues. It is a sign of retrobulbar neuritis.

retrocecal /-sē'kəl/ [L, *retro,* backward, *caecus,* blind], pertaining to the region behind the cecum.

retroclusion /ret'rokloo'zhən/, a method of controlling hemorrhage from an artery by compressing it between tissues on either side. A needle is inserted through the tissues above the bleeding vessel, then turned around and down so it also passes through the tissues beneath the artery.

retroflexion /-flek'shən/ [L, *retro* + *flectere,* to bend], an abnormal position of an organ in which the organ is tilted back acutely, folded over on itself.

retroflexion of the uterus, a condition in which the body of the uterus is bent backward at an angle with the cervix, whose position usually remains unchanged.

retrognathia /ret'rōnā'thē·ə/ [L, retro, backward; Gk, gnathos, jaw], a condition in which either or both jaws recede with respect to the frontal plane of the forehead.

retrognathism /ret'rōnā'this'əm/ [L, retro + Gk, gnathos, jaw], a facial abnormality in which one or both jaws, usually the mandible, are posterior to their normal facial positions.

retrograde /ret'rəgrād/ [L, retro + gradus, step], **1.** moving backward; moving in the opposite direction to that which is considered normal. **2.** degenerating; reverting to an earlier state or worse condition. **3.** catabolic.

retrograde amnesia, the loss of memory for events occurring before a particular time in a person's life, usually before the event that precipitated the amnesia.

retrograde cystoscopy, (in radiology) a technique for examining the bladder in which a catheter is inserted through the urethra into the bladder. A radiopaque medium is introduced, filling the bladder, and the contour of the bladder is observed, using serial x-ray films or fluoroscopy.

retrograde ejaculation [L, retro, backward; gradus, step, ejaculari, to throw out], an ejaculation of semen in a reverse direction into the urinary bladder. The effect is sometimes the result of prostate surgery or a congenital condition.

retrograde filling, a filling placed in the apical part of a tooth root to seal the apical part of the root canal.

retrograde flow [L, retro, backward; AS, flowan], the flow of fluid in a direction other than normal, as in regurgitation.

retrograde infection, an infection that spreads along a tubule or duct against the flow of secretions or excretions, as in the urinary and lymphatic systems.

retrograde menstruation, a backflow of menstrual discharge through the uterine cavity and fallopian tubes into the peritoneal cavity.

retrograde pyelography, a radiologic technique for examining the structures of the collecting system of the kidneys that is especially useful in locating a urinary tract obstruction. A radiopaque contrast medium is injected through a urinary catheter into the ureters and the calyces of the pelves of the kidneys.

retrograde Wenckebach, a progressively lengthening conduction of impulses from the ventricles or atrioventricular junction to the atria until an impulse fails to reach the atria.

retrogression /-gresh'ən/ [L, retro + gradi, to step], a return to a less complex state, condition, or behavioral adaptation; degeneration; deterioration.

retrolental fibroplasia /-len'təl/ [L, retro + lentil, lens, fibra, fiber; Gk, plassein, to mold], a formation of fibrous tissue behind the lens of the eye, resulting in blindness. The disorder is caused by administration of excessive concentrations of oxygen to premature infants.

retromolar pad /-mō'lər/ [L, retro + mola, mill; D, paden, cushion], a mass of soft tissue, usually pear-shaped, that marks the distal termination of the mandibular residual ridge.

retromylohyoid space /ret'rōmī'lōhī'oid/ [L, retro + Gk, myle, mill, hyoeides, U-shaped; L, spatium], the part of the alveolingual sulcus that is distal to the distal end of the mylohyoid ridge.

retroperitoneal /-per'itōnē'əl/ [L, retro + Gk, peri, around, teinein, to stretch], pertaining to organs closely attached to the posterior abdominal wall and partly covered by peritoneum, rather than suspended by that membrane.

retroperitoneal abscess, a collection of pus between the peritoneum and the posterior abdominal wall.

retroperitoneal fibrosis, a chronic inflammatory process, usually of unknown cause, in which fibrous tissue surrounds the large blood vessels in the lower lumbar area. Symptoms include low-back and abdominal pain, weakness, weight loss, fever, and, with urinary tract involvement, frequency of urination, hematuria, polyuria, or anuria.

retroperitoneal lymph node dissection, surgical removal of lymph nodes behind the peritoneum, usually performed in an attempt to eliminate sites of lymphoma or metastases from malignancies originating in pelvic organs or genitalia.

retroperitoneum /-per'itōnē'əm/ [L, retro, backward; Gk, peri + teinein, to stretch], the space behind the peritoneum.

retropharyngeal abscess /-fərin'jē·əl/ [L, retro + Gk, pharynx, throat], a collection of pus in the tissues behind the pharynx accompanied by difficulty in swallowing, fever, and pain. Occasionally the airway becomes obstructed.

retroplacental /-pləsen'təl/, behind the placenta.

retrospective chart audit /-spek'tiv/ [L, retro + spicere, to look], a format for an audit developed by the Joint Commission on the Accreditation of Health Care Organizations. The audit involves several steps that outline a procedure for evaluating the effectiveness of the care given at a particular institution and for correcting any deficiencies found by reviewing the patient's records.

retrospective study, a study in which a search is made for a relationship between one (usually current) phenomenon or condition and another that occurred in the past.

retrosternal /-stur′nəl/ [L, *retro,* backward; Gk, *sternon,* chest], pertaining to the area behind the sternum.

retrouterine /re′trōyoo′tərin/, behind the uterus.

retroversion /-vur′zhən/ [L, *retro* + *vertere,* to turn], **1.** a common condition in which an organ is tipped backward, usually without flexion or other distortion. Uterine retroversion is measured as first-, second-, or third-degree, depending on the angle of tilt with respect to the vagina. **2.** an abnormal condition in which the teeth or other maxillary and mandibular structures are posterior to their normal positions. —**retrovert,** *v.*

retrovirus /-vī′rəs/ [L, *retro* + *virus*], any of a family of ribonucleic acid (RNA) viruses containing an enzyme, reverse transcriptase, in the virion. During replication the viral deoxyribonucleic acid (DNA) becomes integrated into the DNA of the host cell. Retroviruses are enveloped and assemble their capsids in the cytoplasm of the host cell. Human immunodeficiency virus, which causes acquired immunodeficiency syndrome, is a retrovirus.

revaccination /rēvak′sinā′shən/, an immunization that is repeated although the original was successful.

revascularization /rēvas′kyələr′īzā′shən/ [L, *re* + *vasculum,* small vessel; Gk, *izein,* to cause], the restoration by surgical means of blood flow to an organ or a tissue, as in bypass surgery.

reverberation /rivur′bərā′shən/, the phenomenon of multiple reflections within a closed system.

Reverdin's needle /reverdaNz′/ [Jaques L. Reverdin, Swiss surgeon, 1842–1929], a surgical needle with an eye that can be opened and closed with a slide.

reversal film /rivur′səl/, (in radiology) a reverse-tone duplicate of an x-ray image, showing black changed to white and white to black. It is produced by exposing single-emulsion subtraction film through a standard x-ray film.

reverse Barton's fracture /rivurs′/ [L, *revertere,* to turn back; John R. Barton, American surgeon, 1794–1871], a fracture of the volar articular surface of the ra-

dius with associated displacement of the carpal bones and radius.

reverse curve, (in dentistry) a convex curve of occlusion, as viewed in the frontal plane.

reversed bandage /rivurst′/, a roller bandage that is reversed on itself with a half twist so that it lies smoothly, conforming to the contour of the extremity.

reversed phase, a chromatographic mode in which the mobile phase is more polar than the stationary phase.

reverse isolation, isolation procedures designed to protect a patient from infectious organisms that might be carried by the staff, other patients, or visitors or on droplets in the air or on equipment or materials. Handwashing, gowning, gloving, sterilization, or disinfection of materials brought into the area and other details of housekeeping vary with the reason for the isolation and the usual practices of the hospital.

reverse peristalsis [L, *revertere,* to turn back; Gk, *peristellein,* to clasp], peristalsis that propels the contents in a direction opposite to the normal outward direction.

reverse transcriptase (RT), an enzyme that is present in the virion of retroviruses. Reverse transcriptase occurs in leukoviruses, human immunodeficiency virus, and ribonucleic acid tumor viruses of eukaryotic cells.

reverse transcriptase inhibitor, a compound that inhibits the enzyme used by retroviruses to synthesize complementary deoxyribonucleic acid from viral ribonucleic acid inside host cells.

reverse Trendelenburg [Friederich Trendelenberg], a position in which the lower extremities are lower than the body and head.

reversible /rivur′sibəl/, able to return to its original state or condition, as in a chemical reaction.

reversible brain syndrome, any of a group of acute brain disorders characterized by a disruption of cognition, as in delirium. The symptoms widely vary. The disorder is related to a variety of biologic stressors.

reversible vascular hyperplasia, a variation of Kaposi's sarcoma in which human immunodeficiency virus may induce cells to produce a chemical growth factor. The growth factor, in turn, makes lymphatic endothelial cells proliferate. The process may cascade as each new Kaposi's sarcoma cell produces more growth factor.

reversion /rivur′zhən/, **1.** the appearance in offspring of traits expressed in previous but not immediately recent generations. **2.**

R

a return to an original phenotype by mutation or reinstatement of the original genotype.

review of systems (ROS) /rivyo͞o/ [Fr, *revoir,* to see again], (in a health history) a system-by-system review of the body functions. The ROS is begun during the initial interview with the patient and completed during the physical examination as physical findings prompt further questions.

Reye's syndrome /rāz'/ [Ralph D. K. Reye, twentieth-century Australian pathologist], a combination of acute encephalopathy and fatty infiltration of the internal organs that may follow acute viral infections. This syndrome has been associated with influenza B, chickenpox (varicella), the enteroviruses, and the Epstein-Barr virus. It usually affects people under 18 years of age, characteristically causing an exanthematous rash, vomiting, and confusion about 1 week after the onset of a viral illness. In the late stage there may be extreme disorientation followed by coma, seizures, and respiratory arrest. The cause of Reye's syndrome is unknown; however, there appears to be an association with the administration of aspirin. Therefore aspirin is given only if prescribed by a physician for any condition in infants or children.

rf, **1.** abbreviation for **radiofrequency.** **2.** abbreviation for **rheumatic fever.**

Rf, **1.** symbol for the element **rutherfordium.** **2.** (in chromatography) abbreviation for retardation factor.

RF, abbreviation for **rheumatoid factor.**

R factor, an episome in bacteria that is responsible for drug resistance and transmissible to progeny and other bacterial cells by conjugation. The part of the episome involved in replication and transmission is called *resistance transfer factor.*

RFP, abbreviation for **request for proposal.**

RGP, abbreviation for **rigid gas permeable contact lens.**

Rh, **1.** abbreviation for rhesus. **2.** symbol for the chemical element **rhodium.**

r/h, **1.** abbreviation for **relative humidity.** **2.** abbreviation for *roentgens per hour.*

rhabdomyoblast /rab'dōmī'əblast'/ [Gk, *rhabdos,* rod, *mys,* muscle, *blastos,* germ], large round spindle-shaped cells with cross striations, found in some rhabdomyosarcomas.

rhabdomyolysis /rab'dōmī·ol'isis/, a paroxysmal, potentially fatal disease of skeletal muscle characterized by myoglobinuria. It is also associated with acute renal failure in heatstroke.

rhabdomyoma /rab'dōmī·ō'mə/ [Gk, *rhabdos,* rod, *mys,* muscle, *oma*], a tumor of striated muscle that may occur in the uterus, vagina, pharynx, tongue, or heart.

rhabdomyosarcoma /rab'dōmī'ō·särkō'-mə/ [Gk, *rhabdos* + *mys,* muscle, *sarx,* flesh, *oma*], a highly malignant tumor derived from primitive striated muscle cells that occurs most frequently in the head and neck and is also found in the genitourinary tract, extremities, body wall, and retroperitoneum. In some cases the onset is associated with trauma. The initial symptoms depend on the site of tumor development and indicate local tissue or organ destruction such as dysphagia, vaginal bleeding, hematuria, or obstructed flow of urine.

rhabdosphincter /rab'dōsfingk'tər/, a sphincter composed of striated muscle fibers.

rhabdovirus /rab'dōvī'rəs/ [Gk, *rhabdos* + L, *virus,* poison], a member of a family of viruses that includes the organism causing rabies.

rhagades /rag'ədēz/ [Gk, chinks], cracks or fissures in skin that has lost its elasticity, especially common around the mouth.

Rh antiserum [Rh, rhesus; Gk, *anti,* against; L, *serum,* whey], a serum that contains Rh antibodies.

rhd, **1.** abbreviation for *radioactive health data.* **2.** abbreviation for **rheumatic heart disease.**

Rh₀(D) immune globulin, a passive immunizing agent prescribed to prevent Rh sensitization after abortion, miscarriage, ectopic pregnancy, or normal birth to an Rh-negative mother of an Rh-positive infant or fetus.

rhe /rē/, **1.** an absolute unit of fluidity in the centimeter-gram-second (CGS) system. **2.** the reciprocal of the unit of viscosity expressed as 1/poise or 1/centipoise.

rhegmatogenous /reg'mətoj'ənəs/, [Gk, *rhegma,* breakage, *gen,* producing], arising from a tear or rupture in an organ.

rhegmatogenous retinal detachment, a separation of the retina associated with a hole, break, or tear in the sensory layer of the retina. The detachment occurs secondary to the formation of the opening.

rhenium (Re) /rē'nē·əm/ [L, *Rhenus,* Rhine], a hard, brittle metallic element. Its atomic number is 75; its atomic mass (weight) is 186.21. Rhenium has a high melting point and is used in x-ray tube anodes and in thermometers for measuring high temperatures.

rheobase /rē'əbās/, the least amount of electricity that will produce a stimulated response.

rheoencephalogram /rē′ō·ensef′əlōgram′/, a graphic representation of the changes in electrical conductivity of the head caused by blood flowing through vessels in the head.

rheogram /rē′əgram/, a plot of shear stress versus the shear flow of a fluid.

rheology /rē·ol′əjē/, the study of the flow and deformation of matter.

rheometry /rē·om′ətrē/ [Gk, *rheos*, current, *metron*, measure], a technique for measuring the velocity of blood flow.

rheostat /rē′əstat/ [Gk, *rheos*, current, *statikos*, causing to stand], a variable-resistance electrical device that can be adjusted to control the strength of a current.

rheostosis /rē′ostō′sis/, a condition of bone overgrowth marked by streaks in the bones.

rhestocythemia /res′tōsīthē′mē·ə/, the presence of damaged red blood cells in the peripheral circulation.

rheum /rōōm/ [Gk, *rheuma*, flow], a watery or mucous discharge from the skin or mucous membranes.

rheumatic /rōōmat′ik/ [Gk, *rheuma*, flux], pertaining to rheumatism.

rheumatic aortitis, an inflammatory condition of the aorta, occurring in rheumatic fever. It is characterized by disseminated focal lesions that may progressively form patches of fibrosis.

rheumatic arteritis, a complication of rheumatic fever characterized by generalized inflammation of arteries and arterioles. Fibrin mixed with cellular debris may invade, thicken, and stiffen the vessel wall; and the vessel may be surrounded by hemorrhage and exudate.

rheumatic carditis [Gk, *rheuma*, flux, *kardia*, heart, *itis*, inflammation], the pericarditis, myocarditis, and endocarditis that may be associated with acute rheumatic fever.

rheumatic endocarditis [Gk, *rheuma*, flux, *endon*, within, *kardia*, heart, *itis*, inflammation], an inflammation of the endocardium in association with acute rheumatic fever.

rheumatic fever, an inflammatory disease that may develop as a delayed reaction to inadequately treated group A beta-hemolytic streptococcal infection of the upper respiratory tract. This disorder usually occurs in young school-age children and may affect the brain, heart, joints, skin, or subcutaneous tissues. The onset of rheumatic fever is usually sudden, often occurring in from 1 to 5 symptom-free weeks after recovery from a sore throat or scarlet fever. Early symptoms usually include fever, joint pains, nose bleeds, abdominal pain, and vomiting. The major

manifestations of this disease include migratory polyarthritis affecting numerous joints and carditis, which causes palpitations, chest pain, and in severe cases symptoms of cardiac failure. Sydenham's chorea, which may develop, is usually the sole late sign of rheumatic fever and may initially be manifested as an increased awkwardness and an associated tendency to drop objects. As the chorea progresses, irregular body movements may become extensive, occasionally involving the tongue and the facial muscles, resulting in incapacitation of the affected individual.

rheumatic heart disease, damage to heart muscle and heart valves caused by episodes of rheumatic fever. When a susceptible person acquires a group A beta-hemolytic streptococcal infection, an autoimmune reaction may occur in heart tissue, resulting in permanent deformities of heart valves or chordae tendineae. Involvement of the heart may be evident during acute rheumatic fever, or it may be discovered long after the acute disease has subsided.

rheumatic nodules [Gk, *rheuma*, flux; L, *nodulus*, small knot], aggregations of fibroblasts and lymphoid cells that may accumulate in soft tissues and over bony prominences of patients afflicted with rheumatoid arthritis and rheumatic fever.

rheumatic scoliosis [Gk, *rheuma*, flux, *skoliosis*, curvature], a form of scoliosis associated with muscle spasms and acute inflammation.

rheumatid /rōō′mətid/ [Gk, *rheuma*, flux], a skin eruption that sometimes occurs with rheumatic disorders.

rheumatism /rōō′mətiz′əm/ [Gk, *rheuma*, flux], *nontechnical.* **1.** any of a large number of inflammatory conditions of the bursae, joints, ligaments, or muscles characterized by pain, limitation of movement, and structural degeneration of single or multiple parts of the musculoskeletal system. **2.** the syndrome of pain, limitation of movement, and structural degeneration of elements in the musculoskeletal system as may occur in gout, rheumatoid arthritis, systemic lupus erythematosus, ankylosing spondylitis, and many other diseases. **—rheumatic, rheumatoid,** *adj.*

rheumatoid arteritis /rōō′mətoid/ [Gk, *rheuma*, flux, *arteria*, airpipe, *itis*, inflammation], inflammation of the arterial walls associated with a rheumatic disorder.

rheumatoid arthritis [Gk, *rheuma*, flux, *eidos*, form, *arthron*, joint, *itis*, inflammation], a chronic, inflammatory, destructive, sometimes deforming, collagen disease that has an autoimmune component.

R

Rheumatoid arthritis is characterized by symmetric inflammation of the synovium and increased synovial exudate, leading to thickening of the synovium and swelling of the joint. The course of the disease is variable but is most frequently marked by remissions and exacerbation. Clinical data, using mainly radiographic studies and physical examination, classify the progress of rheumatoid arthritis into four stages. Stage I, representing early effects, is based on x-ray films showing the onset of bone changes. Stage II, moderate rheumatoid arthritis, is assigned to cases in which there is evidence of some muscle atrophy and loss of mobility, in addition to x-ray findings. Stage III, severe rheumatoid arthritis, is marked by joint deformity, extensive muscle atrophy, and soft tissue lesions, as well as definite bone and cartilage destruction. Stage IV, the terminal category, includes all the stage III clinical signs plus fibrous or bony ankylosis.

rheumatoid coronary arteritis, an abnormal condition characterized by a thickening of the tunica intima of the coronary arteries, which may produce coronary insufficiency. Rheumatoid coronary arteritis is a collagen disease that affects the connective tissue by inflammation and fibrinoid degeneration.

rheumatoid factor (RF), antiglobulin antibodies often found in the serum of patients with a clinical diagnosis of rheumatoid arthritis. Rheumatoid factors may also be found in such widely divergent diseases as tuberculosis, parasitic infections, leukemia, and connective tissue disorders.

rheumatologist /rōō'mətol'ə'jist/, a specialist in the treatment of disorders of the connective tissue.

rheumatology /-ol'əjē/ [Gk, rheuma, flux, logos, science], the study of disorders characterized by inflammation, degeneration, or metabolic derangement of connective tissue and related structures of the body.

Rh factor, an antigenic substance present in the erythrocytes of 85% of the people. A person having the factor is Rh$^+$ (Rh positive); a person lacking the factor is Rh$^-$ (Rh negative). If an Rh$^-$ person receives Rh$^+$ blood, hemolysis and anemia occur. Rh+ infants may be exposed to antibodies to the factor produced in the Rh$^-$ mother's blood, resulting in red cell destruction and erythroblastosis fetalis. Transfusion, blood typing, and cross-matching depend on Rh$^+$ and ABO classification. The Rh factor was first identified in the blood of a rhesus (Rh) monkey.

Rh genes [Rh, rhesus; Gk, genein, to produce], a series of allelic genes that ac-

count for the various Rh blood groups. The four variations of the Rh$^+$ gene are identified as R^0, R^1, R^2, and R^z, whereas the four types of Rh-gene are designated as r, r', r'', and r$_y$.

Rh immune globulin [Rh, rhesus; L, immunis, free from, globulus], an immune globulin that is administered to all Rh$^-$ mothers after every abortion or birth unless the infant is Rh$^-$ or unless the mother's serum already contains anti-Rh$_0$(D) reagent.

rhinalgia /rīnal'jə/, pain involving the nose.

Rh incompatibility, (in hematology) a lack of compatibility between two groups of blood cells that are antigenically different because of the presence of the Rh factor in one group and its absence in the other.

rhinedema /rī'nedē'mə/, a fluid accumulation in the mucous membrane of the nose.

rhinencephalon /rī'nensef'əlon/, pl. **rhinencephala** [Gk, rhis, nose, encephalon, brain], a part of each cerebral hemisphere that contains the limbic system, which is associated with the emotions. —**rhinencephalic,** adj.

rhinenchysis /rī'nenkī'sis, rīnen'kisis/, douching of the nasal cavity.

rhinitis /rīnī'tis/ [Gk, rhis + itis, inflammation], inflammation of the mucous membranes of the nose, usually accompanied by swelling of the mucosa and a nasal discharge. It may be complicated by sinusitis.

rhinolaryngitis /-ler'inji'tis/ [Gk, rhis, nose, larynx, throat, itis, inflammation], an inflammation of the mucous membranes of the nose and throat.

rhinolith /rī'nəlith/, a concretion in the nasal cavity.

rhinolithiasis /rī'nəlithī'əsis/, the formation of concretions in the nasal cavity.

rhinologist /rīnol'əjist/, a physician who specializes in the diagnosis and treatment of disorders of the nose.

rhinology /rīnol'əjē/, a branch of medicine specializing in the diagnosis and treatment of disorders involving the nose.

rhinomanometer /rī'nōmənom'ətər/, a device for measuring the air pressure in the nose. It is used in the diagnosis of nasal obstruction.

rhinomycosis /rī'nōmīkō'sis/, a fungal infection of the mucous membrane of the nose.

rhinopathy /rīnop'əthē/ [Gk, rhis + pathos, disease], any disease or malformation of the nose.

rhinophycomycosis /rī'nōfī'kōmīkō'sis/, an infection of the nasal and paranasal sinuses caused by the phycomycete *Entomophthora coronata.* The infection often spreads to surrounding tissues, including the eye and brain.

rhinophyma /rī'nōfī'mə/ [Gk, *rhis* + *phyma,* tumor], a form of rosacea in which there is sebaceous hyperplasia, redness, prominent vascularity, swelling, and distortion of the skin of the nose.

rhinoplasty /rī'nəplas'tē/ [Gk, *rhis* + *plassein,* to mold], a procedure in plastic surgery in which the structure of the nose is changed. Bone or cartilage may be removed, tissue grafted from another part of the body, or synthetic material implanted to alter the shape. The procedure is most frequently performed for cosmetic reasons.

rhinorrhagia /rī'nōrā'jə/ [Gk, *rhis,* nose, *rhegnynein,* to gush forth], a profuse nosebleed.

rhinorrhea /rī'nōrē'ə/ [Gk, *rhis* + *rhoia,* flow], **1.** the free discharge of a thin watery nasal fluid. **2.** the flow of cerebrospinal fluid from the nose after an injury to the head.

rhinosalpingitis /rī'nōsal'pinjī'tis/, an inflammation of the mucous membranes of the nose and eustachian tube.

rhinoscleroma /rī'nosklirō'mə/, a chronic inflammation in the nose, spreading to the larynx and pharynx. The cause is an infection of *Klebsiella rhinoscleromatis.*

rhinoscope /rī'nəskōp/, an instrument for examining the nasal passages through the anterior nares or through the nasopharynx.

rhinoscopy /rīnos'kəpē/ [Gk, *rhis* + *skopein,* to look], an examination of the nasal passages to inspect the mucosa and detect inflammation, deformities, or asymmetry, as in deviation of the septum. The nasal passages may be examined anteriorly by introducing a speculum into the anterior nares or posteriorly by introducing a rhinoscope through the nasopharynx. **—rhinoscopic,** *adj.*

rhinosporidiosis /rī'nōspərid'ē-ō'sis/ [Gk, *rhis* + *sporo,* seed, *osis,* condition], an infection caused by the fungus *Rhinosporidium seeberi.* It is characterized by fleshy red polyps on the mucous membranes of the nose, conjunctiva, nasopharynx, and soft palate. The disease may be acquired by swimming or bathing in infected water.

rhinostenosis /rī'nōstənō'sis/, an abnormal narrowing of a nasal passage.

rhinotomy /rīnot'əmē/ [Gk, *rhis* + *temnein,* to cut], a surgical procedure in which an incision is made along one side of the nose, performed to drain accumulated pus from an abscess or a sinus infection.

rhinovirus /rī'nōvī'rəs/ [Gk, *rhis* + L, *virus,* poison], any of about 100 serologically distinct, small ribonucleic acid viruses that cause about 40% of acute respiratory illnesses. Infection is characterized by dry scratchy throat, nasal congestion, malaise, and headache. Fever is minimal. Nasal discharge lasts 2 or 3 days.

rhizoid /rī'zoid/, resembling a root or serving to anchor.

rhizomelia /rī'zōmē'ljə/ [Gk, *rhizo,* root, *melos,* limb], **1.** a disorder of the hips and shoulders. **2.** an anomaly in the length of the arms and legs of an individual.

rhizomelic /rī'zəmel'ik/ [Gk, *rhizo,* root, *melos,* limb], pertaining to the hip and shoulder joints.

rhizomeningomyelitis /rī'zōmining'gōmī'-əlī'tis/, an inflammation of the nerve roots, meninges, and spinal cord.

Rhizopus /rī'zōpəs/, a genus of fungi that includes some species identified as a cause of zygomycosis in humans.

rhizotomy /rīzot'əmē/, the surgical resection of the dorsal root of a spinal nerve, performed to relieve pain.

rho /rō/, P, ρ, the seventeenth letter of the Greek alphabet.

Rhodesian trypanosomiasis /rōdē'zhən/, an acute form of African trypanosomiasis, caused by the parasite *Trypanosoma brucei rhodesiense.* The disease may progress rapidly, causing encephalitis, coma, and death in only a few weeks.

rhodium (Rh) /rō'dē·əm/ [Gk, *rhodon,* rose], a grayish-white metallic element. Its atomic number is 45; its atomic mass (weight) is 102.91.

rhodopsin /rōdop'sin/ [Gk, *rhodon,* rose, *opsis,* vision], the purple pigmented compound in the rods of the retina, formed by a protein, opsin, and a derivative of vitamin A, retinal. Rhodopsin gives the outer segments of the rods a purple color and adapts the eye to low-density light. The compound breaks down when struck by light, and this chemical change triggers the conduction of nerve impulses.

Rhodotorula /rō'dətôr'yələ/, a genus of yeasts, including species such as *R. rubra* that have been identified as causes of endocarditis and septicemia, particularly in immunocompromised patients.

rhoencephalography, a technique for monitoring blood flow in the brain by recording pulsatile changes in the electrical impedance of the brain.

rhombencephalon /rom'bensef'əlon/ [Gk, *rhombos,* parallelogram, *enkephalos,* brain], the most caudal of the three primary vesicles of the embryonic brain.

rhomboid /rom'boid/ [Gk, *rhombos,* rhombus, *eidos,* form], resembling the shape

R

of an oblique equilateral parallelogram, as a rhomboid muscle.

rhomboidal sinus /rom'boidəl/, an opening in the central canal of the lumbar spinal cord.

rhomboideus major /romboi'dē·əs/ [Gk, *rhombos*, rhombus, *eidos*, form], a muscle of the upper back below and parallel to the rhomboideus minor. With the rhomboideus minor, it functions to draw the scapula toward the vertebral column while supporting it and drawing it slightly upward.

rhomboideus minor, a muscle of the upper back, above and parallel to the rhomboideus major. With the rhomboideus major, it acts to draw the scapula toward the vertebral column while supporting the scapula and drawing it slightly upward.

rhombomere /rom'bəmir/, any of the nine segments of the embryonic neural tube.

rhonchi /rong'kī/, *sing.* **rhonchus** /rong'-kəs/ [Gk, *rhonchos*, snore], abnormal sounds heard on auscultation of an airway obstructed by thick secretions, muscular spasm, neoplasm, or external pressure. The continuous rumbling sounds are more pronounced during expiration, and they characteristically clear on coughing.

rhonchus [Gk, *rhonchos*, snore], the sound produced by air moving into and out of the bronchi when there is a partial obstruction.

rhotacism /rō'təsiz'əm/ [Gk, *rho*, letter R], a speech disorder characterized by a defective pronunciation of words containing the sound /r/, or by the excessive use of the sound /r/, or by the substitution of another sound for /r/.

r-HuEPO, abbreviation for *recombinant human erythropoietin*.

rhus dermatitis /rōōs/, [Gk, *rhous*, sumac], a form of contact dermatitis caused by exposure to an allergenic oil, toxicodendrol, present in any part of a plant of the genus *Rhus* such as poison ivy, poison oak, or poison sumac.

rhythm /rith'əm/ [Gk, *rhythmos*], the relationship of one impulse to neighboring impulses as measured in time, movement, or regularity of action.

rhytidoplasty /ritid'ōplas'tē/ [Gk, *rhytis*, wrinkle, *plassein*, to mold], a procedure in reconstructive plastic surgery in which the skin of the face is tightened, wrinkles are removed, and the skin is made to appear firm and smooth.

rhytidosis /rit'idō'sis/ [Gk, *rhytis*, wrinkle, *osis*, condition], a wrinkling, especially of the cornea.

RIA, abbreviation for **radioimmunoassay.**

rib [AS, roof], one of the 12 pairs of arches of bone forming a large part of the thoracic skeleton. The first seven ribs on each side are called true ribs because they articulate directly with the sternum and vertebrae. The remaining five ribs are called false ribs. The first three attach ventrally to ribs above; the last two are free at their ventral extremities and are called floating ribs.

ribavirin /rī'bəvir'in/, an aerosol antiviral drug prescribed for the treatment of respiratory syncytial virus infections for the lower respiratory tract in infants and small children.

rib fracture, a break in a bone of the thoracic skeleton caused by a blow or crushing injury or by violent coughing or sneezing. The ribs most commonly broken are the fourth to eighth; if the bone is splintered or the fracture is displaced, sharp fragments may pierce the lung, causing hemothorax or pneumothorax. The patient with a fractured rib suffers pain, especially on inspiration, and usually breathes rapidly and shallowly. The site of the break is generally very tender to the touch, and the crackling of bone fragments rubbing together may be heard on auscultation.

riboflavin /rī'bōflā'vin/ [*ribose* + L, *flavus,* yellow], a yellow crystalline water-soluble pigment, one of the heat-stable components of the B vitamin complex (vitamin B_2). It combines with specific flavoproteins and functions as a coenzyme in the oxidative processes of carbohydrates, fats, and proteins. It plays an important role in preventing some visual disorders, especially cataracts. Small amounts of riboflavin are found in the liver and kidneys, but it is not stored to any great degree in the body and must be supplied regularly in the diet.

ribonuclear protein /rī'bōnōō'klē·ər/ [ribose; L, *nucleus,* nut kernel; Gk, *proteios,* first rank], a conjugated protein consisting of a protein molecule and nucleic acid.

ribonuclease /-nōō'klē·ās/, a class of endonucleases that hydrolyze ribonucleic acids.

ribonucleic acid (RNA) /rī'bōnōōklē'ik/ [*ribose* + L, *nucleus,* nut kernel, *acidus,* sour], a nucleic acid, found in both the nucleus and cytoplasm of cells, that transmits genetic instructions from the nucleus to the cytoplasm. In the cytoplasm, RNA functions in the assembly of proteins.

ribonucleoside /rī'bōnōō'klē·ɔsīd'/, a nucleoside in which the sugar component is ribose. The ribonucleosides of ribonucleic acid are adenosine, cytidine, guanosine, and uridine.

ribonucleotide /-nōō'klē·ətīd'/, a class of

nucleotides in which the pentose is D-ribose.

ribose /rī′bōs/, a 5-carbon sugar that occurs as a component of ribonucleic acid.

ribosomal RNA (rRNA) /rī′bōsō′məl/, the ribonucleic acid of ribosomes and polyribosomes.

ribosome /rī′bəsōm/ [*ribose* + Gk, *soma,* body], a cytoplasmic organelle composed of ribonucleic acid (RNA) and protein that functions in the synthesis of protein. Ribosomes interact with messenger RNA and transfer RNA to join together amino acid units into a polypeptide chain according to the sequence determined by the genetic code.

ribosome-inactivating proteins (RIPs), N-glycosidases that cleave the N-glycosidic bond of adenine in a specific ribosomal ribonucleic acid (RNA) sequence. Type 1 RIPs are single-chain proteins. Some type 2 RIPs possess a galactose-specific lectin domain that binds to cell surfaces, making them potent toxins, such as ricin.

ribosuria /rī′bəsŏŏr′ē·ə/, the presence of ribose in the urine, usually a sign of muscular dystrophy.

rib shaking, a procedure in physiotherapy involving constant downward pressure with an intermittent shaking motion of the hands on the rib cage over the area being drained. It is done with the flat part of the palm of the hand over the lung segment being drained.

rib vibration, a procedure in physiotherapy similar to rib shaking but done with a downward vibrating pressure with the flat part of the palm during exhalations.

RICE, abbreviation for *rest, ice, compression, elevation,* referring to the treatment for sprains and strains.

rice diet [Gk, *oryza,* rice, *diaita,* way of living], a diet consisting only of rice, fruit, fruit juices, and sugar, supplemented with vitamins and iron. Salt is forbidden. It is prescribed for the treatment of hypertension, chronic renal disease, and obesity.

Richards, Linda (1841–1930), a nurse considered to be the first American-trained nurse, being graduated in the first class of the New England Hospital for Women and Children. She is credited with being the first to keep written records on patients, a practice she started when she worked as night superintendent at Bellevue Hospital in New York under Sister Helen.

Richter's hernia /rik′tərz, rish′tərs/ [August G. Richter, German surgeon, 1742–1812], a small nonpalpable visceral protrusion involving only a part of the intestinal wall.

ricin /rī′sin/, a potent toxin obtained from castor beans (*Ricinus communis*) that produces agglutination of red blood cells and inflammation and hemorrhage of the respiratory and gastrointestinal mucosa.

rickets /rik′əts/ [Gk, *rachis,* backbone, *itis,* inflammation], a condition caused by the deficiency of vitamin D, seen primarily in infancy and childhood and characterized by abnormal bone formation. Symptoms include soft pliable bones, causing such deformities as bowlegs and knock-knees, nodular enlargements on the ends and sides of the bones, muscle pain, enlarged skull, chest deformities, spinal curvature, enlargement of the liver and spleen, profuse sweating, and general tenderness of the body when touched.

Rickettsia /riket′sē·ə/ [Howard T. Ricketts, American pathologist, 1871–1910], a genus of microorganisms that combine aspects of both bacteria and viruses. They also exist as viruslike intracellular parasites, living in the intestinal tracts of insects such as lice. Thus a human infested with lice is also likely to be infected with a form of typhus transmitted by *Rickettsia prowazeki*. Rickettsial diseases have been responsible for many of history's worst epidemics. The various species are distinguished on the basis of similarities in the diseases they cause. —**rickettsial,** *adj.*

rickettsial disease [Howard T. Ricketts; L, *dis* + Fr, *aise,* ease], an infection caused by a species of *Rickettsia.* Examples include Rocky Mountain spotted fever and typhus.

rickettsialpox /riket′sē·əlpoks′/ [Howard T. Ricketts; ME, *pokkes,* pustules], a mild, acute infectious disease caused by *Rickettsia akari* and transmitted from mice to humans by mites. It is characterized by an asymptomatic crusted primary lesion chills, fever, headache, malaise, myalgia, and a rash resembling chickenpox. About 1 week after onset of symptoms, small, discrete maculopapular lesions appear on any part of the body.

rickettsiosis /riket′sē·ō′sis/, *pl.* **rickettsioses** [Howard T. Ricketts; Gk, *osis,* condition], any of a group of infectious diseases caused by microorganisms of the genus *Rickettsia.* Kinds of rickettsioses include a spotted fever group (**boutonneuse fever, rickettsialpox, Rocky Mountain spotted fever**), a typhus group (**epidemic typhus, murine typhus, scrub typhus**), and a miscellaneous group (**Q fever, trench fever**).

rider's bone [AS, *ridan,* to ride, *ban,* bone], a bony deposit that sometimes develops in horseback riders on the inner side of the lower end of the tendon of the adductor muscle of the thigh.

rider's sprain [OFr, *espreindre*, to force out], a sprain of the adductor muscles of the thigh resulting from horseback riding.

ridge /rij/ [AS, *hyrcg*], a projection or projecting structure such as the gastrocnemial ridge on the posterior surface of the femur, giving attachment to the gastrocnemius muscle.

ridge extension, an intraoral surgical operation for deepening the labial, buccal, or lingual sulci.

ridge lap, the part of an artificial tooth that is adjacent to or laps the residual ridge.

Rieder's cell leukemia /rē'dərz/ [Hermann Rieder, German pathologist, 1858–1932], a malignant neoplasm of blood-forming tissues characterized by the presence in blood of large numbers of atypical myeloblasts with immature cytoplasm and relatively mature lobulated, indented nuclei.

Riehl-Sisca, Joan, a nursing theorist who presented her symbolic interactionism theory in Riehl and Sister Callista Roy's book, *Conceptual Models for Nursing* (1980). The Riehl Interaction Model uses the nursing process in implementing nursing care. In symbolic interactionism theory, people interpret each other's actions based on the meaning attached to the action before reacting. It is a process of interpretation between the stimulus and response. Riehl's emphasis is on the assessment and interpretation of the patient's actions by the nurse, who then makes predictions about the patient's behavior.

RIF, abbreviation for **resistance-inducing factor.**

rifampin /rif'əmpin/, an antibacterial prescribed in the treatment of tuberculosis, in meningococcal prophylaxis, and as an antileprotic.

Rift Valley fever, an arbovirus infection of Egypt and east Africa spread by mosquitoes or by handling infected sheep and cattle. It is characterized by abrupt fever, chills, headache, and generalized aching, followed by epigastric pain, anorexia, loss of taste, and photophobia.

RIG, abbreviation for **rabies immune globulin.**

Riga-Fede's disease /rē'gä fā'dā/ [Antonio Riga, Italian physician, 1832–1919; Francesco Fede, Italian pediatrician, 1832–1913], an ulceration of the lingual frenum in some infants, caused by abrasion of the frenum by natal or neonatal teeth.

right atrial catheter, an indwelling intravenous catheter inserted centrally or peripherally and threaded into the superior vena cava and right atrium.

right brachiocephalic vein [AS, *riht* + Gk, *brachion,* arm, *kephale,* head], a vessel, about 2.5 cm long, that starts in the root of the neck at the junction of the internal jugular and subclavian veins on the right side and descends vertically from behind the sternal end of the clavicle to join the left brachiocephalic vein and form the superior vena cava.

right bundle branch block, impaired or absence of transmission of an electrical impulse down the fibers that transmit impulses from the bundle of His to the right ventricle. A right bundle branch block is often associated with right ventricular hypertrophy, especially in athletes and individuals under 40 years of age. In older individuals a right bundle branch block is commonly caused by coronary artery disease.

right common carotid artery, the shorter of the two common carotid arteries, arising from the brachiocephalic trunk, passing obliquely from the level of the sternoclavicular articulation to the upper border of the thyroid cartilage, and dividing into the right carotid arteries.

right coronary artery, one of a pair of branches of the ascending aorta, arising in the right posterior aortic sinus, passing along the right side of the coronary sulcus, dividing into the right interventricular artery and a large marginal branch. It supplies both ventricles, the right atrium, and the sinoatrial node.

right-handedness, a natural tendency to favor the use of the right hand.

right-hand rule, a principle of physics in which the direction of current flow in a wire is related to the position of the imaginary lines of force of the magnetic field about the wire.

right-heart failure, an abnormal cardiac condition characterized by the impairment of the right side of the heart and congestion and elevated pressure in the systemic veins and capillaries. Right-heart failure is often related to left-heart failure; both sides of the heart are part of a circuit; what affects one side will eventually affect the other.

right hepatic duct, the duct that drains bile from the right lobe of the liver into the common bile duct.

righting reflex [AS, *riht* + L, *refectere,* to bend back], any one of the neuromuscular responses to restore the body to its normal upright position when it has been displaced. Any change in the position of the head produces a change in the pressure on the gelatinous membrane of the macula. The fibers of the nerve (vestibular branch of the eight cranial nerve) transmit im-

right lymphatic duct, a vessel that conveys lymph from the right upper quadrant of the body into the bloodstream in the neck at the junction of the right internal jugular and right subclavian veins.

right pulmonary artery, the longer and slightly larger of the two arteries conveying venous blood from the heart to the lungs. It arises from the pulmonary trunk, bends to the right behind the aorta, and divides into two branches at the root of the right lung.

right subclavian artery, a large artery that arises from the brachiocephalic artery. It has several important branches: the axillary, vertebral thoracic, and internal thoracic arteries and the cervical and costocervical trunks, perfusing the right side of the upper body.

right-to-know laws, laws that require employers to inform workers regarding health effects of materials they must handle, including toxic chemicals and radioactive substances. Under the authority of the U.S. Occupational Safety and Health Act of 1970, the National Institute for Occupational Safety and Health periodically revises recommendations or limits of exposure to potentially hazardous substances in the workplace. It also recommends appropriate preventive measures designed to reduce or eliminate adverse health effects of these hazards and publishes its recommendations in a variety of public documents.

right-to-left shunt [ME, *shunten*], a venoarterial shunt in which unoxygenated venous blood passes directly into the arterial system, bypassing the lungs as in the tetralogy of Fallot and other conditions.

right ventricle, the relatively thin-walled chamber of the heart that pumps blood received from the right atrium into the pulmonary arteries to the lungs for oxygenation. The right ventricle is shorter and rounder than the long conical left ventricle.

rigid gas permeable (RGP) contact lens, a hard contact lens that allows oxygen to be transmitted through the lens.

rigidity /rijid′itē/ [L, *rigere,* to be stiff], a condition of hardness, stiffness, or inflexibility. **—rigid,** *adj.*

rigidus /rij′idəs/ [L, stiff], a deformity characterized by limited motion, especially dorsiflexion of the great toe.

rigor /rig′ər/ [L, stiffness], **1.** a rigid condition of the body tissues, as in rigor mortis. **2.** a violent attack of shivering that may be associated with chills and fever.

rigor mortis /môr′tis/, the rigid stiffening of skeletal and cardiac muscle shortly after death.

rim [OE, *rima,* edge], an outer edge, which may be curved or circular, as on an occluding surface built on a temporary or permanent denture base.

rima /rī′mə/, a cleft or fissure.

rimose /rī′mōs/, having many clefts or fissures.

rimula /rim′yələ/ [L, small cleft], a very small fissure in the central nervous system.

ring [AS, *hring*], **1.** a circular band surrounding a central opening. **2.** a closed chainlike linkage of atoms.

ring chromosome [AS, *hring*], a circular chromosome formed by the fusion of the two ends. It is the primary type of chromosome found in bacteria.

ring-down artifact, (in radiography) an echo pattern caused by reverberation in a bubble or other soft tissue entity.

ring-down time, (in ultrasonics) the time required for vibration of the transducer element at its resonance frequency to decrease to a negligible level following excitation.

Ringer's lactate solution, a fluid and electrolyte replenisher prescribed for correction of extracellular volume and electrolyte depletion.

ring removal from swollen finger, a technique for taking off a tightly fitting ring. It consists of slipping the end of a string under the ring while moving the ring toward the hand. The rest of the string is then wound around the swollen part of the finger a number of times, after which the string is unwound from the hand side, gradually easing the ring toward the finger tip.

Rinne tuning fork test /rin′ē/ [Heinrich A. Rinne, German otologist, 1819–1868], a method of distinguishing conductive from sensorineural hearing loss. The test may be performed with tuning forks of 256, 512, and 1024 cycles. The base of the vibrating fork is placed against the patient's mastoid bone. While one ear is tested, the other is masked. In sensorineural loss the sound is heard relatively longer by air conduction; in conductive hearing loss the sound is heard longer by bone conduction.

RIP, abbreviation for **reflex inhibiting pattern.**

ripe cataract [OE, *ripan* + Gk, *katarrhaktes,* portcullis], a mature cataract that produces swelling and opacity of the entire lens.

RIPs, abbreviation for **ribosome-inactivating proteins.**

R

risk-benefit analysis, the consideration as to whether a medical or surgical procedure, particularly a radical approach, is worth the risk to the patient as compared to possible benefits if the procedure is successful.

risk factor [Fr, *risque,* hazard; L, *factor,* maker], a factor that causes a person or a group of people to be particularly susceptible to an unwanted, unpleasant, or unhealthful event such as immunosuppression, which increases the incidence and severity of infection.

Risk Identification, a Nursing Interventions Classification defined as analysis of potential risk factors, determination of health risks, and prioritization of risk reduction strategies for an individual or group.

Risk Identification: Childbearing Family, a Nursing Interventions Classification defined as identification of an individual or family likely to experience difficulties in parenting and prioritization of strategies to prevent parenting problems.

risk management, a function of administration of a hospital or other health facility directed toward identification, evaluation, and correction of potential risks that could lead to injury to patients, staff members, or visitors.

risorius /risôr′ē·əs/ [L, *ridere,* to laugh], one of the 12 muscles of the mouth. It arises in the fascia over the masseter and inserts into the skin at the corner of the mouth. It acts to retract the angle of the mouth, as in a smile.

Risser cast /ris′ər/ [Joseph C. Risser, American surgeon, 1892–1942], an orthopedic device for encasing the entire trunk of the body, extending over the cervical area to the chin. In rare cases it extends over the hips to the knees.

RIST, abbreviation for **radioimmunosorbent test.**

risus caninus /rī′səs/ [L, *risus,* laughter, *caninus,* doglike], a grinning facial distortion caused by tension in the occipitofrontalis and other facial muscles as a result of tetanus.

risus sardonicus /rē′səs särdon′ikəs/ [L, laughter; Gk, *sardonius,* mocking], a wry masklike grin caused by spasm of the facial muscles, as seen in tetanus.

Ritgen maneuver, an obstetric procedure used to control delivery of the fetal head. It involves applying upward pressure from the coccygeal region to extend the head during actual delivery.

ritodrine hydrochloride /rit′ədrēn/, a beta-sympathomimetic amine agent pre-

scribed in pregnancy management to stop the uterus from contracting in preterm labor.

ritonavir, a protease inhibitor prescribed in the treatment of acquired immunodeficiency syndrome, either alone or in combination with nucleoside analogs.

Ritter's disease [Gottfried Ritter von Rittershain, German physician, 1820–1883], a rare, staphylococcal infection of newborns that begins with red spots about the mouth and chin, gradually spreading over the entire body, and followed by generalized exfoliation. Vesicles and yellow crusts may also be present. Ritter's disease is usually fatal unless treated with antibiotics.

ritual /rich′əwəl/, **1.** a mental health disorder characterized by repetitive sequences of stereotyped daily life routines, such as repeated handwashing that interferes with an individual's level of functioning. **2.** a prescribed order of ceremonial acts or series of acts. **3.** a detailed procedure followed faithfully or regularly.

ritual circumcision, a surgical procedure for removing the prepuce of the male or the labia minora of the female as a religious rite in Jewish or Muslim communities. In Jewish families the male circumcision is usually performed on the eighth day after birth. The practice dates back to the ancient Egyptians, and in some societies it is a prerequisite for marriage.

Rivea corymbosa, a twining vine of the botanical family of Convulvaceae. The seeds contain indole alkaloids, a source of lysergic acid diethylamide, which have an effect of altered perception when ingested in large quantities. They have been used in religious ceremonies of indigenous Latin American cultures since the era of the Aztecs.

Rivinus notch /rēvē′nəs/ [Augustus Q. Rivinus, German anatomist, 1652–1723], a deficiency in the tympanic sulcus of the ear that forms an attachment for the flaccid part of the tympanic membrane and the mallear folds.

rivus lacrimalis /rī′vəs/ [L, stream of tears], a channel between the eyelids and the surface of the eye that normally allows a flow of moisture when the eyes are closed.

RK, 1. abbreviation for **radial keratotomy. 2.** abbreviation for **refractive keratotomy.**

R.L.E., abbreviation for *right lower extremity.*

R.L.L., abbreviation for *right lower lobe of lung.*

r-loop, (in molecular genetics) a distinctive loop formation seen under an electron microscope. It is composed of a single helical strand of deoxyribonucleic acid (DNA) wound with a hybrid strand containing another single strand of DNA with a strand of ribonucleic acid.

RLQ, abbreviation for *right lower quadrant.*

RMP, abbreviation for *right mentoposterior presentation* of fetal position.

RMSF, abbreviation for **Rocky Mountain spotted fever.**

RMT, abbreviation for *right mentotransverse* fetal position.

Rn, symbol for the element **radon.**

RN, abbreviation for **registered nurse.**

RNA, abbreviation for **ribonucleic acid.**

RNA polymerase, (in molecular genetics) an enzyme that catalyzes the assembly of ribonucleoside triphosphates into ribonucleic acid, with single-stranded deoxyribonucleic acid serving as the template.

RNase, abbreviation for **ribonuclease.**

RNA splicing, (in molecular genetics) the process by which base pairs that interrupt the continuity of genetic information in deoxyribonucleic acid are removed from the precursors of messenger ribonucleic acid.

RNA virus, any of a group of viruses with the genome as a core of the macromolecule ribonucleic acid. Animal viruses are generally classified as ribonucleic acid (RNA) viruses. RNA viruses include *Arenavirus, Coronavirus, Orthomyxovirus, Picornavirus, Rhabdovirus,* and *Togavirus.*

RN, C, abbreviation for *registered nurse, certified.*

RN, CNA, abbreviation for *registered nurse, certified in Nursing Administration.*

RN, CNAA, abbreviation for *registered nurse, certified in Nursing Administration, Advanced.*

RN, CS, abbreviation for *registered nurse, certified Specialist.*

ROA, abbreviation for *right occipitoanterior* fetal position.

Robb, Isabel Hampton, (1860–1910) a Canadian-born American nursing educator and writer. She was the first to institute a systematic, step-by-step course for nursing students that integrated clinical experience and classwork and the first educator to arrange for the affiliation of her students at other hospitals for specialized training. She was one of the founders of *The American Journal of Nursing* and of the forerunner of the American Nurses Association.

robertsonian translocation /rob′ərtsō′-nē·ən/, the exchange of entire chromosome arms, with the break occurring at the centromere, usually between two nonhomologous acrocentric chromosomes, to form one large metacentric chromosome and one extremely small chromosome that carries little genetic material and through successive cell divisions may be lost.

robotic /rōbot′ik/, pertaining to a robot, a mechanical or electronic device that resembles a human being, operating automatically or by remote control with the ability to perform a variety of complex tasks.

Rochalimaea /rosh′əlimē′ə/, a genus of bacteria resembling *Rickettsia* but found extracellularly in an arthropod host. The type species, *R. quintana,* is a cause of trench fever as transmitted by the body louse. A related bacterium is a cause of bacillary angiomatosis in immunocompromised humans, including those with human immunodeficiency virus infection.

Rochalimaea henselae, a species of the Rickettsiaceae family that is the etiologic agent of cat-scratch disease and bacillary angiomatosis.

rocker knife, a knife that cuts with a rocking motion, designed for patients who have functional use of one extremity.

rocking bed, a device that rocks a patient from 15 to 30 degrees. The rocking moves the abdominal contents, and the resulting diaphragmatic movement assists ventilation of the lungs.

Rocky Mountain spotted fever (RMSF), a serious tickborne infectious disease occurring throughout the temperate zones of North and South America, caused by *Rickettsia rickettsii.* It is characterized by chills, fever, severe headache, myalgia, mental confusion, and rash. Erythematous macules first appear on wrists and ankles, spreading rapidly over the extremities, trunk, and face and usually on the palms and soles. Hemorrhagic lesions, constipation, and abdominal distension are also common. Care must be taken not to crush ticks, because infection may be acquired through skin abrasions.

rocuronium bromide, a nondepolarizing neuromuscular blocking agent prescribed as an adjunct to general anesthesia in pro viding skeletal muscle relaxation.

rod [AS, *rodd*], **1.** a straight cylindric structure. **2.** one of the tiny cylindric elements arranged perpendicular to the surface of the retina. Rods contain the chemical rhodopsin, which adapts the eye to detect low-intensity light and gives the rods a purple color.

rodenticide poisoning /rōden′tisīd/ [L, *rodere,* to gnaw, *caedere,* to kill, *potio,* drink], a toxic condition caused by the ingestion of a substance intended for the control of rodent populations.

rodent ulcer /rō'dənt/ [L, *rodere*, to gnaw, *ilcus*, ulcer], a slowly developing serpiginous ulceration of a basal cell carcinoma of the skin.

rod-monochromat /rod'monəkrō'mət/, a person who is totally color-blind or who lacks retinal cone function.

rods and cones [AS, *rodd* + Gk, *konos*], the light-sensitive cells of the retina. The rods, under the visual purple pigment epithelium, are mainly located around the periphery of the retina. The cones receive color stimuli.

roentgen (R) /rent'gən, ren'jən/ [Wilhelm K. Roentgen, German physicist, 1845–1923], the quantity of x-or gamma radiation that creates 1 electrostatic unit of ions in 1 ml of air at 0° and 760 mm of pressure. In radiotherapy or radiodiagnosis, the roentgen is the unit of the emitted dose.

roentgen fetometry, the use of radiographic techniques to measure the fetus in utero.

Rogers, Martha, a nurse theorist who developed the Science of Unitary Human Beings, a nursing theory introduced in 1970. The Rogers theory has strong ties to the general systems theory with elements of a developmental model. It considers four "building blocks": Energy Fields, Universe of Open Systems, Pattern and Organization, and Four Dimensionality.

Rohrer's constants, the constants in an empiric equation for airway resistance. It is expressed as $R = K_1 + K_2V$, where R is resistance, V is instantaneous volumetric flow rate, K_1 is a constant representing gas viscosity and airway geometry, and K_2 is a constant representing gas density and airway geometry.

Rolando's fissure [Luigi Rolando, Italian anatomist, 1773–1831; L, *fissura*, cleft], the central sulcus of the cerebrum.

Rolando's fracture /rōlan'dōz/ [Luigi Rolando], a fracture of the base of the first metacarpal.

role [Fr, stage character], a socially expected behavior pattern associated with an individual's function in various social groups. Roles provide a means for social participation and a way to test identities for consensual validation by significant others.

role blurring, the tendency for professional roles to overlap and become indistinct.

role change, a situation in which status is retained while role expectations change.

role clarification, gaining the knowledge,

information, and cues needed to perform a role.

role conflict, the presence of contradictory and often competing role expectations.

Role Enhancement, a Nursing Interventions Classification defined as assisting a patient, significant other, and/or family to improve relationships by clarifying and supplementing specific role behaviors.

role model [Fr, *role*, stage character; L, *modus*, small copy], a person who inspires others to imitate his or her persona. The role model may be a real person such as a parent, or a symbolic character as depicted in movies or television programs.

role overload, a condition in which there is insufficient time in which to carry out all of the expected role functions.

role performance, altered, a NANDA-accepted nursing diagnosis of a disruption in the way one perceives one's role performance. Defining characteristics include a change in self-perception of one's role, denial of the role, a change in others' perception of one's role, conflict in roles, a change in physical capacity to resume one's role, lack of knowledge of role, and change in usual patterns of responsibility.

role playing, a psychotherapeutic technique in which a person acts out a real or simulated situation as a means of understanding intrapsychic conflicts.

role reversal, the act of assuming the role of another person to appreciate how the person feels, perceives, and behaves in relation to himself and others.

role strain, stress associated with expected roles or positions, experienced as frustration. Role ambiguity is a type of role strain that occurs when shared specifications set for an expected role are incomplete or insufficient to tell the involved individual what is desired and how to do it. Role incongruence is role stress that occurs when an individual undergoes role transitions requiring a significant modification in attitudes and values. Role overqualification is a type of role stress that occurs when a role does not require full use of a person's resources.

roll [OFr, *rolle*], intrinsic joint movements on an axis parallel to the articulating surface. The axis can remain stationary or move in a plane parallel to the joint surface.

roller bandage, a long, tightly wound strip of material that may vary in width. It is generally applied as a circular bandage wrapped around an extremity or the trunk.

roller clamp, a device, usually made of plastic, equipped with a small roller that may be rolled counterclockwise to close off primary intravenous tubing or clockwise to open it.

rolling effleurage, a circular rubbing stroke used in massage to promote circulation and muscle relaxation, especially on the shoulder and buttocks. It is performed with the hand flat, the palm and closely held fingers acting as a unit.

ROM, 1. abbreviation for *range of motion.* **2.** abbreviation for **rupture of membranes.**

Romberg sign /rom'bərg/ [Moritz H. Romberg, German physician, 1795–1873; L, *signum,* mark], an indication of loss of the sense of position in which the patient loses balance when standing erect, feet together, and eyes closed.

rongeur forceps /rônzhur'′, rôNzhœr′/ [Fr, *ronger,* to gnaw; L, *forceps,* pair of tongs], a kind of biting forceps that is strong and heavy, used for cutting bone.

R-on-T phenomenon, a cardiac event in which a ventricular stimulus causes premature depolarization of cells that have not completed the repolarization process.

rooming-in, (in a hospital) a practice that allows mothers and newborn babies to share accommodations, remaining together in the hospital as they would at home rather than being separated.

room temperature [AS, *rum* + L, *temperatura*], the air temperature as measured in a specific part of a room.

root /r○̄ot, r○̇ot/ [AS, *rot*], the lowest part of an organ or a structure by which something is firmly attached, such as the anatomic root of the tooth, which is covered by cementum.

root canal file, a small metal hand instrument with tightly spiraled blades, used for cleaning and shaping a pulpal canal.

root canal filling, a material placed in the root canal system of a tooth to seal the space previously occupied by the dental pulp.

root curettage, the debridement and planing of the root surface of a tooth to remove accretions and induce the development of healthy gingival tissues.

root furcation, 1. the anatomic area at which the roots of a multirooted tooth divide. **2.** abnormal intraradicular resorption of bone in multirooted teeth, resulting from periodontal disease.

rooting reflex, a normal response in newborns when the cheek is touched or stroked along the side of the mouth to turn the head toward the stimulated side and begin to suck.

root resorption of teeth [AS, *rot* + L,

resorbere, to suck back; AS, *toth*], destruction of the cementum or dentin by cementoclastic. If only the apex is dissolved, it may result in a short blunted root. When resorption occurs in the middle of the root, it generally results in penetration of the pulp canal.

root retention, a technique that removes the crown of a root canal–treated tooth and retains enough of the root and gingival attachment to support a prosthesis.

root submersion, a root retention in which the tooth structure is reduced below the level of the alveolar crest and the soft tissue is allowed to heal over it.

ROP, abbreviation for *right occipitoposterior* fetal position.

Rorschach test /rôr'shäk, rôr'shokh/ [Hermann Rorschach, Swiss psychiatrist, 1884–1922], a projective personality assessment test that consists of 10 pictures of inkblots, five in black and white, three in black and red, and two multicolored, to which the subject responds by telling, in as many interpretations as is desired, what images and emotions each design evokes. The test is designed to assess the degree to which intellectual and emotional factors are integrated in the subject's perception of the environment.

ROS, abbreviation for **review of systems.**

rosacea /rōzā'shē·ə/ [L, *rosaceus,* rosy], a chronic form of acne seen in adults of all ages. It is associated with telangiectasia, especially of the nose, forehead, and cheeks.

rose fever [L, *rosa* + *febris,* fever], a common misnomer for seasonal allergic rhinitis caused by pollen, most frequently of grasses, that is airborne at the time roses are in bloom. Roses are not the cause of common spring and summer allergic reactions; their pollen is not dispersed by the wind.

rose hips, the fruitlike berries of rose bushes, a rich source of vitamin C.

roseola /rōzē'ələ/ [L, *roseus*], any rose-colored rash.

roseola idiopathica, a skin eruption of symmetric reddish patches in a condition not associated with any other well-defined symptoms of disease.

roseola infantum, a benign viral endemic illness of infants and young children of unknown etiology, characterized by abrupt, high, sustained or spiking fever; mild pharyngitis; and lymph node enlargement. Febrile convulsions may occur. After 4 or 5 days the fever suddenly drops to normal; and a faint pink maculopapular rash appears on the neck, trunk, and

R

thighs. The rash may last a few hours to 2 days.

roseola symptomatica, a rose-colored eruption that occurs at the onset of a well-defined febrile illness.

rose spots [L, *rosa* + ME, *spotte*], small erythematous macules occurring on the upper abdomen and anterior thorax and lasting 2 or 3 days, characteristic of typhoid and paratyphoid fevers.

rosette /rōzet′/, **1.** any structure resembling a rose. **2.** a sporulating body of a malarial parasite.

rosette technique, a method of detecting antigen or antibody on a cell surface using antigen-coated or antibody-coated particles, resulting in erythrocytes forming a rosette pattern.

rosin /roz′in/, a solid oleo resin produced by steam distillation of balsam from various species of pine trees. After extraction of turpentine in the process, the rosin remains as an amber mass. It is used in plasters and ointments.

Ross-Jones test [George W. Ross, Canadian physician, 1841–1931; Ernest Jones, British psychiatrist, 1879–1958], a technique for detecting excess globulin in the cerebrospinal fluid.

rostellum /rostel′əm/ [L, *rostrum*, beak], the anterior of a tapeworm scolex, commonly featuring hooklike jaws.

rostral /ros′trəl/, beak-shaped. **—rostrum,** *n.*

rostrum /ros′trəm/ [L, beak], a beaklike projection, as the rostrum of the sphenoid bone.

rot [AS, *rotian*], **1.** to decay. **2.** decomposition.

ROT, abbreviation for *right occipitotransverse* fetal position.

rotary nystagmus /rō′tərē/ [L, *rotare,* to rotate; Gk, *nystagmos,* nodding], a form of nystagmus in which the eyeball makes rotary motions around an axis.

rotating tourniquet /rō′tāting/ [L, *rotare,* to rotate; Fr, *tourniquet,* garrote], one of four constricting devices used in a rotating order to pool blood in the extremities. The purpose is to relieve congestion in the lungs in the treatment of acute pulmonary edema. Use of the rotating tourniquet has declined in recent years.

rotation /rōtā′shən/ [L, *rotare*], **1.** one of the four basic movements allowed by the various joints of the skeleton. It is the gyration of a bone around its central axis, which may lie in a separate bone, as in the pivot formed by the dens of the axis around which the atlas turns. A bone such as the humerus may also rotate around its own longitudinal axis, or the axis of rotation may not be quite parallel to the long axis of the rotating bone. **2.** a turning around an axis. **3.** (in obstetrics) the turning of the fetal head to descend through the pelvis.

rotator /rō′tātər/ [L, *rotare,* to rotate], a muscle that rotates a structure around its axis, as the cervical, thoracic, and lumbar musculi rotatores, which function to extend and rotate the vertebral column toward the opposite side.

rotavirus /rō′təvī′rəs/, a double-stranded ribonucleic acid molecule that appears as a tiny wheel, with a clearly defined outer layer, or rim, and an inner layer of spokes. The organism is a cause of acute gastroenteritis with diarrhea, particularly in infants.

Roth spots /roth, rōt/ [Moritz Roth, Swiss physician and pathologist, 1839–1914], pale-centered oval hemorrhages on the retina, observed in many disorders associated with a vascular trauma.

Rotokinetic treatment table /rō′tōkinet′-ik/, a special bed equipped with an automatic turning device that completely immobilizes patients while rotating them from 90 to 270 degrees around a horizontal axis.

rotor syndrome /rō′tər/, a rare condition of the liver inherited as an autosomal-recessive trait. It is similar to Dubin-Johnson's syndrome but can be distinguished by the normal functioning of the gallbladder and lack of liver pigmentation.

rotoscoliosis /rō′təskō′lē·ō′sis/, a condition in which there is both lateral and rotational spinal deviation.

rouleaux /rōōlō′/, *sing.* **rouleau** [Fr, cylinder], an aggregation of red cells in a roll formation that may be caused by abnormal proteins, as in multiple myeloma or macroglobulinemia, but is most often a microscopic artifact.

round ligament [L, *rotundus,* round, *ligare,* to bind], **1.** a curved fibrous band that is attached at one end to the fovea of the head of the femur and at the other to the transverse ligament of the acetabulum. **2.** a fibrous cord extending from the umbilicus to the anterior part of the liver. **3.** in the female, a fibromuscular band that extends from the anterior surface of the uterus through the inguinal canal to the labium majus. The structure is homologous to the spermatic cord in the male.

rounds, *informal.* a teaching conference or a meeting in which the clinical problems encountered in the practice of nursing, medicine, or other service are discussed.

round window [L, *rotundus* + ONorse, *vindauga*], a round opening in the medial wall of the middle ear leading into the cochlea and covered by a secondary tympanic membrane.

roundworm, any worm of the class Nematoda, including *Ancylostoma duodenale, Ascaris lumbricoides, Enterobius vermicularis,* and *Strongyloides stercoralis.*

Roussy-Lévy's disease /rōōsē′-lēvē′/ [Gustave Roussy, French pathologist, 1874–1948; Gabrielle Lévy, French neurologist, 1886–1935], an inherited cerebellar ataxia associated with muscle wasting of the extremities, absence of tendon reflexes, and foot deformities.

route of administration /rōōt, rout/ [Fr, *route,* course; L, *administrare,* to serve], (of a drug) any one of the body systems in which a drug may be administered, such as intradermally, intrathecally, intramuscularly, intranasally, intravenously, orally, rectally, subcutaneously, sublingually, topically, or vaginally.

Roux-en-Y /rōō′enwī′, rōō′änēgrek′/ [César Roux, Swiss surgeon, 1857–1926], an anastomosis of the small intestine in the shape of the letter Y. The proximal end of the divided intestine is anastomosed end-to-side to the distal loop, and a part of the distal loop is anastomosed to another part of the digestive tract such as the esophagus.

Rovsing's sign /rov′singz/ [Nils T. Rovsing, Danish surgeon, 1862–1927], an indication of acute appendicitis in which pressure on the left lower quadrant of the abdomen causes pain in the right lower quadrant.

Royal College of Physicians (R.C.P.), a professional organization of physicians in the United Kingdom.

Royal College of Physicians and Surgeons of Canada (RCPSC), a national Canadian organization that recognizes and confers membership on certain qualified physicians and surgeons.

Royal College of Surgeons (R.C.S.), a professional organization of surgeons in the United Kingdom.

Roy, Sister Callista, a nursing theorist who introduced the Adaptation Model of Nursing in 1970 as a conceptual framework for nursing curricula, practice, and research. In the Roy model the human is viewed as an adaptive system. Changes occur in the system in response to stimuli. If the change promotes the integrity of the individual, it is an adaptive response. Otherwise it is a maladaptive response.

RPF, abbreviation for **renal plasma flow.**

rpm, abbreviation for *revolutions per minute.*

RQ, abbreviation for **respiratory quotient.**

RR, R.R., abbreviation for **recovery room.**

R.R.A., abbreviation for **registered record administrator.**

R-R interval, the interval from the peak of one QRS complex to the peak of the next as shown on an electrocardiogram.

rRNA, abbreviation for **ribosomal RNA.**

RRT, abbreviation for **registered respiratory therapist.**

RSD, abbreviation for **reflex sympathetic dystrophy.**

RSNA, abbreviation for **Radiological Society of North America.**

RSV, RS virus, abbreviation for **respiratory syncytial virus.**

RT, abbreviation for **respiratory therapy.**

R.T., abbreviation for **registered technologist.**

RTA, abbreviation for **renal tubular acidosis.**

r.t.c., abbreviation for *return to clinic,* noted on the chart, usually followed by a date on which a subsequent appointment has been made for the patient.

Ru, symbol for the element **ruthenium.**

rub [ME, *rubben,* to scrape], the movement of one surface moving over another, thereby producing friction, as when pleural membranes produce friction rub.

rubber-band ligation, a method of treating hemorrhoids by placing a rubber band around the hemorrhoidal part of the blood vessel, causing it to slough off after a period of time.

rubber dam [ME, *rubben,* to scrape; AS, *demman,* to dam up], a thin sheet of latex rubber for isolating one or more teeth during a dental procedure.

rubber dam clamps forceps, (in dentistry) a type of forceps with beaks designed to engage holes in a rubber dam clamp to facilitate its placement over teeth.

rubbing alcohol [ME, *rubben,* to scrape; Ar, *alkohl,* essence], a disinfectant for skin and instruments. It contains 70% isopropyl alcohol by volume, the remainder consisting of water and denaturants, with or without color or perfume. It may cause dryness of the skin. Rubbing alcohol is for external use only and is flammable.

rubefacient /rōō′bəfā′shənt/ [L, *ruber,* red, *facere,* to make], **1.** a substance or agent that increases the reddish coloration of the skin. **2.** increasing the reddish coloration of the skin.

rubefaction /rōō′bəfak′shən/ [L, *ruber,* red, *facer,* to make], a redness of the skin produced by a counterirritant.

rubella /rōōbel′ə/ [L, *rubellus,* somewhat red], a contagious viral disease charac-

R

terized by fever, symptoms of a mild upper respiratory tract infection, lymph node enlargement, arthralgia, and a diffuse fine red maculopapular rash. The virus is spread by droplet infection, and the incubation time is from 12 to 23 days. The symptoms usually last only 2 or 3 days except for arthralgia, which may persist longer or recur. One attack confers lifelong immunity. If a woman acquires rubella in the first trimester of pregnancy, fetal anomalies may result, including heart defects, cataracts, deafness, and mental retardation. An infant exposed to the virus in utero at any time during gestation may shed the virus for up to 30 months after birth. Complications of postnatal rubella are rare.

rubella and mumps virus vaccine, a suspension containing live attenuated mumps and rubella viruses. It is prescribed for immunization against rubella and mumps.

rubella embryopathy, any congenital abnormality in an infant caused by maternal rubella in the early stages of pregnancy.

rubella titer [L, *rubellus,* somewhat red; Fr, *titre,* standard], a serologic test to determine a patient's state of immunity against rubella.

rubella virus vaccine, a suspension containing live attenuated rubella virus. It is prescribed for immunization against rubella.

rubeosis /rōōbē·ō′sis/, a red discoloration of the skin.

rubeosis iridis, the formation of blood vessels on the anterior of the iris. It may be associated with thrombotic glaucoma and diabetes mellitus.

ruber /roo′bər/, (*Latin*) red.

rubescent /rōōbes′ənt/, reddening.

rubidium (Rb) /rōōbid′ē·əm/ [L, *rubidus,* reddish], a soft metallic element of the alkali metals group. Its atomic number is 37; its atomic mass (weight) is 85.47. Slightly radioactive, it is used in radioisotope scanning.

Rubin's test [Isador C. Rubin, American gynecologist, 1883–1958], a test performed in the process of evaluating the cause of infertility by assessing the patency of the fallopian tubes. Carbon dioxide gas (CO_2) is introduced into the tubes under pressure through a cannula inserted into the cervix. The CO_2 is passed through from a syringe connected to a manometer at pressures of up to 200 mm Hg. If the tubes are open, the gas enters the abdominal cavity, and the recorded pressure falls below 180 mm Hg.

rubivirus /rōō′bēvī′rəs/, a member of the togavirus family, which includes the rubella virus.

rubor /rōō′bôr/, redness, especially when accompanying inflammation.

rubratoxin /rōō′brətok′sin/ a mycotoxin produced on cereal grains by certain species of penicillin.

rubricyte /rōō′brisīt/ [L, *ruber,* red; Gk, *kytos,* cell], a nucleated red blood cell; the marrow stage in the normal development of an erythrocyte.

rudiment /rōō′dimənt/ [L, *rudimentum,* beginning], an organ or tissue that is incompletely developed or nonfunctional. **—rudimentary,** *adj.*

rudimentary /rōō′dimen′tərē/, [L, *rudimentum,* beginning], pertaining to something either vestigial or embryonic.

Ruffini's corpuscles /rōōfē′nēz/ [Angelo Ruffini, Italian anatomist, 1864–1929], a variety of oval-shaped nerve endings in the subcutaneous tissue, located principally at the junction of the dermis and the subcutaneous tissue.

ruga /rōō′gə/, *pl.* **rugae** /rōō′jē/ [L, ridge], a ridge or fold, such as the rugae of the stomach, which presents large folds in the mucous membrane of that organ.

rugae of vagina, [L, *ruga,* ridge, *vagina,* sheath], the transverse ridges on the mucous membrane lining the vagina. They allow the vagina to stretch during childbirth.

rugitus /rōō′jitəs/ [L, roaring], the rumbling sound of flatus in the intestines.

rugose /rōō′gōs/, wrinkled or corrugated.

RUL, abbreviation for *right upper lobe* of lung.

rule, a guide for conduct or action.

rule of bigeminy [L, *regula,* model, *bis,* double, *geminus,* twin], (in cardiology) the tendency of a lengthened ventricular cycle to precipitate a ventricular premature complex.

rule of confidentiality, a principle that personal information about others, particularly patients, should not be revealed to persons not authorized to receive such information.

rule of co-occurrence /kō′əkur′əns/, a mandate that a person use the same level of lexic and syntactic structure when speaking.

rule of nines, a formula for estimating the amount of body surface covered by burns by assigning 9% to the head and each arm, twice 9% (18%) to each leg and the anterior and posterior trunk, and 1% to the perineum. This is modified in infants and children because of the different body proportions.

rule of outlet, an obstetric standard for

determining whether the pelvic outlet will allow the passage of a fetus. It is calculated from the sum of the transverse and posterior sagittal diameters of the outlet, which must equal a least 15 cm.

rule of three, (in respiratory therapy) an arterial oxygen tension that is three times the value of the inspired oxygen concentration. It is regarded as an empiric guide to a temporarily acceptable minimal oxygenation or expression of clinical observation and has no scientific basis.

rum, a spirit distilled from fermented products of sugar cane, including molasses. It may contain up to 60% of ethyl alcohol by volume.

ruminant /roo'minənt/ [L, *ruminare,* to chew again], pertaining to animals that chew their cud and to human infants that may regurgitate and reswallow a meal.

rumination /roo'minā'shən/ [L, *ruminare,* to chew again], habitual regurgitation of small amounts of undigested food with little force after every feeding, a condition commonly seen in infants. It may be a symptom of overfeeding, eating too fast, or swallowing air.

runner's high, a feeling of euphoria experienced by some cross-country runners and joggers as they near the end of a run. The feeling of elation is believed to be associated with the body's production of endorphins during physical stress.

Runyan classification system /run'yən/, a system of identifying mycobacteria on the basis of pigmentation and growth condition of the organisms. It includes group I, yellow-pigment photochromogens; group II, yellow-to-orange-to-red pigment scotochromogens; group III, white-to-tan nonphotochromogens; and group IV, rapid-growing saprophytes.

rupia /roo'pē·ə/, a pustular eruption associated with secondary syphilis. It is characterized by encrusted ulcers resembling shells on darkly pigmented skin.

rupture /rup'chər/ [L, *rumpere,* to break], **1.** a tear or break in the continuity or configuration of an organ or body tissue, including instances when other tissue protrudes through the opening. **2.** to cause a break or tear.

ruptured hymen, a hymen that has been torn as a result of injury, coitus, or surgery.

rupture of membranes (ROM) [L, *rumpere,* to break, *membrana*], the rupture of the amniotic sac, usually at the start of labor. It may be spontaneous or artificial.

rupture of uterus in pregnancy, a tear or break in the uterus because of trauma or other causes, possibly accompanied by displacement of the fetus and amniotic sac

into the peritoneal cavity. The patient may experience acute pain because of tissue damage and irritation of the peritoneal tissues. Excessive loss of blood may be marked by hypotension, fluid volume deficit, and altered cardiac output.

RUQ, abbreviation for *right upper quadrant.*

Rural Clinics Assistance Act /roo'rəl/, an act of the U.S. Congress that permitted the establishment of clinics in certain areas designated rural and underserved and in some inner cities. The clinics are designed to provide primary care through teams of physicians and nurse practitioners.

rush /rush/, **1.** a pleasurable feeling experienced by users of recreational drugs following an injection of amphetamine or heroin. An amphetamine rush is described as an abrupt awakening as distinguished from the drowsy drifting rush of heroin use. **2.** a strong wave of contractile activity that travels along the small intestine, usually as a result of irritation or distension.

Russell dwarf [Alexander Russell, twentieth-century Scottish physician; AS, *dweorge*], a person affected with Russell's syndrome, a congenital disorder in which short stature is associated with various anomalies of the head, face, and skeleton and with varying degrees of mental retardation.

Russell's bodies [William Russell, Scottish physician, 1852–1940; AS, *bodig,* body], the mucoprotein inclusions found in globular plasma cells in cancer and inflammations. The bodies contain surface gamma globulins.

Russell's periodontal index, [Albert L. Russell, American dentist, b. 1905], a measure of the extent of periodontal disease in an individual that considers the amount of bone loss around the teeth and the degree of gingival inflammation.

Russell traction [R. Hamilton Russell, Australian surgeon, 1860–1933; L, *trahere,* to pull along], a unilateral or bilateral orthopedic mechanism that combines suspension and traction to immobilize, position, and align the lower extremities in the treatment of fractured femurs, hip and knee contractures, and disease processes of the hip and knee.

Russian bath /rush'ən/, a hot steam bath followed by a cold plunge.

rusts, microbes that are pathogens of plants, particularly cereal grains. They are also important human allergens.

rusty sputum /rus'tē/ [AS, *rust* + L, *sputum,* spittle], sputum that is reddish, indicative of blood.

R

ruthenium (Ru) /rōōthē′nē-əm/ [Ruthenia, region of western Ukraine], a hard, brittle, metallic element. Its atomic number is 44; its atomic mass (weight) is 101.07.

rutherfordium (Rf) [Sir Ernest Rutherford, British physicist, 1871–1937], a transuranic element, and the first transactinide element. Its atomic number is 104; its atomic mass (weight) is 261. It is produced by an induced nuclear reaction.

rutin /rōō′tin/, a bioflavonoid obtained from buckwheat and used in the treatment of capillary fragility.

RV, abbreviation for **residual volume.**

RVC, abbreviation for *responds to verbal commands.*

rxn, RXN, symbol for drug reaction.

S

s, **1.** abbreviation for *second* in SI units. **2.** abbreviation for **steady state. 3.** abbreviation for the Latin word *sinister,* 'left'.

s̄, s, symbol for the Latin *sine,* 'without'.

S, **1.** symbol for **sulfur. 2.** symbol for *saturation of hemoglobin.* **3.** symbol for **siemens.**

S₁, the first heart sound in the cardiac cycle, occurring at the outset of ventricular systole. It is associated with closure of the mitral and tricuspid valves and is synchronous with the apical pulse.

S₂, the second heart sound in the cardiac cycle. It is associated with closure of the aortic and pulmonic valves at the outset of ventricular diastole.

S₃, the third heart sound in the cardiac cycle. Normally it is audible only in children and physically active young adults. In older people it is an abnormal finding and usually indicates myocardial failure.

S₄, the fourth heart sound in the cardiac cycle. It occurs late in diastole on contraction of the atria. Rarely heard in normal subjects, it indicates an abnormally increased resistance to ventricular filling.

S1, S2, . . . , symbols for sacral nerves.

SA, **1.** abbreviation for **sinoatrial. 2.** abbreviation for **surface area. 3.** abbreviation for **surgeon's assistant.**

saber-sheath trachea /sā'bər/, an abnormally shaped trachea caused by chronic obstructive pulmonary disease. The posterior part of the trachea increase in diameter while the lateral dimension decreases.

saber shin, a sharp anterior bowing of the tibia caused by hereditary syphilis.

Sabin-Feldman dye test /sā'binfeld'mən/ [Albert B. Sabin, American virologist, 1906–1993; H. A. Feldman, American epidemiologist, b. 1914; AS, *deag* + L, *testum,* crucible], a serologic test for the diagnosis of toxoplasmosis that depends on the presence of specific antibodies that block the uptake of methylene blue dye by the cytoplasm of the *Toxoplasma* organisms.

sac /sak/ [Gk, *sakkos,* sack], a pouch or a baglike organ, such as the abdominal sac of the embryo that develops into the abdominal cavity.

saccade /sakād'/ [Fr, *saccader,* to jerk],

pertaining to something jerky, broken, or abrupt, such as rapid shift of eye movement or a staccato voice.

saccadic eye movement /sakad'ik/, an extremely fast voluntary movement of the eyes, allowing them to accurately fix on a still object in the visual field as the person moves or the head turns.

saccharide /sak'ərīd'/, any of a large group of carbohydrates, including all sugars and starches. Almost all carbohydrates are saccharides.

saccharin /sak'ərin/ [Gk, *sakcharon,* sugar], **1.** a white crystalline synthetic sweetening agent derived from coal tar. Although it is up to 500 times as sweet as sugar, it has no food value. **2.** having a sweet taste, especially cloyingly sweet.

saccharometabolism /sak'ərōmətab'əliz'-əm/, the functioning of sugar within a living body.

Saccharomyces /sak'ərōmī'sēz/ [Gk, *sakcharon + mykes,* fungus], a genus of yeast fungi that cause such diseases as bronchitis, moniliasis, and pharyngitis.

saccharomycosis /sak'ərōmīkō'sis/ [Gk, *sakcharon + mykes + osis,* condition], infection with yeast fungi such as the genera *Candida* or *Cryptococcus.*

saccular /sak'yələr/ [L, *sacculus,* small bag], pertaining to a pouch, or shaped like a sac.

saccular aneurysm, a localized dilation of an artery in which only a small area of the vessel, not the entire circumference, is distended, forming a saclike swelling or protrusion.

sacculated /sak'yəlā'tid/ [L, *sacculus,* small bag], a condition of small sacs, pouches, or saclike dilations.

sacculated pleurisy /sak'yəlātid/, an inflammation of the pleura with exudate encapsulated in several locations by adhesions.

saccule /sak'yool/ [L, *sacculus*], a small bag or sac, such as the air saccules of the lungs. —**saccular,** *adj.*

sacculus /sak'yoolǝs/, *pl.* **sacculi** ', a little sac or bag, especially the smaller of the two divisions of the membranous labyrinth of the vestibule, which communicates with the cochlear duct through the ductus reuniens in the inner ear.

SA conduction time, the conduction time for an impulse from the sinus node to the atrial musculature. It is measured from the sinoatrial (SA) deflection in the SA nodal electrocardiogram to the beginning of the P wave in a bipolar record, or to the beginning of the high right atrial electrogram in a unipolar record.

sacral /sā′krəl, sak′rəl/ [L, *sacer,* sacred], pertaining to the sacrum.

sacral bone, a composite bone formed by the fusion during maturation of five sacral vertebrae that were separate at birth. The sacrum forms the back of the pelvis.

sacral canal, an extension of the vertebral canal through the sacrum.

sacral foramen, any one of several openings between the fused segments of the sacral vertebrae in the sacrum through which the sacral nerves pass.

sacral nerves, the five segmental nerves from the sacral part of the spinal cord. The first four emerge through the anterior sacral foramina and the fifth from between the sacral foramen and the coccyx.

sacral node, a node in one of the seven groups of parietal lymph nodes of the abdomen and the pelvis, situated within the sacrum.

sacral plexus, a network of motor and sensory nerves formed by the lumbosacral trunk from the fourth and fifth lumbar, and by the first, second, and third sacral nerves. They converge toward the lower part of the greater sciatic foramen and unite to become a large, flattened band, most of which continues into the thigh as the sciatic nerve.

sacral vertebra, one of the five segments of the vertebral column that fuse in the adult to form the sacrum. The ventral border of the first sacral vertebra projects into the pelvis. The bodies of the other sacral vertebrae are smaller than that of the first and are flattened and curved ventrally, forming the convex, anterior surface of the sacrum.

sacrococcygeal /-koksij′ē·əl/ [L, *sacer,* sacred; Gk, *kokkyx,* cuckoo's beak], pertaining to the sacrum and coccyx.

sacrococcygeal teratoma, a common tumor of newborns, found in the primitive pit. It may represent part of the blastopore of lower vertebrates.

sacroiliac /sā′krō·il′ē·ak/ [L, *sacer* + *ilium,* flank], pertaining to the part of the skeletal system that includes the sacrum and the ilium bones of the pelvis.

sacroiliac articulation, an immovable joint in the pelvis formed by the articulation of each side of the sacrum with an iliac bone.

sacroiliac joint, an irregular synovial joint between the sacrum and the ilium on either side.

sacroiliitis /sa′krō·il′ē·ī′tis/, an inflammation of the sacroiliac joint.

sacrosciatic /sā′krōsī·at′ik/, pertaining to the sacrum and ischium.

sacrospinalis /sak′rōspīnal′is/ [L, *sacer* + *spina,* backbone], the superficial longitudinal muscle mass on either side of the vertebral column. It extends and flexes the vertebral column and the head, draws the ribs downward, and bends the trunk to the side.

sacrum /sā′krəm, sak′rəm/ [L, *sacer,* sacred], the large, triangular bone at the dorsal part of the pelvis, inserted like a wedge between the two hip bones. The base of the sacrum articulates with the last lumbar vertebra, and its apex articulates with the coccyx. —**sacral,** *adj.*

SAD, abbreviation for **seasonal affective disorder.**

saddle block anesthesia [AS, *sadol* + Fr, *bloc* + Gk, *anaisthesia,* lack of feeling], a form of spinal nerve block in which the parts of the body anesthetized are those that would touch a saddle, were the patient sitting astride one. It is performed by injecting a local anesthetic into the subarachnoid cerebrospinal fluid space.

saddle embolism, a thrombus that straddles a dividing blood vessel.

saddle joint, a synovial joint in which surfaces of contiguous bones are reciprocally concavoconvex. A saddle joint permits no axial rotation but allows flexion, extension, adduction, and abduction.

saddle nose [AS, *sadol* + *nosu*], a sunken nasal bridge caused by injury or disease and resulting in damage to the nasal septum.

sadism /sā′dizəm, sad′izəm/ [Marquis Donatien A. F. de Sade, French writer, 1740–1814], **1.** abnormal pleasure derived from inflicting physical or psychologic pain or abuse on others; cruelty. **2.** (in psychiatry) a psychosexual disorder characterized by the infliction of physical or psychologic pain or humiliation on another person, either a consenting or a nonconsenting partner, to achieve sexual excitement or gratification. —**sadistic,** *adj.*

sadist /sā′dist/, a person who is afflicted with or practices sadism.

sadomasochism /sā′dōmas′əkiz′əm/ [Marquis de Sade; Leopold von Sacher-Masoch, Austrian author, 1836–1895], a personality disorder characterized by traits of sadism and masochism.

sadomasochist /sā′dōmas′əkist/ [Marquis de Sade; Leopold von Sacher-Masoch], a person who practices sadomasochism.

safe sex, intimate sexual practices between partners who use condoms or other means to prevent the exchange of body fluids that transmit diseases. Although perfect safety is virtually impossible without abstinence, the known risks of infections by human immunodeficiency virus viruses or other organisms transmitted through sexual contact can be reduced by safe sex practices.

safety director /sāf'tē/ [Fr, *sauver,* to save, *directeur,* manager], a member of a hospital staff whose activities are related to safety functions, such as fire prevention, environmental safety, and disaster planning activities.

safety glass, a hard, transparent material that resists shattering on impact. It usually is made as a sandwich of two sheets of glass with an intermediate layer of plastic. Safety glass may also be produced as a tempered material that breaks into rounded granules instead of sharp shards.

safety glasses, impact-resistant lenses that protect the eyes from blows or other kinds of injury. Such lenses are usually made by tempering the glass, substituting plastic for glass, or laminating.

safflower oil /sef'lou·er/, a liquid fat containing polyunsaturated fatty acids, derived from the seeds of the safflower plant, *Carthamus tinctorium.* It is commonly mixed with other edible vegetable oils.

sagittal /saj'ətəl/ [L, *sagitta,* arrow], (in anatomy) pertaining to a suture or an imaginary line extending from the front to the back in the midline of the body or a part of the body, dividing into right and left parts.

sagittal axis, a hypothetic line through the mandibular condyle that serves as an axis for rotation movements of the mandible.

sagittal fontanel, a soft area located in the sagittal suture, halfway between the anterior and posterior fontanels. It may be found in some normal newborns and also some with Down's syndrome.

sagittal plane, the anterioposterior plane, or the section parallel to the median plane of the body.

sagittal section, an anteroposterior cross section produced by slicing, laterally or through imaging techniques, a body or body part in a vertical plane parallel to the median plane.

sagittal sinus [L, *sagitta,* arrow, *sinus,* hollow], either of two venous sinuses of the dura mater. The superior venous sinus begins near the crista galli and drains backward to empty into a confluence of sinuses near the occipital area. The inferior venous sinus begins in the lower margin of the cerebral falx and follows the superior venous sinus, emptying into the straight sinus.

sagittal suture, the serrated connection between the two parietal bones of the skull, coursing down the midline from the coronal suture to the upper part of the lambdoidal suture.

sago spleen /sā'gō/, a form of amyloid spleen that mainly affects the Malpighian bodies.

SaH, SAH, abbreviation for **subarachnoid hemorrhage.**

SAIN, abbreviation for **Society for Advancement in Nursing.**

Saint's triad [Charles F. M. Saint, twentieth-century South African radiologist], a group of three related conditions: cholelithiasis, diverticulosis, and hiatal hernia occurring together.

Saint Vitus' dance /sāntvī'təs/, a motor nerve disorder characterized by irregular involuntary jerky movements of the limbs and facial muscles. Historically the condition was once confused with symptoms of a dance mania that reportedly was cured by a pilgrimage to the shrine of Saint Vitus.

salaam convulsion /säläm'/ [L, *convulsio,* cramp], a violent muscle spasm of the sternomastoid muscles marked by head bobbing or bowing.

salicylanilide /sal'isilan'ilīd/, a topical antifungal prescribed in the treatment of tinea capitis caused by *Microsporum audouinii.*

salicylate /səlis'əlāt/ [Gk, *salix,* willow, *hyle,* matter], any of several widely prescribed drugs derived from salicylic acid. Salicylates exert analgesic, antipyretic, and antiinflammatory actions. The most important is acetylsalicylic acid, or aspirin. Sodium salicylate also has been used systemically, and it exerts similar effects. Methyl salicylate is used topically as a counterirritant in ointments and liniments. Methyl salicylate can be absorbed through the skin in amounts capable of causing systemic toxicity. Another salicylate, salicylic acid, is too irritating to be used systemically and is used topically as a keratolytic agent, for example, for removing warts.

salicylated /səlis'ilā'tid/ [Gk, *salix,* willow, *hyle,* matter], pertaining to a chemical formed as a salt or ester of salicylic acid.

salicylate poisoning, a toxic condition caused by the ingestion of salicylate, most often in aspirin or oil of wintergreen. Intoxication is characterized by rapid breathing, vomiting, headache, irritability, ketosis, hypoglycemia, and, in severe cases, seizures and respiratory failure.

salicylic acid /sal'isil'ik/, a keratolytic

S

agent prescribed in the treatment of hyperkeratotic skin conditions and as an adjunct in fungal infections.

salicylism /sal′isil′izəm/ [Gk, *salix*, willow, *hyle*, matter, *ismos*, practice], a syndrome of salicylate toxicity.

saline /sā′lēn/ [L, *sal*, salt], **1.** pertaining to a substance that contains a salt or salts. **2.** pertaining to something that is salty or has the characteristics of common table salt.

saline cathartic [L, *sal*, salt; Gk, *katharsis*, cleansing], one of a large group of cathartics administered to achieve prompt, complete evacuation of the bowel. A watery semifluid evacuation usually occurs within 3 to 4 hours.

saline enema [L, *sal*, salt; Gk, *enienai*, to send in], a salt-water enema. Hypertonic saline enema is used to treat worm infestations, by inducing peristalsis and evacuation. A normal saline enema of 1 teaspoonful of salt per 0.5 liter of water is instilled slowly and retained as long as possible to combat shock or replace lost fluids.

saline infusion, the therapeutic introduction of a physiologic salt solution into a vein.

saline irrigation, the washing out of a body cavity or wound with a stream of salt solution, usually an isotonic aqueous solution of sodium chloride.

saline solution, a solution containing sodium chloride. Depending on the use, it may be hypotonic, isotonic, or hypertonic with body fluids.

saliva /səlī′və/ [L, spittle], the clear, viscous fluid secreted by the salivary and mucous glands in the mouth. Saliva contains water, mucin, organic salts, and the digestive enzyme ptyalin. It serves to moisten the oral cavity, to initiate the digestion of starches, and to aid in the chewing and swallowing of food.

salivary /sal′iver′ē/ [L, *saliva*, spittle], pertaining to saliva or to the formation of saliva.

salivary duct, any one of the ducts through which saliva passes.

salivary fistula, an abnormal communication from a salivary gland or duct to an opening in the mouth or on the skin of the face or neck.

salivary gland, any one of three pairs of glands secreting into the mouth, thus aiding the digestive process. The salivary glands are the parotid, the submandibular, and the sublingual. They are racemose structures consisting of numerous lobes subdivided into smaller lobules connected by dense areolar tissue, vessels, and ducts.

salivary gland cancer, a malignant neoplastic disease of a salivary gland, occurring most frequently in a parotid gland. About 75% of tumors that develop in the salivary glands are benign, characteristically slow-growing painless mobile masses that are cystic or rubbery in consistency. The most common malignant neoplasms are mucoepidermoid, adenoid cystic, solid, and squamous cell carcinomas.

salivation /sal′ivā′shən/, the process of saliva secretion by the salivary glands.

salivatory /sal′ivatôr′ē/ [L, *saliva*, spittle], stimulating the production of saliva.

sallow /sal′ō/ [ME, *salou*, dirty-gray], sickly in complexion.

salmeterol xinafoate, a sympathomimetic bronchodilator prescribed in the treatment of reversible bronchospasm associated with bronchial and nocturnal asthma.

Salmonella /sal′mənel′ə/ [Daniel E. Salmon, American pathologist, 1850–1914], a genus of motile gram-negative rod-shaped bacteria that includes species causing typhoid fever, paratyphoid fever, and some forms of gastroenteritis.

Salmonella enteritidis [Daniel E. Salmon; Gk, *enteron*, intestine], a species of *Salmonella* causing food poisoning and gastroenteritis in humans.

salmonellosis /sal′mənəlō′sis/ [Daniel E. Salmon; Gk, *osis*, condition], a form of gastroenteritis, caused by ingestion of food contaminated with a species of *Salmonella*. It is characterized by an incubation period of 6 to 48 hours followed by sudden colicky abdominal pain, fever, and bloody, watery diarrhea. Nausea and vomiting are common, and abdominal signs may resemble those of acute appendicitis or cholecystitis. Symptoms usually last from 2 to 5 days, but diarrhea and fever may persist for up to 2 weeks. Dehydration may occur.

salol camphor /sal′ol/, a clear oily mixture of two parts of camphor and three parts of phenyl salicylate, used as a local antiseptic.

salpingectomy /sal′pinjek′təmē/ [Gk, *salpinx*, tube, *ektome*, excision], surgical removal of one or both fallopian tubes. It is performed for removal of a cyst or tumor, excision of an abscess, or, if both tubes are removed, as a sterilization procedure.

salpingemphraxis /salpinj′emfrak′sis/ [Gk, *salpinx*, tube, *emphraxis*, a stoppage], **1.** an obstruction of the eustachian tube of the ear. **2.** an obstruction of a fallopian tube.

salpingitis /sal′pinji′tis/ [Gk, *salpinx* + *itis*, inflammation], an inflammation or infection of the fallopian tube.

salpingography /sal'ping·gog'rəfē/, a radiographic examination of the fallopian tube after injection of a radiopaque contrast medium.

salpingo-oophorectomy /-ō'əfôrek'təmē/, the surgical removal of a fallopian tube and an ovary.

salpingo-oophoritis /-ō'əfôrī'tis/ [Gk, *salpinx*, tube, *oophoron*, ovary, *itis*, inflammation], an inflammation of a fallopian tube and associated ovary.

salpingostomy /sal'ping·gos'təmē/ [Gk, *salpinx* + *stoma*, mouth], the formation of an artificial opening in a fallopian tube. The procedure is performed to restore patency in a tube whose fimbriated opening has been closed by infection or chronic inflammation or to drain an abscess or a fluid accumulation. A prosthesis may be inserted to maintain the patency of the fallopian tube and to direct the route of the ova to assist fertilization.

salpinx /sal'pingks/, *pl.* **salpinges** /salpin'-jēz/ [Gk, tube], a tube, such as the salpinx auditiva or the salpinx uterina. —**salpingian,** *adj.*

salt /sôlt/ [L, *sal*], **1.** a compound formed by the chemical reaction of an acid and a base. Salts are usually composed of a metal cation and a nonmetal anion. **2.** sodium chloride (common table salt). **3.** a substance such as magnesium sulfate (Epsom salt) used as a purgative.

saltation /saltā'shən/ [L, *saltare*, to dance], (in genetics) a mutation causing a significant difference in appearance between parent and offspring or an abrupt variation in the characteristics of the species. —**saltatorial, saltatoric, saltatory** /sal'tətôr'ē/, *adj.*

saltatory conduction /sal'tətôr'ē/ [L, *saltare* + *conducere*, to lead together], impulse transmission that skips from node to node.

saltatory evolution, the appearance of a sudden abrupt change within a species, caused by mutation; the progression of a species by sudden major changes rather than by the gradual accumulation of minor changes.

salt cake, sodium sulfate anhydrous; a technical grade of sodium sulfate used in detergents, dyes, soaps, and other industrial products.

salt depletion, the loss of salt from the body through excessive elimination of body fluids by perspiration, diarrhea, vomiting, or urination, without corresponding replacement.

salted plasma /sôl'tid/, a fluid part of blood that has been treated with sodium or magnesium sulfate to prevent coagulation.

salt fever, an elevated body temperature in an infant that develops after a rectal saline injection.

salt-losing nephritis, a disorder characterized by abnormal kidney loss of sodium chloride, hyponatremia, azotemia, acidosis, dehydration, and vascular collapse. Causes include kidney tubule damage, endocrine dysfunction, and gastrointestinal abnormality.

saltpeter /sôlt'pē'tər/ [L, *sal*, salt, *petra*, rock], common name for potassium nitrate, KNO$_3$, used in gunpowder, pickling substances, and medicines.

salt-poor diet [Gk, *diaita*, way of living], a diet providing 500 mg or less of sodium chloride daily. To ensure that the maximum salt intake does not exceed the limit, it is necessary to record the amount of dietary sodium chloride, including amounts contained in patient medications.

salt substitute, a chemical compound for flavoring foods without adding sodium to the diet. Examples include potassium chloride, monopotassium glutamate, and glutamic acid.

salvage therapy /sal'vij/ [Fr, *sauver*, to save; Gk, *therapeia*, treatment], therapy administered to sites at which previous therapies have failed and the disease has recurred.

samarium (Sm) /səmer'ē·əm/ [Colonel Samarski, nineteenth-century Russian mine official], a metallic rare earth element. Its atomic number is 62; its atomic mass (weight) is 150.35.

SAMHSA, abbreviation for **Substance Abuse and Mental Health Services Administration.**

sample [L, *exemplum*], (in research) a group or part of the whole that can be used to demonstrate characteristics of the whole. Kinds of samples include cluster, convenience, **random,** and **stratified.**

sand bath, the application of warm dry sand or damp sand to the body.

Sandhoff's disease, a variant of Tay-Sachs' disease that includes defects in the enzymes hexosaminidase A and B. It is characterized by a progressively more rapid course and is found in the general population, not restricted as is Tay-Sachs' disease.

Sandoz Clinical Assessment—Geriatric, an examination of psychologic function that is administered to elderly people to assist in the diagnostic process.

sandwich generation, the middle generation who are trying to raise children and help aging parents at the same time.

sandwich technique, a method of identifying antibodies or antibody-synthesizing cells in a tissue preparation. A solution containing a specific antigen is applied to the preparation. If antibodies to the antigen are present in the tissue, they will bind to the antigen. Unbound antigen is washed away, and then a fluorochrome-labeled antibody specific for the antigen is added. The result is a complex of antigen sandwiched between antibodies, which can be detected by fluorescence microscopy.

sanguine /sang'gwin/ [L, *sanguis,* blood], pertaining to abundant and active blood circulation, ruddy complexion, and an attitude full of vitality and confidence.

sanguineous /sang·gwin'ē-əs/ [L, *sanguis,* blood], pertaining to blood or containing blood, such as full-blooded.

sanguinopurulent /sang'gwinōpyŏŏr'ə-lənt/, containing blood and pus.

sanies /sā'ni·ēz/, a thin blood-stained purulent discharge from a wound or ulcer.

sanioserous, containing sanies and serum.

sanious /sā'nē·əs/, pertaining to or resembling sanies.

sanitarian [L, *sanitas,* health], a health professional who is an expert in the science of public health.

sanitarium /san'iter'ē·əm/ [L, *sanitas,* health], a facility for the treatment of patients suffering from chronic mental or physical diseases, or the recuperation of convalescent patients.

sanitary landfill /san'iterē/ [L, *sanitas,* health; AS, *land* + *fyllan,* to fill], a solid waste disposal site. It is usually a swamp area, ravine, or canyon where the waste is compacted by heavy machines and covered with earth.

sanitary napkin, a disposable pad of absorbent material, usually worn to absorb menstrual flow.

sanitation /san'itā'shən/ [L, *sanitas,* health], the science of maintaining a healthful, disease-free, and hazard-free environment.

sanitize /san'itīz/ [L, *sanitas,* health], to take action needed to clean the environment or a part of it, removing or reducing pathogenic microorganisms and their habitats.

San Joaquin fever /san'wôkēn'/ [San Joaquin Valley, California; L, *febris,* fever], the primary stage of coccidioidomycosis.

SaO₂, symbol for the percentage of oxygen *saturation of arterial blood.*

saphenous [Gk, *saphenes,* manifest], pertaining to certain anatomic structures in the leg such as arteries, veins, or nerves.

saphenous nerve /səfē'nəs/ [Gk, *saphenes,* manifest; L, *nervus,* nerve], the largest and longest branch of the femoral nerve, supplying the skin of the medial side of the leg and the skin over the patella.

saponaceous /sap'ənā'shəs/ [L, *sapo,* soap], pertaining to soap.

saponification /sapon'ifikā'shən/ [L, *sapo,* soap, *facere,* to make], the production of soap.

saponified, pertaining to a substance chemically hydrolyzed into soaps or acid salts and glycerol by heating with an alkali.

saponin /sap'ənin/ [L, *sapo,* soap], a soapy material found in some plants, especially soapwort and certain lilies. It is used in demulcent medications to provide a sudsy quality. Natural saponins, which can be hemolytic toxins, have largely been replaced by synthetic preparations.

saprogen /sap'rəjən/, any microorganism that lives on dead organic matter, contributing to decay and putrefaction.

saprophyte /sap'rəfīt/ [Gk, *sapros,* rotten, *phyton,* plant], an organism that lives on dead organic matter. —**saprophytic,** *adj.*

saquinavir, an antiretroviral protease inhibitor prescribed in the treatment of acquired immunodeficiency syndrome.

SAR, abbreviation for **structure-activity relationship.**

saralasin, a competitive antagonist of angiotensin. It is administered by intravenous injection to assess the role of the renin-angiotensin system in the maintenance of blood pressure.

sarcoadenoma /-ad'ənō'mə/ [Gk, *sarx,* flesh, *aden,* gland, *oma,* tumor], a mixed tumor containing both glandular and connective tissue characteristics.

sarcocarcinoma /-kär'sinō'mə/ [Gk, *sarx,* flesh, *karkinos,* crab, *oma,* tumor], a mixed tumor with characteristics of both sarcomas and carcinomas.

sarcoidosis /sär'koidō'sis/ [Gk, *sarx,* flesh, *eidos,* form, *osis,* condition], a chronic disorder of unknown origin characterized by the formation of tubercles of nonnecrotizing epithelioid tissue. Common sites are the lungs, spleen, liver, skin, mucous membranes, and lacrimal and salivary glands, usually with involvement of the lymph glands. The lesions usually disappear over a period of months or years but progress to widespread granulomatous inflammation and fibrosis.

sarcoidosis cordis, a form of sarcoidosis in which granulomatous lesions develop in the myocardium. In severe cases cardiac failure may result.

sarcolemma /-lem'ə/ [Gk, *sarx,* flesh, *lemma,* sheath], a membrane that covers smooth, striated, and cardiac muscle fibers.

sarcoma /särkō'mə/ [Gk, *sarx* + *oma,* tumor], a malignant neoplasm of the soft tissues arising in fibrous, fatty, muscular, synovial, vascular, or neural tissue, usually first manifested as a painless swelling. The tumor is composed of cells in a connective tissue matrix and may be highly invasive. Trauma probably does not play a role in the cause, but sarcomas may arise in burn or radiation scars.

sarcoma botryoides /bot′rē·oi′dēz/, a tumor derived from primitive striated muscle cells, occurring most frequently in young children and characterized by a painful edematous polypoid grapelike mass in the upper vagina or on the uterine cervix or the neck of the urinary bladder.

sarcomagenesis /särkō′məjen′əsis/ [Gk, *sarx + oma + genesis*, origin], the process of initiating and promoting the development of a sarcoma. —**sarcomagenetic,** *adj.*

sarcomere /sär′kōmir/ [Gk, *sarx + meros,* part], the smallest functional unit of a myofibril. Sarcomeres occur as repeating units along the length of a myofibril, occupying the region between Z lines of the myofibril.

sarcopenia /-pē′nē·ə/ [Gk, *sarx,* flesh, *penia,* poverty], a loss of skeletal muscle mass that may accompany aging. Studies indicate that the loss of skeletal muscle for the average normally healthy person amounts to about 20% between about 30 and 70 years of age. The late loss may accelerate as aging progresses. Although men usually have greater muscle mass in their young adult years, the loss over a period is the same as for women. The muscle loss is replaced by fat, usually in a subtle way that is not noticed by the individual, as by padding areas of muscle loss with extra fat. Muscle strengthening and building exercises can prevent or reverse much of this problem.

sarcoplasm /sär′kōplaz′əm/ [Gk, *sarx,* flesh, *plassein,* to mold], the semifluid cytoplasm of muscle cells.

sarcoplasmic reticulum / plas′mik/ [Gk, *sarx + plassein,* to mold; L, *reticulum,* little net], a network of tubules and sacs in skeletal muscle fibers that plays an important role in muscle contraction and relaxation by releasing and storing calcium ions.

Sarcoptes scabiei /särkop′tēz skā′bē·ī/ [Gk, *sarx + koptein,* to cut; L, *scabere,* to scratch], the genus of itch mite that causes scabies.

sartorius /särtôr′ē·əs/ [L, *sartor,* tailor], the longest muscle in the body, extending from the pelvis to the calf of the leg. It acts to flex the thigh and rotate it laterally and to flex the leg and rotate it medially.

satellite cells /sat′əlīt/ [L, *satelles,* attendant, *cella,* storeroom], glial cells that form around damaged nerve cells.

satellite clinic [L, *satelles,* attendant; Gk, *kline,* bed], a health care facility usually operated under the auspices of a large institution but situated in a location some distance from the larger health center.

satiety /sətī′ətē/, a state of being satisfied, as in the feeling of being full after eating.

satiety center, a locus of nerve tissue in the ventromedial nucleus of the hypothalamus that controls the appetite.

saturated /sach′ərā′tid/ [L, *saturare,* to fill], having absorbed or dissolved the maximum amount of a given substance, such as a solution in which no more of the solute can be dissolved.

saturated calomel electrode (SCE), a reference electrode commonly used in polarography and potentiometry.

saturated fatty acid, any of a number of glyceryl esters of certain organic acids in which all the atoms are joined by single bonds. These fats are chiefly of animal origin and include beef, lamb, pork, veal, whole-milk products, butter, most cheeses, and a few plant fats such as cocoa butter, coconut oil, and palm oil.

saturated hydrocarbon, an organic compound that contains the maximum number of hydrogen atoms so that only single valence bonds exist in the carbon chain, as in saturated fatty acids.

saturated solution, a solution in which the solvent contains the maximum amount of solute it can take up.

saturation /sach′ərā′shən/ [L, *saturare,* to fill], **1.** a condition in which a solution contains as much solute as can remain dissolved. **2.** a measure of the degree to which oxygen is bound to hemoglobin, expressed as a percentage of the possible limit. **3.** a chemical compound in which all the valency bonds have been filled.

saturational cuing /such′ərā′shənəl/, a treatment strategy for visuoconstructive disorders by presenting controlled verbal instruction on task analysis and sequence and presenting cues on spatial boundaries.

saturation index of hemoglobin, [L, *saturare,* to fill, *index,* pointer], a measure of the amount of hemoglobin in a given amount of blood, compared with normal.

Saturday night palsy [Gk, *paralyein,* to be palsied], a radial nerve paralysis caused by pressure on the arm after the person has fallen asleep, usually during an alcoholic binge.

saturnine /sat′ərnīn/, pertaining to lead or lead poisoning.

saturnine tremor, a condition of involuntary muscle contractions in the extremities observed in patients with chronic lead poisoning.

satyr ear /sat′ər/, a congenital abnormal-

S

ity in which the helix of the auricle lacks the usual rolled contour and the tubercle is prominent.

satyriasis /sat′irī′əsis/ [Gk, *satyros,* lecherous, *osis,* condition], excessive, pathologic, or uncontrollable sexual desire in the male.

sauna bath /sô′nə/ [Finn, *sauna* + AS, *baeth*], a bath consisting of exposure to hot vapor to induce sweating, followed by rubbing or light beating of the skin.

saxitoxin /sak′sitok′sin/, a powerful neurotoxin found in bivalve mollusks, including mussels, clams, and scallops. It is produced by certain species of dinoflagellates, which are consumed by the mollusks. Saxitoxin may cause a severe food intoxication in humans who eat the contaminated shellfish.

Sayre's jacket /serz/ [Lewis A. Sayre, American surgeon, 1820–1900; ME, *jaket*], a cast applied for support and immobilization in the treatment of certain abnormalities of the spinal column.

Sb, symbol for the element **antimony.**

SBE, 1. abbreviation for **self-breast examination.** 2. abbreviation for **subacute bacterial endocarditis.**

sc, 1. abbreviation for the Latin *sine correctione,* 'without correction.' 2. abbreviation for **subcutaneously.**

Sc, symbol for the element **scandium.**

SCAB, abbreviation for **single-chain antigen-binding protein.**

scabbard trachea /skab′ərd/, a flattening of the trachea caused by lateral compression by swellings or tumors.

scabicide /skab′isīd/ [L, *scabere,* to scratch, *caedere,* to kill], any one of a large group of drugs that destroy the itch mite, *Sarcoptes scabiei.* These drugs are applied topically in a lotion or cream-based preparation. All are potentially toxic and irritating to the skin.

scabies /skā′bēz/ [L, *scabere,* to scratch], a contagious disease caused by *Sarcoptes scabiei,* the itch mite, characterized by intense itching of the skin and excoriation from scratching. The mite, transmitted by close contact with infected humans or domestic animals, burrows into outer layers of the skin, where the female lays eggs. Two to 4 months after the first infection, sensitization to the mites and their products begins, resulting in a pruritic papular rash.

scabietic /skā′bē·et′ik/ [L, *scabere,* to scratch], pertaining to scabies.

scabrities unguium /skabrish′i·ēz/, a very pronounced thickening and distortion of the nails, separating from skin at the base.

scald /skôld/ [L, *calidus,* hot], a burn caused by exposure of the skin to a hot liquid or vapor.

scale [OFr, *escale,* husk], 1. a small thin flake of keratinized epithelium. 2. to remove encrusted material from the surface of a tooth.

scalene /skā′lēn/ [Gk, *skalenos,* uneven], pertaining to one of the scalenous muscles.

scalenus /skālē′nəs/ [Gk, *skalenos*], one of a group of four muscles arising from the cervical vertebrae with insertions on the first or second rib.

scalp [ME], the skin covering the head, not including the face and ears.

scalpel /skal′pəl/ [L, *scalprum,* knife], a small pointed knife with a convex edge. Some scalpels use interchangeable blades for specific surgical procedures such as operating and amputating.

scalp medication, 1. a cream, ointment, lotion, or shampoo used to treat dermatologic conditions of the scalp. 2. the application of a medication to the scalp.

scalp tourniquet [ME, *skalp* + OFr, *tunicle*], a bandage applied to the scalp to restrict blood flow during administration of antineoplastic drugs. The tourniquet controls the hair loss that commonly accompanies use of cancer-suppressing drugs.

scalp vein needle, a thin-gauge needle designed for use in the veins of the scalp or other small veins, especially in infants and children.

scamping speech [ONorse, *skammr,* scant; ME, *speche*], abnormal speech in which consonants or whole syllables are left out of words because of the person's inability to shape the sounds.

scandium (Sc) /skan′dē·əm/ [Scandinavia], a grayish metallic element. Its atomic number is 21; its atomic mass (weight) is 44.956.

scanning [L, *scandere,* to climb], a technique for carefully studying an area, organ, or system of the body by recording and displaying an image of the area. A concentration of a radioactive substance that has an affinity for a specific tissue may be administered intravenously to enhance the image. —**scan,** *n., v.*

scanning electron microscope (SEM), an instrument similar to an electron microscope in that a beam of electrons instead of visible light is used to scan the surface of a specimen. The image produced is less magnified than that produced by an electron microscope, but it appears to be three-dimensional and lifelike.

scanning electron microscopy, the technique using a scanning electron microscope on a specimen.

scanning speech, abnormal speech characterized by a staccato-like articulation in which the words are clipped and broken because the person pauses between syllables.

scanography /skanog′rəfē/ [L, *scandere,* to climb; Gk, *graphein,* to record], a method of producing a radiogram of an internal body organ or structure by using a series of parallel beams that eliminate size distortion.

scan path, distinct eye movement patterns.

Scanzoni's rotation /skanzō′nēz/ [Friedrich W. Scanzoni, German gynecologist, 1821–1891; L, *rotare,* to rotate], an obstetric operation in which forceps having a curved shank are applied to the fetal head while it is still high in the pelvis. The head is displaced upward and rotated to the occiput anterior position.

scapegoating /skāp′gōting/ [ME, *escapen,* to escape, *goot*], the projection of blame, hostility, or suspicion onto one member of a group by other members to avoid self-confrontation.

scaphocephaly /skaf′ōsef′əlē/ [Gk, *skaphe,* skiff, *kephale,* head], a congenital malformation of the skull in which premature closure of the sagittal suture results in restricted lateral growth of the head, giving it an abnormally long narrow appearance with a cephalic index of 75 or less. —**scaphocephalic, scaphocephalous,** *adj.*

scaphoid /skaf′oid/ [Gk, *skaphe,* skiff, *eidos,* form], boat-shaped, such as the scaphoid bone of the wrist.

scaphoid abdomen, an abdomen with a sunken anterior wall.

scaphoid bone [Gk, *skaphe* + *eidos,* form; AS, *ban*], either of two similar bones of the hand and foot. The scaphoid bone of the hand is slanted at the radial side of the carpus. The scaphoid bone of the foot is located at the medial side of the tarsus between the talus and cuneiform bones.

scapula /skap′yələ/, one of the pair of large flat triangular bones that form the dorsal part of the shoulder girdle.

scapular line /skap′yələr/, an imaginary vertical line drawn through the interior angle of the scapula.

scapular reflex, a contraction of the rhomboids and approximation of the scapulae when a stimulus is applied to the midline of the back between the scapulae.

scapulary /skap′yəlerē/, a suspender for holding a body bandage in place.

scapulocostal syndrome /-kos′təl/, a condition in which pain radiates from the upper or posterior shoulder area into the neck and back of the head, down the arm, and around the chest. There may also be a tingling in the fingers. The syndrome is associated with a change in the relationship between the shoulder blade and thorax.

scapulohumeral /-hyoo′mərəl/ [L, *scapula* + *humerus,* shoulder], pertaining to the area around the scapula and humerus.

scapulohumeral reflex, a normal response to tapping the vertebral border of the scapula, resulting in adduction of the arm.

scapus /skā′pəs/ [Gk, *skapos,* rod], a stem or shaft, such as the scapus penis.

scarf skin, the epidermis, including the cuticle.

scarification /sker′ifikā′shən/ [L, *scarifare,* to scratch open], multiple superficial scratches or incisions in the skin, such as those made for the introduction of a vaccine.

scarify /sker′əfī/ [L, *scarifare*], to make multiple superficial incisions into the skin; to scratch. Vaccination against smallpox is achieved by scarifying the skin under a drop of vaccine.

scarlatiniform /skär′lətē′nifôrm/ [It, *scarlattina* + L, *forma,* form], resembling the rash of **scarlet fever.**

scarlet fever /skär′lit/ [OFr, *escarlate* + L, *febris,* fever], an acute contagious disease of childhood caused by an erythrotoxin-producing strain of group A hemolytic *Streptococcus.* The infection is characterized by sore throat, fever, enlarged lymph nodes in the neck, prostration, and a diffuse bright red rash.

scarlet rash [OFr, *escarlate* + *rasche,* scurf], any scarlitini or rosy skin eruption that accompanies an infection, such as scarlet fever or German measles.

scarlet red, an azo dye that has been used to impart color to pharmaceutic preparations.

scatemia /skətē′mē·ə/ [Gk, *skatos,* feces, *haima,* blood], a toxemic condition caused by absorption of poisonous or harmful substances from the intestinal tract.

scatologic /skatəloj′ik/, pertaining to **scatology.**

scatology /skatol′əje/ [Gk, *skatos,* dung, *logos,* science], the science of feces.

scattered radiation /skat′ərd/ [ME, *scateren,* to throw away; L, *radiare,* to emit rays], photons that move in a different direction than the incident photons that produced them, after the interaction of those incident photons.

scattergram /skat′ərgram′/ [ME, *scateren* + Gk, *gramma,* record], a graph representing the distribution of two variables in a sample population. One variable is plotted on the vertical axis; the second on the horizontal axis. A scattergram demonstrates the degree or tendency with which the variables occur in association with each other.

scattering [ME, *scateren*], **1.** (in radiology) an effect produced by the interaction of low-energy x-rays with matter. **2. coherent scattering,** an effect in which an incident photon interacts with matter and excites an atom, causing it to vibrate. The vibration causes the photon to scatter in a direction different from that initially taken by the incident photon. **3. Compton scattering,** a form of scattering that occurs when an incident photon interacts with an orbital electron, transferring some of its energy to that electron. The electron is ejected, and the photon is scattered.

scavenger cell /skav'ənjər/ [ME, *scavager* + L, *cella,* storeroom], a phagocytic cell that removes tissue debris and some invading pathogens. It may or may not be mobile.

Sc.D., abbreviation for *Doctor of Science.*

SCE, abbreviation for **saturated calomel electrode.**

Schedule I, a category of drugs not considered legitimate for medical use. Among the substances so classified by the Drug Enforcement Agency are mescaline, lysergic acid diethylamide, heroin, and marijuana. Special licensing procedures must be followed to use Schedule I substances.

Schedule II, a category of drugs considered to have a strong potential for abuse or addiction but that have legitimate medical use. Among the substances so classified by the Drug Enforcement Agency are morphine, cocaine, pentobarbital, oxycodone, alphaprodine, and methadone.

Schedule III, a category of drugs that have less potential for abuse or addiction than Schedule II or I drugs. Among the substances so classified by the Drug Enforcement Agency are glutethimide and various analgesic compounds containing codeine.

Schedule IV, a category of drugs that have less potential for abuse or addiction than those of Schedules I to III. Among the substances so classified by the Drug Enforcement Agency are chloral hydrate, chlordiazepoxide, meprobamate, and oxazepam.

Schedule V, a category of drugs that have a small potential for abuse or addiction. Among the substances so classified by the Drug Enforcement Agency are many commonly prescribed medications that contain small amounts of codeine or diphenoxylate. The specific drugs in Schedule V vary greatly from state to state.

Schedule of Drugs [L, *scheda,* sheet of paper; Fr, *drogue],* a classification system

that categorizes drugs by their potential for abuse. The schedule is divided into five groups: Schedules I to V. The assignment of drugs to the categories varies from state to state. Schedule I substances are not approved for medical use. All substances in Schedules II to V require a written prescription signed by a physician. Specific regulations for dispensing these substances vary from state to state and from institution to institution.

schema /skē'mə/, an innate knowledge structure that allows a child to organize in his or her mind ways to behave in his or her environment.

schematic /skēmat'ik/, pertaining to a schema, model, or diagram representing, without absolute precision, a structure, strategy, or system. An anatomic chart is an example.

schematic eye, 1. a simplified and enlarged illustration of the eye, featuring its anatomic details. **2.** a graphic illustration of the normal eye, with data for curvatures, indices of refraction, and distances between optical elements.

Scheuermann's disease /shoi'ərmonz/ [Holger W. Scheuermann, Danish surgeon, 1877–1960], an abnormal skeletal condition characterized by a fixed kyphosis that develops at puberty and is caused by wedge-shaped deformities of one or several vertebrae. The onset is insidious and often associated with a history of unusual physical activity or participation in sports. The most frequent symptom is poor posture with accompanying symptoms of fatigue and pain in the involved area. In adults persistent pain in the thoracic area may indicate a degenerative alteration secondary to this disease process.

Schick test /shik/ [Bela Schick, Austrian-American physician, 1877–1967], a skin test to determine immunity to diphtheria in which dilute diphtheria toxin is injected intradermally. A positive reaction, indicating susceptibility, is marked by redness and swelling at the site of injection.

Schick test control [Bela Schick; L, *testum,* crucible; Fr, *controle,* check], a preparation used in carrying out the Schick skin test for determining diphtheria immunity.

Schilder's disease /shil'dərz/ [Paul F. Schilder, Austrian neurologist, 1886–1940], a group of progressive severe neurologic diseases beginning in childhood. All are characterized by demyelination of the white matter of the brain, with muscle spasticity, optic neuritis, aphasia, deafness, adrenal insufficiency, and dementia. Many of the signs resemble those of multiple sclerosis.

Schiller's test /shil′ərz/ [Walter Schiller, Austrian pathologist in the United States, 1887–1960], a procedure for indicating areas of abnormal epithelium in the vagina or on the cervix of the uterus as a guide in selecting biopsy sites for cancer detection. A potassium iodide or aqueous iodine solution is painted on the vaginal walls and cervix under direct visualization. Normal epithelium contains glycogen and stains a deep brown; abnormal epithelium, containing no glycogen, will not stain, and nonstaining sites may then be included in tissue biopsy samples.

Schilling test /shil′ing/ [Robert F. Schilling, American hematologist, b. 1919], a diagnostic test for pernicious anemia in which vitamin B_{12} tagged with radioactive cobalt is administered orally and gastrointestinal absorption is measured by determining the radioactivity of urine samples collected over a 24-hour period.

schindylesis /skin′dilē′sis/ [Gk, splintering], an articulation of certain bones of the skull in which a thin plate of one bone enters a cleft formed by the separation of two layers of another bone.

Schiötz′ tonometer /shē·ets′/ [Hjalmar Schiötz, Norwegian ophthalmologist, 1850–1927; Gk, tonos, stretching, metron, measure], a tonometer used to measure intraocular pressure by observing the depth of indentation of the cornea made by the weighted plunger on the device after a topical anesthetic is applied.

schistocelia /shis′tɔsē′lyə/, a congenital fissure in the wall of the abdomen.

schistocystis /shis′tōsis′tis/ [Gk, schistos, cleft, kystis, bag], a fissure in the bladder.

schistocyte /shis′tōsīt/ [Gk, schistos, cleft, kytos, cell], an erythrocyte cell fragment characteristic of hemolysis or cell fragmentation associated with severe burns and intravascular coagulation.

Schistosoma /shis′tɔsō′mə/ [Gk, schistos, cleft, soma, body], a genus of blood flukes that may cause urinary, gastrointestinal, or liver disease in humans and that requires freshwater snails as intermediate hosts. Schistosoma hematobium, found chiefly in Africa and the Middle East, affects the bladder and pelvic organs, causing painful frequent urination and hematuria. S. japonicum, found in Japan, the Philippines, and Eastern Asia, causes gastrointestinal ulcerations and fibrosis of the liver. S. mansoni, found in Africa, the Middle East, the Caribbean, and tropical America, causes symptoms similar to those caused by S. japonicum.

schistosomiasis /shis′tɔsōmī′əsis/ [Gk, schistos + soma + osis, condition], a parasitic infection caused by a species of fluke of the genus Schistosoma. It is transmitted to humans, the definitive host, by contact with fresh water contaminated by human feces. A single fluke may live in one part of the body, depositing eggs frequently, for up to 20 years. The eggs are irritating to mucous membrane, causing it to thicken and become papillomatous. Symptoms depend on the part of the body infected.

schistosomicide /shis′tɔsō′məsīd/ [Gk, schistos + soma + L, caedere, to kill], a drug destructive to schistosomes, blood flukes transmitted by snails to human hosts. —**schistosomicidal,** adj.

schistothorax /-thôr′aks/, a congenital cleft in the wall of the thorax.

schizencephaly /skiz′ensef′əlē/, an abnormal cleavage or other division of the brain tissues caused by maldevelopment.

schizoaffective disorder /skit′sō-afek′tiv/ [Gk, schizein, to split; L, affectus, state of mind, dis, opposite of, ordo, rank], a syndrome that includes characteristics of schizophrenia and a mood disorder but fails to meet the DSM-IV criteria for either diagnosis.

schizogenesis /skit′səjen′əsis/ [Gk, schizein + genesis, origin], reproduction by fission. —**schizogenetic, schizogenic, schizogenous,** adj.

schizogony /skitsog′ənē/ [Gk, schizein + genein, to produce], **1.** reproduction by multiple fission. **2.** the asexual reproductive stage of sporozoa, specifically the part of the life cycle of the malarial parasite that occurs in the erythrocytes or liver cells. —**schizogonic, schizogonous,** adj.

schizogyria /skit′səjī′rē·ə/, the presence of wedge-shaped cracks in the convolutions of the brain.

schizoid /skit′soid, skiz′oid/ [Gk, schizein, to split, eidos, form], **1.** characteristic of or resembling schizophrenia; schizophrenic. **2.** a person, not necessarily a schizophrenic, who exhibits the traits of a schizoid personality.

schizoid personality, a functioning but maladjusted person whose behavior is characterized by extreme shyness, oversensitivity, introversion, seclusion, and avoidance of close interpersonal relationships.

schizoid personality disorder, a personality disorder (DSM-IV) characterized by a defect in the ability to form interpersonal relationships, as shown by emotional coldness and aloofness, withdrawn and seclusive behavior, and indifference to praise, criticism, and the feelings of others.

schizont /skit′sont/ [Gk, schizein + on, being], the multinucleated cell stage during the sexual reproductive phase in the life cycle of a sporozoon, such as the malarial parasite *Plasmodium.* It is produced by the multiple fission of the trophozoite in a cell of the vertebrate host and subsequently segments into merozoites.

schizonticide /skitson'təsīd/ [Gk, *schizein* + *on,* being; L, *caedere,* to kill], a substance that destroys schizonts. —**schizonticidal,** *adj.*

schizophasia /skit'səfā'zhə, skiz'ə-/ [Gk, *schizein* + *phasis,* speech], the disordered, incomprehensible speech characteristic of some forms of schizophrenia.

schizophrenia /skit'səfrē'nē·ə, skiz'ə-/ [Gk, *schizein,* to split, *phren,* mind], any one of a large group of *DSM-IV* psychotic disorders characterized by gross distortion of reality, disturbances of language and communication, withdrawal from social interaction, and disorganization and fragmentation of thought, perception, and emotional reaction. Apathy and confusion; delusions and hallucinations; rambling or stylized patterns of speech such as evasiveness, incoherence, and echolalia; withdrawn, regressive, and bizarre behavior; and emotional lability often occur. No single cause of the disease is known; genetic, biochemical, psychologic, interpersonal, and sociocultural factors are usually involved.

schizophrenic /skit'səfren'ik, skiz'ə-/, **1.** pertaining to schizophrenia. **2.** a person with schizophrenia.

schizophreniform disorder /-fren'ifôrm/ [Gk, *schizein* + *phren* + L, *forma,* form], a *DSM-IV* psychiatric disorder exhibiting the same symptoms as schizophrenia but characterized by an acute onset with resolution in 2 weeks to 6 months.

schizophrenogenic /skit'səfren'əjen'ik, skiz'ə-/ [Gk, *schizein* + *phren* + *genein,* to produce], tending to cause or produce schizophrenia.

schizotypal personality disorder /skit'-sōtī'pəl/ [Gk, *schizein* + *typos,* mark; L, *personalis,* of a person, *dis,* opposite of, *ordo,* rank], a *DSM-IV* psychiatric disorder characterized by oddities of thought, perception, speech, and behavior that are not severe enough to meet the clinical criteria for schizophrenia. Symptoms may include magical thinking such as superstition, belief in clairvoyance and telepathy, and bizarre fantasies; ideas of reference; recurrent illusions such as sensing the presence of a force or person not actually present; social isolation; peculiar speech patterns, including ideas expressed vaguely or words used deviantly; and exaggerated anxiety or hypersensitivity to real or imagined criticism.

schlieren optics /shlir'ən/ [Ger, *schlieren,*

ulcers, streaks], a system that observes the refractive index gradient in solutions containing macromolecules.

Schneiderian carcinoma /shnīdir'ē·ən/, an epithelial malignancy of the nasal mucosa and paranasal sinuses.

school nurse practitioner (S.N.P.), a registered nurse who is qualified through satisfactory completion of a nurse practitioner program to serve as a nurse practitioner in a school system.

school phobia [AS, *scol* + Gk, *phobos,* fear], an extreme separation anxiety disorder of children, usually in the elementary grades, characterized by a persistent irrational fear of going to school or being in a schoollike atmosphere. Such children are usually oversensitive, shy, timid, nervous, and emotionally immature and have pervasive feelings of inadequacy. They typically try to cope with their fears by becoming overdependent on others, especially the parents.

Schüffner's dots [Wilhelm A. P. Schffner, German pathologist, 1867–1949], coarse pink or red granules seen in the red blood cells of patients with tertiary malaria. They are signs of *Plasmodium vivax* or *P. ovale* and are absent in blood cells of patients infected with other types of malaria.

Schultz-Charlton phenomenon [Werner Schultz, German physician, 1878–1947; Willy Charlton, German physician, b. 1889], a cutaneous reaction to the intradermal injection of scarlatina antiserum in a person who has a scarlatiniform rash. The rash blanches.

Schultze's mechanism, the delivery of a placenta with the fetal surfaces presenting.

Schwann cells /shwon/ [Theodor Schwann, German anatomist, 1810–1882], cells of ectodermal origin that make up the neurilemma.

schwannoma /shwonō'mə/ [Theodor Schwann; Gk, *oma,* tumor], a benign solitary encapsulated tumor arising in the neurilemma (Schwann's sheath) of peripheral, cranial, or autonomic nerves.

schwannosis /shwonō'sis/ [Theodor Schwann; Gk, *osis,* condition], a condition of overgrowth of the neurilemma or sheath of Schwann.

Schwartzman-Sanarelli phenomenon /shvorts'man san'ərel'ē/ [Gregory Schwartzman, American physician, b. 1896; Guiseppe Sanarelli, Italian bacteriologist, 1864–1940], a phenomenon induced experimentally in the investigation of the role of coagulation in renal disease. Animals injected twice with a bacterial endotoxin experience massive disseminated intravascular coagulation with thrombosis of the blood vessels in the kidneys.

sciatic /sī·at′ik/ [Gk, *ischiadikos,* hip joint], pertaining to an area near the ischium such as the sciatic nerve or the sciatic vein.

sciatica /sī·at′ikə/, an inflammation of the sciatic nerve, usually marked by pain and tenderness along the course of the nerve through the thigh and leg. It may result in a wasting of the muscles of the lower leg.

sciatic hernia, a protrusion of tissue through the greater sciatic notch.

sciatic nerve, a long nerve originating in the sacral plexus and extending through the muscles of the thigh, leg, and foot, with numerous branches.

sciatic scoliosis, an abnormal curvature of the spine caused by an asymmetric spasm of the spinal muscles, often resulting in a list to one side.

SCID, abbreviation for **severe combined immunodeficiency disease.**

science /sī′əns/ [L, *scientia,* knowledge], a systematic attempt to establish theories to explain observed phenomena and the knowledge obtained through these efforts. Pure science is concerned with the gathering of information solely for the sake of obtaining new knowledge. Applied science is the practical application of scientific theory and laws.

Science of Unitary Human Beings a conceptual model and theory of nursing proposed by Martha Rogers in 1970. Its four basic concepts focus on the nature and direction of "unitary human development": (1) human and environmental energy fields, (2) complete and continuous openness of the energy fields, (3) human energy fields perceived as single waves that give identity to a field, and (4) "pandimensionality," a nonlinear domain without spatial or temporal attributes.

scientific method /sī′əntif′ik/, a systematic, ordered approach to the gathering of data and solving of problems. The basic approach is the statement of the problem followed by the statement of a hypothesis. An experimental method is established to help prove or disprove the hypothesis. The results of the experiment are observed, and conclusions are drawn from observed results.

scientific rationale, a reason, based on supporting scientific evidence, that a particular action is chosen.

scimitar sign /sim′ətər/, an arteriographic sign of encroachment on the popliteal or femoral lumen in adventitial cystic disease.

scimitar syndrome, a radiographic artifact caused by a congenital disorder in which the right lower pulmonary vein drains into the inferior vena cava. On a chest radiogram the abnormal vessel configuration produces a scimitar-shaped shadow.

scintigram /sin′tigram′/ [L, *scintillare,* to sparkle; Gk, *gramma,* record], (in nuclear medicine) a recording of the radioactivity emitted by a tracer in an organism or organ system.

scintigraph /sin′tigraf′/, a photographic recording produced by an imaging device showing the distribution and intensity of radioactivity in various tissues and organs after the administration of a radiopharmaceutical.

scintillating scotoma /sin′tilā·ting/ [L, *scintillatio,* sparkling; Gk *skotos* dark, *oma* tumor], an abnormal area of the visual field that is positive and luminous, sometimes becoming hemianopic and appearing in a migraine aura.

scintillation detector /sin′tilā′shən/ [L, *scintillatio,* sparkling], **1.** a device that relies on the emission of light or ultraviolet radiation from a crystal subjected to ionizing radiation. The light is detected by a photomultiplier tube and converted to an electrical signal that can be processed further. **2.** a device used to measure the amount of radioactivity in an area of the body.

scintiscan /sin′tiscan′/, a photographic display of the distribution of a radiopharmaceutical within the body.

scirrhous carcinoma /skir′əs/ [Gk, *skirrhos,* hard, *karkinos,* crab, *oma,* tumor], a hard, fibrous, particularly invasive tumor in which the malignant cells occur singly or in small clusters or strands in dense connective tissue.

scissor gait /siz′ər/ [L, *scindere,* to cut; ONorse, *gata,* way], a manner of walking cross-legged, as observed in spastic paraplegia.

scissor legs [L, *scindere,* to cut; ONorse, *leggr*] legs that are crossed because of a disorder of the adductor muscles of the thigh or a deformity of the hip.

scissors [L, *scindere,* to cut], a sharp instrument composed of two opposing cutting blades held together by a central pin on which the blades pivot. The most common dissecting scissors are the straight Mayo, for cutting sutures; the Snowden-Pencer, for deep, delicate tissue; the long curved Mayo, for deep, heavy, or tough tissue; the short curved Metzenbaum, for superficial, delicate tissue; and the long, blunt curved Metzenbaum, for deep, delicate tissue.

SCL, abbreviation for *soft contact lens.*

sclera /sklir′ə/ [Gk, *skleros,* hard], the tough inelastic opaque membrane covering the posterior five sixths of the eyebulb. It maintains the size and form of the bulb

S

and attaches to muscles that move the bulb. Posteriorly it is pierced by the optic nerve and, with the transparent cornea, makes up the outermost of three tunics covering the eyeball.

scleredema /sklir′ədē′mə/ [Gk, *skleros* + *oidema,* swelling], an idiopathic skin disease characterized by nonpitting induration beginning on the face or neck and spreading downward over the body, sparing the hands and feet. There also may be swelling of the tongue, restriction of the movements of the eyes, and pericardial, pleural, and peritoneal effusions.

sclerema neonatorum /sklirē′mə/ [Gk, *skleros* + *neos,* new; L, *natus,* birth], a progressive generalized hardening of the skin and subcutaneous tissue of the newborn. It is usually a fatal condition that results from severe cold stress in severely ill premature infants.

scleritis /sklirī′tis/ [Gk, *skleros,* hard, *itis,* inflammation], an inflammation of the sclera.

scleroconjunctival /-kon′jungtī′vəl/, pertaining to the sclera and conjunctiva.

sclerocornea /-kôr′nēə/, the cornea and sclera of the eye surface considered as a single layer.

sclerodactyly /sklir′ōdak′tilē/ [Gk, *skleros* + *daktylos,* finger], a musculoskeletal deformity affecting the hands of people with scleroderma. The fingers are fixed in a semiflexed position, with tightened skin to the wrist. The fingertips may be ulcerated.

scleroderma /sklir′ōdur′mə/ [Gk, *skleros* + *derma,* skin], chronic hardening and thickening of the skin caused by new collagen formation, with atrophy of pilosebaceous follicles. Scleroderma is most common in middle-aged women. It may occur in a localized form (**morphea**) or as a systemic disease (systemic sclerosis). **Progressive systemic sclerosis (PSS)** is a relatively rare autoimmune disease affecting the blood vessels and connective tissue. The most common initial complaints are changes in the skin of the face and fingers. Raynaud's phenomenon occurs with a gradual hardening of the skin and swelling of the distal extremities. In the early stages the disease may be confused with rheumatoid arthritis or Raynaud's disease. As the disease progresses, deformity of the joints and pain on movement occur. Skin changes include edema, then pallor; then the skin becomes firm; finally it becomes slightly pigmented and fixed to the underlying tissues. At this stage the skin of the face is taut, shiny, and masklike; and the patient may have difficulty in chewing and swallowing.

scleroderma heart, a heart condition characterized by interstitial myocardial fibrosis and thickening of the small blood vessels in progressive systemic sclerosis.

sclerodermatitis /-dur′məti′tis/, an inflammation, thickening, and hardening of the skin.

sclerokeratitis /-ker′ətī′tis/, an inflammation of the sclera and cornea.

scleromalacia perforans /sklir′ōməlā′shə/ [Gk, *skleros* + *malakia,* softening; L, *perforare,* to pierce], a condition of the eyes in which devitalization and sloughing of the sclera occur as a complication of rheumatoid arthritis. The pigmented uvea becomes exposed; and glaucoma, cataract formation, and detachment of the retina may result.

sclerose /sklərōz′/ [Gk, *skleros*], to harden or to cause hardening. —**sclerotic,** *adj.*

sclerosing /sklirō′zing/ [Gk, *skleros,* hard], pertaining to the tissue changes or other factors involved in the progress of sclerosis.

sclerosing hemangioma [Gk, *skleros* + *haima,* blood, *angeion* vessel, *oma* tumor], a solid cellular tumorlike nodule of the skin or a mass of histiocytes, thought to arise from a hemangioma by the proliferation of endothelial and connective tissue cells.

sclerosing keratitis [Gk, *skleros,* hard, *keras,* horn, *itis,* inflammation], **1.** a form of corneal inflammation in which nodular infiltrates appear near the margin of the cornea in association with a ring of anterior scleritis. **2.** a form of corneal inflammation characterized by an opaque triangle in the deep layers of the cornea, with the base of the triangle near the sclerosing area.

sclerosing phlebitis [Gk, *skleros,* hard, *phleps,* vein, *itis,* inflammation], an inflammation of a vein that has become hardened and obstructed.

sclerosing solution [Gk, *skleros* + L, *solvere,* to dissolve], a liquid containing an irritant that causes inflammation and resulting fibrosis of tissues. It may be used in cauterizing ulcers, arresting hemorrhage, and treating hemangiomas.

sclerosis /sklirō′sis/ [Gk, *skleros,* hard], a condition characterized by hardening of tissue resulting from any of several causes, including inflammation, the deposit of mineral salts, and infiltration of connective tissue fibers. —**sclerotic,** *adj.*

sclerotherapy /-ther′əpē/ [Gk, *skleros,* hard, *therapeia,* treatment], the use of sclerosing chemicals to treat varicosities such as hemorrhoids or esophageal varices. The agent produces inflammation and later fibrosis and obliteration of the lumen.

sclerotic /sklirot′ik/ [Gk, *skleros*, hard], pertaining to induration or hardening.

sclerotomal pain distribution /-tō′məl/, the referral of pain from pain-sensitive tissues covering the axial skeleton along a sclerotomal segment.

sclerotome /sklir′ətōm/ [Gk, *skleros* + *temnein*, to cut], (in embryology) the part of the segmented mesoderm layer in the early developing embryo that originates from the somites and gives rise to the skeletal tissue of the body.

sclerotylosis /-tilō′sis/, an inherited condition of atrophic fibrosis of the skin. There is overgrowth of the nails and horny skin covering the palms of the hands and plantar surfaces of the feet. The disorder may be accompanied by cancer of the gastrointestinal tract.

scolex /skō′leks/, *pl.* **scoleces** /skō′ləsēz/ [Gk, worm], the headlike segment or organ of an adult tapeworm that has hooks, grooves, or suckers by which it attaches itself to the wall of the intestine.

scoliometer /skō′lē·om′ətər/ [Gk, *skoliosis*, curvature], a device for measuring the amount of abnormal curvature in the spine.

scoliosis /skō′lē·ō′sis/ [Gk, *skoliosis*, curvature], lateral curvature of the spine, a common abnormality of childhood. Causes include congenital malformations of the spine, poliomyelitis, skeletal dysplasias, spastic paralysis, and unequal leg length. Unequal heights of hips or shoulders may be a sign of this condition.

scoliotic pelvis /skō′lē·ot′ik/ [Gk, *skoliosis*, curvature; L, *pelvis*, basin], an abnormal pelvic area that results when the effects of scoliosis bend the sacrum to one side.

scombroid /skom′broid/ [Gk, *scombros*, mackerel, *eidos*, form], pertaining to fish of the spiny-finned percoid Scombridae and Scomberescidae families, which include skipjack, mackerel, bonito, and tuna.

scombroid poisoning, toxic effects of eating scombroid types of fish (such as bonito or tuna) that have begun bacterial decomposition after being caught. Scombroid fish contain large amounts of free histidine in the muscle tissue, which gives rise to toxic levels of histamine under conditions of histidine decarboxylation by any of a dozen species of bacteria. Scombroid poisoning is not limited to consumption of fresh fish; the problem also may affect commercially canned tuna. Symptoms, which usually last no more than 24 hours, include nausea, vomiting, diarrhea, epigastric pain, and urticaria.

scopolamine /skōpol′əmēn/ [Giovanni A. Scopoli, Italian naturalist, 1723–1788],

an anticholinergic alkaloid obtained from the leaves and seeds of several solanaceous plants. It is a central nervous system depressant. It is prescribed for prevention of motion sickness and as an antiemetic, a sedative in obstetrics, and a cycloplegic and mydriatic.

scopolamine hydrobromide, an anticholinergic prescribed in the treatment of nausea and vomiting, as a sedative and preanesthetic medication, and as a cycloplegic and mydriatic medication in ophthalmic procedures.

scopophilia /skō′pəfil′ē·ə, skop′-/ [Gk, *skopein*, to look, *philein*, to love], **1.** sexual pleasure derived from looking at sexually stimulating scenes or at another person's genitals; voyeurism. **2.** a morbid desire to be seen; exhibitionism. —**scopophiliac, scopophilic, scoptophiliac, scoptophilic,** *adj., n.*

scopophobia /skō′pə-/ [Gk, *skopein* + *phobos*, fear], an anxiety disorder characterized by a morbid fear of being seen or stared at by others. The condition is commonly seen in schizophrenia.

scorbutic gingivitis /skôrbyōo′tik/ [Fr, *scorbutique*, scurvy; L, *gingiva*, gum; Gk, *itis*, inflammation], an abnormal condition characterized by inflamed or bleeding gums and caused by vitamin C deficiency.

scorbutic pose, the characteristic posture of a child with scurvy, with thighs and legs semiflexed and hips rotated outward. The child usually lies motionless in a state of pseudoparalysis, avoiding voluntary movements of the extremities because of the pain that accompanies any motion.

scorpion sting /skôr′pē·on/ [Gk, *skorpios* + AS, *stingan*], a painful wound produced by a scorpion, an arachnid with a hollow stinger in its tail. The stings of many species are only slightly toxic, but some, including *Centruroides sculpturatus* (bark scorpion) of the southwestern United States, may inflict fatal injury, especially in small children. Initial pain is followed within several hours by numbness, nausea, muscle spasm, dyspnea, and convulsion.

scotoma /skōtō′mə/ [Gk, *skotos*, darkness, *oma*, tumor], a defect of vision in a defined area in one or both eyes. A common prodromal symptom is a shimmering film appearing as an island in the visual field.

scotopic vision /skōtop′ik/ [Gk, *skotos*, darkness; L, *visio*, seeing], the ability of the eye to adjust for vision in darkness or dim light.

scratch test [ME, *scratten* + L, *testum*, crucible], a skin test for identifying an allergen, performed by placing a small quantity of a solution containing a sus-

S

pected allergen on a lightly scratched area of the skin. If a wheal forms within 15 minutes, allergy to the substance is indicated.

screening [ME, *scren*], **1.** a preliminary procedure such as a test or examination to detect the most characteristic sign or signs of a disorder that may require further investigation. **2.** the examination of a large sample of a population to detect a specific disease or disorder such as hypertension.

screen memory [ME, *scren* + L, *memoria*], a consciously tolerable memory that replaces one that is emotionally painful to recall.

screw artery /skrōō, a coiled blood vessel in either the uterine mucosa or the retinal macula.

screw clamp [OFr, *escroe*, screw; AS, *clam*, fastener], a device, usually made of plastic, equipped with a screw that can be manipulated to close and open the primary IV tubing for regulating the flow of intravenous solution.

Scribner shunt [Belding S. Scribner, American physician, b. 1921], a type of arteriovenous bypass, used in hemodialysis, consisting of a special tube connection outside the body.

scripting /skrip'ting/, a technique of family therapy involving the development of new family transactional patterns.

scrofula /skrof'yələ/ [L, *scrofa*, brood sow], *archaic;* a form of tuberculosis cutis with abscess formation, usually of the cervical lymph nodes.

scroll ear /skrōl/, a distortion of the ear in which the pinna is rolled forward.

scrotal /skrō'təl/ [L, *scrupus,* sharp stone], pertaining to the scrotum.

scrotal cancer [L, *scrupus,* sharp stone], an epidermoid malignancy of the scrotum, characterized initially by a small sore that may ulcerate. The lesion occurs most frequently in elderly men who have been exposed to soot, pitch, crude oil, mineral oils, polycyclic hydrocarbons, or arsenic fumes from copper smelting. It is the first malignancy shown to be caused by an environmental carcinogen.

scrotal hernia, an inguinal hernia that has descended into the scrotum.

scrotal raphe, a line of union of the two halves of the scrotum. It is generally more highly pigmented than the surrounding tissue.

scrotal septum, an incomplete wall of connective tissue and smooth muscle that divides the scrotum into two compartments, each containing a testis.

scrotal swelling, the earliest enlargement of embryonic tissue that will become half of the scrotum.

scrotal tongue, a nonpathologic condition in which the tongue is deeply furrowed and resembles the surface of the scrotum.

scrotum /skrō'təm/ the pouch of skin containing the testes and parts of the spermatic cords. It is divided on the surface into two lateral parts by a ridge that continues ventrally to the undersurface of the penis and dorsally along the middle line of the perineum to the anus. The two layers of the scrotum are the skin and the dartos tunic. The skin is very thin, has a brownish color, is usually wrinkled, and has thinly scattered kinky hairs. The dartos tunic is composed of a thin layer of unstriated muscular fibers around the base of the scrotum. The tunic projects an internal septum that divides the pouch into two cavities for the testes, extending between the scrotal ridge and the root of the penis. —**scrotal,** *adj.*

scrubbed team members [ME, *scrobben,* to scrub], the surgeons, physicians, nurses, and technicians who are scrubbed for surgical procedures in a sterile environment.

scrub nurse, a registered nurse or operating room technician who assists surgeons during operations.

scrub room, a special hospital area where surgeons and surgical teams use disposable sterile brushes and bactericidal soaps to wash and scrub their fingernails, hands, and forearms before performing or assisting in surgical operations.

scrub typhus, an acute febrile disease caused by several strains of the genus *Rickettsia tsutsugamushi* and transmitted from infected rodents to humans by mites. The clinical course is characterized by a necrotic papule or black eschar at the site of the lesion caused by the bite of the small arachnid. Tender enlarged regional lymph nodes, fever, severe headache, eye pain, muscle aches, and a generalized rash usually occur. In severe cases the myocardium and the central nervous system may be involved.

scruple /skrōō'pəl/ [L, *scrupulus,* small stone], a measure of weight in the apothecaries' system, equal to 20 grains or 1.296 g.

sculpting /skulp'ting/, a technique of family therapy involving construction of a live family portrait that depicts family alliances and conflicts.

scultetus bandage /skəltē'təs/ [Johann Schultes, German surgeon, 1595–1645], a many-tailed binder or bandage with an attached central piece. The tails are overlapped; the last two, tied or pinned, act to secure the others. A scultetus bandage may be opened or removed without moving the bandaged part of the body.

scurvy /skur′vē/ [Scand, *scurfa,* scabby], severe ascorbic acid deficiency. It is characterized by weakness; anemia; edema; spongy gums, often with ulceration and loosening of the teeth; a tendency to mucocutaneous hemorrhages, and induration of the muscles of the legs.

SD, 1. abbreviation for **skin dose. 2.** abbreviation for **standard deviation.**

SDAT, abbreviation for *senile dementia-Alzheimer type.*

SDMS, abbreviation for *Society of Diagnostic Medical Sonographers.*

Se, symbol for the element **selenium.**

S.E., abbreviation for **standard error.**

sea-blue histiocyte syndrome, a condition of spleen enlargement and mild thrombocytopenia. Histiocytes in the bone marrow contain cytoplasmic granules that stain bright blue.

seaborgium (Sg) /sēbôr′gē·əm/ [Glenn T. Seaborg, American chemistry educator, b. 1912], a synthetic radioactive element, with a half-life of 0.9 second. Its atomic number is 106; its atomic mass (weight) is 266. It was first synthesized in 1974 by scientists working independently in the United States and Russia.

sealed source [ME, *seel,* mark; Fr, *sourdre,* to spring], (in radiotherapy) a source of radiant energy in which the radioactive material is permanently encased in a container or bonding material to prevent leakage.

sealer cement, a compound used in filling a root canal. It is applied as a plastic that solidifies after insertion, fills depressions in the surface of the canal, and helps close the apex of the root canal.

seasonal affective disorder (SAD) /sē′-zənəl/, a *DSM-IV* mood disorder associated with the shorter days and longer nights of autumn and winter. Symptoms include lethargy, depression, social withdrawal, and work difficulties. The patients also consume excess amounts of carbohydrates. The symptoms recede in the spring when days become longer. The condition is associated with the effect of light on melatonin secretion.

sea urchin granuloma, a type of foreign body granuloma in which nodules of granulation tissue develop in the skin several months after contact with the silicate in the spines of a sea urchin.

sea urchin sting /ur′chin/ [AS, *sae* + *heri-chon,* hedgehog], an injury inflicted by any of a variety of sea urchins, in which the skin is punctured and, in some species, venom released. A venomous sting is characterized by pain, muscular weakness, numbness around the mouth, and dyspnea.

seawater bath [AS, *sae* + *waeter*], a bath taken in warm seawater or saline solution.

sebaceous /sibā′shəs/ [L, *sebum,* sweat], pertaining to sebum, the substance secreted by glands of the skin.

sebaceous cyst, a misnomer for epidermoid cyst or pilar cyst.

sebaceous epithelioma, a benign yellowish nodular tumor of sebaceous gland epithelium. It usually appears on the neck or face. It may resemble basal cell carcinoma but is composed mainly of baseloid and sebaceous cells.

sebaceous follicle [L, *sebum,* sweat, *folliculus,* small bag], a sebaceous gland that opens into a hair follicle.

sebaceous gland, one of the many small sacculated organs in the dermis. They are located throughout the body in close association with all types of body hair but are especially abundant in the scalp, the face, the anus, the nose, the mouth, and the external ear. Each gland consists of a single duct that emerges from a cluster of oval alveoli. The ducts from most sebaceous glands open into the hair follicles, but some open onto the surface of the skin. The sebum secreted by the glands oils the hair and the surrounding skin, helps prevent evaporation of sweat, and aids in the retention of body heat.

sebaceous horn, a solid tissue outgrowth from a sebaceous cyst.

seborrhea /seb′ərē′ə/ [L, *sebum* + Gk, *rhoia,* flow], any of several common skin conditions in which an overproduction of sebum results in excessive oiliness or dry scales. —**seborrheic** /seb′ərē′ik/, *adj.*

seborrhea capitis [L, *sebum,* sweat; Gk, *rhoia,* flow; L, *caput,* the head], seborrhea of the scalp.

seborrheic /seb′ərē′ik/ [L, *sebum,* sweat], pertaining to or resembling seborrhea.

seborrheic blepharitis, a form of seborrheic dermatitis in which the eyelids are erythematous and the margins are covered with a granular crust.

seborrheic dermatitis, a common chronic inflammatory skin disease characterized by dry or moist greasy scales and yellowish crusts. Common sites are the scalp, eyelids, face, external surfaces of the ears, axillae, breasts, groin, and gluteal folds. In acute stages there may be exudate and infection resulting in secondary furunculosis. In some people seborrheic dermatitis is associated with paralysis agitans, diabetes mellitus, malabsorption disorders, epilepsy, or an allergic reaction to gold or arsenic.

seborrheic keratosis, a benign, well-circumscribed, slightly raised, tan to black, warty lesion of the skin of the face, neck, chest, or upper back. The macules are loosely covered with a greasy crust that leaves a raw pulpy base when removed. Itching is common.

sebum /sē′bəm/ [L, grease], the oily secretion of the sebaceous glands of the skin, composed of keratin, fat, and cellular debris. Combined with sweat, sebum forms a moist oily acidic film that is mildly antibacterial and antifungal and protects the skin against drying.

seclusion /sikloo′zhən/ [L, *secludere,* to isolate], (in psychiatric nursing) the isolation of a patient in a special room to decrease stimuli that might be causing or exacerbating the patient's emotional distress.

Seclusion, a Nursing Interventions Classification defined as solitary containment in a fully protective environment with close surveillance by nursing staff for purposes of safety or behavior management.

secobarbital sodium /sek′obär′bital/, a sedative and hypnotic. It is classified as a controlled substance. It is prescribed in the treatment of insomnia and agitation and as an anticonvulsant and preoperative sedative.

secondary /sek′ənder′ē/ [L, *secundus,* second], second in importance or in incidence or belonging to the second order of sophistication or development, such as a secondary health care facility or secondary education.

secondary allergen, an agent that induces allergic symptoms in a person through cross-sensitivity with an agent to which the person is hypersensitive.

secondary amputation, amputation performed after suppuration has begun after severe trauma.

secondary analysis, the study of a problem using previously compiled data.

secondary antibody response, a rapid production of antibodies in response to an antigen in an individual who was exposed previously to the same antigen.

secondary apnea, an abnormal condition in which respiration is absent and will not begin again spontaneously. Secondary apnea may result from any event that severely impedes the absorption of oxygen into the bloodstream.

secondary areola, a second ring appearing around the areola of the breast during pregnancy that is more pigmented than the areola before pregnancy.

secondary biliary cirrhosis, an abnormal hepatic condition characterized by obstruction of the bile duct with or without infection.

secondary care, 1. the provision of a specialized medical service by a physician specialist or a hospital on referral by a primary care physician. **2.** the retardation of an existing illness or other pathologic condition.

secondary dementia, dementia resulting from another concurrent form of psychosis.

secondary dental caries, dental caries developing in a tooth already affected by the condition; often a new cavity forms adjacent to or beneath the restorative filling of an old cavity.

secondary disease, any disorder of bodily functions that follows or results from an earlier injury or medical episode.

secondary enuresis [L, *secundus,* second; Gk, *enourein,* to urinate], enuresis in an older child who has demonstrated bedtime control for a year or more. It is typically the result of psychologic stress, but it also may be an early sign of an organic disorder such as diabetes mellitus.

secondary fissure, a fissure between the uvula and the pyramid of the cerebellum.

secondary gain, an indirect benefit, usually obtained through an illness or debility. Such gains may include monetary and disability benefits, personal attention, or escape from unpleasant situations and responsibilities.

secondary gangrene [L, *secundus,* second; Gk, *gaggraina*], a form of gangrene in which putrefaction follows the primary tissue necrosis, generating malodorous and toxic products.

secondary gestation [L, *secundus,* second, *gestare,* to bear], a pregnancy in which the ovum becomes displaced from its original site of implantation but continues development at a different location.

secondary glandular failure, the deficiency of a hormone secreted by a particular gland or gland atrophy caused by absence of a stimulus from another gland, as when a pituitary disorder results in hypogonadism.

secondary health care, an intermediate level of health care that includes diagnosis and treatment, performed in a hospital having specialized equipment and laboratory facilities.

secondary hemorrhage [L, *secundus,* second; Gk, *haima,* blood, *rhegnynei,* to burst forth], a hemorrhage that develops 24 hours or more after the original injury or surgery. It is often caused by an infection.

secondary hydrocephalus [L, *secundus,* second; Gk, *hydor,* water, *kephale,* head], hydrocephalus that develops after an injury or infection such as syphilis or meningitis.

secondary hyperaldosteronism, excessive production of aldosterone caused by an extraadrenal disorder such as heart failure, kidney disease, cirrhosis, or hypoproteinemia.

secondary hypertension, elevated blood pressure associated with several primary diseases such as renal, pulmonary, endocrine, and vascular diseases.

secondary immunodeficiency, a loss of immunity caused by a disease process or toxic effect of medication, rather than a failure or defect in T or B lymphocytes.

secondary infection, an infection by a microorganism that follows an initial infection by another kind of organism.

secondary iritis [L, *secundus,* second; Gk, *iris,* rainbow, *itis,* inflammation], an inflammation of the iris that follows an infection or other disorder in a neighboring part of the eye such as the cornea.

secondary lymphoid organ, a source of effector lymphocytes, such as the spleen, lymph nodes, or tonsils.

secondary nutrient, a substance that acts as a stimulant to activate the flora of the gastrointestinal tract to synthesize other nutrients.

secondary occlusal traumatism, occlusal stress that affects previously weakened periodontal structures.

secondary parkinsonism, a disease of the nervous system caused by degeneration of neurons in the corpus striatum that receive dopaminergic input from the substantia nigra. Unlike idiopathic parkinsonism, the disease does not respond to the administration of levodopa (l-dopa).

secondary peritonitis [L, *secundus,* second; Gk, *peri* + *tenein,* to stretch, *itis,* inflammation], inflammation of the peritoneum caused by the spread of infection from neighboring tissue.

secondary pneumonia [L, *secundus,* second; Gk, *pneumon,* lung], pneumonia that develops during the course of another disease such as diphtheria or tularemia.

secondary polycythemia [L, *secundus,* second; Gk, *polys,* many, *kytos,* cell, *haima,* blood], a form of polycythemia that develops as a result of another disorder such as a pulmonary disease.

secondary port, a control device for regulating the flow of a primary and secondary intravenous solution. It consists of a Y-shaped plastic apparatus that attaches to the primary IV tubing and allows the primary and secondary IV solutions to flow separately or to flow simultaneously.

secondary prevention, a level of preventive medicine that focuses on early diagnosis, use of referral services, and rapid initiation of treatment to stop the progress

of disease processes or a handicapping disability.

secondary radiation, radiation that results from the scattering of primary x-rays. Secondary radiation often accounts for fogging of radiographic film.

secondary relationships, relationships with those who provide or accept services or with acquaintances and friends, as distinguished from family members and intimate friends.

secondary sequestrum, a piece of dead bone that partially separates from sound bone during the process of necrosis but may be pushed back into position.

secondary sex characteristic, any of the external physical characteristics of sexual maturity secondary to hormonal stimulation that develops in the maturing individual.

secondary shock, a state of physical collapse and prostration caused by numerous traumatic and pathologic conditions. It develops over time after severe tissue damage and may merge with primary shock, accompanied by various signs such as weakness, restlessness, low body temperature, low blood pressure, cold sweat, and reduced urinary output. Blood pressure drops progressively in this state, and death may occur within a relatively short time after onset unless appropriate treatment intervenes. Secondary shock is often associated with heat stroke, crushing injuries, myocardial infarction, poisoning, fulminating infections, burns, and other life-threatening conditions. The pathologic characteristics of this state reflect changes in the capillaries, which become dilated and engorged with blood.

secondhand smoke, tobacco smoke from the burning end of a cigarette that is inhaled by nonsmokers. The U.S. Environmental Protection Agency in 1992 estimated that secondhand smoke was responsible for 3000 lung cancer deaths each year in nonsmokers. Also in 1992 the American Heart Association estimated that secondhand smoke was implicated in the deaths of 45,000 nonsmokers each year from heart disease and lung cancer.

second-look operation, a surgical opening of the peritoneal cavity performed within a year after removal of intraabdominal cancer to inspect for and/or resect a hidden tumor.

second messenger, a chemical substance inside a cell that carries information farther along the signal pathway from the internal part of a membrane-spanning receptor embedded in the cell membrane.

second opinion [L, *secundus* + *opinari,* to suppose], a patient privilege of requesting an examination and evaluation of a health condition by a second physician to verify or challenge the diagnosis by a first physician.

second-order change, a change that alters the system itself.

second-order kinetics, a chemical reaction in which the rate of the reaction is determined by the concentration of two chemical reactants involved.

second-set rejection, failure of an organ or tissue graft in a host who is already immune to the histocompatibility antigens of the graft because of a previous graft with the same antigenic specificity.

second sight, 1. an improvement in near vision that may develop in aging as a result of increasing refractivity of the lens nucleus. **2.** an early increase in the index of refraction of the lens, resulting in a decrease in hyperopia and an increase in myopia. **3.** clairvoyance, precognition.

second stage of labor [L, *secundus,* second; OFr, *estage* + L, *labor,* work], the period of childbirth from full dilation of the cervix to delivery of the fetus.

secretagogue /sikrē'əgog'/, any agent that induces exocrine, endocrine, or paracrine secretion.

secrete /sikrēt'/ [L, *secernere,* to separate], to discharge a substance into a cavity, vessel, or organ or onto the surface of the skin, as by a gland. —**secretion,** *n.*

secretin /sikrē'tin/ [L, *secernere,* to separate], a digestive hormone that is produced by certain cells lining the duodenum and jejunum when fatty acids of partially digested food enter the intestine from the stomach. It stimulates the pancreas to produce a fluid high in salts but low in enzymes.

secretin test, a test of pancreatic function after stimulation with a hormone, secretin. The test measures the volume and bicarbonate concentration of pancreatic secretions.

secretion /sikrē'shən/ [L, *secernere,* to separate], **1.** the release of chemical substances manufactured by cells of glandular organs. **2.** a substance released.

secretoinhibitory /sikrē'tō·inhib'itôr'ē/ [L, *secernere,* to separate, *inhibere,* to restrain], pertaining to a function of inhibiting secretion.

secretor /sikrē'tər/, **1.** (in genetics) a person who releases A, B, or AB blood group antigens into saliva, gastric juice, or other exocrine secretions. **2.** the autosomal-dominant gene that determines this trait.

secretor factor, a substance that triggers the release of ABO blood group antigens into exocrine secretions.

secretory /sikrē'tərē/ [L, *secernere,* to separate], pertaining to or contributing to the function of secretion.

secretory component deficiency, a failure of gastrointestinal epithelial cells to produce secretory component, a glycopeptide occurring in secretory immunoglobulin A (IgA). It causes a lack of IgA in external secretions (tears, saliva, colostrum), although serum IgA is normal.

secretory duct [L, *secernere*], (of a gland) a small duct that has a secretory function and joins with an excretory duct.

secretory IgA, a dimer of class A immunoglobulins, the principal agents of mucosal immunity. IgA is the only immunoglobulin isotype that can pass through mucosal membranes to reach the lumen of internal organs.

secretory immune system, the part of the immune system that secretes immunoglobulins, primarily immunoglobulin A, onto mucosal surfaces.

secretory phase, the phase of the menstrual cycle after the release of an ovum from a mature ovarian follicle. The corpus luteum develops from the ruptured follicle. It secretes progesterone, which stimulates the development of the glands and arteries of the endometrium, causing it to become thick and spongy. In a negative-feedback response to the increased level of progesterone in the blood, the secretion of LH from the pituitary decreases.

secretory piece, a polypeptide chain attached to an immunoglobulin A molecule. The secretory piece is necessary for secretion of the immunoglobulin molecule into mucosal spaces.

section /sek'shən/ [L, *sectio,* a cutting], **1.** a cut surface or slice of tissue. **2.** the act of cutting tissue.

sectional arch wire /sek'shənəl/ [L, *sectio,* a cutting, *arcus,* bow; AS, *wir*], a wire attached to only a few teeth, usually on one side of a dental arch or in the anterior segment of the arch to cause or guide orthodontic tooth movement.

sector scan /sek'tər/, (in ultrasonics) a scan in which the transducer or ultrasound beam is rotated through an angle, and the center of rotation is near or behind the surface of the transducer.

secundigravida /səkund'dəgrav'idə/ [L, *secundus,* second, *gravidus,* pregnancy], a woman who is pregnant for the second time. —**secundigravid,** *adj.*

secundines /səkun'dīnz/ [L, *secundus*], the placenta, umbilical cord, and membranes of afterbirth.

secundipara /sek'əndip'ərə/ [L, *secundus* + *parere,* to give birth], a woman who has borne two viable children in separate pregnancies.

Security Enhancement, a Nursing Interventions Classification defined as intensifying a patient's sense of physical and psychological safety.

SED, abbreviation for *skin erythema dose.*

sedation /sidā'shən/ [L, *sedatio,* soothing], an induced state of quiet, calmness, or sleep, as by means of a sedative or hypnotic medication.

sedative /sed'ətiv/ [L, *sedatio,* soothing], **1.** pertaining to a substance, procedure, or measure that has a calming effect. **2.** an agent that decreases functional activity, diminishes irritability, and allays excitement.

sedative bath, the immersion of the body in water for a prolonged period, used especially as a calming procedure for agitated patients.

sedative-hypnotic, a drug that reversibly depresses the activity of the central nervous system, used chiefly to induce sleep and allay anxiety. Barbiturates and many nonbarbiturate sedative-hypnotics with diverse chemical and pharmacologic properties share the ability to depress the activity of all excitable tissue, but the arousal center in the brainstem is especially sensitive to their effects. Various sedative-hypnotics and minor tranquilizers with similar effects are used in the treatment of insomnia, acute convulsive conditions, and anxiety states and in facilitation of the induction of anesthesia.

sedentary /sed'əntər'ē/ [L, *sedentarius,* sitting], pertaining to a condition of inaction, such as work or recreation that can be performed in the sitting posture.

sedentary living [L, *sedentarius* + AS, *lif*], a pattern of daily living that requires a minimum amount of physical effort.

sediment /sed'imənt/ [L, *sedimentum,* settling], a deposit of relatively insoluble material that settles to the bottom of a container of liquid.

sedimentation /sed'iməntā'shən/ [L, *sedimentum,* settling], the deposition of insoluble materials to the bottom of a liquid. The process may be accelerated by centrifugation.

sedimentation rate (SR) [L, *sedimentum* + *ratum,* rate], the speed of settling of red blood cells in a vertical glass column of citrated plasma. It is used to monitor inflammatory or malignant disease and to aid in the detection and diagnosis of occult diseases such as tuberculosis.

sed. rate, *informal.* erythrocyte sedimentation rate.

segment /seg'mənt/ [L, *segmentum,* piece cut off], a component, part, or part of a structure, such as a lobe of the liver or part of the intestine.

segmental bronchus /segmen'təl/ [L, *segmentum,* piece cut off], a secondary bronchus branching from a primary bronchus to a tertiary bronchus.

segmental fracture, a bone break in which several large bone fragments separate from the main body of a fractured bone. The ends of such fragments may pierce the skin, as in an open fracture, or may be contained within the skin, as in a closed fracture.

segmental reflex [L, *segmentum* + *reflectere,* to bend back], a reflex that involves a pathway through only a single segment of the spinal cord.

segmental resection, a surgical procedure in which a part of an organ, gland, or other body part is excised, such as a segmental resection of a part of an ovary performed to diminish the gland's hormonal secretion by decreasing the amount of secretory tissue in the gland.

segmentation /seg'məntā'shən/ [L, *segmentum* + *atio,* process], **1.** the repetition of structured parts or the process of dividing into segments or similar parts, such as the formation of somites or metameres. **2.** the division of the zygote into blastomeres; cleavage.

segmentation method, a technique for filling tooth root canals in which a preselected gutta-percha cone is cut into segments and the tip section sealed into the apex of a root. The other sections are usually warmed and condensed against the first piece with a plugger.

segmentation nucleus, the nucleus of the zygote resulting from the fusion of the male and female pronuclei in the fertilized ovum. It is the final stage in fertilization.

segmented hyalinizing vasculitis /segmen'tid/, a chronic relapsing inflammatory condition of the blood vessels of the lower legs associated with nodular or purpuric skin lesions that may become ulcerated and leave scars.

segmented neutrophil, a neutrophil with a filament between the lobes of its nucleus.

segregation /seg'rəgā'shən/ [L, *segregare,* to separate], (in genetics) a principle stating that the pairs of chromosomes bearing genes derived from both parents are separated during meiosis. Chance alone determines which gene, maternal or paternal, will travel to which gamete.

seizure /sē'zhər/ [Fr, *saisir,* to seize], a hyperexcitation of neurons in the brain

S

leading to a sudden, violent involuntary series of contractions of a group of muscles. It may be paroxysmal and episodic, as in a seizure disorder, or transient and acute, as after a head concussion. A seizure may be clonic or tonic, focal, unilateral, or bilateral.

Seizure Management, a Nursing Interventions Classification defined as care of a patient during a seizure and the postictal state.

Seizure Precautions, a Nursing Interventions Classification defined as prevention or minimization of potential injuries sustained by a patient with a known seizure disorder.

seizure threshold, the amount of stimulus necessary to produce a convulsive seizure. All humans can have seizures if the provocation is sufficient.

selection /silek'shən/ [L, *seligere,* to choose], **1.** the act or product of choosing. **2.** (in genetics) the process by which various factors or mechanisms determine and modify the reproductive ability of a genotype within a specific population, thus influencing evolutionary change.

selective abstraction /silek'tiv/ [L, *seligere,* to choose], a type of cognitive distortion in which focus on one aspect of an event negates all other aspects.

selective angiography, a graphic procedure that allows selective visualization of the aorta, the major arterial systems, or a particular vessel. It is performed using a percutaneous catheter. A few milliliters of a radiopaque substance is injected when the catheter is in place.

selective grinding, any modification of the occlusal forms of the teeth, produced by corrective grinding at selected places to improve occlusion and tooth function.

selective IgA deficiency, a familial or acquired disorder characterized by a lack of serum and secretory immunoglobulin A (IgA). The IgA-deficient patient may appear normal or asymptomatic and is diagnosed by demonstration of less than 5 mg/dl of IgA in serum. Patients have an increased risk of respiratory, gastrointestinal, and urogenital infections.

selective immunoglobulin deficiency, a condition characterized by inadequate levels of one of the major classes of immunoglobulins.

selective inattention, the screening out of unwanted stimuli, particularly the part of a message the listener does not want to hear.

selective neuronal necrosis, a widespread destruction of neurons caused by hypoxic or ischemic events. Only a fraction of the neurons in a given region are destroyed, selected apparently at random.

selective serotonin reuptake inhibitor (SSRI), an antidepressant drug, such as fluoxetine and paroxetine, that is relatively free of side effects of incoordination, ataxia, and tremor but may cause insomnia and anorexia. Advantages include fewer anticholinergic side effects (dry mouth, blurred vision, urinary retention) and fewer antihistaminic side effects (sedation, weight gain).

selectivity /silektiv'itē/ [L, *seligere*], the capacity factor ratios of two substances measured under identical chromatographic conditions.

selectivity coefficient, the degree to which an ion-selective electrode responds to a particular ion with respect to a reference ion.

selenium (Se) /silē'nē·əm/ [Gk, *selene,* moon], a metalloid element of the sulfur group. Its atomic number is 34; its atomic mass (weight) is 78.96. Selenium occurs as a trace element in foods, and research continues to determine the most effective daily allowances for different age groups.

selenium sulfide, an antifungal and antiseborrheic prescribed for dandruff and for seborrheic dermatitis of the scalp.

self, *pl.* **selves** /selvz/ [AS], **1.** the total essence or being of a person; the individual. **2.** those affective, cognitive, and spiritual qualities that distinguish one person from another; individuality. **3.** a person's awareness of his or her own being or identity; consciousness; ego.

self-acceptance [AS, *self* + L, *accipere,* to take], the recognition and acceptance of one's own qualities and limitations.

self-actualization, (in humanistic psychology) the fundamental tendency toward the maximum realization and fulfillment of one's human potential.

self-anesthesia, the self-administered inhalation anesthesia in which whiffs of anesthetic gas are inhaled from a hand-held breathing device controlled by the patient. This form of anesthesia is most common in England.

Self-Awareness Enhancement, a Nursing Interventions Classification defined as assisting a patient to explore and understand his or her thoughts, feelings, motivations, and behaviors.

self-breast examination (SBE), a procedure in which a woman examines her breasts and their accessory structures for evidence of change that could indicate a malignant process. The SBE is usually performed 1 week to 10 days after the first day of the menstrual cycle, when the breasts are smallest and cyclic nodularity is least apparent. The techniques are similar to those of the examination of the breast as performed in the health assessment or physical examination.

self-care, 1. the personal and medical care performed by the patient, usually in collaboration with and after instruction by a health professional. **2.** the health care by laypeople of their families, their friends, and themselves, including identification and evaluation of symptoms, medication, and treatment. **3.** personal care accomplished without technical assistance, such as eating, washing, dressing, using the telephone, and attending to one's own elimination, appearance, and hygiene. The goal of rehabilitation medicine is maximal personal self-care.

Self-Care Assistance, a Nursing Interventions Classification defined as assisting another to perform activities of daily living.

Self-Care Assistance: Bathing/Hygiene, a Nursing Interventions Classification defined as assisting a patient to perform personal hygiene.

Self-Care Assistance: Dressing/Grooming, a Nursing Interventions Classification defined as assisting a patient with clothes and makeup.

Self-Care Assistance: Feeding, a Nursing Interventions Classification defined as assisting a person to eat.

Self-Care Assistance: Toileting, a Nursing Interventions Classification defined as assisting another with elimination.

self-care deficit, bathing/hygiene, a NANDA-accepted nursing diagnosis of a state in which the individual experiences impaired ability to perform or complete bathing and hygiene activities for himself or herself. Defining characteristics include inability to wash the body or parts of the body, inability to get or get to water for bathing, and inability to regulate water temperature or flow.

self-care deficit, dressing/grooming, a NANDA-accepted nursing diagnosis of a state in which the individual experiences impaired ability to perform or complete dressing and grooming activities for himself or herself. Defining characteristics include impaired ability to don or to remove necessary items of clothing, to fasten clothing, to obtain or replace articles of clothing, and to maintain a satisfactory appearance.

self-care deficit, feeding, a NANDA-accepted nursing diagnosis of a state in which the individual experiences impaired ability to perform or complete feeding activities for himself or herself. The major defining characteristic is an inability to carry food from a receptacle to the mouth.

self-care deficit, toileting, a NANDA-accepted nursing diagnosis of a state in which the individual experiences impaired ability to perform or complete toileting activities for himself or herself. The critical defining characteristics of a deficit include inability to get to the toilet or to the commode, to sit down on or to arise from the toilet or commode, to get the necessary clothing on or off, and to perform the proper toilet hygiene. In addition, the person may not be able to flush the toilet or to empty the commode.

self-care theory, a model, central to Dorothea Orem's concept of nursing, used to provide a conceptual framework for nursing care directed to self-care by the client to the greatest degree possible. The model requires an assessment of the client's capability for self-care and need for care.

self-catheterization, a procedure performed by a patient to empty the bladder and prevent it from becoming overdistended with urine. The patient who cannot empty the bladder completely but can retain urine for 2 to 4 hours at a time can be taught self-catheterization if he or she is willing to learn and has some manual dexterity and the ability to palpate the bladder.

self-concept, the composite of ideas, feelings, and attitudes that a person has about his or her own identity, worth, capabilities, and limitations.

self-confrontation, a technique for behavior modification that depends on a patient's recognition of and dissatisfaction with inconsistencies in his or her own values, beliefs, and behaviors, or between his or her own personal system and that of a significant other.

self-conscious, 1. the state of being aware of oneself as an individual entity that experiences, desires, and acts. **2.** a heightened awareness of oneself and one's actions as reflected by the observations and reactions of others; socially ill at ease. **—self-consciousness,** *n.*

self-defeating personality disorder, a personality characterized by a type of behavior that inhibits the individual from achieving his or her own desires and goals. It is characterized by involvement in situations that continuously lead to failure, rejection, and loss even when other options for involvement are available.

self-destructive behavior, any behavior, direct or indirect, that if uninterrupted will ultimately lead to the death of the individual.

self-diagnosis, the diagnosis of one's own health problems, usually without direction or assistance from a physician.

self-differentiation, specialization and

diversification of a tissue or part resulting solely from intrinsic factors.

self-disclosure, the process by which one person lets his or her inner being, thoughts, and emotions be known to another. It is important for psychologic growth in individual and group psychotherapy.

self-esteem, the degree of worth and competence one attributes to oneself.

self-esteem, chronic low, a NANDA-accepted nursing diagnosis of long-standing negative self-evaluation/feelings about self or capabilities. Defining characteristics (long-standing or chronic) include self-negating verbalization; expressions of shame/guilt; evaluation of self as unable to deal with events; rationalization/rejection of positive feedback and exaggeration of negative feedback about self; hesitation to try new things/situations, frequent lack of success in work or other life events; overly conforming behavior and dependence on others' opinions; lack of eye contact; non-assertive/passive behavior; indecisive behavior; and excessive seeking of reassurance.

self-esteem disturbance, a NANDA-accepted nursing diagnosis of negative self evaluation/feeling about the self or self capabilities, which may be directly or indirectly expressed. Defining characteristics include self-negating verbalization; expressions of shame/guilt; evaluation of self as unable to deal with events; rationalization/rejection of positive feedback and exaggeration of negative feedback about self; hesitation to try new things/situations; denial of problems obvious to others; projection of blame/responsibility for problems; rationalizing about personal failures; hypersensitivity to slight or criticism; and grandiosity.

Self-Esteem Enhancement, a Nursing Interventions Classification defined as assisting a patient to increase his/her personal judgment of self-worth.

self-esteem, situational low, a NANDA-accepted nursing diagnosis of negative self-evaluation/feelings about self that develop in response to a loss or change in an individual who previously had a positive self-evaluation. Defining characteristics include an episodic occurrence of negative self-appraisal in response to life events in a person with previous positive self-evaluation, verbalization of negative feelings about the self (helplessness, uselessness), self-negating verbalizations; expression of shame/guilt; evaluation of self as unable to handle situations/events; and difficulty making decisions.

self-fulfilling prophecy, a principle that states that a belief in or the expectation of a particular resolution is a factor that contributes to its fulfillment.

self-healing squamous epithelioma, an inherited condition of skin tumors that appear on the head and resolve spontaneously after a few months, leaving deep-pitted scars. The tumors resemble squamous carcinoma or keratoacanthoma.

self-help group, a group of people who meet to improve their health through discussion and special activities. Characteristically self-help groups are not led by a professional.

self-hypnosis [AS, *self* + Gk, *hypnos,* sleep], the process of putting oneself into a trancelike state by autosuggestion, such as concentration on a single thought or object. Some subjects are more susceptible than others.

self-ideal, a perception of how one should behave based on certain personal standards. The standard may be either a carefully constructed image of the kind of person one would like to be or merely a number of aspirations, goals, or values one would like to achieve.

self-image, the total concept, idea, or mental image one has of oneself and of one's role in society; the person one believes oneself to be.

self-insurance, a system whereby hospitals or health professionals may, in lieu of commercial insurance, assume financial responsibility for their liability.

self-limited, (of a disease or condition) tending to end without treatment.

self-limited disease [AS, *self* + L, *limes,* boundary, *dis,* not; Fr, *aise,* ease], a disease restricted in duration by its own pattern of characteristics and not by other influences.

self-management approach, a treatment approach in which patients assume responsibility for their behavior, changing their environment, and planning their future.

Self-Modification Assistance, a Nursing Interventions Classification defined as reinforcement of self-directed change initiated by the patient to achieve personally important goals.

self-monitoring of blood glucose (SMBG), the use of a glucose meter to enable a patient with diabetes mellitus to recognize glycemic variations and adjust medications for maximum compliance. Most self-monitoring systems use the chemical reaction between glucose oxidase and glucose as a basis for measurement. Some devices depend on hydrogen peroxide, which is a product of the same reaction.

self-mutilation, risk for, a NANDA-accepted nursing diagnosis of a state in which an individual is at high risk to injure but not kill himself or herself, and action that produces tissue damage and tension relief. Defining characteristics include an inability to cope with increased psychologic/physiological tension in a healthy manner; feelings of depression, rejection, self-hatred, separation anxiety, guilt, and depersonalization; fluctuating emotions; command hallucinations; need for sensory stimuli; parental emotional deprivation; and a dysfunctional family. Risk factors include being a member of an at-risk group. Groups at risk include clients with borderline personality disorder, especially females 16 to 25 years of age; clients in a psychotic state (frequently males in young adulthood); emotionally disturbed and/or battered children; mentally retarded and autistic children; clients with a history of self-injury; and clients with a history of physical, emotional, or sexual abuse.

self-other, a concept that characterizes people who believe that the source of power is within the self as opposed to those who believe it is in others.

self-radiolysis, a process in which a compound is damaged by radioactive decay products originating in an atom within the compound.

self-recognition, the ability of the body's immune system to recognize self-identifying antigens on the body's own cells.

self-regulation, a plan for patients to eliminate health risk behaviors. It includes self-monitoring, self-evaluation, and self-reinforcement.

self-reinforcing adaptation, (in occupational therapy) a therapeutic technique in which each successful stage of adjustment stimulates the next more complex step.

self-responsibility, a concept of holistic health by which individuals assume responsibility for their own health.

Self-Responsibility Facilitation, a Nursing Interventions Classification defined as encouraging a patient to assume more responsibility for his or her behavior.

self-retaining catheter, an indwelling urinary catheter that has a double lumen. One channel allows urine to drain from the bladder into a collecting bag; the other has a balloon at the bladder end and a diaphragm at the other end. Several centimeters of air or sterile water are injected through the diaphragm to fill the balloon in the bladder and hold the catheter in place.

self-stimulation, a system in which patients control their pain by manipulating an electrical source of nerve stimulation.

self-system, the organization of experiences that acts as a protective mechanism against anxiety.

self-theory, a personality theory that uses one's self-concept in integrating the function and organization of the personality.

self-threading pin, a screwlike object placed into a hole drilled in tooth dentin to improve retention of a restoration.

self-tolerance, (in autoimmunity) the absence of an immune response directed against a person's own native tissue antigens.

self-transcendence, the ability to focus attention on doing something for the sake of others, as opposed to self-actualization, in which doing something for oneself is an end goal.

sella turcica /sel′ə tur′sikə/ [L, *sella,* seat, *turcica,* Turkish], a transverse depression crossing the midline on the superior surface of the body of the sphenoid bone and containing the pituitary gland.

SEM, abbreviation for **scanning electron microscope.**

semantics /siman′tiks/ [Gk, *semantikos,* significant], the study of language with special concern for the meanings of words or other symbols.

semen /sē′mən/ [L, seed], the thick, whitish secretion of the male reproductive organs discharged from the urethra on ejaculation. It contains various constituents, including spermatozoa in their nutrient plasma and secretions of the prostate, seminal vesicles, and various other glands. —**seminal,** *adj.*

semiautomatic external defibrillator /sem′ē-ô′təmat′ik/, a portable apparatus used to restart a heart that has stopped. It is programmed to analyze cardiac rhythms automatically and indicate to a health professional when to deliver a defibrillation shock.

semicanal /-kənal′/, **1.** a canal with an opening on one side. **2.** a deep groove on the edge of a bone that accommodates part of an adjoining bone.

semicircular canal /-sur′kyələr/ [L, *semi,* half, *circulare,* to go around, *canalis,* channel], any of three bony fluid-filled loops in the osseous labyrinth of the internal ear, associated with the sense of balance.

semicircular duct, one of three ducts that make up the membranous labyrinth of the inner ear.

semicomatose /-kō′mətōs/ [L, *semi,* half; Gk, *koma,* deep sleep], pertaining to a condition of stupor from which a patient can be aroused.

semiconductor /-kənduk′tər/, a solid crystalline substance whose electrical conductivity is intermediate between that of a conductor and that of an insulator. An n-type semiconductor has loosely bound electrons that are relatively free to move about inside the material. A p-type semiconductor is one with holes, or positive traps, in which electrons may be bound.

semiconscious /-kon'shəs/, an impaired state of consciousness, characterized by obtundation, stupor, or hypersomnia, from which a patient can be aroused only by energetic stimulation.

semiflexion /-flek'shən/, a condition in which a limb is midway between full flexion and full extension.

semi-Fowler's position /-fou'lərz/ [L, *semi,* half; George R. Fowler, American surgeon, 1848–1906], placement of the patient in an inclined position, with the upper half of the body raised by elevating the head of the bed.

semihorizontal heart /hôr'əzon'təl/, (in an electrocardiogram) an electrical "position" of the heart that lies between the horizontal and intermediate positions when the QRS axis is 0 degrees.

semilunar fold of the conjunctiva, a fold of membrane that extends laterally from the lacrimal caruncle. It has a concave free border directed to the cornea. In some individuals it contains smooth muscular fibers.

semilunar valve /-lōō'nər/ [L, *semi* + *luna,* moon, *valva,* folding door], **1.** a valve with half-moon-shaped cusps, such as the aortic valve and the pulmonary valve. **2.** any one of the cusps constituting such a valve. **3.** simple cuplike valves found in the venous and lymphatic vessels.

semimembranosus /-ēmem'brənō'səs/ [L, *semi* + *membrana,* membrane], one of three posterior femoral muscles. The tendon of insertion forms one of the two medial hamstrings. The muscle functions to flex the leg, rotate it medially after flexion, and extend the thigh.

semimembranous /-mem'brənəs/ [L, *semi,* half, *membrana*], pertaining to a muscle or other tissue that is partly membrane or fascia, such as the semimembranous hamstring muscle.

seminal duct /sem'inəl/ [L, *semen,* seed, *ducere,* to lead], any duct through which semen passes, such as the vas deferens or the ejaculatory duct.

seminal emission [L, *semen,* seed, *emittere,* to send out], a discharge of semen.

seminal fluid test, any of several tests of semen to detect abnormalities in a male's reproductive system and to determine fertility. Some common factors considered are seminal fluid liquefaction time and spermatic quantity, morphologic characteristics, motility, volume, and pH.

seminal vesicle, either of the paired sac-like glandular structures posterolateral to the urinary bladder in the male and functioning as part of the reproductive system. The seminal vesicles produce a fluid that is added to the secretion of the testes and other glands to form the semen.

seminal vesiculitis, inflammation of a seminal vesicle.

semination /sem'inā'shən/, the introduction of semen into the female genital tract.

seminiferous /sem'inif'ərəs/ [L, *semen* + *ferre,* to bear], transporting or producing semen, such as the tubules of the testis.

seminiferous tubules [L, *semen,* seed, *ferre,* to bear, *tubulus*], long threadlike tubes packed in areolar tissue in the lobes of the testes.

seminoma /sem'inō'mə/ [L, *semen* + *oma,* tumor], a malignant tumor of the testis. It is the most common testicular tumor and is believed to arise from the seminiferous epithelium of the mature or maturing testis.

semipermeable /-pur'mē·əbəl/ [L, *semi,* half, *permeare,* to pass through], pertaining to a membrane that allows the passage of some molecules but prevents the passage of others.

semipermeable membrane [L, *semi,* *permeare,* to pass through], a membrane barrier to the passage of substances above a specific size that allows the passage of substances below that size.

semiprone /-prōn'/ [L, *semi,* half, *pronus,* leaning forward], lying on one's side, with the thigh on the upper side flexed against the abdomen and the arm on the lower side extended back.

semirecumbent /-rikum'bənt/, in a reclining position.

semisupine /-səpīn'/, pertaining to a posture that is between a midposition and the supine position.

semisynthetic /-sinthet'ik/ [L, *semi,* half; Gk, *synthesis,* putting together], pertaining to a natural substance that has been partially altered by chemical manipulation.

semitendinosus /sem'iten'dinō'səs/ [L, *semi* + *tendere,* to stretch], one of three posterior femoral muscles of the thigh. It functions to flex the leg, rotate it medially after flexion, and extend the thigh.

semivertical heart /-vur'tikəl/, (in an electrocardiogram) an electrical "position" of the heart that lies between the intermediate and vertical positions when the QRS axis is 60 degrees.

semustine /səmus'tēn/, an antineoplastic prescribed in the treatment of Lewis lung carcinoma, brain tumors, malignant melanoma, and Hodgkin's disease.

sender [AS, *sendan,* to send], (in communication theory) the person by whom a message is encoded and sent.

seneciosis /senes′ē-ō′sis/, a toxic reaction to the ingestion of plants of the genus *Senecio,* which are used to make bush tea. The poison causes liver damage, particularly in malnourished patients. Common *Senecio* species include ragwort and life root, both used in herbal remedies.

senescence /sənes′əns/ [L, *senescere,* to grow old], the state of growing old.

senescent /sənes′ənt/ [L, *senescere,* to grow old], aging or growing old. —**senescence,** *n.*

senescent cell antigen, an antigen that appears on old red blood cells that bind immunoglobulin G autoantibodies. It is also found on lymphocytes, platelets, and neutrophils.

Sengstaken-Blakemore tube [Robert W. Sengstaken, American neurosurgeon, b. 1923; Arthur H. Blakemore, American surgeon, 1897–1970], a thick catheter having a triple lumen and two balloons, used to produce pressure by balloon tamponade to arrest hemorrhaging from esophageal varices. Attached to a tube, one balloon is inflated in the stomach and exerts pressure against the upper orifice. Similarly attached, another longer and narrower balloon exerts pressure on the walls of the esophagus. The third tube is used for withdrawing gastric contents.

senile /sē′nīl/ [L, *senilis,* aged], pertaining to or characteristic of old age or the process of aging. —**senescent,** *adj.,* **senility,** *n.*

senile arteriosclerosis, a hardening of the arteries associated with aging.

senile cataract, a kind of cataract associated with aging in which a hard opacity forms in the nucleus of the lens of the eye.

senile dental caries, tooth decay occurring at an advanced age. Senile dental caries is usually characterized by cavity formation in or around the cementum layer and root surfaces.

senile involution, a pattern of retrograde changes occurring with advancing age and resulting in the progressive shrinking and degeneration of tissues and organs.

senile nanism, dwarfism associated with progeria.

senile psychosis, a chronic progressive dementia associated with brain atrophy of unknown cause. Symptoms include impaired memory, impaired judgment, decreased moral and aesthetic values, inability to think abstractly, and periods of confusion, confabulation, and irritability, all of which may range from mild to severe.

senile tremor [L, *senilis,* aged, *tremor,* shaking], a tremor associated with aging.

senile vaginitis [L, *senilis,* aged, *vagina,* sheath, *itis,* inflammation], a condition of atrophy of the vagina resulting from the postmenopausal loss of estrogen secretion.

senility /sinil′itē/ [L, *senilis,* aged], the general state of reduced mental and physical vigor associated with aging.

senior centers /sē′nyər/, community agencies for older adults. The centers offer nutritional, recreational, educational, health, and legal services.

Senior Companion Program, a service that offers personal assistance and peer support to low-income, home-bound, and chronically ill older people.

senior patient, (in the United States) a Medicare beneficiary enrolled in a health maintenance organization.

senna /sen′ə/ [Ar, *sana*], the dried leaflets or pods of *Cassia acutifolia* or *Cassia augustifolia,* used as a cathartic.

senopia /senō′pē-ə/ [L, *senex,* old man, *opsis,* vision], an improvement in the near vision of the aged caused by the myopia associated with increasing lenticular nuclear sclerosis.

sensate /sen′sāt/, capable of perceiving sensory stimuli.

sensate focus technique, a therapeutic program for the treatment of erectile dysfunction in males.

sensation /sensā′shən/ [L, *sentire,* to feel], **1.** a feeling, impression, or awareness of a body state or condition that results from the stimulation of a sensory receptor site and transmission of the nerve impulse along an afferent fiber to the brain. **2.** a feeling or an awareness of a mental or emotional state, which may or may not result in response to an external stimulus.

sense [L, *sentire,* to feel], **1.** the faculty by which stimuli are perceived and conditions outside and within the body are distinguished and evaluated. The major senses are sight, hearing, smell, taste, touch, and pressure. Other senses include hunger; thirst; pain; temperature; proprioception; and spatial, temporal, and visceral sensations. **2.** the ability to feel; a sensation. **3.** the capacity to understand; normal mental ability. **4.** to perceive through a sense organ.

sensibility /sen′sibil′itē/, the ability to perceive sensations and impressions, both physical and psychologic.

sensible /sen′sibəl/, **1.** capable of sensation. **2.** possessing reason or judgment. **3.** capable of being perceived.

sensible perspiration /sen′sibəl/ [L, *sensibilis,* perceptible], loss of body fluid

S

through the secretory activity of the sweat glands in a quantity sufficient to be observed.

sensitive /sen'sitiv/ [L, *sentire*, to feel], **1.** able to perceive and transmit a sensation or stimulus. **2.** affected by low concentrations of antimicrobial drugs, said of microorganisms. **3.** abnormally susceptible to a subject, such as a drug or foreign protein.

sensitive volume [L, *sentire* + *volumen*, paper roll], (in magnetic resonance imaging [MRI]) the region of the object from which an MRI signal will preferentially be acquired because of strong magnetic field inhomogeneity elsewhere.

sensitivity /sen'sitiv'itē/ [L, *sentire*], **1.** capacity to feel, transmit, or react to a stimulus. **2.** susceptibility to a substance, such as a drug or an antigen. —**sensitive,** *adj.*

sensitivity test, a laboratory method for testing the effectiveness of antibiotics. It is usually done on organisms known to be potentially resistant to antibiotic therapy in vitro. A report of a "resistant" finding means the antibiotic is not effective in inhibiting the growth of a pathogen, whereas use of an effective antibiotic results in a "sensitive" report.

sensitivity training group, a group that offers members a supportive atmosphere in which to experiment with and alter behavior patterns and interpersonal reactions.

sensitization /sen'sitīzā'shən/ [L, *sentire* + Gk, *izein*, to cause], **1.** an acquired reaction in which specific antibodies develop in response to an antigen. This is deliberately caused in immunization by injecting a disease-causing organism that has been altered in such a way that it is no longer infectious yet remains able to cause the production of antibodies to fight the disease. **2.** a photodynamic method of destroying microorganisms by inserting into a solution substances such as fluorescing dyes that absorb visible light and emit energy at wavelengths destructive to the organism. **3.** *nontechnical.* anaphylaxis. —**sensitize,** *v.*

sensitized /sen'sitīzd/, pertaining to tissues that have been made susceptible to antigenic substances.

sensitized vaccine [L, *sentire,* to feel, *vaccinus,* of a cow], a vaccine that is prepared by suspending microorganisms in their own homologous immune serum.

sensor /sen'sər/, an apparatus designed to react to physical stimuli such as temperature, light, or movement.

sensoriglandular /sen'sərēglan'dyələr/, pertaining to the reflexive secretion by glands triggered by sensory stimulation of a nerve.

sensorimotor /sen'sərēmō'tər/ [L, *sentire,* to feel, *moveo,* to move], pertaining to both sensory and motor nerve functions.

sensorimotor phase [L, *sentire* + *moveo,* to move], the developmental phase of childhood, encompassing the period from birth to 2 years of age, according to piagetian psychology.

sensorimotor therapy, therapy designed to enhance the integration of reflex phenomena and the emergence of voluntary motor behaviors concerned with posture and locomotion.

sensorimuscular /-mus'kyələr/, pertaining to contraction of muscles triggered by sensory stimulation.

sensorineural /sen'sərēnŏŏr'əl/ [L, *sentire,* to feel; Gk, *neuron*], pertaining to sensory nerves.

sensorineural hearing loss [L, *sentire* + Gk, *neuron,* nerve], a form of hearing loss in which sound is conducted normally through the external and middle ear but a defect in the inner ear or auditory nerve results in hearing loss.

sensorium /sensôr'ē-əm/, (in psychology) the part of the consciousness that includes the special sensory perceptive powers and their central correlation and integration in the brain. A clear sensorium conveys the presence of a reasonably accurate memory together with a correct orientation for time, place, and person.

sensorivasomotor /-vā'zōmō'tər/, pertaining to the contraction or dilation of a blood vessel in response to a sensory stimulus.

sensory /sen'sərē/ [L, *sentire* to feel], **1.** pertaining to sensation. **2.** pertaining to a part or all of the body's sensory nerve network.

sensory area [L, *sentire,* to feel, *area,* space], the regions of the cerebral cortex that receive impulses from sensory nerves, including thalamic, nucleic, and parietal lobes.

sensory-based language, the use of nonverbal behavior in neurolinguistic communication. Examples include puzzled expressions, scowling, and finger pointing.

sensory deficit, a defect in the function of one or more of the senses.

sensory deprivation [L, *sentire* + ME, *de-priven,* to deprive; L, *atio,* process], an involuntary loss of physical awareness caused by detachment from external sensory stimuli. Such deprivation often results in psychologic disorders such as panic, mental confusion, depression, and hallucinations.

sensory end organ [L, *sentire,* to feel; AS,

ende + Gk, *organon,* instrument], any of the specialized nerve endings devoted to detection of specific environmental stimuli, such as smell, sight, hearing, temperature, or touch.

sensory integration, the organization of sensory input for use, a perception of the body or environment, an adaptive response, a learning process, or the development of some neural function.

sensory integrative dysfunction, a disorder or irregularity in brain function that makes sensory integration difficult. Many, but not all, learning disorders stem from sensory integrative dysfunctions.

sensory integrative therapy, therapy that involves sensory stimulation and adaptive responses to it according to a child's neurologic needs. Treatment usually involves full body movements that provide vestibular, proprioceptive, and tactile stimulation. The goal is to improve the brain's ability to process and organize sensations.

sensory nerve, a nerve consisting of afferent fibers that conduct sensory impulses from the periphery of the body to the brain or spinal cord via the dorsal spinal roots.

sensory nucleus of trigeminal nerve, a collection of nerve cells in the pons that serve as the main nucleus for reception of tactile fibers of the trigeminal area.

sensory overload, a condition in which the central nervous system receives much more auditory, visual, or other environmental stimuli per time frame than it can process effectively.

sensory pathway [L, *sentire,* to feel; AS, *paeth* + *weg*], the route followed by a sensory nerve impulse from an end organ to a reflex center in the brain or spinal cord.

sensory/perceptual alterations (visual, auditory, kinesthetic, gustatory, tactile, olfactory) /pərsep'chōo·əl/, a NANDA-accepted nursing diagnosis of a state in which an individual experiences a change in the amount or patterning of incoming stimuli accompanied by a diminished, exaggerated, distorted, or impaired response to such stimuli. Defining characteristics include disorientation; change in the ability to abstract, conceptualize, or solve problems; change in behavior and in sensory acuity; restlessness; irritability; inappropriate response to stimuli; lack of concentration; rapid mood changes; exaggerated emotional responses; noncompliance; motor incoordination; complaints of fatigue; changes in posture and muscular tension; inappropriate responses, and hallucinations.

sensory receptor [L, *sentire,* to feel, *reci-*

pere, to receive], a specialized nerve ending that, when stimulated, initiates an afferent or sensory nerve impulse.

sensory root [L, *sentire,* to feel], the proximal end of a dorsal afferent nerve as it is attached to the spinal cord.

sensory threshold [L, *sentire,* to feel; AS, *therscold*], the point at which increasing stimuli trigger the start of an afferent nerve impulse. Absolute threshold is the lowest point at which response to a stimulus can be perceived.

sensual /sen'shōo·əl/ [L, *sensualis*], pertaining to a great interest in sex, food, or other sense satisfying topics.

sentient /sen'shənt/ [L, *sentire,* to feel], possessing sensitivity or powers of sensation and perception.

sentinel gland /sen'tinəl/ [Fr, *sentinelle* + L, *glans,* acorn], a node or growth that is associated with the presence of a nearby tumor or ulcer. An example is a supraclavicular node with cancer cells that have metastasized from an undiscovered primary cancer.

SEP, abbreviation for **somatosensory evoked potential.**

separation agent /sep'ərā'shən/, a reagent used to separate bound and free tracers in radioassay.

separation anxiety [L, *separare,* to separate, *atio,* process], fear and apprehension caused by separation from familiar surroundings and significant people. The syndrome occurs commonly in an infant separated from its mother or mothering figure or approached by a stranger.

s-EPO, abbreviation for *serum erythropoietin.*

sepsis /sep'sis/ [Gk, *sepein,* to become putrid], infection, contamination. —**septic,** *adj.*

septal /sep'təl/ [L, *saeptum,* fence], pertaining to a septum.

septal defect [L, *saeptum,* fence, *defectus,* failure], an abnormal, usually congenital defect in the wall separating two chambers of the heart. Oxygenated and deoxygenated blood mix, causing a decrease in the amount of oxygen carried in the blood to the peripheral tissues.

septate /sep'tāt/, pertaining to a structure divided by a septum.

septic /sep'tik/ [Gk, *septikos,* putrid], pertaining to an infection with pyogenic microorganisms.

septic abortion [Gk, *septikos,* putrid], spontaneous or induced termination of a pregnancy in which the mother's life may be threatened because of the invasion of germs into the endometrium, myometrium, and beyond. The woman requires immediate and intensive care, massive an-

S

tibiotic therapy, evacuation of the uterus, and often emergency hysterectomy to prevent death from overwhelming infection and septic shock.

septic arthritis, an acute form of arthritis, characterized by bacterial inflammation of a joint caused by the spread of bacteria through the bloodstream from an infection elsewhere in the body or by contamination of a joint during trauma or surgery. The joint is stiff, painful, tender, warm, and swollen.

septicemia /sep'tisē'mē-ə/ [Gk, *septikos* + *haima*, blood], systemic infection in which pathogens are present in the circulating bloodstream, having spread from an infection in any part of the body. Characteristically septicemia causes fever, chill, prostration, pain, headache, nausea, or diarrhea. —**septicemic,** *adj.*

septicemic plague /sep'tisē'mik/, a rapidly fatal form of bubonic plague in which septicemia with meningitis occurs before buboes have had time to form.

septic fever, an elevation of body temperature associated with infection by pathogenic microorganisms or in response to a toxin secreted by a microorganism.

septic infarct [Gk, *septikos,* putrid; L, *infarcire,* to stuff], an infected segment of dead tissue.

septic shock, a form of shock that occurs in septicemia when endotoxins or exotoxins are released from certain bacteria in the bloodstream. These toxins cause decreased vascular resistance, resulting in a dramatic fall in the blood pressure. Fever, tachycardia, increased respirations, and confusion or coma also may occur. Septic shock is usually preceded by signs of severe infection, often of the genitourinary or gastrointestinal system. Kinds of septic shock include **toxic shock syndrome** and bacteremic shock.

septic sore throat [Gk, *septikos,* putrid; AS, *sar* + *throte*], a severe throat infection, usually caused by a streptococcus strain, resulting in fever and marked exhaustion.

septivalent /sep'tivā'lənt/ [L, *septem,* seven], pertaining to a chemical that has a valence of 7.

septorhinoplasty /sep'tōrī'nəplas'tē/ [L, *saeptum,* fence], the surgical correction of defects in the nasal septum.

septostomy /septos'təmē/, the creation of an opening in a septum by surgery.

septum /sep'təm/, *pl.* **septa** [L, *saeptum,* enclosure], a partition or wall, such as the interatrial septum that separates the atria of the heart.

septuplet /septup'lit/ [L, *septuplum,* group

of seven], any one of seven children born of a single pregnancy.

sequela /sikwē'lə/, *pl.* **sequelae** [L, *sequi,* to follow], any abnormal condition that follows and is the result of a disease, treatment, or injury, such as paralysis after poliomyelitis.

sequence /sē'kwəns/ [L, *sequi,* to follow], an order of arrangement of objects or events, as the sequence of peptides in a protein molecule.

sequential imaging, (in nuclear medicine) a diagnostic procedure in which a series of closely timed images of the rapidly changing distribution of an administered radioactivetracer is used to identify a physiologic process or processes within the body.

sequential line imaging, (in magnetic resonance imaging) techniques in which the image is built up from successive lines through the object.

sequential multiple analysis (SMA), the biochemical examination of various substances in the blood, such as albumin, alkaline phosphatase, bilirubin, calcium, and cholesterol, using a computerized laboratory analyzer that produces a printout showing measured values of the substances tested.

sequential plane imaging, (in magnetic resonance imaging) a technique in which the image of an object is built up from successive planes in the object.

sequential point imaging, (in magnetic resonance imaging) techniques in which the image is built from successive point positions in the object.

sequester /sikwes'tər/ [L, *sequestare,* to lay aside], to detach, separate, or isolate, such as patient sequestration to prevent the spread of an infection.

sequestered antigens theory, a theory of autoimmunity, stressing the relationship between antigen exposure, immunogenic cells, and body cells, maintaining that immunologic tolerance depends on a certain degree of contact between immunologic cells and body cells and on a certain degree of antigen exposure.

sequestered edema, edema localized in the tissues surrounding a newly created surgical wound.

sequestration /sēkwestrā'shən/ [L, *sequestare,* to lay aside], **1.** the isolation of a patient or group of patients. **2.** a method of controlling hemorrhage of the head or trunk by isolating fluid in the arms and legs from the general circulation. **3.** allowing blood from the systemic circulation to perfuse a nonfunctioning part of a lung.

sequestrum /sikwes'trəm/, *pl.* **sequestra** [L, a deposit], a fragment of dead bone that is partially or entirely detached from the surrounding or adjacent healthy bone.

sequestrum forceps, a forceps with small, powerful teeth used for extracting necrotic or sharp fragments of bone from surrounding tissue.

sequoiasis /sikwoi'əsis/ [sequoia (tree) + Gk, *osis,* condition], a type of hypersensitivity pneumonitis common among workers in sawmills where redwood is processed. The antigens are the fungus *Pullularia pullulans* and species of the genus *Graphium,* found in moldy redwood sawdust. Characteristics of the acute disease include chills, fever, cough, dyspnea, anorexia, nausea, and vomiting.

Ser, abbreviation for the amino acid **serine.**

serendipity /ser'əndip'itē/ [Serendip, author Horace Walpole's mythic land of pleasant surprises], the act of accidental discovery. A number of important medications have been created through serendipity, such as the discovery of antidepressant activity in a drug originally developed to treat tuberculosis.

serial /sir'ē-əl/ [L, *series,* in a row], pertaining to a succession, arrangement, or order of items.

serial casting, a sequence of casts used progressively to correct a deformity.

serial determination [L, *series,* in a row, *determinare,* to limit], a laboratory test that is repeated at stated intervals, as in a series of repeated tests for cardiac enzymes in blood samples taken from a patient with suspected myocardial infarction.

serial dilution, a laboratory technique in which a substance, such as blood serum, is decreased in concentration in a series of proportional amounts.

serial extraction, the extraction of selected primary teeth over a period of years, frequently ending with the removal of the first premolar teeth, to relieve crowding of the dental arches during eruption of the lateral incisors, canines, and premolars.

serial section [L, *series,* in a row, *sectio*], one of a number of consecutive slices of tissue.

serial speech, overlearned speech involving a series of words, such as counting or reciting of days of the week.

series /sir'ēs/, *pl.* **series** /sir'ēs/ [L, in a row], a chain of objects or events arranged in a predictable order, such as the series of stages through which a mature blood cell develops.

serine (Ser) /ser'ēn/, a nonessential amino acid found in many proteins in the body (for example, cassein, vitrellin). It is a precursor of the amino acids glycine and cysteine.

seroconversion /-kənvur'zhən/ [L, *serum,* whey, *conversio,* turned about], a change in serologic test results from negative to positive as antibodies develop in reaction to an infection or vaccine.

serodiagnosis /-dī'əgnō'sis/ [L, *serum,* whey; Gk, *dia,* through, *gnosis,* knowledge], the use of serologic tests in the diagnosis of disease.

serofibrinous pericarditis /-fī'brinəs/ [L, *serum,* whey, *fibra,* fibrin; Gk, *peri,* near, *kardia,* heart, *itis,* inflammation], a form of fibrinous pericarditis marked by a serous exudate.

serofibrinous pleurisy, an inflammation of the pleura with a watery effusion and accumulation of fibrin on the pleural membranes.

seroimmunity /sir'ō-imyoo'nitē/, immunity conferred by administration of an antiserum.

serologic /-loj'ik/ [L, *serum,* whey; Gk, *logos,* science], pertaining to the branch of medicine concerned with the study of blood sera.

serologic diagnosis /siroloj'ik/ [L, *serum,* whey; Gk, *dia,* through, *gnosis,* knowledge], a diagnosis that is made through laboratory examination of antigen-antibody reactions in the serum.

serologic test [L, *serum,* whey, *testum,* crucible], any diagnostic test made with serum.

serologist /sirol'əjist/ [L, *serum,* + Gk, *logos,* science], a bacteriologist or medical technologist who prepares or supervises the preparation of sera used to diagnose and treat diseases and to immunize people against infectious diseases.

serology /sirol'əjē/ [L, *serum* + Gk, *logos,* science], the branch of laboratory medicine that studies blood serum for evidence of infection by evaluating antigen-antibody reactions in vitro. **—serologic, serological,** *adj.*

seroma /sirō'mə/, a lump or swelling caused by an accumulation of serum within a tissue or organ.

seronegative /-neg'ətiv/ [L, *serum,* whey, *negare,* to deny], a serologic test with negative results.

seropositive /-pos'itiv/ [L, *serum,* whey, *positivus*], a serologic test with positive results.

seroprevalence /-prev'ələns/, the overall occurrence of a disease within a defined population at one time, as measured by blood tests. An example is human immunodeficiency virus seroprevalence.

seroprophylaxis /-prō′filak′sis/, the administration of a serum to prevent disease.

seropurulent /-pyŏŏ′ələnt/, containing serum and pus.

serosa /sirō′sə/ [L, *serum*], any serous membrane, such as the tunica serosa that lines the walls of body cavities and secretes a watery exudate.

serosanguineous /sir′ōsang·gwin′ē·əs/, (of a discharge) thin and red; composed of serum and blood.

serotonin /ser′ətō′nin, sir′-/ [L, *serum* + Gk, *tonos*, tone], a naturally occurring derivative of tryptophan found in platelets and in cells of the brain and the intestine. It acts as a potent vasoconstrictor and as a neurotransmitter.

serous [L, *serum, whey*], pertaining to, resembling, or producing serum.

serous fluid /sir′əs/ [L, *serum* + *fluere*, to flow], a fluid that has the characteristics of serum.

serous membrane, one of the many thin sheets of tissue that line closed cavities of the body, such as the pleura lining the thoracic cavity, the peritoneum lining the abdominal cavity, and the pericardium lining the sac that encloses the heart. Between the visceral layer of serous membrane covering various organs and the parietal layer lining the cavity containing such organs is a potential space moistened by serous fluid. The fluid reduces the friction of the structures covered by the serous membrane, such as the lungs, which move against the thoracic walls in respiration.

serovaccination /-vak′sinā′shən/, a technique for producing mixed immunity in which a person is first injected with a serum to establish passive immunity, then vaccinated to produce active immunity.

serpent ulcer /sur′pənt/ [L, *serpens,* snake], an ulceration of the skin that heals in one area while extending to another.

serrate /ser′āt/, having an edge with notches or sawlike teeth.

serrated suture /ser′ātid/, a suture with sawlike edges, such as most of the sagittal suture.

Serratia /serā′shə/ [L, *serra,* saw teeth], a genus of motile, gram-negative bacilli capable of causing infection in humans, including bacteremia, pneumonia, and urinary tract infections. *Serratia* organisms are frequently acquired in hospitals.

serratus anterior /serā′təs/ [L, *serra,* saw teeth], a thin muscle of the chest wall extending from the ribs under the arm to the scapula. It acts to rotate the scapula

and raise the shoulder, as in full flexion and abduction of the arm.

Sertoli cell /sertō′lē/ [Enrico Sertoli, Italian histologist, 1842–1910; L, *cella,* storeroom], one of the supporting cells of the seminiferous tubules of the testes. The cytoplasm of the cells contains spermatids.

Sertoli-cell-only syndrome [Enrico Sertoli], a form of male sterility in which only Sertoli cells are present in the seminiferous tubules of the testes. Germinal epithelium is absent, resulting in azoospermia.

serum /sir′əm/, *pl.* **sera** [L, *whey*], **1.** any serous fluid that moistens the surfaces of serous membranes. **2.** any clear watery fluid that has been separated from its more solid elements, such as the exudate from a blister. **3.** the clear, thin, and sticky fluid part of the blood that remains after coagulation. Serum contains no blood cells, platelets, or fibrinogen. **4.** a vaccine or toxoid prepared from the serum of a hyperimmune donor for prophylaxis against a particular infection or poison.

serum albumin, a major protein in blood plasma. It is important in maintaining the osmotic pressure of the blood.

serum bank, a facility for the storage of frozen samples of blood serum. The specimens are used mainly for medical research.

serum creatinine level, the concentration of creatinine in the serum, used as a diagnostic sign of possible renal impairment.

serumfast /sir′əmfast′/, **1.** resistant (as bacteria) to the destructive effects of sera. **2.** having (as a serum) little or no change in antibody titer.

serum globulin [L, *serum, whey, globulus,* small globe], a protein fraction of blood serum with antibody qualities. The several types of fractions, α, β, and γ, have different specific properties.

serum glutamic oxaloacetic transaminase (SGOT), a catalytic enzyme found in various parts of the body, especially the heart, liver, and muscle tissue. Increased amounts of the enzyme occur in the serum as a result of myocardial infarction, acute liver disease, the actions of certain drugs, and any disease or condition in which cells are seriously damaged.

serum glutamic pyruvic transaminase (SGPT), a catalytic enzyme normally found in high concentration in the liver. Greater than normal amounts in the serum indicate liver damage.

serum osmolality [L, *serum, whey;* Gk, *osmos,* impulse], pertaining to the osmotic concentration of blood serum, expressed in terms of ions of solute per unit of solution.

serum protein [L, *serum,* whey; Gk, *proteios,* first rank], any of the proteins in blood serum.

serum shock, a life-threatening reduction in blood volume and blood pressure caused by the injection of an antitoxic or other foreign serum.

serum sickness, an immunologic disorder that may occur 2 to 3 weeks after the administration of an antiserum. It is caused by an antibody reaction to an antigen in the donor serum. The condition is characterized by fever, splenomegaly, swollen lymph nodes, skin rash, and joint pain.

service dogs, dogs trained to aid disabled persons with such tasks as opening or closing doors, picking up dropped items, or pulling a wheelchair.

service of process /sur′vis/ [L, *servus,* a slave, *processus,* going forth], (in law) the delivery of a writ, summons, or complaint to a defendant. Once delivered or left with the party for whom it is intended, it is said to have been served.

servomechanism /sur′vōmek′əniz′əm/, a control system in which feedback is used to correct errors in another system. A biologic example is the mechanism that controls the size of the pupil of the eye as the intensity of light changes.

sesame oil /ses′əmē/, a liquid fat derived from the seeds of a plant, *Sesamum indicum.* The seeds are demulcent and have a laxative effect. Both seeds and oil are used as food flavorings. The oil is also used in skin lotions, as an emollient, and as a parenteral vehicle for intramuscular injections.

sesamoid /ses′əmoid/ [Gk, *sesamon,* sesame, *eidos,* form], nodular objects having the shape and size of sesame seeds.

sesamoid bone [Gk, *sesamon,* sesame, *eidos,* form], any one of numerous small round bony masses embedded in certain tendons that may be subjected to compression and tension. The largest sesamoid bone is the patella, which is embedded in the tendon of the quadriceps femoris at the knee.

sessile /ses′əl/ [L, *sessilis,* sitting], 1. (in biology) attached by a base rather than by a stalk or a peduncle, such as a leaf that is attached directly to its stem. 2. permanently connected.

set, 1. a predisposition to behave in a certain way. 2. to reduce a fracture by moving the bones back into a normal position.

setaceous /sētā′shəs/, having or resembling bristles.

setback, the surgical treatment of a bilateral cleft of the palate.

seton /sē′ton/, thread, gauze, or other material passed through subcutaneous tissue or a cyst to create a sinus or fistula.

settlement [AS, *setlan,* to put in place], (in law) an agreement made between parties to a suit before a judgment is rendered by a court.

setup [AS, *settan,* to set, *up,* on high], 1. an arrangement of artificial teeth on a trial denture base. 2. a laboratory procedure in which teeth are removed from a plaster cast and repositioned in wax. It is used as a diagnostic procedure and in creation of a mold for a positioner appliance.

severe combined immunodeficiency disease (SCID) /sivēr′/ [L, *servus,* slave], an abnormal condition characterized by the complete absence or marked deficiency of B cells and T cells with the consequent lack of humoral immunity and cell-mediated immunity. This disease occurs as an X-linked recessive disorder affecting only males and as an autosomal-recessive disorder affecting both males and females. It results in a pronounced susceptibility to infection and is usually fatal. The precise cause of SCID is not known, but research indicates it may be caused by a cytogenic dysfunction of the embryonic stem cells in differentiating B cells and T cells. The affected individual consequently has a very small thymus and little or no protection against infection.

sex [L, *sexus,* sex], 1. a classification of male or female based on many criteria, among them anatomic and chromosomal characteristics. 2. coitus.

sex chromatin, a densely staining mass within the nucleus of all nondividing cells of normal mammalian females. It represents the facultative heterochromatin of the inactivated X chromosome.

sex chromosome, a chromosome that is responsible for the sex determination of offspring; it carries genes that transmit sex-linked traits and conditions. In humans and other mammals there are two distinct sex chromosomes, the X and the Y chromosomes, which are unequally paired and appear in females in the XX combination and in males as XY.

sex chromosome mosaic, an individual or organism whose cells contain variant chromosomal numbers involving the X or Y chromosomes. Such variations occur in most of the syndromes associated with sex chromosome aberrations, primarily Turner's syndrome, and may be caused by nondisjunction of the chromosomes during the second meiotic division of gametogenesis or by some error in chromosome distribution during cell division of the fertilized ovum.

sex determination [L, *sexus,* sex, *deter-*

S

minare], an examination of the cellular differences between male and female organisms to find the XY chromosome combination in genetic male or the Barr body in genetic female chromosomes. Whole body differences include secondary sexual characteristics and skeletal variations.

sex deviant, a person whose sexual interests differ markedly from what is accepted as the norm.

sex-hormone-binding globulin (SHBG), a protein produced by the liver that binds testosterone and estradiol in the plasma. It has a greater affinity for testosterone. The plasma concentration of SHBG is influenced by liver cirrhosis, hyperthyroidism, obesity (in women), malnutrition, and estrogens.

sex hormones, any of the androgens, estrogens, or steroid substances produced by the testicular, ovarian, or adrenocortical tissues.

sexidigitate /sek′sidij′itāt/ [L, *sex,* six], having six digits on one or both hands and feet.

sex-influenced, pertaining to an autosomal genetic trait or condition, such as patterned baldness or gout, that in one sex is expressed phenotypically in both homozygotes and heterozygotes, whereas in the other a phenotypic effect is produced in homozygotes only.

sexism /sek′sizəm/, a belief that one sex is superior to the other and that the superior sex has endowments, rights, prerogatives, and status greater than those of the inferior sex. Sexism results in discrimination in all areas of life and acts as a limiting factor in educational, professional, and psychologic development. **—sexist,** *n., adj.*

sexivalent /sek′sivā′lənt/, pertaining to a chemical with a valence of 6.

sex-limited, pertaining to an autosomal genetic trait or condition that is expressed phenotypically in only one sex, although the genes for it may be carried by both sexes.

sex-linked, pertaining to genes or to the normal or abnormal characteristics or conditions they transmit. The genes are carried on the sex chromosomes, particularly the X chromosome. **—sex linkage,** *n.*

sex-linked disorder, any disease or abnormal condition that is determined by the sex chromosomes or a defective gene on a sex chromosome. These may involve a deviation in the number of either the X or Y chromosomes, as occurs in Turner's syndrome and Klinefelter's syndrome, most occurrences of which are a result of nondisjunction during meiosis.

sex-linked ichthyosis, a congenital skin disorder characterized by large thick dry scales with dark color; the scales cover the neck, scalp, ears, face, trunk, and flexor surfaces of the body, such as the folds of the arms and the backs of the knees. It is transmitted by females as an X-linked recessive trait and appears only in males.

sex ratio, the proportion of male-to-female progeny, a relationship that varies with the stage of life. The distribution at birth is usually 106 boys to 100 girls, but the ratio shifts in adulthood, so that, because men have a lower life expectancy, the proportion of females is greater. The ratio may also vary with the effects of a particular disease or trait.

sex role, the expectations held by society regarding what behavior is appropriate or inappropriate for each sex.

sex surrogate [L, *sexus* + *surrogare,* substitute], (in sex therapy) a professional substitute trained to help the patient overcome inhibitions.

sextuplet /seks′tup′lit/ [L, *sextus,* six], one of six children born of a single pregnancy.

sexual /sek′shoo·əl/, pertaining to sex.

sexual abuse, the sexual mistreatment of another person by fondling, rape, or forced participation in unnatural sex acts or other perverted behavior.

sexual asphyxia, accidental strangulation by ligature that occurs in an attempt to induce mild cerebral hypoxia during sexual activity for the purpose of enhancing orgasmic pleasure.

sexual assault, the forcible perpetration of an act of sexual contact on the body of another person, male or female, without his or her consent. Legal criteria vary among different communities.

sexual aversion disorder, a persistent or extreme aversion to or avoidance of all or nearly all genital sexual contact with a partner.

Sexual Counseling, a Nursing Interventions Classification defined as use of an interactive helping process focusing on the need to make adjustments in sexual practice or to enhance coping with a sexual event/disorder.

sexual dwarf, an adult dwarf whose genital organs are normally developed.

sexual dysfunction, a NANDA-accepted nursing diagnosis of the state in which an individual experiences a change in sexual function that is viewed as unsatisfying, unrewarding, or inadequate. Defining characteristics include a statement by the client of the perceived dysfunction, a physical alteration or limitation imposed by disease or treatment, a reported inability to achieve sexual satisfaction, an alteration in the sexual relationship with the partner, and a change in interest in oneself or in others.

sexual fantasy, mental images of an erotic nature that can lead to sexual arousal.

sexual generation, reproduction by the union of male and female gametes.

sexual harassment, an aggressive sexually motivated act of physical or verbal violation of a person over whom the aggressor has some power. Sexual harassment may be heterosexual or, as is common in prison, homosexual.

sexual health [L, *sexus* + AS, *haelth*], a condition defined by the World Health Organization as freedom from sexual diseases or disorders and a capacity to enjoy and control sexual behavior without fear, shame, or guilt.

sexual history, (in a patient record) the part of the patient's personal history concerned with sexual function and dysfunction. It may include the age at onset of sexual intercourse, the kind and frequency of sexual activity, and the satisfaction derived from it.

sexual hormones, chemical substances produced in the body that cause specific regulatory effects on the activity of reproductive organs.

sexuality /sek'shoo·al'itē/, **1.** the sum of the physical, functional, and psychologic attributes that are expressed by one's gender identity and sexual behavior, whether or not related to the sex organs or to procreation. **2.** the genital characteristics that distinguish male from female.

sexuality patterns, altered, a NANDA-accepted nursing diagnosis of the state in which an individual expresses concern regarding his or her sexuality. The major defining characteristics include reported difficulties, limitations, or changes in sexual behaviors or activities.

sexually deviant personality /sek'shoo·-əlē/, a sexual behavior that differs significantly from what is considered normal for a society.

sexually transmitted disease (STD), a contagious disease usually acquired by sexual intercourse or genital contact. Historically, the five venereal diseases were gonorrhea, syphilis, chancroid, granuloma inguinale, and lymphogranuloma venereum. To these have been added scabies, herpes genitalis and anorectal herpes and warts, pediculosis, trichomoniasis, genital candidiasis, molluscum contagiosum, nonspecific urethritis, chlamydial infections, cytomegalovirus, and human immunodeficiency virus.

sexual mores, socially acceptable sexual behavior, usually based on fixed morally binding customs governing sexual behaviors that are harmful to others or the group, such as rape, incest, and sexual abuse of children.

sexual orientation, the clear persistent desire of a person for affiliation with one sex rather than the other.

sexual psychopath, an individual whose sexual behavior is openly perverted, antisocial, and criminal.

sexual reassignment, a change in the gender identity of a person by legal, surgical, hormonal, or social means.

sexual reflex, (in males) a reflex in which tactile or cerebral stimulation results in penile erection, priapism, or ejaculation.

sexual reproduction [L, *sexus,* sex, *re* + *producere,* to produce], replication of an organism by the formation of gametes. Generally this requires the fusion of male spermatozoa and female ova; parthenogenesis is an exception.

sexual response cycle, the four phases of biologic sexual response: excitement, plateau, orgasm, and resolution.

sexual selection, the theory that mates are chosen according to the attraction of or preference for certain characteristics, such as coloration or behavior patterns, so that eventually only those particular traits appear in succeeding generations.

sexual tasks, specific skills learned in various phases of development in the life cycle continuum to allow an adult to function normally in the sexual realm.

sexual therapist, a health care professional with specialized knowledge, skill, and competence in assisting individuals who experience sexual difficulties.

sexual therapy, a type of counseling that aids in the resolution of pathologic conditions so that a healthy sexuality can be maintained.

Sézary's syndrome /sāzärēz'/ [A. Sézary, French dermatologist, 1880–1956], a condition of generalized exfoliating erythroderma, lymphadenopathy, and abnormal circulating T cells. The patient experiences pruritus, alopecia, edema, and nail and pigment changes.

sfc, abbreviation for *spinal fluid count.*

SFD, abbreviation for *small for dates.*

Sg, abbreviation for **seaborgium,** element 106.

SGA, abbreviation for **small for gestational age.**

SGOT, abbreviation for **serum glutamic oxaloacetic transaminase.**

SGPT, abbreviation for **serum glutamic pyruvic transaminase.**

shadow /shad'ō/ [AS, *sceadu*], (in psychology) an archetype that represents the unacceptable aspects and components of behavior.

shadowcasting, a technique for enhancing the visualization of a contoured microscopic specimen, in which a chemical film is deposited on it, making it more visible in relief.

shaft, an elongated cylindric object, such as a long bone between the epiphyses.

shaken baby syndrome, a condition of whiplash-type injuries, ranging from bruises on the arms and trunk to retinal hemorrhages, coma, or convulsions, as observed in infants and children who have been violently shaken. This form of child abuse often results in intracranial bleeding from tearing of cerebral blood vessels.

shakes /shāks/, a popular term for the rigor, tremors, or shivering that occurs in intermittent fever or after drug withdrawal.

shake test, a "foam" test for fetal lung maturity. It is more rapid than determination of the lecithin/sphingomyelin ratio.

shallow breathing /shal'ō/ [ME, *schalowe,* little depth], a respiration pattern marked by slow, shallow, and generally ineffective inspirations and expirations. It is usually caused by drugs and indicates depression of the medullary respiratory centers.

shank, 1. the tibia. **2.** the part of a device that connects the functional part to a handle.

shaping [AS, *scieppan,* to shape], a procedure used for conditioning a person undergoing behavior therapy to develop new behavioral responses.

shared governance, an organized, systematic approach to decision making that enables all levels of nurses to participate in the resolution of clinical, professional, and administrative practice issues.

shared paranoid disorder [AS, *scearan,* to shear], a psychopathologic condition characterized by identical manifestations of the same mental disorder, usually ideas, in two closely associated or related people.

shared services, administrative, clinical, or other service functions that are common to two or more hospitals or other health care facilities and that are used jointly or cooperatively by them.

Sharpey's fiber [William Sharpey, Scottish anatomist, 1802–1880], (in dentistry) any one of the many collagenous bundles of fibers of the periodontal ligament that have become embedded in the cementum during its formation.

sharps, any needles, scalpels, or other articles that could cause wounds or punctures to personnel handling them.

shaving stroke [AS, *scafan,* to shave, *stri-can,* to stroke], a phase of the working stroke of a periodontal curet, used for smoothing or planing a tooth or tooth root surface.

SHBG, abbreviation for **sex-hormone-binding globulin.**

SHCC, abbreviation for **Statewide Health Coordinating Committee.**

shear /shir/ [AS, *scearan,* to cut], an applied force or pressure exerted against the surface and layers of the skin as tissues slide in opposite but parallel planes.

shearling /shir'ling/, a sheepskin placed on a bed to help prevent decubitus ulcers.

sheath /shēth/ [AS, *scaeth*], a tubular structure that surrounds an organ or any other part of the body, such as the sheath of the rectus abdominis muscle.

sheath of Schwann [Theodor Schwann, German anatomist, 1810–1882; AS, *scaeth*], a neurilemma sheath of nucleated cells enclosing a nerve fiber.

Sheehan's syndrome [Harold L. Sheehan, English pathologist, b. 1900], a postpartum condition of pituitary necrosis and hypopituitarism after circulatory collapse resulting from uterine hemorrhaging.

sheep cell agglutination test (SCAT), a test for the presence of the rheumatoid factor in blood serum, using red blood cells of sheep that have been sensitized against rabbit antisheep erythrocyte immune globulin. The globulin will be agglutinated if the serum contains the rheumatoid factor.

sheep cell test [AS, *sceap* + L, *cella,* storeroom, *testum,* crucible], a method that mixes human blood cells with the red blood cells of sheep to determine the absence or the deficiency of human T lymphocytes. When mixed with human blood cells, the red blood cells of sheep cluster around the human T lymphocytes and form characteristic rosettes.

sheet bath [AS, *scete* + *baeth*], the application of wet sheets to the body, used primarily as an antipyretic procedure.

sheet wadding, stretchable sheets of cotton padding used to cover the skin before a cast is applied. The stretching allows for some extremity edema without the cast becoming too tight.

shelf [AS, *scylf*], a flat, hard anatomic structure that resembles a ridge or platform.

shell [AS, *scell*], **1.** a hard outer protective covering that encloses material. **2.** an electron orbit surrounding the nucleus of an atom.

shellfish poisoning [AS, *scell* + *fisc*], a toxic neurologic condition that results from eating clams, oysters, or mussels that have ingested the toxin-producing protozoa commonly called the "red tide." The characteristic symptoms appear within a few minutes and include nausea, light-headedness, vomiting, and tingling or numbness around the mouth, followed by paralysis of the extremities and, possibly, respiratory paralysis. Saxitoxin, the causative agent, is not destroyed by cooking.

shell shock [AS, *scell* + Fr, *choc*], any of a number of mental disorders, ranging from extreme fear to dementia, commonly attributed to the noise and concussion of exploding shells or bombs but actually a traumatic reaction to the stress of combat.

shell teeth, a type of dental dysplasia characterized by large pulp chambers, insufficient coronal dentin, and usually no roots.

sheltered workshop [ME, *sheltrun,* body of guards; AS, *werc* + *sceoppa,* stall], a facility or program, either for outpatients or for residents of an institution, that provides vocational experience in a controlled working environment.

shield [AS, *scild*], (in radiation technology) a material for preventing or reducing the passage of charged particles or radiation. A shield may be designated by the radiation it is intended to absorb, such as a gamma ray shield, or according to the kind of protection it is intended to give, such as a background, biologic, or thermal shield.

shift [AS, *sciftan,* to divide], **1.** (in nursing) the particular hours of the day during which a nurse is scheduled to work. The evening shift is also called "relief," presumably because nurses originally worked 12-hour shifts and the evening and night shift was thought to be relief for the day nurse. **2.** an abrupt change in an analytic system that continues at the new level.

Shift Report, a Nursing Interventions Classification defined as exchanging essential patient care information with other nursing staff at change of shift.

shift to the left, (in hematology) a predominance of immature leukocytes, noted in a differential white blood cell count. The term derives from a graph of blood components in which immature cell frequencies appear on the left side of the graph.

shift to the right, (in hematology) a preponderance of polymorphonuclear neutrophils having three or more lobes, indicating maturity of the cell. It indicates a relative lack of blood-forming activity.

Shigella /shigel′ə/ [Kiyoshi Shiga, Japanese bacteriologist, 1870–1957], a genus of gram-negative pathogenic bacteria that causes gastroenteritis and bacterial dysentery, such as *Shigella dysenteriae.*

Shigella dysenteriae, a species of the bacterial family Enterobacteriaceae that causes a severe form of dysentery in humans. The *dysenteriae* subgroup of *Shigella* is most common in Asia and is particularly virulent.

shigellosis /shig′əlō′sis/ [Kiyoshi Shiga, Gk, *osis,* condition], an acute bacterial infection of the bowel, characterized by diarrhea, abdominal pain, and fever. It is transmitted by hand-to-mouth contact with the feces of individuals infected with bacteria of a pathogenic species of the genus *Shigella.* These organisms may be carried in the stools of asymptomatic people for up to several months and may be spread through contact with contaminated objects, food, or flies, especially in poor, crowded areas.

shim, a thin tapered piece of material used to fill a gap.

shin splints [AS, *scinu,* shin; ME, *splinte*], a painful condition of the lower leg caused by strain of the long flexor muscle of the toes after strenuous athletic activity, such as running.

Shirodkar's operation /shir′odkärz′/, [N. V. Shirodkar, Indian obstetrician, 1900–1971], a surgical procedure called a cerclage in which the cervical canal is closed by a purse-string suture embedded in the uterine cervix encircling the canal. It is performed to correct an incompetent cervix that has failed to retain previous pregnancies. If labor begins with the suture in place, the suture is removed promptly, or the infant is delivered by cesarean section, before the uterus ruptures.

shivering /shiv′əring/, involuntary contractions of muscles, mainly of the skin, in response to the chilling effect of low temperatures. Shivering may also occur at the onset of a fever when the body's heat balance is disturbed.

shock [Fr, *choc*], an abnormal condition of inadequate blood flow to the body's peripheral tissues, with life-threatening cellular dysfunction. The condition is usually associated with inadequate cardiac output, hypotension, oliguria, changes in peripheral blood flow resistance and distribution, and tissue damage. Causal factors include hemorrhage, vomiting, diarrhea, inadequate fluid intake, or excessive renal loss, resulting in hypovolemia. Hypovolemic shock is the most common. There is decreased blood flow with a resulting reduction in the delivery of oxygen, nutrients, hormones, and electrolytes to the body's tissues and a concomitant decreased removal of metabolic wastes. Pulse and respirations are increased. Blood pressure may decline after an initial slight increase. The patient often shows signs of restless-

S

ness and anxiety, an effect related to decreased blood flow to the brain. There also may be weakness, lethargy, pallor, and a cool, moist skin. As shock progresses, the body temperature falls, respirations become rapid and shallow, and the pulse pressure (the difference between systolic and diastolic blood pressures) narrows as compensatory vasoconstriction causes the diastolic pressure to be elevated or maintained in the face of a falling systolic blood pressure. Urinary output is reduced. Hemorrhage may be apparent or concealed, although other factors such as vomiting or diarrhea may account for the deficiency of body fluids.

Shock Management, a Nursing Interventions Classification defined as facilitation of the delivery of oxygen and nutrients to systemic tissue with removal of cellular waste products in a patient with severely altered tissue perfusion.

Shock Management: Cardiac, a Nursing Interventions Classification defined as promotion of adequate tissue perfusion for a patient with severely compromised pumping function of the heart.

Shock Management: Vasogenic, a Nursing Interventions Classification defined as promotion of adequate tissue perfusion for a patient with a severe loss of vascular tone.

Shock Management: Volume, a Nursing Interventions Classification defined as promotion of adequate tissue perfusion for a patient with severely compromised intravascular volume.

Shock Prevention, a Nursing Interventions Classification defined as detecting and treating a patient at risk for impending shock.

shock therapy [Fr, *choc* + GK, *therapeia*], a psychotherapeutic procedure for treating depression and other severe disorders by producing an epileptiform convulsion in the patient. The shock is induced by delivering an electric current through the brain.

shock trousers, pneumatic trousers designed to counteract hypotension associated with internal or external bleeding and hypovolemia. Shock trousers may be contraindicated in patients with pulmonary edema, cardiogenic shock, increased intracranial pressure, or eviscerations. The shock trousers are required when the patient loses consciousness, has a decreased or falling blood pressure, and shows signs of respiratory distress such as dyspnea, rapid breathing, a cough, and pink, frothy sputum. The leg pulses may be diminished or absent, and the feet may appear pale, mottled, and cold.

short-acting [AS, *sceort* + L, *agere,* to do], pertaining to or characterizing a therapeutic agent, usually a drug, with a brief period of effectiveness, generally beginning soon after the substance or measure is administered.

short-acting insulin, a clear preparation of regular (crystalline zinc) insulin with an immediate (15 to 30 minutes) onset of action that reaches a peak of action in 2 to 4 hours. The duration of action is 6 to 8 hours. Semilente insulin is another short-acting (rapid-acting) insulin preparation that contains zinc insulin microcrystals in an acetate buffer. Its onset is within 1 hour, with a peak of action in 4 to 6 hours and a duration of action of 12 to 16 hours.

shortage area /shôr'tij/ [AS, *sceort* + L, *acticum,* process], a geographic area, county as a census tract, or area designated by the federal government as being undersupplied with certain kinds of health care services; a shortage area may be eligible for aid under certain federal programs, including the National Health Service Corps or the Rural Clinics Assistance Act.

short-arm cast, an orthopedic cast applied to immobilize the hand or the wrist. The short-arm cast incorporates the hand below the wrist; it is used in treating fractures, for postoperative positioning, and for correction or maintenance of correction of deformities of the hand and the wrist.

short bones, bones that occur in clusters and usually permit movement of the extremities, such as the carpals and tarsals.

short-bowel syndrome [AS, *sceort* + OFr, *boel* + Gk, *syn,* together, *dromos,* course], a loss of intestinal surface for absorption of nutrients caused by the surgical removal of a section of bowel.

short course tuberculosis chemotherapy, a 6-month treatment regimen for patients with tuberculosis who would otherwise continue to receive medications for at least 18 to 24 months after sputum has a negative finding for tubercle bacilli. The short course requires a combination of four drugs: isoniazid, rifampin, pyrazinamide, and either ethambutol, or streptomycin.

short-gut syndrome, a congenital disorder in which an infant's intestine is too short or underdeveloped to allow normal food digestion. The child is maintained on parenteral nutrition until the intestine grows, develops further, or is replaced by surgical transplantation.

shorting [AS, *sceort*], the fraudulent practice of dispensing a quantity of drug less than that called for in the prescription and of charging for the quantity specified in the prescription.

short-leg cast, an orthopedic cast used for immobilizing fractures in the lower extremities from the toes to the knee.

short-leg cast with walker, an orthopedic cast with rubber walkers on the bottom. It immobilizes the leg from the toes to the knee and allows the patient to walk.

Short Portable Mental Status Questionnaire, a 10-item questionnaire used to screen older adults for cognitive impairment. It tests orientation, remote and recent memory, practical skills, and mathematic ability.

short stature [AS, *sceort,* short; L, *statura,* man's height], a body height that is less than 70% of the average for a population of the same age, culture, gender, and other peer factors.

short-term memory, memory of recent events.

short-wave diathermy [AS, *sceort* + *wafian* + Gk, *dia* + *therme,* heat], a method of providing heat deep in the body by short-wave electrical currents. The high-frequency short-wave uses wavelengths of from 3 to 30 meters. It is used to treat chronic arthritis, bursitis, sinusitis, and other conditions.

shotgun therapy [AS, *scot* + ME, *gonne* + Gk, *therapeia,* treatment], *informal.* any treatment that has a wide range of effects and that therefore can be expected to correct an abnormal condition, even though the particular cause is unknown.

shoulder [AS, *sculder*], the junction of the clavicle, scapula, and humerus where the arm attaches to the trunk of the body.

shoulder girdle [AS, *sculder* + *gyrdel*], a partial arch at the top of the trunk formed by the scapula and clavicle.

shoulder-hand syndrome, a neuromuscular condition characterized by pain and stiffness in the shoulder and arm, limited joint motion, swelling of the hand, muscle atrophy, and decalcification of the underlying bones.

shoulder joint, the ball and socket articulation of the humerus with the scapula. The joint includes eight bursae and five ligaments. It is the most mobile joint in the body.

shoulder presentation [AS, *sculder* + L, *praesentare,* to show], the part of the fetus that occupies the center of the birth canal when the presentation is associated with a transverse or oblique lie.

shoulder spica cast, an orthopedic cast applied to immobilize the trunk of the body to the hips, the wrist, and the hand. It is used in the treatment of shoulder dislocations and injuries and in the positioning and immobilization of the shoulder after surgery.

shoulder subluxation, the separation of the humeral head from the glenoid cavity, resulting in strain on the soft tissues surrounding the joint.

shreds [AS, *screade,* piece cut off], glossy filaments of mucus in the urine, indicating inflammation in the urinary tract.

shunt [ME, *shunten*], **1.** to redirect the flow of a body fluid from one cavity or vessel to another. **2.** a tube or device implanted in the body to redirect a body fluid from one cavity or vessel to another.

shu points /sho͞o/, acupressure points.

Shy-Drager's syndrome /shī'drā'gər/ [G. Milton Shy, American neurologist, 1919–1967; Glenn A. Drager, American physician, b. 1917], a rare progressive neurologic disorder of young and middle-aged adults. It is characterized by orthostatic hypotension, bladder and bowel incontinence, atrophy of the iris, anhidrosis, tremor, rigidity, incoordination, ataxia, and muscle wasting.

Si, symbol for the element **silicon.**

SI, abbreviation for *Système International d'Unités,* the French name for the **International System of Units.**

SIADH, abbreviation for **syndrome of inappropriate antidiuretic hormone secretion.**

sialadenitis /sī'əlad'ənī'tis/, any inflammation of one or more of the salivary glands.

sialemesis /sī'ələmē'sis/, vomiting of saliva, or vomiting associated with excessive salivation.

sialidosis /sī'əlidō'sis/, a neuronal storage disease of children caused by a deficiency of the enzyme sialidase (neuraminidase). The condition is characterized by a cherry-red spot on the macula, progressive myoclonus, and seizures. There are two types. Type 1 patients have normal physical features and beta galactosidase levels; type 2 patients also have short stature, bony abnormalities, and beta-galactosidase deficiency.

sialogogue /sī·al'əgog'/ [Gk, *sialon,* saliva, *agogos,* leading], anything that stimulates, promotes, or produces the secretion of saliva.

sialogram /sī·al'əgram'/ [Gk, *sialon,* saliva, *gramma,* record], a radiographic image of the salivary glands and ducts.

sialography /sī·əlog'rəfē/ [Gk, *sialon* + *graphein,* to record], (in radiology) a technique in which a salivary gland is filmed after injection of a radiopaque contrast medium. —**sialographic,** *adj.*

sialolith /sī·al'əlith/ [Gk, *sialon* + *lithos,* stone], a calculus formed in a salivary gland or duct.

sialolithiasis /-lithī'əsis/, a pathologic

S

condition in which one or more calculi or stones are formed in a salivary gland.

sialorrhea /sī·al'ərē'ə/ [Gk, *sialon* + *rhoia,* flow], an excessive flow of saliva that may be associated with various conditions, such as acute inflammation of the mouth, mental retardation, mercurialism, pregnancy, teething, alcoholism, or malnutrition.

Siamese twins /sī'əmēz/ [Chang and Eng, conjoined twins born in Siam (now Thailand) in 1811], conjoined, equally developed twin fetuses produced from the same ovum. The severity of the condition ranges from superficial fusion, such as of the umbilical vessels, to that in which the heads or complete torsos are united and several internal organs are shared.

sib [AS, *sibb,* kin], pertaining to a close blood relationship.

Siberian tick typhus /sībir'ē·ən/ [Siberia], a mild acute febrile illness seen in north, central, and east Asia, caused by *Rickettsia siberica,* transmitted by ticks. It is characterized by a diffuse maculopapular rash, headache, conjunctival inflammation, and a small ulcer or eschar at the site of the tick bite.

sibilant /sib'īlənt/ [L, *sibilare,* to hiss], a hissing sound or one in which the predominant sound is that of *S.*

sibling /sib'ling/ [AS, *sibb,* kin], **1.** one of two or more children who have both parents in common; a brother or sister. **2.** pertaining to a brother or sister.

Sibling Support, a Nursing Interventions Classification defined as assisting a sibling to cope with a brother's or sister's illness.

sibship /sib'ship/ [AS *sibb,* kin, *scieppan,* to shape], **1.** the state of being related by blood. **2.** a group of people descended from a common ancestor who are used as a basis for genetic studies. **3.** brothers and sisters considered as a group.

sic [L], thus.

sicca complex /sik'ə/, abnormal dryness of the mouth, eyes, or other mucous membranes. The condition is seen in patients with Sjögren's syndrome, sarcoidosis, amyloidosis, and deficiencies of vitamins A and C.

siccant /sik'ənt/ [L, *siccus,* dry], **1.** drying, removing moisture. **2.** an agent that promotes drying.

sick, experiencing symptoms of physical illness such as nausea, aches and pains, dizziness, weakness, blurred vision, or malaise.

sick building syndrome, a condition characterized by fatigue, headache, dry eyes, and respiratory complaints affecting workers in certain buildings with limited ventilation. The symptoms seem to be caused by a combination of chemical agents in low concentrations rather than a specific irritant.

sick cell syndrome, a condition characterized by idiopathic hyponatremia in patients with either acute or chronic illness.

sick euthyroid syndrome, a nonthyroidal condition characterized by abnormalities in hormone levels and function test findings related to the thyroid gland. The condition occurs in patients with severe systemic disease.

sickle cell [AS, *sicol,* crescent; L, *cella,* storeroom], an abnormal crescent-shaped red blood cell containing hemoglobin S, characteristic of sickle cell anemia.

sickle cell anemia, a severe chronic incurable hemoglobinopathic anemic condition that occurs in people homozygous for hemoglobin S. The abnormal hemoglobin results in distortion and fragility of the erythrocytes. Sickle cell anemia is characterized by crises of joint pain, thrombosis, and fever and by chronic anemia, with splenomegaly, lethargy, and weakness.

sickle cell crisis, an acute episodic condition that occurs in children with sickle cell anemia. The crisis may be vasoocclusive, resulting from the aggregation of misshapen erythrocytes, or anemic, resulting from bone marrow aplasia, increased hemolysis, folate deficiency, or splenic sequestration of erythrocytes. Painful vasoocclusive crisis is the most common of the sickle cell crises. It is usually preceded by an upper respiratory or gastrointestinal infection without an exacerbation of anemia. The clumps of sickled erythrocytes obstruct blood vessels, resulting in occlusion, ischemia, and infarction of adjacent tissue. Characteristics of this kind of crisis are leukocytosis, acute abdominal pain from visceral hypoxia, painful swelling of the soft tissue of the hands and feet (hand-foot syndrome), and migratory, recurrent, or constant joint pain, often so severe that movement of the joint is limited. Persistent headache, dizziness, convulsions, visual or auditory disturbances, facial nerve palsies, coughing, shortness of breath, and tachypnea may occur if the central nervous system or lungs are affected.

sickle cell dactylitis [AS, *sicol* + L, *cella,* storeroom; Gk, *daktylos,* finger, *itis,* inflammation], a painful inflammation of one or more fingers caused by an attack of sickle cell anemia.

sickle cell thalassemia, a heterozygous blood disorder in which the genes for sickle cell and for thalassemia are both inherited. A mild and a severe form may be identified, depending on the degree of suppression of beta-chain synthesis by the thalassemia gene. In the mild form synthesis is only partially suppressed. In the severe form beta-chain synthesis is completely suppressed, and only hemoglobin S appears in the red cells. The clinical course is generally as severe as in homozygous sickle cell anemia.

sickle cell trait, the heterozygous form of sickle cell anemia, characterized by the presence of both hemoglobin S and hemoglobin A in the red blood cells. Anemia and the other signs of sickle cell anemia do not occur. People who have the trait are informed of and counseled about the possibility of having an infant with sickle cell disease if both parents have the trait.

sickling, the development of sickle-shaped red blood cells, as in sickle cell anemia.

sick role [AS, *seoc* + Fr, stage character], a behavior pattern in which a person adopts the symptoms of a physical or mental disorder to be cared for, sympathized with, and protected from the demands and stresses of life.

sick sinus syndrome (SSS) [AS, *seoc* + L, *sinus,* hollow], a complex of arrhythmias associated with sinus node dysfunction. The condition may result from a variety of cardiac diseases. It is characterized by severe sinus bradycardia alone, sinus bradycardia alternating with tachycardia, or sinus bradycardia with atrioventricular block. The most common symptoms are lethargy, weakness, light-headedness, dizziness, and episodes of near-syncope or actual loss of consciousness.

SICU, abbreviation for *surgical intensive care unit.*

side effect [AS, *side* + L, *effectus*], any reaction to or consequence of a medication or therapy. Usually, although not necessarily, the effect is undesirable and may manifest itself as nausea, dry mouth, dizziness, blood dyscrasias, blurred vision, discolored urine, or tinnitus.

sideroblast /sid′ərōblast′/ [Gk, *sideros,* iron, *blastos,* germ], an iron-rich nucleated red blood cell in the bone marrow.

sideroblastic anemia /sid′ərōblas′tik/ [Gk, *sideros,* iron, *blastos,* germ], a heterogeneous group of chronic hematologic disorders characterized by normocytic or slightly macrocytic anemia, hypochromic and normochromic red blood cells, and decreased erythropoiesis and hemoglobin synthesis. The red blood cells contain a perinuclear ring of iron-stained granules. The condition may be acquired or hereditary, and primary or secondary to another condition.

siderocyte /sid′ərosīt′/ [Gk, *sideros,* iron, *kytos,* cell], an abnormal erythrocyte in which particles of nonhemoglobin iron are visible.

sideroderma /sid′ərōdur′mə/, a bronze skin coloration caused by accumulation of iron from hemoglobin degeneration.

sideropenia /sid′ərōpē′nē-ə/, an abnormally low level of serum iron.

siderosis /sid′ərō′sis/ [Gk, *sideros* + *osis,* condition], **1.** a variety of pneumoconiosis caused by the inhalation of iron dust or particles. **2.** the introduction of color in any tissue caused by the presence of excess iron. **3.** an increase in the amount of iron in the blood.

siderotic granules /sid′ərot′ik/, inclusion bodies seen in the red blood cells of splenectomy patients and in cases of hemoglobin synthesis and hemolytic anemia. The granules contain iron.

siderotic splenomegaly, an enlarged spleen associated with fibrosis and an excessive accumulation of iron and calcium. The condition is seen in sickle cell disease and hematochromatosis.

SIDS, abbreviation for **sudden infant death syndrome.**

SIECUS /sē′kəs/, abbreviation for *Sex Information and Education Council of the United States.*

siemen (S) /sē′mens/ [Sir William Siemens, German-born British engineer, 1823–1883], a unit of electrical conductance of a body with a resistance of 1 ohm, allowing 1 ampere of current to flow per volt applied.

sievert (Sv) /sē′vərt/ [R. M. Sievert, twentieth-century Swedish physicist], a unit-dose-equivalent radiation. The sievert has identical units to the gray and is determined by multiplying the absorbed dose by the quality factor, a number that has been determined to compare the health consequences of that type of radiation with x-rays.

sig., abbreviation for the Latin *signetur,* 'let it be labeled (according to prescription).'

sigh, a deep breath that may be 1.5 times the normal V_t. It plays a role in pulmonary hygiene.

sight /sīt/ [AS, *gesiht*], **1.** the special sense that enables the shape, size, position, and color of objects to be perceived; the faculty of vision. It is the principal function of the eye. **2.** that which is seen.

sigma, /sig′mə/, Σ, σ or **s,** the eighteenth letter of the Greek alphabet.

Sigma Theta Tau International /sig′mə thā′tə tou′/, an international honor society for nurses.

sigmoid /sig′moid/ [Gk, *sigma,* S-shaped, *eidos,* form], **1.** pertaining to an S shape. **2.** the sigmoid colon.

S

sigmoid colon, the part of the colon that extends from the end of the descending colon in the pelvis to the juncture of the rectum.

sigmoidectomy /sig'moidek'təmē/ [Gk, *sigma* + *eidos* + *ektome*, excision], excision of the sigmoid flexure of the colon, most commonly performed to remove a malignant tumor.

sigmoiditis /sig'moidī'tis/, an inflammation of the sigmoid colon.

sigmoid mesocolon /mez'ōkō'lən/ [Gk, *sigma* + *eidos* + *mesos*, middle, *kolon*], a fold of peritoneum that connects the sigmoid colon with the pelvic wall.

sigmoid notch, a concavity on the superior surface of the mandibular ramus between the coronoid and condyloid processes.

sigmoidoscope /sigmoi'dəskōp'/ [Gk, *sigma* + *eidos* + *skopein*, to look], an instrument used to examine the lumen of the sigmoid colon. It consists of a tube and a light, allowing direct visualization of the mucous membrane lining the colon.

sigmoidoscopy /sig'moidos'kəpē/, the inspection of the rectum and sigmoid colon by the aid of a sigmoidoscope.

sigmoidostomy /sig'moidos'təmē/, the surgical creation of an anus in the pelvic colon.

sign /sīn/ [L, *signum*, mark], an objective finding as perceived by an examiner, such as a fever, a rash, or the whisper heard over the chest in pleural effusion. Many signs accompany symptoms; for example, erythema and a maculopapular rash are often seen with pruritus.

signal molecule /sig'nəl/ [L, *signum*, mark], a hormone, neurotransmitter, or other agent that transfers information from one cell or organ to another. Examples include steroid hormones, insulin, and growth factors.

signal-to-noise ratio (SNR), the number used to describe the relative contributions to a detected signal of the true signal and random superimposed signals or "noise."

signature /sig'nəchər/ [L, *signare*, to mark], (in pharmacy) a part of a prescription containing instructions to the patient about dosage and manner and frequency of administration.

significance /signif'ikəns/ [L, *significare*, to signify], **1.** (in research) the statistical probability that a given finding may have occurred by chance alone. **2.** the importance of a study in developing a practice or theory, as in nursing practice.

significant other /signif'ikənt/, a person who is considered by an individual as being special and as having an effect on that individual.

sign language [L, *signum* + *lingua*, tongue], a form of communication often used with and among deaf people consisting of hand and body movements. Many variations exist, including American Sign Language (**Ameslan**). Other forms of manual communication are Signed English and finger spelling.

silanization /sil'ənizā'shən/, (in chromatography) the chemical process of converting the SiOH moieties of a stationary form to the ester form.

silent disease /sī'lənt/ [L, *silens* + *dis* + Fr, *aise*, ease], a disease or other disorder that produces no clinically obvious signs or symptoms.

silent ischemia [L, *silere*, to be silent], an asymptomatic form of myocardial ischemia that may result in damage to heart muscle. The supply of oxygenated blood is most likely to be decreased during the first 6 hours after awakening in the morning.

silent mutation, (in molecular genetics) an alteration in a sequence of nucleotides that does not result in an amino acid change.

silent myocardial infarction, an interruption in blood flow to the coronary arteries without the usual signs and symptoms of a heart attack. Such infarctions may be associated with diabetes.

silent peritonitis [L, *silere* + Gk, *peri* + *tenein*, to stretch, *itis*, inflammation], a case of peritonitis that develops without clinical signs or symptoms.

silhouette sign /sil'oo·et'/, a radiographic artifact caused by an infiltrate that obscures the demarcating line between lung segments.

silica gel /sil'ikə/, a coagulated form of hydrated silica, used as an absorbent of gases and a dehydrating agent.

silicic acid /silis'ik/, hydrated silicon dioxide. It is used in thin-layer and column chromatography.

silicon (Si) /sil'ikon/ [L, *silex*, flint], a nonmetallic element, second to oxygen as the most abundant of the elements in earth's crust. Its atomic number is 14; its atomic mass (weight) is 28.09. It occurs in nature as silicon dioxide and in silicates. The silicates are used as detergents, corrosion inhibitors, adhesives, and sealants.

silicone /sil'ikōn/ [L, *silex*, flint], any of a large group of inert polymers. Siclicones are useful in medicine as adhesives, lubricants, and sealants. They are also used as a substitute for rubber, especially in prosthetic devices.

silicone-gel breast implant, a type of implant used in reconstructive surgery of the breast and made with synthetic polymers.

The implants have been associated with adverse effects on the immune system as well as distorted and painful breasts caused by leakage of the silicone into surrounding tissues. However, a number of statistical studies have not established, such as cause-and-effect relationship.

silicone septum, a vascular access device used in intravenous therapy. It consists of a silicone partition that covers the port chamber housed in the metal or plastic body of an implanted infusion port.

silicosis /sil'ikō'sis/, a lung disorder caused by continued long-term inhalation of the dust of an inorganic compound, silicon dioxide, which is found in sands, quartzes, flints, and many other stones. Silicosis is characterized by the development of nodular fibrosis in the lungs. In advanced cases severe dyspnea may develop.

silk suture [AS, *seolc* + L, *sutura,* seam], a braided fine suture material, usually used to close incisions, wounds, and cuts in the skin. It is not absorbed by the body and is removed after approximately 7 days.

silo filler's disease /sī'lō/ [Fr, *ensilotage,* ensilage; AS, *fyllan,* to fill], a rare acute respiratory condition seen in agricultural workers who have inhaled nitrogen oxide as they work with fermented fodder in closed, poorly ventilated areas such as silos. Characteristically, symptoms of respiratory distress and pulmonary edema occur several hours after exposure. Loss of consciousness may occur.

silver (Ag) [AS, *seolfor*], a whitish precious metal occurring mainly as a sulfide. Its atomic number is 47; its atomic mass (weight) is 107.88. Silver nitrate is also used externally as an antiseptic and astringent, especially in the prevention of ophthalmia neonatorum. It is also used as a lubricant on the bearings of radiography tubes, and silver halides are used in x-ray films. Silver picrate, an ionizable salt of silver, is used in the treatment of trichomoniasis and of moniliasis of the vagina.

silver amalgam [AS, *seolfor* + Gk, *malagma*], an alloy of silver, tin, copper, mercury, and zinc used in dentistry to fill prepared tooth cavities.

silver cone method, (in dentistry) a technique for filling tooth root canals that is outdated because the silver corrodes over time and retreatment is necessary.

Silver dwarf [Henry K. Silver, twentieth-century American pediatrician], a person who has Silver's syndrome, a congenital disorder in which short stature is associated with lateral asymmetry; various anomalies of the head, face, and skeleton; and precocious puberty.

Silverman-Anderson score, a system of assessing the degree of respiratory distress.

silver nitrate, a topical antiinfective. A 1% solution is prescribed for the prevention of gonococcal ophthalmia in newborns and stronger concentrations for use on wet dressings.

silver salts poisoning, a toxic condition caused by the ingestion of silver nitrate, characterized by discoloration of the lips, vomiting, abdominal pain, dizziness, and convulsions.

silver sulfadiazine, a topical antimicrobial prescribed to prevent or treat infection in second-and third-degree burns.

silver-wire arteries, retinal arterioles that appear as white tubes containing a red fluid when viewed through an ophthalmoscope. The condition occurs as replacement fibrosis associated with hypertension continues and the vessel wall obscures the blood column.

simethicone /simeth'ikōn/, an antiflatulent prescribed to decrease excess gas in the gastrointestinal tract.

simian crease /sim'ē·ən/ [L, *simia,* ape; ME, *creste,* crest], a single crease across the palm produced from the fusion of proximal and distal palmar creases, seen in congenital disorders such as Down's syndrome.

simian immunodeficiency virus (SIV), a lentivirus that produces an acquired immunodeficiency syndrome-like disease in primates. The cytopathologic changes caused by SIV are similar to those caused by the human immunodeficiency virus (HIV). SIV also shares with HIV a group of genes lacking in other retroviruses, and animals infected with either virus experience a similar decrease in the number of CD4+ lymphocytes.

simian virus 40, a vacuolating virus isolated from the kidney tissue of rhesus monkeys.

similia similibus curantur, a homeopathic rule that drugs able to produce symptoms in a healthy person will also remove similar symptoms occurring as an expression of disease.

simplate bleeding time test, a blood test for determining how quickly platelets form a plug when exposed to air. Platelet plug formation is the first step in clotting.

simple, 1. describing something composed of only one or a minimum number of parts or elements. **2.** not involved or complicated.

simple angioma [L, *simplex,* not mixed], a tumor consisting of a network of small vessels or distended capillaries surrounded by connective tissue.

S

simple astigmatism [L, *simplex,* not mixed; Gk, *a + stigma,* point], **1.** simple myopic astigmatism in which one principal meridian is in focus on the retina and the other in front of it. **2.** simple hyperopic astigmatism in which one meridian is focused on the retina and the other behind it.

simple cavity, a cavity that involves only one surface of a tooth.

simple diarrhea [L, *simplex,* not mixed; Gk, *dia + rhein,* to flow], a form of diarrhea in which the loose stools contain normal feces.

simple dislocation [L, *simplex,* not mixed, *dis + locare,* to place], dislocation without a penetrating wound.

simple figure-of-eight roller arm sling, a sling prepared by placing the patient in a supine or sitting position with the affected arm flexed adjacent to the chest. The open sling should fit under the arm and over the chest. Finally, the bandage is drawn down over the scapula and across the chest and arm, overlapping and continuing in a figure-of-eight pattern.

simple fracture, an uncomplicated, closed fracture in which the bone does not break the skin.

simple glaucoma [L, *simplex,* not mixed; Gk, *glaucoma,* cataract], chronic openangle glaucoma in which the angle is open when the intraocular fluid pressure is increased but with associated lowered outflow of fluid. There may be visual field loss and optic atrophy.

simple goiter [L, *simplex,* not mixed, *guttur,* sore throat], a goiter not accompanied by signs or symptoms of hyperthyroidism.

Simple Guided Imagery, a Nursing Interventions Classification defined as purposeful use of imagination to achieve relaxation and/or direct attention away from undesirable sensations.

Simple Massage, a Nursing Interventions Classification defined as stimulation of the skin and underlying tissues with varying degrees of hand pressure to decrease pain, produce relaxation, and/or improve circulation.

simple mastectomy, a surgical procedure in which a breast is completely removed and the underlying muscles and adjacent lymph nodes are left intact.

simple phobia, an anxiety disorder characterized by a persistent, irrational fear of specific things such as animals, dirt, light, or darkness.

simple protein, a protein that yields amino acids as the only or chief product on hydrolysis. The class includes albumins, globulins, glutelins, alcohol-soluble proteins, albuminoids, histones, and protamines.

simple reflex [L, *simplex,* not mixed, *reflectere,* to bend back], a reflex with a motor nerve component that involves only one muscle.

Simple Relaxation Therapy, a Nursing Interventions Classification defined as use of techniques to encourage and elicit relaxation for the purpose of decreasing undesirable signs and symptoms such as pain, muscle tension, or anxiety.

simple stomatitis [L, *simplex* + Gk, *stoma,* mouth, *itis,* inflammation], a simple inflammation of the mucous membranes of the mouth with redness, swelling, and an excess of mucus.

simple sugar, a monosaccharide such as glucose.

simple tubular gland, one of the many multicellular glands with only one duct and a tube-shaped part, such as various glands within the epithelium of the intestine.

Sims' position [James M. Sims, American gynecologist, 1813–1883], a position in which the patient lies on the left side with the right knee and thigh drawn upward toward the chest. The chest and abdomen are allowed to fall forward. It is the position of choice for administering enemas or conducting rectal examinations.

simulation /sim′yəlā′shən/ [L, *simulare,* to imitate], a method of representing the actions of one system by those of another, as a computer program that represents the actions of something in the real world. Simulation enables a computer to explore situations that might be too expensive, dangerous, or time consuming in real life.

simultanagnosia /sī′multan′aguō′zhə/, a visual disorder in which a person actually perceives only one element of a picture or object at a time and is unable to absorb the whole.

sinciput /sin′siput/ [L, half a head], the anterior or upper part of the head.

sinew /sin′yōo/ [ME, *sinewe*], the tendon of a muscle, such as the thick, flattened tendon attached to the short head of the biceps brachii.

single-blind study [L, *singulus,* one by one; AS, *blind* + L, *studere,* to be busy], an experiment in which the person collecting data knows whether the subject is in the control or experimental group, but subjects do not.

single-chain antigen-binding protein (SCAB), a polypeptide that joins an antibody's variable sequence to the antibody heavy chain variable sequence. SCABs are used as biosensors, in chemical separations, and in the treatment of can-cers and heart disease.

single component insulin [L, *singulus* + *componere*, to bring together, *insula*, island], any highly purified insulin with less than 10 ppm of proinsulin.

single-locus probe (SLP), a sequence of labeled deoxyribonucleic acid (DNA) or ribonucleic acid that can be used to identify a single locus of variable number of tandem repeats and permit detection of a region of DNA repeats found in the genome only once. It may be used in resolving cases of disputed parentage.

single monster, a fetus with a single body and head but severely malformed or duplicated parts or organs.

single-parent family, a family consisting of only the mother or the father and one or more dependent children.

single-photon emission computed tomography (SPECT), (in nuclear medicine) a variation of computed tomography scanning in which the ray sum is defined by the collimator holes on the gamma-ray detector rotating around the patient. SPECT units usually consist of large crystal gamma cameras mounted on a gantry that permits rotation of the camera around the patient. Multiple detectors are used to reduce the imaging time.

single room occupant (SRO), a single person, usually an elderly individual, who lives alone in a single room of a low-cost hotel or apartment building.

single sweep scan, (in ultrasonics) a scan that is completed in a single sweep of the sensing device across the area being examined.

singleton /sing'gəlton/, an offspring born alone.

singlet state /sing'glit/, a state of an atom or molecule in which all electrons have paired spins.

sinister /sin'istər/ [L], left, at the left side, at the left hand.

sinistral /sinis'trəl,/ [L, *sinister*, left], relating to the left side.

sinoatrial [L *sinus*, hollow, *atrium*, hall], pertaining to the sinus node and atrium.

sinoatrial (SA) block /sī'nō·ā'trē·əl/ [L, *sinus*, hollow, *atrium*, hall; Fr, *bloc*], a conduction disturbance in the heart during which an impulse formed within the SA node is blocked or delayed from depolarizing the atria. There are two types of SA block. Type I (SA Wenckebach) is recognized on the electrocardiogram through the presence of group beating, shortening of PP intervals, and pauses that are less than twice the shortest cycle. Type II SA block is identified on the electrocardiogram by absent P waves without the short-

ening PP intervals. Causes include excessive vagal stimulation, acute infections, and atherosclerosis. SA block also may be an adverse reaction to quinidine or digitalis.

sinoatrial (SA) node, a cluster of hundreds of cells located in the right atrial wall of the heart, near the opening of the superior vena cava. It comprises a knot of modified heart muscle that generates impulses that travel swiftly throughout the muscle fibers of both atria, causing them to contract. Specialized pacemaker cells in the node have an intrinsic rhythm that is independent of any stimulation by nerve impulses from the brain and the spinal cord. The sinoatrial node will normally "fire" at a rhythmic rate of 70 to 75 beats/min. If the node fails to generate an impulse, pacemaker function will shift to another excitable component of the cardiac conduction system, such as the atrioventricular node or Purkinje's fibers.

sinus /sī'nəs/ [L, hollow], a cavity or channel, such as a cavity within a bone, a dilated channel for venous blood, or one permitting the escape of purulent material.

sinus arrest, a heart disorder in which there is a cessation of activity in the sinoatrial node. The ventricles may continue to contract under the control of pacemakers in the atrioventricular node or the ventricles.

sinus arrhythmia, an irregular cardiac rhythm in which the heart rate usually increases during inspiration and decreases during expiration. It is common in children and young adults and has no clinical significance except in elderly patients.

sinus bradycardia, the slow beating of the sinus node at rates of fewer than 60 beats/min.

sinus dysrhythmia, an irregular heart rhythm characterized by alternate speeding up and slowing down of the heart rate. It is often associated with the vagal effects of respiration, with increased rate on inspiration and decreased on expiration.

sinusitis /sīnəsī'tis/ [L, *sinus* + Gk, *itis*, inflammation], an inflammation of one or more paranasal sinuses. It may be a complication of an upper respiratory infection; dental infection; allergy; change in atmospheric pressure, as in air travel or underwater swimming; or a structural defect of the nose. With swelling of nasal mucous membranes, the openings from sinuses to the nose may be obstructed, resulting in an accumulation of sinus secretions, causing pressure, pain, headache, fever, and local tenderness. Complications include cavernous sinus thrombosis and spread of infection to bone, brain, or meninges.

S

sinus node, an area of specialized heart tissue near the entrance of the superior vena cava that generates the cardiac impulse and is in turn controlled by the autonomic nervous system.

sinusoid /sī′nəsoid/ [L, *sinus* + Gk, *eidos*, form], an anastomosing blood vessel, somewhat larger than a capillary, lined with reticuloendothelial cells.

sinus rhythm, a cardiac rhythm stimulated by the sinus (sinoatrial) node. A rate of 60 to 100 beats/min is normal.

sinus tachycardia [L, *sinus,* hollow; Gk, *tachys,* fast, *kardia,* heart], a rapid heartbeat generated by discharge of the sinoatrial pacemaker. The rate is generally 100 to 180 beats/min in the adult, greater than 200 beats/min in an infant, and 140 to 200 beats/min in a child.

si op. sit (in prescriptions), abbreviation for the Latin phrase *si opus sit,* 'if necessary.'

siphonage /sīfənij/, a process of drawing off fluid from a cavity with a tube using atmospheric pressure.

sirenomelia /sī′rənəmē′lē·ə/ [Gk, *seiren,* mermaid, *melos,* limb], a congenital anomaly in which there is complete fusion of the lower extremities and no feet.

sirenomelus /sī′rənom′ələs/, an infant who has sirenomelia.

siriasis /sirī′əsis/ [Gk, *sieros,* scorching], sunstroke.

sister, a term used in the United Kingdom and Commonwealth for a nurse, particularly the head nurse in a hospital, a ward, or an operating room.

Sister Joseph's nodule [Sister Mary Joseph Dempsy, U.S. surgical assistant, 1856–1929], a malignant intraabdominal neoplasm of gastric, ovarian, colorectal, or pancreatic origin and metastatic to the umbilicus.

Sister Kenny's treatment [Elizabeth Kenny, Australian nurse, 1886–1952; Fr, *traitement*], poliomyelitis therapy in which the patient's limbs and back are wrapped in warm, moist woolen cloths and, after the pain subsides, the patient is taught to exercise affected muscles, especially by swimming. Equally important is passive movement of affected limbs with simultaneous stimulation at the site of muscle origins, carried out after hot packs.

site [L, *situs,* location], **1.** location. See also **situs. 2.** a quantum of space occupied and defined by a cluster of people.

site visit, a visit made by designated officials to evaluate or gather information about a department or institution. A site visit is a step in the accreditation of an institution.

sitosterol /sītos′tərôl/ [Gk, *sitos,* food, *stereos,* solid; Ar, *alkohl,* essence], a mixture of sterols derived from plants, such as wheat germ, used for treating hyperbetalipoproteinemia and hypercholesterolemia that are unresponsive to dietary measures. Its use is controversial.

sitotherapy /sī′tōther′əpē/ [Gk, *sitos,* food], a health maintenance system based on food, diet, and nutrition.

sit-to-stand, in the treatment of balance disorders, a movement in which the base of support is transferred from the seat to the feet. The feet begin to accept the weight first by downward pressure through the heels as the pelvis rolls anteriorly. The weight then moves to the front of the feet as the trunk moves forward and the pelvis lifts from the surface.

situational anxiety /sich′o͞o·ā′shənəl/ [L, *situs,* location], a state of apprehension, discomfort, and anxiety precipitated by the experience of new or changed situations or events. Situational anxiety requires no treatment; it usually disappears as the person adjusts to the new experience.

situational crisis, (in psychiatry) an unexpected crisis that arises suddenly in response to an external event or a conflict concerning a specific circumstance.

situational depression, (in psychiatry) an episode of emotional and psychologic depression that occurs in response to a specific set of external conditions or circumstances.

situational loss, the loss of a person, thing, or quality, resulting from alteration of a life situation, including changes related to illness, body image, environment, and death.

situational psychosis, (in psychiatry) a psychotic episode that results from a specific set of external circumstances.

situational supports, people who are available and can be depended on to help a patient solve problems.

situational theory, a leadership theory in which the manager chooses a leadership style to match the particular situation.

situational therapy, (in psychiatry) a kind of psychotherapy in which the milieu is part of the treatment program.

situation relating /sich′o͞o·ā′shən/, (in nursing research) a study design used to explain or predict phenomena in nursing practice in which a relationship is thought to exist among certain practices or characteristics of the population being studied.

situs /sī′təs/ [L, location], the normal position or location of an organ or part of the body.

situs inversus viscerum, the transposition of the abdominal and thoracic organs to opposite sides of the body.

sitz bath /sits, zits/ [Ger, *Sitz,* seat; AS, *bæth*], a bath in which only the rectal and perineal areas are immersed in water or saline solution. The procedure is used after childbirth and after rectal or perineal surgery.

SI units, the international units of physical amounts. Examples of these units are the mass of a kilogram, the length of a meter, and the precise amount of time in a second.

SIV, abbreviation for **simian immunodeficiency virus.**

Sjögren-Larrson's syndrome /shō'-grenlär'sən/ [Torsten Sjögren, Swedish pediatrician, 1859–1939; T. Larsson, twentieth-century Swedish pediatrician], a congenital condition, inherited as an autosomal-recessive trait, characterized by ichthyosis, mental deficiency, and spastic paralysis.

Sjögren's syndrome [Henrik S. C. Sjögren, Swedish ophthalmologist, b. 1899], an immunologic disorder characterized by deficient moisture production of the lacrimal, salivary, and other glands, resulting in abnormal dryness of the mouth, eyes, and other mucous membranes. Atrophy of the lacrimal glands can lead to desiccation of the cornea and conjunctiva. When the lungs are affected, the dryness increases susceptibility to pneumonia and other respiratory infections. Sjögren's syndrome is frequently associated with Raynaud's phenomenon, rheumatoid arthritis, Waldenstr'm's macroglobulinemia, and lymphoma.

SK, abbreviation for **streptokinase.**

skelalgia [Gk, *skelos,* leg], a sensation of pain in the leg.

skeletal fixation /skel'ətəl/ [Gk, *skeletos,* dried up; L, *figere,* to fasten], any method of holding together the fragments of a fractured bone by the attaching of wires, screws, plates, or nails.

skeletal survey, the radiographic study of the skeletal system in a search for possible fractures or tumors.

skeletal system, all of the bones and cartilage of the body that collectively provide the supporting framework for the muscles and organs.

skeletal traction, one of the two basic kinds of traction used in orthopedics for the treatment of fractured bones and the correction of orthopedic abnormalities. Skeletal traction is applied to the affected structure by a metal pin or wire inserted into the tissue of the structure and attached to traction ropes. Skeletal traction is often used when continuous traction is desired

to immobilize, position, and align a fractured bone properly during the healing process. Infection of the pin tract is one of the complications that may develop with skeletal traction.

skeleton /skel'ətən/ [Gk, *skeletos,* dried up], the supporting framework for the body, comprising 206 bones in the adult that protect delicate structures; provide attachments for muscles; allow body movement; serve as major reservoirs of blood; and produce red blood cells, platelets, and most white blood cells. The skeleton is divided into the axial skeleton, which has 74 bones; the appendicular skeleton, with 126 bones; and the 6 auditory ossicles. The four types of bones composing the skeleton are long bones, short bones, flat bones, and irregular bones. The skeleton changes throughout life as bone formation and bone destruction proceed concurrently. —**skeletal,** *adj.*

Skene's glands /skēnz/ [Alexander J. C. Skene, American gynecologist, 1838–1900], the largest of the glands opening into the urethra of women. They contain ducts that open immediately within the urethral orifice.

skew /skyōō/ [ME, *skewen,* to escape], a deviation from a line or symmetric pattern, such as data in a research study that do not follow the expected statistical curve of distribution because of the unwitting introduction of another variable.

skilled nursing facility (SNF) [ME, *skil,* distinction], an institution or part of an institution that meets criteria for accreditation established by the sections of the Social Security Act that determine the basis for Medicaid and Medicare reimbursement for skilled nursing care. Skilled nursing care includes rehabilitation and various medical and nursing procedures. Written policies and protocols are formulated with appropriate professional consultation.

Skillern's fracture /skil'ərnz/ [Penn G. Skillern, American surgeon, b. 1882], an open fracture of the distal radius associated with a greenstick fracture of the distal ulna.

skill play [ME, *skil* + *plega,* sport], a form of play in which a child persistently repeats an action or activity until it has been mastered, such as throwing or catching a ball.

skills training, the teaching of specific verbal and nonverbal behaviors and the practicing of these behaviors by the patient.

skimmed milk [Dan, *skumme,* scum removal; AS, *meolc*], milk from which the fat has been removed. Most of the vitamin

S

A is removed with the cream, although all other nutrients remain.

skimming [Dan, *skumme*], a practice, sometimes used by health programs that receive their income on a prepaid or capitation basis, of seeking to enroll only relatively healthy individuals as a means of increasing profits by decreasing costs.

skimping [Swed, *skrympa*, to shrink], a practice, sometimes used by health programs that receive their income on a prepaid or capitation basis, of delaying or denying services to enrolled members of the program as a means of increasing profits by decreasing costs.

skin [AS, *scinn*], the tough, supple cutaneous membrane that covers the entire surface of the body. It is composed of a thick layer of connective tissue called the dermis and an epidermis made of five layers of cells. The deepest layer is the stratum basale. It anchors the more superficial layers to the underlying tissues, and it provides new cells to replace those lost by abrasion from the outermost layer. The cells of each layer migrate upward as they mature. Above the stratum basale lies the stratum spinosum. As the cells migrate to the next layer, the stratum granulosum, they become flat, lying parallel with the surface of the skin. Over this layer lies a clear, thin band of homogenous tissue called the stratum lucidum. The outermost layer, the stratum corneum, is composed of scaly, squamous plaques of dead cells that contain keratin. This horny layer is thick over areas of the body subject to abrasion, such as the palms of the hands, and thin over other more protected areas. The color of the skin varies according to the amount of melanin in the epidermis. Genetic differences determine the amount of melanin.

skin barrier, an artificial layer of skin, usually made of plastic, applied to skin before the application of tape or ostomy drainage bags. It protects the real skin from chronic irritation.

skin button, a plastic and fabric device that covers the drivelines of an artificial heart at their exit point from the skin. Its purpose is to prevent the transmission of pumping pressure to the surrounding tissues.

skin cancer, a cutaneous neoplasm caused by ionizing radiation, certain genetic defects, or chemical carcinogens, including arsenics, petroleum, tar products, and fumes from some molten metals, or by overexposure to the sun or other sources of ultraviolet light. Skin cancers, the most common and most curable malignancies, are also the most frequent secondary lesions in patients with cancer in other sites. Risk factors are a fair complexion, xeroderma pigmentosa, vitiligo, senile and seborrheic keratitis, Bowen's disease, radiation dermatitis, and hereditary basal cell nevus syndrome. The most common skin cancers are basal cell carcinomas and squamous cell carcinomas.

Skin Care: Topical Treatments, a Nursing Interventions Classification defined as application of topical substances or manipulation of devices to promote skin integrity and minimize skin breakdown.

skin dose (SD), the amount of radiation absorbed by the skin.

skin flap [AS, *scinn* + ME, *flappe*], a layer of skin, usually separated by dissection from deeper layers of tissue.

skinfold calipers, an instrument used to measure the breadth of a fold of skin, usually on the posterior aspect of the upper arm or over the lower ribs of the chest.

skinfold thickness [AS, *scinn* + *fealden* + *thicce*], a measure of the amount of subcutaneous fat, obtained by inserting a fold of skin into the jaws of a caliper. The skinfolds are usually measured on the upper arm, thigh, or upper abdomen, and the caliper measurements are later compared with precalibrated standard tables to assess an individual's body fat content indirectly.

skin graft, a part of skin implanted to cover areas where skin has been lost through burns or injury or by surgical removal of diseased tissue. To prevent tissue rejection of permanent grafts, the graft is taken from the patient's own body or from the body of an identical twin. Skin from another person or animal can be used as a temporary cover for large burned areas to decrease fluid loss. The area from which the graft is taken is called the donor site; that on which it is placed is called the recipient site. Various techniques are used, including pinch, split-thickness, full-thickness, pedicle, and mesh grafts. In pinch grafting, pieces of skin are placed as small islands on the recipient site that they will grow to cover. The split-thickness graft consists of sheets of superficial and some deep layers of skin. The grafts are sutured into place; compression dressings may be applied for firm contact, or the area may be left exposed to the air. A full-thickness graft contains all skin layers and is more durable and effective for weight-bearing and friction-prone areas. A pedicle graft is one in which a part remains attached to the donor site whereas the remainder is transferred to the recipient site. Its own blood supply remains intact, and it is not detached until the new blood supply has fully developed.

skin integrity, impaired, a NANDA-accepted nursing diagnosis of a state in which an individual's skin is adversely altered. Defining characteristics include disruption of the skin surface, destruction of cell layers of the skin, and invasion of body structures through the skin.

skin integrity, impaired, risk for, a NANDA-accepted nursing diagnosis of a state in which an individual's skin is at risk of being adversely altered. Risk factors may be environmental (external) or somatic (internal). Environmental factors include hypothermia or hyperthermia; presence of an injurious chemical substance; shearing force or pressure, restraint, or laceration; radiation; physical immobilization; presence on the skin of excretions or secretions; and abnormally high humidity. Somatic factors include reaction to some medications; obesity or emaciation; an abnormal metabolic state; alteration in circulation, sensory function, or pigmentation; bony prominences; adverse developmental factors; decrease in normal skin turgor; and psychogenic or immunologic abnormalities.

Skinner box [Burrhus F. Skinner, American psychologist, 1904–1990; L, *buxus,* boxwood], a boxlike laboratory apparatus used in operant conditioning in animals, usually containing a lever or other device that, when pressed, reinforces by either giving a reward such as food or an escape outlet or removing a punishment such as an electric shock.

skin pigment [AS, *scinn* + L, *pigmentum,* paint], any skin coloring caused by melanin deposits in skin and hair. The coloring may be modified by substances in the blood, such as the several blood pigments, bile, or malarial parasites.

skin prep, a procedure for cleansing the skin with an antiseptic before surgery or venipuncture. Skin preps are performed to kill bacteria and pathologic organisms and to reduce the risk of infection. Various skin prep devices are available for this procedure. Such devices are commonly constructed of plastic, filled with a specific antiseptic, and equipped with an applicator. The antiseptic is applied by rubbing the device in a circular motion over the skin.

skin self-examination, the practice of studying one's own skin for early signs of premalignant or malignant tumors. A 5-year study by the Sloan-Kettering Cancer Center in New York found that people who examined themselves, looking for moles that change color, shape, or size, were 44% less likely to die of melanoma than those who did not.

Skin Surveillance, a Nursing Interventions Classification defined as collection and analysis of patient data to maintain skin and mucous membrane integrity.

skin test, a test to determine the reaction of the body to a substance by observing the results of injecting the substance intradermally or of applying it topically to the skin. Skin tests are used to detect allergens, determine immunity, and diagnose disease.

skin traction, one of the two basic types of traction used in orthopedics for the treatment of fractured bones and the correction of orthopedic abnormalities. Skin traction applies pull to an affected body structure by straps attached to the skin surrounding the structure.

skin turgor [AS, *scinn* + L, *turgere,* to swell], the resilience of the normal skin when subjected to physical distortion, such as by pinching or pressing. The relative speed with which the skin resumes its normal appearance after stretching or compression is an indicator of skin hydration. Turgor is slower in older people.

skull [ME, *skulle,* shell], the bony structure of the head, consisting of the cranium and the skeleton of the face. The cranium, which contains and protects the brain, consists of 8 bones; the skeleton of the face is composed of 14 bones.

skull shield, a protective plastic plate worn over a cranial defect.

SL, abbreviation for **soda lime.**

slander [Fr, *esclandre,* scandal], any words spoken with malice that are untrue and prejudicial to the reputation, professional practice, commercial trade, office, or business of another person.

slant of occlusal plane [ME, *slenten,* to slope], (in dentistry) the inclination measured by the angle between the extended occlusal plane and the axis-orbital plane.

SLE, abbreviation for **systemic lupus erythematosus.**

sleep [AS, *slaepan,* to sleep], a state marked by reduced consciousness, diminished activity of the skeletal muscles, and depressed metabolism. People normally experience sleep in patterns that follow four observable, progressive stages. During stage 1 the brain waves are of the theta type, followed in stage 2 by the appearance of distinctive sleep spindles; during stages 3 and 4 the theta waves are replaced by delta waves. These four stages represent three fourths of a period of typical sleep and collectively are called *nonrapid eye movement (NREM)* sleep. The remaining time is usually occupied with *rapid eye movement (REM)* sleep, which can be detected with electrodes placed on the skin around the eyes so that tiny electrical discharges from contractions of the eye muscles are transmitted to recording equipment. The REM sleep periods, lasting from a few minutes to half an hour, alternate with the NREM periods. Dreaming occurs during REM time.

sleep apnea, a sleep disorder characterized by periods of an absence of attempts to breathe. The person is momentarily unable to move respiratory muscles or maintain airflow through the nose and mouth.

Sleep Enhancement, a Nursing Interventions Classification defined as facilitation of regular sleep/wake cycles.

sleeping pill, 1. *informal.* a sedative taken for insomnia or for postoperative sedation. **2.** an over-the-counter pill, classified pharmaceutically as an aid to sleeping.

sleep pattern disturbance, a NANDA-accepted nursing diagnosis of disruption of sleep time that causes discomfort or interferes with desired life-style. The critical defining characteristics, at least one of which must be present to make the diagnosis, are difficulty in falling asleep, awakening earlier than usual, interruption of sleep by periods of wakefulness, or not feeling rested after sleep. Other defining characteristics are changes in behavior and performance, including increasing irritability, restlessness, disorientation, lethargy, and listlessness; physical signs such as mild, fleeting nystagmus, slight hand tremor, ptosis of the eyelid, and expressionless face; thick speech with mispronunciation and incorrect words; dark circles under the eyes; frequent yawning; and changes in posture.

sleep terror disorder [AS, *slaepan* + L, *terrere,* to frighten], a condition occurring during stage 3 or 4 of nonrapid eye movement sleep. It is characterized by repeated episodes of abrupt awakening, usually with a panicky scream, accompanied by intense anxiety, confusion, agitation, disorientation, unresponsiveness, marked motor movements, and total amnesia concerning the event. The disorder usually occurs in children.

sleep-wake schedule disorder, a form of dyssomnia caused by a conflict between a person's circadian rhythm and the socioeconomic demands of society, such as work and travel schedules.

slide clamp [AS, *slidan* + *clam,* fastener], a device, usually constructed of plastic, used to regulate the flow of intravenous solution. The slide clamp has a graduated opening through which the intravenous tubing passes.

sliding esophageal hiatal hernia, a protrusion of the cardioesophageal junction and stomach through the esophageal hiatus.

sliding filaments [AS, *slidan* + L, *filamentum,* thread], interdigitated thick and thin filaments of a sarcomere. In muscle contraction they slide past each other so that the sarcomere becomes shorter, although the filament lengths do not change. The action of the sliding filaments contributes to the increased thickness of a muscle in contraction.

sliding hernia, a protrusion of either the cecum or the sigmoid colon into the parietal peritoneum. The protrusion can be either abdominal or esophageal.

sliding hiatal hernia, a protrusion through the diaphragm into the posterior mediastinum.

sliding transfer, the movement of a person in a sitting position from one site to another, such as from a bed to a wheelchair, by sliding him or her along a transfer board.

sling [ME, *slingen,* to hurl], a bandage or device used to support an injured part of the body, especially a forearm.

sling restraint, a therapeutic device, usually constructed of felt, used to assist in the immobilization of patients, especially orthopedic patients in traction. The sling is placed over the pelvis to reduce pelvic motion with lower extremity traction or over the abdominal area as countertraction with Dunlop traction.

slip-on blood pump [ME, *slippen,* slippery, *on*], a plastic mesh device with an attached squeeze bulb, rubber tubing, and pressure gauge, used to help administer large amounts of blood quickly. The plastic mesh slips over the blood bag and applies pressure to it when the bulb is squeezed.

slipped femoral epiphysis, a failure of the femoral epiphyseal plate that tends to occur primarily in overweight adolescents as a result of hormonal changes. Clinical features include hip stiffness and pain, with difficulty in walking. There also may be knee pain and external rotation of the affected leg.

slipping patella [ME, *slippen* + L, *patella,* small dish], a patella that undergoes recurrent dislocation.

slipping rib, a chest pain caused by a loose ligament that allows slippage of one of the lower five ribs. One of the ribs may slip inside or outside an adjacent rib, causing pain or discomfort that may mimic a disorder of the pancreas, gallbladder, or other upper abdominal organ.

slit lamp [AS, *slitan* + Gk, *lampein,* to shine], an instrument used in ophthalmology for examining the conjunctiva, lens, vitreous humor, iris, and cornea. A high-intensity beam of light is projected through a narrow slit, and a cross section of the illuminated part of the eye is examined through a magnifying lens.

slit lamp microscope, a microscope for ophthalmic examination. It permits the viewer to examine the endothelium of the posterior surface of the cornea in a projected band of light that is shaped like a slit.

slit scan radiography, a technique for producing x-rays of body structures without length distortion by scanning a fan-shaped beam through a narrow slit collimator. The beam divergence perpendicular to the scan results in some distortion of width.

slit ventricle syndrome, a condition of chronic headaches and cardiac disorders affecting shunt-dependent patients. Characteristics include small ventricles and slow reflux of the valve mechanism of the shunt.

slough /sluf/ [ME, *sluh*, husk], **1.** to shed or cast off dead tissue, such as cells of the endometrium, shed during menstruation. **2.** the tissue that has been shed.

slow channel, a protein channel that is slow to become activated. An example is the calcium channel. Channel proteins are responsible for transporting solutes across a membrane.

slow diastolic depolarization [AS, *slaw*, dull], the slow loss of negativity that occurs during the resting phase in cardiac cells having automaticity.

slow pain, an unpleasant sensory experience that travels a multisynaptic route to the brain via slow-conducting, nonmyelinated nerve fibers.

slow pulse [AS, *slaw*, dull; L, *pulsare*, to beat], a pulse rate of less than 60 beats/min. The rate is common among older people, conditioned athletes, and patients receiving beta blocker medications.

slow-reacting substance of anaphylaxis (SRS-A), a group of active substances, including histamine and leukotrienes, that are released during an anaphylactic reaction. They cause the smooth muscle contraction and vascular dilation that mark the signs and symptoms of anaphylaxis.

slow response action potential, (in cardiology) an action potential produced when none of the fast sodium channels is available for depolarization and the fiber is activated via slow calcium channels, producing an action potential with a slow upstroke velocity, low amplitude, and consequent slow conduction.

slow stroking, a therapeutic pressure technique of slow continuous movement of the hands over the paravertebral areas along the spine from the cervical through the lumbar region. Usually a lubricant is applied to the skin, and the index and middle fingers are used to stroke both sides of the spinal column simultaneously.

slow-twitch (ST) fiber, a muscle fiber that develops less tension more slowly than a fast-twitch fiber. The ST fiber is usually fatigue resistant and has adequate oxygen and enzyme activity.

slow vestibular stimulation, a feeding therapy technique for disabled children, designed to promote parasympathetic loading.

slow virus, a virus that remains dormant in the body after initial infection. Years may elapse before symptoms occur.

slurred speech /slurd/ [D, *sleuren*, to drag; ME, *speche*], abnormal speech in which words are not enunciated clearly or completely but are run together or partially eliminated. The condition may be caused by weakness of the muscles of articulation, damage to a motor neuron, cerebellar disease, drug use, or carelessness.

slurry /slur'ē/ [ME, *sloor*, mud], a thin suspension of finely divided solids in a liquid.

Sm, symbol for the element **samarium.**

SMA, **1.** trademark for a nutritional supplement for infants. **2.** abbreviation for **sequential multiple analysis.**

small cardiac vein [AS, *smael*], one of the five tributaries of the coronary sinus that drain blood from the myocardium. It conveys blood from the back of the right atrium and the right ventricle.

smallest cardiac vein, one of the tiny vessels that drain deoxygenated blood from the myocardium into the atria. A few of these vessels end in the ventricles.

small for gestational age (SGA) infant, an infant whose weight and size at birth fall below the tenth percentile of appropriate for gestational age infants, whether delivered at term or earlier or later than term. Factors associated with smallness or retardation of intrauterine growth other than genetic influences include any disorder causing short stature such as dwarfism; malnutrition caused by placental insufficiency; and certain infectious agents, including cytomegalovirus, rubella virus, and *Toxoplasma gondii*. Other factors associated with the smallness of an SGA infant include cigarette smoking by the mother during pregnancy, her addiction to alcohol or heroin, and her having received methadone treatment.

small intestine, the longest part of the digestive tract, extending for about 7 m from the pylorus of the stomach to the ileocecal junction. It is divided into the duodenum, jejunum, and ileum. It functions in digestion and is the major organ of absorption of prepared food.

smallpox /smôl′poks/ [AS, *smael* + *pocc*], a highly contagious viral disease characterized by fever, prostration, and a vesicular, pustular rash. It is caused by one of two species of poxvirus, variola minor (alastrim) or variola major. Because human beings are the only reservoir for the virus, worldwide vaccination with vaccinia, a related poxvirus, has been effective in eradicating smallpox.

smallpox vaccine, a vaccine prepared from dried smallpox virus. It is indicated only for laboratory workers exposed to pox viruses.

small sciatic nerve [AS, *smael* + Gk, *ischiadikos,* of the hip joint; L, *nervus*], the posterior femoral cutaneous nerve, which pierces the fascia and subdivides into filaments, supplying the skin from the level of the greater trochanter to the middle of the thigh.

SMBG, abbreviation for **self-monitoring of blood glucose.**

smear [AS, *smeoru,* grease], a laboratory specimen for microscopic examination prepared by spreading a thin film of tissue on a glass slide. A dye, stain, reagent, diluent, or lysing agent may be applied to the specimen.

smegma /smeg′mə/ [Gk, soap], a secretion of sebaceous glands, especially the cheesy, foul-smelling secretion sometimes found under the foreskin of the penis and at the base of the labia minora near the glans clitoris.

smell [ME, *smellen,* to detect odors], **1.** the special sense that allows perception of odors through the stimulation of the olfactory nerves; olfaction. **2.** any odor, pleasant or unpleasant.

smelling salt [ME, *smellen* + AS, *sealt*], aromatized ammonium carbonate to which may be added ammonia. It is used as a stimulant to arouse a person who has fainted.

Smith fracture [Robert W. Smith, Irish surgeon, 1807–1873], a reverse Colles′ fracture of the wrist, involving volar displacement and angulation of a distal bone fragment.

Smith-Petersen nail [Marius N. Smith-Petersen, American surgeon, 1886–1953; AS, *naegel,* nail], a three-flanged stainless steel nail used in orthopedic surgery to anchor the fractured neck of the femur to its head. It is introduced below the prominence of the greater trochanter and

passed through the fractured part into the head of the femur.

smog, a polluting combination of smoke and fog in the atmosphere.

smoke inhalation [AS, *smoca* + L, *in,* within, *halare,* to breathe], the inhalation of noxious fumes or irritating particulate matter that may cause severe pulmonary damage. Respiratory burns are difficult to distinguish from simple smoke inhalation. Chemical pneumonitis, asphyxiation, and physical trauma to the respiratory passages may occur. Characteristics include irritation of the upper respiratory tract, singed nasal hairs, dyspnea, hypoxia, dusty gray sputum, rhonchi, rales, restlessness, anxiety, cough, and hoarseness. Pulmonary edema may develop up to 48 hours after exposure.

smokeless tobacco [AS, *smoca* + Sp, *tabaco*], **1.** chewing tobacco or tobacco powder that allows the stimulating components of tobacco to be absorbed through the digestive tract or through the mucus membrane in the case of snuff. **2.** a transdermal nicotine patch that can be affixed to the upper part of the body to satisfy the person′s craving for nicotine.

Smoking Cessation Assistance, a Nursing Interventions Classification defined as helping a patient to stop smoking.

smooth muscle [AS, *smoth*], one of three kinds of muscle, composed of elongated, spindle-shaped cells in muscles not under voluntary control, such as the smooth muscle of the intestines, stomach, and other viscera. The nucleated cells of smooth muscle are arranged parallel to one another and to the long axis of the muscle they form. Smooth muscle fibers are shorter than striated muscle fibers, have only one nucleus per fiber, and are smooth in appearance.

smooth muscle relaxant, an agent that reduces the tone of smooth muscle, such as a bronchodilator or vasodilator.

smooth pursuit eye movement, the tracking by the eyes of a slowly moving object at a steady coordinated velocity rather than in saccades.

smooth surface cavity, a cavity formed by decay that starts on surfaces of teeth without pits, fissures, or enamel faults.

SMR, abbreviation for **submucous resection.**

smudge cell [ME, *sogen,* to soil], a disrupted leukocyte, sometimes seen during preparation of blood smears.

Sn, symbol for the element **tin.**

S.N., abbreviation for *student nurse,* used in signing nursing notes (in the United States).

SNA, 1. abbreviation for **State Nurses Association. 2.** abbreviation for *Student Nurses Association.*

snail [AS, *snagel,* slug], an invertebrate of the order Gastropoda, several species of which are intermediate hosts of the blood flukes that cause schistosomiasis in humans.

snakebite [AS, *snacan,* to creep, *bitan*], a wound resulting from penetration of the flesh by the fangs of a snake. Bites by snakes known to be nonvenomous are treated as puncture wounds; those produced by an unidentified or poisonous snake require immediate attention.

snake venom [AS, *snacan* + L, *venenum*], a poison produced in glands of certain snakes and injected through fangs into a victim's flesh. The exact composition of snake venoms varies with different species, but generally they are complex mixtures of neurotoxins, proteolytic enzymes, and phosphatases. About 20 of more than 100 North American species of snakes are venomous. A venomous snakebite is considered a medical emergency.

snapping hip [ME, *snappen* + AS, *hype*], a condition in which a tendon slips over the greater trochanter when the hip is moved, possibly producing a loud snapping sound.

snare /sner/ [AS, *sneare,* noose], a device designed for holding a wire noose, used in removing small stalklike growths. The operator tightens the wire around the stalk (peduncle), thus removing the growth.

sneeze [AS, *snesen,* to sneeze], a sudden forceful involuntary expulsion of air through the nose and mouth occurring as a result of irritation to the mucous membranes of the upper respiratory tract, such as by dust, pollen, or viral inflammation.

Snellen chart [Hermann Snellen, Dutch ophthalmologist, 1834–1908], one of several charts used in testing visual acuity. Letters, numbers, or symbols are arranged on the chart in decreasing size from top to bottom.

Snellen's reflex [Hermann Snellen], unilateral congestion of the ear on stimulation of the distal end of the divided great auricular nerve.

Snellen test [Hermann Snellen], a test of visual acuity using a Snellen chart. The person being tested stands 20 feet from the chart and reads as many of the symbols as possible, reading each line and proceeding downward from the top. A score is assigned in the form of a ratio, comparing the subject's performance to that of a statistically normal subject's performance. A person who can read at 20 feet what the

average person can read at this distance has 20/20 vision.

SNF, abbreviation for **skilled nursing facility.**

snore /snôr/, a harsh rough sound of breathing caused by vibration of the ovula and soft palate during sleep.

snout reflex [ME, *snoute,* muzzle], an abnormal sign elicited by tapping the nose, resulting in a marked facial grimace. It usually indicates bilateral corticopontine lesions.

snowball sampling, a method of obtaining subjects for a study by soliciting names of potential subjects from those participating in the study.

snow blindness [AS, *snaw* + *blind*], a condition of photophobia, sometimes accompanied by conjunctivitis, as a result of overexposure of the eyes to the glare of sun on snow.

SNP, abbreviation for **sodium nitroprusside.**

S.N.P., abbreviation for **school nurse practitioner.**

snuff, a powder that is inhaled through the nostrils.

snuff dipping, the practice of extracting juices from moist, fine-cut chewing tobacco placed in the mucobuccal fold of the mouth. The practice has been associated with an increased incidence of leukoplakia, tooth and gum diseases, and oral cancer.

snuffles [D, *snuffelen,* to sniff], a nasal discharge in infancy characteristic of congenital syphilis.

soap [L, *sapo*], a compound of fatty acids and an alkali. Soap cleanses because molecules of fat are attracted to molecules of soap in a water solution and pulled off the dirty surface into the water.

SOAP /sōp′, es′ō′ā′pē′/, (in a problem oriented medical record) abbreviation for *subjective, objective, assessment, and plan,* the four parts of a written account of the health problem.

soapsuds enema (SSE) [L, *sapo* + D, *sudse,* marsh water; Gk, *enienai*], an evacuant enema made of 1 ounce of soft soap dissolved in 2 pints of hot water and administered at a temperature of 100° F (38° C).

SOB, abbreviation for *short of breath.*

socia /sō′shē·ə/, an ectopic or displaced part of an organ, such as an accessory parotid gland.

Social Behavior Assessment Scale /sō′-shəl/, a semistructured interview guide that elicits information from significant others regarding a patient's functioning.

social breakdown syndrome [L, *socius,*

partner; AS, *brecan* + *dune*], the progressive deterioration of social and interpersonal skills in long-term psychiatric patients.

social class, a grouping of people with similar values, interests, income, education, and occupations.

social deviance, behavior that violates social standards, engendering anger, resentment, and a desire for punishment in a significant segment of the society.

social interaction, impaired, a NANDA-accepted nursing diagnosis of the state in which an individual participates in an insufficient or excessive quantity or ineffective quality of social exchange. Major defining characteristics include verbalized or observed discomfort in social situations; verbalized or observed inability to receive or communicate a satisfying sense of belonging, caring, interest, or shared history; observed use of unsuccessful social interaction behaviors; and dysfunctional interaction with peers, family, and/or others. A family report of change of style or pattern of interaction is a minor defining characteristic.

social isolation, a NANDA-accepted nursing diagnosis of a condition in which a feeling of aloneness is experienced that the client acknowledges as a negative or threatening state imposed by others. The defining characteristics may be objective, subjective, or both. Objective characteristics include the absence of family and friends; the absence of a supportive or significant personal relationship with another person; the client's withdrawal and preoccupation with his or her own thoughts and interests; meaningless actions or interests and activities inappropriate to the client's developmental age; a physical or mental handicap or illness; or unacceptable social behavior. Subjective characteristics include verbal expression of feeling different from and rejected by others, acknowledgment of values unacceptable to the dominant cultural group, absence of a significant purpose in life, inability to meet the expectations of others, and the expressed feeling of insecurity in social situations.

socialization /sō′shəlīzā′shən/, **1.** the process by which an individual learns to live in accordance with the expectations and standards of a group or society, acquiring the beliefs, habits, values, and accepted modes of behavior primarily through imitation, family interaction, and educational systems; the procedure by which society integrates the individual. **2.** (in psychoanalysis) the process of adjustment that begins in early childhood by which the individual becomes aware of the need to accommodate inner drives to the demands of external reality.

Socialization Enhancement, a Nursing Interventions Classification defined as facilitation of another person's ability to interact with others.

socialized medicine /sō′shəlīzd/, a system for the delivery of health care in which the expense of care is borne by a governmental agency supported by taxation rather than being paid directly by the client on a fee-for-service or contract basis.

social learning theory, a concept that the impulse to behave aggressively is subject to the influence of learning, socialization, and experience.

social margin, the total of all resources (material, personal, and interpersonal) available to assist an individual in coping with stress.

social medicine, an approach to the prevention and treatment of disease that is based on the study of human heredity, environment, social structures, and cultural values.

social mobility, the process of moving upward or downward in the social hierarchy.

social motivation, an incentive or drive resulting from a sociocultural influence that initiates behavior toward a particular goal.

social network, an interconnected group of cooperating significant others, who may or may not be related, with whom a person interacts.

social network therapy, the gathering together of patient, family, and other social contacts into group sessions for the purpose of problem solving.

social order, the manner in which a society is organized and the rules and standards required to maintain that organization.

social phobia, an anxiety disorder characterized by a compelling desire for the avoidance of and a persistent, irrational fear of situations in which the individual may be exposed to scrutiny by others. Examples of such situations are speaking, eating, or performing in public or using public lavatories or transportation.

social psychiatry, a field of psychiatry based on the study of social, cultural, and ecologic influences on the development and course of mental diseases.

social psychology, the study of the effects of group membership on the behavior, attitudes, and beliefs of the individual.

social readjustment rating scale, a scale of 43 common events associated with some degree of disruption of an individual's life. The scale was developed by the psychologists T. J. Holmes and R. Rahe, who found that a number of serious physical disorders such as myocardial infarction, peptic ulcer, and infections, as well as a variety of psychiatric disorders, were associated with an accumulation of 200 or more points on the rating scale within a period of 1 year. Most disruptive on one's life, according to the psychologists, was the death of a spouse, an event that warranted 100 points. The lowest rated event was a minor law violation, rated at 11 points.

social sanctions, the measures used by a society to enforce its rules of acceptable behavior.

Social Security Act, a U.S. federal statute that provides for a national system of old age assistance, survivors' and old age insurance benefits, unemployment insurance and compensation, and other public welfare programs, including Medicare and Medicaid.

social support programs, services provided older persons, including organizations of volunteers who visit older individuals to decrease loneliness and social isolation, volunteers who telephone older persons for similar purposes, and programs that provide a daily call with emergency procedures that go into effect if the telephone is not answered.

social theories of aging, concepts of social and psychologic adjustment in older persons. The theories include activity expressed in adoption of new roles and continuity, which includes retention of physical and social activities from the middle years.

social worker, a person with advanced education in dealing with social, emotional, and environmental problems associated with an illness or disability. A medical social worker usually has completed a master's degree program that includes experience in counseling patients and their families in a hospital setting. A **psychiatric social worker** may specialize in counseling individuals and families in dealing with social, emotional, or environmental problems pertaining to mental illness.

society /səsī'ətē/, a nation, community, or broad group of people who establish particular aims, beliefs, or standards of living and conduct.

Society for Advancement in Nursing (SAIN), a group established for advancement of the profession of nursing through higher education.

sociobiology /sō'sē·ō'bī·ol'əjē/ [L, *socius,*

companion; Gk, *bios,* life, *logos,* science], the systematic study of biology as a basis for human behavior. Proponents contend that disease, stress, and aggression are natural pressures for maintaining an optimal level of population.

socioeconomic status /sō'sē·ō·ik'ənom'ik/ [L, *socius,* companion, *oeconomicus,* methodical, *status,* state], the position of an individual on a social-economic scale that measures such factors as education, income, type of occupation, place of residence, and in some populations heritage and religion.

sociogenic /-jen'ik/ [L, *socius* + Gk, *genesis,* origin], pertaining to personal or group activities that are motivated by social values and constraints.

sociolinguistics /-ling·gwis'tiks/, the study of the relationship between language and the social context in which it occurs.

sociology /sō'sē·ol'əjē/ [L, *socius* + Gk, *logos,* science], the study of group behavior within a society.

sociopath, popular term for antisocial personality.

sociopathy /sō'sē·op'əthē/ [L, *socius,* companion; Gk, *pathos,* disease], a personality disorder characterized by a lack of social responsibility and failure to adapt to ethical and social standards of the community.

socket, the part of a prosthesis into which the stump of the remaining limb fits. Most modern prosthetic sockets are made of plastic materials, which are odorless, lighter, and easier to clean than traditional leather sockets.

soda [It, *sodo,* solid], a compound of sodium, particularly sodium bicarbonate, sodium carbonate, or sodium hydroxide.

soda lime (SL), a mixture of sodium and calcium hydroxides used to absorb exhaled carbon dioxide in an anesthesia rebreathing system.

sodium (Na) /sō'dē·əm/ [soda + L, *ium* (coined by Sir Humphry Davy, English chemist, b. 1778)], a soft grayish metal of the alkaline metals group. Its atomic number is 11; its atomic mass (weight) is 22.99. Sodium is one of the most important elements in the body. Sodium ions are involved in acid-base balance, water balance, transmission of nerve impulses, and contraction of muscles. Sodium is the chief electrolyte in interstitial fluid, and its interaction with potassium as the main intracellular electrolyte is critical to survival. A decrease in the sodium concentration of the interstitial fluid immediately decreases osmotic pressure, making it hypotonic to intracellular fluid osmotic pressure.

S

sodium arsenite poisoning, a toxic condition caused by the ingestion of sodium arsenite, an insecticide and weed killer. The characteristic symptoms of arsenite poisoning are similar to those of arsenic poisoning.

sodium barbital, the sodium salt of 5,5-diethylbarbituric acid, a hypnotic and sedative drug.

sodium bicarbonate, an antacid, electrolyte, and urinary alkalinizing agent. It is prescribed in the treatment of acidosis, gastric acidity, peptic ulcer, and indigestion.

sodium chloride, common table salt (NaCl), used as a fluid and electrolyte replenisher, isotonic vehicle, irrigating solution, and enema.

sodium fluoride poisoning, a chronic condition of fluorine poisoning that occurs in some communities where the fluorine concentration in the water supply exceeds 1 ppm. Signs of the condition include mottling of tooth enamel and severe osteosclerosis.

sodium hypochlorite solution, a 5% aqueous solution of NaOCl used as a disinfectant for utensils not harmed by its bleaching action.

sodium iodide, an iodine supplement prescribed in the treatment of thyrotoxic crisis and neonatal thyrotoxicosis and in the management of hyperthyroidism before thyroidectomy.

sodium lactate injection, an electrolyte replenisher that has been prescribed for metabolic acidosis.

sodium nitroprusside (SNP), a vasodilator prescribed primarily in the emergency treatment of hypertensive crises and in heart failure.

sodium perborate, an oxygen-liberating antiseptic ($NaBO_2.H_2O_2.3H_2O$) that may be used in treating necrotizing ulcerative gingivitis and other kinds of gingival inflammation and bleaching pulpless teeth.

sodium phenobarbital, the sodium salt of phenylethylbarbituric acid, a long-acting sedative and hypnotic. It can be administered orally or parenterally and is used in the therapeutic management of seizure disorders.

sodium phosphate, a saline cathartic prescribed to achieve prompt, thorough evacuation of the bowel and, in lower dosage, for laxative effect.

sodium phosphate P32, an antineoplastic, antipolycythemic radioactive agent. It is prescribed for polycythemia vera, for neoplasms, including myelocytic leukemia, and for localizing tumors of the eye.

sodium pump, a mechanism for transporting sodium ions across cell membranes against an opposing concentration gradient. Energy for this transport system is obtained from the hydrolysis of adenosine triphosphate by special enzymes.

sodium salicylate, an analgesic, antipyretic, and antirheumatic prescribed to relieve pain and fever.

sodium stibocaptate, an investigational parasiticide for certain schistosomal infections. It is available from the Centers for Disease Control and Prevention.

sodium sulfate, a saline cathartic for chronic constipation caused by peristaltic disorders. It is prescribed to achieve prompt, thorough evacuation of the bowel and, in lower dosage, for laxative effect.

sodomist /sod'əmist/ [Sodom, biblical city in ancient Palestine], a person who practices sodomy.

sodomy /sod'əmē/ [Sodom, biblical city in ancient Palestine], **1.** anal intercourse. **2.** intercourse with an animal. **3.** a vague term for "unnatural" sexual intercourse. —**sodomize,** v.

soft chancre [AS, *softe* + Fr, *canker*], a usually painless local genital ulcer that follows an infection by *Haemophilus ducreyi*. It is accompanied by suppuration of the inguinal lymphatic nodes, or inguinal buboes. Complications may include phimosis, urethral stricture or fistula, and marked tissue destruction.

soft contact lens [AS, *softe* + L, *contingere* + *lentil*], a contact lens made of a flexible plastic material that can be shaped more easily to fit the eyeball than a rigid gas-permeable lens and typically provide good initial comfort. Among the disadvantages of soft lenses are that they are more easily damaged, do not provide vision as sharp as alternative methods, and must be disinfected periodically because they tend to harbor bacteria.

soft data [AS, *softe* + L, *datum,* something given], health information that is mainly subjective as provided by the patient and the patient's family, including pain or other sensations, life-style habits, and family health history.

soft diet, a diet that is soft in texture, low in residue, easily digested, and well tolerated. It provides the essential nutrients in the form of liquids and semisolid foods, such as milk, fruit juices, eggs, cheese, custards, tapioca and puddings, and strained soups and vegetables.

softening of bones /sô'fəning, sof'əning/ [AS, *softe* + *ban*], any disease that results in a loss of the mineral content of the bones.

soft fibroma, a fibroma that contains many cells.

soft neurologic sign, a mild or slight neu-

rologic abnormality that is difficult to detect or interpret.

soft palate, the structure composed of mucous membrane, muscular fibers, and mucous glands, suspended from the posterior border of the hard palate forming the roof of the mouth. When the soft palate rises, as in swallowing and sucking, it separates the nasal cavity and the nasopharynx from the posterior part of the oral cavity and the oral part of the pharynx.

soft radiation, a relatively long wavelength with less penetrating radiation than short wavelength radiation.

soft water [AS, *softe* + *waeter*], water that does not contain salts of calcium or magnesium, which precipitate soap solutions.

sol, a colloidal state in which a solid is suspended throughout a liquid, such as a soap or starch in water. The fluidity of cytoplasm depends on its sol/gel balance.

sol., abbreviation for **solution.**

Solanaceae /sō'lənā'si·ē/, a family of plants that includes the genus *Solanum*, or nightshades, and more than 1800 species, including deadly nightshade (belladonna), henbane, tomatoes, and potatoes.

solanaceous /sō'lənā'shəs/, pertaining to plants of the Solanaceae family or substances derived from them.

solarium /sōler'ē·əm/ [L, terrace exposed to sun], a large, sunny room or area serving as a lounge for ambulatory patients in a hospital.

solar plexus /sō'lər/ [L, *sol*, sun, *plexus*, network], a dense network of nerve fibers and ganglia that surrounds the roots of the celiac and superior mesenteric arteries at the level of the first lumbar vertebra. It is one of the great autonomic plexuses of the body in which the nerve fibers of the sympathetic system and the parasympathetic system combine.

solar radiation, the emission and diffusion of actinic rays from the sun. Overexposure may result in sunburn, keratosis, skin cancer, or lesions associated with photosensitivity.

solar sneeze reflex [L, *sol*, sun; ME, *snesen* + L, *reflectere*, to bend back], a sneeze that may be caused by exposure to bright sunlight.

solar therapy [L, *sol*, sun; Gk, *therapeia*, treatment], the therapeutic use of sunlight.

sole [L, *solea*], the plantar surface of the foot.

soleus /sō'lē·əs/ [L, *solea*, sole of foot], one of three superficial posterior muscles of the leg. It is a broad flat muscle lying just under the gastrocnemius. The soleus plantar flexes the foot.

solid /sol'id/ [L, *solidus*], **1.** a dense body, figure, structure, or substance that has length, breadth, and thickness; is not a liquid or a gas; contains no significant cavity or hollowness; and has no breaks or openings on its surface. **2.** describing such a body, figure, structure, or substance.

solitary coin lesion /sol'iter'ē/ [L, *solitarius*, standing alone, *cuneus*, wedge, *laesus*, injury], a nodule identified on a chest radiographic film by clear normal lung tissue surrounding it. A coin lesion is often malignant.

solitary play, a form of play among a group of children within the same room or area in which each child engages in an independent activity, using toys that are different from the others' and showing no interest in joining in or interfering with the play of others.

soln, abbreviation for **solution.**

solubility /sol'yəbil'itē/ [L, *solubilis*, able to dissolve], **1.** the maximum amount of a solute that can dissolve in a specific solvent under a given set of conditions. **2.** the concentration of a solute in a solvent at its saturation point.

solute /sol'yoot, sō'loot/ [L, *solutus*, dissolved], a substance dissolved in a solution.

solution (sol., soln) /səloo'shən/ [L, *solutus*], a mixture of one or more substances dissolved in another substance. The molecules of each of the substances disperse homogenously and do not change chemically. A solution may be a gas, a liquid, or a solid.

solvent /sol'vənt/ [L, *solvere*, to dissolve], **1.** any liquid in which another substance can be dissolved. **2.** *informal.* an organic liquid such as benzene, carbon tetrachloride, and other volatile petroleum distillates that, when inhaled, can cause intoxication, as well as damage to mucous membranes of the nose and throat and tissues of the kidney, liver, and brain.

soma /sō'mə/ [Gk, body], **1.** the body, as distinguished from the mind or psyche. **2.** the body, excluding germ cells. **3.** the body of a cell. —**somatic** /sōmat'ik/, **somal,** *adj.*

somatic cell /sōmat'ik/, any of the cells of body tissue that have the diploid number of chromosomes, as distinguished from germ cells, which contain the haploid number.

somatic chromosome, any nonsex chromosome in a diploid or somatic cell, as contrasted with those in a haploid or gametic cell; an autosome.

somatic delusion, a false notion or belief concerning body image or body function.

S

somatic mutation [Gk, *soma*, body; L, *mutare*, to change], a sudden change in the chromosomal material in somatic cell nuclei affecting derived cells but not offspring.

somatic therapy, a form of treatment pertaining to the body that affects one's physiologic functioning.

somatist /sō′mətist/, a psychotherapist or other health professional who believes that every neurosis and psychosis has an organic cause.

somatization /sō′mətīzā′shən/ [Gk, *soma*, body], a process whereby a mental event is expressed in a body disorder or physical symptom. Examples include peptic ulcers and asthma.

somatization disorder [Gk, *soma* + *izein*, to cause], a *DSM-IV* psychiatric disorder characterized by recurrent multiple physical complaints and symptoms for which there is no organic cause. It is classified as a somatoform disorder in *DSM-IV*. The symptoms vary according to the individual and the underlying emotional conflict. Some common symptoms are gastrointestinal dysfunction, paralysis, temporary blindness, cardiopulmonary distress, painful or irregular menstruation, sexual indifference, and pain during intercourse.

somatodyspraxia /-disprak′sē·ə/, an impairment in the ability to plan skilled movements that are nonhabitual. Patients may be able to learn specific motor skills with practice but cannot accomplish unfamiliar tasks.

somatoform disorder /sōmat′əfôrm, sō′-mətōfôrm′/ [Gk, *soma* + L, *forma*, form], any of a group of disorders, characterized by symptoms suggesting physical illness or disease, for which there are no demonstrable organic causes or physiologic dysfunctions. The symptoms are usually the physical manifestations of some unresolved intrapsychic factor or conflict. Kinds of somatoform disorders are **conversion disorder, hypochondriasis, psychogenic pain disorder,** and **somatization disorder.**

somatogenesis /sō′matəjen′əsis/ [Gk, *soma* + *genein*, to produce], 1. (in embryology) the development of the body from the germ plasm. 2. the development of a physical disease or of symptoms from an organic pathophysiologic cause. —**somatogenic, somatogenetic,** *adj.*

somatomegaly /sō′matōmeg′əlē/ [Gk, *soma* + *megas*, large], a condition in which the body is abnormally large as a result of an excessive secretion of somatotropin or an inadequate secretion of somatostatin.

somatoplasm /sō′mətōplaz′əm/ [Gk, *soma*

+ *plasma*, something formed], the nonreproductive protoplasmic material of the body cells, as distinguished from the reproductive material of the germ cells.

somatopleure /sō′mətōplŏŏr′/ [Gk, *soma* + *pleura*, side], the tissue layer that forms the body wall of the early developing embryo. —**somatopleural,** *adj.*

somatosensory evoked potential (SEP) /-sen′sərē/ [Gk, *soma* + L, *sentire*, to feel], evoked potential elicited by repeated stimulation of the pain and touch systems. It is the least reliable of the evoked potentials studied as monitors of neurologic function during surgery.

somatosensory system, the components of the central and peripheral nervous systems that receive and interpret sensory information from organs in the joints, ligaments, muscles, and skin. This system processes information about the length, degree of stretch, tension, and contraction of muscles; pain; temperature; pressure; and joint position.

somatosplanchnic /-splangk′nik/ [Gk, *soma* + *splanchna*, viscera], pertaining to the trunk of the body and the viscera.

somatostatin /sō′matōstat′in/, a hormone produced in the hypothalamus that inhibits the factor that stimulates release of somatotropin from the anterior pituitary gland. It also inhibits the release of certain hormones, including thyrotropin, adrenocorticotropic hormone, glucagon, insulin, and cholecystokinin, and of some enzymes, including pepsin, renin, secretin, and gastrin.

somatotherapy /-ther′əpē/, the treatment of physical disorders, as distinguished from psychotherapy.

somatotropic /-trop′ik/ [Gk, *soma*, body, *trope*, a turn], pertaining to an agent that influences the body or body cells.

somatotype /sō′matōtīp′/ [Gk, *soma* + *typos*, mark], 1. body build or physique. 2. the classification of individuals according to body build based on certain physical characteristics. The primary types are **ectomorph, endomorph,** and **mesomorph.**

somatovisceral reflex /-vis′ərəl/, a reflex in which visceral functions are activated or inhibited by somatic sensory stimulation.

somatrem /sō′mətrem/, a synthetic polypeptide growth hormone produced by recombinant deoxyribonucleic acid technology. It is prescribed for patients who do not grow because of limited endogenous growth hormone secretion.

somite /sō′mīt/ [Gk, *soma*, body], any of the paired segmented masses of mesodermal tissue that form along the length of the neural tube during the early stage of embryonic development in vertebrates.

somite embryo, an embryo in any stage of development between the formation of the first and last pairs of somites, which in humans occurs in the third and fourth weeks after fertilization of the ovum.

somnambulism /somnam'byəliz'əm/ [L, *somnus,* sleep, *ambulare,* to walk], **1.** a condition occurring during stage 3 or 4 of nonrapid eye movement sleep that is characterized by complex motor activity, usually culminating in leaving the bed and walking about. The person has no recall of the episode on awakening. The episodes usually last from several minutes to half an hour or longer. **2.** a hypnotic state in which the person has full possession of the senses but no recollection of the episode.

somniloquence /somnil'əkwəns/, talking during sleep or under hypnosis.

somnolent /som'nələnt/ [L, *somnolentia,* sleepy], **1.** the condition of being sleepy or drowsy. **2.** tending to cause sleepiness. —**somnolence,** *n.*

somnolent detachment, (in psychology) a term introduced by H. S. Sullivan for a type of security operation in which a person falls asleep when confronted by a highly threatening, anxiety-producing experience.

Somogyi phenomenon [Michael Somogyi, American biochemist, 1883–1971; Gk, *phainomenon*], a diabetes mellitus rebound effect in which an overdose of insulin induces hypoglycemia. This releases hormones that stimulate lipolysis, gluconeogenesis, and glycogenolysis, leading to hyperglycemia and ketosis.

sonographer /sōnog'rəfər/, an allied health professional with special training in the use of ultrasound equipment for diagnostic and therapeutic purposes.

sopor /sō'pər/ [L, deep sleep], a sleep that is as deep or sound as the state of stupor.

soporiferous /sop'ərif'ərəs/ [L *sopor,* deep sleep, *ferre,* to bear], tending to cause deep sleep, such as an agent that induces deep sleep.

soporific /sop'ərif'ik/ [L, *sopor,* deep sleep, *facere,* to make], **1.** pertaining to a substance, condition, or procedure that causes sleep. **2.** a soporific drug.

sorbent /sôr'bənt/ [L, *sorbere,* to swallow], **1.** an agent that attracts and retains substances by absorption or adsorption. **2.** the property of a substance that allows it to interact with another compound, usually to make it bind.

sorbic acid /sôr'bik/, a compound occurring naturally in berries of the mountain ash. Commercial sorbic acid derived from

acetaldehyde is used in fungicides, food preservatives, lubricants, and plasticizers.

sordes /sôr'dēz/, *pl.* **sordes** [L, *sordere,* to be dirty], dirt or debris, especially the crusts consisting of food, microorganisms, and epithelial cells that accumulate on teeth and lips during a febrile illness or one in which the patient takes nothing by mouth. Sordes gastricae is undigested food and mucus in the stomach.

sore /sôr, sōr/ [AS, *sar*], **1.** a wound, ulcer, or lesion. **2.** tender or painful.

sore throat [AS, *sar* + *throte*], any inflammation of the larynx, pharynx, or tonsils.

Sorrin's operation, a surgical technique for treating a periodontal abscess, used especially when the marginal gingiva appears healthy and provides no access to the abscess. A semilunar incision is made below the abscess area in the attached gingiva, leaving the gingival margin undisturbed. The tissue flap produced by the incision is raised, accessing the abscessed area for curettage, after which the wound is sutured.

s.o.s., abbreviation for the Latin phrase *si opus sit,* 'if necessary.'

souffle /sōō'fəl/ [Fr, breath], a soft murmur heard through a stethoscope. When detected over the uterus in a pregnant woman, it is usually coincident with the maternal pulse and is caused by blood circulating in the large uterine arteries.

soul food [AS, *sawel* + *foda*], food linked with cultural or traditional origins, especially African-American, that produces feelings of emotional significance and personal satisfaction in an individual.

sound [L, *sonus*], an instrument used to locate the opening of a cavity or canal, to test the patency of a canal, to ascertain the depth of a cavity, or to reveal the contents of a canal or cavity.

Souques's sign /sōōks/ [Alexandre A. Souques, French neurologist, 1860–1944], in patients with a disease of the corpus striatum, the failure of a seated patient to extend the legs when the chair is pushed backward. The legs normally would be extended to prevent overbalancing.

source to image receptor distance (SID), (/sôrs, sōrs/ [OFr, *sourse,* origin; L, *imago,* likeness], the distance between the focus of an x-ray beam and the x-ray film as measured along the beam.

Southern blot test /suth'ərn/, a gene analysis method used in identification of specific deoxyribonucleic acid fragments and in diagnosis of cancers and hemoglobinopathies.

Sp, *pl.* **sp., spp.,** abbreviation for **species.**

space [L, *spatium*], an actual or potential

S

cavity of the body, such as the complemental spaces in the pleural cavity that are not occupied by lung tissue and the lymph spaces occupied by lymph.

space adaptation syndrome, the ability to accommodate changes in cardiac function, bone mineral changes, and muscle atrophy while in the weightless state of a space traveler.

space maintainer, a fixed or removable appliance for preserving the space created by the premature loss of one or more teeth.

space medicine, a branch of medicine concerned with the effects of travel in space, beyond the atmosphere and pull of gravity, including weightlessness, motion sickness, and restricted physical activity.

space obtainer, an appliance for increasing the space between adjoining teeth.

space regainer, a fixed or removable appliance for moving a displaced permanent tooth into its normal position in a dental arch.

sparganosis /spär'gənō'sis/ [Gk, _sparganon,_ swaddling clothes, _osis,_ condition], an infection with larvae of the fish tapeworm of the pseudogenus Sparganum. It is characterized by painful subcutaneous swellings or swelling and destruction of the eye. It is acquired by ingesting larvae in contaminated water or in inadequately cooked infected frog flesh.

spasm /spaz'əm/ [Gk, _spasmos_], **1.** an involuntary muscle contraction of sudden onset, such as habit spasms, hiccups, stuttering, or a tic. **2.** a convulsion or seizure. **3.** a sudden transient constriction of a blood vessel, bronchus, esophagus, pylorus, ureter, or other hollow organ.

spasmatic asthma /spazmat'ik/ [Gk, _spasmos + asthma,_ panting], an airway obstruction characterized by paroxysms of wheezing and coughing caused by spasms of the bronchioles and inflammation of the bronchial mucosa.

spasmodic dysmenorrhea /spazmod'ik/, difficult menstruation accompanied by painful contractions of the uterus.

spasmodic dysphonia [Gk, _spasmodes,_ spasms, _dys,_ bad, _phone,_ voice], a speech disorder in which phonation is intermittently blocked by spasms of the larynx.

spasmodic stricture [Gk, _spasmodes_ + L, _strictura,_ compression], a narrowing of a passage in which there is no organic change, merely muscle spasms.

spasmodic tic [Gk, _spasmodes_ + Fr, _tic_], any repetitive movement in which spasmodic muscle group contractions occur at variable intervals.

spasmodic torticollis [Gk, _spasmodes_ + L, _tortus,_ twisted, _collum,_ neck], a form of

torticollis characterized by episodes of spasms of the neck muscles. In some cases, severe stress and muscular spasm may be the cause.

spasmogen /spaz'məjən/, any substance that can produce smooth muscle contractions, as in the bronchioles; examples are histamine, bradykinin, and serotonin.

spastic /spas'tik/ [Gk, _spastikos,_ drawing in], pertaining to spasms or other uncontrolled contractions of the skeletal muscles. **—spasticity,** _n._

spastic aphonia, a condition in which a person is unable to speak because of spasmodic contraction of the abductor muscles of the throat.

spastic bladder, a form of neurogenic bladder caused by a lesion of the spinal cord above the voiding reflex center. It is marked by loss of bladder control and bladder sensation; incontinence; and automatic interrupted, incomplete voiding. It is most often caused by trauma.

spastic constipation [Gk, _spasmos,_ spasm; L, _constipare,_ to crowd together], a form of constipation associated with neurasthenia and constrictive spasms in part of the intestine. The condition may be a sign of lead poisoning.

spastic diplegia, paralysis of corresponding parts on both sides of the body.

spastic dysarthria, a speech or language disorder caused by lesions of the corticobulbar tracts. It affects voluntary movements of the speech mechanism.

spastic dysuria, difficulty in urination caused by bladder spasms.

spastic gait [Gk, _spasmos,_ spasm; ONorse, _gata_], a pattern of walking in which the legs are stiff, the feet plantar-flexed, and movements made by circumduction. The steps also may be accompanied by toe dragging.

spastic hemiplegia, paralysis of one side of the body with increased tendon reflexes and uncontrolled contraction occurring in the affected muscles.

spastic ileus [Gk, _spasmos,_ spasm, _eilein,_ to twist], a form of intestinal obstruction caused by bowel spasms.

spasticity /spastis'itē/ [Gk, _spastikos,_ drawing in], a form of muscular hypertonicity with increased resistance to stretch. It usually involves the flexors of the arms and the extensors of the legs. Moderate spasticity is characterized by movements that require great effort and lack of normal coordination. Slight spasticity may be marked by gross movements that are coordinated smoothly, but combined selective movement patterns are incoordinated or impossible.

spastic paralysis, an abnormal condition

characterized by the involuntary contraction of one or more muscles with associated loss of muscular function.

spastic paraplegia [Gk, *spasmos,* spasm, *para* + *plege,* stroke], a form of partial paralysis mainly affecting older people. It is accompanied by irritability and spastic contractions of the leg muscles.

spastic strabismus [Gk, *spasmos* + *strabismos,* squint], squint caused by spasmodic contractions of ocular muscles.

spatial dance /spā'shəl/ [L, *spatium,* space; ME, *dauncen,* to drag along], the body shifts or movements used by individuals as they try to adjust the distance between themselves and other individuals.

spatial relationships, 1. orientation in space; the ability to locate objects in the three-dimensional external world, using visual or tactile recognition, and to make a spatial analysis of the observed information. **2.** the relative locations of staff and equipment in an operating room, with particular emphasis on what is sterile, clean, or contaminated.

spatial zones, the areas of personal space in which most people interact. Four basic spatial zones are the intimate zone, in which distance between individuals is less than 18 inches; the personal zone, between 18 inches and 4 feet; the social zone, extending between 4 and 12 feet; and the public zone, beyond 12 feet.

SPE, abbreviation for **sucrose polyester.**

Spearman's rho /spir'mənz rō'/ [Charles E. Spearman, English psychologist, 1863–1945; *rho,* 17th letter in the Greek alphabet], a statistical test for correlation between two rank-ordered scales. It yields a statement of the degree of interdependence of the scores of the two scales.

special care unit /spesh'əl/ [L, *specialis,* individual], a hospital unit with the necessary specialized equipment and personnel for handling critically ill or injured patients, such as an intensive care unit, burn unit, or cardiac care unit.

special gene system, a plasmid, transposon or other genetic fragment that is able to transfer genetic information from one cell to another.

specialing /spesh'əling/, *informal.* **1.** (in psychiatric nursing) the constant attendance of a professional staff member on a disturbed patient to protect the patient from harming the self or others and to observe the patient's behavior. **2.** (in nursing) the giving of nursing care to only one person, such as when acting as a private duty nurse or when caring for a patient whose needs are so great that a nurse is required at all times.

specialist /spesh'əlist/, a health care professional who practices a specialty. A specialist usually has advanced clinical training and may have a postgraduate academic degree.

special sense, the sense of sight, smell, taste, touch, or hearing.

specialty /spesh'əltē/ [L, *specialis*], a branch of medicine or nursing in which the professional is specially qualified to practice by having attended an advanced program of study, passed an examination given by an organization of the members of the specialty, or gained experience through extensive practice in the specialty.

specialty care, specialized medical services provided by a physician specialist.

species (Sp) /spē'sēz, spē'shēz/, *pl.* **species (sp., spp.)** /spē'sēz, spē'shēz/ [L, form], the category of living things below genus in rank. A species is a genetically distinct group of demes that share a common gene pool and are reproductively isolated from all other such groups.

species immunity, a form of natural immunity shared by all members of a species.

species-specific [L, *specere,* to see, *facere,* to make], **1.** pertaining to the characteristics of a particular species. **2.** having a characteristic effect on, or interaction with, cells, tissues, or membranes of a particular species; said of an antigen, drug, or infective agent.

species-specific antigen, antigen that is restricted to a single species but occurs in all members of that species.

specific absorption rate (SAR) /spisif'ik/ [L, *species,* form], (in hyperthermia treatment) the rate of absorption of heat energy (W) per unit mass of tissue in units of watts per kilogram (W/kg).

specific activity, 1. (in nuclear medicine) the radioactivity of a radioisotope per unit mass of the element or compound, expressed in microcuries per millimole or disintegrations per second per milligram. **2.** the relative activity per unit mass, expressed as counts per minute per milligram.

specific disease, a disorder caused by a special pathogenic organism.

specific granule, a secondary granule in the cytoplasm of polymorphonuclear leukocytes that contain lysozyme, vitamin B_{12}-binding protein, neutral proteases, and lactoferrin.

specific granule deficiency, an immunodeficiency state associated with pyodermas and abscesses in which neutrophils fail to make specific granules.

specific gravity, the ratio of the density of a substance to the density of another substance accepted as a standard. The

S

usual standard for liquids and solids is water. Thus a liquid or solid with a specific gravity of 4 is four times as dense as water.

specific immune globulin, a special preparation obtained from human blood that is preselected for its high antibody count against a specific disease, such as varicella zoster immune globulin.

specificity /spes´əfis´itē/ [L, *species,* form, *facere,* to make], the quality of being distinctive. Kinds of specificity may include **group, species,** and **type.**

specificity of association, the uniqueness of a relationship between a causal factor and the occurrence of a disease.

specific rates, statistical rates in which the events in both the numerator and the denominator are restricted to a specific subgroup of a population.

specific ulcer [L, *species, facere,* to make, *ilcus*], ulcer associated with a specific disease, as a syphilitic ulcer.

specific viscosity [L, *species + facere,* to make, *viscosus,* sticky], the internal friction of a fluid, which may be measured by comparing the rate of flow of the fluid through a tube with the rate of a standard liquid under standard conditions.

specimen /spes´imən/ *pl.* **specimens** [L, *specere,* to look], a small sample of something, intended to show the nature of the whole, such as a urine specimen.

Specimen Management, a Nursing Interventions Classification defined as obtaining, preparing, and preserving a specimen for a laboratory test.

speckled dystrophy of the cornea /spek´əlt/, a familial condition characterized by irregular mottling of the cornea by spots that vary in shape and size, with clear centers and sharp margins.

speckled pattern, an immunofluorescence pattern produced when serum from a patient with a particular connective tissue disease is placed in contact with human epithelial cells and stained with fluorochrome-labeled animal antisera. Fine, coarse, or large speckles are observed in disorders such as lupus erythematosus and rheumatoid arthritis.

SPECT, abbreviation for *single-photon emission computed tomography.*

spectator ions /spek´tātər/, ions that are not involved in a chemical reaction.

spectinomycin hydrochloride /spek´tinō-mī´sin/, an antibiotic prescribed in the treatment of gonorrhea and certain infections in penicillin-allergic patients.

spectrometer /spektrom´ətər/ [L, *spectrum,* image; Gk, *metron,* measure], an instrument for measuring wavelengths of rays of the spectrum, the deviation of refracted rays, and the angles between faces of a prism.

spectrometry /spektrom´ətrē/, the process of measuring wavelengths of light and other electromagnetic waves. —**spectrometric,** *adj.*

spectrophotometry /spek´trōfətom´ətrē/, the measurement of color in a solution by determining the amount of light absorbed in the ultraviolet, infrared, or visible spectrum, widely used in clinical chemistry to calculate the concentration of substances in solution. —**spectrophotometric,** *adj.*

spectrum /spek´trəm/, *pl.* **spectra** [L, image], **1.** a range of phenomena or properties occurring in increasing or decreasing magnitude. Radiant or electromagnetic energy is arranged on the basis of wavelength and frequency. **2.** the range of effectiveness of an antibiotic. A broad-spectrum antibiotic is effective against a wide range of microorganisms.

speculum /spek´yələm/ [L, mirror], a retractor used to separate the walls of a cavity to make examination possible, such as an ear speculum, an eye speculum, a nasal speculum, or a vaginal speculum.

speech [ME, *speche*], **1.** the utterance of articulate vocal sounds that form words to give expression to one's thoughts or ideas. **2.** communication by means of spoken words. **3.** the faculty of language production, which involves the complex coordination of the muscles and nerves of the organs of articulation.

speech center [AS, *spaec* + Gk, *kentron*], a unilateral area in the posterior part of the inferior frontal gyrus and usually on the side contralateral to the dominant hand. Also associated with articulate speech are Brodmann's areas 44 and 45.

speech dysfunction, any defect or abnormality of speech, including aphasia, alexia, stammering, stuttering, aphonia, and slurring. Speech problems may result from any of a variety of causes, among them neurologic injury to the cerebral cortex; muscular paralysis caused by trauma, disease, or cerebrovascular accident; structural abnormality of the organs of speech; emotional or psychologic tension, strain, or depression; hysteria; and severe mental retardation.

speech-language pathologist, an individual with graduate professional training in human communication, its development, and its disorders. The person specializes in the measurement and evaluation of language abilities, auditory processes and speech production, clinical treatment of children and adults with speech and language disorders, and research methods in the study of communication processes.

speech pathology, 1. the study of abnormalities of speech or organs of speech. **2.** the diagnosis and treatment of abnormalities of speech as practiced by a speech pathologist or a speech therapist.

speech reading, [ME, *reden,* to explain], a method of oral communication in which one uses the visual clues of the speaker's lip and facial movements, along with residual hearing. Gestures and "body language" also are observed.

speech synthesizer [AS, *spaec* + Gk, *synthesis,* placing together], an electronic apparatus with a keyboard that produces sounds that imitate the human voice.

speech therapy [AS, *spaec* + Gk, *therapeia,* treatment], the application of treatments and counseling in the prevention or correction of speech and language disorders.

speed [AS, *spedan,* to hasten], **1.** the rate of change of position with time. **2.** *slang.* any stimulating drug, such as amphetamine. **3.** a reciprocal of the amount of radiation used to produce an image with various components of an x-ray imaging system, such as screens, film, and image intensifiers. A system using little radiation is "fast," whereas one requiring more radiation is "slow." **4.** the amount of exposure of film to light or x-rays needed to produce a desired image.

speed shock, a sudden adverse physiologic reaction to intravenous medications or drugs that are administered too quickly. Some signs of speed shock are a flushed face, headache, a tight feeling in the chest, irregular pulse, loss of consciousness, and cardiac arrest.

sPEEP, abbreviation for **spontaneous PEEP.**

spell of illness [MF, *spel* + *illr,* bad], a period regarded by Medicare rules as the number of days between the admission of an insured patient to a hospital and the day that marks the end of a period during which the insured has not been an inpatient in a hospital or a skilled nursing facility.

sperm antibody /spurm/, a glycoprotein substance that is specific for the head or tail of a spermatozoon. The antibodies are found in a small percentage of infertile males and females and often in vasectomized males.

spermatic cord /spərmat′ik/ [Gk, *sperma,* seed, *chorde,* string], a structure extending from the deep inguinal ring in the abdomen to the testis, descending nearly vertically into the scrotum.

spermatic fistula, an abnormal passage communicating with a testis or a seminal duct.

spermatid /spur′mətid, spəmat′id/ [Gk, *sperma,* seed], a male germ cell that arises from a spermatocyte and becomes a mature spermatozoon in the last phase of the continual process of spermatogenesis.

spermatocele /spərmat′əsēl′, spur′-/ [Gk, *sperma* + *kele,* tumor], a cystic swelling, either of the epididymis or of the rete testis, that contains spermatozoa.

spermatocide /spərmat′əsīd, spur′-/ [Gk, *sperma* + L, *caedere,* to kill], a chemical substance that kills spermatozoa by reducing their surface tension, causing the cell wall to break down by a bactericidal effect or by creation of a highly acidic environment.

spermatocyte /spur′mətōsīt′/ [Gk, *sperma* + *kytos,* cell], a male germ cell that arises from a spermatogonium.

spermatogenesis /spərmat′əjen′əsis, spur′-/ [Gk, *sperma* + *genesis,* origin], the process of development of spermatozoa, including the first stages, in which spermatogonia become spermatocytes that develop into spermatids, and the second stage, called spermiogenesis, in which the spermatids become spermatozoa. —**spermatogenic, spermatogenous** /spur′mətoj′ənəs/, *adj.*

spermatogonium, *pl.* **spermatogonia** /-gō′nē-əm/ [Gk, *sperma* + *gone,* generation], a male germ cell that gives rise to a spermatocyte early in spermatogenesis.

spermatopathia /-path′e·ə/ [Gk, *sperma,* seed, *pathos,* disease], pertaining to diseased sperm or their associated organs.

spermatozoon /spur′mətəzō′ən, spərmat′-/, *pl.* **spermatozoa** /-zō′ə/ [Gk, *sperma* + *zoon,* animal], a mature male germ cell that develops in the seminiferous tubules of the testes. Resembling a tadpole, it is about 50 μm (1/500 inch) long and has a head with a nucleus, a neck, and a tail that provides propulsion.

sperm bank /spurm/ [Gk, *sperma,* seed; It, *banca,* bench], a facility for storage of semen to be used for artificial insemination.

spermicidal /spur′misī′dəl/, destructive to spermatozoa.

SPF, abbreviation for **sunscreen protective factor index.**

sp.gr., abbreviation for **specific gravity.**

sphacelous /sfas′ələs/, pertaining to something that is necrotic or gangrenous.

S-phase, the phase of a cell reproductive cycle in which deoxyribonucleic acid is synthesized before mitosis.

sphenoethmoid recess /sfē′nō·eth′moid/ [Gk, *sphen,* wedge, *eidos,* form; L, *recedere,* to retreat], a narrow opening in the lateral wall of the nasal cavity bounded above by the cribriform plate of the ethmoid and the body of the sphenoid and below by the superior nasal concha. It opens into the sphenoidal sinus of the skull.

sphenoid /sfē′noid/ [Gk, *sphen*, wedge, *eidos*, form], wedge-shaped.

sphenoidal fissure /sfēnoi′dəl/ [Gk *sphen*, wedge, *eidos* form], a cleft between the great and small wings of the sphenoid bone.

sphenoidal sinus, one of a pair of cavities in the sphenoid bone of the skull, lined with mucous membrane that is continuous with that of the nasal cavity.

sphenoid bone, the bone at the base of the skull, anterior to the temporal bones and the basilar part of the occipital bone.

sphenoid fontanel, an anterolateral fontanel that is usually not palpable.

sphenoiditis /sfē′noidī′tis/ [Gk, *sphen*, wedge, *eidos*, form, *itis*, inflammation], an inflammation of the sphenoidal sinus.

sphenomandibular ligament /sfē′nōmandib′yələr/ [Gk, *sphen* + *eidos* + L, *mandere*, to chew], one of a pair of flat, thin ligaments comprising part of the temporomandibular joint between the mandible of the jaw and the temporal bone of the skull.

sphere /sfir/ a globe-shaped object, theoretically generated by a circle revolving on a diameter as its axis.

spherocyte /sfir′əsīt/ [Gk, *sphaira*, sphere, *kytos*, cell], an abnormal spheric red cell that contains more than the normal amount of hemoglobin. —**spherocytic**, *adj.*

spherocytic anemia /sfir′əsit′ik/, a hematologic disorder inherited as an autosomal-dominant trait and characterized by hemolytic anemia caused by the presence of red blood cells that are spheric rather than round and biconcave. The cells are fragile and tend to hemolyze in the oxygen-poor peripheral circulatory system. Episodic crises of abdominal pain, fever, jaundice, and splenomegaly occur.

spherocytosis /sfir′ōsītō′sis/, the abnormal presence of spherocytes in the blood.

spheroidal /sfir′oidəl/ [Gk, *sphaira*, ball, *eidos*, form], ball-shaped.

spherule /sfer′yo͞ol/ [Gk, *sphaira*, ball], a small ball.

sphincter /sfingk′tər/ [Gk, *sphingein*, to bind], a circular band of muscle fibers that constricts a passage or closes a natural opening in the body, such as the hepatic sphincter in the muscular coat of the hepatic veins near their union with the superior vena cava, and the external anal sphincter, which closes the anus.

sphincter ani, a double set of circular muscles at the opening of the anus. One, the sphincter ani internus, consists of a thickened inner circular coat of the bowel smooth muscle; the other, the sphincter ani externus, is a flat sheet of striated, voluntary muscle surrounding the anal orifice.

sphincter choledochus /kōled′əkəs/, a smooth muscle sphincter that encircles the lower end of the bile duct and is part of the sphincter of Oddi.

sphincter of Oddi [Ruggero Oddi, Italian physician, 1864–1913], a band of circular muscle fibers around the lower end of the common bile and pancreatic duct (hepatopancreatic duct).

sphincter pupillae, a muscle that contracts the iris, narrowing the diameter of the pupil of the eye. It is composed of circular fibers arranged in a narrow band about 1 mm wide, surrounding the margin of the pupil toward the posterior surface of the iris.

sphingolipid /sfing′gōlip′id/ [Gk, *sphingein*, to bind, *lipos*, fat], a compound that consists of a lipid and a sphingosine. It is found in high concentrations in the brain and other tissues of the nervous system.

sphingomyelin /sfing′gōmī′əlin/ [Gk, *sphingein* + *myelos*, marrow], any of a group of sphingolipids containing phosphorus. It occurs primarily in the tissue of the nervous system.

sphingomyelin lipidosis, any of a group of diseases characterized by an abnormality in the ability of the body to store sphingolipids. Kinds of sphingomyelin lipidosis include **Gaucher's disease, Niemann-Pick's disease,** and **Tay-Sachs' disease.**

sphingosine /sfing′gōsēn/, a long-chain unsaturated amino alcohol, a major constituent of sphingolipids and sphingomyelin.

sphygmogram /sfig′məgram/ [Gk, *sphygmos*, pulse, *gramma*, record], a pulse tracing produced by a sphygmograph. Sphygmographic abnormalities of rate, rhythm, and form may be diagnostically useful in an assessment of cardiovascular function.

sphygmograph /sfig′məgraf/, an instrument that records the force of the arterial pulse on a tracing, the sphygmogram. —**sphygmographic**, *adj.*

sphygmoid /sfig′moid/ [Gk, *sphygmos*, pulse, *eidos*, form], pertaining to or resembling the pulse.

sphygmomanometer /sfig′mōmənom′ətər/ [Gk, *sphygmos* + *manos*, thin, *metron*, measure], an instrument for indirect measurement of blood pressure. It consists of an inflatable cuff that fits around the arm, a bulb for controlling air pressure within the cuff, and a mercury or aneroid manometer. Pressure in the brachial artery is estimated by the column of mercury it balances when the cuff is inflated.

sphygmoplethysmograph /-pləthis'mə-graf'/ [Gk, *sphygmos,* pulse, *plethysmos,* increase, *graphein,* to record], an instrument for measuring and recording the arterial pulse curve and blood flow in a limb.

spica [L, *spica,* spike, or ear of wheat], a figure-of-eight bandage that, when applied to a joint, resembles the head of a stalk of wheat.

spica bandage /spī'kə/ [L, *spica,* spike of wheat; Fr, *bande,* strip], a figure-of-eight bandage in which each turn generally overlaps the previous to form a succession of V-like designs. It may be used to give support; to apply pressure; or to hold a dressing in place on the chest, limbs, thighs, or pelvis.

spica cast, an orthopedic cast applied to immobilize part or all of the trunk of the body and part or all of one or more extremities. Kinds of spica casts are **bilateral long-leg spica cast, one-and-a-half spica cast, shoulder spica cast,** and **unilateral long-leg spica cast.**

spicule /spik'yool/ [L, *spiculus,* sharp point], a sharp body with a needlelike point.

spider angioma [ME, *spithre* + Gk, *angeion,* vessel, *oma,* tumor], a form of telangiectasis characterized by a central elevated red dot the size of a pinhead from which small blood vessels radiate.

spider bite [ME, *spithre* + AS, *bitan* + L, *potio,* drink], a puncture wound produced by the bite of any of nearly 60 species of venomous spiders found in North America. Most spiders have fangs that are too short or fragile to penetrate the skin, but some are dangerous to humans. These include the black widow, *Lactrodectus mactans;* the brown recluse, *Loxosceles reclusa;* and species of jumping spiders and tarantulas.

spider telangiectasia [ME, *spithre* + Gk, *telos,* end, *angeion,* vessel, *ektasis,* dilation], a branched group of dilated capillary blood vessels forming a spiderlike image on the skin.

spike, the main peak in an electronic recording such as an oscillograph.

spikeboard /spīk'bôrd/, a device that enables people with upper extremity handicaps to stabilize foods for meal preparation, typically used by individuals with functional use of only one hand..

spillway [AS, *spillan,* to destroy, *weg,* wagon track], a channel or passageway through which food normally escapes from the occlusal surfaces of the teeth during mastication.

spin [AS, *spinnan,* to draw threads], **1.**

the intrinsic angular momentum of an elementary particle or a nucleus of an atom. **2.** intrinsic joint movements about an axis perpendicular to the articular surface.

spina /spī'nə/, *pl.* **spinae** [L, backbone], **1.** the spinal column. **2.** a spine or a thornlike projection, such as the bony projection on the anterior border of the ilium, forming the anterior end of the iliac crest.

spina bifida /bif'ədə, bī'fədə/, a congenital neural tube defect characterized by a developmental anomaly in the posterior vertebral arch. It may occur with only a small deformed lamina separated by a midline gap, or it may be associated with the complete absence of laminae surrounding a large area. Spina bifida that does not involve herniation of the meninges or the contents of the spinal canal rarely requires treatment.

spina bifida anterior, incomplete closure along the anterior surface of the vertebral column.

spina bifida cystica, a developmental defect of the central nervous system in which a hernial cyst containing meninges (meningocele), spinal cord (myelocele), or both (myelomeningocele) protrudes through a congenital cleft in the vertebral column. The protruding sac is encased in a layer of skin or a fine membrane that readily ruptures, causing the leakage of cerebrospinal fluid and an increased risk of meningeal infection.

spina bifida occulta, defective closure of the laminae of the vertebral column in the lumbosacral region without hernial protrusion of the spinal cord or meninges. It is identified externally by a skin depression or dimple, dark tufts of hair, telangiectasis, or soft subcutaneous lipomas at the site. Because the neural tube has closed, there are usually no neurologic impairments associated with the defect. However, any abnormal adhesion of the spinal cord to the area of the malformation may lead to neuromuscular disturbances.

spinal /spī'nəl/ [L, *spina*], **1.** pertaining to a spine, especially the spinal column. **2.** *informal.* spinal anesthesia, such as saddle block or caudal anesthesia.

spinal anesthesia [L, *spina,* backbone; Gk, *anaisthesia,* lack of feeling], a state of insensitivity to pain in the lower part of the body produced by injection of a local anesthetic drug into the subarachnoid cerebrospinal fluid space.

spinal aperture, a large opening formed by the body of a vertebra and its arch.

spinal block [L, *spina,* backbone; OFr, *bloc*], an obstruction of cerebrospinal fluid circulation.

spinal canal, the cavity within the vertebral column.

spinal cord, a long, nearly cylindric structure lodged in the vertebral canal and extending from the foramen magnum at the base of the skull to the upper part of the lumbar region. A major component of the central nervous system, the adult cord is approximately 1 cm in diameter, with an average length of 42 to 45 cm and a weight of 30 g. The cord is an extension of the medulla oblongata of the brain that extends at the level of the first or second lumbar vertebra. The cord conducts sensory and motor impulses to and from the brain and controls many reflexes. Thirty-one pairs of spinal nerves originate from the cord: 8 cervical, 12 thoracic, 5 lumbar, 5 sacral, and 1 coccygeal. It has an inner core of gray material consisting mainly of nerve cell bodies. The cord is enclosed by three protective membranes (meninges): the dura mater, arachnoid, and pia mater.

spinal cord compression, an abnormal and often serious condition resulting from pressure on the spinal cord. The symptoms range from temporary numbness of an extremity to permanent quadriplegia, depending on the cause, severity, and location of the pressure. Causes include spinal fracture, vertebral dislocation, tumor, hemorrhage, and edema associated with contusion.

spinal cord injury, any one of the traumatic disruptions of the spinal cord, often associated with extensive musculoskeletal involvement. Common spinal cord injuries are vertebral fractures and dislocations, such as those commonly suffered by individuals involved in car accidents, airplane crashes, or other violent impacts. Such trauma may cause varying degrees of paraplegia and quadriplegia. Injuries to spinal structures below the first thoracic vertebra may produce paraplegia. Injuries to the spine above the first thoracic vertebra may cause quadriplegia. Injuries that completely transect the spinal cord cause permanent loss of motor and sensory functions activated by neurons below the level of the lesions involved. Spinal cord injuries produce a state of spinal shock, characterized by flaccid paralysis and complete loss of skin sensation at the time of injury. Musculoskeletal complications are associated with the neurologic involvement of spinal cord injuries.

spinal cord tumor, a neoplasm of the spinal cord of which more than 50% are extramedullary, about 25% are intramedullary, and the rest are extradural. Symptoms usually develop slowly and may progress from unilateral paresthesia and a dull ache to lancinating pain; weakness in one or both legs; abnormal deep tendon reflexes; and, in advanced cases, monoplegia, hemiplegia, or paraplegia. Function of the autonomic nervous system is sometimes disturbed, causing areas of dry, cold, bluish pink skin or profuse sweating of the lower extremities.

spinal curvature any persistent, abnormal deviation of the vertebral column from its normal position. Kinds of spinal curvature are **kyphoscoliosis, kyphosis, lordosis,** and **scoliosis.**

spinal fusion, the fixation of an unstable segment of the spine. It is accomplished by skeletal traction or immobilization of the patient in a body cast but most frequently by a surgical procedure.

spinal headache, a headache occurring after spinal anesthesia or lumbar puncture, caused by a loss of cerebrospinal fluid from the subarachnoid space, resulting in traction of the meninges on the pressure-sensitive intracranial structures. Severe spinal headache may be accompanied by diminished aural and visual acuity. Meningeal irritation and backache may persist for several days. The incidence of spinal headache is greatest when a large-bore needle is used for the initial anesthetic or diagnostic procedure.

spinal manipulation, the forced passive flexion, extension, and rotation of vertebral segments, carrying the elements of articulation beyond the usual range of movement to the limit of anatomic range.

spinal meningitis, an inflammation of the membranes of the spinal cord.

spinal motion segment, two adjacent vertebrae and the connecting tissues that bind them together.

spinal nerves, the 31 pairs of nerves without special names that are connected to the spinal cord and numbered according to the level of the vertebral column at which they emerge. There are 8 cervical, 12 thoracic, 5 lumbar, 5 sacral, and 1 coccygeal pair. The first cervical pair of nerves emerges from the spinal cord in the space between the first cervical vertebra and the occipital bone. The rest of the cervical pairs and all the thoracic pairs emerge horizontally through the intervertebral foramina of their respective vertebrae. The lumbar, the sacral, and the coccygeal nerve pairs descend from their points of origin at the lower end of the cord before reaching the intervertebral foramina of their respective vertebrae. Each spinal nerve attaches to the spinal cord by an anterior (or ventral) root and a posterior (or dorsal) root. The posterior roots contain sensory neurons and accompany a distended spinal ganglion within the vertebral foramina. The ventral roots contain motor neuron axons. The sacral plexus in the pelvic cavity comprises certain spinal nerve fibers from the lumbar and sacral regions and gives rise to the great sciatic nerve in the back of the thigh.

spinal reflex [L, *spina* + *reflectere*, to bend back], any reflex with a pathway through the spinal cord but not the brain.

spinal segment, a division of the spinal cord containing a bilateral pair of nerve roots. From the anterior to the posterior, the segments are referred to as cervical (C_1-C_8), thoracic (T_1-T_{12}), lumbar (L_1-L_5), sacral (S_1-S_5), and coccygeal (Co_1-Co_3).

spinal shock, a form of shock associated with acute injury to the spinal cord.

spinal tract, any one of the ascending (sensory) and descending (motor) pathways for sensory or motor nerve impulses that is found in the white matter of the spinal cord. Twenty-one different tracts lie within the dorsal, ventral, and lateral funiculi of the white substance. Ascending tracts conduct impulses up the spinal cord to the brain; descending tracts conduct impulses down the cord from the brain. Touch, pressure, proprioception, temperature, and pain are sensory stimuli transmitted via the spinal tracts. Reflex and voluntary motor activity is regulated by motor nerve stimulation from the brain and brainstem to the motor neurons of the spinal cord.

spin density, (in nuclear magnetic resonance [MR] imaging) a measure of the hydrogen concentration. It is a quantity proportional to the number of hydrogen nuclei precessing at the Larmor frequency and contributing to the MR signal.

spindle [AS, *spinel*, to spin], **1.** the fusiform figure of achromatin in the cell nucleus during the late prophase and the metaphase of mitosis. **2.** a type of brain wave, consisting of a short series of changes in electrical potential with a frequency of 14 per second. **3.** any one of the special receptor organs comprising the neurotendinous and neuromuscular spindles distributed throughout the body.

spindle cell carcinoma, a rapidly growing neoplasm composed of fusiform squamous cells.

spine, 1. the vertebral column, or backbone. **2.** descriptive of a spinous process.

spine of scapula [L, *spina,* backbone, *scapulae,* shoulder blades], a sharp-edged plate of bone projecting posteriorly backward from the flattened scapula base.

spinnbarkeit /spin'bärkīt, shpin'-/ [Ger, threadability], the clear slippery elastic consistency characteristic of cervical mu-

cus during ovulation. It has the consistency of an uncooked egg white, and it is a valuable sign of the peak fertile period in a woman's menstrual cycle.

spinocerebellar /spī'nōser'əbel'ər/ [L, *spina* + *cerebellum,* small brain], pertaining to the spinal cord and the cerebellum.

spinocerebellar disorder, an inherited disorder characterized by a progressive degeneration of the spinal cord and cerebellum, often involving other parts of the nervous system as well. These disorders tend to occur within families and can be inherited as dominant or recessive traits. Some kinds of spinocerebellar degeneration are **ataxia-telangiectasia, Charcot-Marie-Tooth disease, Dejerine-Sottas disease, Friedreich's ataxia, olivopontocerebellar atrophy,** and **Refsum's syndrome.**

spinous /spī'nəs/ [L, *spina,* backbone], pertaining to an object that has the shape of a spine or thorn.

spinous process [L, *spina,* backbone, *processus*], a spinelike projection of bony tissue.

spiral bandage /spī'rəl/ [Gk, *speira,* coil; Fr, *bande,* strip], any roller bandage applied around a limb that ascends the body part, with each turn overlapping the previous one by half to two thirds of a bandage width.

spiral fracture [Gk, *speira,* coil], a bone break in which the disruption of bone tissue is spiral, oblique, or transverse to the long axis of the fractured bone.

spiraling /spī'rəling/, the process by which immunodeficiency allows viral replication, which further depresses the immune system, allowing further viral replication, and so on.

spiral reverse bandage, a spiral bandage that is turned and folded back on itself as necessary to make it fit the contour of the body more securely.

spirit /spir'it/ [L, *spiritus,* breath], **1.** any volatile liquid, particularly one that has been distilled. **2.** a volatile substance dissolved in alcohol.

spirit of ammonia [L, *spiritus,* breath; *Ammon,* temple in Libya], a solution of 3% ammonium carbonate in alcohol with flavorings added. It is mixed with water for use as a stimulant and carminative.

spiritual distress (distress of the human spirit) /spir'ichoo·əl/, a NANDA-accepted nursing diagnosis of disruption in the life principle that pervades a person's entire being and that integrates and transcends one's biologic and psychosocial nature. Defining characteristics include stated anger against the deity or

S

questions about the meaning of the suffering being experienced. The client may joke in a macabre fashion, regard the illness as punishment, have nightmares, cry, act in a hostile or apathetic manner, express self-blame or deny all responsibility for the problem, express anger or resentment against religious figures, and cease participation in religious practices.

Spiritual Support, a Nursing Interventions Classification defined as assisting the patient to feel balance and connection with a greater power.

spiritual therapy [L, *spiritus,* breath; Gk, *therapeia,* treatment], a form of counseling or psychotherapy that involves moral and religious influences on behavior and physical health.

spiritual well-being, potential for enhanced, a NANDA-accepted nursing diagnosis of the process of an individual's developing or unfolding of mystery through harmonious interconnectedness that springs from inner strengths. The defining characteristics are inner strengths: a sense of awareness, self-consciousness, sacred source, unifying force, inner core, and transcendence; unfolding mystery: one's experience about life's purpose and meaning, mystery, uncertainty, and struggles; harmonious interconnectedness: relatedness, connectedness, harmony with self, others, higher power or God, and the environment.

Spirochaeta pallida /spī′rəkē′tə/ [Gk, *speira,* coil, *chaite,* hair; L, *pallidus,* pale], a species of flexible spiral motile microorganisms that is the cause of human syphilis.

spirochete /spī′rəkēt′/ [Gk, *speira,* coil, *chaite,* hair], any bacterium of the genus *Spirochaeta* that is motile and spiral-shaped with flexible filaments. Kinds of spirochetes include the organisms responsible for leptospirosis, relapsing fever, syphilis, and yaws. —**spirochetal,** *adj.*

spirochetemia /spī′rōkətē′mē-ə/ [Gk, *speira,* coil, *chaite,* + *haima,* blood], the presence of spirochetal organisms in the blood.

spirogram /spī′rōgram/ [Gk, *speira* + *gramma,* record], a visual record of respiratory movements made by a spirometer, used in the assessment of pulmonary function and capacity.

spirograph /spī′rəgraf/ [Gk, *speira* + *graphein,* to record], a device for recording respiratory movements. —**spirographic,** *adj.*

spirometer /spīrom′ətər/ [Gk, *speira* + *metron,* measure], an instrument that measures and records the volume of in-

haled and exhaled air, used to assess pulmonary function. —**spirometric,** *adj.*

spirometry /spīrom′ətrē/, laboratory evaluation of the air capacity of the lungs by means of a spirometer. —**spirometric,** *adj.*

spironolactone /spī′rənəlak′tōn/, a potassium-sparing aldosterone antagonist diuretic. It is prescribed in the treatment of primary hyperaldosteronism, edema of congestive heart failure, cirrhosis of the liver accompanied by edema, nephrotic syndrome, essential hypertension, and hypokalemia.

spittle [AS, *spittan,* spew], saliva.

splanchnic /splangk′nik/, pertaining to the internal organs; visceral.

splanchnic engorgement, the excessive filling or pooling of blood within the visceral vasculature after the removal of pressure from the abdomen, as in the excision of a large tumor or birth of a child.

splanchnic nerves [Gk, *splanchna,* viscera, *nervus*], a network of nerves, mainly preganglionic fibers, with filaments innervating the penis and clitoris, as well as the uterus, rectum, and other structures of the abdominal cavity.

splanchnocele /splangk′nōsēl′/ [Gk, *splanchna,* viscera, *kele,* hernia], hernial protrusion of any abdominal viscera.

splanchnocoele /splangk′nōsēl′/ [Gk, *splanchna,* viscera, *koilos,* hollow], a part of the embryonic body cavity, or coelom, that gives rise to the abdominal, pericardial, and pleural cavities.

splanchnopleure /splangk′nōplōōr′/ [Gk, *splanchna* + *pleura,* side], a layer of tissue in the early developing embryo, formed by the union of endoderm and splanchnic mesoderm. —**splanchnopleural,** *adj.*

S-plasty /es′plas′tē/, a technique of plastic surgery in which an S-shaped instead of a straight line incision is made to reduce tension and improve healing in areas where the skin is loose.

splay /splā/, **1.** to spread or turn out. **2.** to spread out, as said of the limbs. **3.** to open, as with the end of a tubular structure by making a longitudinal incision. **4.** to dislocate a bone.

splayfoot [ME, *splaien* + AS, *fot*], a foot that is flat and extremely everted, away from the midline.

spleen [Gk, *splen*], a soft, highly vascular, roughly ovoid organ situated between the stomach and the diaphragm in the left hypochondriac region of the body. It is considered part of the lymphatic system because it contains localized lymphatic nodules. It is dark purple and varies in shape in different individuals. Research indicates it performs various tasks such as defense, hemopoiesis, blood storage, and destruction/recycling of red blood cells and platelets. The spleen also produces leukocytes, monocytes, lymphocytes, and plasma cells in response to an infectious agent. If the body suffers severe hemorrhage, the spleen can contract and increase the blood volume from 350 ml to 550 ml in less than 60 seconds. —**splenic** /splen'ik/, adj.

spleen scan, the scan of the spleen after the injection of radioactive red blood cells, performed to detect a tumor, damage, or other problem.

splenectomy /splənek'təmē/ [Gk, splen + ektome, excision], the surgical removal of the spleen.

splenic flexure /splen'ik/ [Gk, splen, spleen; L, flectere, to bend], the left flexure of the colon, as it bends at the junction of the transverse and descending segments of the colon, near the spleen.

splenic flexure syndrome [Gk, splen + L, flectere, to bend], a recurrent pain and abdominal distension in the left upper quadrant of the abdomen caused by a pocket of gas trapped in the large intestine below the spleen, at the flexure of the transverse and descending colon.

splenic puncture, a perforation of the parenchyma of the spleen to obtain pressure data or inject radiopaque material.

splenius capitis /splē'nē·əs/ [Gk, splenion, bandage; L, caput, head], one of a pair of deep muscles of the neck and back. It acts to rotate, extend, and bend the head.

splenius cervicis, one of a pair of deep muscles of the neck and back. It acts to rotate, bend, and extend the head and neck.

splenohepatomegaly /splē'nōhep'ətōmeg'-əlē/ [Gk, splen, spleen, hepar, liver, megas, great], an abnormal simultaneous increase in the sizes of the liver and spleen.

splenomegaly /splē'nōmeg'əlē, splen'-/ [Gk, splen + megas, large], an abnormal enlargement of the spleen, as is associated with portal hypertension, hemolytic anemia, Niemann-Pick's disease, or malaria.

splenosis /splēnō'sis/, multiple splenic growths in the peritoneum resulting from splenic rupture or iatrogenic injury.

splint [D, splinte, piece of wood], **1.** an orthopedic device for immobilization, restraint, or support of any part of the body. It may be rigid (of metal, plaster, or wood) or flexible (of felt or leather). **2.** (in dentistry) a device, usually made of hard acrylic and wire, for anchoring the teeth or modifying the bite.

splinter [D, splinte], a sharp pointed piece of bone or other substance.

splinter fracture [D, splinte], a comminuted fracture with thin, sharp bone fragments.

splinter hemorrhage, linear bleeding under a fingernail or toenail, resembling a splinter.

splinting, the process of immobilizing, restraining, or supporting a body part.

Splinting, a Nursing Interventions Classification defined as stabilization, immobilization, and/or protection of an injured body part with a supportive appliance.

split-brain state, a condition resulting from the disconnection of the two cerebral hemispheres. It is produced when the corpus callosum is surgically divided completely or partially as a treatment for epilepsy. The cognitive effects are identified as a disconnection syndrome.

split gene [D, splitten, to split], (in molecular genetics) a genetic unit whose continuity is interrupted.

split Russell traction, an orthopedic mechanism that combines suspension and traction to immobilize, position, and align the lower extremities in the correction of orthopedic deformities and in the treatment of congenital hip dislocation and hip and knee contractures.

split-thickness skin graft, a tissue transplant involving the epidermis and a part of the dermis. This type of graft is the most commonly used method of covering open burn wounds.

splitting, a primitive defense mechanism that when overused represents a developmental arrest. It is a failure to synthesize the positive and negative experiences and ideas one has of oneself, other people, situations, and institutions.

spondylitic [Gk, sphondylos, vertebra], pertaining to a person afflicted with spondylitis.

spondylitis /spon'dəli'tis/ [Gk, sphondylos, vertebra, itis], an inflammation of any of the spinal vertebrae, usually characterized by stiffness and pain. The condition may follow traumatic injury to the spine, or it may be the result of infection or rheumatoid disease.

spondyloarthropathies /spon'dilo'ärthrop'əthēs/, diseases of the joints and spine. Most commonly affected are the lower extremities, sacroiliac joint, and hip. Pain and restricted motion of the hips and lower back are typical complaints. Many patients also experience eye disorders.

spondylolisthesis /spon'dilo'listhē'sis/ [Gk, sphondylos + olisthanein, to slip], the

S

partial forward dislocation of one vertebra over the one below it.

spondylosis /spon'dilō'sis/ [Gk, *sphondylos* + *osis*], a condition of the spine characterized by fixation or stiffness of a vertebral joint.

spondylous /spon'diləs/ [Gk, *sphondylos*, vertebra], pertaining to a vertebra.

sponge /spunj/ [Gk, *spongia*], **1.** a resilient absorbent mass used to absorb fluids, apply medication, or cleanse. **2.** *informal.* a folded gauze square used in surgery.

sponge bath, the procedure of washing the patient with a damp washcloth or sponge, used when a full bath is not necessary or when lowering of body temperature is required.

spongioblastoma /spun'jē-ōblastō'mə/ [Gk, *spongia* + *blastos*, germ, *oma*, tumor], a neoplasm composed of spongioblasts, embryonic epithelial cells that develop around the neural tube and transform into cells of the supporting connective tissue of nerve cells or cells of lining membranes of the ventricles and the spinal cord canal.

spongioblastoma unipolare, a rare neoplasm composed of parallel spongioblasts. The tumor may occur near the third ventricle, in the pons and brainstem, in basal ganglia, or in the terminal filament of the spinal cord.

spongy /spun'jē/ [Gk, *spoggia*], pertaining to or resembling a sponge.

spontaneous /spontá'nē-əs/ [L, *sponte*, willingly], occurring naturally and without apparent cause, such as spontaneous remission.

spontaneous abortion, a termination of pregnancy before the twentieth week of gestation as a result of abnormalities of the conceptus or maternal environment.

spontaneous delivery, a vaginal birth occurring without the mechanical assistance of obstetric forceps or vacuum aspirator.

spontaneous generation, the theoretic origin of living organisms from inanimate matter; abiogenesis.

spontaneous labor, a labor beginning and progressing without mechanical or pharmacologic stimulation.

spontaneous PEEP (sPEEP), a spontaneous breathing system with end-expiratory pressure.

spontaneous phagocytosis [L, *sponte,* free will; Gk, *phagein,* to eat, *kytos,* cell, *osis,* condition], ingestion of antigenic particles by phagocytes of the reticuloendothelial system.

spontaneous pneumothorax [L, *sponte,* free will; Gk, *pneuma,* air, *thorax,* chest], the presence of air or gas in the intrapleural space as a result of a rupture of the

lung parenchyma and visceral pleura with no demonstrable cause.

spontaneous remission, **1.** the reversal of progress of disease without formal treatment. **2.** the disappearance of symptoms of a mentally ill patient without formal treatment.

spontaneous ventilation, normal unassisted breathing in which the patient creates the pressure gradient through muscle and chest wall movements that move the air into and out of the lungs.

spontaneous version [L, *sponte,* free will], *vertere,* to turn], a change in the lie of a fetus that occurs without manipulation.

spoon nail [AS, *spon* + *naegel*], a nail of the finger or toe that is thin and concave.

sporadic /spôrat'ik/ [Gk, *sporaden,* scattered], (of a number of events) occurring at scattered, intermittent, and apparently random intervals.

spore [Gk, *sporos,* seed], **1.** a reproductive unit of some genera of fungi or protozoa. **2.** a form assumed by some bacteria that is resistant to heat, drying, and chemicals. Diseases caused by spore-forming bacteria include anthrax, botulism, gas gangrene, and tetanus.

sporicidal /spôr'isī'dəl/ [Gk, *sporos,* seed; L, *caedere,* to kill], spore-killing, as are certain chemicals or other agents.

sporicide /spôr'isīd/ [Gk, *sporos* + L, *caedere,* to kill], any agent effective in destroying spores, such as compounds of chlorine and formaldehyde, and the glutaraldehydes.

sporiferous /spôrif'ərəs/, producing or bearing spores.

spork, a spoonlike food utensil with fork tines designed for people with upper extremity disabilities.

sporoblast /spôr'əblast'/ [Gk, *sporos* + *blastos,* germ], any cell that gives rise to a sporozoite or spore during the sexual reproductive phase of the life cycle of a sporozoon. It refers specifically to the cells resulting from the multiple fission of the encysted zygote of the malarial parasite *Plasmodium,* from which the sporozoites develop.

sporocyst /spôr'əsist/ [Gk, *sporos* + *kystis,* bag], **1.** any structure containing spores or reproductive cells. **2.** a saclike structure, or oocyst, secreted by the zygote of certain protista before sporozoite formation. **3.** the second larval stage in the life cycle of parasitic flukes.

sporogenesis /spôr'ōjen'əsis/ [Gk, *sporos* + *genesis,* origin], **1.** also called **sporogeny** /spôroj'ənē/. the formation of spores. **2.** reproduction by means of spores. **—sporogenic,** *adj.*

sporogenous /spôroj'ənəs/ [Gk, *sporos* +

genein, to produce], describing an animal or plant that reproduces by spores.

sporogony /spôrog'ənē/ [Gk, *sporos* + *genesis*, origin], reproduction by means of spores. It refers specifically to the formation of sporozoites during the sexual stage of the life cycle of a sporozoon, primarily the malarial parasite *Plasmodium*.

sporont /spôr'ont/ [Gk, *sporos* + *on*, being], a mature protozoan parasite in the sexual reproductive stage of its life cycle.

sporonticide /spôron'tisīd/ [Gk, *sporos* + *on* + L, *caedere*, to kill], any substance that destroys sporonts, such as chloroquine and other antimalarial drugs.— **sporonticidal,** *adj.*

sporophore /spôr'əfôr/ [Gk, *sporos* + *pherein*, to bear], the part of an organism or plant that produces spores.

sporophyte /spôr'əfīt/ [Gk, *sporos* + *phyton*, plant], the asexual, spore-bearing stage in plants that reproduce by alternation of generations.

sporotrichosis /spôr'ōtrikō'sis/ [Gk, *sporos* + *thrix*, hair, *osis*, condition], a common chronic fungal infection caused by the species *Sporothrix schenckii*. It is usually characterized by skin ulcers and subcutaneous nodules along lymphatic channels. It rarely spreads to involve bones, lungs, joints, or muscles. The fungus is found in soil and decaying vegetation and usually enters the skin by accidental injury.

Sporotrichum /spôrot'rikəm/ [Gk, *sporos* + *thrix*, hair], a genus of soil-inhabiting fungi formerly thought to cause sporotrichosis.

Sporozoa /spôr'əzō'ə/ [Gk, *sporos* + *zoon*, animal], a class of parasite in the phylum Protozoa that is characterized by the absence of any external organs of locomotion. Included in this class are the genera *Toxoplasma* and *Plasmodium*.

sporozoite /spôr'əzō'īt/ [Gk, *sporos* + *zoon*, animal], any of the cells resulting from the sexual union of spores during the life cycle of a sporozoon.

sport [ME, *disporten*, to amuse], **1.** an individual or organism that differs drastically from its parents or others of its type because of genetic mutation; a mutant. **2.** a genetic mutation.

sports medicine, a branch of medicine that specializes in the prevention and treatment of injuries resulting from training for and participation in athletic events. Among the most common sports injuries are shin splints, runner's knee, pulled hamstring muscles, Achilles tendonitis, and ankle sprain.

sporulation /spôr'yəlā'shən/ [Gk, *sporos* + L, *atus*, process], **1.** a type of reproduction that occurs in lower plants and animals such as fungi, algae, and protozoa and involves the formation of spores by the spontaneous division of the cell into four or more daughter cells, each of which contains a part of the original nucleus. **2.** the formation of a refractile body, or resting spore, within certain bacteria that makes the cell resistant to unfavorable environmental conditions.

spot [ME, blot], (in psychotherapy) a small quantum of space that becomes the territorial object and extension of point behavior.

spot film, a radiograph made instantly during fluoroscopy.

spotting [ME, *spot*, blot], the appearance of a blood-stained discharge from the vagina between menstrual periods, during pregnancy, or at the beginning of labor.

sprain [ME], a traumatic injury to the tendons, muscles, or ligaments around a joint, characterized by pain, swelling, and discoloration of the skin over the joint. The duration and severity of the symptoms vary with the extent of damage to the supporting tissues.

sprain fracture, a fracture that results from the separation of a tendon or ligament at the point of insertion, associated with the separation of a bone at the same insertion site.

sprain of ankle or foot [AS, *ancleow* + *fot*], sudden traction on a muscle, ligament, or capsule. The injury is not severe enough to cause a rupture of the tissue.

sprain of back [AS, *baec*], a sudden traction injury to muscles and related tissues of the back. The tissues may have undergone traumatic strain without being ruptured.

spreader bar /spred'ər/, a metal bar with curved hoop areas for attaching hooks or pins for traction.

spring forceps [AS, *springan*, to jump], a kind of forceps that includes a spring mechanism, used for grasping an artery to arrest or prevent hemorrhage.

spring lancet, a very small knife with a spring-triggered blade. It may be used for collecting small specimens of blood for laboratory tests.

sprinter's fracture [Swe, *sprinta*, to spurt; L, *fractura*, to break], a fracture of the anterior superior or the anterior inferior spine of the ilium, caused when a fragment of bone is forcibly pulled by a violent muscle spasm.

sprue /sprōō/ [D, *sprouw*, kind of tumor], a chronic degenerative disorder resulting from malabsorption of nutrients from the small intestine and characterized by a broad range of symptoms, including diarrhea, weakness, weight loss, poor appetite, pallor, muscle cramps, bone pain, ulceration of the mucous membrane lining the digestive tract, and a smooth shiny tongue. It occurs in both tropical and nontropical forms.

SPSS, (in statistics) abbreviation for *Statistical Package for the Social Sciences,* a computer program often used in research in clinical nursing for the analysis of complex data from large samples.

spur [AS, *spura*], a projection of bone or metal from a body structure or appliance.

sputum /spyōo′təm/ [L, spittle], material coughed up from the lungs and expectorated through the mouth. It contains mucus, cellular debris, or microorganisms, and it also may contain blood or pus. The amount, color, and constituents of the sputum are important in the diagnosis of many illnesses.

sputum specimen [L, spittle + *specere,* to look], a sample of material expelled from the respiratory passages taken for laboratory analysis to determine the presence of pathogens.

squama /skwā′mə/, *pl.* **squamae, 1.** a flattened scale from the epidermis. **2.** the thin, expanded part of a bone, especially in the cranial wall.

squamocolumnar junction /skwā′mōkə-lum′nər/, a region of transition from stratified squamous epithelium to columnar epithelium in the cervical canal. It is a location where cells are obtained for Papanicolaou's smears.

squamous [L, *squama,* scale], platelike, scaly, or covered with scales.

squamous cell /skwā′məs/ [L, *squama,* scale, *cella,* storeroom], a flat, scalelike epithelial cell.

squamous cell carcinoma, a slow-growing malignant tumor of squamous epithelium, frequently found in the lungs and skin and occurring also in the anus, cervix, larynx, nose, and bladder. The neoplastic cells characteristically resemble prickle cells and form keratin pearls.

squamous epithelium [L, *squama,* scale; Gk, *epi,* above, *thele,* nipple], a sheet of flattened scalelike cells, attached together at the edges.

square centimeter (cm²) /skwer/, a unit of area measurement equivalent to 1 centimeter in length multiplied by 1 centimeter in width where 1 centimeter equals 0.3937 inch or 0.03281 foot.

square window [OFr, *esquarre* + ME, *wind,* air, *owe,* eye], an angle of the wrist between the hypothenar prominence and forearm. It is used as a reference point for estimating the gestational age of a newborn.

squatting position /skwot′ing/ [Fr, *es-quatir,* to press down], a posture in which the knees and hips are flexed and the buttocks are lowered to the level of the heels. It is a posture adopted by children with certain heart diseases as they seek relief from exercise distress.

squeeze dynamometer /skwēz/ [AS, *cwesan,* to press tightly; Gk, *dynamis,* force, *metron,* measure], a device for measuring the muscular strength of the grip of the hand.

squeeze-film lubrication, the exudation of fluid from the cartilage of joints, forming a film in the transient area of impending contact.

squinting eye /skwin′ting/ [D, *schuinte,* oblique; AS, *eage*], the abnormal eye in a person with strabismus that cannot be focused with the fixated eye.

Sr, symbol for the element **strontium.**

SR, abbreviation for **sedimentation rate.**

sRNA, abbreviation for *soluble ribonucleic acid (RNA).*

SRO, abbreviation for **single room occupant.**

SRS-A, abbreviation for **slow-reacting substance of anaphylaxis.**

SRY, symbol for a "maleness" gene found on the sex-determining region of the Y chromosome. The gene is believed to function as a master control switch with the ability to turn off or on other genes involved in sexual development.

ss, abbreviation for **steady state.**

SSE, 1. abbreviation for **skin self-examination. 2.** abbreviation for **soapsuds enema.**

SSKI, trademark for an expectorant (potassium iodide).

SSRI, abbreviation for **selective serotonin reuptake inhibitor.**

SSS, 1. abbreviation for *sterile saline soak.* **2.** abbreviation for **sick sinus syndrome.**

SSSS, abbreviation for **staphylococcal scalded skin syndrome.**

ST, abbreviation for **slow-twitch.**

stab [ME, *stabbe,* piercing wound], a nonsegmented neutrophil.

stab culture [ME, *stabbe,* piercing wound; L, *colere,* to cultivate], a culture made by dipping a needle into an inoculum and then into a transparent gelatin or agar medium.

stabilization /stab′iləzā′shən/ [L, *stabilis,* firm, *atus,* process], **1.** the physiologic and metabolic process of attaining homeostasis. **2.** the seating of a fixed or removable denture so that it will not tilt or be displaced under pressure. **3.** the control of induced stress loads and the development of measures to counteract such forces so that the movement of the teeth or of a prosthesis does not irritate surrounding tissues.

stabilization exercises, exercises to develop proximal control in symptom (pain)-free positions, such as sitting on a gymnastic ball and extending one knee to maintain balance and control without pain.

stable /stā'bəl/ [L, *stabilis*, firm], remaining unchanged.

stable condition, a state of health or disease from which little if any immediate change is expected.

stable element [L, *stabilis*, firm, *elementum*], a nonradioactive element, one not subject to spontaneous nuclear degeneration. Some kinds of stable elements are calcium, iron, lead, potassium, and sodium.

staccato speech /stəkä'tō/ [It, detached; ME, *speche*], abnormal speech in which the person pauses between words, breaking the rhythm of the phrase or sentence. The condition is sometimes observed in association with multiple sclerosis.

stadium /stā'dē·əm/, *pl.* **stadia** [Gk, *stadion*, racetrack], a significant stage in a fever or illness, such as the fastigium of a febrile illness or the prodromal stage of a viral infection.

staff [AS, *staef*], **1.** the people who work toward a common goal and are employed or supervised by someone of higher rank. **2.** a designation by which a staff nurse is distinguished from a nurse manager or other nurse. **3.** (in nursing education) the nonprofessional employees of the institution such as librarians, technicians, secretaries, and clerks. **4.** (in nursing service administration) the units of the organization that provide service to the line, or administratively defined hierarchy.

staff development, (in nursing) a process that assists individual nurses in an agency or organization in attaining new skills and knowledge, gaining increasing levels of competence, and growing professionally. The process may include such programs as orientation, in-service education, and continuing education.

staffing, the process of assigning people to fill the roles designed for an organizational structure through recruitment, selection, and placement.

staffing pattern, (in hospital or nursing administration) the number and types or categories of staff assigned to the particular units and departments of a hospital or other health care facility. Staffing patterns vary with the unit, department, and shift.

staff of Æsculapius, a staff carried by Æsculapius, the Greek god of medicine. It is used as the traditional symbol of the physician. A single serpent entwines the staff of Æsculapius.

Staff Supervision, a Nursing Interventions Classification defined as facilitating the delivery of high-quality patient care by others.

stage [OFr, *estage*], **1.** a platform. **2.** a period or phase.

stages of dying [OFr, *estage,* stage; ME, *dyen,* to lose life], the five emotional and behavioral stages that may occur after a person first learns of approaching death. The stages, identified and described by Elisabeth Kübler-Ross, are denial and shock, anger, bargaining, depression, and acceptance. The stages may occur in sequence or they may recur, as the person moves forward and backward—especially among denial, anger, and bargaining.

staging /stā'jing, the classification of phases or periods of a disease or other pathologic process, as in the TMN clinical method of assigning numeric values to various stages of tumor development.

stagnant anoxia /stag'nənt/ [L, *stagnum,* standing water; Gk, *a,* without, *oxys,* sharp, *genein,* to produce], a condition in which there is inadequate blood flow in the capillaries, causing low tissue oxygen tension and reduced oxygen exchange.

stain [OFr, *desteindre,* to dye], **1.** a pigment, dye, or substance used to impart color to microscopic objects or tissues to facilitate their examination and identification. **2.** to apply pigment to a substance or tissue to examine it under a microscope. **3.** an area of discoloration.

stained film fault, a defect in a radiograph or developed photographic film that appears as a streaky discoloration or abnormal opacity.

stammering [AS, *stamerian,* to stutter], a speech dysfunction characterized by spasmodic pauses, hesitations, and faltering utterances. The term is not used in the United States but is frequently used synonymously with *stuttering,* especially in Great Britain.

stamp cusp [ME, *stampen* + L, *cuspis,* point], a cusp that works in a fossa, such as any of the maxillary lingual cusps.

stance phase of gait [L, *stare,* to stand; Gk, *phainein,* to show; ME, *gate,* a way], the first phase of the normal gait cycle, which begins with the strike of the heel on the ground and ends with the lift of the toe at the beginning of the swing phase of gait: the brief period in which both feet are on the ground.

standard [OFr, *estandart*], **1.** an evaluation that serves as a basis of comparison for evaluating similar phenomena or substances, such as a standard for the prepara-

S

tion of a pharmaceutic substance or a standard for the practice of a profession. **2.** a pharmaceutic preparation or a chemical substance of known quantity, ingredients, and strength that is used to determine the constituents or the strength of another preparation. **3.** of known value, strength, quality, or ingredients. **4.** predetermined criteria used to provide guidance in the operation of a health care facility to ensure high-quality performance by the personnel. —**standardize,** *v.,* **standardization,** *n.*

standard air chamber, a radiation measuring device used by national and international calibration laboratories to provide exposure calibrations of ion chambers for use in the diagnostic or orthovoltage energy range.

standard bicarbonate, the bicarbonate ion concentration of plasma separated anaerobically from whole blood that has been saturated with oxygen and equilibrated at carbon dioxide pressure of 40 mm Hg at 100° F (38° C). It is a measure of the metabolic disturbance of acid-base balance in a sample of blood after any respiratory disturbance present has been corrected.

standard curve, a graphic plot of tracer binding versus the known concentration of test substances in a set of standards usually prepared by serial dilution or incremental addition.

standard of care, a written statement describing the rules, actions, or conditions that direct patient care. Standards of care guide practice and can be used to evaluate performance.

standard death certificate, a form for a death certificate that is commonly used throughout the United States.

standard deviation (SD), (in statistics) a mathematic statement of the dispersion of a set of values or scores from the mean. Each sample value is subtracted from the sample mean and squared, and the squares are summed. The square root of the summed squares gives a mathematically standardized value so that sample deviations can be compared.

standard error (S.E.), (in statistics) the variability in scores that can be expected if measurements are made on random samples of the same size from the same universe of populations, phenomena, or observations. The standard error provides a framework within which a determination of the difference between groups may be made.

standard hydrogen electrode, a reference electrode that is assigned a value of 0 volt.

standardized death rate, the number of deaths per 1000 people of a specified population during 1 year. This rate is adjusted to prevent distortion by the age composition of the population.

standardized test, any empirically developed examination with established reliability and validity as determined by repeated evaluation of the method and results.

Standard Precautions, guidelines recommended by the Centers for Disease Control and Prevention (CDC) to reduce the risk of transmission of blood-borne and other pathogens in hospitals. The Standard Precautions synthesize the major features of Universal (Blood and Body Fluid) Precautions and Body Substance Isolation (designed to reduce the risk of pathogens from moist body substances) and apply them to all patients receiving care in hospitals, regardless of their diagnosis or presumed infection status. Standard Precautions apply to (1) blood; (2) all body fluids, secretions, and excretions, *excluding sweat,* regardless of whether they contain blood; (3) nonintact skin; and (4) mucous membranes. The Precautions are designed to reduce the risk of transmission of microorganisms from both recognized and unrecognized sources of infection in hospitals.

standard reference gamble, a method of diagnostic testing in which a decision maker is faced with a choice between a certain outcome or intermediate value and a gamble involving a better or worse outcome. The outcomes are assigned arbitrary numeric values of 100 and 0, respectively. All other outcomes can be assigned values relative to the best and worst outcomes.

standards of nursing practice, a set of guidelines for providing high-quality nursing care and criteria for evaluating care. Such guidelines help assure patients that they are receiving high-quality care. The standards are important if a legal dispute arises over the quality of care provided a patient.

standby guardianship, a legal process in the United States that may name an individual to assume specified health care or financial authority for an elderly person who becomes mentally incapacitated.

standing orders [L, *stare,* to stand, *ordo,* rank], a written document containing rules, policies, procedures, regulations, and orders for the conduct of patient care in various stipulated clinical situations. Standing orders usually name the condition and prescribe the action to be taken in caring for the patient, including the dosage and route of administration for a drug or the schedule for the administration of a therapeutic procedure.

stannous fluoride /stan'əs/ [L, *stannum,* tin, *fluere,* to flow], a salt of fluorine and tin used in oral hygiene products to reduce caries activity.

stanozolol /stənō'zəlol/, an androgenic anabolic steroid prescribed in the treatment of aplastic anemia and osteoporosis.

stapedectomy /stā'pədek'təmē/ [L, *stapes,* stirrup; Gk, *ektome,* excision], the removal of the stapes of the middle ear and insertion of a graft and prosthesis, performed to restore hearing in cases of otosclerosis. The stapes that has become fixed is replaced so that vibrations again transmit sound waves through the oval window to the fluid of the inner ear.

stapedius /stəpē'dē·əs/, a small muscle on the wall of the tympanic cavity of the middle ear. With the tensor tympani, it acts reflexively in response to loud sounds to reduce excessive vibrations that could injure the internal ear by pulling the head of the stapes posteriorly out of the oval window.

stapes /stā'pēz/ [L, stirrup], one of the three ossicles in the middle ear, resembling a tiny stirrup. It transmits sound vibrations from the incus to the internal ear.

staphylococcal /-kok'əl/ [Gk, *staphyle,* bunch of grapes + *kokkos,* berry], pertaining to a genus of facultatively anaerobic gram-positive cocci.

staphylococcal infection [Gk, *staphyle,* bunch of grapes, *kokkos,* berry; L, *inficere,* to taint], an infection caused by any one of several pathogenic species of *Staphylococcus,* commonly characterized by the formation of abscesses of the skin or other organs. Staphylococcal infections of the skin include carbuncles, folliculitis, furuncles, and hidradenitis suppurativa. Bacteremia is common and may result in endocarditis, meningitis, or osteomyelitis. Staphylococcal pneumonia often follows influenza or other viral disease and may be associated with chronic or debilitating illness. Acute gastroenteritis may result from an enterotoxin produced by certain species of staphylococci in contaminated food.

staphylococcal pneumonia [Gk, *staphyle* + *kokkos* + *pneumon,* lung], pneumonia caused by a staphylococcus infection.

staphylococcal scalded skin syndrome (SSSS), an infection or mucous membrane colonization with toxin-producing *Staphylococcus aureus.* It is characterized by epidermal erythema, peeling, and necrosis that give the skin a scalded appearance. This disorder primarily affects infants 1 to 3 months of age and other children, but it also may affect adults. De-

ficient immune functions and renal insufficiency may predispose individuals to the disease. SSSS is more common in the newborn because of undeveloped immunity and renal systems.

staphylococcemia, /-koksē'mē·ə/ **1.** the presence of staphylococci in the blood. **2.** septicemia caused by staphylococci.

Staphylococcus /staf'ilōkok'əs/, *pl.* **staphylococci** [Gk, *staphyle* + *kokkos,* berry], a genus of nonmotile spheric grampositive bacteria. Some species are normally found on the skin and in the throat; certain species cause severe purulent infections or produce an enterotoxin, which may cause nausea, vomiting, and diarrhea. Life-threatening staphylococcal infections may arise within hospitals. —**staphylococcal,** *adj.*

Staphylococcus aureus [Gk, *staphyle* + *kokkos* + L, *aurum,* gold], a species of *Staphylococcus* that produces a golden pigment with some color variations. It is also responsible for a number of pyogenic infections such as boils, carbuncles, and abscesses.

staphylokinase /staf'ilōkī'nās/, an enzyme, produced by certain strains of staphylococci, that catalyzes the conversion of plasminogen to plasmin in various animal hosts of the microorganism.

staphyloma /staf'ilō'mə/, a protrusion of eye contents through a thin region of the cornea or sclera.

staple /stā'pəl/, a piece of stainless steel wire used to close certain surgical wounds.

stapling [ME, *stapel,* stake], a method of fastening tissues together at the end of surgery by using a U-shaped piece of wire as a suture. The ends of the wire are bent toward the center to close the staple.

starch [AS, *stearc,* strong], the principal molecule used for the storage of food in plants. Starch is a polysaccharide and is composed of long chains of glucose subunits. In animals excess glucose is stored as glycogen.

Starling's law of the heart [Ernest H. Starling, English physiologist, 1866–1927; AS, *lagu,* law, *heorte,* heart], a general rule that the energy of contraction of the heart is a function of the length of the fibers composing the myocardial walls just before contraction.

Starr-Edwards prosthesis [Albert Starr, American physician, b. 1926; M. L. Edwards, American physician, b. 1906; Gk, *prosthesis,* attachment], an artificial cardiac valve. A caged-ball form of device, it obstructs the valve opening and prevents the backward flow of blood.

start hesitation, a characteristic of parkinsonism in which the patient has diffi-

S

culty initiating walking movements, as if the feet were stuck to the floor.

startle reflex /stär′təl/ [ME, *stertlen,* to rush; Gk, *syn,* together, *dromos,* course], a reflex response to a sudden unexpected stimulus. The reaction may be accompanied by physiologic effects, including increased heartbeat and respiration, closing of the eyes, and flexion of trunk muscles. The reaction is rapid, pervasive, and uncontrollable, regardless of the unexpected stimulus, which may be as simple as a touch.

start point [ME, *sterte* + L, *punctum,* prick], (in molecular genetics) the initial nucleotide transcribed from the deoxyribonucleic acid template in the formation of messenger ribonucleic acid.

starvation /stärvā′shən/ [ME, *sterven,* to die], **1.** a condition resulting from the lack of essential nutrients over a long period and characterized by multiple physiologic and metabolic dysfunctions. **2.** the act or state of starving or being starved.

stasibasiphobia /stas′ibas′ifō′bē·ə/, a mental health condition in which a person is convinced that walking or standing is physically impossible. The person may also express a morbid distrust of his or her ability to stand or walk.

stasis /stā′sis, stas′is/ [Gk, standing], **1.** a disorder in which the normal flow of a fluid through a vessel of the body is slowed or halted. **2.** stillness.

stasis dermatitis, a common result of venous insufficiency of the legs, beginning with ankle edema and progressing to tan pigmentation, patchy erythema, petechiae, and induration. Ultimately there may be atrophy and fibrosis of the skin and subcutaneous tissue, with ulcerations that are slow to heal. The tan pigment is hemosiderin from blood leaking through capillary walls under elevated venous pressure. The involved skin is easily irritated or sensitized to topical medications.

stasis ulcer, a necrotic craterlike lesion of the skin of the lower leg caused by chronic venous congestion. The ulcer is often associated with stasis dermatitis and varicose veins.

stat., abbreviation for the Latin word *statim,* 'immediately.'

state /stāt/ [L, *status,* condition], the circumstances or qualities that characterize a person, thing, or way of being at a particular time.

State Board Test Pool Examination (SBTPE), revised and retitled in 1982 as the NCLEX-RN, an examination prepared by the National Council of State Boards of Nursing for testing the competency of a person to perform safely as a newly licensed registered nurse. Each jurisdiction within the United States and its territories regulates entry into the practice of nursing; each requires the candidate to pass the examination. The content of the examination is planned to test the candidate's knowledge of the nursing process as applied to the broad areas of nursing practice, including maternal and child health, medical and surgical nursing, and psychiatric nursing.

State Nurses Association (SNA), an association of nurses at the state level. The various State Nurses Associations are constituent units of the American Nurses Association.

Statewide Health Coordinating Committee (SHCC), a component of the U.S. national network of Health Systems Agencies.

static /stat′ik/ [Gk, *statikos,* causing to stand], without motion, at rest, in equilibrium.

static cardiac work, the energy transfer that occurs during the development and maintenance of ventricular pressure immediately before the opening of the aortic valve.

static electricity film fault, a defect in a radiograph or a developed photographic film, which appears as lightninglike streaks. It is caused by overly rapid opening of the film packet or transfer of static electricity from the user to the film.

static equilibrium, the ability of an individual to adjust to displacements of his or her center of gravity while maintaining a constant base of support.

static imaging, (in nuclear medicine) a diagnostic procedure in which a radioactive substance is administered to a patient to visualize an internal organ or body compartment. An image or set of images is made of the fixed or slowly changing distribution of the radioactivity.

static labyrinth, the vestibule of the inner ear. It contains two communicating chambers, the saccule and the utricle, and elicits tonic reflexes on postural muscles in response to changes in head and body positions.

static pressure [Gk, *statikos,* causing to stand; L, *premere,* to press], a condition of equalized blood pressure throughout the body when the heartbeat is stopped. A nonmoving fluid exerts a uniform pressure in all directions.

static reflex [Gk, *statikos,* causing to stand; L, *reflectere,* to bend back], a reflex that helps one maintain normal posture and muscle tone when the body is at rest.

static scoliosis [Gk, *statikos,* causing to stand, *skoliosis,* curvature], a form of scoliosis resulting from a difference in the length of the legs.

static tremor, irregular involuntary muscle contractions that occur when a patient makes an effort to hold the trunk or limbs in certain positions.

station /stā'shən/ [L, *stare*, to stand], the level of the biparietal plane of the fetal head relative to the level of the ischial spines of the maternal pelvis. An imaginary plane at the level of the spines is designated "zero station." Higher and lower stations are numbered at intervals of 1 cm and labeled as minus above and plus below.

stationary grid /stā'shəner'ē/ [L, *stare* + ME, *gridere*, gridiron], (in radiography) an x-ray grid that does not move or oscillate during the exposure of a radiographic film.

stationary lingual arch, an orthodontic arch wire that is designed to fit the lingual surface of the teeth and soldered to the associated anchor bands.

statistic /stetis'tik/ [L, *status*, condition], a number that describes a property of a set of data or other numbers.

statistical model of patient evaluation, a system based on gross quantitative measurements of similar cases used to determine payment for services.

statistical significance [L, *status*, condition, *significare*, to signify], an interpretation of statistical data that indicates an occurrence was probably the result of a causative factor and not simply a chance result. Statistical significance at the 1% level indicates a 1 in 100 probability that a result can be ascribed to chance.

statistics /stətis'tiks/, a mathematic science concerned with measuring, classifying, and analyzing objective information.

status /stā'təs, stat'əs/ [L, condition], **1.** a specified state or condition such as emotional status. **2.** an unremitting state or condition such as status asthmaticus.

status asthmaticus, an acute, severe, and prolonged asthma attack. It is caused by critically diminished airway diameter resulting from ongoing bronchospasm, edema, and mucous plugging. Hypoxia, cyanosis, and unconsciousness may follow, and the attack may be fatal.

status epilepticus, a medical emergency characterized by continuous seizures occurring without interruptions. Status epilepticus can be precipitated by the sudden withdrawal of anticonvulsant drugs, inadequate body levels of glucose, a brain tumor, a head injury, a high fever, or poisoning.

status marmoratus, the presence in full-term infants of basal nucleus lesions re-

sulting from acute total asphyxia. The lesions have a marbled appearance caused by neuronal loss and an overgrowth of myelin in the putamen, caudate, and thalamus.

statute of limitations /stach'ōōt/ [L, *statuere*, to place, *limes*, boundary], (in law) a statute that sets a limit of time during which a suit may be brought or criminal charges may be made.

statutory rape /stach'ətôr'ē/ [L, *statuere*, to place, *rapere*, to seize], (in law) sexual intercourse with a female below the age of consent, which varies from state to state.

stavudine, a synthetic thymidine nucleoside analogue. It is prescribed in the treatment of adults with advanced human immunodeficiency virus (HIV) infection who are intolerant of other approved therapies. However, patients should be advised that the product is not a cure for HIV infection, that they may continue to acquire opportunistic infections associated with acquired immunodeficiency syndrome, and that long-term effects of this therapy are unknown.

STD, abbreviation for **sexually transmitted disease.**

steady state (s, ss) /sted'ē/ [AS, *stedefast*, firm in its place; L, *status*, condition], a basic physiologic concept implying that the various forces and processes of life are in a state of homeostasis.

steam sterilization [ME, *steme*, vapor; L, *sterilis*, barren], the destruction of all forms of microbial life on an object by exposing the object to moist heat for 15 minutes at 121° F (49.44° C).

Stearns' alcoholic amentia /sturnz/ [A. Warren Stearns, American physician, 1885–1959; Ar, *alkohl*, essence; L, *ab*, from, *mens*, mind], a form of insanity brought on by alcohol characterized by an emotional disturbance of a less severe nature than that of delirium tremens but of longer duration and with greater mental clouding and amnesia.

stearrhea [Gk, *stear*, fat, *rhoia*, flow], excessive secretion of fat.

stearyl alcohol, a solid substance, prepared by the catalytic hydrogenation of stearic acid, used in various ointments.

steatorrhea /stē'ətərē'ə/ [Gk, *stear*, fat, *rhoia*, flow], greater than normal amounts of fat in the feces, characterized by frothy foul-smelling fecal matter that floats, as in celiac disease, some malabsorption syndromes, and any condition in which fats are poorly absorbed by the small intestine.

Steele-Richardson-Olszewski's syndrome [John C. Steele, Canadian neurologist,

S

1951–1968; J. Clifford Richardson, Canadian neurologist, b. 1909; Jerzy Olszewski, Canadian neurologist, 1913–1966], a rare progressive neurologic disorder of unknown cause, occurring in middle age, more often in men. It is characterized by paralysis of eye muscles, ataxia, neck and trunk rigidity, pseudobulbar palsy, and parkinsonian facies. Dementia and inappropriate emotional responses also are common.

steering wheel injury, a traumatic injury most commonly to the anterior chest wall caused by forward propulsion of the body of an automobile driver into the steering wheel during collision. Injuries include broken ribs and sternum, cardiac and pulmonary damage, and tearing of major blood vessels.

Steinmann /stīn'mən/ [Fritz Steinmann, Swiss surgeon, 1872–1932; AS, *pinn*], a wide-diameter pin used for heavy skeletal traction, as in the tibia or femur.

stellate /stel'it, -āt/ [L, *stella*, star], star-shaped or arranged in the pattern of a star.

stellate fracture, a fracture that involves the central point of impact or injury with numerous fissures radiating throughout surrounding bone tissue.

stellate ganglion [L, *stella,* star; Gk, *gagglion,* knot], a large irregular ganglion on the lowest part of the cervical sympathetic trunk fused with the first thoracic ganglion. Its branches communicate with the seventh and eighth cervical nerves.

stem cell [AS, *stemm,* tree, trunk; L, *cella,* storeroom], a formative cell; a cell whose daughter cells may give rise to other cell types. A pluripotential stem cell is one that has the potential to develop into several different types of mature cells, including lymphocytes, granulocytes, thrombocytes, and erythrocytes.

stem cell leukemia, a neoplasm of blood-forming organs in which the predominant malignant cell is too immature to classify. The acute disease has a rapid, relentless course.

stenosis /stinō'sis/ [Gk, *stenos,* narrow, *osis,* condition], an abnormal condition characterized by the constriction or narrowing of an opening or passageway in a body structure. —**stenotic,** *adj.*

stenotic [Gk, *stenos,* narrow], pertaining to a structure that is narrowed or strictured.

stent [Charles R. Stent, nineteenth-century English dentist], **1.** a compound used in making dental impressions and medical molds. **2.** a mold or device made of stent, used in anchoring skin grafts. **3.** a rod or threadlike device for supporting tubular structures during surgical anastomosis or for holding arteries open during angioplasty.

step-care therapy, a therapeutic program that begins with a simple, conservative type of treatment but may advance to more complex stages as needed to achieve control of a disease or disorder.

steppage gait /step'ij/ [AS, *staepe* + ONorse, *gata,* way], a gait in which the legs are raised abnormally high, as in cases of drop foot.

stepwedge /step'wej/, an aluminum device that, when exposed to x-rays, displays a range of exposure intensities on a radiogram. These exposure "steps" are analyzed to determine the speed characteristics of the radiographic film.

stereognosis /stir'·ē·ōgnō'sis/ [Gk, *stereos,* solid, *gnosis,* knowledge], **1.** the faculty of perceiving and understanding the form and nature of objects by the sense of touch. **2.** perception by the sense of the solidity of objects. —**stereognostic,** *adj.*

stereognostic perception /stir'ē·ognos'tik/ [Gk, *stereos,* solid, *gnosis,* knowledge], the ability to recognize objects by the sense of touch.

stereoisomer /stir'ē·ō·ī'səmər/ [Gk, *stereos,* solid, *isos,* equal, *meros,* part], one of two or more chemical compounds that contain the same atoms linked in the same way but are organized differently in space. For example, one may be the mirror image of the other.

stereoisomeric specificity /-ī'səmer'ik/ [Gk, *stereos* + *isos,* equal, *meros,* part], specificity of an enzyme for one enantiomer of a racemic mix.

stereoophthalmoscope /stir·ē·ō'ofthal'məskōp/ an ophthalmoscope fitted with two eyepieces so the examiner can view the three-dimensional interior of the eye.

stereopsis, binocular perception of depth or three-dimensional space.

stereoradiography /-rā'dē·og'rəfē/ [Gk, *stereos* + L, *radiare,* to emit rays; Gk, *graphein,* to record], a technique for producing radiographs that give a three-dimensional view of an internal body structure.

stereoscopic microscope /-skop'ik/ [Gk, *stereos* + *skopein,* to look], a microscope that produces three-dimensional images through the use of double eyepieces and double objectives.

stereoscopic radiograph, a composite of two radiographs, made by shifting the position of the x-ray tube a few centimeters between each of two exposures. The result is a three-dimensional presentation of the radiograph when viewed through stereoscopic lenses.

stereotaxic instrument /-tak′sik/, an apparatus that fits on the head and helps locate structures in the brain by means of coordinates.

stereotaxic neuroradiography [Gk, *stereos* + *taxis*, arrangement, *neuron*, nerve; L, *radiare*, to emit rays; Gk, *graphein*, to record], a radiographic procedure commonly performed during neurosurgery to guide the insertion of a needle into a specific area of the brain.

stereotype /stir′ē-ətīp/ [Gk, *stereos* + *typos*, mark], a generalization about a form of behavior, an individual, or a group.

stereotypic behavior /stir′ē-ōtip′ik/, a pattern of body movements that has autistic and symbolic meaning for an individual.

stereotypy /ster′ē-ətī′pē/ [Gk, *stereos* + *typos*, mark], the persistent inappropriate mechanical repetition of actions, body postures, or speech patterns, usually occurring with a lack of variation in thought processes or ideas. —**stereotypical**, *adj*.

sterile /ster′il/ [L, *sterilis*, barren], **1.** free of living microorganisms. **2.** barren; unable to produce children because of a physical abnormality, often the absence of spermatogenesis in a man or blockage of the fallopian tubes in a woman. **3.** aseptic. —**sterility**, *n*.

sterile field, **1.** a specified area that is considered free of microorganisms. **2.** an area immediately around a patient that has been prepared for a surgical procedure. The sterile field includes the scrubbed team members, who are properly attired, and all furniture and fixtures in the area.

sterile meningitis [L, *sterilis*, barren; Gk, *meningx*, membrane, *itis*, inflammation], a form of meningitis, usually involving a viral infection, in which there is a primarily lymphocytic response in the cerebrospinal fluid.

sterility /stəril′itē/ [L, *sterilis*, barren], a condition of being unable to conceive or reproduce the species.

sterilization /ster′ilīzā′shən/ [L, *sterilis* + Gk, *izein*, to cause], **1.** a process or act that renders a person unable to produce children. **2.** a technique for destroying microorganisms or inanimate objects, using heat, water, chemicals, or gases. —**sterilize**, *v*.

sterilize /ster′ilīz/ [L, *sterilis*, barren], **1.** to make powerless to reproduce, such as by surgery. **2.** to destroy all living organisms and viruses in a material.

sternal /stur′nəl/ [Gk, *sternon*, chest], pertaining to the sternum.

sternal node [Gk, *sternon*, chest; L, *nodus*,

knot], a node in one of the three groups of thoracic parietal lymph nodes.

sternal puncture [Gk, *sternon*, chest; L, *punctura*], a diagnostic procedure in which a needle is inserted into the marrow of the sternum to remove blood samples for diagnosis.

Sternheimer-Malbin stain /sturn′hīmər-mal′bin/, a crystal violet and safranin stain used in urinalyses to provide additional contrast for certain casts and cells.

sternoclavicular /-klavik′yələr/ [Gk, *sternon*, chest; L, *clavicula*, little key], pertaining to the sternum and clavicle.

sternoclavicular articulation [Gk, *sternon* + L, *clavicula*, little key], the double gliding joint between the sternum and the clavicle.

sternocleidomastoid /-klī′dōmas′toid/ [Gk, *sternon*, chest, *kleis*, key, *mastos*, breast, *eidos*, form], a muscle of the neck that is attached to the mastoid process of the temporal bone and superior nuchal line and by separate heads to the sternum and clavicle. They function together to flex the head.

sternocostal articulation /-kos′təl/ [Gk, *sternon* + L, *costa*, rib], the gliding articulation of the cartilage of each true rib and the sternum, except the articulation of the first rib, in which the cartilage is directly united with the sternum to form a synchondrosis.

sternohyoideus /stur′nōhī·oi′dē·əs/ [Gk, *sternon* + *hyoeides*, upsilon, U-shaped], one of the four infrahyoid muscles. It acts to depress the hyoid bone.

sternothyroideus /stur′nōthīroi′de·əs/ [Gk, *sternon* + *thyreos*, shield, *eidos*, form], one of the four infrahyoid muscles. It acts to depress the thyroid cartilage.

sternum /stur′nəm/ [Gk, *sternon*], the elongated flattened bone forming the middle part of the thorax. It supports the clavicles, articulates directly with the first seven pairs of ribs, and comprises the manubrium, the gladiolus (body), and the xiphoid process.

steroid /stir′oid/ [Gk, *stereos* + *eidos*, form], any of a large number of hormonal substances with a similar basic chemical structure, produced mainly in the adrenal cortex and gonads.

steroid acne [Gk, *stereos*, solid; L, *oleum*, oil; Gk, *eidos*, form, *akme*, point], a form of acne caused by the use of corticosteroids.

steroid cell antibody, an immunoglobulin G glycoprotein molecule that interacts with antigens in the cytoplasm of gonadal or adrenal cells that produce steroids.

steroid hormones [Gk, *stereos*, solid; L, *oleum*, oil; Gk, *eidos*, form, *hormaein*, to set in motion], any of the ductless gland

S

secretions that contain the basic steroid nucleus in their chemical formulae. The natural steroid hormones include the androgens, estrogens, and adrenal cortex secretions.

steroid hormone therapy [Gk, *stereos* + L, *oleum*, oil; Gk, *eidos*, form, *hormaein*, to set in motion, *therapeia*, treatment], treatment with any of the steroid hormones, such as the use of estrogen to reduce symptoms of postmenopausal disorders.

steroidogenesis /stiroi'dōjen'əsis/, the biologic synthesis of steroid hormones.

sterol /stir'ôl/ [Gk, *stereos* + Ar, *alkohl*, essence], a large subgroup of steroids containing an OH group at position 3 and a branched aliphatic side chain of eight or more carbon atoms at position 17. Kinds of sterols include **cholesterol** and **ergosterol.**

stertorous /stur'tərəs/ [L, *stertere*, to snore], pertaining to a respiratory effort that is strenuous or struggling; having a snoring sound.

stethomimetic /steth'ōmimet'ik/, pertaining to any condition causing or associated with a reduction of chest volume below its normal value.

stethoscope /steth'əskōp/ [Gk, *stethos*, chest, *skopein*, to look], an instrument consisting of two earpieces connected by means of flexible tubing to a diaphragm, which is placed against the skin of the patient's chest or back to hear heart and lung sounds. It is also used to hear bowel sounds.

Stevens-Johnson's syndrome [Albert M. Stevens, American pediatrician, 1884–1945; F. C. Johnson, American physician, 1894–1934], a serious, sometimes fatal inflammatory disease affecting children and young adults. It is characterized by the acute onset of fever, bullae on the skin, and ulcers on the mucous membranes of the lips, eyes, mouth, nasal passage, and genitalia. Other complications are pneumonia, pain in the joints, prostration, and perforation of the cornea. It may be an allergic reaction to certain drugs; or it may follow pregnancy, herpesvirus I, or other infection.

Stewart, Isabel Maitland (1878–1963), a Canadian-born American nursing educator and writer. She was the first nurse to receive a master's degree from Columbia University in New York. She was instrumental in upgrading the nursing curriculum and directing educational policies and became an important figure in international nursing affairs.

STH, abbreviation for **somatotropic hormone.**

sthenic fever /sthen'ik/ [Gk, *sthenos,* power; L, *febris,* fever], high body temperature associated with thirst, dry skin, and often delirium.

stibogluconate sodium /stib'ōgloō'kənāt/, an antileishmanial available from the Centers for Disease Control and Prevention. It is a drug of choice for the visceral form of leishmaniasis and has some effect on other forms.

stibophen /stib'əfin/, a schistosomicide prescribed in the treatment of infestations of *Schistosoma japonicum* or *S. haematobium.*

Stieda's fracture /stē'dəz/ [Alfred Stieda, German surgeon, 1869–1945], a fracture of the internal condyle of the femur.

stiff [OE, *stif*], pertaining to a condition of rigidity or muscular inflexibility.

stiff joint [OE, *stif* + L, *jungere*, to join], a rigid or inflexible joint, as may be caused by arthritis or other rheumatic disorders.

stigma /stig'mə/ [Gk, brand], **1.** a moral or physical blemish. **2.** a mental or physical characteristic that serves to identify a disease or condition.

stigmatism /stig'mətiz'əm/ [Gk, *stigma,* brand], **1.** normal visual accommodation and refraction whereby light rays fall onto the retina. **2.** a condition of abnormal skin markings.

stillbirth [AS, *stille* + ME, *burth*], **1.** the birth of a fetus that died before or during delivery. **2.** a fetus, born dead, that weighs more than 1000 g and would usually have been expected to live.

stillborn [AS, *stille* + *boren*], **1.** an infant that was born dead. **2.** pertaining to an infant that was born dead.

stimulant /stim'yələnt/ [L, *stimulare*, to incite], any agent that increases the rate of activity of a body system.

stimulant cathartic, a cathartic that acts by promoting the motility of the bowel, especially the longitudinal peristalsis of the colon. Kinds of stimulant cathartics are **cascara** and **senna.**

stimulate /stim'yəlāt/ [L, *stimulare*, to incite], to excite, as in the process of increasing a vigorous functional activity.

stimulating bath, a bath taken in water that contains an aromatic substance, an astringent, or a tonic.

stimulation /stim'yəlā'shən/ [L, *stimulare*, to incite], the condition of being stimulated.

stimulus, /stim'yələs/ *pl.* **stimuli** [L, *stimulare*, to incite], anything that excites or incites an organism or part to function, become active, or respond. **—stimulate,** *v.*

stimulus control, a strategy for self-modification that depends on manipulating the causes of behavior to increase goals or behaviors desired by a patient while decreasing those that are undesired.

stimulus duration, the length of time a stimulus must be applied for the resulting nerve impulse to produce excitation in the receptor tissue.

stimulus generalization, a type of conditioning in which the reaction to one stimulus is reinforced to allow transfer of the reaction to other occurrences.

sting [AS, *stingan*], an injury caused by a sharp, painful penetration of the skin, often accompanied by exposure to an irritating chemical or the venom of an insect or other animal. Kinds of stings include bee, jellyfish, scorpion, sea urchin, and shellfish stings.

stingray /sting'rā/ [AS, *stingan* + L, *raia*, ray-fish], a flat, long-tailed fish bearing barbed spines on its back that are connected to sacs of venom. Spasm of the skeletal muscles, severe local pain, seizures, and dyspnea may occur if the skin is broken by the spines.

stippling [D, *stippen*, to prick], **1.** the appearance of colored dots in some cells when stained. Red stippling in blood cells stained with eosin hematoxylin is a sign of malaria. **2.** the appearance of the retina, as if dotted with light and dark points.

stitch [ME, *stiche*], **1.** a suture. **2.** a sudden sharp pain.

stitch abscess [ME, *stiche* + L, *abscedere*, to go away], an abscess that develops around a suture.

St. Louis encephalitis /säntloo′is/ [St. Louis, Missouri; Gk, *enkephalon*, brain, *itis*, inflammation], an arbovirus infection of the brain transmitted from birds to humans by the bite of an infected mosquito. It is characterized by headache, malaise, fever, stiff neck, delirium, and convulsions. Sequelae may include visual and speech disturbances, difficulty in walking, and personality changes. Convalescence may be prolonged, and death may result.

stocking aid, a device that enables handicapped people to pull on a pair of stockings although unable to reach their feet. One type consists of a dowel with a cuphook on the end.

stock vaccine, an immunizing agent made from a stock microbial strain.

stoma /stō′mə/ [Gk, mouth], **1.** a pore, orifice, or opening on a surface. **2.** an artificial opening of an internal organ on the surface of the body, created surgically, such as for a colostomy. **3.** a new opening created surgically, between two body structures, such as for a gastroenterostomy.

stomach /stum′ək/ [Gk, *stomakhos*, gullet], the food reservoir and first major site of digestion, located just under the diaphragm and divided into a body and a pylorus. It receives partially processed food and drink funneled from the mouth through the esophagus and gradually feeds liquefied food (chyme) into the small intestine. It is lined with a mucous coat, a submucous coat, a muscular coat, and a serous coat, all richly supplied with blood vessels and nerves and contains fundic, cardiac, and pyloric gastric glands.

stomach ache [Gk, *stomakhos*, gullet; ME, *aken*, pain], pain in the stomach area.

stomach drops, a medication that promotes gastric activity.

stomach pump, a pump for withdrawing the contents of the stomach through a tube passed through the mouth or nose into the stomach.

stomach tube, a tube used to introduce nutrients into the stomach, remove fluids and ingested poisons, or decompress the stomach.

stomal /stō′məl/ [Gk, mouth], pertaining to one or more stomata or mouthlike openings.

stomal peptic ulcer, a marginal peptic ulcer.

stomatitis /stō′mətī′tis/ [Gk, *stoma* + *itis*, inflammation], any inflammatory condition of the mouth. It may result from infection by bacteria, viruses, or fungi; from exposure to certain chemicals or drugs from vitamin deficiency; or from a systemic inflammatory disease.

stomatitis parasitica [Gk, *stoma*, mouth, *itis*, inflammation, *parasitos*, guest], an inflammation of the mucous membranes of the mouth by a yeast fungus, *Candida albicans*, typically expressed by a white coating on the tongue. It may affect infants or immunosuppressed people with human immunodeficiency virus or appear as an outgrowth secondary to antibiotic therapy.

stomatognathic system /stō′mətōnath′ik/ [Gk, *stoma* + *gnathos*, jaw, *systema*], the combination of organs, structures, and nerves involved in speech and reception, mastication, and deglutition of food. This system is composed of the teeth, the jaws, the masticatory muscles, the tongue, the lips, surrounding tissues, and the nerves that control these structures.

stomatology /stō′mətol′əjē/ [Gk, *stoma* + *logos*, science], the study of the morphologic characteristics, structure, function, and diseases of the oral cavity. —**stomatologic, stomatological,** *adj.*

stomion /stō′mē·on/ [Gk, *stoma*], the me-

S

dian point of the oral slit when the mouth is closed.

stomodeum /stom'ədē'əm/, *pl.* **stomodeums, stomodea** [Gk, *stoma* + *odaios,* a way], an invagination in the ectoderm located in the foregut of the developing embryo that forms the mouth. —**stomodeal, stomodaeal, stomadeal,** *adj.*

stone disease, urolithiasis that may have complications when obstructive uropathy or infection develops.

stopcock, a valve or turning plug that controls the flow of fluid from a container through a tube.

stop needle [AS, *stoppian,* to stop, *naedel*], a needle with a shoulder flange that prevents it from penetrating beyond a certain distance.

storage capacity /stôr'ij/, the amount of data that can be held on a computer disk or tape, usually expressed in kilobytes, megabytes, gigabytes, or terabytes (one trillion bytes).

storage disease, a metabolic disorder in which certain cells accumulate excessive amounts of lipids, proteins, or other substances.

storage pool disease, a blood coagulation disorder caused by failure of platelets to release adenosine diphosphate in response to aggregating agents.

stored-energy foot, a lower-limb prosthesis designed to imitate the springlike action of a natural foot and leg. A device stores energy when weight is put on the artificial leg. When the weight is shifted to the other leg, the stored energy is released, returning the prosthesis to its original shape.

storing fermentation [L, *staurare,* to store, *fermentum,* leaven], the rapid gaseous clotting of milk caused by *Clostridium perfringens.*

STP, *slang.* a psychedelic agent, dimethoxy-4-methylamphetamine. STP is an abbreviation for *serenity, tranquillity, and peace.*

STPD, abbreviation for *standard temperature, standard pressure, dry.*

STPD conditions of a volume of gas, (standard temperature, standard pressure, dry) the conditions of a volume of gas at 0° C and 760 mm Hg and containing no water vapor (dry). It should contain a calculable number of moles of a particular gas.

strabismal /strabiz'məl/ [Gk, *strabismos,* squint], pertaining to the condition of strabismus.

strabismus /strəbiz'məs/ [Gk, *strabismos,* squint], an abnormal ocular condition in which the visual axes of the eyes are not directed at the same point. There are two kinds of strabismus, paralytic and non-paralytic. Paralytic strabismus results from the inability of the ocular muscles to move the eye because of neurologic deficit or muscular dysfunction. The muscle that is dysfunctional may be identified by watching as the patient attempts to move the eyes to each of the cardinal positions of gaze. Nonparalytic strabismus is a defect in the position of the two eyes in relation to each other. The condition is inherited. The person cannot use the two eyes together but has to fixate with one or the other. The eye that looks straight at a given time is the fixing eye. Some people have alternating strabismus, using one eye and then the other; some have monocular strabismus, which affects only one eye. Visual acuity diminishes with diminished use of an eye, and suppression amblyopia may develop. —**strabismal, strabismic, strabismical,** *adj.*

straight-leg-raising (SLR) test, a physical examination technique to determine abnormality of the sciatic nerve or tightness of the hamstrings. The presence of sciatica is confirmed by sciatic nerve pain radiating down the limb when the supine person attempts to raise the straightened limb.

straight line blood set /strāt/ [ME, *streght*], a common device, composed of plastic components, for delivering blood infusions. It includes plastic tubing, a clamp, a drip chamber, and a filter.

straight sinus [ME, *streght* + L, *sinus,* hollow], one of the six posterior-superior venous channels of the dura mater, draining blood from the brain into the internal jugular vein. It has no valves and is located at the junction of the falx cerebri with the tentorium cerebelli.

straight wire fixed orthodontic appliance, an orthodontic appliance used for correcting and improving malocclusion. It is designed to decrease arch wire adjustments by reorienting arch wire slots.

strain [ME, *streinen*], **1.** to exert physical force in a manner that may result in injury, usually muscular. **2.** to separate solids or particles from a liquid with a filter or sieve. **3.** damage, usually muscular, that results from excessive physical effort. **4.** a taxon that is a subgroup of a species. **5.** an emotional state reflecting mental pressure or fatigue.

straitjacket /strāt'jakit/ [OFr, *estreit,* strict, *jaquette,* short coat], a coatlike garment of canvas with long sleeves that can be tied behind the wearer's back to prevent arm movement. It is used for restraining violent or uncontrollable people.

strangle /strang'gəl/ [L, *strangulare,* to

choke], to cause an interruption of breathing by compressing or constricting the trachea.

strangulated /strang′gyəlā′tid/ [L, *strangulare,* to choke], pertaining to a constriction or compression of the trachea or other upper airway structure that interrupts the normal flow of air.

strangulated hemorrhoid [L, *strangulare,* to choke; Gk, *haimorrhoise,* vein that discharges blood], a prolapsed hemorrhoid that has become trapped by the anal sphincter, causing the blood supply to become occluded by the sphincter's constricting action.

strangulated hernia [L, *strangulare,* to choke, *hernia,* rupture], a hernia in which the blood vessels have become constricted by the neck of the hernial sac, resulting in ischemia and possible gangrene if blood circulation is not quickly restored.

strangulation /strang′gyəlā′shən/ [L, *strangulare,* to choke], the constriction of a tubular structure of the body such as the trachea, a segment of bowel, or the blood vessels of a limb that prevents function or impedes circulation.

strap [AS, *stropp*], **1.** a band, such as that made of adhesive plaster, that is used to hold dressings in place or to attach one thing to another. **2.** to bind securely.

strapping, the application of overlapping strips of adhesive tape to an extremity or body area to exert pressure and hold a structure in place, performed in the treatment of strains, sprains, dislocations, and certain fractures.

stratified /strat′ifīd/ [L, *stratum + facere,* to make], arranged in layers.

stratified clot, a semisolid mass of coagulated blood that forms in layers within an aneurysm.

stratified epithelium [L, *stratum + facere;* Gk, *epi,* above, *thele,* nipple], closely packed sheets of epithelial cells arranged in layers over the external surface of the body and lining most of the hollow structures. The layers may include stratified squamous, stratified columnar, or stratified columnar ciliated types of cells.

stratiform fibrocartilage /strat′iform/ [L, *stratum,* layer, *forma,* form, *fibra,* fiber, *cartilago,* cartilage], a structure made of fibrocartilage that forms a thin coating of osseous grooves through which tendons of certain muscles glide.

stratum /strā′təm, strat′əm/, *pl.* **strata** [L, layer], a uniformly thick sheet or layer, usually associated with other layers, such as the stratum basale of the epidermis.

stratum basale, 1. the deepest of the five layers of the epidermis, composed of tall cylindric cells. This layer provides new cells by mitotic cell division. **2.** the deepest layers of the uterine decidua, containing uterine gland terminals.

stratum corneum, the horny, outermost layer of the skin, composed of dead flat cells converted to keratin that continually flakes away. The stratum corneum is thick on the palms of the hands and the soles of the feet but relatively thin over most areas.

stratum granulosum, one of the layers of the epidermis, situated just below the stratum corneum except in the thick skin of the palms of the hands and the soles of the feet, where it lies just under the stratum lucidum.

stratum lucidum, one of the layers of the epidermis, situated just beneath the stratum corneum and present only in the thick skin of the palms of the hands and the soles of the feet.

stratum spinosum, one of the layers of the epidermis, composed of several layers of polygonal cells. It lies on top of the stratum basale and beneath the stratum granulosum and contains tiny fibrils within its cellular cytoplasm.

stratum spongiosum, one of the three layers of the endometrium of the uterus, containing tortuous, dilated uterine glands and a small amount of interglandular tissue.

strawberry gallbladder /strô′berē/ [AS, *streawberig + ME, gal,* gall; AS, *blaedre*], a tiny yellow gallbladder spotted with deposits on the red mucous membrane, characteristic of cholesterolosis.

strawberry tongue, a strawberry-like coloration of the inflamed tongue papillae. It is a clinical sign of scarlet fever and is also seen in Kawasaki's disease.

stray light [OFr, *estraier,* to wander; AS, *leoht,* illumination], radiant energy that reaches a photodetector and that consists of wavelengths other than those defined by the filter or monochromator.

streak [AS, *strican,* to stroke], a line or a stripe, such as the primitive streak at the caudal end of the embryonic disk.

street virus, a natural infectious agent such as rabies that may be transmitted from a domestic animal or obtained in the wild, outside the laboratory.

strength [AS, *strengou*], the ability of a muscle to produce or resist a physical force.

strength of association, the degree of relationship between a causal factor and the occurrence of a disease, usually expressed in terms of a relative risk ratio.

strength training, a method of improving muscular strength by gradually increasing the ability to resist force through the use of free weights, machines, or the person's own body weight. Strength training sessions are designed to impose increasingly greater resistance, which in turn stimulates development of muscle strength to meet the added demand.

streptavidin /strep'təvī'din/, a biotin-binding protein isolated from streptomyces and used to identify antigens in surgical pathologic diagnosis.

strep throat [*Streptococcus* + AS, *throte*], *informal.* an infection of the oral pharynx and tonsils caused by a hemolytic species of *Streptococcus,* usually belonging to group A. The infection is characterized by sore throat, chills, fever, swollen lymph nodes in the neck, and sometimes nausea and vomiting. The symptoms usually begin abruptly a few days after exposure to the organism in airborne droplets or after direct contact with an infected person. The throat is diffusely red, and tonsils often are covered with a yellow or white exudate.

Streptobacillus moniliformis [Gk, *streptos,* curved; L, *bacillum,* small rod, *monile,* necklace, *forma,* form], a species of necklace-shaped bacteria that can cause rat-bite fever in humans.

streptococcal [Gk, *streptos,* curved, *kokkos,* berry], pertaining to any of the species of streptococcus.

streptococcal angina /strep'təkok'əl/ [Gk, *streptos* + *kokkos,* berry; L, *angina,* quinsy], a condition in which feelings of choking, suffocation, and pain result from a streptococcal infection.

streptococcal infection, an infection caused by pathogenic bacteria of one of several species of the genus *Streptococcus* or their toxins. The infections occur in many forms, including cellulitis, endocarditis, erysipelas, impetigo, meningitis, pneumonia, scarlet fever, tonsillitis, and urinary tract infection.

streptococcemia /-koksē'mē-ə/ [Gk, *streptos,* curved, *kokkos,* berry], a condition of presence of streptococci bacteria in the blood.

Streptococcus /strep'təkok'əs/ [Gk, *streptos* + *kokkos,* berry], a genus of nonmotile gram-positive cocci classified by serologic types (Lancefield groups A through T), by hemolytic action (alpha, beta, gamma) when grown on blood agar, and by reaction to bacterial viruses (phage types 1 to 86). Many species cause disease in humans. *Streptococcus faecalis,* a penicillin-resistant group D enterococcus and normal inhabitant of the gastrointestinal tract, may cause infection of the urinary tract or endocardium.

streptococcus B-hemolitic, Group B, a strain of streptococcus that causes human infections such as neonatal sepsis, endocarditis, and septic arthritis.

Streptococcus pneumoniae [Gk, *streptos,* curved, *kokkos,* berry, *pneumon,* lung], any of 70 antigenic types of pneumococci that cause pneumonia and other diseases in humans.

Streptococcus pyogenes [Gk, *streptos,* curved, *kokkos,* berry, *pyon,* pus, *genein,* to produce], a species of streptococcus with many strains that are pathogenic to humans. It causes suppurative diseases such as scarlet fever and strep throat.

Streptococcus viridans [Gk, *streptos,* curved, *kokkos,* berry], a species of streptococcus similar to *pyogenes* strains. It produces alpha-hemolysis in cultures and is a common cause of subacute bacterial endocarditis and other infections in humans.

streptokinase /strep'təkī'nās/ [Gk, *streptos* + *kinesis,* motion, (ase) enzyme], a fibrinolytic activator that enhances the conversion of plasminogen to the fibrinolytic enzyme plasmin. It is used in the treatment of certain cases of pulmonary and coronary embolism.

streptokinase-streptodornase /-strep'tō-dôr'nās/, two enzymes derived from a strain of *Streptococcus hemolyticus.* It is prescribed for debridement of purulent exudates, clotted blood, radiation necrosis, or fibrinous deposits resulting from trauma or infection.

streptolysin /streptol'isis/ [Gk, *streptos* + *lysein,* to loosen], a filterable substance, produced by streptococci, that liberates hemoglobin from red blood cells.

streptomycin sulfate /strep'təmī'sin/, an aminoglycoside antibiotic prescribed in the treatment of tuberculosis, endocarditis, and certain other infections.

streptozocin /strep'təzō'sin/, an antineoplastic used in the treatment of neoplasms, including metastatic islet cell tumors of the pancreas. It is an antibiotic substance from *Streptomyces acromogenes.*

stress [OFr, *estrecier,* to tighten], any emotional, physical, social, economic, or other factor that requires a response or change. Examples include dehydration, which can cause an increase in body temperature, and a separation from parents, which can cause a young child to cry. Stress also may be applied therapeutically to promote change, such as implosive therapy for phobic patients.

stress-adaptation theory, a concept that stress depletes the reserve capacity of individuals, thereby increasing their vulnerability to health problems.

stress amenorrhea [OFr, *estrecier,* GK, *a*

+ *men,* month, *rhoia,* to flow], a cessation in menstruation caused by a physical change or mental stress.

stress behavior, a change from a person's normal behavior in response to a stressor.

stress fracture, a fracture, especially of one or more of the metatarsal bones, caused by repeated, prolonged, or abnormal stress.

stress inoculation, a procedure useful in helping patients control anxiety by substituting positive coping statements for statements that bring about anxiety.

stress kinesic, a type of behavioral characteristic of personal conversation, such as the use of body shifts or movements, that marks the flow of speech and generally coincides with linguistic stress patterns.

stress management, methods of controlling factors that require a response or change within a person by identifying the stressors, eliminating negative stressors, and developing effective coping mechanisms. Examples include progressive muscular relaxation, guided imagery, biofeedback, and breathing techniques.

stressor /stres′ər/ [OFr, *estrecier,* to tighten], anything that causes wear and tear on the body's physical or mental resources.

stress radiography, a technique for examining a body area by x-ray for soft tissue tears or ruptures. The image may appear as an abnormal gap between joint surfaces.

stress reaction. an acute maladaptive emotional response to an actual or perceived stressor.

stress test, a test that measures the function of a system of the body when subjected to carefully controlled amounts of physiologic stress, usually exercise but sometimes specific drugs. The data produced allow the examiner to evaluate the condition of the system being tested.

stress ulcer, a gastric or duodenal ulcer that develops in previously unaffected individuals subjected to severe stress, such as a severe burn.

stretching of contractures [AS, *streccan* + L, *contractura,* drawing together], procedures for release of muscle that has been shortened because of paralysis, spasm, or fibrosis. The procedures may include tissue grafts, scar tissue removal, tendon transfer, and incision of a joint capsule.

stretch pressure, a rehabilitation technique in which the thumb, fingertips, or palm of the hand is used to apply quick stretches of a target muscle, followed by briefly maintained pressure.

stretch receptors [AS, *streccan* + L, *recipere,* to receive], specialized sensory nerve endings in muscle spindles or tendons that are stimulated by stretching movements.

stretch reflex [AS, *streccan* + L, *reflectere,* to bend back], a reflex muscle contraction after it is stretched as a result of stimulation of proprioceptors in the muscle. Tendon reflexes function in a similar manner.

stretch release, a rehabilitation technique in which the fingertips are placed over the belly of a large muscle and then spread apart in an effort to stretch the skin and underlying muscle. The stretch is done firmly enough to deform the soft tissue temporarily, stimulating cutaneous and muscle efferents and producing facilitation of the underlying muscle.

stria /strī′ə/, *pl.* **striae** [L, furrow], a streak or a linear scar that often results from rapidly developing tension in the skin, such as seen on the abdomen after pregnancy. Purplish striae are among the classic findings in hyperadrenocorticism.

stria gravidarum, irregular depressions with red to purple coloration that appear in the skin of the abdomen, thighs, and buttocks of pregnant women.

striatal /strī·ā′təl, strī′ətəl/ [L, *striatus,* striped], pertaining to the corpus striatum.

striatal toe, hyperextension of the great toe.

striate /strī′āt/ [L, *striatus,* striped], identifying something that is striped, is marked by parallel lines, or has structural lines.

striated muscle /strī′ātid/ [L, *striatus,* striped, *musculus,* muscle], any muscle, including all the skeletal muscles, in which the fibers are divided by bands of cross striations (stripes) as a result of overlapping of thick and thin myofilaments. Contractions in such muscles are voluntary. The heart, a striated involuntary muscle, is an exception.

stria terminalis, a slender, compact fiber bundle that functions as a limbic pathway running from the amygdaloid complex to the hypothalamus and septum.

stricture /strik′chər/ [L, *stringere,* to tighten], an abnormal temporary or permanent narrowing of the lumen of a hollow organ, such as the esophagus, pylorus of the stomach, ureter, or urethra. It is caused by inflammation, external pressure, or scarring.

strict vegetarian [L, *stringere* + *vegetare,* to grow, *arius,* believer], a vegetarian whose diet excludes the use of all foods of animal origin. Such diets, unless ad-

S

stridor /strī'dôr/ [L, harsh sound], an abnormal high-pitched musical sound caused by an obstruction in the trachea or larynx. It is usually heard during inspiration. Stridor may indicate several neoplastic or inflammatory conditions, including glottic edema, asthma, diphtheria, laryngospasm, and papilloma.

strike [AS, *strican*, to advance swiftly], an action taken by the employees of a company or institution in which they stop reporting for work in an effort to cause the employer to accede to certain demands.

string, a cord, usually made of fiber, configured in a long thin line.

string carcinoma [AS, *strenge,* cord; Gk, *karkinos,* cancer, *oma,* tumor], a malignancy of the large intestine, usually the ascending or transverse colon. On radiologic visualization, it causes the intestine to appear to be tied in segments like a string of large beads.

stringiness /string'inəs/, an abnormal tissue texture caused by fine or stringlike myofascial structures.

string sign, (in radiography) a narrow pyloric canal with congenital pyloric stenosis or a narrowed bowel segment with regional ileitis; use of a radiopaque contrast medium causes it to appear as a thin string radiographically, indicating a narrowed lumen.

striocerebellar tremor /strī'ōser'əbel'ər/, a combination of static, active, and intentional voluntary muscle contractions with both striatal and cerebellar components. It is associated with hereditary ataxia and diffuse degeneration of the central nervous system.

strip membranes [Ger, *strippe,* strap; L, *membrana,* thin skin], (in obstetrics) a procedure in which an examiner, with the fingers, frees the membranes of the amniotic sac from the wall of the lower segment of the uterus in the small area around the cervical os.

stripping, 1. *nontechnical.* a surgical procedure for the removal of the long and short saphenous veins of the legs. **2.** the mechanical removal of a very small amount of enamel from the mesial or distal surfaces of teeth to alleviate crowding.

stroke prone profile [AS, *strac*], a predictive index using a complex of risk factors that indicate susceptibility of a person to cerebrovascular accident (CVA). The factors include advanced age, hypertension, a history of transient ischemic attacks, cigarette smoking, heart disorders, associated embolism, family history of CVA, use of oral contraceptives, diabetes mellitus, physical inactivity, and obesity.

stroke volume, the amount of blood ejected by the ventricle during contraction.

stroke volume index, the stroke volume divided by the body surface area.

stroking /strō'king/, running the entire hand over large parts of the body to relax the muscles reflexively and eliminate muscle spasm, improve circulation, or produce a parasympathetic response.

stroma /strō'mə/ [Gk, covering], the supporting tissue or the matrix of an organ, as distinguished from its parenchyma.— **stromatic,** *adj.*

Strongyloides /stron'jiloi'dēz/ [Gk, *strongylos,* round, *eidos,* form], a genus of parasitic intestinal nematode. A species of *Strongyloides, S. stercoralis,* causes strongyloidiasis.

strongyloidiasis /stron'jəloidī'əsis/, infection of the small intestine by the roundworm *Strongyloides stercoralis.* It is acquired when larvae from the soil penetrate intact skin, incidentally causing a pruritic rash. The larvae pass to the lungs via the bloodstream, sometimes causing pneumonia. They then migrate up the air passages to the pharynx, are swallowed, and develop into adult worms in the small intestine. Bloody diarrhea and intestinal malabsorption may result.

strontium (Sr) /stron'sh(ē)əm/ [Strontian, Scotland], a metallic element. Its atomic number is 38; its atomic mass (weight) is 87.62. Chemically similar to calcium, it is found in bone tissue. Isotopes of strontium are used in radioisotope scanning procedures of bone. Strontium 90, the longest-lived, is the most dangerous constituent of fallout from atomic bomb tests. It can replace some of the calcium in food, become concentrated in teeth and bones, and continue to emit electrons that can cause death in the host. Strontium 90 becomes concentrated in cow's milk.

structural /struk'chərəl/ [L, *structura,* arrangement], pertaining to the arrangement or pattern of component parts of an object or organism.

structural chemistry [L, *structura,* arrangement], the science dealing with the molecular structure of chemical substances.

structural gene, (in molecular genetics) a unit of genetic information that specifies the amino acid sequence of a polypeptide.

structural integration, a technique of deep massage intended to help in the realignment of the body by altering the length and tone of myofascial tissues. The basis of the practice is the belief that misalignment of myofascial tissues may have an overall detrimental effect on a person's energy level, self-image, muscular efficiency, perceptions, and general health.

structural model, a model of family therapy that views the family as an open system and identifies subsystems within the family that carry out specific family functions.

structure /struk'chər/ [L, *structura*], a part of the body, such as the heart, a bone, a gland, a cell, or a limb.

structure-activity relationship (SAR), the relationship between the chemical structure of a drug and its activity.

structured learning therapy /struk'chərt/, a rehabilitation technique used with schizophrenic patients.

Strümpell-Marie's disease /strim'pəlmä-rē′/ [Ernst A. von Strümpell, German neurologist, 1853–1925; Pierre Marie, French neurologist, 1853–1940; L, *dis* Fr, *aise*, ease], ankylosing spondylitis.

strychnine /strik'nin, strik'nīn/ [Gr, *strychnos*, nightshade], a white crystalline alkaloid obtained from the leaves of the *Strychnos nux-vomica* plant. It is extremely toxic to the central nervous system.

strychnine poisoning [Gk, *strychnos* + L, *potio*, a drink], toxic effects of ingesting strychnine, a central nervous system stimulant. Symptoms include restlessness and hyperacuity of hearing and vision. Minor stimuli may produce convulsions, but there may be complete muscle relaxation between convulsions. One classic sign of strychnine poisoning is an arched back.

Stryker wedge frame /strī'kər/, trademark for an orthopedic bed that allows the patient to be rotated as required to either the supine or the prone position. It is used in the immobilization of patients with unstable spines, postoperative management of multilevel spinal fusions, and management of severe burn patients.

S-T segment, an isoelectric line after the QRS complex on the electrocardiogram before the ascent of the T wave. It represents phase 2 of the action potential. Elevation or depression of the S-T segment is the hallmark of myocardial ischemia or injury and coronary artery disease.

stump [ME, *stumpe*], the part of a limb after amputation that is proximal to the part amputated.

stump hallucination, the sensation of the continued presence of an amputated limb.

stunned myocardium, impaired myocardial contractile function, cellular biochemical characteristics, and microvasculature function in the absence of gross myocardial necrosis for minutes to days

caused by ischemia of short duration or in the immediate outlying area of an infarct zone.

stupefacient /st(y)ōō′pəfā′shənt/ [L, *stupere,* to stun, *facere,* to make], a narcotic or other agent that has the effect of making a person stuporous.

stupor /st(y)ōō′pər/ [L, *stupere,* to stun], a state of unresponsiveness in which a person seems unaware of the surroundings. The condition occurs in neurologic and psychiatric disorders.

stuporous /st(y)ōō′pərəs/ [L, *stupere,* to stun], in a state of reduced consciousness and diminished spontaneous movement.

Sturge-Weber's syndrome /sturj′web′ər/ [William A. Sturge, English physician, 1850–1919; Frederick P. Weber, English physician, 1863–1962], a congenital neurocutaneous disease marked by a port wine–colored capillary hemangioma over a sensory dermatome of a branch of the trigeminal nerve of the face. The cerebral cortex may atrophy, and generalized or focal seizures, angioma of the choroid, secondary glaucoma, optic atrophy, and new cutaneous hemangiomas may develop.

stuttering [D, *stotteren*], a speech dysfunction usually characterized by excessive abnormal hesitations, part-word and whole-word repetitions, and audible or silent prolongation of sounds. The cause of stuttering is unknown; it may result from neurologic impairment. Hesitancy and lack of fluency in speech are normal characteristics of normal speech and language development during the preschool years, when a child's physical, psychologic, and speech/language development do not match the linguistic demands of talking.

sty [ME, *styanye,* eyelid tumor], a purulent infection of a meibomian or sebaceous gland of the eyelid, often caused by a staphylococcal organism.

stylet /stī′lət, stīlet′/ [It, *stiletto,* dagger], a thin metal probe for inserting into or passing through a needle, tube, or catheter to clean the hollow bore or for inserting into a soft, flexible catheter to make it stiff as the catheter is placed in a vein or passed through an orifice of the body.

stylohyoideus /stī′lōhī-oi′dē·əs/ [Gk, *stylos,* pillar, *hyoeides,* upsilon, U-shaped], one of four suprahyoid muscles, lying anterior and superior to the posterior belly of the digastricus. It serves to draw the hyoid bone up and back.

stylohyoid ligament /stī′lōhī′oid/, the ligament attached to the tip of the styloid process of the temporal bone and to the lesser cornu of the hyoid bone.

styloid /stī′loid/ [Gk, *stylos,* pillar, *eidos,*

S

form], long and tapered, like a pen or stylus.

styloid process [Gk, *stylos* + *eidos* + L, *processus*], any of several projections of bone tissue, particularly a projection on the temporal bone.

stylomandibular ligament /stī′lōman-dib′yələr/ [Gk, *stylos* + L, *mandere,* to chew, *ligare,* to bind], one of a pair of specialized bands of cervical fascia, forming an accessory part of the temporomandibular joint. It extends from the styloid process of the temporal bone to the ramus of the mandible between the masseter and pterygoideus muscles and separates the parotid gland from the submandibular gland.

stylus /stī′ləs/, **1.** a fine probe. **2.** a wire inserted into a catheter to stiffen it. **3.** a device that imprints electrical activity and wave patterns on electrocardiographic, electroencephalographic, or similar graphic recordings.

styptic /stip′tik/ [Gk, *styptikos,* astringent], **1.** a substance used as an astringent, often to control bleeding. A chemical styptic induces coagulation of blood. A cotton pledget used as a compress to control bleeding is a mechanical styptic. **2.** acting as an astringent or agent to control bleeding.

subacromial /sub′əkrō′mē·əl/ /-əkrō′mē-·əl/ [L, *sub,* beneath; Gk, *akron,* extremity, *omos.* shoulder], pertaining to the area below the acromion process.

subacromial bursa [L, *sub,* under; Gk, *akron,* extremity, *omos,* shoulder, *byrsa,* wineskin], the bursa separating the acromion process and deltoid muscle from the insertion of the supraspinatus muscle and the greater tubercle of the humerus.

subacute /-əkyo͞ot′/ [L, *sub* + *acutus,* sharp], **1.** less than acute. **2.** pertaining to a disease or other abnormal condition present in a person who appears to be clinically well.

subacute bacterial endocarditis (SBE), a chronic bacterial infection of the valves of the heart. It is characterized by a slow, quiet onset with fever, heart murmur, splenomegaly, and development of clumps of abnormal tissue, called vegetations, around an intracardiac prosthesis or on the cusps of a valve. Various species of *Streptococcus* or *Staphylococcus* are commonly the cause of SBE. Dental procedures are associated with infection by *Streptococcus viridans,* surgical procedures with *Streptococcus faecalis,* and self-infection (especially by drug abusers) with *Staphylococcus aureus.*

subacute care, 1. a level of treatment that is between chronic and acute. **2.** treatment of a disease that is of moderate severity or duration.

subacute glomerulonephritis, an uncommon noninfectious disease of the glomerulus of the kidney characterized by proteinuria, hematuria, decreased production of urine, and edema. Of unknown cause, the disease may progress rapidly, and renal failure may occur. Kidney transplantation and dialysis are the only treatments available.

subacute infection [L, *sub,* beneath, *acutus,* sharp, *inficere,* to stain], a disease condition that is not chronic and that runs a rapid and severe, but less than acute, course.

subacute inflammation, a reactive sign of inflammation with a gradual onset, later increasing to a chronic or severe type of reaction.

subacute myelooptic neuropathy (SMON), a condition of muscular pain and weakness, usually below the T12 vertebra; painful dysesthesia of the limbs; and, in some cases, optic atrophy.

subacute sclerosing panencephalitis, an uncommon slow virus infection caused by the measles virus. It is characterized by diffuse inflammation of brain tissue, personality change, seizures, blindness, dementia, fever, and death.

subaortic /-ā-ôr′tik/ [L, *sub* + Gk, *aerein,* to raise], pertaining to the area of the body below the aorta.

subaortic stenosis [L, *sub,* beneath; Gk, *aerein,* to raise, *stenos,* narrow, *osis* condition], a narrowing of the left ventricle outflow tract below the aortic valve.

subapical /-ap′ikəl/, below the peak or apex.

subaponeurotic /-ap′ōnŏŏrot′ik/ [L, *sub,* beneath; Gk, *apo,* from, *neuron* nerve; L, *tendo*], beneath an aponeurosis.

subarachnoid /sub′ərak′noid/ [L, *sub* + Gk, *arachne,* spider, *eidos* form], pertaining to the area under the arachnoid membrane and above the pia mater.

subarachnoid hemorrhage (SaH, SAH), an intracranial hemorrhage into the cerebrospinal fluid–filled space between the arachnoid and pial membranes on the surface of the brain. The hemorrhage may extend into the brain if the force of the bleeding from the broken vessel is sudden and severe. The cause may be trauma, rupture of an aneurysm, or an arteriovenous anomaly. The first symptom of a subarachnoid hemorrhage is a sudden extremely severe headache that begins in one localized area and then spreads, becoming dull and throbbing. Other characteristics of subarachnoid hemorrhage can include dizziness, rigidity of the neck, pupillary inequality, vomiting, seizures, drowsiness, sweating and chills, stupor, and loss of consciousness. A brief period of unconsciousness immediately after the rupture is common; severe hemorrhage may result in continued unconsciousness, coma, and death. Delirium and confusion often persist through the first weeks of recovery, and permanent brain damage is common.

Subarachnoid Hemorrhage Precautions, a Nursing Interventions Classification defined as reduction of internal and external stimuli or stressors to minimize risk of rebleeding prior to aneurysm surgery.

subarachnoid space, the space between the arachnoid and pia mater membranes.

subatomic /-ətom′ik/ [L, *sub,* beneath; Gk, *atmos,* indivisible], pertaining to the particles and phenomena that are within an atom.

subaxillary /-ak′siler′ē/ [L, *sub,* beneath, *axilla,* wing], pertaining to the area beneath the axilla.

subcapital fracture /-kap′itəl/ [L, *sub* + *caput,* head], a fracture of tissue just below the head of a bone that pivots in a ball and socket joint, such as the head of the femur.

subcapsular /-kap′s(y)ələr/ [L, *sub,* beneath, *capsula,* little box], pertaining to the area below a capsule.

subcapsular cataract [L, *sub* + *capsula,* little box], a condition marked by opacity or cloudiness beneath the anterior or posterior capsule of the lens of the eye.

subclavian /səbklā′vē·ən/ [L, *sub* + *clavicula,* little key], situated under the clavicle, such as the subclavian vein.

subclavian artery, one of a pair of arteries passing under the clavicle that vary in origin, course, and the height to which they rise in the neck but have six similar main branches supplying the vertebral column, spinal cord, ear, and brain

subclavian steal syndrome, a vascular syndrome caused by an occlusion in the subclavian artery proximal to the origin of the vertebral artery. It results in a reversal of the normal blood pressure gradient in the vertebral artery and decreased blood flow distal to the occlusion. It is characterized by episodes of flaccid paralysis of the arm, pain in the mastoid and occipital areas, and a diminished or absent radial pulse on the involved side.

subclavian vein, the continuation of the axillary vein in the upper body, extending from the lateral border of the first rib to the sternal end of the clavicle, where it joins the internal jugular to form the brachiocephalic vein.

subclavius /səbklā′vē·əs/ [L, *sub* + *cla-*

vicula], a short muscle of the chest wall. It acts to draw the shoulder down and forward.

subclinical /-klin′ikəl/ [L, *sub* + Gk, *kline,* bed], pertaining to a disease or abnormal condition that is so mild it produces no symptoms.

subcollateral gyrus /-kəlal′ərəl/ [L, *sub* + *con* + *lateralis* + Gk, *gyros,* turn], a convolution below the collateral fissure or sulcus of the cerebrum.

subconscious /-kon′shəs/ [L, *sub* + *conscire,* to be aware], imperfectly or partially conscious. **—subconsciousness,** *n.*

subconscious memory, a thought, sensation, or feeling that is not immediately available for recall to the conscious mind.

subculture /sub′kulchər/ [L, *sub* + *colere,* to cultivate], an ethnic, regional, economic, or social group with characteristic patterns of behavior and ideals that distinguish it from the rest of a culture or society.

subcutaneous /sub′kyo͞otā′nē·əs/ [L, *sub* + *cutis,* skin], beneath the skin.

subcutaneous adipose tissue [L, *sub,* beneath, *cutis,* skin, *adeps,* fat; OFr, *tissu*], fat deposits beneath the skin.

subcutaneous emphysema, the presence of free air or gas in the subcutaneous tissues. The air or gas may originate in the rupture of an airway or alveolus and migrate through the subpleural spaces to the mediastinum and neck. The face, neck, and chest may appear swollen. Skin tissues can be painful and may produce a crackling or popping sound as air moves under them. The patient may experience dyspnea and appear cyanotic if the air leak is severe.

subcutaneous fascia, a continuous layer of connective tissue over the entire body between the skin and the deep fascial investment of the specialized structures of the body, such as the muscles. It comprises an outer normally fatty layer and an inner thin elastic layer.

subcutaneous injection, the introduction of a hypodermic needle into the subcutaneous tissue beneath the skin, usually on the upper arm, thigh, or abdomen.

subcutaneous mastectomy, a surgical procedure in which all the breast tissue of one or both breasts is removed, leaving the skin, areola, and nipple intact. The adjacent lymph nodes, pectoralis major, and pectoralis minor are not removed. It may be performed on women who are at great risk of development of breast cancer.

subcutaneous nodule, a small, solid mass, or node beneath the skin that can be detected by touch.

subcutaneous tunnel, a tunnel under the

skin between the exit site of an atrial catheter and the entrance into the vein.

subcutaneous wound [L, *sub,* beneath, *cutis,* skin; AS, *wund*], an injury to internal organs, such as by crushing or another violent force, without a break in the surface of the skin.

subcuticular suture /-kyo͞otik′yələr/ [L, *sub,* beneath, *cutis,* skin, *sutura*], a continuous suture placed to draw together the tissues immediately beneath the skin. It is frequently a suture of nonabsorbable material that later can be removed by pulling on one end.

subdural /-d(y)o͞o′rəl/ [L, *sub* + *durus,* hard], pertaining to the area under the dura mater and above the arachnoid membrane.

subdural hematoma, an accumulation of blood in the subdural space, usually caused by an injury.

subdural hygroma, a collection of fluid between the dura mater and arachnoid layers, resulting from a spinal fluid leak through a rupture in the arachnoid tissue.

subdural puncture, a perforation of the space between the dura mater and arachnoid membrane to insert a needle for the injection of diagnostic or therapeutic medications or for aspiration of blood or other fluid.

subdural space [L, *sub,* beneath, *dura, mater,* hard mother, *spatium*], the potential space between the dura mater and the arachnoid membrane.

subendocardial infarction /-en′dōkär′-dē·əl/, a myocardial infarction that involves only the innermost layer of the myocardium and in some cases parts of the middle layer of tissue, but does not extend to the epicardial region.

subepidermal /-ep′idur′məl/ [L, *sub,* beneath; Gk, *epi,* above, *derma,* skin], beneath the epidermis.

subgingival calculus /-jinjī′vəl/ [L, *sub* + *gingiva,* gum], a deposit of various mineral salts, such as calcium phosphate and calcium carbonate, that accumulates on the surface of acquired pellicle, with organic matter, bacteria, and oral debris on the teeth or within the gingival crevice, the gingival pocket, or the periodontal pocket. It is usually darker, more pigmented, and denser than supragingival calculus.

subgingival curettage, the debridement of an ulcerated epithelial attachment and subjacent gingival corium to eliminate inflammation and shrink and restore gingival tissue.

subglottic /-glot′ik/, beneath the glottis.

subiculum /səbik′yələm/, a part of the hippocampal formation consisting of the transition zone between the parahippocampal gyrus and Ammon's horn.

subintimal /-in′timəl/ [L, *sub* + *intimus,* innermost], pertaining to the area beneath the intima or membrane lining a blood vessel, usually a large artery.

subjective /-jek′tiv/ [L, *subicere,* to expose], **1.** pertaining to the essential nature of an object as perceived in the mind rather than to a thing in itself. **2.** existing only in the mind. **3.** that which arises within or is perceived by the individual, as contrasted with something that is modified by external circumstances or something that may be evaluated by objective standards. **4.** pertaining to a person who places excessive importance on his own moods, attitudes, or opinions; egocentric.

subjective data collection, the process in which data relating to his or her problem are elicited from a patient. The interviewer encourages a full description of the onset, the course, and the character of the problem and any factors that aggravate or ameliorate it.

subjective sensation, a feeling or impression that is not associated with or does not directly result from any external stimulus.

subjective symptoms [L, *subicere,* to expose; Gk, *symptoma*], symptoms that are observed only by the patient and cannot be objectively confirmed.

subjective vertigo, an inappropriate sensation of bodily movement.

subjects /sub′jekts/, people, animals, or events selected for a study to examine a particular variable or condition such as the effects of a new medication or therapy.

sublethal dose /-lē′thəl/ [L, *sub,* beneath, *letum,* death; Gk, *dosis,* giving], a dose of a potentially lethal substance that is not large enough to cause death.

sublethal gene [L, *sub* + *lethum,* death; Gk, *genein,* to produce], a gene whose presence causes abnormalities or impairs the functioning of an organism but does not cause its death.

sublimate /sub′limāt/ [L, *sublimare,* to lift up], to refine or divert instinctual impulses and energy from an immediate goal to one that can be expressed in a social, moral, or aesthetic manner acceptable to the person and the society.

sublimation /-limā′shən/ [L, *sublimare*], **1.** an unconscious defense mechanism by which an unacceptable instinctive drive is diverted to and expressed through a personally approved, socially accepted means. **2.** (in psychoanalysis) the process of diverting certain components of the sex drive to a socially acceptable, nonsexual goal. **3.** change in a physical state from the solid phase directly to the gas phase.

subliminal /-lim'inəl/ [L, *sub* + *limen*, threshold], taking place below the threshold of sensory perception or outside the range of conscious awareness.

subliminal self [L, *sub*, beneath, *limen*, threshold; AS, *self*], a level of mental activity at which an individual under normal waking conditions may function without consciousness.

sublingual /səbling'gwəl/ [L, *sub* + *lingua*, tongue], pertaining to the area beneath the tongue.

sublingual administration of a medication, the administration of a drug, such as nitroglycerin, usually in tablet form, by placing it beneath the tongue until the tablet dissolves.

sublingual caruncle [L, *sub*, beneath, *lingua*, tongue, *caruncula*, small piece of flesh], a small fleshy growth under the tongue.

sublingual gland, one of a pair of small salivary glands situated under the mucous membrane of the floor of the mouth, beneath the tongue. A narrow, almond-shaped structure, it secretes mucus produced by its alveoli.

subluxation complex /-luksā'shən/, (in chiropractic) a theoretic model of motion segment dysfunction that incorporates the complex interaction of pathologic changes in nerve, muscle, ligamentous, vascular, and connective tissues.

subluxation syndrome, (in chiropractic) an aggregate of signs and symptoms that relate to pathophysiologic characteristics or dysfunction of spinal and pelvic motion segments or to peripheral joints.

submandibular /-məndib'yələr/ [L, *sub* + *mandible*], pertaining to the area below the mandible, or lower jaw.

submandibular duct [L, *sub* + *mandere*, to chew], a duct through which a submandibular gland secretes saliva.

submandibular gland, one of a pair of round walnut-sized salivary glands in the submandibular triangle. The gland secretes both mucus and a thinner serous fluid, which aid the digestive process.

submaxillary /-mak'siler'ē/ [L, *sub* + *maxilla*], pertaining to the area below the maxilla, or upper jaw.

submeatal /-mē-ā'təl/ [l, *sub*, beneath, *meatus*, passage], pertaining to tissues beneath a meatus, such as the mastoid air cells under the acoustic meatus or the hard palate beneath the nasal meatus.

submental /-men'təl/ [L, *sub* + *mentum*, chin], pertaining to the area beneath the chin.

submentovertex /-men'tōvur'teks/ [L, *sub* + *mentum*, chin, *vertex*, peak], a reference point at the base of the skull used in preparing radiographic projections of the skull and its associated structures.

submetacentric /-sub'metəsen'trik/ [L, *sub* + Gk, *meta*, besides, *kentron*, center], pertaining to a chromosome in which the centromere is located approximately equidistant between the center and one end so that the arms of the chromatids are not equal in length.

submucous /m(y)ōō'kəs/, pertaining to a location beneath a mucous membrane.

submucous resection (SMR) [L, *sub* + *mucous* + *re* + *secare*, to cut], a surgical procedure for correcting a deviated nasal septum, leaving the mucous membrane of the septum intact.

subnormal temperature /-nôr'məl/, any degree of sensible heat below the normal body level of 98.6° F (37° C).

suboccipitobregmatic /-aksip'itō'bregmat'ik/ [L, *sub* + *occiput*, back of the head; Gk, *bregma*, front of the head], pertaining to the smallest anteroposterior diameter of an infant's head when the neck is well flexed during labor.

subperiosteal fracture /sub'perē·os'tē·əl/ [L, *sub* + Gk, *peri*, around, *osteon*, bone], a fracture in a bone beneath the periosteum that does not disrupt the periosteal covering.

subphrenic /-fren'ik/ [L, *sub* + Gk, *phren*, diaphragm], pertaining to the area under the diaphragm.

subphrenic abscess [L, *sub*, beneath; Gk, *phren*, diaphragm; L, *abscedere*, to go away], an abscess that develops on or near the undersurface of the diaphragm, usually as a result of peritonitis or from another visceral site.

subpoena /-pē'nə/ [L, *sub* + *poena*, penalty], (in law) a document from a court commanding that a person appear at a certain time and place to testify on a specific matter.

subpoena duces tecum, (in law) a subpoena commanding a person to take books, papers, records, or other items to the court.

subscapularis /-skap'yələr'is/ [L, *sub*, beneath, *scapulae*, shoulder blades], the muscle arising from the subscapular fossa with insertion in the humerus. It functions to rotate the arm medially.

subscriber, (in managed care) an individual, agency, or employer that has contracted for services under a health plan.

subserous fascia /-sir'əs/ [L, *sub* + *serum*, whey, *fascia*, band], one of three kinds of fascia, lying between the internal layer of deep fascia and the serous membranes lining the body cavities. It is thin in some areas, such as between the pleura and the chest wall, and thick in other areas, where it forms a pad of adipose tissue.

subsistence /-sis′təns/ [L, *subsistere,* to stand still], the state of being sustained or remaining alive with a minimum of life essentials.

subspecialty /-spesh′əltē/ [L, *sub* + *specialis,* individual], (in nursing) a nurse's particular highly specialized professional field of practice, such as dialysis, oncology, neurology, or newborn intensive care nursing.

substance /sub′stəns/ [L, *substantia,* essence], **1.** any drug, chemical, or biologic entity. **2.** any material capable of being self-administered or abused because of its physiologic or psychologic effects.

substance abuse, the overindulgence in and dependence on a stimulant, depressant, or other chemical substance, leading to effects that are detrimental to the individual's physical or mental health or the welfare of others.

Substance Abuse and Mental Health Services Administration (SAMHSA), an agency of the United States Department of Health and Human Services with the function of disseminating accurate and up-to-date information about and provide leadership in the prevention and treatment of addictive and mental disorders.

substance dependence, a maladaptive pattern of substance abuse, leading to clinically significant impairment or distress as manifested by three or more episodes within a 12-month period of tolerance, withdrawal, use of larger amounts or over a longer period, a persistent desire or unsuccessful effort to control substance abuse, or investment of a great deal of time in activities necessary to obtain the substance.

substance P, a polypeptide neurotransmitting substance that is synthesized by the body and acts to stimulate vasodilation and contraction of intestinal and other smooth muscles. It also plays a part in salivary secretion, diuresis, and natriuresis, and it affects the function of the peripheral and central nervous systems.

Substance Use Prevention, a Nursing Interventions Classification defined as prevention of an alcoholic or drug use lifestyle.

Substance Use Treatment, a Nursing Interventions Classification defined as supportive care of a patient/family members with physical and psychosocial problems associated with the use of alcohol or drugs.

Substance Use Treatment: Alcohol Withdrawal, a Nursing Interventions Classification defined as care of the patient experiencing sudden cessation of alcohol consumption.

Substance Use Treatment: Drug Withdrawal, a Nursing Interventions Classification defined as care of a patient experiencing drug detoxification.

Substance Use Treatment: Overdose, a Nursing Interventions Classification defined as monitoring, treatment, and emotional support of a patient who has ingested prescription or over-the-counter drugs beyond the therapeutic range.

substandard /-stan′dərd/ [L, *sub,* beneath; OFr, *estandart*], below the predetermined model or measure.

substantia alba /-stan′shə/ [L, *substantia,* essence, *albus,* white], the part of the central nervous system that is enclosed in myelin sheaths. The myelin contributes a white coloring to otherwise gray nerve tissue.

substantia gelatinosa, the apical part of the posterior horn of the spinal cord's gray matter. It appears gelatinous because of its lack of myelinated nerve fibers.

substantia innominata, a region of the forebrain that lies ventral to the anterior half of the lentiform nucleus. It contains the basal forebrain, which receives afferent input from the reticular formation, hypothalamus, and limbic cortex.

substantia nigra [L, *substantia,* essence, *niger,* black], a dark band of gray matter lying between the tegmentum of the midbrain and the crus cerebri.

substantive epidemiology /sub′stəntiv/ [L, *subtantia* + Gk, *epi,* upon, *demos,* people, *logos,* science], the body of knowledge derived from epidemiologic studies, including for each disease the natural history of the disorder, patterns of occurrence, and risk factors for development of the disorder.

substantivity /-stantiv′itē/, the property of continuing therapeutic action despite removal of the vehicle, such as applied to certain shampoos.

substernal /-stur′nəl/ [L, *sub* + Gk, *sternon,* chest], pertaining to the area beneath the sternum.

substernal goiter [L, *sub* + Gk, *sternon,* chest; L, *guttur,* throat], a nonbacterial inflammation of the thyroid gland, often preceded by a viral infection causing fever, tenderness, and enlargement of the thyroid gland.

substitution /-stit(y)o͞o′shən/, a mental defense mechanism, operating unconsciously, by which an unattainable or unacceptable goal, emotion, or object is replaced by one that is more attainable or acceptable.

substitutive therapy /-stit(y)o͞o′tiv/ [L,

substituere, to put in place of; Gk, *therapeia,* treatment], a treatment that effects a condition incompatible with or antagonistic to the condition being treated.

substrate /sub'strāt/ [L, *sub* + *stratum,* layer], a chemical substance acted on and changed by an enzyme in any chemical reaction.

substrate depletion phase, a period during an enzyme assay when the concentration of substrate is falling and the assay is not following zero-order kinetics.

substratum /-strā'təm/ [L, *sub* + *stratum,* layer], any underlying layer; a foundation.

subsystem /sub'sistəm/, a smaller component of a large system composed of individuals or dyads, formed by generation, gender, interest, or function.

subtask work, a part of the whole task in a rehabilitation program but distinguished by changes in speed or direction.

subthalamus /-thal'əməs/ [L, *sub* + Gk, *thalamos,* chamber], a part of the diencephalon that serves as a correlation center for optic and vestibular impulses relayed to the globus pallidus. —**subthalamic,** *adj.*

subtle /sut'əl/ [L, *subtilis*], having a low intensity; not severe and having no serious sequelae, such as a mild infection or inflammation.

subtotal /sub'tōtəl/ [L, *sub,* beneath, *totus,* whole], less than complete.

subtotal hysterectomy [L, *sub* + *totus* + Gk, *hystera,* womb, *extome,* excision], the surgical removal of the body of the uterus without removing the cervix.

subtrochanteric osteotomy /-trō'kəntər'ik/ [L, *sub* + Gk, *trochanter,* runner, *osteon,* bone, *temnein,* to cut], a surgical procedure that divides the shaft of the femur below the lesser trochanter to correct ankylosis of the hip joint.

subungual /səbung'gwəl/ [L, *sub* + *unguis,* nail], under a fingernail or toenail.

subungual hematoma, a collection of blood beneath a nail that usually results from trauma.

subunit vaccine /sub'yoōnit/, a viral immunizing agent that has been treated to remove traces of viral nucleic acid, so that only protein subunits remain. The subunits have little likelihood of causing adverse reactions.

subventricular zone /-ventrik'yələr/, an area located between the ventricular and intermediate zones in the fetal forebrain, in which neurons of the cerebrum are generated.

succinic acid /suksin'ik/, a compound found in certain hydatid cysts and in lichens, amber, and fossils.

succinylcholine chloride /suk'sinilkō'lēn/, a skeletal muscle relaxant prescribed to provide an adjunct to anesthesia, to reduce muscle contractions during surgery or mechanical ventilation, and to facilitate endotracheal intubation.

succus /suk'əs/, *pl.* **succi** /suk'sī/ [L, juice], a juice or fluid, usually one secreted by an organ, such as succus prostaticus of the prostate.

succussion splash /səkush'ən/ [L, *succutere,* to shake up; ME, *plasche,* puddle], the sound elicited by shaking the body of a person who has free fluid and air or gas in a hollow organ or body cavity. This sound may be present over a normal stomach but also may be heard with hydropneumothorax, large hiatal hernia, or intestinal or pyloric obstruction.

suck [L, *sugere,* to suck], **1.** to draw a liquid or semiliquid into the mouth by creating a partial vacuum through motions of the lips and tongue. **2.** to hold on the tongue and dissolve by the movements of the mouth and action of the saliva. **3.** to draw fluid into the mouth, specifically to draw milk from the breast or nursing bottle.

sucking blisters, the pale soft pads on the upper and lower lips of a baby that look like blisters but are not. They seem to augment the seal of the lips around the nipple or breast. Some babies who have sucked on their own fingers, hand, or arm before birth are born with them.

sucking reflex, involuntary sucking movements of the circumoral area in newborns in response to stimulation. The reflex continues throughout infancy and often occurs without stimulation, such as during sleep.

suckle [L, *sugere*], **1.** to provide nourishment, specifically to breast-feed. **2.** to take in nourishment, especially by feeding from the breast.

suckling, an infant that has not been weaned.

sucrose /soō'krōs/ [Fr, *sucre,* sugar], a disaccharide sugar derived from sugar cane, sugar beets, and sorghum.

sucrose polyester (SPE), a synthetic nonabsorbable fat that, when added to the diet, reduces plasma cholesterol levels by increasing the excretion of cholesterol in the feces.

suction /suk'shən/ [L, *sugere,* to suck], the aspiration of a gas or fluid by reducing air pressure over its surface, usually by mechanical means.

suction biopsy [L, *sugere,* to suck; Gk, *bios,* life, *opsis,* view], a procedure for obtaining tissue or fluid samples from lymph nodes or a deep lesion by using suction and a trochar or cannula.

suction curettage, a method of curettage in which a specimen of the endometrium or the products of conception are removed by aspiration.

sudden death [ME, *sodain,* to come up; AS, *death*], death that occurs unexpectedly and from 1 to 24 hours after the onset of symptoms, with or without known preexisting conditions.

sudden infant death syndrome (SIDS) [ME, *sodain,* to come up; L, *infans,* unable to speak; AS, *death* + Gk, *syn,* together, *dromos,* course], the unexpected and sudden death of an apparently normal and healthy infant that occurs during sleep and with no physical or autopsic evidence of disease. Multiple causes have been proposed, including lack of biotin in the diet, abnormality of the endogenous-opioid system, mechanical suffocation, a defect in respiratory mucosal defense, prolonged apnea, an unknown virus, anatomic abnormality of the larynx, and immunoglobulin abnormalities. It is seen more often among babies who have recently had a minor illness such as upper respiratory infection. The syndrome is neither contagious nor hereditary, although there is a greater than average risk of its occurrence within the same family, which may indicate the influence of polygenic factors.

sudor /soō'dôr/ [L, sweat], perspiration.

sudoriferous duct /soō'dərif'ərəs/ [L, *sudor,* sweat, *facere,* to make], a duct leading from a sweat gland to the surface of the skin.

sudoriferous gland, one of about two million tiny structures within the dermis that produce sweat. The average quantity of sweat secreted in 24 hours varies from 700 to 900 g. Most of these glands are eccrine glands, producing sweat that carries away sodium chloride, the waste products urea and lactic acid, and the breakdown products from garlic, spices, and other substances. Each sudoriferous gland consists of a single tube with a deeply coiled body and a superficial duct.

sudorific /soō'dərif'ik/ [L, *sudor,* sweat, *facere,* to make], **1.** pertaining to a substance or condition, such as heat or emotional tension, that promotes sweating. **2.** a sudorific agent. Sweat glands are stimulated by cholinergic drugs.

sufentanil citrate /sufen'tənil/, an intravenous analgesic and anesthetic used as an adjunct to general anesthesia and as a primary anesthetic with 100% oxygen.

suffocation /suf'əkā'shən/ [L, *suffocare,* to choke], an interruption in breathing with oxygen deprivation, usually caused by an obstruction in the airways. The condition may be accidental or intentional or may result from disease or inadequate levels of respirable gases in the atmosphere.

suffocation, risk for, a NANDA-accepted nursing diagnosis of the accentuated risk of accidental suffocation (inadequate air available for inhalation). The risk factors may be internal (individual) or external (environmental). Internal risk factors include reduced olfactory sensation, reduced motor abilities, lack of safety education, lack of safety precautions, cognitive or emotional difficulties, and disease or injury processes. External risk factors include a pillow or a propped bottle placed in an infant's crib, a vehicle warming in a closed garage, children's playing with plastic bags or inserting small objects into their mouths or noses, discarded or unused refrigerators or freezers without removed doors, lack of monitoring of children in bathtubs or pools, household gas leaks, smoking in bed, consumption of overly large mouthfuls of food, use of fuel-burning heaters not vented to the outside, low-strung clotheslines, and a pacifier hung around an infant's neck.

suffocative goiter /suf'əkā'tiv/ [L, *suffocare,* to choke, *guttur,* throat], an enlargement of the thyroid gland causing a sensation of suffocation on pressure.

sugar /shoōg'ər/ [Gk, *sakcharon*], any of several water-soluble carbohydrates. The principal categories of sugars are monosaccharides, disaccharides, and polysaccharides. A monosaccharide is a single sugar such as glucose, fructose, or galactose. A disaccharide is a double sugar such as sucrose (table sugar) or lactose. A polysaccharide is a sugar made up of repeating units of fructose such as cellulose, starch, and glycogen.

sugar alcohol, an alcohol produced by the reduction of an aldehyde or ketone of a sugar.

sugar cataract, a visual disorder associated with diabetes in which sorbitol collects within the lens, causing an osmotic gradient of fluid in the lens. This condition leads to a disruption of the lens matrix and loss of transparency.

suggestibility /səjəs'tibil'itē/, pertaining to a person's susceptibility to having his or her ideas or actions influenced or altered by others.

suggestion /səjəs'chən/ [L, *suggerere,* to propose], **1.** the process by which one thought or idea leads to another, as in the association of ideas. **2.** the use of persuasion, exhortation, or another technique to implant an idea, thought, attitude, or belief in the mind of another as a means of influencing or altering behavior or states of mind. **3.** an idea, belief, or attitude implanted in the mind of another.

suicidal /soo'isī'dəl/ [L, *sui,* of oneself, *caedere,* to kill], of, relating to, or tending toward self-destruction.

suicide /soo'isīd/ [L, *sui,* of oneself, *caedere,* to kill], **1.** the intentional taking of one's own life. **2.** *informal.* the ruin or destruction of one's own interests. **3.** a person who commits or attempts self-destruction.

suicide gesture, (in psychiatric nursing) an apparent attempt by a patient to cause self-injury without lethal consequences and generally without actual intent to commit suicide.

Suicide Prevention, a Nursing Interventions Classification defined as reducing the risk of self-inflicted harm for a patient in crisis or severe depression.

suicide prevention center, a crisis-intervention facility dealing primarily with people preoccupied with suicidal thoughts. Such facilities are usually operated by professional social workers with special training in counseling possible suicide victims in person or by telephone.

suicidology /soo'isīdol'əjē/ [L, *sui* + *caedere* + Gk, *logos,* science], the study of the prevention and causes of suicide. **—suicidologist,** *n.*

sulculus /sul'kyələs/ [L, *sulcus*], a small sulcus.

sulcus /sul'kəs/, *pl.* **sulci** /sul'sī/ [L, furrow], a shallow groove, depression, or furrow on the surface of an organ, such as a sulcus that separates the convolutions of the cerebral hemisphere. **—sulcate,** *adj.*

sulcus pulmonalis, a depression on each side of the vertebral bodies that accommodates the posterior part of the lung.

sulfacetamide /sul'fəset'əmīd/, a topical antibacterial most commonly prescribed for the prophylaxis of infection after injury to the cornea and in the treatment of bacterial conjunctivitis and urinary tract infections.

sulfachlorpyridazine /sul'fəklôr'pirid'ə-zēn/, a sulfonamide antibacterial prescribed in the treatment of infection, particularly of the urinary tract.

sulfacytine /sul'fəs'itēn/, a sulfonamide antibacterial prescribed in the treatment of infection, particularly primary pyelonephritis and cystitis.

sulfadiazine /sul'fədī'əzēn/, a sulfonamide antibacterial prescribed in the treatment of infection of the urinary tract, and in rheumatic fever prophylaxis.

sulfa drugs /sul'fə/, a group of bacteriostatic agents that inhibit the biosynthesis of folic acid.

sulfamethizole /sul'fəmeth'izōl/, a sulfonamide antibacterial prescribed in the treatment of infection, particularly pyelonephritis, pyelitis, and cystitis.

sulfamethoxazole /sul'fəmethok'səzōl/, a sulfonamide antibacterial prescribed in the treatment of otitis media, bronchitis, and certain urinary tract infections.

sulfamethoxazole and trimethoprim /trī-meth'əprim/, a fixed-combination antibacterial prescribed in the treatment of urinary tract infections, otitis media, and shigellosis.

sulfanilic acid /sul'fənil'ik/, a red-tinged white crystalline compound used in the synthesis of sulfonamides and as a reagent in tests for phenol, fecal matter in water, albumin, aldehydes, and glucose.

sulfasalazine /sul'fəsəlaz'ēn/, a sulfonamide; salicylazosulfapyridine prescribed in the treatment of mild to moderate ulcerative colitis and as adjunctive therapy in severe cases.

sulfate /sul'fāt/, a salt of sulfuric acid. Natural sulfate compounds such as sodium sulfate, calcium sulfate, and potassium sulfate are plentiful in the body.

sulfatide lipidosis /sul'fətīd/, an inherited lipid metabolism disorder of childhood caused by a deficiency of cerebroside sulfatase enzyme. It results in an accumulation of metachromatic lipids in tissues of the central nervous system, kidney, spleen, and other organs, leading to dementia, paralysis, and death by 10 years of age.

sulfhemoglobin /sulfhem'əglō'bin/, a form of hemoglobin found in the blood in trace amounts that contains an irreversibly bound sulfur molecule that prevents normal oxygen binding.

sulfhemoglobinemia /-ē'mē·ə/, the presence of abnormal sulfur containing hemoglobin circulating in the blood.

sulfinpyrazone /sul'finpir'əzōn/, a uricosuric prescribed in the treatment of chronic gout and intermittent gouty arthritis.

sulfisoxazole /sul'fisok'səzōl/, a sulfonamide antibacterial prescribed in the treatment of conjunctivitis and urinary tract infections, including vaginitis, cystitis, and pyelonephritis.

sulfiting agents /sul'fīting/, food preservatives composed of potassium or sodium bisulfite or potassium metabisulfite. Sulfiting agents are used in processing of beer, wine, baked goods, soup mixes, and some imported seafoods and by restaurants to impart a "fresh" appearance to salad fruits and vegetables. The chemicals can cause a severe allergic reaction in people who are hypersensitive to sulfites. The reactions are marked by flushing, faintness, hives, headache, gastrointestinal distress, breathing difficulty, and, in extreme cases, loss of consciousness and death.

sulfobromophthalein /sul′fəbrō′məfthal′ēn, -ē·in/, a substance used in its disodium salt form for evaluating the function of the liver.

sulfonamide /səlfon′əmīd/, one of a large group of synthetic bacteriostatic drugs that are effective in treating infections caused by many gram-negative and gram-positive microorganisms. They are bacteriostatic rather than bactericidal. Some sulfonamides are short acting, some are intermediate acting, and some are long acting, depending on the speed with which they are excreted. They are used in treating many urinary tract infections.

sulfonates /sul′fənāts/, a class of anticholinesterase compounds used as insecticides.

sulfonylurea /sul′fənilyŏŏr′ē·ə/, an oral antidiabetic agent that stimulates the pancreatic production of insulin. Hypersensitivity to sulfonamides is a contraindication for using such agents, and ethanol consumption is incompatible with all sulfonylureas. Aspirin or other salicylates taken with any sulfonylurea may intensify the hypoglycemic effect.

sulfosalicylic acid /sul′fōsalisil′ik/, a white or faintly pink crystalline substance that is highly water soluble and is used as a reagent in tests for albumin and as an intermediate compound in the manufacture of dyes and surfactants.

sulfoxone sodium /sulfok′sōn/, a bacteriostatic sulfone derivative prescribed in the treatment of leprosy and dermatitis herpetiformis.

sulfur (S) /sul′fər/ [L], a nonmetallic multivalent tasteless, odorless chemical element that occurs abundantly in yellow crystalline form or in masses, especially in volcanic areas. Its atomic number is 16; its atomic mass (weight) is 32.07. Sulfur has been used in the treatment of gout, rheumatism, and bronchitis and as a mild laxative.

sulfuric acid /sulf(y)ŏŏ′rik/, a clear, colorless, oily highly corrosive liquid that generates great heat when mixed with water. An extremely toxic substance, sulfuric acid causes severe skin burns, blindness on contact with the eyes, serious lung damage if the vapors are inhaled, and death if it is ingested.

sulfurous acid /sul′fərəs/, a weak inorganic acid used as a chemical reducing and bleaching agent. It has been used in medicine in skin lotions and nasal and throat sprays. Sulfites formed by the acid

may be included in antiseptics, antifermentatives, and antizymotics.

sulindac /sulin′dek/, a nonsteroidal antiinflammatory agent prescribed in the treatment of osteoarthritis, rheumatoid arthritis, and ankylosing spondylitis.

sumac [Ar, *summaq*], any of a number of species of trees and shrubs in the Anacardiaceae family, including the Rhus species, that have poisonous properties.

summary judgment [L, *summa*, total, *jus*, law, *dicere*, to state], (in law) a judgment requested by any party to a civil action to end the action when it is believed that there is no genuine issue or material fact in dispute.

summation [L, *summa*, total], **1.** an accumulative effect or action; a total aggregate; totality. **2.** (in neurology) the concentration of a neurotransmitter at a synapse, either by increasing the frequency of nerve impulses in each fiber (temporal summation) or by increasing the number of fibers stimulated (spatial summation), so that the threshold of the postsynaptic neuron is overcome and an impulse is transmitted.

summons /sum′əns/ [OFr, *somondre*, to remind secretly], (in law) a document issued by a clerk of the court on the filing of a complaint. A sheriff, marshal, or other appointed person serves the summons, notifying a person that an action has been begun against him or her.

sump drain, a drainage device consisting of two tubes, one to allow fluid to be drained from a cavity and the other to allow air to enter the cavity to replace the fluid. It may be attached to a suction apparatus.

sunbath [AS, *sunne* + *baeth*], the exposure of the naked body to the sun.

sunburn, a skin injury characterized by redness, tenderness, and possible blistering that results from exposure to actinic radiation from the sun.

sundowning /sun′douning/ [AS, *sunne* + *ofdune*, off the hill], a condition in which persons with cognitive impairment and elderly people tend to become confused or disoriented at the end of the day. With less light, they lose visual cues that help them to compensate for their sensory impairments.

sunrise syndrome, a condition of unstable cognitive ability on arising in the morning.

sunscreen protective factor index (SPF), a system of evaluating the effectiveness of various formulations for protecting the skin from actinic rays of the sun. Protective agents are rated from 1 to 50 by the U.S. Food and Drug Administration. A sun protective factor of 15 means that the sunscreen provides 15 times the protection of unprotected skin.

sun-setting sign, a characteristic of hydrocephalus in which an infant's eyes appear to look only downward, with the sclera prominent over the iris.

sunstroke [AS, *sunne* + *strac,* stroke], a morbid condition caused by overexposure to the sun and characterized by a high temperature and altered level of consciousness.

superantigens, a family of related substances, including staphylococcal and streptococcal exotoxins that can short-circuit the normal sequence of events leading to activation of helper T cells. Superantigens do not require processing and presentation by macrophages to induce a T cell response. They initiate an uncontrolled proliferation of T cells. The result is either an acute and potentially life-threatening disease such as toxic shock syndrome or a chronic inflammatory process such as rheumatic fever.

superego /ē′gō/ [L, *super,* over; Gk, *ego,* I], (in psychoanalysis) that part of the psyche, functioning mostly in the unconscious, that develops when the standards of the parents and of society are incorporated into the ego. The superego has two parts, the conscience and the ego ideal.

superfecundation /-fekəndā′shən/ [L, *super* + *fecundare,* to be fruitful], the impregnation of two or more ova released during the same ovulation by spermatozoa from the successive coital acts.

superfetation /-fētā′shən/ [L, *super* + *fetus,* pregnancy], the fertilization of a second ovum after the onset of pregnancy, resulting in the simultaneous development of two fetuses of different degrees of maturity within the uterus.

superficial /-fish′əl/ [L, *superficies,* surface], **1.** pertaining to the skin or another surface. **2.** not grave or dangerous.

superficial abscess [L, *superficialis* + *abscedere,* to go away], an abscess that develops above the fascia layer.

superficial fading infantile hemangioma, a superficial temporary salmon-colored patch in the center of the forehead, face, or occiput of many newborns.

superficial implantation, (in embryology) the partial embedding of the blastocyst within the uterine wall so that it and later the chorionic sac protrude into the uterine cavity.

superficial inguinal node, a node in one of the two groups of inguinal lymph glands in the upper femoral triangle of the thigh.

superficial reflex, any neural reflex initiated by stimulation of the skin.

superficial sensation, the awareness or perception of feelings in the superficial layers of the skin in response to touch, pressure, temperature, and pain.

superficial spreading melanoma, the most common melanoma that grows outward, spreading over the surface of the affected organ or tissue. It occurs most commonly on the lower legs of women and the torso of men. The lesion is raised and palpable, unevenly pigmented, and irregularly shaped and has an unclear border.

superficial temporal artery, an artery at each side of the head that can be easily felt in front of the ear and is often used for taking the pulse. It is the smaller of the two terminal branches of the external carotid.

superficial vein, one of the many veins between the subcutaneous fascia just under the skin.

superinfection /-infek′shən/ [L, *super* + *inficere,* to stain], an infection occurring during antimicrobial treatment for another infection.

superior /səpir′ē·ər/ [L, higher], situated above or oriented toward a higher place, as the head is superior to the torso.

superior aperture of minor pelvis, an opening bounded by the crest and pecten of the pubic bones, the arch-shaped lines of the ilia, and the anterior margin of the base of the sacrum.

superior aperture of thorax, an elliptic opening at the summit of the thorax bounded by the first thoracic vertebra, the first ribs, and the upper margin of the sternum.

superior carotid triangle [L, *superior,* higher; Gk, *karos,* heavy sleep; L, *triangulus*], a triangle bounded by the sternocleidomastoid muscle, in front and below by the omohyoid muscle, and above by the stylohyoid and digastric muscles.

superior conjunctival fornix, the space in the fold of the conjunctiva created by the reflection of the conjunctiva covering the eyeball and the lining of the upper lid.

superior costotransverse ligament, one of five ligaments associated with each costotransverse joint, except that of the first rib. It passes from the neck of each rib to the transverse process of the vertebra immediately above.

superior gastric node, a node in one of two sets of gastric lymph glands, accompanying the left gastric artery.

superior mediastinum, the upper part of the mediastinum in the middle of the thorax, containing the trachea, esophagus, aortic arch, and origins of the sternohyoidei and the sternothyroidei.

S

superior mesenteric artery, a visceral branch of the abdominal aorta, arising inferior to the celiac artery, dividing into five branches, and supplying most of the small intestine and parts of the colon.

superior mesenteric node, a node in one of the three groups of visceral lymph nodes that serve the viscera of the abdomen and the pelvis.

superior mesenteric vein, a tributary of the portal vein that drains the blood from the small intestine, the cecum, and the ascending and transverse colons.

superior olivary nucleus [L, *supurus* + *oliva* + *nucleus*, nut kernel], a collection of nerve cells appearing as a clump of gray matter in the pons. It assists in the localization of sound by comparing the time difference between sounds received by the left and right ears.

superior sagittal sinus, one of the six venous channels in the posterior of the dura mater, draining blood from the brain into the internal jugular vein.

superior subscapular nerve /səbskap'- yələr/, one of a pair of small nerves on opposite sides of the body that arise from the posterior cord of the brachial plexus. It supplies the superior part of the subscapularis.

superior temporal gyrus, a rounded elevation on the lateral surface of either temporal lobe of the brain.

superior thyroid artery, one of a pair of arteries in the neck, usually arising from the external carotid artery, that supplies the thyroid gland and several muscles in the head.

superior ulnar collateral artery, a long slender division of the brachial artery, arising just distal to the middle of the arm, descending to the elbow, and anastomosing with the posterior ulnar recurrent and inferior ulnar collateral arteries.

superior vena cava, the second largest vein of the body, returning deoxygenated blood from the upper half of the body to the right atrium. The section of the superior vena cava closest to the heart composes about one half of the vessel's length and is within the pericardial sac, covered by the serous pericardium.

superior vena cava syndrome, a condition of edema and engorgement of the veins of the upper body caused by obstruction of the superior vena cava by primary pulmonary tumors or thrombi. Signs and symptoms include a nonproductive cough and breathing difficulty; cyanosis; central nervous system disorders; and edema of the conjunctiva, trachea, and esophagus.

supernatant /-nā'tənt/ [L, *super* + *natare,* to swim], **1.** situated above or on top of something. **2.** the clear upper liquid part of a mixture (a liquid and a solid) after it has been centrifuged.

supernormal excitability /-nôr'məl/, the ability of the myocardium to respond to a stimulus that would be ineffective earlier or later in the cardiac cycle.

supernormal period, a period at the end of phase 3 of the cardiac action potential when activation can be initiated with less stimulus than is required at maximal repolarization.

supernumerary nipples /-nōō'mərer'ē/ [L, *super* + *numerus,* number; ME, *neb,* beak], an excessive number of nipples, which are usually not associated with underlying glandular tissue. They may vary in size from small pink dots to that of normal nipples.

supernumerary tooth [L, *super,* above, *numerus,* number; AS, *toth*], any tooth in addition to the normal 32 teeth in permanent dentition or the 20 teeth in deciduous dentition.

superoxide /-ok'sīd/, a common reactive form of oxygen that is formed when molecular oxygen gains a single electron. Superoxide radicals can attack susceptible biologic targets, including lipids, proteins, and nucleic acids.

superoxide dismutase (SOD), an enzyme composed of metal-containing proteins that converts superoxide radicals into less toxic agents. It is the main enzymatic mechanism for clearing superoxide radicals from the body.

supersaturate /-sach'ərāt/ [L, *super,* above, *saturare,* to fill], a solution that contains solute above the saturation point at a given temperature.

supertwins, multiple births of more than two infants. Children of multiple births are more prone to premature birth and are likely to suffer from congenital defects, according to studies. The rate of cerebral palsy in multiple births is six times that for single births.

supervised fast /sōō'pərvīsd/, a hypoglycemic diagnostic procedure in which glucose levels are measured every 4 to 6 hours in a fasting person until they fall below 50 mg/dl. The fasting person is closely observed, and glucose values are rapidly determined and reported by the laboratory.

supervision /-vizh'ən/, (in psychology) a process whereby a therapist is helped to become a more effective clinician through the direction of a supervisor who provides theoretic knowledge and therapeutic techniques.

supervisor /sōō'pərvī'zər/ [L, *super* + *videre,* to see], (in hospital or public health nursing) the midlevel management position between the chief nurse executive and nurse managers of a division or of several units. In many hospitals *clinical director* or *director* is the preferred term.

supervitaminosis /-vī′təminō′sis/ [L, *super,* above, *vita* + *amine* + Gk, *osis,* condition], a condition of ingesting an excessive amount of vitamins.

supinate /sōō′pənāt/, pertaining to a supine position or upturning of the palm.

supination /sōō′pinā′shən/ [L, *supinus,* lying on the back], **1.** one of the kinds of rotation allowed by certain skeletal joints, such as the elbow and the wrist joints, which allow the palm of the hand to turn up. **2.** the position of lying on the back, face up. —**supinate,** *v.*

supinator longus reflex /sōō′pinā′tər/ [L, *reflectere,* to bend back], a contraction of the brachioradialis muscle, causing flexion at the elbow joint on tapping the point of insertion of the supinator longus muscle at the lower end of the radius.

supine /səpīn′, sōō′pīn/ [L, *supinus*], **1.** position of the arms or body in which the palms of the hands face upward. **2.** lying horizontally on the back.

supine hypotension, a fall in blood pressure that occurs when a pregnant woman is lying on her back. It is caused by impaired venous return that results from pressure of the gravid uterus on the vena cava.

supplemental inheritance /sup′lemen′təl/ [L, *supplere,* to complete, *in,* in, *hereditare,* hereditary], the acquisition or expression of a genetic trait or condition through the presence of two independent pairs of nonallelic genes that interact in such a way that one gene supplements the action of the other.

supplementary gene /sup′ləmen′tərē/ [L, *supplere* + Gk, *genein,* to produce], one of two pairs of nonallelic genes that interact in such a way that one pair needs the presence of the other to be expressed, whereas the second pair can produce an effect independently of the first.

Supply Management, a Nursing Interventions Classification defined as ensuring acquisition and maintenance of appropriate items for providing patient care.

support /səpôrt′/ [L, *supportare,* to bring up], **1.** to sustain, hold up, or maintain in a desired position or condition, as in physically supporting the abdominal muscles with a scultetus binder or emotionally supporting a client under stress. **2.** the assistance given to this end, such as physical support, emotional support, or life support.

Support Group, a Nursing Interventions

Classification defined as use of a group environment to provide emotional support and health-related information for members.

support groups, 1. organizations that serve as a link in the network for family caregivers and patients, such as those who are homebound, mentally ill, elderly, or suicidal or who have a specific disorder such as multiple sclerosis. The groups help families and patients find a balance of responsibility. The groups are supported by various national and local organizations. **2.** organizations for people who share a common problem.

supporting area [L, *supportare* + *area,* space], any of the areas of maxillary or mandibular edentulous ridges that are considered best suited to bear the forces of mastication with functioning dentures.

supportive psychotherapy /səpôr′tiv/, a form of psychotherapy that concentrates on creating an effective means of communication with an emotionally disturbed person rather than on trying to produce psychologic insight into the underlying conflicts.

Support System Enhancement, a Nursing Interventions Classification defined as facilitation of support of a patient by the family, friends, and community.

suppository /səpoz′ətôr′ē/ [L, *sub,* under, *ponere,* to place], an easily melted medicated mass for insertion into the rectum, urethra, or vagina. Theobroma oil, glycerinated gelatin, and high-molecular-weight polyethylene glycols are common vehicles for drugs in suppositories that are cone- or spindle-shaped for insertion into the rectum, globular or egg-shaped for use in the vagina, and pencil-shaped for insertion into the urethra.

suppressant /səpres′ənt/ [L, *supprimere,* to press down], an agent that suppresses or diminishes a physical or mental activity, such as a medication that reduces hyperkinetic behavior.

suppressed menstruation /səprest′/ [L, *supprimere,* to press down, *menstruare*], a failure of menstruation to occur when expected, as in amenorrhea.

suppression /səpresh′ən/ [L, *supprimere*], (in psychoanalysis) the conscious inhibition of or effort to conceal unacceptable or painful thoughts, desires, impulses, feelings, or acts.

suppression amblyopia, a partial loss of vision, usually in one eye, caused by cortical suppression of central vision to prevent diplopia. It occurs commonly in strabismus in the eye that deviates and does not fixate.

suppressor gene /səpres′ər/, (in molecu-

S

lar genetics) a genetic unit that is able to reverse the effect of a specific kind of mutation in other genes.

suppressor mutation, (in molecular genetics) a mutation that partially or completely restores a function lost by a primary mutation occurring in a different genetic site.

suppurate /sup'yərāt/ [L, *suppurare,* to form pus], to produce purulent matter. —**suppuration,** *n.,* **suppurative** /sup'yə-rā'tiv/, *adj.*

suppuration /sup'yərā'shən/ [L, *suppurare,* to form pus], the production and exudation of pus.

suppurative /sup'yərətiv'/ [L, *suppurare,* to form pus], pus-forming.

suppurative arthritis, an inflammation of a joint with exudation of infected cells into the joint fluid.

suppurative fever [L, *suppurare,* to form pus, *febris,* fever], a fever accompanied by pus formation.

suppurative pancreatitis [L, *suppurare,* to form pus; Gk, *pan,* all, *kreas,* flesh, *itis,* inflammation], a form of pancreatic inflammation accompanied by the appearance of small abscesses.

suppurative phlebitis [L, *suppurare,* to form pus; Gk, *phleps,* vein, *itis,* inflammation], a vein inflammation that results from septicemia or a nearby pyogenic infection.

supracallosus gyrus /-kəlō'ses/ [L, *supra,* above, *callosus,* hard; Gk, *gyros,* turn], the gray matter covering the corpus callosum of the brain.

supracervical hysterectomy /-sur'vikəl/ [L, *supra,* above, *cervix,* neck; Gk, *hystera,* womb, *ektome,* excision], a subtotal hysterectomy in which the body of the uterus is removed, leaving the cervix.

supraclavicular /-kləvik'yələr/ [L, *supra,* above, *clavicula,* little key], pertaining to the area above the clavicle, or collar bone.

supraclavicular nerve, one of a pair of cutaneous branches of the cervical plexus, arising from the third and fourth cervical nerves, mostly from the fourth nerve.

supraclavicular triangle [L, *supra,* above, *clavicula,* little key, *triangulus*], the lower and anterior areas of the neck, bounded by the omohyoid muscle above, the sternocleidomastoid muscle in front, and the clavicle below. The first rib is in the base of the triangle.

supracondylar /-kon'dilər/ [L, *supra,* above; Gk, *kondylos,* knuckle], pertaining to an area above a condyle.

supracondylar fracture /sōō'prəkon'dilər/ [L, *supra + kondylos,* knuckle], a fracture involving the area between the condyles of the humerus or the femur.

supragingival calculus /-jinjī'vəl/ [L, *supra + gingiva,* gum], an amorphous deposit composed of various mineral salts, such as calcium phosphate and calcium carbonate, which accumulates on the surface of acquired pellicle with organic matter, bacteria, and oral debris on the teeth occlusal or coronal to the gingival crest.

suprahyoid muscles, a group of four muscles that attach the hyoid bone to the skull.

suprainfection /-infek'shən/ [L, *supra + inficere,* to stain], a secondary infection usually caused by an opportunistic pathogen, such as a fungal infection after the antibiotic treatment of another infection.

supranuclear gaze disturbance /-nōō'-klē-ər/, an inability to direct the eyes to the side contralateral to a lesion in the frontal lobe. If the frontal lobe lesions are bilateral, the patient can maintain fixation and follow visual targets but cannot shift the gaze in any direction in the absence of a target.

supraoptic nucleus /-op'tik/ [L, *supra,* above; Gk, *optikos* + L, *nucleus,* nut kernel], a hypothalamic nucleus that lies above the optic chiasma, with fibers extending to the posterior lobe of the pituitary.

suprapatellar /-pətel'ər/ [L, *supra,* above, *patella,* small dish], pertaining to a location above the patella.

suprapubic /-p(y)ōō'bik/ [L, *supra + pubes,* signs of maturity], pertaining to a location above the symphysis pubis.

suprapubic aspiration of urine, a procedure for draining the bladder by inserting a sterile needle through the skin above the pubic arch and into the bladder. The bladder may also be emptied by inserting a catheter through a suprapubic incision when conditions prohibit use of the conventional insertion.

suprapubic catheter [L, *supra + pubis* + Gk, *katheter,* a thing lowered into], a urinary bladder catheter inserted through the skin above the symphysis pubis.

suprarenal /-rē'nəl/ [L, *supra + ren,* kidney], pertaining to a location above the kidney, such as the suprarenal gland.

suprascapular ligament /-skap'yələr/ [L, *supra,* above, *scapula,* shoulder blade, *ligare,* to bind], a ligament that extends from the base of the coracoid process to the medial end of the suprascapular notch.

suprascapular nerve /sōō'prəskap'yələr/ [L, *supra + scapulae,* shoulder blades], one of a pair of branches from the cords of the brachial plexus.

suprasellar /-sel′ər/, above the sella tur-cica.

supraspinal /-spī′nəl/ [L, *supra,* above, *spina,* backbone], pertaining to an area above the spine.

supraspinal ligament [L, *supra* + *spina,* backbone], the ligament that connects the apices of the spinous processes from the seventh cervical vertebra to the sacrum.

supraspinatus syndrome /-spīnā′təs/, pain and tenderness involving the supraspinatus tendon of the arm, restricting abduction of the shoulder.

supraspinous fossa /-spī′nəs/ [L, *supra,* above, *spina,* backbone, *fossa,* ditch], a depressed area on the dorsal surface of the scapula, above the spine.

suprasternal /-stur′nəl/, pertaining to a location above the sternum, adjacent to the neck.

supratentorial /-tentôr′ē-əl/ [L, *supra,* above, *tentorium,* tent], pertaining to a location above a tentorium.

supravaginal hysterectomy /-vaj′inəl/ [L, *supra,* above, *vagina,* sheath; Gk, *hystera,* womb, *ektome,* excision], a subtotal hysterectomy in which the body of the uterus is removed but the cervix remains.

supraventricular tachycardia (SVT) /-ventrik′yələr/ [L, *supra* + *ventriculus,* little belly], any cardiac rhythm exceeding 100 beats/min that originates above the branching part of the His bundle, that is, in the sinoatrial node, atria, or atrioventricular junction.

suprofen /səprō′fən/, an oral nonsteroidal antiinflammatory analgesic used in the treatment of mild to moderate pain and primary dysmenorrhea.

sural region /sŏŏ′rəl/ [L, *sura,* calf of the leg], the calf of the leg. It is formed by the bellies of the gastrocnemius and soleus muscles.

suramin sodium /sŏŏ′rəmin/, an antilysosomal and an antifilarial available from the Centers for Disease Control and Prevention.

surcharge, (in the United States) an additional fee charged to health plan enrollees for benefits not provided in the health plan contract.

surface anatomy /sur′fəs/ [L, *superficies,* surface], the study of the structural relationships of the external features of the body to the internal organs and parts.

surface area (SA), the total area exposed to the outside environment. The surface area of an object increases with the square of its linear dimensions; volume increases as the cube of the object's linear dimensions.

surface biopsy, the removal of living tissue for microscopic examination by scraping the surface of a lesion.

surface tension, the tendency of a liquid to minimize the area of its surface by contracting. This property causes liquids to rise in a capillary tube, affects the exchange of gases in the pulmonary alveoli, and alters the ability of various liquids to wet another surface.

surface therapy, a form of radiotherapy administered by placing one or more radioactive sources on or near an area of body surface.

surface thermometer, a device that detects and indicates the surface temperature of any part of the body.

surfactant /sərfak′tənt/ [L, *superficies*], **1.** an agent such as soap or detergent dissolved in water to reduce its surface tension or the tension at the interface between the water and another liquid. **2.** certain lipoproteins that reduce the surface tension of pulmonary fluids, allowing the exchange of gases in the alveoli of the lungs and contributing to the elasticity of pulmonary tissue.

surfer's nodules [ME, *suffe,* rush; L, *nodus,* knot], nodules on the skin of the knees, ankles, feet, or toes of a surfer caused by repeated contact of the skin with an abrasive, sandy surfboard.

surgeon /sur′jən/, a physician who treats injuries, deformities, and diseases by operative methods.

Surgeon General, (in the United States) the chief medical officer of the Army, Navy, Air Force, and Public Health Service. In other countries the title may indicate any physician with the rank of general.

surgeon's assistant (SA) /sur′jənz/ [Gk, *cheirourgos,* surgeon; L, *assistere,* to cause to stand], a medical professional trained to assist during surgery and in the preoperative and postoperative periods under the supervision of a licensed physician qualified to practice surgery.

surgery /sur′jərē/ [Gk, *cheirourgia*], the branch of medicine concerned with diseases and trauma requiring operative procedures. **—surgical,** *adj.*

surgical /sur′jikəl/ [Gk, *cheirourgia*], pertaining to the treatment of disease by manipulative and operative methods.

surgical anatomy, (in applied anatomy) the study of the structure and morphologic characteristics of the tissues and organs of the body as they relate to surgery.

Surgical Assistance, a Nursing Interventions Classification defined as assisting the surgeon/dentist with operative procedures and care of the surgical patient.

surgical fever [Gk, *cheirourgia* + L, *febris*], a fever that develops after surgery. As a result of modern aseptic techniques, fever is unlikely to accompany an operation.

surgical ligature, the exposure of an unerupted tooth by placing a metal ligature around its cervix.

surgical menopause [Gk, *cheirourgia* + L, *men,* month; Gk, *pauein,* to cease], the creation of a menopausal state by surgical termination of menstrual function.

surgical neck of humerus [Gk, *cheirourgia* + AS, *hnecca* + L, *humerus,* shoulder], the shaft of the humerus distal to the tuberosities. It is a region particularly vulnerable to fracture and surgical correction.

surgical pathology, the study of disease by the analysis of tissue specimens obtained during surgery. The surgical pathologist often examines specimens during surgery to determine how the operation should be modified or completed. Various techniques are used. The appearance of the specimen is first noted; then slices of the tissue are prepared by the paraffin or frozen section method and microscopically examined.

Surgical Precautions, a Nursing Interventions Classification defined as minimizing the potential for iatrogenic injury to the patient related to a surgical procedure.

Surgical Preparation, a Nursing Interventions Classification defined as providing care to a patient immediately before surgery, verifying required procedures/ tests, and documenting the information in the clinical record.

surgical scrub, 1. a bactericidal soap or solution used by surgeons and surgical nurses before performing or assisting in surgery. 2. the act of washing the fingernails, hands, and forearms.

surgical sectioning, an oral surgery procedure for dividing a tooth to facilitate its removal.

surgical shock [Gk, *cheirourgia* + Fr, *choc*], a condition of shock that may follow surgery, with signs of low blood volume, failure of peripheral circulation, sweating, thirst, restlessness, and cyanosis of the extremities.

surgical suite, a group of one or more operating rooms and adjunct facilities, such as a sterile storage area, scrub room, and recovery room.

surgical technician, an allied health professional who prepares the operating room by selecting and opening sterile supplies; assembles, adjusts, and checks nonsterile equipment to ensure it is in good working order; and operates sterilizers, lights, suction machines, electrosurgical units, and diagnostic equipment. Surgical technicians have primary responsibility for maintaining the sterile field.

surrogate /sur′əgāt/ [L, *surrogare,* to substitute], 1. a substitute; a person or thing that replaces another. 2. a person who represents and acts as a parent, taking the place of the father or mother. 3. (in psychoanalysis) a substitute parental figure, a symbolic image or representation of another, as may occur in a dream.

surrogate parenting, a form of artificial insemination in which a fertile woman who is not the wife of the sperm donor agrees to be impregnated by him and to carry the child to term, at which time the offspring is surrendered to the care of the infertile wife. The surrogate mother usually receives a fee for bearing the child.

surveillance /sərvā′ləns/ [Fr, *surveiller,* to watch over], 1. supervising or observing a patient or a health condition. 2. a detailed examination or investigation for the accurate collection of data to record changes in the character of a population as at a particular time or, in a prospective or longitudinal surveillance, over a period.

Surveillance, a Nursing Interventions Classification defined as purposeful and ongoing acquisition, interpretation, and synthesis of patient data for clinical decision making.

Surveillance: Late Pregnancy, a Nursing Interventions Classification defined as purposeful and ongoing acquisition, interpretation, and synthesis of maternal-fetal data for treatment, observation, or admission.

Surveillance: Safety, a Nursing Interventions Classification defined as purposeful and ongoing collection and analysis of information about the patient and the environment for use in promoting and maintaining patient safety.

surveyed height of contour /sərvād′/ [OFr, *surveir,* to survey; AS, *heah,* high; It, *contornare,* to surround], a line, scribed or marked on a cast, that designates the greatest convexity relative to a selected path of denture placement and removal.

survival curve /sərvī′vəl/ [Fr, *survivre,* to survive; L, *curvus,* bent], a curve obtained by plotting the number or percentage of organisms surviving at different intervals against doses of radiation.

survivor guilt /sərvī′vər/ [OFr, *survivre* + ME, *gilt,* sin], feelings of guilt for surviving a tragedy in which others died. In some cases the person may believe the tragedy occurred because he or she did something bad; in others the person may feel guilty for not taking proper steps to avert the tragedy.

susceptibility /səsep'tibil'itē/ [L, *suscipere,* to undertake], the condition of being vulnerable to a disease or disorder.

susceptible /səsep'tibəl/ [L, *suscipere,* to undertake], being predisposed, liable, or sensitive to effects of an infectious disease, allergen, or other pathogenic agent; lacking immunity or resistance.

suspension /səspen'shən/ [L, *suspendere,* to hang], **1.** a liquid in which small particles of a solid are dispersed, but not dissolved, and in which the dispersal is maintained by stirring or shaking the mixture. **2.** a treatment, used primarily in spinal disorders, consisting of suspending the patient by the chin and shoulders. **3.** a temporary cessation of pain or of a vital process.

suspension sling, a sling usually made of muslin or lightweight canvas and used primarily to provide support.

suspensory ligament /səspen'sərē/ [L, *suspendere,* to hang, *ligare,* to bind], any of a number of ligaments that help support an organ or body structure, such as the suspensory ligaments inside the eye that hold the lens in tension.

sustenance /sus'tənəns/ [L, *sustenare,* to sustain], **1.** the act or process of supporting or maintaining life or health. **2.** the food or nutrients essential for maintaining life.

Sustenance Support, a Nursing Interventions Classification defined as helping a needy individual/family to locate food, clothing, or shelter.

susto /soōs'tō/, a culture-bound syndrome found in Central American populations. It is related to stress engendered by a self-perceived failure to fulfill sex-role expectations.

sutilains /soō'tilänz/, a proteolytic enzyme prescribed for debridement of certain wounds, ulcers, and second-and-third-degree burns.

sutura /soōchoō'rə/, *pl.* **suturae** [L, suture], an immovable fibrous joint in which certain bones of the skull are connected by a thin layer of fibrous tissue.

sutura dentata, an immovable fibrous joint that is one kind of true suture in which toothlike processes interlock along the margins of connecting bones of the skull.

sutura limbosa, an immovable fibrous joint that is one kind of true suture in which beveled and serrated edges of certain connecting bones of the skull such as the parietal and temporal bones overlap and interlock.

sutura plana, a fibrous joint that is one

kind of false suture in which rough contiguous edges of certain bones of the skull such as the maxillae form a connection.

sutura serrata, an immovable fibrous joint that is one kind of true suture in which connecting bones interlock along serrated edges that resemble fine-toothed saws.

sutura squamosa, an immovable fibrous joint that is one kind of false suture in which overlapping beveled edges unite certain bones of the skull, such as the temporal and parietal bone.

suture /soō'chər/ [L, *sutura*], **1.** a border or a joint, such as between the bones of the cranium. **2.** to stitch together cut or torn edges of tissue with suture material. **3.** a surgical stitch taken to repair an incision, tear, or wound. **4.** material used for surgical stitches, such as absorbable or nonabsorbable silk, catgut, wire, or synthetic material.

Suturing, a Nursing Interventions Classification defined as approximating edges of a wound using sterile suture material and a needle.

Sv, abbreviation for **sievert.**

SV40, abbreviation for **simian virus 40.**

SvO₂, symbol for the percentage of oxygen saturation of mixed venous blood.

SVR, abbreviation for **systemic vascular resistance.**

swab /swob/ [D, *swabber,* ship's drudge], a stick or clamp for holding absorbent gauze or cotton, used for washing, cleansing, or drying a body surface; for collecting a specimen for laboratory examination; or for applying a topical medication.

swaddling /swod'ling/ [OE, *swethel,* swaddling band], **1.** long narrow bands of cloth once used to wrap a newborn. **2.** a method of wrapping a newborn, especially a premature or at risk newborn, that provides maximal comfort.

Swain, Mary Ann P. See **Modeling and Role Modeling.**

swallowing /swol'ō·ing/ [AS, *swelgan*], the process that usually involves movement of food from the mouth to the stomach via the esophagus. Coordination of muscles is needed from the tongue to the esophageal sphincter.

swallowing, impaired, a NANDA-accepted nursing diagnosis of the state in which an individual has decreased ability to pass fluids and/or solids from the mouth to the stomach voluntarily. The major defining characteristic is observed evidence of difficulty in swallowing, such as stasis of food in the oral cavity, coughing, or choking. Evidence of aspiration is a minor defining characteristic.

swallowing reflex [AS, *swelgan* + L,

reflectere, to bend back], a sequence of reflexes that begins when a bolus of food is manipulated by the tongue and other oral cavity muscles to the palate or the pharynx.

Swallowing Therapy, a Nursing Interventions Classification defined as facilitating swallowing and preventing complications of impaired swallowing.

Swan-Ganz catheter /swän′ganz′/ [Harold J. C. Swan, American physician, b. 1922; William Ganz, American cardiologist, b. 1919; Gk, *katheter,* something lowered], a long thin cardiac catheter with a tiny balloon at the tip.

swan neck deformity /swän/ [D, *zwaan* + AS, *hnecca,* neck; L, *deformis,* misshapen], **1.** an abnormal condition of the finger characterized by flexion of the distal interphalangeal joint and hyperextension of the proximal interphalangeal joint. The condition is seen most often in rheumatoid arthritis. **2.** a structural abnormality of the kidney tubules associated with rickets. The kidney tubule connecting the glomerulus with the convoluted part of the tubule is narrowed into a configuration referred to as "swan neck."

S wave, the negative component of the QRS complex on the electrocardiogram after an R wave.

sway, to rock, teeter, wobble, or swing back and forth.

sweat bath, a bath given to induce sweating.

sweat test, a method for evaluating sodium and chloride excretion from the sweat glands, often the first test performed in the diagnosis of cystic fibrosis. The sweat glands are stimulated with a drug such as pilocarpine, and the perspiration produced is analyzed. The eccrine glands of patients with cystic fibrosis produce sodium and chloride concentrations that are three to six times normal.

Swedish massage /swē′dish/ [Fr, *masser*], a regimen of massage combined with physical exercises.

sweep tapping, a proprioceptive-tactile treatment technique in which the clinician uses a light-touch sweep pattern over the back of the fingers of one of the hands. The stimulus is applied quickly over a dermatomal area, helping the patient to contract the muscle.

Sweet localization method, a radiographic technique for locating a foreign body in the eye by making two radiographic films of the eye while the patient's head is immobilized. A small metal ball and a cone are placed at precise distances from the center of the cornea as register marks while lateral and perpendicular radiographic views of the eye are made. A three-dimensional view of the eye is constructed from the two films, and, guided by the positions of the ball and cone, the location of the foreign body in the eye is plotted from the intersection of lines through the ball and cone.

swimmer's ear [AS, *swimman,* to swim, *eare*], *informal.* otitis externa resulting from infection transmitted in the water of a swimming pool.

swimmer's itch, an allergic dermatitis caused by sensitivity to schistosome cercariae that die under the skin, leading to erythema, urticaria, and a papular rash lasting 1 or 2 days.

swimming reflex, a primitive fetal activity, marked by well-coordinated movements, that is exhibited when the infant's face is placed in water. It normally disappears at 6 months of age.

swing phase of gait [AS, *swingan* + Gk, *phasis,* appearance; ME, *gata,* a way], one of the two phases in the rhythmic process of walking. The swing phase of gait follows the stance phase and is divided into the initial swing, the midswing, and the terminal swing stages.

switch sites, points on a chromosome where gene segments unite during segment rearrangement, as in the production of immunoglobulins.

swoon [OE, *geswogen,* unconscious], a fainting spell.

sycosis barbae /sikō′sis/ [Gk, *sycon,* fig, *osis,* condition; L, *barba,* beard], an inflammation of hair follicles of skin that has been shaved.

Sydenham's chorea /sid′ənhamz/ [Thomas Sydenham, English physician, 1624–1689; Gk, *choreia,* dance], a form of chorea associated with rheumatic fever, usually occurring during childhood. The cause is a streptococcal infection of the vascular and perivascular tissues of the brain. The choreic movements increase over the first 2 weeks, reach a plateau, and then diminish.

sylvatic plague /silvat′ik/ [L, *sylva,* forest, *plaga,* stroke], an endemic disease of wild rodents caused by *Yersinia pestis* and transmitted to humans by the bite of an infected flea. It is found on every continent except Australia.

sylvian aqueduct /sil′vē·ən/ [Franciscus Sylvius, Dutch anatomist, 1614–1672], L, *aquaductus,* canal], a canal from the third to the fourth ventricle of the midbrain.

sylvian fissure [Franciscus Sylvius; L, *fissura,* cleft], the lateral sulcus of the cerebral hemisphere.

symbiosis /sim′bē·ō′sis/ [Gk, *syn,* together,

bios, life], **1.** (in biology) a mode of living characterized by close association between organisms of different species, usually in a mutually beneficial relationship. **2.** (in psychiatry) a state in which two mentally disturbed people are emotionally dependent on each other. **3.** pathologic inability of a child to separate from its mother emotionally and sometimes physically.

symbiotic /sim'bē·ot'ik/ [Gk, *syn,* together, *bios,* life], characterized by or concerned with symbiosis or living together.

symbiotic phase, in Mahler's system of preoedipal development, the stage between 1 and 5 months when the infant participates in a "symbiotic orbit" with the mother.

symbol /sim'bəl/ [Gk, *symbolon,* sign], **1.** an image, object, action, or other stimulus that represents something else by reason of conscious association, convention, or another relationship. **2.** an object, mode of behavior, or feeling that disguises a repressed emotional conflict through an unconscious association rather than through an objective relationship, as in dreams and anxiety.

symbolism /sim'bəlizəm/, **1.** the representation or evocation of one idea, action, or object by the use of another, as in systems of writing, poetic language, or dream metaphor. **2.** (in psychiatry) an unconscious mental mechanism characteristic of all human thinking in which a mental image stands for but disguises some other object, person, or thought.

symmelia /simē'lyə/ [Gk, *syn,* together, *melos,* limb], a fetal anomaly characterized by the fusion of the lower limbs with or without feet.

symmelus /sim'ələs/, a malformed fetus characterized by symmelia.

symmetric /simet'rik/ [Gk, *syn* + *metron,* measure], (of the body or parts of the body) pertaining to equality in size or shape; very similar in relative placement or arrangement about an axis. —**symmetry,** *n.*

symmetric orientation, (in neonatal care) midline positioning of the head with similar alignment of the trunk and extremities. The orientation helps promote even development of tone and function in both sides of the body.

symmetric tonic neck reflex, a normal response in infants to assume the crawl position by extending the arms and bending the knees when the head and neck are extended.

symmetry /sim'ətrē/ [Gk, *syn,* together, *metron,* measure], (in anatomy) the correspondence of parts on opposite sides of the body, or equality of parts on both sides of a dividing line.

sympathectomize /sim'pəthek'təmiz/ [Gk, *sympathein,* to feel with, *ektome,* excision], to interrupt the conduction of nerve impulses along part of the sympathetic trunk by surgery or drugs.

sympathectomy /sim'pəthek'təmē/ [Gk, *sympathein,* to feel with, *ektome,* excision], a surgical interruption of part of the sympathetic nerve pathways. It is performed for the relief of chronic pain or the promotion of vasodilation in vascular diseases such as arteriosclerosis, claudication, Buerger's disease, and Raynaud's phenomenon. The sheath around an artery carries the sympathetic nerve fibers that control constriction of the vessel. Removal of the sheath causes the vessel to relax and expand and allows more blood to pass through it.

sympathetic /sim'pəthet'ik/ [Gk, *sympathein,* to feel with], **1.** displaying of compassion for another's grief. **2.** pertaining to a division of the autonomic nervous system.

sympathetic ganglion [Gk, *sympathein,* to feel with, *gagglion,* knot], a collection of multipolar nerve cells along the course of the sympathetic trunk. Nearly two dozen of the ganglia serve as "cell stations" on efferent pathways between the cervical and sacral parts of the sympathetic trunk.

sympathetic imbalance [Gk, *sympathein,* to feel with; L, *in* + *balance*], pertaining to vagotonia, or vagus nerve tension, and hyperexcitability of the parasympathetic nervous system, as opposed to the sympathetic nervous system.

sympathetic irritation [Gk, *sympathein,* to feel with; L, *irritare,* to tease], inflammation of one organ after inflammation of a related organ, such as when trauma to an eye is followed by similar symptoms in the uninjured eye.

sympathetic nerve [Gk, *sympathein,* to feel with; L, *nervus*], any nerve of the sympathetic branch of the autonomic nervous system.

sympathetic ophthalmia, a granulomatous inflammation of the uveal tract of both eyes occurring after an injury to the uveal tract of one eye.

sympathetic pain, distress that occurs in the hemiplegic shoulder as a result of muscle imbalance, with a loss of joint range. It results from loss of active and passive motion, loss of ability to bear weight, and long-standing subluxation without support.

sympathetic symptom [Gk, *sympathein,* to feel with, *symptoma,* that which occurs],

S

a symptom occurring in one body area when the causative lesion is actually in another area.

sympathetic trunk, one of a pair of chains of ganglia extending along the side of the vertebral column from the base of the skull to the coccyx. Each trunk is part of the sympathetic nervous system and consists of a series of ganglia connected by various types of fibers. Each sympathetic trunk distributes branches with postganglionic fibers to the autonomic plexuses, the cranial nerves, the individual organs, the nerves accompanying arteries, and the spinal nerves.

sympathizing eye /sim'pəthī'zing/, (in sympathetic ophthalmia) the uninfected eye that becomes infected by lymphatic or blood-borne metastasis of the microorganism.

sympathomimetic /sim'pəthō'mimet'ik/ [Gk, *sympathein* + *mimesis,* imitation], denoting a pharmacologic agent that mimics the effects of stimulation of organs and structures by the sympathetic nervous system. It functions by occupying adrenergic receptor sites and acting as an agonist or by increasing the release of the neurotransmitter norepinephrine at postganglionic nerve endings. Various sympathomimetic agents are used as decongestants of nasal and ocular mucosa, such as bronchodilators in the treatment of asthma, bronchitis, bronchiectasis, and emphysema and vasopressors and cardiac stimulants in the treatment of acute hypotension and shock.

sympathomimetic bronchodilator, a medication that reduces bronchial muscle spasm through action that mimics the sympathetic nervous system in producing smooth muscle relaxation.

sympathy /sim'pəthē/ [Gk, *sympathein*], **1.** an expressed interest or concern regarding the problems, emotions, or states of mind of another. **2.** the relation that exists between the mind and body, causing the one to be affected by the other. **3.** mental contagion or the influence exerted by one individual or group on another and the effects produced, such as the spread of panic, uncontrollable laughter, or yawning. **4.** the physiologic or pathologic relationship between two organs, systems, or parts of the body. —**sympathetic,** *adj.,* **sympathize,** *v.*

symphalangia /sim'falan'jē·ə/ [Gk, *syn,* together, *phalanx,* finger], **1.** a condition, usually inherited, characterized by ankylosis of the fingers or toes. **2.** a congenital anomaly in which webbing of the fingers or toes occurs in varying degrees.

symphocephalus /sim'fōsef'ələs/ [Gk, *symphes,* growing together, *kephale,* head], twin fetuses joined at the head.

symphyseal angle /simfiz'ē·əl/ [Gk, *symphysis,* growing together; L, *angulus,* corner], (in dentistry) the angle of the chin, which may be protruding, straight, or receding, according to type.

symphysic teratism /simfiz'ik/, a congenital anomaly in which there is a fusion of normally separated parts or organs, such as a horseshoe kidney.

symphysis /sim'fəsis/, *pl.* **symphyses** [Gk, growing together], **1.** a line of union, especially a cartilaginous joint in which adjacent bony surfaces are firmly united by fibrocartilage. **2.** *informal.* symphysis pubis. —**symphysic,** *adj.*

symphysis menti, **1.** the junction between the two halves of the mandible. **2.** the prominence of the chin.

sympodia /simpō'dē·ə/ [Gk, *syn,* together, *pous,* foot], a congenital developmental anomaly characterized by fusion of the lower extremities.

symptom /simp'təm/ [Gk, *symptoma,* that which happens], a subjective indication of a disease or a change in condition as perceived by the patient. Many symptoms are accompanied by objective signs such as pruritus, which is often reported with erythema and a maculopapular eruption on the skin. Some symptoms may be objectively confirmed, such as numbness of a body part, which may be confirmed by absence of response to a pin prick. Primary symptoms are symptoms that are intrinsically associated with a disease. Secondary symptoms are a consequence of illness and disease.

symptomatic /simp'təmat'ik/ [Gk, *symptoma,* that which happens], having characteristics of a symptom or indications of a specific disease.

symptomatic esophageal peristalsis, a condition in which peristaltic progression in the body of the esophagus is normal but contractions in the distal esophagus are increased in amplitude and duration.

symptomatic impotence [Gk, *symptoma,* that which happens; L, *in* + *potentia,* power], impotence that is the result of poor health or the use of medications.

symptomatic nanism, dwarfism associated with defects in bone growth, tooth formation, and sexual development.

symptomatic neuralgia [Gk, *symptoma,* that which happens, *neuron,* nerve, *algos,* pain], nerve pain that is secondary to a disease condition.

symptomatic torticollis [Gk, *symptoma* +

L, *tortus,* twisted, *collum,* neck], stiff neck caused by a disease in the neck, such as rheumatoid torticollis or myogenic torticollis.

symptomatology /simp'təmətol'əjē/ [Gk, *symptoma + logos,* science], the science of symptoms of disease in general or of the symptoms of a specific disease.

symptom-bearer, (in psychology) a family member frequently seen as the patient who is functioning poorly because family dynamics interferes with functioning at a higher level.

symptothermal method of family planning /simp'təthur'məl/ [Gk, *symptoma + therme,* heat], a natural method of family planning that incorporates the ovulation and basal body temperature methods of family planning.

sympus /sim'pəs/ [Gk, *syn,* together, *pous,* foot], a malformed fetus in which the lower extremities are completely fused or rotated and the pelvis and genitalia are defective.

sympus dipus /dē'pəs/, a malformed fetus in which the lower extremities are fused and both feet are formed.

sympus monopus /mon'əpəs/, a malformed fetus in which the lower extremities are fused and one foot is formed.

synactive model of infant behavior /sinak'tiv/, a major theoretic framework for establishing physiologic stability as the foundation for the organization of motor, behavioral state, and attentive/interactive behaviors in neonates.

synadelphus /sin'ədel'fəs/, *pl.* **synadelphi** [Gk, *syn + adelphos,* brother], a conjoined twin fetal monster with a single head and trunk and eight limbs.

Synanon, a residential center that provides a therapeutic community approach to rehabilitation of drug abusers.

synapse /sin'aps, sinaps'/ [Gk, *synaptein,* to join], **1.** the region surrounding the point of contact between two neurons or between a neuron and an effector organ, across which nerve impulses are transmitted through the action of a neurotransmitter such as acetylcholine or norepinephrine. Synapses are polarized so that nerve impulses normally travel in only one direction; they are also subject to fatigue, oxygen deficiency, anesthetics, and other chemical agents. **2.** to form a synapse or connection between neurons. **3.** (in genetics) to form a synaptic fusion between homologous chromosomes during meiosis. **—synaptic,** *adj.*

synapsis /sinap'sis/, *pl.* **synapses,** the pairing of homologous chromosomes during the early meiotic prophase stage in gametogenesis to form double or bivalent chromosomes.

synaptic /sinap'tik/ [Gk, *synaptein,* to join], pertaining to or resembling a synapse.

synaptic cleft, the microscopic extracellular space at the synapse that separates the membrane of the terminal nerve endings of a presynaptic neuron and the membrane of a postsynaptic cell.

synaptic junction, the membranes of both the presynaptic neuron and the postsynaptic receptor cell together with the synaptic cleft.

synaptic transmission, the passage of a neural impulse across a synapse from one nerve fiber to another by means of a neurotransmitter.

synaptogenesis /sinap'tōjen'əsis/, the formation of synapses between neurons. In humans it begins early in gestation but occurs most rapidly from 2 months before birth to 2 years after birth.

synaptosome /sinap'təsōm'/, a presynaptic nerve terminal that has been separated from the rest of the neuron and isolated from homogenates of brain tissue. It appears as a membrane-bound structure containing synaptic vesicles.

synarthrosis, any of several immovable articulations.

syncephalus /sinsef'ələs/ [Gk, *syn + kephale,* head], a conjoined twin monster having a single head and two bodies.

synchilia /singkē'lyə/ /singkē'lē-ə/ [Gk, *syn + cheilos,* lip], a congenital anomaly in which there is complete or partial fusion of the lips; atresia of the mouth.

synchondrosis /sing'kondrō'sis/, *pl.* **synchondroses** [Gk, *syn + chondros,* cartilage], a cartilaginous joint between two immovable bones, such as the synchondroses of the cranium.

synchorial /singkôr'ē·əl/ [Gk, *syn + chorion,* skin], pertaining to multiple fetuses that share a common placenta, as in monozygosity.

synchronized intermittent mandatory ventilation (SIMV) /sing'krənīzd/, periodic assisted mechanical breaths occurring at preset intervals. The patient makes an inspiratory effort sensed by the ventilator that results in ventilation. Spontaneous breathing by the patient occurs between the assisted mechanical breaths.

synchronous /sing'krənəs/, occurring at the same time.

synclitism /sing'klitiz'əm/ [Gk, *syn + klinein,* to lean], **1.** (in obstetrics) a condition in which the sagittal suture of the fetal head is in line with the transverse diameter of the inlet, equidistant from the maternal

S

symphysis pubis and sacrum. **2.** (in hematology) the normal condition in which the nucleus and the cytoplasm of the blood cells mature simultaneously and at the same rate.

syncope /sing'kəpē/ [Gk, *synkoptein*, to cut short], a brief lapse in consciousness caused by transient cerebral hypoxia. It is usually preceded by a sensation of light-headedness and often may be prevented by lying down or sitting with the head between the knees.

syncretic thinking /singkret'ik/ [Gk, *synkretismos*, combined beliefs; AS, *thencan*, to think], a stage in the development of the cognitive thought processes of the child. During this phase thought is based purely on what is perceived and experienced. The child is incapable of reasoning beyond the observable or of making deductions or generalizations. —**syncresis,** *n.*

syncytial /sinsish'əl/, pertaining to a syncytium.

syncytial virus a virus that induces the formation of syncytia, particularly in cell cultures. Syncytial viruses are members of the Spumavirinae subfamily of Retroviridae.

syncytiotrophoblast /sinsish'ē·ōtrof'ə-blast'/ [Gk, *syn* + *kytos*, cell, *trophe*, nutrition, *blastos*, germ], the outer syncytial layer of the trophoblast of the early mammalian embryo that erodes the uterine wall during implantation and gives rise to the villi of the placenta. —**syncytiotrophoblastic,** *adj.*

syncytium /sinsit'ē·əm/, *pl.* **syncytia** [Gk, *syn* + *kytos*, cell], a group of cells in which the protoplasm of one cell is continuous with that of adjoining cells.

syndactylus /sindak'tiləs/, a person with webbed fingers or toes.

syndactyly /sindak'təlē/ [Gk, *syn* + *daktylos*, finger], a congenital anomaly characterized by the fusion of the fingers or toes. —**syndactyl, syndactylous,** *adj.*

syndesis /sin'dəsis/ [Gk, *syn*, together, *dein*, to bind], surgical fixation of a joint.

syndesmophyte /sindez'məfīt/, an osseous excrescence or bony growth attached to a ligament. It is found between adjacent vertebrae in ankylosing spondylitis.

syndesmosis /sin'desmō'sis/, *pl.* **syndesmoses** [Gk, *syndesmos*, ligament], a fibrous articulation in which two bones are connected by interosseous ligaments, such as the anterior and the posterior ligaments in the radioulnar and tibiofibular articulations.

syndrome /sin'drəm/ [Gk, *syn*, together, *dromos*, course], a complex of signs and symptoms resulting from a common cause or appearing in combination to present a clinical picture of a disease or inherited abnormality.

syndrome of inappropriate antidiuretic hormone secretion (SIADH), an abnormal condition characterized by the excessive release of antidiuretic hormone that alters the body's fluid and electrolytic balances. It results from various malfunctions, such as the inability to produce and secrete dilute urine, water retention, increased extracellular fluid volume, and hyponatremia. SIADH develops in association with diseases that affect the osmoreceptors of the hypothalamus. Oat cell carcinoma of the lung is the most common cause. Common signs and symptoms of SIADH are weight gain despite anorexia, vomiting, nausea, muscle weakness, and irritability. In some patients SIADH may produce coma and convulsions. Most of the free water associated with this syndrome is intracellular, and associated edema is rare unless excess water volume exceeds 4 mOsm.

syndrome X, a condition characterized by hypertension with obesity, type II diabetes mellitus, hypertrigleceridemia, increased peripheral insulin resistance, hyperinsulinemia, and elevated catecholamine levels.

synechia /sinek'ē·ə/, *pl.* **synechiae** [Gk, continuity], an adhesion, especially of the iris to the cornea or lens of the eye. It may develop from glaucoma, cataracts, uveitis, or keratitis or as a complication of surgery or trauma to the eye. Synechiae prevent or impede flow of aqueous fluid between the anterior and posterior chambers of the eye and may lead rapidly to blindness.

synechiotomy /sinek'ē·ot'əmē/ [Gk, *synechia*, continuity, *temnein*, to cut], the surgical division of an adhesion.

syneresis /siner'əsis/ [Gk, *syn* + *hairein*, to draw], the drawing together or coagulation of particles of a gel with separation from the medium in which the particles were suspended, such as occurs in blood clot retraction.

synergist /sin'ərjist/ [Gk, *syn* + *ergein*, to work], an organ, agent, or substance that augments the activity of another organ, agent, or substance.

synergistic /sin'ərjis'tik/ [Gk, *syn*, together, *ergein*, to work], pertaining to the acting or working together of a number of components, as when groups of muscles function in a coordinated manner.

synergistic agent, a substance that augments or adds to the activity of another substance or agent.

synergistic muscles, groups of muscles that contract together to accomplish the same body movement.

synergy /sin′ərjē/ [Gk, *syn* + *ergein*, to work], **1.** the process in which two organs, substances, or agents work simultaneously to enhance the function and effect of one another. **2.** the coordinated action of a set of muscles that work together to produce a specific movement **3.** a combined action of different parts of the autonomic nervous system, as in the sympathetic and parasympathetic innervation of secreting cells of the salivary glands. **4.** the interaction of two or more drugs to produce a certain effect.

synesthesia /sin′esthē′zhə/, a phenomenon in which sensations of two or more modalities accompany one another, as when a visual sensation is experienced when a particular sound is heard.

syngeneic /sin′jənē′ik/ [Gk, *syn* + *genesis,* origin], **1.** (in genetics) denoting an individual or cell type that has the same genotype as another individual or cell. **2.** (in transplantation biology) denoting tissues that are antigenically similar.

synkinesis /sin′kinē′sis/ [Gk, *syn,* together, *kinesis,* movement], an involuntary movement by one part of the body when an intentional movement is made by another part. In imitative synkinesis, movement may be detected in paralyzed muscles when normal muscles are moved, and vice versa.

synopsis /sinop′sis/ [Gk, *syn,* together, *opsis,* vision], a brief review, condensation, summary, or abridgment.

synostosis /sin′ostō′sis/ [Gk, *syn,* together, *osteon,* bone], the joining of two bones by the ossification of connecting tissues. It occurs normally in the fusion of cranial bones to form the skull.

synostotic joint /sin′ostot′ik/ [Gk, *syn* + *osteon,* bone], a joint in which bones are connected to bones and there is no movement between them, as in the bones of the adult sacrum or skull.

synotia /sīnō′shə/ [Gk, *syn* + *ous,* ear], a congenital malformation characterized by the union or approximation of the ears in front of the neck, often accompanied by the absence or defective development of the lower jaw.

synotus /sīnō′təs/, a fetus with synotia.

synovectomy /sin′ōvek′təmē/ [Gk, *syn* + L, *ovum,* egg; Gk, *ektome,* excision], the removal of a synovial membrane of a joint.

synovia /sinō′vē·ə/ [Gk, *syn* + L, *ovum*], a transparent, viscous fluid, resembling the white of an egg, secreted by synovial membranes and acting as a lubricant for

many joints, bursae, and tendons. It contains mucin, albumin, fat, and mineral salts.

synovial /sinō′vē·əl/ [Gk, *syn,* together; L, *ovum,* egg], pertaining to, consisting of, or secreting synovia, the lubricating fluid of the joints, bursae, and tendon sheaths.

synovial bursa, one of the many closed sacs filled with synovial fluid in the connective tissue between muscles, tendons, ligaments, and bones.

synovial chondroma, a rare cartilaginous growth developing in the connective tissue below the synovial membrane of the joints, tendon sheaths, or bursa.

synovial crypt, a pouch in the synovial membrane of a joint.

synovial joint, a freely movable joint in which contiguous bony surfaces are covered by articular cartilage and connected by a fibrous connective tissue capsule lined with synovial membrane.

synovial membrane, the thin layer of tissue lining the articular capsule surrounding a freely movable joint. The synovial membrane is loosely attached to the external fibrous capsule. It secretes into the joint a thick fluid that normally lubricates the joint but that may accumulate in painful amounts when the joint is injured.

synovial sac, a herniation of the synovium beyond the confines of the joint.

synovial sarcoma, a malignant tumor composed of synovioblasts that begins as a soft swelling and often metastasizes through the bloodstream to the lung before it is discovered.

synovial sheath, any one of the membranous sacs enclosing a tendon of a muscle and facilitating the gliding of a tendon through a fibrous or a bony tunnel, such as that under the flexor retinaculum of the wrist.

synovial tendon sheath, one of the many membranous channels or tubes enclosing various tendons that glide through fibrous and bony tunnels in the body, such as those under the flexor retinaculum of the wrist. One layer of the synovial sheath lines the tunnel; the other covers the tendon. The sheath secretes synovial fluid, which lubricates the tendon.

synovitis /sin′əvī′tis/ [Gk, *syn* + L, *ovum* + Gk, *itis*], an inflammatory condition of the synovial membrane of a joint as the result of an aseptic wound or a traumatic injury, such as a sprain or severe strain. The knee is most commonly affected. Fluid accumulates around the capsule; the joint is swollen, tender, and painful; and motion is restricted.

synovium /sinō′vē·əm/ [Gk, *syn,* together; L, *ovum,* egg], a synovial membrane.

S

syntactic aphasia /sintak′tik/ [Gk, *syn,* together, *taxis,* arrangement, *a, phasis,* not speech], an inability to arrange words in a logical sequence, with the result that what is spoken is not understood.

syntax /sin′taks/ [Gk, *syn + taxis,* arrangement], a property of language involving structural cues for the arrangement of words as elements in a phrase, clause, or sentence.

syntaxic mode /sintaks′ik/, the ability to perceive whole, logical, coherent pictures as they occur in reality, according to the H. S. Sullivan theory of psychology.

synteny /sin′tənē/ [Gk, *syn + taina,* ribbon], (in genetics) the presence on the same chromosome of two or more genes that may or may not be transmitted as a linkage group but that appear to be able to undergo independent assortment during meiosis.

synthermal /sinthur′məl/, possessing the same temperature.

synthesis /sin′thəsis/ [Gk, *synthenai,* to put together], a level of cognitive learning in which the individual puts together the elements of previous learning levels to create a unified whole.

synthesize /sin′thəsīz/ [Gk, *synthesis,* putting together], to form by building, as in forming complex chemical compounds such as proteins from simpler units of amino acids.

synthetic /sinthet′ik/, pertaining to a substance that is produced by an artificial rather than a natural process or material.

synthetic chemistry, the science dealing with the formation of more complex chemical compounds from simpler substances.

synthetic human growth hormone, a synthetic form of somatotropin produced by recombinant deoxyribonucleic acid techniques from a strain of *Escherichia coli* bacteria. The polypeptide hormone consists of 191 amino acid residues in a sequence identical to that of natural human growth hormone.

synthetic insulin [Gk, *synthesis,* putting together; L, *insula,* island], a form of insulin synthesized in a nondisease-producing strain of *Escherichia coli* bacteria or in yeast cells that has been genetically altered by the addition of the human gene for insulin production.

synthetic vaccines, prophylactic immunization substances prepared by artificial techniques, such as through peptide synthesis or cloning of deoxyribonucleic acid.

syntrophism /sin′trafiz′əm/, **1.** mutual dependence for food or other resources. **2.** a condition in which two strains of bacteria can grow together in a mixed culture in a medium that would not support either alone; each strain produces a nutrient required by the other.

syntropy /sin′trəpē/ [Gk, *syn,* together, *trepein,* to turn] a tendency for two diseases to merge into one.

syphilis /sif′ilis/ [from the name of a literary figure (1530) who was thus infected (literally, L, lover of swine)], a sexually transmitted disease caused by the spirochete *Treponema pallidum,* characterized by distinct stages of effects over a period of years. Any organ system may become involved. The spirochete is able to pass through the human placenta, producing congenital syphilis. The first stage (primary syphilis) is marked by the appearance of a small painless red pustule on the skin or mucous membrane between 10 and 90 days after exposure. The lesion may appear anywhere on the body where contact with a lesion on an infected person has occurred, but it is seen most often in the anogenital region. It quickly erodes, forming a painless, bloodless ulcer, called a *chancre,* exuding a fluid that swarms with spirochetes. It heals spontaneously within 10 to 40 days, often creating the mistaken impression that it was not a serious symptom. The second stage (secondary syphilis) occurs about 2 months later, after the spirochetes have increased in number and spread throughout the body. This stage is characterized by general malaise, anorexia, nausea, fever, headache, alopecia, bone and joint pain, or the appearance of a morbilliform rash that does not itch, flat white sores in the mouth and throat, or condylomata lata papules on the moist areas of the skin. The disease remains highly contagious at this stage and can be spread by kissing. The third stage (tertiary syphilis) is characterized by the appearance of soft rubbery tumors, called *gummas,* that ulcerate and heal by scarring. Gummas may develop anywhere on the surface of the body and in the eye, liver, lungs, stomach, or reproductive organs. Tertiary syphilis may be painless, or it may be accompanied by deep, burrowing pain. Various tissues and structures of the body, including the central nervous system, myocardium, and valves of the heart, may be damaged or destroyed, leading to mental or physical disability and premature death. **Congenital syphilis** resulting from prenatal infection may result in the birth of a deformed or blind infant. In some cases the infant appears to be well until, at several weeks of age, snuffles, sometimes with a blood-stained or mucopurulent discharge, and skin lesions, particularly on the palms and soles or in the genital region, are observed. Such children also may have visual or hearing defects, and progeria and poor health may develop.

syphilitic /sif'ilit'ik/, pertaining to, resembling, or infected with syphilis.

syphilitic aortitis, an inflammatory condition of the aorta, occurring in tertiary syphilis. It is characterized by diffuse dilation with gray wheallike plaques containing calcium on the inner coat and scars and wrinkles on the outer coat of the aorta. The middle layer of the vascular wall is usually infiltrated with plasma cells and contains fragments of damaged elastic tissue and many newly formed blood vessels. There may be damage to the cardiac valves, narrowing of the mouths of the coronary arteries, and formation of thrombi. Cerebral embolism may result. Signs of syphilitic aortitis are substernal pain, dyspnea, bounding pulse, and high systolic blood pressure.

syphilitic dementia [L, *de* + *mens*, mind], a form of dementia resulting from a syphilis infection. Specific symptoms may vary from memory impairment to personality changes and are severe enough to interfere with social and occupational activities.

syphilitic endocarditis [L, *endon*, within, *kardia*, heart, *itis*, inflammation], a thickening and stretching of the cusps of the aortic valve, with aortic valve incompetence, caused by a syphilis infection of the aorta.

syphilitic fever [L, *febris*], pyrexia that is caused by a syphilis infection.

syphilitic periarteritis, an inflammatory condition of the outer coat of one or more arteries occurring in tertiary syphilis and characterized by soft gummatous perivascular lesions infiltrated with lymphocytes and plasma cells.

syphilitic retinopathy [L, *rete*, net, Gk, *pa thos*, disease], an invasion of the retina and optic nerve by a spreading syphilis infection. Primary retinal lesions are associated with the blood vessels, and the choroid layer is often affected first. There may be occlusion of the retinal vessels.

syr., abbreviation for the Latin *syrupus*, 'syrup.'

syringe /sərinj', sir'inj/ [Gk, *syrinx*, tube], a device for withdrawing, injecting, or instilling fluids. A syringe for the injection of medication usually consists of a calibrated glass or plastic cylindric barrel having a close-fitting plunger at one end and a small opening at the other to which the head of a hollow-bore needle is fitted. A syringe for irrigating a wound or body cavity or for extracting mucus or another body fluid from an orifice or body cavity is usually larger than the kind used for injection.

syringectomy /sir'injek'təmē/ [Gk, *syrinx*, tube, *ektome*, excision], a surgical procedure for excising the walls of a fistula.

syringoencephalomyelia /siring'gō·ensef'-əlōmī·ē'lyə/, a progressive disorder characterized by cavitation of the spinal cord. It may occur anywhere from the medulla oblongata to the thoracic segments but usually appears in cervical segments.

syringoma, *pl.* **syringomata** /sir'ing·gō'-mə/, a benign tumor derived from an eccrine sweat gland. It appears as a small smooth papule the color of the underlying skin, often on the upper body of a postpubertal woman. Some are typically multiple, often appearing on the lower eyelids.

syringomeningocele /-məning'gōsēl'/ [Gk, *syrinx*, tube, *meningx*, membrane, *kele*, hernia], a meningocele that is connected to the central canal of the spinal cord.

syringomyelia /-mī·ē'lyə/ [Gk, *syrinx*, tube, *myelos*, marrow], a chronic progressive disease of the spinal cord, marked by elongated central fluid-containing cavities, surrounded by gliosis or a proliferation of neurologic tissue. Symptoms begin early in adulthood, usually involving the cervical region with muscular wasting in the upper limbs.

syringomyelocele /siring'gōmī'əlōsēl'/ [Gk, *syrinx* + *myelos*, marrow, *kele*, hernia], a hernial protrusion of the spinal cord through a congenital defect in the vertebral column. The cerebrospinal fluid within the central cavities of the cord is greatly increased so that the cord tissue forms a thin-walled sac that lies close to the membrane of the cavity.

syrup of ipecac /sir'əp/, an emetic preparation of ipecac fluid extract, glycerin, and syrup used to treat certain types of poisonings and drug overdoses.

system /sis'təm/ [Gk, *systema*], a collection or assemblage of parts that, unified, make a whole. Physiologic systems such as the cardiovascular or reproductive system are made up of structures specifically able to engage in processes that are essential for a vital function in the body.

systematic /sis'təmat'ik/ [Gk, *systema*], pertaining to a system.

systematic error [Gk, *systema* + L, *errare*, to wander], a nonrandom statistical error that affects the mean of a population of data and defines the bias between the means of two populations.

systematic heating, the elevation of the temperature of the whole body.

systematic tabulation, (in research) mechanical or manual techniques for record-

S

ing and classifying data for statistical analysis.

systemic /sistem'ik/ [Gk, *systema*], pertaining to the whole body rather than to a localized area or regional part of the body.

systemic circulation [Gk, *systema* + L, *circulare*, to go around], the general blood circulation of the body, not including the lungs.

systemic desensitization, a technique used in behavior therapy for eliminating maladaptive anxiety associated with phobias. The procedure involves the construction by the person of a hierarchy of anxiety-producing stimuli and the general presentation of these stimuli until they no longer elicit the initial response of fear.

systemic heart, pertaining to the normal cardiac function of the left atrium and ventricle, which move aerated blood from the heart into the general circulatory system.

systemic immunoblastic proliferation, a condition of immature lymphocyte production resulting in rash, breathing difficulty, enlarged spleen, lymphadenopathy, and increased incidence of immunoblastic lymphoma.

systemic infection [Gk, *systema* + L, *inficere*, to stain], an infection in which the pathogen is distributed throughout the body rather than concentrated in one area.

systemic lesion [Gk, *systema* + L, *laesio*, attack], a pathologic disturbance that involves a system of tissues with a common function.

systemic lupus erythematosus (SLE), a chronic inflammatory disease affecting many systems of the body. The pathophysiologic characteristics of the disease includes severe vasculitis, renal involvement, and lesions of the skin and nervous system. The primary cause of the disease has not been determined; viral infection or dysfunction of the immune system has been suggested. Adverse reaction to certain drugs also may cause a lupuslike syndrome. Four times more women than men have SLE. The initial manifestation is often arthritis. An erythematous rash ("butterfly rash") over the nose and malar eminences, weakness, fatigue, and weight loss also are frequently seen early in the disease. Photosensitivity, fever, skin lesions on the neck, and alopecia where the skin lesions extend beyond the hairline may occur. The skin lesions may spread to the mucous membranes and other tissues of the body. They do not ulcerate but cause degeneration of the tissues affected. Depending on the organs involved, the patient also may have glomerulonephritis, pleuritis, pericarditis, peritonitis, neuritis,

or anemia. Renal failure and severe neurologic abnormalities are among the most serious manifestations of the disease.

systemic mycosis [Gks, *systema* + *mykes*, fungus, *osis* condition], a fungal infection that involves more than one body system or area.

systemic oxygen consumption, the amount of oxygen consumed by the body's tissues as measured during a period of 60 seconds.

systemic remedy, a medicinal substance that is given orally, parenterally, or rectally to be absorbed into the circulation for treatment of a health problem. Medication administered systemically may have various local effects, but the intent is to treat the whole body.

systemic sclerosis, a form of scleroderma characterized by formation of thickened collagenous fibrous tissue, thickening of the skin, and adhesion to underlying tissues. The disease, which may be preceded by Raynaud's phenomenon, progresses to involve the tissues of the heart, lungs, muscles, genitourinary tract, and kidneys.

systemic vascular resistance (SVR), the resistance against which the left ventricle must eject to force out its stroke volume with each beat. As the peripheral vessels constrict, the SVR increases.

systemic vein, one of a number of veins that drain deoxygenated blood from most of the body. Systemic veins arise in tiny plexuses that receive blood from capillaries and converge into trunks that increase in size as they pass toward the heart. They are larger and more numerous than the arteries, have thinner walls, and collapse when they are empty.

system of care /sis'təm/, a framework within which health care is provided, comprising health care professionals; recipients, consumers, or patients; energy resources or dynamics; organizational and political contexts or frameworks; and processes or procedures.

system overload, an inability to cope with messages and expectations from a number of sources within a given time limit.

systems theory, a holistic medical concept in which the human patient is viewed as an integrated complex of open systems rather than as semiindependent parts.

systole /sis'təlē/ [Gk, *systole*, contraction], the contraction of the heart, driving blood into the aorta and pulmonary arteries. The occurrence of systole is indicated by the first heart sound heard on auscultation, by the palpable apex beat, and by the peripheral pulse.

systolic /sistol′ik/ [Gk, *systole,* contraction], pertaining to or resulting from a heart contraction.

systolic click [Gk, *systole,* contraction; Fr, *cliqueter,* to click], an extra heart sound having a clicklike quality heard in mid-or late systole and believed to originate from the abnormal motion of the mitral valve. The most frequent cause of systolic clicks is prolapse of a mitral valve leaflet.

systolic dysfunction a loss of cardiac muscle with volume overload and decreased contractility.

systolic ejection period, the amount of time spent in systole per minute.

systolic gradient, the difference in pres-sure in the left atrium and left ventricle during systole.

systolic murmur, cardiac murmur occur-ring during systole. Systolic murmurs in-clude ejection murmurs often heard in pregnant women or in people with anemia, thyrotoxicosis, or aortic or pulmonary ste-nosis; pansystolic murmurs heard in people with incompetence of the mitral or tricuspid valve; and late systolic murmurs, also caused by mitral valve incompetence.

systolic pressure, the blood pressure measured during the period of ventricular contraction (systole). In blood pressure readings it is the higher of the two mea-surements.

S

t, symbol for **time.**

T, 1. symbol for **temperature.** 2. abbreviation for **tumor.**

T₁/₂, 1. symbol for half-life of radioactive isotopes. 2. symbol for half-time of radioactive isotopes.

T₃, symbol for **triiodothyronine.**

T₄, symbol for **thyroxine.**

Ta, symbol for the element **tantalum.**

TA, abbreviation for **transactional analysis.**

tabes /tā'bēz/ [L, *tabes,* wasting], a gradual, progressive wasting of the body in any chronic disease.

tabes dorsalis [L, *tabes,* wasting, *dorsum,* the back], an abnormal condition characterized by the slow degeneration of all or part of the body and the progressive loss of deep tendon reflexes. This disease involves the spinal cord and destroys the large joints of affected limbs in some individuals. A wide-base ataxic gait is usually present. It is often accompanied by incontinence, impotence, and severe flashing pains in the abdomen and extremities. The cause of tabes dorsalis is syphilitic.

tabetic crisis /tābet'ik/ [L, *tabes,* wasting; Gk, *krisis,* turning point], an exacerbation of pain in tabes dorsalis because of syphilis.

tabetic gait [L, *tabes,* wasting; ONorse, *gata,* a way], a high-steppage gait associated with the tertiary form of tabes. The condition results from degeneration of the dorsal columns of the spinal cord and of sensory nerve trunks.

tabetic neuritis [L, *tabes,* wasting; Gk, *neuron,* nerve, *itis,* inflammation], a form of neuritis that accompanies a syphilitic infection or tabes dorsalis, involving the dorsal posterior column spinal pathways.

table [L, *tabula*], **1.** any structure with a flat surface. **2.** a chart showing columns of data.

tablespoon (Tbs, tbsp), a household spoon that may be used to measure a dose of liquid medicine, equivalent to about 4 fluid drams or ½ fluid ounce or 15 ml.

tablet /tab'lit/ [Fr, *tablette,* lozenge], a small, solid dosage form of a medication. It may be of almost any size, shape, weight, and color. Most tablets are intended to be swallowed whole; but some may be dissolved in the mouth, chewed, or dissolved in liquid before swallowing; and some may be placed in a body cavity.

taboo /təbōō'/, something that is forbidden by a society as unacceptable or improper. Incest is a taboo common to many societies.

taboparesis /tā'bōpərē'sis/ [L, *tabes,* wasting; Gk, *paralyein,* to be palsied], a form of paralysis associated with cerebral syphilis.

tabula rasa /tä'bōōlä rä'sä, tab'yəle rä'sə/, a term used to describe a child's mind at birth as a receptive 'blank slate.'

tache /täsh/ [Fr], a spot, stain, blot, or mark.

tache noire /täshnô·är'/ [Fr, black spot], a local ulcerous lesion marking the point of infection in certain rickettsial diseases such as African tick typhus and scrub typhus.

tachistoscope /təkis'təskōp'/ [Gk, tachistos, rapid, *skopien,* to view], a device used to increase the speed of visual perception by displaying visual stimuli only extremely briefly.

tachometer /təkom'ətər/, a device for measuring speed, such as the rate of blood flow in a vessel.

tachyarrhythmia /tak'ē·ərith'mē·ə/ [Gk, *tachys,* fast, *a + rhythmos,* rhythm], an abnormally rapid heartbeat accompanied by an irregular rhythm.

tachycardia /tak'ēkär'dē·ə/ [Gk, *tachys,* fast, *kardia,* heart], a condition in which the myocardium contracts at a rate greater than 100 beats/min. The heart rate normally accelerates in response to fever, exercise, or nervous excitement. Pathologic tachycardia accompanies anoxia, such as caused by anemia, congestive heart failure, hemorrhage, or shock. Tachycardia acts to increase the amount of oxygen delivered to the cells of the body by increasing the amount of blood circulated through the vessels.

tachycardiac /-kär'dē·ak/ [Gk, *tachys,* fast, *kardia,* heart], pertaining to or affected by tachycardia.

tachyphagia /-fā'jē·ə/, rapid or hasty eating.

tachyphylaxis /tak'əfəlak'sis/ [Gk, *tachys*

+ *phylax,* guard], **1.** (in pharmacology) a phenomenon in which the repeated administration of some drugs results in a marked decrease in effectiveness. **2.** (in immunology) a rapidly developing immunity to a toxin because of previous exposure, such as from previous injection of small amounts of the toxin.

tachypnea /tak'epnē'ə/ [Gk, *tachys* + *pnoia,* breathing], an abnormally rapid rate of breathing (more than 20 breaths per minute), such as that seen with hyperpyrexia.

tack, the degree of stickiness of an adhesive required to affix a therapeutic foreign substance such as a transdermal delivery device to the skin.

tacrine /tak'rin/, a respiratory stimulant, cognition enhancer, and analeptic. It is also used as an anticholinesterase agent. It may have a role in early Alzheimer's disease to improve some cognitive functions. It does not affect prognosis of the disease.

tacrolimus, an immunosuppressive drug prescribed to suppress the immune system after transplantation of the liver or other organs.

tactile /tak'təl/, tak'tīl/ [L, *tactus,* touch], pertaining to the sense of touch.

tactile amnesia [L, *tactus* + Gk, *amnesia,* forgetfulness], a loss of the ability to determine the shape of objects through the sense of touch.

tactile anesthesia, the absence or lack of the sense of touch in the fingers, possibly resulting from injury or disease. This condition may cause the patient to incur severe burns, serious cuts, contusions, or abrasions.

tactile defensiveness, a sensory integrative dysfunction characterized by tactile sensations that cause excessive emotional reactions, hyperactivity, or other behavior problems.

tactile discrimination [L, *tactus* + *discrimen,* division], the ability to discriminate among objects by the sense of touch.

tactile fremitus, a tremulous vibration of the chest wall during breathing that is palpable on physical examination. It may indicate inflammation, infection, congestion, or consolidation of a lung or a part of a lung.

tactile hair [L, *tactus* + AS, *haer*], a hair shaft that is sensitive to the sensation of touch.

tactile hallucination [L, *tactus* + *alucinare,* to wander in mind], a subjective experience of touch in the absence of tactile stimulation.

tactile hyperesthesia [L, *tactus* + Gk, *hyper,* excessive, *aesthesis,* sensitivity], an abnormal increase in the sense of touch.

tactile image, a mental concept of an object as perceived through the sense of touch.

tactile localization [L, *tactus* + *locus,* place], the ability to identify, without looking, the exact point on the body where a tactile stimulus is applied. The localization test is applied in sensory evaluation tests.

tactile sensation [L, *tactus* + *sentire,* to feel], the sensation of touch.

tactile system [L, *tactus* + Gk, *systema*], the part of the nervous system that is concerned with the sense of touch.

Taenia /tē'nē-ə/ [Gk, *tainia,* ribbon], a genus of large parasitic intestinal flatworm of the family Taeniidae, class Cestoda, having an armed scolex and a series of segments in a chain. Taeniae are among the most common parasites infecting humans.

Taenia saginata, a species of tapeworm that inhabits the tissues of cattle during its larval stage and infects the intestine of humans in its adult form.

taeniasis /tēnī'əsis/ [Gk, *tainia* + *osis,* condition], an infection with a tapeworm of the genus *Taenia.*

Taenia solium, a species of tapeworm that most commonly inhabits the tissues of pigs during its larval stage and infects the intestine of humans in its adult form.

TAF, abbreviation for **tumor angiogenesis factor.**

tag, a small piece of tissue attached by one margin or a pedicle to a main structure.

TAG, abbreviation for *3,4,6-tri-O-acetyl-D-glucal.*

take, a popular term for a satisfactory response, as of a vaccination or tissue graft.

tail, the caudal extremity of an organ or body, such as an axillary tail of a mammary gland.

tail fold [AS, *taegel* + *fealdan,* to fold], a curved ridge formed at the caudal end of the early developing embryo.

tail of Spence, the upper outer tail of breast tissue that extends into the axilla.

Takayasu's arteritis /tä'kəyä'sōoz/ [Mikito Takayasu, Japanese surgeon, 1860–1938], an inflammatory disorder of the aorta, its major branches, and the pulmonary artery. It is characterized by progressive occlusion of the innominate and the left subclavian and left common carotid arteries above their origin in the aortic arch. Signs of the disorder are absence of a pulse in both arms and in the carotid arteries, transient paraplegia, transient blindness, and atrophy of facial muscles.

talbutal /tal'byōotəl/, a barbiturate sedative-hypnotic prescribed as a hypnotic in the treatment of insomnia.

talc /talk/ [Ar, *talq*], a native, hydrous magnesium silicate, sometimes containing a small proportion of aluminum silicate, used as a dusting powder and adsorbent in clarifying liquids.

talcosis /talkō′sis/, a silicosis-like respiratory disorder caused by inhalation of magnesium silicate dust.

talipes /tal′ipēz/ [L, *talus*, ankle, *pes*, foot], a deformity of the foot, usually congenital, in which the foot is twisted and relatively fixed in an abnormal position. Talipes refers to deformities that involve the foot and ankle.

tallow /tal′ō/, **1.** a hard fat obtained from the bodies of ruminant animals such as cattle and sheep and used in soaps and lubricants. **2.** a vegetable fat obtained from plants, such as the wax myrtle.

talofibular /tā′lōfib′yələr/, pertaining to the talus and fibula.

talonavicular /tā′lōnəvik′yələr/ [L, *talon*, bird claw, *naviculus*, scaphoid], pertaining to the talus and the navicular bones.

talus /tā′ləs/, *pl.* **tali** [L, ankle], the second largest tarsal bone. It supports the tibia, rests on the calcaneus, and articulates with the malleoli and navicular bones.

tambour /tam′bo͞or/, a cylindric drumlike device connected to an air tube and stylus, used to record sphygmograph or other physiologic data.

Tamm-Horsfall protein (THP) [Igor Tamm, American virologist, b. 1922; Frank L. Horsfall, American virologist, 1906–1971], a mucoprotein found in the matrix of renal tubular casts. THP is secreted in the loop of Henle.

tamoxifen /təmok′səfin/, a nonsteroidal antiestrogen used in the palliative treatment of advanced breast cancer in premenopausal and postmenopausal women whose tumors are estrogen-dependent.

tampon /tam′pon/ [Fr, plug], a packed cotton, a sponge or other material for checking bleeding or absorbing secretions in cavities or canals or for holding displaced organs in position.

tamponade /tam′pənād′/ [Fr, *tamponner*, to plug up], stoppage of the blood flow to an organ or a part of the body by pressure or by the compression of a part by an accumulation of fluid, such as in cardiac tamponade.

tangentiality /tanjen′chē·al′itē/ [L, *tangere*, to touch], expressions or responses characterized by a tendency to digress from an original topic of conversation. Tangentiality can destroy or seriously hamper the ability of people to communicate effectively.

tangible elements /tan′jibəl/ [L, *tangere* + *elementum*, first principle], objects that can be seen or touched as distinguished from emotions, knowledge, or abstractions.

Tangier disease /tanjir′/ [Tangier Island, Virginia], a rare familial deficiency of high-density lipoproteins, characterized by low blood cholesterol and an abnormal orange or yellow discoloration of the tonsils and pharynx.

tangle /tan′gəl/, a dense mass of interlacing of fibers, sometimes appearing as a loose knot, such as intraneural fibrillary tangle.

tannic acid /tan′ik/ [Celt, *tann*, oak; L, *acidus*, sour], a substance obtained from the bark and fruit of various trees and shrubs, particularly the nutgalls of oak trees. The acid is used as an astringent and protein precipitant.

tanning [Fr, *tanner*, to tan], a process in which the pigmentation of the skin deepens as a result of exposure to ultraviolet light. Skin cells containing melanin darken immediately.

tantalum (Ta) /tan′tələm/ [Gk, *Tantalus*, mythic king of Phrygia], a silvery metallic element. Its atomic number is 73; its atomic mass (weight) is 180.95. Relatively inert chemically, tantalum is used in prosthetic devices such as skull plates and wire sutures.

tantrum /tan′trəm/, a sudden outburst or violent display of rage, frustration, and bad temper, usually occurring in a maladjusted child and certain emotionally disturbed people.

tap [ME, *tappen*], **1.** to strike lightly, as in percussion or testing of reflexes. **2.** to draw off fluid through a small opening.

tape [AS, *taeppe*], a thin flat strip of tisue, a tendon, or other natural or synthetic material, which may be used as a tie or suture.

tape-compression folliculitis, inflammation of the hair follicles caused by tape dressings placed over foam or cotton-ball pads under a graduated compression stocking. The condition is more likely to occur on patients with hairy legs who may perspire during the summer months.

tapering arch /tā′pəring/ [AS, *tapor*, slender, *arcus*, bow], a dental arch that converges from the molars to the central incisors to such a degree that lines passing through the central grooves of the molars and premolars intersect within 1 inch (2.5 cm) anterior to the central incisors.

tapetoretinopathy /tapē′tōret′inop′əthē/, a hereditary visual disorder characterized by degeneration of the sensory retina and pigmentary epithelium. It occurs in pigmentary retinopathy and other eye diseases.

tapetum, 1. a carpetlike layer or covering of tissue. 2. a thin sheet of fibers covering parts of the brain and continuous with the corpus callosum. 3. the reflective part of the choroid coat of the eye in many mammals.

tapeworm /tāp'wurm/ [AS, *taeppe* + *wyrm*], a parasitic intestinal worm belonging to the class Cestoda and having a scolex and a ribbon-shaped body composed of segments in a chain. Humans usually acquire tapeworms by eating the undercooked meat of intermediate hosts contaminated by the cysticercus or larval form of the tapeworm.

tapeworm infection, an intestinal infection by one of several species of parasitic worms, caused by eating raw or undercooked meat infested with tapeworm or its larvae. Tapeworms live as larvae in one or more vertebrate intermediate hosts and grow to adulthood in the intestine of humans. Symptoms of intestinal infection with adult worms are usually mild or absent; but diarrhea, epigastric pain, and weight loss may occur.

tapioca /tap'ē-ō'kə/, tiny starchy balls or flakes made from the dried paste of grated cassava root, *Janipha manihot.* It is used as a thickener in a variety of easily digested food items, particularly cereals, soups, and puddings.

tapotement /täpôtmäN'/ [Fr, *tapoter,* to pat], a type of massage in which the body is tapped in a rhythmic manner with the tips of the fingers or the sides of the hands, using short, rapid, repetitive movements.

tar /tär/ [AS, *teoru*], a dark, viscid organic mixture produced by the distillation of coal, wood, or vegetable matter. Some forms of tar are used to treat eczema and other skin disorders.

tarantula /təran'chələ/, popular name for any of a number of species of large, hairy spiders. Although potentially poisonous, most are relatively harmless to humans. A bite by some species may produce an area of superficial skin destruction.

tardive /tär'div/ [L, *tardus,* late], describing a disease in which a period of time passes between exposure and the first symptoms.

tardive dyskinesia /tär'div/ [L, *tardus,* late; Gk, *dys,* difficult, *kinesis,* movement], an abnormal condition characterized by involuntary repetitious movements of the muscles of the face, limbs, and trunk. This disorder most commonly affects older people who have been treated for extended periods with phenothiazine.

tardy peroneal nerve palsy [L, *tardus* + Gk, *perone,* brooch; L, *nervus* + *paralyein,* to be palsied], an abnormal condition and a type of mononeuropathy in which the peroneal nerve is excessively compressed where it crosses the head of the fibula. Such compression may occur when an individual falls asleep with the legs crossed.

tardy ulnar nerve palsy, an abnormal condition characterized by atrophy of the first dorsal interosseous muscle and difficulty in performing fine manipulations. It may be caused by injury of the ulnar nerve at the elbow and commonly affects individuals with a shallow ulnar groove or those who persistently rest their weight on their elbows. Signs and symptoms of this disorder may include numbness of the small finger, of the contiguous half of the proximal and middle phalanges of the ring finger, and of the ulnar border of the hand.

target /tär'git/ [OFr, *targuete,* small shield], 1. (in radiotherapy) any object area subjected to bombardment by radioactive particles or another form of diagnostic or therapeutic radiation. 2. a device used to contain stable materials and subsequent radioactive materials during bombardment by high-energy nuclei from a cyclotron or other particle accelerator.

target cell, 1. an abnormal red blood cell characterized by a densely stained center surrounded by a pale unstained ring circled by a dark, irregular band. 2. any cell having a specific receptor that reacts with a specific hormone, antigen, antibody, antibiotic, sensitized T cell, or other substance.

target organ, 1. (in radiotherapy) an organ intended to receive a therapeutic dose of irradiation. 2. (in nuclear medicine) an organ intended to receive the greatest concentration of a diagnostic radioactive tracer. 3. (in endocrinology) an organ most affected by a specific hormone such as the thyroid gland, which is the target organ of thyroid-stimulating hormone secreted by the anterior pituitary gland.

target symptoms, symptoms of an illness that are most likely to respond to a specific treatment such as a particular psychopharmacologic drug.

tarsal /tär'səl/ [Gk, *tarsos,* flat surface], pertaining to the tarsus, or ankle bone.

tarsal arches [Gk, *tarsos,* flat surface; L, *arcus,* rainbow], the superior and inferior branches of the palpebral artery supplying the eyelid.

tarsal bone, any one of seven bones making up the tarsus of the foot, consisting of

the talus, calcaneus, cuboid, navicular, and the three cuneiforms.

tarsalgia /tärsal'jə/, a foot pain, usually involving fallen arches.

tarsal gland, any one of numerous modified sebaceous glands on the inner surfaces of the eyelids.

tarsal tunnel syndrome, an abnormal condition and a kind of mononeuropathy characterized by pain and numbness in the sole of the foot. This disorder may be caused by fractures of the ankle that compress the posterior tibial nerve.

tarsometatarsal /tär'sōmet'ətär'səl/ [Gk, *tarsos,* flat surface, *meta,* beyond, *tarsos*], pertaining to the metatarsal bones and the tarsus of the foot.

tarsorrhaphy /tärsôr'əfē/, a surgical procedure for uniting the upper and lower eyelids. It usually is performed in procedures to protect the cornea and may involve only the lateral parts of the eyelids.

tarsus /tär'səs/, *pl.* **tarsi** [Gk, *tarsos,* flat surface], **1.** the area of articulation between the foot and the leg. **2.** any one of the plates of cartilage about 2.5 cm long that form the eyelids. One tarsal plate shapes each eyelid.

tart, abbreviation for the *tartrate carboxylate anion.*

tartar /tär'tär/ [Fr, *tartre*], **1.** a hard gritty deposit composed of organic matter, phosphates, and carbonates that collects on the teeth and gums. **2.** any of several compounds containing tartrate, the salt of tartaric acid.

tartaric acid /tärtär'ik/, a colorless or white powder found in various plants and prepared commercially from maleic anhydride and hydrogen peroxide. It is used in baking powder, certain beverages, and tartar emetic.

tartrate /tä'trāt/, **1.** a dianion of tartaric acid. **2.** any salt or ester of tartaric acid.

Tarui's disease, a form of glycogen storage disease (type VII) in which abnormally large amounts of glycogen are deposited in the skeletal muscle. The disorder is characterized by cramping on exercise but no rise in blood lactate, as well as hemolysis.

task functions, behaviors that focus or direct activities toward movements with work or labor overtones.

task group, a group in which structured verbal or nonverbal exercises are used to help a person gain emotional, physical, and other personal awareness.

task-oriented behavior, actions involving a person's cognitive abilities in an attempt to solve problems, resolve conflicts, and gratify the person's needs to reduce or avoid distress.

taste [ME, *tasten*], the sense of perceiving different flavors in soluble substances that contact the tongue and trigger nerve impulses to special taste centers in the cortex and thalamus of the brain. The four basic traditional tastes are sweet, salty, sour, and bitter. The front of the tongue is most sensitive to salty and sweet substances; the sides of the tongue are most sensitive to sour substances; and the back of the tongue is most sensitive to bitter substances. The middle of the tongue produces virtually no taste sensation. The sense of taste is intricately linked with the sense of smell.

taste bud, any one of many peripheral taste organs distributed over the tongue and the roof of the mouth. Each taste bud rests in a spheric pocket, which extends through the epithelium. Gustatory and supporting cells form each bud, which has a surface opening and an opening in the basement membrane.

taste papilla [OFr, *taster* + L, *papilla,* nipple], small nipplelike elevations on the tongue. They contain sense organs that are sensitive to the chemicals identified with tastes, which vary with their location on the tongue.

TAT, abbreviation for **tetanus antitoxin.**

tattoo /tatōō'/ [Tahitian, *tatau,* marks], a permanent coloration of the skin by the introduction of foreign pigment. A tattoo may be created deliberately or may accidentally occur when a bit of graphite from a broken pencil point is embedded in the skin.—**tattoo,** *v.*

tau /tou,tō/, T, τ, the nineteenth letter of the Greek alphabet.

taurine /tôr'in/, a derivative of the amino acid cysteine. It is present in bile in combination with cholic acid. It is used in the synthesis of bile salts.

Taussig-Bing's syndrome /tô'sig-/ [Helen B. Taussig, American pediatrician, 1898–1986; Richard J. Bing, American cardiologist, b. 1909], a developmental anomaly of the heart, characterized by transposition of the aorta and pulmonary artery. It is accompanied by a subpulmonary ventricular septal defect and ventricular hypertrophy.

tautomer /tôtəmir/, structural isomers that differ only in the position of a hydrogen atom, or proton. Because tautomers can be rapidly interconverted by proton transfer in aqueous solutions, they are usually in equilibrium with one another. Keto and enol isomers are common examples of tautomers.

taxis /tak'sis/, **1.** the movement of cells either away from or toward other cells. **2.** the reduction of a hernia. **3.** a dislocation of a hernia by means of manipulation.

taxonomic /tak'sənom'ik/ [Gk, *taxis*, arrangement, *nomos*, law], pertaining to the orderly classification of organisms into appropriate groups, or taxa, on the basis of interrelationships, with the use of suitable names.

taxonomy /takson'əmē/ [Gk, *taxis*, arrangement, *nomos*, rule], a system for classifying organisms according to their natural relationships based on such common factors as embryology, structure, or physiologic chemistry.—**taxonomic**, *adj.*

Taylor, Effie J. (1874–1970), a Canadian-born American nurse who was graduated from Johns Hopkins School of Nursing and served as a nurse in World War I. She served as president of the International Council of Nurses during World War II.

Taylor brace [Charles F. Taylor, American surgeon, 1827–1899], a padded steel brace used to support the spine.

Tay-Sachs' disease /tā'saks'/ [Warren Tay, English ophthalmologist, 1843–1927; Bernard Sachs, American neurologist, 1858–1944], an inherited, neurodegenerative disorder of lipid metabolism caused by a deficiency of the enzyme hexosaminidase A, which results in the accumulation of sphingolipids in the brain. The condition, which is transmitted as an autosomal-recessive trait, occurs predominantly in families of Eastern European Jewish origin, specifically the Ashkenazic Jews. It is characterized by progressive mental and physical retardation and early death.

Tb, symbol for the element **terbium.**

TB, 1. abbreviation for **tuberculosis.** 2. abbreviation for *tubercle bacillus.*

T bandage, a bandage in the shape of the letter T. It is used for the perineum and sometimes for the head.

TBI, abbreviation for *total body irradiation.*

TBP, 1. abbreviation for **bithionol.** 2. abbreviation for *total bypass.*

Tbs, tbsp, abbreviation for **tablespoon.**

TBSA, abbreviation for *total body surface area.*

TBT, abbreviation for **tracheobronchial tree.**

TBW, abbreviation for **total body water.**

TBZ, abbreviation for **tetrabenazine,** an anesthetic adjuvant.

t.c., abbreviation for *telephone call.*

Tc, symbol for the element **technetium.**

TC, abbreviation for **therapeutic community.**

T cell, a small circulating lymphocyte produced in the bone marrow that matures in the thymus. T cells primarily mediate cellular immune responses such as graft rejection and delayed hypersensitivity.

One kind of T cell, the **helper cell,** affects the production of antibodies by B cells; a *suppressor T cell* suppresses B cell activity.

T cell antigen receptor, a protein present on T cells that combines with antigens to produce discrete immunologic components.

T-4 cell, a thymus-derived lymphocyte of the body's immune system with a role of destroying or neutralizing cells or substances identified as "nonself." T-4 cells are 'helper/inducer' cells that secrete a substance, interleukin-2, which in turn stimulates the activity of natural killer cells, gamma interferon, and suppressor T-8 cells. The human immunodeficiency virus commonly targets the T-4 cells with the result that the body's immune defenses are severely damaged and opportunistic infections are allowed to flourish.

Td, abbreviation for **tetanus and diphtheria toxoids.**

TD, abbreviation for **toxic dose.**

TDD, abbreviation for **transdermal drug delivery.**

tDNA, abbreviation for **transfer DNA.**

t.d.s. abbreviation for Latin phrase *'(ter die sumendum'*, (to be taken) three times a day.

Te, symbol for the element **tellurium.**

tea [Chin, *ch'a*], 1. an herbal beverage prepared from the leaves and leaf buds of an evergreen shrub, *Thea sinensis.* A member of the camellia family, the plant is grown mainly in Asia. Its pharmacologically active components include caffeine, theobromine, theophylline, and tannin. 2. maté tea, a caffeine beverage prepared from the leaves of *Ilex paraguayensis,* a shrub grown in South America.

Teaching: Disease Process, a Nursing Interventions Classification defined as assisting the patient to understand information related to a specific disease process.

Teaching: Group, a Nursing Interventions Classification defined as development, implementation, and evaluation of a patient teaching program for a group of individuals experiencing the same health conditions.

teaching hospital [AS, *taecan,* to show how], a hospital associated with a university that has accredited programs in various specialties of medical practice.

Teaching: Individual, a Nursing Interventions Classification defined as planning, implementation, and evaluation of a teaching program designed to address a patient's particular needs.

Teaching: Infant Care, a Nursing Interventions Classification defined as instruction on nurturing and physical care needed during the first year of life.

Teaching: Preoperative, a Nursing Interventions Classification defined as assisting a patient to understand and mentally prepare for surgery and the postoperative recovery period.

Teaching: Prescribed Activity/Exercise, a Nursing Interventions Classification defined as preparing a patient to achieve and/or maintain a prescribed level of activity.

Teaching: Prescribed Diet, a Nursing Interventions Classification defined as preparing a patient to correctly follow a prescribed diet.

Teaching: Prescribed Medication, a Nursing Interventions Classification defined as preparing a patient to safely take prescribed medications and monitor for their effects.

Teaching: Procedure/Treatment, a Nursing Interventions Classification defined as preparing a patient to understand and mentally prepare for a prescribed procedure or treatment.

Teaching: Psychomotor Skill, a Nursing Interventions Classification defined as preparing a patient to perform a psychomotor skill.

teaching rounds, informal conferences held regularly, often at the beginning of the day. Specific problems in the care of current patients are discussed.

Teaching: Safe Sex, a Nursing Interventions Classification defined as providing instruction concerning sexual protection during sexual activity.

Teaching: Sexuality, a Nursing Interventions Classification defined as assisting individuals to understand physical and psychosocial dimensions of sexual growth and development.

team nursing [AS, *team,* family; L, *nutrix,* nurse], a decentralized system in which the care of a patient is distributed among the members of a group working in coordinated effort. The charge nurse delegates authority to a team leader who must be a professional nurse. The team leader assigns tasks, schedules care, and instructs team members in details of care.

team practice, professional practice by a group of professionals that may include physicians, nurses, and others such as a social worker, nutritionist, or physical therapist who manage the care of a specified number of patients as a coordinated group, usually in an outpatient setting.

tear /ter/ [ME, *teren,* to rend], to rip, rend, or pull apart by force.

teardrop fracture /tir'drop/ [AS, *tear* + *dropa* + L, *fractura,* break], avulsion

fracture of one of the short bones such as a vertebra, causing a tear-shaped disruption of bone tissue.

tear duct /tir/ [AS, *tear* + L, *ducere,* to lead], any duct that carries tears, including the lacrimal ducts, nasolacrimal ducts, and excretory ducts of the lacrimal glands.

tearing /tir'ing/, watering of the eye usually caused by excessive tear production, such as by strong emotion, infection, or mechanic irritation by a foreign body. If the normal amount of fluid tears is produced but not drained into the lacrimal punctum at the nasal border of the eye, tearing will occur.

tears /tirs/ [ME, *tere*], a watery saline or alkaline fluid secreted by the lacrimal glands to moisten the conjunctiva.

tears of the perineum /ters/ [ME, *teren* + Gk, *perineos*], a rending of the tissues between the vulva and anus caused by overstretching of the vagina during child delivery.

teaspoon (tsp), a small spoon that may be used to measure a dose of a liquid medication, equivalent to about 1 fluid dram or 5 ml.

tebutate, a contraction for tertiary butyl acetate.

technetium (Tc) [Gk, *technectos,* artificial], a radioactive, metallic element. Its atomic number is 43; its atomic mass (weight) is 99. Isotopes of technetium are used in radioisotope scanning procedures of internal organs such as the liver and spleen.

technetium-99m, the radionuclide most commonly used to image the body in nuclear medicine scans. It is preferred because of its short half-life and because the emitted photon has an appropriate energy for normal imaging techniques. The "m" indicates that this radionuclide is generated on site from a molybdenum source.

technical [Gk, *technikos,* skillfull], pertaining to a procedure or its results that require special techniques, skills, expertise, or knowledge.

technician /teknish'ən/ [Gk, *technikos,* skillful], a person with special training and experience in some form of technical procedures, usually those involving mechanical adjustments such as maintaining and operating radiologic equipment.

technique /teknēk'/ [Gk, *technikos,* skillful], the method and details followed in performing a procedure, such as those used in conducting a laboratory test, a physical examination, a psychiatric interview, a surgical operation, or any process requiring certain skills or an ordered sequence of actions.

technologist /teknol'əjist/ [Gk, *techne,* art,

logos, science], a person who studies the application of processes for making natural resources beneficial for humans. A medical technologist may work under the supervision of a physician in general clinical laboratory procedures.

technology /teknol′əjē/ [Gk, *techne,* art, *logos,* study], **1.** the application of science or the scientific method to commercial or industrial objectives. **2.** the knowledge and use of science applied to the conversion of natural resources for the benefit of humans.

Technology: Management, a Nursing Interventions Classification defined as use of technical equipment and devices to monitor patient condition or sustain life.

tectonic /tekton′ik/, **1.** pertaining to variations in structure in the cornea or other parts of the eye. **2.** pertaining to plastic surgery or tissue transplants.

tectorial /tektôr′ē·əl/, pertaining to a rooflike structure or cover.

tectorium /tektôr′ē·əm/, a bodily structure that serves as a roof.

teether /tē′thər/, an object such as a plastic or rubber teething ring on which an infant can bite or chew during the teething process.

teething /tē′thing/ [AS, *toth*], the physiologic process of the eruption of the deciduous teeth through the gums. It normally begins around the sixth month of life and occurs periodically until the complete set of 20 teeth has appeared at about 30 to 36 months. Discomfort and inflammation result from the pressure exerted against the periodontal tissue as the crown of the tooth breaks through the membranes. General signs of teething include excessive drooling, biting on hard objects, irritability, difficulty in sleeping, and refusal of food.—**teethe,** *v.*

tegmen /teg′mən/, a covering, such as the bone that covers the tympanic cavity.

tegmental /tegmen′təl/ [L, *tegmentum,* cover], of or relating to an integument.

TEIB, abbreviation for *triethylene-immunobenzoquinone.*

telangiectasia /təlan′jē·ekta′zhə/ [Gk, *telos,* end, *angeion,* vessel, *ektasis,* swelling], permanent dilation of groups of superficial capillaries and venules. Common causes are actinic damage, atrophy-producing dermatoses, rosacea, elevated estrogen levels, and collagen vascular diseases.

telangiectasia lymphatica [Gk, *telos,* end, *angeion,* vessel, *ektasis,* swelling; L, *lympha,* water], a congenital or acquired condition of obstructed dilated lymphatic vessels, resulting in lymphangiomata.

telangiectatic angioma /təlan′jē·ektat′ik/,

a tumor composed of dilated blood vessels.

telangiectatic epulis, a benign red tumor of the gingiva, containing prominent blood vessels. Low-grade or chronic irritation is a risk factor.

telangiectatic glioma, a tumor composed of glial cells and a network of blood vessels, which give the mass a vivid pink appearance.

telangiectatic nevus, a common skin condition of neonates, characterized by flat, deep-pink localized areas of capillary dilation that occur predominantly on the back of the neck, lower occiput, upper eyelids, upper lip, and bridge of the nose.

telangiectatic sarcoma, a malignant tumor of mesodermal cells with an unusually rich vascular network.

telediagnosis /tel′ədī′əgnō′sis/ [Gk, *tele,* far off, *dia,* through, *gnosis,* knowledge], a process whereby a disease diagnosis, or prognosis, is made by the electronic transmission of data between distant medical facilities.

telehealth, the use of telecommunication technologies to provide health care services and access to medical and surgical information for training and educating health care professionals and consumers, to increase awareness and educate the public about health-related issues, and to facilitate medical research across distances.

telekinesis /tel′əkinē′sis/ [Gk, *tele,* far off, *kinesis,* movement], a concept of parapsychology that one can control external events such as the movement of a solid object by the powers of the mind.

telemedicine, the use of telecommunication equipment and information technology to provide clinical care to individuals at distant sites and the transmission of medical and surgical information and images needed to provide that care.

telemetry /telem′ətrē/ [Gk, *tele,* far off, *metron,* measure], the electronic transmission of data between distant points, such as the transmission of cardiac monitoring data.

telencephalization /tel′ensef′əlīzā′shən/, a stage in fetal development in which the forebrain begins to assume control over nervous system functions previously directed by more primitive neural centers.

telencephalon /tel′ensef′əlon/ [Gk, *telos,* end, *egekephalos,* brain], the paired brain vesicles or endbrain from which the cerebral hemispheres are derived.

teleology /tel′ē·ol′əjē/ [Gk, *telos,* end, *logos,* science], **1.** the study of ultimate purpose or design in natural phenomena.

2. a theory that everything is directed toward some final purpose.

telepathist /tǝlep'ǝthist/, **1.** a person who believes in telepathy. **2.** a person who claims to have telepathic powers.

telepathy /tǝlep'ǝthē/ [Gk, *tele*, far off, *pathos*, feeling], the alleged communication of thought from one person to another by means other than the physical senses.—**telepathic**, *adj.*, **telepathize**, *v.*

Telephone Consultation, a Nursing Interventions Classification defined as exchanging information, providing health education and advice, managing symptoms, or doing triage over the telephone.

telephone counseling, a strategy system to provide support by telephone for patients or family caregivers who are homebound. The system may offer safety provisions and social contacts for frail older persons or the visually impaired as well as suicide-prevention counseling.

telereceptive /tel'ǝrisep'tiv/, pertaining to the exteroceptors of hearing, sight, and smell that detect stimuli distant from the body.

teletherapy /tel'ǝther'ǝpē/ [Gk, *tele* + *therapeia*, treatment], radiation therapy administered by a machine that is positioned at some distance from the patient.

telluric /teloo'rik/ [L, *tellus*, earth], pertaining to the soil and its possible pathogenic influence.

tellurium (Te) /teloo'rē·ǝm/ [L, *tellus*, earth], an element exhibiting metallic and nonmetallic chemical properties. Its atomic number is 52; its atomic mass (weight) is 127.60. Inhaling vapors of tellurium results in a garlicky breath.

telocentric /tel'ǝsen'trik/ [Gk, *telos*, end, *kentron*, center], pertaining to a chromosome in which the centromere is located at the end, so that the chromatids appear as straight filaments.

telophase /tel'ǝfāz/ [Gk, *telos* + *phasis*, appearance], the final of the four stages of nuclear division in mitosis and in each of the two divisions in meiosis.

temazepam /temaz'ǝpam/, a benzodiazepine hypnotic agent prescribed for the relief of transient and intermittent insomnia.

temper [L, *temperare*, to moderate], **1.** to moderate or soften the effects. **2.** a state of mind regarding calmness or anger.

temperament /temp'(ǝ)rǝmǝnt/ [L, *temperamentum*, mixture in proper proportions], the features of a persona that reflect an individual's emotional disposition or the way he or she behaves, feels, and thinks.

temperance /tem'pǝrǝns/, behavior that emphasizes moderation and self-restraint, particularly in the use of alcohol.

temperate phage /tem'pǝrit/ [L, *temperare*, to moderate; Gk, *phagein*, to eat], a bacteriophage whose genome is incorporated into the host bacterium.

temperature /tem'pǝ(r)chǝr/ [L, *temperatura*], **1.** a relative measure of sensible heat or cold. **2.** (in physiology) a measure of sensible heat associated with the metabolism of the human body, normally maintained at a constant level of 98.6° F (37° C). **3.** *informal.* a fever.

temperature of infant [L, *temperatura* + *infans*, infant], the neonatal temperature, which normally ranges from 96° to 99.5° F (35.5° to 37.5° C). It is unstable because of immature physiologic mechanisms.

Temperature Regulation, a Nursing Interventions Classification defined as attaining and/or maintaining body temperature within a normal range.

Temperature Regulation: Intraoperative, a Nursing Interventions Classification defined as attaining and/or maintaining desired intraoperative body temperature.

template /tem'plit/ [L, *templum*, section], (in genetics) the strand of deoxyribonucleic acid that acts as a mold for the synthesis of messenger ribonucleic acid.

temporal /tem'pǝrǝl/ [L, *temporalis*, temporary], **1.** pertaining to a limited time. **2.** pertaining to the temporal bone of the skull.

temporal arteritis [L, *temporalis*, temporary, *arteria*, airpipe, *itis*, inflammation], a progressive inflammatory disorder of cranial blood vessels, principally the temporal artery. Symptoms are intractable headache, difficulty in chewing, weakness, rheumatic pains, and loss of vision if the central retinal artery becomes occluded.

temporal artery, any one of three arteries on each side of the head: the superficial temporal artery, the middle temporal artery, and the deep temporal artery.

temporal bone, one of a pair of large bones forming part of the lower cranium and containing various cavities and recesses associated with the ear such as the tympanic cavity and the auditory tube.

temporal bone fracture, a break of the temporal bone of the skull, sometimes characterized by bleeding from the ear.

temporal gyrus [L, *temporalis*, temporary; Gk, *gyros*, turn], any of three convolutions, inferior, middle, or superior, on the lateral surface of the temporal lobe of the brain.

temporalis /tem'pǝral'is/ [L, temporary], one of the four muscles of mastication. It is a broad radiating muscle that acts to close the jaws and retract the mandible.

temporal lobe, the lateral region of the cerebrum, below the lateral fissure.

temporal subtraction, the subtraction of two or more digitized x-ray images that were acquired at different times. The subtraction process eliminates information in the image that was static.

temporary pacemaker /tem´pərer´ē/ [L, *temporalis,* temporary, *passus,* step; ME, *maken*], an artificial electronic heart generator/battery attached outside the patient's body and connected to a transvenous electrode located within the right ventricle of the heart. It is used as an interim treatment when the heart rate is excessively slow.

temporary removable splint [L, *temporalis,* temporary, *remover* + D, *splint*], any of a variety of dental appliances, including occlusal splints, used when limited stability of the teeth is required. It may be placed on or removed from teeth at will.

temporary stopping [L, *temporalis* + AS, *stoppian,* to stop up], a mixture of guttapercha, zinc oxide, white wax, and coloring, used for temporarily sealing dressings in tooth cavities.

temporomandibular /tem´pərō´mandib´-yələr/ [L, *temporalis,* temporary, *mandere,* to chew], pertaining to the articulation between the temporal bone and the condyle of the mandible.

temporomandibular joint (TMJ), [L, *temporalis* + *mandere,* to chew, *jungere,* to join], one of a pair of joints connecting the mandible of the jaw to the temporal bone of the skull. It is a combined hinge and gliding joint, formed by the anterior parts of the mandibular fossae of the temporal bone, the articular tubercles, the condyles of the mandible, and five ligaments.

temporomandibular joint capsule, a fibrous protective sheath enclosing the temporomandibular joint of the lower jaw.

temporomandibular joint (TMJ) pain dysfunction syndrome, an abnormal condition characterized by facial pain and mandibular dysfunction, apparently caused by a defective or dislocated temporomandibular joint. Some common indications of this syndrome are clicking of the joint when the jaws move, limitation of jaw movement, subluxation, and temporomandibular dislocation.

temporomandibular ligament [L, *temporalis* + *mandere,* to chew, *ligare,* to bind], an oblique band of tissue that extends downward and backward from the zygomatic process to the neck of the mandible.

temporomaxillary /-mak´siler´ē/, pertaining to the area of the temporal and maxillary bones.

temporooccipital /tem´pərō·oksip´itəl/, pertaining to the area of the temporal and occipital bones.

temporoparietalis /tem´pərōpərī´ətal´is/ [L, *temporalis* + *paries,* wall], one of a pair of broad, thin muscles of the scalp, divided into three parts, which fan out over the temporal fascia and insert into the galea aponeurotica. The three parts include an anterior temporal part, a superior parietal part, and a triangular part in between. On both sides it acts in combination with the occipitofrontalis to wrinkle the forehead, widen the eyes, and raise the ears. It is innervated by branches of the facial nerve.

TEN, abbreviation for **toxic epidermal necrolysis.**

tenacious /tenā´shəs/ [L, *tenax,* holding fast], pertaining to secretions that are sticky or adhesive or otherwise tend to hold together, such as mucus and sputum.

tenacity /tenas´itē/ [L, *tenax,* holding fast], the ability to be persistent or remain attached.

tenaculum /tənak´yələm/, *pl.* **tenacula** [L, holder], a clip or clamp with long handles used to grasp, immobilize, and hold an organ or a piece of tissue. Kinds of tenacula include the abdominal tenaculum, which has long arms and small hooks, the forceps tenaculum, which has long hooks and is used in gynecologic surgery, and the uterine or cervical tenaculum, which has short hooks or open, eye-shaped clamps used to hold the cervix.

tenalgia /tenal´jə/, pain referred to a tendon.

tender, responding with a sensation of pain to pressure or touch that would not normally cause discomfort.

tendinitis /ten´dənī´tis/ [L, *tendere,* to stretch; Gk, *itis,* inflammation], an inflammatory condition of a tendon, usually resulting from strain.

tendinous /ten´dinəs/ [L, *tendere,* to stretch], pertaining to or resembling a tendon.

tendo /ten´dō/, a tendon, such as the tendo calcaneus, the Achilles tendon.

tendon /ten´dən/ [Gk, *tenon*], any one of many white, glistening bands of dense fibrous connective tissue that attach muscle to bone. Except at points of attachment, tendons are parallel bundles of collagenous fibers sheathed in delicate fibroelastic connective tissue. Tendons are extremely strong, flexible, and inelastic and occur in various lengths and thicknesses.—**tendinous,** *adj.*

tenesmic /tənez´mik/ [Gk, *tenedere,* to stretch], pertaining to or resembling tenesmus.

tenesmus /tənez´məs/ [Gk, *tendere,* to

stretch], persistent, ineffectual spasms of the rectum or bladder, accompanied by the desire to empty the bowel or bladder.

tenia /tē′nē-ə/, **1.** any anatomic bandlike structure, such as a band of muscle fibers. **2.** a bandage or tape.

teniasis /tēnī′əsis/, an infection of intestinal tapeworms of the genus *Taenia.*

tenodesis splint /tənod′əsis, ten′ōdē′sis/, the fixation of a tendon, sometimes performed by suturing one of its ends to a different point.

tenophony /tenof′ənē/, a heart murmur associated with a defect in the chordae tendineae.

tenosynovitis /ten′ōsin′əvī′tis/ [Gk, *tenon,* tendon, *syn,* together; L, *ovum,* egg; Gk, *itis*], inflammation of a tendon sheath caused by calcium deposits, repeated strain or trauma, high levels of blood cholesterol, rheumatoid arthritis, gout, or gonorrhea.

tenotomy /tenot′əmē/ /tənot′əmē/ [Gk, *tenon,* tendon, *temnein,* to cut], the total or partial severing of a tendon, performed to correct a muscle imbalance such as in the correction of strabismus of the eye or in clubfoot.

TENS, abbreviation for **transcutaneous electrical nerve stimulation.**

Tensilon test, a diagnostic technique for verifying the signs of myasthenia gravis by testing the power of skeletal muscles before and after injection of edrophonium hydrochloride.

tensiometer /ten′sē-om′ətər/ [L, *tendere,* to stretch; Gk, *metron,* measure], a device for measuring the surface tension of a liquid.

tension /ten′shən/ [L, *tendere,* to stretch], **1.** the act of pulling or straining until taut. **2.** the condition of being taut, tense, or under pressure. **3.** a state or condition resulting from the psychologic and physiologic reaction to a stressful situation. It is characterized physically by a general increase in muscle tonus, heart rate, respiration rate, and alertness and psychologically by feelings of strain, uneasiness, irritability, and anxiety.

tension headache, a pain that affects the head as the result of overwork or emotional strain and involves tension in the muscles of the neck, face, and shoulder.

tension pneumothorax [L, *tendere,* to stretch; Gk, *pneuma,* air, *thorax*], a condition of air in the intrapleural space of the thorax caused by a rupture through the chest wall or lung parenchyma associated with the valvular opening. Air passes through the valve during coughing but cannot escape on exhalation.

tensor /ten′sər/ [L, *tendere,* to stretch],

any one of the muscles of the body that tenses a structure, such as the tensor fasciae latae of the thigh.

tensor fasciae latae, one of the 10 muscles of the gluteal region. It functions to flex the thigh and rotate it slightly medially.

tent [ME, *tente*], **1.** a transparent cover, usually of plastic, supported over the upper part of a patient by a frame. Used in the treatment of respiratory conditions, it provides a controlled environment into which steam, oxygen, vaporized medication, or droplets of cool water may be sprayed, such as an oxygen tent. **2.** a cone made of various materials inserted into a cavity or orifice of the body to dilate its opening, such as a laminaria tent. **3.** a pack placed in a wound to hold it open to ensure that healing progresses from the base of the wound upward to the skin.

tentative /ten′tətiv/ [L, *tentare,* to touch], not final or definite, such as an experimental finding that has not been validated.

tenth-value layer (TVL) [ME, *tenpe* + L, *valere,* to be worth; AS, *lecgan,* to lie], the thickness of material required to attenuate a beam of radiation to one tenth of its original intensity.

tenting of skin /ten′ting/, a slow return of the skin to its normal position after being pinched, a sign of either dehydration or aging, or both.

tentorial herniation /tentôr′ē-əl/ [L, *tentorium,* tent, *hernia,* rupture], the protrusion of brain tissue into the tentorial notch, caused by increased intracranial pressure resulting from edema, hemorrhage, or a tumor. Characteristic signs are severe headache, fever, flushing, sweating, abnormal pupillary reflex, drowsiness, hypotension, and loss of consciousness.

tentorial notch [L, *tentorium,* tent; OFr, *enochier*], an area occupied by the midbrain and enclosed by the free border of the tentorium cerebelli and the sphenoid bone.

tentorium /tentôr′ē-əm/, *pl.* **tentoria** [L, tent], any part of the body that resembles a tent, such as the tentorium of the hypophysis that covers the hypophyseal fossa.

tentorium cerebelli, one of the three extensions of the dura mater that separates the cerebellum from the occipital lobe of the cerebrum.

tenure /ten′yər/ [L, *tenere,* to hold], (in a university) a faculty appointment with few limits on the number of years it may be held.

tepid, moderately warm to the touch.

teprotide /tep′rōtīd/, a bradykinin-potentiating peptide.

teramorphous [Gk, *teras,* monster, *morphe,* form], of the nature of or characteristic of a monster.

teras /ter′əs/, *pl.* **terata** [Gk, monster], a severely deformed fetus; a monster. —**teratic,** *adj.*

teratism /ter′ətiz′əm/, any congenital or developmental anomaly that is produced by inherited or environmental factors or a combination of the two; any condition in which a severely malformed fetus is produced.

teratoblastoma /ter′ətō′blastō′mə/, a teratoma in which not all germ layers are present.

teratogen /ter′ətəjen′/ [Gk, *teras* + *genein,* to produce], any substance, agent, or process that interferes with normal prenatal development, causing the formation of one or more developmental abnormalities in the fetus. Teratogens act directly on the developing organism or indirectly, affecting such supplemental structures as the placenta or some maternal system. The period of highest vulnerability in the developing embryo is from about the third through the twelfth week of gestation, when differentiation of the major organs and systems occurs. —**teratogenic,** *adj.*

teratogenesis /ter′ətōjen′əsis/, the development of physical defects in the embryo. —**teratogenetic,** *adj.*

teratogenous /ter′ətoj′ənəs/ [Gk, *teras,* monster, *genein,* to produce], developed from fetal membranes.

teratoid /ter′ətoid/ [Gk, *teras* + *eidos,* form], pertaining to abnormal physical development; resembling a monster.

teratologist /ter′ətol′əjist/, one who specializes in the causes and effects of congenital anomalies and developmental abnormalities.

teratology /-tol′əge̅/ [Gk, *teras* + *logos,* science] the study of the causes and effects of congenital malformations and developmental abnormalities. —**teratologic, teratological,** *adj.*

teratoma /ter′ətō′mə/, a tumor composed of different kinds of tissue, none of which normally occur together or at the site of the tumor. Teratomas are most common in the ovaries or testes.

terazosin /ter′əzō′sin/, a drug approved for the treatment of benign prostatic hypertrophy. It acts by relaxing the smooth muscle fibers of the prostate through its alpha receptor blockage mechanisms.

terbium (Tb) /tur′be̅-əm/ [Yterby, Sweden], a rare earth metallic element. Its atomic number is 65; its atomic mass (weight) is 158.294.

terbutaline sulfate /terbyoo̅′tələn/, a beta-adrenergic stimulant prescribed as a

bronchodilator in the treatment of asthma, bronchitis, and emphysema and as a uterine relaxant to treat premature labor.

teres /tir′e̅z, ter′e̅z/, *pl.* **teretes** /ter′ətēz/ [L, rounded], a long cylindric muscle such as the teres minor or the teres major. —**teres,** *adj.*

teres major, a thick flat muscle of the shoulder. It functions to adduct, extend, and rotate the arm medially.

teres minor, a cylindric, elongated muscle of the shoulder. It functions to rotate the arm laterally, weakly adduct the arm, and draw the humerus toward the glenoid fossa of the scapula, strengthening the shoulder joint.

terfenadine /terfen′əde̅n/, a histamine H_1-receptor antagonist used to relieve symptoms of seasonal allergic rhinitis.

term [Gk, *terma,* limit], **1.** a specified period of time. **2.** the normal gestation period.

terminal /tur′minəl/ [L, *terminus,* boundary], (of a structure or process) near or approaching its end, such as a terminal bronchiole or a terminal disease. —**terminate,** *v.,* **terminus,** *n.*

terminal arteriole [L, *terminus,* boundary, *arteriola,* little artery], an arteriole that divides into capillaries.

terminal cancer [L, *terminalis* + *cancer,* crab], an advanced stage of a malignant neoplastic disease with death as the inevitable prognosis.

terminal drop, a rapid decline in cognitive function and coping ability that occurs 1 to 5 years before death.

terminal illness [L, *terminalis* + ME, *yfel,* evil], an advanced stage of a disease with an unfavorable prognosis and no known cure.

terminal insomnia, a chronic sleep disturbance occurring at the end of a sleep period. It may be indicative of an underlying depressive disorder and treated with an antidepressant.

terminal nerve, a small nerve originating in the cerebral hemisphere in the region of the olfactory trigone, classified by most anatomists as part of the olfactory, or first cranial, nerve.

terminal stance, one of the five stages in the stance phase of a walking gait, directly associated with the continuation of single limb support or the period during which the body moves forward on the supporting foot.

terminal sulcus of right atrium, a shallow channel on the external surface of the right atrium between the superior and inferior venae cavae.

termination codon /tur′minā′shən/, (in molecular genetics) a unit in the genetic code that specifies the end of the sequence of amino acids in a polypeptide.

termination phase, the last stage of a therapeutic relationship when attained goals are evaluated and outcomes achieved.

termination sequence, (in molecular genetics) a deoxyribonucleic acid (DNA) segment at the end of a unit that is transcribed to messenger ribonucleic acid from the DNA template.

term infant [Gk, *terma,* limit], any neonate, regardless of birth weight, born after the end of the thirty-seventh and before the beginning of the forty-third week of gestation.

terminus /tur'minəs/ [L, the end], a boundary or limit.

terpin /tur'pin/, **1.** a diterpene alcohol derived from turpentine oil. **2.** an expectorant ingredient produced through the action of nitric and sulfuric acids on pine oil.

terpin hydrate and codeine elixir /tur'-pin/, a preparation of the expectorant terpin hydrate, with sweet orange peel tincture, benzaldehyde, glycerin, alcohol, syrup, water, and the antitussive narcotic codeine.

territorial /ter'ətôr'ē·əl/ [L, *territorium,* district], a type of body movement that aids in communication. A territorial will frame an interaction and define an individual's "territory."

territoriality /ter'itôr'ē·al'itē/, an emotional attachment to and defense of certain areas related to one's existence.

tertian /tur'shən/ [L, *tertius,* third], occurring every 48 hours, including the first day of occurrence, such as vivax or tertian malaria, in which fever occurs every third day.

tertian malaria, a form of malaria caused by the protozoan *Plasmodium vivax* or *P. ovale,* characterized by febrile paroxysms that occur every 48 hours. Vivax malaria, caused by *P. vivax,* is the most common form of malaria; although it is rarely fatal, it is the most difficult form to cure. Relapses are common. Ovale malaria, caused by *P. ovale,* is usually milder and causes only a few short attacks.

tertiary /tur'shē·ərē, tursh'ərē/ [L, *tertius,* third], third in frequency or order of use.

tertiary health care, a specialized, highly technical level of health care that includes diagnosis and treatment of disease and disability in sophisticated, large research and teaching hospitals. It offers highly centralized care to the population of a large region and in some cases to the world.

tertiary prevention, a level of preventive

medicine that deals with the rehabilitation and return of a patient to a status of maximum usefulness with a minimum risk of recurrence of a physical or mental disorder.

tertiary syphilis [L, *tertius,* third], the most advanced stage of syphilis, resulting in infections of the cardiovascular and neurologic systems and marked by destructive lesions involving many tissues and organs. Late-stage syphilis is symptomatic but not contagious.

tesla /tes'lə/ [Nikola Tesla, American engineer, 1856–1943], a unit of magnetic flux density, defined by the International System of Units as 1 weber per square meter, the equivalent of 1 volt/second per square meter, or 10,000 gauss.

test [L, *testum,* crucible], **1.** an examination or trial intended to establish a principle or determine a value. **2.** a chemical reaction or reagent that has clinical significance. **3.** to detect, identify, or conduct a trial.

testa /tes'tə/ [L, a shell], **1.** an eggshell. **2.** powdered oyster shells used in antacids. **3.** the outer coat of a seed.

Testacealobosia /tes'təsē'lōbā'zhə/, a subclass of ameboid protozoa in which the cells are enclosed in chitinous or a complex membrane envelope, vest, or shell. It includes both marine and freshwater forms.

testamentary capacity /tes'təmen'tərē/, a person's competency to make a will, including the requirement that he or she be aware that a will is being made, of the nature and extent of the property covered by the will, and of the identities of the beneficiaries.

testcross [L, *testum* + *crux,* cross], **1.** (in genetics) the cross of a dominant with a recessive phenotype to determine either the degree of genetic linkage or whether the dominant phenotype is homozygous or heterozygous. **2.** the subject undergoing such a test.

testes determining factor (TDF) /tes'tēz/, a Y-chromosome gene that is believed to determine male sexual development.

test for acetone in urine, a part of routine urinalysis. Normal findings are negative, since acetone and other ketones are not normally present in urine. Exceptions include such cases as poorly controlled diabetic patients, alcoholics, and people who may be fasting or on special high-protein diets.

test for lacrimation, a test for possible keratoconjunctivitis sicca conducted by placing a 35-mm long piece of filter paper in the lower fornix of the conjunctiva for 5 minutes. Failure of tears to wet as much as

10 mm of the strip indicates keratoconjunctivitis sicca.

testicular /testik′yələr/ [L, *testiculus,* testicle], pertaining to the testicle.

testicular artery, one of a pair of long, slender branches of the abdominal aorta, arising inferior to the renal arteries and supplying the testis.

testicular cancer, a malignant neoplastic disease of the testis. An undescended testicle is often involved. In many cases the tumor is detected after an injury, but trauma is not considered a causative factor. Patients with early testicular cancer are often asymptomatic, and metastases may be present in lymph nodes, the lungs, and the liver before the primary lesion is palpable. In the later stages there may be pulmonary symptoms, ureteral obstruction, gynecomastia, and an abdominal mass.

testicular hormone, any androgenic steroid hormone secreted by the Leydig cells in the interstitial tissues of the male gonads. Testosterone is the principal hormone secreted by the cells, which are also a source of estrogen, the female sex hormone. Testosterone is a circulating hormone. It also serves as a prohormone for dihydrotestosterone and estradiol. The testicular hormone function is under the control of luteinizing hormone and follicle-stimulating hormone, both secreted by the anterior pituitary gland.

testicular self-examination (TSE), a procedure recommended by the National Institutes of Health for detecting tumors or other abnormalities in the male testes. The TSE is conducted in four simple steps, starting by standing in front of a mirror and looking for any swelling on the skin of the scrotum. Next, each testicle is examined with both hands, placing the fingers under the testicle while the thumbs are placed on top. The testicle is then rolled gently between the thumbs and fingers. In the next step the epididymis, a normal cordlike structure on the top and back of each testicle, should be found. A small pea-sized lump is felt for on the front or side of a testicle. TSE should be performed once a month.

testicular vein, one of a pair of veins emerging from convoluted venous plexuses, forming the greater mass of the spermatic cords.

testimony /tes′timō′nē/ [L, *testimonium,* evidence], the statement of a witness, usually made orally and given under oath, such as at a court trial.

testis /tes′tis/, *pl.* **testes** /tes′tēz/, [L.], one of the pair of male gonads that produce sperm and testosterone. The adult testes are suspended in the scrotum by the spermatic cords. Each testis is a laterally compressed oval body about 4 cm long and 2.5 cm wide and weighs about 12 g. The convoluted epididymis lying on the posterior border of the testis contains a tightly coiled tube that is about 20 feet long and connects with the vas deferens through which spermatozoa pass during ejaculation. Each testis consists of several hundred conical lobules containing the tiny coiled seminiferous tubules, each about 75 mm long, in which spermatozoa develop.

test method, a method chosen for experimental testing or study by means of method evaluation.

test of patency of tear duct, a procedure in which drops of a weak sugar solution are placed in the eye. If the patient then detects a sweet taste, the tear duct is assumed open.

testolactone /tes′təlak′tōn/, an antineoplastic androgen analog prescribed in the treatment of postmenopausal breast cancer and in premenopausal women whose ovarian function has been terminated.

testosterone /testos′tərōn/, a naturally occurring androgenic hormone prescribed for androgen deficiency, female breast cancer, and stimulation of growth, weight gain, and red blood cell production.

testosterone cypionate, a long-acting form of testosterone.

testosterone enanthate, a long-acting form of testosterone.

testosterone propionate, an androgen given intramuscularly.

test tube, a thin glass container with one open end and one closed end. It is used in common laboratory functions.

test tube baby, a popular term for an infant conceived through in vitro fertilization, using an ovum removed from the mother. After fertilization the zygote is transplanted to the mother's uterus to develop normally.

tetanic contraction /tetan′ik/ [Gk, *tetanos,* extreme tension; L, *contractio,* drawing together], a condition of continuous contraction in a voluntary muscle caused by a steady stream of efferent nerve impulses.

tetanic convulsion [Gk, *tetanos,* extreme tension; L, *convulsio,* cramp], **1.** a generalized tonic muscular contraction. **2.** a prolonged violent involuntary muscular contraction.

tetanus /tet′ənəs/ [Gk, *tetanos,* extreme tension], an acute, potentially fatal infection of the central nervous system caused by an exotoxin, tetanospasmin, elaborated by an anaerobic bacillus, *Clostridium tetani.* The toxin is a neurotoxin and one of the most lethal poisons known.

C. tetani infects only wounds that contain dead tissue. The bacillus is a common resident of the superficial layers of the soil and a normal inhabitant of the intestinal tracts of cows and horses. The bacillus may enter the body through a puncture wound, abrasion, laceration, or burn. The infection occurs in two clinical forms: one with an abrupt onset, high mortality, and a short incubation period (3 to 21 days); the other with less severe symptoms, a lower mortality, and a longer incubation period (4 to 5 weeks). Wounds of the face, head, and neck are the ones most likely to result in fatal infection. The disease is characterized by irritability, headache, fever, and painful spasms of the muscles, resulting in lockjaw, risus sardonicus, opisthotonos, and laryngeal spasm; eventually every muscle of the body is in tonic spasm. The motor nerves transmit the impulses from the infected central nervous system to the muscles. There is no lesion; even at autopsy no organic lesion is seen, and the cerebrospinal fluid is clear and normal.

tetanus and diphtheria toxoids (Td), an active immunizing agent containing detoxified tetanus and diphtheria toxoids that slowly produce an antigenic response to the diseases. It is prescribed for immunization against tetanus and diphtheria in children under 7 years of age when pertussis vaccine present in the usual diphtheria, pertussis, and tetanus trivalent vaccine is contraindicated.

tetanus antitoxin (TAT), a tetanus immune serum that neutralizes exotoxins in tetanus infection. It is prescribed for short-term immunization against tetanus after possible exposure to the organism and in tetanus treatment.

tetanus immune globulin (TIG), an injectable solution prepared from the globulin of an immune human. It is effective and much safer than tetanus antitoxin. It is prescribed for short-term immunization against tetanus after possible exposure to the organism and tetanus treatment.

tetanus toxoid, an active immunizing agent prepared from detoxified tetanus toxin that produces an antigenic response in the body, conferring permanent immunity to tetanus infection. It is prescribed for primary active immunization against tetanus.

tetany /tet′ənē/ [Gk, *tetanos,* extreme tension], a condition characterized by cramps, convulsions, twitching of the muscles, and sharp flexion of the wrist and ankle joints. These symptoms are sometimes accompanied by attacks of stridor. Tetany is a manifestation of an abnormality in calcium metabolism, which can oc-

cur in association with vitamin D deficiency, hypoparathyroidism, alkalosis, or the ingestion of alkaline salts.

tetrabasic /tet′rəbā′sik/, **1.** describing a compound that has four acidic hydrogen atoms replaced by metal ions. **2.** an alcohol containing four hydroxyl groups.

tetracaine hydrochloride, a local anesthetic used for spinal nerve blockage and topical anesthesia.

tetrachloroethane /-klôr′ō·eth′ān/, a potentially toxic solvent with a sweet, chloroform-like odor. It is used to dissolve fats, waxes, oils, and resins and in the manufacture of paints, varnishes, and rust removers. Symptoms of overexposure include nausea, vomiting, abdominal pain, finger tremors, skin disorders, and liver damage.

tetracycline /tet′rəsī′klēn/, a broad-spectrum antibiotic prescribed for the treatment of many bacterial and rickettsial infections.

tetracycline hydrochloride, a tetracycline antibiotic prescribed in the treatment of infections.

tetrad /tet′rad/ [Gk, *tetra,* four], (in genetics) a group of four chromatids of a synapsed pair of homologous chromosomes during the first meiotic prophase stage of gametogenesis.—**tetradic,** *adj.*

tetradactyly /-dak′tilē/ [Gk, *tetra* + *dactylos*], the presence of only four fingers on each hand or four toes on each foot.

tetraethyl lead /tet′rə·eth′il led/, a potentially toxic, anti-knock gasoline additive. Effects of overexposure include insomnia, lassitude, anxiety, nausea, tremor, pallor, hypothermia, anorexia, and psychosis.

tetrahydrocannabinol (THC) /-hi′drō-kənab′inol/, the active principle, occurring as two psychomimetic isomers, in the hemp plant *Cannabis sativa,* used in the preparation of marijuana, hashish, bhang, and ganja. THC, a rapidly metabolized beta-adrenergic agonist, increases pulse rate; causes conjunctival reddening and a feeling of euphoria; and has variable effects on blood pressure, respiratory rate, and pupil size. The drug affects memory, cognition, and the sensorium; decreases motor coordination; and increases appetite.

tetrahydrozoline hydrochloride /-hīdroz′-əlēn/, an adrenergic vasoconstrictor prescribed for the treatment of nasal and nasopharyngeal congestion and as an ophthalmic vasoconstrictor.

tetralogy /tetrol′əjē/ [Gk, *tetra,* four, *logos,* word], any group of four writings, symptoms, or other related factors.

tetralogy of Fallot /falō′/ [Gk, *tetra,* four, *logos,* word; Etienne-Louis A. Fallot,

French physician, 1850–1911], a congenital cardiac anomaly that consists of four defects: pulmonic stenosis, ventricular septal defect, malposition of the aorta so that it arises from the septal defect or the right ventricle, and right ventricular hypertrophy. The primary symptoms in the infant are cyanosis and hypoxia, difficulty in feeding, failure to gain weight, and poor development. In older children a typical squatting position and clubbing of the fingers and toes are evident.

tetramer /tet′rəmer/ [Gk, *tetra* + *meros,* part], something that is composed of four parts, such as a protein composed of four polypeptide subunits.

tetraodon poisoning, a reaction caused by a toxin in puffer fish and marine sunfish. It may result in myalgia, paresthesia, and other neuromuscular disorders. Death may result from respiratory paralysis.

tetrapeptide /-pep′tīd/, a compound formed by four amino acids united by peptide links.

tetraplegia /-plē′jə/ [Gk, *tetra,* four, *plege,* stroke], paralysis of both arms and both legs.

tetraploid (4n) /tet′rəploid/ [Gk, *tetraploos,* fourfold, *eidos,* form], **1.** pertaining to an individual, organism, strain, or cell that has four complete sets of chromosomes. **2.** such an individual, organism, strain, or cell.

tetraploidy /tet′rəploi′dē/, the state or condition of having four complete sets of chromosomes.

tetrasaccharide /-sak′ərīd/, a sugar containing four molecules of monosaccharide.

tetrascelus /tetras′ēləs/, a fetal anomaly with four legs.

tetravalent /-vā′lənt/, pertaining to a chemical with a valency of four.

TFIIE, a general transcription factor involved in complementary deoxyribonucleic acid encoding. TFIIE consists of two subunits, TFIIE-alpha and TFIIE-beta.

T fracture /tē′frakchər/, an intercondylar fracture in which the fracture lines are T-shaped.

TGF, abbreviation for **transforming growth factor.**

Th, symbol for the element **thorium.**

thalamic /thalam′ik/ [Gk, *thalamos,* chamber], pertaining to the thalamus.

thalamic peduncle [Gk, *thalamos,* chamber; L, *pes,* foot], a group of fibers linking the thalamus with the hypothalamus.

thalamic syndrome [Gk, *thalamos* + *syn,* together, *dromos,* course], a vascular disorder involving the ventral and posterolateral nuclei of the thalamus and related nerve fibers. It causes disturbances of sensation and partial or complete paralysis of one side of the body. A major effect is an increased threshold to all stimuli on the opposite side of the body so that any stimuli may cause an exaggerated response.

thalamotomy /thal′əmot′əmē/, the surgical production of lesions within the nuclei of the thalamus, generally performed to treat diseases of the basal ganglia.

thalamus /thal′əmas/, *pl.* **thalami** [Gk, *thalamos,* chamber], one of a pair of large oval nervous structures forming most of the lateral walls of the third ventricle of the brain and part of the diencephalon. It relays sensory information, excluding smell, to the cerebral cortex. It is composed mainly of gray substance and translates impulses from appropriate receptors into crude sensations of pain, temperature, and touch. It also participates in associating sensory impulses with pleasant and unpleasant feelings, in the arousal mechanisms of the body, and in the mechanisms that produce complex reflex movements.—**thalamic,** *adj.*

thalassemia /thal′əsē′mē-ə/ [Gk, *thalassa,* sea, *a* + *haima,* without blood], a hemolytic hemoglobinopathy anemia characterized by microcytic, hypochromic, and short-lived red blood cells caused by deficient hemoglobin synthesis. The disease occurs in two forms. Thalassemia major (Cooley's anemia), the homozygous form, evident in infancy, is recognized by anemia, fever, failure to thrive, and splenomegaly and is confirmed by characteristic changes in the red blood cells on microscopic examination. The spleen may become so enlarged that respiratory excursion is impeded and the abdominal organs are crowded. Headache, abdominal pain, fatigue, and anorexia often occur. Thalassemia minor, the heterozygous form, is characterized only by a mild anemia and minimal red blood cell changes. Thalassemia minima is a form that lacks clinical symptoms, although patients show hematologic evidence of the disease.

thalassotherapy /thalas′ōther′əpē/ [Gk, *tahassa,* sea], a treatment system based on sea bathing and exposure to sea air.

thalidomide /thalid′əmīd/, a sedative-hypnotic, withdrawn from general use because of its potential for teratogenic effects, particularly phocomelia, when taken during pregnancy. It is sometimes prescribed for treatment of leprosy.

thallium (Tl) /thal′ē-əm/ [Gk, *thallos,* green line], a soft, bluish-white metallic element that exhibits some nonmetallic chemical properties. Its atomic number is 81; its atomic mass (weight) is 204.38. Many of its compounds are highly toxic.

thallium poisoning, a toxic condition caused by the ingestion or absorption through the skin of thallium salts, especially thallium sulfate. Characteristic of the condition are abdominal pain, vomiting, bloody diarrhea, tremor, delirium, and alopecia.

thanatology /than'ətol'əjē/ [Gk, *thanatos,* death, *logos,* science], the study of death and dying.—**thanatologist,** *n.*

thanatomania /than'ətōmā'nē·ə/ [Gk, *thanatos,* death, *mania,* frenzy], an obsession with death, dying, or suicide.

thanatophoric dwarf /than'ətōfôr'ik/ [Gk, *thanatos* + *phoros,* bearer; AS, *dweorge*], an infant with severe micromelia, the limbs usually extending straight out from the trunk, an extremely narrow chest, and flattened vertebral bodies with wide intervertebral spaces.

Thanatos /than'ətəs/ [Gk, death], a freudian term for the death instinct.

THC, abbreviation for **tetrahydrocannabinol.**

theater /thē'ətər/, **1.** an operating room or suite of rooms. **2.** a large room used for lectures and demonstrations.

thebesian foramen /thəbē'zē·ən, tābā'zē·ən/ [Adam C. Thebesius, German physician, 1686–1732], any of the openings of the venae cordis minimae, or small veins, into the right atrium.

thebesian vein [Adam C. Thebesius], any of the smallest cardiac veins.

the blues, *informal.* a designation for Blue Cross (an insurance system that pays the costs of treatment by a hospital or clinic) and Blue Shield (an insurance system that pays the costs of treatment by a professional).

theca /thē'kə/, *pl.* **thecae** /thē'sē/, a sheath or capsule, such as the theca cordis or pericardium.

theca cell tumor [Gk, *theke,* sheath; L, *cella,* storeroom; *tumor,* swelling], an uncommon benign fibroid tumor of the ovary, composed of theca cells and usually containing granulosa (follicular) cells.

thecal /thē'kəl/ [Gk, *theke,* sheath], pertaining to a theca or sheath.

Theden's bandage /tā'dənz/ [Johann C. A. Theden, German surgeon, 1714–1797], a roller bandage applied below the injury and continued upward over a compress, used to stop bleeding.

thelarche /thilär'kē/ [Gk, *thele,* nipple, *archaios,* beginning], the beginning of female pubertal breast development normally occurring between 9 and 13 years of age. Premature thelarche is precocious breast development in a female without other evidence of sexual maturation.

thenar /thē'när/ [Gk, palm of the hand], **1.** the ball of the thumb. **2.** pertaining to the thumb side of the palm.

thenar eminence [Gk, *thenar,* palm of the hand; L, *eminentia,* projection], a raised rounded area on the palm of the hand near the base of the thumb.

theobroma oil /thē'ōbrō'mə/, a liquid fat derived from seeds of *Theobroma cacao,* the cocoa plant. It contains a number of fatty acids used in suppositories, ointments, and lubricants.

theobromine /thē'əbrō'min/, a substance (methylxanthine) that is related chemically to caffeine and theophylline and differs from them by the number and distribution of methyl groups. Theobromine occurs naturally in cocoa, cola nuts, and tea. It acts as a diuretic, vasodilator, cardiac stimulant, and smooth muscle relaxant.

thecoma, a tumor derived from ovarian mesenchyme, consisting of spindle-shaped cells that may contain fat droplets. It is sometimes associated with excessive estrogen production and precocious sexual development in prepubertal girls.

theophylline /thē·əfil'ēn/ [L, *thea,* tea; Gk, *phyllon,* leaf], a bronchodilator prescribed to relax the smooth muscle of the bronchial passages in the treatment of bronchospasm in bronchial asthma, bronchitis, and emphysema.

theorem /thē'ərəm/ [Gk, *theorein,* to look at], **1.** a proposition to be proved by a chain of reasoning and analysis. **2.** a rule expressed by symbols or formulae.

theoretic effectiveness /thē·əret'ik/ [Gk, *theorein* + L, *efficere,* to do], (of a contraceptive method) the effectiveness of a medication, device, or method in preventing pregnancy if used consistently and exactly as intended, without error.

theoretic plate number (N), a number defining the efficiency of a chromatographic column.

theory /thē'ərē/ [Gk, *theorein,* to look at], an abstract statement formulated to predict, explain, or describe the relationships among concepts, constructs, or events. Theory is developed and tested by observation and research, using factual data.

theotherapy /thē'ōther'əpē/ [Gk, *theos,* god, *therapeia,* treatment], a therapeutic approach to the prevention, diagnosis, and treatment of disease and dysfunction based on religious or spiritual beliefs.

therapeutic /ther'əpyoo'tik/ [Gk, *therapeuein,* to treat], **1.** beneficial. **2.** pertaining to a treatment.

therapeutic abortion, 1. a termination of early pregnancy deemed necessary by a physician. **2.** *informal.* any legal induced abortion.

therapeutic communication, a process in which the nurse consciously influences a client or helps the client to a better understanding through verbal or nonverbal communication.

therapeutic community (TC), (in mental health) a treatment facility in which the entire milieu is part of the treatment. The physical environment, the other clients, the staff, and the policies of the facility influence the function of the individual in the activities of daily living in the community.

therapeutic dose [Gk, *therapeia,* treatment, *dosis,* giving], the dose that may be required to produce a desired effect.

therapeutic equivalent, a drug that has essentially the same effect in the treatment of a disease or condition as one or more other drugs.

therapeutic exercise, any exercise planned and performed to attain a specific physical benefit, such as maintenance of the range of motion, strengthening of weakened muscles, increased joint flexibility, or improved cardiovascular and respiratory function.

therapeutic gain, the ratio of the biologic effect of a therapy on a tumor compared with the effect on surrounding normal tissue.

therapeutic index, the difference between the minimum therapeutic and minimum toxic concentrations of a drug.

therapeutic pneumothorax [Gk, *therapeia,* treatment, *pneuma,* air, *thorax*], the intentional introduction of air in the intrapleural space, causing partial collapse of the lung. It was used in the 1940s for treatment of certain cases of tuberculosis.

therapeutic radiopharmaceutical, a radioactive drug administered to a patient to deliver radiation to body tissues internally, such as iodide 131, which is used to ablate thyroid tissue in hyperthyroid patients.

therapeutic recreation, an allied health group, staffed by people with expertise in organizing and supervising recreational activities designed to accelerate recovery from mental or physical disorders.

therapeutic recreation specialist, a person who assists patients in their recovery or rehabilitation after physical or emotional illness or disability by planning and supervising recreation programs.

therapeutics /ther′əpyōō′tiks/ [Gk, *therapeia,* treatment], a branch of health care that is concerned with the treatment of disease, seeking to relieve symptoms or produce a cure.

therapeutic temperature, (in hyperthermia treatment) temperatures between 107° to 113° F (42° to 45° C).

Therapeutic Touch, a Nursing Interventions Classification defined as directing one's own interpersonal energy to flow through the hands to help or heat another.

therapist /ther′əpist/, a person with special skills, obtained through education and experience, in one or more areas of health care.

therapy /ther′əpē/ [Gk, *therapeia*], the treatment of any disease or a pathologic condition, such as inhalation therapy, which administers various medicines for patients suffering from diseases of the respiratory tract.

Therapy Group, a Nursing Interventions Classification defined as application of psychotherapeutic techniques to a group, including the use of interactions between members of the group.

thermal /thur′məl/ [Gk, *therme,* heat], pertaining to the production, application, or maintenance of heat.

thermal burn, tissue injury, usually of the skin, caused by exposure to extreme heat.

thermal field size, the area over which therapeutic heating is likely to be produced.

thermalgesia /thur′məljē′zhə/ [Gk, *therme,* heat, *algos,* pain], pain caused by exposure to high temperatures.

thermalgia /thurmal′jə/, a sensation of intense burning pain sometimes experienced following nerve injuries.

thermal radiation [Gk, *therme,* heat; L, *radiare,* to shine], the emission of energy in the form of heat.

thermic sense [Gk, *therme,* heat; L, *sentire,* to feel], the network of sense organs and connecting pathways that allow an appreciation of temperature changes.

thermistor /thərmis′tər/ [Gk, *therme* + L, *resistere,* to withstand], a kind of thermometer for measuring minute changes in temperature.

thermocautery /thur′mōkô′tərē/ [Gk, *therme* + *kauterion,* branding iron], the use of a needle or snare heated by direct flame, a heated hydrocarbon vapor, or an electrical current in the destruction of tissue.

thermochemistry /-kem′istrē/ [Gk, *therme,* heat, *chemia,* alchemy], a branch of chemistry that is concerned with the heat changes involved in chemical reactions.

thermocoagulation /-kō·ag′yəlā′shən/ [Gk, *therme,* heat; L, *coagulare*], the use of high-frequency electrical currents to destroy tissue through heat coagulation.

thermocouple /thur′məkup′əl/ [Gk, *therme* + Fr, *couple,* pair], a temperature-measuring device that relies on the production of a temperature-dependent voltage at the junction of two dissimilar metals.

thermodilution /-dilyōō′zhən/, a method of cardiac output determination. A bolus of solution of known volume and temperature is injected into the right atrium, and the resultant cooling of blood temperature is detected by a thermistor previously placed in the pulmonary artery with a catheter.

thermodynamics /-dīnam′iks/ [Gk, *therme,* heat, *dynamis,* power], the science of the interconversion of heat and work.

thermogenesis /thur′mōjen′əsis/ [Gk, *therme* + *genesis,* origin], production of heat, especially by the cells of the body. —**thermogenetic,** *adj.*

thermograph /thur′məgraf′/ [Gk, *therme* + *graphein,* to record], **1.** a photographic record of the amount of heat radiated from the surface of the body, revealing 'hot spots' of potential tumors or other disorders. **2.** a device consisting of a thermometer, inked stylus, and chart for continuous recording of the ambient temperature.

thermography /thərmog′rəfē/, a technique for sensing and recording on film hot and cold areas of the body by means of an infrared detector that reacts to blood flow.—**thermographic,** *adj.*

thermointegrator /thur′mō·in′təgrā′tər/, an instrument used to create a thermal model of an environment, measuring the warmth and coldness as it might be experienced by a living organism in that environment.

thermokeratoplasty /-ker′ətōplas′tē/, a procedure to correct myopia by applying heat to flatten the cornea. The heat shrinks the collagen in the substantia propria layer of the cornea.

thermolabile /thur′məlā′bəl/ [Gk, *therme* + L, *labilis,* slipping], easily destroyed or altered by heat.

thermoluminescent dosimetry /-lōō′-mines′ənt/ [Gk, *therme* + L, *lumen,* light; Gk, *dosis,* something given, *metron,* measure], a method of measuring the ionizing radiation to which a person is exposed by a device that stores the radiant energy and releases it later as ultraviolet or visible light.

thermomassage /-məsäzh′/, a physical therapy technique that combines heat and massage.

thermometer /thermom′ətər/ [Gk, *therme* + *metron,* measure], an instrument for measuring temperature. It usually consists of a sealed glass tube, marked in degrees of Celsius or Fahrenheit and containing liquid such as mercury or alcohol. The liquid rises or falls as it expands or contracts according to changes in temperature.

thermoneutral environment /-nōō′trəl/ [Gk, *therme* + L, *neutralis,* neutral; ME, *environ,* around], **1.** an environment that keeps body temperature at an optimum point at which the least amount of oxygen is consumed for metabolism. **2.** an environment that enables a neonate to maintain a body temperature of 97.7° F (36.5° C) with a minimal requirement of energy and oxygen.

thermonuclear /-nōō′klē·ər/ [Gk, *therme,* heat; L, *nucleus,* nut kernel], pertaining to a reaction in which isotopes of hydrogen (protium, deuterium, or tritium) can be fused at temperatures of nearly 100,000,000° C into heavier nuclei of helium atoms. The process is the source of energy of the sun and is used in the explosion of thermonuclear weapons.

thermopenetration /-pen′ətrā′shən/ [Gk, *therme* + L, *penetrale,* passing through], the use of diathermic techniques to produce warmth within the body tissues for therapeutic purposes.

thermophilic /-fil′ik/ [Gk, *therme,* heat, *philein,* to love], pertaining to organisms that thrive in warmth of up to 70° C, well above the normal human body temperature of 37° C.

thermophore /thur′məfôr/, a procedure in which heat is applied locally to a body part.

thermoradiotherapy /-rā′dē·ōther′əpē/, a therapeutic process that applies ionizing radiation to any part of the body in which the temperature has been raised by artificial means.

thermoreceptor /-risep′tər/ [Gk, *therme,* heat; L, *recipere,* to receive], nerve endings that are sensitive to heat or a rise in body temperature.

thermoregulation /-reg′yəlā′shən/ [Gk, *therme* + L, *regula,* rule], the control of heat production and heat loss, specifically the maintenance of body temperature through physiologic mechanisms activated by the hypothalamus.

thermoregulation, ineffective, a NANDA-accepted nursing diagnosis of the state in which an individual's temperature fluctuates between hypothermia and hyperthermia. The critical defining characteristic is the fluctuation in body temperature above or below the normal range.

thermoregulatory centers /reg′yələtôr′ē/ [Gk, *therme,* heat; L, *regula,* rule; Gk, *kentron,* center], centers located in the hypothalamus concerned mainly with the regulation of heat production, heat inhibition, and heat conservation to maintain a normal body temperature.

thermoresistance /-ris'is'təns/, an ability to tolerate heat, such as certain bacteria that can withstand high temperatures.

thermostable /-stā'bəl/, unaffected by or resistant to change by an increase in temperature.

thermostasis /-stā'sis/, maintenance of a stable body temperature, as in warm-blooded animals.

thermostat /thur'məstat/ [Gk, *therme* + *statos,* standing], a device for the automatic control of a heating or cooling system.—**thermostatic,** *adj.*

thermotaxis /-tak'sis/ [Gk, *therme* + *taxis,* arrangement], **1.** the normal adjustment and regulation of body temperature. **2.** the movement of an organism in response to heat, either toward the stimulus (positive thermotaxis) or away from the stimulus (negative thermotaxis).

thermotherapeutic penetration /-ther'-əpyoo'tik/, the depth to which heating to therapeutic temperatures is likely to extend.

thermotherapy /-ther'əpē/ [Gk, *therme* + *therapeia,* treatment], the treatment of disease by the application of heat. Thermotherapy may be administered as dry heat with heat lamps, diathermy machines, electrical pads, or hot water bottles or as moist heat with warm compresses or immersion in warm water.—**thermotherapeutic,** *adj.*

theta /thē'tə, thā'tə/, Θ, θ, the eighth letter of the Greek alphabet.

theta wave [Gk, *theta,* eighth letter of Greek alphabet; AS, *wafian*], one of the several types of brain waves, characterized by a relatively low frequency of 4 to 7 Hz and a low amplitude of 10 μV. Theta waves are the 'drowsy waves' of the temporal lobes of the brain.

thiabendazole /thī'əben'dəzōl/, an anthelmintic prescribed in the treatment of worm infestations, including hookworms, roundworms, and pinworms.

thiamin /thī'əmin/ [Gk, *theion,* containing sulfur, *amine,* ammonia], a water-soluble, crystalline compound of the B vitamin complex, essential for normal metabolism and health of the cardiovascular and nervous systems. Thiamin plays a key role in the metabolic breakdown of glucose to yield energy in body tissues. A deficiency of thiamin affects chiefly the nervous system, the circulation, and the gastrointestinal tract. Symptoms include irritability, emotional disturbances, loss of appetite, multiple neuritis, increased pulse rate, dyspnea, reduced intestinal motility, and heart irregularities. Severe deficiency causes beriberi.

thiaminase, /thī·am'inās/ an enzyme present in raw fish that destroys thiamin. A diet containing a substantial amount of raw fish could result in a thiamin deficiency because of the enzyme.

thiemia /thī·ē'mē·ə/ [Gk, *theion,* sulfur, *haima,* blood], an excess of sulfur in the blood.

thiethylperazine /thī·eth'ilper'əzēn/, a phenothiazine antiemetic prescribed to control nausea and vomiting.

thigh [AS, *theoh*], the section of the lower limb between the hip and the knee.

thinking [AS, *thencan,* to think], **1.** the cognitive process of forming mental images or concepts. **2.** the process of cognitive problem solving through the sorting, organizing, and classification of facts.

thin-layer chromatography (TLC), a method of separating two or more chemical compounds in a solution through their differential migrations across a thin layer of adsorbent spread over a glass or plastic plate.

thioamide derivative /thī'ō·am'īd/, one of a group of antithyroid drugs prescribed in the treatment of hyperthyroidism. Thioamide drugs act by inhibiting the synthesis of thyroid hormone.

thioctic acid /thī·ok'tik/, a pyruvate oxidation factor found in liver and yeast, used in bacterial culture media.

thioester /thī'ō·es'tər/, an important group of biologic chemicals formed by the hydrosulfides and carboxylic acids and identified by an ester bond involving the -SH radical. Examples include the coenzyme A thioesters.

thioethanolamine acetyltransferase /thī'-ō·eth'ənol'əmin/, an enzyme that catalyzes the transfer of acetyl groups from acetyl CoA to the sulfur atom of thioethanolamine, producing CoA and S-acetylthioethanolamine.

thioflavine 1 /thī·ōflā'vin/, a yellow dye used as a fluorochrome in histopathology.

thioguanine /thī'ōgwä'nēn/, an antineoplastic prescribed in the treatment of a variety of malignant neoplastic diseases, including the acute leukemias.

thiopental sodium / pen'təl/, a potent ultrashort-acting barbiturate used as a general anesthetic induction agent. By depressing the central nervous system, thiopental sodium induces hypnotic sleep in less than 1 minute after injection. It has no analgesic properties and therefore must be supplemented by analgesics.

thioridazine hydrochloride /-rid'əzēn/, a phenothiazine antipsychotic prescribed in the treatment of childhood behavioral disorders, geriatric mental disorders, depression, and alcohol withdrawal.

thiotepa /thī'ōtep'ə/, an antineoplastic alkylating agent prescribed in the treatment of malignant neoplastic diseases, including adenocarcinoma of the breast and ovary and urinary bladder carcinomas.

thiothixene /-thī'ksēn/, a thioxanthene antipsychotic prescribed in the treatment of acute agitation and mild-to-severe psychotic disorders.

thiouracil /thī'ōyŏŏr'əsil/ [Gk, theion, sulfur, ouron, urine], a chemical compound derived from thiourea that inhibits the formation of thyroxine in the thyroid gland and is used to treat hyperthyroidism.

thioxanthene derivative /thī-oksan'thēn/, any one of a group of antipsychotic drugs, each of which is similar to the phenothiazenes in indication, action, and adverse effects.

third-party reimbursement, reimbursement for services rendered to a person in which an entity other than the receiver of the service is responsible for the payment.

third stage of labor, the expulsion of the placenta, membranes, and a small amount of blood and amniotic fluid, occurring within 5 to 30 minutes after delivery of the fetus.

third ventricle [Gk, triotus, below second rank; L, ventriculus, little belly], a cavity of the brain bounded on each side by a thalamus and the hypothalamus. It communicates anteriorly with the lateral ventricles and posteriorly with the aqueduct of the midbrain.

third ventriculostomy /ventrik'yəlos'-təmē/ [L, tertius, three, ventriculus, little belly; Gk, stoma, mouth], a surgical procedure for draining cerebrospinal fluid into the cisterna chiasmatis of the subarachnoid space in hydrocephalus, usually in the newborn.

thirst /thurst/ [AS, Thurst], a perceived desire for water or other fluid. The sensation of thirst is usually referred to the mouth and throat.

Thiry-Vella fistula /thī'rĭvel'ə/ [Ludwig Thiry, Austrian physiologist, 1817–1897; Luis Vella, Italian physiologist, 1825–1886], an artificial passage from the abdominal surface of an experimental animal to an isolated intestinal loop, created surgically for the study of intestinal secretions.

thixotropy /thiksot'rəpē/ [Gk, this, touch, terpin, to turn], a property of certain gels or colloids that become less viscous when shaken or agitated but revert to their original viscosity after standing.

Thomas's splint [Hugh O. Thomas, English surgeon, 1834–1891], **1.** a rigid splint constructed of steel bars that are curved to fit the involved limb and held in place by a cast or a rigid bandage. **2.** a rigid metal splint that extends from a ring at the hip to beyond the foot.

thoracentesis /thôr'əsentē'sis/ [Gk, thorax + centesis, puncture], the surgical perforation of the chest wall and pleural space with a needle to aspirate fluid for diagnostic or therapeutic purposes or to remove a specimen for biopsy.

thoracic /thôars'ik/, pertaining to the thorax.

thoracic aorta [Gk, thorax, chest, aerein, to raise], the large upper part of the descending aorta, starting at the lower border of the fourth thoracic vertebra, dividing into seven branches, and supplying many parts of the body such as the heart, ribs, chest muscles, and stomach.

thoracic cage [Gk, thorax, chest; L, cavus, hollow], the bony framework that surrounds the organs and soft tissues of the chest. It consists of 12 thoracic vertebrae, 12 pairs of ribs, and the sternum.

thoracic cavity [Gk, thorax, chest; L, cavum], the cavity enclosed by the ribs, the thoracic part of the vertebral column, the sternum, the diaphragm, and associated muscles.

thoracic duct, the common trunk of all the lymphatic vessels in the body, except those on the right side of the head, the neck, and the thorax, the right upper limb, the right lung, the right side of the heart, and the diaphragmatic surface of the liver.

thoracic fistula, an abnormal opening in the chest wall that ends blindly or communicates with the thoracic cavity.

thoracic medicine, the branch of medicine concerned with the diagnosis and treatment of disorders of the structures and organs of the chest, especially the lungs.

thoracic nerves, the 12 pairs of spinal nerves emerging from the spinal cord at the level of the thorax, including 11 intercostal nerves and one subcostal nerve. They are distributed mainly to the walls of the thorax and the abdomen. The first two intercostal nerves innervate the upper limb and the thorax; the next four supply only the thorax; and the lower five supply the walls of the thorax and the abdomen.

thoracic outlet syndrome, an abnormal condition and a type of mononeuropathy characterized by paresthesia. It may be caused by a nerve root compression by a cervical disk.

thoracic parietal node, one of the lymph glands in the thorax, associated with various lymphatic vessels and divided into sternal nodes, intercostal nodes, and diaphragmatic nodes.

thoracic surgery [Gk, thorax, chest, cheirourgia, surgery], the branch of medicine that deals with disease and injuries of the thoracic area by manipulative and operative methods.

thoracic vertebra, one of the 12 bony segments of the spinal column of the upper back designated T1 to T12. T1 is just below the seventh cervical vertebra (C7), and T12 is just above the first lumbar vertebra (L1). The thoracic part of the spine is flexible and has a concave ventral curvature.

thoracic visceral node, a node in the three groups of lymph nodes connected to the part of the lymphatic system that serves certain structures within the thorax such as the thymus, pericardium, esophagus, trachea, lungs, and bronchi.

thoracodorsal nerve /thôr'əkōdôr'səl/ [Gk, *thorax* + L, *dorsum,* back], a branch of the brachial plexus, usually arising between the two subscapular nerves. It courses along the posterior wall of the axilla and terminates in branches that supply the latissimus dorsi.

thoracodynia /-din'ē-ə/ [Gk, *thorax,* chest, *odyne,* pain], chest pain.

thoracolumbar fascia /thôr'əkōlum'bər/, a noncontractile structure that functions in a manner similar to a ligament in the lumbar area. It extends from the iliac crest and sacrum to the thoracic cage and envelops the paravertebral musculature.

thoracopathy /thôr'əkop'əthē/, any disorder involving the thorax or the organs it contains.

thoracoplasty /thôr'əkoplas'tē/, the surgical reduction in the size of abnormal spaces in the thoracic cavity, such as may result from a collapsed lung.

thoracostomy /thôr'əkos'təmē/ [Gk, *thorax* + *stoma,* mouth], an incision made into the chest wall to provide an opening for the purpose of drainage.

thoracostomy tube, a catheter inserted through the chest wall to drain fluid from the pleural space.

thoracotomy /thôr'əkot'əmē/ [Gk, *thorax* + *temnein,* to cut], a surgical opening into the thoracic cavity.

Thoraeus filters /thôrē'əs/, combinations of metals, usually tin, copper, and aluminum, used to modify the quality of orthovoltage x-ray beams to improve the penetrating ability.

thorax /thôr'aks/, *pl.* **thoraxes, thoraces** [Gk, chest], the cage of bone and cartilage containing the principal organs of respiration and circulation and covering part of the abdominal organs. It is formed ventrally by the sternum and costal cartilages and dorsally by the 12 thoracic vertebrae and the dorsal parts of the 12 ribs.

thorium (Th) /thôr'ē-əm/ [ONorse, *Thor,* god of thunder], a heavy grayish radioactive metallic element. Its atomic number is 90; its atomic mass (weight) is 232.04. Thorium is used in nuclear medicine and radiation therapy.

thought broadcasting /thôt/ [AS, *thot*], a symptom of psychosis in which the patient believes that his or her thoughts are "broadcast" beyond the head so that other people can hear them.

thought insertion, a belief by some mentally ill patients that thoughts of other people can be inserted into their own minds.

thought processes, altered, a NANDA-accepted nursing diagnosis of a state in which an individual experiences a disruption in cognitive operations and activities. The defining characteristics are inaccurate interpretation of environment, cognitive dissonance, distractibility, memory deficit/ problems, egocentricity, and hypervigilance or hypovigilance. Another possible characteristic is inappropriate nonreality-based thinking.

Thr, abbreviation for **threonine.**

thready pulse /thred'ē/ [AS, *thraed* + L, *pulsare,* to beat], an abnormal pulse that is weak, somewhat difficult to palpate, and often fairly rapid; the artery does not feel full, and the rate may be difficult to count.

threatened abortion /thret'ənd/ [AS, *threat,* coercion; L, *ab,* away from, *oriri,* to be born], a condition in pregnancy before the twentieth week of gestation characterized by uterine bleeding and cramping sufficient to suggest that miscarriage may result.

3-methyl fentanyl, a potent heroin substitute and so-called designer drug. It is an analog of fentanyl.

three-point gait [Gk, *treis* + L, *pungere,* to prick; ONorse, *gata,* way], a pattern of crutch walking in which the crutches and affected leg are advanced first with each step.

threonine(Thr), an essential amino acid needed for proper growth in infants and maintenance of nitrogen balance in adults.

threshold /thresh'ōld/ [AS, *therscold*], the point at which a stimulus is great enough to produce an effect; for example, a pain threshold is the point at which a person becomes aware of pain.

threshold dose [AS, *therscold* + Gk, *dosis,* giving], a measure of a dose of radiation exposure defined in terms of conditions needed to produce a visible erythema in a given proportion of people exposed.

threshold limit values, the maximum concentration of a chemical to which workers can be exposed for a fixed period, such as 8 hours per day, without developing a physical impairment.

T

threshold of consciousness [AS, *therscold* + L, *conscire*, to be aware], the lowest limit of perception of a stimulus.

threshold stimulus [AS, *therscold* + L, *stimulare*, to incite], a stimulus that is just sufficient to produce a response. Below that level, no action or response is likely without additional intensity of the stimulus.

thrill [AS, *thyrlian*, to pierce], a fine vibration, felt by an examiner's hand on a patient's body over the site of an aneurysm or on the precordium, indicating the presence of an organic murmur of grade 4 or greater intensity.

thrix /thriks/ [GK], hair.

throb [ME, *throbben*, to beat intensely], a deep, pulsating kind of discomfort or pain.—**throbbing,** *adj., n.*

thrombasthenia /throm′basthē′nē·ə/ [Gk, *thrombos,* lump, *a* + *sthenos,* not strength], a rare hemorrhagic disease characterized by a defect in plateletmediated hemostasis caused by an abnormality in the membrane surface of the platelet. The platelets do not aggregate, a clot does not form, and hemorrhage ensues.

thrombectomy /thrombek′təmē/ [GK, *thrombos* + *ektome,* excision], the removal of a thrombus from a blood vessel, performed as emergency surgery to restore circulation to the affected part.

thrombin /throm′bin/, an enzyme formed from prothrombin, calcium, and thromboplastin in plasma during the clotting process. Thrombin causes fibrinogen to change to fibrin, which is essential in the formation of a clot.

thromboangiitis /throm′bō·an′jē·ī′tis/, an inflammation of the blood vessels associated with thrombosis and accompanied by destruction of the intima.

thromboangiitis obliterans [Gk, *thrombos* + *angeion,* vessel, *itis,* inflammation; L, *obliterare,* to cancel], an occlusive vascular condition, usually of a leg or a foot, in which the small and medium-sized arteries become inflamed and thrombotic. Early signs of the condition are burning, numbness, and tingling of the foot or leg distal to the lesion. Phlebitis and gangrene may develop as the disease progresses. Pulsation in the limb below the damaged blood vessels is often absent.

thromboarteritis /throm′bō·är′tərī′tis/, arterial inflammation with thrombus formation.

thrombocyst /throm′bəsist/, a membranous sac enclosing a thrombus.

thrombocytopathy /throm′bōsītop′əthē/ [Gk, *thrombos* + *kytos,* cell, *pathos,* disease], any disorder of the blood coagula-

tion mechanism caused by an abnormality or dysfunction of platelets.—**thrombocytopathic,** *adj.*

thrombocytopenia /throm′bōsī′təpē′nē·ə/ [Gk, *thrombos* + *kytos* + *penia,* poverty], reduction in the number of platelets. There may be decreased production of platelets, decreased survival of platelets, and increased consumption of platelets or splenomegaly. Thrombocytopenia is the most common cause of bleeding disorders.

thrombocytopenic purpura /-sī′təpē′nik/ [Gk, *thrombos* + *kytos,* cell, *penia,* poverty; L, *purpura,* purple], a bleeding disorder characterized by a marked decrease in the number of platelets, resulting in multiple bruises, petechiae, and hemorrhage into the tissues. Etiologies include infection and drug sensitivity and toxicity.

thrombocytosis /throm′bōsītō′sis/ [Gk, *thrombos* + *kytos* + *osis,* condition], an abnormal increase in the number of platelets in the blood. **Benign thrombocytosis,** or **secondary thrombocytosis,** is asymptomatic. **Essential thrombocythemia** is characterized by episodes of spontaneous bleeding alternating with thrombotic episodes.

thromboembolism /-em′bəliz′əm/ [Gk, *thrombos* + *embolos,* plug], a condition in which a blood vessel is blocked by an embolus carried in the bloodstream from the site of formation of the clot. The area supplied by an obstructed artery may tingle and become cold, numb, and cyanotic. An embolus in the lungs causes a sudden sharp thoracic or upper abdominal pain, dyspnea, cough, fever, and hemoptysis. Obstruction of the pulmonary artery or one of its main branches may be fatal.

thrombogenesis /-jen′əsis/, formation of a thrombus or blood clot.

thrombogenic /-jen′ik/ [Gk, *thrombos* + *genein,* to produce], pertaining to a thrombus or a factor causing a thrombus or clot.

thromboid /throm′boid/, **1.** clotlike. **2.** resembling a thrombus.

thrombolysis /thrombol′isis/, the dissolution of a thrombus.

thrombolytic /-lit′ik/ [Gk, *thrombos* + *lysis,* a loosening], pertaining to a drug or other agent that dissolves thrombi.

thrombolytic therapy (TT), administration of a thrombolytic agent such as tissue plasminogen activator, urokinase, or streptokinase to dissolve an arterial clot, such as a clot in a coronary artery in a patient with an acute myocardial infarction. TT is also used to dissolve clots (thrombus) in venous access devices.

thrombopathy /thrombop′əthē/, a condition in which there is a deficiency of clotting ability for reasons other than thrombocytopenia.

thrombophlebitis /-fləbī'tis/ [Gk, *thrombos* + *phleps*, vein, *itis*], inflammation of a vein, often accompanied by formation of a clot. It occurs most commonly as the result of trauma to the vessel wall; hypercoagulability of the blood; infection; chemical irritation; postoperative venous stasis; prolonged sitting, standing, or immobilization; or a long period of intravenous catheterization. Thrombophlebitis of a superficial vein is generally evident; the vessel feels hard and thready or cordlike and is extremely sensitive to pressure; the surrounding area may be erythematous and warm to the touch, and the entire limb may be pale, cold, and swollen. Deep vein thrombophlebitis is characterized by aching or cramping pain, especially in the calf when the patient walks or dorsiflexes the foot (Homans' sign).

thrombophlebitis purulenta, an inflammation of a vein associated with the formation of a soft purulent thrombus that infiltrates the wall of the vein.

thromboplastic /-plas'tik/, **1.** causing clot formation. **2.** pertaining to the role of thromboplastin in forming a clot.

thromboplastin /throm'bóplas'tin/ [Gk *thrombos* + *plassein*, to mold], a complex substance that initiates the clotting process by converting prothrombin to thrombin in the presence of calcium ion.

thrombosed /throm'bōst/, **1.** clotted. **2.** pertaining to a blood vessel in which a thrombus has formed.

thrombosis /thrombō'sis/, *pl.* **thromboses,** an abnormal vascular condition in which a clot (thrombus) develops within a blood vessel of the body.

thrombotic /thrombot'ik/ [Gk, *thrombos,* lump], caused or characterized by thrombosis.

thrombotic thrombocytopenic purpura (TTP) [Gk, *thrombos,* lump, *thrombos* + *kytos,* cell, *penia,* poverty; L, *purpura,* purple], a disorder characterized by thrombocytopenia, hemolytic anemia, and neurologic abnormalities. It is accompanied by a generalized purpura with the deposition of microthrombi within the capillaries and smaller arterioles.

thromboxane A₂ (TXA₂) /thrombok'sān/, a highly unstable, biologically active compound derived from the endoperoxide prostaglandin G_2. It increases concentration after injury to blood vessels and stimulates the primary hemostatic response and irreversible platelet aggregation.

thromboxane-A synthase, an enzyme that catalyzes the conversion in platelets of prostaglandin G_2 to thromboxane A_2. A deficiency of the enzyme causes a defect in the release of platelets.

thromboxane B₂ (XB₂), a stable metabolite of thromboxane A_2 that has some kind of effect on polymorphonuclear cells and may possess chemotactic activity. It is released during anaphylaxis in laboratory animals.

thromboxanes, compounds synthesized by platelets and other cells that cause platelet aggregation and vasoconstriction.

thrombus /throm'bəs/, *pl.* **thrombi** [Gk, *thrombos,* lump], an aggregation of platelets, fibrin, clotting factors, and the cellular elements of the blood attached to the interior wall of a vein or artery, sometimes occluding the lumen of the vessel.

through-and-through drainage /throō/ [ME, *thurgh* +S, *drachen,* tear drop], a method of irrigating a body organ by inserting two tubes, one to introduce the fluid and another to drain the fluid that accumulates within the organ.

through transmission, (in ultrasonography) the process of imaging by transmitting the sound field through a specimen and picking up the transmitted energy on a far surface or receiving transducer.

thrush [Dan, *troeske,* dryness], candidiasis of the tissues of the mouth. The condition is characterized by the appearance of creamy white patches of exudate on an inflamed tongue or buccal mucosa. It is usually a benign condition in normal children but may be a sign of human immunodeficiency virus infection in young adults.

thulium (Tm) /thoō'lē·əm/ [L, *Thule,* northern island], a rare earth metallic element. Its atomic number is 69; its atomic mass (weight) is 168.93.

thumb /thum/ [AS, *thuma*], the first and shortest digit of the hand, classified by some anatomists as one of the fingers because its metacarpal bone ossifies in the same manner as those of the phalanges. Other anatomists classify the thumb separately, noting that it has a much different articulation with the metacarpal bone (a saddle joint) and is composed of one metacarpal bone and only two phalanges.

thumb forceps, a surgical instrument used to grasp soft tissue, especially while suturing.

thumb sign [AS, *thuma* + L, *signum*], the flexing of the terminal phalanx of the thumb against the flexed index finger, as in holding a piece of paper. It is observed in patients who are unable to adduct the thumb because of an ulnar lesion.

thumbsucking, the habit of sucking the thumb for oral gratification. It is normal in infants and young children as a pleasure-seeking or comforting device, especially when the child is hungry or tired. The habit reaches its peak when the child is between 18 and 20 months of age, and it normally disappears as the child develops and matures.

thumps, **1.** hiccups. **2.** spasmodic contractions of the diaphragm.

thyme /tīm, thim/ [Gk, *thymon*], the dried leaves and flowering tops of an herb, *Thymus vulgaris,* which produces a pungent mintlike aroma. It is the source of a volatile oil, tannin, and gum but is used mainly as a flavoring agent.

thymectomy /thīmek′təmē/ [Gk, *thymus*], the surgical removal of the thymus.

thymi. See **thymus.**

thymic /thī′mik/, pertaining to the thymus gland.

thymidine (dThd) /thī′mədēn/, one of the four major nucleosides in deoxyribonucleic acid. It is formed by the condensation of thymin with deoxyribose.

thymin /thī′mīn/, a major pyrimidine base found in nucleotides and a fundamental constituent of deoxyribonucleic acid.

thymol /thī′mol/, a synthetic or natural thyme oil, used as an antibacterial and antifungal, that is an ingredient in some over-the-counter preparations for the treatment of hemorrhoids, acne, and tinea pedis.

thymoma /thīmō′mə/ [Gk, *thymos,* thyme, flowers, *oma* tumor], a usually benign tumor of the thymus gland that may be associated with myasthenia gravis or an immune deficiency disorder.

thymosin /thī′məsin/, **1.** a naturally occurring immunologic hormone secreted by the thymus gland. It is present in greatest amounts in young children and decreases in amount throughout life. **2.** an investigational drug derived from bovine thymus extracts and prescribed as an immunomodulator in experimental treatments.

thymus /thī′məs/, *pl.* **thymuses, thymi** [Gk, *thymos,* thyme, flowers], a single unpaired gland that is located in the mediastinum, extending superiorly into the neck to the lower edge of the thyroid gland and inferiorly as far as the fourth costal cartilage. The thymus is the primary central gland of the lymphatic system. The T cells of the cell-mediated immune response develop in this gland before migrating to the lymph nodes and spleen. The gland consists of two lateral lobes closely bound by connective tissue, which also encloses the entire organ in a capsule.

thymus-dependent antigen, an antigen that requires the interaction between T and B cells to initiate antibody production.

thymus-independent antigen, an antigen

that induces antibody (IgM) production without direct cooperation from T cells.

thyroaplasia /thī′rō·aplā′zhə/, variations in any of several defects in the thyroid gland and deficiencies of its secretions.

thyrocervical trunk /-sur′vikəl/ [Gk, *thyreos,* shield, *eidos,* form; L, *cervix,* neck, *truncus*], one of a pair of short thick arterial branches arising from the first part of the subclavian arteries close to the medial border of the scalenus anterior and supplying numerous muscles and bones in the head, neck, and back.

thyrocricotomy /-krīkot′əmē/ [Gk, *thyreos,* shield, *eidos,* form, *krikos,* ring, *temnein,* to cut], a tracheotomy procedure in which the cricovocal membrane is divided.

thyrogenic /-jen′ik/ [Gk, *thyreos,* shield, *eidos,* form, *genein,* to produce], pertaining to an origin in the thyroid gland.

thyroglobulin /-glōb′yəlin/, a purified extract of porcine thyroid prescribed in the treatment of cretinism, myxedema, goiter, and other hypothyroid states.

thyroglossal /-glos′əl/, pertaining to an embryonic duct connecting the thyroid gland and the tongue.

thyroid acropathy /thī′roid/ [Gk, *thyreos,* shield, *eidos,* form, *akron,* extremity, *pathos,* disease], swelling of subcutaneous tissue of the extremities and clubbing of the digits, occurring rarely in patients with thyroid disease and usually associated with pretibial myxedema or exophthalmos.

thyroid cancer, a neoplasm of the thyroid gland, usually characterized by slow growth and a slower and more prolonged clinical course than that of other malignancies. The first sign of cancer may be an increased size of the thyroid gland, a palpable nodule, hoarseness, dysphagia, dyspnea, or pain on pressure. More than half of thyroid malignancies are papillary carcinomas, about one third are follicular carcinomas, and the rest consist of rapidly growing invasive anaplastic carcinomas; medullary carcinomas that secrete calcitonin; and metastatic lesions from primary tumors in the breast, kidneys, or lungs.

thyroid cartilage, the largest cartilage of the larynx, consisting of two laminae fused together at an acute angle in the midline of the anterior neck to form the Adam's apple.

thyroid crisis [Gk, *thyreos,* shield, *eidos,* form, *krisis,* turning point], a sudden exacerbation of symptoms of thyrotoxicosis characterized by fever, sweating, tachycardia, extreme nervous excitability, and pulmonary edema. It usually occurs in a patient whose thyrotoxicosis treatment is inadequate, and the paroxysm is triggered by a stressful infection or injury. If untreated, the crisis is often fatal.

thyroid dermoid cyst, a tumor derived from embryonal tissues that is believed to have developed in the thyroid gland or in the thyrolingual duct.

thyroidectomized /thī'roidek'təmīzd/ [Gk, *thyreos,* shield, *eidos,* form, *ektome,* excision], pertaining to a patient or condition in which the thyroid gland has been removed.

thyroidectomy /thī'roidek'təmē/ [Gk, *thyreos* + *eidos,* form, *ektome,* excision], the surgical removal of the thyroid gland. It is performed for colloid goiter, tumors, or hyperthyroidism that does not respond to iodine therapy and antithyroid drugs. All but 5% to 10% of the gland is removed; regrowth usually begins shortly after surgery, and thyroid function may return to normal. For cancer of the thyroid, the entire gland is removed, along with surrounding structures from neck to collarbone, in a radical neck dissection.

thyroid function test, any of several laboratory tests performed to evaluate the function of the thyroid gland. Thyroid function tests include protein-bound iodine, butanol-extractable iodine, T_3, T_4, free thyroxine index, thyroxin-binding globulin, thyroid-stimulating hormone, long-acting thyroid stimulator, radioactive iodine uptake, and radioactive iodine excretion.

thyroid gland [Gk, *thyreos,* shield, *eidos,* form], a highly vascular organ at the front of the neck, usually weighing about 30 g, consisting of bilateral lobes connected in the middle by a narrow isthmus. It is slightly heavier in women than in men and enlarges during pregnancy. The majority of the thyroid gland secretes the hormone thyroxin, and other clusters of cells produce the hormone calcitonin. These hormones are secreted directly into the blood; thus the thyroid is part of the endocrine system of ductless glands. It is essential to normal body growth in infancy and childhood, and its removal greatly reduces the oxidative processes of the body, producing a lower metabolic rate characteristic of hypothyroidism.

thyroid hormone, an iodine-containing compound secreted by the thyroid gland, predominantly as thyroxine (T_4) and in smaller amounts as four times–more potent triiodothyronine (T_3). These hormones increase the rate of metabolism; affect body temperature; regulate protein, fat, and carbohydrate catabolism in all cells; maintain growth hormone secretion, skeletal maturation, and the cardiac rate, force, and output; promote central nervous system development; stimulate the synthesis of many enzymes; and are necessary for muscle tone and vigor. Derivatives of thyronine, T_4 and T_3, are synthesized in the thyroid gland by a complex process involving the uptake, oxidation, and incorporation of iodide and the production of thyroglobulin, the form in which the hormones apparently are stored in thyroid follicular colloid.

thyroiditis /thī'roidī'tis/, inflammation of the thyroid gland. Acute thyroiditis caused by staphylococcal, streptococcal, or other infections is characterized by suppuration and abscess formation and may progress to subacute diffuse disease of the gland. Subacute thyroiditis is marked by fever, weakness, sore throat, and a painfully enlarged gland containing granulomas composed of colloid masses surrounded by giant cells and mononuclear cells. Chronic lymphocytic thyroiditis (Hashimoto's disease), characterized by lymphocyte and plasma cell infiltration of the gland and diffuse enlargement, seems to be transmitted as a dominant trait and may be associated with various autoimmune disorders. Another chronic form of thyroiditis is Riedel's struma, a rare progressive fibrosis, usually of one lobe of the gland but sometimes involving both lobes; the trachea; and surrounding muscles, nerves, and blood vessels. Radiation thyroiditis occasionally occurs 7 to 10 days after the treatment of hyperthyroidism with radioactive iodine 131.

thyroid notch, 1. (superior) a separation above the anterior border of the thyroid cartilage. **2.** (inferior) a depression in the middle of the lower border of the thyroid cartilage.

thyroid-stimulating hormone (TSH), a substance secreted by the anterior lobe of the pituitary gland that controls the release of thyroid hormone and is necessary for the growth and function of the thyroid gland. The secretion of TSH is regulated by thyrotropin-releasing factor, elaborated in the median eminence of the hypothalamus.

thyroid storm, a crisis in uncontrolled hyperthyroidism caused by the release into the bloodstream of increased amounts of thyroid hormones. The storm may occur spontaneously or be precipitated by infection, stress, or a thyroidectomy performed on a patient who is inadequately prepared with antithyroid drugs. Characteristic signs are fever that may reach 106° F, a rapid pulse, acute respiratory distress, apprehension, restlessness, irritability, and prostration. The patient may become delirious, lapse into a coma, and die of heart failure.

thyroliberin /thī′rōlib′ərin/, a tripeptide hormone produced by the hypothalamus that stimulates the anterior pituitary gland to release thyrotropin.

thyromegaly /-meg′əlē/ [Gk, *thyreos,* shield, *eidos,* form, *megas,* large], enlargement of the thyroid gland.

thyrotoxic myopathy /-tok′sik/, a condition in thyrotoxicosis consisting of severe weakness in the limb and trunk muscles, including those used in speech and swallowing.

thyrotoxin /-tok′sin/, a theoretic cytotoxin of the thyroid gland, assumed to be a cause of the signs and symptoms of thyrotoxicosis.

thyrotrophic /-trof′ik/ [Gk, *thyreos,* shield, *eidos,* form, *trophe,* nutrition], influencing the thyroid gland, such as the thyroid-stimulating hormone.

thyrotropin (systemic) /-trō′pin/, a preparation of bovine thyroid-stimulating hormone that increases the uptake of radioactive iodine in the thyroid and the secretion of thyroxine by the thyroid. It is prescribed in diagnostic tests and in the treatment of thyroid cancer.

thyrotropin-releasing hormone, a substance produced in the hypothalamus that stimulates the release of thyrotropin (thyroid-stimulating hormone) from the anterior lobe of the pituitary gland.

thyroxine (T₄) /thīrok′sēn/, a hormone of the thyroid gland, derived from tyrosine, that influences metabolic rate.

thyroxine-binding globulin, a plasma protein that binds with and transports thyroxine in the blood.

Ti, symbol for the element **titanium.**

TI, abbreviation for *therapeutic index.*

TIA, abbreviation for **transient ischemic attack.**

tibia /tib′ē·ə/ [L, shin bone], the second longest bone of the skeleton, located at the medial side of the leg. It articulates with the fibula laterally, the talus distally, and the femur proximally, forming part of the knee joint.

tibial /tib′ē·əl/ [L, *tibia,* shin bone], pertaining to the largest long bone of the lower leg.

tibialis anterior /tib′ē·ā′lis/ [L, *tibia* + *anticus,* in front], one of the anterior crural muscles of the leg, situated on the lateral side of the tibia. It dorsiflexes and supinates the foot.

tibial torsion [L, *tibia* + *torquere,* to twist], a lateral or a medial twisting rotation of the tibia on its longitudinal axis.

tibia valga [L, *tibia,* shin bone, *valgus,* bowlegged], a bowed tibia with the convex surface toward the outside of the leg.

ticarcillin /tik′ärsil′in/, an antibiotic prescribed in the treatment of bacterial septicemia, as well as skin, soft tissue, and respiratory infections caused by both gram-negative and gram-positive organisms.

tic douloureux /tikdōōlōōroe′/ [Fr, painful spasm], a brief extremely painful attack of trigeminal neuralgia. It is unilateral and limited to the distribution of the trigeminal (fifth cranial) nerve. An attack is easily and unexpectedly provoked by any stimulus of the facial muscles, from touching to speaking, and may occur repetitively.

tick bite [ME, *tike* + AS, *bitan,* to bite], a puncture wound produced by the toothed beak of a blood-sucking tick, a small, tough-skinned, arachnid. Ticks transmit several diseases to humans, and a few species carry a neurotoxin in their saliva that may cause ascending paralysis beginning in the legs. Nervousness, loss of appetite, tingling, and headache, followed by muscle pain and in extreme cases respiratory failure, may occur.

tick-borne rickettsiosis [ME, *tike* + *beren* + *Rickettsia* + Gk, *osis,* condition], any disease transmitted by Ixodid ticks carrying the *Rickettsia* pathogens, microorganisms smaller than bacteria but larger than viruses. A common infectious species in North America is *Rickettsia rickettsii,* the cause of Rocky Mountain spotted fever.

tickling, a gentle stimulation of the skin surface that produces pleasurable reflexes.

tick paralysis, a rare progressive reversible disorder caused by several species of ticks that release a neurotoxin that causes weakness, incoordination, and paralysis. The tick must feed on the host for several days before the symptoms appear, and removal of the tick leads to rapid recovery.

t.i.d., (in prescriptions) abbreviation for the Latin phrase *ter in die* /dē′ä/, 'three times a day.'

tidal /tī′dəl/ [AS, *tid,* time] pertaining to an alternating process, such as a rise-and-fall, ebb-and-flow, or periodic lapse of time.

tidal volume (TV) [AS, *tid,* time; L, *volumen,* paper roll], the amount of air inhaled and exhaled during normal ventilation. Inspiratory reserve volume, expiratory reserve volume, and tidal volume make up vital capacity.

tide [AS, *tid*], a variation, increase or decrease, in the concentration of a particular component of body fluids, such as acid tide, fat tide.—**tidal,** *adj.*

tidemark, a transitional zone, appearing as a wavy line, that marks the junction between calcified and uncalcified cartilage.

Tietze's syndrome /tēt′sēz/ [Alexander Tietze, German surgeon, 1864–1927], **1.** a disorder characterized by nonsuppurative swellings of one or more costal cartilages causing pain that may radiate to the neck, shoulder, or arm and mimic the pain of coronary artery disease. **2.** albinism, except for normal eye pigment, accompanied by deaf mutism and hypoplasia of the eyebrows.

TIG, abbreviation for **tetanus immune globulin.**

tight junction /tīt/ [ME, *thight,* strong; L, *jungere,* to join], the zonula occludens of the junctional complex between cells in which the plasma membranes of adjacent cells are in direct contact and where there is no intercellular space.

tilt table [AS, *tealt,* unsteady; Fr, *tablette*], an examining table that allows the patient to be raised to an approximate 60-degree angle during study of the response of a patient's circulatory system to gravitational forces.

timbre /tim′bər/ [Fr], **1.** a characteristic sound quality of a voice or musical instrument, as determined by harmonics of the sound and distinguished from intensity and pitch. **2.** a second metallic sound heard in aortic dilation.

time (t) [AS, *tima*], **1.** a measure of duration. **2.** an interval separating two points in a continuum between the past and future.

time constant, (in pulmonary physiology) the factors determining rate of flow in the airways.

timed collection, the collection of a specimen such as a urine or stool sample for a specific period of time.

time delay, a period between the application of an input and the beginning of the response.

timed vital capacity [AS, *tima* + L, *vita,* life, *capacitas*], a diagnostic test of certain lung disorders determined by the percentage of predicted vital capacity that adults can expire forcefully for at least 3 seconds after a maximal inspiration.

timolol maleate /tim′əlōl/, a beta adrenergic receptor blocking agent prescribed for reducing intraocular pressure in chronic open-angle, aphakic, and secondary glaucoma.

tin (Sn) [AS], a whitish metallic element. Its atomic number is 50; its atomic mass (weight) is 118.69. Tin oxide is used in dentistry as a polishing agent for teeth and in some restorative procedures.

tinct., abbreviation for tincture.

tincture (tinct). /tingk′chər/, a substance in a solution that is diluted with alcohol.

tine, a sharp projecting point, as a prong of a fork.

tinea /tin′ē·ə/ [L, worm], a group of fungal skin diseases caused by dermatophytes of several kinds. The condition is characterized by itching, scaling, and sometimes painful lesions.

tinea capitis, a superficial fungal infection of the scalp, most common in children. Most infections are caused by species of *Trichophyton.* The infection may lead to hair loss and become secondarily infected with bacteria, causing a severe inflammation. Symptoms include severe itching and scaling of the scalp.

tinea corporis, a superficial fungal infection of the nonhairy skin of the body, most prevalent in hot, humid climates and usually caused by species of *Trichophyton* or *Microsporum.*

tinea cruris /krōō′ris/, a superficial fungal infection of the groin caused by species of *Trichophyton* or *Epidermophyton floccosum.* It is most common in the tropics and among males.

tinea pedis, a chronic superficial fungal infection of the foot, especially of the skin between the toes and on the soles. It is common worldwide and is usually caused by *Trichophyton mentagrophytes, T. rubrum,* and *Epidermophyton floccosum.*

tinea unguium /un′gwē·əm/, a superficial fungal infection of the nails caused by various species of *Trichophyton* and occasionally by *Candida albicans.* It is more common on the toes than the fingers and can cause complete crumbling and destruction of the nails.

tinea versicolor, a fungal infection of the skin caused by *Malassezia furfur* and characterized by finely desquamating, pale tan patches on the upper trunk and upper arms that may itch and do not tan. The fungus fluoresces under Wood's light and may be easily identified in scrapings viewed under a microscope.

Tinel's sign /tinelz′/ [Jules Tinel, French neurosurgeon, 1879–1952], an indication of irritability of a nerve, resulting in a distal tingling sensation on percussion of a damaged nerve.

tine test /tīn/ [ME, *tind,* rake tooth; L, *testum,* crucible], a tuberculin skin test in which a small disposable disk with multiple tines bearing tuberculin antigen is used to puncture the skin. The method is widely used to test for sensitivity to the tuberculin antigen. Induration around the puncture site indicates previous exposure or active disease, requiring further testing.

tingling [ME, *tinklen,* to tinkle], a prickly sensation in the skin or a body part, ac-

tinnitus /tinī'təs/ [L, *tinnire,* to tinkle], a subjective noise sensation, often described as ringing, heard in one or both ears. It may be a sign of acoustic trauma, Ménière's disease, otosclerosis, presbycusis, or an accumulation of cerumen impinging on the eardrum or occluding the external auditory canal.

tint, a shade or gradation of a color, usually a pale or less saturated version of the basic shade.

tinted denture base, a denture base that resembles the coloring of natural oral tissue.

tip, 1. the end of a pointed object. **2.** an attachment fitted to the end of something else. **3.** a point.

tipped uterus /tipt/ [ME, *tipen,* upset; L, *uterus,* womb], a uterus that is displaced from its normal position.

tip pinch, a grasp in which the tip of the thumb is pressed against any or each of the tips of the other fingers.

tipping, a tooth movement in which the angle of the tooth's long axis is changed.

tip seal, the closure of an ampule accomplished by melting a bead of glass at the neck of the ampule.

tisane /tizän', tizän'/, a tealike infusion or light drink of a vegetable herb consumed for a claimed medicinal effect.

tissue /tish'oo/ [Fr, *tissu,* fabric], a collection of similar cells acting together to perform a particular function.

tissue bank, a facility for storing and maintaining a collection of tissues for future use in transplants.

tissue-base relationship, (in dentistry) the relationship of the bottom of a removable prosthesis to underlying structures.

tissue committee, a group that evaluates all surgery performed in a hospital or other health care facility.

tissue culture [OFr, *tissu* + L, *colere,* to cultivate], the maintenance of growth in vitro, under artificial conditions, of tissue or organ specimens.

tissue dose, (in radiotherapy) the amount of radiation absorbed by tissue in the region of interest, expressed in rad.

tissue fixation, a process in which a tissue specimen is placed in a fluid that preserves the cells as nearly as possible in their natural state.

tissue fixative, a fluid that preserves cells in their natural state so they may be identified and examined.

tissue integrity, impaired, a NANDA-accepted nursing diagnosis of a state in which an individual experiences damage to mucous membrane, corneal, integumen-tary, or subcutaneous tissue. The principal characteristic is damaged or destroyed tissue.

tissue macrophage [OFr, *tissu* + Gk, *makros,* large, *phagein,* to eat], a large mobile, highly phagocytic cell derived from monocytes. These cells become mobile when stimulated by inflammation, migrating to the affected area.

tissue perfusion, altered (renal, cerebral, cardiopulmonary, gastrointestinal, peripheral), a NANDA-accepted nursing diagnosis of a state in which an individual experiences a decrease in nutrition and oxygenation at the cellular level caused by a deficit in capillary blood supply. Defining characteristics include coldness of the affected extremity, paleness on elevation of the extremity, diminished arterial pulses, and changes in the arterial blood pressure when measured in the affected extremity. Claudication, gangrene, brittle nails, slowly healing ulcers or wounds, shiny skin, and lack of hair are also common.

tissue plasminogen activator (TPA), a clot-dissolving substance produced naturally by cells in the walls of blood vessels. TPA activates plasminogen to dissolve clots and has been used therapeutically to dissolve blood clots blocking coronary arteries.

tissue response, any reaction or change in living cellular tissue when it is acted on by disease, toxin, or other external stimulus. Some kinds of tissue responses are **immune response, inflammation,** and **necrosis.**

tissue review, a review of the surgery performed in a hospital or other health care facility. The evaluation is usually made on the basis of the extent of agreement of the preoperative, postoperative, and pathologic diagnoses and on the relevance and acceptability of the diagnostic procedures.

tissue typing, a systematized series of tests to evaluate the intraspecies compatibility of tissues from a donor and a recipient before transplantation.

titanium (Ti) /tītā'nē-əm/ [Gk, *Titan,* mythic giant], a grayish brittle metallic element. Its atomic number is 22; its atomic mass (weight) is 47.88. Titanium dioxide is the active ingredient in a number of topical ointments and lotions.

titer /tī'tər/ [Fr, *titre,* to make a standard] **1.** the normality of a solution or substance, determined by titration to find the equivalence of two reactants. **2.** the extent to which an antibody can be diluted before losing its power to react with a specific antigen. **3.** the highest dilution of a serum that causes clumping of bacteria.

titillation /tit′ilā′shən/ [L, *titillare,* to tickle], tickling.

Title [L, *titulus,* title], a section of the Social Security Act that provides for the establishment, funding, and regulation of a service to a specific segment of the population. Examples include Title XIX, which includes medical coverage under Medicaid.

titration /tī′trā′shən/, a method of estimating the amount of solute in a solution. The solution is added in small, measured quantities to a known volume of a standard solution until a reaction occurs, as indicated by a change in color or pH or the liberation of a chemical product.

titubation /tich′əbā′shən/ b [L, *titubare,* to stagger], unsteady posture characterized by a staggering or stumbling gait and a swaying head or trunk while sitting. It may be a manifestation of cerebellar disease.

Tl, symbol for the element **thallium.**

TLC, 1. abbreviation for **total lung capacity. 2.** *informal.* abbreviation for *tender loving care.*

TLI, abbreviation for **total lymphoid irradiation.**

TLR, abbreviation for **tonic labyrinthine reflex.**

Tm, symbol for the element **thulium.**

TM, abbreviation for **transcendental meditation.**

TMJ, abbreviation for **temporomandibular joint.**

TMP/SMX, abbreviation for *trimethoprim sulfamethoxazole.*

TNF, abbreviation for **tumor necrosis factor.**

TNM, a system for staging malignant neoplastic disease.

t.n.t.c., abbreviation for *too numerous to count,* usually applied to organisms or cells viewed on a slide under a microscope.

t.o., abbreviation for *telephone order.*

toadstool poisoning /tōd′stōol/ [AS, *tadige* + *stol* + L, *potio,* drink], a toxic condition caused by ingestion of certain varieties of poisonous mushrooms.

tobacco /təbak′ō/ [Sp, *tabaco*], a plant whose leaves are dried and used for smoking and chewing, and in snuff.

tobacco withdrawal syndrome, a change in mood or performance associated with the cessation of or reduction in exposure to nicotine. Symptoms may range from lack of concentration to anxiety and temper outbursts.

TOBEC, abbreviation for **total body electrical conductivity.**

tobramycin sulfate /tō′brəmī′sin/, an aminoglycoside antibiotic prescribed in the treatment of external ocular infection, septicemia, and lower respiratory tract and central nervous system infections.

Tobruk plaster /tō′brŏŏk/, a plaster cast splint with tapes for skin traction coming through openings in the plaster and connected with Thomas' splint. It covers and immobilizes the leg from foot to groin.

tocainide hydrochloride /tōkā′nīd/, an oral lidocaine-type antiarrhythmic prescribed for the suppression of symptomatic ventricular arrhythmias.

tocodynamometer /tō′kōdī′nəmom′ətər/ [Gk, *tokos,* birth, *dynamis,* force, *metron,* measure], an electronic device for monitoring and recording uterine contractions in labor. It consists of a pressure transducer that is applied to the fundus of the uterus by means of a belt, which is connected to a machine that records the duration of the contractions and the interval between them on graph paper.

tocolytic drug /-lit′ik/, any drug used to suppress premature labor.

tocopherolquinone (TQ) /tōkof′ərōlkwī′-nōn/, an oxidized form of tocopherol, or vitamin E.

tocotransducer /-transd(y)ōō′sər/ [Gk, *tokos* + L, *trans,* through, *ducer,* to lead], an electronic device used to measure uterine contractions.

toddler [ME, *toteren,* to walk unsteadily], a child between 12 and 36 months of age. During this period of development the child acquires a sense of autonomy and independence through the mastery of various specialized tasks such as control of body functions, refinement of motor and language skills, and acquisition of socially acceptable behavior.

toddlerhood /tod′lərhŏŏd′/, the state or condition of being a toddler.

Todd's paralysis [Robert Bentley Todd, English physician, 1809–1860; Gk, *paralyein,* to be palsied], a transient postictal paralysis of a limb or limbs.

toe, any one of the digits of the feet.

toe clonus [AS, *tá* + Gk, *klonos*], an increased reflex activity in the large toe caused by a sudden extension of the first phalanx.

toe drop [AS, *tá* + *dropa*], a condition in which the toes droop and cannot be lifted because of paralysis of the tibial muscles.

toenail [AS, *ta* + *naegel*], one of the heavy ungual structures covering the terminal phalanges of the toes.

togaviruses /tō′gəvī′rəsəs/ [L, *toga,* cloak, *virus,* poison], a family of arboviruses that includes the organisms causing encephalitis, dengue, yellow fever, and rubella.

toilet training, the process of teaching a child to control the functions of the bladder and bowel. Training often begins around 24 months of age, when voluntary control of the anal and urethral sphincters is achieved by most children. Nighttime bladder control may not be achieved until the child is 4 or 5 years of age or older.

token economy [AS, *tacen,* to show; Gk, *oikonomia,* household management], a technique of reinforcement used in behavior therapy in the management of a group of people, such as in hospitals, institutions, or classrooms. Individuals are rewarded for specific activities or behavior with tokens they can exchange for desired objects or privileges.

tolazamide /tolaz′əmid/, an oral sulfonylurea antidiabetic prescribed in the treatment of stable or noninsulin-dependent diabetes mellitus and for some patients sensitive to other types of sulfonylureas or who have failed to respond to other similar drugs.

tolazoline hydrochloride /tolaz′əlēn/, a peripheral vasodilator prescribed in the treatment of spastic peripheral vascular disorders, including Buerger's disease, Raynaud's disease, and scleroderma.

tolbutamide /tolbōō′təmīd/, an oral sulfonylurea antidiabetic prescribed in the treatment of stable noninsulin-dependent diabetes mellitus uncontrolled by diet alone and for some patients changing from insulin to oral therapy.

tolerance /tol′ərəns/ [L, *tolerare,* to endure], a phenomenon by which the body becomes increasingly resistant to a drug or other substance through continued exposure to exposure to the substance. A kind of tolerance is **work tolerance.**

tolerance test, 1. an investigation of the ability of a body to metabolize a drug or nutrient, such as a glucose tolerance test. 2. a physical activity drill administered to evaluate the efficiency of blood circulation or other body system.

tolmetin sodium /tol′mətin/, a nonsteroidal antiinflammatory agent prescribed primarily in the treatment of rheumatoid arthritis, juvenile rheumatoid arthritis, and osteoarthritis.

tolnaftate /tolnaf′tāt/, an antifungal prescribed in the treatment of superficial fungus infections of the skin, including tinea pedis, tinea cruris, and tinea versicolor.

toluene (C₇H₈) /tol′yōō-ēn/, an aromatic colorless flammable liquid produced from coal tar, petroleum, or Peruvian tolu balsam. It is used in dyes, explosives, gums, and lacquers and in the manufacture of

drugs and the extraction of organic chemicals from plants.

Tomlin, Evelyn M. See **Modeling and Role Modeling.**

tomogram /tō′məgram′/ [Gk, *tome,* section, *gramma,* record], a radiograph produced by tomography.

tomograph /tō′məgraf′/ [Gk, *tome,* section, *graphein,* to record], a radiographic apparatus that makes an image of layers of body tissues at various depths.

tomographic DSA /-graf′ik/, the visualization of blood vessels in the body in three dimensions.

tomography /təmog′rəfē/ [Gk, *tome* + *graphein,* to record], 1. sectional imaging. 2. a radiographic technique in which the tube and film are made to move synchronously during exposure, producing a blurred radiograph in which objects within the focal plane are seen better than objects outside the focal plane. 3. a radiographic technique that produces a film representing a detailed cross section of tissue structure at a predetermined depth. It is a valuable diagnostic tool for the discovery and identification of space-occupying lesions such as might be found in the brain, liver, pancreas, and gallbladder.

tone deafness [Gk, *tonos,* stretching; AS, *deaf*], an inability to detect the pitch or changing pitch of a musical note or a voice change.

tongue /tung/ [AS, *tunge*], the principal organ of the sense of taste that also assists in the mastication and deglutition of food. It is located in the floor of the mouth within the curve of the mandible. Its root is connected to the hyoid bone posteriorly. It is also connected to the epiglottis, soft palate, and pharynx. The use of the tongue as an organ of speech is not anatomic but a secondary acquired characteristic.

tongue-thrust swallow, an immature form of swallowing in which the tongue is projected forward instead of retracted during the act of swallowing. It may result in forward displacement of the maxilla with consequent malocclusion of the teeth.

tonic /ton′ik/, pertaining to a type of afferent or sensory nerve receptor that responds to length changes placed on the noncontractile part of a muscle spindle. It may be triggered by a mechanical external force such as positioning or by an internal stretch caused by intrafusal muscle contraction.

tonic-clonic seizure, an epileptic seizure characterized by a generalized involuntary muscular contraction and cessation of respiration followed by tonic and clonic spasms of the muscles. Breathing resumes with noisy respirations. The teeth may be clenched, the tongue bitten, and control of the bladder or bowel lost. As this phase of the seizure passes, the person may fall asleep or experience confusion. Usually the person has no recall of the seizure on awakening. A sensory warning, or aura, can precede each tonic-clonic seizure.

tonic convulsion [Gk, *tonos*, stretching; L, *convulsio*, cramp], a prolonged generalized contraction of the skeletal muscles.

tonicity /tōnis′itē/ [Gk, *tonikos*, stretching], the quality of possessing tone, or tonus.

tonic labyrinthine reflex [Gk, *tonikos* + *labyrinthos*, maze; L, *reflectere*, to bend back], a normal postural reflex in animals, abnormally accentuated in decerebrate humans, characterized by extension of all four limbs when the head is positioned in space at an angle above the horizontal in quadripeds or in the neutral erect position in humans.

tonic neck reflex, a normal response in newborns to extend the arm and leg on the side of the body to which the head is quickly turned while the infant is supine and to flex the limbs of the opposite side. The reflex prevents the infant from rolling over until adequate neurologic and motor development occurs.

tonic spasm [Gk, *tonos,* stretching, *spasmos*], a sustained contraction of a muscle as distinguished from a transient clonic contraction.

tonitrophobia /tonit′rōfō′bē-ə/, an abnormal fear of thunder.

tonoclonic /ton′əklon′ik/ [Gk, *tonos,* stretching, *klonos,* tumult], pertaining to muscular spasms that are tonic and then clonic.

tonofibril /ton′əfī′bril/ [Gk, *tonos,* stretching, *fibrilla,* small fiber], a bundle of fine filaments found in the cytoplasm of epithelial cells. The individual strands, or **tonofilaments,** spread throughout the cytoplasm and extend into the intercellular bridge to converge at the desmosome.

tonofilament /ton′ōfil′əmənt [Gk, *tonos,* stretching], a proteinaceous fiber found in epithelial cells. Bundles of tonofilaments form a tonofibril, which has a supporting function.

tonograph /ton′əgraf/, an apparatus that makes a record of tension measurements.

tonography /tōnog′rəfē/, 1. the measurement of intraocular pressure. 2. the measurement of tension.

tonometer /tōnom′ətər/ [Gk, *tonos* + *metron,* measure], an instrument used in measuring tension or pressure, especially intraocular pressure.

tonometry /tōnom′ətrē/, the measuring of intraocular pressure by determining the resistance of the eyeball to indentation by an applied force. The air-puff tonometer, which does not touch the eye, records deflections of the cornea from a puff of pressurized air. The Schiötz impression and the applanation tonometers record the pressure needed to indent or flatten the corneal surface.

tonoscillograph /ton′əsil′əgraf′/, an apparatus that records arterial and capillary pressures with a corresponding pulse tracing.

tonsil /ton′səl/ [L, *tonsilla*], a small rounded mass of tissue, especially lymphoid tissue, such as that composing the palatine tonsils in the oropharynx.

tonsillar /ton′silər/ [L, *tonsilla*] pertaining to the palatine tonsil.

tonsillar crypt [L, *tonsilla* + Gk, *kryptos,* hidden], a small tubular invagination on the surface of a palatine or pharyngeal tonsil.

tonsillar herniation [L, *tonsilla* + *hernia,* rupture], the herniation of tonsils of the cerebellum through the foramen magnum of the skull. It may occur as a result of intracranial pressure from an injury or tumor.

tonsillectomy /ton′silek′təmē/ [L, *tonsilla* + Gk, *ektome,* excision], the surgical excision of the palatine tonsils, performed to prevent recurrent tonsillitis.

tonsillitis /-ī′tis/, an infection or inflammation of a tonsil. Acute tonsillitis, frequently caused by *Streptococcus* infection, is characterized by severe sore throat, fever, headache, malaise, difficulty in swallowing, earache, and enlarged tender lymph nodes in the neck. Acute tonsillitis may accompany scarlet fever.

tonsilloadenoidectomy /ton′silō·ad′ənoidek′təmē/ [L, *tonsilla* + Gk, *aden,* gland, *eidos,* form, *ektome,* excision], the surgical removal of tonsil and adenoid tissues.

tonus /tō′nəs/ [Gk, *tonos,* stretching], 1. the normal state of balanced tension in the body tissues, especially the muscles. Partial contraction or alternate contraction and relaxation of neighboring fibers of a group of muscles hold the organ or the part of the body in a neutral functional position without fatigue. 2. the state of the body tissues being strong and fit.

tooth, *pl.* **teeth** [AS, *toth*], any one of numerous dental structures that develop in the jaws. Each tooth consists of a crown, which projects above the gum; two to four roots embedded in the alveolus; and a neck, which stretches between the crown and the root. Each tooth also contains a cavity filled with pulp, richly supplied with blood vessels and nerves that enter the cavity through a small aperture at the base of each root. The solid part of the tooth consists of dentin, enamel, and a thin layer of bone on the surface of the root. The dentin composes the bulk of the tooth. The enamel covers the exposed part of the crown. Two sets of teeth appear at different periods of life: the 20 deciduous teeth appear during infancy, the 32 permanent teeth during childhood and early adulthood.

tooth abscess [AS, *toth* + L, *abscedere,* to go away], a collection of pus, usually close to the root of a tooth and often the result of an untreated cavity. If untreated, the pressure of the abscess may destroy the alveolar bone and adjoining soft tissues.

toothache /tōō'thāk/ [AS, *toth* + *aeca*], a pain in a tooth, usually caused by caries that has extended into the dentin or pulp or by traumatic occlusion.

tooth alignment, the arrangement of the teeth in relation to their supporting bone or alveolar process, adjacent teeth, and opposing dentitions.

tooth bleaching, the process of removing stains or color from teeth by applying chemicals such as hydrogen peroxide.

tooth-borne, describing a dental prosthesis or part of a prosthesis that depends entirely on abutment teeth for support.

tooth-borne base, a denture base restoring an edentulous area that has abutment teeth at each end for support.

toothbrush, an implement of various designs, with bristles fixed to a head at the end of a handle, used for brushing and cleaning the teeth and cleaning and massaging the gingival tissues.

tooth form, the identifying curves, lines, angles, and contours of a tooth that differentiate it from other teeth.

tooth fulcrum, axis of movement of a tooth subjected to lateral forces, considered to be at the middle third of the part of the tooth root embedded in the alveolus.

tooth germ, a primitive cell in the embryo that is the precursor of a tooth.

tooth inclination, the angle of slope of a tooth or teeth from the vertical plane, such as mesially, distally, lingually, buccally, or labially inclined.

tooth rotation [AS, *toth* + L, *rotare,* to rotate], **1.** the malposition of a tooth that has turned around its longitudinal axis or that has been turned by an orthodontic appliance to a normal position. **2.** the process by which the tooth is turned.

TOP, abbreviation for **temporal, occipital, and parietal** bones of the skull.

tophaceous /tōfā′shəs/, pertaining to the presence of tophi.

tophaceous gout [L, *tufa,* porous rock], a form of purine metabolism disorder characterized by formation of chalky deposits of sodium biurate under the skin and in the joints. If untreated, the deposits may eventually destroy the involved joints.

tophus /tō′fəs/, *pl.* **tophi** [L, *tufa,* porous rock], a calculus containing sodium urate deposits that develops in periarticular fibrous tissue, typically in patients with gout.

topical /top′ikəl/ [Gk, *topos,* place], **1.** pertaining to the surface of a part of the body. **2.** pertaining to a drug or treatment applied topically.

topical anesthesia, surface analgesia produced by application of a topical anesthetic in the form of a solution, gel, or ointment to the skin, mucous membrane, or cornea.

topognosis /top′ognō′sis/ [Gk, *topos* + *gnosis,* recognition], the ability to recognize tactile stimuli.

topogometer /top′ōgom′ətər/, [Gk, *topos,* place, *gonia,* angle, *metron,* measure], a movable fixation target attached to an instrument for measuring the radius of curvature of the cornea. It is used in fitting contact lenses of correct curvature.

topographic /top′əgraf′ik/, (in psychiatry) pertaining to a freudian conceptualization of the layers of human consciousness.

topographic anatomy [Gk, *topos,* place, *graphein,* to record, *ana* + *temnein,* to cut], the study of a specific region of a body structure such as a lower leg, including all of the systems in the part and their relationship to each other.

topographic disorientation, a psychiatric disorder based on Freud's topographic model of the mental apparatus, consisting of conscious, preconscious, and unconscious systems for interpreting perceptions of the outside world and internal perceptions.

topography /təpog′refē/ [Gk, *topos,* place, *graphein,* to record], the anatomic description of a body part in terms of the region in which it is located.

topology /topol′əjē/, **1.** orientation of the presenting part of a fetus. **2.** the study of special regions of anatomy. **3.** the science of properties of geometric configuration.

TOPV, abbreviation for *trivalent oral polio vaccine.*

TORCH /tôrch/, abbreviation for *toxoplasmosis, other, rubella virus, cytomegalovirus, and herpes simplex viruses,* a group of agents that can infect the fetus or the newborn, causing a constellation of morbid effects called the TORCH syndrome.

TORCH syndrome, infection of the fetus or newborn by one of the TORCH agents. The outcome of a pregnancy complicated by a TORCH agent may be abortion, stillbirth, intrauterine growth retardation, or premature delivery. At delivery and during the first days after birth an infant infected with any one of the organisms may demonstrate various clinical manifestations such as fever, lethargy, poor feeding, petechiae on the skin, purpura, and pneumonia. Each of the agents is associated with several other abnormal clinical findings involving abnormal immune response, cataracts, glaucoma, vesicles, ulcers, and congenital cardiac defects.

torose /tôr′ōs/ [L, *torosus,* bulging], knoblike, knobby, or bulging.

torpor /tôr′pər/, **1.** a state of mental or physical inactivity. **2.** an absence or slowness of response to a stimulus.

torque /tôrk/ [L, *torquere,* to twist], **1.** a twisting force produced by contraction of the medial femoral muscles that tend to rotate the thigh medially. **2.** (in dentistry) a force applied to a tooth to rotate it on a mesiodistal or buccolingual axis. **3.** a rotary force applied to a denture base.

torr /tôr/ [Evangelista Torricelli, Italian physicist, 1608–1647], a unit of pressure equal to 1333.22 dynes/cm2, or 1.33322 millibars. One torr is the pressure required to support a column of mercury 1 mm high when the mercury is of standard density and subjected to standard acceleration.

torsades de pointes /tôrsäd′ depô·aNt′, tôr′säd dəpoint′/ [Fr, *torsader,* to twist together, *pointes,* tips], a type of ventricular tachycardia with a spiral-like appearance ("twisting of the points") and complexes that at first look positive and then negative on an electrocardiogram. It is precipitated by a long QT interval, which often is drug induced, but which may be the result of hypokalemia or profound bradycardia.

torsiometer /tôr′sē·om′ətər/, a device for measuring the amount of torsion of an eye around its anteroposterior axis.

torsion /tôr′shən/ [L, *torquere,* to twist], **1.** the process of twisting in a positive (clockwise) or negative (counterclockwise) direction. **2.** the state of being turned. **3.** (in dentistry) the twisting of a tooth on its long axis.

torsion fracture, a spiral fracture, usually caused by a torsion injury.

torsion of the testis, the axial rotation of the spermatic cord that cuts off the blood supply to the testicle, epididymis, and other structures. Complete ischemia for 6 hours may result in gangrene of the testis.

Partial loss of circulation may result in atrophy.

torso /tôr′sō/ [L, *thyrsus,* stem], the body excluding the limbs.

tort [L, *tortus,* twisted], (in law) a civil wrong, other than a breach of contract. Torts include negligence, false imprisonment, assault, and battery. The elements of a tort are: a legal duty owed by the defendant to the plaintiff, a breach of duty, and damage from the breach of duty.—**tortious,** *adj.*

torticollis /tôr′tikol′is/ [L, *tortus,* twisted, *collum,* neck], an abnormal condition in which the head is inclined to one side as a result of the contraction of the muscles on that side of the neck. It may be congenital or acquired.

tortipelvis /-pel′vis/ [L, *tortus,* twisted, *pelvis,* basin], a form of muscular dystonia resulting in a distortion of the pelvis or the spine and hips.

tortuous /tôr′cho͞o·əs/ [L, *tortus,* twisted], having or making twists and turns.

torulopsosis /tôr′yəlopsō′sis, tôr′yo͞olop′-səsis/ [L, *torulus,* small swelling; Gk, *opsis,* appearance, *osis,* condition], an infection with the yeast *Torulopsis glabrata,* a normal inhabitant of the oropharynx, gastrointestinal tract, and skin that causes disease in severely debilitated patients or in those with impaired immune function.

torus palatinus [L, *torus,* swelling, *palatum,* palate], a bony ridge along the hard palate at the line of fusion of the left and right jawbone segments. It is a hereditary feature.

total allergy syndrome, a condition of hypersensitivity to a wide range of substances, natural and synthetic, including pesticides, insecticides, pharmaceuticals, certain metals, and chemicals used in the manufacture of plastics and epoxy resins.

total anomalous venous return [L, *totus,* whole; Gk, *anomalos,* uneven; L, *vena,* vein; ME, *retourner,* to turn back], a rare congenital cardiac anomaly in which the pulmonary veins attach directly to the right atrium or to various veins draining into the right atrium rather than directing flow to the left atrium. Clinical manifestations include cyanosis, pulmonary congestion, and heart failure.

total body electrical conductivity (TOBEC), a method of measuring body composition by the differences in electrical conductivity of fat, bone, and muscle. It is used in clinical studies of weight control in which physicians want to determine if weight loss is caused by fat, water, or other tissues.

total body radiation, radiation that exposes the entire body so that, theoretically, all cells in the body receive the same radiation.

total body water (TBW), all the water within the body, including intracellular and extracellular water plus the water in the gastrointestinal and urinary tracts.

total cleavage, mitotic division of the fertilized ovum into blastomeres.

total communication, the combined use of oral language and manual communication by a person with hearing loss.

total hip replacement, a surgical procedure to correct a hip joint damaged by degenerative disease, often arthritis. The head of the femur and the acetabulum are replaced with metal components. The acetabulum is plastic coated to avoid metal-to-metal articulating surfaces.

total iron, the total iron concentration in the blood. The normal concentrations in serum are 50 to 150 μg/dl.

total joint replacement, a surgical procedure for the treatment of severe arthritis and other disorders in which the normal articulating surfaces are replaced by metal and plastic prostheses. The operation most commonly involves replacement of the hip joint with a metallic femur head and a plastic-coated metal acetabulum.

total lung capacity (TLC), the volume of gas in the lungs at the end of a maximum inspiration. It equals the vital capacity plus the residual capacity.

total lymphoid irradiation (TLI), a method of inducing a strong immunosuppressive effect in patients undergoing bone marrow transplants, treatment of certain lymphomas, or other therapies requiring immunosuppression. TLI involves exposing all lymph nodes, the thymus, and spleen to a total of 2000 rad in 100 rad doses from a linear accelerator.

total macroglobulins, the heavy serum macroglobulins that are elevated in various diseases such as cancer and infections.

total nitrogen, the nitrogen content of the feces, measured to detect various disorders such as pancreatic insufficiency and impaired protein digestion. The normal amount in a 24-hour fecal specimen is 10% of intake, or 1 to 2 g.

total parenteral nutrition (TPN), the administration of a nutritionally adequate hypertonic solution consisting of glucose, protein hydrolysates, minerals, and vitamins through an indwelling catheter into the superior vena cava. The procedure is used in prolonged coma, severe uncontrolled malabsorption, extensive burns, gastrointestinal fistulas, and other conditions in which feeding by mouth cannot provide adequate amounts of the essential nutrients.

Total Parenteral Nutrition (TPN) Administration, a Nursing Interventions Classification defined as preparation and delivery of nutrients intravenously and monitoring of patient responsiveness.

total peripheral resistance, the maximum degree of resistance to blood flow caused by constriction of the systemic blood vessels.

total renal blood flow (TRBF), the total volume of blood that flows into the renal arteries. The average TRBF in a normal adult is 1200 ml per minute.

totem /tō′təm/, an animal, plant, force of nature, or inanimate object that represents the tribal ancestor of a clan. It also serves as a tutelary spirit and protector and may communicate through oracles.

totipotency /tō′tipō′tənsē/, the ability of a cell, particularly a germ cell, to differentiate into any of a number of specialized cells and thus form a new organism or regenerate a body part.

touch /tuch/ [Fr, *toucher*, to touch], **1.** the ability to feel objects and distinguish their various characteristics; the tactile sense. **2.** the ability to perceive pressure when it is exerted on the skin or mucosa of the body. **3.** to palpate or examine with the hand, such as the digital examination of the abdomen, rectum, or vagina.

Touch, a Nursing Interventions Classification defined as providing comfort and communication through purposeful tactile contact.

touch deprivation, a lack of tactile stimulation, especially in early infancy. If continued for a sufficient length of time, it may lead to serious developmental and emotional disturbances such as stunted growth, personality disorders, and social regression.

touch receptors [Fr, *toucher* + L, *recipere*, to receive], specialized sensory nerve endings that are sensitive to tactile stimuli.

tourniquet /tur′nikit, tōōr′-/ [Fr, turnstile], a device used in controlling hemorrhage, consisting of a wide constricting band applied to the limb proximal to the site of bleeding. The use of a tourniquet is a drastic measure and is to be used only if the hemorrhage is life-threatening and if other safer measures have proved ineffective.

tourniquet infusion method, a technique of intraarterial regional chemotherapy used in the treatment of osteogenic sarcoma. The technique uses one or two external tourniquets, depending on the location of the tumor, that slow or interrupt the blood flow to a limb temporarily while an anticancer drug such as adriamycin is infused into the area.

tourniquet test, a test of capillary fragility in which a blood pressure cuff is applied for 5 minutes to a person's arm and inflated to a pressure halfway between the diastolic and systolic blood pressure. The number of petechiae within a circumscribed area of the skin may be counted.

Toxascaris leonina /toksas′kəris/, a species of nematode found mainly in domestic animals. It differs from related species in that it spends its entire developmental cycle in the digestive tract, rather than migrating through the lungs.

toxemia /toksē′mē·ə/ [Gk, *toxikon,* poison, *haima,* blood], the presence of bacterial toxins in the bloodstream.—**toxemic,** *adj.*

toxic /tok′sik/ [Gk, *toxikon*], **1.** pertaining to a poison. **2.** (of a disease or condition) severe and progressive.

toxic albuminuria [Gk, *toxikon,* poison; L, *albus,* white; Gk, *ouron,* urine], a condition of serum albumin in the urine caused by the presence of toxic substances in the body.

toxic amblyopia, partial loss of vision because of retrooptic bulbar neuritis, resulting from poisoning with quinine, lead, wood alcohol, nicotine, arsenic, or certain other poisons.

toxicant /tok′sikənt/, any poisonous agent.

toxic delirium [Gk, *toxikon,* poison; L, *delirare,* to rave], a symptom of disordered mental status as a result of poisoning.

toxic dementia, dementia resulting from excessive use of or exposure to a poisonous substance.

toxic dilation of colon [Gk, *toxikon* + L, *dilatare,* to widen; Gk, *kolon*], a condition of transverse colon dilation as a complication of amebic colitis, ulcerative colitis, or other bowel disease. Symptoms may include cramping, fever, rapid heartbeat, and mental confusion.

toxic dose (TD), (in toxicology) the amount of a substance that may be expected to produce a toxic effect.

toxic encephalitis [Gk, *toxikon,* poison, *enkephalos,* brain, *itis,* inflammation], encephalitis caused by heavy metal poisoning. It is characterized by convulsions and cerebral edema.

toxic epidermal necrolysis (TEN), a rare skin disease, characterized by epidermal erythema, superficial necrosis, and skin erosions. This condition, which affects mainly adults, makes the skin appear scalded, often leaving scars. TEN may result from toxic or hypersensitive reactions. It is commonly associated with drug reactions. The disease also has been associated with airborne toxins such as carbon monoxide. TEN also may indicate an immune response, or it may be associated with se-

vere physiologic stress. Early signs of the condition include inflammation of the mucous membranes, fever, malaise, a burning sensation in the conjunctivae, and pervasive tenderness of the skin. The first phase of TEN is manifested by diffuse erythema. The second phase involves vesiculation and blistering. The third phase is marked by extensive epidermal necrolysis and desquamation.

toxic erythema [Gk, *toxikon* poison, *erythema,* redness], an inexact term sometimes applied to reddish skin eruptions of undetermined origin.

toxic goiter, an enlargement of the thyroid gland associated with exophthalmia and systemic disease.

toxicity /toksis′itē/ [Gk, *toxikon*], **1.** the degree to which something is poisonous. **2.** a condition that results from exposure to a toxin or to toxic amounts of a substance that does not cause adverse effects in smaller amounts.

toxic neuritis [Gk, *toxikon,* poison, *neuron,* nerve, *itis,* inflammation], a painful nerve inflammation caused by a metallic, bacterial, or other poison.

toxic nodular goiter, an enlarged thyroid gland characterized by numerous discrete nodules and hypersecretion of thyroid hormones. Typical signs of thyrotoxicosis such as nervousness, tremor, weakness, fatigue, weight loss, and irritability are usually present, but exophthalmia is rare; anorexia is more common than hyperphagia, and cardiac arrhythmia or congestive heart failure may be a predominant manifestation.

Toxicodendron /tok′sikōden′dron/, a genus of plants that includes poison ivy, poison oak, and poison sumac. The toxic agent in the plants is a nonvolatile oil, toxicodendrol.

toxicokinetics /tok′nikō′kinet′iks/, the passage through the body system of a toxic agent or its metabolites, usually in an action similar to that of pharmacokinetics.

toxicologist /tok′sikol′əjist/, a specialist in poisons, their effects, and antidotes.

toxicology /-ol′əjē/, the scientific study of poisons, their detection, their effects, and methods of treatment for conditions they produce.—**toxicologic, toxicological,** *adj.*

toxic or drug-induced hepatitis, hepatitis resulting from a chemical, parasitic, or metabolic poison.

toxicosis /tok′sikō′sis/ [Gk, *toxikon,* poison, *osis,* condition], a disease condition caused by the absorption of metabolic or bacterial poisons.

toxic psychosis, psychosis that results from the poisonous effects of chemicals or drugs, including those produced by the body itself.

toxic shock syndrome (TSS), a severe acute disease caused by infection with strains of *Staphylococcus aureus,* phage group I, that produces a unique toxin, enterotoxin F. It is most common in menstruating women using high-absorbency tampons but has been seen in newborns, children, and men. The onset of the syndrome is characterized by sudden high fever, headache, sore throat with swelling of the mucous membranes, diarrhea, nausea, and erythroderma. Acute renal failure, abnormal liver function, confusion, and refractory hypotension usually follow; and death may occur.

toxic substance [Gk, *toxikon,* poison; L, *substantia,* essence], any poison.

toxin /tok′sin/, a poison, usually one produced by or occurring in a plant or microorganism.

toxin-antitoxin [Gk, *toxikon,* poison, *anti,* against, *toxikon*], a mixture of toxin and antitoxin. Diphtheria toxin-antitoxin was formerly used for active immunization.

toxinology /tok′sinol′əjē/, the study of poisons, with particular emphasis on relatively unstable proteinaceous substances.

Toxocara /tok′səker′ə/, a genus of ascarid nematodes. *T. canis* affects mainly dogs. *T. mustax* affects cats but may also infect humans, particularly children, causing intestinal and respiratory symptoms and damage to the spleen and liver.

toxocariasis /tok′sōkərī′əsis/ [Gk, *toxo,* bow, *kara,* head, *osis,* condition], infection with the larvae of *Toxocara canis,* the common roundworm of dogs and cats. Human ingestion of viable eggs, commonly found in soil, leads to the spread of tiny larvae throughout the body, resulting in respiratory symptoms, enlarged liver, skin rashes, eosinophilia, and delayed ocular lesions. Children who eat dirt are particularly subject to this disease.

toxoid /tok′soid/ [Gk, *toxikon,* poison, *eidos,* form], a toxin that has been treated with chemicals or heat to decrease its toxic effect but that retains its antigenic power. It is given to produce immunity by stimulating the creation of antibodies.

toxophore /tok′səfôr′/, the part of a toxic molecule that is responsible for the poisonous effect.

Toxoplasma /tok′sōplaz′mə/ [Gk, *toxikon* + *plasma,* something formed], a genus of protozoa with only one known species, *Toxoplasma gondii,* an intracellular parasite of cats and other hosts that causes toxoplasmosis in humans.

toxoplasmosis /tok′sōplazmō′sis/ [Gk, *toxikon* + *plasma* + *osis,* condition], a common infection with the protozoan intracellular parasite *Toxoplasma gondii.* The congenital form is characterized by liver and brain involvement with cerebral calcification, convulsions, blindness, microcephaly or hydrocephaly, and mental retardation. The acquired form is characterized by rash, lymphadenopathy, fever, malaise, central nervous system disorders, myocarditis, and pneumonitis.

TPA, abbreviation for **tissue plasminogen activator.**

TPN, abbreviation for **total parenteral nutrition.**

TPR, abbreviation for *temperature, pulse, respiration.*

TQ, symbol for **tocopherolquinone.**

trabecula carnea /trəbek′yələ/, *pl.* **trabeculae carneae** [L, little beam, *carneus,* flesh], any one of the irregular bands and bundles of muscle projecting from the inner surfaces of the ventricles of the heart.

trabeculae, (in ophthalmology) the part of the eye in front of the canal of Schlemm and within the angle created by the iris and cornea.

trabecular pattern /trəbek′yələr/ [L,little beam], an irregular meshwork of stress and stress-related struts within a cancellous bone.

trabeculectomy /trəbek′yəlek′təmē/ [L, *trabecula* + Gk, *ektome,* excision], the surgical removal of a section of corneoscleral tissue to increase the outflow of aqueous humor in patients with severe glaucoma.

trabeculoplasty trabek′yəlōplśtē/, a plastic surgery procedure used in the treatment of glaucoma. An argon laser beam is used to blanch the trabecular network of the eye, thereby permitting drainage of the excess fluid causing increased pressure within the eyeball.

trabeculotomy /-ot′əmē/, a surgical opening in an orbital trabecula to increase the outflow of aqueous humor.

trace element [L, *trahere,* to draw, *elementum,* first principle], an element essential to nutrition or physiologic processes, found in such minute quantities that analysis yields a presence of virtually zero amounts.

trace gas, a gas or vapor that escapes into the atmosphere during an anesthetic procedure.

tracer [L, *trahere,* to draw], **1.** a radioactive isotope that is used in diagnostic x-ray techniques to allow a biologic process to be seen. The tracer, which is introduced into the body, binds with a specific substance and is followed with a scanner or fluoroscope. **2.** a device that graphically records the outline or movements of an object or part of the body. **3.** a dissecting instrument that is used to isolate vessels and nerves.—**trace,** *v.*

tracer depot method, (in nuclear medicine) a technique used to determine local skin or muscle blood flow, based on the rate at which a radioactive tracer deposited in a tissue is removed by diffusion into the capillaries and washed out by the local blood supply.

trachea /trā′kē·ə/ [Gk, *tracheia,* rough artery], a nearly cylindric tube in the neck, composed of cartilage and membrane, that extends from the larynx at the level of the sixth cervical vertebra to the fifth thoracic vertebra, where it divides into two bronchi. The trachea conveys air to the lungs.—**tracheal,** *adj.*

tracheal /trā′kē·əl/ [Gk, *tracheia,* rough artery], pertaining to the trachea.

tracheal breath sound, a normal breath sound heard in auscultation of the trachea. Inspiration and expiration are equally loud; the expiratory sound is heard during the greater part of expiration, whereas the inspiratory sound stops abruptly at the height of inspiration.

tracheal tugging [Gk, *tracheia,* rough artery; ME, *toggen*], an effect of an aortic aneurysm in which the trachea is tugged downward with each heart contraction.

tracheitis /trā′kē·ī′tis/, any inflammatory condition of the trachea. It may be acute or chronic, resulting from infection, allergy, or physical irritation.

tracheobronchial tree (TBT) /-brong′-kē·əl/ [Gk, *tracheia* + *bronchos,* windpipe], an anatomic complex that includes the trachea, bronchi, and bronchial tubes. It conveys air to and from the lungs.

tracheobronchitis /trā′kē·ōbrongkī′tis/, inflammation of the trachea and bronchi, a common form of pulmonary infection.

tracheobronchomegaly /-brong′kōmeg′-əlē/, an abnormally large upper airway, in which the trachea may be as wide as the spinal column.

tracheoesophageal fistula /trā′kē·ō·ē′-səfā′jē·əl/, [Gk, *tracheia* + *osophagos,* gullet], a congenital malformation in which there is an abnormal tubelike passage between the trachea and the esophagus.

tracheoesophageal shunt, a surgical procedure enabling a laryngectomee to speak by constructing a passageway between the trachea and the esophagus. The operation results in an ability to produce esophageal speech with normal respiration as a source of air and without the need to belch to produce voice sounds.

tracheolaryngeal /-lerin′jē·əl/, pertaining to the trachea and larynx.

tracheomalacia /trā′kē·ōmələā′shə/, an eroding of the trachea, usually caused by excessive pressure from a cuffed endotracheal tube.

tracheopharyngeal /-ferin′jē·əl/, pertaining to the trachea and pharynx.

tracheoplasty /trā′kē·ōplas′tē/, plastic surgery of the trachea.

tracheostenosis /-stənō′sis/, constriction of the lumen of the trachea.

tracheostomy /trā′kē·os′təmē/ [Gk, *tracheia* + *stoma,* mouth], an opening through the neck into the trachea through which an indwelling tube may be inserted. The patient is reassured that the tube is open and that air can pass through it. The tube is suctioned frequently to keep it free from tracheobronchial secretions using a suction catheter attached to a Y-connector. The patient is taught to cough to move secretions up and out of the bronchi. If the procedure was done as an emergency, the tracheostomy is closed after normal breathing is restored. If the tracheostomy is permanent, such as with a laryngectomy, the patient is taught self-care.

tracheostomy care [Gk, *tracheia,* rough artery, *stoma,* mouth], care of the tracheostomy patient, consisting of maintenance of a patent airway, adequate humidification, aseptic wound care, and sterile tracheal aspiration. Complications can include injury to the vocal cords, gastric distension and regurgitation, occlusion of the endotracheal tube, and an increased risk of infection.

tracheotomy /trā′kē·ot′əmē/ [Gk, *tracheia* + *temnein,* to cut], an incision made into the trachea through the neck below the larynx, performed to gain access to the airway below a blockage with a foreign body, tumor, or edema of the glottis. The opening may be made as an emergency measure at an accident site, at a hospitalized patient's bedside, or in the operating room.

tracheotomy tube [Gk, *tracheia,* rough artery, *temnein,* to cut; L, *tubus*], a curved hollow tube of rubber, metal, or plastic surgically inserted in the trachea to relieve a breathing obstruction.

trachoma /trəkō′mə/ [Gk, roughness], a chronic infectious disease of the eye caused by the bacterium *Chlamydia trachomatis.* It is characterized initially by inflammation, pain, photophobia, and lacrimation. If untreated, follicles form on the upper eyelids and grow larger until the granulations invade the cornea, eventually causing blindness.

tracing [L, *trahere,* to draw], a graphic record of a physical event, such as an electrocardiograph tracing made by pens on a moving sheet of paper while recording the electrical impulses of heart muscle contractions.

tract [L, *tractus,* trail], **1.** an elongate group of tissues and structures that function together as a pathway, such as the digestive tract or the respiratory tract. **2.** (in neurology) the neuronal axons that are grouped together to form a pathway.

traction /trak′shən/ [L, *trahere,* to draw], **1.** (in orthopedics) the process of putting a limb, bone, or group of muscles under tension by means of weights and pulleys to align or immobilize the part or to relieve pressure on it. **2.** the process of pulling a part of the body along, through, or out of its socket or cavity, such as axis traction with obstetric forceps in delivering an infant.

traction frame, an orthopedic apparatus that supports the pulleys, ropes, and weights by which traction is applied to various parts of the body or by which various parts of the body are suspended. The main components of a traction frame are metal uprights that attach to the bed and support an overhead metal bar.

Traction/Immobilization Care, a Nursing Interventions Classification defined as management of a patient who has traction and/or a stabilizing device to immobilize and stabilize a body part.

traction, 90-90, an orthopedic mechanism, used especially in pediatrics, that combines skeletal traction and suspension with a short-leg cast or a splint to immobilize and position the lower extremity in the treatment of a displaced fractured femur.

traction response, the response to traction applied to the spine. Alterations of certain signs and symptoms of a musculoskeletal disorder may be revealed by traction tests.

trademark, a word, symbol, or device assigned to a product by its manufacturer, registered or not registered, as a part of its identity.

tragacanth /trag′əkanth/, a white tasteless vegetable gum derived from a shrub, *Astragalus gummifer,* and related species. It is used as a suspending agent in pharmaceutical preparations, particularly powders and tinctures.

tragal /trā′gəl/ [Gk, *tragos,* goat], pertaining to the tragus.

tragus /trā′gəs/, *pl.* **tragi** /trā′jī/ [Gk, *tragos,* goat], a small extension of the auricular cartilage of the ear, anterior to the external meatus.

trainable /trā′nəbəl/ [L, *trahere,* to draw], pertaining to a mentally retarded person who is capable of some degree of self-care

and social adjustment in a supervised setting but would not benefit from formal education.

traineeship /trānē′ship/ [L, *trahere,* to draw; AS, *scieppan,* to shape], a grant of money allocated to an individual for advanced study in a given field.

training effect, a rehabilitation influence effect for heart patients that can be measured by changes in cardiac function.

training grant, a grant of money or other resources to provide training in a particular field.

trait [Fr, trace], **1.** a characteristic mode of behavior or any mannerism or physical feature that distinguishes one individual or culture from another. **2.** any characteristic quality or condition that is genetically determined and inherited as a specific genotype.

trance [L, *transire,* to pass across], **1.** a sleeplike state characterized by the complete or partial suspension of consciousness and loss or diminution of motor activity. **2.** a dazed or bewildered condition; stupor. **3.** a state of detachment from one's immediate surroundings, such as in deep concentration or daydreaming.

tranquilizer /trang′kwilī′zər/ [L, *tranquillus,* calm], a drug prescribed to calm anxious or agitated people, ideally without decreasing their consciousness. Major tranquilizers such as derivatives of phenothiazine, butyrophenone, and thioxanthene are generally used in the treatment of psychoses. Minor tranquilizers usually prescribed for the treatment of anxiety, irritability, tension, or psychoneurosis include chlordiazepoxide, diazepam, and hydroxyzine. Tranquilizers tend to induce drowsiness and have the potential for causing physical and psychologic dependence.

transabdominal /-abdom′inəl/ [L, *trans,* across, *abdomen,* belly], pertaining to a procedure through the abdominal wall.

transactional analysis (TA) /-ak′shənəl/ [L, *transigere,* to drive through; Gk, *analyein,* to loosen], a form of psychotherapy developed by Eric Berne, based on a theory that three different coherent organized egos exist throughout life simultaneously in every person, representing the child, the adult, and the parent. Interactions between people are transactions, originating from a person in one of the ego states and received by another person who may be in a complementary or a crossed ego state.

transaminase /transam′inās/ [L, *trans,* across, *amine,* ammonia; Fr, *diastase,* enzyme], an enzyme that catalyzes the transfer of an amino group from an alpha-amino acid to an alpha-keto acid, with pyridoxal phosphate and pyridoxamine phosphate acting as coenzymes.

transamination /-am′inā′shən/, the reaction between an amino acid and an alpha-ketoacid in which the enzyme transaminase induces transfer of the amino group to the alpha-ketoacid.

transanimation /-an′imā′shən/, the resuscitation effort to induce a newborn to breathe.

transaortic /-ā-ôr′tik/ [L, *trans,* across; Gk, *aerein,* to raise], pertaining to a procedure through the aorta.

transcellular water /-sel′yələr/ [L, *trans + cella,* storeroom], the part of extracellular water that is enclosed by an epithelial membrane and whose volume and composition are determined by the cellular activity of that membrane.

transcendence /transen′dəns/ [L, *trans + scandere,* to climb], the rising above one's previously perceived limits or restrictions.

transcendental meditation (TM), a psychophysiologic exercise designed to lower levels of tension and anxiety and increase tolerance of frustration. TM has been described as a state of consciousness that does not require any physical or mental control. During meditation, the person enters a hypometabolic state in which there is reduced activity of the adrenergic component of the autonomic nervous system.

transcervical fracture /transur′vikəl/ [L, *trans,* across, *cervix,* neck, *fractura*], a fracture through the neck of the femur.

transcondylar fracture /transkon′dilər/ [L, *trans + Gk, kondylos,* condyle], a fracture that occurs transversally and distal to the epicondyles of any one of the long bones.

transconfiguration /-kənfig′yərə′shən/ [L, *trans + configurare,* to form from], **1.** (in genetics) the presence of the dominant allele of one pair of genes and the recessive allele of another pair on the same chromosome. **2.** the presence of at least one mutant gene and one wild-type gene of a pair of pseudoalleles on each chromosome of a homologous pair.

transcortin /-kôr′tin/, a diglobulin protein that binds a majority of cortisol in the plasma.

transcriptase /transkrip′tās/, an enzyme that induces transcription.

transcription /transkrip′shən/ [L, *trans + scribere,* to write], (in molecular genetics) the process by which messenger ribonucleic acid is formed from a deoxyribonucleic acid template in the process of manufacturing a protein.

transcultural nursing /-kul′chərəl/ [L, *trans + colere,* to cultivate, *nutrix,* nurse], a field of nursing in which the nurse transcends ethnocentricity and practices nursing in other cultural environments.

transcutaneous /-k(y)ootā′nē·əs/ [L, *trans + cutis,* skin], pertaining to a procedure that is performed through the skin.

transcutaneous electrical nerve stimulation (TENS), a method of pain control by the application of electrical impulses to the nerve endings. This is done through electrodes that are placed on the skin and attached to a stimulator by flexible wires. The electrical impulses generated are similar to those of the body, but different enough to block transmission of pain signals to the brain.

Transcutaneous Electrical Nerve Stimulation (TENS), a Nursing Interventions Classification defined as stimulation of skin and underlying tissues with controlled low-voltage electrical vibration via electrodes.

transcutaneous oxygen/carbon dioxide monitoring, a method of measuring the oxygen or carbon dioxide in the blood by attaching electrodes to the skin. Oxygen is commonly measured through an oximeter, which contains heating coils to raise the skin temperature and increase blood flow at the surface. Transcutaneous carbon dioxide electrodes are similar to blood gas electrodes.

transdermal drug delivery (TDD) /-dur′-məl/ [L, *trans + Gk, derma,* skin], a method of applying a drug to unbroken skin. The drug is absorbed continuously through the skin and enters the systemic system.

transdermal scopolamine, a method of administration of the motion sickness drug by application of a skin patch containing the medication.

transducer /-d(y)oo′sər/ [L, *trans + ducere,* to lead], (in ultrasound) a handheld device that sends and receives a soundwave signal.

transductant /-duk′tənt/, a cell that has acquired a new character by the transfer of genetic material.

transduction /-duk′shən/, (in molecular genetics) a method of genetic recombination by which deoxyribonucleic acid is transferred from one cell to another by a viral vector.

transect /transekt′/ [L, *trans + secare,* to cut], to sever or cut across, as in preparing a cross section of tissue.

transfection /-fek′shən/ [L, *trans + inficere,* to taint], (in molecular genetics) the process by which a bacterial cell is infected with purified deoxyribonucleic acid or ribonucleic acid isolated from a virus or a viral vector.

transfer, to move a person or object from one site to another.

transfer agreement /trans′fur/ [L, *transferre,* to carry over, *ad,* toward, *gratus,* pleasure], a written hospital agreement between two health care institutions for the transfer of patients from one to another and the orderly exchange of pertinent clinical information on the patients transferred.

transferase /trans′fərās/ [L, *transferre* + Fr, *diastase,* enzyme], any of a group of enzymes that catalyzes the transfer of a chemical group or radical, such as the phosphate, methyl, amine, or keto groups, from one molecule to another.

transfer DNA (tDNA), (in molecular genetics) DNA transferred from its original source and present in transformed cells.

transference /-fur′əns/ [L, *transferre*], **1.** the shifting of symptoms from one part of the body to another, as occurs in conversion disorder. **2.** (in psychiatry) an unconscious defense mechanism whereby feelings and attitudes originally associated with important people and events in one's early life are attributed to others in current interpersonal situations. **3.** (in psychoanalysis and psychotherapy) the feelings of a patient for the analyst to whom the patient has attributed or assigned the qualities, attitudes, and feelings of a person or people significant in his or her emotional development, usually a figure from childhood.

transference love, (in psychoanalytic therapy) a projection of libidinal drives expressed by the patient for the psychoanalyst who has "unconsciously" come to represent a person from the patient's past.

transfer factor, a leukocyte extract that transfers delayed hypersensitivity from one person to another.

transferrin /transfer′in/, a trace protein present in the blood that is essential in the transport of iron from the intestine into the bloodstream.

transferring /-fur′ing/ [L, *trans,* across, *ferre,* to bring], relocating a person in need from one location to another.

transfer RNA (tRNA), (in molecular genetics) a kind of ribonucleic acid that carries the anticodon (consisting of three nitrogenous bases). Each anticodon specifies a particular amino acid. There are 64 possible anticodons and about 20 to 24 amino acids. This means that several anticodons may refer to the same amino acid.

transfixation /-fiksā′shən/, a surgical procedure in which, in an amputation, the soft tissues are cut through from one side

to the other, close to the bone. The muscles are then divided from within outward.

transformation /-fôrmā′shən/ [L, *transformare,* to change shape], (in molecular genetics) the process in which exogenous genes are integrated into chromosomes in a form that is recognized by the replicative and transcriptional apparatus of the host cell.

transformer /-fôr′mər/ [L, *transformare,* to change shape], an electrical apparatus that changes alternating current of one voltage into a different voltage of the same frequency.

transforming growth factor (TGF), a group of proteins produced by the cells of a tumor that, when inoculated into a normal cell culture, causes a disorderly increase in the number of cells in the culture.

transfuse /-fyoo̅z′/, to transfer blood or blood components from one person to another.

transfusion /-f(y)oo̅′zhən/ [L, *trans* + *fundere,* to pour], the introduction into the bloodstream of whole blood or blood components such as plasma, platelets, or packed red cells. Whole blood may be infused into the recipient directly from a donor matched for the ABO blood group and antigenic subgroups, but more frequently the donor's blood is collected and stored by a blood bank.

transfusion reaction, a systemic response by the body to the administration of blood incompatible with that of the recipient. The causes include red cell incompatibility; allergic sensitivity to the leukocytes, platelets, plasma protein components of the transfused blood; or potassium or citrate preservatives in the banked blood. Fever is the most common transfusion reaction; urticaria is a relatively common allergic response. Asthma, vascular collapse, and renal failure occur less commonly. A hemolytic reaction from red cell incompatibility is serious and must be diagnosed and treated promptly. Symptoms develop shortly after beginning the transfusion, before 50 ml have been given, and include a throbbing headache, sudden deep severe lumbar pain, precordial pain, dyspnea, and restlessness. Objective signs include ruddy facial flushing followed by cyanosis and distended neck veins; rapid, thready pulse; diaphoresis; and cold, clammy skin. Profound shock may occur within 1 hour.

transgene /trans′jēn/, a newly introduced gene.

transgenic /-jen′ik/, pertaining to the transfer of new deoxyribonucleic acid material into one genome from a different genome.

transient /tran'shənt, tran'zē·ənt/ [L, *transire,* to go through], pertaining to a condition that is temporary, such as transient ischemic attack.

transient global amnesia (TGA) [L, *transire,* to go through, *globus,* ball; Gk, *amnesia,* forgetfulness], a temporary short-term memory loss followed by full recovery. The disorder tends to affect middle-aged adults and may be attributed to cerebral ischemia. It is usually not accompanied by other mental deficiencies.

transient ischemic attack (TIA), an episode of cerebrovascular insufficiency, usually associated with partial occlusion of an artery by an atherosclerotic plaque or an embolism. The symptoms vary with the site and the degree of occlusion. Disturbance of normal vision in one or both eyes, dizziness, weakness, dysphasia, numbness, or unconsciousness may occur. The attack is usually brief, lasting a few minutes; rarely symptoms continue for several hours.

transient myopia [L, *transire,* to go through; Gk, *myops,* nearsighted], a temporary change in visual accommodation secondary to trauma, high blood sugar level, sulfanilamide therapy, and other conditions.

transillumination /-iloo'minā'shən/ [L, *trans,* through, *illuminare,* to light up], **1.** the passage of light through a solid or liquid substance. **2.** the passage of light through body tissues for the purpose of examining a structure interposed between the observer and the light source.

transition /tranzish'ən/ [L, *transire,* to go through], the last phase of the first stage of labor, sometimes indicated by cervical dilation of 8 to 10 cm.

transitional /tranzish'ənl/ [L, *transire,* to go through] between a previous and a succeeding state, or in a state of becoming something else.

transitional cell carcinoma, a malignant, usually papillary tumor derived from transitional stratified epithelium, occurring most frequently in the bladder, ureter, urethra, or renal pelvis. The majority of tumors in the collecting system of the kidney are of this kind.

transitional object, an object used by a child to provide comfort and security while he or she is away from a secure base, such as mother or home.

transitional zone [L, *transire,* to go through; Gk, *zone,* belt], a part of the crystalline lens of the eye where epithelial-capsule cells change into lens fibers.

transitory mania /tran'sitôr'ē/ [L, *transire,* to go through; Gk, *mania,* madness], a mood disorder characterized by the sudden onset of manic reactions that are of short duration, usually lasting from 1 hour to a few days.

translation /-lā'shən/ [L, *translatio,* handing over], (in molecular genetics) the process in which the genetic information carried by nucleotides in messenger ribonucleic acid directs the amino acid sequence in the synthesis of a specific polypeptide.

translocation /-lōkā'shən/ [L, *trans* + *locus,* place], (in genetics) the rearrangement of genetic material within the same chromosome or the transfer of a segment of one chromosome to another nonhomologous one.

translucent /-loo'sənt/ [L, *trans,* across, *lucens,* shining], pertaining to a medium through which light can pass in a diffused manner so that a field is illuminated but objects cannot be seen distinctly.

transmethylation /-meth'ilā'shən/, the transfer of a methyl group from one compound to another.

transmigration /-mīgrā'shən/ [L, *trans* + *migrare,* to migrate], a movement from one side to another, from inside to outside, or from outside to inside.

transmissible /-mis'ibəl/ [L, *transmittere,* to transmit], capable of being passed from one person or place to another, as in the transmission of a disease.

transmission /-mish'ən/ [L, *transmittere,* to transmit], the transfer or conveyance of a thing or condition, such as a neural impulse, an infectious or genetic disease, or a hereditary trait, from one person or place to another.**—transmissible,** *adj.*

transmission-based precautions, safeguards designed for patients documented or suspected to be infected with highly transmissible or epidemiologically important pathogens for which additional precautions beyond standard precautions are needed to interrupt transmission in hospitals. There are three types of transmission-based precautions: airborne precautions, droplet precautions, and contact precautions. They may be combined for diseases that have multiple routes of transmission. When used either singularly or in combination, they are to be used in addition to standard precautions.

transmission scanning electron microscope, an instrument that transmits a highly magnified, well-resolved, three-dimensional image on a television screen, thus combining the advantages of the electron and the scanning electron microscopes.

transmission scanning electron microscopy (TSEM), a technique using a transmission scanning electron microscope in which the atomic number of the part of the sample being scanned is determined and used to modulate a beam of electrons in a cathode-ray tube and in the beam scanning the sample.

transmitted light [L, *transmittere,* to transmit; AS, *leoht*], light that has been transmitted through a transparent medium.

transmural /-m(y)oo͞o′rəl/ [L, *trans + murus,* wall], pertaining to the entire thickness of the wall of an organ, such as a transmural myocardial infarction.

transmural infarction, the death of myocardial tissue that extends from the endocardium to the epicardium as a result of a myocardial infarction.

transmutation /-m(y)oo͞otā′shən/ [L, *transmutare,* to change], **1.** a mutation, as when a significant species change occurs during evolution. **2.** the conversion of one chemical element into another by radioactive bombardment.

transovarial transmission /-ōver′ē·əl/ [L, *trans + ovum,* egg], the transfer of pathogens to succeeding generations through invasion of the ovary and infection of the egg.

transparent /-per′ənt/ [L, *trans,* across, *parere,* to appear], pertaining to a clear medium that allows for the transmission of light so that objects on the other side are distinguishable.

transpeptidase /-pep′tidās/, an enzyme that catalyzes the transfer of an amino group from one peptide chain to another.

transpeptidation /-pep′tidā′shən/, the transfer of an amino acid from one peptide chain to another.

transplacental /trans′pləsen′təl/ [L, *trans + placenta,* flat cake], across or through the placenta, specifically in reference to the exchange of nutrients, waste products, and other material between the developing fetus and the mother.

transplant /trans′plant, transplant′/ [L, *transplantare*], **1.** to transfer an organ or tissue from one person to another or from one body part to another to replace a diseased structure, restore function, or change appearance. Skin and kidneys are the most frequently transplanted structures; others include cartilage, bone, bone marrow, corneal tissue, parts of blood vessels and tendons, hearts, lungs, and livers. Preferred donors are identical twins or people having the same blood type and immunologic characteristics. **2.** any tissue or organ that is transplanted. **3.** pertaining to a tissue or organ that is transplanted, a recipient of a donated tissue or organ, or

a phenomenon associated with the procedure.

transplantation /-plantā′shən/ [L, *transplantare,* to transplant], the transfer of tissue from one site to another or from one person or organism to another.

transplantation endometriosis [L, *transplantare,* to transplant; Gk, *endon,* within, *metra,* womb, *osis,* condition], endometrial tissue that is accidentally transplanted to the incision wound during pelvic surgery.

transport /trans′pôrt/ [L, *trans,* across, *portare,* carry], the movement or transference of biochemical substances from one site to another. Active transport involves an expenditure of energy, whereas passive transport allows movement down a gradient without an energy expenditure.

Transport, a Nursing Interventions Classification defined as moving a patient from one location to another.

transposable element /-pō′zəbəl/ [L, *transponere,* to transpose, *elementum,* first principle], (in molecular genetics) a deoxyribonucleic acid fragment or segment that can move or be moved from one site in the genome to another.

transposase /trans′pəzās/, (in molecular genetics) an enzyme involved in the movement of a deoxyribonucleic acid fragment or segment from one site in the genome to another.

transposition /-pəsish′ən/ [L, *transponere*], **1.** an abnormality occurring during embryonic development in which a body part normally on the left is found on the right or vice versa. **2.** the shifting of genetic material from one chromosome to another at some point in the reproductive process.—**transpose,** *v.*

transposition of the great vessels, a congenital cardiac anomaly in which the pulmonary artery arises from the left ventricle and the aorta from the right ventricle so that there is no communication between the systemic and pulmonary circulations. The primary symptoms are cyanosis and hypoxia, especially in infants with small septal defects, although cardiomegaly is usually evident a few weeks after birth. Signs of congestive heart failure develop rapidly, especially in infants with large ventricular septal defects.

transposon /transpō′sən/ [L, *transponere + on*], a gene or group of genes that are mobile and, like plasmids, act to transfer genetic instructions from one place to another. Transposons travel piggyback from virus to virus on bacteriophages.

transpulmonary pressure /-pul′mɔner′ē/, the difference between intraalveolar and intrapleural pressure, or the pressure acting across the lung from the intrapleural space to the alveoli.

transsection /transek′shən/ [L, *trans,* across, *sectio*], a cross-section of a biologic specimen or a cut across the long axis.

transseptal fiber /transep′təl/ [L, *trans* + *saeptum,* wall], (in dentistry) any one of the many filamentous tissues of the gingival system that extends mesially from the supraalveolar cementum of one tooth, through the interdental-attached gingiva above the septum of the alveolar bone, to the distal cementum of an adjacent tooth.

transsexual /transek′choo·əl/, a person whose gender identity is opposite his or her biologic sex.

transsexualism /-iz′əm/, a condition in which a person has an intense desire to discard one's biologic sex and live as a member of the opposite sex. It is considered a psychiatric disorder if the condition continues for more than 2 years. Some transsexual individuals crossdress and seek medical or surgical help to change their physical sex characteristics.

transexual surgery /transek′shoo·əl/, the surgical alteration of external sexual characteristics so that they resemble those of the opposite sex.

transtentorial herniation /trans′tentôr′-ē·əl/ [L, *trans* + *tentorium,* tent, *hernia,* rupture], a bulge of brain tissue out of the cranium through the tentorial notch, caused by increased intracranial pressure.

transthoracic /trans′thôras′ik/, across or passing through the thorax.

transthoracic pacemaker /-thôras′ik/ [L, *trans,* across; Gk, *thorax,* chest; L, *passus,* step; ME, *maken*], a permanent heart pacemaker with the pulse generator located in the abdominal wall and the pacing wires attached directly to the epicardium.

transtracheal oxygen /-trā′kē·əl/ [L, *trans,* across; Gk, *tracheia,* rough artery, *oxys,* sharp, *genein,* to produce], a method of administering oxygen to a patient requiring oxygen therapy by establishing a low-flow catheter route directly into the trachea. It is a sometimes preferred alternative to the administration of oxygen through a nasal cannula.

transtrochanteric osteotomy /-trō′kəntər′-ik/ [L, *trans* across; Gk, *trochanter,* runner, *osteon* + *temnein,* to cut], a surgical division of the upper end of the femur through the area of the trochanters.

transubstantiation /trans′əbstan′chē·ā′-shən/, the replacement or substitution of tissue of one kind for another.

transudate /trans′yədāt/ [L, *trans* + *sudare,* to sweat], a fluid passed through a membrane or squeezed through a tissue or into the space between the cells of a tissue.

transudation /-yədā′shən/, **1.** the passage of a substance through a membrane as a result of a difference in hydrostatic pressure. **2.** the passage of a fluid through a membrane with nearly all the solutes of the fluid remaining in solution or suspension.

transudative ascites /transyoo′dətiv/, an abnormal accumulation in the peritoneal cavity of a fluid that characteristically contains scant amounts of protein and cells.

transurethral resection (TUR) /trans′-yoorē′thrəl/ [L, *trans* + Gk, *ourethra,* urethra; L, *re,* again, *secare,* to cut], a surgical procedure through the urethra, such as in transurethral prostatectomy.

transverse /-vurs′/ [L, *transversus,* oblique], at right angles to the long axis of any common part, such as the planes that cut the long axis of the body into upper and lower parts and are at right angles to the sagittal and frontal planes.

transverse colon, the segment of the colon that extends from the end of the ascending colon at the hepatic flexure on the right side across the midabdomen to the beginning of the descending colon at the splenic flexure on the left side.

transverse fissure, a fissure dividing the dorsal surface of the diencephalon and the ventral surface of the cerebral hemisphere.

transverse foramen [L, *transversus* + *foramen,* hole], an opening through the transverse process of a cervical vertebra.

transverse fracture, a fracture that occurs at right angles to the longitudinal axis of the bone involved.

transverse lie, abnormal presentation of a fetus in which the long axis of the baby's body is across the long axis of the mother's body.

transverse ligament of the atlas, a thick, strong ligament stretched across the ring of the atlas, holding the dens against the anterior arch.

transverse mesocolon /mez′ōkō′lən/, a broad fold of the peritoneum connecting the transverse colon to the dorsal wall of the abdomen.

transverse myelitis [L, *transversus* + Gk, *myelos,* marrow, *itis,* inflammation], an acute attack of spinal cord inflammation involving both sides of the cord.

transverse palatine suture, the line of junction between the processes of the maxilla and the horizontal parts of the palatine bones that form the hard palate.

transverse plane, any one of the planes cutting across the body perpendicular to the sagittal and frontal planes, dividing the body into superior and inferior parts.

transverse presentation [L, *transversus* +

praesentare, to show], a presentation of the fetal body in an oblique or transverse position across the birth canal.

transverse sinus, one of a pair of large venous channels in the posterior superior group of sinuses serving the dura mater.

transversus abdominis /-vur′səs/, one of a pair of transverse abdominal muscles that are the anterolateral muscles of the abdomen, lying immediately under the internal abdominal oblique. It serves to constrict the abdomen and, by compressing the contents, to assist in micturition, defecation, emesis, parturition, and forced expiration.

transvestism /-ves′tizəm/, a tendency to achieve psychic and sexual relief by dressing in the clothing of the opposite sex.

tranylcypromine sulfate /tran′əlsip′rə-mēn/, a monoamine oxidase inhibitor that acts as an antidepressant. It is prescribed in the treatment of severe reactive or endogenous mental depression.

trapeze bar /trapēz′/, a triangular metal apparatus above a bed, used to help support the weight of a patient during transfer or position change.

trapezium /trəpē′zē-əm/, *pl.* **trapeziums, trapezia** [Gk, *trapezion,* small table], a carpal bone in the distal row of carpal bones. The trapezium articulates with the scaphoid proximally, the first metacarpal distally, and the trapezoideum and second metacarpal medially.

trapezius /trəpē′zē-əs/ [Gk, *trapezion,* small table], a large, flat triangular muscle of the shoulder and upper back. It acts to rotate the scapula, raise the shoulder, and abduct and flex the arm.

trapezoid /trap′əzoid/ [Gk, *trapezion,* small table, *eidos,* form], having the shape of a trapeze, an irregular four-sided figure with one set of parallel sides.

trapezoidal arch /trap′əzoidəl/ [Gk, *trapezion + eidos,* form; L, *arcus,* bow], a dental arch that has slightly less convergence than that of a tapering arch.

trapezoid bone [Gk, *trapezion + eidos +* AS, *ban*], the smallest carpal bone, located in the distal row of carpal bones between the trapezium and the capitate.

trauma /trou′mə, trô′mə/ [Gk, wound], **1.** physical injury caused by violent or disruptive action or by the introduction into the body of a toxic substance. **2.** psychic injury resulting from a severe emotional shock.—**traumatic,** *adj.,* **traumatize,** *v.*

trauma center, a service providing emergency and specialized intensive care to critically ill and injured patients.

trauma registry, a repository of data on the incidence, diagnosis, and treatment of acute trauma victims treated by emergency service personnel.

trauma, risk for, a NANDA-accepted nursing diagnosis of the accentuated risk of accidental tissue injury such as a wound, burn, or fracture. The risk factors may be internal (individual) or external (environmental). Internal risk factors include weakness; poor vision; balancing difficulties; reduced temperature or tactile sensation; reduced muscle or eye-hand coordination; lack of safety education, precautions, or equipment; cognitive or emotional difficulties; and history of previous trauma. External risk factors include slippery floors, stairs, or walkways; a bathtub without hand grip or antislip equipment; unsteady chairs or ladders; defective electric wires or appliances; obstructed passageways; potential igniting gas leaks; unscreened fires or heaters; inadequately stored combustibles or corrosives; contact with intense cold or heat (such as very hot water); overexposure to sun, sunlamps, or radiotherapy; and exposure to dangerous machinery.

Trauma Score, a system of combining cardiopulmonary assessment with the Glasgow Coma Scale in estimating the degree of injury and the prognosis in a patient who has suffered a head injury. Cardiopulmonary factors include respiratory rate and chest expansion, systolic blood pressure, and capillary refill. The neurologic factors are eye opening, verbal response, and motor response.

traumatic /trômat′ik/ [Gk, *trauma,* wound], pertaining to an injury, usually a serious and unexpected injury.

traumatic abscess, a pus collection that develops in tissue that has been damaged by a wound or injury.

traumatic anesthesia [Gk, *trauma + anaisthesia,* lack of feeling], a total lack of normal sensation in a part of the body, resulting from injury, destruction of nerves, or interruption of nerve pathways.

traumatic aphasia, aphasia that results from a head injury.

traumatic delirium, delirium after severe head injury, characterized by alertness and consciousness, with disorientation, confabulation, and amnesia apparent.

traumatic dislocation [Gk, *trauma,* wound; L, *dis + locare*], a dislocation caused by an injury.

traumatic epilepsy [Gk, *trauma,* wound, *epilepsia,* seizure], a form of motor or sensory seizures caused by a brain injury.

traumatic fever, an elevation in body temperature secondary to mechanic trauma, particularly a crushing injury. The increased body temperature may help provide resistance to subsequent infection, and increased wound temperature may accelerate local healing.

traumatic gangrene [Gk, *trauma*, wound, *gaggraina*], gangrene that follows a severe injury resulting in damage to blood vessels.

traumatic herpes [Gk, *trauma*, wound, *herpein*, to creep], herpes that develops at the site of an injury.

traumatic meningitis [Gk, *trauma*, wound, *menigx*, membrane, *itis*, inflammation], meningitis that develops as a result of injury to the skull or spinal column.

traumatic myelitis [Gk, *trauma*, wound, *myelos*, marrow, *itis*, inflammation], a spinal cord inflammation resulting from an injury.

traumatic myositis, an inflammation of the muscles resulting from a wound or other trauma.

traumatic neuritis [Gk, *trauma*, wound, *neuron*, nerve, *itis*, inflammation], neuritis that is caused by injury to a nerve.

traumatic neuroma, a mass of nerve elements and fibrous tissue produced by the proliferation of Schwann cells and fibroblasts after severe injury to a nerve.

traumatic occlusion, a repeated excessive force in closure of the teeth that injures the teeth, the periodontal tissues, the residual ridge, or other oral structures.

traumatic psychosis [Gk, *trauma*, wound, *psyche*, mind, *osis*, condition], a psychiatric disorder that results from injury to the head, with symptoms usually indicating brain trauma. It is differentiated from psychic trauma in which personality damage can be traced to an unpleasant experience such as sexual assault.

traumatic rhabdomyolysis, a condition of skeletal muscle destruction following a crush injury. During reperfusion of the damaged tissue, after crushing pressure has been removed, myoglobin, potassium, and phosphorus are released into the circulation, causing symptoms of renal failure, hypovolemic shock, and hyperkalemia.

traumatic shock [Gk, *trauma*, wound; Fr, *choc*], the emotional or psychologic state after trauma that may produce abnormal behavior. The most common types are hypovolemic shock from blood loss and neurogenic shock caused by a disruption of the integrity of the spinal cord.

traumatic thrombosis [Gk, *trauma*, wound, *thrombos*, lump, *osis*, condition], intravascular coagulation of a vein or other blood vessel after injury or irritation. The condition may develop as an adverse effect of an intravenous injection that damages the wall of a vein.

traumatology /trô′mətol′əjē/ [Gk, *trauma* + *logos*, science], **1.** the study of wounds and injuries. **2.** a surgical specialty dealing with the treatment of wounds, injuries, and resulting disabilities.—**traumatologic, traumatological,** *adj.*

traumatopathy /trô′mətop′əthē/ [Gk, *trauma* + *pathos*, disease], a pathologic condition resulting from a wound or injury.—**traumatopathic,** *adj.*

traumatophilia /trô′mətōfil′ē-ə/ [Gk, *trauma* + *philein*, to love], a psychologic state in which the individual derives unconscious pleasure from injuries and surgical operations.—**traumatophiliac,** *n.,* **traumatophilic,** *adj.*

traumatopnea /trô′mətop′nē-ə/ [Gk, *trauma* + *pnein*, to breathe], partial asphyxia with collapse of the patient, caused by a penetrating thoracic wound permitting air to enter the pleural space and compress the lungs.

traumatopyra /trô′mətōpī′rə/ [Gk, *trauma* + *pyr*, fire], an elevated temperature resulting from a wound or injury.

traumatotherapy /-ther′əpē/ [Gk, *trauma* + *therapeia*, treatment], the medical, surgical, and psychologic treatment of wounds, injuries, and disabilities resulting from trauma.—**traumatotherapeutic,** *adj.*

traumatropism /trômat′rəpiz′əm/ [Gk, *trauma* + *trepein*, to turn], the tendency of damaged tissue to attract microorganisms and promote their growth, frequently causing infections after injuries, especially burns.

travail /trəvāl′/ [OFr, *travaillier,* to work], **1.** physical or mental exertion, especially when distressful. **2.** (in obstetrics) the effort of labor and childbirth.

Travelbee, Joyce (1926-1973), a nursing theorist who developed the Human-to-Human Relationship Model and Theory, presented in her book *Interpersonal Aspects of Nursing,* (1966, 1971). Travelbee based the assumptions of her theory on the concepts of logotherapy, first proposed by Viktor Frankel, a survivor of Auschwitz, in his book *Man's Search for Meaning* (1963). Travelbee believed nursing is accomplished through human-to-human relationships that begin with the original encounter and then progress through stages of emerging identities, developing feelings of empathy and later of sympathy.

traveler's diarrhea [OFr, *travaillier,* to work; Gk, *dia,* through, *rhein,* to flow], any of several diarrheal disorders commonly seen in people visiting regions of the world other than their own. Some strains of *Escherichia coli,* which produce a powerful exotoxin, are the common cause. Other causative organisms include *Giardia lamblia* and species of *Salmonella* and *Shigella*. Symptoms last for a few days and include abdominal cramps, nausea, vomiting, slight fever, and watery stools.

traverse /travurs'/, 1. to travel or pass across, over, or through. 2. (in computed tomography) a single complete movement of the x-ray tube around the object being scanned.

TRBF, abbreviation for **total renal blood flow.**

Treacher Collins' syndrome [Edward Treacher Collins, English ophthalmologist, 1862–1919], an inherited disorder, characterized by mandibulofacial dysostosis.

treatment [Fr, *traitement*], 1. the care and management of a patient to combat, ameliorate, or prevent a disease, disorder, or injury. 2. a method of combating, ameliorating, or preventing a disease, disorder, or injury. Active or curative treatment is designed to cure; palliative treatment is directed to relieve pain and distress; prophylactic treatment is for the prevention of a disease or disorder; and causal treatment focuses on the cause of a disorder. Treatment may be pharmacologic, using drugs; surgical, involving operative procedures; or supportive, building the patient's strength.

treatment guardian, a person who is appointed by the court for the purpose of consenting to or refusing medical treatment for a patient.

treatment plan [Fr, *traitement* + L, *planta*], (in dentistry) a schedule of procedures and appointments designed to restore, step by step, a patient's oral health. The plan contains the advantages, disadvantages, costs, alternatives, and sequelae of treatment. It must be presented to the patient for approval.

treatment room, a room in a patient care unit, usually in a hospital, in which various treatments or procedures requiring special equipment are performed, such as removing sutures.

Trechona /trikon'ə/, a genus of spiders, family Dipluridae, the bite of which is toxic and irritating to humans.

tree [AS, *treow*], 1. (in anatomy) an anatomic structure with branches that spread out like those of a tree, such as the bronchial tree. 2. a pattern of searching for information in a computer data base, following a series of branching options from a general category to reach specific desired items.

Trematoda /trem'ətōdə/, a class of flatworms, Platyhelminthes, that includes flukes. The adults are external or internal parasites of vertebrates. Intestinal infections in North America are rare except through flukes in foods imported from Asia or the tropics.

trematode /trem'ətōd/ [Gk, *trematodes,* pierced], any species of flatworm of the class Trematoda, some of which are parasitic to humans, infecting the liver, the lungs, and the intestines.

trembles /trem'bəls/, a toxic reaction experienced by cattle that have eaten white snakeroot or rayless goldenrod, pasture weeds that contain tremetone, a ketone. The toxic chemical is eliminated in the milk of the cows, causing sickness in humans who drink the milk.

tremor /trem'ər, trē'mər/ [L, shaking], rhythmic, purposeless, quivering movements resulting from the involuntary alternating contraction and relaxation of opposing groups of skeletal muscles occurring in some elderly individuals, certain families, and patients with various neurodegenerative disorders.

tremulous /trem'yələs/ [L, *tremulare,* to tremble], pertaining to tremors, or involuntary muscular contractions.

tremulous pulse [L, *tremulare,* to tremble, *pulsare,* to beat], a feeble fluttering pulse.

trench fever [OFr, *trenchier,* to cut; L, *febris,* fever], a self-limited infection, caused by *Rochalimaea quintana,* a rickettsial organism transmitted by body lice, characterized by weakness, fever, rash, and leg pains.

trench foot [OFr, *trenchier,* to cut; AS, *fot*], a condition of moist gangrene of the foot caused by the freezing of wet skin.

Trendelenburg gait /trendel'ənbərg, tren'-d(e)lənburg'/ [Friederich Trendelenburg, German surgeon, 1844–1924], an abnormal gait associated with a weakness of the gluteus medius. The Trendelenburg gait is characterized by the dropping of the pelvis on the unaffected side of the body at the moment of heelstrike on the affected side.

Trendelenburg operation [Friederich Trendelenburg], the ligation of varicose veins whose valves are ineffective, performed to remove weakened parts of tissues in which thrombi might lodge. During surgery the saphenous vein is ligated at the groin, where it joins the femoral vein. A wire device, called a stripper, is threaded through the lumen of the vein from groin to ankle. The wire and the vein are then pulled from the groin incision.

Trendelenburg position [Friederich Trendelenburg], a position in which the head is low and the body and legs are on an inclined plane. It is sometimes used in pelvic surgery to displace the abdominal organs upward, out of the pelvis, or to increase the blood flow to the brain in hypotension and shock.

Trendelenburg test [Friederich Trendelenburg], a simple test for incompetent valves in a person who has varicose veins. The person lies down and elevates the leg to empty the vein, then stands, and the vein is observed as it fills. If the valves are incompetent, the vein fills from above; if the valves are normal, they do not allow backflow of blood, and the vein fills from below.

trephination /trif´inā´shən/, the surgical excision of a circular piece of bone or other tissue accomplished with a cylindric saw.

trephine /trifīn´, trifēn´/ [Gk, trypan, to bore], a circular sawlike instrument used in removing pieces of bone or tissue, usually from the skull.

trepidation /trep´idā·shən/ [L, trepidare, to tremble], a state of anxiety.

Treponema /trep´onē´mə/ [Gk, trepein, to turn, nema, thread], a genus of spirochetes, including some pathogenic to humans, such as the organisms causing bejel, pinta, syphilis, and yaws.

Treponema pallidum, an actively motile, slender spirochetal organism that causes syphilis.

treponematosis /trep´onē´mətō´sis/, pl. **treponematoses** [Gk, trepein + nema + osis, condition], any disease caused by spirochetes of the genus Treponema. All these infections are effectively treated with penicillin.

tretinoin /tret´inō´in/, a keratolytic prescribed in the topical treatment of acne vulgaris.

TRF, abbreviation for *thyrotropin-releasing factor.*

TRH, abbreviation for **thyrotropin-releasing hormone**

triacetin /trī·as´itin/, an antifungal prescribed in the treatment of superficial fungus infections of the skin, including athlete's foot.

triad /trī´əd/ [Gk, trias, three], a combination of three, such as two parents and a child.

triage /trē·äzh´/ [Fr, trier, to sort out], **1.** (in military medicine) a classification of casualties of war and other disasters according to the gravity of injuries, urgency of treatment, and place for treatment. **2.** a process in which a group of patients is sorted according to their need for care. **3.** (in disaster medicine) a process in which a large group of patients is sorted so that care can be concentrated on those who are likely to survive.

Triage, a Nursing Interventions Classification defined as establishing priorities of patient care for urgent treatment while allocating scarce resources.

trial, a process of quality testing.

trial forceps /trī´əl/ [Fr, trier, to sort out], an obstetric operation consisting of an attempt to deliver an infant with obstetric forceps. The forceps are applied to the baby's head, and moderate traction is applied. The delivery is continued only if the trial indicates that delivery can be accomplished safely.

trial of labor [Fr, trier, to sort out; L, labor, work], childbirth in which there is doubt as to whether the head of the fetus will pass through the pelvic brim. The situation must be monitored and assessed carefully to avoid fetal or maternal distress.

triamcinolone /trī´amsin´əlōn/, a glucocorticoid prescribed as an antiinflammatory agent in the treatment of dermatoses, stomatitis, and lichen planus lesions.

triamterene /trī·am´tərēn/, a potassium-sparing diuretic usually prescribed alone or with another diuretic in the treatment of edema, hypertension, and congestive heart failure.

triangle [L, triangulus, three-cornered], a predictable emotional process that takes place when there is difficulty in a relationship. The three corners of a triangle can be composed of three people or two people and an object, group, or issue.

triangular bandage /trī·ang´gyələr/, a square of cloth folded or cut into the shape of a triangle. It may be used as a sling, a cover, or a thick pad to control bleeding.

triangular bone, the pyramidal carpal bone in the proximal row on the ulnar side of the wrist.

triazolam /tri·az´əlam/, a benzodiazepine hypnotic agent prescribed in the short-term treatment of insomnia.

tribe [L, tribus], a taxonomic division of organisms, subordinate to a family and superior to a genus, or subtribe.

tribology /tribol´əjē/ [Gk, tribo, to rub, logos, science], the study of friction, wear, and lubrication of articulating surfaces.

TRIC /trik/, abbreviation for *trachoma inclusion conjunctivitis* agent, which refers to *Chlamydia trachomatis*, the organism that causes both inclusion conjunctivitis and trachoma.

triceps brachii /trī´seps brak´ē·ī/ [L, three-headed, brachium, arm], a large muscle that extends the entire length of the posterior surface of the humerus. It functions to extend the forearm and to adduct the arm.

triceps reflex, a deep tendon reflex elicited by tapping sharply the triceps tendon

T

proximal to the elbow with the forearm in a relaxed position.

triceps skinfold, the thickness of a fold of skin around the triceps muscle. It is measured primarily to estimate the amount of subcutaneous fat.

triceps surae limp, an abnormal action in the walking or gait cycle, associated with a deficiency in the elevating and propulsive factors on the affected side of the body, especially a deficiency of the triceps surae. Such a deficiency prevents the triceps surae from raising the pelvis and carrying it forward during the walking cycle.

trichiasis /trikī'əsis/ [Gk, *thrix,* hair, *osis,* condition], an abnormal inversion of the eyelashes that irritates the eyeball. It usually follows infection or inflammation.

trichinosis /trik'inō'sis/ [Gk, *thrix + osis,* condition], infestation with the parasitic roundworm *Trichinella spiralis,* transmitted by eating raw or undercooked pork or bear meat. Early symptoms of infection include abdominal pain, nausea, fever, and diarrhea; later, muscle pain, tenderness, fatigue, and eosinophilia are observed. Light infections may be asymptomatic.

trichlormethiazide /trī'klôrməthī'əzīd/, a thiazide diuretic and antihypertensive prescribed in the treatment of hypertension and edema.

trichloroethylene /trīklôr'ō·eth'ilēn/, a general anesthetic, administered by mask with N_2O, for dentistry, minor surgery, and the first stages of labor. It is not currently used in clinical anesthesia practice in developed countries.

trichoepithelioma /trik'ō·ep'ithē'lē·ō'mə/ [Gk, *thrix + epi,* above, *thele* nipple, *oma* tumor], a cutaneous tumor derived from the basal cells of the follicles of fine body hair.

trichoid /trik'oid/, resembling a hair.

trichologia /trik'əlō'jē·ə/ [Gk, *thrix + legein,* to pull], an abnormal condition in which a person pulls out his or her own hair, usually seen only in delirium.

trichology /trikol'əjē/, the study of the anatomy, development, and diseases of the hair.

trichomatous /trikom'ətəs/ [Gk, *trichoma,* hairy, growth], **1.** pertaining to an introversion of the margin of the eyelid. **2.** pertaining to matted or ingrowing hair.

trichomonacide /trik'ōmon'əsīd/ [Gk, *thrix + monas,* unit; L, *caedere,* to kill], an agent destructive to *Trichomonas vaginalis,* a parasitic protozoan flagellate that causes a refractory type of vaginitis, cystitis, and urethritis.—**trichomonacidal,** *adj.*

Trichomonas /trik'əmon'əs/, a genus of flagellate protozoa, which includes many species that are parasitic. Some live in the mouth of humans and are found around carious teeth; other species are found in the vagina and urethra of women. They are a cause of trichomoniasis.

Trichomonas tenax, a species of protozoa that is found in the human mouth, particularly in cases of pyorrhea.

Trichomonas vaginalis [Gk, *thrix + monas* + L, *vagina,* sheath], a motile protozoan parasite that causes vaginitis with a copious malodorous discharge and pruritus.

trichomoniasis /trik'əmənī'əsis/ [Gk, *thrix + monas + osis,* condition], a vaginal infection caused by the protozoan *Trichomonas vaginalis.* It is characterized by itching, burning, and frothy, pale yellow to green, malodorous vaginal discharge. Infection is transmitted by sexual intercourse, rarely by moist washcloths, or, in newborns, by passage through the birth canal.

trichuriasis, an infection of the large intestine by the nematode *Trichuris trichiura,* or whipworm.

Trichuris trichiura, a species of whipworms, commonly found in warm, moist regions of the world. Ingestion of whipworm eggs results in infection in humans; the parasites live mainly in the cecum or large intestine. Heavy infections cause symptoms of abdominal pain and diarrhea; very heavy infections may result in anemia because of intestinal blood loss.

trichopathy /trikop'əthē/ [Gk, *thrix,* hair, *pathos,* disease], any disease condition involving the hair.

Trichophyton /trikof'iton/ [Gk, *thrix + phyton,* plant], a genus of fungi that infects skin, hair, and nails.

trichosis /trikō'sis/ [Gk, *thrix,* hair, *osis,* condition], any abnormal condition of hair growth, including alopecia, excessive female hair growth, or abnormal hair color.

trichosporosis [Gk, *thrix,* hair, *spora,* seed, *osis,* condition], a fungus disease of the hair shaft, giving the hair a metallic appearance and caused by *Trichosporon biegetii.*

trichostrongyliasis /trik'ōstron'jəlī'əsis/ [Gk, *thrix + strongylos,* round, *osis,* condition], infestation with *Trichostrongylus,* a genus of nematode worm.

Trichostrongylus /trik'ōstron'jiləs/ [Gk, *thrix + strongylos*], a genus of roundworm, some species of which are parasitic to humans, such as *T. orientalis.*

trichotillomania /trik'ōtil'ōmā'nē·ə/ [Gk, *thrix + tillein,* to pull, *mania* madness], an impulse disorder characterized by a desire to pull out one's hair, frequently seen in cases of severe mental retardation and delirium.—**trichotillomanic, tricho-manic,** *adj.*

trichuriasis /trik´yərī´əsis/ /trik´yŏŏrī´əsis/ [Gk, *thrix* + *oura,* tail, *osis,* condition], infestation with the roundworm *Trichuris trichiura.* The condition is usually asymptomatic, but heavy infestation may cause nausea, abdominal pain, diarrhea, and occasionally anemia and rectal prolapse.

Trichuris /trikyŏŏr´is/ [Gk, *thrix* + *oura*] a genus of parasitic roundworms of which the species *T. trichiura* infects the intestinal tract.

tricrotic pulse /trīkrot´ik/, an abnormal pulse that has three peaks of elevation on a sphygmogram, representing the pressure wave from the heart in systole followed by two pressure waves in diastole.

tricuspid /trīkus´pid/ [Gk, *treis,* three; L, *cuspis,* point], **1.** pertaining to three points or cusps. **2.** pertaining to the tricuspid valve of the heart.

tricuspid area [Gk, *treis,* three; L, *cuspis,* point], a region of the chest near the left lower sternum and opposite the fourth and fifth costal cartilages, where sounds of the tricuspid heart valve are best heard by auscultation.

tricuspid atresia, a congenital cardiac anomaly characterized by the absence of the tricuspid valve so that there is no opening between the right atrium and right ventricle. Clinical manifestations include severe cyanosis, dyspnea, anoxia, and signs of right-sided heart failure.

tricuspid murmur [Gk, *treis,* three; L, *cuspis* point, *murmur,* humming], one of the heart murmurs caused by a defective tricuspid valve. The tricuspid diastolic and systolic murmurs resemble mitral valve diastolic and systolic murmurs.

tricuspid stenosis, narrowing or stricture of the tricuspid valve. It is relatively uncommon and usually associated with lesions of other valves caused by rheumatic fever. Clinical characteristics include diastolic pressure gradient between the right atrium and ventricle, jugular vein distension, pulmonary congestion, and in severe cases hepatic congestion and splenomegaly.

tricuspid tooth [Gk, *treis,* three; L, *cuspis,* point; AS, *toth*], a tooth with three points or cusps, rare in humans.

tricuspid valve, a valve with three main cusps situated between the right atrium and right ventricle of the heart. As the right and left ventricles relax during the diastolic phase of the heartbeat, the tricuspid valve opens, allowing blood to flow into the ventricle. In the systolic phase of the heartbeat, both blood-filled ventricles contract, pumping out their contents, while the tricuspid and mitral valves close to prevent any backflow.

tricyclic compound /trīsik´lik/ [Gk, *treis* + *kyklos,* circle; L, *componere,* to put together], a chemical substance containing three rings in the molecular structure, especially a tricyclic antidepressant drug such as imipramine, amitriptyline, doxepin, and nortriptyline used in the treatment of reactive or endogenous depression.

tridihexethyl chloride /trī´dīhek´səthil/, an anticholinergic prescribed in the treatment of gastrointestinal (GI) muscle spasm and to reduce gastric secretion and GI motility.

trientine hydrochloride /trī·en´tēn/, an oral medication for treatment of an inherited defect in copper metabolism. It is prescribed for the relief of symptoms of Wilson's disease.

triethanolamine polypeptide oleate-condensate /trī·eth´ənol´əmēn/, a ceruminolytic agent prescribed to reduce excessive earwax, used as a solution in propylene glycol.

trifluoperazine hydrochloride /trī´flŏŏ·ōper´əzēn/, a phenothiazine tranquilizer prescribed in the treatment of anxiety, schizophrenia, and other psychotic disorders and as an antiemetic.

trifluorothymidine /trīflŏŏr´ōthī´mədēn/, an antiviral prescribed in the treatment of keratoconjunctivitis, herpetic keratitis, and other forms of keratitis caused by herpes simplex virus.

triflupromazine hydrochloride /trī´fluprō´məzēn/, a phenothiazine tranquilizer prescribed in the treatment of severe agitation and other psychotic disorders and for the control of severe vomiting.

trifocal lens /trīfō´kəl/ [Gk, *treis,* three; L, *focus,* hearth, *lens,* lentil], an eyeglass lens ground for viewing objects at three different distances—near, intermediate, and far.

trifurcation /-furkā´shən/ [Gk, *treis,* three; L, *furca,* fork], pertaining to a vessel or other structure with three branches.

trigeminal /trījem´inəl/ [Gk, *treis,* three; L, *geminus,* twins], pertaining to the three-branch trigeminal (fifth cranial) nerve innervating the face, eyes, nose, mouth, and jaws.

trigeminal nerve [Gk, *treis* + *geminus,* twin], either of the largest pair of cranial nerves, essential for the act of chewing, general sensibility of the face, and muscular sensibility of the obliquus superior.

trigeminal neuralgia, a neurologic condition of the trigeminal facial nerve, characterized by paroxysms of flashing, stab-like pain radiating along the course of a branch of the nerve from the angle of the jaw. It is caused by degeneration of the nerve or pressure on it. Any or all of the three branches of the nerve may be affected. Neuralgia of the first branch results in pain around the eyes and over the forehead; of the second branch, in pain in the upper lip, nose, and cheek; of the third branch, in pain on the side of the tongue and lower lip. The momentary bursts of pain recur in clusters lasting many seconds; paroxysmal episodes of the pains may last for hours.

trigeminal pulse, an abnormal pulse in which every third beat is absent.

trigeminy /trījem'inē/ [Gk, *treis* + L, *geminus,* twin], **1.** a grouping in threes. **2.** a cardiac arrhythmia characterized by the occurrence of three heartbeats, two normal beats coupled to an ectopic beat or two ectopic beats coupled to a normal beat in a repeating pattern.—**trigeminal,** *adj.*

trigger [D, *trekker,* that which pulls], a substance, object, or agent that initiates or stimulates an action.

triggered activity [D, *trekker,* that which pulls; L, *activus*], rhythmic cardiac activity that results when a series of afterdepolarizations reach threshold potential.

trigger finger, a phenomenon in which the movement of a finger is halted momentarily in flexion or extension and then continues with a jerk.

trigger point, a point on the body that is particularly sensitive to touch and, when stimulated, becomes the site of a painful neuralgia.

triglyceride /trīglis'ərīd/, a simple fat compound consisting of three molecules of fatty acid (e.g., oleic, palmitic, or stearic) and glycerol. Triglycerides make up most animal and vegetable fats and are the principal lipids in the blood, where they circulate, bound to a protein, forming high-and low-density lipoproteins.

trigone /trī'gōn/ [Gk, *trigonos,* threecornered], **1.** a triangle. **2.** the first three dominant cusps, considered collectively, of an upper molar.

trigonelline /trig'ōnel'ēn/, an alkaloid derived from various kinds of plant products, including coffee beans, fenugreek, and seeds of *Cannabis sativa,* as well as from sea urchins and jellyfish. Trigonelline is used in the manufacture of poultices and other medicinals.

trigonitis /trī'gənī'tis/, inflammation of the trigone of the bladder, which often accompanies urethritis.

trigonum vesicae /trīgō'nəm/, a triangular area of the bladder between the opening of the ureters and the orifice of the urethra.

trihexyphenidyl hydrochloride /trīhex'-ifen'idil/, an anticholinergic agent prescribed in the treatment of Parkinson's disease and to control drug-induced extrapyramidal reactions.

trihybrid /trīhī'brid/ [Gk, *treis* + *hybrida,* mixed offspring], (in genetics) pertaining to or describing an individual, organism, or strain heterozygous for three specific traits that is the offspring of parents differing in three specific gene pairs.

trihybrid cross, (in genetics) the mating of two individuals, organisms, or strains that have different gene pairs that determine three specific traits or in which three particular characteristics or gene loci are being followed.

trihydric alcohol /trīhid'rik/, an alcohol containing three hydroxyl groups.

triiodothyronine (T₃) /trī'ī-ō'dōthī'rənēn/, a hormone that helps regulate growth and development, helps control metabolism and body temperature, and, by a negative-feedback system, acts to inhibit the secretion of thyrotropin by the pituitary gland.

trilaminar blastoderm /trīlam'inər/ [Gk, *treis* + L, *lamina,* plate; Gk, *blastos,* germ, *derma,* skin], the stage of embryonic development in which all three of the primary germ layers, the ectoderm, mesoderm, and entoderm, have formed.

trill [It, *trillare* to make a ringing sound], a vibratory, quavering, warbling sound, as produced by human voice, birds, insects, or musical instruments.

trilogy of Fallot /tril'əjē, falō'/ [Gk, *treis* + *logos,* word; Etienne-Louis A. Fallot, French physician, 1850–1911], a congenital cardiac anomaly consisting of the combination of pulmonic stenosis, interatrial septal defect, and right ventricular hypertrophy.

trilostane /tril'əstān/, a synthetic steroid that inhibits the synthesis of adrenal steroids. It is prescribed for the treatment of Cushing's syndrome.

trimeprazine tartrate /trīmep'rəzēn/, an antipruritic prescribed in the treatment of pruritus and hypersensitivity reactions of the skin.

trimester /trīmes'tər, trī'-/ [L, *trimestris,* three months], one of the three periods of approximately 3 months into which pregnancy is divided. The first trimester includes the time from the first day of the last menstrual period to the end of 12 weeks. The second trimester, closer to 4 months in length than 3, extends from the twelfth to the twenty-eighth week of gestation. The third trimester begins at the twenty-eighth week and extends to the time of delivery.

trimethadione /trī'methədī'ōn/, an anticonvulsant prescribed to prevent seizures in petit mal epilepsy, particularly seizures that are resistant to other therapies.

trimethaphan camsylate /trīmeth'əfan/, a ganglionic blocking agent prescribed to produce controlled hypotension during surgery and to lower blood pressure in hypertensive emergencies.

trimethobenzamide hydrochloride /trī-meth'ōben'zəmid/, an antiemetic prescribed for the relief of nausea and vomiting.

trimethoprim /trīmeth'əprim/, an antibacterial prescribed in the treatment of infections, particularly of the urinary tract, middle ear, and bronchi.

trimipramine maleate /trimip'rəmēn/, an antidepressant prescribed in the treatment of anxiety, depression, and insomnia.

trinucleotide /trīnōō'klē·ətīd'/, a combination of three adjacent nucleotide units used to identify a specific amino acid in a genome.

trioxsalen /trī·ok'sələn/, a melanizing agent prescribed to enhance pigmentation, for repigmentation of the skin in idiopathic vitiligo, and to increase tolerance to sunlight.

tripelennamine hydrochloride /trī'pelen'-əmēn/, an antihistamine prescribed in the treatment of rhinitis and hypersensitivity reactions of the skin.

tripe palms, a condition of thickened velvet or moss-textured palms with pronounced skin ridge patterns. It has been associated with certain malignancies, including lung and stomach cancers and pulmonary carcinomas.

triphasic /trifā'zik/ [Gk, *treis,* three, *phasis,* appearance], having three phases or stages.

triple-dye treatment, a therapy for burns in which three dyes, 6% gentian violet, 1% brilliant green, and 0.1% acriflavine base, are applied.

triplegia /trīplē'jə/ [Gk, *treis,* three, *plege,* stroke], a condition of paralysis on one side of the body plus paralysis of an arm or leg on the opposite side.

triple lumen catheter [L, *triplus,* triple; L, *lumen,* light; Gk, *katheter,* a thing lowered into], any catheter with three separate passages. In a triple-lumen urinary catheter, one passage is for irrigation, one for drainage, and one for inflation of the bulb.

triple point, a situation in which a given substance may exist in solid, liquid, and vapor forms at the same time. Every substance has a theoretic triple point, which depends on ideal conditions of temperature and pressure.

triple response, a triad of phenomena that occur in sequence after the intrader-

mal injection of histamine. First, a red spot develops, spreading outward for a few millimeters, reaching its maximal size within 1 minute and then turning bluish. Next, a brighter red flush of color spreads slowly in an irregular flare around the original red spot. Finally, a wheal filled with fluid forms over the original spot.

triple sugar iron reaction, any one of several reactions seen in certain bacterial cultures growing on triple sugar iron agar, a culture medium used to aid in the identification of *Escherichia coli, Proteus, Salmonella, Shigella,* and other pathogenic enteric bacteria.

triplet /trip'lit/ [L, *triplus*], **1.** any one of three offspring born of the same gestation period during a single pregnancy. **2.** (in genetics) the unit of three consecutive bases in one polynucleotide chain of deoxyribonucleic acid or ribonucleic acid that codes for a specific amino acid.

triploid (3n) /trip'loid/ [L, *triplus* + *eidos*], **1.** pertaining to an individual, organism, strain, or cell that has three complete sets of chromosomes. In humans the triploid number is 69, found in rare cases of aborted or stillborn fetuses. **2.** such an individual, organism, strain, or cell.

triploidy /trip'loidē/, the state or condition of having three complete sets of chromosomes.

tripod /trī'pod/ [Gk, *treis,* three, *pous,* foot], any object with three legs or three feet.

tripodial symmelia /trīpō'dē·əl/ [Gk, *treis,* three, *pous,* foot, *syn,* together, *melos,* limb], a fetal anomaly characterized by the fusion of the lower extremities and the presence of three feet.

triprolidine hydrochloride /trī·prol'idēn/, an antihistamine prescribed in the treatment of hypersensitivity reactions, including rhinitis, skin rash, and pruritus.

tripsis /trip'sis/ [Gk rubbing], **1.** massage. **2.** the process of reducing the particle size of a substance by grinding it with a mortar and pestle.

trisaccharide /trīsak'ərīd/ [Gk, *treis,* three, *sakcharon,* sugar], a carbohydrate composed of three monosaccharide units linked together.

trismus /triz'məs/ [Gk, *trismos,* gnashing], a prolonged tonic spasm of the muscles of the jaw.

trisomy /trī'səmē/ [Gk, *treis* + *soma,* body], a chromosomal aberration characterized by the presence of one more than the normal number of chromosomes in a diploid complement; in humans the trisomic cell contains 47 chromosomes and is designated $2n + 1$.—**trisomic,** *adj.*

trisomy 8, a congenital condition associated with the presence of an extra chromosome 8 within the C group. Those with the condition are slender and of normal height and have a large asymmetric head, prominent forehead, deep-set eyes, low-set prominent ears, and thick lips. There is mild to severe mental and motor retardation, often with delayed and poorly articulated speech. Skeletal anomalies and joint limitation, especially permanent flexion of one or more fingers, may occur. There are unusually deep palmar and plantar creases, which are diagnostically significant. Most trisomy 8 individuals are mosaic.

trisomy 13, a congenital condition caused by the presence of an extra chromosome in the D group, predominantly chromosome 13, although in rare instances chromosome 14 or 15. It occurs in approximately 1 in 5000 births and is characterized by multiple midline anomalies and central nervous system defects, including holoprosencephaly, microcephaly, myelomeningocele, microphthalmos, and cleft lip and palate. There is also severe mental retardation; polydactyly; deafness; convulsions; and abnormalities of the heart, viscera, and genitalia.

trisomy 18, a congenital condition caused by the presence of an extra chromosome 18, characterized by severe mental retardation and multiple deformities. Among the most common defects are scaphocephaly or other skull abnormalities; micrognathia; abnormal facies with low-set malformed ears and prominent occiput; cleft lip and palate; clenched fists with overlapping fingers, especially the index over the third finger; clubfeet; and syndactyly. Ventricular septal defect, patent ductus arteriosus, atrial septal defect, and renal anomalies are also common.

trisomy 22, a congenital condition caused by the presence of an extra chromosome 22 in the G group, characterized by psychomotor retardation and various developmental anomalies. Common defects include microcephaly, micrognathia, hypotonia, hypertelorism, abnormal ears with preauricular tags or fistulas and congenital heart disease. In partial trisomy 22 the extra chromosome is much smaller than the normal pair and causes coloboma of the iris, anal atresia, or both, as well as various other defects.

trisomy syndrome, any condition caused by the addition of an extra member to a normal pair of homologous autosomes or to the sex chromosomes or by the translocation of a part of one chromosome to another. Most trisomies occur as a result of

complete or partial nondisjunction of the chromosomes during cell division.

trisplanchnic /trīsplangk′nik/, pertaining to three major body cavities: skull, thorax, and abdomen.

trisulfapyrimidines /trīsul′fəpirim′idīnz/, three antibacterials in combination (sulfadiazine, sulfamerazine, and sulfamethazine), rarely prescribed today.

tritium (3H) /trit′ē·əm, trish′əm/ [Gk, tritos, third], the radioactive isotope of the hydrogen atom, used as a tracer; a b emitter.

trivalence /trīvā′ləns/ [Gk, treis + L, valere, to be worth], a triple state, an ability of a group of atoms to replace three monovalent elements in a compound.

trivalent /trīvā′lənt/ [Gk, treis + L, valere, to be worth], **1.** pertaining to an atom or group of atoms with the capability of bonding with or replacing three monovalent elements. **2.** designating a vaccine that can prevent diseases or conditions.

trivial name /triv′ē·əl/, a chemical name that lacks a systematic notation that would indicate its molecular structure or other information about its relationship to other chemicals. The name may be accepted as an official nonproprietary designation because of common usage. Examples include caffeine, folic acid, and aspirin.

tRNA, abbreviation for **transfer RNA.**

trocar /trō′kär/ [Fr, trois, three, carres, sides], a sharp, pointed rod that fits inside a tube. It is used to pierce the skin and the wall of a cavity or canal in the body to aspirate fluids, to instill a medication or solution, or to guide the placement of a soft catheter.

trochanter /trōkan′tər/ [Gk, runner], one of the two bony projections on the proximal end of the femur that serve as the point of attachment of various muscles.

trochanter major [Gk, trochanter, runner; L, major, great], a large projection from the proximal end of the shaft of the femur. It is a point of attachment for the gluteus minimus and gluteus medius muscles.

troche /trō′kē/ [Gk, trochos, lozenge], a small oval, round, or oblong tablet containing a medicinal agent incorporated in a flavored, sweetened mucilage or fruit base that dissolves in the mouth, releasing the drug.

trochlea /trok′lē·ə/, a pulley-shaped part or structure.—**trochlear,** adj.

trochlear /trok′lē·ər/ [L, trochlea, pulley], **1.** pertaining to a trochlea or something that is pulley shaped. **2.** relating to the trochlear (fourth cranial) nerve.

trochlear nerve [L, trochlea, pulley; nervus, nerve], either of the smallest pair of cranial nerves, essential for eye movement and eye muscle sensibility.

trochlear notch of ulna, a large depression in the ulna, formed by the olecranon and coronoid processes, that articulates with the trochlea of the humerus.

trolamine /trol'əmēn/, a contraction for *triethanolamine.*

troleandomycin /trol'ē·an'dōmī'sin/, a macrolide antibiotic prescribed in the treatment of certain infections, including pneumococcal pneumonia and group A streptococcal infections of the upper respiratory tract.

Trombiculidae /trom'bikyōo'lidē/, a family of mites, including harvest mites, red bugs, and chiggers. The larvae are parasitic, and the adults are free-living. The mites are disease vectors of typhus, rickettsiae, scrub itch, tsutsugamushi disease, and other infections.

trombiculosis /trombik'yəlō'sis/ [Gk, *tromein,* to tremble, *osis,* condition], an infestation with mites of the genus *Trombicula,* some species of which carry scrub typhus.

trophic /trof'ik/ [Gk, *trophe,* nutrition], pertaining to a nutritive effect on or quality of cellular activity.

trophic action [Gk, *trophe,* nutrition; L, *agere,* to do], the stimulation of cell reproduction and enlargement by nurturing and causing growth.

trophic fracture, a fracture resulting from the weakening of bone tissue caused by nutritional disturbances.

trophic hormones, hormones secreted by the adenohypophysis that stimulate target organs.

trophic ulcer, a pressure ulcer caused by external trauma to a part of the body that is in poor condition resulting from disease, vascular insufficiency, or loss of afferent nerve fibers.

trophism /trof'izəm/ [Gk, *trophe,* nutrition], the influence of nourishment.

trophoblast /trof'əblast'/ [Gk, *trophe* + *blastos,* germ], the layer of tissue that forms the wall of the blastocyst of placental mammals in the early stages of embryonic development. It functions in the implantation of the blastocyst into the uterine wall and in supplying nutrients to the embryo.—**trophoblastic,** *adj.*

trophoblastic cancer /-blas'tik/, a malignant neoplastic disease of the uterus derived from chorionic epithelium, characterized by the production of high levels of human chorionic gonadotropin (HCG). The tumor may be an invasive hydatid mole (chorioadenoma destruens) formed by grossly enlarged vesicular chorionic villi or a malignant uterine choriocarcinoma that arises from nonvillous chorionic epithelium. Initial symptoms are vaginal bleeding and a profuse, foul-smelling discharge; a persistent cough or hemoptysis signals pulmonary involvement. As the disease progresses, there may be frequent hemorrhage, weakness, and emaciation.

trophotropic /trof'ətrop'ik/ [Gk, *trophe* + *trepein,* to turn], pertaining to a combination of parasympathetic nervous system activity, somatic muscle relaxation, and cortical beta rhythm synchronization, such as in a resting or sleep state.

trophotropism /trof'ətrop'izəm/, a tropism in which cells migrate toward or away from nutrient sources.

trophozoite /trof'əzō'it/ [Gk, *trophe* + *zoon,* animal], an immature ameboid protozoon. When fully developed, a trophozoite may be identified as a schizont.

tropical acne /trop'ikəl/, a form of acne that is caused or aggravated by high temperature and humidity. It is characterized by large nodules or pustules on the neck, back, upper arms, and buttocks.

tropical medicine [Gk, *tropikos,* of the solstice; L, *medicina*], the branch of medicine concerned with the diagnosis and treatment of diseases commonly occurring in tropic and subtropic regions of the world, generally between 30 degrees north and south of the equator.

tropical sprue, a malabsorption syndrome of unknown cause that is endemic in the tropics and subtropics. It is characterized by abnormalities in the mucosa of the small intestine, resulting in protein malnutrition and multiple nutritional deficiencies, often complicated by severe infection. Symptoms include diarrhea, anorexia, and weight loss. Megaloblastic anemia may result from folic acid and vitamin B_{12} deficiency.

tropocollagen /trop'əkol'əjən/ [Gk, *trepein,* to turn, *kolla,* glue, *genein,* to produce], fundamental units of collagen fibrils obtained by prolonged extraction of insoluble collagen with dilute acid.

tropomyosin /trop'əmī'əsin/ [Gk, *trepein* + *mys,* muscle], a protein component of sarcomere filaments, which, together with troponin, regulates interactions of actin and myosin in muscle contractions.

troponin /trō'pənin/ [Gk, *trepein,* to turn], a protein in the striated cell ultrastructure that modulates the interaction between actin and myosin molecules.

trough /trôf/ [AS, *trog*], a groove or channel, such as the gingival trough around the neck of a tooth.

T

Trousseau's sign /troॊosōz'/ [Armand Trousseau, French physician, 1801–1867; L, *signum*, mark], **1.** a test for latent tetany in which carpal spasm is induced by inflating a sphygmomanometer cuff on the upper arm to a pressure exceeding systolic blood pressure for 3 minutes. **2.** a reddened streak, the result of drawing a finger across the skin. It is seen with a variety of nervous system disorders.

Trousseau's syndrome [Armand Trousseau], superficial migratory thrombophlebitis associated with visceral cancer.

Trp, abbreviation for **tryptophan.**

true ankylosis [ME, *treue*, faith; Gk, *anklosis*, joint stiffness], an abnormal fusion or union of the separate bones that usually form a joint.

true birth rate [ME, *treue*, faith, *burthe* + L, *reri*, to calculate], the ratio of total births to the total female population of childbearing age, between 15 and 45 years of age.

true conjugate, a radiographic measurement of the distance from the upper margin of the symphysis pubis to the sacral promontory. It is usually 1.5 to 2 cm less than the diagonal conjugate.

true denticle, a calcified body composed of irregular dentin found in the pulp chamber of a tooth.

true diverticulum [ME, *treue*, faith; L, *diverticulare*, to turn aside], diverticulum that includes all the same tissue layers as the organ from which it originates.

true hermaphroditism [ME, *treue*, faith; Gk, *Hermaphroditos*, son of Hermes and Aphrodite], a condition in which an individual is born with both male and female gonads.

true labor, uterine contractions that result in a change in the cervix and birth of an infant.

true neuroma, any neoplasm composed of nerve tissue.

true oxygen, the calculated concentration as either a percentage or a fraction that, when multiplied by the expiratory minute volume at STP, gives oxygen uptake.

true suture, an immovable fibrous joint of the skull in which the edges of bones interlock along a series of processes and indentations.

true value, (in statistics) a value that is closely approximated by the definitive value and somewhat less closely by the reference value.

true vocal cords [ME, *treue*, faith; L, *vocalis*, of the voice; Gk, *chorde*, string], the vocal folds of the larynx (plicae vocales), as distinguished from the vestibular folds (plicae vestibulares), called false vocal cords.

truncal /trung'kəl/ [L, *truncus*], pertaining to the trunk of the body.

truncal ataxia. a loss of coordinated muscle movements for maintaining normal posture of the trunk.

truncal obesity, obesity that preferentially affects or is located in the trunk of the body as opposed to the extremities.

truncated /trung'kātid/, **1.** amputated from the trunk. **2.** cut across at right angles to the long axis.

truncus /trung'kəs/ [L, trunk], the main stem of an anatomic part from which branches may arise, such as the sympathetic nerve chain or jugular lymph trunk.

truncus arteriosus [L, trunk; Gk, *arteria*, airpipe], the embryonic arterial trunk that initially opens from both ventricles of the heart and later divides into the aorta and the pulmonary trunk, the two parts separated by the bulbar septum.

truncus brachiocephalicus, a branch of the aorta that divides into the right common carotid and right subclavian arteries.

trunk [L, *truncus*], **1.** the main stalk of an anatomic structure with many branches, such as an artery or nerve. **2.** the body, excluding the head and appendages.

trunk balance, the ability to maintain postural control of the trunk, including the shifting and bearing of weight on each side to free an extremity for a particular function such as reaching and grasping. Weight shifting can be anterior, posterior, lateral, or diagonal and involve righting, equilibrium, and protective reactions. Head and neck control allows for dissociation of the shoulder and pelvic girdles from the trunk.

truss [Fr, *trousser*, to pack up], an apparatus worn to prevent or retard the herniation of the intestines or other organ through an opening in the abdominal wall.

trust [ME, protection], a risk-taking process whereby an individual's situation depends on the future behavior of another person.

truth [AS, *treowo*], a rule or statement that conforms to fact or reality.

truth serum, a common name for any of several sedatives, such as the short-acting barbiturates, that have been administered intravenously in subjects to elicit information that may have been repressed. It has been used successfully in helping to identify amnesia victims.

Truth Telling, a Nursing Interventions Classification defined as use of whole truth, partial truth, or decision delay to promote the patient's self-determination and well-being.

Trypanosoma /trip'ənōsō'mə/ [Gk, *tryp-*

anon, borer, *soma,* body], a genus of parasitic organisms, several species of which can cause significant diseases in humans. Most *Trypanosoma* organisms live part of their life cycle in insects and are transmitted to humans by insect bites.

trypanosome /trip'ənōsōm', tripan'-/, any organism of the genus *Trypanosoma.*—**trypanosomal,** *adj.*

trypanosomiasis /trip'ənō'sōmī'əsis/ [Gk, *trypanon* + *soma* + *osis,* condition], an infection by an organism of the *Trypanosoma* genus. Kinds of trypanosomiasis are **African trypanosomiasis** and **Chagas' disease.**

trypanosomicide /trip'ənōsō'misīd/ [Gk, *trypanon* + *soma* + L, *caedere,* to kill], a drug destructive to trypanosomes, especially the species of the protozoan parasite transmitted to humans by various insect vectors common in Africa and Central and South America.—**trypanosomicidal,** *adj.*

trypsin /trip'sin/ [Gk, *tripsis,* rubbing], a proteolytic digestive enzyme produced by the exocrine pancreas that catalyzes in the small intestine the breakdown of dietary proteins to peptones, peptides, and amino acids.

trypsin, crystallized, a proteolytic enzyme from the pancreas of the ox, *Bos taurus,* that has been used as a debriding agent for open wounds and ulcers.

trypsin inhibitor, one of a group of peptides present in such varied sources as soybeans, egg white, and human colostrum, which mask or inhibit the active site of the trypsin molecule.

trypsinogen /tripsin'əjən/ [Gk, *tripsis* + *genein,* to produce], the inactive precursor form of trypsin. Trypsinogen is secreted in pancreatic juice and converted to active trypsin through the action of enterokinase in the intestine.

tryptophan (Trp) /trip'təfan/ an amino acid essential for normal growth in infants and nitrogen balance in adults. Tryptophan is the precursor of several substances, including serotonin and niacin.

TSEM, abbreviation for **transmission scanning electron microscopy.**

tsetse fly /tset'sē, tsē'tsē/ [Afr, *tsetse* + AS, *flyge*], a blood-sucking fly found in regions of Africa. It is an insect of the *Glossina* genus and a secondary host of trypanosomes, which cause African sleeping sickness and other diseases in humans.

TSH, abbreviation for **thyroid-stimulating hormone.**

tsp, abbreviation for **teaspoon.**

TSS, abbreviation for **toxic shock syndrome.**

TSTA, abbreviation for *tumor-specific transplantation antigen.*

TT, abbreviation for **thrombolytic therapy.**

t test, a statistic test used to determine whether there are differences between two means or between a target value and a calculated mean.

TTP, abbreviation for **thrombotic thrombocytopenic purpura.**

T tube, **1.** a tubular device in the shape of a T, inserted through the skin into a cavity or a wound, used for drainage. **2.** an apparatus used to connect a source of humidified oxygen to the endotracheal tube so that a spirometer can be attached for the evaluation of tidal volume and appropriate removal of the endotracheal tube.

T tubule cholangiography, a type of biliary tract radiographic examination in which a water-soluble iodinated contrast medium is injected into the bile duct through an indwelling T-tube.

T tubule system, a system of tubular invaginations along the surface of all striated muscle cell membranes, providing an extension of the membrane into the cells. The system is believed to be part of an extensive endomembrane system involved in storing calcium ions and in the movement of action potentials into the cells.

T.U., **1.** abbreviation for *toxic unit.* **2.** abbreviation for *toxin unit.* **3.** abbreviation for **tuberculin unit.**

tubal abortion /t(y)ōō'bəl/ [L, *tubus* + *ab,* away from, *oriri,* to be born], a condition of pregnancy in which an embryo, ectopically implanted, is expelled from the uterine tube into the peritoneal cavity. Tubal abortion is often accompanied by significant internal bleeding, causing acute abdominal and pelvic pain.

tubal dermoid cyst, a tumor derived from embryonal tissues that develops in an oviduct.

tubal ligation, one of several sterilization procedures in which both fallopian tubes are blocked to prevent conception from occurring.

tubal pregnancy, an ectopic pregnancy in which the conceptus implants in the fallopian tube. The most important predisposing factor is prior tubal injury. Pelvic infection, scarring and adhesions from surgery, or intrauterine device complications may result in damage that diminishes the motility of the tube. Transport of the ovum through the tube after fertilization is slowed, and implantation takes place before the conceptus reaches the uterine cavity.

tube /t(y)ōōb/ [L, *tubus*], a hollow, cylindric piece of equipment or structure of the body.

Tube Care, a Nursing Interventions Classification defined as management of a patient with an external drainage device exiting the body.

Tube Care: Chest, a Nursing Interventions Classification defined as management of a patient with an external water-seal drainage device exiting the chest cavity.

Tube Care: Gastrointestinal, a Nursing Interventions Classification defined as management of a patient with a gastrointestinal tube.

Tube Care: Umbilical Line, a Nursing Interventions Classification defined as management of a newborn with an umbilical catheter.

Tube Care: Urinary, a Nursing Interventions Classification defined as management of a patient with urinary drainage equipment.

Tube Care: Ventriculostomy/Lumbar Drain, a Nursing Interventions Classification defined as management of a patient with an external cerebrospinal fluid drainage system.

tube feeding, the administration of nutritionally balanced liquefied foods or nutrients through a tube inserted into the stomach, duodenum, or jejunum. The conditions for which tube feeding is administered include after mouth or gastric surgery, in severe burns, in paralysis or obstruction of the esophagus, in severe cases of anorexia nervosa, and for unconscious patients or those unable to chew or swallow.

tube feeding care, the nursing care and management of a patient receiving nourishment through a nasogastric tube.

tube gain, the overall electron gain of a photomultiplier tube, calculated as gn, where g is the dynode gain and n is the number of dynodes in the tube.

tuber /t(y)ōō′bər/, a knoblike localized swelling.

tubercle /t(y)ōō′bərkəl/ [L, *tuber,* swelling], 1. a nodule or a small eminence, such as that on a bone. 2. a nodule, especially an elevation of the skin that is larger than a papule. 3. a small rounded nodule produced by infection with *Mycobacterium tuberculosis,* consisting of a gray translucent mass of small spheric cells surrounded by connective cells.

tubercles of Montgomery [William Featherstone Montgomery, Irish gynecologist, 1797–1859], small papillae on the surface of nipples and areolas that secrete a fatty lubricating substance.

tubercular /t(y)ōō bur′kyələr/ [L, *tuber,* swelling], pertaining to or resembling tuberculosis.

tuberculid /t(y)ōōbur′kyəlid/, a condition in tuberculous patients characterized by skin or mucous membrane lesions in which the tubercle bacillus is absent. It is the result of sensitivity to mycobacterial antigens.

tuberculin purified protein derivative /tōōbur′kyōōlin/, a solution containing a purified protein fraction derived from isolated culture filtrates of strains of *Mycobacterium tuberculosis.* It is used as an aid in the diagnosis of tuberculosis, in the Mantoux test, and, for the same purpose in a dried form, in multiple puncture devices.

tuberculin test [L, *tuber + testum,* crucible], a test to determine past or present tuberculosis infection based on a positive skin reaction, using one of several methods. A purified protein derivative of tubercle bacilli, called *tuberculin,* is introduced into the skin by scratch, puncture, or intradermal injection. If a raised, red, or hard zone forms surrounding the tuberculin test site, the person is said to be sensitive to tuberculin, and the test is read as positive. Kinds of tuberculin tests include **Heaf test, Mantoux test, Pirquet's test,** and **tine test.**

tuberculin tine test /t(y)ōōbur′kyəlin/ [L, *tuber + ME, tind + L, testum,* crucible], a test for the presence of tubercle bacilli. It is performed by applying a device with multiple sharp prongs to the skin. The prongs penetrate the skin and inject tuberculin, a purified protein derivative tubercle bacilli. A hardened raised area at the test site 48 to 72 hours later indicates the presence of the pathogens in the blood. Because of variations in sensitivity and strength of tuberculin units administered, a negative test result does not necessarily exclude a diagnosis of tuberculosis.

tuberculoma /t(y)ōōbur′kyəlō′mə/ /tōōbur′kyōōlō′mə/ [L, *tuber + Gk, oma,* tumor], a rare tumorlike growth of tuberculous tissue in the central nervous system, characterized by symptoms of an expanding cerebral, cerebellar, or spinal mass.

tuberculosis (TB) /t(y)ōōbur′kyəlō′sis/ [L, *tuber + Gk, osis,* condition], a chronic granulomatous infection caused by an acid-fast bacillus, *Mycobacterium tuberculosis.* It is generally transmitted by the inhalation or ingestion of infected droplets and usually affects the lungs, although infection of multiple organ systems occurs. Listlessness, vague chest pain, pleurisy, anorexia, fever, and weight loss are early symptoms of pulmonary tuberculosis. Night sweats, pulmonary hemorrhage, expectoration of purulent sputum, and dyspnea develop as the disease progresses.

The lung tissues react to the bacillus by producing protective cells that engulf the disease organism, forming tubercles. Untreated, the tubercles enlarge and merge to form larger tubercles that undergo caseation, eventually sloughing off into the cavities of the lungs. Hemoptysis occurs as a result of cavitary spread.

tuberculous /t(y)ō̄obur′kyələs/ [L, *tuber*], pertaining to tuberculosis.

tuberculous arthritis, a joint inflammation caused by invasion of the joint by tuberculosis bacilli that have migrated from a primary infection, usually in the chest.

tuberculous lymphadenitis [L, *tuber* + *lympha*, water; Gk, *aden*, gland, *itis*, inflammation], an inflammation of the lymph glands caused by the presence of *Mycobacterium tuberculosis.*

tuberculous peritonitis [L, *tuber* + Gk, *peri* + *teinein*, to stretch, *itis*, inflammation], an inflammation of the peritoneum that is secondary to a tuberculous infection in the viscera.

tuberculous pneumonia [L, *tuber* + Gk, *pneumon*, lung], a complication of tuberculosis in which caseous material is inhaled into the bronchi, leading to bronchopneumonia or lobar pneumonia.

tuberculous spondylitis, a rare, grave form of tuberculosis caused by the invasion of *Mycobacterium tuberculosis* into the spinal vertebrae. The intervertebral disks may be destroyed, resulting in the collapse and wedging of affected vertebrae and the shortening and angulation of the spine.

tuberculum /t(y)ō̄obur′kyələm/, a tubercle, nodule, or rounded elevation.

tuberosity /t(y)ō̄o′bərōs′itē/ [L, *tuber*], an elevation or protuberance, especially of a bone.

tuberosity of the tibia, a large oblong elevation at the proximal end of the tibia to which the ligament of the patella attaches.

tuberous carcinoma /t(y)ō̄o′bərəs/ [L, *tuber* + Gk, *karkinos*, crab, *oma*, tumor], a scirrhous carcinoma of the skin, characterized by nodular projections.

tuberous sclerosis, a familial, neurocutaneous disease characterized by epilepsy, mental deterioration, adenoma sebaceum, nodules and sclerotic patches on the cerebral cortex, retinal tumors, depigmented leaf-shaped macules on the skin, tumors of the heart or kidneys, and cerebral calcifications.

tuboabdominal gestation /-abdom′inəl/ [L, *tubus* + *abdomen*, belly; L, *gestare*, to bear], an ectopic pregnancy in which the embryo develops while partly in the abdominal cavity and partly in the fallopian tube. The condition usually begins as a

tubal pregnancy and extends into the abdomen as development continues.

tubo-ovarian /t(y)ō̄obō·ōver′ē·ən/ [L, *tubus* + *ovum*, egg], pertaining to the ovary and fallopian tube.

tubo-ovarian abscess [L, *tubus* + *ovum* + *abscedere*, to go away], an abscess involving the ovary and fallopian tube. It is commonly associated with salpingitis.

tubo-ovarian cyst [L, *tubus* + *ovum* + Gk, *kystis*, bag], a cyst that forms by adhesion of the ovary at the fimbriated end of the fallopian tube.

tubo-ovarian gestation [L, *tubus* + *ovum* + *gestare*, to bear], an ectopic pregnancy that develops partly in the fallopian tube and partly in the ovary.

tuboplasty /t(y)ō̄o′bōplas′tē/ [L, *tubus*, tube; Gk, *plassein*, to mold], a surgical procedure in which severed or damaged fallopian tubes are repaired in hopes of restoring fertility.

tubular necrosis [L, *tubulus*, little tube; Gk, *nekros*, dead, *osis*, condition], the death of cells in the small tubules of the kidneys as a result of disease or injury.

tubule /t(y)ō̄o′byool/ [L, *tubulus*], a small tube, such as one of the collecting tubules in the kidneys, the seminiferous tubules of the testes, or Henle's tubules between the distal and proximal convoluted tubules.—**tubular,** *adj.*

tuft [Fr, *touffe*, a tuft], an object resembling a tassel, such as a tuft of hair.

tuft fracture [Fr, *touffe*, tuft; L, *fractura*, break], fracture of any one of the distal phalanges.

tug [ME, *toggen*, to pull], a dragging or hauling movement or sensation.

tularemia /tō̄o′lərē′mē·ə/ [Tulare, California; Gk, *haima*, blood], an infectious disease of animals caused by the bacillus *Francisella (Pasteurella) tularensis,* which may be transmitted by insect vectors or direct contact. It is characterized in humans by fever, headache, and an ulcerated skin lesion with localized lymph node enlargement or by eye infection, gastrointestinal ulcerations, or pneumonia, depending on the site of entry and the response of the host.

tumescence /t(y)ō̄omes′əns/ [L, *tumescere*, to begin to swell], a state of swelling or edema.

tumescent anesthesia, administration of a local infiltration anesthetic (lidocaine) through the use of large volumes of fluid. The technique is applied in liposuction surgery, varicose vein treatment, scalp surgery, dermabrasion, and soft tissue reconstruction.

tumor /t(y)ō̄o′mər/ [L]. **1.** a swelling or enlargement occurring in inflammatory conditions. **2.** a new growth of tissue characterized by progressive, uncontrolled proliferation of cells. The tumor may be localized or invasive, benign or malignant. A tumor may be named for its location, for its cellular makeup, or for the person who first identified it.

tumor albus, a white swelling occurring in a tuberculous bone or joint.

tumor angiogenesis factor (TAF), a protein that stimulates the formation of blood vessels in tumors.

tumoricide /t(y)ōōmôr′isīd/, a substance capable of destroying a tumor.—**tumoricidal,** *adj.*

tumorigenesis /t(y)ōō′mərijen′əsis/, the process of initiating and promoting the development of a tumor.—**tumorigenic,** *adj.*

tumorigenic /-jen′ik/ [L, *tumor,* swelling; Gk, *genein,* to produce], capable of producing tumors.

tumor marker, a substance in the body that may be associated with the presence of a cancer.

tumor necrosis factor (TNF), a natural body protein, also produced synthetically, with anticancer effects. The body produces it in response to the presence of toxic substances such as bacterial toxins.

tumor registry, a repository of data on the incidence of cancers and personal characteristics, treatment, and treatment outcomes of patients diagnosed with cancer.

tumor-specific antigen, an antigen produced by a particular type of tumor that does not appear on normal cells of the tissue in which the tumor developed.

tumor viruses [L, *tumor,* swelling, *virus,* poison], viruses that are capable of directly or indirectly inducing tumor formation. Direct tumor formation may result from inoculation of living cells with tumorigenic viruses. Tumor formation may result from the influence of the virus on normal cells that are transformed into tumor cells.

tumor volume, a part of an organ or tissue that includes both the tumor and adjacent areas of invasion.

tungsten (W) /tung′stən/ [SW, *tung,* heavy, *sten,* stone], a metallic element. Its atomic number is 74; its atomic mass (weight) is 183.85. It has the highest melting point of all metals and is used as a target material in x-ray tubes.

tunica /t(y)ōō′nikə/ [L, *tunic*], an enveloping coat or covering membrane.

tunica adventitia, the outer layer or coat of an artery or other tubular structure.

tunica albuginea [L, *tunic* + *albus,* white], a tissue covering of white collagenous fi-

bers, such as the sclerotic coat of the eyeball.

tunica intima, the membrane lining an artery.

tunica media, a muscular middle coat of an artery.

tunica vaginalis testis, the serous membrane surrounding the testis and epididymis.

tuning fork /t(y)ōō′ning/ [Gk, *tonos,* stretching; L, *furca,* fork], a small metal instrument consisting of a stem and two prongs that produces a constant pitch when either prong is struck. It is used by physicians as a screening test of air and bone conduction.

tunnel [OFr, *tonnel*], a canal or passage, such as the carpal tunnel.

tunnel vision [OFr, *tonnel,* fowl trap; L, *videre,* to see], a defect in sight in which there is a great reduction in the peripheral field of vision, as if looking through a hollow tube or tunnel. The condition occurs in advanced chronic glaucoma.

tunnel wound [OFr, *tonnel* + AS, *wund*], a break in the surface of the body or an organ in which the entry and exit wounds are the same size.

TUR, abbreviation for **transurethral resection.**

turban tumor /tur′bən/ [Turk, *tulbend,* headdress; L, *tumor,* swelling], a benign neoplasm consisting of pink or maroon nodules that may cover the entire scalp, trunk, and extremities.

turbid /tur′bid/ [L, *turbidus,* confused], clouded or obscured, as in solids in suspension in a solution.

turbidimetry /tur′bidim′ətrē/ [L, *turbidus,* confused; Gk, *metron,* measure], measurement of the turbidity (cloudiness) of a solution or suspension in which the amount of transmitted light is quantified with a spectrophotometer or estimated by visual comparison with solutions of known turbidity.

turbidity /tərbid′itē/ [L, *turbidus*], a condition of light scattering in a liquid resulting from the presence of suspended particles in the fluid.

turbinate /tur′binit/ [L, *turbinum,* top-shaped], **1.** pertaining to a scroll shape. **2.** pertaining to the concha nasalis.

turgid /tur′jid/ [L, *turgidus*], swollen, hard, and congested, usually as a result of an accumulation of fluid.—**turgor,** *n.*

turgor /tur′gər/ [L, *turgere,* to be swollen], the expected resiliency of the skin caused by the outward pressure of the cells and interstitial fluid. An evaluation of the skin turgor is an essential part of physical assessment.

turnbuckle cast [AS, *tyrnan* + ME, *bocle,*

small shield; ONorse, *kasta*], an orthopedic device used to encase and immobilize the entire trunk, one upper arm to the elbow and the opposite upper leg to the knee. It is constructed of plaster of Paris or fiberglass and incorporates hinges as part of its design in the treatment of scoliosis. The hinges are placed at the level of the apex of the curvature.

Turner's syndrome [Henry H. Turner, American endocrinologist, 1892–1970], a chromosomal anomaly seen in about 1 in 3000 live female births, characterized by the absence of one X chromosome; congenital ovarian failure; genital hypoplasia; cardiovascular anomalies; dwarfism; short metacarpals; "shield chest"; extosis of tibia; and underdeveloped breasts, uterus, and vagina. Spatial disorientation and moderate degrees of learning disorders are common.

tussis /tus′is/ [L, *tussis*, cough], a cough or pertussis.

tussive fremitus /tus′iv/ [L, *tussis,* cough, *fremitus,* murmuring], a vibratory cough that can be felt by a hand over the chest of the patient.

TV, abbreviation for **tidal volume.**

TVL, abbreviation for **tenth-value layer.**

T wave, the component of the cardiac cycle shown on an electrocardiogram as a short, inverted, U-shaped curve after the ST segment.

Tweed triangle [Charles Tweed, American dentist, 1895–1970; L, *triangulus,* three-cornered], a triangle used as a diagnostic aid, formed by the mandibular plane, the Frankfort plane, and the long axis of the lower central incisor.

24-hour clock system, a method of designating time by using the numeric sequence from 00 to 23 for the hours and the numbers 00 to 59 for the minutes in a daily cycle beginning with 0000 (midnight) and ending with 2359 (1 minute before the next midnight).

twilight state [Ger, *Zwielicht,* twilight; L, *status*], an impaired state of consciousness in which the patient may experience visual or auditory hallucinations and responds to them with irrational behavior. The person may be unaware of the surroundings at the time of the experience and have no memory of it later, except perhaps to recall a related dream.

twin [AS, *twinn,* double], either of two offspring born of the same pregnancy and developed from either a single ovum or from two ova that were released from the ovary simultaneously and fertilized at the same time. The incidence of twin births is approximately 1 in 80 pregnancies.

twinge /twinj/ [ME, *twengen,* to pinch], a sudden brief darting pain.

twinning [AS, *twinn*], **1.** the development of two or more fetuses during the same pregnancy, either spontaneously or through external intervention for experimental purposes in animals. **2.** the duplication of like structures or parts by division.

twin-wire fixed orthodontic appliance, an orthodontic appliance developed by J. E. Johnson typically using a pair of 0.01-inch (0.25-mm) wires to form the midsection of the arch wire. It is used to correct or improve malocclusion.

twitch [AS, *twiccian*], **1.** the contraction of small muscle units, manifested as a quick, simple, spasmodic contraction of a muscle. **2.** to jerk convulsively.

twitching [AS, *twiccian*], a series of contractions by small muscle units. Twitching that involves large groups of muscle fibers is identified as *fascicular twitching.*

two-point discrimination test, a test of the ability of a person to differentiate touch stimuli at two nearby points on the body at the same time. It is used in studies of possible damage to the parietal regions of the brain.

two-point gait [OE, *twa* + L, *punctus,* pricked; ONorse, *gata,* way], a pattern of crutch-walking with crutches in which the right foot and left crutch advance first, the step being completed by advancing the left foot and right crutch.

two-way catheter [AS, *twa* + *weg* + Gk, *katheter,* something lowered], a catheter that has a double lumen, one channel for injection of medication or fluids and the other for removal of fluid or specimens.

TXA₂, abbreviation for **thromboxane A₂.**

TXB₂, abbreviation for **thromboxane B₂.**

tylosis /tīlō′sis/, formation of a callus.

tyloxapol /tīlok′səpôl/, a respiratory tract detergent prescribed for bronchitis, emphysema, pulmonary abscess, bronchiectasis, or atelectasis.

tympanectomy /tim′pənek′təmē/ [Gk, *tympanon,* drum, *ektome*], the surgical removal of the tympanic membrane.

tympanic /timpan′ik/ [Gk, *tympanon,* drum], pertaining to a structure that resonates when struck; drumlike, such as a **tympanic abdomen** that resonates on percussion because the intestines are distended with gas.—**tympanum** /tim′pənəm (*pl.* **tympana**), *n.*

tympanic antrum, a relatively large, irregular cavity in the superior anterior part of the mastoid process of the temporal bone, communicating with the mastoid air cells and lined by the extension of the mucous membrane of the tympanic cavity.

tympanic membrane, a thin semitransparent membrane in the middle ear that transmits sound vibrations to the internal ear by means of the auditory ossicles. It is nearly oval in form, with a vertical diameter of about 10 mm, and separates the tympanic cavity from the bottom of the external acoustic meatus.

tympanic membrane thermometer, a device that measures the temperature of the tympanic membrane by detecting infrared radiation from the tissue. Results are obtained within 2 seconds and directly reflect the body's core temperature.

tympanic reflex, the reflection of a beam of light shining on the eardrum. In a normal ear a bright, wedge-shaped reflection is seen; its apex is at the end of the malleus, and its base is at the anterior inferior margin of the eardrum.

tympanic resonance [Gk, *tympanon* + L, *resonare,* to sound again], a drumlike or hollow sound heard over a large air space of the body such as the pneumothorax.

tympanic sulcus [Gk, *tympanon,* drum; L, *sulcus,* furrow], a narrow circular groove at the medial end of the osseous part of the external acoustic meatus that holds the tympanic membrane.

tympanic temperature, the body temperature as measured electronically at the tympanic membrane.

tympanogram /timpan′əgram/, a graphic representation of the acoustic impedance and air pressure of the middle ear and mobility of the tympanic membrane, measured as part of the audiologic test battery. Various middle ear pathologies such as otitis media, otosclerosis, or tympanic membrane perforations each yield distinctive tympanograms.

tympanoplasty /timpan′əplas′tē/ [Gk, *tympanon* + *plassein,* to mold], any of several operative procedures on the eardrum or ossicles of the middle ear designed to restore or improve hearing in patients with conductive hearing loss. These operations may be used to repair a perforated eardrum, for otosclerosis, or for dislocation or necrosis of one of the small bones of the middle ear.

tympany /tim′pənē/ [Gk, *tympanon,* drum], a relatively low-pitched resonant sound heard on percussion over a pneumothorax or distended abdomen.

type A personality [Gk, *typos,* mark], a parent ego state characterized by a behavior pattern described by Meyer Friedman and Ray Rosenman as associated with individuals who are highly competitive and work compulsively to meet deadlines. The behavior also is associated with a higher than usual incidence of coronary heart disease.

type B personality, a child ego state characterized by a form of behavior associated by Friedman and Rosenman with people who appear free of hostility and aggression and who lack a compulsion to meet deadlines, are not highly competitive at work and play, and have a lower risk of heart attack.

type E personality, a term introduced by Harriet Braiker to describe professional women who fit neither type A nor type B personality categories, but who have a marked sense of insecurity and strive to convince themselves that they are worthwhile.

type I diabetes mellitus. See **insulin-dependent diabetes mellitus.**

type II diabetes mellitus. See **non-insulin-dependent diabetes mellitus.**

type I error, in a test of a statistical hypothesis, the probability of rejecting the null hypothesis when it is true and should be accepted.

type II error, in a test of a statistical hypothesis, the probability of accepting the null hypothesis when it is false and should be rejected.

type I hypersensitivity. See **anaphylactic hypersensitivity.**

type II hypersensitivity. See **cytotoxic hypersensitivity.**

type III hypersensitivity. See **immune complex hypersensitivity.**

type IV hypersensitivity. See **cell-mediated immune response.**

typhoid /tī′foid/ [Gk, *typhos,* fever, *eidos,* form], pertaining to or resembling typhus.

typhoid carrier, a person without signs or symptoms of typhoid fever who carries on his or her body the bacteria that cause the disease and sheds the pathogens in body excretions. The typical typhoid carrier is one who has recovered from an attack of the disease.

typhoid fever [Gk, *typhos,* fever, *eidos,* form; L, *febris,* fever], a bacterial infection usually caused by *Salmonella typhi,* transmitted by contaminated milk, water, or food. It is characterized by headache, delirium, cough, watery diarrhea, rash, and a high fever. The incubation period may be as long as 60 days. Characteristic maculopapular rosy spots are scattered over the skin of the abdomen and chest. Splenomegaly and leukopenia develop first. The disease is serious and may be fatal. Complications include intestinal hemorrhage or perforation and thrombophlebitis. Some people who recover from the disease continue to be carriers and excrete the organism, spreading the disease.

typhoid nodules [Gk, *typhos*, fever; L, *nodulus*, small knot], a liver nodule consisting of a cluster of monocytes and lymphocytes surrounding the typhoid fever pathogen, *Salmonella typhi*.

typhoid pellagra, a form of pellagra in which the symptoms also include continued high temperatures.

typhoid vaccine, a bacterial vaccine prepared from an inactivated dried strain of *Salmonella typhi*. It is prescribed for primary immunization against typhoid fever for adults and children.

typhomania /tīfōmā'nē-ə/, a condition characterized by coma and delirium associated with typhus, typhoid fever, and similar febrile infections.

typhous /tī'fəs/ [Gk, *typhos*, fever], pertaining to typhus fever.

typhus /tī'fəs/ [Gk, *typhos*, fever], any of a group of acute infectious diseases caused by various species of *Rickettsia* and usually transmitted from infected rodents to humans by the bites of lice, fleas, mites, or ticks. These diseases are all characterized by headache, chills, fever, malaise, and a maculopapular rash.

typhus vaccine, any one of three vaccines, each of which is prepared for the different rickettsial organisms that cause epidemic typhus, murine typhus, or Brill-Zinsser's disease. Each of the vaccines is prescribed for immunization against a form of typhus.

typical /tip'ikəl/ [L, *typicus*, characteristic of a kind], a representative example.

typing [Gk, *typos*, mark], the process of classifying a specimen of blood, tissue, or other substance according to common traits or characteristics.

Tyr, abbreviation for **tyrosine.**

tyramine /tī'rəmēn/ [Gk, *tyros*, cheese, *amine*, ammonia], an amino acid synthesized in the body from the essential acid tyrosine. Tyramine stimulates the release of the catecholamines epinephrine and norepinephrine. It is important that people taking monoamine oxidase inhibitors avoid the ingestion of foods and beverages containing tyramine.

tyroma /tīrō'mə/ [Gk, *tyros* + *oma*, tumor], a new growth or nodule with a caseous or cheesy consistency.

tyromatosis /tī'rōmətō'sis/ [Gk, *tyros* + *oma* + *osis*, condition], a process in which necrotic tissue is broken down and degenerates to a granular, amorphous, caseous mass.

tyrosine (Tyr) /tī'rəsēn/ [Gk, *tyros*], an amino acid synthesized in the body from the essential amino acid phenylalanine. Tyrosine is found in most proteins and is a precursor of melanin and several hormones, including epinephrine and thyroxin.

tyrosinemia /tī'rōsinē'mē-ə/ [Gk, *tyros* + *haima*, blood], **1.** a benign, transient condition of the newborn, especially premature infants, in which an excessive amount of the amino acid tyrosine is found in the blood and urine. The disorder is caused by an anomaly in amino acid metabolism, usually delayed development of the enzymes necessary to metabolize tyrosine. **2.** a hereditary disorder involving an inborn error of metabolism of the amino acid tyrosine. The condition is caused by an enzyme deficiency and results in liver failure or hepatic cirrhosis, renal tubular defects that can lead to renal rickets and renal glycosuria, generalized aminoaciduria, and mental retardation.

tyrosinosis /tīrōsinō'sis/ [Gk, *tyros* + *osis*, condition], a rare condition resulting from a defect in amino acid metabolism. It is characterized by the excretion of an excessive amount of parahydroxyphenylpyruvic acid, an intermediate product of tyrosine, in the urine.

tyrosinurea /tī'rōsinōōr'e-ə/ [Gk, *tyros* + *ouron*, urine], the presence of tyrosine in the urine.

Tzanck test /tsangk/ [Arnault Tzanck, Russian dermatologist in France, 1886–1954], a microscopic examination of cellular material from skin lesions to help diagnose certain vesicular diseases.

T

u, symbol sometimes used to stand for **micro-**(properly μ), as in "ul" or "um," representing μl or μm.

U, 1. abbreviation for **unit.** 2. symbol for the element **uranium.**

UAO, abbreviation for **upper airway obstruction.**

ubiquinone /yo͞obik'winōn/, a quinone derivative that occurs in the lipid core of mitochondrial membranes and functions in the electron transport chain as a carrier.

ubiquitin /yo͞obik'witin/, a small polypeptide that is involved in histone modification. It is found in all cells of higher organisms.

UGI, abbreviation for **upper GI.**

UICC, abbreviation for *International Union Against Cancer, Unión internacional contra el cancer, Union internationale contre le cancer, Unio internationalis contra cancrum,* or *Unione internazionale contro il cancro.*

ulcer /ul'sər/ [L, *ulcus,* a sore], a circumscribed, craterlike lesion of the skin or mucous membrane resulting from necrosis that accompanies some inflammatory, infectious, or malignant processes. An ulcer may be shallow, involving only the epidermis, as in pemphigus, or deep, as in a rodent ulcer.—**ulcerate,** *v.,* **ulcerative** /ul'sərā'tiv/, *adj.*

ulcerate /ul'sərāt/ [L, *ulcus,* a sore], to form an ulcer.

ulceration /ul'sərā'shən/ [L, *ulcus,* a sore], the process of ulcer formation.

ulcerative blepharitis /ul'sərā'tiv, ul'-sərətiv'/ [L, *ulcus + atus,* relating to; Gk, *blepharon,* eyelid, *itis,* inflammation], a form of blepharitis in which a staphylococcal infection of the follicles of the eyelashes and glands of the eyelids results in sticky crusts forming on the lid margins. If the crusts are pulled off, the skin beneath bleeds. Tiny pustules develop in the follicles of the eyelashes and break down to form shallow ulcers.

ulcerative colitis, a chronic, episodic, inflammatory disease of the large intestine and rectum. It is characterized by profuse watery diarrhea containing varying amounts of blood, mucus, and pus. Some of the many systemic complications of ulcerative colitis include peripheral arthritis, ankylosing spondylitis, kidney and liver disease, and inflammation of the eyes, skin, and mouth. People with severe disease may develop toxic megacolon, a dangerous complication that may lead to perforation of the bowel, septicemia, and death. The attacks of diarrhea are accompanied by tenesmus, severe abdominal pain, fever, chills, anemia, and weight loss. Children with the disease may suffer retarded physical growth. The debilitating symptoms often prevent people with ulcerative colitis from carrying on the normal activities of daily living.

ulcerative inflammation [L, *ulcus + inflammare,* to set afire], the development of an ulcer over an area of inflammation.

ulcerative stomatitis [L, *ulcus + Gk stoma,* mouth, *itis,* inflammation], an infectious disease of the mouth characterized by swollen spongy gums, ulcers, and loose teeth.

ulcerogenic drug /ul'sərōjen'ik/, a drug that produces or exacerbates peptic ulcers, such as aspirin and NSAID medications.

ulceromembranous /ulsərōmem'brənəs/, describing an ulcer with a membranous exudation.

ulcerous /ul'sərəs/, pertaining to ulcers.

ULD, abbreviation for **upper level discriminator.**

ulegyria /yo͞o'ləjī'rē·ə/, a cerebral cortex abnormality in which the gyri are narrow and distorted by scars.

ulerythema /yo͞o'lərithē'mə/, a skin eruption characterized by redness and scarring.

ulna /ul'nə/ [L, elbow], the bone on the medial or little finger side of the forearm, lying parallel with the radius. The ulna articulates with the humerus, the carpals, and the radius.

ulnar /ul'nər/ [L, *ulna,* elbow], pertaining to the long medial bone of the forearm.

ulnar artery, a large artery branching from the brachial artery, supplying muscles in the forearm, wrist, and hand. Arising near the elbow, it passes obliquely in a distal direction to become the superficial palmar arch.

ulnar drift [L, *ulna,* elbow; AS, *drifan,* to drive], a joint change in the metacarpophalangeal joints because of rheumatoid arthritis and chronic synovitis. The long axis of the fingers makes an angle with the long axis of the wrist so that fingers are deviated to the ulnar side of the hand.

ulnar nerve, one of the terminal branches of the brachial plexus that arises on each side from the medial cord of the plexus. It receives fibers from both cervical and thoracic nerve roots and supplies the muscles and skin on the ulnar side of the forearm and hand. It can be easily palpated as the 'funny bone' of the elbow.

ulnocarpal /ul'nōkär'pəl/, pertaining to the ulna and carpus or ulnar area of the wrist.

ulnoradial /ul'nōrā'dē·əl/, pertaining to the ulna and radius and the ligaments associated with them.

ulocarcinoma /yōō'lōkär'sinō'mə/ [Gk, *oule,* scar, *karkinos,* crab, *oma,* tumor], any malignant neoplasm of the gums that is classified as a carcinoma.

ulodermatitis /yōō'lōdur'mətī'tis/, dermatitis resulting in the destruction of tissue and scar formation.

uloid /yōō'loid/, resembling scar tissue.

ulterior transactions /ultir'ē·ər/, (in transactional analysis), communication that is bilevel. The first level is overt (social), usually of relevant verbal statements. The second level is usually covert (psychologic) and nonverbal and has hidden psychologic meaning.

ultimate strain /ul'timit/, the strain at the point of failure.

ultimate stress, the highest load that can be sustained by a material at the point of failure.

ultrabrachycephalic /-brak'ēsəfal'ik/, describing an extremely short, broad skull.

ultracentrifuge /ul'trəsen'trifyōōj/ [L, *ultra,* beyond; Gk, *kentron,* center; L, *fugere,* to flee], a high-speed centrifuge with a rotation rate fast enough to produce sedimentation of viruses, even in blood plasma.

ultradian /rā'dē·ən/ [L, *ultra* + *dies,* day], pertaining to a biorhythm that occurs in cycles of less than 24 hours.

ultrafilter /-fil'tər/, a semipermeable membrane with pores of a known diameter used to separate colloids and large molecules from water and other small molecules.

ultrafiltrate /-fil'trāt/ [L, *ultra* + Fr, *filtre,* filter], a solution that has passed through a semipermeable membrane with very small pores.

ultrafiltration /-filtrā'shən/, a type of filtration, sometimes conducted under pressure, through filters with very small pores, such as used by an artificial kidney. Ultra-

filtration can separate large molecules from smaller molecules in body fluids.

ultra-high-speed handpiece, a device for holding rotary instruments, such as burs, that permits rotational speeds of 100,000 to 300,000 rpm. It is used primarily for tooth cavity preparation.

ultraligation /-līgā'shən/, tying or closing off a blood vessel beyond the point where it branches.

ultramicrotome /-mī'krətōm'/, a microtome that cuts very thin slices for examination by electron microscopy.

ultrasonic /ul'trəson'ik/ [L, *ultra,* beyond + *sonus,* sound], pertaining to ultrasound, or sound frequencies so high (greater than 20 kilohertz) that they cannot be perceived by the human ear.

ultrasonic cleaning, the use of high-frequency vibrations to dislodge deposits from teeth or other objects.

ultrasonic nebulizer, a humidifier in which an electric current is used to produce high-frequency vibrations in a container of fluid. The vibrations break up the fluid into aerosol particles.

ultrasonics /-son'iks/, the science dealing with sound waves having frequencies above the approximately 20-kHz range of human hearing. Ultrasound evolved from the World War II SONAR underwater detection apparatus and was first adapted for medical diagnostic purposes in the 1950s. It uses a transducer and generates very short pulses of high-frequency sound that are transmitted into the body. Echoes from interfaces within the body are displayed on a cathode ray tube so that images of normal and abnormal structures can be viewed.

ultrasonic wave [L, *ultra,* beyond, *sonus,* sound], a sound wave transmitted at a frequency greater than 20,000 per second, or beyond the normal hearing range of humans. The specific wavelength is equal to the velocity divided by the frequency.

ultrasonography /-sənog'rəfē/ [L, *ultra* + *sonus,* sound; Gk, *graphein,* to record], the process of imaging deep structures of the body by measuring and recording the reflection of pulsed or continuous high-frequency sound waves.

Ultrasonography: Limited Obstetric, a Nursing Interventions Classification defined as performance of ultrasound examinations to determine ovarian, uterine, or fetal status.

ultrasound /ul'trəsound/ [L, *ultra* + *sonus*], sound waves at the very high frequency of over 20,000 kHz (vibrations per second). Ultrasound has many medical applications, including fetal monitoring, imaging of internal organs, and, at an ex-

U

tremely high frequency, the cleaning of dental and surgical instruments.—**ultrasonic,** *adj.*

ultrasound imaging, the use of high-frequency sound (several MHz or more) to image internal structures by the differing reflection signals produced when a beam of sound waves is projected into the body and bounces back at interfaces between those structures.

ultrastructure /-struk′chər/, a structure so small it can be viewed only with an ultramicroscope or electron microscope.

ultraviolet (UV) /-vī′ələt/ [L, *ultra* + Fr, *violette*], light beyond the range of human vision, at the short end of the spectrum, or that part of the electromagnetic spectrum with wavelengths between about 10 and 400 nm. It occurs naturally in sunlight; it burns and tans the skin and converts precursors in the skin to vitamin D. Ultraviolet lamps are used in the control of infectious airborne bacteria and viruses and in the treatment of psoriasis and other skin conditions. Black light is ultraviolet light used in fluoroscopy.

ultraviolet lamp /-vī′ələt/, a lamp that emits electromagnetic radiation in a range between 4 and 400 nm, or beyond the violet spectrum of visible light. Equipped with a nickel oxide filter, an ultraviolet lamp radiating at wavelengths around 360 nm can be used to examine hairs infected with certain agents. The pathogens reflect the ultraviolet light with a greenish-yellow fluorescence.

ultraviolet rays [L, *ultra,* beyond; OFr, *violette* + L, *radius*], electromagnetic radiations found just beyond the violet edge of the visible spectrum, with wavelengths extending to the beginning of x-rays. The wavelengths range from 390 to 290 nm for near ultraviolet rays to 290 to 20 nm for far ultraviolet wavelengths. Ultraviolet radiation in the region of 260 nm can distort deoxyribonucleic molecules, causing mutations and destroying microorganisms, including bacteria and viruses. About 5% of the radiation from the sun is in the ultraviolet range, but little of this type of energy reaches the earth because much is absorbed by oxygen and ozone in the atmosphere. In medicine ultraviolet radiation is used in the treatment of rickets and certain skin conditions. Milk and some other foods become activated with vitamin D when exposed to this type of energy.

ultraviolet therapy [L, *ultra,* beyond; OFr, *violette* + Gk, *therapeia,* treatment], the therapeutic application to the body of electromagnetic radiations in the ultraviolet region of the spectrum. This therapy is useful in the control of infectious airborne bacteria and viruses and in the treatment of psoriasis and other skin conditions.

umbilical /umbil′ikəl/ [L, *umbilicus,* navel], **1.** pertaining to the umbilicus. **2.** pertaining to the umbilical cord.

umbilical artery catheter [L, *umbilicus,* navel; Gk, *arteria,* airpipe, *katheter,* a thing lowered], a catheter inserted into the umbilical artery of a newborn.

umbilical catheterization, a procedure in which a radiopaque catheter is passed through an umbilical artery to provide a newborn with parenteral fluid, to obtain blood samples, or both, or through the umbilical vein for an exchange transfusion or the emergency administration of drugs, fluids, or volume expanders.

umbilical cord, a flexible structure connecting the umbilicus with the placenta in the gravid uterus and giving passage to the umbilical arteries and vein. In the newborn it is about 2 feet long and ½ inch in diameter.

umbilical fissure, a groove on the inferior surface of the liver that holds the ligamentum teres and separates the right and left lobes of the liver.

umbilical fistula, an abnormal passage from the umbilicus to the intestine or more frequently to the remnant of the canal in the median umbilical ligament that connects the fetal bladder with the allantois.

umbilical hernia, a soft, skin-covered protrusion of intestine and omentum through a weakness in the abdominal wall around the umbilicus. It usually closes spontaneously within 1 to 2 years.

umbilical region, the part of the abdomen surrounding the umbilicus, in the middle zone between the right and left lateral regions.

umbilical vasculitis, an inflammation of the umbilical cord and its blood vessels.

umbilical vein, one of a pair of embryonic vessels that return the blood from the placenta and fuse to form a single trunk in the body stalk.

umbilical vesicle, a pear-shaped structure formed from the yolk sac at about the fourth week of prenatal development that protrudes into the cavity of the chorion and connects to the developing embryo by the yolk stalk at the region of the future midgut.

umbilication /um′bilikā′shən/ [L, *umbilicus,* navel], the process of becoming dimpled or pitted or acquiring a depressed area.

umbilicus /umbilī′kəs, umbil′ikəs/ [L, navel], the point on the abdomen at which the umbilical cord joined the fetal abdomen. In most adults it is marked by a depression; in some it is marked by a small protrusion of skin.

umbo [L, knob], a projection on any rounded surface, such as the inner surface of the tympanic membrane where the malleus is attached.

umbrella filter /umbrəl´ə/, a small, porous, umbrella-shaped device that can be inserted into the vena cava or other blood vessels to trap blood clots.

uncal [L, *uncus,* hook], pertaining to the uncus.

uncal herniation /ung´kəl/ [L, *uncus,* hook, *hernia,* rupture], a condition in which the medial part of the temporal lobe protrudes over the tentorial edge as a result of increased intracranial pressure. A dilated pupil on the side of the herniation is a diagnostic sign of the disorder.

Uncinaria /un´siner´ē·ə/ [L, *uncinus,* hook], a genus of nematode that causes hookworm in dogs, cats, and other carnivores.

uncinate /un´sināt/, having hooks or barbs.

uncipressure /un´sipresh´ər/, pressure with a hook to control a hemorrhage.

uncompensated care /unkom´pənsā´tid/ [ME, *un,* against, not; L, *compendere,* to be equivalent], services provided by a hospital or physician or other health care professional for which no charge is made and for which no payment is expected.

uncompetitive inhibitor /un´kəmpet´itiv/ [ME, *un* + L, *competere,* to compete, *inhibere,* to restrain], an enzymatic inhibitor that appears to bond only to the enzyme substrate complex and not to free enzyme molecules.

uncomplemented, not united with proteins of the body's immune defense system and therefore inactive.

unconditioned response /un´kəndish´ənd/ [ME, *un* + L, *conditio,* condition, *respondere,* to reply], a normal, instinctive, unlearned reaction to a stimulus; one that occurs naturally and is not acquired by association and training.

unconjugated monoclonal antibodies /unkon´jəgā´tid/, hybrid antibodies of a single antigenic specificity used for highly selective targeting of tumor cells. These antibodies can destroy malignant cells by direct lysis, by binding to cell receptors, and by mobilization of effector cells.

unconscious /unkon´shəs/ [ME, *un* + L, *conscire,* to be aware], **1.** unaware of the surrounding environment; insensible; incapable of responding to sensory stimuli. **2.** (in psychiatry) the part of the mental function in which thoughts, ideas, emotions, or memories are beyond awareness and rarely subject to ready recall.

unconsciousness /unkon´shəsnəs/, a state of complete or partial unawareness or lack of response to sensory stimuli as a result of hypoxia caused by respiratory insufficiency or shock; from metabolic or chemical brain depressants such as drugs, poisons, ketones, or electrolyte imbalance; or from a form of brain pathologic condition such as trauma, seizures, cerebrovascular accident, brain tumor, or infection. Various degrees of unconsciousness can occur during stupor, fugue, catalepsy, and dream states.

uncus /ung´kəs/ [L, hook], **1.** the hook-like anterior end of the hippocampal gyrus on the temporal lobe of the brain. **2.** a hook-shaped structure.

undecylenic acid /un´desilen´ik/, an antifungal agent prescribed in the treatment of athlete's foot and ringworm.

undercut, the part of a tooth or artificial crown that lies between the gingiva and the height of contour.

underdamping /un´dərdam´ping/ [AS, *under,* beneath, *dampen,* to check], (in cardiology) the transmission of all frequency components without a reduction in amplitude.

underlying assumption /un´dərlī´ing/, a set of rules one holds about oneself, others, and the world. These rules are regarded by the individual as unquestionably true.

undernutrition /-nōōtrish´ən/, malnutrition caused by an inadequate food supply or an inability to use the nutrients in food.

underwater exercise /un´dərwô´tər/ [AS, *under* + *woeter*], any physical activity performed in a pool or large tub, such as a Hubbard tank, where the buoyancy of the water facilitates the movement of weak or injured muscles.

underwater seal, a seal formed by water allowed to flow over a tube that exits from the chest cavity of a patient. The water acts as a one-way valve and permits the outflow of air but prevents the ingress of air.

underweight /un´dərwāt/ [AS, *under* + *wiht*], less than normal in body weight after adjustment for height, body build, and age.

undifferentiated cell /undif´əren´shē·ā´tid/ [AS, *un* not; L, *differentia,* difference, *cella,* storeroom], an embryonic-type cell that has not yet expressed signs of its future special type at maturity.

undifferentiated family ego mass, an emotional fusion in a family in which all members are similar in emotional expression.

undifferentiated malignant lymphoma [ME, *un* + L, *differe,* to differ, *atus,* process, *malignus,* evil, *lympha,* water; Gk, *oma,* tumor], a lymphoid neoplasm containing stem cells that have large nuclei, a small amount of pale cytoplasm, and ill-defined borders.

undifferentiation /un'difəren'shē·ā'shən/, the lack or absence of normal cell differentiation into an identifiable cell type.

undisplaced fracture /un'displāst, un'dis-plāst'/, a bone break in which cracks in the osseous tissue may radiate in several directions without the separation or displacement of fragmented sections.

undoing /undoo'ing/ [ME, *un* + AS, *don*], the performance of a specific action that is intended to negate in part a previous action or communication. According to some psychologists, undoing is related to the magical thinking of childhood.

undulant /un'dyələnt/ [L, *unda,* wave], wavelike, such as a vibration, fluctuation, or oscillation.

undulate /un'dyəlit/, to have wavelike fluctuations or oscillations.

undulating pulse /un'dyəlā'ting/, a pulse characterized by a succession of waves without force.

unengaged head /un'engājd'/ [ME, *un* + Fr, *engager,* to involve; AS, *heafod*], the head of a floating fetus.

unequal cleavage /une'kwəl/ [ME, *un* + L, *aequare,* to make equal; AS, *cleofan,* to split], mitotic division of the fertilized ovum into blastomeres that are larger near the yolk part of protoplasm, or vegetal pole, and smaller near the nucleus, or animal pole.

unequal pulse [AS, *un,* not; L, *aequare,* to make equal, *pulsare,* to beat], a pulse in which the beats vary in intensity.

unequal twins, two nonjoined fetuses born of the same pregnancy in which only one of the pair is fully formed, with the other showing various degrees of developmental defects.

unfinished business /unfin'isht/, the concerns of a dying patient that require resolution before death can be accepted by the patient.

ung., abbreviation for the Latin word *unguentum,* 'unguenta', 'or ointment.'

ungual /ung'gwəl/, pertaining to the fingernails.

uniaxial joint /yoo'nē·ak'sē·əl/ [L, *unus,* one, *axis,* axle, *jungere,* to join], a synovial joint in which movement is only in one axis, such as a pivot or hinge joint.

UNICEF /yoo'nisef'/, abbreviation for **United Nations International Children's Emergency Fund.**

unicellular reproduction /-sel'yələr/ [L, *unus* + *cella,* storeroom, *re,* again, *producere,* to produce], the formation of a

new organism from a female egg that has not been fertilized; parthenogenesis.

unidirectional block /-direk'shənəl/ [L, *unus* + *dirigere,* to direct; Fr, *bloc*], a pathologic failure of cardiac impulse conduction in one direction while conduction is possible in the opposing direction.

unidisciplinary health care team /-dis'i-pliner'ē/, a group of health care workers who are members of the same discipline.

unification model /-kā'shən/ [L, *unus* + *ficare,* to make whole, *atus,* process, *modulus,* small measure], a theoretic framework based on the close relationship of nursing education and clinical nursing service at the University of Rochester (New York). The faculty of the school of nursing hold joint appointments to the school and the hospital, teaching nursing students and providing clinical leadership in nursing service in the hospital.

uniform /yoo'nifôrm/, **1.** having only one form or shape. **2.** distinctive clothing worn by members of a group.

uniform reporting, the reporting of service and financial data by a hospital in conformance with prescribed standard definitions to permit comparisons with other health facilities.

unilaminar /-lam'inər/, composed of only one layer.

unilateral /-lat'ərəl/ [L, *unus,* one, *latus,* side], involving only one side.

unilateral hypertrophy [L, *unus* + *latus,* side; Gk, *hyper,* above, *trophe,* nourishment], enlargement of one side or a part of one side of the body.

unilateral long-leg spica cast, an orthopedic cast applied to immobilize one leg and the trunk of the body cranially as far as the nipple line.

unilateral neglect, a NANDA-accepted nursing diagnosis of a state in which an individual is perceptually unaware of and inattentive to one side of the body. Defining characteristics include consistent inattention to stimuli on the affected side, inadequate self-care (as in positioning and/or safety precautions in regard to the affected side), lack of looking toward the affected side, and leaving food on the plate on the affected side.

Unilateral Neglect Management, a Nursing Interventions Classification defined as protecting and safely reintegrating the affected part of the body while helping the patient adapt to disturbed perceptual abilities.

unilobular /-lob'yələr/, having only one lobe.

unilocular /-lok'yələr/, having only one locus, chamber, or cell.

uninterrupted suture /unin'tərup'tid/ [AS,

un, not; L, *interrumpere,* to sever, *sutura*], a continuous suture running forward and backward without interruption.

uniovular /yōō′nē-ov′yələr/ [L, *unus* + *ovum,* egg], developing from a single ovum, as in monozygotic twins as contrasted with dizygotic twins.

unipolar /-pō′lər/ [L, *unus,* one, *polus*], pertaining to a nerve cell with only one pole, such as a nerve cell in which the axon and dendrite are fused into a single process a short distance from the cell body.

unipolar depression a major disorder of mood that is characterized by symptoms of depression only.

unipolar lead [L, *unus* + *polus,* pole; AS, *laedan,* to lead], **1.** an electrocardiographic conductor in which the exploring electrode is placed on the precordium or a limb while the indifferent electrode is in the central terminal. **2.** *informal.* a tracing produced by such a lead on an electrocardiograph.

unique radiolytic product /yōōnēk′/, a product such as a food substance that has undergone chemical changes as a result of exposure to ionizing radiation.

uniseptate /-sep′tāt/, having only one septum.

unisex /yōō′niseks/ [L, *unus,* one, *sexus,* sex], **1.** concerning only one sex or having reproductive organs of only one sex. **2.** an interchange of sex roles in clothing and hair styles, work assignments, shared restrooms, and activities such as encouraging boys to play with dolls.

unit (U) /yōō′nit/ [L, *unus*], **1.** a single item. **2.** a quantity designated as a standard of measurement. **3.** an area of a hospital that is staffed and equipped for treatment of patients with a specific condition or other common characteristics.

unitary human conceptual framework /yōō′niter′e/, a complex theory in nursing that emphasizes the importance of holistic health care and an understanding of the human being in relation to the universal environment.

unit clerk, a person who performs routine clerical and reception tasks in a hospital inpatient care unit.

unit dose, a method of preparing medications in which individual doses of patient medications are prepared by the pharmacy and delivered in individual labeled packets to the patient's unit to be administered by the nurses on the ordered schedule.

unit dose system, a system of drug distribution in which a portable cart containing a drawer for each patient's medications is prepared by the hospital pharmacy with a 24-hour supply of the medications.

United Nations International Children's Emergency Fund (UNICEF) /yōō′-nisef′/, a fund established by the General Assembly of the United Nations in 1946 to aid children in devastated areas of the world.

United Network for Organ Sharing (UNOS), a national organization for the collection and distribution of body organs that can be used in transplants. Hospitals advise relatives of newly deceased patients about the availability of UNOS service in arranging organ donations.

United States Pharmacopeia (USP), a compendium recognized officially by the Federal Food, Drug, and Cosmetic Act that contains descriptions, uses, strengths, and standards of purity for selected drugs and for all of their forms of dosage.

United States Public Health Service (USPHS), an agency of the federal government responsible for the control of the arrival from abroad of any people, goods, or substances that may affect the health of U.S. citizens. The agency sets standards for the domestic handling and processing of food and the manufacture of serums, vaccines, cosmetics, and drugs.

unit of blood, a standard measure of approximately 1 pint of whole blood.

unit of service, any individual, family, aggregate, organization, or community given nursing care.

univalent /yōō′nivāl′ənt, yōōniv′ələnt/ [L, *unus* + *valere,* to be worth], referring to a chemical valency of one, or the capacity of one atom of a chemical element to attract one atom of hydrogen or to displace one atom of hydrogen.

univalent reduction, a phenomenon during intracellular metabolism involving oxygen-reduction reactions in which superoxide radicals are produced because oxygen accepts electrons only one at a time.

universal /yōō′nivur′səl/ [L, *universus,* whole world], occurring everywhere and in all things.

universal antidote [L, *universus,* whole world; Gk, *anti,* against, *dotos,* something given], a mixture of 50% activated charcoal, 25% magnesium oxide, and 25% tannic acid, formerly thought to be useful as an antidote for most types of acid, heavy metal, alkaloid, and glycoside poisons. It is now believed that the mixture is no more effective than activated charcoal given with water.

universal cuff, an adaptive device worn on the hand to hold items such as utensils, shaver, or pencil, allowing a patient with a weak grasp to participate more in self-care.

U

universal donor, a person with type O, Rh factor–negative red blood cells. Packed red blood cells of this type may be used for emergency transfusion with minimal risk of incompatibility.

universalizability principle /yōō′nivur′səlī′zəbil′itē/, a principle that an act is good if everyone should, in similar circumstances, do the same act without exception.

universal numbering system, a system for identifying and referring to teeth that assigns numbers 1 to 32 to the permanent teeth and the letters A to T (or the numbers 1 to 20 plus the letter d) to the primary teeth.

universal precautions, an approach to infection control designed to prevent transmission of blood-borne diseases such as human immunodeficiency virus and hepatitis B in health care settings. Universal precautions were initially developed in 1987 by the Centers for Disease Control and Prevention in the United States and in 1989 by the Bureau of Communicable Disease Epidemiology in Canada. The guidelines for universal precautions include specific recommendations for use of gloves and masks and protective eyewear when contact with blood or body secretions containing blood is anticipated.

universal qualifiers, (in neurolinguistic programming) the use of terms that give general impressions of limitations, such as all, common, every, only, and never.

universal recipient [L, *universus* + *recipere,* to receive], a person with blood type AB who can receive a transfusion of blood of any group type without agglutination or precipitation effects.

unlicensed assistive personnel, health care workers who are not licensed and who are prepared to provide certain elements of patient care under the supervision of a registered nurse. Unlicensed assistive personnel include patient care technicians, nurses' aides, and certified nursing assistants.

unmyelinated /unmī′əlinā′tid/ [AS, *un,* not; Gk, *myelos,* marrow], describing a nerve fiber that is not coated with a myelin sheath. An unmyelinated fiber, lacking the whitish sheath, appears as gray matter in the brain.

Unna's paste boot /ōō′nəz/ [Paul G. Unna, German dermatologist, 1850–1929; L, *pasta,* paste; ME, *bote*], a dressing for varicose ulcers formed by applying a layer of a gelatin-glycerin-zinc oxide paste to the leg and then a spiral bandage covered with successive coats of paste to produce a rigid boot.

UNOS, /yōō′nos/, abbreviation for **United Network for Organ Sharing.**

unresolved grief /un′rizolvd′/, a severe, chronic sorrow reaction in which a person does not complete the resolution stage of the mourning process within a reasonable time.

unsaturated /unsach′ərātid/ [ME, *un* + L, *saturare,* to fill], describing a solution that is capable of dissolving more of the solute; not saturated.

unsaturated alcohol, an alcohol derived from an unsaturated hydrocarbon such as an alkene or olefin.

unsaturated compound [AS, *un,* not; L, *saturare,* to fill, *componere,* to put together], a chemical compound that contains double or triple bonds.

unsaturated fatty acid, any of a number of glyceryl esters of certain organic acids in which some of the atoms are joined by double or triple valence bonds. Monounsaturated fatty acids have only one double or triple bond per molecule and are found in such foods as fowl, almonds, pecans, cashew nuts, peanuts, and olive oil. Polyunsaturated fatty acids have more than one double or triple bond per molecule.

unsaturated hydrocarbon, unsaturated hydrocarbon; an organic compound in which two or more carbon atoms are united by double or triple valence bonds, as in unsaturated fatty acids.

unscrubbed team members /unskrubd′/, the members of a surgical team, including the anesthetist and circulating nurse, who wear surgical attire but are not gowned or gloved and do not enter the sterile field.

unsocialized aggressive reaction /unsō′shəlīzd/ [ME, *un* + L, *socialis,* companion, *aggressio,* an attack, *re* + *agere,* again to act], a behavior disorder of childhood characterized by overt and covert hostility, disobedience, physical and verbal aggression, vengefulness, quarrelsome behavior, and destructiveness, often manifested in acts such as lying, stealing, temper tantrums, vandalism, and physical violence against others.

unstable /unstā′bəl/, **1.** in an excited or active state, such as an atom with a nucleus possessing excess energy. **2.** easily broken down.

unstable angina [AS, *un,* not, *stabilis,* firm, *angina,* quinsy], a form of pain that is prodromal to acute myocardial infarction. It typically has a sudden onset, sudden worsening, and stuttering recurrence over days and weeks. It carries a more severe short-term prognosis than stable chronic angina.

Unverricht's disease /un′vərikts, ŏŏn′ferishts/ [Heinrich Unverricht, German physician, 1853–1912], an inherited condition characterized by progressive degeneration of gray matter, resulting in myoclonic epilepsy. It appears in patients 8 to 13 years old and is marked by general neurologic and intellectual decline.

upper airway obstruction (UAO), any abnormal condition of the mouth, nose, or larynx that interferes with breathing when the rest of the respiratory system is functioning normally.

upper extremity suspension, an orthopedic procedure used in the treatment of bone fractures and the correction of orthopedic abnormalities of the upper limbs. The procedure uses traction equipment, including metal frames, ropes, and pulleys, to relieve the weight of the upper limb involved rather than to exert traction.

upper GI, pertaining to the upper gastrointestinal tract, from the esophagus to and including the duodenum. The term is commonly applied to radiographic or fluoroscopic diagnostic views after ingestion of a barium sulfate solution. Normal findings include normal size, contour, patency, filling, positioning, and transmission of barium through the lower esophagus, stomach, and duodenum.

upper level discriminator (ULD), an electronic device used to discriminate against all pulses that have heights above a given level.

upper motor neuron paralysis, an injury to or lesion in the brain or spinal cord that causes damage to the cell bodies, axons, or both of the upper motor neurons, which extend from the cerebral centers to the cells in the spinal column. Clinical manifestations include weakness or paralysis, increased muscle tone and spasticity of the muscles involved with little or no atrophy, hyperactive deep tendon reflexes, diminished or absent superficial reflexes, the presence of pathologic reflexes such as Babinski's and Hoffmann's reflexes, and no local twitching of muscle groups.

upper respiratory tract (URT), one of the two divisions of the respiratory system. The URT consists of the nose, nasal cavity, ethmoidal air cells, frontal sinuses, sphenoidal sinuses, maxillary sinus, larynx, and trachea. The URT conducts air to and from the lungs and filters, moistens, and warms the air during each inspiration.

upsilon /yŏŏp′silon, up′-/, Υ, υ, the twentieth letter of the Greek alphabet.

uptake /up′tāk/ [AS, *uptacan*], the drawing up or absorption of a substance.

UR, abbreviation for **utilization review.**

urachus /yōōr′əkəs/ [Gk, *ourachos,* urinary tract], an epithelial tube connecting the apex of the urinary bladder with the allan-

tois. Its connective tissue forms the median umbilical ligament.

uracil, a major pyrimidine base found in nucleotides, and a fundamental component of ribonucleic acid.

uragogue, an agent that increases production of urine.

uranium (U) /yŏŏrā′nē-əm/ [planet Uranus], a heavy, radioactive metallic element. Its atomic number is 92; its atomic weight (mass) is 238.03. Uranium is the heaviest of the natural elements.

uranoschisis /yŏŏ′rənos′kisis/, [Gk, *ouranos,* palate, *schisis,* fissure], cleft palate.

uranostaphyloplasty /-staf′ilōplas′tē/ [Gk, *ouranos,* palate, *staphyle,* uvula, *plassein,* to mold], the surgical repair of a cleft palate.

uranostaphyloschisis /yŏŏ′rənostaf′ilos′-kisis/, a fissure that extends from the hard to the soft palate.

urarthritis, inflammation of a joint caused by gout.

urate /yŏŏr′āt/, any salt of uric acid, such as sodium urate. Urates are found in the urine, blood, and tophi or calcareous deposits in tissues. They also may be deposited as crystals in body joints.

uraturia /yŏŏr′ətŏŏr′ē-ə/, the presence of uric acid salts in the urine.

urceiform /ōōrsē′ifôrm/, pitcher-shaped.

Ur-defenses /ōōr′dəfen′səs/, a set of three fundamental beliefs essential for psychologic integrity of the individual, as proposed by Jules Masserman. They are a delusion of invulnerability and immortality, faith in a celestial order, and a wishful fantasy that fellow human beings are potential friends available for mutual service.

urea /yŏŏr′ē-ə/ [Gk, *ouron,* urine], a systemic osmotic diuretic and topical keratolytic. It is prescribed to reduce cerebrospinal and intraocular fluid pressure and is used topically as a keratolytic agent.

urea cycle, a series of enzymatic reactions by which ammonia is detoxified in the liver. In the series of steps for disposing of the ammonia molecule, a waste product of protein metabolism, five enzymatic reactions occur as NH_2 radicals are combined with carbon and oxygen atoms from carbon dioxide to form urea, which is excreted.

ureagenesis /yŏŏr′ē-əjen′əsis/, the process by which urea becomes the final waste product of amino acid metabolism and the detoxification of ammonia from the blood.

Ureaplasma urealyticum /-plaz′mə/, a sexually transmitted microorganism that is a common inhabitant of the urogenital systems of men and women in whom infection is asymptomatic. Neonatal death, pre-

U

maturity, and perinatal morbidity are statistically associated with colonization of the chorionic surface of the placenta by *Ureaplasma urealyticum.*

urease /yŏŏr′ē-ās/, **1.** an enzyme used in the determination of urea in the blood or urine. **2.** an enzyme that catalyzes the hydrolysis of urea to carbon dioxide and ammonia. **3.** an antitumor enzyme.

uremia /yŏŏrē′mē-ə/ [Gk, *ouron* + *haima,* blood], the presence of excessive amounts of urea and other nitrogenous waste products in the blood, as occurs in renal failure.

uremic /yŏŏrē′mik/ [Gk, *ouron,* urine, *haima,* blood], pertaining to a toxic level of urea in the blood.

uremic coma [Gk, *ouron,* urine, *koma,* deep sleep], a stuporous condition resulting from acidosis and the toxic effects of uremia with the retention in the blood of metabolic end products that normally would be excreted through the kidneys.

uremic convulsion, an episode of involuntary muscle contractions caused by uremia or retention in the blood of substances that would normally be excreted by the kidneys.

uremic frost, a pale frostlike deposit of white crystals on the skin caused by kidney failure and uremia. Urea compounds and other waste products of metabolism that cannot be excreted by the kidneys into the urine are excreted through the small superficial capillaries into the skin, where they collect on the surface.

ureter /yŏŏr′ətər, yŏŏrē′tər/ [Gk, *oureter*], one of a pair of tubes, about 30 cm long, that carries urine from the kidney into the bladder. Each tube is composed of a fibrous, a muscular, and a mucous coat and divides into an abdominal part and a pelvic part. The ureter enters the bladder through a tunnel that functions as a valve to prevent backflow of urine into the ureter when the bladder contracts. Connecting with the kidneys, the ureters expand into funnel-shaped renal pelves that branch into calyces. Urine is pumped through the ureters by peristaltic waves that occur an average of three times a minute.—**ureteral** /yŏŏrē′terəl/, *adj.*

ureteral dysfunction /yŏŏrē′terəl/ [Gk, *oureter* + *dys,* bad; L, *functio,* performance], a disturbance of the normal peristaltic flow of urine through a ureter, resulting from dysfunction of ureteral motor nerves.

uretercystoscope /yŏŏr′ētər-sis′təskōp′/ [Gk, *oureter,* ureter, *kystis,* bladder, *skopein,* to view], a cystoscope equipped with ureteric catheters that can be inserted into either ureter.

ureteritis /yŏŏre′tərī′tis/ [Gk, *oureter* + *itis*], an inflammatory condition of a ureter caused by infection or by the mechanic irritation of a stone.

ureterocele /yŏŏrē′tərōsēl′/ [Gk, *oureter* + *kele,* hernia], a prolapse of the terminal part of the ureter into the bladder. The condition may lead to obstruction of the flow of urine, hydronephrosis, and loss of renal function.

ureterodialysis /-dī-al′isis/ [Gk, *oureter,* ureter, *dialysis,* a breaking], the rupture of a ureter.

ureterography /yŏŏrē′tərog′rəfē/ [Gk, *oureter* + *graphein,* to record], the radiologic imaging of a ureter, usually conducted as part of an examination of the urinary tract. The examination may involve injection of a radiopaque medium through a urinary catheter.

ureteroplasty /yŏŏrē′tərōplas′tē/ [Gk, *oureter* + *plassein,* to mold], a surgical procedure performed to restructure a ureter, such as when a stricture blocks the normal flow of urine.

ureteropyelonephritis /-pī′əlō′nəfrī′tis/ [Gk, *oureter* + *pyelos,* pelvis, *nephros,* kidney, *itis,* inflammation], an inflammation of the kidney, pelvis, and ureter.

ureterosigmoidostomy /-sig′moidos′təmē/ [Gk, *oureter* + *sigma,* S-shaped, *eidos,* form, *stoma,* mouth], a surgical procedure in which a ureter is implanted in the sigmoid flexure of the intestinal tract.

ureterostomy /-os′təmē/ [Gk, *oureter* + *stoma,* mouth], the surgical creation of a new opening from a ureter to the surface of the body or into another outlet, such as the rectum.

ureterotomy, an incision into a ureter.

ureterovaginal /-vaj′inəl/, pertaining to the ureters and vagina.

urethra /yŏŏrē′thrə/ [Gk, *ourethra*], a small tubular structure that drains urine from the bladder. In women it is about 3 cm long and lies directly behind the symphysis pubis, anterior to the vagina. In men it is about 20 cm long and begins at the bladder, passes through the center of the prostate gland, goes between two sheets of tissue connecting the pubic bones, and finally passes through the urinary meatus of the penis. In men the urethra is joined by the ejaculatory duct and serves as a passageway for semen during ejaculation, as well as a canal for urine during voiding.

urethral /yŏŏrē′thrəl/, pertaining to the urethra.

urethral caruncle [Gk, *ourethra* + L, *caruncula,* small piece of flesh], a small painful growth in the mucous membrane of the female urethral meatus. It may be a source of bleeding.

urethral hematuria [Gk, *ourethra* + *haima,* blood, *ouron,* urine], blood in the urine as a result of a urethral lesion.

urethral orifice, 1. a slitlike opening of the male urethra in the glans penis. **2.** the external orifice of the female urethra in the vestibule. **3.** an internal opening of the urethra at the anterior and inferior angle of the trigone.

urethral sphincter, the voluntary muscle at the neck of the bladder that relaxes to allow urination.

urethral swab [Gk, *ourethra* + D, *zwabber*], an absorbent pad on a slender rod used to treat lesions or to remove secretions.

urethritis /yŏŏr′ithrī′tis/, an inflammatory condition of the urethra that is characterized by dysuria, usually the result of an infection in the bladder or kidneys.

urethrocele /yŏŏrē′thrə′sēl/ [Gk, *urethra* + *kele,* hernia], (in women) a herniation of the urethra. It is characterized by a protrusion of a segment of the urethra and the connective tissue surrounding it into the anterior wall of the vagina.

urethrocystitis /yŏŏrē′thrōsistī′tis/, an inflammation of the urethra and bladder.

urethrodynia /-din′ē·ə/, pain in the urethra.

urethrography /yŏŏr′ēthrog′rəfē/, the radiologic examination of the urethra after the injection of a radiopaque agent into the urethra, usually through a catheter.

urethroplasty /yŏŏrē′thrəplastē/, a surgical procedure for the repair of a urethra, as in the correction of hypospadias.

urethroscope /-skōp′/ [Gk, *ourethra,* urethra, *skopein,* to view], an instrument used to examine the internal surfaces of the urethra.

urethrospasm /-spaz′əm/, a spasm of the musculature of the urethra.

urethrostenosis /-stənō′sis/ [Gk, *ourethra,* urethra, *stenosis,* a narrowing], a stricture of the urethra.

urgency /ur′jensē/ [L, *urgere,* to drive on], a feeling of the need to void urine immediately.

URI, abbreviation for **upper respiratory infection.**

uric acid /yŏŏr′ik/, a product of the metabolism of protein present in the blood and excreted in the urine.

uricaciduria /yŏŏr′ikas′idŏŏr′ē·ə/ [Gk, *ouron* + L, *acidus,* sour; Gk, *ouron*], a greater than normal amount of uric acid in the urine, often associated with urinary calculi or gout.

uricosuric drugs /yŏŏr′ikōsŏŏr′ik/ [Gk, *ouron* + L, *acidus,* sour; Gk, *ouron* + Fr, *drogue*], drugs administered to relieve the pain of gout or to increase the elimination of uric acid.

urinal /yŏŏr′inəl/, a plastic or metal receptacle for collecting urine from males.

urinalysis /yŏŏr′inal′isis/ [Gk, *ouron* + *analysein,* to loosen], a physical, microscopic, or chemical examination of urine. The specimen is physically examined for color, turbidity, specific gravity, and pH. Then it is spun in a centrifuge to allow collection of a small amount of sediment that is examined microscopically for blood cells, casts, crystals, pus, and bacteria. Chemical analysis may be performed for the identification and quantification of any of a large number of substances but most commonly for ketones, sugar, protein, and blood.

urinary /yŏŏr′iner′ē/, pertaining to urine or the formation of urine.

urinary albumin [Gk, *ouron,* urine; L, *albus,* white], the presence of albumin, a protein, in the urine. Normally protein is not found in the urine because the spaces in the glomerular membrane of the kidney are too small to allow escape of protein molecules. If the membrane is damaged, as in some kidney diseases, albumin molecules can leak through into the urine. Normal findings are: none or as high as 8 mg/dl; 50 to 80 mg/24 hours at rest; less than 250 mg/24 hours after strenuous exercise.

urinary bladder [Gk, *ouron* + AS, *blaedre*], the muscular membranous sac in the pelvis that stores urine for discharge through the urethra. It is connected anteriorly with the two ureters and posteriorly with the urethra.

Urinary Bladder Training, a Nursing Interventions Classification defined as improving bladder function for those with urge incontinence by increasing the bladder's ability to hold urine and the patient's ability to suppress urination.

urinary calculus, a calculus formed in any part of the urinary tract. Calculi may be large enough to obstruct the flow of urine or small enough to be passed with the urine.

urinary casts [Gk, *ouron,* urine; ONorse, *kasta*], cells or particles excreted in the urine having the shape of renal-collecting tubule cells.

Urinary Catheterization, a Nursing Interventions Classification defined as insertion of a catheter into the bladder for temporary or permanent drainage of urine.

Urinary Catheterization: Intermittent, a Nursing Interventions Classification defined as regular periodic use of a catheter to empty the bladder.

urinary elimination, altered, a NANDA-accepted nursing diagnosis of the state in which an individual experiences a disturbance in urine elimination. The defining characteristics are dysuria, urinary frequency, urinary hesitancy, urinary incontinence, nocturia, urinary retention, and urinary urgency.

Urinary Elimination Management, a Nursing Interventions Classification defined as maintenance of an optimum urinary elimination pattern.

urinary frequency, a greater than normal frequency of the urge to void without an increase in the total daily volume of urine. The condition is characteristic of bladder or urethral inflammation or of diminished bladder capacity or other structural abnormalities.

Urinary Habit Training, a Nursing Interventions Classification defined as establishing a predictable pattern of bladder emptying to prevent incontinence for persons with limited cognitive ability who have urge, stress, or functional incontinence.

urinary hesitancy, a decrease in the force of the stream of urine, often with difficulty in beginning the flow. Hesitancy is usually the result of an obstruction or stricture between the bladder and the urethral opening; in men it may indicate an enlargement of the prostate gland, in women stenosis of the urethral opening.

urinary ileostomy [Gk, *ouron,* urine; L, *ilia,* intestines; Gk, *stoma,* mouth], the surgical creation of a passage between the urinary bladder and the ileum for the diversion of urinary flow from the ureters.

urinary incontinence, involuntary passage of urine, with the failure of voluntary control over bladder and urethral sphincters.

Urinary Incontinence Care, a Nursing Interventions Classification defined as assistance in promoting continence and maintaining perineal skin integrity.

Urinary Incontinence Care: Enuresis, a Nursing Interventions Classification defined as promotion of urinary incontinence in children.

urinary meatus, the external opening of the urethra.

urinary output, the total volume of urine excreted daily, normally between 700 and 2000 ml. Various metabolic and renal diseases may change the normal urinary output.

urinary overflow, a condition that occurs when a patient's bladder is extremely distended with urine and the patient voids in amounts of 100 ml.

urinary retention, a NANDA-accepted nursing diagnosis of the state in which an individual experiences incomplete emptying of the bladder. Defining characteristics include bladder distension, small, infrequent voiding or absence of urine output, a sensation of bladder fullness, dribbling, residual urine, dysuria, and overflow incontinence.

Urinary Retention Care, a Nursing Interventions Classification defined as assistance in relieving bladder distension.

urinary sediment [Gk, *ouron,* urine; L, *sedimentum,* a settling], solid matter that settles to the bottom of a urine sample that has been allowed to stand for several hours.

urinary system, all of the organs involved in the secretion and elimination of urine. These include the kidneys, ureters, bladder, and urethra.

urinary system assessment, an evaluation of the condition and functioning of the kidneys, bladder, ureters, and urethra and an investigation of concurrent and previous disorders that may be factors in abnormalities in the urinary system. The patient is asked whether painful urination, frequency or burning on urination, dribbling, a decreased urinary stream, nocturia, stress incontinence, headache, back pain, or increased thirst has occurred. The color, odor, and amount of urine voided and obtained via catheter are determined. Diagnostic procedures may include cystoscopy, excretory and intravenous urography, renal angiography, retrograde studies, and x-ray film of the kidneys, ureters, and bladder.

urinary tract, all organs and ducts involved in the secretion and elimination of urine from the body.

urinary tract infection (UTI), an infection of one or more structures in the urinary tract. Most of these infections are caused by gram-negative bacteria, most commonly *Escherichia coli* or species of *Klebsiella, Proteus, Pseudomonas,* or Enterobacter. UTI is usually characterized by urinary frequency, burning, pain with voiding, and, if the infection is severe, visible blood and pus in the urine. Kinds of urinary tract infections include **cystitis, pyelonephritis,** and **urethritis.**

urinate /yŏŏr′ināt/[Gk *ouron* urine], to excrete urine from the bladder.

urination /yŏŏr′inā′shən/ [Gk, *ouron* + L, *atus,* process], the act of passing urine.

urine /yŏŏr′in/ [Gk *ouron*], the fluid secreted by the kidneys, transported by the ureters, stored in the bladder, and voided through the urethra. Normal urine is clear, straw-colored, and slightly acid and has the characteristic odor of urea. Its normal constituents include water, urea, sodium chloride and potassium chloride, phosphates, uric acid, organic salts, and the pigment urobilin.

urine osmolality, the osmotic pressure of urine. The normal values are 500 to 800 mOsm/L.

urine pH, the hydrogen ion concentration of the urine, or a measure of its acidity or alkalinity. The normal pH value for urine is 4.6 to 8.0.

urine specific gravity, a measure of the degree of concentration of a sample of urine. The normal range of urine specific gravity is 1.003 to 1.035, depending on the patient's previous fluid intake, renal perfusion, and renal function.

urinoma /yōōr′inō′mə/, a cyst filled with urine.

urinometer /yōōr′inom′ətər/ [Gk, *ouron* + *metron,* measure], any device for determining the specific gravity of urine.

urobilin /yōōr′əbī′lin/, a brown pigment formed by the oxidation of urobilinogen, normally found in feces and in small amounts in urine.

urobilinogen /yōōr′əbīlin′əjən/, a colorless compound formed in the intestine after the breakdown of bilirubin by bacteria.

urobilinuria /yōō′ōbī′linōōr′ē-ə /, a condition of excess urobilin in the urine.

urodynamics /-dīnam′iks/ [Gk, *ouron,* urine, *dynamis,* force], the study of the hydrology and mechanics of urinary bladder filling and emptying.

urogenital /yōōr′ōjen′itəl/ [Gk, *ouron* + L, *genitalis,* fruitful], pertaining to the urinary and the reproductive systems.

urogenital sinus, one of the elongated cavities, formed by the division of the cloaca in early embryonic development, into which opens the ureter, mesonephric and paramesonephric ducts, and bladder.

urogenital system, the urinary and genital organs and the associated structures that develop in the fetus to form the kidneys, ureters, bladder, urethra, and genital structures of the male and female. In women these structures are the ovaries, uterine tubes, uterus, clitoris, and vagina. In men these are the testes, seminal vesicles, seminal ducts, prostate, and penis.

urogram /yōōr′əgram′/, an x-ray film of the urinary tract, obtained by urography.

urography /yōōrog′rəfē/ [Gk, *ouron* + *graphein,* to record], any of a group of x-ray techniques used to examine the urinary system. A radiopaque substance is injected, and radiographs are taken as the substance is passed through or excreted from the part of the system being studied.

urokinase /yōōr′əkī′nās/, an enzyme produced in the kidney and found in urine that is a potent plasminogen activator of the fibrinolytic system.

urolagnia /yōōr′əlag′nē-ə/, sexual stimulation gained from acts involving urine, such as watching people urinate or being urinated on.

urologic /-loj′ik/ [Gk, *ouron,* urine, *logos,* science], pertaining to the scientific study of the urinary tract.

urologist /yōōrol′əjist/, a licensed physician who has completed an approved residency program and who specializes in the practice of urology.

urology /yōōrol′əjē/ [Gk, *ouron* + *logos,* science], the branch of medicine concerned with the study of the anatomy and physiology, disorders, and care of the urinary tract in men and women and of the male genital tract.

urometer /yōōrom′ətər/ [Gk, *ouron,* urine, *metron,* measure], a type of hydrometer used to measure the specific gravity of a urine sample.

uropathy /yōōrop′əthē/ [Gk, *ouron* + *pathos,* disease], any disease or abnormal condition of any structure of the urinary tract.—**uropathic,** *adj.*

uroporphyria /yōōr′ōpôrfir′ē-ə/ [Gk, *ouron* + *porphyros,* purple], a rare genetic disease characterized by excessive secretion of uroporphyrin in the urine, blistering dermatitis, photosensitivity, splenomegaly, and hemolytic anemia.

uroporphyrin /yōōr′ōpôr′firin/, a porphyrin normally excreted in the urine in small amounts.

uroradiology /-rā′dē-ol′əjē/, the radiologic study of the urinary tract.

urorectal septum /-rek′təl/ [Gk, *ouron* + L, *rectus,* straight, *saeptum,* wall], a ridge of mesoderm covered with endoderm that in the early developing embryo divides the endodermal cloaca into the urogenital sinus and the rectum.

uroscopy /yōōros′kəpē/ [Gk, *ouron,* urine, *skopein,* to view], diagnostic examination of urine samples.

urostomy /yōōros′təmē/, the diversion of urine away from a diseased or defective bladder through a surgically created opening, or stoma, in the skin.

urotoxicity /yōōr′ōtoksis′itē/, toxicity of urine.

ursodeoxycholic acid /ur′sōdē-ok′sikol′-ik/, a secondary bile salt. It is used in vivo to dissolve cholesterol gallstones.

urticaria /ur′tiker′ē-ə/ [L, *urtica,* nettle], a pruritic skin eruption characterized by transient wheals of varying shapes and sizes with well-defined erythematous margins and pale centers. It is caused by capillary dilation in the dermis that results

U

from the release of vasoactive mediators.—**urticarial**, *adj.*

urticaria bullosa [L, *urtica,* nettle, *bulla,* bubble], a skin eruption in which the lesions are capped by blisters.

urticaria maculosa [L, *urtica,* nettle, *macule,* spot], a chronic skin eruption in which red lesions form with little or no edema present.

urticaria medicamentosa [L, *urtica,* nettle, *medicina*], a form of skin eruption that follows the use of certain medications, including those containing quinine.

urticaria papulosa [L, *urtica,* nettle, *papula,* pimple], a form of skin eruption affecting mainly children and characterized by reddish macules on which papules develop.

urticaria pigmentosa, an uncommon form of mastocytosis characterized by pigmented skin lesions that usually begin in infancy and become urticarial on mechanical or chemical irritation.

urushiol /əroo′she·ôl/, a toxic resin in the sap of certain plants of the genus *Rhus,* such as poison ivy, poison oak, and poison sumac, that produces allergic contact dermatitis in many people.

USAN /yoo′san, yoo′es′ā′en′/, abbreviation for *United States Adopted Names,* an organization that works with pharmaceutical manufacturers to designate names for nonproprietary drugs.

use effectiveness [L, *usus,* make use of, *efficere,* to produce], (of a contraceptive method) the actual effectiveness of a medication, device, or method in preventing pregnancy.

useful radiation, the part of direct radiation that is permitted to pass from an x-ray tube housing through the tube head port, aperture, or collimator.

user friendly, presenting operating information or instructions in a form that is familiar and easy to understand.

use test, a procedure used to identify offending allergens in foods, cosmetics, or fabrics by the systematic elimination and addition, one at a time, of specific items associated with the life-style of the patient involved.

U-shaped arch, a dental arch in which there is little difference in width between the first premolars and the last molars and the curve from canine to canine is abrupt and U shaped.

Usher's syndrome, an inherited disorder characterized by retinitis pigmentosa and a sensorineural hearing deficit.

USP unit, a dose unit as recommended by the *United States Pharmacopoeia,* the primary legally recognized national drug-standard compendium.

USPHS, abbreviation for **United States Public Health Service.**

uta /yoo′tə/ [Sp, facial ulcers], a mild cutaneous form of American leishmaniasis, occurring in the Andes of Peru and Argentina, caused by *Leishmania peruana.* The lesions are small and usually occur on the exposed surfaces of the skin.

ut dict., abbreviation for the Latin phrase *ut dictum,* 'as directed.'

utend., abbreviation for the Latin phrase *utendus,* 'to be used.'

uterine /yoo′tərən/ [L, *uterus,* womb], pertaining to the uterus.

uterine anteflexion [L, *uterus,* womb, *ante,* before, *flectere,* to bend], an abnormal position of the uterus in which the uterine body is bent forward on itself at the juncture of the isthmus of the uterine cervix and the lower uterine segment.

uterine anteversion, a position of the uterus in which the body of the uterus is directed ventrally. Mild degrees of anteversion are of no clinical significance.

uterine bleeding [L, *uterus* + ME, *blod*], any loss of blood from the uterus.

uterine bruit, a sound made by the passage of blood through the arteries of the pregnant uterus. The sounds are synchronized with the maternal heart rate.

uterine cancer, any malignancy of the uterus, including the cervix or endometrium.

uterine colic [L, *uterus* + Gk, *kolikos,* pain in the colon], a spasmodic pain originating in the uterus. It is usually caused by dysmenorrhea or extrusion of a fibroid polyp.

uterine fibroid [L, *uterus* + *fibra,* fiber; Gk, *eidos,* form], a growth of fibrous tissue in the uterus, usually a fibroma, fibromyoma, or leiomyofibroma.

uterine fibroma, a benign encapsulated uterine tumor. It affects about 20% of women over the age of 30. The tumor may develop in the wall of the uterus or be attached to a stalk of tissue originating in the wall. Symptoms may include menstrual disorders and are also likely to be related to the location of the tumor with respect to neighboring organs.

uterine hemorrhage, bleeding from the uterus. Types of uterine hemorrhage include fetomaternal hemorrhage, in which fetal blood cells leak into the maternal circulation; postmenopausal bleeding; and dysfunctional uterine bleeding.

uterine inertia, abnormal relaxation of the uterus during labor, causing a lack of obstetric progress, or after childbirth, causing uterine hemorrhage.

uterine ischemia, a decreasing or ineffective blood supply to the uterus.

uterine prolapse, the falling, sinking, or sliding of the uterus from its normal location in the body.

uterine retroflexion, a position of the uterus in which its body is bent backward on itself at the isthmus of the cervix and the lower uterine segment. This condition has no clinical significance.

uterine retroversion, a position of the uterus in which the body of the uterus is directed away from the midline, toward the back. Severe retroversion may be accompanied by vague persistent pelvic discomfort and dyspareunia and may prevent the fitting and use of a contraceptive diaphragm.

uterine sinus, one of the small irregular vascular channels in the endometrium of the pregnant uterus.

uterine souffle, a soft, blowing sound made by the blood in the arteries of a pregnant uterus. It is synchronized with the maternal pulse.

uterine subinvolution [L, *uterus* + *sub,* under, *involere,* to roll up], delayed or absent involution of the uterus during the postpartum period. The causes of subinvolution include retained fragments of placenta, uterine fibromyomas, and infection. Regardless of the cause of the condition, it is characterized by longer and heavier bleeding after childbirth and, on pelvic examination, a larger and softer uterus than would be expected at that time.

uterine swab [L, *uterus* + D, *zwabber*], an absorbent material on a rod or flattened wire used to obtain specimens or to remove secretions from the uterus.

uterine tetany, a condition characterized by uterine contractions that are extremely prolonged.

uteroabdominal pregnancy /yōō′tərō′-abdom′inəl/ [L, *uterus* + *abdomen* + *pregnans*], a twin pregnancy in which one fetus develops in the uterus and the other develops in the abdomen.

uteroovarian varicocele /yōō′tərō-′ōver′-ē-ən/ [L, *uterus* + *ovum,* egg, *varix,* varicose vein; Gk, *kele,* tumor], a swelling of the veins of the pampiniform plexus of the female pelvis.

uteroplacental sinus /yōō′tərōpləsen′təl/, one of the spaces in the zone of the placenta and the uterine wall where blood is exchanged between the circulations of the fetus and the mother.

uterosalpingography /yōō′tərō-sal′ping-gog′rəfē/ [L, *uterus* + Gk, *salpinx,* tube, *graphein,* to record], a radiographic examination of the uterus and fallopian tubes.

uterotomy /yōō′tərot′əmē/ [L, *uterus* + Gk, *temnein,* to cut], a surgical incision into the uterus, such as in a cesarean section.

uterovaginal /yōō′tərovaj′inəl/, pertaining to the uterus and vagina.

uterus /yōō′tərəs/ [L, womb], the hollow pear-shaped internal female organ of reproduction in which the fertilized ovum is implanted and the fetus develops and from which the decidua of menses flows. Its anterior surface lies on the superior surface of the bladder. Its posterior surface, also covered with peritoneum, is adjacent to the sigmoid colon and some of the coils of the small intestine. The uterus is composed of three layers: the endometrium, the myometrium, and the parametrium. The endometrium lines the uterus and becomes thicker and more vascular in pregnancy and during the second half of the menstrual cycle under the influence of the hormone progesterone. The myometrium is the muscular layer of the organ. The parametrium is the outermost layer of the uterus. It is composed of serous connective tissue and extends laterally into the broad ligament. The uterus has two parts: a body and a cervix. The body extends from the fundus to the cervix, just above the isthmus. The cavity within the body is only a potential space. The walls of the body touch, unless the woman is pregnant. The cervix has a vaginal part, protruding into the vagina, and a supravaginal part at the juncture of the lower uterine segment.

uterus bicornis [L, *uterus* + *bis* + *cornu,* horn], a uterus that is divided into two parts, usually separate at the upper end and joined at the lower end.

UTI, abbreviation for **urinary tract infection.**

utilitarianism /yōō′tiliter′ē-əniz′əm/ [L, *utilis,* useful, *isma,* practice], a doctrine of ethics that the purpose of all action should be to bring about the greatest happiness for the greatest number of people and that the value of anything is determined by its utility.

utilization review (UR) /yōō′tilīzā′shən/ [L, *utilis* + *atus,* process], an assessment of the appropriateness and economy of an admission to a health care facility or a continued hospitalization.

utricle /yōō′trikəl/ [L, *utriculus,* small bag], the larger of two membranous pouches in the vestibule of the membranous labyrinth of the inner ear. It is an oblong structure that communicates with the semicircular ducts by five openings and receives utricular filaments of the vestibular branch of the vestibulocochlear nerve.

utriculosaccular duct /yōōtrik′yəlōsak′-yələr/ [L, *utriculus* + *sacculus,* small sack, *ducere,* to lead], a duct connecting the utricle with an endolymphatic duct of the membranous labyrinth.

UV, abbreviation for **ultraviolet.**

uvea /yo͞o′vē·ə/ [L, *uva,* grapes], the fibrous tunic beneath the sclera that includes the iris, the ciliary body, and the choroid of the eye.—**uveal,** *adj.*

uveitis /yo͞o′vē-ī′tis/ [L, *uva* + Gk, *itis*], inflammation of the uveal tract of the eye, including the iris, ciliary body, and choroid. It may be characterized by an irregularly shaped pupil, inflammation around the cornea, pus in the anterior chamber, opaque deposits on the cornea, pain, and lacrimation.

uvula /yo͞o′vyələ/, *pl.* **uvulae** [L, *uva,* grape], the small cone-shaped process suspended in the mouth from the middle of the posterior border of the soft palate.— **uvular,** *adj.*

uvular /yo͞o′vyələr/ [L, *uva,* grape], pertaining to the palatine uvula.

uvulectomy /yo͞o′vyəlek′təmē/ [L, *uva,* grape; Gk, *ektome,* excision], the surgical removal of the uvula.

uvulitis /yo͞o′vyəlī′tis/, an inflammation of the uvula. Common causes are allergy and infection.

uvulotomy /yo͞o′vyəlot′əmē/, the surgical removal of all or part of the uvula.

U wave, (in electrocardiography) a small, rounded wave that follows the T wave.

v, **1.** abbreviation for **vein.** **2.** abbreviation for **venous blood.**

V, **1.** symbol for the element **vanadium.** **2.** symbol for *ventilation capacity of the lung.*

V̇, symbol for *rate of gas flow.*

V_{max}, the maximum rate of catalysis.

VAC, an anticancer drug combination of vincristine, dactinomycin, and cyclophosphamide.

vacc, abbreviation for **vaccination.**

vaccination (vacc) /vak′sinā′shən/ [L, *vaccinus,* relating to a cow], any injection of attenuated microorganisms, such as bacteria, viruses, or rickettsiae, administered to induce immunity or to reduce the effects of associated infectious diseases.—**vaccinate,** *v.*

vaccine /vaksēn′, vak′s̄, -sin/ [L, *vaccinus*], a suspension of attenuated or killed microorganisms administered intradermally, intramuscularly, orally, or subcutaneously to induce active immunity to infectious disease.

vaccinia /vaksin′ē·ə/ [L, *vaccinus*], an infectious disease of cattle caused by a poxvirus that may be transmitted to humans by direct contact or deliberate inoculation as a protection against smallpox. A pustule develops at the site of infection, usually followed by malaise and fever that last for several days. After 2 weeks the pustule becomes a crust that eventually drops off, leaving a scar.

vaccinia immune globulin, a hyperimmune gamma globulin developed for treatment of skin reactions to vaccinia immunization.

vaccinotherapeutics /vak′sinōther′ə-pyoo′tiks/, a form of therapy that involves injections of bacterial antigens.

vacuole /vak′yoo·ōl/ [L, *vacuus,* empty], **1.** a clear or fluid-filled space or cavity within a cell, such as occurs when a droplet of water is ingested by the cytoplasm. **2.** a small space in the body enclosed by a membrane, usually containing fat, secretions, or cellular debris.—**vacuolar, vacuolated,** *adj.*

vacuum aspiration /vak′yoo·əm/ [L, *vacuus,* empty, *aspirare,* to breathe upon], a method of removing tissues from the uterus by suction for diagnostic purposes or to remove elements of conception.

VAD, abbreviation for **vascular access device.**

vade mecum /vā′dē mē′kəm/ [L, go with me], something carried by a person for constant use.

vagal /vā′gəl/ [L, *vagus,* wandering], pertaining to the vagus nerve.

vagal tone [L, *vagus,* wandering; Gk, *tonos,* stretching], **1.** pertaining to the hyperexcitability of the parasympathetic nervous system. **2.** pertaining to the inhibitory control of the vagus nerve over heart rate and atrioventricular conduction.

vagina /vəjī′nə/ [L, sheath], the part of the female genitalia that forms a canal from the orifice through the vestibule to the uterine cervix. It is behind the bladder and in front of the rectum. The canal is actually a potential space; the walls usually touch. The muscles of the vagina are innervated by the pudendal nerve and perfused by the vaginal artery.

vaginal atrophy, a postmenopausal condition of gradually declining tissue activity in the female reproductive tract. It is caused by a cessation of follicular inhibin and estrogen secretion. This leads to decreased negative feedback on the release of follicle-stimulating hormone and luteinizing hormone by the anterior pituitary gland. Tissue effects related to estrogen deficiency include atrophy and dystrophy of the vulva and vagina, pruritus vulvae, dyspareunia, cystourethritis, ectropion, and uterovaginal prolapse.

vaginal bleeding /vaj′ənəl/, an abnormal condition in which blood is passed from the vagina, other than during the menses. It may be caused by abnormalities of the uterus or cervix. The following terms are commonly used in describing the approximate amount of vaginal bleeding: heavy vaginal bleeding, which is greater than heaviest normal menstrual flow; moderate vaginal bleeding, which is equal to heaviest normal menstrual flow; light vaginal bleeding, which is less than heaviest normal menstrual flow; vaginal staining, which is a very light flow of blood barely requiring the use of a sanitary napkin or tampon; vaginal spotting, which is the passage vaginally of a few drops of blood; bloody show, which is an episode of light vaginal bleeding as often occurs in early labor, during labor, and, particularly, at the time of full dilation of the cervix at the end of the first stage of labor.

vaginal cancer, a malignancy of the vagina occurring rarely as a primary neoplasm and more often as a secondary lesion or extension of vulvar, cervical, endometrial, or ovarian cancer. Clear cell adenocarcinoma occurs in young women exposed in utero to diethylstilbestrol, given to their mothers to prevent abortion. A predisposing factor is cervical carcinoma. Vaginal leukoplakia, erythematosus, erosion, or granulation of the mucosa may prove to be carcinoma in situ. Symptoms of invasive lesions are postmenopausal bleeding, purulent discharge, pain, and dysuria.

vaginal cornification test, a test for the level of estrogen in a urine sample of a woman. Confirmation is indicated by the appearance of cornified epithelial cells in a vaginal smear of a laboratory animal.

vaginal cyst [L, *vagina,* sheath; Gk, *kytis,* bag], an abnormal closed sac or pouch in the vaginal tissues.

vaginal delivery, birth of a fetus through the vagina.

vaginal discharge, any discharge from the vagina. A clear or pearly-white discharge occurs normally. The discharge is largely composed of secretions of the endocervical glands. Inflammatory conditions of the vagina and cervix often cause an increase in the discharge, which may then have a foul odor and cause pruritus of the perineum and external genitalia.

vaginal fornix, a recess in the upper part of the vagina caused by the protrusion of the uterine cervix into the vagina.

vaginal hernia, 1. a hernia into the vagina. **2.** a downward protrusion of the cul-de-sac of Douglas between the posterior vaginal wall and the rectum.

vaginal hysterectomy [L, *vagina,* sheath; Gk, *hystera,* womb, *ektome,* excision], the surgical removal of the uterus through the vagina.

vaginal instillation of medication, the instillation of a medicated cream, suppository, or gel into the vagina, usually to treat a local infection of the vagina or uterine cervix.

vaginal jelly, a contraceptive product containing a spermicide in a jelly medium. It is usually used in conjunction with a contraceptive diaphragm or cervical cap. Some antimicrobial medications are also supplied in the form of a vaginal jelly.

vaginal lubricant, an ointment or cream used to reduce friction in the vagina.

vaginal mucification test /myoo′sifikā′shən/, a test for the presence of progestins in a urine sample of a woman. Confirmation is indicated by the stimulation of mucus production in the vaginal epithelium of a laboratory animal.

vaginal speculum [L, *vagina,* sheath; L, *speculum,* mirror], a bivalved instrument, with two opening blades used for inspection of the vaginal cavity.

vaginismus /vaj′iniz′məs/ [L, *vagina* + *spasmus,* spasm], a psychophysiologic genital reaction of women, characterized by intense contraction of the perineal and paravaginal musculature, tightly closing the vaginal introitus. It occurs in response to fear of painful intercourse before coitus or pelvic examination. Vaginismus is considered abnormal if it occurs in the absence of genital lesions and if it conflicts with a woman's desire to participate in sexual intercourse or to permit examination, but it may be a normal or physiologic response if painful genital conditions exist or if forcible or premature intromission is anticipated.

vaginitis /vaj′inī′tis/, an inflammation of the vaginal tissues, such as trichomonas vaginitis.

vaginography /vaj′inog′rəfē/, the radiologic examination of the vagina after injection of a radiopaque contrast medium.

vaginolabial hernia /vaj′inōlā′bē·əl/, an inguinal hernia that reaches the tissue of the labium majus.

vaginoperineoplasty /vaj′inōper′inē′əplas′te/, plastic surgery of the vagina and perineum.

vagosympathetic /vā′gōsim′pəthet′ik/ [L, *vagus,* wandering; Gk, *sympathein,* to feel with] pertaining to the vagus nerve and the cervical part of the sympathetic nervous system.

vagotomy /vāgot′əmē/ [L, *vagus,* wandering, *temnein,* to cut], the cutting of certain branches of the vagus nerve, performed with gastric surgery, to reduce the amount of gastric acid secreted and lessen the chance of recurrence of a gastric ulcer. Because peristalsis will be diminished, a pyloroplasty or an anastomosis of the stomach to the jejunum may be done to ensure proper emptying of the stomach.

vagotonus /vā′gəto′nəs/ [L, *vagus* + Gk, *tonos,* tension], an abnormal increase in parasympathetic activity caused by stimulation of the vagus nerve, especially bradycardia with decreased cardiac output, faintness, and syncope.

vagovagal reflex /vā′gōvā′gəl/ [L, *vagus* + *vagus* + *reflectere,* to bend backward], a stimulation of the vagus nerve by reflex in which irritation of the larynx or trachea results in slowing of the pulse rate.

vagueness /văg'nəs/, a communication pattern involving the use of global pronouns and loose associations that lead to ambiguity and confusion in communication.

vagus nerve /vā'gəs/ [L, *vagus,* wandering, *nervus,* nerve], either of the longest pair of cranial nerves mainly responsible for parasympathetic control over the heart and many other internal organs, including thoracic and abdominal viscera.

vagus pulse [L, *vagus,* wandering, *pulsare,* to beat], a slow, regular pulse caused by overactivity of the vagus nerve.

Val, abbreviation for **valine.**

valence /vāl'əns/ [L, *valere,* to be strong], **1.** (in chemistry) a numeric expression of the capability of an element to combine chemically with atoms of hydrogen or their equivalent. A negative valence indicates the number of hydrogen atoms to which one atom of a chemical element can bond. A positive valence indicates the number of hydrogen atoms that one atom of a chemical element can displace. **2.** (in immunology) an expression of the number of antigen-binding sites for one molecule of any given antibody or the number of antibody-binding sites for any given antigen.

valence electron, any of the electrons in the highest principal energy level of an atom. They are responsible for the bonding of atoms to form crystals, molecules, and compounds.

valeric acid /vəler'ik/, an organic acid with a foul odor found in the roots of *Valeriana officinalis.*

valgus /val'gəs/ [L, bent], an abnormal position in which a part of a limb is bent or twisted outward, away from the mid line, such as the heel of the foot in talipes valgus.

validation /val'idā'shən/, an agreement of the listener with certain elements of the patient's communication.

validity /valid'itē/, (in research) the extent to which a test measurement or other device measures what it is intended to measure.

valine (Val) /val'ēn/, an essential amino acid needed for optimal growth in infants and nitrogen equilibrium in adults.

vallecula /vəlek'yələ/ [L, little valley], any groove or furrow on the surface of an organ or structure.—**vallecular,** *adj.*

vallecula epiglottica, a furrow between the glossoepiglottic folds of each side of the posterior oropharynx.

vallecular dysphagia /vəlek'yələr/, diffi-

culty or pain on swallowing caused by inflammation of the vallecula epiglottica.

valproic acid /valprō'ik/, an anticonvulsant prescribed to prevent certain types of seizure activity, particularly complex absence and petit mal seizures.

Valsalva maneuver /valsal'və/ [Antonio M. Valsalva, Italian surgeon, 1666–1723; OFr, *maneuvre,* work done by hand], any forced expiratory effort against a closed airway, such as when an individual holds the breath and tightens the muscles in a concerted, strenuous effort to move a heavy object or change position in bed. Most healthy individuals perform Valsalva maneuvers during normal daily activities without any injurious consequences; but such efforts are dangerous for many patients with cardiovascular diseases.

Valsalva's test [Antonio Valsalva; L, *testum,* crucible], a method for testing the patency of the eustachian tubes. With mouth and nose kept tightly closed, the patient makes a forced expiratory effort; if the eustachian tubes are open, air will enter into the middle ear cavities, and the subject will hear a popping sound.

value /val'yoo/ [L, *valere,* to be strong], a personal belief about the worth of a given idea or behavior.

values clarification, a method whereby a person can discover his or her own values by assessing, exploring, and determining what those personal values are and how they affect personal decision making.

Values Clarification, a Nursing Interventions Classification defined as assisting another to clarify her or his own values in order to facilitate effective decision-making.

value system, the accepted mode of conduct and the set of norms, goals, and values binding any social group.

valve /valv/ [L, *valva,* folding door], a natural structure or artificial device in a passage or vessel that prevents reflux of the fluid contents passing through it. —**valvular,** *adj.*

valve of lymphatics, any one of the tiny semilunar structures in the vessels and trunks of the lymphatic system that helps regulate the flow of lymph and prevents venous blood from entering the system. There are no valves in the capillaries of the system, but there are many in the collecting vessels.

valvotomy /valvot'əmē/ [L, *valva* + Gk, *temnein,* to cut], the incision into a valve, especially one in the heart, to correct a defect and allow proper opening and closure.

valvular endocarditis /val'vyələr/ [L, *valva,* folding door; Gk, *endon,* within, *kardia,* heart, *itis,* inflammation], a form

V

of chronic inflammation of the lining membrane of the heart in which the valves are stenotic or incompetent.

valvular heart disease [L, *valva* + AS, *hoert* + L, *dis*, opposite of; Fr, *aise*, ease], an acquired or congenital disorder of a cardiac valve. It is characterized by stenosis and obstructed blood flow or by valvular degeneration and regurgitation of blood. Diseases of aortic and mitral valves are most common and may be caused by congenital defects, bacterial endocarditis, syphilis, or, most frequently, rheumatic fever. Valvular dysfunction results in changes in intracardiac pressure and pulmonary and peripheral circulation. It may lead to cardiac arrhythmia, heart failure, and cardiogenic shock.

valvular regurgitation [L, *valva*, folding door, *re* + *gurgitare*, to flow], a circulatory backflow that occurs when the heart contracts and the heart valves fail to close properly, allowing blood to be squeezed back into the atria from the ventricles.

valvular stenosis, a narrowing or constricture of any of the heart valves. The condition may result from a congenital defect, or it may be caused by some disease process.

valvulitis /val'vyəlī'tis/, an inflammatory condition of a valve, especially a cardiac valve. Inflammatory changes in the aortic, mitral, and tricuspid valves of the heart are caused most commonly by rheumatic fever and less frequently by bacterial endocarditis and syphilis.

valvuloplasty /val'vyəlōplas'tē/ [L, *valva*, folding door; Gk, *plassein*, to shape], the use of a balloon-tipped catheter to dilate a cardiac valve.

VAMP /vamp/, abbreviation for a combination drug regimen, used in the treatment of cancer, containing three antineoplastics (vincristine sulfate, methotrexate, and mercaptopurine) and a glucocorticoid (prednisone).

vanadium (V) /vənā'dē·əm/ [ONorse, *Vanadis*, (Freya) goddess of fertility], a grayish metallic element. Its atomic number is 23; its atomic weight (mass) is 50.942. Absorption of vanadium compounds results in a condition called **vanadiumism,** characterized by anemia, conjunctivitis, pneumonitis, and irritation of the respiratory tract.

van Bogaert's disease /vanbō'gərts/ [Ludo van Bogaert, Belgian neurophysiologist, b. 1897], a rare familial disorder of lipid metabolism in which the substance cholestanol is deposited in the nervous system, blood, and connective tissue. Individuals with the disease develop progressive ataxia and dementia, premature athero-

sclerosis, cataracts, and xanthomas of the tendons.

vancomycin /van'kōmī'sin/, an antibiotic prescribed in the treatment of infections, particularly staphylococcal infections resistant to other antibiotics.

Van Deemter's equation /vandēm'tərz/, an expression of a gas chromatography relationship between the height equivalent to the theoretic plate and linear velocity of the carrier gas.

Van de Graaff generator /van'dəgräf'/ [Robert J. Van de Graaff, American physicist, 1901–1967], an electrostatic machine in which electronically charged particles are sprayed on a moving belt and carried by it to build up a high potential on an insulated terminal. The generator often is used to inject particles into a larger accelerator.

van den Bergh's test /van'dənburgs'/ [Albert A. H. van den Bergh, Dutch physician, 1869–1943], a test for the presence of bilirubin in the blood serum. Blood is obtained from a patient who has fasted overnight, and the diluted serum is added to diazo reagent. A blue or violet color indicates the presence of bilirubin.

van der Waals forces /van'derwäls', fän-/ [Johannes D. van der Waals, Dutch physicist and Nobel laureate, 1837–1923], weak attractive forces between neutral atoms and molecules. They occur because a fluctuating dipole moment in one molecule induces a dipole moment in another. The activity accounts for some deviation from Boyle's law at very low temperatures or very high pressures.

vanillylmandelic acid (VMA) /vənil'-ilmandel'ik/, a urinary metabolite of epinephrine and norepinephrine. A greater than normal amount of VMA is characteristic of a pheochromocytoma and neuroblastomas.

vanishing twin /van'ishing/, a twin embryo or fetus that is aborted during pregnancy.

vanity surgery /van'itē/, plastic surgery performed primarily to make the patient appear more youthful.

Van Rensselaer, Euphenia /vanren'səlir/, (1840–1912), an American nurse who designed the first nurses' uniform, a blue and white seersucker dress with collar and cuffs, apron, and cap. She organized the Seton Hospital for Tuberculosis in New York.

vapor bath /vā'pər/, the exposure of the body to vapor, such as steam.

vaporization /vā'pərīzā'shən/ [L, *vapor*, steam], the changing of a liquid or solid (such as dry ice) to a gaseous state.

vaporizer, a device for reducing medicated liquids to a vapor useful for inhalation or application to accessible mucous membranes.

vapor pressure depression, a phenomenon in which the addition of a solute molecule to a solvent will decrease the vapor pressure of the solvent in equilibrium with the vapor phase and the liquid phase.

vapor therapy, the therapeutic use of vapors or sprays.

variability /ver′ē·əbil′itē/ [L, *variare*, to diversify], the degree of divergence or ability of an object to vary from a given standard or average.

variable /ver′ē·əbəl/, a factor in an experiment or scientific test that tends to vary, or take on different values, while other elements or conditions remain constant.

variable behavior [L, *variare*, to diversify; AS, *bihabban*, to behave], a response, activity, or action that may be modified by individual experience.

variable interval (VI) reinforcement, reinforcement that is offered after varying lapses of time.

variable ratio (VR) reinforcement, reinforcement that requires variable numbers of responses.

variable region, the N-terminal part of an immunoglobulin polypeptide chain whose amino acid sequence can change. The region includes the antigen combining site.

variance /ver′ē·əns/ [L, *variare*], **1.** (in statistics) a numeric representation of the dispersion of data around the mean in a given sample. It is represented by the square of the standard deviation and is used principally in performing an analysis of variance. **2.** *nontechnical.* the general range of a group of findings.

variant /ver′ē·ənt/ [L, *variare*, to diversify], the differences between individuals or subpopulations of a species, as the notypic or genotypic traits of mutants.

varicella gangrenosa /ver′isel′ə/, a potentially fatal form of varicella characterized by gangrenous lesions. A fulminating subvariety of the skin disorder may become fatal within a few hours if complicated by hemolytic streptococcus.

varicella-zoster immune globulin (VZIG) /zos′tər/ [L, *varius*, diverse; Gk, *zoster*, girdle; L, *immunis*, free from, *globulus*, small globe], an immune globulin obtained from the blood of normal people with high levels of varicella-zoster antibodies. The immune globulin can be administered to people exposed to chickenpox to prevent or modify symptoms of the infection.

varicella zoster virus (VZV) [L, *varius*, diverse; Gk, *zoster*, girdle; L, *virus*, poison], a member of the herpesvirus family, which causes the diseases varicella (chickenpox) and herpes zoster (shingles). The virus has been isolated from vesicle fluid in chickenpox, is highly contagious, and may be spread by direct contact or droplets. Dried crusts of skin lesions do not contain active virus particles. Herpes zoster is produced by reactivation of latent varicella virus, usually several years after the initial infection.

varicelliform /ver′isel′ifôrm/, resembling the rash of chickenpox.

varicocele /ver′əkōsēl′/ [L, *varix*, varicose vein; Gk, *kele*, tumor], a dilation of the pampiniform venous complex of the spermatic cord. The varicocele forms a soft, elastic swelling that can cause pain.

varicose /ver′əkōs/ [L, *varix*], **1.** (of a vein) exhibiting varicosis, or a varicosity. **2.** abnormally and permanently distended, such as the bulging veins in some individuals.

varicose aneurysm, a blood-filled, saclike projection that connects an artery and one or several veins and that is formed from a localized dilation of the adjoining vessels.

varicose vein, a tortuous, dilated vein with incompetent valves. Causes include congenitally defective valves, thrombophlebitis, pregnancy, and obesity. Varicose veins are common, especially in women. The saphenous veins of the legs are most often affected.

varicosis /ver′ikō′sis/ [L, *varix* + Gk, *osis*, condition], a common condition characterized by one or more tortuous, abnormally dilated, or varicose veins, usually in the legs or the lower trunk. Varicosis may be caused by congenital defects of the valves or walls of the veins or by congestion and increased intraluminal pressure resulting from prolonged standing, poor posture, pregnancy, abdominal tumor, or chronic systemic disease. Symptoms include pain and muscle cramps with a feeling of fullness and heaviness in the legs. Dilation of superficial veins is often evident before the condition produces discomfort.

varicosity /ver′ikos′itē/, **1.** an abnormal condition, usually of a vein, characterized by swelling and tortuosity. **2.** a vein in this condition.

variegate /ver′ē·əgāt′/ [L, *varius*, diverse], having characteristics that vary, especially as to color.

variegate porphyria, an uncommon form of hepatic porphyria, characterized by skin lesions and photosensitivity. The condition may be congenital or acquired.

varioloid /ver′ē·əloid′/ [L, *varius* + Gk, *ei-*

V

dos, form], **1.** resembling smallpox. **2.** a mild form of smallpox in a vaccinated person or one who has previously had the disease.

varix /ver′iks/, *pl.* **varices** /ver′əsēz/ [L, varicose vein], **1.** a tortuous dilated vein. **2.** an enlarged tortuous artery or a distended twisting lymphatic.

varnish /vär′nish/, (in dentistry) a solution of natural resins and gums used as a protective coating over the surfaces of a dental cavity preparation before restorative material is applied or on a tooth surface after sealing and root planing.

varus /ver′əs/ [L, bent], an abnormal position in which a part of a limb is turned inward toward the midline, such as the heel and foot in **talipes varus.**

vas /vas/, *pl.* **vasa** /vā′sə/ [L, vessel], any one of the many vessels of the body, especially those that convey blood, lymph, or spermatozoa.

vasa vasorum [L, *vas,* vessel], small blood vessels that supply the walls of the arteries and veins.

vascular /vas′kyələr/ [L, *vasculum,* little vessel], pertaining to a blood vessel.

vascular access device (VAD), an indwelling catheter, cannula, or other instrumentation used to obtain venous or arterial access.

vascular insufficiency, inadequate peripheral blood flow caused by occlusion of vessels with atherosclerotic plaques, thrombi, or emboli; damaged, diseased, or intrinsically weak vascular walls, arteriovenous fistulas, or hematologic hypercoagulability; or heavy smoking. Signs of vascular insufficiency include pale, cyanotic, or mottled skin over the affected area; swelling of an extremity; absent or reduced tactile sensation; tingling; diminished sense of temperature; muscle pain such as intermittent claudication in the calf; and in advanced disease atrophy of muscles of the involved extremity.

vascularity /vas′kyəler′itē/ [L, *vasculum,* little vessel], the state of blood vessel development and functioning in an organ or tissue.

vascularization /vas′kyələr′īzā′shən/, the process by which body tissue becomes vascular and develops proliferating capillaries. It may be natural or induced by surgical techniques.—**vascularize,** *v.*

vascular leiomyoma, a neoplasm that has developed from smooth muscle fibers of a blood vessel.

vascular sclerosis [L, *vasculum* + Gk, *skerosis,* hardening], a condition of hyaline degeneration of the blood vessels with hypertrophy of the media and subintimal fibrosis. Along with fibrosis and intimal

thickening, there may be weakening and loss of elasticity in the artery walls.

vascular tumor, an aneurysm.

vasculature /vas′kyəlā′chər/ [L, *vasculum*], the distribution of blood vessels in an organ or tissue.

vasculitis /vas′kyəli′tis/, an inflammatory condition of the blood vessels that is characteristic of certain systemic diseases or caused by an allergic reaction.

vasculogenic impotence /vas′kyəlōjen′ik/ [L, *vasculum,* little vessel; Gk, *genein,* to produce; L, *in* + *potentia,* power], an inability to perform the male sexual act because of an inadequate supply of arterial blood to the penis.

vasculomotor /-mō′tər/ [L, *vasculum* + *movere,* to move], pertaining to the system of controlling constriction and dilation of blood vessels.

vas deferens /def′ərənz/, *pl.* **vasa deferentia** /def′əren′ shē·ə/ [L, *vas* + *deferens,* carrying away], the extension of the epididymis of the testis that ascends from the scrotum and joins the seminal vesicle to form the ejaculatory duct.

vasectomy /vasek′təmē/ [L, *vas* + Gk, *ektome,* excision], a procedure for male sterilization involving the bilateral surgical removal of a part of the vas deferens. Vasectomy is most commonly performed at an outpatient surgery center using local anesthesia.

vasectomy reversal, a surgical procedure for rejoining the sections of the vas deferens previously severed to render the male infertile. Reanastomosis success varies from 45% to 60%, and in some cases the severed ends of the vas deferens rejoin spontaneously.

vas afferens, a small arteriole that supplies blood to a renal glomerulus.

vasoactive /vā′zō·ak′tiv/ [L, *vas* + *activus,* active], (of a drug) tending to cause vasodilation or vasoconstriction.

vasoactive intestinal polypeptide (VIP), a glucagon-secretin hormone found in the pancreas, intestine, and central nervous system. The hormone stimulates insulin and glucagon release. Gastric secretion, gastric motility, and peripheral vasodilation, as well as hyperglycemia by hepatic glycogenolysis, are inhibited.

vasoconstriction [L, *vas* + *constrigere,* to tighten], a narrowing of the lumen of any blood vessel, especially the arterioles and veins in the blood reservoirs of the skin and the abdominal viscera. It is accomplished by various mechanisms that together control blood pressure and distribution of blood throughout the body.

vasoconstrictive /-kənstrik′tiv/ [L, *vas,*

vessel, *constringere,* to draw tight], able to cause a constriction of blood vessels.

vasoconstrictor /-kənstrik′tər/ [L, *vas* + *constringere*], **1.** pertaining to a process, condition, or substance that causes the constriction of blood vessels. **2.** an agent that promotes vasoconstriction. Cold, fear, stress, and nicotine are common exogenous vasoconstrictors. Internally secreted epinephrine and norepinephrine cause blood vessels to contract by stimulating adrenergic receptors of peripheral sympathetic nerves.

vasodepressor syncope, a sudden loss of consciousness, resulting from cerebral ischemia; secondary to decreased cardiac output, peripheral vasodilation, and bradycardia. The condition may be triggered by pain, fright, or trauma and accompanied by symptoms of nausea, pallor, and perspiration.

vasodilation /-dīlā′shən/ [L, *vas* + *dilatare*], an increase in the diameter of a blood vessel. It is caused by inhibition of its constrictor nerves or stimulation of dilator nerves.

vasodilator /vā′zōdī′lātər/ [L, *vas* + *dilatare*], **1.** a nerve or agent that causes dilation of blood vessels. **2.** pertaining to the relaxation of the smooth muscle of the vascular system. **3.** producing dilation of blood vessels.

vasoganglion /-gang′glē·on/, a mass of small blood vessels that form a ball.

vasogenic shock /-jen′ik/ [L, *vas* + *genein,* to produce; Fr, *choc*], shock resulting from peripheral vascular dilation produced by factors such as toxins that directly affect the blood vessels.

vasohypertonic /-hī′pərton′ik/, causing constriction of blood vessels.

vasoinhibitor /vas′ō·inhib′itər/, an agent that opposes the action of vasomotor nerves, thereby causing arterial dilation and reduced blood pressure.

vasoinhibitory /vas′ō·inhib′itôr′ē/, inhibiting the activity of vasomotor nerves.

vasomotor /-mō′tər/ [L, *vas* + *movere,* to move], pertaining to the nerves and muscles that control the caliber of the lumen of the blood vessels. Circularly arranged fibers of the muscles of arteries can contract, causing vasoconstriction, or they can relax, causing vasodilation.

vasomotor center, a collection of cell bodies in the medulla oblongata of the brain that regulates or modulates blood pressure and cardiac function primarily via the autonomic nervous system.

vasomotor epilepsy, a form of epilepsy characterized by episodes of autonomic dysfunction and extreme contractions of the arteries.

vasomotor paralysis, hypotonia of blood vessels caused by blockage of activity in nerves that produce vascular constriction.

vasomotor reflex [L, *vas,* vessel, *movere,* to move, *reflectere,* to bend back], any reflex response of the circulatory system caused by stimulation of vasodilator or vasoconstrictive nerves.

vasomotor rhinitis, chronic rhinitis and nasal obstruction, without allergy or infection, characterized by sneezing, rhinorrhea, nasal obstruction, and vascular engorgement of the mucous membranes of the nose.

vasomotor spasm [L, *vas,* vessel, *movere,* to move; Gk, *spasmos,* to wrench], an involuntary contraction of the muscles of the small arteries.

vasomotor system, the part of the nervous system that controls the constriction and dilation of the blood vessels.

vasoparesis, a mild form of vasomotor paralysis.

vasospasm /vas′ōspaz′əm/, a spasm in a blood vessel.

vasospastic /-spas′tik/, **1.** relating to a spasmodic constriction of a blood vessel. **2.** any agent that produces spasms of the blood vessels.

vasospastic angina, an ischemic myocardial chest pain caused by spasms of the coronary arteries. It has features that differ from exertional angina.

vasostimulation /-stim′yəlā′shən/ [L, *vas,* vessel, *stimulare,* to incite], the promotion of vasomotor activity.

vasovagal reflex, a stimulation of the vagus nerve by reflex in which irritation of the larynx or the trachea results in slowing of the pulse rate.

vasovasostomy /vā′zōvəsos′təmē/ [L, *vas* + *vas* + Gk, *stoma,* mouth], a surgical procedure in which the function of the vas deferens on each side of the testes is restored, having been cut and ligated in a preceding vasectomy. The procedure is performed if a man wants to regain his fertility.

vastus intermedius /vas′təs/ [L, *vastus,* enormous, *inter,* between, *mediare,* to divide], one of the four muscles of the quadriceps femoris group, situated in the center of the thigh. It functions with the other three muscles of the quadriceps to extend the leg.

vastus lateralis, the largest of the four muscles of the quadriceps femoris group, situated on the lateral side of the thigh. It functions to help extend the leg.

vastus medialis, one of the four muscles of the quadriceps femoris group, situated in the medial part of the thigh. It functions

V

in combination with other parts of the quadriceps femoris to extend the leg.

Vater-Pacini corpuscles /fä'tərpäsē'nē/ [Abraham Vater, German anatomist, 1684–1751; Filippo Pacini, Italian anatomist, 1812–1883], kinesioceptors located in joint capsules and ligaments.

Vater's ampulla /fä'tərz/ [Abraham Vater; L, *ampulla,* jug], a flask-shaped dilation at the end of the common bile duct where the duct joins with the duodenum.

VBP, an anticancer drug combination of vinblastine, bleomycin, and cisplatin.

VC, abbreviation for **vital capacity.**

Vco$_2$, symbol for carbon dioxide output per unit of time.

VD, abbreviation for *venereal disease.*

V deflection (HBE) /diflek'shən/, a deflection on the HIS electrogram that represents ventricular activation.

VDRL, abbreviation for *Venereal Disease Research Laboratories.*

VDRL test, abbreviation for *Venereal Disease Research Laboratory test,* a serologic flocculation test for syphilis. It is also positive in other treponemal diseases such as yaws.

VDT, abbreviation for **video display terminal.**

V̇e, symbol for *expired volume.*

V̇E, symbol for *volume expired in 1 minute.*

vector /vek'tər/ [L, carrier], **1.** a quantity having direction and magnitude, usually depicted by a straight arrow; the length of the arrow represents magnitude, and the head represents direction. **2.** a carrier, especially one that transmits disease. A biologic vector is usually an arthropod in which the infecting organism completes part of its life cycle. A mechanical vector transmits the infecting organism from one host to another but is not essential to the life cycle of the parasite. **3.** a retrovirus that has been modified by alteration of its genetic component. Through recombinant deoxyribonucleic acid techniques, genes that cause harmful effects such as cancer are removed, and genes that mediate synthesis of essential enzymes are added. The vector then can be injected into a patient who suffers from an enzyme deficiency.—**vector,** *v.,* **vectorial,** *adj.*

vectorcardiogram /-kär'dē·əgram'/ [L, *vector,* carrier; Gk, *kardia,* heart, *gramma,* record], a tracing of the direction and magnitude of the electrical forces of a heart's activity during a cardiac cycle. It is produced by the simultaneous recording of three standard leads, using an oscilloscope.

vectorcardiography /-kär'dē·og'rəfē/ [L, *vector,* carrier; Gk, *kardia,* heart,

graphein, to record], a method of recording the magnitude and direction of electrical forces acting on the heart as P-, QRS-, and T-wave vectors, using a continuous loop for each vector.

vecuronium bromide /vek'yərō'nē·əm/, an intravenous neuromuscular blocking drug. It is used as an adjunct to general anesthesia, to facilitate endotracheal intubation, and to relax skeletal muscles during surgery or mechanical ventilation.

VEE, abbreviation for *Venezuelan equine encephalitis.*

veganism /vej'əniz'əm/ [L, *vegetare,* to grow, *ismus,* practice], the adherence to a strict vegetarian diet, with the exclusion of all protein of animal origin.

vegetable albumin /vej'(i)təbəl/, albumin protein produced in plants.

vegetal pole /vej'ətəl/ [L, *vegetare* + *polus,* pole], the relatively inactive part of the ovum protoplasm where the food yolk is situated, usually opposite the animal pole.

vegetarian /vej'əter'ē·ən/ [L, *vegetare*], a person who eats only foods of plant origin, including fruits, grains, and nuts. Many vegetarians eat eggs and milk products but avoid all animal flesh. Kinds of vegetarians are **lacto-ovo-vegetarian, lacto-vegetarian, ovo-vegetarian,** and **strict vegetarian.**

vegetarianism /vej'əter'ē·əniz'əm/, the theory or practice of eating only foods of plant origin, including fruits, grains, and nuts.

vegetation /vej'ətā'shən/, an abnormal growth of tissue around a valve, composed of fibrin, platelets, and bacteria.

vegetative /vej'ətā'tiv, vej'ətətiv'/ [L, *vegetare*], **1.** pertaining to nutrition and growth. **2.** pertaining to the plant kingdom. **3.** denoting involuntary function, as produced by the parasympathetic nervous system. **4.** resting, not active; denoting the stage of the cell cycle in which the cell is not replicating. **5.** leading a secluded, dull existence without social or intellectual activity. **6.** (in psychiatry) emotionally withdrawn and passive, as may occur in schizophrenia and depression or in unipolar depression in severe cases.—**vegetate,** *v.*

vegetative endocarditis [L, *vegetare,* to grow; Gk, *endon,* within, *kardia,* heart, *itis,* inflammation], a subacute form of bacterial endocarditis characterized by vegetation on the heart valves. The vegetation may cause ulceration and perforation of the heart valve cusps.

vegetative state, a physical condition in which a previously comatose patient continues to be unable to communicate or respond to stimuli. The eyes may be open, but, because of senile brain disease, cerebral arteriosclerosis, or injury to the cerebral cortex, the patient remains immobile and must be fed and toileted, and all other physical needs attended to.

vehicle /vē′ikəl/ [L, *vehiculum*, conveyance], **1.** an inert substance with which a medication is mixed to facilitate measurement and administration or application. **2.** any fluid or structure in the body that passively conveys a stimulus. **3.** any substance, such as food or water, that can serve as a mode of transmission for infectious agents.

Veillonella /vā′yənel′ə/ [Adrien Veillon, French bacteriologist, 1864–1931], a genus of gram-negative anaerobic bacteria. The species *Veillonella parvula* is normally present in the alimentary tract, especially in the mouth.

Veillon tube /vāyōn′/, a transparent tube, the ends of which are closed with removable stoppers, one cotton and one rubber. It is used for the laboratory growth of bacteriologic cultures.

vein (v) /vān/ [L, *vena*], any one of the many vessels that convey blood from the capillaries as part of the pulmonary venous system, the systemic venous network, or the portal venous complex. Most of the veins of the body are systemic veins that convey blood from the whole body (except the lungs) to the right atrium of the heart. Each vein is a macroscopic structure enclosed in three layers of different kinds of tissue homologous with the layers of the heart. Deep veins course through the more internal parts of the body, and superficial veins lie near the surface, where many of them are visible through the skin. Veins have thinner coatings and are less elastic than arteries and collapse when cut. They also contain semilunar valves at various intervals.

vein ligation and stripping, a surgical procedure consisting of the ligation of the saphenous vein and its removal from groin to ankle.

vein lumen, the central opening through which blood flows in a vein.

veins of the vertebral column, the veins that drain the blood from the vertebral column, adjacent muscles, and meninges of the spinal cord.

velocity /vəlos′itē/ [L, *velox*, quick], the rate of change in the position of a body moving in a particular direction. Velocity along a straight line is linear velocity. Angular velocity is that of a body in circular motion.

velocity of growth, the rate of growth or change in growth measurements over a period of time.

velocity of ultrasound, the speed of ultrasound energy, measured in meters per second (m/sec), in a particular medium. The velocity varies from 331 m/sec in air to 1450 m/sec in fat, 1570 m/sec in blood, and 4080 m/sec in the skull.

velocity spectrum rehabilitation, a rehabilitation program that uses strength training at multiple speeds of movement from slow to fast.

velopharyngeal insufficiency, an abnormal condition resulting from a congenital defect in the structure of the velopharyngeal sphincter. Closure of the oral cavity beneath the nasal passages is not complete. Food may be regurgitated through the nose, and speech is impaired.

Velpeau's bandage /velpōz′/ [Alfred A. L. M. Velpeau, French surgeon, 1795–1867], a roller bandage that immobilizes the elbow and shoulder by holding the brachium against the side and the flexed forearm on the chest.

vena cava /vē′nə kā′və/, *pl.* **venae cavae** [L, *vena*, vein, *cavum*, cavity], one of two large veins returning blood from the peripheral circulation to the right atrium of the heart.—**vena caval,** *adj.*

vena caval foramen, an opening in the diaphragm through which the inferior vena cava and vagus nerve pass.

vena comes /kō′mēz/, *pl.* **venae comites** /kom′itēz/, one of the deep paired veins that accompany the smaller arteries on each side of the artery. The three vessels are wrapped together in one sheath.

veneer /vənir′/ [Fr, *fournir*, to furnish], **1.** (in dentistry) a layer of tooth-colored material, usually porcelain or acrylic, attached to the surface of a crown or artificial tooth by direct fusion. **2.** a thin, tenacious film of *calculus* found subgingivally and discolored blue-black.

venereal /vənir′ē·əl/ [L, *Venus,* goddess of love], pertaining to or caused by sexual intercourse or genital contact.

venereal bubo [L, *Venus,* goddess of love; Gk, *boubon,* groin], a swollen, inflamed lymph gland or node, usually in the groin and sometimes purulent. It is associated with a sexually transmitted disease.

venereal urethritis, an inflammation of the male urethra caused by sexually transmitted microorganisms.

venereologist /vənir′ē·ol′əjist/ [L, *Venus,* goddess of love; Gk, *logos,* science], a health professional who specializes in the study of the causes and treatments of venereal diseases.

venereology /-ol′əjē/, the study of the causes and treatments of venereal diseases.—**venereologic, venereological,** *adj.,* **venereologist,** *n.*

venerupin poisoning /ven′ərōō′pin/, a potentially fatal form of shellfish poisoning that results from ingestion of oysters or clams contaminated with venerupin, a toxin that causes impaired liver functioning, gastrointestinal distress, and leukocytosis. The shellfish toxin occurs in waters around Japan.

venipuncture /ven′əpungk′chər/ [L, *vena* + *pungere,* to prick], the transcutaneous puncture of a vein by a sharp rigid stylet or cannula carrying a flexible plastic catheter or by a steel needle attached to a syringe or catheter. It is done to withdraw a specimen of blood, perform a phlebotomy, instill a medication, start an intravenous infusion, or inject a radiopaque substance for radiologic examination of a part or system of the body. Aseptic technique is required to avoid infection. A quick, skillful insertion is nearly painless for the patient. Specific sequelae to venipuncture vary with the techniques and equipment used.

venoatrial /vē′nō·ā′trē·əl/, pertaining to either vena cava and the right atrium.

venom /ven′əm/ [L, *venenum,* poison], a toxic fluid substance secreted by some snakes, arthropods, and other animals and transmitted by their stings or bites.

venom extract therapy, the administration of antivenin as prophylaxis against the toxic effects of the bite of a specific poisonous snake or spider or other venomous animal.

venom immunotherapy, the reduction of sensitivity to the bite of a venomous insect or animal by the serial administration of gradually increasing amounts of the specific antigenic substance secreted by the insect or animal.

venomous snake /ven′əməs/, a snake that secretes a poison.

venospasm /vēn′əspaz′əm/ [L, *vena,* vein; Gk, *spasmos,* spasm], a spasmodic contraction of a vein.

venothrombotic /vē′nəthrombot′ik/, producing a venous thrombus.

venotomy /vēnot′əmē/, the surgical opening of a vein.

venous /vē′nəs/, pertaining to a vein.

venous access device, a catheter designed for continuous access to the venous system. Such devices may be required for long-term parenteral feeding or the administration of intravenous fluids or medications for a period of several days.

Venous Access Devices (VAD) Maintenance, a Nursing Interventions Classification defined as management of the patient with prolonged venous access via tunneled, non-tunneled catheters, and implanted ports.

venous blood (v) [L, *vena,* vein; AS, *blod*], dark red blood that has been deoxygenated during passage from the left ventricle through the systemic circulation, en route to the right atrium.

venous blood gas [L, *venosus,* full of veins; AS, *blod* + Gk, *chaos,* gas], the oxygen and carbon dioxide in venous blood measured by various methods to assess the adequacy of oxygenation and ventilation and to determine the acid-base status. The oxygen tension of venous blood normally averages 40 mm Hg; the dissolved oxygen, 0.1% by volume; the total oxygen content, 15.2%; and the oxygen saturation of venous hemoglobin, 75%. The carbon dioxide tension normally averages 46 mm Hg; the dissolved carbon dioxide, 2.9% by volume; and the total carbon dioxide content, 50%. The normal average pH of venous plasma is 7.37.

venous capillaries [L, *vena,* vein, *capillaris,* hairlike], capillaries that terminate in venules.

venous circulation [L, *vena,* vein, *circulare,* to go around], the movement of blood from the venules, which drain deoxygenated blood from the cells, through the veins to the vena cava, and from there through the right atrium and ventricle to the pulmonary circulation of the lungs.

venous cutdown, a small surgical incision made in a vein of a patient who has suffered vascular collapse to permit the introduction of intravenous fluids or drugs. A cutdown also may be performed for the insertion of a cannula for the withdrawal of blood.

venous hemorrhage, the escape of blood from a vein.

venous hum, a continuous musical murmur heard on auscultation over the major veins at the base of the neck. It is audible particularly when the patient is anemic, upright, and looking to the contralateral side.

venous insufficiency, an abnormal circulatory condition characterized by decreased return of the venous blood from the legs to the trunk of the body. Edema is usually the first sign of the condition; pain, varicosities, and ulceration may follow.

venous pressure, the stress exerted by circulating blood on the walls of veins; it is elevated in congestive heart failure, acute or chronic constrictive pericarditis, and venous obstruction caused by a clot or external pressure against a vein. Indications of increased pressure are continued distension of veins on the back of the hand when it is raised above the sternal notch and distension of the neck veins when the individual is sitting with the head elevated 30 to 45 degrees.

venous pulse, the pulse of a vein usually palpated over the internal or external jugular veins in the neck. The pulse in the jugular vein is taken to evaluate the pressure of the pulse and the form of the pressure wave.

venous return, the return of the blood to the heart via vena cavae and coronary sinus.

venous sinus, any one of many sinuses that collect blood from the dura mater and drain it into the internal jugular vein. Each sinus is formed by the separation of the two layers of the dura mater.

venous stasis, a disorder in which the normal flow of blood through a vein is slowed or halted.

venous thrombosis, a condition characterized by the presence of a clot in a vein in which the wall of the vessel is not inflamed. Pain, swelling, and inflammation may follow if the vein is significantly occluded.

ventilate /ven'tilāt/ [L, *ventilare, to fan*], **1.** to provide with fresh air. **2.** to provide the lungs with air from the atmosphere and to aerate or oxygenate blood in the pulmonary capillaries. **3.** (in psychiatry) to open discussion of something, such as to ventilate feelings.

ventilation /ven'tilā'shən/ [L, *ventilare*], the process by which gases are moved into and out of the lungs.—**ventilatory,** *adj.*

Ventilation Assistance, a Nursing Interventions Classification defined as promotion of an optimal spontaneous breathing pattern that maximizes oxygen and carbon dioxide exchange in the lungs.

ventilation, inability to sustain spontaneous, a NANDA-accepted nursing diagnosis of a state in which the response pattern of decreased energy reserves results in an individual's inability to maintain breathing adequate to support life. Defining characteristics include dyspnea, increased metabolic rate, increased restlessness, apprehension, increased use of accessory muscles, decreased tidal volume, increased heart rate, decreased pO_2 level, increased pCO_2 level, decreased cooperation, and decreased SaO_2 level.

ventilation lung scan, a radiographic examination of the lungs, performed while the patient inhales a radioactive gas as a contrast medium and the lungs are scanned to detect nonfunctional or impaired lung areas or other abnormalities.

ventilation perfusion defect, a disorder in which one or more areas of the lung receive ventilation but no blood flow, or blood flow but no ventilation.

ventilation/perfusion (V/Q) ratio, the ratio of pulmonary alveolar ventilation to pulmonary capillary perfusion, both measured quantities being expressed in the same units.

ventilator /ven'tilātər/, any of several devices used in respiratory therapy to provide assisted respiration and intensive positive-pressure breathing.

ventilatory compliance /ven'tilətôr'ē/, the sum of dynamic compliance of the lung and the compliance of the thoracic cage.

ventilatory rate [L, *ventilare*, to fan, *ratum*, to calculate], the volume of air passing through the lungs per minute.

ventilatory standstill [L, *ventilare*, to fan; AS, *standan + stille*], the complete cessation of breathing activity.

ventilatory weaning process, dysfunctional (DVWR), a NANDA-accepted nursing diagnosis of a state in which an individual cannot adjust to lowered levels of mechanical ventilatory support, which interrupts and prolongs the weaning process. DVWR may be classified as mild, moderate, or severe. For mild DVWR, the major defining characteristic is a response to lowered levels of mechanical ventilator support with restlessness or a respiratory rate slightly increased from baseline. For moderate DVWR, the major defining characteristic is a response to lowered levels of mechanical ventilator support with a slight increase from baseline blood pressure (less than 20 mm Hg), a slight increase from baseline heart rate (less than 20 beats/min), and a baseline increase in respiratory rate (less than 5 breaths per minute). For severe DVWR, the major defining characteristic is a response to lowered levels of mechanical ventilator support with agitation, deterioration in arterial blood gas levels from current baseline, increase from baseline blood pressure of greater than 20 mm Hg, increase from baseline heart rate of greater than 20 beats/min, and significant increase in respiratory rate.

venting [Fr, *vent*, breath], (in intravenous therapy) a method for allowing air to enter the vacuum of the intravenous bottle and displace the intravenous solution as it flows out. Glass intravenous bottles are usually equipped with a venting tube attached to the primary intravenous (IV) tubing or to a vent port incorporated with the bottle stopper.

ventral /ven'trəl/ [L, *venter*, belly], pertaining to a position toward the anterior surface of the body; frontward.

ventral horn [L, *venter*, belly, *cornu*], the anterior columns of the gray substance of the spinal cord.

ventral recumbent [L, *venter*, belly, *recumbere*, to lie down], a prone position of lying face down.

ventral root [L, *venter*, belly; AS, *rot*], the anterior or motor division of each spinal nerve.

ventricle /ven′trikəl/ [L, *ventriculus*, little belly], a small cavity, such as the right and left ventricles of the heart or one of the cavities filled with cerebrospinal fluid in the brain.

ventricular /ventrik′yələr/ [L, *ventriculus*, little belly], pertaining to a ventricle.

ventricular aneurysm, a localized dilation or saccular protrusion in the wall of the ventricle, occurring most often after a myocardial infarction. Scar tissue is formed in response to the inflammatory changes of the infarction. This tissue weakens the myocardium, allowing its walls to bulge outward when the ventricle contracts.

ventricular bigeminy [L, *ventriculus* + *bis* + *geminus*, twin], an arrhythmia in which every other beat is caused by a premature ventricular beat.

ventricular block [L, *ventriculus* + OFr, *bloc*], an obstruction of the flow of cerebrospinal fluid. The condition results in a distension of the brain ventricles because of an increased accumulation of cerebrospinal fluid.

ventricular compliance, a property of a heart ventricle in its resting state that determines the relation between the filling of the ventricle and its diastolic pressure.

ventricular dysfunction, abnormalities in contraction and wall motion within the ventricles.

ventricular ejection [L, *ventriculus* + *ejicere*, to cast out], a forceful expulsion of blood from the ventricles to the main arteries.

ventricular escape [L, *ventriculus* + OFr, *escaper*], the discharge of a normal His-Purkinje pacemaker fiber when the sinus or junctional rate of discharge fails or falls below that of ventricular pacemaker cells.

ventricular extrasystole, a premature beat arising from the ventricle.

ventricular fibrillation (VF), a cardiac arrhythmia marked by rapid disorganized depolarizations of the ventricular myocardium. The condition is characterized by a complete lack of organized electric activity, as well as ventricular contraction. Blood pressure falls to zero, resulting in unconsciousness. Death may occur within 4 minutes. Cardiopulmonary resuscitation must be initiated immediately, with defibrillation and resuscitative medications given per advanced cardiac life support protocol.

ventricular flutter, a condition of very rapid contracting of the ventricles of the heart. Electrocardiograms show poorly defined QRS complexes occurring at a rate of 250 beats/min or higher. The condition is fatal if untreated.

ventricular gallop, an abnormal low-pitched extra heart sound (S_3) heard early in diastole. When it is heard in an older person with heart disease, it indicates myocardial failure.

ventricular gradient, the algebraic sum of the areas within the QRS complex and within the T wave in the electrocardiogram.

ventricular hypertrophy [L, *ventriculus* + Gk, *hyper*, excessive, *trophe*, nourishment], an abnormal enlargement of the heart ventricles. It is often caused by hypertension or a valvular disease.

ventricular remodeling, progressive myocardial ventricular dilation, eccentric hypertrophy, and distortion of left ventricular geometry that persist in the noninfarcted myocardium after a myocardial infarction has healed. It is associated with impaired functional capacity, congestive heart failure, and premature death.

ventricular rhythm [L, *ventriculus* + Gk, *rhythmos*] the beating of the ventricles, normal or abnormal.

ventricular septal defect (VSD), an abnormal opening in the septum separating the ventricles. It permits blood to flow from the left to the right ventricle and to recirculate through the pulmonary artery and lungs. It is the most common congenital heart defect.

ventricular standstill, a complete cessation of electrical and mechanical activity in the ventricles of the heart.

ventricular systole [L, *ventriculus* + Gk, *systole*, contraction], the contraction of the heart ventricles. It begins with the first heart sound.

ventricular tachycardia, tachycardia of at least three consecutive ventricular complexes with a rate of more than 100 beats/min. It usually originates in a focus distal to the branching part of the bundle of His.

ventriculoatrial shunt /ventrik′yəlō·ā′-trē·əl/ [L, *ventriculus* + *atrium*, hall; ME, *shunten*], a surgically created passageway, consisting of plastic tubing and one-way valves, implanted between a cerebral ventricle and the right atrium of the heart to drain excess cerebrospinal fluid from the brain in hydrocephalus.

ventriculocisternostomy /-sis′tərnos′təmē/ [L, *ventriculus* + *cisterna*, vessel; Gk, *stoma,* mouth], a surgical procedure performed to treat hydrocephalus. An opening is created that allows cerebrospinal fluid to drain through a shunt from the ventricles of the brain into the cisterna magna.

ventriculofallopian tube shunt /-fəlō'-pē-ən/, a surgical procedure with limited effectiveness for diverting cerebrospinal fluid into the peritoneal cavity. This procedure is used to correct both the obstructive and the communicating types of hydrocephalus.

ventriculogram /ventrik'yəlōgram'/, a radiograph of the cerebral ventricles or the ventricles of the heart.

ventriculography /ventrik'yəlog'rəfē/ [L, *ventriculus* + *graphein,* to record], **1.** a radiographic examination of a ventricle of the heart after injection of a radiopaque contrast medium. **2.** radiography of the head following cerebrospinal fluid removal from the cerebral ventricles and its replacement by a contrast medium, usually air.

ventriculoperitoneal shunt /-per'itənē'əl/ [L, *ventriculus* + Gk, *peri,* around, *teinein,* to stretch; ME, *shunten*], a surgically created passageway consisting of plastic tubing and one-way valves between a cerebral ventricle and the peritoneum for the draining of excess cerebrospinal fluid from the brain in hydrocephalus.

ventriculoperitoneostomy /ventrik'yəlōper'itō'nē·os'təmē/ [L, *ventriculus* + Gk, *peri,* around, *teinein,* to stretch, *stoma,* mouth], a surgical procedure for temporarily diverting cerebrospinal fluid in hydrocephalus, usually in the newborn. In this procedure a polyethylene tube is passed from the lateral ventricle subcutaneously down the dorsal spine and is reinserted into the peritoneal cavity, where the diverted fluid is absorbed.

ventriculopleural shunt /-ploor'əl/ [L, *ventriculus* + Gk, *pleura,* rib; ME, *shunten*], a surgical procedure for diverting cerebrospinal fluid from engorged ventricles in hydrocephalus, usually in the newborn. In this procedure cerebrospinal fluid is diverted from the lateral ventricle into the pleural cavity.

ventriculoureterostomy /ventrik'yəlō'-yōōrē'təros'təmē/ [L, *ventriculus* + Gk, *oureter,* ureter, *stoma,* mouth], a surgical procedure for directing cerebrospinal fluid into the general circulation. It is performed in the treatment of hydrocephalus, usually in the newborn. In this procedure a polyethylene tube is passed from the lateral ventricle down the dorsal spine subcutaneously to the twelfth rib; the tube is in-

serted through the paraspinal muscles into a ureter.

ventrolateral /ven'trōlat'ərəl/, pertaining to the part of the body opposite the back and away from the midline.

ventromedial /ven'trōmē'dē·əl/, pertaining to the part of the body opposite the back and near the midline.

Venturi effect /ventōō'rē/ [Giovanni B. Venturi, Italian physicist, 1746–1822], a modification of the Bernoulli effect in which there is dilation of a gas passage just beyond an obstruction or restriction. The principle is used in respiratory therapy equipment for mixing medical gases.

Venturi mask, a respiratory therapy face mask designed to allow entrained air to mix with oxygen, which is supplied through a jet at a fixed concentration.

venule /ven'yōōl/ [L, *venula,* small vein], any one of the small blood vessels that gather blood from the capillary plexuses and anastomose to form the veins.—**venular,** *adj.*

VEP, abbreviation for **visual evoked potential.**

verapamil /verap'əmil/, a calcium channel blocker prescribed for the treatment of vasospastic and exertional angina, supraventricular tachycardia, atrial fibrillation, and atrial flutter.

Veratrum /vərā'trəm/ [L, hellebore], a genus of poisonous herbs of the lily family. The dried rhizomes of the British and American hellebore provide alkaloids that are used as antihypertensive agents.

verbal language /vur'bəl/ [L, *verbum,* a word, *lingua,* tongue], a culturally organized system of vocal sounds that communicates meaning between individuals.

vergence /ver'jəns/, movement of the two eyes in opposite directions.

vermicide /vur'misīd/ [L, *vermis,* worm, *caedere,* to kill], an agent that kills worms, particularly those in the intestine.

vermicular /vərmik'yələr/ [L, *vermis,* worm], resembling a worm.

vermicular pulse, a small rapid pulse that feels like a writhing worm when the pulse is monitored with the fingers.

vermiform /vur'mifôrm/ [L, *vermis,* worm, *forma,* form], resembling a worm.

vermiform appendix [L, *vermis* + *forma,* form, *appendix,* appendage], a wormlike blunt process extending from the cecum. Its length varies from 7 to 15 cm, and its diameter is about 1 cm.

vermifuge /vərmifyōōj'/ [L, *vermis* + *fugare,* to chase away], an agent that causes the evacuation of intestinal parasitic worms.

vermilion border /vərmil'yən/ [L, *vermil-*

lium, bright red; OFr, *bordure,* frame], the external pinkish-to-red area of the upper and lower lips. It extends from the junction of the lips with the surrounding facial skin on the exterior to the labial mucosa within the mouth.

vermin /vur'min/ [L, *vermis,* worm], any parasitic insects, such as lice and bedbugs, regarded as destructive or disease-carrying pests.

vermis /vur'mis/, *pl.* **vermes** [L], **1.** a worm. **2.** a structure resembling a worm, such as the median lobe of the cerebellum.—**vermiform,** *adj.*

vernal conjunctivitis /vur'nəl/ [L, *vernare,* springlike, *conjunctivus,* connecting; Gk, *itis,* inflammation], a chronic, bilateral form of conjunctivitis, thought to be allergic in origin, that occurs most frequently in young men under 20 years of age during the spring and summer months. Most common symptoms include intense itching and crusting discharge.

Vernet's syndrome /vernāz'/ [Maurice Vernet, French neurologist, b. 1887], a neurologic disorder caused by injury to the ninth, tenth, and eleventh cranial nerves as they pass through the jugular foramen when leaving the skull. The patient experiences dysphagia, the voice is nasal and hoarse, and there may be some loss of taste sensations.

vernix caseosa /vur'niks kas'ē·ō'sə/ [Gk, resin; L, *caseus,* cheese], a grayish-white cheeselike substance, consisting of sebaceous gland secretions, lanugo, and desquamated epithelial cells, that covers the skin of the fetus and newborn.

verruca /vəroo'kə/ [L, wart], a benign viral warty skin lesion with a rough papillomatous surface. It is caused by a common contagious papovavirus.—**verrucose, verrucous,** *adj.*

verruca plana, a small, slightly elevated, smooth tan or flesh-colored wart, sometimes occurring in large numbers on the face, neck, back of the hands, wrists, and knees, especially in children.

verrucous carcinoma /vəroo'kəs/, a well-differentiated squamous cell neoplasm of soft tissue of the oral cavity, larynx, or genitalia. A slow-growing tumor with displacement of surrounding tissue rather than invasion or metastasis occurs.

verrucous endocarditis [L, *verruca,* wart; Gk, *endon,* within, *kardia,* heart, *itis,* inflammation], a form of heart inflammation characterized by the development of wartlike growths on the heart valves.

verrucous dermatitis, any skin rash with wartlike lesions.

version /vur'zhən/ [L, *vertere,* to turn],

the changing of the fetal position in the uterus, usually done to facilitate delivery.

version and extraction, an obstetric operation in which a fetus presenting head first is turned and delivered feet first. It is performed by reaching deeply into the uterus, grasping the feet and pulling them down, and extracting the infant. The procedure is considered outmoded and hazardous.

vertebra /vur'təbrə/*pl.* **vertebrae** [L, joint], any one of the 33 bones (26 in the adult) of the spinal column, comprising the 7 cervical, 12 thoracic, 5 lumbar, 5 sacral (1 in adult), and 4 coccygeal vertebrae (1 in adult). The vertebrae, with the exception of the first and second cervical vertebrae, are much alike and are composed of a body, an arch, a spinous process for muscle attachment, and pairs of pedicles and processes. The first cervical vertebra is called the atlas and has no vertebral body. The second cervical vertebra is called the axis and forms the pivot on which the atlas rotates, permitting the head to turn. The body of the axis also extends into a strong, bony process (the dens).

vertebral /vur'təbrəl/ [L, *vertebra,* joint], pertaining to one or more vertebrae.

vertebral angiography [L, *vertebra* + Gk, *angeion* + *graphein,* to record], the diagnostic study of blood circulation in the spinal area after the injection of radiopaque medium.

vertebral arch [L, *vertebra,* joint, *arcus,* bow], the arch formed on the back of the vertebral body by the pedicles and laminae.

vertebral artery, one of a pair of arteries branching from the subclavian arteries, arising deep in the neck from the cranial and dorsal subclavian surfaces. Each vertebral artery divides into two cervical and five cranial branches, supplying deep neck muscles, the spinal cord and spinal membranes, and the cerebellum.

vertebral-basilar system, an arterial complex in which two vertebral arteries join at the base of the skull to form the basilar artery.

vertebral body, the weight-supporting, solid central part of a vertebra. The pedicles of the arch project from its dorsolateral surfaces.

vertebral canal [L, *vertebra,* joint, *canalis*], the passage formed anterior to the vertebral arches and posterior to the vertebral bodies and occupied by the spinal cord.

vertebral column, the flexible structure that forms the longitudinal axis of the skeleton. In the adult it includes 26 vertebrae arranged in a straight line from the base of the skull to the coccyx. The vertebrae are separated by intervertebral disks. They provide attachment for various muscles such as the iliocostalis thoracis and the longissimus thoracis that give the column strength and flexibility. In the adult the five sacral and four coccygeal vertebrae fuse to form the sacrum and the coccyx.

vertebral foramen [L, *vertebra,* joint, *foramen,* a hole], the opening between the neural arch and the body of a vertebra through which the spinal cord passes.

vertebral groove [L, *vertebra,* joint; D, *groeve*], a shallow depression on each side of the spinous processes of the vertebrae, occupied by the deep back muscles.

vertebral notch [L, *vertebra,* joint; OFr, *enochier,* notch], either of the concavities on the lower or upper border of a vertebral pedicle.

vertebral rib, one of two lower ribs on either side that are not attached anteriorly.

vertebral-venous system, a group of four interconnected venous networks surrounding the vertebral column.

vertebrate [L, *vertebra,* joint], pertaining to any animal possessing a backbone and thus being a member of the subphylum *Vertebrata.* The group includes fish, amphibians, birds, reptiles, and mammals.

vertebrochondral /vur′təbrōkon′drəl/, pertaining to a vertebra and a costal cartilage.

vertebrocostal /-kos′təl/, pertaining to a vertebra and a rib or a vertebra and a costal cartilage.

vertebrocostal rib, one of the eighth, ninth, and tenth ribs on either side that articulate posteriorly with the vertebrae and have their costal cartilages connected anteriorly by capsular ligaments.

vertebrosternal rib /-stur′nəl/, one of the seven upper ribs on either side that have cartilage articulating directly with the sternum.

vertex /vur′teks/ [L, summit], **1.** the top of the head; crown. **2.** the apex or highest point of any structure.

vertex presentation, (in obstetrics) a fetal presentation in which the vertex of the fetus is the part nearest to the cervical os and can be expected to be born first.

vertical /vur′tikəl/ [L, *vertex,* summit], perpendicular or at a right angle to the plane of the horizon.

vertical angulation [L, *vertex* + *angulus,* corner], (in dentistry) the measured angle within the vertical plane at which the central beam of an x-ray is projected relative to a reference in the horizontal or occlusal plane.

vertical coordination, a system of community health nurses who serve as links between their level in the organization and those above and below their level.

vertical diplopia [L, *vertex* + Gk, *diploos,* double, *opsis,* vision], a form of double vision in which one image is displaced vertically above the other.

vertical-integrated health care, a health delivery system in which the complete spectrum of care, including financial services, is provided within a single organization, such as a health maintenance organization.

vertical nystagmus, a visual abnormality in which the eyes involuntarily move up and down.

vertical resorption, a pattern of bone loss in which the alveolar bone adjacent to the affected tooth is destroyed without simultaneous crestal loss.

vertical strabismus [L, *vertex* + Gk, *strabismos,* squint], a deviation of one eye in a vertical direction from a point of fixation. A common cause is overaction by the inferior oblique muscles, resulting in a quick vertical movement of the eyeball on adduction.

vertical transmission, the transfer of a disease, condition, or trait from one generation to the next, either genetically or congenitally, such as the spread of an infection through breast milk or through the placenta.

vertical vertigo, a sense of instability caused by looking up or down.

verticosubmental /vur′tikō′submen′təl/ [L, *vertex* + *sub,* below, *mentum,* chin], pertaining to a radiographic projection of the head in which the central ray passes from the vertex of the skull through its base.

vertigo /vur′tigō, vurtī′gō/, a sensation of instability, giddiness, loss of equilibrium, or rotation, caused by a disturbance in the semicircular canal of the inner ear or the vestibular nuclei of the brainstem. The sensation that one's body is rotating in space is called subjective vertigo, whereas the sensation that objects are spinning around the body is termed objective vertigo.

very low–density lipoprotein (VLDL), a plasma protein that is composed chiefly of triglycerides with small amounts of cholesterol, phospholipid, and protein. It transports triglycerides primarily from the liver to peripheral sites in the tissues for use or storage.

vesical /ves′ikəl/ [L, *vesica,* bladder], pertaining to a fluid-filled sac, usually the urinary bladder.

vesical fistula [L, *vesica,* bladder, *fistula,*

pipe], an abnormal passage communicating with the urinary bladder.

vesical hematuria [L, *vesica,* bladder; Gk, *haima,* blood + *ouron,* urine], blood in the urine caused by bleeding in the bladder. The urine is bright red.

vesical reflex, the sensation of a need to urinate when the bladder is moderately distended.

vesical sphincter, a circular muscle surrounding the opening of the urinary bladder.

vesicant /ves'ikənt/, a drug capable of causing tissue necrosis when extravasated.

vesicle /ves'ikəl/ [L, *vesicula*], a small bladder or blister, such as a small, thin-walled raised skin lesion containing clear fluid.—**vesicular,** *adj.*

vesicle calculus, a concretion occurring in the bladder.

vesicoabdominal /ves'iko·abdom'inəl/, pertaining to the urinary bladder and abdominal wall.

vesicoureteral reflux /ves'ikōyŏŏrē'tərəl/ [L, *vesica* + Gk, *oureter,* ureter; L, *refluxus,* backflow], an abnormal backflow of urine from the bladder to the ureter, resulting from a congenital defect, obstruction of the outlet of the bladder, or infection of the lower urinary tract. Reflux increases the hydrostatic pressure in the ureters and kidneys. The condition is characterized by abdominal or flank pain, enuresis, pyuria, hematuria, proteinuria, and bacteriuria accompanied by persistent or recurrent urinary tract infections.

vesicouterine /ves'ikōyŏŏ'tərin, -ēn/ [L, *vesica* + *uterus,* womb], pertaining to the bladder and uterus.

vesicovaginal /ves'ikōvaj'inəl/, pertaining to the urinary bladder and vagina.

vesicula /vəsik'yələ/ [L], a vesicle or small bladder.

vesicular /vesik'yələr/, pertaining to a blisterlike condition.

vesicular appendix, a cystic structure on the fimbriated end of each of the fallopian tubes. It represents a remnant of the mesonephric ducts.

vesicular breath sound, a normal sound of rustling or swishing heard with a stethoscope over the lung periphery, characteristically higher pitched during inspiration and fading rapidly during expiration.

vesiculitis /vəsik'yəlī'tis/, an inflammation of any vesicle, particularly the seminal vesicles.

vesiculography /vəsik'yəlog'rəfē/, the radiologic examination of the seminal vesicles and adjacent structures, usually conducted by injecting a radiopaque medium into the deferent ducts or by catheterization of the medium into the ejaculatory ducts.

vessel /ves'əl/ [L, *vascellum,* small vase], any one of the many tubules throughout the body conveying fluids such as blood and lymph. The main kinds of vessels are the arteries, veins, and lymphatic vessels.

vestibular /vestib'yələr/, [L, *vestibulum,* courtyard], pertaining to a vestibule, such as the vestibular part of the mouth, which lies between the cheeks and the teeth.

vestibular apparatus, the inner ear structures that are associated with balance and position sense. They include the vestibule and semicircular canals.

vestibular function, the sense of balance.

vestibular gland, any one of four small glands, two on each side of the vaginal orifice. The vestibular glands secrete a lubricating substance.

vestibular nerve [L, *vestibulum,* courtyard, *nervus*], a branch of the eighth cranial nerve associated with the sense of equilibrium. It arises in the vestibular ganglion (Scarpa's ganglion) of the ear.

vestibular neuronitis, a sudden, severe attack of vertigo without symptoms of deafness or tinnitus. It usually affects young or middle-aged adults, is temporary, and follows an upper respiratory infection.

vestibular toxicity, toxic effects (commonly of drugs) on the vestibule of the ear, resulting in dizziness, vertigo, and loss of balance.

vestibule /ves'tibyŏŏl/ [L, *vestibulum,* courtyard], a space or cavity that serves as the entrance to a passageway, such as the vestibule of the vagina or the vestibule of the ear.

vestibule of the ear, the central part of the inner ear, within the osseous labyrinth, involved with the sensation of position and movement.

vestibulocochlear nerve, either of a pair of cranial nerves composed of fibers from the cochlear nerve and the vestibular nerve in the inner ear, conveying impulses of both the sense of hearing and the sense of balance.

vestibuloocular reflex /vestib'yəlō·ok'-yələr/, a normal reflex in which eye position compensates for movement of the head. It is induced by excitation of the vestibular apparatus.

vestibuloplasty /vestib'yələplas'tē/ [L, *vestibulum,* courtyard; Gk, *plassein,* to shape], plastic surgery of the oral vestibule, particularly modification of the gingival tissues.

vestige /ves'tij/ [L, *vestigium,* trace], an imperfectly developed, relatively useless organ or other structure of the body that had a vital function at an earlier stage of life or in a more primitive form of life.— **vestigial,** *adj.*

veterinarian /vet′əriner′ē·ən/ [L, *veterinarius,* beasts of burden], a health professional who specializes in the causes and treatment of diseases and disorders of domestic and wild animals.

veterinary medicine /vet′əriner′ē/, the field of medicine concerned with the health and diseases of animals other than humans.

VF, 1. abbreviation for **ventricular fibrillation. 2.** abbreviation for **visual field. 3.** abbreviation for **vocal fremitus.**

VH, abbreviation for **viral hepatitis.**

VI, abbreviation for *variable interval.*

via /vī′ə, vē′ä/ [L, a way], any passage or course, such as the esophagus or trachea.

viable /vī′əbəl/ [Fr, likely to live], capable of developing, growing, and otherwise sustaining life, such as a normal human fetus at 24 weeks of gestation.— **viability,** *n.*

viable infant, an infant who at birth weighs at least 500 g or is 24 weeks or more of gestational age.

viability /vī′əbil′itē/ [L, *vita,* life], the ability to continue living.

vial /vī′əl/, a glass container with a metal-enclosed rubber seal.

vibration /vībrā′shən/ [L, *vibrare,* to vibrate], a type of massage administered by quickly tapping with the fingertips or alternating the fingers in a rhythmic manner or by a mechanical device.

vibratory /vī′brətôr′ē/ [L, *vibrare,* to vibrate], causing vibrations or a state of vibration.

vibratory massage, the manipulation of body surfaces with an instrument that produces a rapid tapping sensation.

vibratory sense [L, *vibrare,* to vibrate, *sentire,* to feel], the ability to perceive vibratory sensations. Vibration receptors in the body are found in a variety of locations, from the skin surface to the membranes covering bones. Some respond only to certain vibration frequencies.

vibrio /vib′rē·ō/ [L, *vibrare*], any bacterium that is curved and motile, such as those belonging to the genus *Vibrio.* Cholera and several other epidemic forms of gastroenteritis are caused by members of the genus.

Vibrio cholerae, the species of comma-shaped, motile bacillus that is the cause of cholera.

vibrio gastroenteritis, an infectious disease caused by *Vibrio parahaemolyticus* acquired from contaminated seafood. It is characterized by nausea, vomiting, ab-

dominal pain, and diarrhea. Headache, mild fever, and bloody stools also may be present.

Vibrio parahaemolyticus /per′əhē′mōlit′-ikəs/, a species of microorganisms of the genus *Vibrio,* the causative agent in food poisoning associated with the ingestion of raw or undercooked shellfish, especially crabs and shrimp. Thorough cooking of seafood prevents the infection associated with *Vibrio parahaemolyticus,* which causes watery diarrhea, abdominal cramps, vomiting, headache, chills, and fever.

vicarious menstruation /vīker′ē·əs/ [L, *vicarius,* substituted, *menstruare,* to menstruate], discharge of blood from a site other than the uterus at the time when the menstrual flow is normally expected. Such bleeding is usually caused by the increased capillary permeability that occurs during menstruation.

vidarabine /vider′əbēn/, an antiviral agent used systemically to treat herpes simplex encephalitis and locally to treat herpesvirus type 1 keratoconjunctivitis and keratitis.

video display terminal (VDT) [L, *videre,* to see, *displicare,* to scatter, *terminus,* end], a cathode-ray tube device with a surface similar to a television screen, used in word processors, computer terminals, and similar equipment. Use of video display terminals has been associated with a variety of environmental health complaints, including burning and itching eyes, headaches, and back and arm pain. Published studies indicate the health effects are caused by inadequate or improper office environments, such as unsuitable furniture or light levels, rather than VDT radiation.

vigilambulism /vij′ilam′byəliz′əm/, a condition in which walking or other motor acts are performed in an unconscious but waking state.

vigilance /vij′iləns/ [L, *vigil,* awake], a state of being attentive or alert.

vigil coma /vij′əl/ [L, *vigil* + Gk, *koma,* deep sleep], a semiconscious state of delirium in which the patient may appear awake, with eyes open and staring, and may make verbal sounds.

villoma /vilō′mə/ [L, *villus,* hair; Gk, *oma,* tumor], a villous neoplasm or papilloma, occurring in the bladder or rectum.

villous adenoma /vil′əs/ [L, *villus,* hair], a slow-growing, soft, spongy, potentially malignant papillary growth of the mucosa of the large intestine.

villous carcinoma, an epithelial tumor with many long velvety papillary outgrowths.

V

villous papilloma, a benign tumor with long, slender processes, usually occurring in the bladder, breast, or a cerebral ventricle.

villus /vil'əs/, *pl.* **villi** [L, shaggy, hair], one of the many tiny projections, barely visible to the naked eye, clustered over the entire mucous surface of the small intestine. The villi are covered with epithelium that diffuses and transports fluids and nutrients. Each villus has a core of delicate areolar and reticular connective tissue supporting the epithelium, various capillaries, and often a single lymphatic lacteal that fills with milky white chyle during the digestion of a fatty meal.—**villous,** *adj.*

vinblastine sulfate /vinblas'tēn, -tin/, an antineoplastic prescribed in the treatment of many neoplastic diseases such as choriocarcinoma, testicular carcinoma, Hodgkin's disease, and non-Hodgkin's lymphoma.

Vincent's stomatitis [Henri Vincent, French physician, 1862–1950; Gk, *stoma,* mouth, *itis,* inflammation], an infection of the mouth.

vincristine sulfate /vinkris'tēn, -tin/, an antineoplastic prescribed in the treatment of many neoplastic diseases such as leukemia, neuroblastoma, lymphomas, and sarcomas.

vindesine sulfate /vin'dəsēn/, an antineoplastic prescribed in the treatment of acute lymphoblastic leukemia, breast cancer, malignant melanoma, lymphosarcoma, and nonsmall-cell lung carcinoma.

Vineberg's operation /vī'burg/ [Arthur M. Vineberg, Canadian thoracic surgeon, b. 1903], a technique in which the internal mammary artery is implanted into the myocardium to improve blood flow to the heart. Common in the 1950s, the procedure has been replaced by others such as saphenous vein grafting.

vinorelbine tartrate, an anticancer mitotic inhibitor prescribed in the treatment of nonsmall cell lung cancer.

violence, risk for: directed at others, a NANDA-accepted nursing diagnosis of behaviors in which an individual demonstrates that he or she can be physically, emotionally, and/or sexually harmful to others. Risk factors include history of violence: (1) against others; (2) threats; (3) against self; (4) social; (5) indirect. Many other factors may be present, including neurologic impairment; cognitive impairment; history of childhood abuse; history of witnessing family violence; cruelty to animals; fire-setting; prenatal and perinatal complications/abnormalities; history of drug/alcohol abuse; and pathologic intoxication.

violence, risk for: self-directed, a NANDA-accepted nursing diagnosis of behaviors in which an individual demonstrates that he or she can be physically, emotionally, and/or sexually harmful to himself or herself. Risk factors may include age, marital status, employment, occupation, interpersonal relationships, family background, sexual orientation, physical health, mental health, emotional status, suicidal ideation, suicidal plan, lethality, personal resources, social resources, verbal clues, and persons who engage in autoerotic sexual acts.

viosterol /vī·os'tərōl/, synthetic vitamin D_2 in an oil base.

VIP, 1. abbreviation for **vasoactive intestinal polypeptide. 2.** abbreviation for *very important person.* A VIP suite in a hospital is one reserved for such people.

vipoma /vipō'mə/, a type of pancreatic tumor that causes changes in secretion of vasoactive intestinal polypeptide (VIP). VIP causes dilation of blood vessels throughout the body and secretion of fluid and salt in the intestinal tract, resulting in diarrhea.

viral dysentery /vī'rəl/ [L, *virus,* poison; Gk, *dys,* bad, *enteron,* intestine], a form of dysentery caused by a virus and usually characterized by an acute watery diarrhea.

viral gastroenteritis, an inflammation of the intestine caused by a virus. The symptoms usually include abdominal cramps, diarrhea, nausea, and vomiting.

viral hepatitis (VH) a viral inflammatory disease of the liver caused by one of the hepatitis viruses, A, B, C, or delta. All have chronic forms except hepatitis A. The disease is transmitted sexually and through blood transfusions and is common among people with behavior risks of human immunodeficiency virus infection. Speed of onset and probable course of the illness vary with the kind and strain of virus, but the characteristics of the disease and its treatment are the same.

viral infection, any of the diseases caused by one of approximately 200 viruses pathogenic to humans. Some are the most communicable and dangerous diseases known; some cause mild and transient conditions that pass virtually unnoticed. If cells are damaged by the viral attack, disease exists. After the virus enters the body, the first step in the cycle is its attachment to a susceptible cell and the cell's adsorption of the virus. This is followed by penetration of the viral nucleic acid into the parasitized cell. At this point the dissembled virus causes no symptoms and cannot be recovered from the cells in infectious form. The virus begins to mature within the cell and, carrying its own genetic information, begins to replicate itself, using chemical building blocks and energy available in the parasitized cell. The virus has now taken over the cell. After a variable period of time, masses of fully grown viruses appear, each able to survive outside the cell until more susceptible cells are found. In many viral diseases, including mumps, smallpox, and measles, one attack confers permanent immunity. In others immunity is short-lived. The incubation period for viral infection is usually short, the viruses do not circulate in the bloodstream, antibodies do not form, and most often immunity does not develop.

viral keratoconjunctivitis [L, *virus,* poison; Gk, *keras,* horn; L, *conjunctivus,* connecting; Gk, *itis,* inflammation], a combination of inflammation of the cornea and conjunctiva caused by a viral infection.

viral load test, a method for measuring the amount of human immunodeficiency virus in the blood. The U. S. Food and Drug Administration approved the test to guide decisions about starting treatment and to monitor patients periodically to make sure the infection has not progressed.

viral marker, a marker for human immunodeficiency virus infection progress as determined by the quantity of the virus in a blood sample. This marker is believed to be more useful than the CD4 lymphocyte count to measure disease progression.

viral pneumonia, pulmonary infection caused by a virus.

viral therapy, the use of genetically altered viruses to deliver genes to specific sites.

Virchow's node /fer′shōz/ [Rudolf L. K. Virchow, German pathologist, 1821–1902] a firm supraclavicular lymph node, particularly on the left side, that is so enlarged that it is palpable.

viremia /vīrē′mē·ə/ [L, *virus* + Gk, *haima,* blood], the presence of viruses in the blood.

virgin /vur′jən/, **1.** a person who has never had sexual intercourse. **2.** uncontaminated.

virginity /vurjin′itē/, the state of being a virgin.

virile /vir′əl/ [L, *virilis,* masculine], **1.** pertaining to or characteristic of an adult male; masculine; manly. **2.** possessing or exhibiting masculine strength, vigor, force, or energy. **3.** pertaining to the male sexual functions; capable of procreation.—**virility,** *n.*

virilism /vir′əliz′əm/ [L, *virilis* + *ismus,* practice], **1.** pseudohermaphroditism in

a female. **2.** premature development of masculine characteristics in the male.

virilization /vir′əlīzā′shən/ [L, *virilis* + *atus,* process], a process in which secondary male sexual characteristics are acquired by a female, usually as the result of adrenal dysfunction or hormonal medication.

virion /vir′ē·on, vī′rē·on/ [L, *virus,* poison], a rudimentary virus particle with a central nucleoid surrounded by a protein sheath or capsid. The complete nucleocapsid with a nucleic acid core may constitute a complete virus, such as the adenoviruses and the picornaviruses, or it may be surrounded by an envelope, as in the herpesviruses and the myxoviruses.

virocytes /vī′rəsīts/ [L, *virus* + Gk, *kytos,* cell], lymphocytes altered in appearance and staining that are seen in blood smears from patients with viral diseases.

viroid /vī′roid/, a small infective segment of nucleic acid, usually ribonucleic acid (RNA). It is not translated and is replicated by host cell enzymes. Viroids include segments that are complementary to introns and may bind to intron RNA.

virologist /vīrol′əjist, vir-/, a specialist who studies viruses and diseases caused by viruses.

virology /-l′əjē/ [L, *virus* + Gk, *logos,* science], the study of viruses and viral diseases.—**virologic, virological,** *adj.*

virtual reality /vur′choo·əl/, a system of computer-generated, three-dimensional, imaginary environments with which a person can subjectively interact. It is used in medical research to monitor brain activity in the hippocampus of subjects trying to solve maze problems.

virucidal /vī′rəsī′dəl/, pertaining to the destruction of viruses.

virucide /vī′rəsīd/ [L, *virus* + *caedere,* to kill], any agent that destroys or inactivates a virus.

virulence /vir′yələns/, [L, *virulentus,* poisonous], the power of a microorganism to produce disease.

virulent /vir′yələnt/, [L, *virulentus*], pertaining to a very pathogenic or rapidly progressive condition.

virus /vī′rəs/ [L, poison], a minute parasitic microorganism much smaller than a bacterium that, having no independent metabolic activity, may replicate only within a cell of a living plant or animal host. A virus consists of a core of nucleic acid (deoxyribonucleic acid or ribonucleic acid) surrounded by a coat of antigenic protein sometimes surrounded by an envelope of lipoprotein. The virus provides the genetic code for replication, and the host cell provides the necessary energy and raw materials. More than 200 viruses have been identified as capable of causing disease in humans. Some kinds of viruses are **adenovirus,** *Arenavirus,* **enterovirus, herpesvirus,** and **rhinovirus.—viral,** *adj.*

virus shedding, the movement by any route of a virus from an infected host.

virustatic /vī′rəstat′ik/, pertaining to the inhibition of the growth and development of viruses, as distinguished from their destruction.

vis /vis, vēs/ [L, force], energy or power.

viscera /vis′ərə/, *sing.* **viscus** /vis′kəs/ [L, *viscus,* internal organs], the internal organs enclosed within a body cavity, including the abdominal, thoracic, pelvic, and endocrine organs.

visceral /vis′ərəl/ [L, *viscus,* internal organs], pertaining to the viscera, or internal organs, in the abdominal cavity.

visceral afferent fibers, the nerve fibers of the visceral nervous system that receive stimuli, carry impulses toward the central nervous system, and share the sensory ganglia of the cerebrospinal nerves with the somatic sensory fibers. Some of the parts of the body with visceral afferent fibers are the face, scalp, nose, mouth, descending colon, lungs, abdomen, and rectum.

visceral cavity [L, *viscus,* internal organs, *cavum*], **1.** the abdominal cavity containing the viscera. **2.** the cavity of any viscus, such as the stomach.

visceral efferent system [L, *viscus,* internal organs, *effere,* to bear out; Gk, *systema*], the part of the autonomic nervous system that supplies efferent nerve fibers from the central nervous system to the visceral organs.

visceral larva migrans, infestation with parasitic larvae, *Toxocara,* or, occasionally, *Ascaris, Strongyloides,* or other nematodes.

visceral lymph node, a small oval nodular gland that filters lymph circulating in the lymphatic vessels of the thoracic, abdominal, and pelvic viscera.

visceral nervous system, the visceral part of the peripheral nervous system that comprises the whole complex of nerves, fibers, ganglia, and plexuses by which impulses travel from the central nervous system to the viscera and from the viscera to the central nervous system.

visceral pain, abdominal pain caused by any abnormal condition of the viscera. It is characteristically severe, diffuse, and difficult to localize.

visceral pericardium [L, *viscus* + Gk, *peri,* around, *kardia,* heart], the surface of the pericardial membrane that is in direct contact with the heart.

visceral peritoneum, one of two parts of the largest serous membrane in the body that invests the viscera. The free surface of the visceral peritoneum is a smooth layer of mesothelium exuding a serous fluid that lubricates the viscera and allows them to glide freely against the wall of the abdominal cavity or over each other.

visceral pleura, the inner layer of pleura that is adjacent to the external lung tissue.

visceral protein status, the amount of protein that is contained in the internal organs.

visceral skeleton [L, *viscus* + Gk, *skeletos,* dried up], the part of the skeleton, including sternum, ribs, pelvis, and vertebrae, that enclose the viscera.

visceral swallow, an immature swallowing pattern of an infant, resembling wavelike contractions of peristalsis.

visceromotor /vis′ərōmō′tər/, **1.** pertaining to nerve impulses that control visceral smooth muscle. **2.** pertaining to movement of the viscera.

viscerosomatic reaction /vis′ərō′sōmat′ik/ [L, *viscus* + Gk, *soma,* body; L, *re* + *agere,* to act], a muscular response to stimulation of a nerve-receptor organ in a visceral organ.

viscid /vis′id/ [L, *viscidus,* sticky], sticky or glutinous.

viscoelasticity /vis′kō-ē′lastis′itē/, the quality or condition of being both viscous and elastic.

viscosity /viskos′itē/ [L, *viscosus,* sticky], the ability or inability of a fluid solution to flow easily. A solution that has high viscosity is relatively thick and flows slowly because of the adhesive effect of adjacent molecules.

viscous /vis′kəs/ [L, *viscosus,* sticky], pertaining to something thick, viscid, sticky, or glutinous.

viscous fermentation [L, *viscosus*], the formation of viscous material in milk, urine, and wine by the action of various bacilli.

visibility /vis′əbil′itē/ [L, *visibilitas,* being seen], a condition of being visible under the circumstances of light, distance, and other factors.

visible /viz′ibəl/ [L, *visibilis,* visible], perceptible to the eye.

visible light [L, *visus,* sight; AS, *leoht*], the radiant energy in the electromagnetic spectrum that is visible to the human eye. The wavelengths cover a range of approximately 390 to 780 nm.

visible radiation [L, *visibilis,* vision, *radiare,* to shine], electromagnetic radiation in the wavelengths between infrared and ultraviolet that can be perceived by most normal humans.

visible spectrum [L, *visibilis,* vision, *spectrum,* image], the colors of the spectrum that can be observed by most people, from violet at about 4000 angstrom units (400 nm) through blue, green, yellow, and orange, to red, at about 6500 angstrom units (650 nm).

vision /vizh′ən/ [L, *visus,* vision], the capacity for sight.

visit /viz′it/ [L, *visitare,* to see often], **1.** a meeting between a practitioner and a client or patient. In the hospital and home the practitioner visits the patient; in the clinic or office the patient visits the practitioner. **2.** (of a patient) to meet a practitioner to obtain professional services or (of a practitioner) to see a patient or client to render a professional service.

Visitation Facilitation, a Nursing Interventions Classification defined as promoting beneficial visits by family and friends.

visiting nurse, a nurse who is responsible for a group of patients in a home setting, usually in a defined geographic area. The nurse makes visits to provide skilled nursing care as prescribed by a physician, particularly for persons unable to leave home for professional care, and to educate patients in matters of self-care.

visual /vizh′ōō·əl/ [L, *visus,* vision], pertaining to the sense of sight.

visual accommodation, a process by which the eye adjusts and is able to focus, producing a sharp image at various, changing distances from the object seen. The convexity of the anterior surface of the lens may be increased or decreased by contraction or relaxation of the ciliary muscle.

visual acuity [L, *visus,* vision, *acuitas,* sharpness], **1.** a measure of the resolving power of the eye, particularly with its ability to distinguish letters and numbers at a given distance. **2.** the sharpness or clearness of vision.

visual agnosia, an inability to recognize objects by sight, although vision is intact.

visual amnesia [L, *visus,* vision; Gk, *amnesia,* forgetfulness], an inability to recognize objects, including written words, previously seen.

visual angle [L, *visus,* vision, *angulus*], the angle between two lines passing from the extremities of an object looked at, through the nodal point of the eye.

visual aphasia [L, *visus,* vision; Gk, *a + phasis,* not speech], the inability to understand written language caused by a lesion in the left visual cortex and the connections between the right visual cortex and the left hemisphere.

visual center, the center of the brain concerned with vision.

visual center of the cornea, the point of intersection of the line of sight with the cornea.

visual evoked potential (VEP), an evoked potential elicited by a repeatedly flashing light or a pattern stimulus. It may be used to confirm optic nerve or visual pathway damage.

visual field (VF), the area of physical space visible to an eye in a given position. The average VF is 65 degrees upward, 75 degrees downward, 60 degrees inward, and 90 degrees outward.

visual field defect, one or more spots or defects in the vision that move with the eye, unlike a floater. This fixed defect is usually caused by damage to the retina or visual pathways, such as by chorioretinitis, traumatic injury, macular degeneration, glaucoma, or a vascular occlusion of the eye or the brain.

visual hallucinations [L, *visus,* vision, *alucinari*], a subjective visual experience in the absence of objective evidence of a corresponding stimulus. Such hallucinations are most likely to be associated with acute organic disorders such as toxic confusional psychoses, delirium, and focal brain diseases and may occur with any stage of schizophrenia.

visualization /vizh′ōō·əlīzā′shən/, an effective means of deepening relaxation and desensitizing a real-life situation that is generally met with stress and tension. The imagery combines positive experiences with actual or perceived negative events or situations in an effort to desensitize the person to the trauma.

visual memory, the ability to create an eidetic image of past visual experiences.

visual-motor coordination, the ability to coordinate vision with the movements or parts of the body.

visual-motor function, the ability to draw or copy forms or to perform constructive tasks.

visual pathway, a pathway over which a visual sensation is transmitted from the retina to the brain. A pathway consists of an optic nerve, the fibers of an optic nerve traveling through or along the sides of the optic chiasm to the lateral geniculate body of the thalamus, and an optic tract terminating in an occipital lobe. Each optic nerve contains fibers from only one retina. The optic chiasm contains fibers from the nasal parts of the retinas of both eyes; these fibers cross to the opposite side of the brain at the optic chiasm.

visual plane, the plane in which the two optic axes lie.

visual-spatial agnosia, an inability to analyze spatial relationships or to perform

V

simple constructional tasks under visual control.

visuospatial /vizh′o͞o·ōspā′shəl/, pertaining to the ability to comprehend visual representations and their spatial relationships.

vital /vī′təl/ [L, *vita,* life], pertaining or contributing to life forces.

vital capacity (VC) [L, *vita,* life, *capacitas,* capacity], a measurement of the amount of air that can be expelled at the normal rate of exhalation after a maximum inspiration, representing the greatest possible breathing capacity. The vital capacity equals the inspiratory reserve volume plus the tidal volume plus the expiratory reserve volume.

vitality test /vītal′itē/, a group of thermal, transillumination, and electrical tests used to evaluate the health of dental pulp.

vital signs, the measurements of pulse rate, respiration rate, and body temperature. Although not strictly a vital sign, blood pressure is also customarily included.

Vital Signs Monitoring, a Nursing Interventions Classification defined as collection and analysis of cardiovascular, respiratory, and body temperature data to determine and prevent complications.

vital stain [L, *vita,* life; OFr, *desteindre,* to dye], any dye used to impart color to tissues or cells of living organisms.

vital statistics, data relating to births or natality, deaths or mortality, marriages, health, and disease or morbidity.

vital ultraviolet, the ultraviolet wavelengths between 320.0 and 290.0 nm, which are believed to be necessary or helpful for normal growth and health.

vitamin /vī′təmin/ [L, *vita* + *amine,* ammonia], an organic compound essential in small quantities for normal physiologic and metabolic functioning of the body. With few exceptions, vitamins cannot be synthesized by the body and must be obtained from the diet or dietary supplements. No one food contains all the vitamins. Vitamin deficiency diseases produce specific symptoms usually alleviated by the administration of the appropriate vitamin. Vitamins are classified according to their fat or water solubility, their physiologic effects, or their chemical structures; they are designated by alphabetic letters and chemical or other specific names. The fat-soluble vitamins are A, D, E, and K; the B complex and C vitamins are water soluble.

vitamin A, a fat-soluble, solid terpene alcohol essential for skeletal growth, maintenance of normal mucosal epithelium, and visual acuity. It is derived from various carotenoids, mainly beta-carotene, and is present in leafy green vegetables, yellow fruits and vegetables, fish liver oils, liver, milk, cheese, butter, and egg yolk. Deficiency leads to atrophy of epithelial tissue resulting in keratomalacia, xerophthalmia, night blindness, and lessened resistance to infection of mucous membranes.

vitamin A₁, one of the two forms of vitamin A that occur in nature. It is a fat-soluble unsaturated alcohol formed by hydrolysis of beta-carotene, one molecule of which yields two molecules of vitamin A₁. Natural sources include fish-liver oils, butterfat, and egg yolk. The vitamin is needed for healthy vision and skin epithelium.

vitamin A₂, an alternative form of vitamin A found in the tissues of freshwater fish but not in mammals or saltwater fish. Differences in ultraviolet light absorption spectra are used to distinguish the vitamin A forms.

vitamin B₁. See thiamin.

vitamin B₂. See riboflavin.

vitamin B₆. See pyridoxine.

vitamin B₁₂. See cyanocobalamin.

vitamin B₁₇. See laetrile.

vitamin B complex, a group of water-soluble vitamins differing from each other structurally and in their biologic effect. All of the B vitamins are found in large quantities in liver and yeast, and they are present separately or in combination in many foods.

vitamin C. See ascorbic acid.

vitamin D, a fat-soluble vitamin chemically related to the steroids and essential for the normal formation of bones and teeth and for the absorption of calcium and phosphorus from the gastrointestinal tract. The vitamin is present in natural foods in small amounts, and requirements are usually met by artificial enrichment of various foods, especially milk and dairy products, and exposure to sunlight. Ultraviolet rays activate a form of cholesterol in an oil of the skin and convert it to a form of the vitamin, which is then absorbed. The natural foods containing vitamin D are of animal origin and include saltwater fish, especially salmon, sardines, and herring; organ meats; fish-liver oils; and egg yolk. Deficiency of the vitamin results in rickets in children, osteomalacia, osteoporosis, and osteodystrophy.

vitamin D₂. See calciferol.

vitamin D₃, an antirachitic white odorless crystalline unsaturated alcohol that is the predominant form of vitamin D of animal origin. It is found in most fish-liver oils, butter, brain, and egg yolk and is formed in the skin, fur, and feathers of animals and birds exposed to sunlight or ultraviolet rays.

vitamin deficiency, a state or condition resulting from the lack of or inability to use one or more vitamins. The symptoms and manifestations of each deficiency vary, depending on the specific function of the vitamin in promoting growth and development and maintaining body health.

vitamin D-resistant rickets, a disease clinically similar to rickets but resistant to treatment with large doses of vitamin D. It is caused by a congenital defect in renal tubular resorption of phosphate and usually occurs in men.

vitamin E, any or all of the group of fat-soluble vitamins that consist of the tocopherols and are essential for normal reproduction, muscle development, resistance of erythrocytes to hemolysis, and various other biochemical functions. It is an intracellular antioxidant and acts in maintaining the stability of polyunsaturated fatty acids and other fatlike substances, including vitamin A and hormones of the pituitary, adrenal, and sex glands. Deficiency results in muscle degeneration, vascular system abnormalities, megaloblastic anemia, hemolytic anemia, infertility, creatinuria, and liver and kidney damage and is associated with the aging process.

vitamin H. See **biotin.**

vitamin K, a group of fat-soluble vitamins known as quinones that are essential for the synthesis of prothrombin in the liver and of several related proteins involved in the clotting of blood. It is also involved with the process of phosphorylation and electron transport. The vitamin is widely distributed in foods and is synthesized by the bacterial flora of the gastrointestinal tract. Deficiency results in hypoprothrombinemia, characterized by poor coagulation of the blood and hemorrhage, and usually occurs from inadequate absorption of the vitamin from the gastrointestinal tract or the inability to use it in the liver.

vitamin K₁, a yellow, viscous, oil-soluble vitamin, occurring naturally, especially in alfalfa, and produced synthetically. It is used as a prothrombinogenic agent.

vitamin K₂, a pale yellow fat-soluble crystalline vitamin of the vitamin K group that is more unsaturated than vitamin K₁ and slightly less active biologically. It is isolated from putrefied fish meal and synthesized by various bacteria in the gastrointestinal tract.

vitamin K₃. See **menadione.**

vitamin loss [L, *vita,* life, *amine*], reduction in vitamin content of food resulting

from the handling and preparation of fresh foods during harvesting, heating, pickling, salting, milling, canning, and other food-processing techniques. Further vitamin losses can occur because of digestive disorders that prevent nutrient absorption and the use of drugs such as isoniazid that are vitamin antagonists.

vitaminology /vī′təminol′əjē/ [L, *vita* + *amine* + Gk, *logos,* science], the study of vitamins, including their structures, modes of action, and function in maintaining body health.

vitamin P. See **bioflavonoid.**

vitamin supplements, any vitamins or provitamins consumed in addition to nutrients in the food eaten.

vitellin /vitel′in/ [L, *vitellus,* yolk], a phosphoprotein containing lecithin, found in the yolk of eggs.—**vitelline** /-ēn/, *adj.*

vitelline artery /vitel′in, -ēn/ [L, *vitellus* + Gk, *arteria,* airpipe], any of the embryonic arteries that circulate blood from the primitive aorta of the early developing embryo to the yolk sac.

vitelline circulation, the circulation of blood and nutrients between the developing embryo and the yolk sac by way of the vitelline arteries and veins.

vitelline duct, (in embryology) the narrow channel connecting the yolk sac with the intestine.

vitelline membrane, the delicate cytoplasmic membrane surrounding the ovum.

vitelline vein, any of the embryonic veins that return blood from the yolk sac to the primitive heart of the early developing embryo.

vitellogenesis /vitel′ōjen′əsis/ [L, *vitellus* + Gk, *genein,* to produce], the formation or production of yolk.—**vitellogenetic,** *adj.*

vitellus /vitel′əs, vī-/ [L, yolk], the yolk of an ovum.

vitiligo /vit′ilē′gō/, /-ī′gō/ [L, *vitium,* blemish], a benign acquired skin disease of unknown cause, consisting of irregular patches of various sizes totally lacking in pigment and often having hyperpigmented borders. Exposed areas of skin are most often affected.—**vitiliginous,** *adj.*

vitrectomy /vitrek′təmē/ [L, *vitreus,* glassy; Gk, *ektome,* excision], a surgical procedure for replacing the contents of the vitreous chamber of the eye.

vitreous /vit′rē-əs/ [L, *vitreus,* glassy], pertaining to the vitreous humor of the eye located in the posterior chamber of the eye.

vitreous cavity [L, *vitreus,* glassy, *cavum,* cavity], the cavity in the eye posterior to the lens that contains the vitreous body and vitreous membrane and is transected

V

by the vestigial remnants of the hyaloid canal.

vitreous degeneration [L, *vitreus,* glassy, *degenerare,* to deviate from kind], a form of hyaline degeneration; the formation of glassy material in the connective tissue of blood vessels and other tissues.

vitreous hemorrhage, a hemorrhage into the vitreous humor of the eye.

vitreous humor, a transparent, semigelatinous substance contained in a thin hyoid membrane filling the cavity behind the crystalline lens of the eye.

vitreous membrane, a membrane that lines the posterior cavity of the eye and surrounds the vitreous body.

vitrification /vit'rifikā'shən/ , the conversion of a silicate material by heat and fusion to a glassy substance. Heat converts the material into a viscous liquid, which hardens on cooling.

viviparous /vivip'ərəs/ [L, *vivus,* alive, *parere,* to bear], bearing living offspring rather than laying eggs, such as most mammals and some fish and reptiles.

vivisection /viv'əsek'shən [L, *vivus,* alive, *secare,* to cut], the performance of surgical operations on living animals, particularly experimental surgery for the purpose of research.

VLDL, abbreviation for **very low–density lipoprotein.**

VMA, abbreviation for **vanillylmandelic acid.**

VNA, abbreviation for *Visiting Nurses Association.*

VO$_2$, symbol for *oxygen uptake.*

vocal apparatus /vō'kəl/ [L, *vocalis,* voice, *ad + parare,* to prepare], the larynx, pharynx, and oral and nasal cavities involved in the production of sound.

vocal cord [L, *vocalis,* voice; Gk, *chorde,* string], one of a pair of strong bands of yellow elastic tissue in the larynx enclosed by membranes called vocal folds and attached ventrally to the angle of the thyroid cartilage and dorsally to the vocal process of the arytenoid cartilage.

vocal cord nodule, a small inflammatory or fibrous growth that develops on the vocal cords of people who constantly strain their voices.

vocal cues, a category of nonverbal communication that includes all the noises and sounds that are extra-speech sounds.

vocal folds [L, *vocalis* + AS, *fealdan*], the true vocal cords.

vocal fremitus (VF), the vibration of the chest wall as a person speaks or sings that allows the person's voice to be heard by the examiner during auscultation of the chest with a stethoscope. Vocal fremitus is decreased in emphysema, pleural effusion,

pulmonary edema, or bronchial obstruction.

vocal paralysis, paralysis of the vocal cords.

vocal resonance [L, *vocalis* + *resonare,* to sound again], **1.** auscultation. **2.** modification of the laryngeal tone as it passes through the pharynx and oral cavity to produce an increase in the intensity and quality of the sound.

voice, the acoustic component of speech that is normally produced by vibration of the vocal folds of the larynx.

voiceprint /vois'print/, a graphic representation of a person's speech pattern electronically recorded. Like a fingerprint, the speech pattern for any individual is distinctive.

void /void/ [ME, *voide,* empty], to empty, or evacuate, such as urine from the bladder.

voiding urethrography [ME, *voide,* empty; Gk, *ourethra* + *graphein,* to record], radiography of the urethra during micturition after the introduction of a radiopaque fluid into the bladder.

vol., abbreviation for **volume.**

vol.%, abbreviation for *volume percent.*

volar /vō'lər/ [L, *vola,* palm, sole], pertaining to the palm of the hand or the sole of the foot.

volatile /vōl'ətəl/ [L, *volatilis,* flying], (of a liquid) easily vaporized.

volatile solvent, an easily vaporized solvent.

Volhard's test /vol'ärdz, fōl'härts/ [Franz Volhard, German physician, 1872–1950], a renal function test in which the patient drinks 1500 ml of water after liquids have been withheld for a period of time. After 4 hours the specific gravity of the urine is measured. If kidneys are normal, specific gravity of the urine will be 1.001 to 1.004.

volition /vōlish'ən/ [L, *voluntas,* inclination], **1.** the act, power, or state of willing or choosing. **2.** the conscious impulse to perform or abstain from an act.—**volitional,** *adj.*

volitional /vōlish'ənəl/ [L, *velle,* to wish], pertaining to the use of one's own will in performing or abstaining from an action.

volitional tremor [L, *velle,* to wish, *tremor,* shaking], a trembling that begins during voluntary effort, sometimes spreading throughout the body. It may occur in multiple sclerosis and cerebellar disorders.

Volkmann's canal /fōlk'munz/ [Alfred W. Volkmann, German physiologist, 1800–1877], any one of the small blood vessel canals connecting haversian canals in bone tissue.

Volkmann's contracture [Richard von Volkmann, German surgeon, 1830–1889], a serious persistent flexion contraction of forearm and hand caused by ischemia. A pressure or crushing injury in the region of the elbow usually precedes this condition, and pressure from a cast or tight bandage about the elbow is a common cause.

Volkmann's splint [Richard von Volkmann; AS, *splinte,* thin board], a splint that supports and immobilizes the lower leg. It has a footpiece attached to two sides that extends from the foot to the knee, allowing ambulation.

volsella forceps /volsel'ə/ [L, *vosella,* tweezers, *forceps,* tongs], a kind of forceps having a small, sharp-pointed hook at the end of each blade.

volt (V) /vōlt/ [Alessandro Volta, Italian physicist, 1745–1827], the unit of electrical potential. In an electric circuit a volt is the force required to send 1 ampere of current through 1 ohm of resistance, or the difference in potential between two points on a conductor carrying a charge of 1 ampere when there is a dissipation of 1 watt between them.

voltage /vō'tij/ [Alessandro Volta], an expression of electromotive force in terms of volts.

voltammetry /voltam'ətərē/, the measurement of an electric current as a function of potential.

voltmeter /vōlt'mētər/, an instrument such as a galvanometer that measures in volts the differences in potential between different points of an electric circuit.

volume (vol.) /vol'yəm,-yo͞om/ [L, *volumen,* paper roll], the amount of space occupied by a body, expressed in cubic units.

volume ATPS, abbreviation for ambient temperature, ambient pressure, saturated with water vapor conditions of a volume of gas. The conditions exist in a water-sealed spirograph or gasometer when the water temperature equals ambient temperature.

volume BTPS, abbreviation for body temperature, ambient pressure, saturated with water vapor conditions of a volume of gas. For humans normal respiratory tract temperature is measured at 37° C, the pressure as ambient pressure, and the partial pressure of water vapor at 37° C as 47 mm Hg.

volume control fluid chamber, any one of several types of transparent plastic reservoirs with graduated volumetric markings, used to regulate the flow of intravenous solutions.

volume imaging, magnetic resonance (MR) imaging techniques in which MR signals are gathered from the whole object volume to be imaged at once. Many sequential plane imaging techniques can be generalized to volume imaging, at least in principle.

volumetric flow rate /vol'yəmet'rik/, the rate at which a volume of fluid flows past a designated point, usually measured in liters per second.

volumetric glassware, (in chemistry) glassware designed and marked to contain or deliver specific volumes of liquid solutions.

volume unit (VU), a unit of a logarithmic scale for expressing the power level of a complex audio-frequency electrical signal such as that transmitting sound.

volume ventilator, a ventilator that delivers a predetermined volume of gas with each cycle.

voluntary /vol'ənter'ē/ [L, *voluntas,* inclination], referring to an action or thought originated, undertaken, controlled, or accomplished as a result of a person's free will or choice.

voluntary agency, a service agency legally controlled by volunteers rather than by owners or a paid staff.

voluntary hospital system, a nationwide complex of autonomous, self-established, and self-supported private not-for-profit and investor-owned hospitals in the United States.

volunteer /vol'əntir'/ [Fr, *volontaire*], a person who serves without pay, augmenting but not replacing paid personnel and professional staff members.

volvulus /vol'vyələs/ [L, *volvere,* to turn], a twisting of the bowel on itself, causing intestinal obstruction. The condition is frequently the result of a prolapsed segment of mesentery and occurs most often in the ileum, the cecum, or the sigmoid parts of the bowel. If it is not corrected, the obstructed bowel becomes necrotic, and peritonitis and rupture of the bowel occur.

volvulus neonatorum, an intestinal obstruction in a newborn resulting from a twisting of the bowel caused by malrotation or nonfixation of the colon. Typical symptoms include abdominal distension; persistent regurgitation, often accompanied by fecal vomiting; and nonpassage of stools.

vomer /vō'mər/ [L, plowshare], the bone forming the posterior and inferior part of the nasal septum and having two surfaces and four borders.

vomeronasal organ, a structure on each side of the nasal septum believed to be a chemical sensory center for "sixth sense" detection of pheromones.

vomit /vom'it/ [L, *vomere,* to vomit], **1.** to expel the contents of the stomach through the esophagus and out of the mouth. **2.** the material expelled.

vomiting [L, *vomere,* to vomit], the forcible voluntary or involuntary emptying of the stomach contents through the mouth.

vomiting of pregnancy, vomiting that occurs during the early months of pregnancy. Factors contributing to the condition include delayed stomach emptying during pregnancy, relaxation of the esophageal sphincter at the opening into the stomach, and relaxation of the diaphragmatic hiatus, which increase the risk of gastric reflux.

vomitus /vom'itəs/ [L, *vomere,* to vomit], the material expelled from the stomach during vomiting. Vomitus is sometimes classified by color or other appearances as an indicator of the cause of illness, such as a 'coffee-ground' vomitus being a clinical sign of peptic ulcers.

VON, abbreviation for *Victorian Order of Nurses.*

von Gierke's disease /fôngir'kəz/ [Edgar von Gierke, German pathologist, 1877–1945], a form of glycogen storage disease in which abnormally large amounts of glycogen are deposited in the liver and kidneys. The disorder is characterized by hypoglycemia, ketoacidosis, and hyperlipemia.

von Hippel-Lindau disease [Eugen von Hippel, German ophthalmologist, 1867–1939; Arvid Lindau, Swedish pathologist, 1892–1958], a hereditary disease characterized by congenital, tumorlike vascular nodules in the retina and hemangioblastomas of the cerebellar hemispheres. Similar spinal cord lesions; cysts of the pancreas, kidneys, and other viscera; seizures; and mental retardation may be present.

von Willebrand's disease [Erick A. von Willebrand, Finnish physician, 1870–1949], an inherited disorder characterized by abnormally slow coagulation of the blood and spontaneous epistaxis and gingival bleeding caused by a deficiency of a component of factor VIII.

voracious [L, *vorax*], greedy or gluttonous, with an insatiable appetite.

vortex, *pl.* **vortexes, vortices** [L, whirl], a whirlpool effect produced by the whirling of a more or less cylindric mass of fluid (liquid or gas).

vox /voks'/ [L], voice, such as **vox choleraica,** the barely audible, hoarse voice of a patient in an advanced and severe case of cholera.

voxel /vok'səl/, abbreviation for *vo*lume *el*ement, the three-dimensional version of a pi*x*el.

voyeur /voiyur'', vô·äyœr'/ [Fr, *voir,* to see], one whose sexual desire is gratified by the practice of voyeurism.

voyeurism /voi'yəriz'əm, voiyur'izəm/ [Fr, *voyeur* + L, *ismus,* practice], a psychosexual disorder in which a person derives sexual excitement and gratification from looking at the naked bodies and genital organs or observing the sexual acts of others, especially from a secret vantage point.

VP-L-asparaginase, an anticancer drug combination of vincristine, prednisone, and asparaginase.

V/Q, abbreviation for *ventilation/perfusion.*

VR, abbreviation for *variable ratio.*

V.S., 1. abbreviation for **vesicular sound. 2.** abbreviation for *Veterinary Surgeon.* **3.** abbreviation for **vital signs. 4.** abbreviation for *volumetric solution.*

VSD, abbreviation for **ventricular septal defect.**

V_t, abbreviation for *tidal volume,* the amount of air in milliliters per breath.

VU, abbreviation for **volume unit.**

vulgaris /vulger'is/ [L, *vulgus,* common people], common or ordinary.

vulnerable /vul'nərəbəl/ [L, *vulnus,* wound], being in a dangerous position or condition and thereby susceptible to being infected or injured.

vulnerable period, a short period in the cardiac cycle during which activation may result in ectopy. The ventricular vulnerable period corresponds to the apex of the T wave toward its ascending side.

vulvar /vul'vər/, pertaining to the vulva.

vulvar dystrophy, a disorder characterized by skin eruptions of white atrophic pustules, squamous cell hyperplasia, and lichen sclerosis et atrophicus.

vulvectomy /vulvek'təmē/ [L, *vulva,* wrapper; Gk, *ektome,* excision], the surgical removal of part or all of the tissues of the vulva, performed most frequently in the treatment of malignant or premalignant neoplastic disease. Simple vulvectomy includes the removal of the skin of the labia minora, labia majora, and clitoris. Radical vulvectomy involves excision of the labia majora, labia minora, clitoris, surrounding tissues, and pelvic lymph nodes.

vulvitis /vulvi'tis/ [L, *vulva,* wrapper; Gk, *itis,* inflammation], an inflammation of the vulva.

vulvocrural /vul'vōkrōō'rəl/ [L, *vulva* + *crus,* leg], pertaining to the vulva and the thigh.

vulvodynia /vul'vōdin'ē·ə/, chronic pain and discomfort in the female external genitals.

vulvovaginal /vul'vōvaj'inəl/ [L, *vulva* + *vagina,* sheath], pertaining to the vulva and vagina.

vulvovaginitis /vul'vōvaj'inī'tis/, an inflammation of the vulva and vagina, or of the vulvovaginal glands.

vv, **1.** an abbreviation for *veins.* **2.** an abbreviation for *vice versa.*

v/v, **1.** symbol for *volume of dissolved substance per volume of solvent.* **2.** symbol for *volume per volume.*

v/w, symbol for *volume of substance per unit of weight of another component.*

V-Y plasty /vē′wī′plas′tē/, a surgical incision made in a V shape and sutured in a Y shape to lengthen the tissue area. In a variation of the procedure, the incision is made in a Y shape and sutured in a V shape to shorten the tissue area.

VZIG, abbreviation for **varicella-zoster immune globulin.**

VZV, abbreviation for **varicella zoster virus.**

V

w, the amount of energy required to ionize a molecule of air, as expressed by w = 33.85 eV/ion pair. This is an important quantity for radiation dosimetry because it allows the extraction of dose from ionization measurements.

W, symbol for the element **tungsten.**

waddling gait /wod'ling/ [ME, *wade,* to wade; ONorse, *gata,* way], a gait observed in patients with progressive muscular dystrophy characterized by exaggerated lateral trunk movements and hip elevations.

Wagstaffe's fracture /wag'stafs/ [William Wagstaffe, English surgeon, 1834–1910; L, *fractura,* break], a fracture characterized by separation of the internal malleolus.

waiting list, a roll of persons waiting to fill a vacancy, such as a list of candidates waiting for an organ transplant.

wakefulness /wāk'fulnəs/, **1.** an alert state of mind. **2.** sleeplessness or insomnia.

waking imagined analgesia (WIA) [AS, *wacian,* to awaken; L, *imaginari,* to picture oneself; Gk, *a + algos,* without pain], the pain relief experienced by a patient who uses the psychologic technique, usually with the help of an attending nurse or a hospital aide, of concentrating on previous pleasant personal experiences that produced tranquillity. This technique is often effective in reducing mild to moderate pain.

Wald /wôld/, **Lillian** (1867–1940), an American public health nurse who was instrumental in establishing the school nursing system, the federal government's Children's Bureau, and the Nursing Service Division of the Metropolitan Life Insurance Company. She was the first nurse to be elected into the Hall of Fame for Great Americans.

Waldeyer's throat ring /wäl'dī·ərz/ [Heinrich W. G. von Waldeyer, German anatomist, 1836–1921; AS, *hring*], the palatine, pharyngeal, and lingual tonsils that encircle the pharynx.

walker /wô'kər/ [AS, *wealcan,* to roam], an extremely light, movable apparatus, about waist high, made of metal tubing, used to aid a patient in walking. It has four widely placed sturdy legs. The patient holds onto the walker and takes a step, then moves the walker forward and takes another step.

walking belt, a leather or nylon device with handles that fastens around the patient's waist and assists the health care provider with the patient's ambulation.

walking cast [AS, *wealcan,* to roam;, ONorse, *kasta*], a cast that permits a patient to walk. A short-leg walking cast has an attached rubber walker to accept a cast shoe for foot or ankle injuries. A long-leg walking cast covers the leg from the upper thigh to the toes, with an attached rubber sole device called a walker.

walking heel, a plastic or rubber heel placed in the sole of a leg cast to allow weight-bearing.

walking program, an aerobic exercise regimen of walking 30 to 45 minutes a day 5 or 6 days a week. It may be part of a program to condition the heart or lower blood pressure.

walking reflex, a series of steplike motions of an infant's legs when the infant is held under the arms and with the feet in contact with a surface. The reflex disappears at approximately 4 to 8 weeks of age.

walking rounds [AS, *wealcan* + Fr, *rond*], rounds in which the clinician responsible leads a group of junior clinicians on a tour to visit the patients for whom they are collectively responsible.

walking typhoid [AS, *wealcan,* to roam; Gk, *typhos,* fever, *eidos,* form], an ambulatory subclinical case of typhoid fever. The person may be infected with typhoid but have mild symptoms that do not interfere with the activities of daily living.

walking wounded [AS, *wealcan,* to roam, *wund*], a triage term for an injured person who is ambulatory and has minor injuries.

wall [L, *vallum,* palisade], a limiting structure within the body, such as the wall of the abdominal, thoracic, or pelvic cavities or the wall of a cell.

wallerian degeneration /waler'ē·ən/ [Augustus V. Waller, English physician, 1816–

1870; L, *degenerare*, to degenerate], the fatty degeneration of a nerve fiber after it has been severed from its cell body.

wall stress, the tension within the wall of the left ventricle. It is determined by the pressure in the ventricle, the internal radius of the ventricle, and the thickness of the wall.

wander /won'dər/ [AS, *wandrian*], **1.** to move about purposelessly. **2.** to cause to move back and forth in an exploratory manner.

wandering abscess [AS, *wandrian* + L, *abscedere*, to go away], an abscess that moves through tissue openings to a point some distance from its origin.

wandering atrial pacemaker [AS, *wandrian* + L, *passus* + ME, *maken*], a sinus arrhythmia with an atrial or junctional escape rhythm during the slow phase of the sinus rhythm. Frequently there are atrial fusion beats when the two pacing sources collide within the atrial chamber. An accelerated junctional rhythm that competes with the sinus rhythm is often mislabled 'wandering pacemaker.'

Wangensteen apparatus /wang'ənstēn/ [Owen H. Wangensteen, American surgeon, 1898–1981; L, *ad* + *parare*, to prepare], a nasogastroduodenal catheter and suction apparatus used for constant gentle drainage and decompression of the stomach or duodenum.

Wangensteen tube [Owen H. Wangensteen], the catheter part of a Wangensteen apparatus.

ward /wôrd/ [AS, *weard*, guard], a hospital room designed and equipped to house more than four patients.

warfarin poisoning /wôr'fərin/ [Wisconsin Alumni Research Foundation + coumarin], a toxic condition caused by the ingestion of warfarin accidentally in the form of a rodenticide or by overdose with the substance in its pharmacologic anticoagulant form. The poison accumulates in the body and results in nosebleed, bruising, hematuria, melena, and internal hemorrhage.

warfarin sodium, an oral anticoagulant prescribed for the prophylaxis and treatment of thrombosis and embolism.

warm-blooded [AS, *wearm* + *blod*], having a relatively high and constant body temperature, such as the temperatures maintained by humans, other mammals, and birds, despite changes in environmental temperatures. Heat is produced in the warm-blooded human body by the catabolism of foods in proportion to the amount of work performed by the tissues in the body. Heat is lost from the body by evaporation, radiation, conduction, and convec-

tion. The average temperature of the healthy human is 98.6° F (37° C). The human body's tolerance for change in its temperature is very small, and significant changes can have drastic, even fatal, consequences.

warmup, light calisthenics and stretching exercises intended to increase flexibility, minimize risk of musculoskeletal complications, and gradually increase heart rate before the start of strenuous athletic activity.

washout /wosh'out/ [AS, *wascan*, to wash; ME, *oute*], the elimination or expulsion of one gas or volatile anesthetic agent by the administration of another.

wasp /wosp/ [L, *vespa*], a slender, narrow-waisted hymenopteran insect with two pairs of membranous wings that are folded lengthwise when at rest like parts of a fan. Many species of wasps can give painful stings that produce severe effects in hypersensitive individuals.

Wassermann blood test. /was'ərmən, vos'ərmun/ [August P. von Wassermann, German bacteriologist, 1866–1925], the first standard diagnostic blood test (no longer used) for syphilis based on the complement fixation reaction.

wasted ventilation, the volume of air that ventilates the physiologic dead space in the respiratory system.

waste products [L, *vastare*, to destroy, *producere*, to produce], the products of metabolic activity after oxygen and nutrients have been supplied to a cell. These include mainly carbon dioxide and water, along with sodium chloride and soluble nitrogenous salts, which are excreted in feces, urine, and exhaled air.

wasting [L, *vastare*, to destroy], a process of deterioration marked by weight loss and decreased physical vigor, appetite, and mental activity.

wasting syndrome, a condition characterized by weight loss associated with chronic fever and diarrhea. Over a period of 1 month, the patient may lose 10% of baseline body weight. In cases of human immunodeficiency virus infection, the malnutrition of wasting exacerbates the condition.

watchfulness /woch'fəlnes/, continuous supervision provided either openly or unobtrusively as the situation indicates.

water (H_2O) /wô'tər/ [AS, *waeter*], a chemical compound, one molecule of which contains one atom of oxygen and two atoms of hydrogen. Almost three quarters of the earth's surface is covered by water. Essential to life as it exists on this planet, water makes up more than 70% of living things. Pure water freezes at

32° F (0° C) and boils at 212° F (100° C) at sea level.

waterbed, a closed rubber bag filled with water and used as a mattress to prevent or treat pressure sores by equalizing the patient's weight against the support. For infants waterbeds provide a soft, intermittently oscillating surface that helps increase vestibular and proprioceptive stimulation and decrease apnea.

waterborne, carried by water, such as a waterborne epidemic of typhoid fever.

water-hammer pulse [AS, *waeter* + Gk, *akme*, point; L, *pulsare*, to beat], a large-amplitude pulse associated with aortic regurgitation. It is characterized by a full, forcible impulse and immediate collapse, causing a jerking sensation.

Waterhouse-Friderichsen's syndrome /wô′tərhous′ frid′ərik′sən/ [Rupert Waterhouse, English physician, 1873–1958; Carl Friderichsen, Danish physician, b. 1886], overwhelming cerebrospinal meningitis, characterized by the sudden onset of fever, cyanosis, petechiae, and collapse from massive bilateral adrenal hemorrhage. It requires immediate emergency treatment, hospitalization, and intensive care.

water intoxication, an increase in the volume of free water in the body, resulting in dilutional hyponatremia. Clinical manifestations are abdominal cramps, nausea, vomiting, lethargy, and dizziness.

water pollution, the contamination of lakes, rivers, and streams by industrial or community sources of pollutants.

water purification, emergency, methods of purifying unclean water for drinking purposes in emergencies. The three basic techniques include boiling the water and straining it through a cloth, adding 3 drops of tincture (alcoholic solution) of iodine per each quart of the water, and adding 10 drops of 1% chlorine bleach per each quart of water. When purifying chemicals are added, they should be thoroughly mixed with the water, and the mixture allowed to stand for 30 minutes.

watershed infarct /wô′tərshed/, an insufficiency of blood in an area of the brain where the distributions of cerebral arteries overlap. The condition resembles that of an agricultural field irrigation system in which the most distant sections may not be irrigated if there is a fall in water pressure.

water-soluble contrast medium, an iodinated contrast medium that is absorbed by the blood and excreted by the kidneys. Among the advantages of a water-soluble contrast medium are that it does not need

to be removed after a procedure and it may reduce the length of the procedure.

Watson-Crick helix /wôt′sənkrik′/ [John Dewey Watson, American geneticist, b. 1928; Francis H. Crick, British biochemist, b. 1916; Gk, *helix*, coil], a model of the deoxyribonucleic acid (DNA) molecule proposed by Watson and Crick as two right-handed polynucleotide chains coiled around the same axis as a double helix. The purine and pyrimidine bases of each strand are on the inside of the double helix and paired according to a Watson-Crick base-pairing rule. Variations in the sequences of the bases determine the genetic information transmitted by the DNA molecule. Watson and Crick received the Nobel Prize in 1962.

Watson, Jean, a nursing theorist who proposed a philosophy and science of caring in 1979 in an effort to reduce the dichotomy between theory and practice. Her Theory of Human Caring reflects an existential phenomenologist's view of psychology and humanities. Caring is a universal social phenomenon that is only effectively practiced interpersonally. Thus nursing concerns itself with health promotion, restoration, and prevention of illness as opposed to curing. Clients require holistic care that promotes humanism, health, and quality of living.

watt /wot/ [James Watt, Scottish engineer, 1736–1819], the unit of electric power or work in the meter/kilogram/second system of notation. The watt is the product of the voltage and the amperage. One watt of power is dissipated when a current of 1 ampere flows across a difference in potential of 1 volt.

watt per square centimeter (W/cm²), a unit of power density or intensity used in ultrasonography.

wave [AS, *wafian*, to fluctuate], a periodic disturbance in which energy moves through a medium without permanently altering the constituents of the medium.

waveform, 1. the graphic representation of a wave, derived by plotting a characteristic wave against time. **2.** the form of an arterial pressure pulse or displacement wave. **3.** the representation of a neuromuscular electrical stimulation unit, which is usually a symmetric or asymmetric biphasic pulse with two phases in each pulse. The two phases continually alternate or reverse in direction between positive and negative polarity.

wavelength, the distance between a given point on one wave cycle and the corresponding point on the next successive wave cycle.

WBC, abbreviation for white blood cell. See **leukocyte.**

wbt, abbreviation for *wet bulb thermometer.*

wc, abbreviation for **wheelchair.**

W chromosome and Z chromosome, the sex chromosomes of certain insects, birds, and fishes. Females of such species are heterogametic and have one W and one Z chromosome, whereas males are homogametic and have two Z chromosomes. The ZZ-ZW system of nomenclature was chosen to differentiate the chromosomes from the XX-XY type, which occurs in humans and various other animals and in which the female is homogametic and the male is heterogametic.

W/cm², abbreviation for **watt per square centimeter.**

W/D, abbreviation for *well developed,* often used in the initial identifying statement in a patient record.

weakness /wēk'nəs/, a condition of being feeble, fragile, frail, or decrepit or lacking physical strength, energy, or vigor. Specific patterns of weakness may vary with the site of a nerve injury. Partially denervated muscle shows some degree of weakness, whereas completely denervated muscle becomes flaccid. Concomitant with partial denervation is a patient's complaint of rapid fatigue and diminished capacity to perform activities of daily living. Deep tendon reflexes are diminished or absent, and electromyographic readings are abnormal.

wean [AS, *wenian,* to accustom], **1.** to induce a child to give up breastfeeding and accept other food in place of breast milk. **2.** to withdraw a person from something on which he is dependent. **3.** to remove a patient gradually from dependency on mechanical ventilation.

weanling, a child who has recently been weaned.

wear-and-tear theory /wer/, one theory of biologic aging in which structural and functional changes occur during the aging process (e.g., osteoarthritis).

weaver's bottom [AS, *wefan,* to weave, *botm,* undersurface], a form of bursitis affecting the ischial bursae of the hips of people whose work requires prolonged sitting in one position.

web, a network of fibers and cells forming a tissue or membrane.

webbed neck /webd/, a congenital thick fold of skin and fascia that stretches from the mastoid process to the clavicle on the lateral aspect of the neck. It occurs in such genetic conditions as Noonan's syndrome and Turner's syndrome.

webbed toes [AS, *wefan,* to weave, *tá*], an abnormality in which the toes are connected by webs of skin.

webbing, skinfolds connecting adjacent structures such as fingers or toes or the neck from the acromion to the mastoid, associated with genetic anomalies.

Weber (Wb), a unit of magnetic flux equal to m²kg/s²A.

Weber's sign [Hermann D. Weber, English physician, 1823–1918], ipsilateral oculomotor nerve paresis and contralateral paralysis of the face, tongue, and extremities caused by a midbrain lesion.

Weber's tuning fork test /web'ərz/, a method of screening auditory acuity. The test is performed by placing the stem of a vibrating tuning fork in the center of the person's forehead, or the midline vertex. The loudness of the sound is equal in both ears if hearing is normal.

web of causation, an interrelationship of multiple factors that contribute to the occurrence of a disease.

Wechsler intelligence scales /weks'lər/ [David Wechsler, American psychologist, b. 1896], a series of standardized tests designed to measure the intelligence at several age levels from preschool through adult by means of questions that examine general information, arrangement of pictures and objects, vocabulary, memory, reasoning, and other abilities.

wedge fracture /wej/ [AS, *wecg,* peg; L, *fractura,* break], a fracture of the vertebral body with anterior compression.

wedge pressure, the capillary pressure in the left atrium, determined by measuring the pressure in a cardiac catheter wedged in the most distal segment of the pulmonary artery.

wedge resection, the surgical excision of part of an organ, such as part of an ovary containing a cyst. The segment excised may be wedge-shaped.

WEE, abbreviation for *western equine encephalitis.*

weeping [AS, *wepan,* to cry], **1.** crying, lacrimating. **2.** oozing or exuding fluid, such as a sore or rash.

weeping eczema [AS, *wepan,* to cry; Gk, *ekzein,* to boil over], an inflammatory form of skin disease marked by a fluid exudate.

weeping lubrication, a form of hydrostatic lubrication in which the interstitial fluid of hydrated articular cartilage flows onto its surface when a load is applied.

Wegener's granulomatosis /wā'gənərz/ [Friedrich Wegener, German pathologist, 1907–1990; L, *granulum,* little grain; Gk, *oma,* tumor, *osis,* condition], an uncom-

W

mon disease characterized by a granulomatosis vasculitis of the upper and lower respiratory tract, a necrotizing glomerulonephritis, and varying degrees of small vessel vasculitis. Depending on the organ involved, symptoms may include sinus pain; a bloody, purulent nasal discharge; saddle-nose deformity; chest discomfort and cough; weakness; anorexia; weight loss; and skin lesions.

weight (wt) /wāt/ [AS, *gewiht*], the force exerted on a body by gravitational attraction. As a body moves away from the earth, the weight of the body decreases, but the mass remains constant. Weight is sometimes measured in units of force such as newtons or poundals, but it is usually expressed in pounds or kilograms, as is mass.

Weight Gain Assistance, a Nursing Interventions Classification defined as facilitating gain of body weight.

weight holder, a metal T-shaped bar that holds weights for traction.

weightlessness [AS, *gewiht* + ME, *les*], a state of absence of apparent weight, as in being beyond the effects of gravitational force in space travel.

weightlifter's headache, a type of headache sometimes experienced by weightlifters and others engaged in resistance forms of exercise. The headache is commonly occipital or upper cervical and comes on suddenly while straining, perhaps as a result of cervical ligament damage. The pain may be severe, steady, burning, or boring and may last for days.

weightlifting, a resistance form of exercise that involves the lifting of maximum heavy weights in a prescribed manner.

weight loss, a reduction in body weight. The loss may be the result of a change in diet or life-style or a febrile disease. To lose 1 pound a week a person must consume 500 fewer calories daily.

Weight Management, a Nursing Interventions Classification defined as facilitating maintenance of optimal body weight and percent body fat.

weight per volume (W/V) solution, the relationship of a solute to a solvent expressed as grams of solute per milliliter of the total solution. An example is 50 g of glucose in 1 L of water, considered a 5% W/V solution, even though it is not a true percent solution.

Weight Reduction Assistance, a Nursing Interventions Classification defined as facilitating loss of weight and/or body fat.

weights and measures, a system of establishing units or parts of quantities of substances, including standards of mass or volume.

weight traction [AS, *gewiht* + L, *trahere,* to draw], traction applied to a limb or part of a limb by means of a suspended weight.

weight training, a type of resistance training exercise using barbells, dumbbells, or machines to increase muscle strength.

weismannism /vīs′muniz′əm/ [August F. L. Weismann, German biologist, 1834–1914; L, *ismus,* practice], the basic concepts of heredity and development as proposed by A. Weismann. These state that the vehicle of inheritance is the germ plasm, which is distinct from the somatoplasm and transmitted from one generation to the next, and that changes in somatoplasm do not affect germ plasm, so that acquired characteristics cannot be inherited.—**weismannian,** *adj., n.*

well baby care [AS, *wyllan,* to wish; ME, *babe* + L, *garrire,* to chatter], periodic health supervision for infants and children to promote optimal physical, emotional, and intellectual growth and development. Such health care measures include routine immunizations to prevent disease, screening procedures for early detection and treatment of illness, and parental guidance and instruction in proper nutrition, accident prevention, and specific care and rearing of the child at various stages of development.

well baby clinic, a clinic that specializes in medical supervision and services for healthy infants.

well-being [AS, *wyllan* + *beon,* to be], achievement of a good and satisfactory existence as defined by the individual.

well-differentiated lymphocytic malignant lymphoma /-dif′əren′shē-ā′tid/, a lymphoid neoplasm characterized by the predominance of mature lymphocytes.

Wellens syndrome, in patients with unstable angina, the electrocardiographic signs of critical proximal left anterior descending coronary artery stenosis.

wellness, a dynamic state of health in which an individual progresses toward a higher level of functioning, achieving an optimum balance between internal and external environments.

welt [OE, *wealtan,* to roll], a raised ridge on the skin, usually caused by a blow.

Wenckebach heart block /veng′kəbäk, -bäkh/ [Karel F. Wenckebach, Dutch-Austrian physician, 1864–1940], a form of second-degree atrioventricular block with a progressive beat-to-beat prolongation of the PR interval, finally resulting in a nonconducting P wave.

Werdnig-Hoffmann's disease /verd′nig-hôf′mun/ [Guido Werdnig, Austrian neurologist, 1844–1919; Johann Hoffman, German neurologist, 1857–1919], a genetic disorder beginning in infancy or young childhood, characterized by progressive atrophy of the skeletal muscle resulting from degeneration of the cells in the anterior horn of the spinal cord and the motor nuclei in the brainstem. Symptoms include congenital hypotonia; absence of stretch reflexes; flaccid paralysis, especially of the trunk and limbs; lack of sucking ability; fasciculations of the tongue and sometimes of other muscles; and often dysphagia.

Werner's syndrome /wur′nərz, wer′nərz/, an inherited condition of progeria with scleroderma, juvenile cataracts, diabetes, and hypogonadism.

Wernicke-Korsakoff's syndrome, the coexistence of Wernicke's encephalopathy and Korsakoff's syndrome.

Wernicke's aphasia [Karl Wernicke, Polish neurologist, 1848–1905], a form of aphasia with impairment in the comprehension of written and spoken words, possibly caused by a lesion in Wernicke's center. The client may articulate normally, but speech is incoherent, with malformed or substitute words and grammatic errors.

Wernicke's center [Karl Wernicke; Gk, *kentron,* center], a sensory speech center located in the posterior temporal gyrus and adjacent angular gyrus in the dominant hemisphere. Wernicke observed in 1874 that patients with brain damage in that area also suffered a loss of speech comprehension.

Wernicke's encephalopathy /ver′nikēz/ [Karl Wernicke], an inflammatory, hemorrhagic, degenerative condition of the brain. It is characterized by lesions in several parts of the brain, including the hypothalamus, mammillary bodies, and tissues surrounding ventricles and aqueducts; double vision; involuntary and rapid movements of the eyes; lack of muscular coordination; and decreased mental function, which may be mild or severe. Wernicke's encephalopathy is caused by a thiamin deficiency and is seen in association with chronic alcoholism.

Westermark's sign, [Neil Westermark, German radiologist, b. 1904], the absence of blood vessel markings beyond the location of a pulmonary embolism as seen on a radiograph.

Western blot test, a laboratory blood test to detect the presence of antibodies to specific antigens. It is regarded as more precise than the enzyme-linked immunosorbent assay (ELISA) and is sometimes used to check the validity of ELISA tests.

West nomogram, a graph used in estimating the body surface area.

West's syndrome, an infantile encephalopathy characterized by spasms, arrest of psychomotor development, and an electroencephalogram abnormality of random high-voltage slow waves and spikes from multiple loci.

wet-and-dry-bulb thermometer, an instrument used to measure the relative humidity of the atmosphere. It consists of a thermometer with a bulb that is wet or moist and one that is kept dry. The relative humidity is calculated from the difference in readings of the thermometers when water evaporates from the wet bulb, decreasing its temperature.

wet dressing [AS, *waet* + Ofr, *dresser,* to arrange], a moist dressing used to relieve symptoms of some skin diseases. As the moisture evaporates, it cools and dries the skin, softens dried blood and sera, and stimulates drainage.

wet lung, an abnormal condition of the lungs, characterized by a persistent cough and crackles at the lung bases. It occurs in workers exposed to pulmonary irritants.

wet nurse, a woman who cares for and breastfeeds another's infant.

wet pack [AS, *waet,* moist; ME, *pakke*], a therapy that involves wrapping the patient in wet sheets with a top covering of a dry blanket, usually to reduce fever.

wet pleurisy [AS, *waet* + Gk, *pleuritis*], pleurisy in which the inflammation has progressed to an effusive state, with the fluid having a high specific gravity because of the presence of blood clots and fibrin.

wetting agent, a detergent such as tyloxapol used as a mucolytic in respiratory therapy.

W/F, abbreviation for *white female,* often used in the initial identifying statement in a patient record.

Wharton's jelly /wôr′tənz/ [Thomas Wharton, English anatomist, 1614–1673; L, *gelare,* to congeal], a gelatinous tissue that remains when the embryonic body stalk blends with the yolk sac within the umbilical cord.

wheal /wēl/ [AS, *walu,* pimple], an individual lesion of urticaria.

wheal-and-flare reaction [AS, *walu* + *flare* + ME, *fleare,* to blaze up; L, *re,* again, *agere,* to act], a skin eruption that may follow injury or injection of an antigen. It is characterized by swelling and redness caused by a release of histamine. The reaction usually occurs in three stages, beginning with the appearance of an erythematous area at the site of injury, followed by development of a flare sur-

W

rounding the site. Finally a wheal forms at the site as fluid leaks under the skin from surrounding capillaries.

wheat weevil disease, a hypersensitivity pneumonitis caused by allergy to weevil particles found in wheat flour.

wheel, **1.** a rigid circular frame designed to revolve about an axis in the center of the disk. **2.** a round cutting or polishing dental instrument.

wheelchair (wc), a mobile chair equipped with large wheels and brakes.

wheelie /wē′lē/, a term used to describe a wheelchair mobility skill in which the front casters are raised and balance is maintained over the large rear wheels. it is used for negotiating steep ramps, steps, curbs, and other rough terrain.

wheeze [AS, *hwesan,* to hiss], **1.** a form of rhonchus, characterized by a high-pitched or low-pitched musical quality. It is caused by a high-velocity flow of air through a narrowed airway and is heard during both inspiration and expiration. **2.** to breathe with a wheeze.

whiplash injury [ME, *whippen* + *lasshe* + L, *ijuria*], *informal.* an injury to the cervical vertebrae or their supporting ligaments and muscles marked by pain and stiffness, usually resulting from sudden acceleration or deceleration, such as in a rear-end car collision that causes violent back and forth movement of the head and neck.

Whipple's disease [George Hoyt Whipple, American pathologist, 1878–1976], a rare intestinal disease characterized by severe intestinal malabsorption, steatorrhea, anemia, weight loss, arthritis, and arthralgia. People with the disease are severely malnourished and have abdominal pain, chest pain, and a chronic nonproductive cough.

whirlpool bath /(h)wurl/, the immersion of the body or a part of the body in a tank of hot water agitated by a jet of equally hot water and air.

whispered pectoriloquy, the transmission of a whisper through the pulmonary structures so that it is heard as normal audible speech on auscultation.

white cell, *informal.* white blood cell.

white fibrocartilage [AS, *hwit* + L, *fibra,* fiber, *cartilago*], a mixture of tough, white fibrous tissue and flexible cartilaginous tissue.

white gold, a gold alloy with a high content of palladium or platinum used in dental restorations such as prepared tooth cavities and gold crowns.

white infarct [AS, *hwit* + L, *infarcire,* to stuff], an infarct that is white because of an absence of blood.

white noise, a sound in which the intensity is the same at all frequencies within a designated band.

white radiation, a form of radiation that results from the rapid deceleration of high-speed electrons striking a target, such as when the electron beam of a tungsten cathode strikes the tungsten or molybdenum target of the anode in an x-ray tube.

white spots film fault, a defect in a radiograph or a developed photographic film that appears as scattered white spots throughout the image area.

white substance, the tissue of the central nervous system and much of the part of the cerebrum, consisting mainly of myelinated nerve fibers, but with some unmyelinated nerve fibers, embedded in a spongy network of neuroglia. It is subdivided in each half of the spinal cord into three funiculi: anterior, posterior, and lateral white column. Each column subdivides into tracts that are closely associated in function.

white thrombus, **1.** an aggregation of blood platelets, fibrin, clotting factors, and cellular elements containing few or no erythrocytes. **2.** a thrombus composed chiefly of white blood cells. **3.** a thrombus composed primarily of blood platelets and fibrin.

whitlow /(h)wit′lō/ [Scand, *whick,* nail, *flaw,* crack], an inflammation of the end of a finger or toe that results in suppuration.

WHO, abbreviation for **World Health Organization.**

whole blood /hōl/ [AS, *hal* + *blod*], blood that is unmodified except for the presence of an anticoagulant. Whole blood may be used for transfusion.

whole blood clot retraction test, a procedure to determine if a bleeding disorder is caused by a decreased platelet count. The test measures the progress of blood clot retraction, which should be complete in 4 to 24 hours. If thrombocytopenia exists, clot retraction will be slower, and the clot will remain soft and watery.

whole-body irradiation, ionizing radiation exposure that affects the entire body. Short-term whole-body exposure to ionizing radiation can cause injury or death in humans, mainly from damage to the gastrointestinal tract and the bone marrow. This occurs only in doses far beyond the diagnostic range, such as with exposure to nuclear weapons. The absorbed dose equivalent limit for whole-body occupational exposure is 5 rem per year. For other persons in the community the absorbed dose equivalent limit is 0.5 rem per year.

whole bowel irrigation, a method of treating poison patients by flushing large volumes of fluid through the gastrointestinal tract.

whole milk, milk from which no constituent such as fat has been removed. To be called whole milk it must contain 3.5% fat, 8.5% nonfat milk solids, and 88% water.

wholistic health /hōlis'tik/ [AS, *hal*, whole, *haelth*], a concept that concern for health requires a perspective of the individual as an integrated system rather than one or more separate parts.

whoop /ho͞op, (h)wo͞op/, a noisy spasm of inspiration that terminates a coughing paroxysm in cases of pertussis. It is caused by a sudden sharp increase in tension on the vocal cords.

whorl /(h)wurl/ /wurl, hwurl/ [ME, *hwarwy*], a spiral turn, such as one of the turns of the cochlea or of the dermal ridges that form fingerprints.

WIA, abbreviation for **waking imagined analgesia.**

wick humidifier, a respiratory care device in which a piece of paper, sponge, or similar material that absorbs water by capillary action is inserted in the path of the air flow. With the addition of heat, high levels of humidity can be achieved.

Widal's test /vēdäls'/ [Georges F. I. Widal, French physician, 1862–1929], an agglutination test used to aid in the diagnosis of *Salmonella* infections such as typhoid fever.

Wiedenbach /wē'dənbak/, **Ernestine** (b. 1900), a German-born American nursing educator and writer. She was a leader in family-centered maternity nursing and developed the full range of the art and science of obstetric nursing.

wild-type gene [AS, *wilde*, untamed; Gk, *typos*, mark, *genein*, to produce], a normal or standard form of a gene, as contrasted with a mutant form.

will [AS, *wyllan*], **1.** the mental faculty that enables one consciously to choose or decide on a course of action. **2.** the act or process of exercising the power of choice. **3.** a wish, desire, or deliberate intention. **4.** a disposition or attitude toward another or others. **5.** determination or purpose; willfulness. **6.** (in law) an expression or declaration of a person's wishes as to the disposition of property to be performed or take effect after death.

Wilms' tumor /vilms/ [Max Wilms, German surgeon, 1867–1918], a malignant neoplasm of the kidney occurring in young children before the fifth year in 75% of the cases. The most frequent early signs are hypertension, a palpable mass, pain, and hematuria. The tumor, an embryonal adenomyosarcoma, is well encapsulated in the early stage, but it may extend into lymph nodes, the renal vein, or the vena cava and metastasize to the lungs or other sites.

Wilson's disease [Samuel A. K. Wilson, English neurologist, 1878–1937], a rare inherited disorder whereby a decrease in ceruloplasmin causes copper to accumulate slowly in the liver to then be released and taken up in other parts of the body. Hemolysis and hemolytic anemia occur as the copper accumulates in the red blood cells. Accumulation in the brain destroys certain tissue and may cause tremors, muscle rigidity, poorly articulated speech, and dementia. Kidney function is diminished; the liver becomes cirrhotic.

windburn /wind'burn/ [AS, *wind*, air, *baernan*], a skin disorder caused by exposure to winds.

windchill /win'chil/, the loss of heat from the body when it is exposed to wind of a given speed at a given temperature and humidity.

windchill factor [AS, *wind*, air, *cele*, cold], the amount of chilling of the body, beyond that resulting from a cold ambient temperature, because of exposure to cool air currents. The windchill factor is expressed in degrees Celsius or Fahrenheit as the effective temperature felt by a person exposed to the weather. Because windchill factors are based on exposure of dry skin to cool air currents, air blowing at the same speed over a wet skin surface would cause additional loss of body heat and a greater windchill.

wind chill index, a chart that compares temperatures of the atmosphere with various wind speeds, enabling one to calculate the windchill factor. The comparison is expressed in kilocalories per hour per square meter of skin surface.

winding sheet /wīn'ding/, a shroud for wrapping a dead body.

window [AS, *wind*, air, *owe*, eye], **1.** a surgically created opening in the surface of a structure or an anatomically occurring opening in the surface or between the chambers of a structure. **2.** a specific time period during which a phenomenon can be observed, a reaction monitored, or a procedure initiated.

windowed /win'dōd/, (of an orthopedic cast) having an opening, especially to relieve pressure that may irritate and inflame the skin.

winegrower's lung /wīn'grō·ərs/, a type of hypersensitivity pneumonitis caused by contact with mold on grapes.

winged scapula /wingd/ [ONorse, *vaengr*

W

+ L, *scapulae,* shoulderblades], an abnormal prominence of the scapula caused by either projection of posterior angles of the ribs in a flat chest or paralysis of the serratus anterior muscle.

wink reflex, an automatic closure of the eyelids in response to an appropriate stimulus.

winter cough [AS, *winter* + *cohhetan*], *nontechnical.* a chronic condition characterized by a persistent cough occasioned by cold weather.

winter itch, pruritus occurring in cold weather in people who have dry skin, particularly in those who have atopic dermatitis.

wire suture [AS, *wir* + L, *sutura*], a stainless steel or silver wire used for uniting bone fracture fragments or in dentistry.

wiry pulse /wī′(ə)re/ [AS, *wir* + L, *pulsare,* to beat], an abnormal pulse that is strong but small.

wisdom tooth [AS, *wisdom* + *toth*], either of the last teeth on each side of the upper and lower jaw. These are third molars and are the last teeth to erupt, usually between 17 and 25 years of age, often causing considerable pain, dental problems, and the need for extraction.

wish fulfillment [AS, *wiscan,* to wish, *fullfyllan,* to fill full], **1.** the gratification of a desire. **2.** (in psychology) the satisfaction of a desire or the release of emotional tension through such processes as dreams, daydreams, and neurotic symptoms. **3.** (in psychoanalysis) one of the primary motivations for dreams in which an unconscious desire or urge is given expression.

wishful thinking [AS, *wiscan* + *thencan,* to think], the interpretation of facts or situations according to one's desires or wishes rather than as they exist in reality, usually used as an unconscious device to avoid painful or unpleasant feelings.

Wiskott-Aldrich's syndrome /wis′kotôl′drich/ [Alfred Wiskott, German pediatrician, 1898–1978; Robert Anderson Aldrich, American pediatrician, b. 1917], an immunodeficiency disorder inherited as a recessive X-linked trait, characterized by thrombocytopenia; eczema; inadequate T and B cell function; and an increased susceptibility to viral, bacterial, and fungal infections and cancer.

witch doctor, a shamanistic healer whose primary function is to cure the sick members of the community. The healing system is based on a belief that illness is the result of an evil object entering the body or the soul of the patient being stolen. Treatment involves removing the evil object from the patient's body or finding the lost soul and returning it to its owner.

witch hazel [AS, *wican,* to bend; Ger, *hasel*], **1.** a shrub, *Hamamelis virginiana,* indigenous to North America, from which an astringent extract is derived. **2.** a solution comprising the extract, alcohol, and water, used as an astringent.

witch's milk, a milklike substance secreted from the breast of the newborn, caused by circulating maternal lactating hormone.

withdrawal /withdrô′əl/ [ME, *with* + *drawen,* to take away], a common response to physical danger or severe stress characterized by a state of apathy, lethargy, depression, retreat into oneself, and in grave cases catatonia and stupor.

withdrawal behavior, the physical or psychologic removal of oneself from a stressor.

withdrawal bleeding, the passage of blood from the uterus, associated with the shedding of endometrium that has been stimulated and maintained by hormonal medication. It occurs when the medication is discontinued.

withdrawal method, a contraceptive technique in coitus wherein the penis is withdrawn from the vagina before ejaculation. It is not reliable because small amounts of seminal fluid carrying millions of spermatozoa may be emitted without sensation before full ejaculation.

withdrawal symptoms, the unpleasant, sometimes life-threatening physiologic changes that occur when some drugs are withdrawn after prolonged, regular use.

withdrawal syndrome [ME, *with* + *drawen,* to take away; Gk, *syn,* together, *dromos,* course], a physical and mental response after cessation or severe reduction in intake of a substance such as alcohol or opiates that has been used regularly to induce euphoria, intoxication, or relief from pain or distress. The body tissues become dependent on the regular reinforcing effect of the chemical so that interruption of the dosage induces an organic mental state characterized by anxiety, restlessness, insomnia, irritability, impaired attention, and often physical illness.

withdrawn behavior, a condition in which there is a blunting of the emotions and a lack of social responsiveness.

witness, a person who is present and can testify that he or she has personally observed an event, such as the signing of a will or consent form.

W/M, abbreviation for *white male,* often used in the initial identifying statement in a patient record.

W/N, abbreviation for *well nourished,* often used in the initial identifying statement in a patient record.

WOB, abbreviation for **work of breathing.**

wobble /wob'əl/, an eccentric rotation that permits increased resolution of tomographic imaging devices composed of discrete detector systems.

Wolff-Chaikoff effect /wōolf'chī'kəf/, the decreased formation and release of thyroid hormone in the presence of an excess of iodine.

wolffian cyst /wôl'fē·ən/ [Kaspar F. Wolff, German anatomist, b. 1733–1794; Gk, *kystis,* bag], **1.** a cyst of the wolffian duct. **2.** a cyst of a broad ligament of the uterus.

Wolff-Parkinson-White's syndrome /wōolf'pär'kinsən-(h)wīt'/ [Louis Wolff, American physician, 1898–1972; John Parkinson, English cardiologist, 1885–1976; Paul Dudley White, American cardiologist, 1886–1973], a disorder of atrioventricular (AV) conduction, characterized by two AV conduction pathways.

Wolff's law /wôlfs/ [Julius Wolff, German anatomist, 1836–1902], the principle that changes in the form and function of a bone are followed by changes in its internal structure.

Wolf-Herschorn's syndrome, a genetic disorder of infants characterized by psychomotor and growth retardation, hypertonicity, seizures, and microcephaly. Other features include craniofacial anomalies, ocular malformations, cleft lip or palate, heart malformations, and scoliosis.

woman, an adult female human.

woman-year [AS, *wifman* + *gear*], (in statistics) 1 year in the reproductive life of a sexually active woman; a unit that represents 12 months of exposure to the risk of pregnancy.

Wood's lamp [Robert W. Wood, American physicist, 1868–1955; AS, *glaes*], an illuminating device with a nickel oxide filter that holds back all light except for a few violet rays of the visible spectrum and ultraviolet wavelengths of about 365 nm. It is used extensively to help diagnose fungus infections of the scalp and erythrasma.

wood tick [AS, *wudu* + ME, *tike*], a hardshelled tick of the Ixodidae family and a natural reservoir of *Rickettsia rickettsii.* One species of wood tick, *Dermacentor andersoni,* is the principal vector in western North America of **Rocky Mountain spotted fever,** transmitted by *R. rickettsii.*

wool fat, a fatty substance obtained from sheep's wool and of which lanolin is a common chemical component.

woolsorter's disease [AS, *wull* + Fr, *sorte*

+ L, *dis,* opposite of; Fr, *aise,* ease], the pulmonary form of anthrax, so named because it is an occupational hazard to those who handle sheep's wool. Early symptoms mimic influenza, but the patient soon develops high fever, respiratory distress, and cyanosis.

word blindness [AS, *word* + *blind*], an inability to understand written language; a form of receptive aphasia caused by lesions in the parietal or parietal-occipital areas of the brain. The condition may be congenital or acquired as a result of disease or injury.

word salad, a jumble of words and phrases that lacks logical coherence and meaning, often characteristic of disoriented individuals and persons with schizophrenia.

working occlusion [AS, *weorc* + L, *occludere,* to shut], the occlusal contacts of teeth on the side of the jaw toward which the mandible is moved.

working phase, (in psychology) the second stage of the therapist-client relationship. During this stage clients explore their experiences. Therapists assist clients in this process by helping them to describe and clarify their experiences, to plan courses of action and try out the plans, and to begin to evaluate the effectiveness of their new behavior.

working pressure, a recommended working pressure of about 50 pounds per square inch, gauge (psig) for oxygen or compressed air leaving a cylinder; it is reduced by a pressure regulator for clinical use in respiratory therapy.

working through, a process by which repressed feelings are released and reintegrated into the personality.

workload, an amount of work to be performed within a specific time period.

work of breathing (WOB), the effort required to inspire air into the lungs. WOB accounts for 5% of total body oxygen consumption in a normal resting state but can increase dramatically during acute illness.

work of worrying, a coping strategy in which inner preparation through worrying increases the level of tolerance for subsequent threats.

workout, 1. a test of ability and endurance. **2.** a physical exercise session.

work simplification, the use of special equipment, ergonomics, functional planning, and behavior modification to reduce the physical and psychologic stresses of home maintenance for disabled people or their family members.

workstation, 1. an area, as in an office equipped with a computer or computer terminal. **2.** an electronic monitor such as a

work therapy [AS, *weorc* + Gk, *therapeia*, treatment], a therapeutic approach in which the client performs a useful activity or learns an occupation, as in occupational therapy.

work tolerance, the kind and amount of work that a physically or mentally ill person can or should perform.

work-up, the process of performing a complete patient evaluation, including history, physical examination, laboratory tests, and x-ray or other diagnostic procedures to acquire an accurate data base on which a diagnosis and treatment plan may be established.

World Health Organization (WHO), an intergovernmental organization within the United Nations system. Its purpose is to aid in the attainment of the highest possible level of health by all people. Its programs include education for current health issues, proper food supply and nutrition, safe water and sanitation, maternal and child health, immunization against major infectious diseases, and prevention and control of diseases. WHO is coordinating global strategies to control and prevent acquired immunodeficiency syndrome.

worm /wurm/ [AS, *wyrm*], any of the soft-bodied, elongated invertebrates of the phyla Annelida, Nemathelminthes, or Platyhelminthes. Some kinds of worms parasitic for humans are **hookworm,** pinworm, and **tapeworm.**

wormian bone /vôr′mē·ən/ [Olaus Worm, Danish anatomist, 1588–1654; AS, *ban*], any of several tiny smooth bones, usually found at the serrated borders of the sutures between the cranial bones.

worthlessness /wurth′ləsnəs/, a component of low self-esteem, characterized by feelings of uselessness and inability to contribute meaningfully to the well-being of others or to one's environment.

wound /wōōnd/ [AS, *wund*], **1.** any physical injury involving a break in the skin, usually caused by an act or accident rather than by a disease, such as a chest wound, gunshot wound, or puncture wound. **2.** to cause an injury, especially one that breaks the skin.

Wound Care, a Nursing Interventions Classification defined as prevention of wound complications and promotion of wound healing.

Wound Care: Closed Drainage, a Nursing Interventions Classification defined as maintenance of a pressure drainage system at the wound site.

wound healing, a process to restore to a state of soundness any injury that results in an interruption in the continuity of external surfaces of the body.

wound irrigation, the rinsing of a wound or the cavity formed by a wound using a medicated solution, water, or antimicrobial liquid preparation.

Wound Irrigation, a Nursing Interventions Classification defined as flushing of an open wound to cleanse and remove debris and excessive drainage.

Wright's stain /rīts/ [James H. Wright, American pathologist, 1869–1928; Fr, *teindre,* to dye], a stain containing methylene blue and eosin that is used to color blood specimens for microscopic examination, such as for complete blood count and particularly for malarial parasites.

wrinkle test /ring′kəl/ [AS, *gewrinclian,* to wind; L, *testum,* crucible], a test for nerve function in the hand by observing the presence of skin wrinkles after the hand has been placed in warm water for 20 to 30 minutes. Denervated skin does not wrinkle.

wrist clonus reflex /rist/, a sustained clonic muscle spasm caused by the sudden hyperextension of the wrist joint.

wrist drop [AS, *wrist* + *dropa*], a condition caused by paralysis of the extensor muscles of the hand and fingers or by injury to the radial nerve, resulting in flexion of the wrist.

wrist ganglion, a cystic enlargement of a tendon sheath on the back of the wrist.

writer's cramp [AS, *writan,* to write, *crammian,* to fill], a painful involuntary contraction of the muscles of the hand when attempting to write. It often occurs after long periods of writing.

wrongful birth /rông′fəl/ [OE, *wrang,* twisted; ME, *burth*], a belief that a birth could have been avoided if the parents had been properly advised by a physician that a pregnancy could occur or that a fetus would be deformed.

wrongful death statute [AS, *wrang* + *death* + L, *statuere,* to set up], (in law) a statute existing in all states that provides that the death of a person can give rise to a cause of legal action brought by the person's beneficiaries in a civil suit against the person whose willful or negligent acts caused the death.

wrongful life action, (in law) a civil suit usually brought against a physician or health facility on the basis of negligence that resulted in the wrongful birth or life of an infant. The parents of the unwanted child seek to obtain payment from the defendant for the medical expenses of pregnancy and delivery, for pain and suffering, and for the education and upbringing of the child.

wt., abbreviation for **weight.**

Wuchereria /vo͞o′kərē′rē·ə/ [Otto Wucherer, German physician, 1820–1873], a genus of filarial worms found in warm, humid climates. *Wuchereria bancrofti,* transmitted by mosquitoes, is the cause of elephantiasis.

W/V, abbreviation for *weight per volume.*

w/w, abbreviation for *weight per weight.*

W

xanthelasmatosis /zan′thilaz′mətō′sis/ [Gk, *xanthos,* yellow, *elasma,* plate, *osis,* condition], a disseminated, generalized form of planar xanthoma frequently associated with reticuloendothelial disorders, especially multiple myeloma.

xanthene /zan′thēn/ [Gk, *xanthos,* yellow], a crystalline organic compound in which two benzene rings are fused to a central pyran ring. The pyran oxygen bridges the two benzene rings. It is a parent chemical structure of many medicinal elements.

xanthine /zan′thīn/ [Gk, *xanthos,* yellow], a nitrogenous by-product of the metabolism of nucleoproteins. It is normally found in the muscles, liver, spleen, pancreas, and urine. —**xanthic,** *adj.*

xanthine base [Gk, *xanthos,* yellow], a purine compound occurring in plants and animals as a metabolite of adenine and guanine. It is the parent structure of the methyl xanthine alkaloids that include caffeine in coffee, theophylline in tea, and theobromine in cocoa.

xanthine derivative, any one of the closely related alkaloids caffeine, theobromine, and theophylline. They are found in plants widely distributed geographically and are variously ingested as components in beverages such as coffee, tea, cocoa, and cola drinks. The xanthine derivatives or methylxanthines have pharmacologic properties that stimulate the central nervous system, produce diuresis, and relax smooth muscles.

xanthinuria /zan′thinyŏŏr′ē-ə/ [Gk, *xanthos* + *ouron,* urine], **1.** the presence of excessive quantities of xanthine in the urine. **2.** a rare disorder of purine metabolism, resulting in the excretion of large amounts of xanthine in the urine because of the absence of an enzyme, xanthine oxidase, that is necessary in xanthine metabolism.

xanthism /zan′thizəm/, a genetic pigment anomaly characterized by yellow or yellowish-red hair, copper-red skin, and reddish-brown irises.

xanthochromia /zan′thəkrō′mē-ə/, a pale yellow or straw-colored discoloration of cerebrospinal fluid. It is caused by the presence of hemoglobin breakdown products.

xanthochromic /zan′thəkrō′mik/ [Gk, *xanthos* + *chroma,* color], having a yellowish color, such as cerebrospinal fluid that contains blood or bile.

xanthoderma /zan′thədur′mə/, skin that has a yellow coloration, as in jaundice.

xanthogranuloma /zan′thəgran′yəlō′mə/ [Gk, *xanthos* + L, *granulum,* little grain; Gk, *oma,* tumor], a tumor or nodule of granulation tissue containing lipid deposits. A kind of xanthogranuloma is **juvenile xanthogranuloma.**

xanthoma /zanthō′mə/ [Gk, *xanthos* + *oma,* tumor], a benign fatty fibrous yellowish plaque, nodule, or tumor that develops in the subcutaneous layer of skin, often around tendons.

xanthoma disseminatum, a benign chronic condition in which small orange or brown papules and nodules develop on many body surfaces, especially on the mucous membrane of the oropharynx, larynx, and bronchi.

xanthoma palpebrarum, a soft yellow spot or plaque usually occurring in groups on the eyelids.

xanthomasarcoma /zan′thōməsärkō′mə/ [Gk, *xanthos* + *oma* + *sarx,* flesh, *oma,* tumor], a giant cell sarcoma of the tendon sheaths and aponeuroses that contains xanthoma cells.

xanthoma striatum palmare, a yellow or orange flat plaque or slightly raised nodule occurring in groups on the palms of the hands.

xanthoma tendinosum, a yellow or orange elevated or flat round papule or nodule occurring in clusters on tendons, especially the extensor tendons of the hands and feet, of individuals with hereditary lipid storage disease.

xanthomatosis /zan′thōmətō′sis/ [Gk, *xanthos* + *oma* + *osis,* condition], an abnormal condition in which there are deposits of yellowish fatty material in the skin, internal organs, and reticuloendothelial system.

xanthomatosis bulbi, a fatty degeneration of the cornea.

xanthoma tuberosum, a yellow or orange flat or elevated round papule occurring in clusters on the skin of joints, especially the elbows and knees, usually in people who have a hereditary lipid storage disease.

Xanthomonas /zan'thəmon'əs/, a genus of gram-negative rod-shaped aerobic bacteria that produces a yellow pigment.

Xanthomonas maltophilia, a species of *Xanthomonas* bacteria commonly found in water, milk, and frozen food and in the upper respiratory tract, blood, and urine of humans. It is an opportunistic cause of infections in hospitalized and immunocompromised patients.

xanthopsia /zanthop'sē·ə/ [Gk, *xanthos* + *opsis,* sight], an abnormal visual condition in which everything appears to have a yellow hue.

xanthosis /zanthō'sis/ [Gk, *xanthos* + *osis,* condition], **1.** a yellowish discoloration sometimes seen in degenerating tissues of malignant diseases. **2.** a reversible yellow discoloration of the skin most commonly caused by the ingestion of large amounts of yellow or orange leafy vegetables containing carotene pigment.

xanthosis of retina, a generalized yellow discoloration of the posterior pole of the fundus, sometimes found in diabetic retinopathy.

xanthurenic acid /zan'thŏŏrē'nik/, a metabolite of tryptophan that occurs in normal urine and in elevated levels in patients with vitamin B_6 deficiency.

xanthurenic aciduria, a genetic disorder of tryptophan metabolism characterized by a deficiency of the kynureninase liver enzyme. It is also seen in vitamin B deficiency.

X chromosome, a sex chromosome that in humans and many other species is present in both sexes, appearing singly in the cells of normal males and in duplicate in the cells of normal females. The chromosome is carried as a sex determinant by all of the female gametes and one half of all male gametes.

Xe, symbol for the element **xenon.**

xenoantibody, an antibody produced in one species to an antigen derived from a different species.

xenoantigen /zē'nō·an'təjən/, an antigen that occurs in organisms of more than one species.

xenobiotic /-bī·ot'ik/ [Gk, *xenos,* strange, *bios,* life], pertaining to organic substances that are foreign to the body, such as drugs or organic poisons.

xenodiagnosis, /-dī·agnō'sis/ a method of diagnosing a vector-transmitted infection such as Chagas' disease, in which a laboratory-reared, pathogen-free insect is allowed to suck blood from a patient. The intestinal contents of the insect are

then examined for the presence of the pathogen.

xenogeneic /-jənē'ik/ [Gk, *xenos* + *genein,* to produce], **1.** (in genetics) denoting individuals or cell types from different species and different genotypes. **2.** (in transplantation biology) denoting tissues from different species that are therefore antigenically dissimilar.

xenogenesis /-zen'əjen'əsis/, **1.** alternation of traits in successive generations; heterogenesis. **2.** the theoretic production of offspring that are totally different from both of the parents.—**xenogenetic, xenogenic,** *adj.*

xenograft /zen'əgraft'/ [Gk, *xenos* + *graphion,* stylus], tissue from another species used as a temporary graft in certain cases, as in treating a severely burned patient when sufficient tissue from the patient or from a tissue bank is not available.

xenology /zēnol'əjē/ [Gk, *xenos,* stranger, *logos,* science], the study of parasites.

xenoma /zēnō'mə/, a tumor that develops on tissue infected with certain parasites.

xenon (Xe) /-zen'on, zē'non/ [Gk, *xenos,* strange], a nonreactive gaseous nonmetallic element. Its atomic number is 54; its atomic mass (weight) is 131.30.

xenon-133 [Gk, *xenos,* strange], a radioactive isotope of zenon gas, used in radiographic studies of the lung.

xenoparasite /-per'əsīt/, an ectoparasite that has become pathogenic as a result of weakened resistance of the host.

xenophobia /-fō'bē·ə/ /zen'ə-, zē'nə-/ [Gk, *xenos* + *phobos,* fear], an anxiety disorder characterized by a pervasive, irrational fear or uneasiness in the presence of strangers, especially foreigners, or in new surroundings.

Xenopsylla /zen'ōsil'ə/, a genus of parasitic fleas responsible for the transmission of bubonic plague and other infections. Many of more than 30 species of *Xenopsylla* are vectors of pathogens, including *X. cheopis,* a rat flea found worldwide. It is a vector of *Yersinia pestis,* the bacterial source of murine typhus, as well as of the plague.

xenotype /zen'ətīp/, molecular variations based on differences in structure and antigenic specificity, such as immunoglobulins from different species.

xeroderma /zir'ədur'mə/ [Gk, *xeros,* dry, *derma,* skin], a chronic skin condition characterized by dryness and roughness.

xeroderma pigmentosum (XP), a rare, inherited skin disease characterized by extreme sensitivity to ultraviolet light, exposure to which results in freckles, telangiectases, keratoses, papillomas, carcinoma, and possibly, melanoma. Keratitis and tumors developing on the eyelids and cornea may result in blindness.

xerogram /zir′əgram′/ [Gk, *xeros* + *gramma*, record], an x-ray image produced by xeroradiography.

xeromammogram /-mam′əgram′/, a type of breast radiograph.

xeromammography /-mamog′rəfē/, the use of xerographic methods to produce radiographic images of the breasts.

xerophthalmia /zir′ofthal′mē-ə/ [Gk, *xeros* + *ophthalmos*, eye], a condition of dry and lusterless corneas and conjunctival areas, usually the result of vitamin A deficiency and associated with night blindness.

xeroradiography /-rā′dē·og′rəfē/ [Gk, *xeros* + L, *radiare*, to emit rays; Gk, *graphein*, to record], a diagnostic x-ray technique in which an image is produced electrically rather than chemically, permitting lower exposure times and radiation of lower energy than that of ordinary x-rays. The latent image is made visible with a powder toner similar to that used in a copying machine. Xeroradiography is used primarily for mammography.

xerostomia /zir′əstō′mē-ə/ [Gk, *xeros* + *stoma*, mouth], dryness of the mouth caused by cessation of normal salivary secretion. The condition is a symptom of various diseases such as diabetes, acute infections, hysteria, and Sjögren's syndrome and can be caused by paralysis of facial nerves.

xerotic keratitis /zirot′ik/ [Gk, *xeros*, dry, *keras*, horn, *itis*, inflammation], an inflammation of the cornea resulting from dryness of the conjunctiva. Underlying causes may be malnutrition, a deficiency of vitamin A, or autoimmune diseases.

Xi /zī, sī/, Ξ, ξ, the fourteenth letter of the Greek alphabet.

xiphisternal articulation /zif′istur′nəl/ [Gk, *xiphos*, sword, *sternon*, chest; L, *articulare*, to divide into joints], the cartilaginous connection between the xiphoid process and the body of the sternum.

xiphodynia /zī′fōdin′ē-ə/, a pain in the xiphoid process.

xiphoid /zif′oid/ [Gk, *xiphos*, sword, *eidos*, form], shaped like a sword; the xiphoid process of the sternum.

xiphoid process /zif′oid/ [Gk, *xiphos* + *eidos*, form; L, *processus*, going forth], the smallest of three parts of the sternum, articulating with the inferior end of the body of the sternum above and laterally with the seventh rib.

xiphopagus /zīfop′əgəs/, conjoined twins united at the xiphoid process of the sternum.

X-linked /eks′lingkt/, pertaining to genes

or to the characteristics or conditions they transmit that are carried on the X chromosome.—**X linkage,** *n.*

x-linked disorders, diseases and disorders associated with genetic abnormalities on the x-chromosomes. Examples are the muscular dystrophies and hemophilias.

X-linked dominant inheritance, a pattern of inheritance in which the transmission of a dominant gene on the X chromosome causes a characteristic to be manifested. X-linked dominant inheritance closely resembles autosomal-dominant inheritance.

x-linked bulbospinal neuropathy, a hereditary disorder of the spinal cord and medulla oblongata in males, with associated endocrine features, including azoospermia, gynecomastia, glucose intolerance, and feminized skin changes.

X-linked inheritance, a pattern of inheritance in which the transmission of traits varies according to the sex of the person, because the genes on the X chromosome have no counterparts on the Y chromosome. The inheritance pattern may be recessive or dominant. The characteristic determined by a gene on the X chromosome is always expressed in males.

x-linked lymphoproliferative syndrome, a type of infectious mononucleosis in x-linked immunodeficiency patients with Epstein-Barr nuclear antigen. It is a potentially fatal disease associated with an inability to resist Epstein-Barr virus.

X-linked recessive inheritance, a pattern of inheritance in which transmission of an abnormal recessive gene on the X chromosome results in a carrier state in females and characteristics of the condition in males.

XO, (in genetics) the designation for the presence of only one sex chromosome; either the X or Y chromosome is missing so that each cell is monosomic and contains a total of 45 chromosomes.

XP, abbreviation for **xeroderma pigmentosum.**

x radiation [*X*, an unknown quantity], radiation of electromagnetic energy in the wavelengths of 10^{-8} meters, longer than gamma rays but shorter than ultraviolet rays.

x-ray, 1. electromagnetic radiation of shorter wavelength than visible light. X-rays are produced when electrons traveling at high speed strike certain materials, particularly heavy metals such as tungsten. They can penetrate most substances and are used to investigate the integrity of certain structures, to therapeutically destroy diseased tissue, and to make photographic images for diagnostic purposes, as in radiography and fluoroscopy. Discrete x-rays are those with precisely fixed energies that are characteristic of differences between electron binding energies of a particular element. **2.** a radiograph made by projecting x-rays through organs or structures of the body onto a photographic film. **3.** to make a radiograph.—**x-ray,** *adj.*

x-ray dermatitis, a skin inflammation caused by exposure to x-rays. Excessive exposure to x-rays can lead to skin cancer.

x-ray fluoroscopy, real-time imaging using an x-ray source that projects through the patient onto a fluorescent screen or image intensifier. Image-intensified fluoroscopy has replaced conventional fluoroscopy in current practice.

x-ray microscope, a microscope that produces images by x-rays and records them on fine-grain film or projects them as enlargements.

x-ray pelvimetry, a radiographic examination used to determine the dimensions of the bony pelvis of a pregnant woman and, if possible, the biparietal diameter of her baby's head. It is performed when doubt exists as to whether the head can pass safely through the pelvis in labor.

x-ray tube, a large vacuum tube containing a tungsten filament cathode and an anode that often is a rotating tungsten disk. When heated to incandescence, the cathode emits a cloud of electrons that produce x-rays when they strike the surface of the anode at high speed. The anode is designed to deflect the x-rays toward the object being radiographed.

X-tra densities /ek′strə/, images on x-ray film caused by the presence of foreign objects such as bullets or surgical clips in the patient's body.

XX /ekseks′/, (in genetics) the designation for the normal sex chromosome complement in the human female.

XXX syndrome /trip′əleks′/, a human sex chromosomal aberration characterized by the presence of three X chromosomes and two Barr bodies instead of the normal XX complement, so that somatic cells contain a total of 47 chromosomes; trisomy X.

XXXX, XXXXX /fôreks′, fīveks′/, (in genetics) the designation for an abnormal sex chromosome complement in the human female in which there are, respectively, four or five instead of the normal two X chromosomes so that each somatic cell contains a total of 48 or 49 chromosomes.

XXXY, XXXXY, XXYY /thrē′ekswī, fôr′ekswī, dob′əleks′dob′əlwī′/, (in genetics) the designation for an abnormal sex chromosome complement in the human male in which there are more than the normal one X chromosome, resulting in a total of 48, 49, or more chromosomes in each somatic cell.

XY /ekswī′/, (in genetics) the designation for the normal sex chromosome complement in the human male.

xylitol /zī′litôl/, a sweet crystalline pentahydroxy alcohol obtained by the reduction of xylose and used as a sweetener.

xylometazoline hydrochloride /zī′lō-metaz′əlēn/, an adrenergic vasoconstrictor prescribed in the treatment of nasal congestion in colds, hay fever, sinusitis, and other upper respiratory allergies.

xylose /zī′lōs/, an aldopentose sugar produced by hydrolyzing straw and corn cobs. It is incompletely absorbed when taken by mouth and is used in diagnostic studies of the digestive tract.

xylose absorption test, a laboratory test for intestinal absorption of the monosaccharide D-xylose. Absorption of D-xylose occurs readily in the normal intestine but is diminished in malabsorption patients.

xysma /zis′mə/, membranous shreds sometimes found in the feces of patients with diarrhea.

XYY syndrome /eks′dob′əlwī′/, the phenotypic manifestation of an extra Y chromosome, which tends to have a positive effect on height and may have a negative effect on mental and psychologic development. However, the anomaly also occurs in normal males.

X

Y, symbol for the element **yttrium.**

YACs, abbreviation for **yeast artificial chromosomes.**

YAG, abbreviation for *yttrium aluminum garnet,* a crystal used in some types of lasers.

Yallow, Rosalyn Sussman [U.S. medical physicist, b. 1921], co-winner with Roger Guillemin and Andrew Schally of the 1977 Nobel prize for medicine or physiology for her work in endocrinology and development of the radioimmunoassay technique.

yang, a polarized aspect of ch'i that is active or positive energy.

Yankauer suction catheter, a rigid hollow tube with a curve at the distal end to facilitate the removal of thick pharyngeal secretions during oral pharyngeal suctioning.

yaw /yô/ [Carib, *ïaïa*], a lesion of the syphilis-like tropical disease of yaws. The initial lesion or primary sore is identified as the mother yaw.

yawn /yôn/ [AS, *geonian*], an involuntary act of opening the mouth wide and taking a deep breath. It tends to occur when a person is bored, drowsy, or depressed and may be accompanied by upper body movements or the act of stretching to aid chest expansion.

yaws /yôs/ [Afr, *yaw,* raspberry], a nonvenereal infection caused by the spirochete *Treponema pertenue,* transmitted by direct contact. It is characterized by chronic, ulcerating sores anywhere on the body with eventual tissue and bone destruction, leading to crippling if untreated. All serologic tests for syphilis may be positive in yaws.

Yb, symbol for the element **ytterbium.**

Y-cartilage, a Y-shaped band of connective tissue that extends through the acetabulum to join the ilium, ischium, and pubis.

Y chromosome, a sex chromosome that in humans and many other species is present only in the normal male. It is carried as a sex determinant by one half of the male gametes and none of the female gametes, is morphologically much smaller than the X chromosome, and has genes associated with triggering the development and differentiation of male characteristics.

years of potential life lost (YPLL), an evaluation of the economic, social, and other consequences of premature death in a population from injury or disease as compared to the potential productivity of the deceased if they had lived normal lifespans.

yeast /yēst/ [AS, *gist*], any unicellular, usually oval, nucleated fungus that reproduces by budding. *Candida albicans* is a kind of pathogenic yeast.

yeast artificial chromosomes (YACs), yeast chromosomes used in recombinant deoxyribonucleic acid (DNA) procedures. They carry large segments of foreign DNA in the sequencing of nucleic acids.

yellow fever, an acute arbovirus infection transmitted by mosquitoes. It is characterized by headache, fever, jaundice, vomiting, and bleeding. Recovery is followed by lifelong immunity. Immunization for travelers to endemic areas is advised.

yellow fever vaccine, a vaccine produced from live, attenuated yellow fever virus grown in chick embryos. It is prescribed for immunization against yellow fever.

yellow jacket venom, a toxin injected by the stings of wasps and hornets. It can induce potentially fatal anaphylactic shock.

yellow marrow, bone marrow in which the fat cells predominate in the meshes of the reticular network.

yellow nail syndrome, a condition in which there is complete or almost complete cessation of nail growth and loss of cuticle. They become thickened, convex, opaque, and pale yellow to yellowish green. It is associated with pulmonary disorders and lymphedema.

Yersinia /yersin′ē-ə/ [Alexandre E. J. Yersin, French bacteriologist, 1862–1943], a genus of nonmotile ovoid or rod-shaped gram-negative bacteria of the *Enterobacteriaceae* family. The genus includes *Y. pestis,* which causes plague in rats and humans; *Y. enterolitica,* a cause of enterocolitis and other diseases; and *Y. pseudotuberculosis,* a cause of pseudotuberculosis.

Yersinia **arthritis** [Alexandre E. J. Yersin], a polyarticular inflammation occurring a few days to 1 month after the onset of infection caused by *Yersinia enterocolitica* or *Y. pseudotuberculosis* and usually persisting longer than 1 month. Knees, ankles, toes, fingers, and wrists are most often affected. The clinical presentation may mimic juvenile rheumatoid arthritis, rheumatic fever, or Reiter's syndrome.

Yersinia pestis [Alexandre E. J. Yersin; L, *pestis,* plague], a small gram-negative bacteria that causes plague. The primary host is the rat, but other small rodents also harbor the organism.

Y fracture, a Y-shaped intercondylar fracture.

yield, 1. an amount or quantity produced in return for an effort or investment. **2.** the energy released by a nuclear reaction.

yin, a polarized aspect of ch'i that is passive or negative energy.

Y-linked /wī'lingkt/, pertaining to genes or to the characteristics or conditions they transmit that are carried on the Y chromosome.—**Y linkage,** *n.*

yoga, a discipline that focuses on the body's musculature, posture, breathing mechanisms, and consciousness. The goal of yoga is attainment of physical and mental well-being.

yogurt /yō'gərt/ [Turk, *yoghurt*], a slightly acid, semisolid, curdled milk preparation made from either whole or skimmed cow's milk and milk solids by fermentation with organisms from the genus *Lactobacillus.* It is rich in B complex vitamins and a good source of protein. It also provides a medium in the gastrointestinal tract that retards the growth of harmful bacteria and aids in mineral absorption.

yoke /yōk/ [L, *jungere,* to join], a connector used to link small cylinders of medical gases, such as portable oxygen tanks, to respiratory equipment.

yolk /yōk,yelk/ [AS, *geolca*], the nutritive material rich in fats and proteins that is contained in the ovum to supply nourishment to the developing embryo. In humans and most mammals the yolk is absent or greatly diffused through the cell, because embryos absorb nutrients directly from the mother through the placenta.

yolk sac, a structure that develops in the inner cell mass of the embryo and expands into a vesicle with a thick part that becomes the primitive gut and a thin part that grows into the cavity of the chorion. After supplying the nourishment for the embryo, the yolk sac usually disappears during the seventh week of pregnancy.

yolk stalk, the narrow duct c\ the yolk sac with the midgut of t bryo during the early stages of prenatu velopment.

young and middle adult, the stages o. life from 22 to 65 years of age.

Young-Helmholtz theory of color vision [Thomas Young, English physician, 1773–1829; Hermann L. F. von Helmholtz, German physician, physicist, and physiologist, 1821–1894], the concept that all color sensations are mediated by three types of retinal receptors, which correspond to three primary colors: red, green, and blue-violet. By their individual and combined activities, the receptors produce the perception of all visible hues.

Young prostatic tractor [Hugh H. Young, American urologist, 1870–1945], a short straight surgical instrument with blades operated by a knob, for use in open perineal prostatectomy. The device can be inserted through the prostatic urethra and by direct traction used to draw down the prostate gland into the operative field.

Young's operation [Hugh S. Young, U.S. urologist, 1870–1945], **1.** the surgical construction of a new urethra to repair a structural defect of the penis. **2.** perineal prostatectomy.

Y-plasty /wī'plas'tē/, a method of surgical revision of a scar, using a Y-shaped incision to reduce scar contractures.

YPLL, abbreviation for **years of potential life lost.**

Y-set, a device composed of plastic components, used for delivering intravenous fluids through a primary intravenous line connected to a combination drip chamber filter section from which two separate plastic tubes lead to fluid sources. The Y-set also includes three clamps, one for the primary intravenous line and one for each of the two separate tubes. It is often used to transfuse packed blood cells that must be diluted with saline solution to decrease their viscosity.

ytterbium (Yb) /itur'bē·əm/ [Ytterby, Sweden], a rare earth metallic element. Its atomic number is 70; its atomic mass (weight) is 173.04.

yttrium (Y) /it're·əm/ [Ytterby, Sweden], a scaly, grayish metallic element. Its atomic number is 39; its atomic mass (weight) is 88.905. Radioactive isotopes of yttrium have been used in cancer therapy.

Y

Z

Zakrzewski /zakshef′skē/, **Marie** (1829–1902), a Polish-German-American midwife who studied medicine in Berlin and in 1872 organized the first successful American school of nursing at the New England Hospital for Women and Children.

zalcitabine, an antiretroviral nucleoside analog prescribed in the treatment of human immunodeficiency virus infections.

Zeeman effect /sē′man, tsä′mon/ [Pieter Zeeman, Dutch physicist and Nobel Laureate, 1865–1945], a splitting of spectral lines of an emission spectrum into three or more symmetrically placed lines when the radiation source is in a magnetic field.

ZEEP, abbreviation for **zero-end expiratory pressure.**

Zeitgeist /tsīt′gīst/ [Ger], literally, the spirit of the time, a climate of opinion, a convention of thought, or implicit assumptions.

Zenker's diverticulum /tseng′kerz/ [Friedrich A. Zenker, German pathologist, 1825–1898; L, *diverticulare,* to turn aside], a circumscribed herniation of the mucous membrane of the pharynx as it joins the esophagus. Food may become trapped in the diverticulum and can be aspirated.

zeolites, hydrated silicates of aluminum used in ion exchange water softeners. Synthetic zeolites are used as porous molecular containers for reagents and drugs.

zeranol /zer′ənol/, an estrogenic substance used to fatten livestock. Consumption of beef from zeranol-treated cattle has been associated with precocious puberty in some boys and girls.

zero /zir′ō/ [Ar, *sifr,* cipher], **1.** a symbol for nothing. **2.** the point on most scales from which measurements begin. **3.** absolute zero (0 K) on the Kelvin scale, the temperature at which there is no molecular movement, corresponding to $-273.15°$ C on the Celsius scale or $-459.67°$ F.

zero dose, the absence of added ligand.

zero-end expiratory pressure (ZEEP) [Ar, *zefiro* + ME, *ende*], pressure that has returned to ambient or atmospheric level at the end of exhalation.

zero fluid balance, a state in which the amount of fluid intake is equal to the amount of fluid output.

zero gravity, a physical state of weightlessness in space or during flight when the centrifugal thrust on a body in a parabolic glide exactly counteracts the force of gravity.

zero order kinetics, a state at which the rate of an enzyme reaction is independent of the concentration of the substrate.

zero population growth (ZPG), a situation in which there is no population increase during a given year because the total of live births is equal to the total of deaths.

zero-to-three infant stimulation groups, groups that provide therapeutic services for children from birth to 3 years of age, an age group not yet eligible for public school placement.

zero V/Q, an intrapulmonary shunt in which blood passes through the lungs without entering alveolar capillaries, causing hypoxemia.

zeta /zē′tə,zā′tə/, Z, ζ, the sixth letter of the Greek alphabet.

zeta potential [Gk, *zeta,* sixth letter of Greek alphabet; L, *potentia,* power], the potential produced by the effective charge of a macromolecule, usually measured at the boundary between what is moving in a solution with the macromolecule and the rest of the solution.

zeugmatography /zo͞og′mətog′rəfē/ [Gk, *zeugnynai,* to join, *graphein,* to record], another name for MR imaging suggesting the role of the gradient magnetic field in joining the radiofrequency magnetic field to a desired local spatial region through nuclear magnetic resonance.

zidovudine (ZDU) /zīdov′ədēn/, a pyrimidine nucleoside analogue active against human immunodeficiency virus (HIV). Its function is to inhibit the reverse transcriptase of human immunodeficiency disease. It is used in the management of patients with HIV infection who have some evidence of impaired immunity. It also may be used for prophylaxis after exposure to HIV.

Ziehl-Neelsen test /zēl′nēl′sən/ [Franz Ziehl, German bacteriologist, 1857–1926; Friedrich K. A. Neelsen, German pathologist, 1854–1894], one of the most widely used methods of acid-fast staining, commonly used in the microscopic examination of a smear of sputum suspected of containing *Mycobacterium tuberculosis.*

Zieve's syndrome [Lieslie Zieve, American physician, b. 1915], a mild spherocytic anemia with transient jaundice and hyperlipidemia found in patients with acute alcoholism and liver cirrhosis.

ZIG, abbreviation for **zoster immune globulin.**

Zimmermann reaction /zim'ərman, tsim'ərmon/ [Wilhelm Zimmermann, German physician, b. 1910], a standard chromogen reaction for detecting androgens with the 17-keto configuration. It involves a reaction between an alkaline solution of meta-dinitrobenzene and an active methylene group.

zinc (Zn) /zingk/ [Ger, *Zink*], a bluish-white crystalline metal commonly associated with lead ores. Its atomic number is 30; its atomic mass (weight) is 65.38. Zinc is an essential nutrient in the body and is used in numerous pharmaceutics such as zinc acetate, zinc oxide, zinc permanganate, and zinc stearate. Zinc acetate is used as an emetic, a styptic, and an astringent. Zinc oxide is used internally as an antispasmodic and as a protective in ointments. Zinc permanganate is used as an astringent and in the treatment of urethritis by injection or douche in a 1:4000 solution. Zinc stearate is used as a water-repellent protective agent in the treatment of acne, eczema, and other skin diseases.

zinc deficiency, a condition resulting from insufficient amounts of zinc in the diet. It is characterized by abnormal fatigue, decreased alertness, a decrease in taste and odor sensitivity, poor appetite, retarded growth, delayed sexual maturity, prolonged healing of wounds, and susceptibility to infection and injury.

zinc finger, a loop or sequence of transcription factor subunits with a zinc atom linked to four carbon atoms at the base of a sequence. It is an important step in the cloning and sequencing of human general transcription factors.

zinc gelatin, a topical protectant for varicosities and other lesions of the lower limbs.

zinc ointment [Ger, *Zink* + OFr, *oignement*], a preparation of 20% zinc oxide in mineral oil or a white petrolatum semisolid base, used as a local surface treatment for various skin disorders.

zinc oxide, a topical protectant prescribed for a wide range of minor skin irritations.

zinc oxide and eugenol (ZOE), a dental cement composed primarily of zinc salts, eugenol, and rosin, used chiefly in temporary tooth fillings. It has low relative strength and abrasion resistance, but its nearly neutral pH causes minimal irritation to dental pulp. It is intended as a sedative dressing until pain subsides and a more permanent filling can be inserted.

zinc phosphate dental cement, a material for luting or attaching of dental inlays, crowns, bridges, and orthodontic appliances and for some temporary restorations of teeth.

zinc salt poisoning, a toxic condition caused by the ingestion or inhalation of a zinc salt. Symptoms of ingestion include a burning sensation of the mouth and throat, vomiting, diarrhea, abdominal and chest pain, and in severe cases shock and coma.

zinc sulfate, an ophthalmic astringent given in drops for nasal congestion or irritation of the eye, applied topically in deodorants, and given orally in tablets to promote healing and as a dietary supplement.

ZIP, abbreviation for *zoster immune plasma.*

zirconium (Zr) /zərkō'nē·əm/ [Ar, *zarqun*, zircon], a steel-gray, tetravalent metallic element. Its atomic number is 40; its atomic mass (weight) is 91.22.

zirconium granuloma, an inflammatory lesion, usually occurring in the axilla as a reaction to zirconium salts in antiperspirants.

Z line, a narrow, darkly-staining cross-striation that bisects the I band of skeletal muscles. The distance between Z lines is the length of the sarcomere.

Zn, symbol for the element **zinc.**

zoacanthosis /zō'akanthō'sis/, a dermatitis caused by retention in the skin of foreign bodies such as insect stingers, animal hairs, or bristles.

zoanthropy /zō·an'thrəpē/ [Gk, *zoon*, animal, *anthropos*, human], the delusion that one has assumed the form and characteristics of an animal.—**zoanthropic,** *adj.*

ZOE, abbreviation for **zinc oxide and eugenol.**

Zollinger-Ellison syndrome /zol'injərel'-isən/ [Robert M. Zollinger, American surgeon, 1903–1992; Edwin H. Ellison, American physician, 1918–1970], a condition characterized by severe peptic ulceration, gastric hypersecretion, elevated serum gastrin, and gastrinoma of the pancreas or the duodenum.

zombie /zom'bē/, a supernatural power that supposedly can enter into and reanimate a corpse.

zona /zō'nə/, *pl.* **zonae** [Gk, *zone*, belt], a zone, or girdlelike segment of a rounded or spheric structure.

Z

zona fasciculata, the middle part of the adrenal cortex, which is the site of production of glucocorticoids and sex hormones.

zona glomerulosa, the outer part of the adrenal cortex, where mineralocorticoids are produced.

zona pellucida /pəloo'sidə/, the thick transparent noncellular membrane that encloses the mammalian ovum. It is secreted by the maturing oocyte during its development in the ovary and is retained until near the time of implantation.

zona radiata, a zona pellucida that has a striated appearance caused by radiating canals within the membrane.

zona reticularis, the innermost part of the adrenal cortex, which borders on the adrenal medulla part of the gland. It acts in consort with the zona fasciculata in producing various sex hormones and glucocorticoids.

zonate /zō'nāt/, having ringed layers with differing colors of textures.

zone [Gk, belt], an area with specific boundaries and characteristics, such as the epigastric, mesogastric, and hypogastric zones of the abdomen.

zone of equivalence, a region of an antibody-antigen reaction in which concentrations of both reactants are equal.

zonesthesia /zō'nesthē'zhə/ [Gk, zone + aisthesis, feeling], a painful sensation of constriction, as of a bandage bound too tightly, especially experienced around the waist or abdomen.

zone therapy, the treatment of a disorder by mechanical stimulation and counterirritation of a body area in the same longitudinal zone as the affected organ or region.

zonifugal /zōnif'yəgəl/ [Gk, zone, belt; L, fugere, to flee], moving from within a zone or area outward.

zonography /zōnog'rəfē/ [Gk, zone + graphein, to record], an x-ray imaging technique used to produce films of body sections similar to those made by tomography.

zonula /zōn'yələ/, pl. **zonulae** [Gk, zone, belt], a small zone.

zonula adherens [L, zone, belt, adhaerere, to stick], a continuous zone running around the outer surface of a cell in which there is an intercellular space of about 15 to 20 nm width. A component of the junctional complex between cells, the zone contains dense filamentous material.

zonula ciliaris, a ligament composed of straight fibrils radiating from the ciliary body of the eye to the crystalline lens, holding the lens in place and relaxing by the contraction of the ciliary muscle. Relaxation of the ligament allows the lens to become more convex.

zonula occludens [L, zona, belt, occludere, to close up], a component of the junctional complex between cells in which there is no intercellular space and the plasma membranes of adjacent cells are in direct contact.

zoobiology /-bī·ol'əjē/ [Gk, zoon, animal, bios, life, logos, science], the biology of animals.

zoochemistry /-kem'istrē/ [Gk, zoon, animal, chemeia, alchemy], the biochemistry of animals.

zoogenous /zō-oj'ənəs/ [Gk, zoon, animal, genein, to produce], acquired from or originating in animals.

zoograft /zō'əgraft/ [Gk, zoon + graphion, stylus], tissue of an animal transplanted to a human, such as a heart valve from a pig to replace a damaged heart valve in a human.

zoologist /zō-ol'əjist/ [Gk, zoon, animal, logos, science], a person concerned with the scientific study of animals.

zoology /zō-ol'əjē/, the study of animal life.

zoom /zoom/, a system of camera lenses that allows an object to remain in focus when the camera approaches or recedes or when the object is viewed close-up or at a distance.

zoomania /zō-əmā'nē-ə/ [Gk, zoon + mania, madness], a psychopathologic state characterized by an excessive fondness for and preoccupation with animals.—**zoomaniac,** *n.*

zoonosis /zō-on'əsis, zō'ənō'sis/ [Gk, zoon + nosis, disease], a disease of animals that is transmissible to humans from its primary animal host. Some kinds of zoonoses are **equine encephalitis, leptospirosis, rabies,** and **yellow fever.**

zooparasite /zō-əper'əsīt/ [Gk, zoon + parasitos, guest], any parasitic animal organism. Kinds of zooparasites are **arthropods, protozoa,** and **worms.**—**zooparasitic,** *adj.*

zoopathology /-pəthol'əjē/, the study of the diseases of animals.

zoophilia /zō-əfil'ē-ə/ [Gk, zoon + philein, to love], **1.** an abnormal fondness for animals. **2.** (in psychiatry) a psychosexual disorder in which sexual excitement and gratification are derived from the fondling of animals or from the fantasy or act of engaging in sexual activity with animals.—**zoophile,** *n.,* **zoophilic, zoophilous,** *adj.*

zoophobia /-fō'bē-ə/ [Gk, zoon + phobos, fear], an anxiety disorder characterized by a persistent, irrational fear of animals, particularly dogs, snakes, insects, and mice.

zoopsia /zō-op'sē-ə/ [Gk, zoon + opsis, vision], a visual hallucination of animals or insects, often occurring in delirium tremens.

zootoxin /zō′ətok′sin/ [Gk, *zoon* + *toxikon*, poison], a poisonous substance from an animal, such as the venom of snakes, spiders, and scorpions.—**zootoxic**, *adj.*

zoster auricularis /zos′tər/, an acute earache with herpetic blebs on the eardrum and external auditory meatus.

zosteriform /zoster′ifôrm/ [Gk, *zoster*, girdle; L, *forma*, form], resembling the pocks seen in herpes zoster infection.

zoster immune globulin (ZIG) [Gk, *zoster* + L, *immunis*, freedom, *globulus*, small sphere], a passive immunizing agent currently in limited experimental use for preventing or attenuating herpes zoster virus infection in immunosuppressed individuals who are at great risk of severe herpes zoster virus infection.

zoster ophthalmicus [Gk, *zoster*, girdle; *ophthalmos*, eye], a herpes infection of the eye, particularly of the optic nerve. The infection frequently involves the cornea. There may be lid edema, ciliary and conjunctival involvement, and pain. Keratitis may be severe. Scarring and glaucoma are common sequelae.

ZPG, abbreviation for **zero population growth.**

Z-plasty /zē′plas′tē/, a method of surgical revision of a scar or closure of a wound using a Z-shaped incision to reduce contractures of the adjacent skin.

Zr, symbol for the element **zirconium.**

Z-track, a technique for injecting irritating preparations into muscle without tracking residual medication through sensitive tissues.

Zung Self-Rating Depression Scale, a 'self-report test' of 20 descriptors of depression on which clients rate themselves on a four-point scale ranging from 'a little of the time' to 'most of the time.' The scale is useful in determining the depth or intensity of a client's depression.

zwieback /zwī′bak, zwē′-/ [Ger, *zwie*, twice, *backen*, to bake], a sweetened bread that is enriched with eggs and baked, then sliced and toasted until dry and crisp. It is used as a snack food for children, especially teething infants.

zwitterion /svit′ərī′ən/, a molecule that has regions of both negative and positive charge. Amino acids such as glycine are almost always present as zwitterions when in neutral solutions.

zygogenesis /zī′gōjen′əsis/ [Gk, *zygon*, yoke, *genesis*, origin], **1.** the formation of a zygote. **2.** reproduction by the union of gametes.—**zygogenetic, zygogenic,** *adj.*

zygoma /zīgō′mə, zig-/ [Gk, *zygon*, yoke],

1. a long slender zygomatic process of the temporal bone, arising from the lower part of the squamous part of the temporal bone, passing forward to join the zygomatic bone, and forming part of the zygomatic arch. **2.** the zygomatic bone that forms the prominence of the cheek.

zygomatic /-mat′ik/ [Gk, *zygon,* yoke], pertaining to the zygoma, or malar bone of the face.

zygomatic arch [Gk, *zygon* + L, *arcus,* bow], an arch formed by the temporal process of the zygomatic bone with the zygomatic process of the temporal bone. The tendon of the temporal muscle passes beneath it.

zygomatic bone [Gk, *zygon* + *ban*], one of the pair of bones that forms the prominence of the cheek, the lower part of the orbit of the eye, and parts of the temporal and infratemporal fossae.

zygomaticofacial /zī′gōmat′ikōfā′shəl/, pertaining to the facial surface of the zygomatic bone.

zygomatic process [Gk, *zygon* + L, *processus*], **1.** a projection of the frontal bone forming the lateral boundary of the superciliary arch. **2.** a process of the maxilla. **3.** a process of the temporal bone.

zygomatic reflex [Gk, *zygon* + L, *reflectere,* to bend back], movement of the lower jaw toward the percussed side when the zygoma is tapped lightly but sharply.

zygomaticus major /zī′gōmat′ikəs/, one of the 12 muscles of the mouth. It acts to draw the angle of the mouth up and back to smile or laugh.

zygomaticus minor, one of the 12 muscles of the mouth. It acts to deepen the nasolabial furrow in a sad facial expression.

zygomycosis /zī′gōmīkō′sis/ [Gk, *zygon* + *mykes,* fungus], an acute, often fulminant, and sometimes fatal fungal infection caused by a class of Phycomycetal water molds. It occurs primarily in patients with chronic debilitating diseases. It begins with fever, pain, and discharge in the nose and paranasal sinuses that progresses to invade the eye and lower respiratory tract. The fungus may enter blood vessels and spread to the brain and other organs.

zygonema /zī′gənē′mə/ [Gk, *zygon* + *nema,* thread], the synaptic chromosome formation that occurs in the zygotene stage of the first meiotic prophase of gametogenesis.—**zygonematic,** *adj.*

zygopodium /zī′gōpō′dē·əm/, the part of an embryonic limb consisting of the radius and ulna or the tibia and fibula.

zygosis /zīgō′sis/, a form of sexual reproduction in unicellular organisms, consist-

Z

ing of the union of the two cells and fusion of the nuclei.—**zygotic** /zīgot'ik/, *adj.*

zygosity /zīgos'itē/, the characteristics or conditions of a zygote. The form occurs primarily as a suffix combining form to denote genetic makeup, referring specifically to whether the paired alleles determining a particular trait are identical (homozygosity) or different (heterozygosity).

zygospore /zī'gōspôr'/ [Gk, *zygon* + *sporos*, seed], the spore resulting from the conjugation of two isogametes, as in certain fungi and algae.

zygote /zī'gōt/ [Gk, *zygon*, yoke], (in embryology) the combined cell produced by the union of a sperm pronucleus and the "egg" pronucleus at the completion of fertilization until first cleavage.

zygotene /zī'gətēn/ [Gk, *zygon* + *tainia*, band], the second stage in the first meiotic prophase of gametogenesis in which synapsis of homologous chromosomes occurs.

zymogen granules /zi'məjən/ [Gk, *zyme*, ferment, *genein*, to produce; L, *granulum*, little grain], granules found in some secretory exocrine cells. They contain the precursors of enzymes that become active after the granules leave the cell.

zymoprotein /-prō'tēn/ [Gk, *zyme*, ferment, *proteios*, first rank], **1.** a yeast protein. **2.** any protein that functions as an enzyme.

zymorphic /zīmôr'fik/ [Gk, *zyme*, ferment, *morphe*, form], pertaining to fermentation properties.

Z.Z'.Z.'', symbol for increasing strength or intensity of contraction.

Commonly Used Abbreviations—cont'd

KUB	Kidney, ureter, and bladder	NS	Normal saline
KVO	Keep vein open	NSAID	Nonsteroidal anti-inflammatory drug
L	Left; liter; length; lumbar; lethal; pound	NSR	Normal sinus rhythm
lab	Laboratory	O_2	Oxygen; both eyes
L & D	Labor and delivery	OB	Obstetrics
LDL	Low-density lipoprotein	OBS	Organic brain syndrome
LE	Lower extremity; lupus erythematosus	OD	Optical density; overdose; right eye (*Oculus dexter*)
LLE	Left lower extremity	OOB	Out of bed
LLL	Left lower lobe	OR	Operating room
LLQ	Left lower quadrant	ORIF	Open reduction and internal fixation
LMP	Last menstrual period		
LOC	Level/loss of consciousness	OS	Left eye (*Oculus sinister*)
LP	Lumbar puncture	OT	Occupational therapy
LR	Lactated Ringer's	OTC	Over-the-counter
LUE	Left upper extremity	OU	Each eye (*Oculus uterque*)
LUL	Left upper lobe	oz	Ounce
LUQ	Left upper quadrant	p̄	After
LV	Left ventricle	P-A; PA; P/A	Posterior-anterior
LVH	Left ventricular hypertrophy	PALS	Pediatric advanced life support
L & W	Living and well	Para I, II, etc.	Unipara, bipara, tripara, etc.
MAP	Mean arterial pressure	PAT	Paroxysmal atrial tachycardia
MCH	Mean corpuscular hemoglobin	PCA	Patient-controlled analgesia
MCHC	Mean corpuscular hemoglobin concentration	PCWP	Pulmonary capillary wedge pressure
MCV	Mean corpuscular volume	PDA	Patent ductus arteriosus
MD	Muscular dystrophy	PE	Physical examination
MDI	Medium dose inhalant; metered dose inhaler	PEEP	Positive end-expiratory pressure
mEq	Milliequivalent	PEFR	Peak expiratory flow rate
MI	Myocardial infarction	PERRLA	Pupils equal, regular, react to light and accommodation
mm Hg	Millimeters of mercury		
MMR	Maternal mortality rate; measles-mumps-rubella	PET	Positron emission tomography
MRI	Magnetic resonance imaging	PICC	Percutaneously inserted central catheter
MS	Multiple sclerosis	PID	Pelvic inflammatory disease
MVA	Motor vehicle accident	PKU	Phenylketonuria
N/A	Not applicable	PM	Postmortem; evening
Na	Sodium	PMH	Past medical history
NaCl	Sodium chloride	PMI	Point of maximal impulse
N & V, N/V	Nausea and vomiting	PMN	Polymorphonuclear neutrophil leukocytes (polys)
NG, ng	Nasogastric		
NICU	Neonatal intensive care unit	PMS	Premenstrual syndrome
NIDDM	Noninsulin-dependent diabetes mellitus	PND	Paroxysmal nocturnal dyspnea
		PO; p.o.	Orally (*per os*)
NKA	No known allergies	PPD	Purified protein derivative (TB test)
NPO; n.p.o	Nothing by mouth (*non per os*)		